MAYO CLINIC
FAMILY HEALTH BOOK

Scott C. Litin, M.D.
Medical Editor

Sanjeev Nanda, M.D.
Associate Medical Editor

Fifth Edition

Published by Mayo Clinic

Mayo Clinic Family Health Book, Fifth Edition, provides reliable, practical, comprehensive, easy-to-understand information on issues relating to good health. The information in this book is true and complete to the best of our knowledge. This book is intended to supplement the advice of your personal physician, whom you should consult about your individual medical condition. The information in this book is offered with no guarantees. The author and publisher disclaim all liability in connection with this book. *Mayo Clinic Family Health Book* does not endorse any company or product.

For bulk sales to employers, member groups and health-related companies, contact Mayo Clinic, 200 First St. SW, Rochester, MN 55905, call 800-430-9699, or send an e-mail to *SpecialSalesMayoBooks@Mayo.edu.*

ISBN: 978-1-945564-02-4

Library of Congress Control Number: 2017955624

Fifth Edition

Printed in USA

1 2 3 4 5 6 7 8 9 10

A Note to Readers

In this book, we commonly use the term *doctor* when referring to an interaction between a health care professional and a patient. However, we are well aware that health care today is often provided by individuals who aren't medical doctors. Other talented providers such as physician assistants, nurse practitioners, clinical nurse specialists and nurse midwives are taking on an increasing role in medicine, especially in providing primary care. We use the term *doctor* as an umbrella term that encompasses medical doctors and other certified health professionals who are licensed to provide medical care. For space reasons and for ease of reading, using one word to describe this group of individuals was preferable.

Photo Credits

The individuals pictured in the lifestyle photos are models, and the photos are used for illustrative purposes only. There is no correlation between the individuals portrayed and the condition or subject being discussed. All photographs and illustrations are copyright of MFMER, except for the following:

Preface

The field of medicine is ever-changing. Advances in technology and diagnostic and surgical techniques, and the development of new medications, continue to provide doctors and scientists with ever-more-powerful tools for diagnosing and treating disease. What this means for you and me is a better chance of living a longer, healthier life.

However, medical advances alone can't guarantee good health. You still play a crucial role in determining your future health and wellness. Even more important than the ability to treat disease is the ability to prevent it. And that's where your actions can pay off the most. Healthy lifestyle habits, such as exercising daily, eating well and seeing your doctor for appropriate preventive care, are still your best bet for enjoying a long and productive life.

Mayo Clinic Family Health Book, Fifth Edition, is based on the premise that knowledge gives you the tools needed to maintain good health. This new edition of *Mayo Clinic Family Health Book* was created by revising and rewriting much of the information in the previous edition. It's our hope that this fully updated fifth edition will serve not only as a reference during times of illness but also as a guide in helping you and your family adopt healthy lifestyle practices.

The information provided in this book isn't a substitute for seeing a doctor. No book can replace the advice of a doctor who has evaluated your overall health. The intent of this book is to help you better understand various symptoms, diseases, tests and treatments so that you can communicate more effectively with your doctor and the two of you can work together to manage your health.

Mayo Clinic Family Health Book is based on the expertise of hundreds of Mayo Clinic health care professionals and the advice they give their patients day in and day out. A special thanks goes out to many Mayo Clinic staff members who took time from their busy schedules to offer their advice and guidance as we prepared this new edition.

This book could not have been completed without the dedication and efforts of Associate Editor Sanjeev Nanda, M.D., and Senior Editor Karen Wallevand.

I also want to thank the marvelous colleagues, nurses and support staff with whom I work, especially my administrative teammate Amy Clark, who have made my Mayo Clinic career so gratifying. They all care for our patients as they would their own families.

A final thank you goes to my wife, Jolene, my son, Sam, my daughter, Cassie, and her husband, Chad, and my sister Nancie. They have taught me the true meaning and importance of the word *family*.

All of us involved in the development of this book hope you find the information that it contains to be useful and that this great resource will help you and your family stay healthy.

Scott C. Litin, M.D.
Medical Editor

Editorial Staff

Medical Editor	Scott C. Litin, M.D.
Associate Medical Editor	Sanjeev Nanda, M.D.
Editorial Director	Paula M. Marlow Limbeck
Senior Editor	Karen R. Wallevand
Senior Product Manager	Christopher C. Frye
Art Director	Stewart Jay Koski
Medical Illustrators	David J. Cheney
	David A. Factor
	Stephen Graepel
	John Hagen
	Joanna R. King
	Michael A. King
	Margaret Alice McKinney
	James Postier
Photographers	Michael J. Cleary
	Jodi O'Shaughnessy Olson
Production	Kent McDaniel
	Gunnar T. Soroos
Editorial Research Manager	Deirdre A. Herman
Editorial Research Librarians	Abbie Y. Brown
	Erika A. Riggin
	Katie J. Warner
Proofreaders	Miranda M. Attlesey
	Alison K. Baker
	Julie M. Maas
Indexer	Steve Rath
Administrative Assistant	Terri L. Zanto Strausbauch

Assistant Editors

Jayanth Adusumalli, M.B.B.S., M.P.H., General Internal Medicine

Paldeep S. Atwal, M.B., Ch.B., Clinical Genomics

Sophie J. Bakri, M.D., Ophthalmology

Brent A. Bauer, M.D., General Internal Medicine

Tracy M. Berg, R.Ph., Pharmacy Services

Crystal R. Bonnichsen, M.D., Cardiovascular Diseases

Barbara K. Bruce, Ph.D., L.P., Psychology

Lisa K. Buss Preszler, R.Ph., Pharmacy Services

Alan B. Carr, D.M.D., Dental Specialties

Bart L. Clarke, M.D., Endocrinology

Walter J. Cook, M.D., Pediatrics

John M. Davis III, M.D., Rheumatology

Stephanie S. Faubion, M.D., Women's Health Clinic

Debbie L. Fuehrer, L.P.C.C., General Internal Medicine

Lawrence E. Gibson, M.D., Dermatology

John B. Hagan, M.D., Allergic Diseases

Stephanie L. Hansel, M.D., Gastroenterology

Donald D. Hensrud, M.D., M.P.H., Preventive Medicine

LaTonya J. Hickson, M.D., Nephrology

Jeffrey R. Janus, M.D., ENT

Mary J. Kasten, M.D., General Internal Medicine

Cassie C. Kennedy, M.D., Pulmonary Medicine

Kelsey M. Klaas, M.D., Pediatrics

Esther H. Krych, M.D., Pediatrics

Edward R. Laskowski, M.D., Physical Medicine and Rehabilitation

Melissa C. Lipford, M.D., Sleep Medicine

Margaret E. Long, M.D., Obstetrics and Gynecology

David D. McFadden, M.D., General Internal Medicine

Timothy J. Moynihan, M.D., Oncology

Todd B. Nippoldt, M.D., Endocrinology

Laura J. Odell, R.Ph., Pharmacy Services

Sandhya Pruthi, M.D., Breast Diagnostic Clinic

S. Vincent Rajkumar, M.D., Hematology

Joyce L. Sanchez, M.D., Infectious Diseases

Benjamin J. Sandefur, M.D., Emergency Medicine

Rebecca A. Sanders, M.D., Pain Medicine

Terry D. Schneekloth, M.D., Psychiatry

Jacob J. Strand, M.D., Palliative Medicine

Bruce Sutor, M.D., Psychiatry

R. Houston Thompson, M.D., Urology

Farris K. Timimi, M.D., Cardiovascular Diseases

Matthew K. Tollefson, M.D., Urology

Landon W. Trost, M.D., Urology

Myra J. Wick, M.D., Ph.D., Obstetrics and Gynecology

Nathan P. Young, D.O., Neurology

Debra A. Zillmer, M.D., Orthopedics

Additional Contributors

Nusheen Ameenuddin, M.D., M.P.H., Pediatrics

Herjot K. Atwal, R.Ph., Pharmacy Services

Patrick R. Blackburn, Ph.D., Genetics and Genomics

Judy C. Boughey, M.D., Surgery

Bryan J. Buechel, Pharmacy Services

Petra M. Casey, M.D., Obstetrics and Gynecology

Anna L. Cavallo, Global Business Solutions

Charles C. Coddington III, M.D., Reproductive Endocrinology and Infertility

Valeria Cristiani, M.D., Pediatrics

Susanne M. Cutshall, APRN, CNS, D.N.P., General Internal Medicine

Donald Chris Derauf, M.D., Pediatrics

Amanda J. Ewald, R.Ph., Pharmacy Services

Alice Gallo De Moraes, M.D., Pulmonary Medicine

Jennifer M. Gass, Ph.D., Genetics and Genomics

Gretchen E. Glaser, M.D., Gynecologic Surgery

Tara L. Henrichsen, M.D., Radiology

Matthew R. Hopkins, M.D., Obstetrics and Gynecology

Robert M. Jacobson, M.D., Pediatrics

Yogish C. Kudva, M.B.B.S., Endocrinology

Brenda S. Lindsay, Creative Media

Sarah K. Macklin, M.S., CGC, Clinical Genomics

Meghna P. Mansukhani, M.D., Family Medicine

Dietrich Matern, M.D., Ph.D., Laboratory Genetics

Angela C. Mattke, M.D., Pediatrics

Lonzetta Neal, M.D., Breast Diagnostic Clinic

Rose J. Prissel, M.S., RDN, LD, Clinical Nutrition

Kathryn J. Ruddy, M.D., Oncology

Jordan Rullo, Ph.D., L.P., Psychiatry

Emanuel C. Trabuco, M.D., Gynecologic Surgery

Maria G. Valdes, M.D., Pediatrics

Stephanie K. Vaughan, Global Business Solutions

Laura Hamilton Waxman

Tomohiko Yamada, O.D., Ophthalmology

Contents

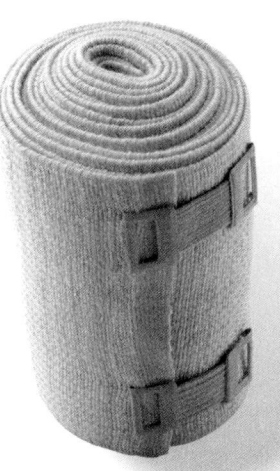

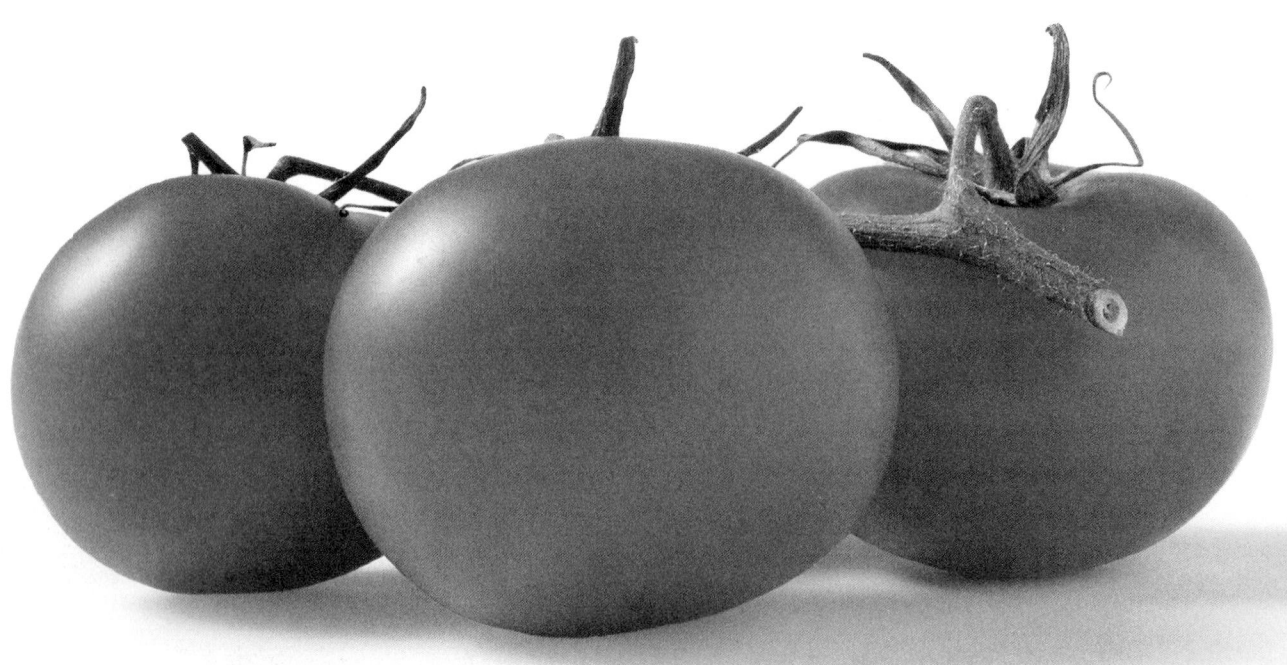

Experts.
Answers.

Mayo Clinic.

Learn more at **MayoClinic.org**.

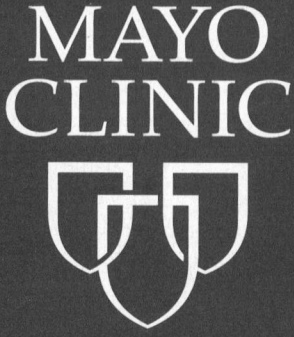

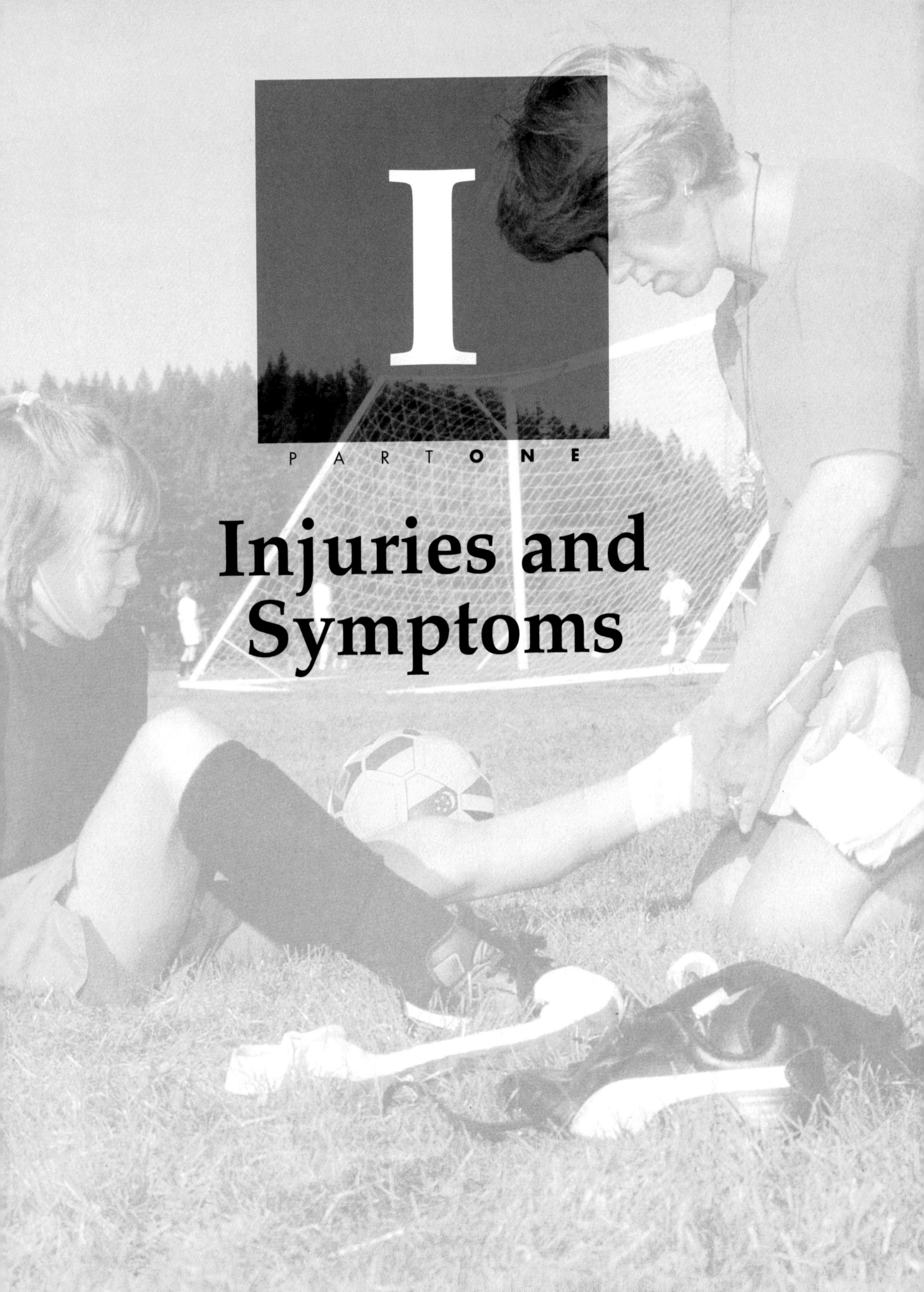

PART ONE

Injuries and Symptoms

First Aid and Emergency Care

Emergencies don't happen often, but when they do, you don't have much time to seek out first-aid information. First aid comprises knowing when emergency care is needed, how to provide care appropriate to your level of knowledge and skill, and how to recognize your limitations and call for help when needed. In order to react effectively, it's important to know what actions to take when a person appears injured, seriously ill or in distress. Your skills and knowledge could someday mean the difference between life and death for another human being.

This chapter provides valuable information on how to react in various emergency situations. You might also consider taking a certified first-aid course to learn lifesaving skills, such as the Heimlich maneuver, cardiopulmonary resuscitation (CPR), and how to respond to a heart attack, stroke or cardiac arrest.

To find out more about first-aid courses offered in your community, check with your local hospital, Red Cross office, county emergency services office or American Heart Association chapter.

Choking and the Heimlich Maneuver

Choking is caused by a blockage of the respiratory passage in the throat (larynx) or windpipe (trachea). The flow of air to the lungs is blocked. This in turn reduces the supply of oxygen-rich blood to the brain and other organs. If the problem isn't corrected promptly, choking can be fatal.

Choking is often due to a large piece of inadequately chewed food that becomes lodged in the throat or windpipe. Solid foods such as meat are usually

Emergency Warning Signs

If you're experiencing any of the following signs or symptoms, call for emergency medical help — 911 is the emergency phone number in most regions — or go immediately to the emergency department at the nearest hospital:
- Sudden or severe pain
- Pain or pressure in the chest, back or upper abdominal area, which can signal a heart attack
- Difficulty breathing or shortness of breath
- Sudden dizziness, a sudden severe headache or a change in vision or speech
- Sudden weakness or partial paralysis
- Severe or persistent vomiting or diarrhea
- Significant bleeding
- Suicidal or homicidal feelings

The Universal Choking Sign

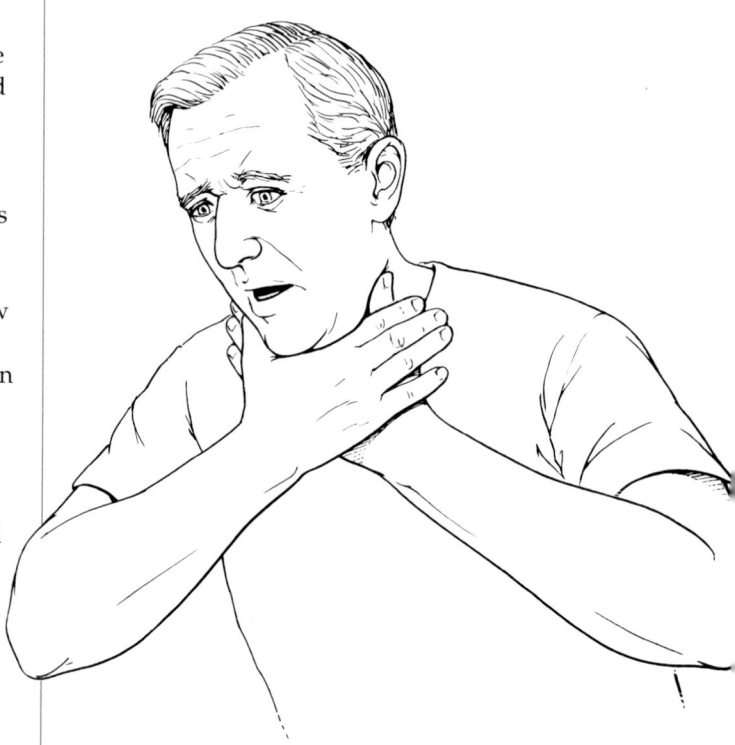

A person who's choking is unable to communicate except by hand motions. The universal signal for choking is hands clutched to the throat, with thumbs and fingers extended. If the person doesn't give the signal, look for these indicators:
- **Inability to speak**
- **Difficulty breathing or noisy breathing**
- **Inability to cough forcefully or a silent cough**
- **Skin, lips and nails turning blue or dusky**
- **Loss of consciousness**

The Finger Sweep

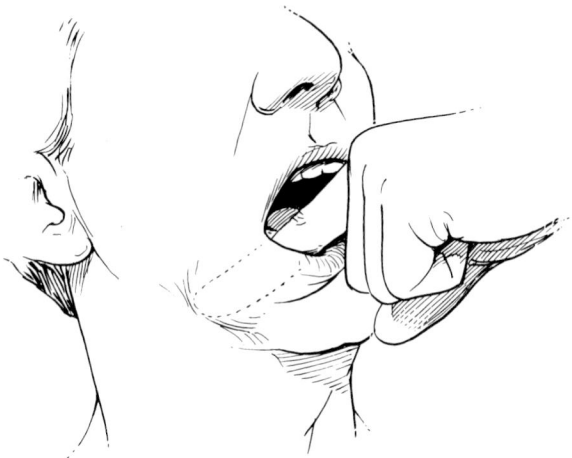

The simplest method for clearing an obstructed airway of an unresponsive person is to reach a finger into the back of the throat and sweep out the cause of the blockage, if it can be seen and reached.

The Heimlich Maneuver

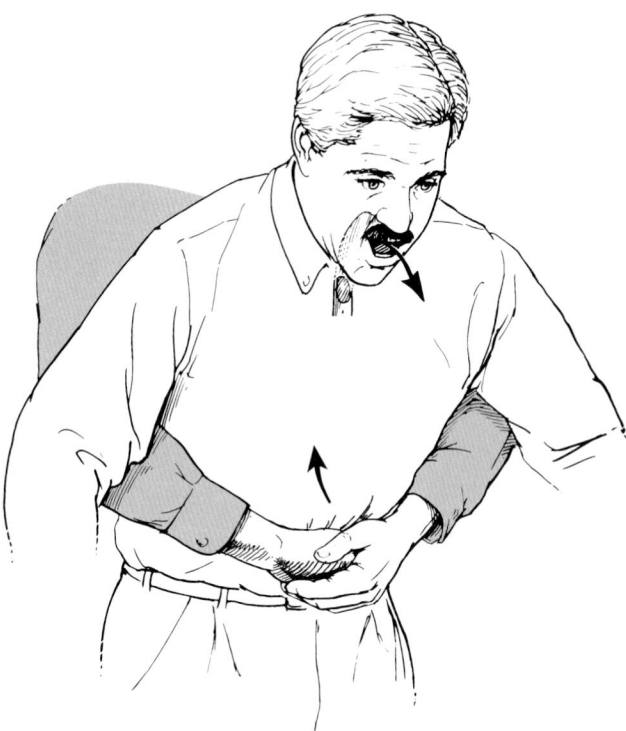

The Heimlich maneuver should be performed if the person is unable to speak, cough or effectively exchange air.

the cause. Often, people who are choking had been talking while chewing a large piece of meat. False teeth also can increase the risk of choking because they interfere with how food feels in the mouth, making it harder to tell if the food is fully chewed. In addition, people with false teeth can't chew food as thoroughly as they could with natural teeth because false teeth exert less pressure.

Other common causes of choking include:

- Excessive consumption of alcohol (Alcohol is a sedative. It dulls the nerves that help you swallow and sense how well your food has been chewed.)
- Eating too fast
- Eating while laughing or talking hurriedly
- Eating while walking, running or playing

Panic is often the first response of someone choking. The person's face often assumes an expression of terror and then takes on a bluish or ashen color as he or she stops breathing. The person may wheeze or gasp.

Coughing vs. choking

If a morsel of food "goes down the wrong pipe," the coughing reflex will often quickly solve the problem. In fact, a person isn't choking if he or she is able to cough freely and has normal skin color. But if the cough is more like a gasp or is silent, he or she is probably choking and needs immediate help.

Ask the person if he or she is choking. If the person indicates yes by nodding his or her head without speaking, he or she is choking. If the person can talk, then the airway is not completely blocked, and oxygen is reaching the lungs.

How to clear an obstructed airway

For most cases of choking in a person who is responsive and older than age 1, the obstruction can be cleared by performing abdominal thrusts, known as the Heimlich maneuver.

If you're the only rescuer, attempt to clear the obstruction by performing abdominal thrusts before calling 911 or your local emergency number. If another person is available, have that person call for help immediately while you perform first aid.

In an unresponsive person, the simplest method for clearing an obstructed airway is to sweep out the cause of the blockage. However, often the blockage is too far down the throat to be seen.

If you can see the food or object causing the blockage and it's at the back of the throat or high in the throat, sweep a finger into the back of the person's throat to clear the airway. Be careful not to push the food or object deeper into the airway, which can happen easily in young children. If the cause of the obstruction can't be seen, don't blindly insert your finger.

Performing the Heimlich maneuver

You've seen it displayed on posters and acted out on television, but do you know how to perform the Heimlich maneuver on someone who's choking?

The Heimlich maneuver is perhaps the best known technique for clearing an obstructed airway. It should be performed on someone only if there's complete or near-complete blockage of the airway.

Indications that a person is choking and needs help generally include the following: The person is unable to speak, has a silent cough, or is making squeaky or gurgling sounds with great effort. The person's face may turn blue, gray or ashen.

Performing the Heimlich maneuver on a conscious person age 1 or older

1. Stand behind the choking person and wrap your arms around his or her waist. Tip the person slightly forward.
2. Make a fist with one hand and position it slightly above the person's navel.
3. Grasp the fist with the other hand and press hard into the abdomen with a quick, upward thrust — as if you were trying to lift the person up. This action raises the diaphragm, putting pressure on the lungs and forcing air out of the lungs.
4. Perform abdominal thrusts in rapid succession until the obstruction is cleared or the person loses consciousness.
5. If the person becomes unresponsive, begin cardiopulmonary resuscitation (CPR).

Performing the Heimlich maneuver on yourself

If you're alone and choking, you can still perform abdominal thrusts to dislodge the object:

1. Make a fist and place it above your naval, with the thumb side toward your abdomen.
2. Grasp your fist with the other hand and bend over a hard surface — a chair or countertop will do.
3. Shove your fist inward and upward. Continue to do so until the object dislodges.

Performing the Heimlich maneuver on someone who is pregnant or obese

The abdomen of a pregnant or obese person can prevent the effective use of the Heimlich maneuver abdominal thrust.

1. Position your hands higher than with the normal Heimlich maneuver, at the base of the breastbone, just above the joining of the lowest ribs.
2. Proceed as with the Heimlich maneuver, carefully and forcefully pressing into the chest with a quick thrust.
3. Continue chest thrusts until the blockage is dislodged or the person becomes unconscious.
4. If the person becomes unresponsive, begin CPR.

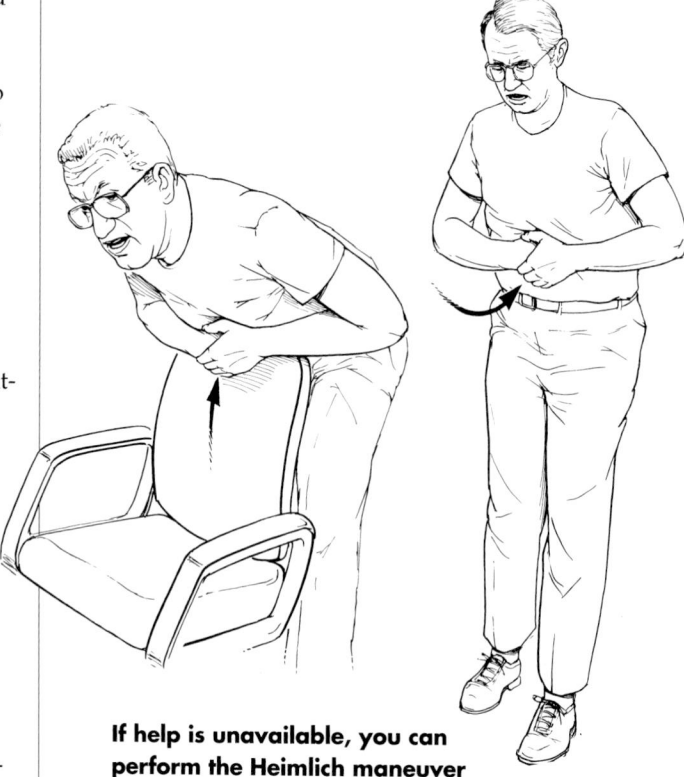

If help is unavailable, you can perform the Heimlich maneuver on yourself.

Clearing the airway of an unconscious person

If the individual becomes unconscious:

1. Lower the person on his or her back to the floor.
2. If there's a visible blockage at the back of the throat or high in the throat, reach a finger in and sweep out the cause of the blockage. Be careful not to push the food or object deeper in the airway. If you don't see the cause of the blockage, don't blindly place your finger in the person's mouth.
3. If the object remains lodged and the person remains unconscious, begin CPR. The chest compressions used in CPR may dislodge the object.

Clearing the airway of an infant younger than age 1

1. Assume a seated position and hold the infant facedown on your forearm, which is resting on your thigh. The infant's head should be slightly lower than his or her chest.
2. Thump the infant gently but firmly five times between the shoulder blades using the heel of your hand. The combination of gravity and the back blows should release the object blocking the airway.
3. If the back blows are unsuccessful, hold the infant faceup on your forearm with the head lower than the trunk. Using two fingers placed at the center of the infant's breastbone, give five quick chest compressions. Abdominal thrusts aren't recommended for infants younger than age 1.
4. Repeat the cycle of five back blows and five chest thrusts if breathing doesn't resume. If the infant becomes unresponsive, start CPR with chest compressions and call for emergency medical help.

Cardiopulmonary Resuscitation

Cardiopulmonary resuscitation (CPR) is a lifesaving technique that's useful in a wide range of emergencies that can lead to cardiac arrest, such as a heart attack or drowning, in which someone's breathing or heartbeat has stopped.

Basic Life Support

Basic life support is a crucial and potentially lifesaving sequence of events and actions taken in the event of a sudden cardiac arrest. It includes:

- Immediate recognition of sudden cardiac arrest
- Immediate activation of the emergency response system (911 or local emergency response number)
- Early cardiopulmonary resuscitation (CPR)
- Rapid defibrillation

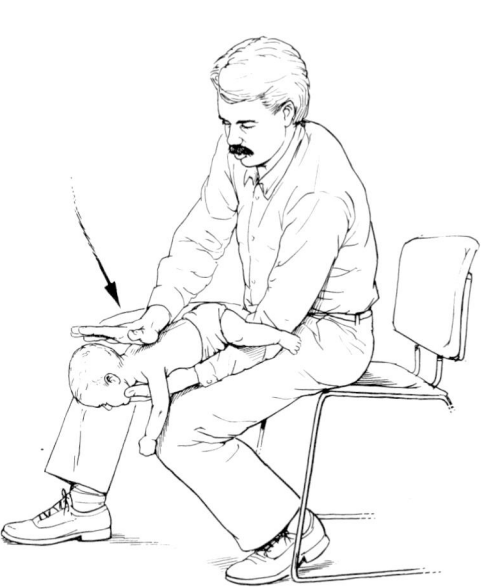

Gentle but firm thumps on the back can help clear the airway of a choking infant.

CPR involves two elements: chest compressions combined with mouth-to-mouth rescue breathing. However, what you as a bystander should do in an emergency situation really depends on your knowledge and comfort level.

The bottom line is that it's far better to do something than to do nothing at all, even if you're fearful that your knowledge or abilities aren't 100 percent complete. The difference between your doing something and doing nothing could be someone's life. CPR can keep oxygenated blood flowing to the brain and other vital organs until emergency response personnel arrive.

Below is advice from the American Heart Association on how to respond to an adult who needs CPR. In all circumstances, call 911 or your local emergency response number and follow the dispatcher's instructions:

- **Untrained layperson.** If you're not trained in CPR, then provide hands-only CPR. That means uninterrupted chest compressions of about two per second until paramedics arrive. You don't need to do rescue breathing. Just push hard and fast.
- **Trained layperson.** If you have trained in CPR and are confident in your ability, follow one of two approaches: A. Alternate between 30 chest compressions and two rescue breaths or B. Just do chest compressions.
- **Trained layperson, but rusty.** If you've received CPR training but you're not confident in your abilities, it's fine to do compression-only CPR.

To learn CPR properly, take an accredited basic life support course that includes CPR and how to use an automated external defibrillator (AED).

The following discussion is meant to guide you if you're an untrained layperson or if you've had prior CPR training.

Before you begin

Before starting CPR, assess the situation:
- Quickly scan the scene to make sure there aren't any imminent hazards to your personal health.
- Check if the person is responsive or unresponsive. Tap his or her shoulder and shout, "Are you OK?"
- If the person is unresponsive (doesn't answer, moan or move), immediately activate the emergency response system by calling 911.
- Check if the person is breathing or if his or her breathing is abnormal (such as gasping).
- If the person is unresponsive and isn't breathing or has abnormal breathing, the person is likely in cardiac arrest. Immediately begin CPR. It's not necessary to check for a pulse if you're a layperson.
- If an AED is immediately available and you're trained in how to use it or you're being guided by an emergency dispatcher, deliver one shock if advised by the device, then begin CPR.

Cardiopulmonary Resuscitation (CPR)

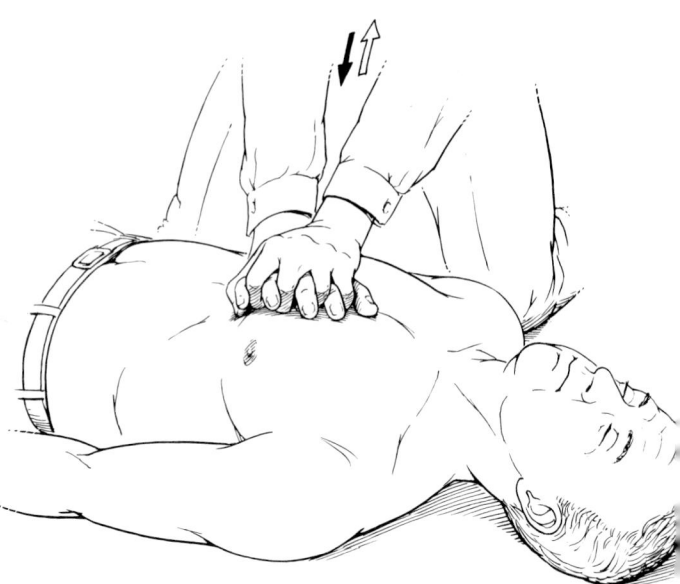

Perform chest compressions by placing one hand over the center of the person's chest and placing your other hand on top of the first hand. Push hard and fast.

Using an AED

If you've been trained in CPR you should be familiar with the proper use of an automated external defibrillator (AED). Attach the device to the individual who isn't breathing and use it as soon as possible.

If you're not trained in the use of an AED but one is available, alert the emergency dispatcher and follow his or her instructions.

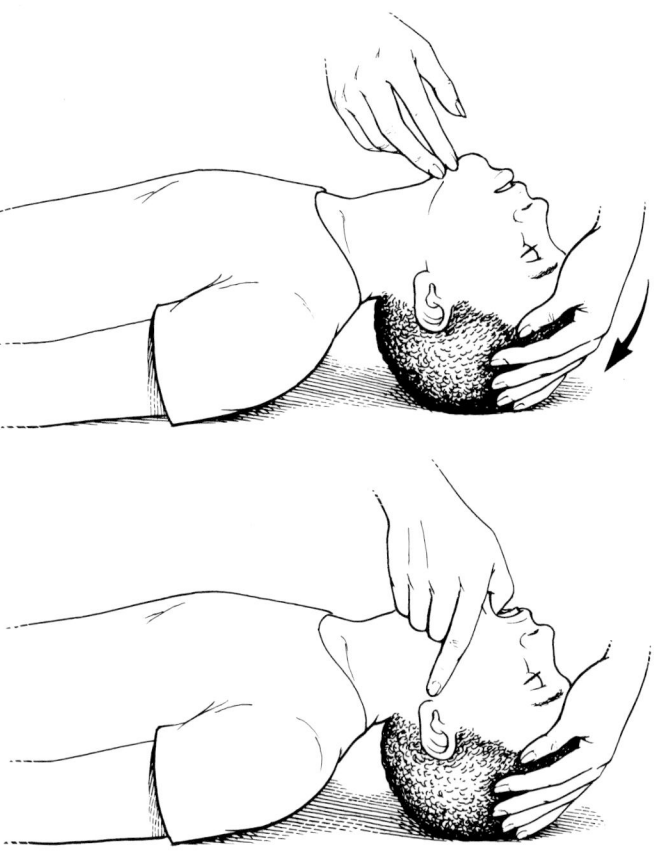

To open the airway, first tilt the head and lift the chin (head tilt-chin lift).

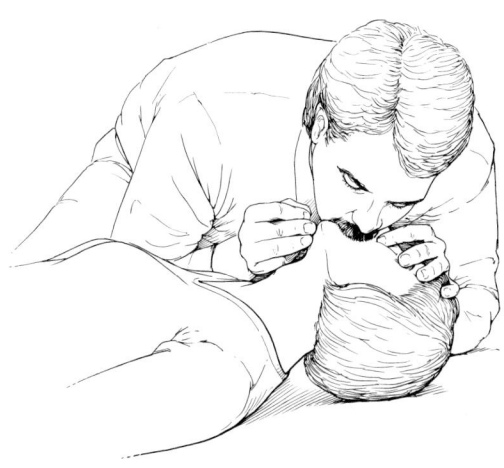

Effective rescue breathing should cause the chest to visibly rise.

How to perform CPR

When performing CPR, the first and most important step is to do chest compressions.

Begin chest compressions

The most important component of CPR is the forceful, rhythmic compression of the chest. Chest compressions should be started as soon as possible when cardiac arrest is suspected, and interruptions should be minimized.

When you perform chest compressions, you're acting as a heart pump to push blood and oxygen to the heart muscle (myocardium) and brain.

1. Place the person on his or her back on a firm surface.
2. Kneel next to the person's chest.
3. Place the heel of one hand over the center of the person's chest, between the nipples. Place your other hand on top of the first hand. Keep your elbows straight and position your shoulders directly above your hands.
4. Use your upper body weight (not just your arms) as you push straight down on (compress) the chest 2 inches (approximately 5 centimeters). Push hard and push fast — give two compressions per second, or about 120 compressions per minute.
5. If you're an untrained layperson, continue performing hands-only CPR using continuous hard and fast chest compressions until help arrives.
6. If you have CPR training and are able to perform rescue breaths, perform 30 chest compressions followed by two rescue breaths.
7. Continue CPR until there are signs of movement or until someone arrives with an AED or emergency medical personnel take over.

Open the airway

1. If you're a trained CPR layperson, open the person's airway using the head tilt-chin lift maneuver. Put your palm on the person's forehead and tilt the head back. With the other hand, tilt the chin forward to open the airway. Don't press deeply into the soft tissue below the chin.
2. If a spinal injury is suspected, don't manipulate the neck. If another person is available, have that person stabilize the head and neck.
3. Perform the airway maneuvers quickly, so that interruptions in chest compressions are minimized.

Breathe for the person

1. With the airway open (using the head tilt-chin lift maneuver) pinch the nostrils shut for mouth-to-mouth breathing and cover the person's mouth, making a seal.
2. Give the first rescue breath — lasting more than one second — with enough air to make the chest visibly rise. If it does, give a second rescue breath,

also lasting more than one second. If the chest doesn't rise, repeat the head tilt-chin lift maneuver and then give another breath.

3. If there's no breathing, coughing or movement, resume chest compressions.

Performing CPR on a child

The procedure for giving CPR to children age 1 through puberty is essentially the same as that for adults, with a few differences:

• The same as adults, if you're not trained in CPR and you don't know how to perform rescue breaths, do hands-only CPR. If you do know how to perform rescue breaths, infants and children may benefit from this step because cardiac arrest in children is frequently due to a breathing problem.

• You may use one or two hands to perform chest compressions. Depending on the size of the child, push down on the chest at least one-third its depth, or about 2 inches.

• Breathe more gently, but make sure the child's chest rises. Each breath should take about one second.

• As with adults, alternate between 30 chest compressions and two rescue breaths.

• If you're alone and no one else is able to call 911 to activate the emergency response system, perform five cycles of compressions and breaths on the child (this should take about two minutes) before leaving the child to alert emergency medical personnel.

• After five cycles (about two minutes) of CPR, if there's no response and an AED is available and you are able to use it, apply it and follow the prompts. Use pediatric pads if available. If pediatric pads aren't available, use adult pads.

Continue performing continuous CPR until the child moves or help arrives.

Performing CPR on an infant

Most cardiac arrests in infants occur from lack of oxygen, such as from drowning or choking. If you know the infant has an obstructed airway, perform first aid for choking. If you don't know why the infant isn't breathing, perform CPR.

To begin, assess the situation. Stroke the baby and watch for a response, such as movement, but don't shake the child. If there's no response, follow the steps listed and time the emergency call for help as follows:

• If you're the only rescuer and CPR is needed, do CPR for two minutes (about five cycles) before calling 911 or your local emergency number.

• If another person is available, have that person call for help immediately while you attend to the infant.

Begin chest compressions

1. Place the infant on his or her back on a firm, flat

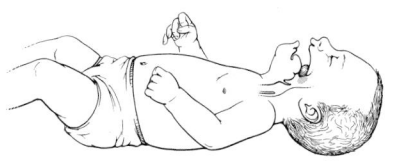
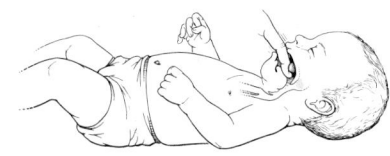

Before giving mouth-to-mouth resuscitation to an infant, tilt the child's head back to open the airway (top). If you see food or a foreign object in the infant's mouth, remove it with a sweep of your finger (bottom). Be careful not to push the food or object deeper into the child's airway.

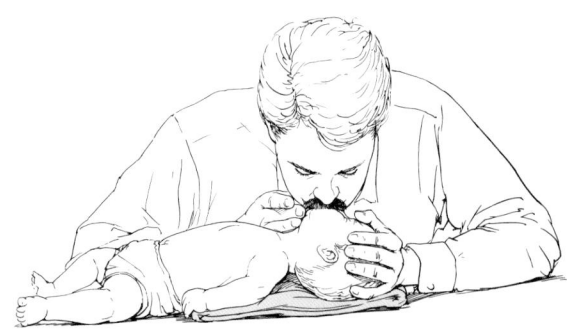

To perform mouth-to-mouth resuscitation on an infant, cover the baby's mouth and nose with your mouth. Using the strength of your cheeks, give two rescue breaths.

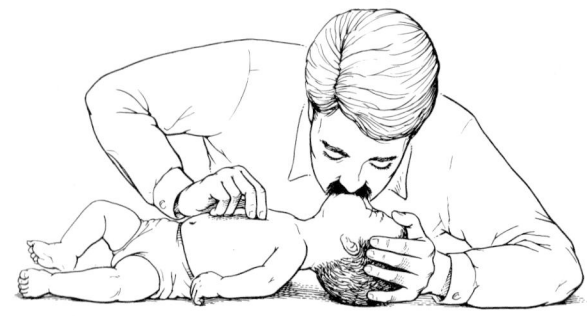

To perform cardiopulmonary resuscitation (CPR) on an infant, alternate compression of the baby's chest with gentle breaths from your mouth.

Sudden Infant Death Syndrome (SIDS)

SIDS is an unexpected and unexplained death occurring in infancy. The American Academy of Pediatrics recommends the following steps to reduce the risk of death from SIDS:

- "Back to Sleep." Every time a child sleeps, including naps, place the child on his or her back. Infants who sleep on their stomachs are at greater risk of SIDS.
- Have the child sleep on a firm mattress, free of soft bedding materials, crib bumpers and soft toys. A child can suffocate if his or her face comes into contact with these objects.
- For at least the first six months of life, a child should sleep in his or her parents' room, close to the parents' bed but not in the parents' bed.
- Breast-feeding has been shown to reduce the risk of SIDS, as has the use of a pacifier. Not smoking and avoiding alcohol during pregnancy also reduces the risk of SIDS.

surface, such as a table. The ground will also do.

2. Imagine a horizontal line drawn between the baby's nipples. Place two fingers of one hand about one finger-width below this line, in the center of the chest.
3. Compress the chest to at least one-third its depth, or about 1½ inches.
4. As with adults and children, give two compressions per second, or about 120 compressions per minute.
5. If you're able, give two breaths after every 30 chest compressions. If you're unable to perform rescue breaths, maintain continuous hands-only CPR until emergency medical help arrives.

Clear the airway

1. Gently tip the infant's head back by tilting the chin with one hand and pushing down on the baby's forehead with the other hand (head tilt-chin lift).

Breathe for the infant

1. Cover the baby's mouth and nose with your mouth.
2. Give two rescue breaths. Use the strength of your cheeks to deliver gentle puffs of air (instead of deep breaths from your lungs) to slowly breathe into the baby's mouth. Take one second for each breath. Watch to see if the baby's chest rises. If it does, give a second rescue breath. If the chest

Breathing Worries

Several disorders of the upper respiratory tract can produce difficulty breathing, especially in children. The most common include croup, epiglottitis and bronchitis. Noisy breathing may be common to all three of these conditions.

Croup

Croup is caused by a virus that infects the voice box (larynx) and windpipe (trachea). It's most likely to affect children between the ages of 6 months and 3 years.

Signs and symptoms include fever, hoarseness and cough. The cough often sounds like a bark (see page 450). Seek immediate medical attention if there's noisy breathing when a child breathes in (stridor).

Epiglottitis

The epiglottis is the lidlike cartilage that covers the windpipe during swallowing. When it becomes inflamed, the condition is called epiglottitis. Signs and symptoms often include a very sore throat, fever, drooling, hoarseness, voice change, difficulty swallowing saliva due to pain, and noisy breathing (see page 654).

Epiglottitis is a medical emergency requiring immediate treatment.

Bronchitis

Bronchitis is characterized by a cough that's often accompanied by the production of sputum (see page 763). Bronchitis usually is caused by a viral infection of the passages that carry air to the lungs (bronchi). It usually isn't associated with significant shortness of breath and it often doesn't pro-

duce a fever. Most people improve without treatment.

Getting treatment

Be concerned if your child's symptoms include voice changes, drooling, difficulty breathing and noisy breathing. These signs and symptoms can mean severe swelling of the tissues that line the airways. Call for emergency help or take the child to the nearest emergency department. Perform CPR if the child stops breathing.

For croup and bronchitis, exposure to warm, humid air may provide relief. You could seat your child in the bathroom and quickly humidify the air by closing the door and filling the bathtub with hot water. Breathing cold air during the night by opening a window or door also may help.

doesn't rise, repeat the head tilt-chin lift maneuver and give the second breath.

3. If the chest still doesn't rise, examine the mouth to make sure no foreign material is inside. If an object can be seen, sweep it out with your finger.

4. Continue with cycles of chest compressions and rescue breaths until help arrives.

CPR and specific emergencies

CPR can save lives in many kinds of emergencies. Some situations in which it may be necessary to provide breathing assistance, as well as chest compressions, include heart attack, smoke inhalation, carbon monoxide poisoning, drowning and electrical injury.

Heart attack

A heart attack occurs when one or more coronary arteries that supply oxygen-rich blood to the heart muscle become blocked. When deprived of blood, portions of the heart muscle gradually die.

A heart attack may be preceded by intermittent pain, occurring during exertion or even rest. This is known as angina. Sometimes, a heart attack will occur without any previous pain.

A heart attack is a medical emergency. If you think that you're having a heart attack:

1. Get immediate medical attention. Call 911 for emergency medical help or have someone take you to the nearest emergency department. Don't drive yourself. Delaying medical treatment is a mistake that costs thousands of lives every year.

2. While waiting for emergency help to arrive or while traveling to the emergency facility, chew and swallow an aspirin tablet (one 325-milligram tablet or four 81-milligram tablets). Aspirin helps prevent further blood clotting in the heart arteries. Chewing the tablet before swallowing it speeds its action.

If you're with an individual having a heart attack and the person becomes unresponsive and stops breathing, perform CPR.

Severe asthma attack

People with asthma may experience occasional or even frequent asthma attacks. Often, the individual's asthma medication is all that's needed to improve symptoms.

Occasionally, more serious or even life-threatening asthma attacks may occur. Signs and symptoms of a serious asthma attack may include extreme difficulty in breathing, a bluish cast to the person's face and lips, severe anxiety, a rapid pulse and excessive perspiration.

1. Establish that the problem isn't a choking emergency. People with asthma, like the rest of us, can

Is It a Heart Attack?

A heart attack may cause one or more of the following signs and symptoms. If you experience any of these, call for emergency medical help.

- Chest pain, at times intense or prolonged, that's often described as heavy pressure under the breastbone or a weight upon the chest. The pain may extend beyond your chest, radiating to your shoulder and arm, both arms, your back and even your teeth, jaw, and neck. Sometimes, radiating pain may occur without chest pain. At times the pain may occur in the upper abdomen and feel much like severe indigestion. The pain may come on suddenly or gradually, with exertion or at rest.
- Nausea, with or without vomiting.
- Shortness of breath.
- Unexplained sweating.
- Weakness, restlessness and anxiety.

Women, older adults and people with diabetes, are more likely to experience atypical symptoms, which may include no chest pain at all. Occasionally, the only sign is cardiac arrest.

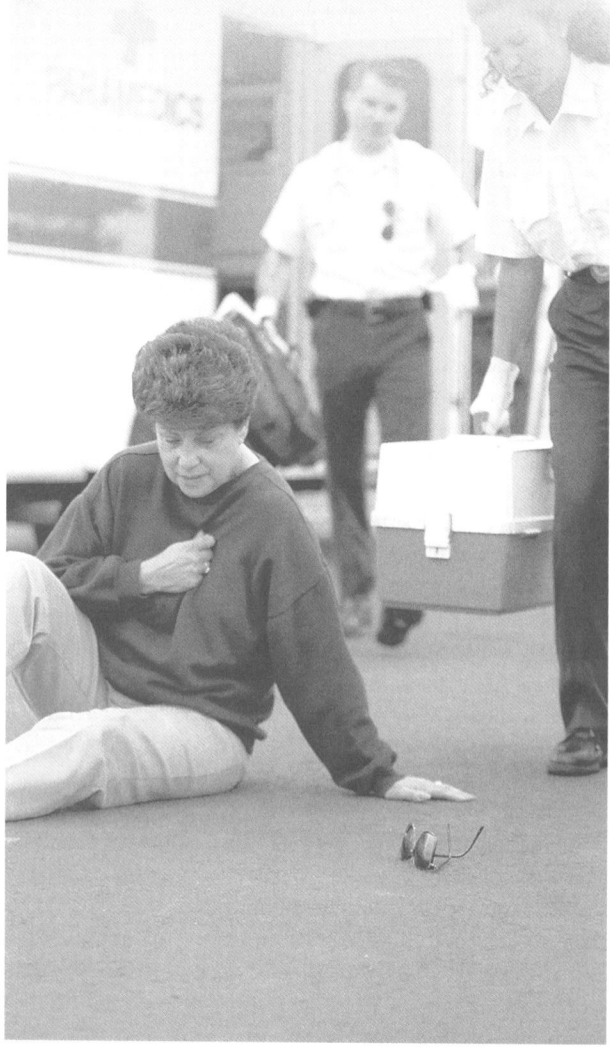

choke on food or other foreign objects that block the airway.
2. Call 911 for emergency medical help.
3. If the person has an inhaled bronchodilator device, such as an albuterol inhaler, help the person use it.
4. If the person becomes unresponsive and stops breathing, begin CPR.

Smoke inhalation

Fire produces smoke that may contain poisons. When burned, plastics, synthetic fabrics, wood, chemicals and other flammable materials can generate toxic gases, including carbon monoxide and cyanide.

Inhaled smoke from these burning substances can cause severe illness due to the toxic nature of these gases or breathing problems resulting from heat damage to your airways and lungs.

The key signs and symptoms of smoke inhalation are irritated eyes, soot around the nose or mouth, difficulty breathing, noisy breathing, or gasping for breath. Any sign of breathing difficulty — even a cough — should be treated as an emergency because the problem will often get worse. To treat smoke inhalation:
1. Move the victim to a smoke-free area a safe distance from the fire or source of smoke.
2. Once the person is clear of the smoke, check for breathing. If the person is unresponsive and isn't breathing, begin CPR.
3. If the person is breathing, loosen any tight clothing, make the person as comfortable as possible and summon emergency medical help.

Hyperventilation

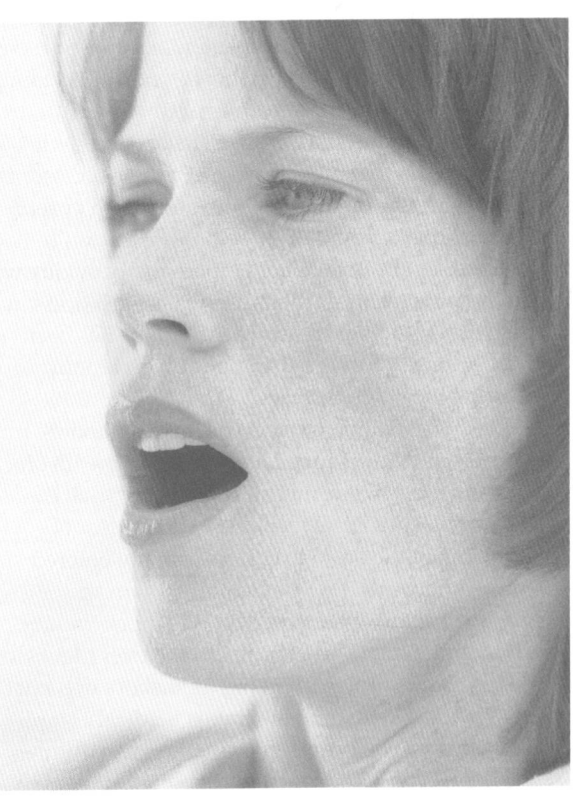

Fear or panic attacks can cause hyperventilation — over-breathing that results from taking too many breaths or breathing too deeply. Even though you're taking in extra air, you may feel as though you're not getting enough.

Hyperventilation can cause tingling and spasms of the hands, in which the fingers are extended while the thumb and fifth finger are involuntarily drawn together. Your feet may also have similar muscle spasms. Other symptoms include lightheadedness, a woozy feeling and tingling around the mouth. These symptoms result from rapid, shallow breathing, causing too much carbon dioxide to be exhaled. This creates a chemical imbalance in your body, leading to symptoms of hyperventilation.

Treatment of hyperventilation consists of reassuring the individual that everything is OK and persuading the person to breathe more normally. Make sure to talk to the individual in a calm tone of voice.

If the person hasn't had such an incident before, he or she should see a doctor to be sure the episode isn't something dangerous that's mimicking a panic attack.

Carbon monoxide poisoning

One byproduct of fire is carbon monoxide. Carbon monoxide is colorless, odorless and causes death without warning. When inhaled, carbon monoxide takes the place of oxygen in your bloodstream and reduces the supply of oxygen to your body's cells. Typical signs and symptoms of carbon monoxide poisoning are headache, nausea, vomiting and confusion. Loss of consciousness, seizures and death may occur when levels of carbon monoxide in the blood become high.

Inadequately vented furnaces and wood- or coal-burning stoves, among other things, can result in carbon monoxide accumulation in the home.

1. If you wake up at night with a headache — especially if another member of your family complains of headache or nausea or is hard to rouse — have everyone exit the house immediately. Go to a neighbor's home and call for emergency medical assistance.
2. If you're with someone who's been exposed to carbon monoxide, check to see if he or she is responsive and breathing. If not, begin CPR.
3. If the person is breathing, loosen any tight clothing and make the individual as comfortable as possible. Summon emergency medical help, even if the person seems recovered. He or she will benefit from high-flow oxygen as soon as it's available from responding emergency medical personnel.

Drowning

If you find an individual floundering or submerged in water and you believe that you're strong enough and sufficiently trained to rescue the person, do so immediately. If you're not a strong swimmer or are unsure that you can manage the person by yourself, get help.

To treat someone rescued from drowning:

1. Once the individual has been rescued, call for emergency medical help if you're alone. Check if the person is breathing. If the person isn't breathing and is unresponsive, begin CPR. If you're not alone, send someone for help as you provide care. This may mean starting the breathing process in shallow water even before the person has been positioned on shore. Throughout, make sure your safety isn't compromised.
2. Don't waste time trying to drain the person's lungs of water. Immediately begin to breathe for the person. Air should still be able to reach the lungs in spite of any residual water. Most of the time little or no water has actually entered the lungs.
3. Clear the airway and deliver two quick breaths. Continue to breathe for the person every few seconds while moving him or her to shore or a boat.
4. Drowning can result in various medical complications, so seek emergency medical care for the victim even after a successful rescue.

To prevent carbon monoxide poisoning, purchase carbon monoxide detectors for your home. Carbon monoxide detectors should be battery operated or have a battery backup and they should be located near every sleeping area in the home.

The detectors sound a warning when carbon monoxide levels in a home or other building exceed an unsafe level. Look for the code UL 2034 on the box. This indicates the detector meets an industry standard that requires alarms to sound before a typical, healthy adult begins to experience symptoms.

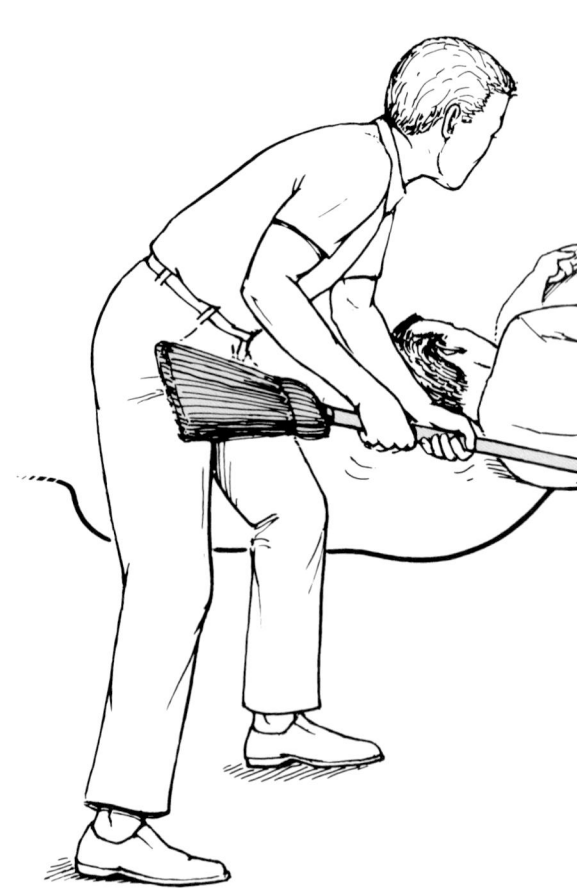

Electrical injury

Most people experience minor electrical shocks now and again. Such shocks are usually more surprising than dangerous because a reflex action almost instantly jerks you away from the source of electricity. Under certain circumstances, though, even small amounts of electricity can result in heart rhythm problems, respiratory failure, numbness and tingling, seizures, unconsciousness, or cardiac arrest.

If you notice any of these signs or symptoms, call 911 or your local emergency number.

To treat someone with an electrical injury:

1. Look first, don't touch. The person may still be in contact with the electrical source. Touching the person may pass the current through you.
2. Turn off the source of electricity if possible. If that isn't possible, move the source of the electricity away from the victim. Use a dry, non-conducting object, such as plastic, rubber or fiberglass. Wood and cardboard were previously recommended, but they may be wet and may conduct electricity. Don't use a metal object.
3. Don't move the person if you don't have to. Unless the person is in immediate danger, treat the person in the location in which you found him or her.
4. Once the person is removed from the electrical source, check if the person is responsive and breathing. If he or she is not, begin CPR.
5. Prevent shock. Lay the person down if possible and position his or her head slightly lower than the trunk, with the legs elevated.

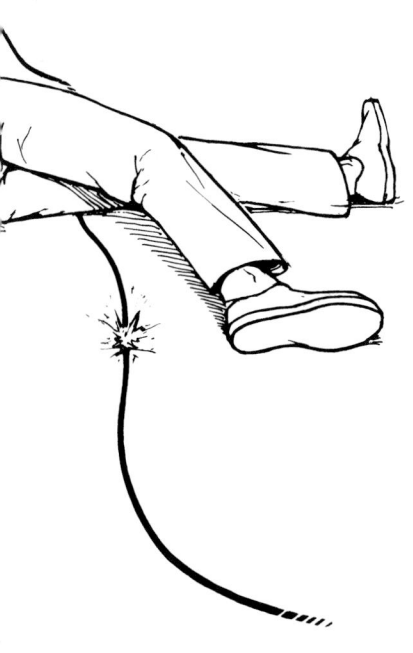

Use a nonconducting object — such as a plastic or fiberglass broom handle — to pull or push a victim of electrical shock away from the live electrical source.

Chest Pain

Causes of chest pain can vary from minor problems, such as indigestion or muscle strain, to serious medical emergencies, such as a heart attack or pulmonary embolism. The specific cause of chest pain is often difficult to interpret. As with other sudden, unexplained pains, chest pain is a signal for you to seek medical help. Use the following information to help you determine whether your chest pain is a medical emergency. If you're uncertain, seek emergency care.

Heart attack

A heart attack occurs when an artery that supplies oxygen to your heart muscle becomes blocked. A heart attack generally causes chest pain that lasts longer than 15 minutes. But a heart attack can also be silent and produce no signs or symptoms.

Many people who have a heart attack have warning symptoms hours, days or weeks in advance. The earliest predictor may be recurrent chest pain triggered by exertion and relieved by rest, often called angina.

Someone having a heart attack may experience any or all of the following:

- Uncomfortable pressure, fullness or squeezing pain in the center of the chest lasting more than a few minutes.
- Pain spreading to the shoulders, neck or arms.
- Lightheadedness, fainting, sweating, nausea or shortness of breath.

If you or someone else may be having a heart attack:

- **Call 911 or emergency medical assistance.** Don't attempt to "tough out" the symptoms of a heart attack. If you don't have access to emergency medical services, have someone such as a neighbor or friend drive you to the nearest emergency department. Drive yourself only if there are absolutely no other options. Driving yourself puts you and others at risk if your condition suddenly worsens.
- **Chew a regular-strength aspirin.** Aspirin can inhibit blood clotting. However, you shouldn't take aspirin if you're allergic to aspirin, have bleeding problems or have been told by your doctor not to do so.
- **Take nitroglycerin, if prescribed.** If you think you're having a heart attack and your doctor has previously prescribed nitroglycerin for you, take it as directed. Do not take anyone else's nitroglycerin.
- **Begin CPR.** If the person suspected of having a heart attack becomes unconscious, begin CPR. If you're not trained, a dispatcher can instruct you what to do until emergency help arrives.

Pulmonary embolism

An embolus is an accumulation of foreign material — usually a blood clot — that becomes lodged in an artery, blocking blood flow. When an artery becomes blocked, tissue that normally receives blood and nutrients from that artery can be damaged due to the sudden loss of blood. This can cause tissue death.

Pulmonary embolism is the term used to describe a condition that occurs when a clot — usually from the veins of your leg or pelvis — breaks loose and lodges in an artery of your lung, preventing the lungs from supplying adequate oxygen to the bloodstream and body tissues.

Signs and symptoms include:

- Sudden, unexplained shortness of breath, even without pain
- Sudden, sharp chest pain that begins or worsens with a deep breath or a cough
- Cough that may produce blood-streaked sputum
- Rapid heartbeat
- Anxiety and excessive perspiration
- Momentary loss of consciousness

As with a suspected heart attack, call 911 or emergency medical assistance immediately.

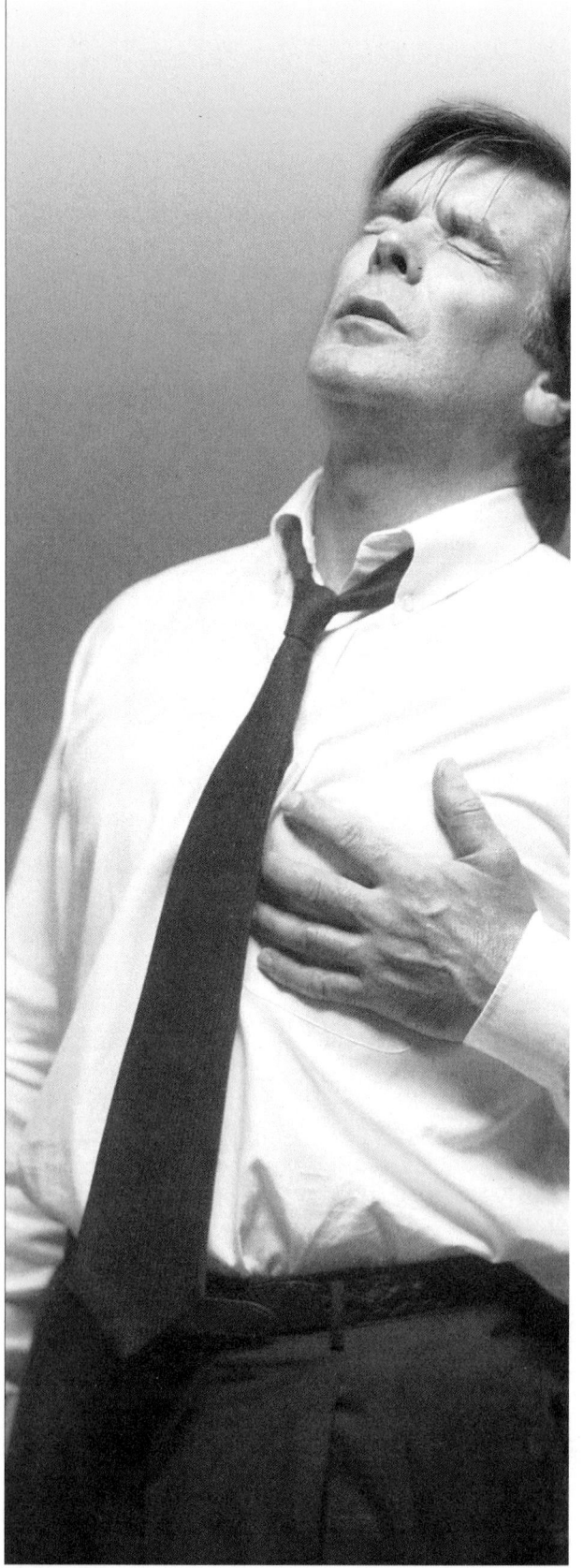

Pneumonia and pleurisy

Frequent signs and symptoms of pneumonia are a cough that may produce sputum, shortness of breath, chills, fever and chest pain. When pneumonia occurs with an inflammation of the membranes that surround the lung (pleura), you may have considerable chest discomfort when inhaling or coughing. This condition is called pleurisy.

One sign of pleurisy is that the pain is usually relieved temporarily by holding your breath or putting pressure on the painful area of your chest. This isn't true of a heart attack. See your doctor if you have a cough and a fever or chills with chest pain.

Chest wall pain

A harmless form of chest pain is what's called costochondritis, a type of pain that originates in the chest wall. It consists of pain and tenderness in and around the cartilage that connects your ribs to your breastbone (sternum). If the pressure of a finger placed on a few points along the margin of the sternum reproduces the pain, chest wall pain is a likely cause.

Other causes of chest pain include:
- Strained chest muscles from overuse or excessive coughing
- Chest muscle bruising from minor trauma
- A rib bruise or fracture in the setting of an injury
- Pain from the gastrointestinal tract, such as esophageal reflux, peptic ulcer pain or gallbladder pain

Severe Bleeding

When an injury results in bleeding, you need to take steps to stop the loss of blood. Most injuries don't cause life-threatening bleeding, but if substantial

Types of Bleeding

When you're assisting someone who's bleeding, it's often helpful to distinguish the type of bleeding that's occurring because treatment varies from one type to another. The three main classifications are:

Capillary bleeding
Capillaries are the most numerous and smallest blood vessels in the body. When a minor cut or skin scrape opens some capillaries, the bleeding is usually slow and small in content. The body's normal clotting action generally stops the bleeding in a matter of minutes.

Venous bleeding
Deeper cuts often open veins, releasing blood that's on its way back to the heart. Having delivered its load of oxygen to the cells, the blood is dark red. It flows steadily but relatively slowly. Placing firm, direct pressure on the wound will usually stop the blood flow.

Arterial bleeding
The least common but most serious type of bleeding is caused by injury to an artery. The blood that's released is bright red and often spurts with each contraction of the heart. If a major artery is severed and not treated promptly, it's possible to bleed to death in as little as a few minutes. In most cases, though, direct, firm pressure on the wound will stop arterial bleeding.

amounts of blood are lost, shock, unconsciousness and death can result. Appropriate care must be taken to stop the bleeding and also to avoid infection and other complications. The information that follows discusses appropriate emergency procedures to accomplish these goals.

Stopping severe bleeding

To stop severe bleeding from an injury:

1. **Lay the bleeding person down.** If possible, elevate the legs. This position helps reduce the chances of fainting by increasing blood flow to the brain.
2. **Don't remove any objects impaled in the person.** Don't probe the wound or attempt to clean it at this point. Your main concern is to stop the bleeding.
3. **Apply firm pressure directly on the wound.** Use a sterile bandage, clean cloth or even a piece of clothing. If nothing else is available, use your hand. Continuous firm and direct pressure is your best tool to stop the bleeding.
4. **Maintain pressure until the bleeding stops.** Hold continuous pressure for at least 20 minutes without looking to see if the bleeding has stopped. Maintain pressure afterward, if possible, by binding the wound tightly with a bandage or piece of clean clothing and adhesive tape.
5. **Don't remove the gauze or bandage.** If the bleeding continues and seeps through the gauze or other material that you're holding on the wound, don't remove it. Instead, add more absorbent material on top of it and maintain firm, direct pressure.
6. **Squeeze a main artery if necessary.** If the bleeding doesn't stop with direct pressure, you may need to make a tourniquet from cloth or a belt and apply it to the affected limb above the wound to stop the bleeding until emergency medical care arrives.
7. **Immobilize the injured area once the bleeding has stopped.** Leave the bandages in place and get the injured person to an emergency department as soon as possible.

Bleeding from an open wound

Bleeding from the surface of your body can range from very minor, such as a needle prick, to major, as with a deep gash in which an artery is severed. All wounds require appropriate care and treatment. Inadequate wound care can result in serious infection. One important precaution against infection is to make sure your tetanus immunization is always kept up-to-date.

Severe cuts

If your cut is serious — the bleeding doesn't stop on its own in a few minutes or the cut is large or deep — seek emergency medical care. First stop the bleeding by applying pressure directly to the injury, using a

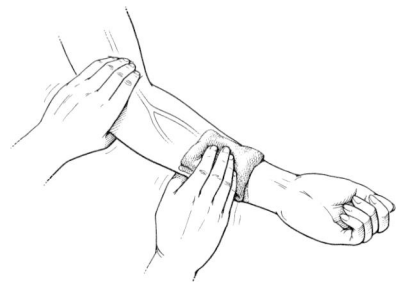

To stop bleeding, apply pressure directly to the wound, using sterile gauze or a clean cloth.

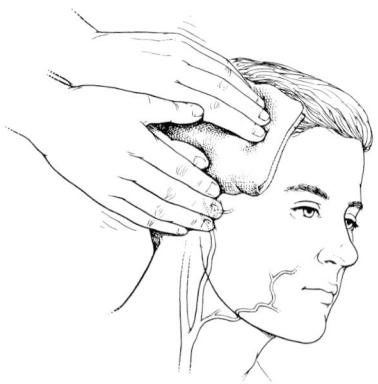

If bleeding continues despite pressure applied directly to the wound, maintain pressure and also apply pressure to the nearest major artery between the injury and the heart.

Tetanus Immunizations

A cut, laceration, bite or other wound, even if minor, can lead to tetanus, an infection that occurs days or even weeks later. Tetanus, also called lockjaw, causes stiffness of jaw muscles and other muscles. Other signs and symptoms may include irritability, sweating and breathing problems. The disease can be fatal.

Tetanus bacteria usually are found in the soil but can occur just about anywhere. If their spores enter a wound beyond the reach of oxygen, they germinate and produce a toxin that interferes with the nerves controlling your muscles. For more information on tetanus, see page 454.

Immunization for tetanus is important for everyone. The tetanus vaccine usually is given to children as a DTaP shot, in which diphtheria and whooping cough (pertussis) vaccines are included with the tetanus vaccine. Adults generally need a tetanus booster shot (Tdap or Td) every 10 years. You may also get a booster shot if you suffer a deep or dirty wound and your most recent booster was more than five years ago. Boosters should be given as soon as possible after the injury.

If you haven't had a tetanus immunization previously, your doctor may administer tetanus immune globulin. It provides immediate protection, but it lasts only a few weeks. Several antibiotics can help eliminate the tetanus bacterium, but the best protection is proper care of the wound and staying up-to-date on your vaccinations.

sterile gauze pad or a clean cloth. Maintain pressure until the bleeding stops.

Bruises

Bruises (contusions) usually result from a blow or fall. Bleeding beneath the skin produces an accumulation of blood (hematoma). To reduce discomfort, elevate the injured area and apply ice or cold packs for 20 minutes at a time several times a day.

Punctures

Stepping on a nail is a common way to get a puncture wound. Such a wound usually doesn't result in excessive bleeding. A little blood flows and the wound seems to close almost instantly. This doesn't mean that treatment is unnecessary.

Puncture wounds are dangerous because of the risk of infection. The object that caused the wound, especially if it has been exposed to soil, may carry spores of tetanus or other bacteria. These can result in serious infections. A puncture wound through a shoe is particularly prone to serious bacterial infection.

If you sustain a puncture wound, stop the bleeding, if necessary, by applying pressure with a sterile gauze pad or clean cloth. Then seek emergency treatment to prevent infection. If the bleeding is minor, some doctors recommend allowing the wound to bleed for a short period of time to help flush it out. When the bleeding is stopped, apply an antibiotic cream to the wound, cover it with a bandage or dressing, and watch for signs of infection.

If an animal inflicted the wound, you may have been exposed to rabies and your doctor may suggest a rabies vaccination series (see page 458). The type of animal inflicting the wound and the location of the wound will determine the need for antibiotic treatment.

Soft tissue injuries

With a soft tissue injury, the skin is damaged, as are underlying tissues such as muscle, supporting structures and blood vessels. These injuries can occur when an area is hit, when an area is badly cut, when skin is separated from the underlying tissues or when skin is forcefully torn away. Soft tissue injuries require emergency medical care. Apply pressure to the wound to stop bleeding and seek emergency care immediately.

Abdominal wounds

Because of possible injury to internal organs, any wound that penetrates the abdominal wall is a potentially serious injury. If you or someone with you sustains an abdominal wound, seek emergency care.

Before moving someone with an abdominal wound, position the person on his or her back. If no internal organs protrude through the wound, use a gauze pad or sterile cloth and exert pressure on the injury to stop bleeding. When the blood flow has stopped, tape the bandage in place. If organs have been displaced, don't try to replace them in the abdominal cavity. Cover the injury with a dressing.

Bleeding from body openings

Bleeding from body openings can result from an internal injury or disease. Internal bleeding may accompany seemingly superficial injuries. For example, a blow to the head that produces minor bleeding from or under the skin may result in much more dangerous internal bleeding. In some cases, an internal injury may show no signs of external bleeding.

If the person has sustained an injury, such as during a fall, an automobile accident or an event involving violence, he or she may be bleeding internally.

Vomiting of blood
Vomiting of blood can occur as the result of injury to or disease of the throat, esophagus, stomach or first portion of the small intestine (duodenum).

Call for emergency assistance. While waiting for help to arrive, have the person lie down with legs elevated, if possible. The person shouldn't eat or drink anything. Food or liquids can worsen the problem. If the person is unconscious or having trouble breathing, position the person on his or her side to prevent choking.

Coughing up blood
When a person coughs up blood, the source of the blood is usually the lungs or windpipe. The blood that appears is usually frothy and bright red. Some possible causes include a lung infection, a blood clot in the lung, an injury to the chest or lung cancer.

Seek emergency help if the person coughs up large amounts of blood. While waiting for help to arrive, keep the individual's head elevated slightly and supported by pillows. Loosen clothing that's tight around the person's throat and chest.

Rectal bleeding
Bleeding from the anus can be the result of various problems. Hemorrhoids can cause bright red blood in the toilet bowl or on the toilet paper. Black, tarry stools, maroon stools or large amounts of bright red blood in the stool may suggest serious bleeding in the gastrointestinal tract.

If the bleeding is minimal and you feel fine, make an appointment to see your doctor. If rectal bleeding occurs in moderate to large amounts, or you're experiencing weakness or abdominal pain, seek emergency care.

Vaginal bleeding
Vaginal bleeding is a normal part of menstruation. However, bleeding from the vagina may also signal a wide range of gynecological and other medical prob-

Detecting Internal Bleeding

In the event of a traumatic injury, internal bleeding may not be immediately apparent. Consider it a possibility if you observe any of the following signs or symptoms:
- Bleeding from the ears, nose, rectum or vagina
- Vomiting or coughing up blood
- Bruising on the neck, chest or abdomen
- Wounds that have penetrated the skull, chest or abdomen
- Abdominal tenderness, possibly accompanied by rigidity of the abdominal muscles
- Fractures

Internal bleeding may produce shock. If the volume of blood in the body decreases, the person may feel weak, anxious, thirsty or lightheaded. In addition, the skin may feel cool. Other signs and symptoms of shock from internal bleeding include shallow and rapid breathing, a rapid and weak pulse, trembling, and restlessness. The person may faint when standing or even while seated but soon recover when allowed to lie down. Elevating the person's legs may help.

If you suspect internal bleeding, request immediate emergency help. Try to keep the person still and loosen the person's clothing. In case of internal bleeding in an extremity, stop the bleeding by applying pressure directly to this area or manually compressing the major artery between the heart and the fracture or bruise.

Basic First-Aid Supplies

Keep your medicine cabinet or first-aid kit well stocked. Include the following basic supplies:
- Instant cold packs
- Gauze wrappings or pads in several sizes
- Bandages
- Adhesive tape
- A sharp scissors, tweezers and a needle
- Soap or hand sanitizer
- Cotton balls or cotton-tipped swabs
- Antibiotic ointment
- Hydrocortisone cream (for stings or contact rashes)
- Aspirin (especially for chest pain)
- Ibuprofen or acetaminophen (for pain and fever)
- A thermometer
- Sterile eyewash, such as saline solution
- Petroleum jelly or other lubricant
- Tissues
- Disposable latex or synthetic gloves
- A first-aid manual

Other medications that you may want to have on hand include antihistamine tablets, antacids and reserve supplies of medications taken by family members, such as insulin for diabetes or medication for high blood pressure. If you or a family member has a severe allergy such as a nut allergy or bee allergy, make sure that your first-aid kit includes a syringe or autoinjector containing the medication epinephrine.

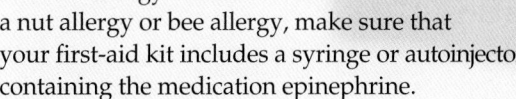

lems. See your doctor if you experience unexpected vaginal bleeding, especially if you've gone through menopause. If you have low-abdominal pain and unexpected vaginal bleeding, seek emergency care.

Blood in urine

Blood in urine can be frightening because it can appear as if you're bleeding more than you really are. A relatively small amount of bright red blood in the toilet may make the bowl appear to be full of blood. But chances are you've lost relatively little blood. See your doctor as soon as possible to determine the cause, even if the bleeding has subsided.

Nosebleeds

A nosebleed usually involves bleeding from one nostril. It may result from trauma, dry air, allergies or for no apparent reason.

Most nosebleeds come from the septum, the cartilage that separates the nasal chambers and is lined with fragile blood vessels. This form of nosebleed isn't serious and is usually easy to stop. In some people, nosebleeds may begin farther back in the nose. These nosebleeds, which are less common, are often harder to stop.

To stop the flow of blood:
1. Sit or stand upright, with your head tilted slightly down. Don't tip your head back.
2. Pinch your nose with your thumb and index finger and breathe through your mouth. Do this for five to 10 minutes without releasing pressure.
3. If you stop the flow of blood, there's no need to see a doctor. If the bleeding proves hard to stop, seek emergency medical care.
4. To prevent re-bleeding, don't blow or pick your nose and try not to bend down for several hours after the bleeding episode.
5. Seek medical care if the bleeding lasts for more than 20 minutes or if it follows an accident, such as a fall.

Treating Minor Burns at Home

To treat a minor burn:
1. Cool the burn by holding it under cold, running water for 15 minutes. If this isn't possible, immerse the burn in cold water or cover it with cold compresses. Don't put ice directly on the burn. Doing so can cause further damage.
2. Once the burn is cooled, apply a lotion or moisturizer to soothe the area and prevent dryness.
3. Cover the burn with a sterile gauze bandage. Wrap it loosely to avoid putting pressure on the burn.
4. Fluid-filled blisters sometimes form. If they do, don't break the blisters. If they break by themselves, wash the area with mild soap and water. Then apply an antibiotic ointment and gauze bandage. You can gently trim away dead skin from popped blisters.
5. Acetaminophen (Tylenol, others) or ibuprofen (Advil, Motrin IB, others) may help relieve pain and swelling.

Burns

Burns come from many sources, including fire, the sun, steam, electricity, chemicals, and hot liquids or objects. Burns may cause only minor injury that you can treat on your own or life-threatening emergencies that require intensive medical treatment.

Burn classifications

To distinguish a minor burn from a serious burn, the first step is to determine the degree and the extent of damage to body tissues. The traditional burn classification — first-degree burn, second-degree burn and third-degree burn — has been replaced by a new system indicating the need for specialized care. The severity of your wound, based on depth, will determine your care:

Superficial burns
Superficial burns, previously called first-degree burns, are the least serious burns, involving only the outer layer of skin (epidermis). The skin is usually dry and red, and it may be slightly swollen and painful. The outer layer of skin hasn't been burned through, and the skin doesn't blister. Superficial burns can generally be cared for at home.

Partial-thickness burns
When the first layer of skin has been burned through and the second layer of skin (dermis) also is burned, the injury is a partial-thickness burn. Symptoms depend on the depth of the burn. Superficial partial-thickness burns cause blisters, deep red skin color that lightens with pressure, weeping and intense pain. Deep partial-thickness burns may appear wet or waxy, vary in color, don't lighten as much with pressure and are less painful. If a partial-thickness burn is limited to an area no larger than 2 to 3 inches in diameter, you may be able to treat it at home. If the burned area of skin is larger or if the burn occurred on the hands, feet, face, groin, buttocks or over a joint, seek emergency medical care.

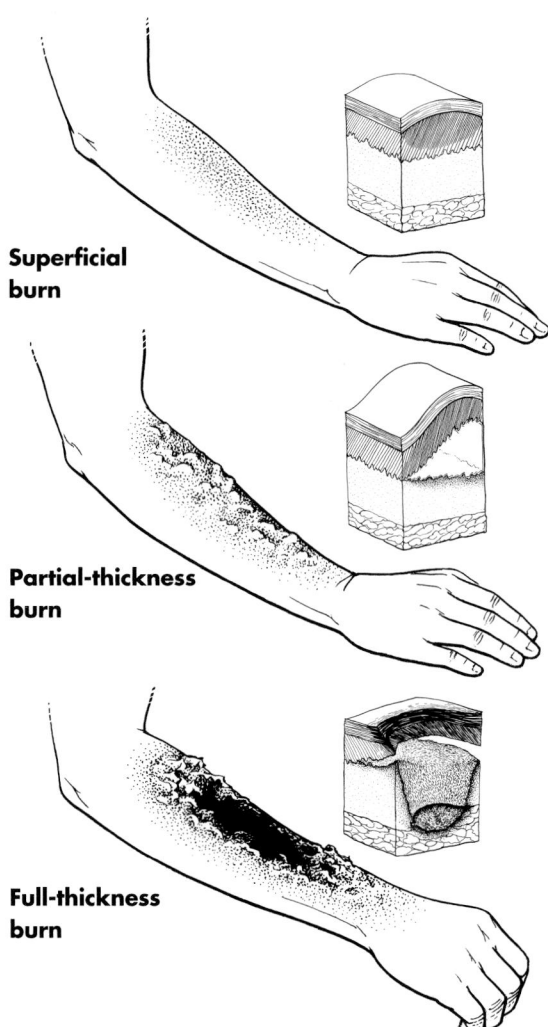

Superficial burn

Partial-thickness burn

Full-thickness burn

Burns are classified according to the degree of damage to skin and body tissue.

Treating Major Burns

Call for emergency medical assistance for all major burns. While waiting for help to arrive:
1. Make sure the cause of the burn has been extinguished or removed. Don't remove burned clothing that adheres to the skin, but check that the person isn't in contact with harmful smoldering materials.
2. Make certain the individual is breathing. If the individual is unresponsive and breathing has stopped, begin cardiopulmonary resuscitation (CPR).
3. If the individual appears to be in shock, take steps to treat the shock. Don't immerse severe burns in cold water. This could cause hypothermia.
4. Cover the area of the burn with a dry, sterile bandage or clean cloth. Don't use a blanket or towel because of the fabric's tendency to stick to burns. A light cotton sheet will do if the burned area is large. Don't apply ointments and try not to break burn blisters.

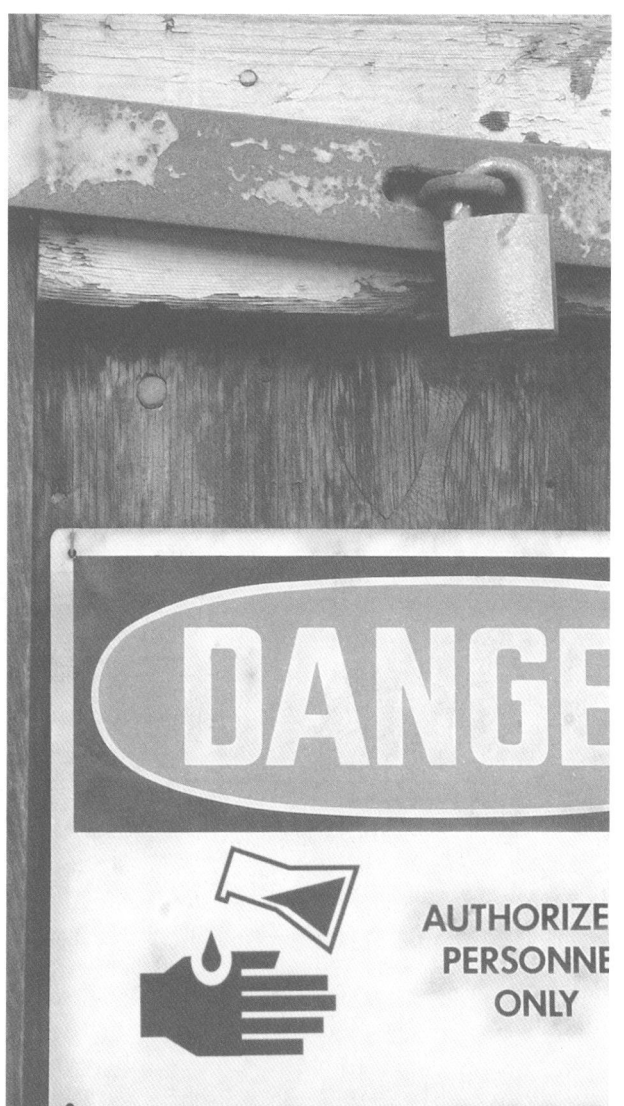

Full-thickness burns

Full-thickness burns involve all of the layers of skin — and sometimes deeper tissue, such as fat or muscle — and they cause permanent tissue damage. Full-thickness burns usually have areas that are charred black, or they may appear dry and waxy white. Blisters don't develop. Because nerve damage is substantial, there's minimal pain or none at all. These burns need emergency care and often require surgical intervention.

Burns caused by fire

Burns caused by direct contact with fire — such as those that happen around campfires and among children playing with matches — should be treated according to the degree and extent of the burn. Some superficial burns may be treated as minor burns. Burns that are extensive or that extend to deeper layers of tissue may require a visit to your doctor's office or local emergency department. Seek medical attention if the burn involves the face, hands, feet or groin.

Electrical burns

Any electrical burn should be examined by a doctor. An electrical burn may appear minor, but the damage can extend deep into the tissues beneath the skin. Electrical shocks can sometimes result in a heart rhythm disturbance, cardiac arrest or other internal damage from electrical current passing through the body. Sometimes, the jolt associated with the electrical injury can cause the person to be thrown or to fall, resulting in fractures or other injuries.

Call for emergency medical assistance if the person who has been burned is in pain, is confused or is experiencing changes in his or her breathing, heartbeat or consciousness. In addition, turn off the source of electricity if possible. If not, move the source away from both you and the injured person with a nonconducting object made of plastic or fiberglass.

Chemical burns

If a chemical burns the skin, follow these steps:
1. Stop the burning by removing contaminated clothing and jewelry and flushing the chemicals off the skin surface with cool, running water. Do this for 20 minutes or more. If the burning chemical is a powderlike substance, brush it off the skin before flushing.
2. If the chemical entered the eyes, immediately flush the eyes with tap water for 15 minutes.
3. Wrap the burned area loosely with a dry, sterile dressing or clean cloth.
4. Seek emergency assistance if the person displays signs of shock, such as fainting or shallow breathing, or if the burn is extensive or involves the eyes.

Blisters, Bruises and Cuts

These types of injuries generally don't require emergency care, but it's important to know how to care for blisters, bruises and cuts to promote healing and prevent them from recurring or becoming more serious.

Blisters

Common causes of blisters include friction and burns. If the blister isn't too painful, do everything possible to keep it intact. Unbroken skin over a blister provides a natural barrier to bacteria and decreases the risk of infection. Cover a small blister with an adhesive bandage, and cover a large one with a porous, plastic-coated gauze pad that absorbs moisture and allows the wound to breathe.

Don't puncture a blister unless it's painful or prevents you from walking or using one of your hands. If you have diabetes or poor circulation, contact your doctor before performing self-care measures.

To relieve blister-related pain, drain the fluid while leaving the overlying skin intact.

1. Wash your hands and the blister with soap and warm water.
2. Swab the blister with iodine or rubbing alcohol.
3. Sterilize a clean, sharp needle by wiping it with rubbing alcohol.
4. Use the needle to puncture the blister. Aim for several spots near the blister's edge. Let the fluid drain, but leave the overlying skin in place.
5. Apply an antibiotic ointment to the blister and cover it with a bandage or gauze pad.
6. After several days, cut away all the dead skin, using tweezers and scissors sterilized with rubbing alcohol. Apply more ointment and a bandage.

Call your doctor if you see signs of infection — pus, redness, increasing pain or warm skin.

Prevention tips

To prevent a blister, use gloves, socks, a bandage or similar protective covering over the area being rubbed. Special athletic socks are available that have extra padding in critical areas. And remember the following when you shop for shoes:

- Shop during the middle of the day when your feet may be more swollen to give you the best fit.
- Wear the same socks you'll wear when walking, or bring them with you to the store.
- Measure both feet and try on both shoes. If your feet differ in size, buy the larger size.
- Go for flexible, but supportive, shoes with cushioned insoles.
- Leave toe room. Be sure that you can comfortably wiggle your toes.

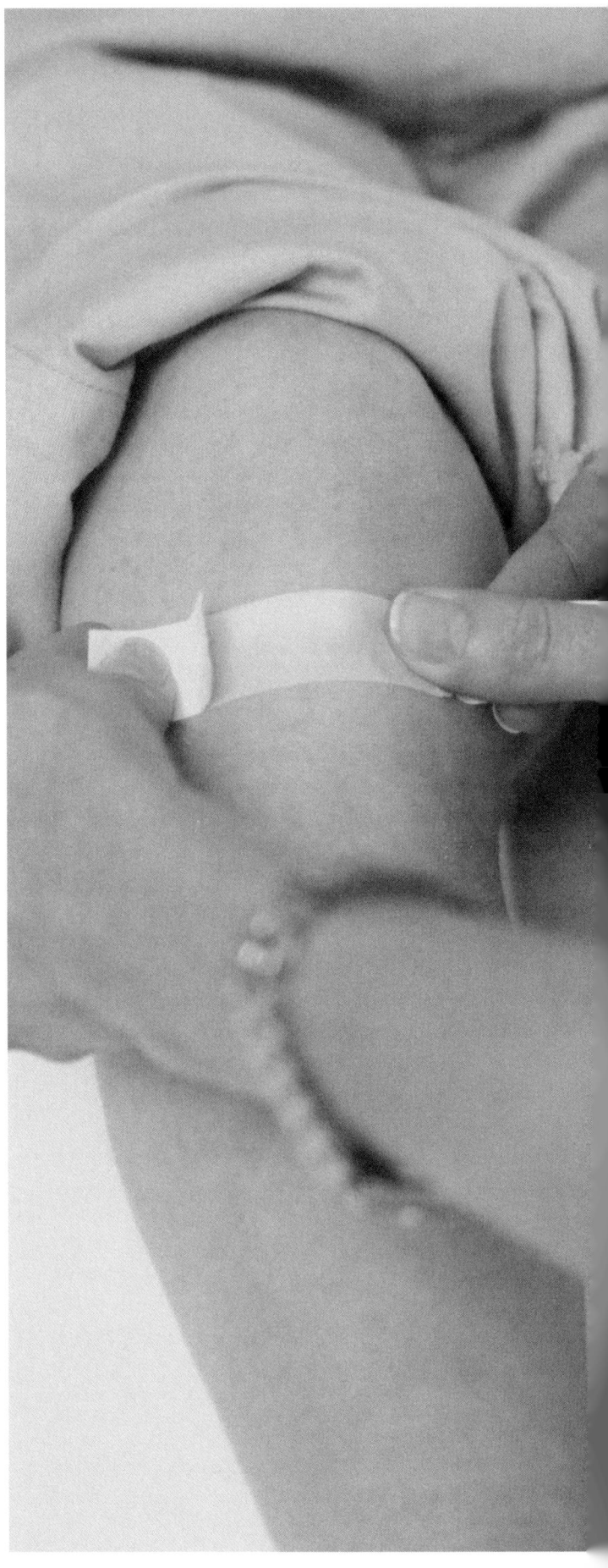

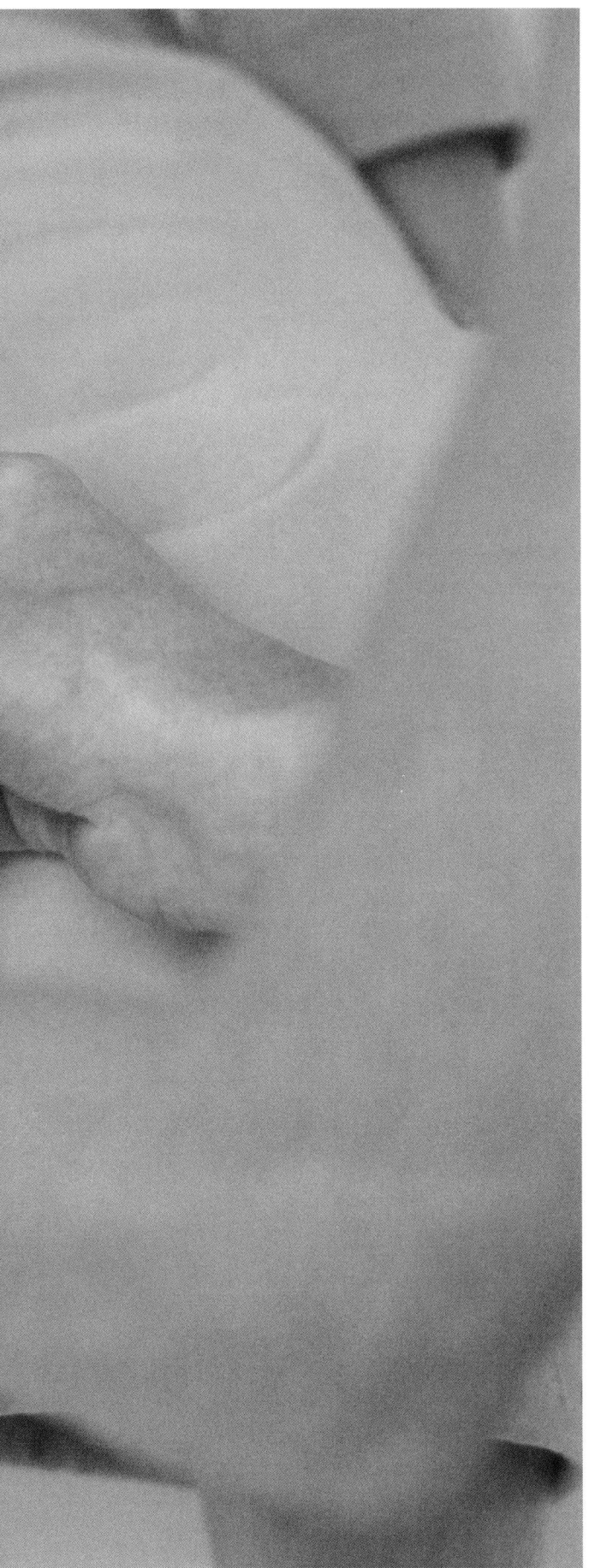

Bruises

A bruise forms when a blow breaks small blood vessels near your skin's surface, allowing a small amount of blood to leak out into the tissues under your skin. The trapped blood appears as a black-and-blue mark. Sometimes, there also are tiny red dots or red splotches.

If your skin isn't broken, you don't need a bandage. You can, however, enhance bruise healing with these simple techniques:
- Elevate the injured area.
- Apply ice or a cold pack several times a day for a day or two after the injury.
- Rest the bruised area, if possible.
- Take acetaminophen (Tylenol, others) for pain relief.

See your doctor if:
- You have unusually large or painful bruises, particularly if they seem to develop for no known reason.
- You bruise easily and you're experiencing abnormal bleeding elsewhere, such as your nose or gums, or you notice blood in your eyes, stool or urine.
- You have no history of bruising, but suddenly experience bruises.

These signs and symptoms may indicate a more serious problem, such as a blood-clotting problem or blood-related disease. Bruises accompanied by persistent pain also may indicate a more serious underlying illness requiring medical attention.

Cuts

Seek a doctor for a wound that is deep, is gaping, or has fat or muscle protruding. It may need medical care, including stitches. If your wound is deep or dirty and your last tetanus shot was more than five years ago, ask your doctor if you need a booster shot.

Minor cuts and scrapes usually don't require a trip to the emergency department. Yet proper care is essential to avoid complications. To care for simple wounds:

1. **Stop the bleeding.** Minor cuts and scrapes usually stop bleeding on their own. If they don't, apply gentle pressure with a clean cloth or bandage. Hold the pressure continuously for 20 to 30 minutes. Don't keep checking to see if the bleeding has stopped because this may damage or dislodge the fresh clot that's forming and cause bleeding to resume. If the blood spurts or continues to flow after continuous pressure, seek medical assistance.

2. **Clean the wound.** Rinse out the wound with lukewarm water. Soap can irritate the wound, so try to keep it out of the actual wound. If dirt or debris remains in the wound after washing, use tweezers cleaned with alcohol to remove the particles. If debris remains embedded in the wound after cleaning, see a doctor. Thorough wound irrigation with water reduces the risk of infection and tetanus. To clean the area around the wound,

use soap and a washcloth. There's no need to use hydrogen peroxide, iodine or an iodine-containing cleanser. They may damage healthy tissues.

3. **Apply an antibiotic.** After you clean the wound, apply a thin layer of an antibiotic cream or ointment to help keep the surface moist and reduce the risk of infection. Ingredients in some ointments can cause a mild rash in some people. If a rash appears, stop using the ointment.

4. **Cover the wound.** Bandages can help keep the wound clean and keep harmful bacteria out.

5. **Change the dressing.** Change the dressing at least daily or whenever it becomes wet or dirty. See a doctor if you notice any redness, increasing pain, drainage, warmth or swelling.

Types of Fractures

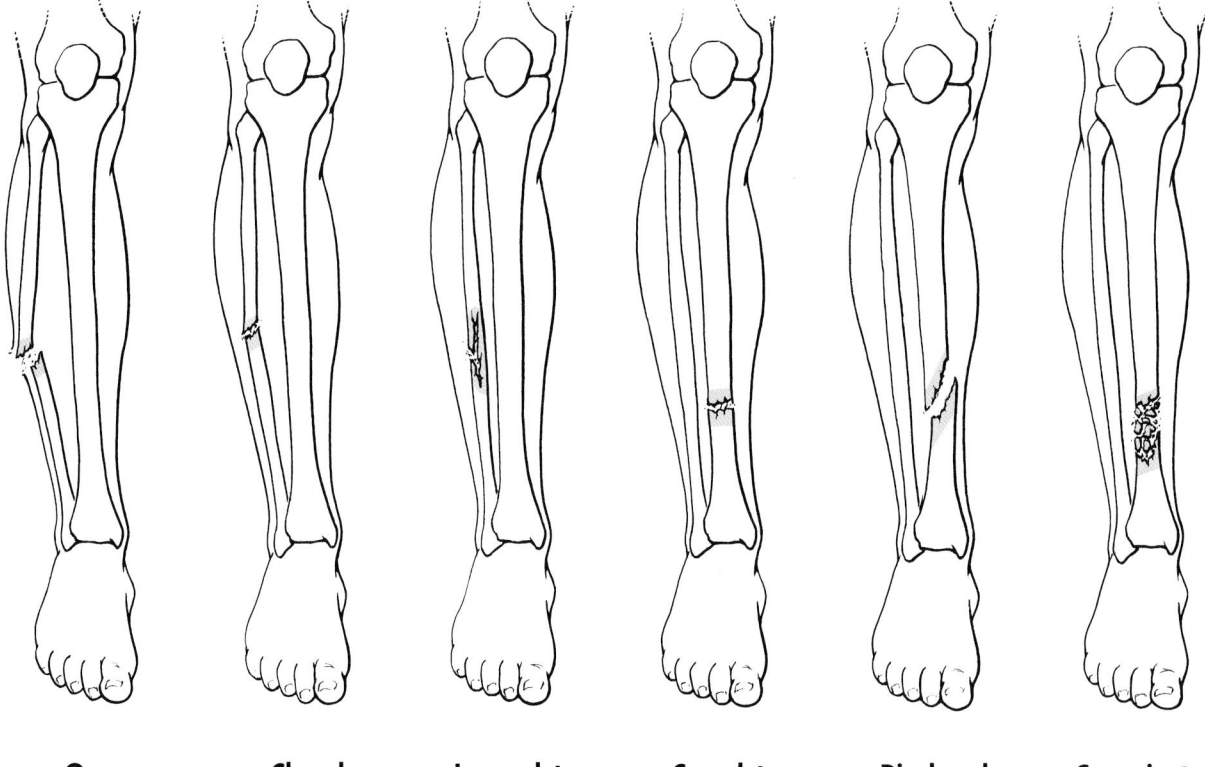

| Open | Closed | Incomplete | Complete | Displaced | Comminuted |

Open. The fracture communicates with the outside environment through a disruption of the skin.

Closed. There's no communication of the broken bone and the outside environment. Generally, the skin is intact.

Incomplete. The bone is fractured but isn't separated into two parts.

Complete. The bone is broken into two or more parts.

Displaced. The two bone ends no longer line up.

Comminuted. The bone is splintered or broken into more than two pieces.

Other types of fractures

Impacted. One fragment of bone is embedded into another fragment of bone.

Pathologic. This type of fracture involves a bone break in a person whose bones are weakened by disease. Such a break may occur in an individual with decreased bone mass (osteoporosis) or cancer involving bone. The break is called a pathologic fracture because an underlying disease is the main cause of the break.

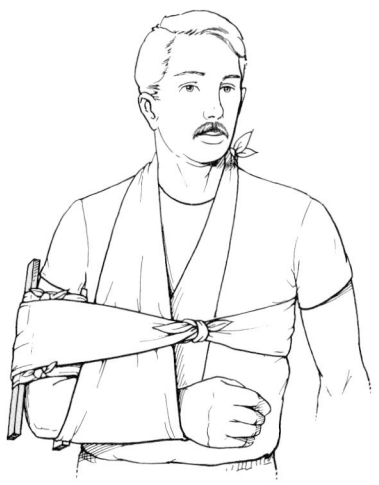

If professional help is unavailable, immobilize an upper arm fracture with a splint and a sling.

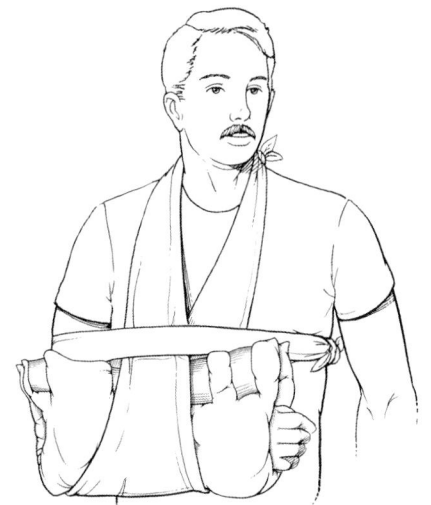

A pillow can serve as an effective temporary splint for a fracture of the lower arm. Use adhesive tape to hold the ends of the pillow closed.

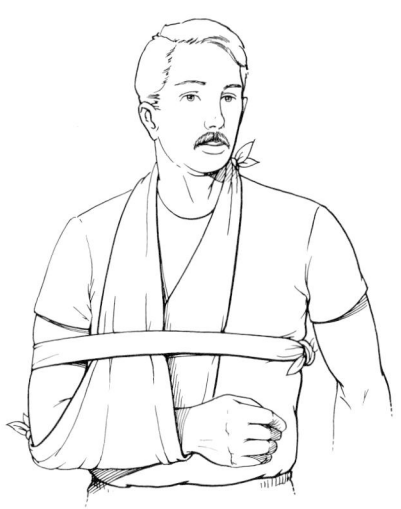

A simple sling can effectively immobilize an injured elbow or shoulder.

Trauma

A traumatic wound is a physical injury caused by external force. A broken bone, a severe blow to the head and a knocked-out tooth are all examples. Broken bones (fractures) are among the most common traumatic injuries. The term *sprain* is frequently used to describe a wide range of injuries, but a sprain involves damage to the ligaments that connect the bones, not the bone itself.

Fractures, severe sprains, dislocations, and other serious bone and joint injuries usually require professional medical care. You risk permanent disability, deformity and, in the case of head, neck and spinal injuries, even death if you don't get prompt medical care. Likewise, eye injuries and tooth loss should receive appropriate emergency treatment.

Fractures

A fracture usually occurs as a result of a fall, blow or other traumatic event. If you suspect a fracture, protect the injured area from further damage. Don't try to align the broken bone. Signs and symptoms of a fracture may include:

- Swelling or bruising over a bone
- Deformity of the affected limb
- Localized pain that's intensified when the injured area is moved or pressure is put on it
- Loss of function in the area of the injury
- A broken bone protruding from the skin

Treatment

To help protect against further injury from the fracture:

1. **Check for a pulse below the fracture.** Make sure that the wound is between the person's heart and the place where you're checking for the pulse. This will help you determine whether blood is still flowing past the break. If there's no pulse, blood may not be flowing past the injury and the person is at risk of losing the fractured limb. Seek emergency medical help.
2. **Stop the bleeding.** If the break is an open fracture, apply pressure to stop the bleeding. Place pressure directly on the wound with a sterile bandage, a clean cloth or even a piece of clean clothing. If nothing else is available, use your hand, but don't injure yourself on sharp bone fragments. Maintain pressure until the bleeding stops. Elevate the site of the fracture to reduce blood flow.
3. **Immobilize the injured area.** If you've been trained in how to splint an injury and professional help isn't available, apply a splint to the area.
4. **Apply ice to limit swelling and relieve the pain.** Don't apply ice directly to the skin. Wrap the ice in a towel, piece of cloth or some other material before placing it on the injured area.

CHAPTER 1: First Aid and Emergency Care **37**

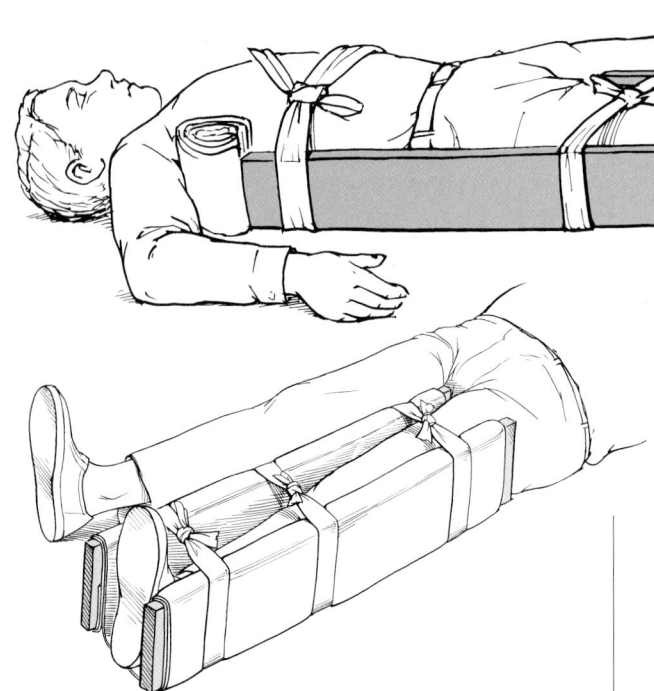

A leg splint can effectively immobilize a fracture of the lower leg (left). A fracture of a thighbone requires splinting of the trunk and lower leg (above).

5. **Treat for shock.** If the person is faint, pale or breathing in a notably shallow, hurried fashion, treat him or her for shock. Lay the person down with the legs elevated.

Splinting or immobilizing fractures

Splints can be made of wood, plastic, metal or another rigid material. Pad the splint with gauze or some other cloth, then apply it to the limb. The splint should be longer than the bone it's splinting and extend below and above the injury. Fasten the splint to the limb with gauze or strips of cloth, tape or other material. Splint the limb firmly to prevent motion but not so tightly that blood flow is stopped. A simple splint that works well is to put one or more pillows around the limb and tape across the pillows.

How to splint the fracture depends on the location of the break. A spinal injury or hip or pelvic fracture can't be splinted and must be immobilized in another way.

Arm fractures

Place one or more pillows around the injured limb and tape across the pillows. Rolled magazines or newspapers also can be tied around a broken lower arm. A sling over the shoulder and a band around the sling and arm can help immobilize the limb and shoulder.

Leg fractures

If a lower leg is broken, place the entire leg between two splints. Another option is to place pillows around the leg and tape across the pillows. If no splints are available, the healthy leg can be used as a splint to limit movement of the broken one. A broken thighbone requires that the hip joint also be immobilized.

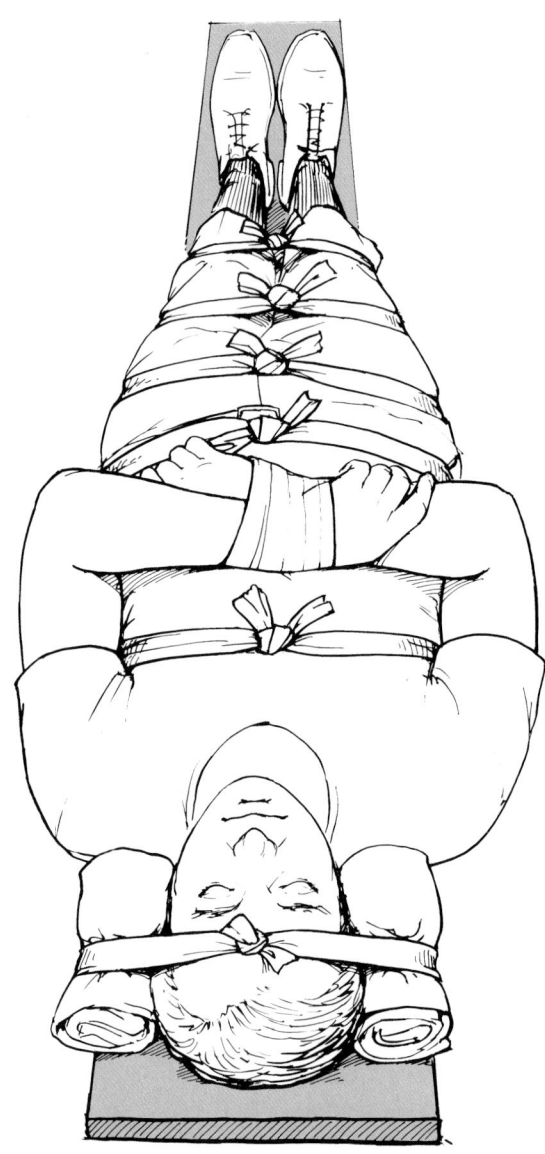

Neck and back injuries require special precautions. If medical help is unavailable and the injured person must be moved, recruit several people to help. Neck and back injuries can lead to permanent paralysis. Proper use of a backboard immobilizes the victim's head, neck and spine.

Spinal injuries

If you suspect a neck or spinal injury, don't move the injured person. Permanent paralysis and other serious complications can result from moving a person with a spinal injury. The broken spine, if moved, could accidentally injure or sever the spinal cord.

Assume the person has a spinal injury if:

- There's evidence of a head injury.
- There's an ongoing change in the person's level of consciousness.
- The person complains of pain in the neck or back.
- The injury resulted in substantial force on the back, neck or head.
- The person complains of tingling, numbness, weakness, paralysis or lack of control of the limbs, bladder or bowel.
- The neck or back is twisted or positioned oddly
  If you suspect a spinal injury:
- Call for emergency medical help.
- Keep the person still and don't try to move him or her.

Amputation

When a finger, toe or larger body part is severed, life-threatening risks can include blood loss, shock and infection. Call for emergency medical help immediately. It's important that you quickly get the injured person and the severed part to a hospital, where the limb may possibly be reattached. Until help arrives:

Stop the bleeding

The first goal of emergency treatment is to stop blood loss. Whether the amputation involves an extremity as small as a toe or as large as a leg, apply pressure on the wound with a sterile bandage, clean cloth or piece of clothing. If possible, have the individual lie down. The limb with the injury should be slightly elevated. When the bleeding is under control, wrap the wound with additional layers.

If the bleeding continues

If a hand, foot, leg or an arm has been amputated, the bleeding may be hard to stop. First apply pressure to the artery that feeds the injured area. If that fails, application of a tourniquet may be necessary.

To apply a tourniquet, wrap a necktie or other piece of cloth around the tissue immediately above — but not touching — the wound. The cloth must be long enough to wrap around the area twice with enough material left for a knot. Tie a half-knot first, then place a screwdriver, stick, dowel rod or similar object on top of the knot and tie the second half-knot. Twist the object to tighten the tourniquet. Tighten the cloth

only as much as is required to stop the flow of blood. Note the time at which you applied the tourniquet. Tie the object in place with the cloth once bleeding has stopped.

Treat other injuries

When you have the bleeding at the site of the amputation under control, examine the person for other signs of injury you may not have noticed.

Save the severed part

Once the person is stable, carefully put the amputated body part in a clean plastic bag or wrap it in a clean cloth. If ice is available, place the bag with the severed body part in it inside a second bag that contains ice and water. Don't put the ice and water in direct contact with the severed part and don't use dry ice. If ice isn't available, use very cold water.

Remarkable advances have been made in reattaching fingers, hands and even severed limbs. The results depend on many factors, but if you care for the severed body part and a qualified surgeon is readily available, reattachment may be possible.

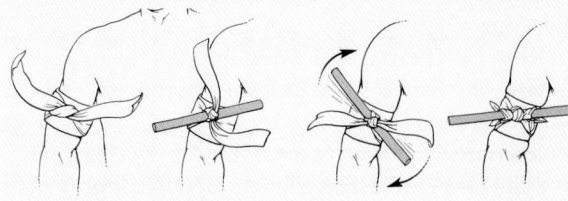

If all other methods to stop bleeding fail, apply and tighten a tourniquet.

- Provide as much first aid as possible without moving the person's head or neck.

If you must move the person because of choking or immediate danger, use at least two people and try to keep the person's head, neck and back carefully aligned.

Hip or pelvic fractures

Hip or pelvic fractures usually occur as a result of a fall or an accident. In some people whose bones are weakened from osteoporosis or bone cancer, such breaks can occur spontaneously. Suspect a broken pelvis or hip if the person complains of:

- Pain in the hip, lower back or groin area
- Pain in these areas that worsens with movement of one or both legs

As with a spinal injury, call for emergency assistance and don't move the individual. If you need to move the person, gently reposition him or her on a board or a flat surface, just as you would a person with a spinal injury. Don't try to straighten an injured leg or hip that seems oddly positioned.

Other broken bones

When a fracture occurs in a bone in a finger, toe, rib or the face, splinting prior to seeking medical care is usually unnecessary. Make sure to stop any bleeding.

Sprains

A sprain occurs when trauma such as a violent twist or stretch causes the joint to move beyond its normal range of motion, tearing ligaments attached to bone.

Usual indications of a sprain include:

- Pain and tenderness in the affected area
- Rapid swelling, sometimes accompanied by discoloration of the skin
- Impaired joint function

Treatment

If a popping sound and immediate difficulty in using the joint accompany the injury, this could indicate a fracture or sprain. If you suspect bone or ligament damage in the joint, seek medical care as soon as possible. Also seek care if you don't begin to see improvement after two or three days.

For minor sprains, you can probably treat the injury yourself with rest, ice, compression and elevation (R.I.C.E.):

1. **Rest.** Don't avoid all activity, but rest the injured limb. Increase activity and weight bearing slowly as tolerated.
2. **Ice.** Immediately apply ice to decrease swelling and pain. Don't use it for too long or apply it directly to the skin, as this could cause tissue damage.
3. **Compression.** Compress the area with an elastic bandage or wrap. Compressive wraps or sleeves made from elastic or neoprene are best.

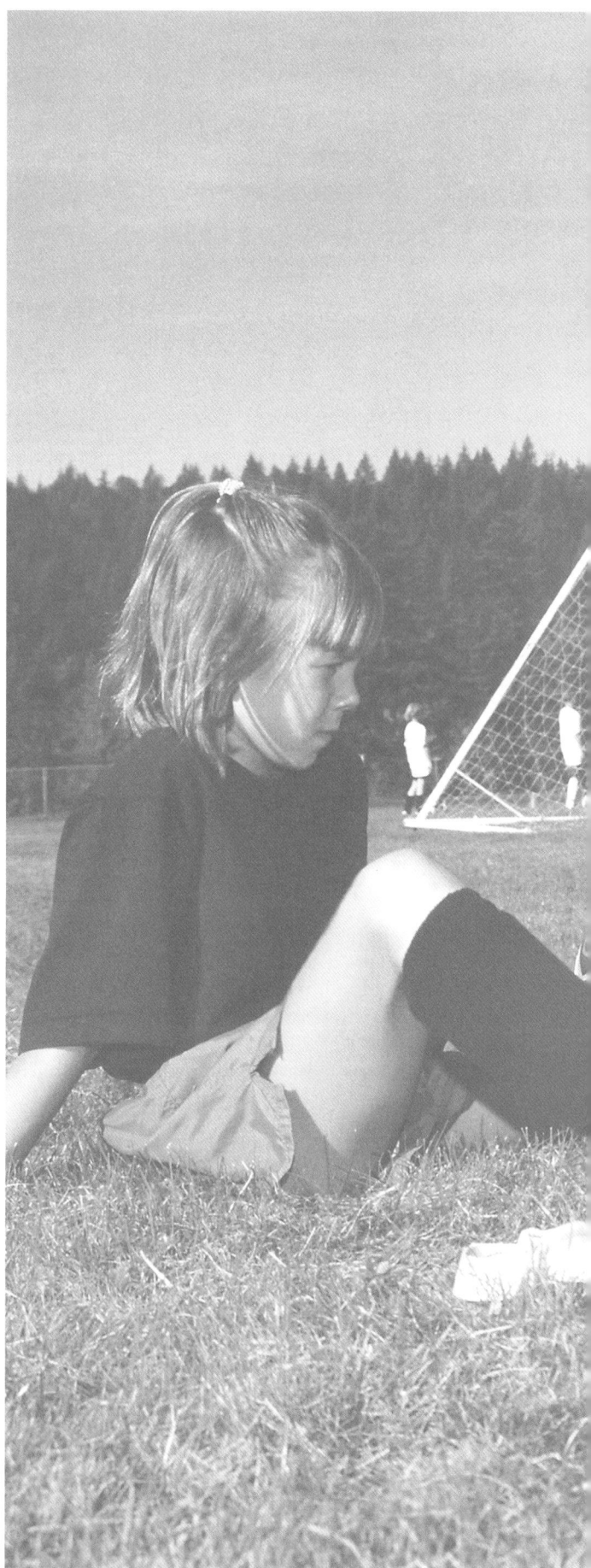

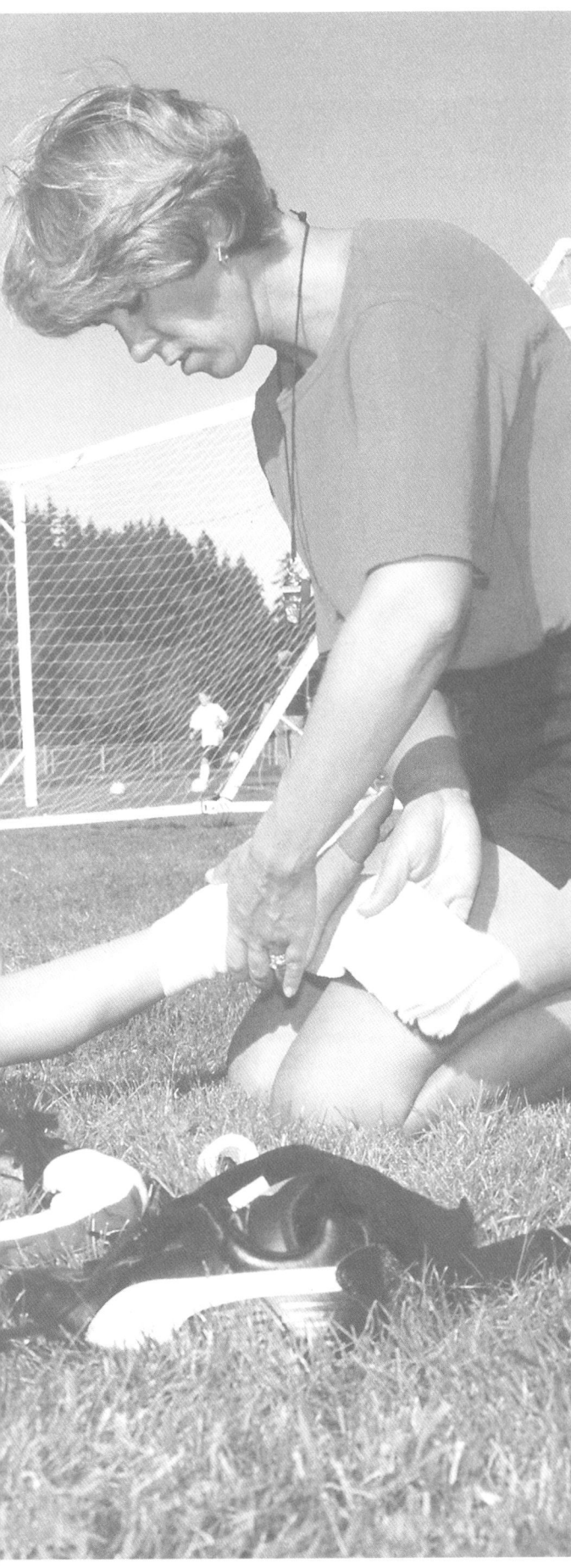

4. **Elevation.** Raise the swollen arm or leg joint above the level of your heart when able to help reduce swelling. This is especially important at night.

Dislocations

A dislocation is an injury in which the ends of bones are forced from their normal positions. A blow, fall or other form of trauma can cause a dislocation. One of the most common dislocation injuries is caused by trauma to the shoulder. In some cases, an underlying disease such as rheumatoid arthritis, a congenital weakness or a joint weakened by previous dislocations may be responsible.

The usual signs of dislocation are:
- Swelling and intense pain
- A joint that's visibly out of position, misshapen and difficult to move

Treatment

Don't try to return the joint to its proper position unless you're trained to do so. Doing so can damage the joint and surrounding muscles, ligaments, nerves or blood vessels. Splint the affected joint and put ice on the injury site. Ice helps reduce swelling. Seek medical care as soon as possible. If you also suspect a neck or spinal injury, don't move the injured person. Call for emergency medical care.

Head injuries

Most head injuries are minor because the skull provides considerable protection to the brain. Only about 10 percent of all head injuries require hospitalization. Seek emergency medical care if any of the following signs or symptoms are apparent:
- Absence of breathing
- Seizures
- Severe head or facial bleeding
- Bleeding or leakage of clear fluid from the nose or ears
- Change in level of consciousness — confusion, lethargy or loss of consciousness, even if the person regains consciousness quickly
- Slurred speech
- Loss of balance, weakness or an inability to use an arm or leg
- Vomiting
- Severe headache
- Vision changes
- Black-and-blue discoloration below the eyes or behind the ears

If severe head trauma occurs:
1. **Keep the person still.** Until medical help arrives, keep the injured person lying down and quiet. For a severe head injury, assume the spine may be

injured as well. Don't move the person unless necessary.

2. **Stop any bleeding.** Apply firm pressure to the wound with a clean cloth. Don't apply direct pressure to the wound if you suspect a skull fracture.

3. **Watch for changes in breathing and alertness.** If the person stops breathing, begin cardiopulmonary resuscitation (CPR) right away, while trying to keep the neck as still as possible.

Concussions

When the head sustains a hard blow from being struck or from a fall, a concussion may result. The impact causes the brain to strike the inside of the skull.

A concussion, also called mild traumatic brain injury, may or may not cause loss of consciousness. It can produce confusion, headache, loss of memory, dizziness or nausea. More-serious head injuries can cause a prolonged loss of consciousness or persistent symptoms of a concussion, such as confusion or a headache. A concussion requires emergency medical evaluation.

Intracranial hematoma

An intracranial hematoma results when a blood vessel — either an artery or a vein — ruptures between the skull and brain. Blood leaks between the brain and skull and forms an accumulation of blood (hematoma) that presses on the brain tissue.

The most common cause of a hematoma is a strong blow to the head, such as from being hit by a baseball, falling off a stepladder or being in a car accident. Signs and symptoms may develop a few moments to several weeks after the head injury. They can include headache, nausea, vomiting, change in consciousness and pupils of unequal size.

The condition can be rapidly fatal if not treated. Treatment may involve surgery to stop the bleeding and remove the excess blood.

Skull fractures

Visible bone fragments or brain matter are obvious signs of a skull fracture. Other, less noticeable signs of a possible skull fracture include:

- Bruising or discoloration behind the ear or around the eyes
- Blood or watery fluid leaking from the ears or nose

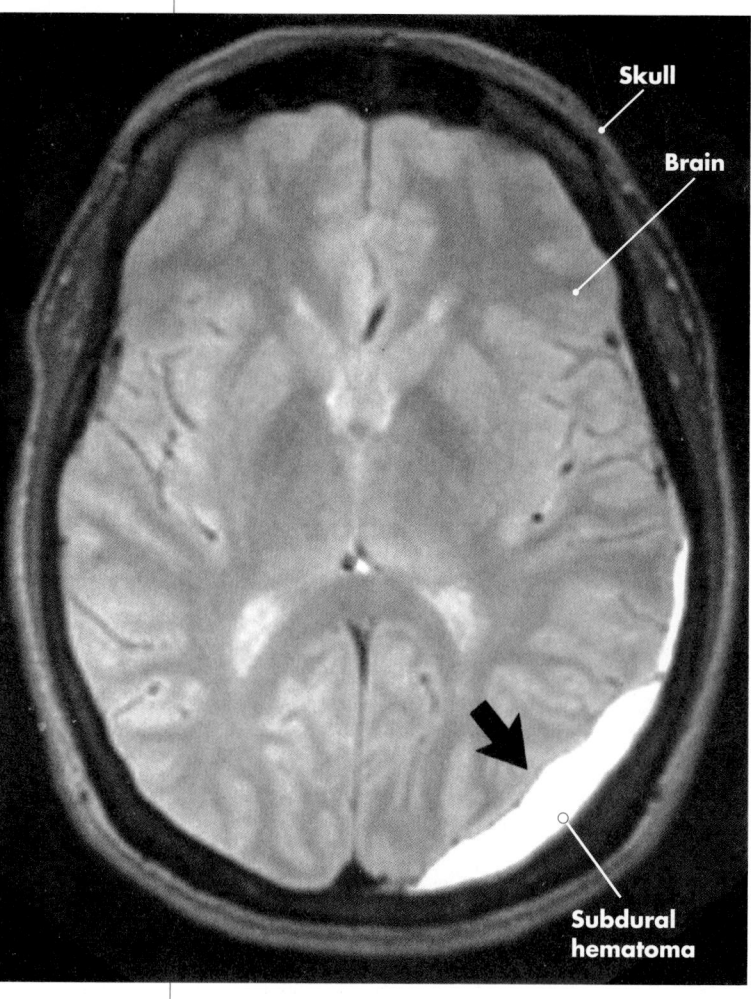

Skull

Brain

Subdural hematoma

Hematomas are detected most often with the help of a computerized tomography (CT) scan or magnetic resonance imaging (MRI). This MRI scan shows a subdural hematoma.

- Pupils of unequal size, accompanied by a change in mental status, such as confusion or unconsciousness
- Deformity of the skull, including swelling or depressions

A skull fracture is a medical emergency and must be treated promptly to avoid further brain damage and even death.

Eye injuries

Potential traumatic injuries to the eye include corneal abrasions, blood in an eye, black eye and eyelid lacerations (see page 595 for additional eye injuries).

Corneal abrasion

The most common types of eye injuries affect the cornea — the clear, protective structure overlying the front of your eye. The cornea refracts light to the retina at the rear of your eye. It is easily injured — a speck of sand or dirt or even a contact lens that's worn for too long can scratch it, causing corneal abrasion.

Because the cornea is extremely sensitive, abrasions can be very painful. Instantaneous pain at the moment of the injury followed by persistent pain and redness are key signs and symptoms of a corneal abrasion. Some corneal abrasions can become infected and result in a corneal ulcer, which is a serious problem.

Steps you can take to care for a corneal abrasion are to:

- **Use saline solution, if available, or clean water to rinse the eye.** Use an eyecup or small, clean glass positioned with its rim resting on the bone at the base of your eye socket. If your work site has an eye-rinse station, use it. Rinsing the eye may wash out an offending foreign body.
- **Blink several times.** This movement may remove small particles of dust or sand.
- **Pull the upper eyelid over the lower eyelid.** The lashes of your lower eyelid can brush a foreign body from the undersurface of your upper eyelid.

Take caution to avoid certain actions that may aggravate the injury:

- Don't try to remove an object that's embedded in your eye.
- Don't rub your eye after an injury. Touching or pressing on your eye can worsen a corneal abrasion.
- Don't touch your eyeball with tweezers, cotton swabs or other instruments. This can aggravate a corneal abrasion.

Blood in an eye

Blood visible in the front chamber of the eye, in front of the iris, is called a hyphema. It can result from a blow to the eye or an injury that perforates the eye. Certain medical conditions also can cause the problem. See an ophthalmologist or seek emergency medical care if you experience this condition.

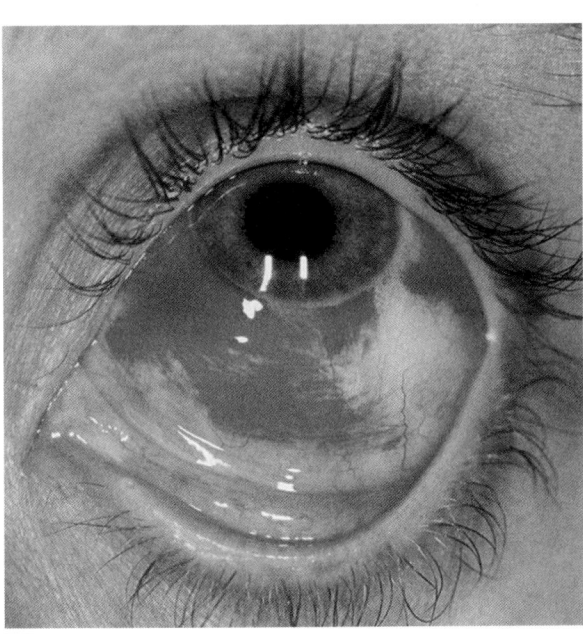

A subconjunctival hemorrhage occurs when a tiny blood vessel breaks just underneath the clear surface of your eye (conjunctiva). Subconjunctival hemorrhages are usually painless, cause no vision changes and resolve on their own.

Hyphema is different from the relatively harmless problem of bloodshot eyes, which are caused by broken surface blood vessels in the white part of the eyes. A very red, bloodshot eye may also result from subconjunctival hemorrhages, blotchy red spots that occur when small blood vessels break between the white of the eye and the membranes of the eyelid (conjunctiva). Subconjunctival hemorrhages are usually painless, cause no vision changes and resolve on their own.

Black eye

A so-called black eye is caused by bleeding beneath the skin around the eye. Most black eyes aren't serious, but sometimes a black eye indicates a more extensive injury, such as a facial or skull fracture, particularly if the area around both eyes is bruised or if further signs indicate a head injury.

To take care of a black eye, using gentle pressure, apply a cold pack or a cloth filled with ice to the area around the eye to reduce swelling. Take care not to press on the eye itself.

Seek immediate medical care if you experience vision problems, such as double vision or blurring, or you have severe pain or bleeding in an eye or from the nose.

Eyelid laceration

If an eyelid is cut, apply clean gauze to the eye without applying pressure and seek emergency medical care.

Tooth loss

When a permanent tooth is accidentally knocked out in one piece, it can sometimes be reimplanted, but only if you act quickly. A broken tooth can't be reimplanted, and a primary (baby) tooth shouldn't be reimplanted because doing so could damage the developing permanent tooth.

Treatment

If a permanent tooth is knocked out, save the tooth and seek emergency dental care immediately. Successful reimplantation depends on how quickly the tooth is replaced in the socket. Within five minutes is ideal. Longer than one hour after the injury may be too long.

1. Handle the tooth by the crown only. Don't touch the root.
2. Don't rub or scrape the tooth to remove debris. This damages the root surface, making the tooth less likely to survive reimplantation.
3. Gently rinse the tooth in tap water or saline. Don't hold it under running water.
4. Try to gently replace the tooth in the socket. If it doesn't go all the way into place, bite down gently on gauze or a moistened tea bag to help hold the tooth in place until you see a dentist.

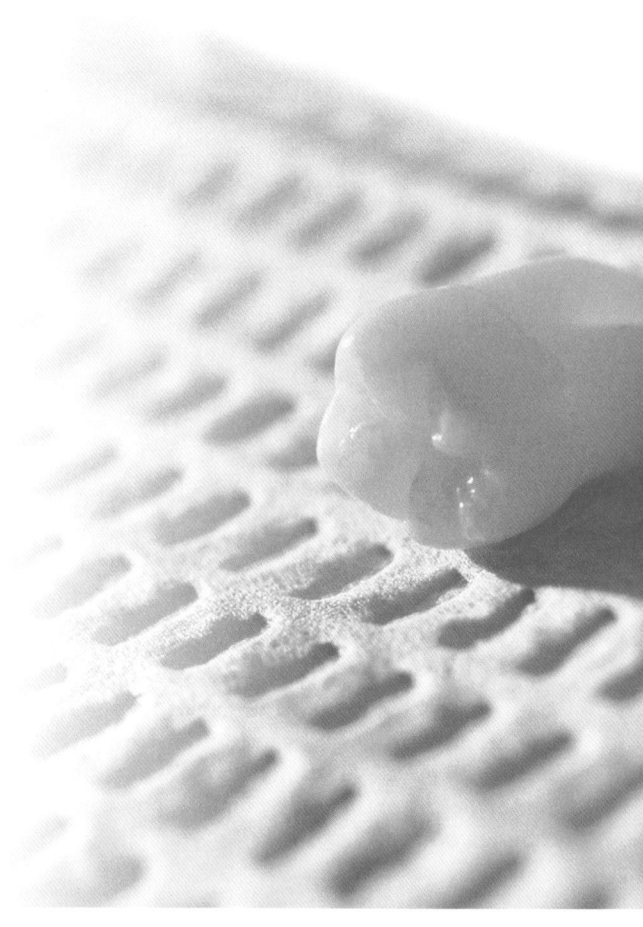

Recognizing and Treating Shock

Before you can effectively treat a person in shock, you need to recognize its signs and symptoms.

Recognizing shock

The following signs and symptoms may indicate the presence of shock in an ill or injured person:

Change in skin color and feel
The skin may appear pale or gray and feel cool and clammy. In some forms of shock the skin remains warm.

Rapid pulse and breathing
The heartbeat is weak and rapid and is accompanied by hurried breathing, which may be shallow or deep. Blood pressure drops and may not be measurable.

Staring eyes
The eyes may appear dull, and the person appears to be staring, due to an alteration of mental status. He or she may also have large (dilated) pupils, making the black center of each eye look large.

Unconsciousness, dizziness, agitation and thirst
The person may feel faint, dizzy or weak. He or she may become agitated, confused or even unresponsive. Many people in shock complain of thirst and a dry mouth.

Treating shock

Seek emergency medical help if you observe the signs and symptoms of shock. While waiting for medical help to arrive:

Have the person lie down
Lay the person down on his or her back with his or her feet elevated 6 to 12 inches from the ground. Elevating the feet on a cushion or another prop is often the easiest way to establish this position. If the person has sustained an injury in which raising the legs will cause pain or further injury, leave the person flat on his or her back. Try to keep movement to a minimum.

Keep the person warm and comfortable
Loosen tight collars, belts or other constricting clothing. Cover the person with a blanket if the temperature is cold. If the floor or ground is cold, put a blanket beneath the victim. If it's hot, place the person in the shade or a cool area, if possible.

Check for signs of respiration
Look for breathing, coughing or movement. If the person stops breathing, begin cardiopulmonary resuscitation (CPR).

Take steps to prevent choking
If the person is vomiting or bleeding from the mouth, position the person on his or her side. This helps prevent choking or inhaling (aspirating) the vomit or blood.

Treat injuries
If an injury has occurred, treat it if you can. Immobilize a fracture or take other appropriate first-aid steps. Be careful when immobilizing someone who may have a spinal injury so that you don't further injure the spinal cord.

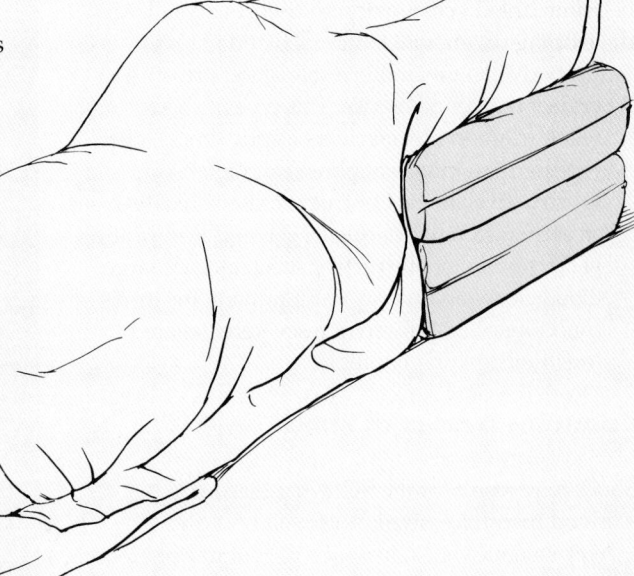

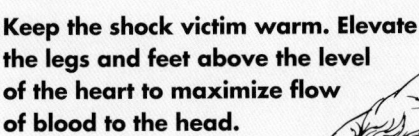

Keep the shock victim warm. Elevate the legs and feet above the level of the heart to maximize flow of blood to the head.

5. If the tooth can't be replaced in the socket, immediately place it in cold whole milk or a small container of your own saliva.

Shock

Shock is a common complication of blood loss, infection, severe burns and other medical problems. It's a condition in which there's a reduction of blood flow throughout your body. This produces a decrease in your blood pressure and a reduction in the supply of oxygen to your tissues. This decrease may produce various signs and symptoms, including pale skin, severe sweating, lightheadedness, confusion and a rapid, weak pulse. Shock can come on suddenly or gradually and can be life-threatening.

Types of shock

Shock is divided into four broad categories:
1. **Hypovolemic shock.** In hypovolemic shock there's too little blood volume for the heart to effectively pump blood to body tissues. This form of shock is associated with serious bleeding or severe dehydration resulting from loss of fluids, often due to vomiting or diarrhea. Severe hypovolemic shock may cause death in a matter of minutes if left untreated.
2. **Cardiogenic shock.** Cardiogenic shock is brought on by a heart that doesn't function properly. Causes of this type of shock include a heart attack, a very slow heart rate or an extremely rapid heart rate.
3. **Distributive shock.** Distributive shock occurs when blood vessels become abnormally enlarged (dilated). Even with a normal blood volume, the body can't maintain a safe blood pressure to deliver oxygen to tissues. This type of shock can result from severe infections (septic shock), allergic reactions (anaphylactic shock) and toxins.
4. **Obstructive shock.** Obstructive shock results from an obstruction (impairment) of blood flow to the heart. Causes of obstructive shock include large blood clots in blood vessels supplying the lungs (pulmonary embolism) or a severely deflated lung (tension pneumothorax).

Common causes of shock

Shock may result for the following reasons:
• **Blood loss.** Excessive loss of blood produces hypovolemic shock, in which the volume of blood falls below a healthy amount. The bleeding may be external, as with a severe cut, or internal, as with a fractured pelvis or rupture of an organ.

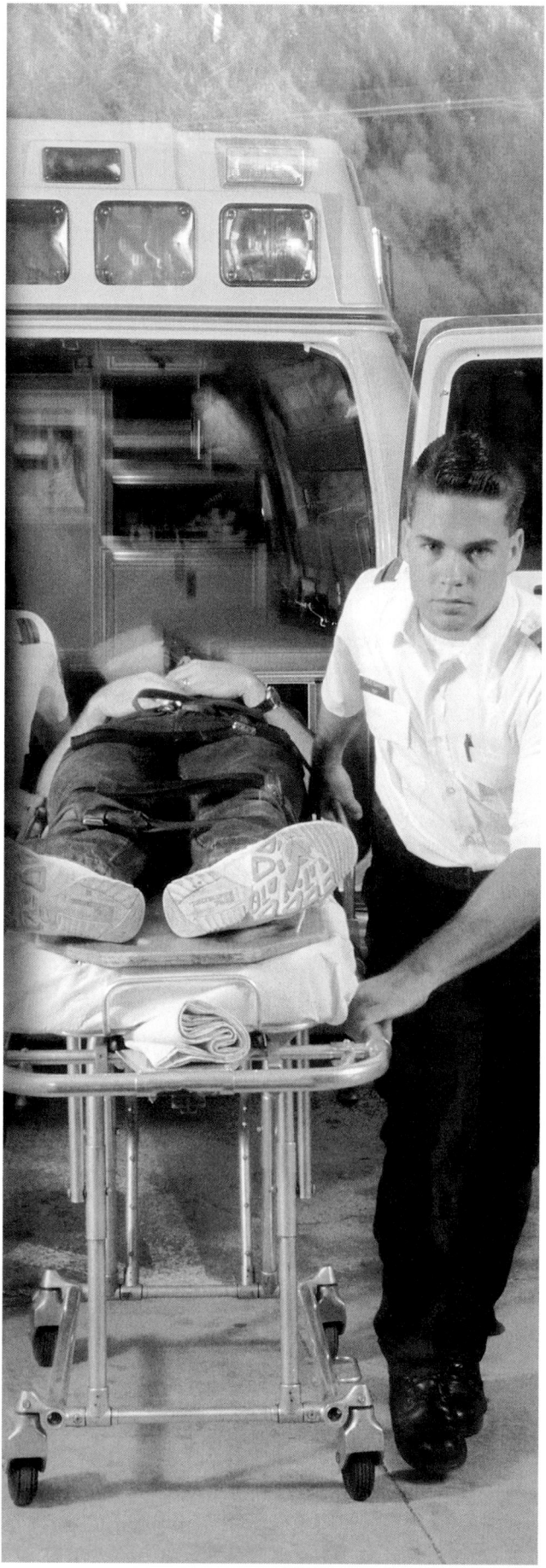

- **Dehydration.** A reduction in body fluids from vomiting, diarrhea and decreased fluid intake also can lead to hypovolemic shock.
- **Heart conditions.** Certain conditions such as a heart attack can reduce the heart's ability to circulate blood. Tissue cells don't have enough oxygen for normal functioning, resulting in cardiogenic shock.
- **Infection.** Severe infections can overwhelm your body's immune defenses and produce septic shock, a type of distributive shock. Symptoms may include fever, flushed skin that is warm to the touch, and shaking chills that can give way to cool, clammy skin, a drop in blood pressure, shortness of breath and even respiratory failure. Septic shock is more common among older individuals, the very young and people with underlying illnesses, such as diabetes and liver disease.
- **Severe allergic reaction (anaphylaxis).** Some people react more strongly than others to certain allergens, and the introduction of the allergen into their systems can produce anaphylactic shock (anaphylaxis). A form of distributive shock, anaphylaxis is most frequent in people with a history of allergies.

Anaphylactic shock

You should suspect anaphylactic shock if symptoms develop within minutes after the person is stung or bitten by a bee or an insect or after the person has ingested a food that may contain an ingredient to which he or she is allergic. Some medications also can produce anaphylactic shock. In sensitive people, a severe allergic reaction can occur within minutes. Signs and symptoms usually include:
- Skin that's warm to the touch
- Reddish skin or itchy hives
- Swelling of the face, eyes, lips or throat
- Wheezing and difficulty breathing
- Increased pulse and low blood pressure
- Nausea, vomiting, diarrhea and abdominal cramps

Death from anaphylactic shock is most commonly due to severe breathing difficulty. Swelling of tissues in the throat may block the airway. If you observe someone who may be having an allergic reaction:

1. Call 911 or your local emergency number.
2. Check for medication the person might be carrying to treat a severe allergic reaction, such as an autoinjector of epinephrine. Administer the drug as directed — usually by pressing the autoinjector against the person's thigh and holding it in place for several seconds. Then massage the injection site for 10 seconds to enhance absorption.
3. Have the person take an antihistamine pill if he or she is able to without choking.
4. If the person is able to, have him or her lie still on his or her back with the feet elevated.

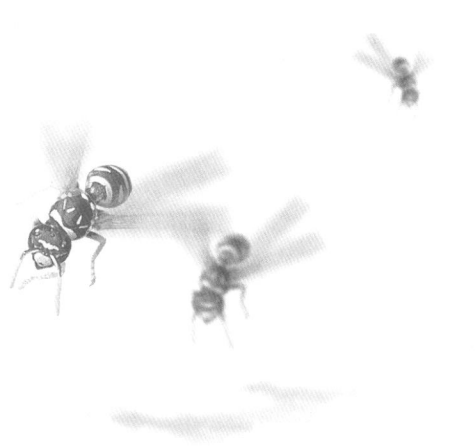

PREVENTION TIP

If you or a member of your family is severely allergic to bees, insects or certain foods, keep a properly equipped emergency kit available. The kit should include epinephrine that can be administered with a hypodermic needle or a single-dose autoinjector in case of anaphylactic shock. Epinephrine can quickly open swollen airways and reverse anaphylactic shock, which can be lifesaving. You can obtain this type of kit with a prescription from your doctor.

5. Loosen tight clothing and cover the person with a blanket.
6. If the individual stops breathing, begin CPR.

Fainting, Seizure, Stroke and Diabetic Emergency

Sudden loss of consciousness is an alarming medical event that may occur for several reasons. Basic fainting spells are the least serious cause of loss of consciousness. For example, some perfectly healthy people faint at the sight of blood and recover completely in a matter of minutes. But all losses of consciousness, seizures and strokes must be treated as potentially serious medical emergencies, and the person should receive immediate medical care.

Fainting

A person faints when the supply of blood to his or her brain temporarily decreases and he or she loses consciousness. Often, within a moment of lying flat, blood flow is restored, and he or she regains consciousness.

Fainting spells can have no medical significance, or they can be a sign of a serious illness. Several serious

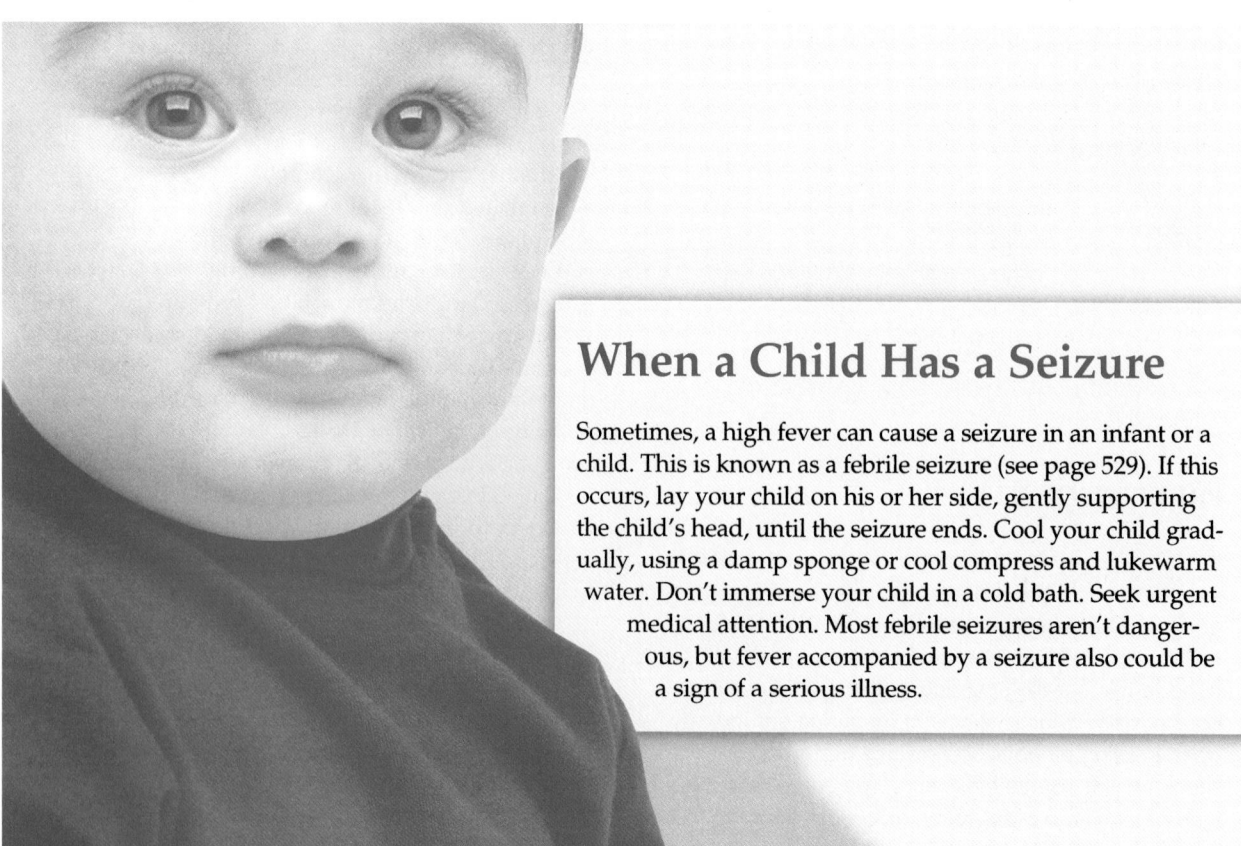

When a Child Has a Seizure

Sometimes, a high fever can cause a seizure in an infant or a child. This is known as a febrile seizure (see page 529). If this occurs, lay your child on his or her side, gently supporting the child's head, until the seizure ends. Cool your child gradually, using a damp sponge or cool compress and lukewarm water. Don't immerse your child in a cold bath. Seek urgent medical attention. Most febrile seizures aren't dangerous, but fever accompanied by a seizure also could be a sign of a serious illness.

When a Fever Becomes an Emergency

Even when you're well, your body temperature varies, and that variation is normal. Doctors usually consider 98.6 F a healthy body temperature. But your normal temperature may differ by a degree or more. In the morning, your temperature is generally lower, and in the afternoon it's somewhat higher.

Fever itself isn't an illness, but it's often a sign of one. A fever tells you that something is happening inside your body. Most likely your body is fighting an infection caused by either a virus or a bacterium.

Often, a fever isn't anything to worry about, but sometimes a fever should be evaluated, especially if it's accompanied by other severe symptoms. Contact a doctor in any of the following situations:

- A child or adult with a temperature of more than 103 F
- A child or adult with a temperature of more than 101 F for more than three days
- An infant younger than 3 months with a rectal temperature of 100.4 F or higher
- An infant older than 3 months with a temperature of 102 F or higher

Seek emergency medical care if any of these signs or symptoms accompany a fever:

- Severe headache
- Severe swelling of the throat
- Unusual skin rash
- Unusual eye sensitivity to bright light
- A stiff neck and significant neck pain when you bend your head forward
- Confusion or severe drowsiness
- Persistent vomiting or abdominal pain
- Difficulty breathing or chest pain
- Extreme listlessness, irritability or poor eye contact
- A seizure
- A bulging soft spot on a baby's head

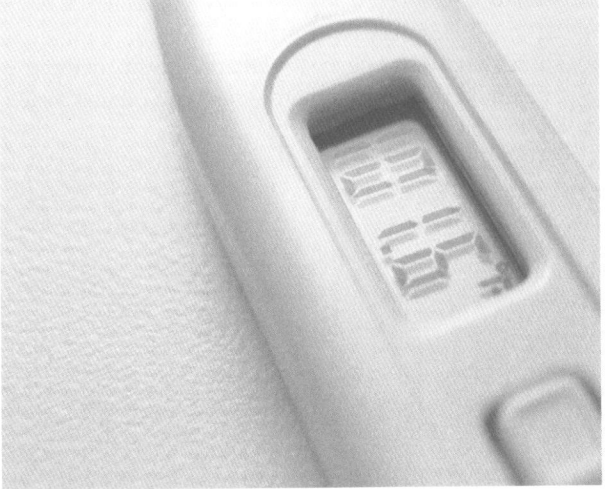

medical disorders, including life-threatening heart rhythm disturbances and sudden internal blood loss, can produce fainting. Some people faint when they're extremely tired, they receive upsetting news or they see something disturbing, such as blood. The person's heart rate temporarily slows and blood pressure falls. Often, it's the fall during a fainting spell that causes the most serious injury.

Treatment

You can do several things to help a person who has fainted or feels as if he or she is about to faint:

1. **Have the person lie down.** If someone complains of faintness or dizziness while sitting or standing, have the person lie down. If there isn't space to do so, have the individual lean forward while seated and put his or her head between the knees. This will help increase circulation to the brain. If a person faints, yet remains seated, quickly lay the individual on the floor on his or her back or side.
2. **Check the person's airway to be sure it's clear.** People who lose consciousness sometimes vomit. If they do vomit, turn them on their side so they don't choke.
3. **Check for signs of circulation.** This includes breathing, coughing and movement. If the person isn't breathing, begin cardiopulmonary resuscitation (CPR) and have someone call for emergency medical help.
4. **Help restore blood flow.** If the person is breathing, raise the person's legs above the level of his or her head. The person should revive quickly.
5. **Check for other signs and symptoms.** Does the person have chest pain or head pain? Does the person complain of numbness or continuing weakness? These may be signs of an underlying medical emergency. If any of these signs and symptoms develop, seek emergency medical help.
6. **Encourage the person to rest.** After a fainting spell is over, the person's facial color should return to normal. He or she may feel weak afterward, so lying quietly for a few minutes is a good idea.
7. **Treat injuries.** If the person was injured in a fall associated with the faint, treat any injuries.

Seizure

Normally, brain cells produce coordinated electrical discharges. When electrical discharges become disorganized, a seizure can occur. A grand mal seizure, also called a convulsion, is an involuntary episode of alternating muscular contractions and relaxations accompanied by loss of consciousness.

Seizures caused by epilepsy are perhaps the most familiar kind, but several other disorders also can produce them. These conditions include kidney failure, meningitis, toxemia of pregnancy, head injury, sudden withdrawal from certain medications and illegal use of some drugs. In rare cases, a seizure is the first sign of a brain tumor.

Treatment

When you're with a person having a seizure:

1. **Keep the person from injuring himself or herself.** If vomiting occurs, try to turn the person's head so that the vomit is expelled and isn't breathed in (aspirated) to the windpipe or lungs. Clear the area around the person of furniture or other objects to reduce his or her risk of injury during uncontrolled body movements. Although the person may briefly stop breathing — and may turn bluish from lack of oxygen — breathing almost invariably returns without the need for cardiopulmonary resuscitation (CPR).

2. **Position the individual on his or her side.** Once the seizure is over, position the person on his or her side. This allows for normal breathing and lets vomit or fluids drain from the mouth and airway. The person may have blood coming from the mouth if he or she bit the tongue or cheek. After the seizure, the person may be confused for a while. Watch the person until there's a complete return of mental function.

3. **Seek emergency help, if necessary.** Call for emergency medical help if someone is having a seizure and any one of these is true:
   - The person has never had a seizure before.
   - The episode lasts more than a few minutes.
   - The seizure is an unexpected recurrence.

4. **Treat injuries.** If the person is injured in a fall associated with the seizure, treat any injuries.

Stroke

A stroke is a condition that results from bleeding into the brain (hemorrhagic stroke) or blockage of normal blood flow to the brain (ischemic stroke). Within minutes of being deprived of essential nutrients, brain cells begin dying — a process that may continue over several hours.

A stroke is a medical emergency. Seek immediate medical treatment the moment you notice signs and symptoms. The sooner treatment is given, the more likely that damage can be minimized.

Signs and symptoms of stroke include:

- Sudden numbness, weakness or paralysis of the face, arm or leg, usually on one side of the body
- Slurred speech, trouble understanding speech or trouble talking (incomprehensible or inappropriate words)
- Sudden dimness, blurring or loss of vision, usually in one eye
- A sudden, severe headache with no apparent cause that may be accompanied by vomiting

Think F.A.S.T.

If you think an individual may be having a stroke, use the F.A.S.T. acronym:

Face. Ask the person to smile. Does one side of the face droop?

Arm. Ask the person to raise both arms. Does one arm drift downward?

Speech. Ask the person to repeat a simple sentence, such as, "The sky is blue." Is the speech slurred? Can the person repeat the sentence correctly?

Time. If you observe any of these signs, call 911 immediately. Try to determine when the signs and symptoms began. When emergency medical personnel arrive, tell them when you first noticed something was wrong.

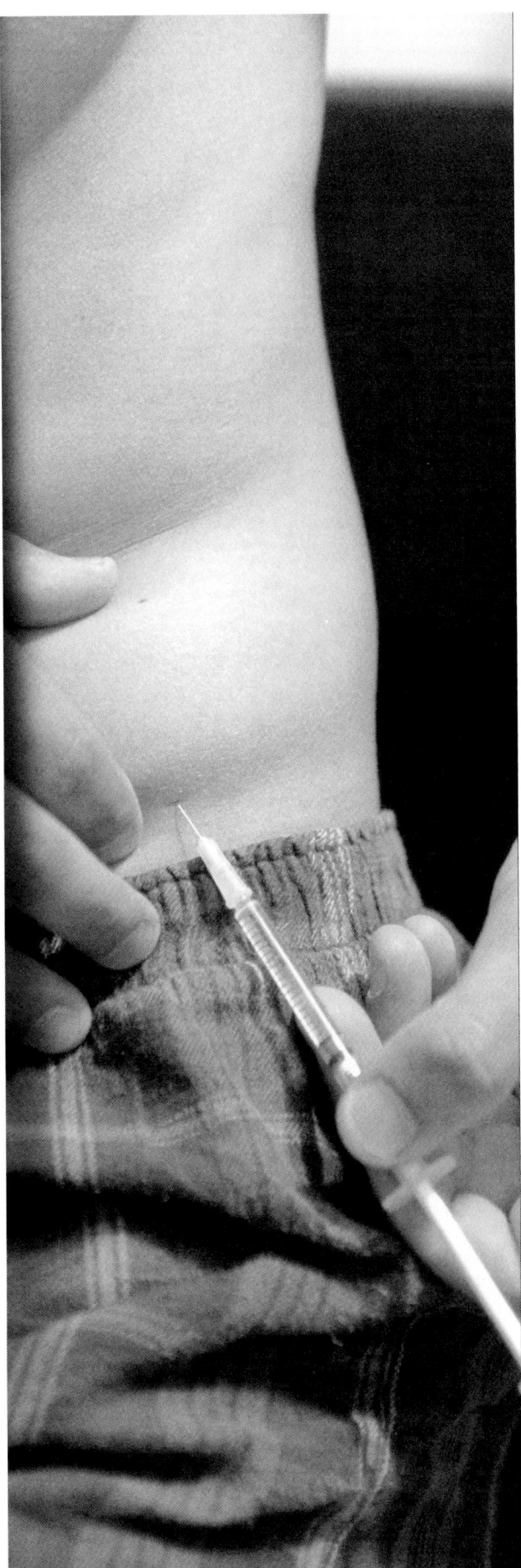

- Unexpected dizziness, loss of balance or loss of coordination
- Sudden confusion or a change in consciousness
 Signs and symptoms of a stroke may last only a few minutes, or they may persist for several hours. Even short-term warning signs should be taken seriously.

Treatment
Call 911 or your local emergency number. While waiting for emergency medical help, pay attention to the person's breathing.
- If breathing stops, begin cardiopulmonary resuscitation (CPR).
- Watch for vomiting. If vomiting occurs, turn the person on his or her side so that the vomit can drain out the mouth instead of being breathed into the lungs. Don't allow the person to eat or drink anything.
- If paralysis is present, protect the paralyzed limbs from injury that might occur when the person moves about or is transported.

Diabetic emergency

People with diabetes may experience several types of medical emergencies. Among them is low blood sugar (hypoglycemia), which may produce confusion, loss of consciousness or a seizure. This condition is treated differently from other similar emergencies.

Hypoglycemia
Hypoglycemia is also referred to as an insulin reaction or low blood sugar. It results from too much insulin and too little sugar (glucose) in your blood. Low blood sugar is most common among people with diabetes who take insulin. Rarely, an individual who isn't known to have diabetes may experience low blood sugar.

Signs and symptoms vary, but they may include nervousness, feelings of apprehension, confusion or altered behavior, cold and clammy skin, sweating, loss of consciousness, or a seizure. This progression of signs and symptoms may take place in less than an hour.

Treatment
If you know the person's symptoms are a result of low blood sugar, give him or her glucose tablets or some kind of sugar, if possible, without causing choking. Fruit juices, candy or sugar-containing soft drinks are effective. The person may stubbornly resist taking the food because low blood sugar has left him or her confused.

If the person is unable to cooperate in swallowing, you can try putting a teaspoonful of a syrup or cake icing in his or her cheek at intervals of a few minutes, but take caution to avoid aspiration into the lungs.

If the person is unconscious, he or she may need an injection of glucagon to reverse the signs and symptoms. If the person has this medication with him or her and you're trained in how to administer it, carefully do so. Seek emergency medical attention if recovery isn't prompt. Remain with the person for an hour or so after the apparent recovery because full mental function sometimes takes that long to return.

Poisoning

Any substance swallowed, inhaled, injected or absorbed by the body that interferes with the body's normal functioning is, by definition, a poison. Some poisons are well-known: pesticides, animal poisons and household chemicals bearing printed warnings. But there are many other less familiar poisons.

In fact, almost any nonfood substance is poisonous if taken in large enough doses. Analgesic medications, such as aspirin and acetaminophen (Tylenol, others), are excellent examples of nonfood substances that you might not think of as poisonous. These useful medications are found in most homes and are safe when used properly. Yet each year more children die of analgesic overdoses than of overdoses of more familiar poisons, such as household cleaners or antifreeze.

When you suspect poisoning

Sometimes, poisoning is obvious. There's no denying it when a child is seated on the floor, surrounded by aspirin tablets, some half-chewed and others crammed like candy into the mouth. Many times, however, it's hard to tell whether someone has been poisoned.

Look for these signs if you suspect poisoning:
- Burns or redness around the mouth and lips
- Breath that smells like chemicals, such as gasoline or paint thinner
- Burns, stains and odors on the person, on his or her clothing, or on the furniture, floor, rugs or other objects in the area in which he or she was playing or working
- Difficulty breathing
- Vomiting, sleepiness, confusion or other unexpected signs

Many conditions mimic the signs and symptoms of poisoning, such as seizures, intoxication and hypoglycemia. Regardless, call for emergency medical help.

Treatment

If someone is unconscious and you think that he or she has ingested a poison, call 911 for emergency medical help. If the person is awake and alert, take the following steps:

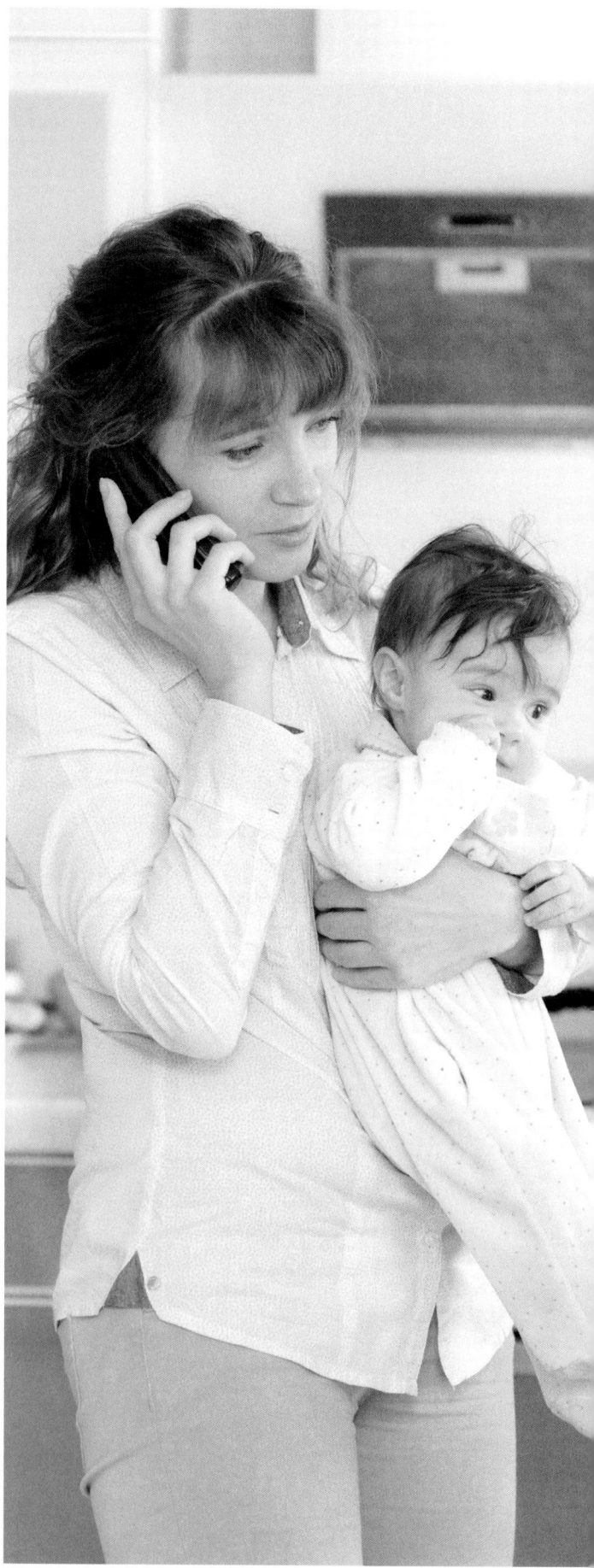

1. If the person has been exposed to poisonous fumes, such as carbon monoxide, get him or her into fresh air immediately.
2. Call a poison center. In the U.S., the toll-free Poison Help line is 800-222-1222. If you can't call a poison center, call for emergency medical assistance or get the person to the nearest emergency department as quickly as possible.
3. When you call a poison center or other emergency assistance, have the following information ready, if possible:
   • The poisoned person's condition, age and weight
   • The ingredients listed on the product container
   • The approximate time the poisoning took place
   • Your name, phone number and location
4. Follow the treatment directions that are given by the poison center.
5. Don't administer ipecac syrup. The American Academy of Pediatrics says there's no good evidence to its effectiveness and it may do more harm than good if the person aspirates while vomiting.
6. Monitor vital signs. Be alert for changes in the person who has been poisoned. If breathing stops, begin cardiopulmonary resuscitation (CPR). Watch for symptoms of shock.
7. If the poison has spilled on the person's clothing, skin or eyes, remove the clothing and flush the skin or eyes with plenty of water. You may need to hold the person's eyelids open while flushing the eyes.
8. Take the container or packaging in which the poison was stored with you to the hospital.

Poisonous plants

Many plants — both cultivated and wild — are poisonous if swallowed. Be aware of plants in your home, garden and neighborhood and know which ones are poisonous. For example, lilies of the valley are poisonous, as are daffodil bulbs, the foxglove plant, and some types of mushrooms.

PREVENTION TIP

Overdoses of seemingly harmless medications, such as the common painkillers aspirin and acetaminophen (Tylenol, others), take many lives each year. Numerous other over-the-counter (nonprescription) drugs also are dangerous if taken in large doses, especially by a child or an older adult. These include sedatives, antihistamines, and iron and vitamin supplements.

Keep all of your prescription and nonprescription drugs and vitamins stored out of the reach of children. Don't put them out where they'll be available to a toddler, such as on a kitchen counter, on a bedside table or in a purse. Buy childproof packages. If you have medications that must be refrigerated, put them on a high shelf out of reach and sight of children. If medications are placed in drawers, lock them or install a latch that toddlers can't open.

Poison Centers

A poison center isn't a hospital or treatment center. It's essentially a call center and library staffed by experts on poisoning. The information it can offer may be crucial to delivering fast and appropriate treatment in a poisoning emergency.

Poison centers are often affiliated with large hospitals or emergency departments. Most states have at least one regional center required to meet reference material and personnel standards established by the American Association of Poison Control Centers. The toll-free number to reach a poison center in the U.S. is 800-222-1222.

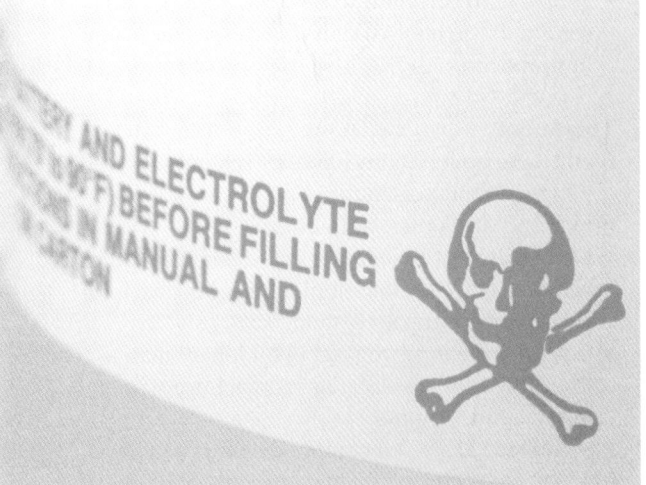

Signs and symptoms that can result from eating a poisonous plant include:
- Burning pain in the mouth and throat
- Swelling in the throat that may lead to difficulty breathing
- Vomiting
- Abdominal pain or other gastrointestinal distress
- Hallucinations
- Seizures
- Unconsciousness

If you think that someone has ingested a poisonous plant, seek emergency medical help. If the person is conscious, get a sample of the plant or take a photo of the leaves or berries, if there are any. Then call the nearest poison center for instructions. If the person is unconscious, call for emergency medical help or get the person and a sample of the plant to the nearest emergency department.

Foodborne illness

All foods naturally contain small amounts of bacteria. But poor handling of food, inadequate cooking or improper storage can result in bacteria multiplying in large enough numbers to cause illness.

Parasites, viruses, toxins and chemicals also can contaminate food. Foodborne illness from these sources, however, is less common than is foodborne illness caused by bacteria.

Signs and symptoms of food poisoning vary with the sources of contamination. Generally, diarrhea, nausea, abdominal pain and, sometimes, vomiting occur within hours after eating contaminated food.

Whether you become ill after eating contaminated food depends on the organism, the amount of exposure, your age and your health. High-risk groups include:
- Older adults. As you get older, your immune system may not respond as quickly and as effectively to infectious organisms as when you were young.
- Infants and young children. Their immune systems haven't fully developed.
- People with chronic diseases. Having a chronic condition, such as AIDS or diabetes, reduces your immune response.

Treatment
If you develop foodborne illness — commonly referred to as food poisoning:
- Rest and drink plenty of liquids.
- Don't use over-the-counter anti-diarrheal medicines because they can slow elimination of the bacteria and toxins from your system.
- Call your doctor if you feel ill for longer than two or three days. Foodborne illness often improves on its own within 48 hours.
- Seek medical assistance immediately if you have severe signs and symptoms, such as watery diarrhea

Common Plants That May Cause Illness

Name	Poisonous parts
Apricot	Pits
Daffodils	Bulbs
Dieffenbachia	Leaves and stems
English ivy	Entire plant
Foxglove (digitalis)	Entire plant
Holly	Leaves and berries
Jimson weed (thorn apple)	Entire plant
Lily of the valley	Entire plant
Mistletoe	Leaves and berries
Mushrooms, some (especially amanita)	Entire plant
Oleander	Leaves
Philodendron	Entire plant
Potatoes	Sprouts, roots and vines
Rhododendron	Entire plant
Rhubarb	Leaves

Source: FDA Poisonous Plant Database

Troublesome Bacteria and How You Can Stop Them

Keep hot food hot. Keep cold food cold. And keep everything — especially your hands — clean. If you follow these three basic rules, you'll be less likely to get food poisoning.

Bacterium	How it's spread	Signs and symptoms	To prevent its spread
Campylobacter jejuni	Contaminates meat and poultry during processing if poultry feces contact meat surfaces. Other sources: unpasteurized milk, untreated water.	Severe diarrhea (sometimes bloody), abdominal cramps, chills and generalized aches. Symptoms begin (onset) within 1 to 7 days. Lasts 1 to 2 weeks.	Cook meat and poultry thoroughly. Wash knives and cutting surfaces after contact with raw meat. Don't drink unpasteurized milk or untreated water.
Clostridium perfringens	Meats, stews and gravies. Commonly spreads when serving dishes don't keep food hot enough or when food is chilled too slowly.	Watery diarrhea, nausea and abdominal cramps. Fever is rare. Onset within 1 to 16 hours. Lasts 1 to 2 days.	Keep hot food hot. Hold cooked meats above 140 F. Reheat to at least 165 F. Chill foods quickly. Store foods in small containers.
Escherichia coli (E. coli) O157:H7	Contaminates beef during slaughter. Spreads mainly by undercooked ground beef. Other sources: unpasteurized milk, unpasteurized apple cider, human feces and contaminated water.	Watery diarrhea may turn bloody within 24 hours. Severe abdominal cramps, nausea and vomiting. Usually no fever. Onset within 1 to 8 days. Lasts 5 to 8 days.	Cook beef to an internal temperature of 160 F. Don't drink unpasteurized milk or unpasteurized apple cider. Wash your hands after using the bathroom.
Salmonella	Raw or contaminated meat, poultry, milk and egg yolks. Spreads by knives, cutting surfaces or infected people who don't wash their hands before handling food.	Severe diarrhea, watery stools, nausea, vomiting and fever of 101 F or more. Onset within 8 to 72 hours. Lasts 4 to 10 days.	Cook meat and poultry thoroughly. Don't drink unpasteurized milk. Don't eat raw or undercooked eggs. Keep hands, utensils and cutting surfaces clean. Wash hands after bathroom use.
Staph (*Staphylococcus aureus*)	Spreads by hand contact, coughing and sneezing. Grows on meats and prepared salads, cream sauces and cream-filled pastries.	Nausea, vomiting and abdominal cramps, sometimes with fever and diarrhea. Onset within 1 to 6 hours. Lasts 1 to 2 days.	Don't leave high-risk foods, such as potato salads and creamed sauces, at room temperature for more than 2 hours. Wash hands and utensils before preparing food.
Vibrio vulnificus	Raw oysters and raw or undercooked mussels, clams and whole scallops.	Chills, fever and skin lesions. Onset 1 hour to 1 week. May be fatal in people with liver disease or weakened immunity.	Avoid eating raw oysters. Make sure all shellfish is thoroughly cooked.

that turns very bloody. Also see a doctor immediately if you suspect *E. coli* poisoning (see page 453).

Prevention

To prevent foodborne illness, take the following steps when handling food:

- Thaw meats and other frozen foods in the refrigerator, not on the countertop.
- Don't buy food in dented cans or in jars with bulging lids.
- Before preparing food, wash your hands with soap and water. Rinse produce thoroughly or peel off the skin or outer leaves. Wash knives and cutting surfaces frequently, especially after handling raw meat and before preparing other foods that will be eaten raw.
- When cooking meat, use a meat thermometer. Cook red meat to an internal temperature of 160 F, poultry to 165 F. Cook fish until it flakes easily with a fork. Cook eggs until the yolks are firm.
- Always check the expiration date on food.

Bites and Stings

A cat, dog, spider, snake or even another person can deliver dangerous bites. And a bee, jellyfish or scorpion can pack a potent sting. Every one of these injuries should be treated promptly to minimize risks of infection, an allergic reaction or other complications.

Animal bites

Most animal bites are from household pets. However, stray dogs and wild animals such as skunks, raccoons and bats also bite thousands of people each year. Animals living in the wild are especially dangerous because they're more likely to carry rabies than are household pets.

Any animal — household, stray or wild — that bites a human should be impounded and observed or checked for rabies.

Treatment

If an animal bites you or someone you know:

- **For minor wounds.** If the bite barely breaks the skin and there is no danger of rabies, treat it as you would a minor wound. Wash the wound thoroughly with soap and water. Apply an antibiotic cream to prevent infection and cover the bite with a clean bandage.
- **For deep wounds.** If the animal bite creates a deep puncture of the skin or the skin is badly torn and bleeding, apply pressure with a clean, dry cloth to stop the bleeding and see your doctor.

Poison-Proofing Your Home

You can take several steps to protect your children from common household products that could poison them.

- Keep all medicine and poisonous household items, such as bathroom cleaners, in their original containers for easy identification.
- Lock poisons and medicine — especially acetaminophen (Tylenol, others), aspirin and iron supplements — out of sight and reach of children.
- Keep purses and diaper bags containing medicine out of reach of children.
- Put child-resistant locks on cabinet doors.
- Don't tell your children that their medicine tastes like candy.
- Keep poisonous plants out of reach of children.
- Keep the Poison Help number (800-222-1222) on or near your phone.

- **For infection.** If you notice signs of infection, such as swelling, redness, increased pain or oozing, see your doctor immediately.
- **For suspected rabies.** If you suspect the bite was caused by an animal that might carry rabies, see your doctor immediately.

Human bites

Human bites can be as dangerous as animal bites, or even more so, because of the types of bacteria and viruses contained in the human mouth. If someone cuts his or her knuckles on another person's teeth, as might happen in a fight, this is also considered a human bite.

Risk of Rabies

Many wild animals carry rabies, but so can the usually friendly pooch next door, especially if it comes in contact with wild animals and hasn't been immunized for rabies.

Rabies is caused by a virus that affects the brain. It's most often transmitted to humans by the saliva of an infected animal. However, a bite isn't necessary to transmit the virus. Even a licking from an infected animal can spread the disease if the animal's saliva comes in contact with an existing wound.

The rabies virus often takes one to three months to produce symptoms, and it can take much longer. If you think you may have been exposed to rabies, consult your doctor or health department right away. For more information on rabies, see page 458.

In the event of a bite by an animal, the animal should be caught, confined and observed by a veterinarian or animal control professional for up to 10 days. If you can't catch the animal — as is often the case with wild animals — then contact your local health department, natural resources or law enforcement officials. The animal may have to be killed, and in such a way that its brain isn't damaged. Health or law enforcement officials will arrange testing of the animal for rabies. If the animal isn't caught, presume that it has rabies and seek medical care accordingly.

Symptoms

Often the first symptom of rabies is a tingling sensation that develops at the site of the animal bite. Skin at the site often becomes very sensitive. An infected person may develop a fever, chills, fatigue, vomiting and headache. As the virus spreads, the person may develop a fear of water (hydrophobia). Foaming at the mouth may occur — a consequence of

excess saliva that can't be swallowed. Severe muscle contractions can develop, and some people develop paralysis. Left untreated, the infection almost inevitably leads to death. In later stages, the virus may be present in the person's saliva and can infect others.

Treatment

Extensive cleaning of the wound with soap and water, followed by irrigation of the wound by a health care professional, should be carried out as soon as possible after the bite. Your doctor then must decide whether to treat you for rabies. Treatment consists of a series of shots to prevent the rabies virus from infecting you. First is a fast-acting shot (rabies immune globulin). Part of this injection is given near the area where the animal bit you, if possible. This is followed by a series of rabies vaccines to help your body identify and fight the rabies virus. The vaccines are given as injections in your arm. You receive four injections over 14 days.

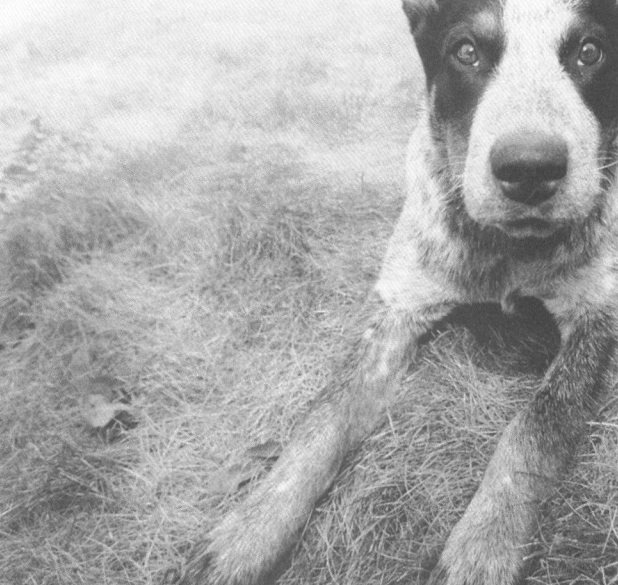

Treatment

If you are bitten by another human, and the bite breaks the skin:

- Stop the bleeding by applying pressure.
- Wash the wound thoroughly with soap and water.
- Apply an antibiotic cream to prevent infection.
- Apply a clean bandage.
- Seek medical care. If you haven't had a tetanus shot within five years, your doctor may recommend a booster. You should have a booster within 48 hours of the injury.

Insect and spider bites and stings

Venom, saliva or other toxins injected into your skin are what cause the symptoms of an insect or spider bite or sting. With minor bites the reaction is temporary and limited to the area of the bite. A bump rises on your skin, the area may itch or hurt for a few hours, and then over a period of days the skin irritation and discomfort disappear. Typically, the bites of insects such as mosquitoes, fleas, flies, bedbugs, ants and chiggers follow this course.

However, your entire body can be affected if the venom is potent, as is the case with certain spiders and scorpions, or if you are hypersensitive to bee, wasp and yellow jacket stings.

Signs and symptoms of a severe reaction include:

- Swelling, particularly the face or mouth, and hives
- Difficulty breathing
- Abdominal pain
- Shock

Spider bites

Only a few spiders are dangerous to humans. Two found in the contiguous United States and more common in the southern states are the black widow and brown recluse. Both types of spiders prefer warm and dark, dry places where flies are plentiful. They may live in woodpiles, closets and under sinks.

If you're bitten by one of these spiders:

- Elevate the limb if possible, if the bite is on an arm or leg.
- Apply to the bite location a cloth dampened with cold water or filled with ice.
- Seek immediate medical attention. Depending on the severity, the bite may require medication.

Black widow

The bite of the black widow spider causes little more than a pinprick-like sensation — some people aren't even aware of the bite. At first you may experience only slight swelling and faint red marks where you were bitten. Within a few hours, you'll begin to feel intense pain and stiffness. Other signs and symptoms include chills, fever, nausea and severe abdominal pain. The bite of a black widow spider is rarely lethal.

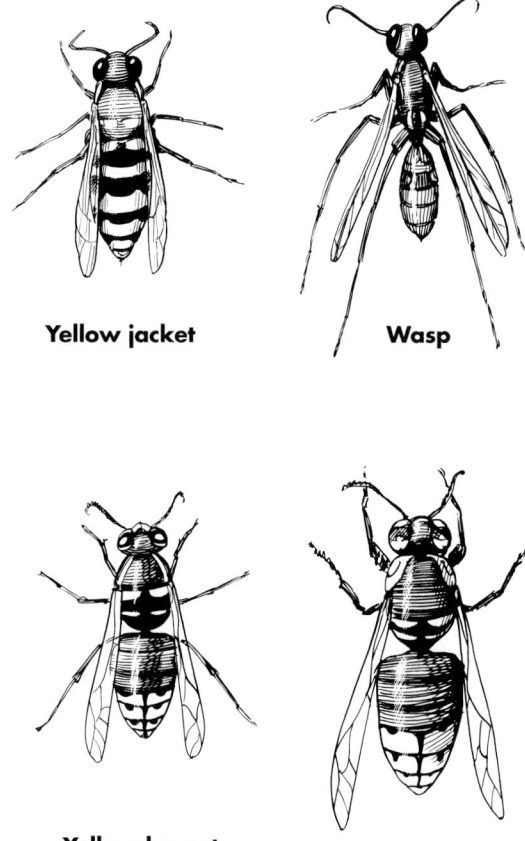

Yellow jacket   **Wasp**

Yellow hornet   **White-faced hornet**

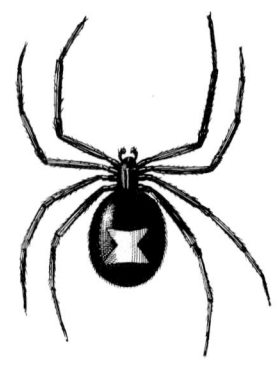

**Black widow
(viewed from below)**

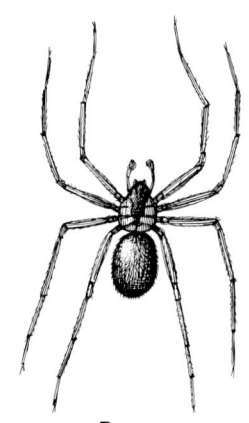

**Brown
recluse**

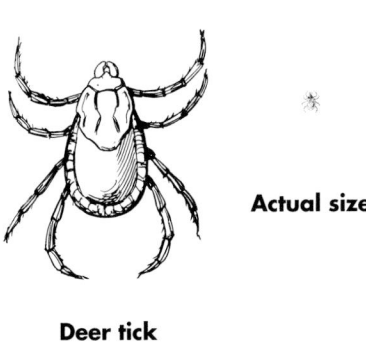

Actual size

Deer tick

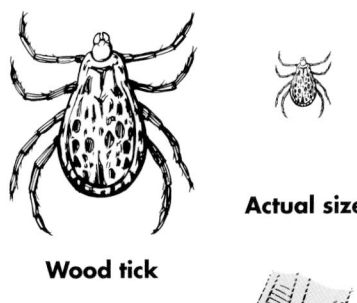

Actual size

Wood tick

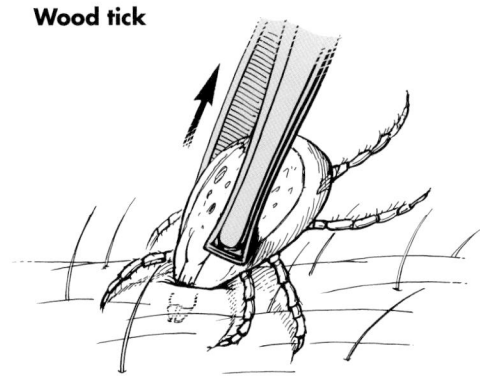

To remove a tick, use tweezers to slowly and steadily pull the tick away from the skin.

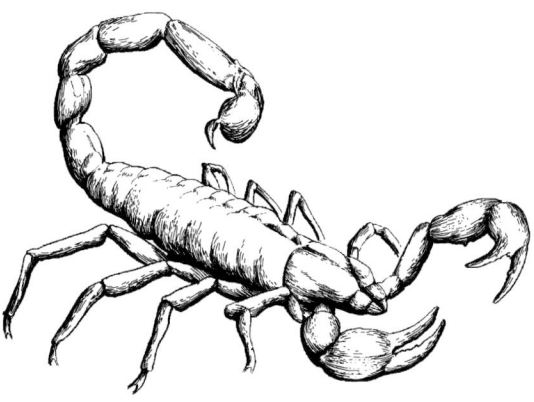

Scorpion

Distinctive marks of individual insects are emphasized to help identify them.

You can identify this spider by the red hourglass marking on its belly.

Brown recluse
If you're bitten by a brown recluse spider, you'll experience mild stinging, followed by local redness and increasing pain. A fluid-filled blister may form at the site, and if the bite is severe, it may develop into a deep, growing ulcer. Your body's reactions can vary from a mild fever and rash to nausea and listlessness. Rarely, death can result.

Tick bites

Ticks can be a threat to human health because some carry infections that can be transmitted to humans by a bite. American dog ticks and Rocky Mountain wood ticks can carry Rocky Mountain spotted fever. Deer ticks — which are much smaller than wood ticks — can carry Lyme disease and anaplasmosis.

Rocky Mountain spotted fever can produce chills and fever, severe headaches, widespread aches, restlessness, and a red rash occurring between days two and six of the onset of fever (see page 467). Lyme disease may produce symptoms of fatigue, headache, muscle and joint pain, along with a characteristic non-painful rash, often with a target or bull's-eye appearance (see page 465). Anaplasmosis may cause fever, malaise, headache and general body aches.

If you receive a tick bite:
- Remove the tick promptly and carefully using a tweezers to grasp the tick near its head. Pull gently to remove the whole tick without crushing it.
- If possible, seal the tick in a jar or storage container. If you develop signs or symptoms of illness after the bite, your doctor may want to see the tick.
- Wash the area around the tick bite and your hands with soap and water.
- Call your doctor if you can't completely remove the tick, or if you develop a rash, fever, stiff neck, muscle aches, joint pain, swollen lymph nodes or flu-like symptoms.

Scorpion stings

Scorpions are found in the southwestern United States. Some scorpions have potentially lethal venom that's injected by a sting. Because it's difficult to distinguish the highly poisonous scorpions from the nonpoisonous ones, all scorpion stings are treated as emergencies.

Other stings

Some people are allergic to the venom of bees, wasps, hornets, yellow jackets or fire ants. For such sensitive individuals, getting stung can cause a life-threatening allergic response called anaphylactic shock (see page 47). Signs and symptoms include:
- Constriction of airways, including swelling of the mouth, tongue or throat, causing breathing difficulty

- Shock associated with an abrupt decrease in blood pressure
- Rapid heart rate
- Hives and welts below the skin surface
- Nausea, vomiting or diarrhea
- Dizziness, mental confusion, slurred speech or extreme anxiety
- Swelling of the lips and around the eyes
- Flushing of skin and intense itching

Treatment

While waiting for medical help to arrive:

1. Check for special medications the person may be carrying to treat a severe allergic reaction, such as an autoinjector of epinephrine (EpiPen, Adrenaclick). Administer the medication as recommended — usually by pressing the autoinjector against the person's thigh and holding it in place for several seconds. Massage the injection site afterward to enhance absorption of the medication.
2. After administering epinephrine, have the person take an antihistamine pill containing diphenhydramine (Benadryl), if he or she is able to do so without choking.
3. Have the person lie still on his or her back and loosen tight clothing.
4. If the person stops breathing, begin administering cardiopulmonary resuscitation (CPR).

Snakebites

Most North American snakes aren't poisonous, but a few are — such as rattlesnakes, coral snakes, water moccasins and copperheads.

If you're bitten by a snake, it's important to determine whether the snake is poisonous. If it is, you'll need emergency treatment. Most poisonous snakes in North America, with the exception of the coral snake, have slit-like (elliptical) eyes. Their heads are triangular with a pit (depression) midway between the eyes and nostrils on both sides of the head.

Other characteristics are unique to certain poisonous snakes:

- Rattlesnakes make a rattling sound by shaking the rings at the end of their tails.
- Water moccasins have a whitish, cottony lining in their mouths.
- Coral snakes have red, yellow and black rings along the length of their bodies.

Treatment

Take these steps if you're bitten by a snake:

- Remain calm.
- Don't try to capture the snake.
- Immobilize the bitten arm or leg and try to stay quiet.
- Remove jewelry because swelling tends to progress rapidly.

PREVENTION TIP

When walking in wooded or grassy areas, wear shoes, long pants tucked into socks and long-sleeved shirts. This can help prevent tick bites. In addition, stick to trails and avoid walking through bushes and tall grass.

Insect repellents will often repel ticks. Among the longest lasting and most effective are products containing DEET. The American Academy of Pediatrics recommends that repellents used on children contain no more than 30 percent DEET, and that DEET not be used on children younger than 2 months of age.

DEET concentrations of 10 percent and 30 percent are similarly effective, but higher concentrations last longer. Ten percent DEET will protect you for about two hours, while 30 percent DEET will protect your for about five hours. Use the lowest concentration for the amount of time you'll need protection.

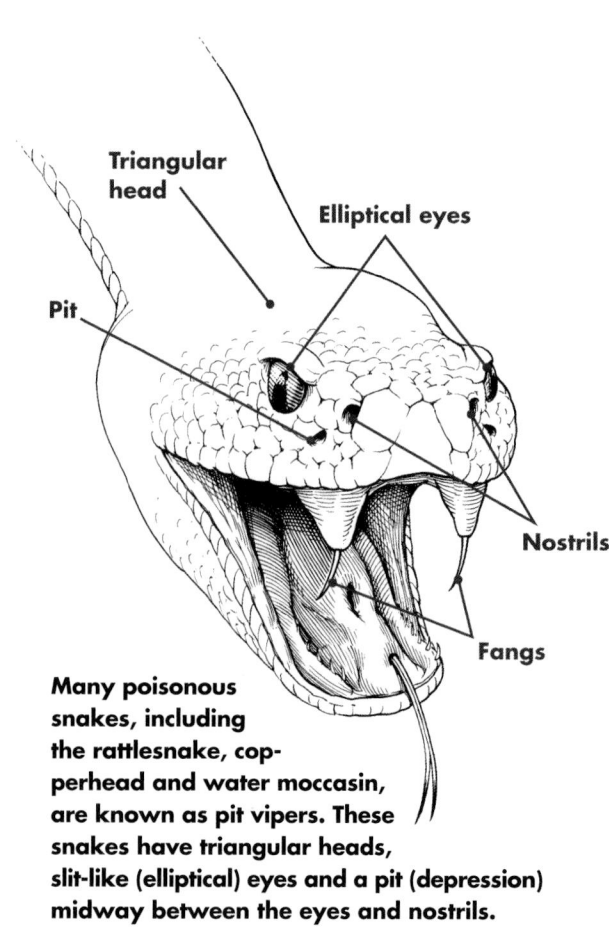

Triangular head

Elliptical eyes

Pit

Nostrils

Fangs

Many poisonous snakes, including the rattlesnake, copperhead and water moccasin, are known as pit vipers. These snakes have triangular heads, slit-like (elliptical) eyes and a pit (depression) midway between the eyes and nostrils.

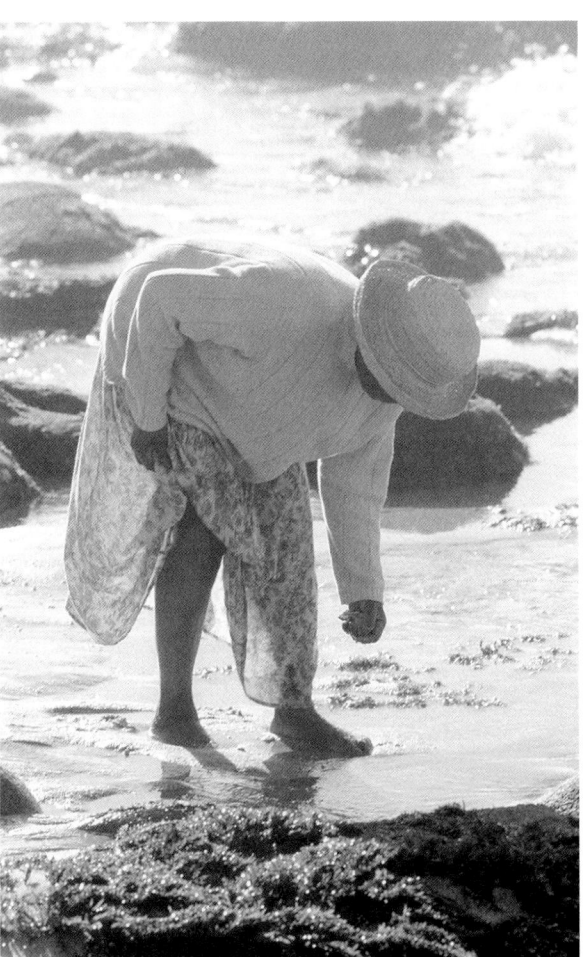

- Apply a splint to reduce movement of the affected area and make sure it is loose enough not to restrict blood flow.
- Don't use a tourniquet or apply ice.
- Don't cut the wound or attempt to remove the venom.
- Seek medical attention as soon as possible, especially if the bitten area changes color, begins to swell or is painful.

Sea organism stings

Several sea organisms, including the jellyfish and Portuguese man-of-war, carry venom in their tentacles. This venom can be discharged on contact, in some cases even after the animals are dead.

Stinging and pain are the key symptoms, along with a red, hive-like line of lesions. If a considerable amount of venom is injected, you may also experience shortness of breath, nausea and stomach cramps. Severe stings can lead to muscle cramps, fainting, coughing, vomiting, difficulty breathing and, in rare cases, death.

Treatment
If you're stung by a jellyfish or Portuguese man-of-war:
1. Get out of the water. Pain and cramps can be disabling, and you could drown.
2. Promptly remove any stinging tentacles with a plastic object, such as a driver's license or credit card. It's best to wear gloves or use a towel when removing the Portuguese man-of-war debris. You can also use salt water to wash off the tentacles.
3. Immerse or shower the area in hot water for 20 minutes.
4. Don't immerse the wound in cold or cool fresh water and don't rub the skin because either action could trigger discharge of more venom.
5. Urinating on the wound isn't recommended.
6. Apply over-the-counter hydrocortisone ointment to reduce redness and swelling. A calamine-type lotion and oral antihistamines, such as diphenhydramine, can help reduce itching.
7. For severe stings, seek emergency medical care.

Foreign Bodies

Children and adults alike occasionally get foreign objects in body openings — especially the eyes, ears and nose. Sometimes, you can get the objects out without the help of a doctor. Other cases require a doctor's expertise and equipment.

In the eyes

An eye often clears itself of foreign airborne objects, such as specks of dirt, by automatically tearing up and blinking. If you have something in your eye and tearing and blinking aren't enough to get rid of it, treat the condition promptly to avoid damage that can be caused by scratches, infection or exposure to chemicals.

Clearing your own eye

If an object is lodged in your eye and no one is available to help you, try to remove the foreign matter yourself by flushing the eye with clear water or saline solution:

- Fill an eyecup or small juice glass with clean water or saline solution.
- Position the eyecup or glass with its rim resting on the bone at the base of your eye socket and pour the water in, keeping the eye open.

Even if you think the object has been removed, flush your eye if it still hurts and looks red. If you don't succeed in clearing the eye, seek emergency medical help.

Clearing someone else's eye

To clear someone else's eye:

1. Wash your hands before examining the eye.
2. Seat the person in a well-lighted area.
3. Gently examine the eye to find the object. Pull the lower lid downward and instruct the person to look up. Then hold the upper eyelid while the person looks down.
4. If the object is floating in the tear film on the surface of the eye, try flushing it out. If you're able to remove the object, flush the eye with clear, lukewarm water or a saline solution.
5. Don't rub the eye or try to remove an object that's embedded into the eyeball or makes closing the eye difficult. Seek emergency medical care.

In the ears

Children often insert objects into their ears, such as erasers, beads or tiny toys. Sometimes, an insect will accidentally enter the ear.

Treatment

If an object becomes lodged in an ear:

- Don't probe the ear with any tool. This includes a cotton swab or any other tool. You could push the object farther into the ear and damage the fragile structures of the middle ear.
- If the object is clearly visible, is pliable and can be easily grasped with a tweezers, gently remove it.
- Try using gravity. Tilt the head to the affected side to try to dislodge the object.
- If the object is an insect, tilt the person's head so that the ear with the insect is up. You can try to float the insect out by pouring a small amount of warm — not hot — mineral oil, olive oil or baby oil into the

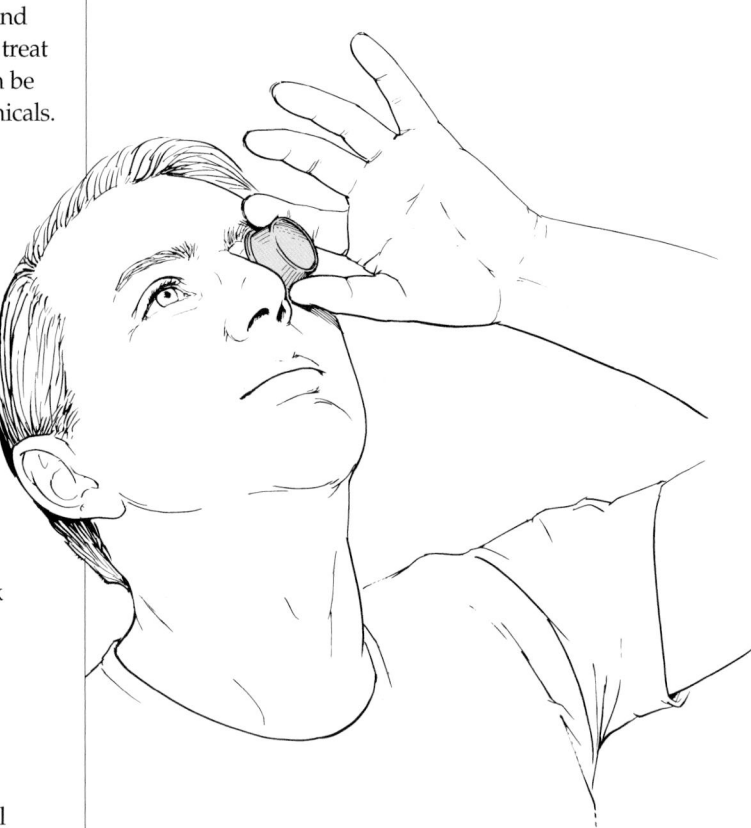

To remove a small object from your eye, flush it with a small amount of clean water or saline solution.

A few simple steps can go a long way toward avoiding eye injuries:
- Wear goggles when working with tools, especially saws and grinders.
- Wear safety glasses for sports.
- Pick up sticks and other loose objects on the lawn before mowing.
- Don't lean over a battery when attaching jumper cables.
- Store household chemicals out of reach of children.
- Supervise children at play, especially when they're playing with toys that can cause eye injuries, such as spring-loaded toys.

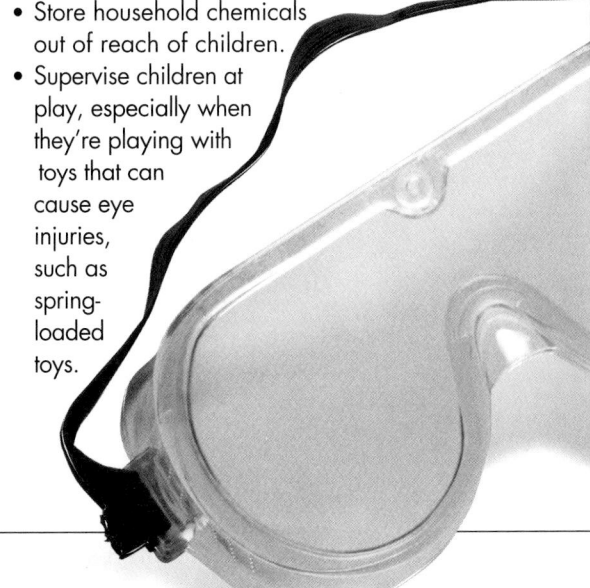

Children and Button Batteries

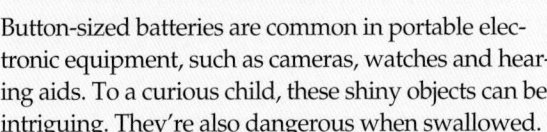

Button-sized batteries are common in portable electronic equipment, such as cameras, watches and hearing aids. To a curious child, these shiny objects can be intriguing. They're also dangerous when swallowed.

Button batteries can cause damage to fragile gastrointestinal tract tissues through electrical discharge. They also contain dangerous alkali fluids. If released into the stomach or intestine, the battery fluid may eat through the lining, producing signs and symptoms such as chest pain, abdominal pain, vomiting and fever.

If your child swallows a button battery, seek emergency medical care. Depending on the location of the battery and the child's symptoms, a procedure to remove the battery may be necessary.

Store unused batteries out of reach of children. When disposing of used batteries, don't toss them into a wastebasket that a toddler can easily explore.

ear. Ease the entry of the oil by straightening the ear canal: Pull the ear gently backward and upward. The insect should suffocate and may float out in the oil bath. Don't use oil to remove any other object.
- If these methods fail and the person continues to experience pain or reduced hearing, see a doctor.

In the nose

The nose is a favorite place for children and grown-up jokesters to insert things, such as a drinking straw, marble or piece of candy. Sometimes the object gets stuck.

Treatment
If a foreign object becomes lodged in your nose:
- Don't probe at the foreign object with a cotton swab, a matchstick or other tool. This risks pushing the object farther into the nose.
- Don't try to inhale the object by forcefully breathing in. Instead, breathe through your mouth until the object is removed.
- Blow your nose with short, firm puffs of air while gently applying pressure to the opposite nostril to close the nostril.
- If the object is clearly visible, is pliable and can be easily grasped with tweezers, gently try to remove it.

If an object is lodged in your child's nose, attempt to remove it with the "parent's kiss." Place gentle pressure on the unaffected nostril to close it. Then firmly seal your mouth around your child's mouth and deliver short puffs of air into the child's mouth. This may dislodge the object.

See a doctor as soon as possible if these methods fail.

In the windpipe or lungs

When an object is accidentally inhaled, sometimes it lodges in the windpipe (trachea) or the lungs. If an inhaled object causes choking, use the Heimlich maneuver to try to dislodge it (see page 14). If that doesn't work, seek emergency medical help.

In some cases, a foreign body lodged in the windpipe or the bronchial tubes doesn't inhibit breathing, but it does constitute a health hazard. If you or someone with you inhales a foreign object, see a doctor.

Swallowed

If you swallow a foreign object, it will usually pass through the digestive system without causing a problem, but sometimes an object can become lodged. Seek emergency help if the following signs or symptoms appear:
- Difficulty swallowing
- Spitting up saliva
- Chest pain
- Abdominal pain or vomiting

In the skin

It's common for an object to become embedded in your skin. If a foreign object is partially embedded, take the following steps:

- Wash your hands and clean the area well with soap and water.
- Use tweezers to remove splinters of wood, fiberglass, small pieces of glass or other foreign objects. If the object is completely embedded:
- Wash your hands and clean the area well with soap and water.
- Sterilize a clean, sharp needle by wiping it with rubbing alcohol. If rubbing alcohol isn't available use soap and water.
- Use the needle to gently break the skin over the object and lift the tip of the object out.
- Use a tweezers to remove the object. A magnifying glass may help you see the object better.
- Wash and pat dry the area and apply antibiotic ointment.
- Seek medical help if the object doesn't come out easily or is close to an eye.

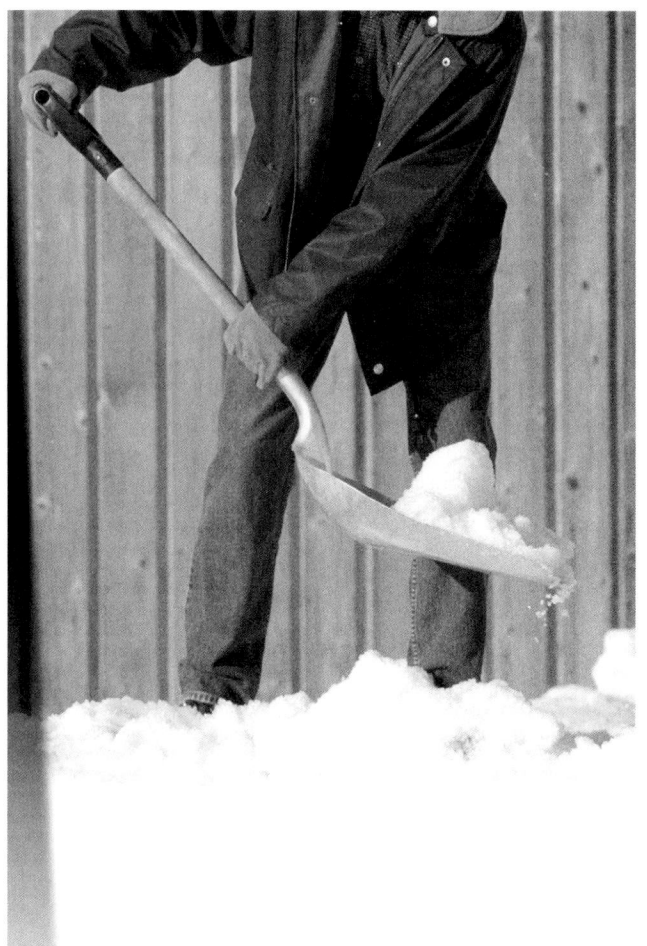

Cold-Related Emergencies

Overexposure to cold and damp weather can lead to frostbite or hypothermia.

PREVENTION TIP

You can do several things to prevent injury from frostbite and hypothermia:

Stay dry
Your body loses heat faster when your skin is wet from rain, snow or sweat.

Protect yourself from the wind
Exposed skin is especially vulnerable and can freeze in minutes when wind combines with sub-freezing temperatures. Here's an example of what the wind can do. An outdoor temperature of minus 20 F combined with a 10 mph wind produces a wind chill factor of minus 41 F.

Wear warm clothing
Choose clothes that both shield and breathe. Layers are often best. Layers of light, loosefitting clothes trap air, which adds insulation. As an outer layer, make sure to wear something that's water-repellent and windproof.

Cover your head, neck and face
Much of your body heat is lost as it rises from the top of your body. Cap the heat in.

Wear warm socks and mittens
If you're going to be in subfreezing temperatures for more than a few minutes, wear two layers of socks. In addition, wear mittens, which protect your fingers more effectively than do gloves.

Stay alert to numbness
If part of your body gets so cold that it starts feeling painful or numb, that's a clue your skin is beginning to freeze. Take time to rewarm yourself.

Frostbite

When your skin is exposed to very cold temperatures, your skin and the underlying tissues may freeze, resulting in frostbite. Frostbite can affect any part of your body, but your hands, feet, nose and ears are most susceptible because they're small and often exposed.

Anyone can get frostbite, but people with circulatory problems, such as peripheral vascular disease, are at greater risk. Excessive consumption of alcohol or other drugs also puts you at increased risk of frostbite.

You can identify frostbite by the pale and cold quality of skin that's been exposed to the cold. The skin may feel numb and hard to the touch. As the area thaws, the flesh becomes red and painful. Large, clear or bloody blisters may develop.

Treatment

The first step in treating frostbite is to warm the affected skin:

- If possible, get out of the cold.
- Warm the affected skin by immersing it in warm, but not hot, water. The temperature should feel comfortable to skin that's not affected.
- If you can't immerse the injured skin in warm water, you can warm your hands by tucking them under your arms. If your nose, ears or face is frostbitten, warm the area by covering it with dry, gloved hands. If your feet are affected, don't walk, unless you must do so to escape the cold.
- Expect some discomfort. Frostbitten areas will turn red and throb, or they'll burn with pain as they thaw. Even with mild frostbite, normal sensation may not return immediately.
- Don't rub the affected area. Doing so can damage frozen tissues. Never rub snow on frozen skin.
- If there's a chance of refreezing, don't thaw out the affected areas. If they're already thawed out, wrap them up so that they don't refreeze.
- If your symptoms don't improve after taking these steps, seek emergency medical care.

Altitude Sickness

If you live at a low altitude and make a trip to an altitude of more than 8,000 feet, you might experience high-altitude illness. The condition is sometimes called acute mountain sickness. It can cause headache, nausea, fatigue, sleeplessness, shortness of breath and loss of appetite. It usually develops several hours after arriving at a high altitude, and gradually resolves within a day if you don't go any higher. Skiers who travel to mountain slopes from lower elevations are commonly affected.

More-serious forms of altitude sickness can produce severe breathing distress or severe brain illness that can become fatal if not treated.

Treatment

You can minimize the effects of mild altitude sickness by making a gradual ascent. Your doctor may prescribe certain medications if you know that your travel plans will rapidly take you to high altitudes. For serious altitude sickness, you'll need to descend to a lower altitude. Oxygen and rest also are helpful.

Prevention

To keep your kids from getting frostbite, make sure their skin is covered when outside. Watch for wet chin straps on caps and snowsuits because the skin under the strap can easily freeze. Teach your child to avoid touching cold metal with bare hands or licking cold metal objects.

Hypothermia

Under most conditions your body is able to maintain a steady and healthy temperature. However, when you're exposed for prolonged periods to cold temperatures or a cool, damp environment — particularly if your clothing is wet or damp — the body's temperature control mechanisms may fail. When you lose more heat than your body can generate, hypothermia can result.

Wet or inadequate clothing, falling into cold water or even having an uncovered head during cold weather can increase your chances of hypothermia.

Hypothermia is defined as having an internal body temperature of less than 95 F. A normal body temperature is 98.6 F. Other signs and symptoms of hypothermia — which tend to develop slowly — include:

- Shivering
- Slurred speech
- An abnormally slow rate of breathing
- Cold, pale skin
- Loss of coordination
- Tiredness, lethargy or apathy
- Confusion or memory loss

People with hypothermia typically experience gradual loss of mental acuity and physical ability, so they may be unaware that they need medical treatment.

Older adults, young children, very thin people and people who are intoxicated are at particular risk of hypothermia. Malnutrition, cardiovascular disease and an underactive thyroid also can increase your risk of hypothermia.

Treatment

To treat hypothermia:

1. Call for emergency medical assistance. While waiting for help to arrive, monitor the person's breathing. If breathing stops, begin cardiopulmonary resuscitation (CPR) immediately.
2. If possible, get the person with hypothermia out of the cold. If going indoors isn't possible, get the person out of the wind, cover his or her head and insulate him or her from the cold ground.
3. Remove the person's wet clothes and cover him or her with dry, warm clothes or blankets.
4. Don't apply direct heat, such as hot water or a heating pad, to warm the person. Instead, apply warm compresses to the neck, chest wall and groin. Don't attempt to warm the arms and legs.

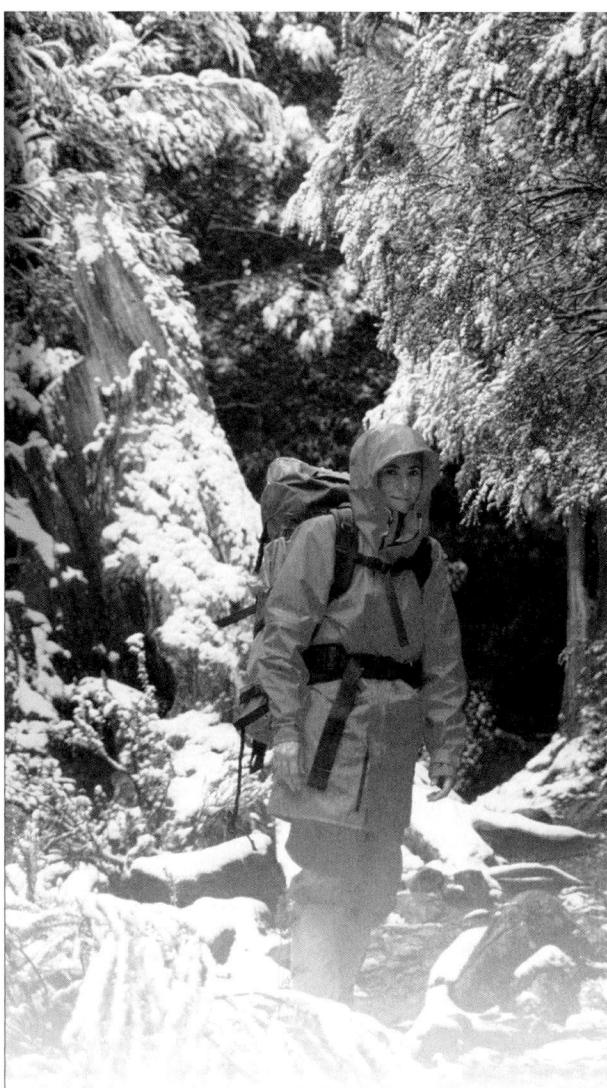

Damage to your skin from recurrent sunburns is cumulative, and continued overexposure to ultra-violet radiation can produce long-term problems. These may include skin discolorations, premature aging of your skin, increased wrinkling and skin cancer. To reduce your risk of these conditions, try to avoid being outside for long periods when the sun's ultraviolet radiation is at its peak — between 10 a.m. and 3 p.m.

When you're outside for more than a few minutes, cover exposed areas of skin, wear a broad-brimmed hat and use a water-resistant, broad-spectrum sunscreen with a sun protection factor (SPF) of 30 or higher. Apply sunscreen every two hours while in the sun.

To beat the heat:

Stay out of the sun
Avoid going outside during the hottest part of the day, from noon to 4 p.m.

Limit physical activity
Reserve vigorous exercise for early morning or the evening.

Dress for the heat
Wear clothes that are light colored, lightweight and loosefitting.

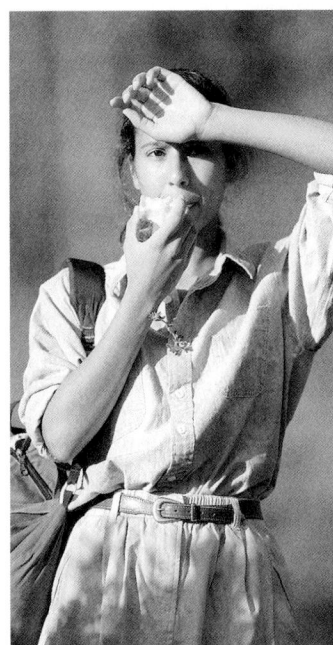

Drink lots of liquids
Drink lots of liquids, but avoid excess alcohol and caffeine because they can cause dehydration.

Avoid hot and heavy meals
Smaller meals supplemented with healthy snacks are a good idea when the weather gets hot.

Heat applied to the arms and legs forces cold blood back toward the heart, lungs and brain, causing the core body temperature to drop. This can be fatal.

5. Don't give the person alcohol. Give the person warm nonalcoholic drinks, unless he or she is vomiting.
6. Don't massage or rub the person. Handle him or her gently, because a hypothermic person is at risk of developing cardiac arrest.

Heat-Related Emergencies

Excessive sun exposure or heat can damage your skin and cause your body to overheat.

Sunburn

Prolonged exposure to the sun's ultraviolet rays produces red, tender or swollen skin, which can blister. The swelling and redness of a sunburn are due to inflammation of the damaged skin. Severe sunburn may also cause headache, fever, nausea and fatigue.

Treatment
If you have a sunburn:
- Aloe vera lotion, cool compresses or calamine lotion may relieve mild discomfort.
- Don't break water blisters because they help protect against infection and speed healing. If they burst, apply an antibacterial ointment on the open areas.
- Take ibuprofen (Advil, Motrin IB, others) to control the pain and to reduce inflammation.

If sunburn is severe, with severe blistering or headache, vomiting, and fever, contact your doctor.

Heat stress

Under normal conditions, your body's natural control mechanisms help you adjust to the heat. Porous skin allows excessive heat to escape, and perspiration generates a cooling evaporation. However, when you're exposed to high temperatures for long periods — especially when there's little breeze and high humidity — your body's normal control mechanisms may get overwhelmed. They simply can't handle the amount of intense heat bearing down on you. When that happens, problems develop. One of the most serious is heatstroke, which can be fatal.

Heatstroke
The three key features of heatstroke are:
- A temperature of 104 F or higher

- Altered mental status
- Exposure to excessive heat (classic heatstroke) or to exertion (exertional heatstroke)

Other signs and symptoms may include:

- Hot, flushed skin, which may be dry or moist
- Rapid heartbeat
- Rapid and shallow breathing
- Stopping (cessation) of sweating
- Feeling dizzy or lightheaded
- Headache
- Nausea
- Weakness or fainting, which may be the first sign in older adults

Those most at risk are older adults and the very young. Others at high risk are people with previous heat-related illness and people who are dehydrated, who have heart disease and who drink excessive amounts of alcohol.

Certain medicines also can increase your chances of getting heatstroke. Some medications for motion sickness and depression can impair your ability to sweat.

Treatment

If you suspect heatstroke:

- Move the person out of the sun and into a shady or air-conditioned place.
- Call 911 or your local emergency number.
- While you're waiting for the emergency help to arrive, cool the person by spraying him or her with cool water. Use a fan to blow air over the moistened skin. Placing towels wet with ice water on the individual also can be effective.
- Have the person drink cool water, if he or she is able to do so.

Heat exhaustion

Heat exhaustion is more common. It isn't as dangerous as heatstroke because its symptoms don't include confusion or altered consciousness (central nervous system dysfunction). However, heat exhaustion can quickly evolve into heatstroke if steps aren't taken to treat it.

Signs and symptoms of heat exhaustion often begin suddenly. They may include:

- Inability to continue with exercise
- Feeling faint or dizzy
- Nausea, vomiting or diarrhea
- Heavy sweating
- Rapid, weak heartbeat
- Low blood pressure
- An ashen appearance
- Cold, clammy skin, chills and goose bumps
- Muscle cramps
- Headache
- Fatigue
- Dark-colored urine

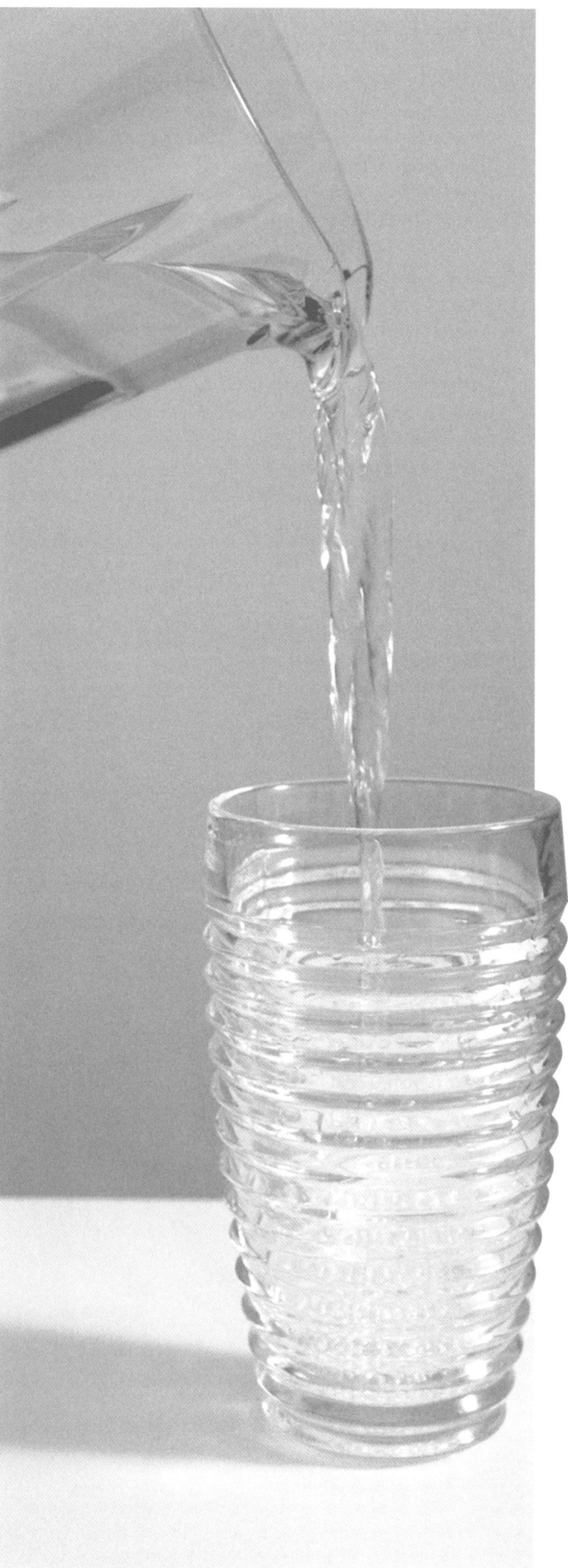

Treatment

If you suspect that someone has heat exhaustion:
- Get him or her out of the heat and into a shady or air-conditioned location.
- Lay the person down and elevate the legs.
- Loosen or remove most of the person's clothing.
- Have the person drink a carbohydrate-electrolyte solution found in some sports drinks.
- Cool the person by spraying or sponging him or her with cool water and using a fan to blow air over the moistened skin.
- If signs of heatstroke appear, seek emergency medical care.

Heat cramps

Heat cramps are painful muscle spasms that can occur after vigorous exercise and profuse sweating. Your legs, abdominal muscles and other muscles that you use during exercise are most often affected. Heat cramps usually happen in warm environments, but they can also occur in cooler surroundings.

Treatment

Take these steps if you experience heat cramps:
- Rest briefly and cool down.
- Drink a carbohydrate-electrolyte solution found in some sports drinks to replenish lost electrolytes, such as sodium.
- Practice gentle, range-of-motion stretching and gentle massage of the affected muscles.
- If the cramps don't go away in an hour, call your doctor.

Mental Health Emergencies

Situations affecting an individual's mental health can also create medical emergencies. Similar to a physical injury, a mental illness may require immediate, professional medical intervention.

Alcohol intoxication and withdrawal

Alcohol is a drug that depresses your central nervous system by acting as a sedative. In some people, the first reaction may be stimulation, but as drinking continues, sedating effects set in.

At first, alcohol affects mainly your thoughts, emotions and judgment. But if you continue drinking, the alcohol impairs your speech and muscle coordination. Taken in large enough quantities, it can lead to a coma by depressing the vital centers of your brain.

The signs of alcohol intoxication range from slurred speech, uncoordinated movements and loud, unruly behavior to vomiting, lethargy and unconsciousness. An individual who is intoxicated may appear flushed and give off a noticeable odor of alcohol.

Serious symptoms can also occur when a habitual drinker suddenly stops drinking. Physical symptoms of withdrawal may occur within hours or several days of stopping drinking.

The person may act strangely, hallucinate, become confused or agitated, and develop a noticeable trembling in the hands. These signs and symptoms are sometimes called delirium tremens (DTs). Without medical treatment, seizures and even death can occur.

Treatment

If you're trying to help someone who you think is intoxicated or experiencing symptoms of alcohol withdrawal, if possible try to determine if his or her symptoms are caused by drinking alcohol or by withdrawal from it. Ask the person about this in a nonthreatening way. You're more likely to get an honest answer if you appear calm and nonjudgmental instead of angry and condemning.

Also ask whether he or she has taken any medications while drinking. Mixing alcohol with certain drugs can cause the person's condition to quickly deteriorate and become life-threatening.

If the person vomits, try to prevent him or her from inhaling (aspirating) vomit into the lungs by bending the head between the knees or, if the person is lying down, by turning the head to one side.

If you observe any of the following circumstances, seek emergency medical assistance:
- The person is withdrawing from habitual alcohol use.
- The person shows no evidence of alcohol consumption, but his or her behavior is unusual.
- The person is unconscious or has inhaled vomit.
- There's evidence that the person has consumed dangerous excessive amounts of alcohol along with other drugs.

Intoxication from other drugs

Many drugs — even prescription medications — can cause serious effects in people who are sensitive to the chemicals in the drug. Mixing drugs, such as alcohol and certain medications or illegally used drugs, can cause interactions that are particularly dangerous and potentially lethal.

Prescription medications

If you experience signs or symptoms that are concerning or worrisome after taking any medication, stop taking it and contact your doctor for advice. More serious signs and symptoms, such as loss of consciousness or seizures, indicate a need for emergency medical attention.

Treating a Hangover

A lot of hangover remedies have been tried, but there isn't much evidence that they help. And some may hurt. Alcohol dehydrates you, as do caffeine drinks that are sometimes used to fight a hangover. If you have a hangover:
- Rest and drink plenty of bland liquids, such as water, sports drinks, low-acid fruit juices and broth. Avoid drinks with lots of citric acid or caffeine.
- Take ibuprofen (Advil, Motrin IB, others) or another nonprescription pain medication.

Suicidal Thoughts and Behavior

It's commonly said that people who talk about suicide don't do it. That's an old cliché that simply isn't true. No two people with suicidal thoughts are alike, but people thinking about suicide often express themselves with similar behavior. Here are some of those behaviors — common warning signs of potential suicide:

Suicidal threats

Sometimes, an individual will tell others outright that he or she is thinking of suicide. Or the person might try a less direct approach, such as saying that everyone would be better off if he or she had never been born or was dead. Take such words as a sign that he or she needs professional help.

Withdrawing from others

People at risk of suicide may be less willing to talk with others or may want to be left alone. Trouble at work or poor grades in school can be other signs of withdrawal.

Moodiness

We all have our ups and downs. But drastic mood swings — an emotional high on one day and deep discouragement the next — aren't normal. A sense of profound hopelessness should prompt an evaluation by a mental health professional.

Illegal drugs

Signs of illegal drug use vary according to the type of drug. With a drug such as marijuana, the effects may be subtle. You might notice redness about the eyes of the user, abnormal eye movements or dryness around the mouth. You may also notice that the person's speech is slurred.

Some street drugs, such as methamphetamine, produce profound changes in mood and thought processes, often resulting in hallucinations. Acute, severe agitation may occur, as may a rapid heart rate, high blood pressure, and tremors or other abnormal movements. Methamphetamine intoxication can cause a person to become a danger to themselves and others. When there's a loss of contact with reality (acute psychosis), the person is at high risk of suicide or violence toward others.

Other street drugs, such as heroin, may lead to a slower pulse, slower breathing and slurred speech. Various street drugs can cause drooling, vomiting, stupor or a coma.

Treatment

Call for emergency help if you suspect a person has taken an overdose of drugs or is acutely intoxicated and is a danger to themselves or others. Concerning signs and symptoms include:

- A loss of consciousness
- Breathing that has stopped or seems dangerously slow
- Behavior that's aggressive, fearful, panicky, hostile, delusional or violent

In case of an overdose, call the a poison center while awaiting for emergency medical help to arrive (see page 53).

People who use drugs habitually may experience withdrawal if they suddenly quit taking the drug. Proper detoxification often takes a week or more of treatment, ideally guided by medical or mental health professionals.

Sudden personality changes

Sudden personality changes can result from drug use or from mental illness. A quiet and thoughtful person can become disoriented or violent, and a previously gregarious person can become withdrawn, depressed or suicidal.

If you find yourself dealing with a person who's acting or talking in a bizarre way, ensure your safety at all times and call for emergency help. It may help to try to talk calmly to that person. Attempt to reassure the individual that you're there to help. Listen and respond gently, in a nonthreatening manner, while always ensuring that you have an exit route if you need to move to safety quickly.

If the person has threatened suicide or harm to others and you believe the person is armed, remove

Personality changes

A person at risk of suicide may have changes in his or her personality and routines, such as eating or sleeping patterns. The individual may demonstrate feelings of hopelessness or become withdrawn.

Risk taking

Uncharacteristically dangerous activities or impulsivity — such as high-speed driving, unsafe sex or drug use — may be a sign of an emerging desire to die and is a risk factor for suicide.

Personal crisis

A major life setback, such as a divorce, a lost job or the death of a loved one, can be difficult for anyone to manage. Among people who are depressed, such a crisis can push them over the edge, triggering a suicide attempt.

Depression

Another warning sign is deep depression. Sometimes, the person is so depressed that he or she has difficulty functioning socially or in the workplace.

Gift giving

Sometimes before suicide, a depressed individual will give away his or her cherished possessions, believing that they won't be needed any longer.

yourself from the situation immediately and call for emergency help. Also don't attempt to restrain a violent person unless you have proper training. A person in a disturbed state — especially if it's induced by drugs — can be more dangerous and stronger than you may imagine.

Call for emergency help if the person is disoriented, agitated or poses a danger to himself or herself or others. Also seek help if you're unable to communicate with the person. A person reacting in this manner needs immediate medical attention.

Treatment

If a friend or a family member talks about dying by suicide or behaves in a way that leads you to believe that suicide is a possibility, treat the person with respect and seriousness and seek professional help as soon as possible.

Contact your family doctor, a mental health professional or a local suicide hot line. They will be able to suggest where you can get immediate help for the person and help you determine if you need to call for immediate emergency assistance. In the meantime, keep a close eye on the individual to prevent an opportunity for suicide.

If you encounter a person who has just attempted suicide, seek emergency medical help. If the person has stopped breathing, begin assisting the breathing with mouth-to-mouth resuscitation. If the person is bleeding, try to stop the bleeding. If it appears the person has ingested a poison or taken an overdose of pills, try to find out what the person has taken and how much. Call a poison center while you're waiting for emergency medical personnel to arrive. ■

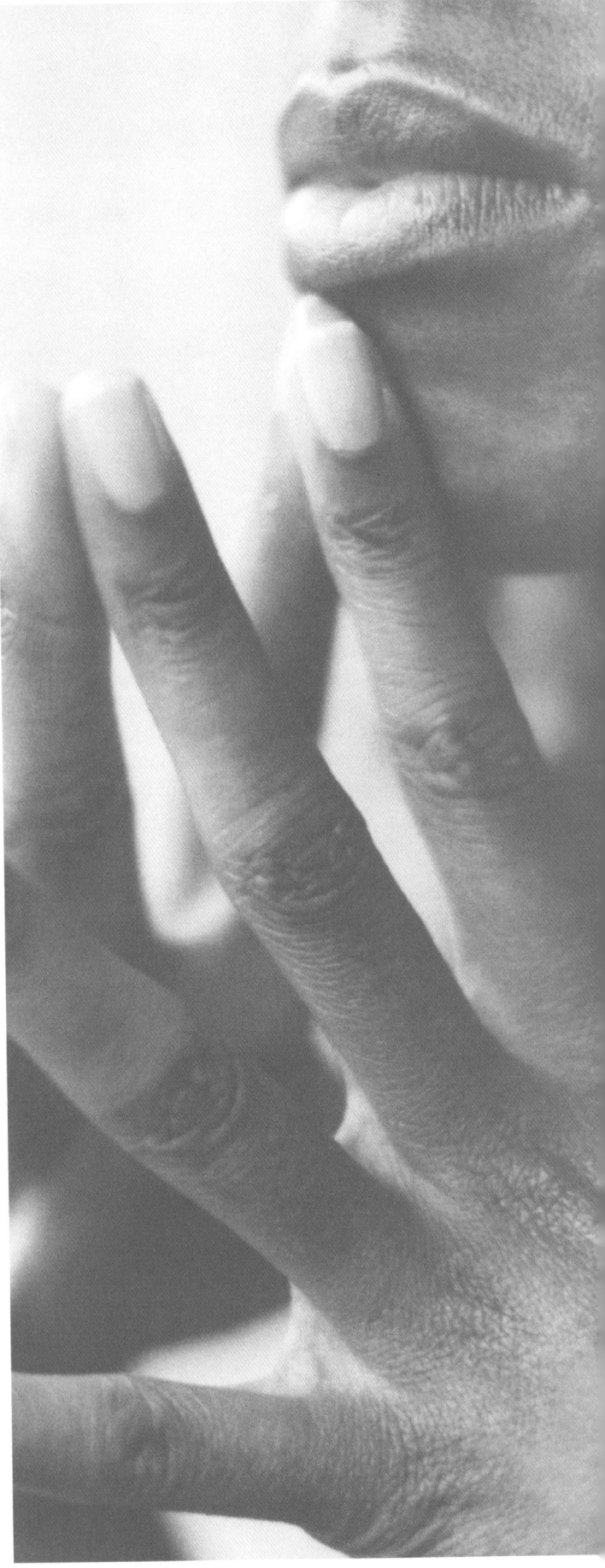

Making Sense of Your Symptoms

The human body usually operates effectively and reliably. At times, though, you may experience a breakdown in one of the body systems. Or an invader, such as a virus or a bacterium, may affect normal functioning. When this happens, your body usually gives off one or more signals to alert you that something is wrong. These are commonly referred to as signs and symptoms. A sign is an indication of illness that's noticeable to others, such as a cough or a red eye. A symptom is a sensation that only you can perceive, such as pain or stiffness.

Many times, it's easy to figure out what's triggering your signs and symptoms. Sneezing, a sore throat and a runny nose are usually indications of a common cold or an allergy. A deep, throbbing ache in a tooth is often associated with a dental abscess. Other times, it can be difficult to make sense of what your body is telling you. You may worry that a sign or symptom is a warning of one condition but later find out that it's really related to another. Or, you may be at a loss for what's causing it.

This section is intended to help you better understand what may be triggering a certain complaint. Following each sign or symptom is a list of diseases and disorders frequently associated with that sign or symptom. They are listed in alphabetical order, not by importance or frequency of occurrence.

By reading about each of the conditions listed, you may be able to better identify possible causes of the problem. Keep in mind, though, that the following information is only a guide. It may help you better understand the problem and assist you in communicating with your or your child's doctor so that he or she can more quickly get to the root of the ailment. Reading this section is *not* a replacement for seeing a doctor. In many cases, it's important that you get an expert opinion to be certain that what you think might be the cause of your sign or symptom is in fact the true culprit.

Signs and Symptoms Common in Adults

Listed here are 25 signs and symptoms commonly experienced by adults. These are some of the most frequent reasons that men and women see their doctors.

Abdominal pain

Abdominal pain can occur alone or with other signs and symptoms, such as nausea and vomiting. Occasional episodes of abdominal pain may be related to a bacterial or viral infection (gastroenteritis) or result from overeating or eating too much of the wrong foods

Warning!

If you or someone you know is experiencing signs and symptoms that might be a warning of a medical emergency, such as a heart attack or stroke, don't take time to read this section. Call for emergency medical help or have someone take you or the person in distress to the nearest hospital emergency department immediately. In a true emergency, time is of the essence. If you're not certain whether you're dealing with a medical emergency, call your doctor's office or the emergency department at your local hospital and describe the signs and symptoms being experienced by you or the person you're helping.

— fatty or gas-producing foods or, for people with intolerance to some sugars, milk and dairy products. Abdominal pain that's recurrent, persistent or severe may signal a variety of other conditions. Abdominal pain is often associated with one of the following causes:

- **Abdominal wall pain (see page 968)**
  The pain is nagging and accompanied by tenderness in the abdominal muscles that increases when the muscles are tensed, such as when sitting up from a lying position. A specific spot (tender trigger point) can be located where the pain is worse with abdominal muscle tension.
- **Acute pancreatitis (see page 870)**
  Mild to severe pain in the upper abdomen or midabdomen may radiate through to the back. The pain may persist for hours or days without relief and be accompanied by nausea and vomiting. Alcohol and food may increase the pain. Bending forward or curling up in the fetal position may relieve it.
- **Appendicitis (see page 840)**
  Signs and symptoms often start with a loss of appetite, a low-grade fever, and nausea with or without vomiting. The pain is initially located around the navel and later moves to the lower right abdomen.
- **Diverticulitis (see page 849)**
  The pain typically comes on suddenly and is accompanied by a fever and nausea. The signs and symptoms are similar to those of appendicitis, except that the pain is usually located in the lower left side of the abdomen instead of the lower right.
- **Gallbladder attack (see "Gallstones," page 866)**
  The pain is usually in the upper right abdomen or right midabdomen, and it may radiate to the back or right shoulder. It's unrelieved by changing positions or taking an antacid or pain medication. The pain often occurs one to two hours after eating, and it may be associated with nausea and vomiting.
- **Inflammatory bowel disease (see page 842)**
  The pain is caused by inflammation of the intestines.

It may be accompanied by cramping, diarrhea, weight loss, fatigue and intermittent fever.

- **Intestinal obstruction (see page 853)**
The cramping, colicky abdominal pain comes and goes. It may be associated with visible bloating, bowel noise, nausea and vomiting and, if the obstruction is complete or near complete, an inability to pass gas (flatus) or stool.
- **Irritable bowel syndrome (see page 850)**
This chronic condition is often associated with periods of pain or diarrhea alternating with constipation and uncomfortable abdominal cramping and bloating. Irritable bowel syndrome isn't associated with a fever, weight loss or bleeding.
- **Kidney stones (see page 897)**
In this condition, the pain usually begins in the back or side and radiates around to the front, moving downward to the groin, vulva or testicles. You may also have a persistent urge to urinate.
- **Malabsorption disorder (see page 838)**
An intestinal sensitivity to a dietary protein, such as the gluten found in wheat and other grains, may result in abdominal pain, bloating, gas and diarrhea. A common malabsorption disorder is lactose intolerance, caused by an inability to digest the sugar in milk (lactose).
- **Peptic ulcer (see page 828)**
The pain is gnawing and often located in the upper abdomen between the navel and breastbone. It's generally worse when the stomach is empty and tends to flare during sleep. Eating temporarily relieves the pain. You may have black or bloody stools or vomiting.
- **Shingles (see page 1097)**
Symptoms may begin as itching or burning, tingling, or knifelike pain on one side of your abdomen. The pain typically wraps around from the spine, following a nerve pathway. One to five days later, groupings of blisters appear in the same location.

Ankle and foot pain

Nearly everyone experiences an occasional episode of foot or ankle pain. Often, the pain is the result of a misstep that causes a sprain or fracture, or it's associated with a common problem such as a corn or callus. Many times, ankle and foot pain result from one of the following conditions:

- **Achilles tendinitis (see page 938)**
The pain is located where the heel cord (Achilles tendon) meets the heel bone and in the Achilles tendon itself. The heel cord is tender to the touch.
- **Bone fracture (see page 921)**
The pain is caused by a broken bone in a foot or ankle. Such injuries may occur during a misstep or accident.
- **Bunion (see page 942)**
A bunion is a common deformity of the big toe joint.

It causes painful swelling at the bump on the base of the big toe.

- **Gout (see page 982)**
Acute gout causes excruciating pain, often in the joint at the base of the big toe. The pain comes on rapidly and occurs with any movement of the affected joint. Even a bedsheet rubbing over an affected joint can be painful.
- **Metatarsalgia (see page 940)**
The pain occurs on the bony prominences of the balls of the feet when you walk or stand.
- **Morton's neuroma (see page 941)**
A burning or sharp pain is felt between the third and fourth toes. The pain is often worse when you wear tight shoes.
- **Osteoarthritis (see page 970)**
The pain is chronic and slowly progressive. It may be worse with weight-bearing activity.
- **Plantar fasciitis (see "Heel pain," page 938)**
The pain is located under the heel and is often most severe with the first steps out of bed in the morning or with the first steps after being seated for a while. Walking often improves the pain.
- **Sprain (see page 929)**
A sprain occurs when a joint moves beyond its normal range of motion, stretching or tearing ligaments. The resulting pain is often accompanied by swelling.
- **Tendinitis (see page 964)**
The pain is caused by an inflamed tendon in a foot or ankle.

Back pain

Low back pain not only is very common but also can result from injuries and diseases that range from minor to extremely serious. Back pain is often related to one of the following conditions:

- **Bone cancer (see "Bone tumors," page 960)**
This is a rare cause of back pain. The pain is in the bone and is deep and aching. It's often worse with rest than during activity.
- **Bone infection (see "Osteomyelitis," page 960)**
The pain is sudden and remains severe. It's often associated with a fever.
- **Herniated disk (see page 949)**
The pain is typically in the lower back, and it may be accompanied by numbness or tingling that radiates into the buttocks and down a leg.
- **Muscle strain (see page 927)**
Muscle stain is a common cause of sudden (acute) low back pain. Certain movements of the lower back worsen the pain.
- **Osteoarthritis (see page 970)**
This common cause of back pain results from deterioration of bony joints. The pain is long term (chronic) and may worsen with weight-bearing activity and certain movements.

• **Osteoporotic compression fracture (see "Osteoporosis," page 953)**

Sudden, severe back pain in a person with osteoporosis may be due to one or more fractures in a spinal vertebra.

Chest pain

Chest pain may be a warning of a heart attack, but it can also occur for a number of other reasons. It may be caused by some other heart condition, or it may be associated with a chest wall or lung disorder or a gastrointestinal problem. Often, chest pain is related to one of the following conditions:

• **Angina (see page 722)**

Discomfort, tightening or pressure occurs in the chest due to lack of blood flow to the heart muscle. Pain may also be felt in the jaw and inner left arm or, occasionally, both arms. The discomfort typically develops with physical exertion or high emotional stress. When you stop an activity or relax, symptoms often improve.

• **Chest wall pain (see page 968)**

This is a common, harmless pain caused by muscle or cartilage tenderness in the chest wall. Pushing on a tender area in your chest reproduces the pain.

• **Esophageal spasm (see "Swallowing difficulties," page 822)**

Tight, severe pressure develops under the breastbone, often after drinking a large gulp of cold or carbonated fluid. The pain usually improves in seconds. If prolonged, it can mimic a heart attack.

• **Gastroesophageal reflux disease (see page 818)**

A warm, burning sensation (heartburn) develops in the upper part of the abdomen and the lower chest under the breastbone. You may get a sour taste in your mouth. Drinking a liquid antacid or chewing antacid pills usually relieves the discomfort.

• **Heart attack (see page 723)**

Severe pain or pressure can be felt in the chest, neck, jaw or arms. It may be accompanied by shortness of breath, sweating, nausea and vomiting.

• **Pneumonia (see page 766)**

Pneumonia is associated with a fever and a cough that may bring up colored sputum. You might experience shortness of breath and sharp chest pain when taking a deep breath.

• **Pneumothorax (see page 783)**

Abrupt chest pain and shortness of breath are the most common symptoms of a collapsed lung.

• **Pulmonary embolism (see page 792)**

Attempting to take a deep breath produces sharp chest pain. This may be accompanied by sudden shortness of breath and the coughing up of blood.

• **Rib fracture**

A rib fracture can result from an injury or from severe coughing. Applying pressure to the fractured rib produces intense pain.

Involuntary Weight Loss

For many people who struggle to shed pounds, unintentional weight loss might seem like a gift. However, significant loss of weight that occurs without trying can signify a serious medical disorder, and it should be investigated.

Involuntary weight loss is defined as a loss of more than 5 percent of your body weight over a six-month span. For a 160-pound individual, a 5 percent loss would be 8 pounds. If you're unsure about your original weight, other signs can help pinpoint if significant loss has occurred. Your clothes may fit more loosely, or you may be fastening your belt at a tighter notch. Friends and family members may comment that you've lost weight.

Questions

If you've lost weight without trying, ask yourself:

• Is the weight loss truly unintentional or have you modified your diet or activity level? Even small changes in either can cause weight loss if sustained over several months.

• How much weight have you lost and over how long of a period? This can help your doctor determine the potential seriousness of the problem.

• Is your appetite normal or has it decreased? Making this distinction can narrow the list of possible causes.

• Do you have other signs and symptoms? Other signs and symptoms can also help narrow the list of possible causes.

Causes of involuntary weight loss

The list of potential causes for involuntary weight loss is extensive. Although many people worry most

• **Shingles (see page 1097)**

Symptoms may begin as itching or burning, tingling or knifelike pain on one side of the abdomen. The pain typically wraps around from the spine, following a nerve pathway. One to five days later, groupings of blisters appear in the same location.

Cough

Occasional coughing is a normal part of everyday life. A cough that's severe or persists may be a sign of a variety of conditions, ranging from a medication side effect to lung cancer. A cough is often associated with one of the following conditions or medications:

• **Angiotensin-converting enzyme (ACE) inhibitors (see page 1281)**

These medications are used to treat high blood pres-

about cancer, the majority of people who experience unintentional weight loss don't have cancer. The largest studies of unintentional weight loss have shown that in nearly a quarter of the participants, no cause for the weight loss was found despite an extensive search.

Major causes of weight loss include:
- Cancer, most often of the lung or gastrointestinal tract
- Depression and other mental health conditions
- Dementia
- Hyperthyroidism
- A gastrointestinal disorder, such as an ulcer, a malabsorption disorder or an inflammatory disorder
- Chronic lung disease
- Uncontrolled diabetes
- Some chronic infections, such as tuberculosis and human immunodeficiency virus (HIV)
- Alcoholism or substance misuse
- Certain medications, such as selective serotonin reuptake inhibitors (SSRIs) and nonsteroidal anti-inflammatory drugs (NSAIDs)

In addition, long-term (chronic) pain for almost any reason can cause weight loss. Pain and many of the medicines used to treat it decrease appetite.

When to see your doctor

If you've unintentionally lost more than 5 percent of your original body weight over a six-month period, see your doctor. In preparing for the visit, list other signs or symptoms that you've been experiencing.

Your doctor will likely ask you a number of questions related to your weight loss and your overall health and conduct a physical examination. If you and your doctor think that the weight loss is significant, you may need to undergo diagnostic testing.

sure or heart-related illnesses. In some people, they can cause a bothersome, dry cough.
- **Asthma (see page 495)**
  Shortness of breath, wheezing and tightness in the chest, as well as a cough are common signs and symptoms. Asthma may be triggered by allergies, a respiratory infection, cold air or exercise.
- **Bronchitis (see page 763)**
  The cough produces sputum, and it may be accompanied by wheezing.
- **Cold (see page 445)**
  The cough is often accompanied by a stuffy nose, a sore and often scratchy throat, fatigue, and a fever.
- **Foreign body (see page 825)**
  The cough follows inhalation of a foreign body, such as a piece of food, into the windpipe (trachea) or a bronchial tube.

- **Gastroesophageal reflux disease (see page 818)**
  The cough is typically accompanied by heartburn (acid reflux) and sometimes a sour taste in your mouth.
- **Pneumonia (see page 766)**
  The cough is associated with a lung infection and may produce colored sputum. Other signs and symptoms include shortness of breath, a fever and sharp pain when taking a deep breath.
- **Postnasal drip (see page 652)**
  Excess production of mucus that drains into the back of the throat causes the throat to feel full or "funny." Coughing is an attempt to relieve the sensation.

Diarrhea

Everyone has loose, watery stools at one time or another. Often, diarrhea is a result of a viral or bacterial infection (gastroenteritis) or a side effect of medication. As the infection clears or your body becomes accustomed to the medication, the diarrhea usually stops. Persistent diarrhea generally indicates a gastrointestinal disorder. Diarrhea is often associated with one of the following conditions:
- **Antibiotic-associated diarrhea (see page 838)**
  Antibiotics can kill bacteria that normally live in the digestive tract, replacing them with diarrhea-causing bacteria. Up to 20 percent of people taking antibiotics experience this problem. Usually, the diarrhea is mild and of short duration. Occasionally, a serious colon infection can result, causing severe diarrhea.
- **Gastroenteritis (see "Gastrointestinal infections," page 834)**
  This condition is the most common cause of sudden, severe diarrhea. Other signs include nausea and vomiting.
- **Inflammatory bowel disease (see page 842)**
  Diarrhea may be accompanied by weight loss, fatigue, cramping, abdominal pain and intermittent fever. In some cases, the diarrhea may be bloody.
- **Intestinal obstruction (see page 853)**
  Diarrhea is accompanied by a cramping and colicky pain that comes and goes. Other signs and symptoms include visible bloating, bowel noise (rushes and gurgling), nausea and vomiting.
- **Lactose intolerance (see page 840)**
  This common malabsorption disorder is caused by an inability to digest sugar in milk (lactose).
- **Malabsorption disorder (see page 838)**
  An intestinal sensitivity to a dietary protein, such as the gluten found in wheat and other grains, may result in abdominal pain, bloating, gas and diarrhea.

Dizziness

Dizziness has many causes. Fortunately, most dizziness is mild, brief and harmless. The term *dizziness* may be used to describe lightheadedness and a feeling of faintness. Other times, it's used to describe a feeling of imbalance — like walking in a rocking boat. More often it's used to describe the sensation that you or your surroundings are spinning (vertigo). To help your doctor understand your condition, it's important to clarify the type of dizziness you're experiencing. A spinning sensation is often caused by one of the following conditions:

- **Benign paroxysmal positional vertigo (see page 643)**
  Momentary dizziness occurs when turning your head from side to side, rolling over in bed or looking up suddenly. Intermittent episodes of these symptoms may occur over the years.
- **Labyrinthitis (see page 642)**
  Caused by an inner ear infection, this condition can produce vertigo with nausea and vomiting. Decreased hearing may result in the affected ear.
- **Meniere's disease (see page 638)**
  In addition to severe dizziness, signs and symptoms include ringing in the ear, pressure in the ear and hearing loss. The signs and symptoms come and go and might be recurrent every few months or years.
- **Middle ear infection (see page 630)**
  Dizziness, pain and a plugged ear are signs and symptoms of middle ear infection (otitis media).
- **Stroke (see page 534)**
  Accompanying signs and symptoms often include numbness, tingling, weakness on one side of the body, difficulty speaking, double vision and facial droop. Seek emergency care with these symptoms.
- **Transient ischemic attack (see page 531)**
  Often a precursor to a stroke, this condition can cause dizziness, numbness, tingling, weakness on one side of the body, difficulty speaking, double vision and facial droop. Unlike a stroke, the signs and symptoms usually last only a short time and then fully resolve.

Eye discomfort and redness

Many of the most common eye conditions don't pose a serious threat to vision, but they can be uncomfortable. Eye discomfort and redness are often associated with one of the following conditions:

- **Allergies (see "Respiratory allergies," page 490)**
  Airborne allergens, such as pollen, dust and smog, can produce itchy, pink-colored eyes.
- **Corneal abrasion (see page 596)**
  An injury to the cornea causes pain and a persistent feeling that you have something in your eye. Blinking makes it worse. Covering the eye improves the signs and symptoms.
- **Pink eye (see "Conjunctivitis," page 604)**
  The white of the eye (sclera) has a pinkish discoloration. Other symptoms include itchiness and a gritty feeling in the eye when you blink. The eyelids may stick together while you sleep.

- **Subconjunctival hemorrhage (see "Blood in an eye," page 596)**
  A broken blood vessel causes a painless but alarming bright red area within the white of the eye. The condition is generally harmless.
- **Uveitis (see page 605)**
  The middle layer of tissue between the retina and sclera, including the iris, becomes inflamed. Signs and symptoms may appear suddenly and include eye pain, redness, blurred vision and sensitivity to light. Left untreated uveitis can cause eye damage.

Headache

Headaches are common and usually not due to a serious cause. But some headaches can be a warning of a serious problem. Types of headaches and some conditions that can cause headaches include the following:

- **Brain tumor (see page 548)**
  A brain tumor is a rare cause of headache. Pressure from a tumor may cause chronic or persistent headaches in a person not prone to headache. Associated signs and symptoms may include weakness, clumsiness, vision changes, personality changes and vomiting.
- **Cranial (giant cell) arteritis (see page 622)**
  The headache may be mild or severe. The skin on one side of your face near the ear and temple is tender to the touch. Other signs and symptoms include a fever and aching of the shoulder and hip muscles.
- **Encephalitis (see page 542)**
  A headache associated with encephalitis is usually accompanied by a fever and sometimes pain behind the eyes. Signs and symptoms may be aggravated by light. You may feel lethargic, confused and experience an altered mental state.
- **Medication side effects (see "Medications Guide," page 1267)**
  Headaches are a side effect of a number of medications. Examples include nitrates, some antibiotics and oral contraceptives.
- **Meningitis (see page 540)**
  Meningitis is a life-threatening cause of headache. This type of headache is associated with a fever, a stiff neck and altered mental status. Attempting to bend the neck increases the pain.
- **Migraine attacks (see page 520)**
  Nausea and light sensitivity often accompany the headache. A migraine may be preceded by visual symptoms such as bright or colored light patterns or zigzags in the visual field (auras).
- **Occipital neuralgia (see "Neck Pain," page 931)**
  With this condition, shooting pain in the back of the neck often travels up behind an ear to one side of the scalp. The discomfort can often be reproduced by firmly pressing on the bony bump in the back of the neck, where the occipital nerve is located.

- **Pain relievers (see "Effects of Too Much Medication," page 518)**
  Pain relievers offer quick help for an occasional headache but if you take them too often — more than two or three days a week — they can cause medication overuse headaches.
- **Sinusitis (see page 649)**
  Sinusitis often follows an upper respiratory infection. In addition to a headache, signs and symptoms include nasal congestion, a runny nose, facial pain and pressure in the affected sinus. Head pain often increases when bending over or straining.
- **Subarachnoid hemorrhage (see "Hemorrhagic stroke," page 535)**
  Headache associated with this condition is often described as the "worst headache of my life." Severe pain comes on suddenly and lasts hours to days. It's often associated with nausea, vomiting and a stiff neck.
- **Temporomandibular joint disorder (see page 683)**
  This condition can cause facial pain, ear pain or a headache. Other signs and symptoms may include clicking or catching of the jaw and soreness of the chewing muscles.
- **Tension headaches (see page 518)**
  Tension-type headaches are a common type of headache. The muscles of the back of the neck or scalp feel tight and squeezing.
- **Tooth abscess (see page 667)**
  Throbbing around an abscessed tooth and gum may be mistaken for a headache.

Hip pain

Pain in the hip region is often related to one of the following conditions:
- **Bursitis or tendinitis (see pages 984 and 964)**
  An aching pain is present in the outer hip region. Discomfort often worsens when you lie on the affected side or climb stairs. Sometimes, hip pain is referred, and the pain feels as if it's in the knee.
- **Claudication (see "Arteriosclerosis," page 753)**
  Pain develops in a hip or the buttocks or, more commonly, the thigh or calf muscles, when you walk. The pain goes away when you stand still.
- **Hip fracture (see page 923)**
  The pain often occurs following trauma, such as a fall. Any movement of the hip produces severe pain.
- **Osteoarthritis (see page 970)**
  Aching or stiffness in the hip area may be felt in the groin. The pain worsens when you walk, climb stairs or stand for a prolonged period.
- **Sciatica (see "Radicular pain," page 1315)**
  Sciatic pain actually occurs in the buttocks, but many people refer to it as hip pain. It may be accompanied by muscle weakness and by numbness or tingling that radiates down a leg.

Knee pain

Knee pain can seriously impair walking and exercise. It's often related to one of the following conditions:
- **Cartilage tear (see "Knee injury," page 935)**
  The pain often develops after an injury in which the knee joint twists. The pain can be felt when pressing on the joint. It may be accompanied by swelling.
- **Gout (see page 982)**
  The pain is sudden and severe and worsens when you move your knee. The knee is usually swollen and tender to the touch.
- **Osteoarthritis (see page 970)**
  Slowly progressive discomfort occurs in the knee. The pain worsens when you walk, squat or stand for prolonged periods.
- **Patellar tendinitis (see "Jumper's knee," page 934)**
  The pain is accompanied by swelling and tenderness in the tendon below the kneecap.
- **Sprain (see "Knee injury," page 935)**
  A minor to severe tear of a knee ligament causes pain that may be associated with tenderness, swelling and loss of knee stability. A sprain is generally associated with trauma to the knee.

Lower gastrointestinal bleeding

Lower gastrointestinal bleeding, such as rectal bleeding, can be alarming. Frequently, the bleeding is due to a minor problem, such as hemorrhoids or an anal fissure. Other times, it may be a warning sign of a more serious condition, such as an ulcer or cancer. Lower gastrointestinal bleeding may be associated with one of the following conditions:
- **Anal fissure (see page 863)**
  The bleeding stems from a small tear in the anal tissue and may be accompanied by anal pain. The blood is typically bright red and seen on toilet tissue or in the toilet bowl following a bowel movement.
- **Colon polyps (see page 855)**
  Small, precancerous growths in the colon may bleed occasionally. The blood may be bright red in the toilet or mixed in with stool.
- **Colorectal cancer (see page 856)**
  Blood, which may appear maroon colored, may be mixed into the stool or show up in the toilet bowl. Other signs and symptoms include changes in bowel habits, cramping and weight loss.
- **Diverticular disease (see page 849)**
  Blood may be mixed in the stool or show up in the toilet bowl. The bleeding may be quite heavy.
- **Gastrointestinal infection (see page 834)**
  Some gastrointestinal infections cause cramping and bloody diarrhea.
- **Hemorrhoids (see page 860)**
  Hemorrhoids are the most frequent cause of rectal

bleeding. Bright red blood usually shows up on toilet tissue or in the toilet bowl after a bowel movement. Bleeding may be accompanied by anal itching or discomfort.

- **Inflammatory bowel disease (see page 842)**
  Blood may be bright red or dark and mixed in with stool. Other signs and symptoms include a fever, cramps, diarrhea and weight loss.
- **Peptic ulcer (see page 828)**
  Bleeding from the upper gastrointestinal tract may cause stools to appear black or tarry. You may have gnawing pain in the upper abdomen. The pain is worse when the stomach is empty. Eating may temporarily relieve the pain.

Nasal congestion

Nasal congestion is a common sign of a cold or an allergy, but it can also occur for other reasons. Nasal congestion is often associated with one of the following:

- **Cold (see page 445)**
  A cold is a viral infection in the upper respiratory tract. In addition to nasal congestion, signs and symptoms include a runny nose, a sore or scratchy throat, fatigue, a cough, and a low-grade fever.
- **Hay fever (see page 490)**
  Other signs and symptoms typically include sneezing and watery mucus from the nose. Itching of the nose, throat and eyes also is common.
- **Medication side effects (see "Medications Guide," page 1267)**
  Certain medications, such as the alpha-adrenergic blockers used to treat enlargement of the prostate gland, can cause mild nasal congestion as a side effect. Overuse of nonprescription nasal decongestant sprays also may result in a worsening of signs and symptoms, what's known as the rebound effect.
- **Nasal polyps (see page 493)**
  Small growths in the nasal cavities can obstruct airways, leading to congestion. Polyps are most common in people with hay fever, aspirin-induced asthma and long-term (chronic) sinusitis.
- **Sinusitis (see page 649)**
  Inflammation of sinus membranes can cause nasal congestion. Sinusitis often follows an upper respiratory infection.
- **Vasomotor rhinitis (see page 648)**
  This condition mimics allergic rhinitis, with nasal congestion, sneezing and coughing due to phlegm in the throat. Other allergy symptoms — an itchy nose, eyes and throat — are absent. Triggers include cold air and strong smells.

Neck pain

Neck pain may be a short-term (acute) problem that improves on its own, or it may be long term (chronic)

and disabling. Neck pain is often associated with one of the following conditions:

- **Herniated disk (see page 949)**
  The pain begins in the neck and may radiate to a shoulder and down the arm. Other symptoms include numbness, tingling or weakness in the arm or hand.
- **Muscle strain (see page 927)**
  This is a common cause of sudden and sometimes severe neck pain. Moving your neck muscles produces pain.
- **Occipital neuralgia (see "Neck Pain," page 931)**
  Shooting pain in the back of the neck travels behind an ear to one side of the scalp. The discomfort can often be reproduced by firmly pressing on the bony bump in the back of the neck, where the occipital nerve is located.
- **Osteoarthritis (see page 970)**
  The pain is chronic and slowly progressive and may be accompanied by neck stiffness.

Numbness or tingling in a hand

Numbness or tingling in a hand is often associated with one of the following conditions:

- **Brachial plexus injury**
  Weakness, numbness and tingling develop in an arm and hand. This type of pain results from a shoulder or underarm injury that affects the network of nerves called the brachial plexus.
- **Carpal tunnel syndrome (see page 962)**
  Numbness and tingling may occur at night and radiate up an arm. The thumb, index finger and long finger are most often affected. Hand weakness may occur.
- **Herniated disk (see page 949)**
  A compressed or damaged nerve in the neck can cause numbness and tingling that radiates down a shoulder into the arm, hand and fingers.
- **Peripheral neuropathy (see page 572)**
  A crawling sensation or numbness and tingling or are felt in both hands or both feet.
- **Stroke (see page 534)**
  Weakness or tingling occurs in an arm or hand and is usually accompanied by other symptoms, such as numbness and weakness in the face or a leg. Seek emergency medical care.
- **Ulnar nerve dysfunction (see page 965)**
  Trauma to the ulnar nerve at the elbow causes tingling and numbness from the elbow to the little finger and part of the ring finger. Bumping the area is painful. You may also have hand weakness.

Palpitations

Palpitations are an uncomfortable awareness of your heartbeat or a thumping sensation within your chest.

They're often associated with one of the following conditions:

- **Anxiety and panic attacks (see "Anxiety disorders," page 1130)**
  Sudden episodes of intense fear prompt physical reactions, such as a racing heart, a flushed face, trouble breathing, dizziness, nausea and a sense of being out of control.
- **Atrial fibrillation (see page 733)**
  This condition is characterized by an irregular and often rapid heartbeat (arrhythmia).
- **Hyperthyroidism (see page 1016)**
  In addition to a rapid heartbeat, hyperthyroidism can cause weight loss, nervousness and tremor.
- **Premature contractions (see page 736)**
  Premature heartbeats (contractions) are often described as a skipped heartbeat or a feeling that the heart turns over. They're usually harmless.
- **Tachycardia (see pages 733 and 735)**
  Tachycardia is most often used to describe a racing, usually regular, heartbeat.

Shortness of breath

Shortness of breath is common after running hard, climbing a steep hill or exerting yourself in other ways. When you become short of breath without an obvious cause, you should seek medical attention. Shortness of breath is often associated with one of the following conditions:

- **Anxiety and panic attacks (see "Anxiety disorders," page 1130)**
  Sudden episodes of intense fear prompt physical reactions in your body such as rapid and shallow breathing, a racing heart, a flushed face, dizziness, nausea and a sense of being out of control.
- **Asthma (see page 495)**
  Breathing difficulty is often associated with a tight feeling in the chest, wheezing and coughing. It may be triggered by allergies, a respiratory infection, cold air or exercise.

- **Chronic obstructive pulmonary disease (see page 775)**
  In addition to shortness of breath, signs and symptoms of this condition include a barrel chest, minimal wheezing and, sometimes, pursing of the lips to help exhale.
- **Congestive heart failure (see page 728)**
  Shortness of breath may be worse when lying down and with exertion. Other signs and symptoms include fatigue and swelling with accumulation of fluid (edema) in the feet, legs and trunk.
- **Pneumonia (see page 766)**
  Shortness of breath may be accompanied by a fever and sharp chest pain when you take a deep breath. Typically, pneumonia causes a cough that brings up colored sputum.
- **Pneumothorax (see page 783)**
  Abrupt chest pain and shortness of breath are the most common symptoms.
- **Pulmonary embolism (see page 792)**
  Along with sudden shortness of breath, you may cough up blood and have stabbing chest pain when you take a deep breath.

Shoulder pain

Pain that occurs when you move your shoulder is often due to a mechanical problem in the shoulder joint. Sometimes, illnesses in other parts of your body can cause shoulder pain (see "Referred Shoulder Pain," below). In such situations, moving the shoulder doesn't increase the pain. Shoulder pain is often associated with one of the following conditions:

- **Dislocation (see page 925)**
  The pain generally follows trauma to the shoulder. It improves with rest and worsens with movement. External rotation of the shoulder — such as when you swim the backstroke or cock your arm back to throw a football — can cause the head of the upper arm bone to slip out of the shoulder socket.

Referred Shoulder Pain

A number of conditions that occur in parts of the body other than the shoulder can cause pain that's felt in the shoulder. This is called referred shoulder pain. These conditions include:

- **Diaphragm irritation**
  The pain may be felt on the top of the shoulder and worsen when pushing on the abdomen or during a deep breath. The diaphragm is the thick, dome-shaped muscle separating the chest and abdomen. When the muscle is irritated, as with lower lobe pneumonia, pain can result.
- **Gallbladder attack (see "Gallstones," page 866)**
  In addition to experiencing pain in the upper right abdomen, you may feel it around the shoulder blade or top of the shoulder.
- **Heart attack (see page 723)**
  The pain may occur in the left shoulder, along with tight pressure in the chest, neck, jaw or arm.

- **Frozen shoulder (see page 984)**
  Symptoms include pain and tenderness with shoulder motion. Range of motion of the shoulder is severely limited.
- **Osteoarthritis (see page 970)**
  Osteoarthritis of the shoulder joint is relatively uncommon. Pain generally improves with rest and increases with activity. A grinding sensation or sound may occur with shoulder movement.
- **Rotator cuff injury (see page 986)**
  This is the most common source of shoulder pain, especially in older adults. Pain occurs with shoulder movement, especially when reaching overhead, or with internal rotation of the shoulder. A tear in the cuff muscles may cause upper arm pain and weakness in the shoulder.

Sore throat

Everyone knows what a sore throat feels like. Often, it's not an indication of a serious problem, but sometimes a sore throat requires medical attention. A sore throat is commonly associated with one of the following conditions:

- **Cold (see page 445)**
  An upper respiratory infection, such as a cold, is the most common cause of a sore throat. Other signs and symptoms include a cough, runny nose, scratchy throat and hoarse voice.
- **Epiglottitis (see page 654)**
  This condition generally causes a severe sore throat accompanied by a fever. You may drool or spit into a cup to avoid swallowing. Seek emergency care.
- **Infectious mononucleosis (see page 451)**
  Signs and symptoms generally include a severe sore throat, fever, fatigue, headache, and enlarged lymph glands in the front and back of the neck.
- **Strep throat (see page 449)**
  Other signs and symptoms include a fever, chills, fatigue and a headache. Lymph glands in the front of the neck may be painful. A cough is absent.
- **Tonsillitis (see page 653)**
  Other signs and symptoms are a fever, chills, fatigue and painful glands in the neck. On examination, tonsils appear red and inflamed and may have a white covering.

Swallowing difficulties

Occasional difficulty in swallowing (dysphagia) isn't usually a serious problem and may simply stem from eating too fast or not chewing your food well enough. Difficulty swallowing may be associated with one of the following conditions:

- **Achalasia (see page 823)**
  The lower esophageal muscle (sphincter) doesn't relax properly to let food enter the stomach. This can cause regurgitation of retained "sweet tasting" food not mixed with stomach contents.
- **Aging (see "Swallowing difficulties," page 822)**
  With age the esophagus tends to lose some muscular coordination needed to push food to the stomach.
- **Esophageal stricture (see page 825)**
  Narrowing of the esophagus (stricture) causes large chunks of food to get hung up. Narrowing may result from formation of scar tissue or tumors.
- **Esophageal tumors (see page 825)**
  Difficulty swallowing gets progressively worse over several months. Other signs and symptoms include chest pain and weight loss.
- **Foreign body (see page 825)**
  An object becomes lodged in the esophagus, which causes pain and swallowing difficulty.
- **Gastroesophageal reflux disease (see page 818)**
  Damage to esophageal tissues from stomach acid backing up (refluxing) into the esophagus can lead to scarring, narrowing and spasm of the lower esophagus, making swallowing difficult.
- **Neuromuscular problems (see "Pharyngeal paralysis," page 824)**
  You may be unable to initiate swallowing despite repeated attempts. Food or fluid may enter the windpipe (trachea) or come out the nose.
- **Pharyngeal diverticula (see page 823)**
  A small pouch forms in the throat. Food particles collect in this pouch, causing swallowing difficulty, gurgling sounds, bad breath, and repeated throat clearing, coughing or choking.

Swelling of the feet and legs

Swelling (edema) of the feet and legs is common after long periods of sitting, such as when you're on a long airplane flight. When the swelling occurs without an obvious cause, it may be a sign of a more serious problem. Swelling of the feet and legs is often associated with one of the following conditions:

- **Cellulitis (see page 1095)**
  This form of skin infection commonly causes redness, swelling, warmth and tenderness. It may be accompanied by a fever.
- **Congestive heart failure (see page 728)**
  Swelling occurs in both legs. It may be accompanied by abdominal swelling and shortness of breath with exertion and when lying down.
- **Deep vein thrombosis (see "Thrombophlebitis," page 757)**
  This condition typically causes sudden swelling of the lower leg accompanied by pain and tenderness behind the knee and calf. The leg may also appear dusky in color.
- **Lymphedema (see page 759)**
  Swelling occurs in one or both lower extremities and may extend to the toes and top of the feet.

- **Superficial thrombophlebitis (see page 757)**
  Pain, swelling, redness and tenderness occur near the surface of the skin in a leg vein — typically in a varicose vein.
- **Venous insufficiency (see "Varicose veins," page 757)**
  Swelling is typically worse when standing for a long time and better in the morning. You may also notice heaviness or aching in your lower legs, thickened, hardened skin and brownish skin pigmentation on an ankle.

Upper gastrointestinal bleeding

Upper gastrointestinal bleeding can manifest itself in several ways. Blood may be present in vomit and either be bright red or look like coffee grounds (digested blood). Upper gastrointestinal bleeding may also cause passage of black, tarry stools due to blood passing slowly from the stomach to the colon. If the bleeding is massive, stools may be maroon in color. Upper gastrointestinal bleeding is often caused by one of the following conditions:

- **Esophageal trauma (see page 827)**
  Bleeding may occur from a tear in the esophagus, often caused by vigorous vomiting or gagging.
- **Esophageal tumor (see page 825)**
  Bleeding is accompanied by progressive difficulty in swallowing. You may experience chest pain and weight loss.
- **Esophagitis (see page 822)**
  An inflamed lining of the esophagus may bleed.
- **Gastritis (see page 831)**
  An inflamed lining of the stomach may bleed.
- **Peptic ulcer (see page 828)**
  Bright red blood may appear in vomit, or blood may appear in stool, causing it to be black and tarry. Gnawing pain in the upper abdomen between the navel and breastbone is common. The pain is generally worse with an empty stomach.

Urinary problems

Signs and symptoms associated with urinary difficulties vary from frequent, painless urination to the severe pain that accompanies passage of a kidney stone. Urinary difficulties are often associated with one of the following conditions:

- **Benign prostatic hyperplasia (see page 1247)**
  This condition affects men and is characterized by progressive slowing of the urinary stream, stopping and starting of the stream, an urgency to void, and frequent urination during the night.
- **Kidney stones (see page 897)**
  Passage of a kidney stone or the lodging of a stone in the lower urinary tract may cause a constant feeling of the need to urinate. Kidney stone pain is felt in the lower abdomen. In men it may radiate to the tip of the penis or to the testicles. In women it may spread to the vaginal area.
- **Medication side effects (see "Medications Guide," page 1267)**
  Some medications interfere with the ability to urinate. For example, in some men with benign prostatic hyperplasia, drugs found in some cold and allergy medications, such as pseudoephedrine or diphenhydramine, can accentuate slowed urination or even cause an inability to void.
- **Overactive bladder (see page 917)**
  The bladder muscle becomes hyperactive, causing bladder spasm. You have an urgent, frequent need to urinate, even with an empty or near-empty bladder.
- **Prostatitis (see page 1246)**
  Urination is painful and may be accompanied by a fever and by pain in the pubic area and pelvic floor muscles.
- **Urinary tract infection (see page 909)**
  This condition causes an urgent and frequent sensation that you need to urinate and a painful, burning sensation on urination. The urine may be cloudy or blood tinged.

Vomiting

Vomiting may stem from a gastrointestinal infection (gastroenteritis) or a more serious problem. It may be associated with one of the following conditions:

- **Appendicitis (see page 840)**
  Vomiting is generally accompanied by a loss of appetite, nausea and a low-grade fever. Pain begins around the navel and settles into the lower right abdomen.
- **Gallbladder attack (see "Gallstones," page 866)**
  Pain often begins one or two hours after a meal and may be accompanied by nausea and vomiting. The pain is often directly below the breastbone and may radiate to the back or to the right shoulder.
- **Gastrointestinal infection (see page 834)**
  A viral infection of the gastrointestinal tract is a common cause of vomiting, which may be accompanied by diarrhea. Such infections usually improve in one to three days.
- **Intestinal obstruction (see page 853)**
  Nausea and vomiting are accompanied by cramping, colicky abdominal pain that comes and goes. Other signs and symptoms include visible bloating, bowel noise (rushes and gurgling) and, if obstruction is complete or near complete, passage of little or no gas or stool.
- **Medication side effects (see "Medications Guide," page 1267)**
  In some people, medications such as antibiotics, codeine and morphine can cause nausea and vomiting.

Wheezing

Wheezing is a whistling sound heard when you breathe out (expire) through an obstructed airway. It's often associated with one of the following conditions:

- **Asthma (see page 495)**
  Wheezing may be accompanied by breathing difficulty, a tight feeling in the chest and coughing. It may be triggered by allergies, respiratory infection, cold air or exercise.
- **Bronchitis (see page 763)**
  Wheezing is generally accompanied by a cough that produces sputum.
- **Congestive heart failure (see page 728)**
  Fluid accumulation in the lungs resulting from heart failure can cause wheezing (cardiac asthma).

Signs and Symptoms Common in Children

Following are 15 signs and symptoms common to children and some of the most frequent reasons that children and adolescents see their doctors. Teenagers may also experience signs and symptoms that result from conditions similar to those that affect adults. If the signs and symptoms are severe, such as difficulty breathing or severe distress, seek emergency care.

Abdominal pain

Occasional episodes of abdominal pain may be related to anxiety or a bacterial or viral infection (gastroenteritis). Abdominal pain that's recurrent, persistent or severe may signal a variety of other conditions. Abdominal pain is often associated with one of the following causes:

- **Antibiotic reaction (see "Antibiotic-associated diarrhea," page 838)**
  Some antibiotics cause abdominal pain. All antibiotics are capable of causing loose stools or diarrhea.
- **Anxiety (see "Fears and phobias," page 188, and "Anxiety disorders," page 1130)**
  Many children experience anxiety — often when they experience a new situation or encounter a frightening situation. Anxiety can lead to various physical symptoms, one of them being abdominal pain.
- **Appendicitis (see page 840)**
  Infection or obstruction of the appendix typically causes pain starting around the bellybutton (umbilicus) and settling in the lower right abdomen.
- **Attention-seeking behavior**
  For whatever reason, a child may feel a need for more attention and may find that saying "My stomach hurts" produces a quick response from parents.

- **Constipation (see pages 159 and 196)**
  Trouble passing stool can cause diffuse abdominal pain before a bowel movement and painful struggling during the bowel movement. This is one of the most frequent causes of abdominal pain in children.
- **Gas**
  Gas that's retained within the intestinal system is another common cause of abdominal pain in children from infancy through the elementary school years.
- **Gastroenteritis (see "Gastrointestinal infections," page 834)**
  Children often experience infection of the stomach or intestines due to a virus or, less commonly, a bacterium or a parasite. In addition to abdominal pain, common signs and symptoms include nausea, vomiting and diarrhea. These typically improve in a day or two. See a doctor if they persist.
- **Malabsorption disorders (see page 838)**
  An intestinal sensitivity to a dietary protein, such as the gluten found in wheat and other grains, may result in abdominal pain, bloating, gas and diarrhea. A common malabsorption disorder is lactose intolerance, which is caused by an inability to digest the sugar in milk (lactose).
- **School phobia (see page 188)**
  A child who fears school or wants to avoid it may have poorly described abdominal pain that isn't associated with any other sign or symptom of illness and magically disappears if the child is allowed to stay home from school.

Constipation

Constipation in children is common and only rarely due to a serious problem. It may be related to one of the following conditions:

- **Congenital malformations (see "Congenital digestive and respiratory disorders," page 169)**
  Some babies are born with incomplete formation of

Other Important Concerns

Many times, parents make an appointment with their child's doctor not because their child is sick but because they're concerned about the child's behavior or eating or sleeping habits. Sometimes, the problem is a normal part of growth and development, and it improves on its own. Other times, it's more serious and requires treatment.

Because behavioral, eating and sleeping problems occur for various reasons and their characteristics vary considerably, it's difficult to include them in this brief overview of common childhood signs and symptoms. For more information on these conditions and how they affect children at different stages of life, see Chapters 4 to 6.

part of the small intestine, which can cause intestinal obstruction. Constipation is one of the primary signs.

- **Functional stool holding**
  In some toilet-trained children, constipation may be a sign of a larger behavioral problem. The child may be reluctant to have bowel movements or to soil his or her underwear.
- **Hypothyroidism (see page 1018)**
  Infrequently, constipation is associated with an underactive thyroid gland.
- **Intussusception (see page 841)**
  Intussusception is a telescoping of a segment of the intestines into itself that obstructs normal bowel flow. This generally causes sudden, severe abdominal pain, which may be accompanied by constipation.
- **Lack of dietary fiber and inadequate water consumption (see "Nutrition," page 188)**
  The most common causes of childhood constipation are inadequate water intake and lack of fiber in the diet. Eating too many fatty animal-based foods is another cause.

Cough

Cough is common and is often due to one of the following conditions:

- **Asthma (see page 495)**
  Asthma may cause coughing alone or coughing with other signs, such as wheezing.
- **Cold (see page 445)**
  The common cold often causes nasal mucus to drip into the throat, which can cause a cough.
- **Croup (see page 450)**
  Viral inflammation of the voice box (larynx) and windpipe (trachea) can cause a barky, harsh upper airway cough that may be accompanied by a high-pitched sound on inspiration (stridor). Seek immediate care if stridor is present.
- **Foreign body (see page 63)**
  Toddlers are at high risk of placing objects into their mouths, which then enter their airways, producing a cough and breathing difficulty. This requires immediate medical care.
- **Habitual cough**
  School-age or teenage children may cough out of habit. During sleep the cough isn't present. A habitual cough is diagnosed by excluding other possible causes.
- **Nasal allergies (see "Hay fever," page 490)**
  In addition to a cough, nasal allergies commonly cause nasal congestion and a runny nose. Nasal allergies are most common during warm weather that occurs during the pollen season.
- **Pneumonia (see page 766)**
  Pneumonia typically causes a cough that brings up colored sputum. The cough is usually accompanied by a fever.

- **Secondhand smoke (see page 313)**
  When a child's airway is irritated from breathing in tobacco smoke, cough is common, especially if the child has asthma.
- **Sinusitis (see page 649)**
  Older children can get bacterial infections of the sinuses, although not as often as do adults. Cough that's accompanied by full or painful sinuses may be associated with sinusitis.

Decreased hearing

Decreased hearing may simply be due to a child's inattention, or it may be associated with one of the following conditions:

- **Fluid in the middle ear (see "Middle ear infections," page 630, and "Chronic ear infections," page 632)**
  The most common reason for poor hearing is a temporary collection of fluid behind the eardrum within the middle ear, leading to diminished hearing in that ear. Fluid buildup can lead to infection in the middle ear (otitis media).
- **Nerve damage or dysfunction (see "Hearing problems," pages 143 and 203)**
  Infectious diseases or a congenital deformity of the nerve that carries sound signals may cause hearing loss. Decreased hearing can also result from damage due to loud noise.
- **Selective hearing**
  This is a normal condition that occurs at several ages and stages of life. When a child is intently focused on something or isn't interested in the topic being discussed, he or she may tune out, creating the impression of hearing loss.

Diarrhea

Diarrhea is common in childhood and is often due to one of the following conditions:

- **Antibiotic reaction (see "Antibiotic-associated diarrhea," page 838)**
  Antibiotics can kill bacteria that normally live in the digestive tract, replacing them with diarrhea-causing bacteria. Up to 20 percent of people taking antibiotics experience this problem. Usually, the diarrhea is mild and of short duration. Occasionally, a serious colon infection can result, causing severe, bloody diarrhea. This requires prompt medical attention.
- **Cystic fibrosis (see page 780)**
  Inadequate absorption of food due to this disease can result in fatty, malodorous, loose stools.
- **Eating disorders (see page 225)**
  Eating disorders are most common in teenagers. Anorexia nervosa and bulimia are associated with self-induced vomiting and use of laxatives as a means of losing weight. Laxatives cause diarrhea.

- **Gastroenteritis (see "Gastrointestinal infections," page 834, and "Diarrhea," page 196)**
  Children often experience intestinal infections due to a virus or, less commonly, a bacterium or a parasite. The diarrhea usually stops in a day or two, but it can persist a week or more. Diarrhea associated with a fever and with blood in the stool should receive prompt medical attention.
- **Inflammatory bowel disease (see page 842)**
  Teenagers are more likely than are younger children to develop inflammatory bowel disease. The condition is often associated with bloody diarrhea, weight loss, abdominal cramping and other symptoms.
- **Intestinal obstruction (see page 853 and "Congenital digestive and respiratory disorders," page 169)**
  Blockages due to twisting or telescoping of the intestines can produce vomiting, diarrhea or constipation, as well as abdominal pain.
- **Malabsorption disorders (see page 838)**
  Chronic diarrhea can stem from an inability to digest milk sugar (lactose) or from an intestinal sensitivity to a dietary protein, such as the gluten found in wheat and other grains. Other signs and symptoms include abdominal pain and bloating. Some children and teenagers get diarrhea from sorbitol, a sugar substitute found in many diet foods.

Earache

Earache is very common in childhood and often occurs with head colds. Other causes of earache include:
- **Ear infection (see pages 630 and 632)**
  Middle ear infection (otitis media) is common in children ages 4 months to 4 years. In addition to ear pain, common signs and symptoms include trouble sleeping, irritability and a fever. Older children will complain of ear pain and plugging of the ear.
- **Ear trauma (see "Ruptured eardrum," page 628)**
  Trauma that causes severe pain with bloody discharge from the ear requires immediate attention.
- **Swimmer's ear, or otitis externia (see "Outer ear infections," page 626)**
  This condition is due to infection in the outer ear canal. Moving the ear or pressing on the entrance to the ear canal is painful. The condition is most common among children who spend a lot of time swimming.
- **Tonsillitis (see page 653)**
  It can produce distant (referred) pain in an ear.

Eye discomfort and redness

Red- or pink-colored eyes are often associated with an eye infection, but they can also result from other causes:
- **Allergies (see "Respiratory allergies," page 490)**
  Airborne allergens, such as pollen, dust and smog, can produce itchy, pink-colored eyes.

- **Marijuana use (see page 325)**
  Chronically red eyes may be associated with marijuana smoking.
- **Pink eye (see "Conjunctivitis," page 604)**
  The white of the eye (sclera) has a pinkish discoloration. Other symptoms include itchiness and a gritty feeling with blinking. The eyelids may stick together at night.
- **Secondhand smoke (see page 313)**
  Secondhand tobacco smoke can irritate a child's eyes as well as cause respiratory problems.

Headache

It's not uncommon for a child to experience a mild headache, especially during the adolescent and teenage years. However, head pain that's persistent or severe requires prompt attention. Head pain may be associated with one of the following conditions:
- **Attention-seeking behavior**
  If a parent has headaches, a child may complain of a headache to get attention or support.
- **Headaches (see pages 201 and 217)**
  School-age and teenage children experience tension-type headaches or migraines, although not as commonly as do adults. A headache may be associated with an infection or other causes, such as stress or reaction to a medication.
- **Increased intracranial pressure (see "Structural disorders," page 545, "Intracranial hematoma," page 538)**
  Injury or certain conditions may lead to increased pressure on the brain and cause head pain, vomiting, and other signs and symptoms.
- **Neck injury (see "Neck pain," page 931)**
  What presents as a pain in the head may actually originate from the neck.
- **School troubles (see pages 188 and 222)**
  A child who is fearful of or trying to avoid school may complain of poorly described head pain that

Fever

Every child experiences a fever at some point. A fever may be associated with infection of any body organ. Low-grade fevers commonly occur with an upper respiratory infection, such as the common cold, and aren't to be feared.

A high fever — 103 F or higher — may suggest a more serious infection, especially if it persists. Seek prompt medical attention.

When a fever is long term (chronic) or recurrent without evidence of an infection, a doctor may look for other conditions that can cause a fever. These include rheumatic disorders, some vascular diseases and cancer.

magically disappears if he or she is allowed to stay home from school. The pain isn't associated with any other evidence of illness.

- **Sinusitis (see page 649)**
  Sinus congestion or a sinus infection can cause head pain that's typically accompanied by pain in the sinus cavities or facial pain or pressure when bending down.

Muscle and joint pain

Pain in a child's muscles and joints is often related to a child's active lifestyle or to one of the following causes:

- **Growing pains (see page 202)**
  Whether growth of long bones in the legs and arms actually produces pain isn't certain. During the years when children grow at a rapid pace, the most common reason for a child to complain of muscle or joint pain is simply that he or she is physically active, providing a challenging workout of his or her muscles and skeleton. This is sometimes called overuse syndrome.
- **Rheumatic disorders (see "Juvenile idiopathic arthritis," page 977)**
  Childhood rheumatoid arthritis and related disorders can produce painful, stiff, inflamed joints on a chronic or recurrent basis.
- **Sprain (see page 929)**
  Pain occurs when a joint moves beyond its normal range of motion, stretching or tearing ligaments. It's often accompanied by swelling.
- **Tendinitis (see page 964)**
  Repetitive motions such as those done while participating in athletics or playing a musical instrument can irritate and inflame one or more tendons. In addition to being painful, the joint may be stiff and tender to the touch.

Nasal congestion

A stuffy nose is a common part of childhood. Nasal congestion may stem from a variety of conditions:

- **Cold (see page 445)**
  Common signs and symptoms of a cold are nasal congestion, drainage of clear, gray mucus and a mild fever. Other signs and symptoms include irritability, lack of appetite and poor sleep.
- **Large adenoids (see "Adenoid and tonsil removal," page 653)**
  Snoring is the most common sign of enlarged adenoids. In addition to a stuffy nose, swollen adenoids may give the voice a nasal quality.
- **Sinusitis (see page 649)**
  Prolonged nasal congestion with greenish or yellowish nasal discharge, facial pain, headache, bad breath, cough and a low-grade fever are common signs and symptoms of sinusitis.

Sore throat

An occasional sore throat is a normal part of growing up. All children experience a sore throat at some point. But not all sore throats are trivial. A sore throat in children may be associated with one of the following conditions:

- **Cold (see page 445)**
  An upper respiratory infection, such as a cold, is the most common cause of sore throats. Other signs and symptoms may include a cough, runny nose, scratchy throat and hoarse voice.
- **Strep throat (see page 449)**
  Strep throat is the most common bacterial throat infection, generally occurring in children ages 5 to 15. In addition to a sore throat, signs and symptoms may include a fever, headache, abdominal pain, rash and swollen lymph glands in the front of the neck.
- **Throat infection (see "Sore throat," page 652)**
  A bacterium or a virus can produce a painful throat infection. Even if a child's tonsils have been removed, the throat can become infected and produce signs and symptoms similar to those of tonsillitis.
- **Tonsillitis (see page 653)**
  Tonsillitis is an infection of the tonsils. In addition to a sore throat, other signs and symptoms include trouble swallowing, abdominal pain and a fever.

Urinary problems

Urinary problems may be associated with disorders and diseases that range from minor to serious. Urinary problems in children often are related to one of the following conditions:

- **Diabetes (see page 994)**
  A child's first signs and symptoms of diabetes generally include increased thirst and frequent voiding of large volumes of urine. Some children begin wetting the bed at night.
- **Incontinence after toilet training (see "Bed-wetting," page 194)**
  If a toilet-trained child begins to wet the bed, either the passage of time or medical interventions may resolve the problem. Involuntary loss of urine during the day should be investigated by a doctor.
- **Urinary tract infection (see pages 202 and 217)**
  A urinary tract infection generally causes frequent or painful urination. Other signs and symptoms may include discolored urine, abdominal pain, a fever and chills.
- **Urine color change (see "Injury and inflammation," page 905, and "Urinary tract infections," page 909)**
  Certain kidney disorders, such as an infection, inflammation or injury, may produce cloudy or dark urine. Swelling of the face and legs also may result.

Vision problems

Diagnosing vision problems in very young children can be difficult. As children get older, some of the following conditions may become more apparent:

- **Blurred vision (see "Common vision problems," page 584)**
  School-age children may develop visual disorders requiring corrective lenses. Typically, the child complains of trouble seeing and may squint to see better.
- **Color deficiency (see "Colorblindness," page 601)**
  This inherited condition usually occurs in males. People with this condition generally have trouble recognizing the colors red or green or both.
- **Double vision**
  Double vision can occur for a variety of reasons, some of them serious. See a doctor immediately.
- **Misaligned eyes (see page 602)**
  The eyes don't move in parallel motion. Instead, one eye turns inward or outward, either constantly or intermittently.

Vomiting

Vomiting in infants and young children is most often related to eating too much or to a mild intestinal infection. It may occur for the following reasons:

- **Congenital malformation (see "Congenital digestive and respiratory disorders," page 169)**
  Incomplete or incorrect formation of the small intestine can occur at the upper or lower ends of the intestinal tract, resulting in vomiting or constipation.
- **Eating disorders (see page 225)**
  Eating disorders are most common in teenagers. Anorexia nervosa and bulimia are associated with self-induced vomiting as a means of losing weight.
- **Excess consumption (see "Spitting up and vomiting," page 158)**
  Some infants eat more than their stomachs can hold and spit up the excess.
- **Gastroenteritis (see "Gastrointestinal infections," page 834)**
  Children often experience infection of the stomach or small intestine due to a virus or, less commonly, a bacterium or a parasite. Signs and symptoms commonly include nausea, vomiting, abdominal pain and diarrhea. They typically improve in a day or two. See a doctor if they don't.

Wheezing

Labored breathing with high-pitched sounds — usually during expiration — may represent asthma. But as an old saying goes "All that wheezes is not asthma." A variety of airway or pulmonary problems may produce wheezing. If a child seems to be experiencing respiratory distress — having difficulty breathing — seek emergency care. The distress may be related to one of the following:

- **Asthma (see page 495)**
  Wheezing associated with asthma is often accompanied by breathing difficulty, a tight feeling in the chest and coughing. It may be triggered by an allergy, respiratory infection, cold air or exercise.
- **Bronchiolitis (see page 763)**
  The smallest airways in the lung can become infected with a virus, which may produce wheezing, a cough and rapid breathing. This condition is different from bronchitis, which in children usually causes croup.
- **Hyperventilation (see page 23)**
  When some children become excited, anxious or fearful, they breathe too fast and produce a sound similar to wheezing.
- **Respiratory syncytial virus (see page 765)**
  This respiratory infection, commonly known as RSV, occurs mostly in children under age 4. In addition to wheezing, it causes a congested or runny nose, a cough and a low-grade fever. ■

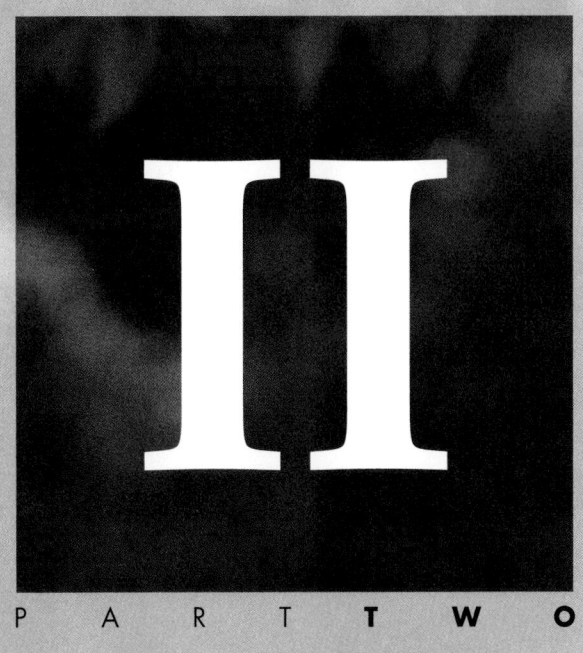

PART TWO

Pregnancy and Healthy Children

CHAPTER **3** PART II

Pregnancy and Childbirth

Pregnancy is one of life's most treasured times for many women. As they anticipate the upcoming birth, many women eat better, exercise more and pay better attention to their health than ever before. But however short nine months may appear to some, it can seem very long if the pregnancy is difficult or the outcome uncertain.

While pregnancy will always involve risks to mother and baby, medical advances have taught us much about how to minimize those risks and how to better deal with unavoidable problems. With proper care and regular visits to your doctor or other health care professionals, chances are you and your baby will be strong and healthy.

Preparing for Pregnancy

Before attempting to become pregnant, it's a good idea to see your doctor for a thorough medical history and physical examination. This is important because many conditions that are initially without symptoms can complicate pregnancy. Diabetes, high blood pressure and anemia are just a few common conditions that can be detected easily during a comprehensive general examination.

If your doctor discovers a health condition, in most cases it doesn't mean that you can't have a child.

But you'll want to have the problem under control before attempting pregnancy. Some pregnant women with chronic diseases such as diabetes might see a high-risk pregnancy specialist (maternal-fetal pregnancy specialist) who has expertise in high-risk pregnancies.

A pre-pregnancy physical is also a good time to ask questions of your doctor or discuss concerns you may have. A particular disease or genetic abnormality may run in your family. Or maybe you're older than 35 and worried about potential complications related to your age. Maybe you've been pregnant before and had a problem, such as miscarriage, and you're worried about a recurrence. A frank discussion with your doctor can provide helpful information about your chances of having a healthy baby.

During your pre-pregnancy physical, your doctor will likely recommend a multivitamin with folic acid. Whenever possible, women should take folic acid from at least one month before conception through the first three months of pregnancy. Folic acid has been shown to prevent birth defects in early fetal development (neural tube defects), and it's generally a good idea for women of childbearing age to take folic acid because many pregnancies are unplanned.

Before conception is also a good time to re-examine your lifestyle. If you're overweight and want to lose weight, do it before you become pregnant. Pregnancy isn't the time to begin a diet. If you smoke, quit. Women who smoke during pregnancy tend to have babies with lower birth weights than do nonsmokers, and these babies may have developmental problems. In addition, smokers have a higher incidence of miscarriages, stillbirths and other pregnancy complications.

Don't use alcohol or illegal drugs during pregnancy. If you take medication — prescription or over-the-counter — ask your doctor about whether you may continue to take it before you try to become pregnant.

Prenatal Care

One of the most important things you can do for you and your baby is to arrange for prenatal care as soon as you realize that you're pregnant. By the time most women call for an appointment with a doctor, they already know they're pregnant — a home pregnancy test was positive, and they're starting to experience signs and symptoms of pregnancy. If your pregnancy hasn't been confirmed, you can have this done at your doctor visit.

Many doctors advise that you seek prenatal care as soon as you've missed a period, especially if you're trying to conceive. At the very latest, wait no longer than two missed periods before seeing a doctor.

Many women receive prenatal care from a doctor specially trained in the care of pregnant women and the delivery of babies (obstetrician). Some family doctors also offer this service to their patients. In some communities, licensed, certified nurse-midwives also provide maternity care.

A certified nurse-midwife has, at a minimum, a master's degree in nursing, specializing in obstetrics and gynecology, and has passed several examinations to receive certification. Nurse-midwives provide complete obstetric care for normal, healthy pregnancies and are trained to screen mothers for potential problems. In case of a problem, the mother is referred to a doctor.

In most states, nurse-midwives are permitted to prescribe medications and vitamins, but they don't perform cesarean deliveries or operative vaginal deliveries. Most nurse-midwives attend births in hospitals or birthing centers. Some with private, solo practices assist in births in the home. All nurse-midwives are legally required to be associated with a backup doctor or group of doctors they can call on in case a problem develops.

During your first visit with your doctor, you may be asked to fill out a detailed health form. He or she will also ask questions about your family health history and overall health to determine if you might have pre-existing conditions that could cause problems or that require special measures during the pregnancy.

To try to determine when your baby will be born (due date), it's important to identify when you conceived, so you'll likely be asked when you had your last menstrual period. The due date is only an approximation, however. Few babies are born on the precise date they're expected. It's perfectly normal for a baby to be born anywhere from three weeks before to two weeks after the due date.

After taking your medical history, the next step of the first prenatal visit is often a physical examination and a pelvic examination, which may include a pap test if you're due for one. Blood and urine tests also are generally done during the first visit.

You may have an ultrasound exam. An ultrasound may be used early in pregnancy to confirm the gestational age of the fetus.

A member of your health care team may discuss important issues of pregnancy with you, such as nutrition, weight gain, exercise and signs of potential complications. Prenatal visit schedules are evolving and may vary depending on patient needs and presence of pregnancy complications.

After the initial visit, regular visits usually begin with your weight and blood pressure measurements. Your doctor also will want to know if you're having any problems or concerns.

After about 10 to 12 weeks of gestation, an exciting part of the visit is listening to your baby's heartbeat, which can be detected with a Doppler instrument or ultrasound. Your doctor may also examine your abdomen to determine whether the baby is growing properly.

Pregnancy and Nutrition

The best time to start thinking about good nutrition is before you plan to become pregnant. Then

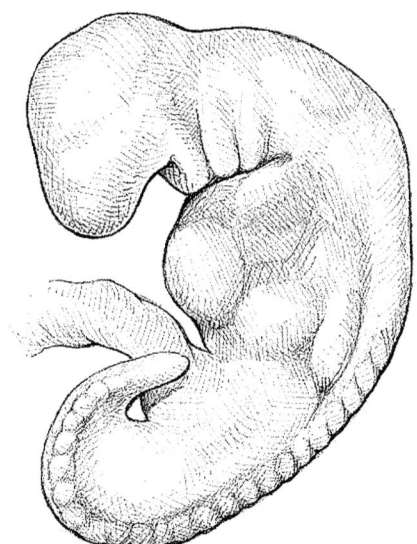
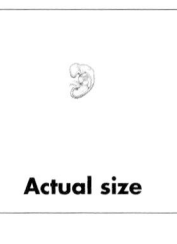

Actual size

Four weeks after conception, an embryo is no longer microscopic but is still less than ¼ inch in length. Growth is rapid during the fourth week. The embryo triples in size.

Pregnancy Tests

The earliest way to know for sure if you're pregnant is to have a pregnancy test. By 4 days of age, a fertilized egg begins to secrete a hormone called human chorionic gonadotropin (HCG). This hormone spreads into the mother's tissues. Initially, it can be detected in the blood and shortly thereafter in the urine.

Most home pregnancy tests are conducted with a sample of urine, because urine can be easily obtained at home. Many types of urine tests are used to detect the presence of HCG. Most depend on a reaction between the HCG and an anti-HCG antibody. A second reaction indicates if the first reaction took place. Often, the second reaction is a color change. Most home pregnancy tests are easy to use and quite accurate if you follow the instructions carefully and correctly.

How accurate are pregnancy tests?
Keep in mind that the accuracy of any pregnancy test depends on the timing of the test and how closely you follow the instructions. A test taken on the first day of your missed period is likely to be between 54 and 97 percent accurate, depending on the sensitivity of the pregnancy test you use. You'll get a more accurate reading if you wait another week to take the test.

If the test is performed in the very early days of pregnancy, it may indicate you're not pregnant when in fact you are. This is called a false-negative test result. This type of result can occur because early in pregnancy the levels of HCG may be low enough to go undetected. For this reason, a negative result from a pregnancy test is less reliable than a positive result.

If your test result is negative, but you have symptoms or signs of pregnancy, try the test again a week later or consult your doctor. If the result is positive, see your doctor for prenatal care. To confirm that you're pregnant, your doctor may get a blood sample for an HCG blood test.

you can be sure that your baby will have all of the essential nutrients from the moment of conception. Improvements that you make in your own diet can also spark a healthy change for the family.

Nutrition risk factors

If you have a history of healthy-eating habits, you begin your pregnancy with optimal amounts of most of the nutrients needed for your baby's growth and development. A history of chronic dieting, skipping meals, fasting or eating a limited variety of foods can put you and your baby at nutritional risk. Other factors that put you at increased risk of poor nutrition include using cigarettes, alcohol or illegal drugs; carrying more than one baby; having a chronic disease that limits your body's ability to utilize nutrients, such as malabsorption; and being significantly underweight or overweight at the time of conception.

Extremely poor eating habits before or during pregnancy can harm both you and your baby. If you eat too few calories or nutrients, fetal development can be less than ideal, and your baby may be underweight at birth. A baby with a low birth weight has an increased risk of short- and long-term health problems.

In the first weeks of your pregnancy — perhaps even before you know you're pregnant — most of your baby's major organs are forming. That's why it's so critical to make nutritious eating habits and folate a part of your decision to begin a new life.

Weight gain

Pregnancy may be the one time in your life when you're encouraged to gain weight. But weight gain in pregnancy doesn't mean eating whatever you want. Your weight increases for various physical reasons, including the weight of the baby you'll deliver.

Over the years, the recommended amount of weight to gain during pregnancy has varied dramatically.

Twenty or 30 years ago, minimal weight gain was thought to be best for mother and baby. Now research indicates that women who are normal weight at the time of conception have the healthiest pregnancies and babies if they gain approximately 25 to 35 pounds. Women who are overweight or underweight at the start of pregnancy or who are pregnant with twins will have different weight gain targets.

During pregnancy, you want to eat normally and as healthfully as you can. Your doctor may recommend how much weight you should gain. Individual recommendations vary based on factors such as your pre-pregnancy weight, your medical history and your health.

How much weight you gain during your pregnancy partly determines your baby's weight, and a normal birth weight is important for good health. A desirable weight for a full-term newborn is between 6½ and 9 pounds. Babies born at these healthy weights have:

- A lower rate of infant death
- Fewer mental and physical handicaps
- Fewer serious childhood illnesses

Keep in mind that each woman gains at different rates. Here are some general guides to weight gain:

- First trimester: 1 to 1½ pounds a month
- Second trimester: ½ to ¾ pound a week
- Third trimester: ¾ to 1 pound a week

Calorie needs

Your developing fetus depends on the calories you provide through eating and drinking. However, this doesn't mean that you should eat excessively.

During the first trimester, you don't need to consume any extra calories over your normal daily intake. You may find, though, that some of the discomforts of early pregnancy — feelings of hunger or nausea and vomiting — are often relieved by intermittent snacking. If you feel more comfortable snacking, eat smaller meals to avoid excessive weight gain.

During your second and third trimesters, you'll need a total of

Where the Weight Goes

Your baby	6½-9 pounds
Placenta	1½ pounds
Amniotic fluid	2 pounds
Breast enlargement	1-3 pounds
Uterus enlargement	2 pounds
Fat stores and muscle development	4-8 pounds
Increased blood volume	3-4 pounds
Increased fluid volume	2-3 pounds
Total	22-32½ pounds

340 to 450 extra calories a day beyond your normal pre-pregnancy diet. This amount will provide for the recommended pregnancy weight gain each month. It's important that these calories and nutrients come from foods that offer the most nutrition for you and your baby. Keep in mind that these extra calories aren't a big increase. For example, two slices of whole-grain bread, 8 ounces of skim milk and 2 ounces of lean meat will add about 340 calories.

The more active you are, the more calories you'll need. Even with this demand for more calories, you shouldn't need to force yourself to eat more because your appetite almost always guides you to enough calories.

Food choices

While you're pregnant, you don't have to keep a food diary or analyze your meals and snacks, but do pay attention to some basic guidelines. Regularly eating a variety of foods is best for staying healthy. Try to eat the following types and amounts of food every day. Listed are the minimum daily servings:

- **Grains: 6 servings.** Grains — whole grain cereals, breads, rice and pasta — are rich in energy-filled complex carbohydrates and provide important nutrients as well as fiber. Along with fruits and vegetables, grains should form the foundation of your diet.
- **Vegetables: At least 3 servings.** Vegetables are naturally low in calories and almost fat-free. They provide fiber, vitamins and minerals.
- **Fruits: At least 2 servings.** Fresh fruits generally have few calories and little or no fat, and they contain beneficial fiber, vitamins and minerals.
- **Dairy products: At least 3 servings.** Milk, yogurt and cheese are outstanding sources of calcium and vitamin D, which help

Vitamin and Mineral Supplements

Pregnant women need more of almost every vitamin and mineral than do women who aren't pregnant.

If you eat a balanced diet, you may not need supplements. However, many pregnant women can't eat enough foods high enough in iron and folate to meet recommendations, and some women can't or won't eat enough high-calcium foods to meet the increased need for this mineral. Multivitamins that include folic acid taken a month or more before conception and early in pregnancy may help prevent birth defects and provide insurance that you get enough vitamins and minerals in your daily diet.

In some cases, your doctor may recommend that you take additional supplements, such as vitamin B-12, zinc, vitamin D or choline. This may be especially true if you're not getting the recommended nutrients due to food insecurity, substance dependence, anemia or a vegan, or vegetarian diet. If you have lactose intolerance, a gastrointestinal condition or an eating disorder, additional supplementation may be recommended. Talk to your doctor if you have any concerns about your nutrition during pregnancy. He or she may refer you to a dietitian for additional guidance.

Folic Acid: A Pregnancy Must

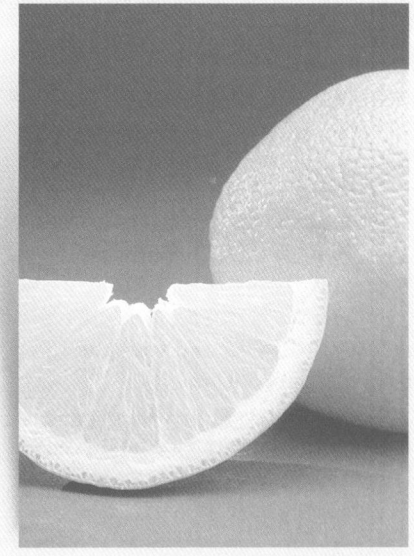

Folic acid is a synthetic form of folate, a vitamin found naturally in certain foods. It's an important nutrient, but never so much so as when you're considering becoming pregnant.

Some very important development takes place in the first several weeks of pregnancy. If you're planning on becoming pregnant or have the potential to become pregnant, take folic acid daily. Taking the supplements can help to avoid serious birth defects. In fact, the U.S. Public Health Service recommends that all women of childbearing age wanting to conceive children consume 400 to 800 micrograms (mcg) of folic acid daily as a means of reducing their risk of having a pregnancy with neural tube defects (NTDs), such as spina bifida. If you've had a pregnancy that resulted in a fetus with an NTD, you may decrease the risk of having a second affected pregnancy by about 70 percent if before conceiving again you take 4 milligrams (mg) of folic acid a day before conception and continuing through the first 12 weeks of pregnancy. Talk with your doctor about when to start taking folic acid.

Folic acid is vital for cell growth and function and for the synthesis of DNA, the building blocks of your genetic code. You'll find folate in citrus fruits, beans, nuts, seeds, liver and dark green leafy vegetables such as spinach. But to get the recommended amount of folic acid, you'll need a supplement.

your body absorb calcium. They also provide protein needed to build and maintain body tissues. Choose low-fat dairy products.

- **Meat, fish, eggs and dry beans (legumes): At least 3 servings.** These foods are rich sources of protein with B vitamins, iron and zinc. Seafood also contains omega-3 fatty acids, which are important to fetal brain development. Select lean varieties of meat and poultry to reduce fat and cholesterol. Legumes — beans, dried peas and lentils — are low in fat, without any cholesterol and the best source of plant protein.

- **Fats and sweets: Sparingly.** Certain fats are healthy during pregnancy, including omega-3 fatty acids from foods such as salmon, eggs and walnuts. However, saturated fats and sugars should be limited. Foods containing hydrogenated oil, a form of trans fat, are best avoided altogether.

Key Nutrients in Pregnancy

More than 50 nutrients are essential for good health when you're pregnant. Here's a summary of those that are important for a healthy pregnancy diet:

Nutrient	Why you and your baby need it	Best sources
Protein	Main building block for your baby's cells. Provides reserves you'll need for labor.	Eggs, lean meats, poultry, fish, cheese, milk, dried peas, beans
Carbohydrate	Provides energy for you and your baby. Allows protein to be used for tissue growth.	Whole-grain and fortified breads and cereals, fruits, vegetables, rice, pasta, potatoes
Fat	Provides long-term energy for growth. Critical for the development of your baby's brain.	Lean meat, fish, poultry, eggs, nuts, seeds, nut butters, oils, avocado, soft-tub margarine
Fluid	Helps increase fluid volume. Prevents constipation and dry skin. Needed for amniotic fluid.	Water, soup, milk
Vitamin A	Promotes healthy skin, eyesight and bone growth.	Sweet potatoes, carrots, dark leafy greens, cantaloupe, apricots, black-eyed peas
Vitamin C	Forms healthy gums, teeth and bones for you and your baby. Improves iron absorption.	Citrus fruits, broccoli, tomatoes, peppers, berries, melons, dark leafy greens, potatoes with skin
Folate	Helps blood cell and hemoglobin formation. Early in pregnancy, it may prevent birth defects.	Dark leafy greens, dried peas and beans, fortified whole-grain breads and cereals, citrus fruits, bananas, cantaloupe, tomatoes
Calcium	Helps form strong bones and teeth.	Milk, cheese, yogurt, collard greens, kale, sardines and canned salmon with the bones, broccoli, dried beans, tofu made with calcium sulfate
Iron	A component of hemoglobin in red blood cells needed to deliver oxygen to your baby.	Lean red meat, spinach, tofu, dried fruits, whole-grain and fortified breads and cereals
Iodine	Makes thyroid hormones, which regulate the body's metabolism and other important functions. Promotes proper bone and brain development in your baby.	Iodized salt (not sea salt), seafood, milk, cheese, yogurt, fruits, vegetables

Vegetarian diets

If you're following a well-balanced vegetarian diet, you can continue your diet throughout your pregnancy and have a healthy baby. Keep in mind, though, that vegetarians are more likely to have difficulty consuming adequate amounts of iron, choline, and vitamins D and E. Getting enough calcium, vitamin B-12 and omega-3 fatty acids also can be a challenge, especially if you're vegan. Take time to review your food intake regularly, and eat a wide variety of foods each day. If you include fish, milk and eggs in your diet, it's easier to balance your nutritional intake. If you're concerned about getting the right amount of nutrients, talk to your doctor and, if recommended, see a dietitian.

Snacks

Healthy snacking is the perfect way to add the extra calories and nutrients essential during pregnancy.

Well-planned snacks are also helpful for the times when you can't eat a full meal. In the early part of your pregnancy, frequent, small meals and snacks can help control nausea. During the last weeks, the pressure of your baby on your stomach may limit the amount of food you can comfortably eat at one time. Snacking may be more feasible.

Salt

Pregnant women were once encouraged to limit their sodium intake. New research suggests that limiting sodium intake isn't necessary. During the last few weeks of pregnancy, almost all women have some swelling (edema) in their ankles, legs, fingers or face. Cutting back on salt to reduce this swelling causes your body to conserve sodium and water, actually making the swelling worse. In fact, the recommended amount of sodium for women before and during pregnancy is the same as it is for the general population — less than 2,300 mg daily.

Artificial sweeteners

More than 1,500 artificially sweetened foods line the shelves of your local grocery store. They include chewing gum, soft drinks, pudding, gelatin, drink mixes, yogurt and candy. Although there's no conclusive evidence to support a recommendation either for or against the use of artificial sweeteners, pregnant women might want to consider limiting the amount in their diets. In all things, moderation.

Caffeine

Caffeine is a drug that has been part of the human diet for thousands of years. It's found naturally in coffee, tea, chocolate and cocoa. Caffeine is frequently added to soft drinks and over-the-counter medications, including some headache and cold tablets and allergy remedies.

Research on the effects of caffeine during pregnancy is ongoing, but the general recommendation is to consume no more than 200 to 300 mg daily.

Coffee is the most common source of caffeine. Drinking more than 12 ounces of coffee a day isn't recommended. But don't assume switching to an herbal tea is safe. Because little is known about herbs and their effect on pregnancy, avoid herbal teas. One exception is ginger tea, which may ease symptoms of nausea.

Pregnancy and Exercise

Today, an increasing number of health-conscious women are exercising throughout their pregnancies.

This isn't to say that pregnancy is the time to embark on a vigorous fitness regimen, especially if you haven't been physically active before. However, if you've been exercising regularly before pregnancy, you can continue to do so unless your doctor advises against it. Doctors even recommend that previously sedentary women begin some form of mild to moderate exercise during pregnancy.

The long-term benefits of a regular exercise program for men and women are well-known. For pregnant women in particular, it may increase maternal stamina.

Smart Snacking

Here are some examples of healthy snacks:

Crunchy
- Raw vegetables
- Whole-grain crackers

Sweet
- Fresh fruit
- Dried fruit
- Low-fat yogurt

Thirst quenchers
- Ice water or sparkling bottled water
- Fruit juice fizz, which is made from juice and sparkling water
- A fruit shake made with skim milk
- Vegetable juice

Hearty
- A fruit muffin or bread
- Cereal with low-fat yogurt
- Vegetable soup
- A tuna sandwich

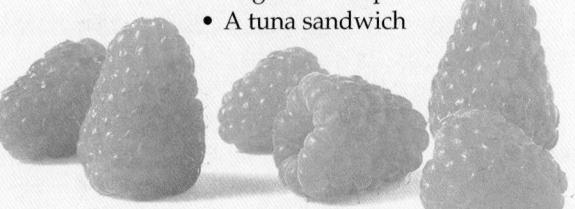

The result of this increased stamina may be a successful vaginal delivery, possibly due to increased cardiorespiratory fitness and better endurance. Endurance is particularly valuable when a mother is pushing the baby out during delivery. Women who exercise regularly can often push for longer periods without fatigue.

Exercise, though, with caution. Because of physical and hormonal changes in your body, you're more vulnerable to injury. Your joints are less stable and more easily injured because your connective tissues now stretch more easily. Moreover, as you become larger, your center of gravity shifts, and you may find yourself losing your balance. Pay attention to your changing body.

Many sports and exercises are suitable for pregnant women. One of the best exercises during pregnancy is swimming. It provides a good cardiovascular workout with minimal risk of injury because of the water's buoyancy.

Low-impact aerobics are also fine, and in many communities low-impact aerobic classes for expectant mothers are available.

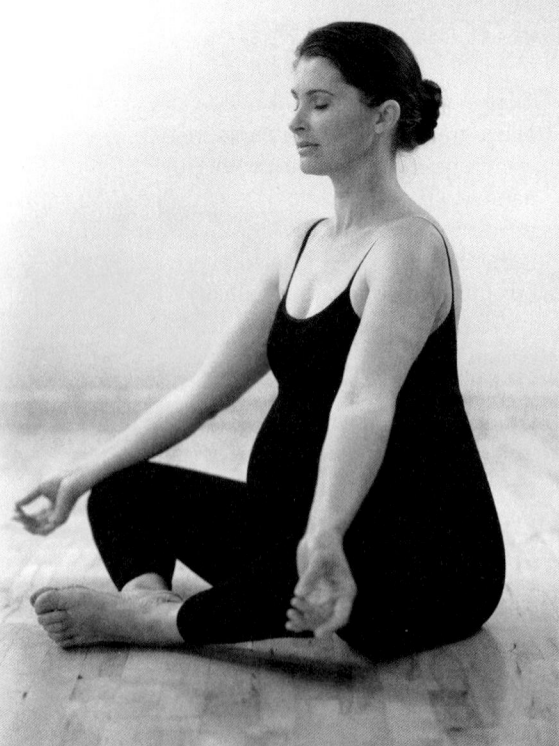

Pregnancy and Fish

Seafood can be a great source of protein, iron and omega-3 fatty acids, important nutrients to your baby's health. But some types of seafood — particularly large, predatory fish such as swordfish, shark, king mackerel and tilefish — contain potentially high levels of mercury and should be avoided. So should orange roughy, marlin and bigeye tuna. Although the mercury in seafood isn't a concern for most adults, special precautions apply if you're pregnant or planning to become pregnant. During pregnancy, go ahead and eat fish — many types of seafood contain very little mercury — but avoid species with potentially high mercury levels. Also be sure to avoid raw or undercooked fish.

It's recommended that pregnant women eat 8 to 12 ounces weekly of low-mercury-containing fish. The Food and Drug Administration, Environmental Protection Agency, and American Congress of Obstetricians and Gynecologists say pregnant women can safely eat up to 12 ounces a week (approximately three meals) of these fish:

Anchovy	Atlantic croaker
Atlantic mackerel	Black sea bass
Butterfish	Catfish
Clams	Cod
Crab	Crawfish
Flounder	Haddock
Hake	Herring
Lobster (American and spiny)	Mackerel
Oyster	Pacific chub
Perch, freshwater and ocean	Pickerel
Plaice	Pollock
Salmon	Sardine
Scallops	Shad
Shrimp	Skate
Smelt	Sole
Squid	Tilapia
Trout, freshwater	Tuna, canned light (includes skipjack)
Whitefish	Whiting

If you eat fish from local waters, pay attention to local fish advisories. Larger game fish contaminated with chemical pollutants could potentially harm a developing baby. If no advice is available, limit consumption.

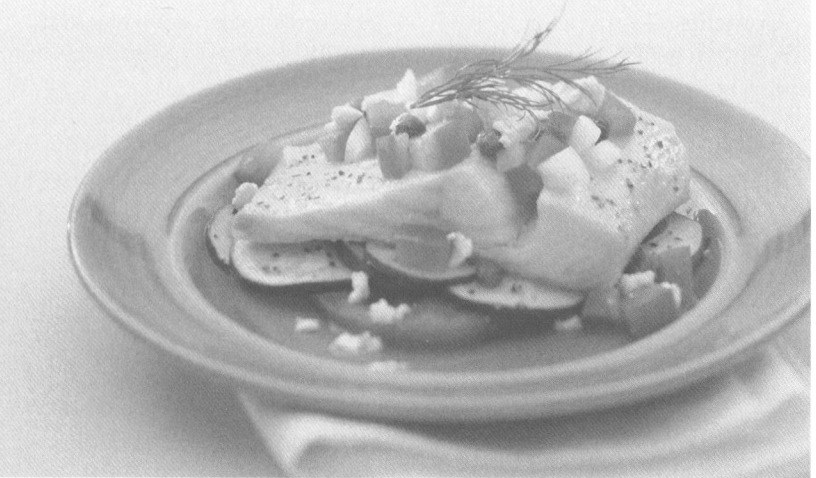

Jogging and cycling also are good if you took part in these activities before conception. You'll want to use caution, though, with any type of exercise that could lead to falling or cause trauma to your abdomen. You may also need to decrease your activity level if you find yourself becoming more fatigued than usual. Walking during pregnancy is often recommended, and it's usually the first exercise advised for previously inactive pregnant women who want to begin exercising. Another good option is yoga, which has many health benefits for pregnant women.

No matter what exercise you choose, check with your doctor before you begin. Although it's safe for most women to exercise during pregnancy, some pregnant women have medical problems that may make exertion inadvisable. In addition, never exercise to the point of exhaustion. Drink plenty of fluids, especially water, to prevent dehydration during a workout.

Common Concerns

Most women come through pregnancy and childbirth healthy and with reason to celebrate. Still, few women escape without at least some discomfort. And along the way, they often have many concerns. Most doctors who deliver babies are accustomed to pregnant women asking questions — lots of them. Keep a notebook in which you can jot down questions as they come up, and bring it with you to your checkups.

Morning sickness

Morning sickness is the term used to describe the queasiness, nausea or vomiting that about half of all pregnant women have during the first 12 weeks of pregnancy.

Although these conditions tend to be worse in the morning, they can occur at any point throughout the day. It's not understood why some women have nausea and vomiting. Hormonal changes may be responsible. Although morning sickness is certainly unpleasant, it's rarely dangerous.

If you experience morning sickness, you can do certain things to minimize your symptoms, although nothing is 100 percent effective. Many women find that the nausea is worse when their stomach is empty. By the time you feel hungry, it may be too late, and you may already feel the nausea creeping up on you. Make it a point to eat several small meals a day. Try keeping crackers at your bedside and eating a few before getting up in the morning. Keep stashes of nutritious foods that you can tolerate in strategic locations — your car, desk drawer or purse.

You may find the smell of certain foods give you an upset stomach. If this happens, avoid that particular food. On the other hand, eat whatever sounds good for your queasy stomach. If plain water upsets your stomach, try crushed ice, fruit juice or ice pops.

If these techniques don't work, talk to your doctor. Some medications may be effective for reducing the symptoms of morning sickness. If you have a history of gastric reflux, treatment may improve the symptoms of morning sickness. In general, most women will find that these symptoms go away about 12 weeks into the pregnancy.

Constipation

Constipation is marked by hard and occasionally painful bowel movements, a diminished frequency of bowel movements, and difficulty in expelling stool. Constipation is a common problem during pregnancy. If you're normally constipated, you may find that the problem worsens during your pregnancy.

To alleviate the problem, drink plenty of fluids, exercise daily, and make sure your diet contains several servings of high-fiber vegetables, fruits (prunes are particularly good) and whole grains, such as oatmeal and whole-wheat crackers. Over-the-counter bulk-formers that contain psyllium also can be helpful. Don't take a laxative unless you check with your doctor.

Heartburn

The burning sensation in the middle of your chest and the bad taste in your mouth that sometimes accompanies it are the result of stomach acid refluxing into your lower esophagus. It occurs when the muscle that closes off the stomach from the esophagus (esophageal sphincter) relaxes, allowing stomach juices to flow back up and irritate the esophagus.

Heartburn is common in pregnancy. It often worsens as the pregnancy advances because the stomach is displaced by the enlarging uterus, which delays the emptying of the stomach contents.

If you have heartburn, try eating smaller meals at more frequent intervals. Eat slowly, and avoid greasy foods. Try drinking fluids separately from meals to avoid filling your stomach too quickly. Avoid using straws when you drink, and take small sips. Both regular and decaffeinated coffee may aggravate heartburn, as can carbonated beverages. Because heartburn is often worse when you lie flat, try not to eat two to three hours before bedtime. When you go to bed, use extra pillows to prop up your head. If these practices don't help, talk to your doctor, who may recommend an antacid. Calcium carbonate (Tums) may be safe to use in limited amounts and with your doctor's permission.

Backache

Low back pain is common during pregnancy. Often, it occurs when you're tired or have been bending, lifting or walking a lot.

When you're pregnant, your ligaments are more elastic, which allows your pelvis to expand during the birth of your baby. Although this is necessary, it makes your joints more prone to strain and injury. During pregnancy, as your center of balance changes, so does your posture, inflicting more strain than ever on your already vulnerable back.

Often, the pain is in the lower back. Some women experience pain that starts at the lower back and radiates down one or both legs (sciatica).

Most women also have pain on the sides of the abdomen because of the stretching of the abdominal ligaments by the expanding uterus. Imagine your uterus being anchored by ligaments that extend down the sides of your abdomen. As your uterus grows, the ligaments stretch to accommodate it. This pain is generally worse during the second trimester. Lying on your left side may ease the strain.

Try not to gain more weight than is recommended because excess weight stresses your back. Backache can usually be relieved by eliminating as much strain as possible. Sometimes a garment that provides back support can help. Ice applied for five to 10 minutes several times a day can provide some relief over time. Your doctor may recommend exercises to relieve the pain. If the pain is severe, your doctor may recommend further evaluation to determine if an underlying problem is causing the pain.

Varicose veins

Varicose veins usually become worse later in pregnancy and are more pronounced in older mothers and in women who stand for long periods. Heredity also plays a role. The condition tends to appear earlier and is more pronounced with each pregnancy.

When you're pregnant, your blood vessels must accommodate an increased blood volume to supply the needs of your baby. Your uterus enlarges, and the flow of blood from your leg veins to your pelvis decreases. This combination can cause the veins in your legs to become swollen, creating leg discomfort.

If you have varicose veins, try to keep off your feet and elevate them when possible. Don't wear clothing that's tight around the thighs or waist. Support hose can help relieve the pain and swelling. Many doctors recommend that you put on support hose first thing in the morning and keep them on until just before you go to bed.

Surgery to treat varicose veins generally isn't recommended during pregnancy, and rarely is the problem so severe that it becomes necessary. After pregnancy, surgery may be an option if varicose veins remain a problem.

Hemorrhoids

Hemorrhoids occur when the veins in the anal canal become enlarged due to pressure, similar to varicose veins. When you strain during a bowel movement, the veins may protrude through the anus and cause pain and itching. Generally, they become worse during pregnancy and often occur in conjunction with constipation.

Prevention is the best treatment. Avoid becoming constipated to the point where you need to strain to expel stool. Eating food high in fiber, drinking plenty of water and exercising daily help prevent constipation.

If you feel pain during a bowel movement and feel a swollen mass near your rectum, you probably have a hemorrhoid. To ease the discomfort, take frequent warm-water baths. A cotton pad soaked with cold witch hazel cream and applied to the hemorrhoidal area also may help. Many women find relief with over-

the-counter rectal suppositories that reduce the hemorrhoid and lubricate the anal canal.

Sleep difficulties

Sleep difficulties often occur during the later months of pregnancy. The frequent urge to urinate contributes to lack of sleep. The movement of your baby also may keep you awake. Some women simply have so much on their minds that sleep eludes them.

What should you do if you find yourself staring at the ceiling half the night? Avoid coffee, tea or cola drinks because they contain caffeine, which can keep you awake. In addition, don't eat a large meal just before bedtime.

Some doctors recommend exercising a little more so that you'll be more tired and more apt to fall asleep. But be sure to finish exercising several hours before bedtime.

For some pregnant women, a warm bath helps. If these ideas don't work, get up — read a book, pay some bills or catch up on household tasks. Try sleeping later.

If your lack of sleep becomes significant, talk to your doctor. Don't take any medications unless he or she recommends it.

Swelling

Swelling (edema) is common during pregnancy. Approximately one-quarter of your weight gain during pregnancy is fluid, which tends to collect in various parts of your body, including the lower legs, feet and hands. You may notice swelling in your legs, ankles and feet after you've been standing for long periods.

The problem is usually worse at the end of the day and in warm weather. After a night of rest, the legs and feet return to their usual size in most women.

The fingers are also a common site for swelling. You may wake up in the morning with your fingers so stiff that you can't button your clothing. Your fingers may also be puffy.

Some women experience facial swelling. If your face becomes extremely swollen over a day or two, contact your doctor.

Lying down and elevating your legs for an hour in midafternoon may reduce the swelling in your legs. Swimming and treading water also may temporarily relieve swelling in your legs and feet. Even standing in a pool can help.

Travel

There's no reason why you can't travel during your pregnancy unless your doctor advises against it.

Before you contemplate a cross-country car trip or a two-week cruise, however, consider how you're going to feel. Many women, particularly during the first three months of pregnancy, have frequent bouts of nausea or morning sickness. Travel during this period may make the nausea worse.

A potential risk of traveling while pregnant is a blood clot in a vein (thrombophlebitis), often in a leg, which can result from sitting for long periods of time. While traveling, get up and walk around for a few minutes every couple of hours to activate your leg muscles and increase blood flow. It's also a good idea to wear compression stockings when you travel.

Another consideration is the proximity to your due date. Most doctors advise against traveling during the last weeks of pregnancy. Also consider that many airlines won't allow you to fly if you're close to your due date. If you're in your second trimester or beyond, cruise lines might require a letter from your doctor and some international flights may have certain restrictions.

When traveling by car, remember to always wear your seat belt. Fasten a lap belt below your uterus, and place a shoulder harness between your breasts and to the

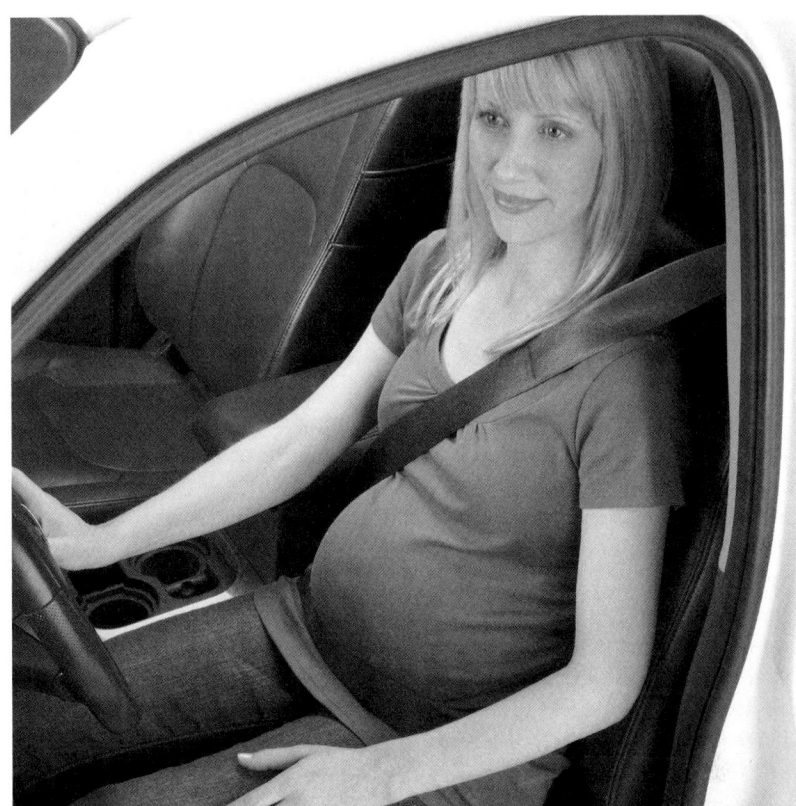

Place the lap portion of the seat belt below your abdomen and across your upper thighs. Position the shoulder strap between your breasts and to the side of your abdomen.

side of your abdomen. You may find it helpful to put a pillow in the small of your back to prevent low back pain. Stop every couple of hours to get out and walk.

Something else to keep in mind when planning travel in the second half of your pregnancy is the availability of obstetric and neonatal care. While most women do not have preterm labor, it's a good idea to be prepared, particularly in remote areas of the United States or other locales that might be somewhat isolated.

Medical Problems of Pregnancy

Most women go through pregnancy without any major complications. For a small percentage of women, however, this nine-month experience isn't without problems.

This section explores some of the more common medical problems that can complicate pregnancy.

Anemia

Anemia occurs when a protein in blood that carries oxygen throughout the body (hemoglobin) falls below usual levels. A small decrease in hemoglobin is normal during pregnancy. Usually, anemia in pregnancy is due to an iron deficiency or an inadequate supply of folate.

If you have mild anemia, you may not have any signs or symptoms, and the condition may only be discovered during a routine blood test. Pregnant women who are anemic are less able to tolerate blood loss than are women with adequate hemoglobin.

Your doctor may recommend iron and folic acid supplements to prevent anemia. You can help prevent the condition by eating a diet rich in iron. Iron is found in foods such as liver, dried fruit, whole grains and beef. Dark leafy greens are a good source of folate. If you're taking the recommended amount of folic acid for early pregnancy, this should also be enough to prevent anemia.

Diabetes

Having diabetes doesn't preclude you from becoming pregnant. In fact, if you have diabetes, you have an excellent chance of having a healthy baby. However, before conception and during pregnancy, it's extremely important to keep your blood sugar (glucose) level under control through careful monitoring. A satisfactory glucose level at the outset of pregnancy decreases your baby's risks of birth defects, particularly those affecting the heart, spine and brain.

If your blood sugar isn't well-controlled, the excess sugar in your blood will travel through the placenta and cause an increase in your baby's blood sugar level. This activates the fetal pancreas to produce insulin, which acts as a growth hormone. Babies born to mothers whose diabetes is out of control may be large, a characteristic that complicates labor and delivery. The baby also may be at risk of serious birth defects, including abnormalities of the heart and brain. Babies born to mothers with uncontrolled diabetes also tend to have more congenital defects and are predisposed to diabetes.

For a pregnant mother with diabetes, the risks associated with the disease include infection, postpartum bleeding, heart and lung problems, and a fourfold greater risk of preeclampsia than in mothers who don't have diabetes.

Women with diabetes prior to becoming pregnant should seek the care of an obstetrician who specializes in high-risk pregnancies.

Gestational diabetes
Sometimes, women who don't have diabetes develop a condition called gestational diabetes during pregnancy. This form of diabetes also requires careful blood sugar control. Changes in your diet are the first step in treatment.

Your doctor may prescribe a medication called glyburide (DiaBeta, Glynase). It can prevent or forestall the need for insulin. Gestational diabetes usually goes away after the baby is born, but it increases your risk of developing diabetes later in life. A dietitian can provide other guidelines and recommendations.

Your doctor will likely recommend a blood glucose screening test 24 to 28 weeks into your pregnancy to check for gestational diabetes. Pregnant women with certain risk factors for gestational diabetes may be tested much earlier in pregnancy.

Asthma

Asthma is a chronic respiratory disease, and the course of asthma during pregnancy can be difficult to predict. In some women, the disease worsens with pregnancy. In others, it improves or remains the same.

If you have asthma, you may be more prone to respiratory infections during pregnancy. However, most women with asthma carry a baby to term safely. Many women with asthma require medication. Most asthma medication is safe to use during pregnancy.

High blood pressure

High blood pressure is a potentially dangerous problem during pregnancy. Pregnant women with high blood pressure tend to have small placentas, and their infants are more likely to be small at birth. The incidence of fetal death is higher in pregnant women with high blood pressure than it is in pregnant women without high blood pressure.

Some pregnant women have pre-existing high blood pressure (chronic hypertension), which means that they had it before they became pregnant. In others, high blood pressure develops during pregnancy (gestational hypertension). The condition is easily detected during a routine blood pressure check, which is a part of every prenatal visit.

If your blood pressure is high enough, your doctor may prescribe medication. Any medication you take during pregnancy can affect your baby. Although some medications used to lower blood pressure are considered safe during pregnancy, others — such as angiotensin-converting enzyme (ACE) inhibitors, angiotensin II receptor blockers (ARBs) and renin inhibitors — are not. Discuss your medications with your doctor before becoming pregnant.

Some women with mild pre-existing high blood pressure have no major problems during pregnancy. In others, their blood pressure continues to increase, and protein is detected in their urine, which is a sign of preeclampsia. This serious medical condition typically occurs in the second half of pregnancy and can develop in women with or without pre-existing high blood pressure (see page 121).

If you have high blood pressure, your doctor will likely request blood and urine tests to determine if your kidneys are functioning properly. During pregnancy, your doctor may also recommend additional laboratory tests and monitoring of your baby.

Heart disorders

Although potentially serious, many women with pre-existing heart disorders have successful pregnancies and healthy babies.

Pregnancy makes your heart and other organs work harder. Thus, if you already have a heart disorder, the extra stress of pregnancy can cause complications. Excessive weight gain, anemia and abnormal retention of fluid can be particularly dangerous for women with heart disorders. Make sure you discuss the risks of pregnancy and delivery with your doctor before you become pregnant. If you have a cardiac condition, you may be managed by both an obstetrician who specializes in high-risk pregnancy and a cardiologist.

Seizure disorders

If you take medication for a seizure disorder, such as epilepsy, you'll need special attention during pregnancy.

Severe nausea and vomiting during early pregnancy may interfere with your ability to take your anticonvulsant medication. Expansion of your blood volume and increase in your weight may change the levels of medication in your blood. These changes can increase the risk of seizures.

Some medications used to control seizures cause birth defects, with certain medications more likely to cause problems than others. Uncontrolled seizures in pregnancy also can pose a risk to you and your baby if you discontinue your seizure medication. If you have a seizure disorder and you're contemplating pregnancy, make sure to discuss your condition and medication with your doctor.

Skin disorders

Skin pigmentation changes often occur during pregnancy. You may notice brownish spots on your face or on other parts of your body. This discoloration on your face is sometimes called the mask of pregnancy (chloasma). The pigmentary changes usually fade after the baby is born.

Other conditions that affect pregnant women are a type of hives (urticaria) and cholestasis. Hives are raised, red, often itchy welts of various sizes that appear and disappear on the skin. They may result from medications, allergic reactions or chemicals in foods, but often the cause is unknown.

Cholestasis is a condition that occurs when the flow of bile from the liver to the intestine is reduced or interrupted. Bile pigment (bilirubin) is deposited in skin tissues, causing itching. Itching without a rash generally occurs all over the body. In pregnant women, cholestasis is often due to hormonal changes and requires medical attention. See your doctor promptly.

Avoid scratching, which may cause infection. Wash with a mild soap. If your symptoms are severe, talk to your doctor, who may be able to provide some suggestions for relief.

Infectious diseases

Some common diseases that seem to do little more than make a pregnant woman miserable can, in fact, do irreparable damage to the fetus, depending on when in fetal development they strike.

German measles
German measles (rubella) is usually a mild viral disease that causes a mild, itchy rash and fever. If contracted during the first 12 weeks of pregnancy, however, the virus can cross the placenta and infect the fetus. Up to 85 percent of newborns born to women who have the virus during early pregnancy are infected with rubella, which can cause congenital malformations such as cataracts, deafness, hernias, heart defects and defects of the central nervous system.

When contracted in later pregnancy, rubella doesn't cause congenital defects, but the infant is born with the virus, which can cause serious illness. Many of these babies later develop diabetes.

Your best defense against rubella is immunization. Most women in the United States have been vaccinated against German measles. However, if you haven't been vaccinated and you haven't had the illness, get vaccinated before you become pregnant.

Chickenpox
If you've never had chickenpox, consider getting the chickenpox vaccine before you become pregnant.

Bleeding During Pregnancy

Bleeding from the vagina during pregnancy can be an indication that something may be wrong. In the first 20 weeks of pregnancy, bleeding may be associated with a miscarriage, an ectopic pregnancy or another condition.

Bleeding during a miscarriage may be slight or heavy. You may have no warning of vaginal bleeding, or you may first notice some brownish discharge.

Approximately 25 percent of all pregnant women have some bleeding in early pregnancy, but only about half of those pregnancies end in miscarriage. So don't necessarily assume the worst, but do check with your doctor and have the bleeding evaluated.

After the 20th week of pregnancy, bleeding is much less common than in early pregnancy. Causes include placenta previa — a condition in which the placenta covers the cervical opening — the onset of premature labor and the separation of the placenta from the uterine wall (placental abruption).

Most often the bleeding is mild. However, a severe episode of bleeding (hemorrhage) can endanger your life and your baby's. If you begin bleeding after the first 12 weeks of pregnancy, see your doctor immediately.

Chickenpox (varicella) can be a serious disease in pregnant women, and it can be dangerous to the fetus. While in the uterus, the fetus may actually develop pocks. If these occur early in pregnancy, the pockmarks may cause some limb deformities.

The greatest risk to the baby seems to be exposure to the virus just before delivery. If the infant is delivered before receiving your antibodies against the virus, he or she may develop the disease. Immediate treatment may prevent serious complications or death in a newborn.

If you're exposed to the chickenpox virus during pregnancy and haven't had the virus, your doctor may recommend an injection of vericella-zoster immune globulin.

Fifth disease

Fifth disease is an infection most common among school-age children. The disease is also known as erythema infectiosum. The most noticeable part of the infection is a bright red rash prominent on the cheeks, giving the impression of slapped cheeks. A lacy, red rash may also appear on the legs, trunk and neck.

Pregnant women are susceptible to developing fifth disease. In the majority of cases, the mother delivers a normal, healthy baby. However, in some cases, fifth disease in a mother can lead to severe, even fatal, anemia in the fetus. This can result in congestive heart failure in the fetus.

Sometimes, it's possible to try to correct the anemia and heart failure with a fetal blood transfusion or administration of medication to the mother. The medication passes through the placenta to the fetus.

If you're pregnant and think you've been exposed to fifth disease, contact your doctor.

Toxoplasmosis

Toxoplasmosis is a disease that results from contact with the parasite Toxoplasma gondii. It's contracted by eating infected, undercooked meat or through contact with infected cat feces. The disease can be passed from an infected pregnant mother to her baby. If you're pregnant, be careful to not come in contact with cat feces. Wear gloves while gardening or cleaning the litter box and wash your hands thoroughly afterward.

More than 30 million men, women and children in the United States carry the organism, though most don't have symptoms. Common symptoms are fatigue and muscle pain. You may feel like you have the flu. If you have toxoplasmosis, your doctor will likely prescribe a medication to treat the infection.

Most infants born with toxoplasmosis don't immediately show evidence of having been infected, but many doctors advise treatment with antibiotics anyway. In addition, most infants are not infected despite maternal infection. Of those who are, most have only minor symptoms. A few, however, eventually develop neurological problems and partial blindness. A small percentage of these infants die of the disease.

Group B streptococci

Group B streptococci are bacteria that can be transmitted to the fetus during childbirth. About 1 out of every 4 pregnant women carry group B strep bacteria in the rectum or vagina but experience no symptoms. If these bacteria are identified, you'll be treated with antibiotics during labor to prevent transmission of the bacteria to the baby as the baby travels through the vagina.

The risk of group B streptococcal disease in infants is small. If an infant is infected with the disease, symptoms such as breathing problems and shock usually arise within 48 hours after delivery. Occasionally, an infant will be a week old before symptoms develop. Immediate treatment with antibiotics is necessary for infants with this infection.

Genital herpes

Genital herpes is a sexually transmitted infection (STI) that appears as painful blisters on the genitals. The cervix or upper vagina also may have blisters, which may not produce symptoms. In a newborn, herpes can cause serious damage to the eyes and central nervous system or, rarely, death.

There's no cure for genital herpes. After one attack, it may be a month or years before the next. Some women carry the virus but never have symptoms. If you have confirmed herpes or suspect that you have the virus, tell your doctor.

The danger to the baby is generally thought to result from exposure to the virus during an active (primary) infection in the mother as the baby travels down the birth canal. If an examination or test confirms that you have active herpes near your delivery time, your doctor may recommend cesarean delivery. Women with herpes may be given preventive medications during the last three weeks of pregnancy to prevent a herpes outbreak during delivery.

Hepatitis B

Hepatitis B is a liver infection caused by the hepatitis B virus. This virus is transmitted through the exchange of bodily fluids. If you have the hepatitis B virus, it can be transmitted to your fetus through the placenta. Risk of premature birth is higher among women who have hepatitis B. In addition, a newborn baby can become infected by the virus.

A test for hepatitis B is generally done as part of prenatal care. If you have hepatitis B, your infant can be given an injection of antibodies against the virus after delivery. Because the hepatitis virus also may be found in breast milk, a mother with hepatitis B shouldn't breast-feed.

Syphilis

Syphilis is a serious sexually transmitted infection that can be passed from a pregnant mother to her baby. If you have syphilis, you may see one or more lesions (chancres) on your genitals. Sometimes, they may go unnoticed. The lesions occur 10 to 90 days after exposure. About six weeks later, you may notice a rash.

During your first prenatal visit, you'll be tested for syphilis, as required by law. The disease can be treated with penicillin. At birth, your infant will be tested. If the baby has congenital syphilis, treatment is initiated immediately.

Gonorrhea

Gonorrhea is another sexually transmitted infection that can be effectively treated with antibiotics. However, if you have untreated gonorrhea, your baby will be exposed during the birth process.

Infection with gonorrhea may result in damage to your baby's eyes. For this reason, all newborns receive preventive treatment immediately after birth. This consists of an antibiotic ointment applied under the baby's eyelids.

Chlamydia

Chlamydia, another sexually transmitted infection, can cause an eye infection (conjunctivitis) in a newborn. This usually appears during the second week of life. If treated with antibiotics, the infection doesn't have any long-term adverse effects. The antibiotic ointment used to treat gonorrhea usually prevents this eye infection as well.

Cytomegalovirus

Cytomegalovirus (CMV) is the most common virus affecting the fetus. Each year, less than 1 percent of newborns are born infected with this virus.

Fortunately, most of these babies don't develop problems. But some do experience disabilities from the virus. It can cause death or numerous birth defects, such as blindness, deafness, seizures, anemia and neurological disorders. There's no effective treatment.

CMV is acquired by contact with saliva, urine or other bodily fluids, often in a child care setting. Careful attention to hygiene is important for protection in this setting. CMV infection brings the risk of hearing loss in otherwise healthy babies.

Human papillomavirus

Human papillomavirus (HPV) causes warts on the skin or cervix. Such warts found on the genitals are called venereal warts (condyloma acuminatum). They're highly infectious, sexually transmitted and occasionally painful. The warts tend to grow faster during pregnancy. Usually, treatment during pregnancy isn't necessary and often isn't effective.

HIV

Pregnant women can be infected by the human immunodeficiency virus (HIV) that causes AIDS through sexual intercourse with infected partners, by injecting drugs with contaminated needles, through artificial insemination with semen containing the virus or by a blood transfusion. Because of improved screening measures, acquiring HIV through a blood transfusion is now rare.

If you have HIV or AIDS and are pregnant, you can pass the disease to your baby. However, if you receive appropriate medication starting early in pregnancy, the risk of transmission may be reduced to as low as 1 percent. In some instances, cesarean delivery rather than a vaginal delivery also may reduce the risk of transmission.

Zika virus

The Zika virus is transmitted by certain species of mosquitoes that are found only in specific regions of the world. Some people infected with Zika virus have no signs or symptoms, while others may report mild symptoms. If a pregnant individual contracts Zika virus, it may cause a serious congenital brain abnormality called microcephaly. Zika may also be associated with other birth defects. Scientists and clinicians are still learning details about Zika and possible pregnancy complications.

Presently, no vaccine exists to prevent Zika virus, and there's no effective antiviral treatment. If you're pregnant, it's recommended that you avoid traveling to places where Zika virus has spread. The Centers for Disease Control and Prevention (CDC) website provides regular updates on locations where Zika virus has been confirmed.

Pregnancy Risk Factors

Most pregnant women deliver healthy babies at or near term. Some factors, however, tend to increase the chances of complications such as miscarriage, stillbirth and premature birth. Some of these factors are to a large extent beyond your control. Others are dangerous practices you should avoid.

Age

Age is especially worthy of some attention because many women are delaying pregnancy until their 30s and even 40s. Most healthy women older than age 35 have uneventful pregnancies. Because many of these women have planned their pregnancies, they're often highly motivated and take especially good care of themselves. There remains, however, an increased risk for mother and child.

Pregnant women older than age 35 are at greater risk of developing gestational diabetes and high blood pressure. The rates of miscarriage and stillbirth also are slightly higher because there's an increased risk of chromosomal abnormalities in the fetus. Placenta previa — a condition in which the placenta covers the opening of the cervix — is more common among older mothers. Labor also tends to be slightly longer in older first-time mothers.

Teenagers also are at higher risk of complications of pregnancy. The risk may not be so much age-related as the result of the mother being less likely to seek prenatal care. Too frequently, pregnant teens have poor diets, engage in illegal use of drugs and alcohol, and get little or no prenatal care. They have higher rates of miscarriage, stillbirths and premature births than do women a few years older.

Diet

An inadequate diet increases your risk of giving birth to an infant with a low birth weight, which makes the infant more vulnerable to infection, disease and death. Failure to gain an adequate amount of weight during pregnancy can adversely affect your baby. If you've been poorly nourished most of your life, the effects may be felt by your baby. However, these effects will be reduced with improved nutrition during pregnancy.

Smoking

Smoking is a difficult habit to break, but it's not impossible, as millions of Americans can attest. Studies show that mothers who smoke a pack or more of cigarettes a day consistently have smaller babies than do nonsmokers.

A small baby is generally weaker and more vulnerable to illness than one of average size. Moreover, smokers are more apt to experience serious conditions during pregnancy, including placental abruption, breaking of water (premature rupture of membranes) and placenta previa. Smokers are also at increased risk of miscarriage or stillbirth or having a baby who dies of sudden infant death syndrome (SIDS) .

Alcohol

Alcohol use during pregnancy is the leading preventable cause of intellectual disability in infants. Because there's no known safe level of alcohol use during pregnancy, you shouldn't drink alcohol at all during your pregnancy.

If you drink excessive alcohol, your baby may be born with fetal alcohol syndrome. It's characterized by prenatal and postnatal growth restriction, facial abnormalities, heart defects, joint and limb problems, and intellectual impairments. The more alcohol you drink, the greater the risk of having a child with fetal alcohol syndrome or other problems.

Illegal use of drugs

More infants are being born with both drug addiction and associated health problems. Pregnant women who use heroin or cocaine are two to six times more likely to have a baby who's born prematurely or at a low birth weight. The pregnancy is also more likely to be complicated by high blood pressure or vaginal bleeding. Babies born to mothers who abuse certain prescription medications, such as oxycodone or other opiates, are exposed to similar risks.

Infants who are born to addicted mothers may also be addicted to drugs. These infants must go through the process of withdrawal under doctor supervision. Often, this takes place in a hospital's neonatal intensive care unit (NICU) or a special care nursery. Medications may be given to the infant to help with symptoms of withdrawal.

Medications

Medications taken during pregnancy may affect your baby too.

As a general rule, it's best to use caution and avoid use of medications during pregnancy. Some drugs can cause an early miscarriage or harm the developing fetus. Very few medications have been proved to be completely safe in pregnancy, but many have been found to be safe enough that their benefits outweigh any tiny, unknown risk.

Before you take any medication — prescription or over-the-counter — check with your doctor for specific advice based on your health history and the medication in question. A pharmacist also can provide general guidelines.

If you have a health concern that requires regular medication, or if you were taking medication regularly before getting pregnant, your doctor will evaluate whether it's safest for you to continue taking the medication, discontinue it, or switch to a different medication that poses less risk to you and your baby.

Often, a medication that was important for your health before pregnancy will be important during pregnancy too.

Radiation

While high levels of radiation are best avoided during pregnancy, low levels of radiation from X-rays won't harm your fetus. Airport scanners, for example, are safe during pregnancy. If possible, avoid medical X-rays directed at the abdomen during pregnancy. Despite the risk, sparing use of

X-rays may be necessary when a serious condition threatens the health of the mother.

Doctors are clearly aware of the potential risks of cumulative radiation to a fetus. Equipment also has improved so that less radiation is needed during diagnostic tests. These factors combine to make X-ray examinations relatively safe when a pregnant woman has a medical condition that requires them.

If you're pregnant, it's safe to have an X-ray of your teeth, head or extremities. Modern techniques protect your abdomen, and the radiation is confined to the area on which the X-ray is focused. If methods that don't require radiation are effective, they should be chosen.

Prenatal Tests

Pregnancy is a time of great anticipation. Will you have a girl or a boy? Will the baby inherit your sense of humor or your partner's compassion? You may have moments of doubt and anxiety as well. Will you experience complications? Will the baby be healthy?

Take comfort in the fact that most babies are born healthy. Still, you may want additional details about your baby's health. Prenatal screening and testing can provide additional information before your baby is born or to help you make decisions about pregnancy management. Most of conditions described in this section are rare sporadic genetic conditions with a low risk of occurring. Your provider may refer you to a genetics professional who will provide more information about genetic screening or testing.

Types

Prenatal testing includes both screening tests and diagnostic tests:

- **Screening tests.** Prenatal screening tests — such as blood tests and ultrasounds — are routine in most pregnancies. Screening tests can identify whether your baby has increased risk of certain conditions, but screening tests can't make a definitive diagnosis. Screening tests pose few or no risks to you or your baby.
- **Diagnostic tests.** If a screening test indicates a possible problem — or your age or family history puts you at increased risk of having a baby with a genetic problem — you may consider a more invasive prenatal diagnostic test, such as chorionic villus sampling or amniocentesis. These procedures carry a very small risk of miscarriage.

Questions to consider

Prenatal testing is optional. It's important to make an informed decision about prenatal testing,

Intrauterine Growth Restriction

An infant who's born extremely small for its gestational age — below the 10th percentile — is considered to be growth restricted. Intrauterine growth restriction often occurs when the fetus doesn't get adequate nourishment from the mother through the placenta.

An infant born small for gestational age doesn't have the amount of body fat that a normal-sized newborn does. Thus, the infant has difficulty maintaining a normal body temperature and blood sugar level. Moreover, many infants who are growth restricted grow slowly throughout at least early childhood. They may also have some delayed intellectual development.

Many conditions and lifestyle characteristics can produce intrauterine growth restriction. Women who smoke, use drugs illegally or drink large amounts of alcohol are more likely to produce a small infant. A mother who is malnourished or fails to gain adequate weight also is in danger of giving birth to a small infant. Certain chronic diseases, such as cardiovascular disease, lupus or high blood pressure, also place the mother at risk.

Conditions related to pregnancy also can cause growth restriction. These include abnormalities of the placenta and umbilical cord, fetal infections or malformations, and the presence of more than one fetus.

When a fetus isn't growing at a proper rate because of smoking, a poor diet, or alcohol or illegal drug use, a change to a healthier lifestyle might help. If the fetus is still far from term, the risk of early delivery must be weighed against the risk of leaving it in the womb and allowing further malnutrition.

Congenital Defects

Birth defects, the leading cause of infant mortality in the United States, affect about 3 percent of pregnancies and account for about 20 percent of all infant deaths.

Some defects correlate with the age of the mother. For example, a woman's chances of giving birth to a child with Down syndrome increases with age because older eggs have a greater risk of improper chromosome division. Pregnant women who take certain medications or have diseases such as diabetes or alcoholism also are at increased risk of giving birth to a child with birth defects, as are women who have intrauterine infections.

especially if you're screening for fetal conditions that can't be treated.

- **What will you do with the test results?** Normal results can ease your anxiety. But if prenatal testing indicates that your baby may have a birth defect, you may be faced with wrenching decisions — such as whether to continue the pregnancy. On the other hand, you may welcome the opportunity to plan for your baby's care in advance.
- **Will the information shape your prenatal care?** Some prenatal tests detect problems that can be treated while you're pregnant. In other cases, prenatal testing alerts your doctor to a condition that requires immediate treatment after birth.
- **How accurate are the results?** Prenatal testing isn't perfect. The proportion of false-negative and false-positive results varies from test to test. In addition, screening and testing cannot rule out all birth defects and genetic disorders.
- **What are the risks?** Weigh the risks of specific prenatal tests —

such as anxiety, pain or possible miscarriage — against the value of knowing the results.

- **What is the expense?** Insurance coverage for prenatal testing varies. If the test you're considering isn't covered by your insurance plan, are you willing and able to cover the cost of the test on your own?

Prenatal testing can provide information that influences your prenatal care. But some screening tests introduce the need for careful personal decisions. Ultimately, the decision to pursue prenatal testing is up to you. If you're concerned about prenatal testing, discuss the risks and benefits with your health care professional.

Ultrasound

An ultrasound exam may be the prenatal screening test you've heard the most about. Ultrasound imaging creates a picture of your unborn

baby to help determine how your pregnancy is progressing.

You may receive one of two kinds of fetal ultrasounds. During a transabdominal ultrasound, sound waves are directed at the tissues in your abdominal area. These sound waves bounce off the tissues in your body, including your baby. The sound waves are translated into a pattern of light and dark areas, creating images of your baby on a monitor. Usually, you're able to watch the monitor and see images of your baby while the test is being done.

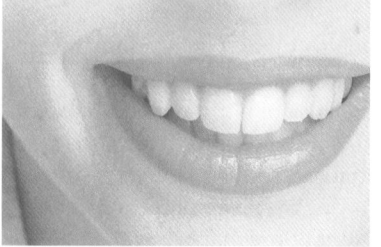

Question and Answer

Is it OK to go to the dentist while I'm pregnant?

You don't want to neglect your teeth during pregnancy. Some women notice that their gums get more sensitive and bleed more easily during pregnancy. It's a good idea to visit your dentist right before you become pregnant and once during your pregnancy for a regular checkup and cleaning.

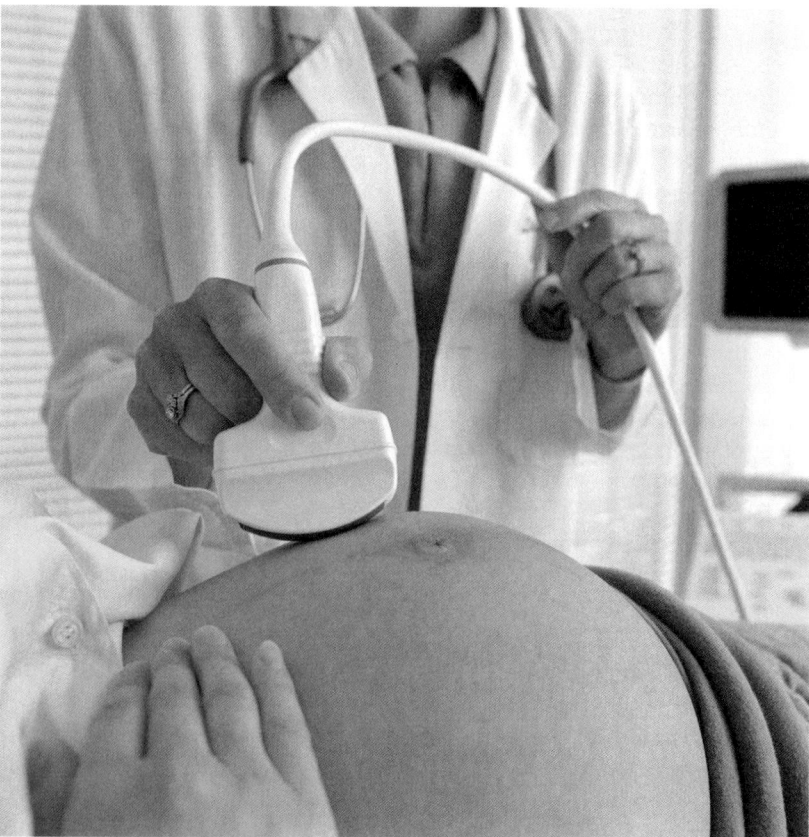

Ultrasound examination painlessly reveals the shape of the fetus within the uterus. Fetal age can be determined by measuring the width of the skull.

During a transvaginal ultrasound, a wandlike device is placed in your vagina to send out sound waves and gather the reflections. Transvaginal ultrasounds are used most often during early pregnancy, when the uterus and fallopian tubes are closer to the vagina than to the abdominal surface.

Why are fetal ultrasounds done?

Your doctor may use a fetal ultrasound to:

- **Confirm the pregnancy and its location.** Some embryos develop in the fallopian tube instead of in the uterus. An ultrasound exam can help detect and treat a tubal (ectopic) pregnancy before it endangers your health.
- **Determine your baby's gestational age.** Knowing the baby's age can help your doctor more accurately determine your due date and track various milestones throughout your pregnancy.
- **Confirm the number of babies.** If a multiple pregnancy is suspected, an ultrasound may be done to resolve the question.
- **Evaluate your baby's growth.** Your doctor can use ultrasound to determine whether your baby is growing at a normal rate. Ultrasound can be used to monitor your baby's movement, breathing and heart rate as well.
- **Study the placenta.** The placenta provides your baby with vital nutrients and oxygen-rich blood. Any problems with the placenta need special attention.
- **Identify possible fetal abnormalities.** An ultrasound can help identify many congenital abnormalities. An early diagnosis may lead to early interventions that help save or improve a baby's life.
- **Screen for Down syndrome and other chromosome problems.** Together with certain blood tests, ultrasound can be used between the 11th and 14th week of pregnancy as an initial screening test for Down syndrome,

a genetic disorder that causes intellectual disability and other problems. Using ultrasound, a health care provider measures a specific region on the back of your baby's neck (nuchal translucency screening test). This screening, in combination with a blood test, can evaluate the risk of Down syndrome, as well as trisomy 13 and 18 syndromes, conditions that cause severe intellectual disability or severe physical defects. If the results of the ultrasound and the blood tests suggest a high risk of these disorders, further testing can be used to confirm the results.

- **Investigate bleeding and other worrisome signs or symptoms.** If you're bleeding or having other complications, an ultrasound may help your doctor determine the cause.
- **Perform other prenatal tests.** An ultrasound may be used during certain prenatal tests to guide placement of the needle, such as when obtaining a sample of amniotic fluid for specific genetic problems (amniocentesis) or obtaining a biopsy of the placenta to test for genetic abnormalities (chorionic villus sampling).

When are ultrasounds done?

Fetal ultrasound can be done at any point during pregnancy.

If your doctor suspects an ectopic pregnancy or other problems, you may need an ultrasound soon after you find out you're pregnant.

Routine fetal ultrasounds are typically done between 19 and 20 weeks, when most anatomic details are visible. If your baby's health needs to be monitored more closely, ultrasounds may be repeated throughout the pregnancy.

Cell-free DNA screening

Prenatal cell-free DNA (cfDNA) screening, also known as non-invasive prenatal screening, is a

method to screen for specific chromosomal abnormalities during pregnancy. It involves taking a sample of the mother's blood. The blood contains DNA from both the mother and the placenta. The DNA from the placenta usually contains the same genetic material as the fetus. This DNA sample can be used to analyze for chromosome problems in the fetus.

Prenatal cell-free DNA screening can be done as early as week 10 of pregnancy. It may be more sensitive and specific than traditional first and second trimester screening tests, such as the first trimester screen and the quad screen. However, cell-free DNA screening has limitations in some situations, such as for a mother who's obese or a mother pregnant with twins.

Why it's done

Prenatal cell-free DNA screening can be used to screen for fetal sex, fetal rhesus (Rh) blood type and:

- **Down syndrome (trisomy 21).** Down syndrome is a genetic condition that causes intellectual disability and other medical problems.
- **Trisomy 13 and 18.** Trisomy 13 and 18 are conditions that cause severe intellectual defects or severe physical defects. These conditions are often fatal during pregnancy or in early infancy.

Other prenatal cell-free DNA screening tests are available, but data regarding the accuracy and sensitivity of certain cfDNA tests is still being evaluated. These tests may be used to screen for increased risk of the following conditions:

- **Trisomy 16 and 22.** Trisomy 16 and 22 are rare chromosome problems that usually result in miscarriage.
- **Triploidy.** Triploidy is a rare chromosome condition that causes severe physical defects. This condition usually leads to miscarriage or fetal death during the early second trimester of pregnancy.

- **Sex chromosome aneuploidy.** Sex chromosome aneuploidy is an abnormality in the number of sex chromosomes. Some of these conditions have no symptoms, while others are associated with risk of infertility, mild intellectual disability or cardiac abnormalities.
- **Specific microdeletion syndromes.** These are rare chromosomal disorders caused by a small segment of chromosome that's missing (chromosome deletion) or an extra copy of a small segment of a chromosome (chromosome duplication). One of the more familiar microdeletion syndromes is 22q11.2 deletion syndrome, also known as DiGeorge syndrome.
- **Certain single gene disorders.** Some laboratories are offering cell-free DNA screening for specific disorders caused by mutations in a single gene, such as disorders associated with abnormalities of the skeleton or bones.

First trimester screen

First trimester screening involves a blood test and an ultrasound exam. The blood test measures levels of two pregnancy-specific proteins, pregnancy-associated plasma protein A (PAPP-A) and beta human chorionic gonadotropin (beta-HCG). The ultrasound is done to measure the size of the clear space in the tissue at the back of a baby's neck (nuchal translucency).

Typically, first trimester screening is done between weeks 11 and 14 of pregnancy.

Why it's done
The first trimester screen is done to evaluate increased risk of chromosomal problems, including:
- **Down syndrome (trisomy 21).** Down syndrome is a genetic condition that causes intellectual disability and other medical problems.

- **Trisomy 18.** Trisomy 18 is a condition that causes severe intellectual disability. It is often fatal in early infancy.

Remember, prenatal screening is optional — and test results only indicate whether you have an increased risk of carrying a baby who has certain developmental or chromosomal conditions, not whether your baby actually has the condition.

Quad screen

The quad screen, also referred to as the second trimester screen, measures levels of four substances in a your blood:
- Alpha-fetoprotein (AFP), a protein produced by the baby's liver
- Human chorionic gonadotropin (HCG), a hormone produced by the placenta
- Estriol, another pregnancy-related hormone
- Inhibin A, another pregnancy-related protein

Typically, the quad screen is done between weeks 15 and 20 of pregnancy. Because other tests are more sensitive and specific, the quad screen is used less often than in the past.

Why it's done
The quad screen, like the first trimester screen, evaluates the risk of certain chromosomal conditions, including Down syndrome and trisomy 18. In addition, it can evaluate the risk of certain developmental conditions, including:
- **Spina bifida.** Spina bifida is a serious birth defect that occurs when the tissue surrounding a baby's developing spinal cord doesn't close properly.
- **Anencephaly.** Anencephaly is an underdeveloped brain and an incomplete skull. A baby born with anencephaly may be stillborn or die within a few hours or days after birth.

Spina bifida, anencephaly and defects in the fetus's abdominal

wall also may be detected by an ultrasound examination during the second trimester.

Like the first trimester screen, test results only indicate whether you have an increased risk of carrying a baby who has certain congenital or chromosomal conditions.

Chorionic villus sampling

Chorionic villus sampling (CVS) is a prenatal test in which a small sample of the placenta (chorionic villi) is sampled for genetic testing. The tissue is sampled using a small tube (catheter) guided through the cervix or through the abdomen to the placenta.

During pregnancy, the placenta provides oxygen and nutrients to the growing baby and removes waste products from the baby's blood. The chorionic villi are wispy projections that make up most of the placenta and share the baby's genetic makeup.

Chorionic villus sampling can reveal whether a baby has a chromosomal abnormality, such as Down syndrome. Chorionic villus sampling can also be used to test for most genetic disorders, such as Tay-Sachs disease and cystic fibrosis.

Why it's done
Generally, chorionic villus sampling is offered after abnormal genetic screening or if there is concern for a single gene disorder that can be detected through DNA testing. The test is usually done between the 11th and 14th weeks of pregnancy — earlier than other prenatal diagnostic tests, such as amniocentesis.

You may consider chorionic villus sampling if:
- **You had abnormal results from a prenatal screening test.** If the results of a screening test — such as cfDNA or the first trimester screen — are positive or worrisome, you may opt for chorionic villus sampling to confirm or rule out a diagnosis.

- **You had a previous pregnancy with chromosomal abnormality.** If a previous pregnancy was affected by specific chromosomal abnormalities, this pregnancy may be at higher risk too.
- **You're age 35 or older.** Women age 35 and older have a higher risk of chromosomal abnormalities, such as Down syndrome.
- **You have a family history of a specific genetic disorder, or you or your partner is a known carrier of a genetic disorder.** In addition to identifying Down syndrome, chorionic villus sampling can be used to diagnose other chromosomal abnormalities and most single gene disorders. Chorionic villus sampling cannot detect congenital malformations such as cleft lip and palate or spina bifida.

Risks

Chorionic villus sampling carries various risks, including:

- **Miscarriage.** Overall, chorionic villus sampling has a 0.22 percent risk of miscarriage.
- **Cramping and vaginal bleeding.** You may feel cramping after the test. Vaginal bleeding also is possible, especially if the cell sample was taken through your cervix rather than the abdominal wall.
- **Rh sensitization.** Chorionic villus sampling may cause some of the baby's blood cells to enter your bloodstream. If you have Rh negative blood type, you'll be given a medication called Rh immunoglobulin after the test to prevent you from producing antibodies against your baby's blood cells.
- **Infection.** Very rarely, chorionic villus sampling results in a uterine infection.

Some older studies suggested that chorionic villus sampling may cause defects in a baby's limbs. However, the risk appears to be a concern only if the procedure is done before the ninth week of pregnancy.

Remember, chorionic villus sampling is typically offered when there is significant concern for a genetic disorder and test results may impact the management of the pregnancy.

Amniocentesis

Amniocentesis is a test that you may choose to have performed early in the second trimester of pregnancy, usually after the 14th week of pregnancy. The test is used to check for certain abnormalities, such as chromosomal problems, single gene disorders, spinal bifida and abdominal wall defects.

During amniocentesis, a doctor inserts a long, thin needle, guided by ultrasonography, into your uterus. A small amount of amniotic fluid is withdrawn, and the needle is removed. The fluid contains fetal cells with fetal DNA, which can be used for genetic testing.

Why it's done

You may consider genetic amniocentesis if:

- **You had abnormal results from a prenatal screening test.** If the results of a screening test — such as the first trimester screen, cfDNA or quad marker screen — are positive or worrisome, you may opt for amniocentesis to confirm or rule out a diagnosis.
- **You had a chromosomal abnormality or neural tube defect in a previous pregnancy.** If a previous pregnancy was affected by Down syndrome or a neural tube defect — a serious abnormality of the brain or spinal cord — this pregnancy may also be at higher risk.
- **You're age 35 or older.** Babies born to women age 35 and older have a higher risk of chromosomal abnormalities, such as Down syndrome.
- **You have a family history of a specific genetic disorder, or you or your partner is a known carrier of a genetic disorder.** In addition to identifying Down syndrome and spina bifida, amniocentesis can be used to diagnose many single gene disorders.
- **You have a suspected uterine infection or complications of red cell antigen incompatibility.**

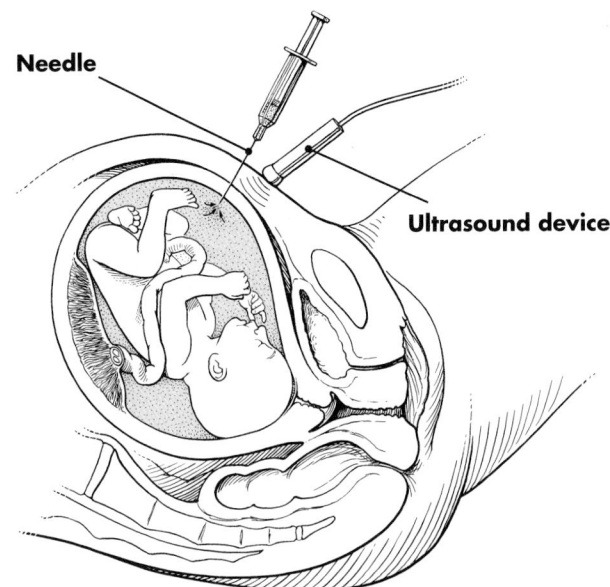

Amniocentesis involves removal of a small amount of amniotic fluid from the sac containing the fetus. Guided by an ultrasound image, a doctor inserts a long, thin needle into the uterus and withdraws fluid. Laboratory analysis of the fluid can reveal such things as your baby's sex, development and chromosome pattern.

Less often, amniocentesis is used later in pregnancy to examine specific concerns, such as uterine infections, fetal lung maturity, or complications of red cell antigen incompatibility — an uncommon condition in which a mother's immune system produces antibodies against a specific protein on the surface of the baby's blood cells.

Risks

Amniocentesis carries various risks, including:

- **Miscarriage.** Early amniocentesis carries a slight risk of miscarriage, often due to rupture of the amniotic sac. This risk is approximately 0.11 percent, which is slightly lower than the risk associated with chorionic villus sampling.
- **Cramping and vaginal bleeding.** Cramping is possible after amniocentesis. Some women experience a small amount of vaginal bleeding.
- **Needle injury.** During amniocentesis, the baby may move an arm or leg into the path of the needle. Serious needle injuries are rare because ultrasound is used to guide and monitor the needle during the procedure.
- **Leaking amniotic fluid.** Rarely, amniotic fluid leaks through the vagina after amniocentesis. If the leak seals, the pregnancy may proceed normally.
- **Rh sensitization.** Rarely, amniocentesis may cause the baby's blood cells to enter the mother's bloodstream. If you have Rh negative blood, you'll be given a medication called Rh immunoglobulin (Rhogam) after amniocentesis to prevent you from producing antibodies against your baby's blood cells.
- **Infection.** Very rarely, amniocentesis may trigger a uterine infection.
- **Preterm labor.** When amniocentesis is used later in pregnancy such as for determination of fetal lung maturity, associated

Red Cell Antigen Incompatibility

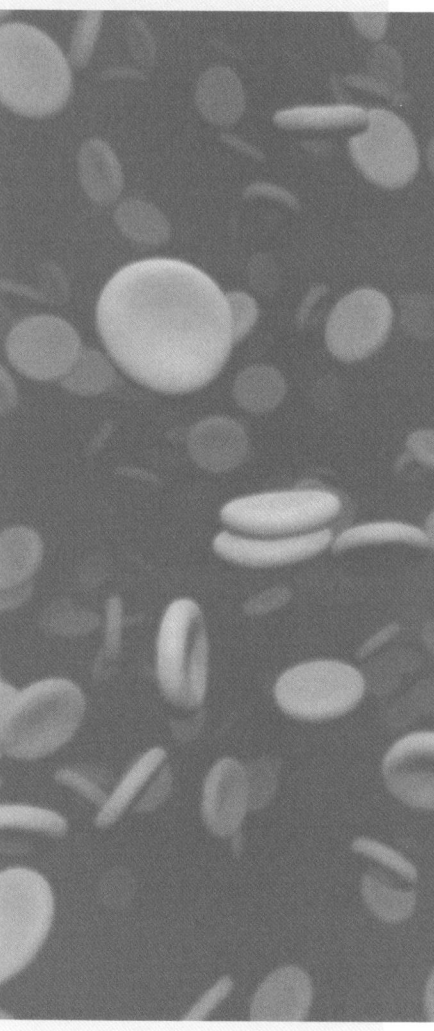

During pregnancy and especially at birth, some of your baby's blood can enter your bloodstream. If your blood type and that of your child are compatible, no problem occurs. Sometimes, though, your baby inherits a blood type from the father that differs from yours. If your and your baby's blood types are incompatible in specific ways, you can develop red cell antibodies that may be harmful to your baby.

Your body makes antibodies in response to certain proteins (antigens) on the surface of your red blood cells. The antigens in your blood and your baby's blood are based on your blood types. If your immune system detects a foreign antigen in your baby's blood, it may produce an antibody that could attack the red cells of the fetus. This can result in severe anemia in the fetus. In very complicated cases, the incompatibility can cause fetal death.

There are more than 50 blood group antigens. An incompatibility in certain blood groups, such as those involving the Rhesus (Rh) factor and Kell blood groups, is associated with particularly harmful antibodies. The most common of these is Rh factor incompatibility, which doesn't usually affect first pregnancies but can affect subsequent pregnancies if the same incompatibility exists. Fortunately, complications from Rh incompatibility have become rare because of more-thorough screening techniques and the use of a medication (RhGam) that prevents the mother from developing damaging antibodies. The medication is delivered as a shot at 28 to 30 weeks and is also given to mothers who are Rh-negative after delivery if the baby is Rh positive. In addition, there's now more effective therapy for infants who are affected by the mother's Rh-negative antibodies.

Blood type and antibody screening is generally done at your first prenatal visit. This will determine whether any red cell antibodies are present. If such antibodies are detected, it's recommended that you have periodic blood tests throughout your pregnancy to monitor antibody levels. If the level increases above a critical point, treatment may be necessary.

If red cell antibodies have developed during pregnancy, the result may be mild or severe anemia in the fetus, and an early delivery may be necessary. In certain cases, the infant may be given a blood transfusion while still in the womb. This is done to buy time until the baby's lungs are developed enough so that he or she can be delivered without severe complications. After birth, additional blood transfusions will be needed.

complications include rupture of membranes or preterm labor. However, infants delivered after 34 weeks gestation generally have good outcomes.

Remember, genetic amniocentesis is most typically offered when there is significant concern for a genetic condition in the fetus and test results may impact pregnancy management. Ultimately, the decision to have genetic amniocentesis is up to you. Your doctor or genetic counselor can help you weigh all the factors in the decision.

Chromosome analysis

Chromosome analysis, also called karyotype analysis, is used to examine a baby's chromosomes. It can detect duplicate or missing chromosomes. The specimen used for chromosome analysis is obtained while you're undergoing amniocentesis or chorionic villus sampling.

Chromosome analysis can identify chromosomal abnormalities such as Down syndrome as well as trisomy 13 and 18, which are rare conditions that cause severe intellectual disability or severe physical defects and are often fatal in early infancy.

Why it's done
- **You're at increased risk.** Certain factors, such as your age, can affect your risk of having a baby with specific genetic abnormalities. If you're at an increased risk of carrying a baby with these conditions, a chromosome analysis may be performed.
- **You're undergoing amniocentesis or chorionic villus sampling.** If you're having other diagnostic testing for certain genetic conditions, your doctor may also recommend chromosome analysis.
- **Your ultrasound exam identified the possibility of Down syndrome.** A chromosome analysis may be recommended if your ultrasound exam raises concerns

about Down syndrome and certain other genetic disorders.

FISH

One of the difficulties of chromosome analysis is the wait that's required for the results. If you undergo chromosome analysis, you'll have to wait one to two weeks to learn if your baby has a detectable problem.

A test called fluorescence in situ hybridization (FISH) uses cells retrieved while you're undergoing chorionic villus sampling or amniocentesis. The test can identify certain specific chromosomal abnormalities such as Down syndrome, trisomy 13 and 18 and monosomy X (Turner syndrome) in as little as one or two days. Because FISH is more targeted, the test is usually followed up with chromosomal analysis or chromosomal microarray. It uses a sample from chorionic villus sampling or amniocentesis.

Why it's done
The FISH test uses cells collected during CVS or amniotic fluid collected during amniocentesis and so is performed in conjunction with the specific procedure.

FISH is highly accurate, but not perfect, in identifying specific chromosomal defects. Both positive and negative results are usually followed up with the chromosomal microarray test.

Chromosomal microarray

Chromosomal microarray (CMA) prenatal testing provides a detailed look at a baby's chromosomes. Chromosomal microarray is used to detect small segments (portions) of a chromosome that are deleted (microdeletions) or duplicated (microduplications). This test is higher resolution than chromosome analysis and may detect small deletions or duplications that cannot be detected with standard chromosome analysis.

Microdeletions may be associated with specific genetic syndromes, some of which are associated with intellectual disability, physical disability or congenital problems such as heart defects.

Like chromosome analysis and FISH, chromosomal microarray uses a sample from chorionic villus sampling or amniocentesis to identify chromosome aberrations, including Down syndrome, trisomy 13 and trisomy 18. Trisomy 13 and 18 are rare genetic disorders usually involving severe intellectual disability and severe physical defects. These conditions are often fatal in early infancy.

Why it's done
Your doctor can discuss with you any risks associated with the procedure. You may consider chromosomal microarray testing if:
- **Your ultrasound examination detected one or more structural abnormalities in the fetus.** If the results of your ultrasound examination identify a structural abnormality, such as a heart defect or brain abnormality, and amniocentesis or chorionic villus sampling testing is warranted, your doctor may recommend analyzing a sample by chromosomal microarray analysis.
- **You're undergoing amniocentesis or chorionic villus sampling.** If you're having other diagnostic testing for certain genetic conditions, your doctor may also recommend chromosomal microarray testing.
- **Your pregnancy ended in a miscarriage or stillbirth.** A chromosomal microarray analysis may be able to help your doctor determine the cause of fetal death during pregnancy.

Fetal surveillance

Under certain circumstances, your doctor may recommend tests to check on the overall health of your baby later in your pregnancy. Also called antenatal fetal testing, these tests include the biophysical profile, the nonstress test, the contraction stress test and umbilical artery Doppler analysis. The tests are used for patients with complications of pregnancy, such as growth problems of the fetus, hypertension in pregnancy and diabetes in pregnancy

Biophysical profile scoring

A biophysical profile combines an ultrasound exam with or without a nonstress test. Four or five factors of the fetus are monitored for a period of time, usually 30 minutes:

• Breathing
• Body movement
• Muscle tone
• Amount of amniotic fluid
• Nonstress test

Each of these factors is given a score, and all are added together for a final score. Each of the five factors is given a score of 2 or 0. If all five components are included, a perfect score is 10. If the nonstress test is not included in the evaluation a score of 8 is considered a perfect score. A score of 6 or less may be cause for concern.

Nonstress test

During the nonstress test, you typically recline in a chair while a recording device connected to an electronic monitor is attached to your abdomen. Fetal heart rate, uterine contractions and fetal movements are recorded.

Contraction stress test

A contraction stress test may be done to evaluate whether a fetus will tolerate labor (contractions) or for further evaluation after a mildly abnormal nonstress test or biophysical profile If your doctor recommends this test, you'll be given a medication that stimulates contractions. The effect of the contractions on the fetus is then monitored.

Umbilical artery Doppler analysis

Umbilical artery Doppler analysis is another method to evaluate your baby's health late in pregnancy. It's used to monitor blood flow through your baby's blood vessels. Doppler testing may be used to determine where and how fast the baby is distributing blood flow throughout its body, the umbilical cord and the placenta.

First Trimester

The first trimester of pregnancy can be difficult for an expectant mother and is the time when a developing embryo is most vulnerable. Virtually every organ in your baby's body is being formed during the first three months of pregnancy. Thus, the embryo is particularly sensitive.

It's difficult to comprehend how something as complex as a human being can emerge from the joining of a single egg and sperm. Every aspect of this process, from the creation of the smallest fingernail to the brain itself, is set into an exquisitely scripted timetable that's usually without complication. If complications occur, they can result in miscarriage or birth defect.

Changes in you

For you, the first three months of your pregnancy can seem like riding a roller coaster. You're delighted yet have some fears. If the pregnancy was unplanned, you may be losing sleep figuring out how you'll cope with this enormous change in your life. Physically, you may feel drained and find yourself napping whenever you get the opportunity. Rest assured that these weeks will pass quickly and so will most of the symptoms.

The first sign of pregnancy for most women is a missed menstrual period. If your periods are usually regular and suddenly you're a week late and you've had intercourse during your cycle, take a home pregnancy test. Sometimes, a woman will have what appears to be a period even though she is pregnant. However, the bleeding is usually light.

Many pregnant women experience breast tenderness. Your breasts may seem fuller and have a tingling sensation. Your nipples may be extremely sensitive. Sometimes the breasts actually hurt. Many pregnant women experience morning sickness, which may range from a slightly upset

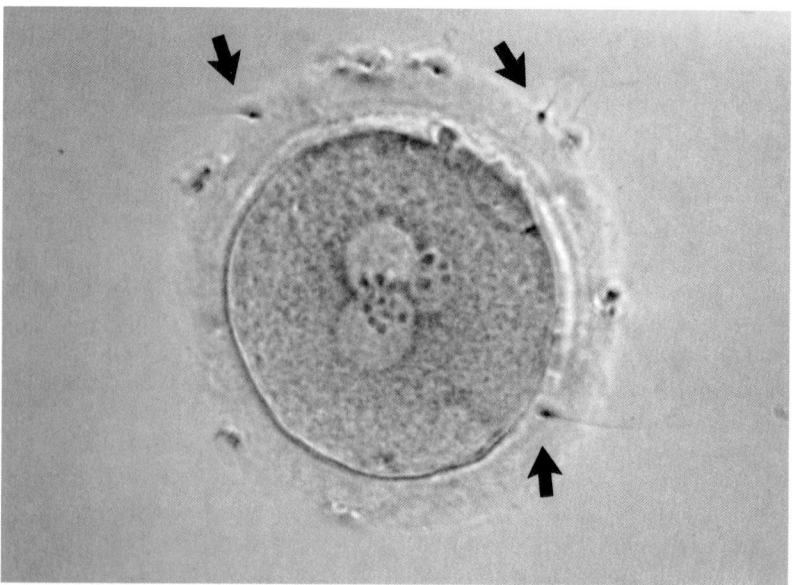

A recently fertilized ovum in an early stage of cell division. Some sperm entered the capsule but did not penetrate the egg (see arrows).

stomach to incessant vomiting. This often begins a few days after the first missed period.

Fatigue is common during early pregnancy. If you're home during the day, you'll probably find yourself lying down for a nap. If you work outside the home, you may arrive home so tired you can't wait to go to bed.

Frequent urination is another sign of pregnancy. This occurs because the growing uterus exerts pressure on the bladder in the pelvis. As the size of your uterus begins to increase in your abdomen, this symptom will diminish. However, in the final weeks of pregnancy it returns. Many women have difficulty sleeping through the night because of the need to urinate.

If you've missed a period and experienced some of these other signs and symptoms, give yourself a home pregnancy test.

Baby's development

So much happens to the fetus in the first three months. Still, the fetus is so small that a pregnant mother may not appear pregnant during the first trimester.

Fertilization

The process of fertilization begins with the penetration of the egg by a single sperm, one of the millions that traveled up the female reproductive system. Enzymes in the head of the sperm allow it to penetrate the firm capsule (zona pellucida) of the egg.

Swimming in an indirect path, the sperm swarm around the egg. Several sperm may begin to enter the outer egg capsule, but ultimately only one will enter the egg itself.

The egg and sperm each bring to the union 23 chromosomes containing thousands of genes. In these 46 chromosomes (23 from you and 23 from the father) is the genetic material that determines sex, physical characteristics —

such as eye, hair and skin color, body size and type, and facial features — creativity, and, to a large extent, intellectual capabilities and even personality. After the sperm penetrates to the center of the egg and the sperm and egg merge, fertilization is complete.

Cell division

The next step in the process is cell division. Within 12 hours, the new cell has divided into two cells, each of which then becomes two cells, and so on, with the number of cells doubling every 12 hours. It's now called a zygote.

The new zygote continues to make its way slowly down the fallopian tube to the uterus, regularly doubling its cell numbers and becoming a bit larger and much more complex. Within four to five days after fertilization, the zygote — by this time made up of 500 cells — reaches its destination inside the uterus.

By the time the zygote reaches the uterus, it has changed considerably from a solid mass of cells to a group of cells arranged around a fluid-filled cavity called a blastocyst. One section of the blastocyst contains a compact mass of cells that will ultimately produce an embryo. The outer layer of cells (trophoblast) will produce the placenta, which provides nourishment.

While all this has been taking place, the rest of the female reproductive system hasn't been idle. The ovaries have been secreting the hormone progesterone into the bloodstream. The result of this hormonal surge is a uterine lining that creates a perfect environment for implantation to take place.

Initially, the blastocyst doesn't bury deeply into the uterus. It clings to the surface of the uterus for a few days. Then the blastocyst releases an enzyme that allows the embryo to drop deeper into the lining,. Eight days have passed since fertilization took place. By

the 12th day, the blastocyst will be firmly embedded in its new home.

At this point, you're pregnant, although it's too early for you to have missed a period or to have any other symptoms of pregnancy. In some cases, a miscarriage can occur in these initial days and weeks after fertilization, often before a woman knows she was pregnant.

Organ formation

By the time the zygote burrows into the uterus, the placenta has begun to form. In another week, the rudiments of a spinal cord are evident and, within days, five to eight vertebrae are in place. In addition, the eyes and heart have begun to form.

It's during the third week after fertilization that the embryonic period begins. If you take a pregnancy test, the results will probably be positive.

Over the next few weeks, the components of a human being develop, although at first the human baby is similar in appearance to the developing babies of some other mammals. The head begins to form, as does the intestinal tract.

At the end of the sixth week, the brain becomes more noticeable, and arm and leg buds begin to appear.

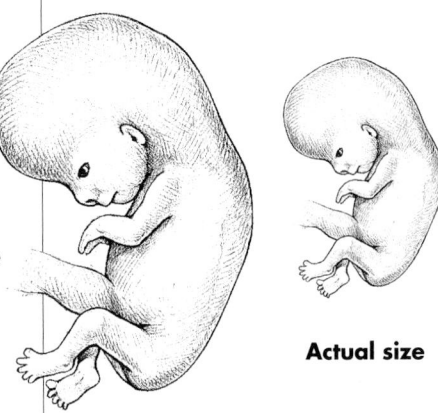

Actual size

At eight weeks after conception, all of the major body organs are formed and growing. The embryo is about 1½ inches long from head to rump and weighs less than half an ounce.

Cells that will later become either ovaries or testicles have appeared. By the seventh week, the chest and abdomen are fully formed, and the lungs are beginning to develop. The embryo measures slightly more than ½ inch and weighs a fraction of an ounce.

Your baby's face and features are forming in the eighth gestational week. Fingers and toes are beginning to develop, as are the ovaries or testicles. If the embryo is a male, his penis begins to appear at this time, though it's too early to see on an ultrasound. At the end of the second month of pregnancy, your baby looks much like a human infant, albeit in miniature.

By the 10th week, your baby's face is well-developed. The heart has four chambers and beats 120 to 160 times a minute. Using a Doppler instrument, your doctor often can hear the heartbeat between 10 and 12 weeks. At this point, the embryo is referred to as a fetus.

By the end of the first trimester, the fetus has a head that's disproportionately large compared with the rest of its body. Your baby is about 3 inches long and weighs little more than 1 ounce.

Possible problems

Having a baby today is safer than at any other time in history. We now know that a lot of problems can be prevented with good nutrition and regular prenatal care. But forming a new human being is still complex, and complications and problems do arise. Following are some of the troubles most common in the first trimester:

Miscarriage
Aside from the initial discomfort of pregnancy, the greatest threat in the first trimester is miscarriage (spontaneous abortion). Miscarriage and abortion refer to the ending of a pregnancy before 20 weeks. A fetus that is lost after 20 weeks and delivered after passing away is termed stillborn.

Some fertilized eggs spontaneously abort before a woman is aware she's pregnant. The percentage of miscarriages in women who know they're pregnant is as high as 20 percent. About 80 percent of these miscarriages occur during the first trimester. Factors associated with miscarriage include older maternal age, difficulty in becoming pregnant and a history of miscarriage.

In the first trimester, miscarriage almost always occurs after the death of the embryo or fetus. Why does an embryo pass away in the uterus? The most common cause of miscarriage — an estimated 60 percent — is an abnormality in development, usually as a result of chromosome problems. Other possible causes include infections, unrecognized diabetes in the mother and defects in the uterus.

Women who experience a miscarriage tend to blame themselves. It's natural to seek an explanation when a miscarriage occurs, but try not to blame yourself. Almost never is miscarriage the result of stress or trauma.

The first symptom of a potential miscarriage is usually vaginal bleeding that may occur with or without cramping.

Approximately 1 in 5 women have some vaginal bleeding or bloody discharge during the first trimester, and less than half of these women lose their babies. If you're bleeding but your cervix hasn't begun to dilate, this is called a threatened miscarriage. Such pregnancies often proceed without any further problems. However, if you have any bleeding, call your doctor immediately.

When the embryo or fetus dies, miscarriage is inevitable. An inevitable miscarriage is usually accompanied by pain in the lower abdomen or back. The pain may be dull and relentless or sharp and intermittent. Bleeding may be heavy and include passage of tissue. The tissue may include the embryo and placenta.

If all the pregnancy tissues pass through the vagina, it's considered a complete miscarriage. Sometimes, though, only some of the products of conception are expelled. When this occurs, it's called an incomplete abortion, and the pain and bleeding can continue for several days. If there's no bleeding — neither the fetus nor the placenta is expelled — but the fetus has died, it's termed a missed abortion. You may feel pregnant

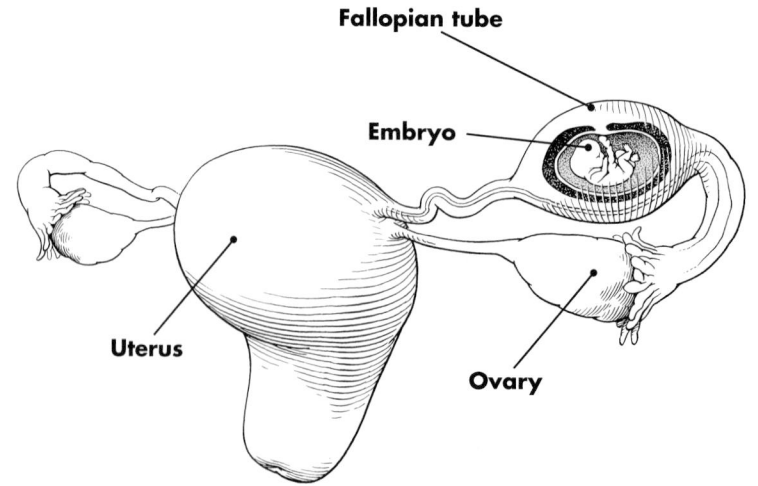

Potentially life-threatening, a tubal pregnancy occurs when a fertilized egg implants itself in the fallopian tube rather than the uterus. As the embryo develops, it causes the tube to expand beyond its capacity, causing bleeding (hemorrhaging) and potentially serious medical consequences.

and have no idea of a problem during a missed abortion, but the symptoms of pregnancy will eventually disappear. Your doctor may suspect miscarriage when your uterus fails to grow or when he or she can't detect a heartbeat during a visit. An ultrasound exam is often used to determine if you've experienced a missed abortion.

Once it starts, nothing can be done to prevent an inevitable, incomplete or missed abortion. With the use of vaginal ultrasound after spotting occurs, a doctor can usually tell if a miscarriage is inevitable.

When a miscarriage is inevitable, the mother has three options. The first is to wait for nature to take its course and the miscarriage to occur. This could take several weeks. Another option is a surgical procedure called a dilation and curettage (D&C), in which the deceased embryo and placenta are removed. Or, the mother can take the medication misoprostol (Cytotec), which will provoke a miscarriage.

Ectopic pregnancy

An ectopic (tubal) pregnancy is one in which a fertilized egg attaches itself in a place other than inside the uterus. The vast majority of ectopic pregnancies occur in a fallopian tube. They can also occur in the abdomen, ovary or cervix. Because the fallopian tube is too narrow to hold a growing baby, ectopic pregnancies can't proceed normally. Eventually, the walls of the fallopian tube stretch and burst, putting the mother in danger of life-threatening blood loss.

Pain and bleeding are usually the first signs of an ectopic pregnancy. You may feel sharp, stabbing pain in your pelvis, abdomen, or even your shoulder and neck. It may come and go, or get better and worse. Other warning signs of ectopic pregnancy include gastrointestinal symptoms, dizziness and lightheadedness. If you experience any of these signs or

Twins and Multiple Pregnancies

A multiple pregnancy occurs when more than one egg is fertilized (dizygotic, nonidentical or fraternal twins) or one egg splits after fertilization (monozygotic or identical twins). The majority of twins are fraternal. Having fraternal twins may run in some families. As the mother, your genes and family history will determine whether you have twins. The father's family history doesn't play a role.

Abnormal weight gain or size, an excessive amount of movement, and the detection of two heartbeats are common clues that you're carrying twins. Your doctor will discuss recommended weight gain and risks associated with a twin pregnancy. It will be important for you to adhere to the recommended prenatal checkup schedule. Regular prenatal care is especially important because twin pregnancies have a higher risk of growth problems, hypertensive problems during pregnancy (preeclampsia, gestational hypertension) and gestational diabetes.

Multiple pregnancies tend to be shorter, an average of 21 days shorter for women delivering twins. Unless there's a medical reason to indicate cesarean delivery, twins can be delivered vaginally. Women with twins who want to breast-feed can do so.

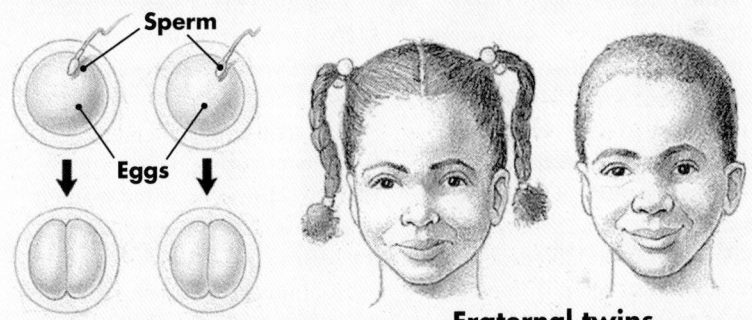

Fraternal twins

Fraternal twins (dizygotic or non-identical), the most common kind, occur when two eggs are fertilized by two different sperm, leading to two individuals who are no more closely related than other brothers and sisters in a family.

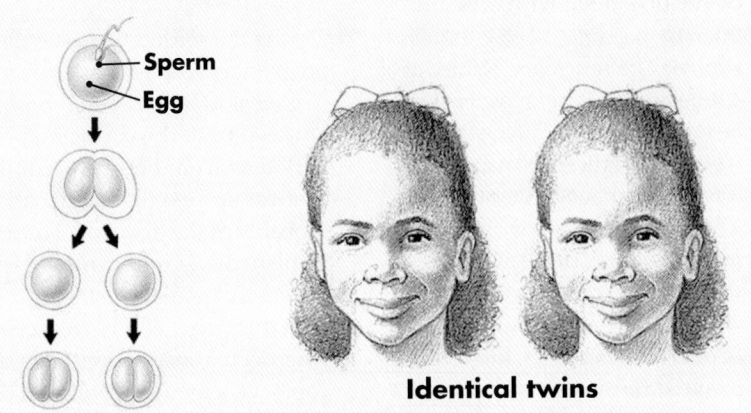

Identical twins

Identical twins (monozygotic) occur when a single fertilized egg, for reasons that are unclear, splits and develops into two individuals who are genetically identical.

symptoms, contact your doctor right away. There may be other possible causes for the signs and symptoms, but your doctor may first want to rule out an ectopic pregnancy.

Certain medical conditions tend to be associated with a higher risk of ectopic pregnancy. These include tubal adhesions caused by infection, appendicitis, endometriosis and the absence of one ovary. Women who've undergone in vitro fertilization (IVF) may also be more likely to experience an ectopic pregnancy.

If you have an ectopic pregnancy, initially you may not know that anything is wrong. If your doctor suspects an ectopic pregnancy, he or she will first do a pelvic examination to check for any abnormalities. An ultrasound examination or minimally invasive (laparoscopic) surgery may be done to confirm the presence of a mass.

If not detected early, an ectopic pregnancy may be very dangerous and is a leading cause of pregnancy-related death. Ectopic fetuses seldom develop beyond three months.

If you have an ectopic pregnancy, your doctor may want to operate immediately. If the embryo is still small and the fallopian tube hasn't been ruptured, the embryo may be cut out without further injury to the tube. Some doctors favor removing the injured part of the tube. If you've had heavy internal bleeding, a blood transfusion may be necessary. Removal of a tube and even of an ovary may be necessary.

Another option for managing ectopic pregnancy consists of using a powerful medication called methotrexate (Trexall, Xatmep) which causes embryonic cells to stop growing and eventually disappear. In most cases, this replaces the need for surgery.

Women who've had one or more previous ectopic pregnancies are at increased risk for having another one. If ectopic pregnancies have significantly injured both fallopian tubes but you still want to become pregnant, in vitro fertilization (see page 1188) may be an option.

Second Trimester

The middle part of the pregnancy is often the time when women feel their best. Usually, the morning sickness is improved, you have more energy, and you start looking pregnant and feeling better. This is also the time when you'll start to feel those gentle flutters that will soon turn into strong kicks and elbowing from your growing baby.

Although the second trimester is the easiest part of pregnancy for most women, it's not without risks.

Miscarriage is no longer the risk that it was during the first three months. However, some women begin premature labor during the second trimester, although it most often occurs during the third trimester. A fetus delivered before 23 weeks isn't mature enough to survive. Rest assured, though, that pregnancy loss in the second trimester is considered rare.

Changes in you

During the second trimester of pregnancy, your abdomen is enlarging slowly, and you'll probably need to start wearing maternity clothes. Your body is becoming rounder around the middle and probably at the hips, too. For most women, the second trimester is uneventful and enjoyable.

At this stage, you're still seeing your doctor once a month, unless you have a medical condition that warrants more-frequent visits. You're taking iron and folic acid supplements, and you're continuing to eat a balanced diet containing protein-rich foods, including milk products, fruits, vegetables and grains.

If you've been contemplating travel, now is probably the best time during pregnancy to take a trip. As your due date approaches, your increased size will tax your energies, and you may be more comfortable staying closer to home.

Baby's development

During the second trimester, the fetus grows, and the organs that formed during the previous weeks mature. At about 13 weeks, the fetus has tiny fingernails. The genitals are fully formed, and the sex can be determined with certain prenatal tests. The fetus can kick and move its toes. The mouth can open and close, and the fetus is able to bend its arms and make a fist.

By the end of the fourth month, you're likely to feel the first signs of life in your abdomen. The fetus's skin is pink and less transparent than it was previously. Fine hair covers the entire body. The first eyelashes and eyebrows begin to appear.

At 20 weeks, the fetus may have hair on its head. Fat deposits begin to appear beneath the wrinkled skin. The fetus is now 12 inches long and weighs about 1 pound. If it's born at this time, it will attempt to breathe but will not have a chance of surviving unless it's born at or after 23 weeks.

Possible problems

As your pregnancy progresses, sometimes new problems can emerge. While risks of miscarriage are greatly reduced, the concern now shifts to keeping the fetus growing and healthy in the uterus for the full term of the pregnancy.

Premature labor
Normally, labor occurs about 40 weeks (280 days) after the first day of your last period. If your baby is born between 37 and 42

weeks, delivery is considered to be at term. Sometimes, labor begins before term. You may have vaginal bleeding, mild to severe abdominal contractions, increased vaginal discharge, or a gush or trickle of fluid from your vagina as your membranes rupture (water breaks).

Most often the precise cause of midpregnancy labor is never determined. However, the following conditions are associated with premature (preterm) labor: spontaneous rupture of membranes, cervical infection, incompetent cervix, abnormal uterus, polyhydramnios, abnormal fetus or placenta, placenta previa — a condition in which the placenta covers the cervix — a retained intrauterine contraceptive device, preeclampsia and eclampsia, death of the fetus, history of premature delivery, multiple fetuses, cigarette smoking, bleeding (hemorrhaging), drug use (cocaine), serious maternal disease, and age. Teenagers and women older than age 40 are more likely to have premature labor.

Rupture of your membranes usually occurs after labor has begun, but occasionally it's the first sign of labor. If you have contractions that last for at least 30 seconds and occur every 10 minutes, and if your cervix is thinning and dilating, you're in labor.

Premature labor can be an ominous sign. The less time your infant has had in your womb, the less its chances of survival. In recent years, however, major advances have been made in the care of seriously ill or premature infants. Babies as small as 1 pound now have a chance of survival when cared for in specialized neonatal units.

A reasonable chance for survival of the baby is now being realized as early as 23 weeks of gestation. Still, these babies often have serious, lifelong physical and intellectual developmental problems.

The treatment for premature labor varies and depends on the age of the fetus. Initially, getting rest and drinking plenty of fluid may help. This precaution alone is sometimes successful in stopping contractions. Cultures from the cervix and preventive antibiotics also may be considered because infection is believed to be one cause of premature labor.

There's no specific medication that's always successful in stopping premature labor. But several have had some degree of success. Under most circumstances, medications that can delay delivery are used only long enough to prepare for the delivery, such as getting the mother to a hospital equipped to care for premature babies. The drugs aren't used long term because they may pose risks and aren't effective over the long term.

Women at high-risk of premature labor and with a history of preterm delivery are sometimes given weekly shots of a form of the hormone progesterone. Studies have found the hormone can reduce the risk of early labor in some women.

If you have a history of premature labor resulting from a shortened cervix, sometimes an operation can be done to reduce the chances of premature labor. A procedure called cerclage involves placing surgical stitches (sutures) around the cervix so that the infant can stay in the uterus until term.

Another cause of prematurity occurs when your doctor needs to induce labor early because the uterine environment appears to be increasingly harmful to your baby and its chances of survival are better outside the uterus. This is rare in the second trimester and, if it does occur, usually doesn't happen until after 28 weeks of gestation.

Placenta previa

In placenta previa, the placenta is located partially or completely over the cervix. You may have painless bleeding from your vagina, usually at the end of the second trimester or later.

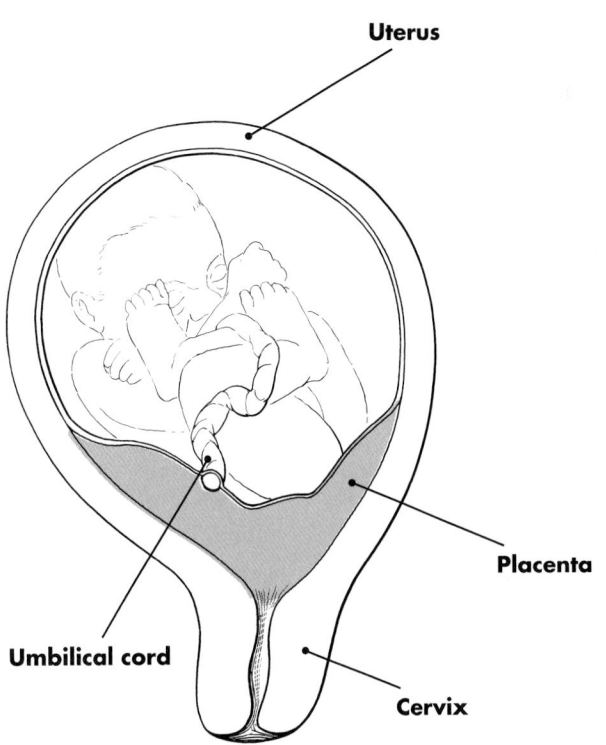

In a condition called placenta previa, the placenta is located over the cervix. Painless bleeding may occur. If you have bleeding in pregnancy, contact your doctor immediately.

Approximately 1 in 200 pregnancies that go beyond the seventh month have placenta previa. Uncommon in first pregnancies, placenta previa is more likely to occur in women who have had more than one cesarean delivery, who have experienced placenta previa in previous pregnancies or who have had several previous births. Women who smoke also are at increased risk of this condition.

If your doctor suspects placenta previa, he or she may request an ultrasound examination. Occasionally, magnetic resonance imaging (MRI) is necessary.

Bleeding with placenta previa can be severe and threaten the life of the mother and baby. If there are two or more episodes of bleeding prior to 36 weeks, you may be hospitalized for the duration of the pregnancy.

Polyhydramnios

Polyhydramnios refers to a condition in which an increased amount of amniotic fluid surrounds the baby. It occurs in about 1 to 2 percent of pregnancies. Polyhydramnios can increase the risk of preterm labor. Severe cases may be caused by certain birth defects in the fetus, particularly with malformations of the central nervous system and gastrointestinal or genitourinary tract. Women with diabetes and those carrying multiple fetuses have a higher incidence of experiencing mild polyhydramnios than do other pregnant women.

Mild cases of polyhydramnios may resolve on their own. Severe polyhydramnios may require treatment, such as draining the excess amniotic fluid.

Incompetent cervix

If you have an incompetent cervix, the lower portion of your uterus opens during the second trimester or early part of the third trimester. The result is a miscarriage or premature delivery.

If your medical history indicates a possible incompetent cervix, a cerclage may be placed to hold the cervix closed during pregnancy. Cerclage placement is a surgical procedure that involves placement of a strong suture in a purse-string fashion to prevent early opening of the cervix. Usually, the cerclage is removed late in pregnancy or at the time of delivery.

Third Trimester

During the third trimester of pregnancy, what seemed so far off just a few months ago is now close! If you haven't done so yet, it's a good time to start practicing relaxation techniques for labor. Toward the end of this trimester, your baby has less room to move around and often settles down into position for labor.

The vast majority of women deliver near term and have no major complications. The problem of premature labor may occur in the third trimester as well as in the second, but the later in pregnancy it occurs, the better the outlook for the infant.

Some serious conditions are associated with late pregnancy. Preeclampsia and eclampsia are dangerous conditions that, when not detected early, can cause both fetal and maternal complications. Your doctor will watch for other conditions including bleeding, premature rupture of membranes and intrauterine growth restriction. Should these occur, specific recommendations for further evaluation and management will be made.

Changes in you

No matter how good you've felt, this is probably the point when you may becoming tired of pregnancy. Your maternity clothes are getting tight. Your walk has given way to the pregnant waddle. You may notice stretch marks on your breasts and abdomen. Your feet and ankles may be swollen. You may be exhausted.

You can't seem to get comfortable at night, and when you do the baby starts kicking. Finally, the kicking stops and you sleep an hour or two, and then you wake up with a strong urge to urinate. You may awaken the next morning feeling like you've been up all night.

During the last trimester of pregnancy, many couples attend classes in preparation for childbirth. These classes teach you about the birth process, about exercises you can do to strength-

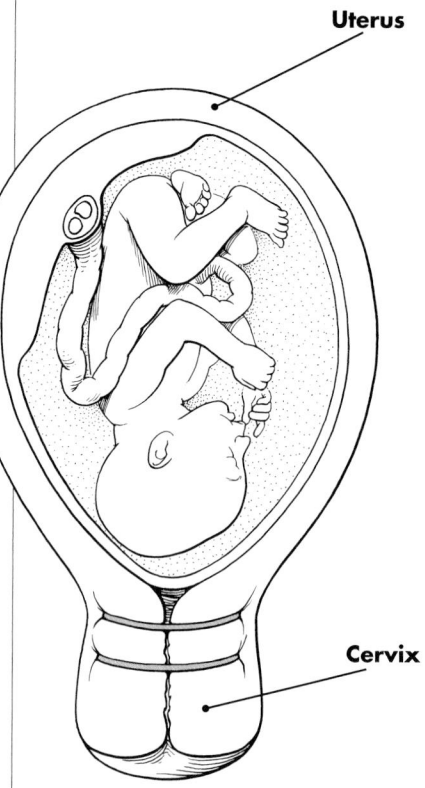

Uterus

Cervix

If the lower portion of your uterus (cervix) shortens during pregnancy, a surgical procedure may be done to prevent premature delivery of your baby. Called cerclage, this procedure involves stitching the cervix closed to prevent opening of the cervix and early delivery of the fetus.

en your pelvic muscles, enabling you to push more effectively, and about relaxation and breathing techniques that may help to relieve some of the pain during labor. These classes are beneficial for all first-time parents!

Many women, particularly those who've previously miscarried in early pregnancy, understandably are relieved to reach the late stage of pregnancy. With proper treatment in a specialized neonatal unit, babies born after 30 weeks have a good chance of survival. But there's no substitute for a full-term pregnancy. Therefore, one of your doctor's goals is to prevent premature labor whenever possible.

Your visits to the doctor after 36 weeks will be every one to two weeks until delivery, unless you have a medical problem that warrants more-frequent visits.

Baby's development

The fetus gains most of its weight after 27 weeks. At the beginning of this last phase of development, the fetus weighs almost 2 pounds. The average baby is born 12 weeks later weighing an average of 7½ pounds.

When you're 28 weeks pregnant, your baby is covered with a thick, white protective coating called vernix. The infant is able to blink its eyes, and an infant born at this time can cry weakly and move its limbs. Although infants born at this stage weigh about only 2 pounds and may experience significant medical problems, the vast majority of them survive because of advances in the care of premature and ill newborns.

One month later, the male infant's testicles descend into the scrotum. The infant now weighs about 3 pounds, 12 ounces. With proper care, most of these infants do well.

An infant born at term, 40 weeks after the mother's last menstrual period, has more body fat and is less wrinkled than babies born preterm or before 37 weeks gestational age. The skin may or may not still be covered with vernix. Most of the fine body hair is gone, although the shoulders and arms may still have a light covering. The fingernails and toenails may be long enough to trim.

Possible problems

Chances are, especially if you've been healthy to this point, the third trimester will be medically uneventful for you and your baby. But some serious problems of pregnancy do occur in the third trimester, and it's important to be aware of them.

Preeclampsia and eclampsia
Preeclampsia is a serious complication of pregnancy. It's critical to address preeclampsia, or it may cause harm to you, to your baby or to both of you. The signs and symptoms are:

Preeclampsia
• High blood pressure
• Excessive protein in the urine (proteinuria)
• Pain in the upper right side of the abdomen
• Severe headache
• Vision disturbances, including seeing flashing lights
Eclampsia is preeclampsia with:
• Convulsions
• Unconsciousness
Preeclampsia can be a serious disease of late pregnancy that must be treated. In the United States, preeclampsia occurs in about 3 to 6 percent of all pregnancies.

Preeclampsia and eclampsia are likely related to an abnormal growth of the placenta, in which the placenta attaches abnormally into the wall of the uterus. The only known treatment for preeclampsia and eclampsia is delivery of the baby.

If preeclampsia develops, you may not know it. Initially, you may feel fine because high blood

? **Question and Answer**

What's the difference between pre-labor contractions and true labor?

Many women have one or more bouts of false labor before real labor begins. False labor is more likely to occur in the final weeks of pregnancy and in women who have already born a child.

How can you distinguish false labor from true labor? With false labor you'll have contractions, but they'll usually be irregular and won't increase in frequency and intensity, as true contractions do. Moreover, the pain will be in the lower abdomen and groin, whereas true labor pains begin higher in the uterus and radiate down the abdomen and lower back.

When your labor is false, walking may stop the contractions, whereas with true labor, walking generally has no effect.

If you have doubts about your labor symptoms, seek medical advice. Many pregnant women have postponed going to the hospital, convinced it was only a false alarm, only to give birth before reaching the hospital.

pressure and protein in the urine usually don't cause any symptoms. This is one reason it's so important to keep your prenatal appointments.

Preeclampsia can have severe consequences, including eclampsia, growth restriction of the baby, placental abruption, uncontrolled hypertension, fluid in the lungs (pulmonary edema) and coagulation problems in the mother. Teenage mothers, women older than age 40, women in their first pregnancy, women with a history of high blood pressure, women who are carrying twins and women who are carrying a pregnancy conceived with a donor egg are all are at higher risk of preeclampsia and eclampsia.

If you develop very mild preeclampsia, your doctor will monitor your fetus closely and may give you instructions and precautions for outpatient management until 37 weeks gestation. This may be all the treatment that's necessary.

If the condition is more serious, you may require hospitalization, during which you may be given medications to control your blood pressure and prevent seizures. The best treatment for severe preeclampsia is delivery of the baby. If you're at or beyond 34 weeks of pregnancy, your doctor may recommend delivery of your baby. If you're less than 37 weeks gestation, your doctor may recommend that you receive steroids to help with development of your baby's lungs before delivery. You and your baby will be monitored carefully to make sure neither of you is in danger.

After delivery, symptoms of preeclampsia usually become less severe, although in some women preeclampsia or eclampsia can still develop during the first 24 hours after delivery and rarely, later. Eclampsia isn't as frequent as it once was. If it does occur, your doctor will likely recommend delivery after your condition is stable. Because of improved prenatal care, the vast majority of women with preeclampsia never progress to eclampsia.

Antepartum bleeding

If you have vaginal bleeding (hemorrhage) after the fifth month of pregnancy, you're experiencing pre-birth (antepartum) bleeding. Many conditions can cause antepartum bleeding in middle or late pregnancy, including placenta previa — a condition in which the placenta covers the cervix — cervical damage or separation of the placenta from the uterine wall.

Report any bleeding during pregnancy to your doctor immediately. He or she will try to determine the cause of the problem. You may need to be hospitalized for examination and tests.

Most often, antepartum bleeding is mild and no damage is done. However, if bleeding becomes heavy, it can be dangerous for both you and your baby. If the bleeding poses a threat, early delivery of the infant may be warranted.

Premature rupture of membranes

Normally, the membranes that surround the fetus rupture either just before or during labor. Occasionally, though, these membranes rupture weeks or months before the anticipated delivery date. If you feel a gush or a constant dribble of fluid from your vagina, your membranes may have ruptured, an event commonly referred to as your water breaking.

No one knows why membranes rupture prematurely, although growing data point to infection as a main cause. Call your doctor immediately. You'll likely be hospitalized. Amniocentesis or collection of vaginal fluid may be done to determine if your infant's lungs are mature enough for it to survive an early delivery.

When premature rupture of your membranes occurs, there's a high risk that your labor will begin within a few days. In addition, there's a risk of infection once the membranes have ruptured.

If you're at or beyond 34 weeks of pregnancy, your doctor will recommend delivery. If you're less than 34 weeks gestational age, there are no signs of infection, and your baby is stable, you will be given antibiotics to prevent infection and steroids to help your baby's lungs mature. This can delay delivery, but risk of serious infection remains, so your condition must be monitored closely.

Placental abruption

Separation of the placenta from the uterine wall (placental abruption) before labor begins can decrease or interrupt the flow of oxygen-rich blood to the baby. Separation may be partial, involving only a part of the placenta, such as an edge, or the entire placenta may be separated from the uterine wall.

Women who have high blood pressure during their pregnancies — whether the condition first developed while they were pregnant or was present before — are more prone to placental abruption.

Placental abruption is one the leading causes of fetal death in the third trimester. It can also cause the mother to have severe circulatory problems or go into shock as a result of severe bleeding. Fortunately, with close monitoring of the mother and baby and prompt delivery at signs of trouble, the outlook for both is good.

Intrauterine death

Most fetal deaths occur as miscarriages in the first weeks of pregnancy. Occasionally, though, a fetus will die after the fifth month of gestation. In the United States, approximately 6 stillbirths occur for every 1,000 live births.

Several conditions may be associated with intrauterine death, including preeclampsia and eclampsia, maternal diabetes, antepartum bleeding, genetic conditions, severe congenital abnormalities, and postmaturity.

The causes of many fetal deaths remain unknown.

Usually, the death of a fetus is silent. One day you may notice that you don't feel the baby move as you used to. When the doctor fails to detect a heartbeat, he or she will likely use ultrasound to determine if the fetus is still alive. Your doctor may want to do an amniocentesis to see if the cause of death can be determined.

Most often, labor begins within two weeks after fetal death, although it may be longer in middle pregnancy. If your labor doesn't begin on its own, you may be given medications to induce it.

In most cases, the outlook for future pregnancies is the same as for first pregnancies. The biggest hurdle is the grief that every couple must work through after an intrauterine death.

Prolonged pregnancy

The average pregnancy lasts 40 weeks from the onset of the last menstrual period. Prolonged pregnancy (postmaturity) describes a pregnancy that lasts beyond 42 weeks.

As with prematurity, postmaturity is associated with certain risks. These include a slightly increased risk of fetal death, a newborn who is significantly larger than normal (macrosomia), low amniotic fluid (oligohydramnios) and the fetus's passage of stool (meconium) into the amniotic fluid.

Occasionally in a postmaturity baby, fetal growth may be halted altogether, and the infant may no longer be receiving the needed nutrients from the placenta. As a result, the stillbirth rate of these babies is twice that of those babies born after a pregnancy of normal length.

If your pregnancy extends beyond 41 weeks, your doctor may recommend fetal surveillance testing, such as fetal nonstress and biophysical profile scoring. Your doctor will probably induce labor, provided he or she is sure that the baby is indeed overdue and there hasn't been a mistake in calculating the time of conception.

Labor and Delivery

For many women, labor and delivery is the part of pregnancy that they look to with anticipation and, often, nervousness. If you've never been through labor before, you may wonder what it will be like and you may worry how you'll make it through.

Try to relax. Most women make it through labor without any problem because women's bodies are made to accommodate labor and delivery. Although giving birth can be difficult work, learning more about the process and practicing relaxation techniques can help make your birthing experience go smoothly.

First signs of labor

"How will I know when labor begins?" That's sometimes a difficult question to answer because each woman and each pregnancy are different. Maybe this is your first child, and you're confused by the advice of friends and relatives. Some people tell you that labor will be the toughest hours of your life, and others say that it won't be so bad. Perhaps you've already delivered a child and you expect this labor to be similar to your previous one.

Whatever you expect, expect the unexpected. Every labor is different. But some good indicators can let you know that labor is beginning or about ready to begin:
1. A few days or hours before labor actually begins, you may have what's called bloody show. This is the discharge of a small amount of blood-tinged mucus. It often occurs due to early changes of the cervix.
2. The membranes that surround the amniotic fluid may rupture at the beginning of labor or as the labor progresses. When your water breaks (membranes rupture), you may feel a gush or slow trickle of fluid from your vagina. Contact your provider if your water breaks.
3. Contractions may or may not be a sign that you're in labor. Throughout pregnancy, you may have noticed your uterus contracting. These contractions are called Braxton Hicks contractions, and they usually don't cause discomfort until the last weeks of pregnancy. Many women have these contractions and believe they're in labor. It's often difficult for pregnant women to distinguish between Braxton Hicks contractions and those of real labor.

As a rule, the contractions of real labor occur at regular intervals. The period between contractions slowly begins to get shorter, and the contractions become longer and more intense. The pain usually begins high in the uterus and radiates down the abdomen and to the lower back. Real labor contractions don't go away if you lie down and relax. If your contractions get longer, stronger and more frequent, chances are they're the real thing.

If you have any of these symptoms, notify your doctor or go to the hospital. Your doctor will likely want to examine you to see if your cervix is dilating and thinning (effacing), signs that the baby is getting ready to be born. If your membranes rupture, your doctor probably will want you to go to the hospital as soon as possible.

Abnormal fetal positions

Between 32 and 34 weeks, most babies will settle into the headfirst position in preparation for labor. During a normal labor, the infant will deliver headfirst (cephalic or vertex), with the baby facing toward the mother's back This position is called occiput anterior. Occasionally, however, a baby enters the world in another position. If your baby is in an abnormal position, this may cause problems during labor and may warrant special care through delivery.

Occiput posterior
Occiput posterior position is when the infant's head is positioned near

the cervix (cephalic presentation), but its face is toward the mother's front. This presentation can make it difficult for the infant to travel down the birth canal.

This position can delay delivery, especially if the infant is large. Your doctor may try to manually rotate the infant to the occiput anterior position. Forceps may also be used for delivery.

Breech
Breech presentation occurs when the infant's buttocks or one or both feet are closest to the cervix. It's the most common of the abnormal presentations. If your baby is breech, it's positioned with its buttocks near your cervix. Thus,

either the buttocks or feet emerge first instead of the head.

Factors associated with breech presentation include preterm delivery, uterine abnormalities, placenta previa and multiple gestation (twins, triplets). Breech delivery can cause problems for you and your baby, including the umbilical cord dropping into the vagina ahead of the baby (umbilical cord prolapse) and entrapment of the baby's head in the birth canal. In general, cesarean delivery is the safer option for babies in breech presentation. One exception is breech delivery of the second twin after cephalic delivery of the first twin.

If your infant is in the breech position in the last weeks of pregnan-

cy (generally 37 to 39 weeks), your doctor may attempt to turn the baby externally. This is referred to as external cephalic version (ECV). If the baby doesn't turn before labor, your doctor will recommend a cesarean delivery.

Transverse
Transverse presentation occurs when the infant lies crosswise in the uterus, usually with the shoulder over the birth canal. This presentation is more common in women who have had four or more children. Prematurity and placenta previa are other conditions associated with the transverse presentation.

Vaginal delivery isn't possible in the transverse position, as an infant can't move through the birth canal in this position. If your baby is transverse at 37 weeks, your doctor may attempt ECV. If your baby remains transverse at 39 weeks, cesarean delivery likely will be scheduled.

Facing up
The facing up position occurs when a baby is facing up rather than down after descending to the midpelvis. It is also known as the occiput posterior position. Intense back labor and prolonged labor may accompany this position.

Your doctor might have you change your position to help your uterus drop forward and help the baby rotate. He or she might also try to rotate the baby manually during vaginal examination. If these techniques aren't successful, you may need to undergo a cesarean delivery. Most babies can be born faceup, but it may take a bit longer.

Abnormal angle
Abnormal angle presentation occurs when a baby enters the birth canal with the top of the head, the forehead or the face presenting first — none of which is a preferred position. If your baby's head moves through your pelvis

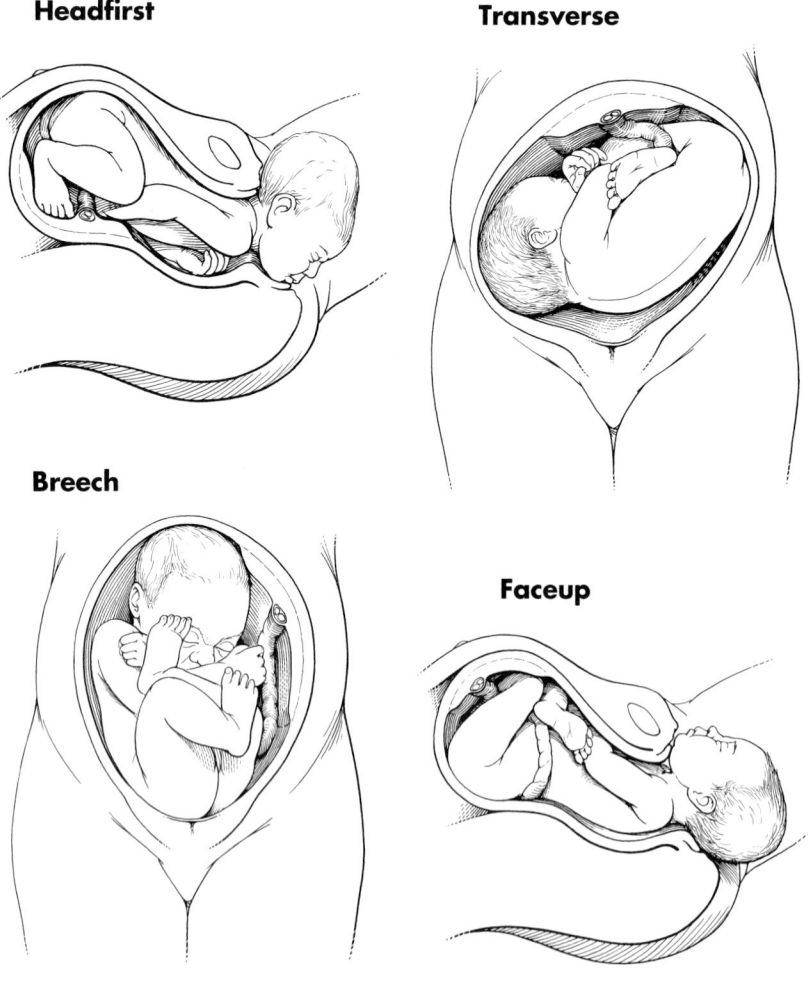

Headfirst

Transverse

Breech

Faceup

At the time of delivery, the normal position for the unborn baby is headfirst, with the face toward the mother's back. This position is called occiput anterior. Other presentations include transverse, breech and occiput posterior.

at an abnormal angle, it can affect the location and intensity of your discomfort and the length of your labor.

A cesarean delivery may be necessary if your baby isn't progressing down the birth canal or shows signs he or she isn't tolerating labor.

Stages of labor

As a rule, labor is usually longer with first babies. The cervix and birth canal of a first-time mother are less flexible, and therefore it takes longer for labor and birth. A first-time mother generally can expect about 14 hours to pass between the time she goes into active labor and the birth of her baby. Some women, however, are in labor much longer. For women who have previously given birth, the average time is between four and eight hours. Labor is divided into three stages:

First stage
The first stage of labor is the longest. During this stage, your cervix — the narrow passageway between your uterus and vagina — opens so that the baby can pass into the birth canal. When labor begins, the cervix is about 3 to 4 centimeters (1½ inches) in length and almost closed.

Contractions cause the cervix to open (dilate) by creating pressure within the uterus. This force is strong and is directed through the uterus in two ways. The contractions cause the cervix to thin (efface) and pull up around the baby's head. Repeated contractions eventually stretch the cervix open. The cervix is fully dilated when it's open to a diameter of 10 centimeters.

During the first stage of labor, contractions become more frequent and last longer. Once you're admitted to labor and delivery, fetal monitors may be used to monitor contractions and your baby's heart rate. Your doctor or

a nurse periodically does a pelvic examination to determine how you're progressing. If the contractions aren't forceful enough to open the cervix, he or she may recommend a medication to help with contractions.

Sometimes, labor doesn't progress normally. When this occurs, it can be because the contractions are poorly coordinated or not strong enough. If the cause is inadequate contractions, the uterus can be stimulated to contract by the intravenous infusion of a medication such as oxytocin (Pitocin). In most cases, this is successful. If not, a cesarean delivery may be necessary.

Conditions that can obstruct delivery include a head that's too large to pass down the birth canal or the positioning of the baby's head.

Second stage
The second stage of labor is when your baby is born. Your cervix is now fully dilated and effaced. This is the baby's signal to start the journey down the birth canal.

Once the cervix no longer offers resistance, each contraction serves to propel the infant downward. You may feel a strong urge to push, similar to that of a bowel movement. Sometimes, this urge occurs before the cervix is fully dilated. Your doctor will check your cervix to make sure that it's time to push. Push only when you're having a contraction. In this way, two forces — that of the contraction and your pushing — combine to move the baby and conserve your energy.

Both the first and the second stages of labor are longer for first-time mothers. On average, it takes about two hours to push a first baby out, whereas women who have previously given birth usually complete the second stage in 15 to 60 minutes.

As you push and the baby begins to move, the vaginal opening becomes more and more dilated

and begins to bulge. It takes several more minutes for the vulva to stretch to allow delivery.

After you've pushed the baby's head out, you may be instructed to stop pushing for a moment while your doctor makes sure that the umbilical cord is not wrapped around the baby. Then, you're encouraged to push again and with just a few more pushes, your baby is born.

Unless there's a problem, your baby is placed in your arms. The umbilical cord that connects the baby to the placenta may be cut shortly after. After delivery, your baby will be weighed and examined. If you and your baby are doing well, this can be delayed until after you have had "skin-to-skin" time with your new baby.

Third stage
The third stage of labor is delivery of the placenta. Your uterus continues to contract to expel the placenta, but you'll likely feel mild pain or no pain. The uterus continues to contract after expelling the placenta, but these are generally milder contractions.

Pain relief

Some women go through the entire labor process with no pain medication. Many women, however, choose pain relief. The decision to use medication for pain relief during labor is yours, but you should discuss medications for labor with your doctor.

What you decide to use, if anything, depends on your preferences, your doctor's recommendations, what's available at the medical facility you've chosen and the specific character of your labor.

Learn about the different options ahead of time so that you can make knowledgeable choices regarding pain medication. Be sure to remain flexible, however, because you may need to change your mind if things don't go as you planned.

Narcotics

Various narcotics may be injected into a muscle in your thigh or buttock or given through an intravenous (IV) catheter. If you have an IV, you may be able to control your dosage. The medication takes effect in minutes.

Narcotics decrease the perception of pain for two to six hours. They promote rest without causing muscle weakness. They may, however, cause sleepiness and temporarily depress breathing for you or your baby. Your baby may experience temporarily slowed reflexes as well. For these reasons, narcotic pain medications are typically not administered during the second stage of labor when delivery is near.

Local anesthetics

A local anesthetic is a medication that's injected directly into tissues, much as a dentist numbs your mouth before drilling. The simplest local anesthetic used during the birthing process is one that numbs you before an episiotomy is made or a tear is repaired. It doesn't provide pain relief during labor.

Pudendal block

A pudendal block is injected into the vaginal wall. This type of pain relief may be used shortly before delivery to block pain between the vagina and anus (perineum). Because it affects just the vagina and rectum, it gives no relief to pain caused by contractions.

Epidurals, spinal blocks and combined spinal epidurals

Epidurals, spinal blocks and combined spinal epidurals involve an injection of narcotics, an anesthetic or a combination of the two into the space surrounding the spinal nerves. These procedures temporarily block pain from the chest level down. They can be used for labor as well as for an episiotomy and a cesarean birth. Their use, however, requires the services of an anesthesiologist.

Epidurals, spinal blocks, and combined spinal epidurals are the most effective forms of anesthesia for childbirth. You can receive good pain relief but still be awake and alert, able to push, and able to enjoy your baby's birth.

Electronic fetal monitoring

Electronic fetal monitoring is commonly used to record the unborn baby's heart rate during labor. It allows your doctor to pick up heartbeat irregularities that may indicate concern. Monitoring can be done externally before or during labor. Internal monitoring may be done during labor after your water breaks.

External monitoring

In external monitoring, two wide straps are placed around the mother's abdomen. One measures and records the length and frequency of contractions. A second monitor is used to check the baby's heart rate. It holds a transducer that records the baby's heart rate. The gauge and transducer are connected to a monitor that displays and prints out both tracings simultaneously so that their interaction can be observed.

Internal monitoring

If more detailed monitoring is necessary during labor, or if there are difficulties with external monitoring, your doctor may recommend internal monitoring. Internal monitoring involves placing a tiny electrode on the baby's head to monitor its heart rate. This is done after the water has broken (membranes have ruptured).

A narrow, pressure-sensitive tube (intrauterine pressure catheter, or IUPC) may also be inserted between the wall of your uterus and the baby to measure the strength of your contractions. Your contractions and the response of the baby's heart to these contractions are then recorded. If the baby's heart rate indicates possible distress, your doctor may use measures such as oxygen or repositioning of the mother to improve the baby's response to contractions. The monitoring may also help to determine if the baby is not tolerating labor and needs to be delivered by cesarean section.

Procedures

Sometimes labor fails to start or progress. If labor is prolonged or complications develop, you may require some medical assistance.

Induction of labor

Sometimes, it's necessary to initiate (induce) labor. Most labor inductions occur because there is concern about the mother or baby's health.

The most common medical reasons for inducing labor include preeclampsia and premature rupture of the membranes. In addition, labor may be induced when the doctor has a concern about the health of the fetus or the baby is overdue.

Synthetic forms of the natural chemicals that trigger contractions in your uterus (prostaglandins) can be used to soften and dilate your cervix. Misoprostol (Cytotec) is one such drug. Dinoprostone (Cervidil, Prepidil, Prostin E2) is another.

Episiotomy

An episiotomy is an incision made in the tissue of the perineum during childbirth. The episiotomy may be easier to repair than an extensive tear. Although an episiotomy was once a routine part of childbirth, that's no longer the case. Research has found that a routine episiotomy does not reduce problems such as extensive tearing.

Researchers say there's no need for a routine episiotomy, but the procedure is still warranted in some cases. Your health care provider may recommend an episiotomy if:

- Extensive vaginal tearing appears very likely
- Your baby is in an abnormal position
- Your baby needs to be delivered quickly
- Your doctor is performing assisted (operative) vaginal delivery (use of forceps or vacuum)

If you need an episiotomy, you'll receive an injection of a local anesthetic to numb the tissue if you haven't had any other type of anesthesia or your anesthesia is no longer numbing the area. You won't feel your doctor making the incision or repairing it later.

To soften the vaginal tissues for delivery, some doctors suggest massaging the area between the vaginal opening and anus in the last weeks of pregnancy. This is known as perineal massage. Although there are no guarantees — and you don't have to do it if the idea makes you uncomfortable — stretching the tissues may reduce vaginal trauma during delivery.

Assisted (operative) vaginal delivery

Sometimes your doctor may use assisted (operative) vaginal delivery methods in the second stage of labor (the pushing stage), after the cervix is fully dilated. This may be done when labor stops progressing or when there are signs that the baby isn't tolerating labor.

Forceps

Forceps are shaped like a pair of spoons that, when attached to each other, look like a pair of salad tongs. They're used to assist vaginal delivery of the infant when the delivery isn't progressing as it should or when signs of fetal stress are evident.

Forceps may be used when labor stops progressing in the second stage, when the baby is abnormally positioned or when there are signs that the baby isn't tolerating labor. Sometimes, use of forceps may be necessary if the mother doesn't have the strength to push the baby out or if the mother has a health condition that limits the amount of pushing recommended (such as a maternal cardiac condition). The chance for vaginal tearing is associated with the use of forceps, and your doctor may recommend an episiotomy with a forceps delivery.

Complications from forceps deliveries are relatively rare. Occasionally, temporary bruises to an infant's face can occur.

Vacuum-assisted vaginal delivery

A vacuum may be used instead of forceps. Your doctor will decide if forceps or vacuum is more appropriate for your specific situation. A flexible cup is fitted near the crown of the baby's head, a pump creates suction, and your doctor gently guides the instrument to ease the baby down the birth canal while the mother pushes. The vacuum extractor cup doesn't take as much room as forceps and is associated with fewer injuries to the mother.

Cesarean delivery

A cesarean delivery is a surgical procedure used to deliver your baby through an incision in your abdomen. Cesarean delivery today accounts for approximately 30 percent of all births in the United States.

When is cesarean delivery necessary?

Cesarean delivery may be performed for many different reasons. In some situations — such as breech presentation, placental problems, multiples (twins, triplets), certain maternal health conditions or uterine abnormalities — a woman may know that she's going to have a cesarean delivery. In other situations, a cesarean delivery can't be predicted, such as when there's an abnormal fetal heart rate pattern during labor or when labor doesn't progress normally.

After one cesarean delivery, the need for a cesarean delivery with subsequent pregnancies will depend on the type of uterine incision that was made in the uterus to deliver the baby. Your doctor will review details of the cesarean delivery and determine whether you're a candidate for future vaginal deliveries.

The procedure

Knowing what to expect during a cesarean delivery can help decrease any fear or anxiety. A cesarean delivery is performed in an operating room. An operating room is a busy place, with teams from anesthesia, obstetrics, pediatrics, and nurses taking care of you and your baby. In most cases, epidural or spinal anesthesia is used so that you're awake for the delivery of your baby.

In some situations, such as an emergency cesarean delivery, general anesthesia will need to be used, and you'll be asleep. Usually, a catheter is placed in your bladder before surgery and is removed as soon as you're able to walk to the bathroom. If you have a planned cesarean birth, you'll receive instructions about fasting before your delivery.

It usually takes a little less than an hour to perform a normal cesarean delivery. Two types of incisions on the skin may be used. One is the so-called bikini cut (Pfannenstiel incision), which is a horizontal incision near the pubic hair line; this is the most commonly used incision. The other is a vertical cut from the navel to the pubis.

An incision is also made on the uterus in one of two ways. The most common method is a horizontal incision in the lower part of the uterus, called a low transverse uterine incision. This incision heals better and is associated with less chance of uterine rupture with a subsequent pregnancy.

On occasion, a doctor will use a vertical incision to open the uterus.

This incision allows more access to your baby, for example, when an infant is premature and in an abnormal position.

The uterine incision determines whether or not you might be able to try for a vaginal birth in the future. If the incision extends into the portion of the uterus that contracts during labor, it will be recommended that you not attempt trial of labor in the future.

After the uterus is opened, the baby is delivered, the umbilical cord is cut, the placenta is delivered, and the uterine and abdominal incisions are stitched closed.

Complications

Although cesarean delivery is safe and most women have no complications, any surgical procedure may be at risk of complications. These complications may include excessive bleeding, sometimes requiring a blood transfusion; infections such as infection of the uterus or of the skin incision; and internal injury, such as injury to the bladder. Your doctor will address any operative complications immediately.

Skin incision infections usually occur after you've been discharged from the hospital. Your doctor will instruct you to call if the incision is red and warm or if there's drainage from the incision that appears to be infected.

Recovery

After surgery, you'll be taken to a recovery room for an hour or two before moving to a room in the maternity unit of the hospital. You'll be allowed to eat soon after surgery, as long as you're not experiencing nausea. You'll likely also be encouraged to take a brief walk.

If you're planning to breast-feed your baby, you may be able to do it for the first time in the recovery room. However, if you've had general anesthesia, you may be groggy and uncomfortable initially. You may want to wait until you're more awake and you've received pain medication before beginning breast-feeding. Women who have a cesarean delivery generally need to stay in the hospital for three days, although some women are discharged as early as two days after surgery.

Future pregnancies

Many women who have had a cesarean delivery are candidates for trial of labor after cesarean (TOLAC), also referred to as vaginal birth after cesarean (VBAC). Your doctor will talk with you about details of the delivery, and whether you're a candidate for future TOLAC. He or she may also use a VBAC calculator, which evaluates information about you and your obstetric history to determine the probability of successful TOLAC in the future.

If you had an incision into the portion of the uterus that contracts during labor, repeat cesarean delivery will be recommended. This is because such an incision increases the risk of a tear in the wall of the uterus (uterine rupture) where the incision was made.

Some birthing centers don't offer TOLAC. In general, it's recommended that TOLAC be done in a medical facility where there is immediate access to the surgical and the anesthesia teams. This will allow for quick delivery in the case of the need for an emergency delivery during TOLAC.

Post-delivery problems

Post-delivery problems are relatively uncommon but do happen in a small percentage of cases. Problems may arise after either a vaginal or cesarean delivery.

Retained placenta

Normally, the placenta is delivered within 30 minutes after the baby. Your doctor may gently massage your uterus to help expel the placenta. A retained placenta is one that's still attached to the wall of the uterus after delivery.

In some situations, your provider may have to gently separate the placenta from the wall of the uterus after placing his or her hand inside the uterus. This is called a manual extraction. If there's still a problem, a surgical procedure called a dilation and curettage (D&C) may be necessary to remove the placenta. This procedure is done in the operating room.

Postpartum bleeding

Postpartum hemorrhage is excessive bleeding from the uterus after delivery. It's often caused by an inability of the uterus to contract enough to control the bleeding that occurs when the placenta separates from the uterus. This is referred to as uterine atony.

Causes of uterine atony include delivering a large infant, long labor or induction, multiple gestation (twins, triplets), a history of postpartum hemorrhage with a previous pregnancy, abnormalities of the placenta, or a retained placenta. Other causes of postpartum bleeding include trauma to the vaginal wall from an episiotomy, lacerations of the vagina or cervix, or uterine rupture.

Postpartum bleeding can usually be controlled with medications that make the uterus contract. If this treatment doesn't stop the bleeding, your doctor may recommend other treatments including D&C or a Bakri balloon, which involves placing a silicone, fluid-filled balloon inside the uterus for several hours.

Rarely, an abdominal operation may be necessary if the bleeding can't be controlled. Treatment options may include tying off or blocking (embolizing) the major blood vessels that supply the uterus, or putting a suture around the uterus to compress the uterus (B-Lynch suture). If the hemorrhage continues, the uterus must be removed (hysterectomy), though this is also quite rare.

After Pregnancy

If you've experienced an uncomplicated labor and delivery, no doubt you'll feel a great sense of relief after giving birth to a healthy baby. Accompanying that relief, however, is a whole new set of responsibilities and worries. There are decisions to make and more than a few problems and hurdles to deal with during the ensuing months.

In Chapter 4, "Infant and Toddler Years," several health matters concerning your baby are discussed in detail. However, you also may confront some issues pertaining largely to your health.

Breast-feeding

The feeding of your newborn baby occupies a considerable portion of your time. In Chapter 4, breast-feeding and bottle-feeding are discussed in more detail.

Breast-feeding provides many benefits for both your baby and for you. Breast milk has the right amount of nutrients for your baby's growth and development. It may also protect your baby from certain illnesses and allergies and may lower the risk of sudden infant death syndrome (SIDS).

After delivery, breast-feeding can help your uterus return to its normal size more quickly and reduce or stop postpartum bleeding. You might find that breast-feeding helps you lose your pregnancy weight more easily, and it may lower the risk of breast cancer and ovarian cancer.

Most women are physically capable of breast-feeding. Some small-breasted women may think they won't be able to produce enough milk. This isn't true, because breast-feeding has very little to do with breast size.

During pregnancy, your breasts are preparing to produce milk. The hormones estrogen and progesterone are produced by the placenta and promote the growth of special breast tissue designed to produce milk. Your breasts slowly increase in size, and the nipples change, becoming darker in color and more prominent.

After your baby is born, you'll probably be able to breast-feed immediately. The baby's suckling stimulates production of the pituitary hormone oxytocin, which stimulates contraction of the muscles that surround the milk ducts. This contraction, called the let-down reflex, releases colostrum, a thin, sticky fluid, into storage areas behind the nipples. Later on, colostrum is replaced by milk.

After the delivery of the placenta, release of the hormone prolactin is triggered, which in turn stimulates milk secretion. About one or two days after delivery, your breasts may feel engorged and uncomfortable. They'll be much larger than usual, tender and firm. You may notice prominent veins appearing. These are normal changes caused by an increased blood flow and the production of milk. The best cure for this discomfort is a hungry baby.

The initial days and weeks of breast-feeding can be challenging as you and your baby adjust. If you're having trouble, get help from someone with experience in breast-feeding. Many hospitals have lactation specialists who can help you get through the first couple of weeks as you and your baby learn to breast-feed. Once you grow accustomed to the routine of breast-feeding, take advantage of its soothing effect on you and your baby.

Nutrition

During pregnancy, your body prepares for breast-feeding by storing additional nutrients and sources of energy. After your baby arrives, you may notice an increase in your appetite and thirst and a change in your dietary preferences. Most important is that you eat a variety of foods during your meals, eat nutritious snacks between meals and drink plenty of fluids to satisfy your thirst. You don't need to drink milk to make milk, but you do need to consume 1,200 milligrams of calcium daily.

Be sure to continue taking your prenatal vitamins during lactation. Avoid fad diets to lose weight. Gradual weight loss is the best route.

Breast problems

While breast-feeding, you may encounter the following problems:

Engorgement

Engorged breasts are breasts that are overly full with milk. Early and frequent nursing helps prevent engorgement. Some engorgement is normal. However, increased fluid and accumulation of milk in the breasts can lead to significant discomfort. Hard, swollen, painful breasts can result. If your breasts are only moderately engorged, carefully position your baby and increase feedings.

For severe engorgement, applying a warm washcloth compress and expressing milk by hand or with a breast pump may soften your breast and help to get your baby attached for feeding. You may also want to try expressing milk while a taking warm shower. Cold packs between feedings can help reduce swelling. For unmanageable engorgement, contact your doctor or a lactation consultant.

Sore nipples

Sore nipples, including cracked, bruised or blistered nipples, most often occur because of problems with the way the baby is latching on or how the baby is positioned during breast-feeding. Talk to a lactation consultant about the best way to hold your baby while breast-feeding. Correcting the position problem is the first step for healing.

Applying expressed breast milk to the damaged areas aids

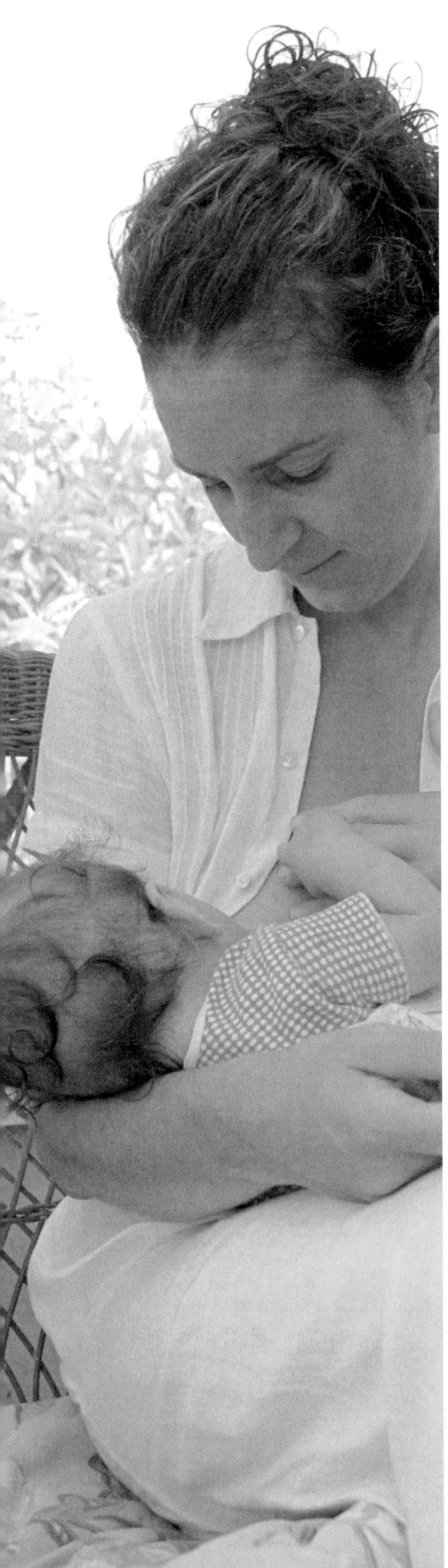

healing and provides antibacterial protection. Cool compresses may provide relief too. Your doctor also may recommend application of a topical antibiotic ointment in between feedings. For unmanageable nipple cracks or nipple pains, contact your doctor or a lactation specialist.

Blocked milk duct

A blocked milk duct leads to a small, hard lump in your breast. Sometimes, the lump will disappear on its own, or you can use hot water compresses, massage your breast and extend the length of breast-feeding sessions on the affected side. If it doesn't disappear, call your doctor.

Mastitis

Mastitis occurs when bacteria, most commonly *Staphylococcus aureus*, enter the breast. Part of the breast becomes red, hard and hot. You may feel unusually tired and have chills and a fever. If you have these signs and symptoms, contact your doctor.

Mastitis is treated with antibiotics. You'll likely receive antibiotics that are safe to use during breast-feeding. It's also safe to use analgesics such as acetaminophen (Tylenol, others) and ibuprofen (Advil, Motrin IB, others) for mastitis associated pain and fever. Continue breast-feeding and increase fluids and rest. You may be more comfortable breast-feeding your baby more often.

With treatment, mastitis usually clears up within a few days.

Postpartum blues, depression and mood disorders

After having a baby, it's important to monitor your mental health and be aware if you may need help.

Depressive disorders after pregnancy, sometimes called postpartum blues, are common.

Contributing factors may include personal history of depression, hormone changes, a perceived unsatisfactory birth experience, a sense of loss in no longer being pregnant, your level of marital satisfaction, a baby with a high level of needs, lack of social support, exhaustion or a family history of postpartum depression.

The transition from pregnancy to parenthood can be difficult. Experiencing depression, whether mild or severe, doesn't mean you've failed as a person or a parent. Expect to recover as you learn new ways to balance your daily life and responsibilities.

The blues

Having a baby is a powerful, exciting, frightening, joyous and awe-inspiring event. In the days that follow the delivery, you may be surprised and confused about the many and varied emotions you experience.

As a new parent you may feel overwhelmed with new responsibilities. Be patient with yourself as you make this transition, and give yourself credit for how well you're doing.

Up to 80 percent of new mothers experience mild depression called the baby blues. This mild form of distress usually occurs a few days to weeks after birth. It's generally self-limiting, resolving spontaneously in a few weeks.

During this time, you may have feelings of sadness, anger, anxiety, irritability and incompetence. New mothers often experience crying for no identifiable reason.

Some mothers are surprised by occasional negative thoughts they may have about their babies and may interpret this as being a bad mother. It can be comforting to know that the baby blues are normal. It's also important to take care of yourself.

Get adequate rest

Listen and respond to your body's cues for rest. Adequate rest has a significant effect on your emotional and physical well-being.

Try sleeping during the day when your baby sleeps, to synchronize your rest periods. You'll know you need more rest when things that didn't bother you before are now perceived as insurmountable events.

Eat a nutritious diet
Good nutrition provides what your body needs during recovery from childbirth. Several small meals a day may be more comfortable for you than three large meals. Fruits and vegetables are healthy snacks that also help with weight control.

Exercise
Light exercise can be helpful. Take a brisk, 30-minute walk as many days of the week as you can. You may enjoy your walk more if you take your baby with you in a baby carrier. Stretching and flexing as you play and talk to your baby will help tone your muscles. Your mind will be more at ease when your body feels good.

Socialize
Spending time with others you enjoy makes you feel good. Having family and friends who truly listen and accept your feelings can greatly lessen depressive symptoms.

Postpartum depression
A more severe form of the blues, called postpartum depression, occurs in approximately 15 percent of new mothers. Symptoms are more intense and longer lasting than those of the blues and can occur anytime within the first year.

Additional symptoms may include constant fatigue, lack of joy in life, a sense of emotional numbness, withdrawal from family and friends, lack of concern for self or baby, severe insomnia, excessive concern for the baby, loss of sexual responsiveness, and severe mood swings. You may have high expectations and be over-demanding, have difficulty making sense of things or feel trapped.

Tell your doctor early on if your family or friends notice these symptoms. Early intervention may result in a more rapid recovery from postpartum depression. Treatment varies according to each individual's needs, but it may include behavior therapy and anti-depressant medication. You might also ask about a support group in your area.

Post-traumatic stress disorder
Post-traumatic stress disorder can occur after the birth of a child. It may be a response to a real or perceived traumatic childbirth, or it may arise from an unresolved past trauma that was triggered during childbirth.

Symptoms are similar to those of postpartum depression, but the cause is trauma related. When identified early, counseling, sometimes in combination with medication and stress-reduction education, generally leads to recovery.

Postpartum psychosis
Fortunately, this condition is rare. Symptoms, which may begin days or weeks after childbirth, may include severe depression, along with acute anxiety, racing thoughts, fear of harming yourself or your baby, hallucinations, irrational thoughts, paranoia, or hysteria.

The goal of treatment is to keep you and your baby safe and to preserve your sense of competence as a parent while you recover.

Contraception

If you're within the first six months of delivery, are breast-feeding exclusively and have experienced a total absence of menstruation (amenorrhea), you may be temporarily protected from pregnancy. In fact, if all three of these conditions are met, breast-feeding in the early post-partum months can be 98 percent effective as a form of birth control.

If this doesn't describe your situation, you'll want to consider your options. Choices for contraception are basically the same after delivery as they were before pregnancy. For more on contraception, see Chapter 33 "Women's Health."

Sex After Childbirth

Many couples want to know when they can resume sexual intercourse after the birth of a baby. The vagina of a woman who has just given birth has been through some trauma. Under the best of circumstances, it's bound to be tender. If you're breast-feeding, vaginal atrophy — thinning and drying of vaginal tissues — may occur as the result of less estrogen in your system.

Many doctors recommend waiting six weeks, or after the new mother has a postpartum examination. During this examination, you and your doctor can discuss contraceptive methods so that you're not faced with an untimely pregnancy.

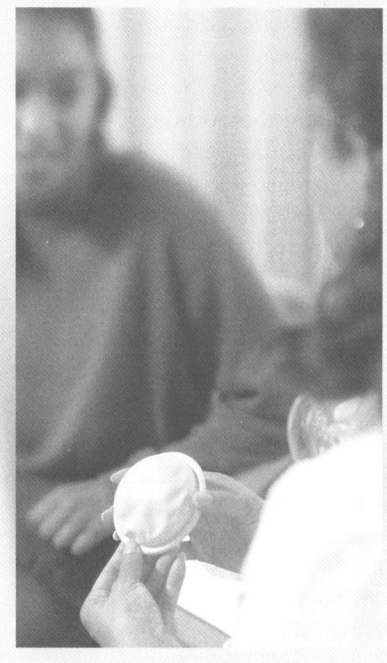

Intrauterine device (IUD)

An intrauterine device can be inserted immediately after the birth of your baby. However, immediate postpartum insertion is associated with increased risk of expulsion (the IUD "falls out"). More commonly, the IUD is inserted at the time of your postpartum visit. Your provider will discuss the risks and benefits of IUD placement, along with timing of the IUD placement.

Oral contraceptives

Many women want to resume taking birth control pills but wonder if it's safe for a breast-feeding mother. Birth control pills containing only progestin can be taken immediately after birth. Pills containing the combination of estrogen and progestin can be started six weeks after delivery if you're breast-feeding and 21 days after delivery if you're not breast-feeding.

Natural methods

Several natural methods of contraception depend in part on a regular menstrual cycle. If you were using these methods before you became pregnant, it might be a good idea to use another method for the first few months after birth because your cycle may be irregular for a while.

Permanent methods

If you're sure you don't want to be pregnant again, you may be able to choose from a few sterilization options, including tubal ligation — a surgical procedure — and the Essure procedure, which permanently blocks the fallopian tubes.

Vasectomy

For men, vasectomy is the only option for sterilization. During this straightforward surgery, the tubes that carry sperm into the semen are cut and sealed. After a successful vasectomy, a man isn't able to father a child. ■

Infant and Toddler Years

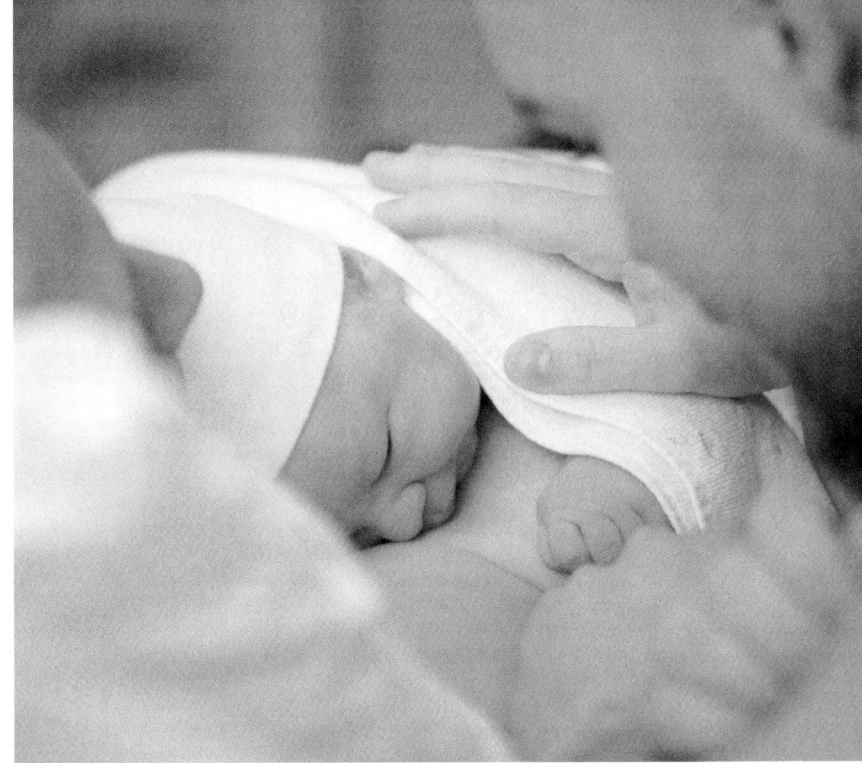

Getting acquainted with a minutes-old newborn is an especially joyous occasion.

After nine months of anticipation, the day finally arrives. Your daughter or son is born and takes her or his first breath. And so begins a new chapter in your life and the life of your child.

The first months of life are an exciting and challenging time, even for experienced parents, because every baby is different. Some babies nurse well from the beginning, and other babies seem to prefer feeding from a bottle. Some babies cry only when hungry, wet or tired, and other babies spend hours crying for no apparent reason. Some babies sleep through the night, and other babies prefer to take frequent catnaps.

As you and your baby adjust to being home together, life usually gets easier. During the first month, your baby may begin to fall into a somewhat predictable schedule of eating, sleeping and soiling diapers. This isn't to say that the schedule won't change. It frequently does during the first year of life. But among all of the changes, a sense of predictability begins to emerge as you learn what to expect from your baby each day.

The first year of life is a time of continuous and rapid change. Your baby will go from a diet of breast milk or formula to table food and drinking from a cup. The young infant who spends a good part of each day sleeping becomes the 11-day-old who is active the whole day except for an afternoon nap. Your baby will progress from being able to sit up on his or her own to crawling and then to walking, which generally occurs between 9 and 16 months of age. You'll watch your baby progress from communicating only by crying to cooing and squealing with pleasure when you walk into the room, and later to saying *mama* and *dada* and waving bye-bye.

Remember that not all babies develop at the same pace. If your baby doesn't reach a developmental milestone within the usual time frame, this doesn't necessarily mean that anything is wrong. Talk to your baby's doctor if you have concerns or questions about your baby's development.

Surviving the First Month

The first month of a baby's life is a period of adjustment and challenge for both baby and parents. It can be exhausting, so take one day at a time. Here are some survival tips:

- Nap when your baby naps.
- Keep meal preparation simple.
- Let a few dust balls accumulate.
- Don't feel obligated to entertain all visitors.
- Accept offers of help with household tasks.
- Ask for assistance from family and friends if you need it.

A Healthy Baby

During your baby's first year, it's natural to worry whether your baby is developing normally, even though serious abnormalities are uncommon. Many parents, especially first-time parents, have questions concerning their baby's weight, posture, skin color, vision, hearing, feeding, bowel movements, crying and sleeping.

Growth

The average newborn weighs between $5\frac{1}{2}$ and 10 pounds and is between 18 and 22 inches long. Within the first week after birth, a baby commonly loses up to 10 percent of its birth weight because of normal fluid loss.

By the time your baby is a month old, he or she likely has gained 1 to 3 pounds over his or her birth weight and grown 1 or 2 inches longer. Your baby may double his or her birth weight by the age of 5 months and triple it by the first birthday. Your baby's height will increase about 10 to 12 inches during the course of the year. The circumference of your baby's head will increase approximately 4 or 5 inches.

Posture and motor capabilities

The posture of your newborn simulates the fetal position. At birth, your baby's head will flop forward or backward and needs to be supported. When placed on a firm surface, he or she can move the head from side to side. If held upright over an adult's shoulder, your newborn can lift his or her head for a short time. On his or her stomach, your baby may lie in

Apgar Score

Apgar scores are used to evaluate the general health of newborns at one minute and again at five minutes after birth. Five areas are assessed: heart rate, respiration, muscle tone, reflexes and color. Each area is rated on a scale of 0 to 2, and the numbers are totaled. The highest possible score is a 10.

A score of 8 to 10 indicates that the baby is in excellent condition. The heart rate is more than 100 beats a minute. The baby is breathing well and crying, is active, coughs or sneezes when the nose is suctioned, and has good skin color. Most newborns have a score of 7 to 9 and require nothing more than having mucus suctioned from the airway to improve breathing. Newborns with a score of 4 or less at one minute after delivery require immediate assistance with their breathing. The heartbeat is slow or inaudible, the baby appears pale or even blue, and reflex responses may be absent or depressed.

a frog-like position or rolled in a ball. The hands are clenched into fists in these early days.

At one month your baby's head still needs support, though he or she may hold the head steady for longer periods. When the infant's fingers are pried open, they can grasp a rattle, but he or she may drop it quickly and won't yet be able to bring it toward the mouth.

By 4 months, infants can sit with some assistance and maintain good head control. When on his or her stomach, your baby may rock, rolling from side to side. Some infants at this age can roll from their stomachs or sides to their backs, or transfer an object from one hand to the other.

Your baby may begin to crawl by 8 months of age. Some infants of this age can even stand when leaning against something. By the time many children have their first birthday, they're walking, although crawling still may be the preferred method of getting around. Your child may even be climbing and going down stairs or climbing out of the crib. And with better hand coordination, babies at this age may point with an index finger or take the covers off containers.

Skin color

Immediately after birth your baby's skin color may be dusky blue. This is the normal color for an infant before birth. During the first few minutes after birth, the normal increase of oxygen in their heart and lungs causes infants of all races to become increasingly pinkish, especially the tongue, lips, palms and soles of the feet.

Some infants may be born with or soon develop a yellowish discoloration of the skin and whites of the eyes (jaundice). More than half of all full-term newborns and 80 percent of premature newborns who are otherwise healthy develop jaundice in the first few days of life. This is known as physiologic jaundice.

Jaundice isn't a disease; rather it's the inability of the immature liver of an infant to break down bilirubin. Bilirubin is a molecule that forms when the body recycles red blood cells. Bilirubin in the skin gives it a yellowish tint.

The American Academy of Pediatrics recommends bilirubin screening for all newborns before leaving the hospital, when bilirubin levels may still increase. This screening helps your baby's care team to identify risk level and assess what follow-up is needed.

Most infants with physiologic jaundice require only observation. Generally, the condition resolves within a week or two. The severity of physiologic jaundice is often influenced by race. East Asian and American Indian newborns are often affected more severely. Jaundice may be worse in babies who are premature, aren't eating well or are having fewer bowel movements.

If your baby has a significantly increased amount of bilirubin, he or she may be placed under a high-intensity light, a procedure called phototherapy. Bilirubin absorbs light and is then converted into a form that can be excreted in the bile and urine. This treatment is continued until the amount of bilirubin has been reduced. Possible side effects of phototherapy include loose stools, rash and dehydration.

If jaundice develops or persists after the second week of life, it may be due to some other liver malfunction, a severe infection, an enzyme deficiency or an abnormality of red blood cells. Jaundice present at birth or that appears within the first 24 hours may be the result of several problems, including bleeding, an infection in the blood (sepsis), or a blood incompatibility between the baby and mother. In such cases, special blood tests may be done.

Vision

A newborn's vision is still relatively poor, as the visual system is not yet fully developed. Your baby will probably keep his or her eyes shut much of the time. Infants are attracted to black-and-white patterns more than to colors, and they also enjoy looking at faces, particularly making eye contact with their mother or father.

Many infants have difficulty coordinating their eye movements during the initial months after birth. At times your baby's eyes may seem to turn in or out. This often improves in the first few months.

Most infants and young children are somewhat farsighted. But as healthy babies grow, their eyes change, allowing them to see both near and far objects more clearly. In most infants, the ability to see things clearly progresses rapidly. By the time most children are 3 years old, their vision will range from 20/25 to 20/40. Some babies, however, particularly those born prematurely, are nearsighted and will be unable to see far-away objects clearly as the eyes develop.

Sometimes a significant visual problem surfaces during infancy. As is often the case, the earlier the diagnosis, the better the chances that treatment will be successful. If you have any concerns about your baby's vision, talk to your baby's doctor (see page 143).

Hearing

Infants generally are born with a good sense of hearing. A healthy newborn blinks and startles in response to a loud sound and can distinguish differences in volume. Soft noises may produce something akin to a smile, and harsh or loud sounds may cause your newborn to cry. Your newborn may develop sound preferences, favoring a high-pitched voice over lower pitches.

Hearing is essential in the acquisition of speech and language. Even minor hearing loss can have a significant effect on your baby's ability to understand and to communicate. Without proper screening, hearing loss may go undetected until the child is 18 to 24 months old, when it leads to speech problems. Most newborns are now screened for hearing loss while in the hospital (see page 143).

Language

Your newborn's main method of communication is crying. Between 1 and 3 months, your baby's verbal repertoire is expanded with small throaty sounds, coos, squeals, chuckles, whimpers and vowel-like sounds such as *ooh* and *ah*. You'll learn your baby's different cries for hunger, pain and other needs, too. Your child's language comprehension is limited to recognizing and responding to familiar voices.

Between 4 and 6 months old is the babbling stage — complete with sighing, grunting, gurgling and laughing. Your child vocalizes both for pleasure and displeasure.

From 7 to 9 months, your baby repeats syllables and babbles in a singsong manner. He or she may produce as many as 12 distinct sounds, particularly the *p, d, b* and *m* sounds. Your child may use different vowels, and he or she may use sounds as a means of play. Toward the end of this period, you'll hear your baby imitating the intonation and speech sounds made by others. Children at this age will search for sources of sound, listen intently to speech and nonspeech sounds and recognize *dada, mama* and *bye-bye*. Your baby is able to differentiate friendliness and anger from the tone and inflection of people's voices and may recognize his or her own name.

Between 10 and 12 months of age, the babbling may take on the melody of actual speech. Your child enjoys repeating sounds made by others, vocalizing considerably during play. Almost all of the consonant and vowel sounds are used. In some children the first words emerge during this period. Your child's comprehension also is improved by this time. He or she can respond to simple requests and recognize the names of family members and some objects.

Nutrition

It's not uncommon for an infant to show little interest in feeding during the first couple of days after birth. By the end of the first week, most infants eat every two to three hours, with rare stretches of up to five hours. At 2 weeks of age, your newborn may take in about 18 ounces of milk a day. By 1 month that may increase to about 25 ounces a day.

The frequency of feedings depends on your baby's needs and the method of feeding. Breast-fed babies typically eat more frequently than formula-fed infants; however, a newborn is hungry at irregular intervals whether receiving breast milk or formula.

At 1 month, feeding is still somewhat disorganized. Babies may eat as often as every two to three hours during the day and one or more times in the night. Gradually over the course of the first month, the number of feedings over a 24-hour period may be reduced from eight or 12 to six or eight. The length of feedings also is erratic. One day a breast-fed infant might want to nurse for 40 minutes at each breast, and the next day he or she may nurse for only 10 minutes.

A baby between 1 and 3 months old probably will want five to six feedings a day, eventually eating every three hours, except for a longer stretch at night. As the baby grows, the number of feedings is reduced. Typically, a 5-month-old is down to four or five feedings, and by 9 months old the child may have only three milk feedings. Each baby's needs for growth are different, so follow your baby's cues to determine feeding frequency and volume.

Breast-feeding
Breast-feeding has proved to be the ideal feeding method for infants because of its nutritional and

immunological advantages as well as its emotional benefits.

Most infants are offered a chance to nurse for the first time shortly after birth. Breast-feeding facilitates closeness between a mother and child, and the infant gets the health benefit of the mother's colostrum, a rich, lemon-colored breast milk that helps protect the baby against disease. As colostrum transitions to mature milk over approximately the first two weeks, frequent, lengthy breast-feeding sessions are important in establishing a good milk supply.

Newborn Nutrition

Whether the source is breast milk or formula, the basic diet of a newborn includes the following components:

Calories

Calories are a measurement of the energy content of food. Everything we eat and much of what we drink contains calories. Human milk has about 15 to 25 calories per ounce. Its nutritional content varies from person to person and over time, but on average about 5 percent of its energy comes from protein, 50 percent from carbohydrates and 45 percent from fats. Standard infant formula contains 19 to 20 calories an ounce, with 9 percent from protein, 44 percent from carbohydrates and 47 percent from fats.

Protein

Protein is essential for growth and for cell repair. Most of the major body organs are composed mainly of protein. Without adequate protein intake, the body begins to break down its muscles to supply protein for essential body needs. Severe protein deprivation causes lethargy, a distended abdomen and swelling, but this is rare outside of developing countries.

Doctors recommend that a newborn be allowed to determine the schedule of feedings, at least to some degree. Many newborns are content to be fed every four hours, while others want more-frequent feedings.

Even if your infant has been on a three-hour feeding routine, the rules may suddenly change — often due to growth spurts — and he or she may shorten the time between feedings. Be prepared for some changes and unpredictability during the first months of life. There also may be periods of

Carbohydrates

Carbohydrates supply most of the body's energy needs. When the body doesn't receive enough carbohydrates, it compensates by using protein and fats for energy. Carbohydrates are stored in the liver and muscles, although an infant's reserve is a fraction of that of an adult.

Fats

Fats are a concentrated source of energy. They help protect body organs, vessels and nerves; insulate against changes in temperature; act as a vehicle for vitamin absorption; and delay the time it takes for the stomach to empty, giving a sensation of fullness. Infants and young children shouldn't be on a fat-restricted or low-fat diet.

Water

Water is essential for human life. Water accounts for 70 to 75 percent of your newborn's body weight, compared with only 50 to 60 percent of an adult's body weight. To remain healthy an infant must take in 10 to 15 percent of his or her weight in water daily.

Fortunately, if an infant is feeding well, the amount of water in breast milk or formula is adequate. Water itself is seldom needed unless the baby has a fever or diarrhea or is in a location of high heat.

cluster (bunched) feedings during which your baby may feed hourly for several hours.

It's important for a nursing mother to feel at ease while breast-feeding. Make sure you're comfortable, either lying down or sitting in a comfortable chair, preferably one with an armrest. Support the baby with his or her face held close to your breast. With the other hand you might want to support the breast so that the nipple is easily accessible to the infant's mouth. Allow your baby

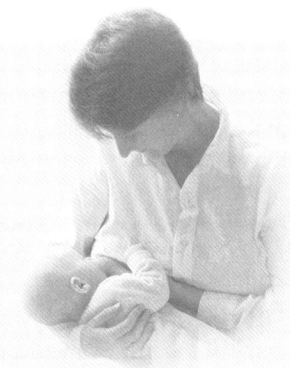

Minerals

Minerals are important to the structure and function of virtually every part of the body. For example, calcium and fluoride are necessary for the formation of strong bones and teeth, copper and iron are required for the production of red blood cells, and sodium is needed to maintain the water balance in the body.

Vitamins

Vitamins in food are needed for your organs to work properly. Vitamin A is important for healthy eyes and the linings of the bronchial, urinary and intestinal tracts. Vitamin C is needed for bone, teeth and tissue development. Vitamin D also is essential to bone and teeth development. However, breast milk alone does not supply enough of this vitamin. Infants who are exclusively breast-fed or who drink less than 32 ounces of formula a day should receive vitamin D supplementation of 400 international units (IU) daily.

to finish feeding on one breast before you offer the other. Alternate which breast you offer first at each feeding to keep milk production even. After each feeding, burp your infant: Set the baby upright or against your shoulder and gently pat or rub his or her back for a few minutes.

Initially, a nursing mother may have tender nipples. Keep your nipples as dry as possible between feedings. Position your baby comfortably at your breast and rotate positions to help prevent cracked nipples. There are various ways to position your baby when breast-feeding. If a particular position isn't comfortable, try another. Contact your baby's doctor or a lactation consultant if soreness persists.

If you're breast-feeding your baby, pay special attention to your own diet and habits. Eat a healthy diet that includes plenty of water. Be wary of taking any medication unless it's approved by your doctor. Avoid smoking and consume only a little, if any, alcohol.

Some women who decide to breast-feed need more flexibility than the method may allow, so they also introduce the infant to the bottle. After the first few weeks, if you want to supplement one or more breast-feedings a day with a bottle, you can pump your breasts and store the milk for later use. Have your baby's doctor or a lactation consultant demonstrate the proper procedure for pumping. Highly efficient breast pumps are now available to enable you to provide breast milk for your baby regardless of your circumstances. They are covered by most insurance plans.

Bottle-feeding

Although no infant formula can match all of the nutritional benefits of breast milk, bottle-feeding is an acceptable alternative in most instances. Infant formula is similar to breast milk and contains the nutrients your baby needs to develop and grow.

Most bottle-fed babies have their first feeding within six hours after delivery. A bottle-fed baby probably will need between six and nine feedings in a 24-hour period by the end of the first week of life.

The setting for bottle-feeding is similar to that for breast-feeding. A bottle should never be propped up against the infant. Rather, a parent should take the time to hold the child closely during the feeding and enjoy the closeness.

The formula should be warmed to body temperature, and the temperature tested by dropping a bit on your wrist. A perfect temperature is one that's neither hot nor cold and barely sensed at all. A word of caution: Don't warm the bottle in a microwave oven, because the formula can become unevenly hot and severely burn your infant.

Bottle-feeding may last from five to 25 minutes, depending on the eagerness and sucking ability of the infant. Burp your baby after each feeding.

Solids

Parents always ask when they should offer their baby solids. This is a difficult question and one that has no shortage of opinions.

For several months the neuromuscular development of infants is geared toward sucking and swallowing liquids. The infant isn't ready for other foods until he or she can hold his or her head up-

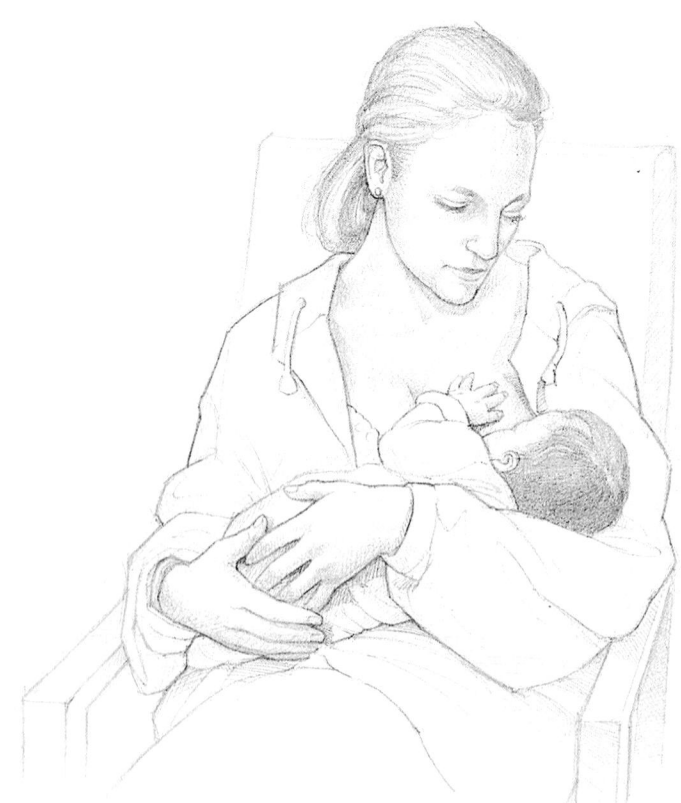

Making the Most of Feedings

Personal interaction is an important factor in your baby's development. Aside from providing the nutrients your baby needs to grow and develop, feeding time is an opportunity for you and your baby to get better acquainted. Your baby can learn about you, how the two of you relate, and the security and love you provide.

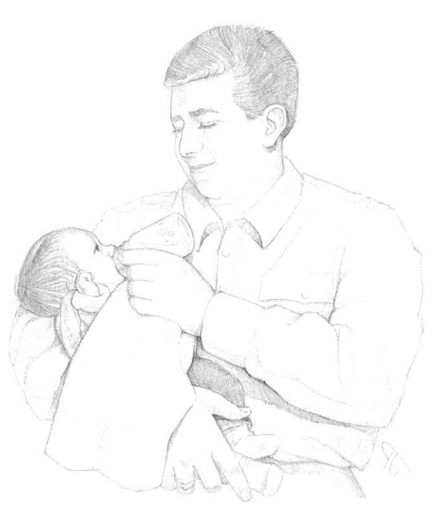

right and sit up, recognize a spoon, keep food in his or her mouth, and swallow appropriately. This usually occurs around 6 months. Also, before the age of 4 to 6 months, your baby's gastrointestinal system may be unable to digest solids efficiently. Introducing solids before then may increase your infant's risk of developing food allergies, too.

Many doctors recommend starting babies on solids between 4 and 6 months of age. From a nutritional standpoint, though, your baby gets everything he or she needs from breast milk or formula for the first six months.

As you start to expand your baby's diet, introduce just one new food at a time. Wait several days before trying another to make sure no signs of an allergy or intolerance develop.

Cereal

When it's time to offer your baby solids, many doctors recommend starting with a cereal. Single-grain cereal especially made for babies is often used as baby's first solid food because it's easy to digest. Cereal is also a good source of iron, which infants need. Mix 1 tablespoon of cereal with 4 or 5 tablespoons of breast milk or formula. Initially, babies generally respond better to solids if the solids are thin rather than thick. Put some food on the tip of a small spoon and place it in your baby's

mouth. Don't be surprised if it comes back out. Babies often need multiple exposures to a food before they develop a taste for it. They also are learning how to use their tongues in a different manner.

Be patient. Don't put solids in a bottle or a syringe-type feeder. The former can encourage your baby to overeat, and the latter can cause choking.

Pureed foods

After your baby is acquainted with cereal, your next step might be a pureed fruit or vegetable. At 8 months of age, most infants are ready to try pureed meats, but breast milk or formula continues to provide ample amounts of protein.

New research suggests introducing peanut butter around 6 months of age may dramatically reduce your child's risk of developing a peanut allergy. If your child has moderate to severe eczema, discuss when and how to do this with your medical provider. For others, introducing peanut butter at 6 months is recommended. Try feeding your baby a small amount of peanut butter thinned with water. If he or she tolerates this without developing signs of an allergic reaction, continue to do this at least three times per week to maintain oral tolerance and potentially prevent a peanut allergy from forming.

Finger foods

After 8 months, most babies are able to eat small pieces of table food. Toast, bits of cheese, pieces of scrambled egg, dry cereals, crackers, mashed potatoes and well-cooked pasta are good finger foods. Avoid foods that could choke your baby, such as hot dogs, grapes, popcorn, nuts, raisins and raw carrots.

Bowel movements

Infants usually have a bowel movement within 24 hours after birth. Called a meconium stool, it's composed of intestinal secretions

Is Your Baby Getting Enough to Eat?

Many parents wonder whether their baby is getting enough to eat. The best answer to that question is to trust your baby. Babies are able to regulate their intake amazingly well. They'll eat as much as is needed, regardless of how much is left. When it's time to eat again, the baby will usually let you know.

If a baby doesn't get enough to eat, you'll soon know. He or she will cry until you offer more food. An infant who needs more food than is being given will awaken more often at night and will decrease rather than increase the time between feedings. You may even observe the baby chewing his or her fist more than usual.

The best early indication that your baby is receiving the necessary nourishment is weight gain. Keep in mind that some babies gain weight slowly, and others gain rapidly.

By the time your infant is between 6 and 8 months old, he or she may be eating 3 to 4 ounces — about 5 to 8 tablespoons — of solid food at each of three meals. A good diet for an infant of this age might include cereal and fruit for breakfast, cereal and fruit or vegetables for lunch, and cereal, fruit and vegetables for supper. Although drinking patterns vary widely, many babies eating this diet reduce their milk consumption to about 16 ounces a day. Many babies also need a midmorning and midafternoon snack, which should be something nutritious such as fruit or yogurt.

In your baby's second six months, you may need to increase feedings with cereal to meet his or her needs for an adequate supply of iron. Sometimes, a baby's diet needs to be supplemented with vitamins and minerals. Consult your child's doctor.

After his or her first birthday, your baby may be eating table food exclusively.

and amniotic fluid and is dark green. As your baby begins to drink breast milk or formula, the next few stools may be greenish brown and contain milk curds. After a few days, the stool resembles the bowel movement of an older infant.

By the end of the first week, most infants pass between three and five stools a day, although it's not uncommon for a baby, especially one that is breast-fed, to have more bowel movements each day. If your newborn goes for several days without a bowel movement, don't panic. This doesn't necessarily mean that the baby is constipated (see page 159).

The stool of a breast-fed baby is odorless and mushy. The stool of a formula-fed baby has a characteristic fecal smell and is usually more formed. One month after birth most babies have three or four bowel movements a day, often after a feeding. However, some infants,

Can You Spoil Your Baby?

If you're concerned about spoiling your newborn with too much love and attention, don't be. Following your instinct to respond to your baby's cry will not spoil him or her. In fact, infants who receive responses consistently and quickly early on cry less in later months than do those left to cry. It seems that an important task for your infant to learn is that others will respond in a caring and predictable way. This helps your baby develop confidence and trust.

especially some nursing babies, may not have a bowel movement for two to 10 days. This is normal and not a cause for concern if the baby appears well and consistency of the stool seems normal.

Crying

The amount a newborn cries, like many other aspects of development, varies. Some infants cry only when hungry or wet. Others cry more often.

On some days your baby may cry for 20 to 30 minutes four or five times — typically before eating, sleeping or having a bowel movement. On other days he or she may cry for hours. Crying usually peaks at about 6 weeks of age and tapers off by 3 or 4 months of age. In premature newborns the peak is typically six weeks after your due date.

What causes excessive crying during the first months of life? There's no easy answer because every baby and every day are different. If your crying baby can't be consoled for more than a few moments by any method, your baby may have colic (see page 160).

Trying to figure out what your baby is signaling with his or her cries requires some detective work. Hunger, discomfort, boredom, fear, loneliness, overstimulation or being overly tired are common reasons babies cry. Babies lack experience in reacting to the many new and confusing situations outside the womb. Although some make the transition easily, most need lots of cuddling and human contact day and night in those important first few months.

As the baby grows and matures, you'll begin recognizing different cries for different needs. You'll soon learn how to distinguish your baby's cries by trying different things and seeing what works and what doesn't. And with time and familiarity, your understanding of your baby's needs will improve.

Circumcision

Circumcision is a procedure in which the foreskin — the sheath of tissue covering the head of the penis — is removed. The practice has been performed since ancient times, and many parents today have their sons circumcised for religious or other reasons, including health and hygiene concerns.

Recent research shows that benefits of circumcision include lower risk of infection and certain types of cancer. However, the benefits are not great enough to recommend circumcision for all newborn boys.

Like any minor surgery, circumcision poses some risk to the newborn. Local anesthesia may be used to lessen the pain for the baby. If you choose circumcision, it's usually done a few days after birth. An uncircumcised penis requires no special care beyond regular hygiene.

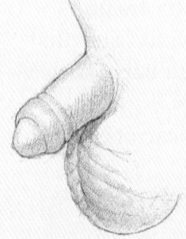

Before circumcision, the foreskin of the penis extends over the end of the penis, or glans (left). After the brief operation, the glans is exposed (right).

Sleep Patterns

| 3 months | 6 months | 12 months | 18 months |

asleep **awake**

The sleep cycles of babies vary. This example shows how sleep is often erratic in the first months of life. With time, children generally settle into a routine.

Sleeping

The average newborn spends more time sleeping than doing any other activity. A newborn often has an alert period immediately after birth. After one to two hours of alertness, the baby sinks into a quiet sleep. During the next several days, most newborns sleep from 14 to 18 hours a day and are alert for only short periods.

A 1-month-old baby spends most of the time sleeping, usually at least 14 hours a day. Generally, toward the end of the first month, parents observe that seven or eight daily sleep periods are reduced to three or four daily naps and a five- or six-hour block of sleep at night. Sleep patterns, however, are highly variable, and your baby may sleep more or less.

Sleep is divided into active and quiet sleep. Rapid eye movement (REM) sleep is when dreaming takes place. In the REM phase, the baby can be easily awakened. During this lighter sleep, babies may toss and turn, suck, and gurgle. In the early months newborns have more of this lighter sleep than deeper sleep. Deeper sleep, or quiet sleep, is referred to as non-REM sleep. As babies mature, they begin to have more quiet sleep, similar to adults.

You'll also find that your infant often is an active sleeper. Even though the baby is asleep, you may see him or her grimace, cry out, startle and move about without waking up.

By 6 months of age some babies are taking one or more daytime naps and may sleep six to eight hours at a time. Be patient with your baby, as he or she will reach this milestone of sleeping throughout the night on his or her own time. Throughout the first few years, there will be many nights of interrupted sleep from teething, illness and dreams.

An older infant is able to sleep through the night only when he or she no longer needs night feedings and has learned how to fall back to sleep without help.

Newborn Screening Tests

Each state requires routine screening for certain disorders that aren't apparent at birth. The U.S. Secretary of Health and Human Services recommends screening for more than 30 conditions as part of states' universal newborn screening programs. Screening tests use a few drops of blood, typically collected on the second day of life, on filter paper that is sent to a state laboratory for analysis. Early detection is important so that measures can be taken to prevent future health problems.

Newborn screening varies by state and is subject to change, especially given advancements in technology and treatments for rare genetic diseases. Your child's doctor or the nursing staff at the hospital where your child is born will inform you of screening tests required or available in your state.

The disorders listed here are the ones typically included in newborn screening programs.

- **Phenylketonuria (PKU).** PKU is a congenital deficiency of a specific enzyme. Infants born with PKU are often normal at birth. The condition disrupts normal metabolism and may lead to intellectual disability if the child's diet isn't carefully regulated beginning in early infancy. Modern screening tests also allow for detection of many similar disorders that affect protein metabolism. When any of these disorders is detected early, feeding an infant a special formula low in phenylalanine or other amino acids can prevent intellectual disability. Special diets and treatments will need to be followed throughout life.

- **Congenital hypothyroidism.** Hypothyroidism is a deficiency in the production of thyroid hormone, which is essential for mental and physical growth and development. If children with hypothyroidism are untreated, they usually have developmental disabilities and short stature. Early treatment with thyroid hormone leads to normal growth and development.

- **Galactosemia.** Galactosemia is an enzyme deficiency that affects the body's ability to metabolize galactose, one of the sugars normally present in milk. If left untreated, it can cause developmental delay, cataracts, and kidney and liver problems. When the diagnosis is made early, such medical problems can be prevented through a diet restricted in galactose content. Several less severe forms of galactosemia may be detected by newborn screening and may not require any intervention.

- **Sickle cell disease.** Sickle cell disease is an inherited blood disease in which red blood cells are abnormally crescent-shaped instead of round. It can cause episodes of pain, damage to vital organs including the lungs and kidneys, and even death. Young children with sickle cell disease are especially prone to certain dangerous bacterial infections, such as pneumonia and meningitis. The screening test also can detect other disorders affecting the blood's hemoglobin.

- **Biotinidase deficiency.** Babies with this condition don't have enough biotinidase, an enzyme that recycles one of the B vitamins (biotin) in the body. The deficiency may cause seizures, poor muscle control, hearing loss, intellectual disability, coma and even death. If the deficiency is detected early, problems can be prevented by routinely giving the baby extra biotin.

- **Congenital adrenal hyperplasia.** This is a group of disorders involving a deficiency of certain hormones produced by the adrenal gland. The condition can affect the development of the genitals and it may cause death due to loss of salt from the kidneys. A blood test in the first days of life can identify the condition before serious symptoms develop. Treatment is very effective and usually consists of medications and sometimes surgery.

- **Maple syrup urine disease (MSUD) and other organic acid disorders.** Babies with MSUD are missing an enzyme needed to process three amino acids that are essential for normal growth. Other enzymes are deficient in similar disorders, known as organic acid disorders. When amino acids are not processed properly, they can build up in the body with some byproducts,

causing urine to smell. In MSUD the urine smells like maple syrup or sweet, burnt sugar. Babies with these disorders usually have little appetite and are extremely irritable. If not detected and treated early, these disorders can cause intellectual and physical disabilities and even death. Medications and a carefully controlled diet that excludes certain high-protein foods can prevent these outcomes.

- **Cystic fibrosis.** Cystic fibrosis is an inherited disorder that causes cells to release a thick mucus, which can lead to chronic respiratory disease, problems with digestion and poor growth. Detecting cystic fibrosis early may help doctors reduce lung and nutritional problems, but there is no known cure for the disease. Traditionally, treatment is limited to trying to prevent the lung infections associated with it and providing good nutrition. New treatments are helping patients to live longer, healthier lives.

- **Medium-chain acyl-CoA dehydrogenase (MCAD) deficiency and other fatty acid oxidation disorders.** These disorders result from the lack of different enzymes required to convert fat to energy. Serious life-threatening signs and symptoms can occur. Treatment may be as simple as avoidance of fasting, but some

Preventing Disease

Most of the medical care a newborn infant receives is geared toward the prevention of disease. Occasionally, bacteria in the birth canal cause serious eye infections in a newborn. Therefore, immediately after birth every newborn's eyes are protected with an antibiotic.

A dose of vitamin K usually is given after birth in shot (intramuscular) form. It prevents potentially life-threatening bleeding due to vitamin K deficiency in newborns. One shot is enough to sustain an infant through the first weeks of life.

Babies may also receive the hepatitis B vaccine before leaving the hospital to protect them from any possible contact with hepatitis B, a viral infection that

affects the liver. In addition, routine screening tests for congenital problems are typically performed at the hospital on the second day of life.

It is wise to continue to limit your newborn's visitors for a while after you take your baby home. In particular, avoid crowds. Remember, colds and other illnesses that may be considered minor in an older baby pose greater risks during the first month of life.

All infants should be seen regularly by a health professional. Before you go home from the hospital, your baby's doctor will discuss this schedule with you. The first follow-up visit typically occurs within a week. Some physicians recommend monthly visits during the first year. Others prefer to see the baby every two months, provided everything is going well, to monitor the baby's development and administer vaccinations.

of these conditions require special diets and medications. With early detection and monitoring, most children with these disorders can lead normal lives.

- **Lysosomal storage disorders (LSDs).** A diverse group of inherited diseases, lysosomal storage disorders are caused by defects in enzymes that play a role in the normal degradation of molecules in the body's cells. Some LSDs predominantly affect the heart or brain, while most affect several different organs. Others cause problems with the skeletal system. Treatment options may include medication and bone marrow transplantation.

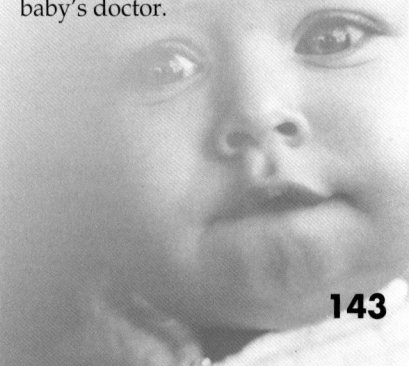

- **X-linked adrenoleukodystrophy (X-ALD).** Because of its inheritance pattern, this condition primarily affects boys in childhood. Most affected girls will develop symptoms as adults. Some of the symptoms of X-ALD are treated with lifelong hormone replacement, though boys with X-ALD usually also require a bone marrow transplant during their second or third year of life to prevent symptoms affecting the brain. Recently recommended as part of universal newborn screenings, X-ALD is now screened in several states.

Blood glucose

In the womb, an infant's blood sugar (glucose) level remains normal because nutrition is being supplied from the placenta. After birth, a newborn must develop the ability to regulate his or her own blood sugar level.

Low blood sugar (hypoglycemia) occurs in some infants whose bodies are not yet able to regulate their own blood sugar levels. Infants whose mothers have diabetes are at greater risk of hypoglycemia be-

cause they're born with increased levels of insulin in their bodies.

Uncommon problems include difficulty breathing or seizures. The risk of seizures is of special concern because seizures caused by low blood sugar increase the risk of lasting neurological or developmental problems.

For newborns with risk factors for hypoglycemia, blood glucose level is commonly measured during the hours after birth to make certain that it's in the normal range. Feeding the baby breast milk, formula or dextrose gel usually helps return low levels to normal.

Hearing

Significant hearing loss in both ears affects approximately 1 in 1,000 newborns in the United States. Infants at risk of hearing loss include those born with infections, such as rubella, cytomegalovirus, syphilis and herpes; those who have head or neck injuries, severe jaundice, or a family history of hearing loss during childhood; and those born prematurely.

Hearing loss is a problem that may not be apparent at first and might go undetected until the child is 24 to 30 months of age, when concerned parents become aware that their child isn't developing normal speech. Hence, all newborns, including healthy babies, should be screened for hearing loss. Most hospitals now test each newborn's hearing before the baby leaves the hospital.

One simple, noninvasive screening test is the otoacoustic emissions (OAE) test. The OAE test measures sound waves generated in the inner ear (cochlea) in response to clicks or tone bursts. The waves are recorded, analyzed by a computer and interpreted by an audiologist.

However, none of the current hearing tests routinely used on newborns can detect slight hearing loss or minimal loss that will

Does Your Infant See Properly?

Some infants are born with partial or total loss of vision. Common causes include brain malformations, damage to the eyes due to infection, birth trauma, a significant loss of oxygen (hypoxia), and genetic diseases that affect either an eye or the nerves to the brain's vision center.

Although an important part of a newborn's initial physical examination includes a check for any apparent vision defects, it's not uncommon for some visual problems to go undetected during early infancy. Often the problem is discovered later by the parents when the child seems unusually clumsy.

You can watch for certain developmental signs to determine whether your baby's vision is indeed within the normal range. When your infant is between 4 and 6 weeks old, try the following test: Bring your face within 20 inches of your baby's. This should elicit a smile. By the time your infant is 3 months old, he or she should be able to visually follow a toy dangling in front of his or her face. The infant should also attempt to reach for a toy or rattle. A baby this age can see objects at least several feet away.

By the time your infant is 4 months old, his or her vision capabilities — the ability of the eye to distinguish color, adjust itself to various distances, see one image instead of two, perceive depth and orient itself to moving images — are near those of an adult. If you suspect that your baby's visual development is slow, consult your baby's doctor.

progress as the child grows. If hearing loss is suspected, your infant should have a follow-up hearing test between the ages of 3 and 6 months.

Certain types of hearing loss can be corrected. When the loss is related to recurrent ear infections, antibiotics can treat the infections so that the ear can function normally. Surgery may correct congenital malformations of the ear.

Four types of hearing loss are found in infants and children:

Conductive hearing loss

Conductive hearing loss involves interference with the external ear's ability to receive sound or to transmit it from the external ear to the inner ear. The most common causes are congenital abnormalities of the ear and ear infections. Often these problems can be treated with medication or surgery.

Sensorineural hearing loss

Sensorineural hearing loss results from abnormalities of the auditory hair cells or of the auditory nerve. About 50 percent of cases of sensorineural hearing loss are hereditary. Other causes include severe jaundice, infection while in the uterus and some medications.

Sensorineural hearing loss is usually permanent; however, cochlear implants may allow young children to develop normal auditory perception and oral language.

Mixed hearing loss

Mixed hearing loss occurs when a child has both conductive and sensorineural hearing loss. This type of loss may be severe. Medication or surgery or both may restore a portion of the child's hearing loss.

Central auditory processing disorders

Central auditory processing disorders result from a problem in the central auditory nervous system, the ear's nerve linkage with the brain. Children with these disorders hear sound only as a jumble of noise.

Getting Vaccinated

Prevention is crucial to good health. It's far better to prevent a disease than to treat it. The best way to protect yourself and your family from many diseases is to get vaccinated. Immunization is the best line of defense against diseases such as chickenpox (varicella), measles (rubeola), mumps, rubella, tetanus, hepatitis, influenza, polio and many other infections. Vaccination stimulates your body's natural defense mechanisms to resist infectious disease, destroying the virus or bacteria before you become sick.

Thanks to vaccines, many infectious diseases that were once common in the United States are now rare or nonexistent. Parents no longer have to fear that their children will die of or become disabled by diphtheria, whooping cough (pertussis) or measles. And children don't have to keep away from water fountains and swimming pools to avoid getting polio.

Since coming into widespread use during the 20th century, vaccinations have saved billions of lives worldwide. However, despite the availability of vaccines, many people remain undervaccinated. One reason is that some people have concerns about the safety and risks of vaccines. These concerns are often the result of incorrect information.

How vaccines work

Every day, your body is threatened by bacteria, viruses and other germs. When a disease-causing microorganism enters your body,

Vaccine Immunity

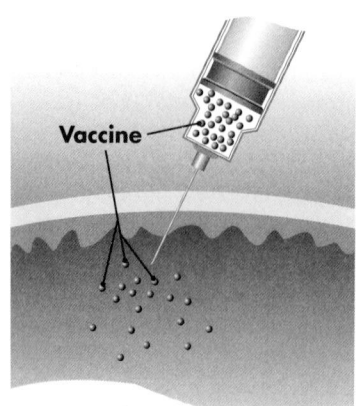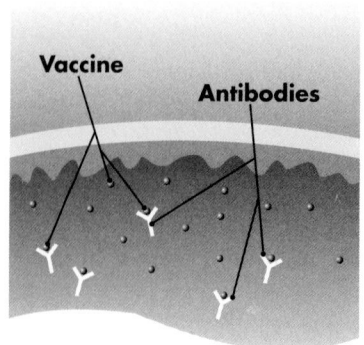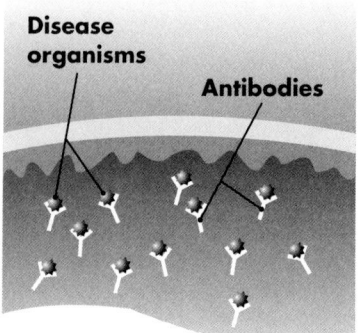

A vaccine with dead or harmless forms of a virus, bacterium or other organism is injected into an individual (left). The vaccine stimulates the immune system to produce antibodies against the organism (center). In any subsequent exposure to this organism, the antibodies attack and stop the infection (right).

your immune system mounts a defense, producing proteins called antibodies to fight off the invader. The goal of your immune system is to neutralize or destroy the foreign invader, preventing you from getting sick.

Your body's immune system fights off foreign invaders and protects you from disease in the following two ways:

Post-exposure immunity

Post-exposure immunity develops after you've been exposed to a certain organism. Your immune system puts into play a complex array of defenses to prevent you from getting sick again from that type of virus or bacterium.

Exposure to a foreign invader (antigen) activates the production of certain white blood cells in your body called B cells (B lymphocytes). B cells produce plasma cells, which in turn produce a huge number of antibodies designed specifically to fight that particular invader. These antibodies circulate in your body's fluids. The next time the antibodies encounter that invader in your body, they recognize it and destroy it. And if needed, your body can rapidly resume production of an antibody it has made before.

In addition to the work of B cells, white blood cells called macrophages confront and destroy foreign invaders. The macrophages "process" the invaders, figuring out if they present a threat. If your body encounters a germ that it has never been exposed to before, information about the germ is relayed to white blood cells called helper T cells. These cells aid in the development of other infection-fighting cells, including memory T cells.

Once you've been exposed to a specific virus or bacterium, the next time you encounter it, antibodies and memory T cells go to work. They immediately react to the organism, attacking it before disease can develop. Your immune system can recognize and effectively combat thousands of different organisms.

Vaccine immunity

Vaccine immunity results from injection of a vaccine, which contains a harmless dead or weakened form of an infectious germ. When given to an individual who's healthy, the vaccine triggers an immune response. The vaccine makes your body think that it's being invaded by a specific organism, and your immune system goes to work to destroy the invader and prevent it from infecting you again.

If you're exposed to a disease for which you've been vaccinated, the invading germs are met by antibodies prepared to destroy them, just as with immunity acquired from natural infection. For some diseases, the vaccine may be better at creating immunity than a natural infection would be. And vaccines work without the risk of serious effects from a disease.

Several doses of a vaccine may be needed for a full immune response. Some people fail to build immunity from the first doses of a vaccine but often respond to later doses. In addition, the immunity provided by some vaccines, such as tetanus and pertussis, isn't lifelong. Because the immune response may decrease over time, you may need another dose of a vaccine (booster) to restore or increase your immunity.

Types of vaccines

Vaccines are prepared in different ways. However, for each type, the goal is the same — to stimulate an immune response without causing disease.

Live, weakened (attenuated)

Some vaccines, such as those for measles-mumps-rubella and chickenpox (varicella), use live viruses that have been weakened (attenuated).

Inactivated

Other vaccines use dead (inactivated) bacteria or viruses. The inactivated polio vaccine (IPV) and the influenza vaccines are made this way.

Toxoid

Some types of bacteria cause disease by producing toxins that invade the bloodstream. Toxoid vaccines, such as those for diphtheria and tetanus, use bacterial toxins that have been rendered harmless.

Subunit and conjugate

These types of vaccines are made by using only part of the virus or bacterium. The hepatitis and *Haemophilus influenzae* type b (Hib) vaccines are made in this way.

Benefits of vaccines

Because many vaccine-preventable diseases are now uncommon in the United States, some people feel less urgency about getting themselves or their children immunized. Few people today have ever seen a case of diphtheria, polio or tetanus. Some may feel cleanliness and sanitation are enough to prevent disease.

? Question and Answer

Won't breast-feeding provide my child with natural immunity? Is vaccination necessary?

Proteins in a mother's milk do offer protection against some infections, such as colds, ear infections and diarrhea. This immunity generally lasts for only a month to about a year. And breast-feeding doesn't give a child any immunity against a number of serious contagious diseases, such as whooping cough (pertussis).

If you're wondering if it's necessary to keep up with vaccinations, the answer is yes. Many infectious diseases that have virtually disappeared in the United States can reappear quickly. The germs that cause the diseases still exist and can be acquired by people who aren't protected by vaccination.

? Question and Answer

Are there times when my child shouldn't be vaccinated?

In a few circumstances, vaccination should be postponed or avoided. Talk to your doctor if you question whether your child should be vaccinated.

Immunization may be inappropriate if a child:
- Has had a serious reaction to a previous dose of that vaccine
- Has a known, significant allergy to a vaccine component, such as chicken eggs or gelatin
- Has a medical condition, such as AIDS or cancer, that's compromised the child's immune system

Vaccinations may need to be deferred if a child:
- Has a moderate to severe illness
- Has taken steroid medications in the last three months
- Has received a transfusion of blood or plasma or been given blood products within the past year

Immunization shouldn't be delayed because a child has a minor illness, such as a common cold, an ear infection or mild diarrhea. The vaccine will still be effective, and it won't make your child sicker.

As travelers unknowingly carry disease from one country to another, a new outbreak in the United States may be only a plane trip away. From a single entry point, an infectious disease can spread quickly among unprotected individuals. U.S. outbreaks of mumps and measles have occurred this way in the 21st century.

The persistent threat of disease is just one reason public health officials recommend vaccinations. Vaccines provide a number of benefits to individuals, communities and the world population.

Safety

Many people have questions and concerns about vaccine safety. A common fear is that ingredients in vaccines may trigger serious side effects or even cause disease. Parents may worry after hearing or seeing reports about a severe reaction that occurs shortly after a child's immunization visit and is ascribed to a side effect or complication of the vaccine. Stories about vaccination fears frequently circulate on the internet.

In fact, vaccines are extremely safe. Before they can be used, they must meet strict safety standards set by the Food and Drug Administration (FDA). Meeting these standards requires a lengthy development process of up to 10 years followed by three phases of clinical trials.

Once vaccines are licensed and made available to the general public, the FDA and the Centers for Disease Control and Prevention (CDC) continue to monitor their safety. Furthermore, vaccines are subject to ongoing research, review and refinement by doctors, scientists and public health officials.

Your chances of being harmed by a disease are far greater than your chances of being harmed by a vaccine used to prevent disease.

Effectiveness

Vaccines are highly effective. Most childhood vaccines are effective in 85 to 99 percent or more of children who receive them. For example, a full series of measles vaccine protects 97 out of 100 children from measles, and a polio vaccine series protects 99 out of 100 children from polio.

In some instances a vaccine provides only partial immunity. It doesn't prevent the disease, but it often lessens the duration of the illness and the severity of the symptoms.

A reduction in suffering and disability

In addition to being potentially fatal, many infectious diseases can cause permanent harm. Polio can cause paralysis. Meningitis can cause deafness. Measles can cause brain damage and death. Hepatitis can cause liver damage. Vaccines prevent these serious complications.

One example is the *Haemophilus influenzae* type b (Hib) vaccine. Before the vaccine became available in 1987, the bacterium caused about 20,000 serious infections in U.S. infants and children each year. Hib meningitis killed 1,000 children annually and left many survivors with deafness, seizures or intellectual disability.

Protection of community health

Vaccination protects not only your health and your child's but also the health of your community. In any community there are some people who shouldn't be vaccinated for certain diseases — for example, newborns, individuals who are allergic to an ingredient in a vaccine or those with a condition that precludes certain vaccinations.

These people depend on community immunity (herd immunity). If 95 percent of the people in a community are immunized, there is little opportunity for an outbreak. Unprotected individuals are much less likely to be exposed to the germ, so they have a smaller chance of becoming infected.

Eradication of disease worldwide

Vaccination protects more than one city, one country and one generation. The long-term goal of an immunization program is to completely eliminate a disease. At least in one instance, this goal has become a reality. The worldwide eradication of smallpox is a success story of modern medicine.

Smallpox was devastating to humankind for centuries. It spread in epidemics and killed about 30 percent of people who contracted it. The disease caused severe headache, fever and a red, blistering rash that often left disfiguring scars on its survivors. Some were blinded from corneal infection.

At the end of the 18th century, Edward Jenner, an English physician, discovered that inoculating individuals with cowpox virus — similar to smallpox but usually harmless — prevented them from getting smallpox. Campaigns in the United States and in Europe began to immunize people against smallpox. In 1967, the World Health Organization (WHO) launched a global campaign to eliminate smallpox. The last reported case occurred in 1977, signaling the end of one of the deadliest diseases in history. As a result, smallpox vaccination is no longer necessary.

Global efforts to eradicate other infectious diseases continue. Polio has been wiped out from the Western Hemisphere, and the number of cases worldwide has dropped dramatically through an ongoing global initiative.

Vaccine Additives

In addition to the dead or weakened microorganisms that make up vaccines, small amounts of other substances may be added to enhance the immune response, prevent contamination, and stabilize the vaccine against temperature variations and other conditions. Vaccines may also contain small amounts of materials used in the manufacturing process, such as gelatin.

A preservative called thimerosal, a derivative of mercury, has received public attention in recent years. Thimerosal has been used in medical products since the 1930s and is in small amounts in some vaccines to prevent bacterial contamination. A large body of evidence supports the safety of such mercury use in vaccines, with no ill effects other than a minor local reaction around a shot. Nonetheless, all vaccines recommended for children 6 years old and under are now available without thimerosal.

Side effects of vaccines

Vaccines are considered very safe. But just like medications, they may cause side effects. Most side effects are minor and temporary, such as a sore arm, a mild fever or swelling at the injection site. Rarely, a child may experience a severe allergic reaction or a neurological side effect, such as a seizure.

According to the Centers for Disease Control and Prevention (CDC), serious side effects occur on the order of 1 per thousand to 1 per million of doses. The risk of death from a vaccine is so slight that it can't be accurately determined. When any serious reactions are reported, they receive careful scrutiny from the Food and Drug Administration and the CDC.

Some vaccines have been blamed for chronic illnesses, such as autism or diabetes. But decades of vaccine use in the United States and scientific study of outcomes have provided no credible evidence that vaccines cause these illnesses. Researchers have on occasion reported a link between vaccine use and chronic illness. But when other researchers have tried to duplicate those results — a test of good scientific research — they haven't been able to do so.

One of the greatest controversies regarding autism centers on whether a link exists between the disorder and childhood vaccines. Despite extensive research, no reliable study has shown a link between autism spectrum disorder and any vaccines. In fact, the original study that ignited the debate years ago has been retracted due to poor design and questionable research methods.

Signs of autism may appear at about the same time children receive certain vaccines — such as the measles-mumps-rubella (MMR) vaccine — however this appears to be simply a coincidence.

Although rare serious side effects are a concern, vaccines are much safer than the diseases they prevent.

Weighing the risks and benefits

The consequences of acquiring a disease that can be prevented by

Signs of a Severe Reaction

After vaccination, watch for any unusual conditions, such as a serious allergic reaction, high fever or behavior changes. Signs and symptoms of a serious allergic reaction include difficulty breathing, hoarseness or wheezing, hives, paleness, weakness, a fast heartbeat, dizziness, and swelling of the throat. If you think that your child may be experiencing a severe reaction, call your child's doctor or seek emergency assistance immediately.

Well-Child Vaccination Schedule

The following chart lists the recommended routine childhood vaccinations. Vaccine guidelines for children change fairly often as new vaccines are developed, recommendations on timing and dosages are revised, and more combination vaccines are created. For information on vaccines for children age 7 and older, see page 215.

Health insurance usually covers most of the cost of immunizations. A federal program called Vaccines for Children provides free vaccines to children who lack health insurance coverage and to other specific groups of children. Ask your health care provider about it.

Recommended Vaccination Schedule for Children Ages 0 to 6 Years

▓ Range of recommended ages

Vaccine ▼ / Age ▶	Birth	1 month	2 months	4 months	6 months	12 months	15 months	18 months	19-23 months	2-3 years	4-6 years
Hepatitis B	HepB	HepB			HepB						
Rotavirus			RV	RV	RV						
Diphtheria, tetanus, pertussis			DTaP	DTaP	DTaP		DTaP				DTaP
***Haemophilus influenzae* type b**			Hib	Hib	Hib	Hib					
Pneumococcal conjugate vaccine			PCV	PCV	PCV	PCV					
Inactivated poliovirus			IPV	IPV	IPV						IPV
Influenza (flu)					Influenza (Yearly)*						
Measles-mumps-rubella						MMR					MMR
Varicella (chickenpox)						Varicella					Varicella
Hepatitis A						HepA (2 Doses)**					

* Two doses are recommended at least four weeks apart for children up to age 8 getting the flu vaccine for the first time.

** The first dose of HepA vaccine should be given between 12 and 23 months of age. The second dose should be given six to 18 months later.

Source: Advisory Committee on Immunization Practices, Centers for Disease Control and Prevention, 2017

---

vaccination are far greater than the extremely rare risk of a serious side effect that may result from vaccine use.

For example, if your child gets the mumps, the risk of developing encephalitis, a brain inflammation that can cause serious brain damage, is as high as 1 in 300. For measles, the risk is about 1 in 1,000. If a child gets serious Hib disease, the chances of death are approximately 1 in 20.

In contrast, the risk of contracting encephalitis from the mumps and measles vaccines is less than 1 in 1 million. And the vaccine for Hib disease hasn't been associated with any serious adverse reactions and is highly effective.

Childhood Vaccinations

Many of the most familiar diseases of childhood — measles, mumps and chickenpox — are highly infectious ailments that can be passed easily from person to person. Fortunately, many of them can be prevented through immunization. For more information on many of the diseases that follow, see Chapter 16, "Infectious Diseases."

Chickenpox (varicella)

Chickenpox (varicella) is a common childhood disease, although its incidence has dropped sharply since a vaccine was introduced in the U.S. in 1995. It may also affect adults who aren't immune. The disease can be serious, especially for babies, adults and people with weakened immune systems.

The chickenpox virus is spread by breathing in infected droplets or by direct contact with fluid from the rash, which is the best known sign of the disease. The rash begins as superficial spots on the face, chest, back and other areas of the body. The spots quickly fill with a clear fluid, rupture and turn crusty.

Recommendation
Children should receive one dose of the chickenpox vaccine between 12 and 15 months of age or at any age after that if they haven't had the disease. A second dose should follow at 4 to 6 years of age, before the child starts school (or at least 3 months after the first dose). Adults without immunity should receive two doses, 4 to 8 weeks apart.

Diphtheria

Diphtheria is a bacterial infection that spreads from person to person through airborne droplets. It causes a thick coating (membrane) to develop in the back of the throat and can lead to severe breathing problems, paralysis, heart failure and death. The disease is rare in the United States.

Recommendation
The diphtheria vaccine typically is given in combination with the tetanus and pertussis vaccines (a DTaP shot). Vaccination should begin when a child reaches 2 months of age. A child should receive five shots in the first six years of life and a booster of tetanus, diphtheria and pertussis (Tdap) at age 11 or 12. An adult booster (Td) should then follow every 10 years.

Flu (influenza)

The influenza vaccine is now recommended yearly for infants and children, beginning at age 6 months. For more information on the vaccine, see page 237.

German measles (rubella)

German measles (rubella) — a disease that spreads through the air — is typically a mild infection that causes a rash and slight fever. However, if a woman develops rubella during pregnancy, she may have a miscarriage, or the baby could be born with birth defects.

Recommendation
Usually, two doses of the combination measles-mumps-rubella (MMR) vaccine are given, the first at ages 12 to 15 months and the second at ages 4 to 6 years. A note for older children: In the event this schedule isn't followed, girls should receive the live weakened (attenuated) vaccine before their first period to avoid the risk of contracting rubella during pregnancy.

Haemophilus influenzae type b disease

Haemophilus influenzae type b (Hib) disease is primarily a childhood illness, but it can also affect some adults. It's caused by bacteria that spread from person to person through the air. This infection can cause serious and potentially fatal problems, including meningitis, sepsis, severe swelling in the throat, and infections of the blood, joints, bones and membrane around the heart (pericarditis).

Recommendation
The Hib conjugate vaccine is given to children at ages 2 months, 4 months, 6 months, and 12 to 15 months. The vaccine typically is given at the same time as other vaccines. Children over 5 years of age usually don't need the Hib vaccine. But some older children and adults with special health conditions should receive it. Such people include those with sickle cell disease, human immunodeficiency virus (HIV), AIDS or no spleen, and those who have undergone a bone marrow transplant or cancer treatment.

Hepatitis A

Hepatitis A is a liver disease caused by the hepatitis A virus. It's usually spread by eating or drinking contaminated food or water or by close personal contact.

Recommendation
The two-dose series of the hepatitis A vaccine is recommended for all children in the United States. The first dose is given at 12 months and the second dose at 24 months.

Hepatitis B

The hepatitis B virus can cause a short-term (acute) illness marked by loss of appetite, fatigue, diarrhea, vomiting, jaundice and pain in muscles, joints and the abdomen. More rarely it can lead to long-term (chronic) liver damage or liver cancer.

The virus is spread through contact with the blood or other body fluids of an infected person. This can happen by sharing a toothbrush, having unprotected sex, sharing needles when injecting illicit drugs, or during birth, when the virus passes from an infected mother to her baby. However, over one-third of people who have hepatitis B in the United States don't know how they got it.

Recommendation
The hepatitis B vaccine is given to children in three doses — at birth, at least one month later (1 to 2 months of age) and then at 6 to 18 months.

Measles (rubeola)

Measles (rubeola) is primarily a childhood illness, although adults also are susceptible. It's extremely contagious. The measles virus is transmitted through the air in droplets, such as from a sneeze.

Signs and symptoms include rash, fever, cough, sneezing, runny nose, eye irritation and a sore throat. Measles can lead to an ear infection, pneumonia, seizures, brain damage and death.

Recommendation

A live, weakened measles vaccine is given to children at 12 to 15 months of age, usually in combination with the mumps and rubella vaccines (MMR). A second dose is given at 4 to 6 years of age. If the immunization schedule is missed, older children and adults can be safely inoculated with a live vaccine.

However, since the vaccine includes a live virus, children who have leukemia or another severe illness and whose immune systems are impaired shouldn't be vaccinated, on the small chance that the weakened virus in the vaccine could cause disease.

Mumps

Mumps is a childhood disease that can also occur in adults. Mumps is caused by a virus that's acquired by inhaling infected droplets. The disease causes fever, headache, fatigue and swollen, painful salivary glands. It can lead to deafness, meningitis, and inflammation of the testicles or ovaries, with the possibility of sterility.

Recommendation

Two doses of the MMR vaccination are given, at ages 12 to 15 months and then at 4 to 6 years. Use of this vaccine has markedly decreased the incidence of mumps in the United States.

Pneumococcal disease

Pneumococcal disease is the leading cause of bacterial meningitis among children under 5 years old, and is a common source of early-childhood ear infections. It can also cause blood infections and pneumonia. Children under the age of 2 are at greatest risk of the most serious complications of this disease.

Pneumococcal disease is caused by *Streptococcus pneumoniae* bacteria. The bacteria spread from person to person through physical contact or by inhaling droplets released into the air when a person with the infection coughs or sneezes. Because many strains of the bacterium have become resistant to antibiotics, the disease can be difficult to treat.

Recommendation

Pneumococcal conjugate vaccine (PCV) can help prevent serious pneumococcal disease and one cause of ear infections. The vaccine is given to all children in four doses between ages 2 and 15 months. It's also recommended for children between ages 2 and 5 years who haven't had the pneumococcal vaccine series and are at high risk of the disease. This includes children without a spleen and children who have sickle cell disease, chronic heart or lung disease, human immunodeficiency virus (HIV), AIDS, or other diseases that may affect the immune system, such as cancer or diabetes. Children who take medications that affect the immune system, such as chemotherapy or steroids, also should be vaccinated.

In addition to PCV, pneumococcal polysaccharide vaccine (PPSV) is recommended for certain high-risk individuals. A first dose may be given as early as age 2, and a second dose five years later may be recommended.

Polio

Polio is caused by a virus (poliovirus) that enters the body through the mouth. Polio affects the brain and spinal cord, often resulting in paralysis or death. Polio vaccination began in the United States in 1955.

No U.S. polio cases have been reported for many years, but the disease is still common in a few parts of the world, and the virus could be brought into the United States. For that reason, getting children vaccinated against polio continues to be important.

Recommendation

The vaccine, called inactivated polio vaccine (IPV), is given in four doses, at ages 2 months, 4 months, 6 to 18 months and at 4 to 6 years. This last vaccination is a booster dose. Contradictory to the fears of some people, the shots can't cause polio.

Rotavirus

Rotavirus is the most common cause of severe diarrhea among infants and children globally. Almost all children are infected with rotavirus before their fifth birthdays. The infection is often accompanied by vomiting and fever.

Since the introduction of a vaccine in 2006, hospitalizations due to rotavirus in the United States have dropped significantly.

? **Question and Answer**

What should I do if my child misses a vaccination?

If your child falls behind on vaccinations, catch-up immunization schedules can address the problem. Contact your child's doctor to determine the vaccinations your child needs and when he or she should receive them.

An interruption in the schedule doesn't require a child to start a series over or redo any doses. But until your child receives the entire vaccine series, he or she won't have maximum possible protection against diseases.

Recommendation

The rotavirus vaccine is a swallowed (oral) vaccine, not a shot. The vaccine won't prevent diarrhea or vomiting caused by other germs, but it's very good at preventing diarrhea and vomiting caused by rotavirus.

There are two brands of rotavirus vaccine. A baby should get either two or three doses, depending on which brand is used. The first dose is given at 2 months, the second at 4 months and the third dose, if needed, at 6 months.

Tetanus

Tetanus causes painful tightening of the muscles, usually all over the body. It can be difficult to open your mouth (lockjaw) or swallow. Tetanus isn't a contagious disease. The tetanus bacteria enter the body through deep or dirty cuts or wounds.

Recommendation

The tetanus vaccine typically is given in combination with those for diphtheria and pertussis (DTaP vaccine). Vaccination should start when a child reaches 2 months of age. The vaccine is administered in a series of five shots in the first six years of life.

Starting at age 11, people should continue to get vaccinated every 10 years with the adult forms of the vaccine — Tdap or Td.

Whooping cough (pertussis)

Whooping cough (pertussis) is a disease that causes severe coughing spells, making it hard for infants and toddlers to eat, drink or even breathe. The word *pertussis* is from the Latin word for "cough." These coughing spells can last for weeks and can lead to pneumonia, seizures, brain damage and death. Severe whooping cough primarily occurs in children younger than 2 years and is contracted by inhaling infected droplets, often coughed into the air from an adult with a mild case of the disease.

Recommendation

The DTaP immunization combines vaccines for diphtheria, tetanus and pertussis. It's given as a series of five shots beginning when the infant is 2 months old and continuing to between ages 4 and 6. The *a* in DTaP stands for "acellular," meaning that only specific parts of the pertussis bacteria are used in the vaccine.

Following up with a form of the vaccine for adolescents and adults, called Tdap, is recommended at age 11 or 12.

Personality, Behavior and Development

Your newborn is a unique human being. From one healthy baby to the next, the variations are infinite. Part of the wonder of parenting is watching, recognizing and reinforcing the changes, development and behaviors as your infant's personality emerges.

Reflexes and responses

Your newborn's movements are governed by reflexes. Stroke your baby's cheek, and your baby will likely root and try to suck. Prick the soles of the feet, and the knees and feet flex. Make a sudden noise, and your baby may startle.

All healthy babies are born with reflexes that disappear in a predictable order as voluntary control of motor functions takes over. The absence of a newborn's natural reflexes and responses may indicate a neurological problem. Part of your newborn's hospital examination includes attempts to elicit various reflexes and responses. This includes:

? **Question and Answer**

Is it safe to give multiple vaccines at once? Isn't that a lot for a child's immune system to handle?

Some childhood vaccines are given in a mixed shot, such as those for measles-mumps-rubella (MMR) and those for diphtheria, tetanus and pertussis (DTaP). In addition, the recommended schedule for vaccinating children involves giving up to four vaccines at the same time.

Many parents worry that the baby's immune system will be overloaded, with damaging effects. But a child isn't harmed by receiving more than one vaccination at a time. Consider that every day children survive exposure to many different germs. For example, a strep throat infection exposes a child to more than 100 different antigens.

A large number of studies show that simultaneous immunization with multiple vaccines is convenient, safe and effective. Giving several vaccinations at once means fewer office visits, which saves time and money for parents and may be less traumatic for the child. It also helps meet the goal of vaccinating children as early as possible to protect them during the vulnerable early months of their lives.

Is Your Baby Warm Enough?

How can you tell whether your baby needs extra clothing? Don't go by the warmth of your baby's hands. The hands aren't a good indicator of how warm a baby is because they tend to be cool even when the body is warm. The legs, arms and neck are better indicators. Your infant's face also can be a guide. A good rule of thumb is to dress your infant in one more layer of clothing than you wear.

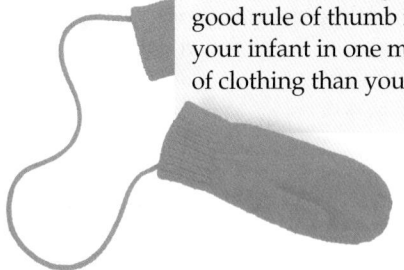

The startle reflex
The startle reflex (Moro reflex) is one of the most frequent and dramatic newborn responses. It occurs when your infant hears a loud noise, has an abrupt change in position or is handled roughly.

The startle reflex causes an infant to arch his or her back and throw his or her head back. At the same time, the infant throws out his or her arms and legs and brings them abruptly back toward the body. The infant cries, then startles and then cries because of the startle. The reflex is often strong enough to make the child fall off something if he or she is not being watched. The startle reflex gradually disappears by the third month of life.

The grasp reflex
Stroking your infant sets off several responses. When you stroke the palm of his or her hand, your baby grasps your finger (palmar reflex). When you stroke the sole of your baby's foot, you'll see the toes turn downward, as if trying to grasp something (plantar reflex). The palmar reflex disappears at about age 6 months. The plantar reflex continues until 10 months of age.

The rooting and sucking reflexes
Rooting and sucking are two of your infant's important reflexes. Stroking the baby's cheek or lips with a nipple or finger produces the rooting reflex. The baby turns toward the stroking object and tries to bring it near the mouth. The sucking reflex is initiated once the object is taken into the baby's mouth.

Sucking and rooting reflexes usually diminish by the time the infant is 4 months old, although these reflexes can often be produced in a sleeping infant until the seventh month.

The tonic neck reflex
The tonic neck reflex occurs when an infant's head is turned to the side while the infant is on his or her back. The baby arches his or her body away from the face side, extends the arm on the face side, flexes the other arm and draws up the legs. This reflex is more prominent in the 2-month-old infant and usually disappears by the sixth month.

The orienting response
The orienting response of your newborn is a response to a change in the environment. When an infant hears or sees something new, he or she becomes more alert and less active. His or her head may turn toward the stimulus, and the baby's heart rate increases. When the infant is adapting to a familiar stimulus, the heartbeat may slow.

The gag and blink reflexes
An infant is able to protect itself because of several responses and reflexes. Because of a strong gag reflex, your newborn is able to spit up mucus to help clear his or her windpipe. A strong blink reflex protects the newborn's eyes from glaring light. And in older infants, when a part of the body is exposed to cold air, his or her skin color appears mottled, limbs pull in close to the body to reduce the exposed surface, and he or she begins to shiver and cry in an attempt to stay warm.

Even though your newborn's reflexes will disappear — most of them during the first year of life — their usefulness seems to be more than short term. Studies indicate that your baby's brain stores information learned from these early reflexes.

Behavior

Your baby's sleeping, crying and eating patterns, and how he or she responds to stimuli such as your touch and voice, define your infant's behavior. A baby that sleeps easily, cries very little, eats predictably, and responds consistently to a parent's touch and communication may seem easier to care for. The irritable, fretful baby that feeds irregularly and sleeps little requires more attention. Typical infant behavior covers a wide range of patterns.

Your baby's behavior will influence how you parent. Initially, a newborn responds primarily to his or her immediate physical needs. But a newborn's emotional needs are equally important. Newborns need comforting and holding. They need the sound of your voice and the sight of your smile.

Prevailing wisdom used to be that a newborn could easily be spoiled. Babies were put on strict schedules and handled only when necessary. If a newborn cried for any reason other than hunger or a diaper change, the wails often were ignored. Experts now know that responsiveness is a better approach.

Research shows that the longer a parent takes to answer a baby's cry, the longer it takes to soothe the baby. Babies whose cries are answered quickly in the early months of their development may cry less often and for shorter periods in later months. Instead of becoming clingy toddlers, these babies are more likely to demonstrate healthy independence.

Keeping flexible schedules allows for considering the needs of the baby and your family. By observing what works and what doesn't, over time you'll discover many things about your baby's behavior. What does your baby enjoy? How much stimulation does your baby need? How can you help quiet your baby?

Parents often underestimate their baby's ability to calm down without help from mom or dad. Examples of such skills include sucking a finger or knuckle, listening to a repetitive noise, or watching an interesting object. As your baby starts to demonstrate these skills, it's important to learn when to intervene during a fussy spell and when to let your baby try to calm himself or herself down.

Bonding

Bonding between parent and child begins long before the baby is born or adopted. When parents-to-be first learn that they're expecting a child — whether through pregnancy or an adoption — they may begin to look through books for a name for their child. They may furnish a nursery. They hear their baby's heartbeat at a prenatal visit or receive a photograph of the child they'll be adopting. They plan and dream, worry, and hope. And finally they're rewarded with the arrival of the baby.

Bonding is the complex array of emotional ties and commitments that characterize the parent-child relationship. By the time a baby arrives, there's already a strong emotional link on the parents' part, a link that feels stronger for some parents than for others. Over the course of the next few months, the infant begins to develop an attachment to the person or people with whom he or she learns to associate protection, love and guidance.

Bonding begins immediately. Most babies have an alert period for one to two hours after delivery, making it a particularly good time for parents and infant to become acquainted. The key isn't when bonding happens but that it does.

How does a parent bond with an infant? There's no easy recipe for bonding, just as there's no way to tell someone how to love. Bonding occurs during the day-to-day exchange of affectionate actions between parent and child.

A mother gently touches her infant, and that touch is pleasurable to the new baby. When the baby's cheek is touched, the infant turns toward the mother's face or toward the breast and begins to nuzzle and nurse. This not only stimulates the production of milk but also is a powerful emotional stimulant. The baby gazes into the mother's eyes during breast- or bottle-feeding. The infant cries and the parent picks up the baby, strokes his or her cheek, and speaks in a soft and soothing voice.

The importance of bonding is well-recognized by hospitals and health professionals. Thus most hospitals encourage new parents to spend time close-up with their newborn, and parents adopting newborns will enjoy the same.

If your infant is born prematurely or is seriously ill, your baby will probably be placed in an incubator and connected to machines to monitor vital signs. Initially, you may not be able to hold or even feed your infant. However, you'll still be encouraged to spend as much time as possible with your newborn. You can stroke the baby's skin, hold his or her tiny hand, and provide comfort with your voice. Even this limited contact is important and beneficial for both you and your baby.

It's not uncommon for parents to wonder before their baby arrives whether they'll be able to love this new person who is about to enter and change their lives. Even after birth or adoption, many parents have looked at the new baby expecting to feel a rush of love and, instead, felt nothing or disappointment or, at times, even dislike.

Don't be too hard on yourself if you don't immediately fall in love with your infant. Parenting is never easy, and at times it can be downright trying. Love for your baby sometimes comes gradually. As you get to know each other, as you see your baby's eyes light up when you come into the room, or when he or she smiles at you for the first time, you'll soon find your affection growing.

Sibling relationships

Much attention has been devoted to sibling rivalry — the hostilities and insecurities aroused in the older child by the birth of a sibling. But what about the infant and his or her relationship with big brother or sister?

Life isn't always cozy for the infant with a sibling. This baby is apt to be poked and jabbed more than once, especially as he or she becomes more mobile. You have to monitor their play and make sure your infant isn't endangered.

On the positive side, watch your 5-month-old's delight when he or she is included in a game with an older sibling. Play with a sibling is so rewarding for the baby that he or she is sometimes willing to put up with a little roughness.

Besides the simple enjoyment of having a brother or sister to play with, your baby's mental and social development benefits from exposure to an older child. The infant learns self-protection, cooperation, imagination and how to get along with others. Moreover, the bond between your children is developed, and they gradually grow to love each other.

Don't feel guilty that your second and subsequent children don't get undivided attention, as did your first child. Remember, your first child didn't reap the benefits of an older brother or sister. There will be times when your baby actually prefers a brother or sister to you, or when a sibling's request that baby eat his or her cereal is quickly granted — whereas your efforts were met with resolute rejection.

Look for creative ways to involve older brothers or sisters in caring for the baby. Make a special effort to give your older children individual attention too. Encourage friends and family members to do the same. Your older children need to understand that you care about them as much as you care about the baby.

Be prepared for the "low point" in family relationships. It often occurs about two months after the baby's arrival. The novelty of a new baby is gone and so are your helpers.

At around 9 months, some babies have trouble getting along with a sibling who only weeks before was an object of admira-

Developmental Milestones

During the first 12 months of life, your baby works harder than at any other stage of his or her existence. In the course of this incredible first year, your infant goes from being totally dependent to walking, feeding himself or herself, and even speaking a few words. Every baby's developmental achievements are different, but the following month-by-month milestones can be used as a general guide.

1 month — First smile
A momentous occasion during the early weeks of life is your baby's first smile. Although you'll often see a smile on your newborn, an infant generally doesn't have what is called a social or responsive smile until after the first month, usually by the eighth week.

2 months — Voice recognition
By the second month of life, your baby can tell people are different from objects, with the former eliciting a more immediate response. Your infant is beginning to recognize your voice. Thus you may find that the baby who screams with a babysitter calms immediately when a parent enters the room and talks in a soothing voice.

3 months — Independent play
An infant at 3 months of age can play for perhaps 10 or 15 minutes at a time, with minimal parental involvement. The infant at this age is more easily distracted and will even interrupt nursing to look at or listen to something that catches his or her attention. The baby will spend time staring at things — a picture, a mobile, his or her own hand.

4 months — Mirror play
A milestone during this period is your baby's behavior in front of a mirror. Hold him or her in front of the mirror and watch the infant smile. When the image smiles back, the baby will become very excited and begin to babble. It will puzzle him or her to see two of you, and he or she will repeatedly look back at you and then at the mirror.

5 months — Stranger anxiety
At 5 months old your baby definitely knows the difference between his or her parents and strangers. For the first time, you may notice your baby is more cautious around strangers.

6 months — Finger foods
A 6-month-old infant is alert for half of his or her waking hours. By this age, solid foods may be a part of his or her diet. Gone are the days when your baby was content to have you do all of the feeding. Now that the infant's dexterity is improved, he or she wants to pick up pieces of food and put them in his or her own mouth (and anywhere else mood dictates).

tion. Babies at this age are intent on battling their own insecurities and fears. An older sibling who loves to tease or assert authority is just too much sometimes. If this happens to your infant, don't worry. Like other stages, this one will eventually pass as well.

Common Conditions and Concerns

As a parent of a newborn, you'll spend many waking and sleeping hours worrying about your baby's health. You may have questions about blemishes on your baby's skin or have concerns if your baby is crying excessively. Birthmarks and excessive crying (colic) are two concerns you may want to discuss with your baby's doctor. Other common newborn health concerns include spitting up, teething, fever, ear infections, diarrhea and constipation.

7 months — More mobility
Increased motor skills give an infant of 7 months a taste of freedom. At the same time that your baby longs to test his or her wings, however, he or she only wants to do it within sight of your reassuring presence. Don't be surprised if every time you leave the room your baby cries. The infant who has been content up until now to spend time in a playpen may suddenly rebel unless you're in the same room.

8 months — Separation anxiety
An 8-month-old baby is clearly attached to the parent providing most of his or her care. Separation anxiety often occurs at this age, and you may find that you can't leave the room without sending your baby into a panic. The baby who previously wasn't bothered by strangers suddenly may fear the next-door neighbor or even a grandparent. Or the infant may cry uncontrollably when the babysitter arrives, even when the caregiver is someone the baby knows. This reaction is a normal part of development and isn't something to be concerned about. Cuddle your child and reassure him or her that you will return soon. Always tell your infant that you're leaving and you will return.

9 months — New games
At 9 months, an infant is sophisticated enough to be bored. This is because his or her memory is more developed. Thus the infant is constantly searching for new stimulation, and the nightly game that has amused him or her for the past month suddenly has become uninteresting.

10 months — Imitation
A 10-month-old may begin to say no. Your child is also developing a sense of possession and may for the first time distinguish between his or her toys and those belonging to a sibling. You'll also notice how imitation plays a role in your infant's learning. During a meal the baby may offer you bits of food. Afterward he or she may attempt to wash your face and hands.

11 months — Testing authority
Although not always cooperative, your 11-month-old baby seeks your approval and will try to avoid your disapproval. Still, the infant can't avoid testing your authority. After you've put your son or daughter to bed, he or she may summon you every five minutes. At the same time, your every request is apt to be met with a resounding no. At this age, no sometimes means yes.

12 months — Temper tantrum
At 12 months, some infants begin to have tantrums. Your eager eater may become picky. Bedtime problems are common at this age.

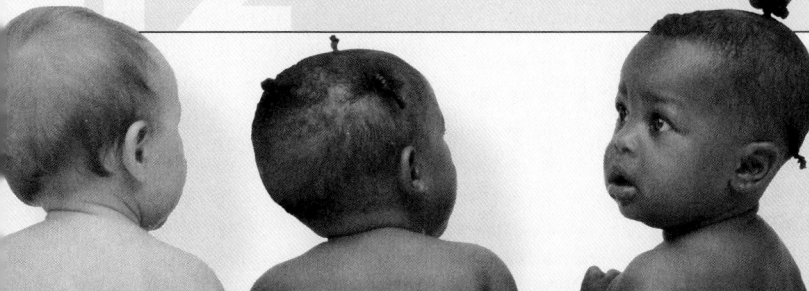

Birthmarks

Birthmarks are common among newborns. Most are harmless and don't require treatment. It's not known what causes birthmarks to occur or why they appear where they do.

Salmon patches
Often called stork bites or angel kisses, salmon patches are small, light pink, flat spots that commonly appear on newborns. They're collections of small blood vessels (capillaries) close to the skin. Occurring most frequently on the eyelids, upper lip, area between the eyebrows, and the back of the neck, salmon patches become more noticeable during crying bouts or when the temperature changes. Salmon patches often seem brighter in a child's first few months and then fade by 1 year of age.

Hemangiomas
Hemangiomas are noncancerous (benign) tumors made of newly formed blood vessels. Characteristically, hemangiomas are bright-red, elevated, sharply demarcated lesions. They usually appear on the face, scalp, back or chest, but may develop anywhere on the body. More common in girls, strawberry hemangiomas are seldom present at birth, but usually appear within the first two months of life.

Most hemangiomas grow rapidly, then remain at a fixed size and finally begin to disappear. Usually, no special care or treatment is recommended, and they're no longer noticeable by the time a child is 9 years old. Hemangiomas developing on the face need closer observation for possible treatment. Some children have some discoloration or a slight puckering of the skin after the mark is gone.

Port-wine stains
A port-wine stain is a flat hemangioma that consists of dilated capillaries. It often appears on the face. The size of the hemangioma varies. Occasionally, half the body surface may be affected. This is a permanent condition. Laser therapy has become the treatment of choice, but it's most successful on older children and adults.

Rashes

Rashes are common in infancy. The vast majority aren't serious and often can be managed at home. But a rash can be a sign of an infectious disease, such as chickenpox or measles. Have your baby examined if you notice a rash that is purple, crusty and weepy, or has blisters. A child who has a fever and rash may also need evaluation.

Diaper rash
Most infants develop a diaper rash at some time or another. Diaper rash can have many causes. The typical diaper rash is the reaction of the newborn's sensitive skin to contact with moisture and irritants. This rash often goes away in a couple of days with exposure to air and more-frequent diaper changes.

If your baby has diaper rash, change his or her diaper more often and gently wash the skin every time the diaper is changed. To clean the baby's bottom, use plain water, which is less irritating than baby wipes. Each time you change your infant, place him or her on his or her tummy for a while and let the rash "air out."

If you've been putting plastic pants over the baby's diaper, stop using them until the rash disappears. Petroleum jelly, zinc oxide paste or lubricating cream can be applied to the rash several times a day. Mild rashes don't require ointment unless the skin is dry and cracked. Cornstarch or talcum powder shouldn't be used because it can worsen the condition.

If the rash is particularly persistent and severe, a combination cream may be recommended to treat the rash and protect the skin. For persistent diaper rash, many doctors recommend taking the baby's diaper off and exposing the affected area to air as often as possible.

If your baby's rash doesn't improve, it could mean the child has a yeast infection. The infection may appear on the buttocks and genitals as bright red spots that come together to form a solid red area with a scalloped border. This type of rash can be treated with an anti-yeast cream or ointment and lots of airing.

If the rash is so severe that it interferes with your child's sleep, is a solid, bright-red color, causes fever, results in blisters or boils, or drains pus, call your child's doctor.

Cradle cap
Cradle cap (seborrheic dermatitis) is a common problem that can occur at any age, but it's most common during infancy and again during adolescence. Cradle cap often begins during the infant's first month of life and may continue to be a problem throughout the first year. Its cause is unknown.

If your infant has cradle cap, you probably first will notice dry, scaly patches on the scalp that give it a dirty appearance. A thick, yellow crust may form over the scales. You may notice some scaly patches around the hairline, eyebrows, eyelids, nose and behind the ears. Sometimes, the rash affects the entire body.

Cradle cap usually has a shorter course than many other rashes, and it responds to simple treatment. Without treatment it will go away over a period of a few months.

For cradle cap, avoid the temptation to wash your baby's hair frequently with baby shampoo. Once a week is often enough. After lathering, massage the scaly scalp with a soft toothbrush for a few minutes. If the scalp is very crusty, you can rub in mineral or baby oil an hour before you shampoo. If the rash is red and irritated, apply a 0.5 percent hydrocortisone cream, available without a prescription, once a week. Use of an anti-dandruff shampoo also may provide relief. A particularly stubborn case should be evaluated by your infant's doctor.

Drool rash

Many infants develop a rash on their cheeks and chin. The rash, which is caused by contact with food and regurgitated stomach contents, comes and goes. Gently cleansing the skin after a feeding is generally the only treatment generally required.

Heat rash

Heat rash causes tiny pink bumps on the skin and usually occurs on the back of the neck and upper back. It's the result of blocked sweat glands. Typically, the rash occurs during hot, humid weather, although an infant who is overdressed or who has a fever may develop a heat rash at any time.

Treatment involves letting the skin dry on its own and dressing your infant in as few clothes as necessary. Use a fan while the child is sleeping. Cool rinses also may help.

Infantile eczema

Infantile eczema (atopic dermatitis) is a rough, red, patchy rash usually associated with extremely dry, sensitive skin. The most common areas for eczema are the cheeks and forehead. The problem may spread to the neck and behind the ears.

Eczema is more likely to occur in infants with a family history of allergies. These infants also have a tendency to develop asthma and seasonal allergies later in their lives. If your infant has eczema, you may first notice light red or tannish-pink patches of rough, scaly skin. The patches later become red (see the illustration on page 396). Your baby may seem restless or irritable due to itching.

Soft Spots

Every baby is born with soft spots (fontanels) on the top of the head. During birth it's necessary for the baby's relatively large head to move down a narrower birth canal. To do so, the head must adapt itself to this smaller space. A completely formed skull couldn't do so. Thus, skull bones aren't tightly joined, and babies have spots on the top part of the skull where the bones haven't yet come together.

The size of fontanels varies. Generally, the larger they are, the longer they take to close. In some babies, the bones come together nine months after birth. In others, the process may take two years. The average is between 12 and 18 months.

New parents often are particularly concerned about soft spots. Some mothers are afraid to shampoo an infant's hair for fear they'll harm the brain. In fact, the baby's brain is well-protected from normal handling by a tough, protective membrane over soft spots. Parents shouldn't be afraid of causing harm by simply touching the top of the baby's head.

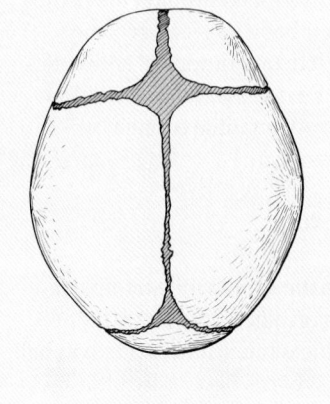

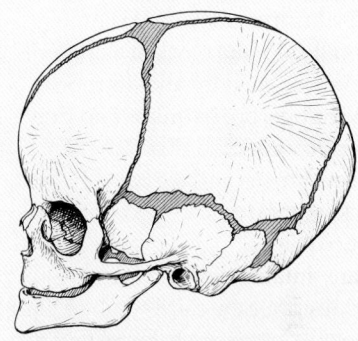

Your child's tiny skull consists of not one but several separate bones. During the first one to two years of life, these bones fuse to form a single protective bone mass. Until then there will be soft spots (fontanels) at the main junctures of the bones.

Occasionally, the rash begins to ooze and crust over. Infection of the skin may follow.

In some infants, the rash can be traced to diet or a change in formula. Sometimes, the offender may be a laundry detergent, a fabric such as wool or excessive perspiration during hot weather. Rarely, eczema may be a sign of a serious disease. Often the cause is hard to identify.

The main complication of eczema is infection of the lesions. Infants with eczema shouldn't be exposed to people with cold sores (herpes simplex).

To decrease the chance of more bacteria being introduced into the open skin, keep your baby's nails clipped as short as possible. If your baby will tolerate them, a

pair of cotton mittens worn especially during sleep, which is when most of the scratching usually occurs, helps prevent further skin damage and infection.

Avoid temperature extremes. Most babies with eczema do better in a mild climate with moderate humidity because sweating seems to aggravate the rash. Avoid wool clothing, and don't lay the baby on wool carpeting. Keep baths to a minimum, and use bath oil to lubricate the dry skin.

If the eczema is particularly severe, your child's doctor may recommend use of dressings soaked in a special solution to ease the redness and itching.

Corticosteroid lotions and creams can be applied after the dressing is removed. Antihistamines are often effective for controlling the itching. If your baby's lesions become infected, oral or topical antibiotics may be necessary. Most children outgrow infantile eczema by 3 to 5 years of age.

Milia

Milia are small white bumps or cysts on a newborn's face that resemble whiteheads. More than half of newborns have these little spots.

By the time the infant is 2 months old, the blocked skin pores generally open up and disappear. The bumps are harmless and don't need treatment.

Baby acne

Many infants develop acne, usually after the third week of life. The cause appears to be related to maternal hormones that cross the placenta before birth.

The presence of acne can be disturbing, but it's only temporary. In some infants, the acne disappears within weeks. In others, it persists for up to six months. Generally, no treatment is necessary other than gently washing your baby's face daily with plain water and once or twice a week with a mild soap.

Thrush

Thrush is a mild yeast infection of the mouth that looks like whitish patches. The patches may be on the tongue and roof of the mouth and stuck to the inside of the cheeks. If the white spots don't come off when gently rubbed with a cotton swab, your baby may have thrush. Consult your child's doctor.

Thrush in healthy newborns generally resolves on its own, but treatment with an anti-yeast medication can hasten the process, particularly if the thrush is extensive. A breast-feeding mother also may need treatment if her nipples are sore or cracked.

An anti-yeast cream may be necessary to treat diaper rash that

can accompany thrush. Exposing infected areas to air may also be helpful in clearing the rash.

Umbilical hernia

An infant with an umbilical hernia has a soft bulge of tissue around the navel (umbilicus) that may protrude more when the baby cries, coughs or strains. It's caused by failure of the tissue ring around the navel to close. As a result, a portion of the small intestine slips through the enlarged umbilical opening.

Unlike other hernias, umbilical hernias have little danger associated with them. Most infant umbilical hernias disappear by the time the baby is a year old. Surgery is rarely necessary unless the hernia becomes progressively larger, fails to heal by the time the child is age 5, or causes an intestinal obstruction.

Spitting up and vomiting

Spitting up usually isn't a cause for concern, but vomiting may be.

Spitting up
Infants often spit up after a feeding. Spitting up is the gentle spilling of what's typically a small amount of milk from the baby's mouth. This shouldn't be confused with vomiting, during which the contents of the baby's stomach are ejected forcefully from its mouth.

One newborn may spit up after every feeding, and another may spit up only infrequently. The reason babies spit up isn't completely understood, but it's likely related to immature digestive systems. Unlike an older child or adult, the muscle between a baby's esophagus and the upper portion of the stomach isn't yet adept at holding contents in the stomach. Thus, any movement, even something as gentle as laying a child down, can cause the milk to be regurgitated.

Spitting up is messy for the parents, but it rarely signifies a serious problem. It gradually resolves

by the time the child is between 6 months and a year old. Burping the baby after each feeding is important and can help reduce spitting up. Place the infant upright on your shoulder and rub his or her back for a few minutes.

Immediately after a feeding, some babies do better sitting upright in an infant seat. If your baby is a natural spitter, the problem may continue no matter what you do. If your baby seems healthy and is gaining weight, there's little cause for concern.

Vomiting
Vomiting can be the result of milk intolerance, or it can be a sign of another illness. Notify your care provider if your infant vomits, but as long as the baby seems healthy and is gaining weight, there's probably no reason to be alarmed.

A newborn may vomit mucus, often streaked with blood, a few hours after birth. Typically, this is blood from the mother that the infant swallowed during delivery and is normal. Usually, this vomiting subsides after a few feedings. If it continues, it can signify an obstruction in the esophagus or intestines that warrants further evaluation. If your baby has blood in his or her vomit or is vomiting persistently, he or she should be seen immediately for further evaluation.

Loose stools or diarrhea

The stool of a breast-fed newborn is naturally mushy. If the mother uses laxatives or eats food with laxative properties, the baby's stools may become even looser. Bottle-fed babies generally have firmer stools than do breast-fed babies.

If your baby has diarrhea during the first month, it may be caused by an infection. The stool is apt to be greenish and watery, and the curds normally found in the stool of a breast-fed newborn will be absent. There may be an unpleasant odor.

If your newborn has persistent diarrhea, contact his or her doctor. If your baby has only a mild case of diarrhea, you may need to change the frequency or amount of your baby's feedings. Let your baby continue feeding, but be aware that he or she may take less than usual. Occasionally, a prepared fluid mixture to prevent dehydration may be suggested for a short time. If the diarrhea is more severe or your doctor thinks the baby is becoming dehydrated, he or she may need to be hospitalized.

Constipation

Don't be concerned if your baby misses a bowel movement or even goes for several days without one. The consistency of the stool is what indicates constipation, not the frequency of bowel movements. A baby who passes hard, pellet-like stools is constipated.

If your infant becomes constipated, it may be due to inadequate fluid or food intake. Constipation rarely occurs in breast-fed infants, but if it does, try more-frequent feedings.

If constipation is present from birth, your baby's doctor may want to examine the infant's rectum to make sure there's no obstruction or congenital abnormality.

Failure to gain weight

Babies undergo dramatic growth in the first days and months of life. The most common reason for slow weight gain is insufficient intake of milk. If you're breast-feeding, your baby's doctor or a lactation consultant may be able to suggest helpful changes in breast-feeding techniques or patterns. If you're bottle-feeding, sometimes a change in formula or an increase in the number of feedings will resolve the problem. Occasionally, failure to gain weight indicates medical problems that need further investigation.

Teething

Your infant will likely develop a first tooth between age 5 and 9 months. Most babies have between six and eight teeth by the time they're a year old.

Many babies breeze through teething. Their only symptoms are increased drooling and an insatiable need to chew on things. For others, the process is fraught with discomfort, daytime restlessness and crankiness. Your child may take to thumb sucking as never before, rub his or her gums, and temporarily lose his or her appetite.

If your baby is among those with teething discomfort, try the following techniques:
- Massage the swollen gum for a couple of minutes with or without a piece of ice. Some babies voluntarily or involuntarily tend to bite a parent's fingers in an attempt to relieve their discomfort.
- Offer a cold teething ring. Never tie a teething ring around your baby's neck because it could cause strangulation. An older baby or toddler can have some ice, an ice pop, or a slice of frozen banana to gnaw on.
- Use acetaminophen (Tylenol, others) to reduce discomfort if needed. Don't use products that contain benzocaine, an agent that could numb the throat and cause your baby to choke.

Fever

Fever in a newborn is defined as a rectal temperature of more than 100.4 F. Fever most commonly results from the body's response to infection. Keep in mind that in the first few months of life, particularly in premature infants, an infection may not cause a fever.

The key is how your baby acts. If he or she seems more listless than usual, contact your baby's doctor. Also contact your child's doctor if the fever is accompanied by a rash.

Febrile seizures

A seizure (convulsion) occurs as a result of abnormal activity in the brain's nerve cells. Typically, an infant having a seizure suddenly becomes unconscious, with his or her arms and legs held rigid. After a few seconds, the limbs and face may begin to twitch rhythmically.

The majority of childhood seizures are caused by fevers and are called febrile seizures. When seizures are recurrent and not related to fever, a child is said to have a seizure disorder.

A febrile seizure most often occurs in children between 6 months

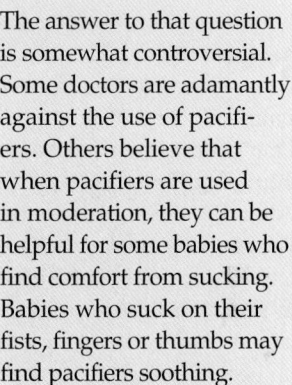

? Question and Answer

Should I give my baby a pacifier?

The answer to that question is somewhat controversial. Some doctors are adamantly against the use of pacifiers. Others believe that when pacifiers are used in moderation, they can be helpful for some babies who find comfort from sucking. Babies who suck on their fists, fingers or thumbs may find pacifiers soothing.

Pacifiers shouldn't be introduced to breast-fed newborns until a nursing routine is well-established.

If you give your infant a pacifier, the most important thing is to use it properly:
- Don't pop it into your baby's mouth every time it opens.
- Encourage your baby to go to sleep without the pacifier.
- Find other methods for calming your crying baby.
- Take the pacifier away as soon as your baby's need for extra sucking is gone, usually between 12 and 15 months of age.

and 4 years of age who develop a sudden fever. Sometimes, a febrile seizure is the first indication that a child is ill. Febrile seizures occur in about 4 percent of children before the age of 4 years. Many children have no recurrence after the initial episode.

Febrile seizures typically are short — usually less than five minutes. It was once believed that a child who had a febrile seizure risked brain damage. This is rarely so. Seizures can be frightening for a parent, but in most cases the child is fine after the seizure.

If your infant with a fever has a febrile seizure, these steps can help him or her avoid injury during the seizure:

- Place your child on his or her stomach or side, not on the back.
- Remove any hard or sharp objects near your child.
- Loosen tight or restrictive clothing that your child is wearing.
- Don't restrain or interfere with your child's movements.
- Don't attempt to put anything in your child's mouth.
- After the seizure is over and your baby is awake, notify your child's doctor. If you're unable to contact his or her primary care provider, take your baby to an urgent care center or a hospital emergency department for an examination.

Excessive crying (colic)

A colicky baby is one who's healthy and well-fed but has predictable periods of crying — usually at about the same time each day and most often in the evening — that may last for minutes or may continue for two or more hours. Colic occurs with equal frequency in male and female babies, firstborns and subsequent babies, and bottle-fed and breast-fed babies.

There are many theories as to the cause of colic, but the reasons for it remain unknown. Colicky spells usually begin within a few weeks of birth and usually disappear in the baby's third or fourth month. The baby can't be consoled for more than a few moments by any method. The crying has an effect on parent-child interaction and is a potential source of family disruption. A colicky baby is at greater risk of child abuse because overwhelmed parents may take out their frustration and anger on the crying child.

If your baby has colic, the weeks of crying can seem like an eternity. When you can't end the crying episodes by the usual consoling methods, you'll need to shift your tactics and concentrate on finding ways to survive the colicky weeks. Here are some suggestions:

- Rock your baby back and forth in a hammock motion.
- Try white noise. For example, turn on a vacuum cleaner, a hair dryer, radio static or any similar sound while rocking your baby.
- Go for a car ride.
- Put your crying baby in a sling or stroller and go for a brisk walk.
- Leave your baby with a supportive caregiver so that you can take a nap or get out of the house for a while.

- If no one is available, lay the baby down for five or 10 minutes and do some on-the-spot stretching or vigorous exercises to re-energize yourself.

Although your attempts to console your baby may be unsuccessful, he or she still needs the reassurance of your presence. Support from your partner, family and friends also is essential during this time.

If you're worried at any time that your baby is sick, or if you or others caring for your baby are starting to feel out of control with anger because of the excessive crying, bring your baby to the doctor's office or a hospital emergency department.

Sleep difficulties

Drooping eyelids, rubbing the eyes and inconsolable fussiness are the usual signs of fatigue in a baby. Many babies cry when they're put down for sleep, but if left alone, most will eventually quiet themselves. It often takes 20 minutes of restlessness for a baby to fall asleep.

The following steps may help your baby learn how to fall asleep

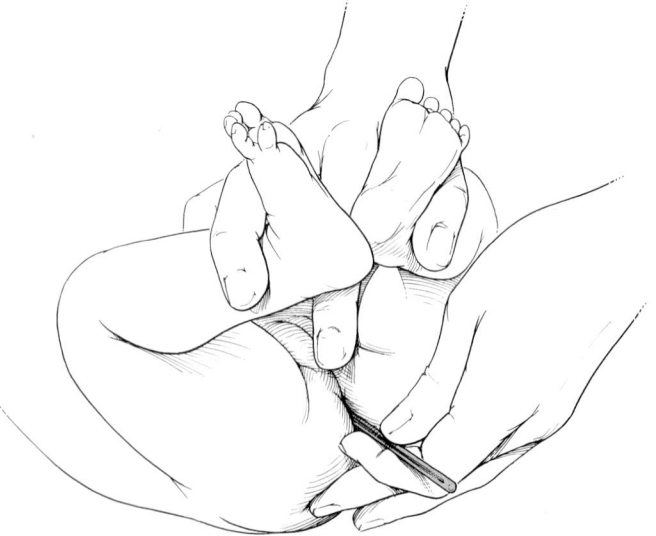

To take a newborn's temperature with a rectal thermometer, insert the lubricated thermometer approximately an inch (though if you feel resistance, never push farther). Hold the thermometer there for three minutes, and do not let go of it while it's in your child.

and get back to sleep if he or she awakes:

- Put your baby to bed drowsy but awake. A baby who habitually falls asleep in someone's arms may wake up in the night and not be able to fall asleep without being held.
- When your baby needs care or feeding in the night, use a soft voice and subtle body language to let the baby know it's nighttime, not playtime. Be businesslike and boring. Let your baby know this isn't the time for fun activities such as walking, rocking and playing.
- Think about your own sleep habits. When you awaken in the night, it takes a couple of minutes to find a comfortable position, settle in and fall back asleep. The same is true of your baby. Unlike you, however, one of the only comforting mechanisms your baby has is crying. Expect some crying as your baby tries to fall back to sleep.
- Make sure your baby is comfortable and safe. If you've made sure the crib and area around it are safe, you won't immediately become concerned about your baby's safety if you hear cries.
- Establish a bedtime routine — a winding down of the day's activities. You may want to turn off the television and have a quiet time 30 minutes before you put your baby to bed.

Ear infections

Middle ear infections (otitis media) are one of the most common illnesses affecting infants and young children. Seven out of 10 children will have at least one middle ear infection by age 3. Although ear infections often recur, most children stop having multiple ear infections by the time they reach school age.

Ear infections often follow a cold, which causes fluid to build up behind a child's eardrum. The trapped fluid is an ideal breeding ground for bacteria or viruses that cause infection. In addition to having an earache or a feeling of pressure and blockage in the ear, some children become very irritable, lose their appetite or develop a fever. Some children may experience temporary hearing loss, but most ear infections don't result in permanent hearing loss.

Most ear infections clear on their own without antibiotics. But your doctor may prescribe antibiotics if the infection is severe or if your child has recurrent ear infections. If your child doesn't respond to antibiotics, his or her doctor may recommend surgically inserting a small drainage tube into the eardrum to help prevent fluid buildup (see page 632).

Toilet training

Toilet training can be a difficult time in the lives of a child and his or her parents. But when handled properly, it can be simply one in a series of many milestones.

The first question most parents ask is, "When is the right time to attempt toilet training?" That's not an easy question to answer. One child's readiness for toilet training may be different from that of another. Some are toilet trained within 24 hours around age 2, and others still balk at the idea near their third birthday.

Unless a child appears extremely interested in being trained, most doctors usually advise waiting until between 2 and 2^1/$_2$ years. Bladder control through the night comes later. Most children continue to wear underwear-type absorbent pants at night for several months afterward.

Signs your child is ready
No rule says that training will be successful immediately. Try it for a few days and if your child clearly isn't interested or protests, put the plan off for a few weeks.

Here are some indications your child may be ready:

Baby-Proofing Your Home

Your infant is particularly susceptible to injury in the home when he or she begins to crawl. It only takes a second for your baby to get into trouble, so it's important to be alert and to take extra safety measures.

- Never leave your infant unattended on a bed or table or in the bath.
- If you have stairs in your home, make sure you have gates at the top and bottom of all stairways.
- Cover your unused electrical outlets with protective covers.
- Keep pull cords for windows out of reach.
- Make sure that all cleaning solutions, insecticides and medications are stored well out of your infant's reach. If you don't have a high shelf or cupboard, you can buy locks that make it difficult for a child to open a cabinet.
- Keep plastic bags away from your baby. They can quickly smother a baby.
- Avoid scalds by lowering the temperature of the water heater in your dwelling.
- Keep kettles and pots on the back burners of stoves, if possible.
- Don't drink hot beverages or foods, such as coffee or soup, while holding your baby.
- Check your houseplants. Be familiar with the toxic plants in and around your home, and make sure that they're well out of reach of your baby.

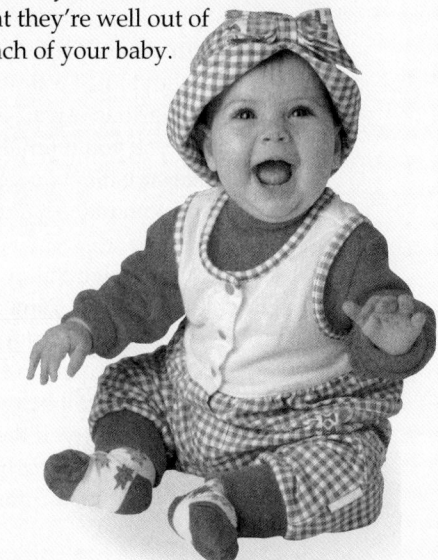

- Your child uses bathroom words such as *potty*, *pee-pee* or *poo-poo*.
- Your child has watched others use the toilet.
- Your child indicates when he or she is wet or dirty and wants to be changed.
- Your child can briefly control his or her bowel and bladder.
- Your child can pull his or her pants down and up.

Supplies

Once you determine that the time may be right, you'll need some supplies:

- A small potty chair that sits on the floor. Some children's toilet seats are designed to fit on a regular toilet, but many children prefer the floor type. A floor type not only allows the child to get on and off at will but also enables the child to push better because his or her feet are on the floor. Purchase the potty a few weeks before you're ready to begin training so that your child becomes familiar with it.
- Training pants, which are heavy, more-absorbent underwear.
- Stickers, if you want to use tangible rewards in addition to your praise. Always reward your child for showing interest in using the toilet and not for what comes out when on the toilet. Your praise is the best reward you can give your child. Don't use food as a reward for using the toilet.

How to train your child

You can go about toilet training your child in various ways. No matter which one you ultimately choose, make sure that you don't turn the bathroom into a battle-ground.

Many doctors suggest allowing the child to become trained according to his or her own free will. This means no coercion whatsoever. Ask your child if he or she wants to sit on the potty. If the answer is no, don't pressure him or her. If your child sits a minute but doesn't do anything, let him or her get off the potty when ready. If your child urinates or has a bowel movement, be free with your praise. But when the inevitable "accident" occurs, don't scold or shame your toddler.

Other methods use similar principles but require more parental involvement. For example, bring your child to the potty chair at appropriate intervals and ask him or her to pee-pee. If your child is reluctant to cooperate, try entertaining him or her with books or games while he or she is seated on the potty chair. If your child doesn't urinate within five minutes, try again later. When your child does use the potty chair, offer praise.

For some children, bowel and bladder control occur simultaneously. Others achieve one before the other. If your attempts at toilet training don't go well, it may be an indication that your child is too young, and you should probably try again in a few weeks or months.

If your child is older than $2\frac{1}{2}$ years and still isn't trained after two months of trying, he or she may be resisting toilet training. The most common cause of this resistance is too much parental pressure. Often, these children have been reminded too much or been forced to sit for long periods on the potty chair.

In trying to train a resistant child, shift the responsibility to him or her. Tell your child that you're not going to remind him or her to go to the bathroom and that he or she must decide when to go. Use positive reinforcement and incentives to reward your toddler for a day without wet or dirty pants. If your child has an accident, change him or her and then involve the toddler in cleaning up the mess. Don't punish or criticize. Try to be patient, however difficult that may be.

Several months after daytime control is achieved, try putting your child to bed without a diaper.

Taking your child to the bathroom just before he or she goes to bed may hasten night training.

Swallowing objects

Young children are naturally curious and are not averse to putting coins, safety pins, buttons, fruit pits and other things into their mouths. Keep these and other small objects out of reach.

In addition to a fondness for small objects, some children chronically ingest non-nutrient substances such as dirt, plaster, clay and ashes. This eating disorder, called pica, may occur during the first two years, when your child's natural curiosity compels him or her to sample everything. If your child persists with this practice, talk to a doctor. Pica may be a sign of an iron deficiency.

A watchful parent may be able to retrieve an object before it's swallowed. When your child swallows an object, it usually passes through the digestive system un-eventfully. A good rule is that if a swallowed object passes into your child's stomach, it will usually pass the rest of the way through the intestines.

However, objects can lodge in the esophagus. If your child has difficulty with breathing or swallowing or if he or she is spitting up saliva, the swallowed object may have become stuck in the esophagus. If this occurs, call for emergency assistance or go to the emergency department at your local hospital.

If your child stops breathing because of an obstruction, try the Heimlich maneuver (see page 14). Indications that an object may be lodged in your child's throat include chest pain, abdominal pain and vomiting.

If your child swallows a button battery, such as those found in watches, cameras and hearing aids, contact a doctor right away or take your child to a hospital emergency department. Button batteries contain dangerous alkali fluids. If the battery gets lodged in the esophagus, the battery fluid can cause severe burns in only two hours.

Special Concerns

Most infants are born fully developed, healthy and ready to be taken home. Unfortunately, a few babies don't follow this pattern. Newborns requiring special care include premature babies, those with birth injuries, some congenital disorders or breathing difficulties, and babies born to mothers dependent on drugs.

Premature babies

A baby born too soon hasn't had time for adequate development of body systems essential to life. Premature infants commonly need monitoring and systems support.

A premature baby is commonly defined as one born before 37 weeks of gestation. The word *premature* may concern some expectant parents because not long ago the survival rates for premature infants were much lower than those for full-term babies. However, recent advances in the care of low birth weight, premature infants have greatly improved their chances of survival.

Risk factors

Many factors contribute to prematurity. Women who are undernourished, anemic or have had little or no prenatal care are more likely to give birth prematurely. A history of infertility, stillbirth and other premature births can increase the chance of premature birth, as can teenage pregnancy and smoking or drug use during pregnancy.

Often the stimulus for early labor comes from factors such as premature separation of the placenta, uterine abnormalities or a cervix that's too weak to bear the weight of the developing fetus. In addition, severe urinary tract infections in the mother may lead to a premature delivery. To reduce the likelihood of premature delivery, seek early and regular prenatal care.

Premature labor

If you go into premature labor, decisions involved in trying to stop your labor are complex. A doctor will assess your health, your baby's health, how your placenta and cervix are functioning, risks of infection, and how far along you are in your pregnancy.

After taking these factors into consideration, your doctor can evaluate whether an attempt should be made to stop preterm labor and what these efforts might be. Interventions may include bed rest, intravenous fluids and medications to help you stop preterm labor. You may also be given antibiotics to prevent the risk of infection.

Babies born after 23 weeks of gestation have a good chance of surviving with the help of newborn intensive care. As a rule, the longer the baby is in the womb, the better able he or she is to live outside with fewer complications and without long-term disabilities.

If your membranes have ruptured, a sample of amniotic fluid can predict the maturity of your baby's lungs and indicate whether there's infection in the amniotic fluid. If the membranes haven't ruptured, amniotic fluid can be collected by an amniocentesis test. If your baby's lungs aren't mature enough, you may be given steroids to enhance the maturation of the baby's lungs before birth.

Complications

One of the most serious and common complications of premature birth is underdeveloped lungs.

A baby with breathing difficulty may require breathing assistance from a ventilator connected to a tube that's placed down the windpipe (trachea). The goal is to maintain adequate oxygen in the blood, blood circulation and nutrition while the baby's lungs mature.

Other problems associated with premature birth include heart problems, bleeding in the brain, pneumonia, low blood sugar concentration (hypoglycemia), anemia and infection.

The combination of very little body fat and immature skin prevents a premature infant from maintaining normal body heat. Babies born prematurely are taken to special units where they're placed under warmers or in incubators to help maintain normal body temperature.

Nutrition

Premature newborns often receive their initial nutrition intravenously. This is called total parenteral nutrition, which is used until the newborn is more stable and ready to start breast milk or formula feedings. Many premature infants haven't developed the sucking reflex or are too weak to suck. These infants may be fed through a tube inserted through their mouths and into their stomachs. After these early feedings are well-established, the infants begin feeding by breast or bottle. Antibodies in breast milk are important to premature babies.

Bonding

The trend in neonatal nurseries is toward greater parental involvement. Parents are encouraged to spend time with their infant and to touch and caress him or her even when tubes, wires and other equipment make cuddling difficult. Whenever practical, parents are encouraged to feed the child and to change a diaper. Some parents bring books and read to their baby or play music.

Birth injuries

A birth injury is a trauma incurred by an infant during labor and delivery. Most often the injury occurs despite excellent obstetric care.

Certain conditions make the possibility of a birth injury more likely. Prematurity, an abnormal fetal position, prolonged pregnancy, an unusually large fetus and a small maternal pelvis are some conditions that can increase the risk of birth trauma.

Forceps sometimes are associated with birth injuries. Forceps are used to assist in difficult vaginal births. Forceps injuries generally are minor, involving facial or scalp abrasions. Often, forceps delivery is the safest way to end a labor that may threaten the health or life of the mother or child.

Another technique used to assist in difficult deliveries is vacuum extraction. In this method a rubber or plastic cap is placed on the head of the baby while the baby is in the birth canal. The doctor applies suction with a pump and then gently pulls on the instrument to help ease the baby down the birth canal. Newer methods that prevent excessive suction help protect the baby from injury.

Some common birth injuries include the following:

A swollen scalp
Swelling of the tissues of the scalp (caput succedaneum) occurs because of pressure on the head as it makes its way through the birth canal. The swelling usually disappears after a few days, and the baby's head soon assumes a normal shape.

A bruise under the scalp
A bruise under the scalp (cephalohematoma) is caused by slow bleeding. The swelling usually isn't visible until several hours after birth. This type of injury usually resolves within two weeks to

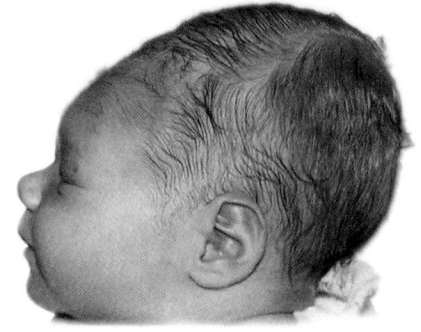 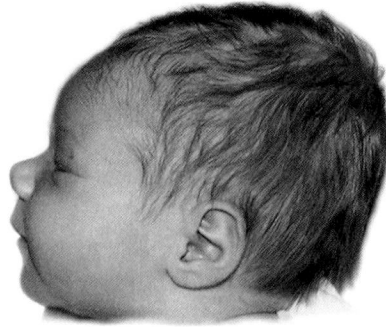

After traveling down the birth canal, a newborn commonly develops swelling of the scalp (left). The swelling isn't harmful and usually disappears in a few days when the baby's head assumes its normal shape (right).

three months. Treatment is rarely required.

A fractured collarbone
A fracture of the collarbone (clavicle) is the most frequent bone injury during labor and delivery. An infant with this injury is reluctant to move the arm on the affected side. The collarbone heals surprisingly quickly in an infant. Usually, the only treatment required is pain relief.

A dislocated nasal septum
Dislocation of the nasal septum, the cartilage between nasal passages, can cause the nose to appear asymmetric and flattened. The infant may have difficulty nursing and some problems breathing through his or her nose. Most nasal flattening resolves spontaneously. More severe flattening may require a minor procedure to reposition the dislocated septum.

Facial nerve palsy
Pressure over the facial nerve during labor or birth can cause weak-to-absent movement of a baby's facial muscles. The condition may involve an entire side of the infant's face. When the infant cries, the affected side of the face doesn't move, and the mouth is drawn to one side. The eye on the weak side can't close, and the corner of the mouth droops. Usually, improvement is rapid and complete.

Respiratory problems

At birth, a newborn must rapidly fill its lungs with air while at the same time clearing them of fluid. Simultaneously, the infant needs to increase the circulation of blood through his or her lungs.

A newborn must breathe without the lungs completely collapsing every time he or she exhales. Most full-term infants are able to accomplish this because the lungs have had time to develop fully and have enough of a liquid substance called surfactant. Surfactant helps reduce surface tension and prevents collapse of the lungs' small air spaces. However, many premature infants and even some full-term babies have problems breathing because their lungs initially lack surfactant.

Breathing problems in newborns include:

Respiratory distress syndrome
Respiratory distress syndrome (RDS) is characterized by difficulty breathing, breathing that's harsh and irregular with grunting, nasal flaring and perhaps a dusky blue skin color. RDS is a specific diagnosis that refers to a lack of surfactant. The severity of RDS correlates with the infant's gestational age and birth weight. The smaller and more premature the infant, the greater the chance he or she will have RDS. This

disorder is rarely found in infants born at full term. Boys have this condition more often than do girls, and white babies are affected more often than are black babies.

RDS generally is recognized within minutes after birth. In some babies the distress at birth is so severe that resuscitation is necessary. Blood tests and an X-ray of the lungs can establish the diagnosis.

If your child is born with RDS, he or she will need to be in a newborn intensive care unit, where his or her vital signs will be monitored constantly. Nutrition and fluids may be given intravenously. Many infants with this condition require help in breathing. A breathing tube attached to a ventilator may be inserted down the mouth into the baby's trachea to provide assistance with breathing. Some babies are helped with a tube in the nose or a mask on the face to provide continuous positive airway pressure.

Infants with severe RDS may be given surfactant directly into their lungs. Other medications used in babies with RDS include diuretics to increase urine output and rid the body of extra water, corticosteroids to reduce inflammation in the lungs, bronchodilators to reduce wheezing, and theophylline or caffeine to stimulate breathing.

The goal in caring for infants with respiratory distress syndrome is to keep them complication-free until the lungs have had time to develop. With the advent of special neonatal units and specially trained pediatricians (neonatologists), nurses and respiratory therapists, the mortality rate for infants with RDS has declined steadily.

Transient tachypnea

Transient tachypnea is a form of respiratory distress that can occur after an uneventful vaginal delivery or cesarean section and in both premature and full-term infants.

Infants born with this form of respiratory distress often have no signs of trouble other than rapid, shallow breathing. In some babies, the skin may have a bluish tinge, which can be alleviated with small amounts of inhaled oxygen.

Unlike infants with RDS, these infants rarely appear severely ill and most recover within three days. Treatment may include giving oxygen until the breathing improves, often within 12 to 24 hours. If the baby is breathing too fast to be fed orally, it may be necessary to use intravenous feeding. Usually, no other treatment is necessary.

Pneumothorax

Every infant is born with collapsed lungs. One of the miracles of birth is that within a few breaths the lungs inflate and the baby begins breathing. However, considerable pressure changes are needed to inflate the lungs that first time.

Occasionally, the lungs don't inflate evenly, and the pressure differences can cause a condition called pneumothorax, a condition that ruptures air sacs (alveoli) of the tiny lungs.

These ruptures allow air to leak out into the spaces between the thin membranes lining the lungs (pleurae) and the inner wall of the chest. This area is called the pleural space. If a small amount of air leaks, the infant will have shortness of breath, rapid or grunting breathing, and perhaps bluish lips and fingernail beds (cyanosis). If a large amount of air leaks, the infant may suddenly develop severe breathing difficulty.

Pneumothorax can be very serious if a lung collapses suddenly, but in most cases the leakage of air is small, and the air is reabsorbed on its own. Sometimes, no specific treatment is necessary. Pneumothorax may be treated by giving the infant extra oxygen to breathe for several hours. In the case of severe pneumothorax, the air that has leaked into the chest may need to be removed by inserting a tube into the space between the ribs (chest wall) and the lungs.

Bronchopulmonary dysplasia

Breathing difficulties associated with premature birth generally improve within several days to weeks. Premature babies who still require assistance with ventilation or supplemental oxygen after a month are often described as having bronchopulmonary dysplasia (BPD).

Signs and symptoms of BPD include rapid breathing, wheezing, coughing, and bluish lips and fingernail beds (cyanosis). BPD is often suspected in infants with RDS who don't recover quickly.

Babies with BPD need supplemental oxygen for an extended period and may need several medications. Most recover slowly over several months.

Drug withdrawal

The infant of a mother who took addicting drugs frequently during her pregnancy may go through withdrawal at birth. Drugs that can cause withdrawal in infants include cocaine, narcotics (heroin, morphine, methadone), barbiturates (especially phenobarbital), prescription pain medications (analgesics), tranquilizers, sedatives, amphetamines and phencyclidine (PCP).

The infant may develop irritability, a high-pitched cry, sleeping and feeding problems, diarrhea, vomiting, and convulsions. If the mother was addicted to barbiturates, withdrawal symptoms in the infant may not appear until seven to 10 days after birth. The infant may be at risk of other problems due to poor intrauterine growth.

If withdrawal symptoms are mild, they're treated simply by providing a quiet, comforting environment, with swaddling, gentle handling and frequent feedings. If symptoms are severe, medications may be required. The smallest dose that will relieve the symptoms is given. After the newborn has had no symptoms for several days, the dose will be decreased until symptoms have disappeared without medication.

Central nervous system disorders

The central nervous system consists of the brain and spinal cord. Three important congenital disorders of the central nervous system are spina bifida, hydrocephalus and cerebral palsy.

Spina bifida

Spina bifida is a defect in the formation of a portion of the backbone and surrounding tissues. The defect can occur at any level but is most common at the base of the back. Approximately 2 in every 10,000 infants born in the United States have spina bifida.

Babies born with spina bifida typically have an outpouching of membranes covering the spinal cord (myelomeningocele) that causes a loss of neurological control of the legs, bladder or bowel.

Surgery is performed soon after birth. The baby's back is closed to minimize the risk of infection and to preserve existing function to the spinal cord. More surgeries and other forms of medical treatment may be needed because of hydrocephalus and paralysis resulting from spina bifida.

Some children with spina bifida may have learning problems, but early intervention can help prepare them for school. Other children may experience problems with mobility and may need crutches, braces or wheelchairs.

Hydrocephalus

Hydrocephalus is an excessive accumulation of water in the brain due to an imbalance between the brain's production of cerebrospinal fluid (CSF) and its ability to absorb it. Sometimes, the cause is a blockage of the normal fluid pathways. Hydrocephalus in a young infant can result in an extremely large head.

In the United States, congenital hydrocephalus occurs in about 6 of every 10,000 live births. An abnormally large head is the most obvious sign. If the head of the fetus is so large that a vaginal delivery is impossible, the baby is delivered by cesarean section. In some cases, the head may be normal at birth but then grow at an abnormally rapid rate.

Hydrocephalus may be detected during a routine prenatal ultrasound, but it's often discovered during infancy or early childhood. Computerized tomography (CT) or magnetic resonance imaging (MRI) is useful for differentiating hydrocephalus from other disorders and for finding the cause of the hydrocephalus.

The goal of treatment is to establish equilibrium between the production and the absorption of cerebrospinal fluid. Sometimes, medication is effective, but hydrocephalus often requires the surgical placement of a shunt system. This system diverts CSF from within the brain to another area of the body where it can be more readily absorbed. Shunts usually are needed for life. Complications may occur, such as mechanical failure of the shunt or infections.

Although hydrocephalus poses risks to both cognitive and physical development, with medical treatment many children live normal lives with few limitations.

Cerebral palsy

Cerebral palsy is one of the more common chronic health problems in children. It refers to abnormalities of motor control caused by injuries to the infant's brain during early development. The injury can occur before or during birth or during the first few months after birth.

Each year approximately 8,000 infants in the United States are diagnosed with cerebral palsy. There are many causes of cerebral palsy. One possible cause is inadequate circulation of blood in brain tissue. Abnormal brain growth and development early in the pregnancy is increasingly recognized as a cause of cerebral palsy. Injury to the brain during labor and delivery may be a cause. Others include infection in or beside the brain or bleeding in the brain. Often there's no obvious explanation.

Cerebral palsy isn't life-threatening, but it may require long-term care. There's no cure for cerebral palsy, but in some cases surgery may help reduce spasticity and resulting deformities. Treatment involves several techniques: aids such as braces and walkers to improve mobility, special education to help compensate for the child's motor difficulties and any learning disabilities, and early stretching exercises to help the muscles stay limber and prevent contractures. A contracture shortens the muscles or related tissues, making it difficult to flex the affected muscles.

Cerebral palsy is classified into the following four broad categories:

Spastic cerebral palsy

Spastic cerebral palsy is the most common type of this disorder. An infant with spastic cerebral palsy has an abnormal persistence of

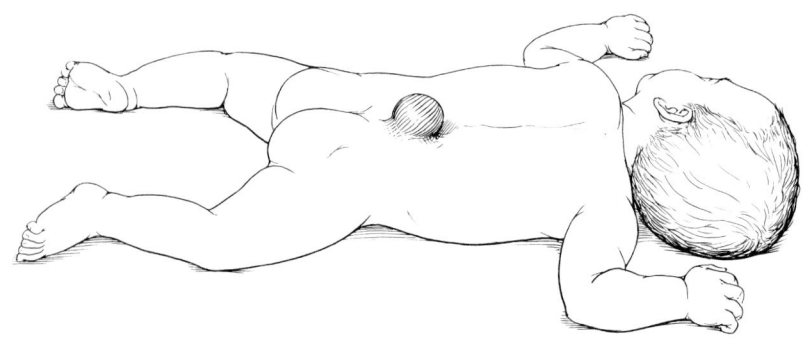

An outpouching of membranes covering the spinal cord (myelomeningocele) occurs in newborns with spina bifida.

some newborn reflexes. A hyperactive grasp reflex leaves the infant's hands in a tight fist. As the infant grows, the limbs become more spastic and stiff.

All four limbs may be involved (spastic quadriplegia). When this occurs, there's often some degree of intellectual disability as well.

Convulsions are more common. When the arms are affected to a lesser degree, the condition is called diplegia. Children with diplegia may acquire good use of their hands. Their intelligence is often normal or near normal, but they may have some difficulties drawing and writing.

Children with paralysis on one side of the body only (spastic hemiplegia) tend to have intelligence in the low-normal range, although some have average or above-average intelligence.

Athetoid cerebral palsy
Athetoid (dyskinetic) cerebral palsy is characterized by uncontrolled, slow, writhing movements. These abnormal movements usually affect the hands, feet, arms or legs and, in some cases, the muscles of the face and tongue, causing grimacing or drooling. Children with this form of cerebral palsy also may have problems coordinating the muscle movements needed for speech. Athetoid cerebral palsy affects about 10 to 20 percent of children with cerebral palsy.

Ataxic cerebral palsy
Ataxic cerebral palsy is rare. It affects balance and depth perception. Individuals with this form of cerebral palsy often have poor coordination and walk unsteadily with a wide-based stance, placing their feet unusually far apart. They may also have difficulty with quick or precise movements such as writing or buttoning a shirt.

Mixed forms
It's common for children with cerebral palsy to have more than one of the three previous forms. The most common mixed form includes spasticity and athetoid movements.

Congenital heart disorders

Approximately 1 of every 125 newborns are born with a congenital heart disorder. The heart defects range from mild to severe, with most cases being mild. The risk of having a baby with heart disease may be higher if you or other family members have had a baby with a birth defect.

The precise cause of a congenital heart disorder is rarely found. Genetic defects and certain viral infections during pregnancy may possibly be causes. Some chromosome abnormalities, such as the one that causes Down syndrome, are associated with heart defects. Infections such as German measles (rubella), contracted by the mother during the first two months of pregnancy, also increase the risk of congenital heart defects.

With recent advances in heart surgery, many of these heart defects can be successfully treated.

Ventricular septal defect
Ventricular septal defect (VSD) is the most common heart malformation, accounting for 20 to 25 percent of all congenital heart disease. An infant born with this condition has an opening between the lower chambers (ventricles) of his or her heart, causing increased blood flow under high pressure to the lungs.

Symptoms of VSD depend on the size of the defect. The problem may be discovered during a routine physical examination when a doctor detects a distinctive heart murmur. Babies born with large defects develop pulmonary hypertension, feeding difficulties, profuse perspiration, poor growth rates, recurrent pulmonary infections and cardiac failure in early infancy. Children with small defects may have no symptoms.

Small ventricular septal defects may close on their own without treatment.

Treatment depends on the size of the defect. If medications are unsuccessful, an operation to close the defect may be done before the baby is a year old.

Atrial septal defect
Atrial septal defect (ASD) is an opening high in the heart between the upper chambers (atria), which produces abnormal blood flow. It's more common in female infants than in male infants, and it often occurs in children with Down syndrome. ASD accounts for approximately 8 percent of congenital heart disease. Children with the condition frequently have no symptoms. Surgical closure is the recommended treatment. This is generally done around age 4.

Patent ductus arteriosus
The ductus arteriosus is a vessel that leads from the pulmonary

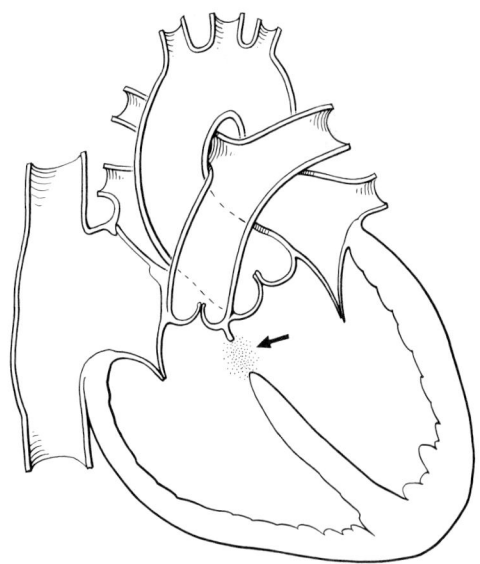

An opening between two of the chambers of the heart — ventricular septal defect (see arrow) — allows blood to flow under high pressure to the lungs. In many cases, the defect resolves itself, but in some instances, surgical correction is required.

artery to the aorta while the infant is in the womb. This opening normally closes immediately after birth. When it doesn't, blood flows between the pulmonary artery and the aorta. Patent ductus arteriosus (PDA) accounts for 6 to 8 percent of cases of congenital heart disease.

In babies born prematurely, the ductus is less apt to close spontaneously. PDA occurs more often in female infants, in babies born at high altitude and in the offspring of women who had German measles (rubella) during the first three months of pregnancy.

When the ductus is small, often no symptoms are present. A large ductus will produce a heart murmur, pulmonary hypertension and growth restriction. In a premature infant, the ductus often closes spontaneously within weeks or months. In infants whose ductus fails to close, surgery may be necessary.

Constriction of the aorta

Constriction (coarctation) of the aorta results in increased blood pressure above the obstruction. Initially, no symptoms may be evident. Significant obstructions should be surgically relieved in early childhood to help prevent future complications. In severe cases, surgery may be necessary in infancy.

Aortic stenosis

Aortic stenosis is a narrowing of the valve through which blood leaves the heart to enter the aorta. Severe stenosis, which may be accompanied by breathing difficulties, is generally detected in early infancy. Mild or moderate stenosis may not present any noticeable symptoms, but during a routine physical examination a doctor may detect a heart murmur. The condition is more common in males.

Surgery is needed to treat severe stenosis. Children with mild or moderate obstruction should have periodic re-examinations because of the possibility of an increase in the obstruction.

Tetralogy of Fallot

Tetralogy of Fallot consists of a large ventricular septal defect, obstruction of blood flow from the heart's right ventricle to lung (pulmonary) arteries and a shift of the aorta to the right side of the heart. In addition, the right ventricle is enlarged. The result is decreased blood flow to the lungs.

The main sign of this disorder is a bluish cast to the skin (cyanosis). The manifestations of tetralogy of Fallot often begin slowly during the first year of life. Sometimes, the problem is apparent at birth.

The goal of treatment is to provide an increase in blood flow to the lungs. A heart operation is the usual treatment once your child is past infancy, but sometimes it's required sooner.

Pulmonary stenosis

Pulmonary stenosis is an obstruction in blood flow from the heart to the pulmonary artery. Mild or moderate obstruction may cause no symptoms. A newborn with a severe obstruction has a bluish cast to the skin and shows signs of heart failure. In severe cases, congestive heart failure can occur during the first month of life. Children with mild to moderate stenosis can lead a normal life, but they should have regular follow-ups by a doctor. Those with more-severe stenosis may require a procedure to open the valve.

Transposition of the great vessels

Transposition of the great vessels is a complex condition in which

SIDS

Sudden infant death syndrome (SIDS) is the sudden and unexplained death of an apparently healthy infant. More often than not, there are no signs that anything is wrong with the infant's health.

SIDS rarely occurs before 2 weeks or after 6 months of age, and the peak incidence is between the second and third months of life. The number of SIDS deaths annually has declined in recent years to about 1,600 in the United States. Males are more likely to die of SIDS than are females, and the syndrome seems to occur more often during cold weather.

Researchers studying SIDS deaths have noted that many of these children weren't really as healthy as they appeared to be. Some evidence suggests that infants with SIDS may have had subtle abnormalities of the cardiac system or central nervous system.

Doctors now know that certain infants may be at greater risk than others. Those at higher risk include premature or low birth weight babies, babies of smokers or drug users, babies who've had a sibling die of SIDS, babies who have stopped breathing and been resuscitated, and babies with low Apgar scores at birth.

Some conditions associated with a higher risk of SIDS are beyond your control. However, the following recommendations may help reduce the risk:

Sleep position

For the first year of life, put your baby to sleep resting on his or her back, not the stomach. At the age when babies begin to move about in the crib while they sleep, parents become concerned about maintaining a back-sleeping position. However, by the time your baby has learned to roll over from back to front or front to back, the baby can be allowed to remain in the sleep position that he or she assumes.

the two arteries arising from the heart are reversed. Blood returning to the heart from the body is pumped back to the body without passage through the lungs. Infants with this condition are often dusky blue (severely cyanotic) and must have immediate medical care. Several surgical procedures are available to treat the problem.

Congenital digestive and respiratory disorders

There are many congenital disorders of the digestive tract, some of which can cause partial or complete obstruction of passage of food or stool. The most common obstructions involve the first section of the small intestine (duodenum) or the lower portion of the gastrointestinal tract (rectum and anus).

Pyloric stenosis
Pyloric stenosis is a narrowing of the pylorus, the outlet of the stomach through which food and other stomach contents enter the small intestine. Although the precise cause is unknown, a family history of the condition may be a factor in its development. Pyloric stenosis occurs more often in males, affecting approximately 2 in 1,000 babies.

If your infant develops pyloric stenosis, the symptoms usually begin during the second or third week of life. The initial signs and symptoms include regurgitation and possibly vomiting, and at times, forceful vomiting. About a week after the initial signs and symptoms, the infant generally begins to vomit more forcefully (projectile vomiting). Rarely, the vomit will contain blood. Vomiting typically occurs during or shortly after a feeding, but it may be delayed for hours. After vomiting, the baby is hungry and wants another feeding.

An infant with pyloric stenosis has very small stools because little food is reaching the intestines. The baby may lose weight and become dehydrated. The infant's eyes may appear sunken, and the cheeks may be wrinkled. Infants with pyloric stenosis may appear uncomfortable but are not in great pain.

Pyloric stenosis usually can be diagnosed from the child's feeding history and from the identification of a pyloric mass on examination of the abdomen. An ultrasound examination is sometimes done. The condition usually requires an operation after rehydration with intravenous fluids. Within six

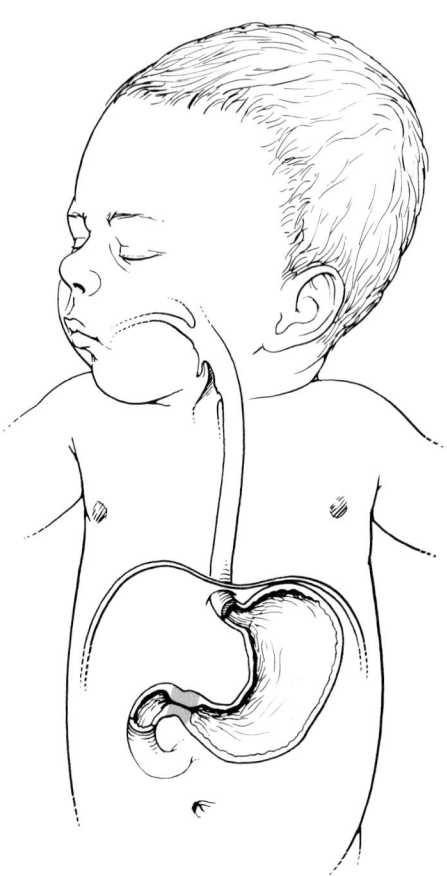

Pyloric stenosis is a narrowing of the outlet of the stomach (pylorus) through which stomach contents pass into the small intestine. The condition generally requires surgical treatment.

Some babies have medical conditions that require sleeping on their stomachs. If your baby's doctor recommends this position, it's usually best to follow that advice. Sleeping tummy-down hasn't been shown to cause SIDS, but it may increase risk of the syndrome.

Bedding
Babies should sleep on a firm mattress. Avoid thick, fluffy padding under the baby. Soft bedding materials may cause your baby to sink in and have difficulty breathing.

Diet
Breast-feeding may reduce the risk of SIDS.

Sleep location
It's recommended infants sleep in their parents' bedroom — close to the parents' bed but not in the bed — for at least six months and ideally for the first year.

Secondhand smoke
Provide a smoke-free environment for your baby. This measure is as important after your baby is born as it was during pregnancy.

Room temperature
Research suggests an increased risk of SIDS with overheating. Set the temperature in your home to be comfortable for you, and it should be comfortable for your baby.

Electronic monitoring
Electronic monitoring of heart rate and breathing may be useful in dealing with some infants at high risk of SIDS. It's still uncertain whether electronic monitoring has any protective value. Babies have died suddenly and unexpectedly even while being monitored. If electronic monitoring is used, special training for the baby's caregivers is often required.

hours after the operation, babies usually can resume oral feedings. The amount of the feeding is increased gradually. Most infants can go home about two days after the operation. A nonsurgical approach involving endoscopic balloon dilation may be another option. The prognosis for an infant with pyloric stenosis is generally very good, depending on how early the diagnosis is made and the overall health of the infant.

Esophageal atresia

In an infant born with esophageal atresia, the tube leading from the throat to the stomach (esophagus) isn't properly connected. This condition can be accompanied by other disorders, which often involve the tube from the larynx into the lungs (trachea).

Signs and symptoms of esophageal atresia often are detected soon

Genetic Conditions

Whether your baby is born healthy or with a genetic disorder is determined by the interaction of the baby's genes (segments of DNA) and the environment in which the child develops. Genes determine many of your child's characteristics, which are passed from one generation to another. Usually this occurs uneventfully. Sometimes unexpected changes called genetic alterations (mutations) occur or are inherited from a parent.

Although most causes of genetic alterations are largely unknown, various environmental agents, such as radiation, viruses and chemicals, are among some of the factors that have been identified. For more information on genetics, see Chapter 14, "Genetics and Disease."

after birth. The infant may have an unusually large amount of secretions coming from its mouth, or it may choke, cough or turn blue when attempting to feed. Infants with this condition require surgery. If the underdeveloped segment is short, repair can be attempted immediately. If the segment is long, further growth of the esophagus may be necessary before attempting repair. In this event, a tube is temporarily placed through the abdominal wall into the stomach for feeding.

Biliary atresia

Biliary atresia is obstruction of the bile ducts. It affects an estimated 1 in 15,000 newborns. Infants with biliary atresia have persistent jaundice and an increased incidence of other abdominal abnormalities. The stools are pale to white, and the liver may be enlarged.

If an infant has biliary atresia, his or her doctor may recommend a procedure called the Kasai operation, which connects the liver to the small intestine, bypassing the malformed ducts. Children with biliary atresia often have persistent inflammation of the liver even after surgery. Some may ultimately require liver transplantation.

Intestinal atresia

Intestinal atresia involves an obstruction of the intestine that can occur anywhere in the intestines. A high obstruction is located just beyond the outlet of the stomach or in the upper small intestine. It causes vomiting, which tends to be persistent even when feedings have been discontinued. An infant with an obstruction in the lower small intestine or colon may have a distended abdomen, often accompanied later by vomiting. Vomiting of yellow-green material (bile) should always be investigated by a doctor.

An infant with an intestinal obstruction generally doesn't have a bowel movement, although

meconium stools may pass during the first days of life if the obstruction is high in the small intestine. An obstruction may be complete or partial. When the baby has a partial obstruction, symptoms may not be immediately apparent.

Treatment depends on the type of obstruction. A complete obstruction requires prompt surgery to prevent severe complications. A partial obstruction may require surgery as well, but minor obstructions may not. With a prompt diagnosis and proper treatment, most infants recover from intestinal atresia completely.

Hirschsprung's disease

An infant born with Hirschsprung's disease gradually develops an abnormally large (dilated) colon. This condition, also called congenital megacolon, is due to a failure of the muscles of the colon to propel stool through the anus. Hirschsprung's disease occurs in about 1 in 5,000 newborns.

Early signs may include a delay of or failure to pass meconium stool or have a bowel movement, vomiting, and abdominal distention. After a rectal examination, the baby may have a large bowel movement. Dehydration and weight loss also are common. Many infants with Hirschsprung's disease have alternating constipation and diarrhea.

Treatment for Hirschsprung's disease typically begins with an operation during which an opening on the outside of the abdomen (colostomy) is created so that the stool can pass into a disposable pouch. This is a temporary measure. The opening is closed during another operation in which the abnormal portion of the colon is removed — typically when the child is between 12 and 18 months old — and the colon rejoined. The treatment is highly successful in restoring normal bowel movements, although continued bouts of diarrhea or constipation can sometimes be a problem.

Imperforate anus

Congenital disorders of the anus and rectum are fairly common, occurring in 1 out of 5,000 newborns. Children born with anal and rectal problems have a higher incidence of other birth defects such as urinary tract disorders.

An infant born with an imperforate anus has an obstructed anal opening, preventing passage of stool. An imperforate anus is sometimes readily apparent on an examination, or it may be suspected when a baby fails to pass a meconium stool within the first few days after birth.

Treatment depends on the location of the obstruction. If the anal opening is simply narrowed, an instrument can be used to dilate the opening. More typically, surgery is required. The higher the obstruction, the more major the surgical procedure. Some children require complete reconstruction of the anus. Others need a temporary opening on the outside of the body (colostomy) for the first six to 12 months of life.

Children with low anal obstruction generally do well after surgery and develop normal bowel control. When the obstruction is higher, there may be some uncontrolled passage of stool.

Diaphragmatic hernia

A diaphragmatic hernia occurs when an opening in the diaphragm enables some abdominal contents to pass into the chest cavity. In severe cases, the entire stomach and much of the intestines can displace the heart and lungs.

This condition typically is a life-threatening situation soon after birth and requires emergency surgery. A rare, later-appearing diaphragmatic hernia might be suspected in a baby who develops vomiting, severe colicky pain, discomfort after eating and constipation. Very rarely the condition causes only minimal symptoms and is discovered incidentally on a routine X-ray.

Omphalocele and gastroschisis

During normal fetal development, the abdominal organs initially develop outside the abdominal cavity and then move into the abdomen in an orderly fashion. In both omphalocele and gastroschisis, one or more of the abdominal organs (intestines, stomach, liver and spleen) remain outside the abdomen at birth.

When the organ or organs are contained in a protective envelope of tissue protruding through the umbilicus, the condition is called omphalocele. When they protrude through an opening beside the umbilicus, it's called gastroschisis. With both conditions, surgery must be performed immediately and recovery can be slow.

Congenital emphysema

Congenital emphysema (infantile emphysema) occurs when a portion of a lung doesn't form properly. Air enters an infant's lungs but has trouble leaving. The affected part of the lung becomes overinflated, and air may leak out into the space around the lungs. In most cases, only one lobe is affected, usually an upper lobe.

Congenital lobar emphysema is almost always detected during the first two weeks of life. Signs and symptoms include persistent shortness of breath with wheezing and a bluish tinge to the lips and fingernail beds (cyanosis). In most cases, no cause can be identified. The infant's lungs may not have developed completely, or something may be obstructing the airway. A chest X-ray shows overinflation of the involved lobe of the lung and may reveal blockage of an air passage. If the baby's symptoms are severe, it may be necessary to remove the affected lobe.

Other congenital disorders

Some children are born with a congenital disorder that's physically apparent. For example, features such as a small head, small ears, flat face and upward slanting eyes are characteristic of a child with Down syndrome.

Down syndrome

Down syndrome results from extra genetic material from chromosome number 21, creating three versions of this chromosome instead of the normal two. Down syndrome is the most common chromosomal disorder. An estimated 1 in every 700 infants are born with this condition.

A woman's chances of giving birth to a child with Down syndrome increases with age. For a 25-year-old woman, the chance of having a baby with this syndrome is 1 in 1,340. For a 35-year-old woman, the chance is 1 in 350, and for a 40-year-old woman, 1 in 85.

An infant born with Down syndrome may have a number of distinctive characteristics such as a small head, small ears, flat face and upward slanting eyes. The child's fingers often are relatively short, and the hands often have a single crease in the palms.

Infants born with Down syndrome may be of average size but then grow slowly and remain small. They have developmental delays that range from mild to severe. They also have an increased risk of congenital heart defects and gastrointestinal problems.

Babies with Down syndrome are at increased risk of problems such as respiratory infections, vision impairment, underactive thyroid and leukemia.

There's no specific treatment for Down syndrome. Heart or other associated conditions often can be repaired successfully with surgery. Many children with Down syndrome are happy, affectionate and easygoing. Many go to school, learn to read and write, find jobs, and eventually live independent or semi-independent lives.

Upper extremity disorders

Sometimes, a baby is born with

extra, missing or deformed hands, arms or fingers.

Total or partial absence of upper extremities

A child may be born without part of a finger, or in rare cases, an entire arm may be missing. As disheartening as this may be for parents, the child may actually do quite well. Just as with adults who are missing limbs, prosthetic limbs for infants and young children also are available. Once a baby with one arm is able to sit, a prosthesis usually can be fitted. Many such children do exceptionally well with no further treatment.

Polydactylism

Polydactylism is the presence of an extra finger or fingers, most commonly a fifth finger or an extra thumb. Frequently, the extra digit consists of only skin and soft tissue and can be removed easily. If the extra finger contains bone or cartilage, removal may also require surgery on adjacent structures and is usually performed after the infant is a few months old.

Syndactylism of the fingers

Syndactylism of the fingers is a webbing of the fingers. Because the bones in the fingers are of various lengths, the joints of the fused fingers don't line up and the fingers are difficult to use. The condition is corrected surgically. Without surgery, the child probably won't acquire significant use of the fingers.

Clubhand

Clubhand, a rare abnormality, is due to the absence of the bone on the thumb side of the forearm (radius) or the larger bone on the opposite side of the forearm (ulna). Treatment includes stretching the soft tissues of the arm during infancy. A later operation is necessary to reposition the bone, but retaining the new position can be a

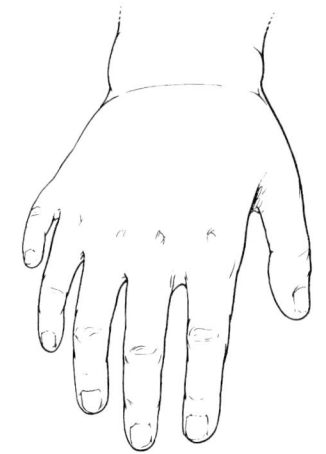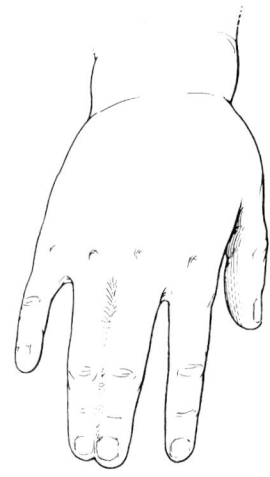

Both polydactylism, a congenital deformity of the hand in which the newborn has an extra finger, and syndactylism, webbing of the fingers, can be effectively treated surgically.

problem. Several operations may be necessary during childhood. Children with this condition also have a higher incidence of heart disease and blood problems.

Lower extremity disorders

A newborn's feet are proportionately longer and thinner than those of an older child, and the joints of the ankle and foot are extremely flexible. Often, normal feet may appear to be in abnormal positions.

Intoeing and out-toeing

Intoeing and out-toeing are common problems in which the foot or leg turns inward or outward. The condition is aggravated if the infant sleeps facedown. Both are usually positional or postural deformities that improve spontaneously during growth and development. Treatment is rarely required.

Syndactylism of the toes

Syndactylism of the toes is a webbing of the toes. It's rarely more than a cosmetic problem. The scars and distortions of surgery may be more unsightly than the webbed toes. In contrast to webbed fingers, webbed toes usually function normally.

Clubfoot

Clubfoot refers to several congenital foot abnormalities in which the foot is twisted out of shape or position. In most cases, the forefoot is twisted downward and inward, the arch is increased, and the heel is turned inward. About half of all infants with clubfoot have abnormalities in both feet.

Early treatment is essential and should begin soon after birth. The foot is manipulated to the normal position and then held there by a cast. This process is typically repeated every few days during the first two weeks of treatment and then at one- to two-week intervals. If this method is successful, corrective shoes may then maintain this position. If this method doesn't correct the problem, an operation, usually between 4 and 18 months of age, may be necessary.

Although the position of the corrected clubfoot may look relatively normal, the foot may never have completely normal contours, and the calf on the affected leg may be thinner than that on the normal leg. Orthopedic care throughout childhood is often necessary.

Extra toes

Extra toes can make it difficult to find shoes that fit. Most of the time

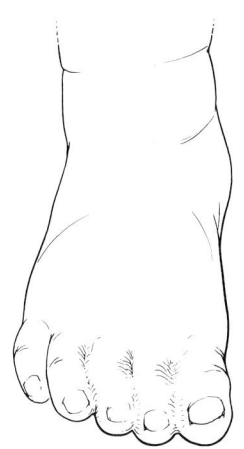
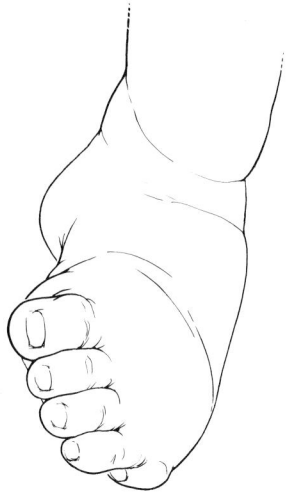

Webbing of the toes (syndactylism) is rarely more than a cosmetic problem, requiring no treatment. In contrast, clubfoot, in which the foot is twisted out of shape or position, requires therapy soon after birth.

the extra toes are surgically removed. The operation shouldn't be performed until the structures are large enough to be easily operated on, yet it should be done before the child begins to walk and needs shoes.

Congenital hip dislocation

Congenital hip dislocation, also known as developmental dysplasia of the hip, is the result of abnormal development of the hip joint. The problem may be detected during initial examination at birth or in the first weeks to months of life.

A newborn with congenital hip dislocation is fitted with a brace or splint-like device to hold the head of the thighbone (femur) in the hip socket (acetabulum). This condition can be treated successfully immediately or shortly after birth.

Dwarfism

Dwarfism (skeletal dysplasia) may be due to several skeletal abnormalities, including disproportionate lengths of limbs and trunk. Sometimes, the infant's limbs are short initially. As the child grows, the trunk also becomes disproportionately short. Other problems may include hearing impairment and joint problems. There's no

cure for the actual skeletal disorder, but many of the accompanying problems can be treated.

Treatment for dwarfism involves a combination of orthopedic techniques to maximize the child's mobility and function and, when possible, to correct malformations of the limbs and spine.

Funnel chest

Funnel chest (pectus excavatum) is a major indentation of the breastbone (sternum). The lower part of the bone is depressed toward the spine, and the chest has a funneled or hollow appearance. This is

usually a congenital problem, although it may be caused by rickets or a chronic airway obstruction. Some inherited muscle diseases are associated with this condition.

Babies and children with funnel chest usually have normal lung function. Only rarely is heart function adversely affected. Surgery is recommended in severe cases with definite cardiac or respiratory abnormalities. Ideal candidates for treatment are children between the ages of 8 and 12. Successful treatment may result in the disappearance of the indentation. For mild to moderate cases, surgery often isn't necessary but may be performed for cosmetic reasons.

Lip and palate disorders

Cleft lip and cleft palate are separate birth defects that sometimes occur together. More than 5,000 infants in the United States are born with cleft malformations each year. Genetics seem to be more of a factor in cleft lip, with or without cleft palate, than in cleft palate alone.

An infant born with a cleft malformation, especially only a cleft palate, has a higher incidence of other problems, including hearing impairment. An infant born with a cleft lip has an elongated opening (fissure) where the upper lip failed to fuse. This can vary from a small notch at the top of the lip to

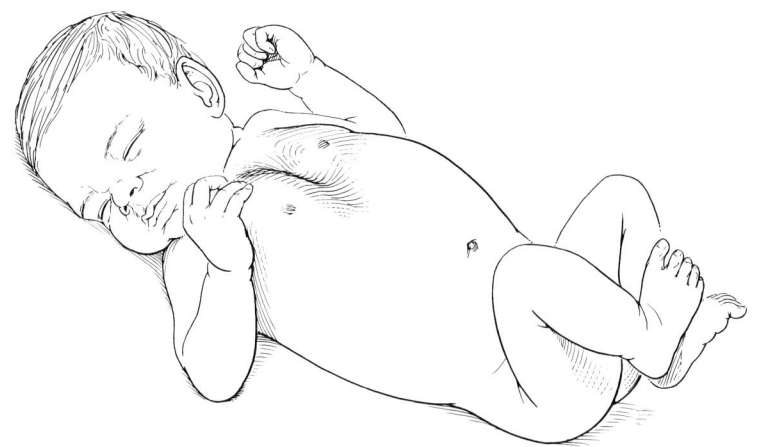

Funnel chest (pectus excavatum) is a congenital indentation of the chest. In severe cases, it can cause cardiac or respiratory problems. Mild cases generally don't require treatment.

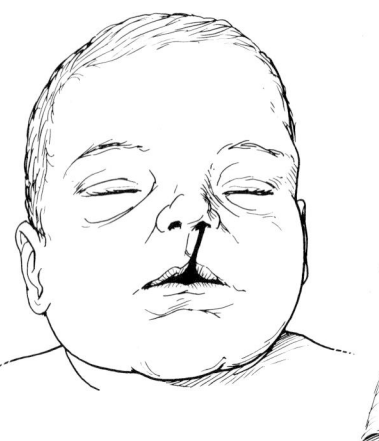

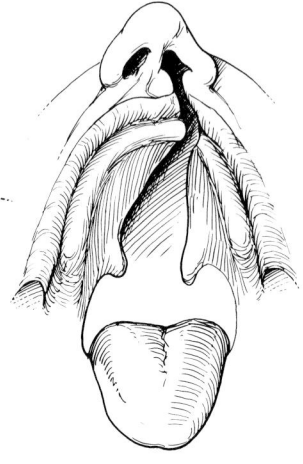

Failure of the lip to fuse together results in a condition called cleft lip. When the roof of the mouth fails to fuse together, it's termed cleft palate. These conditions require surgical correction.

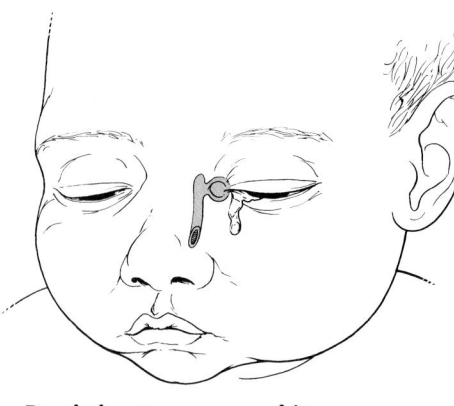

Persisting tears or a white or yellow discharge on the cheek of your infant may indicate an obstruction of the nasolacrimal duct.

a complete separation extending to the nose. If the palate is also cleft, the roof of the baby's mouth has failed to form properly.

With either or both conditions, the most immediate problem is feeding. Soon after birth, a specially designed prosthesis (obturator) can be fitted over the palate so that the baby can eat. Because the infant is growing rapidly, this device will have to be replaced every few weeks.

A baby with a cleft lip typically has an operation to close the lip at 1 or 2 months of age. Frequently, nasal widening is associated with cleft lip deformities. Closure of the cleft lip helps narrow the base of the nose. A nasal operation usually is deferred until the child has reached adolescence. The cosmetic results depend on the severity of the malformation, the absence of infection and the surgeon's skill.

A cleft palate generally is closed within the first year of life to enhance normal speech development. The goals of surgery are to make it possible for the child to speak in a normal voice and to minimize nasal regurgitation. If a child doesn't have the operation by age 3, a prosthesis may be used to help the child develop better speech.

Complications of cleft lip or cleft palate include recurring ear infections, hearing loss, an excessive number of dental cavities and displacement of the teeth, requiring orthodontic correction. Some children continue to have speech problems even after surgery because of muscle problems in the palate.

Tear duct disorders

Congenital obstruction of the nasolacrimal duct results from incomplete development of the tear drainage system. Normally, tears and secretions from the eye drain from the tear ducts, which lead from two small openings at the inner corner of the eyelids into the nasal cavity. If this drainage system is partially or completely obstructed, tears can't drain from the eyes into the nose.

The problem usually becomes apparent within the first days or weeks after birth. A cold or exposure to wind or low temperature often aggravates the problem. The first sign a parent typically notices is the presence of tears in the baby's eyes, ranging from a pool of tears to tears spilling onto the baby's cheeks. There also may be some white or yellow discharge in the corners of the eyes and some

crusting that glues the eyes shut while the baby sleeps.

Sometimes, infants with nasolacrimal duct obstruction develop inflammation in the duct area, causing the area to become swollen, red and tender. They may also have a fever and be irritable. The condition rarely harms the eyes, even when it persists for several months.

Treatment mainly involves cleansing the infant's lids with warm water and massaging the area between the infant's nose and the affected eye two or three times a day. Antibacterial drops or ointment may be used to prevent infection. If the condition persists throughout the first year, a doctor may need to surgically widen (dilate) the duct. Rarely is insertion of tubes or a reconstructive operation necessary.

Male genital conditions

The scrotum in a full-term newborn boy is relatively large. The scrotum may also look especially swollen after a breech birth. The scrotum of newborns with darker pigmentation usually is dark before the rest of the skin darkens during infancy. The foreskin in a newborn normally covers the end of the penis and should never be forced back. None of these char-

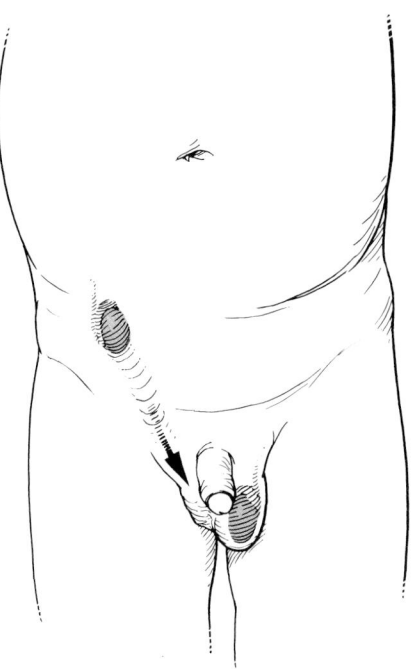

If one or both testicles fail to travel from the abdomen to the scrotum, the condition is termed undescended testicle.

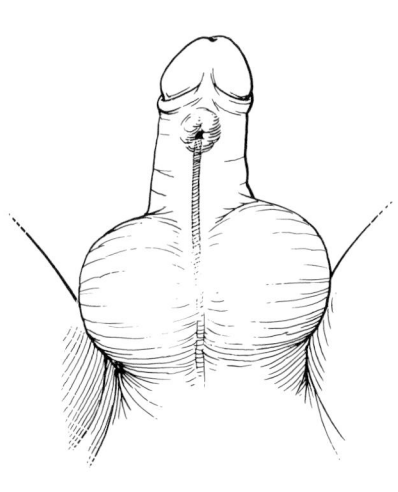

Hypospadias is a condition in which the urethral opening isn't located at its normal position at the end of the penis.

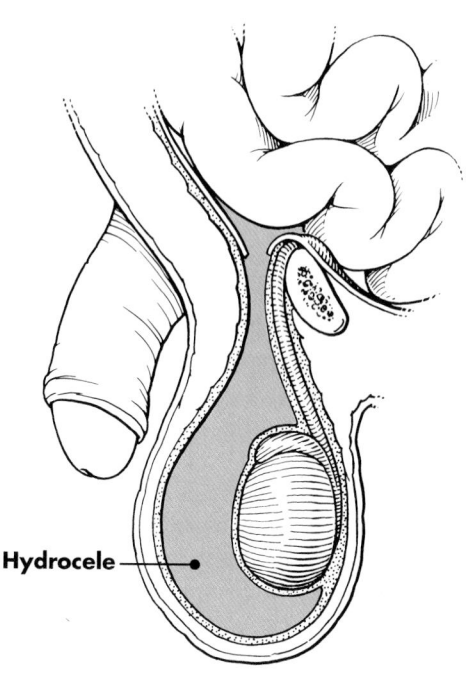

Hydrocele

A common problem in newborns is an accumulation of fluid near the testicles (hydrocele).

acteristics is cause for alarm. Some genital conditions, however, do require treatment.

An undescended testicle
An undescended testicle is the absence at birth of one or both testicles from the scrotum. The testicle may be within the abdomen or be absent altogether. The latter condition is rare and usually occurs in a child born with ambiguous sex characteristics.

About a month before birth, the testicles normally descend from an area near the kidney through a small opening in the abdominal muscles into their normal position in the scrotum. Just under 5 percent of boys are missing one or both testicles from the scrotum at birth. The incidence of undescended testicles is up to 30 percent in premature infants and up to 100 percent in infants weighing less than 2 pounds, because the testicles don't fully descend until after the seventh month of gestation.

In most cases, the testicle descends into the scrotum during the first few months of life, without

any medical intervention. Sometimes, hormones are given to bring the undescended testicle into place. If it hasn't descended by the child's first birthday, it won't do so spontaneously, and the condition is commonly treated surgically.

Surgery is also important because often a boy with an undescended testicle has a hernia due to the failure of the opening in the abdominal muscles to close properly. In such cases, the intestines may slip through the muscle opening and become trapped. Often the operation can be done on an outpatient basis. Occasionally, a testicle has shrunk (atrophied) so severely that removal is indicated.

Left untreated, an undescended testicle might not produce sperm later in life, though if the other testicle functions normally it will produce enough sperm to maintain fertility. A boy born with an undescended testicle also has an increased risk of testicular cancer. Correction doesn't reduce this risk, but it does allow for better examination and earlier detection should a tumor develop.

Hypospadias
Hypospadias is a congenital defect. The urethral opening isn't in its normal position near the end of the penis. In its mildest form, the opening is just on the underside of the glans. In its most severe form, it may be as far back as the scrotum. The more severe the degree of hypospadias, the more downward-curved the penis. This curving of the penis is called chordee.

Hypospadias is treated surgically. Circumcision shouldn't be done because the foreskin is used in the surgical repair. The more severe the condition, the greater the need for surgery because of urination and sexual problems. Unless the problem is corrected, the boy won't be able to stand while urinating and will have difficulty with sexual function later in life. The psychological consequences of having malformed genitals also are a factor in the consideration of surgery.

Many pediatric urologists believe the ideal age for surgery is during the first year, certainly before the child is toilet trained. A surgical procedure can bring the opening closer to the tip of the penis and also help straighten the penis.

Hydrocele

A hydrocele is an accumulation of fluid in the sheath around the testicle. Hydroceles may occur on one or both testicles. This condition is common in newborn boys. If the testicle can be examined easily and the amount of fluid remains constant, treatment is unnecessary. Small hydroceles usually disappear during the first year. However, if the sac changes size during the day, it may mean there's direct contact with the abdominal cavity, which generally requires surgery.

Female genital conditions

Hormonal changes in the mother before birth can cause changes in the breasts and genitals of her newborn daughter. Although these changes may be disturbing to new parents, they're generally temporary and often require no treatment.

Enlarged clitoris

The clitoris of the newborn girl is often enlarged, especially in premature babies, as a result of hormonal changes that affect the genital area. The size decreases after birth. If the clitoris seems unusually large, tests may be performed to confirm the child's sex.

Vaginal discharge

Vaginal discharge sometimes occurs in newborn girls. During the first three weeks, many mothers notice a thick, white discharge or a tinge of blood from the baby's vagina. Treatment is unnecessary and the bleeding often resolves. Vaginal bleeding is sometimes a newborn girl's response to the absence of the maternal hormone estrogen after birth.

Ambiguous genitals

Ambiguous genitals refers to the uncertain appearance of the baby's external sexual features. Sometimes, a female with normal ovaries who has been exposed to an excess of male hormones in the womb is born with male-like genitals (female pseudohermaphroditism). A male may be born with testicles but with ambiguous or completely female genitals (male pseudohermaphroditism). Some newborns have both ovaries and testicles and ambiguous genitals (true hermaphroditism). Causes of ambiguous genitals include tumors, chromosome abnormalities, and hormone excesses or deficiencies.

When a newborn's sex is in question, only thorough testing and evaluation can establish the correct diagnosis, including the infant's sex. Ambiguous genitals is a serious problem that bears a significant impact on a child's future life and emotional health. Treatment may include hormone therapy and reconstructive surgery.

Nipple disorders

Rarely, an infant is born with one or more extra (supernumerary) nipples. The nipples may occur with or without breast tissue and are usually located in the breast area.

Sometimes, the nipple doesn't have an areola — the darker pigment that surrounds a nipple. The condition occurs equally in males and females and may be associated with urinary problems.

Supernumerary nipples rarely present a medical problem, although they can respond to hormonal changes that occur during puberty, menstruation and pregnancy. When this happens, the nipples may enlarge and become painful. The presence of a third breast can be emotionally traumatic. Moreover, a supernumerary nipple is at the same risk as a normal nipple of developing disorders such as mastitis, abscesses and cancer. If your newborn has supernumerary nipples, they can be removed for cosmetic purposes.

An infant can also be born with the absence of a breast or nipple.

Sometimes, the muscle underlying the breast also has failed to develop. When this occurs, nothing should be done during infancy or early childhood. An operation can be performed for cosmetic reasons when the child reaches puberty. ■

Preschool and Early School Years

The transition from toddlerhood to school-age self-sufficiency is an exciting and challenging time. During the preschool years, your child may sometimes be caught between wanting to "do it myself" and longing for the safety net that only you can provide. You'll probably have some anxieties during this time about issues as diverse as monsters hiding under the bed, toilet training and sibling rivalry. But you'll also enjoy seeing your child learn about communicating, socializing and becoming more self-reliant.

These years can be very satisfying for both you and your child as he or she develops his or her own personality and the relationship between the two of you grows.

Some amazing developmental changes occur during this time. For example, your 2-year-old, who proudly knows 50 words, becomes a 3-year-old who can carry on a conversation. Whether mastering the art of language or learning to use a new toy, preschoolers bring tremendous determination to acquiring new skills.

Age 6 usually marks the start of your child's formal education, but education starts much earlier. Before kindergarten many children already have attended nursery school or child care — a time to play and enjoy the informal learning that occurs in these years. This dynamic time is full of change and development.

This is a time when children are generally healthy, active and enthusiastic. Not surprisingly, it's often hard for them to control their energy and exuberance. If your child has deficits in vision or learning, these may become more apparent as he or she grows.

Witnessing your child's achievements and integration into this wider world can be a great source of pride. At the same time, these new horizons may provoke anxiety for both you and your child.

As your child moves in directions that are new or unfamiliar

or of which you don't approve, you may sense waning control. But you still have a crucial role to play in guiding your child through these years of development.

Growth and Development

During the preschool years and near the end of the preteen years, as your child is approaching adolescence, rapid changes occur in growth and development. In the middle, changes are often slow and steady.

Normal changes

The rapid weight gains during a child's first two years begin to level off around age 2. Your child's physical changes involve a transition from the plumpness of babyhood to the leaner body of a preschooler.

Although your son or daughter may not have a large vocabulary, he or she develops an increasing ability to understand language. This passive learning lays the groundwork for the explosion of language between ages 2 and 3. Your child's communication may include reading and writing by age 5.

As your child becomes more mobile, safety becomes vitally

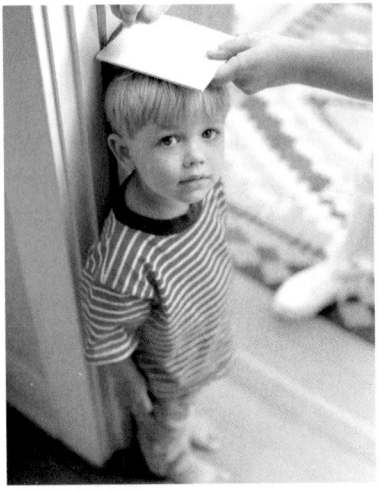

important. Your preschooler will constantly explore by mouthing, touching, grabbing and climbing, with no curiosity left unsatisfied.

You will see improvement in your child's motor skills, but not until between the ages of 6 and 12 do motor skills become more refined. During this period, his or her running, jumping and throwing show steady improvement. To enhance this important process, continue to encourage your child to be physically active.

You and your child may enjoy tracking his or her progress on a growth chart at home. Ask your health care provider for a copy of your child's growth chart. Your provider will also keep track of your child's height and weight. Abnormalities on your child's growth chart can provide early evidence of some serious diseases. For instance, when children develop chronic illnesses, their weight often stays the same or even decreases, and their height may not increase at the expected rate.

If you think your child seems unusually short or tall, you can ask his or her doctor about it. The doctor may obtain an X-ray of the hand and wrist to determine whether your child's bones are developing within a normal time frame (bone age). By comparing this X-ray with a standardized set of tables, your doctor can determine how well your child's bone age correlates with his or her actual age. If bone age is lagging behind chronological age, a child will often catch up. However, if bone age is ahead of chronological age, a child may have a growth-related problem.

Delayed psychomotor development

In most children, development of motor skills proceeds smoothly. Occasionally, though, a child will fall behind his or her peers.

Psychomotor development includes:

- **Gross motor function.** Gross motor function involves the larger muscles used for walking, jumping and skipping. Children who are clumsy or who have delayed gross motor skills, such as an inability to skip or jump, often feel self-conscious and humiliated. These are the children who are often the last ones picked to be on an athletic team. They may develop a poor self-image as a result.
- **Fine motor function.** Fine motor function involves the muscles used for hand dexterity. Some types of fine motor dysfunction may make it difficult for a preschooler to draw or color or cause delay in learning to tie shoes. Some children show impairments in hand-eye coordination. Because of their problems with fine motor skills, these children often have difficulty when they enter school.

The cause for delayed psychomotor development is generally unknown, although it may run in families. If you suspect that your child may have a delay in psychomotor development, discuss your concerns with your health care provider. Tests can determine if there's a problem.

If your child experiences a developmental delay in motor skills, he or she may lose an important area from which to draw for building self-esteem. As a parent, you need to preserve your child's sense of self-esteem by being understanding and patient with his or her progress. If you're impatient, even though your child ultimately will catch up, his or her self-esteem may suffer in the process. Most children do catch up and aren't impaired at a later age.

Growth disorders

Children vary widely in height and weight during their preschool years. Your child's size generally depends on heredity. Large parents are more likely to have a child who falls near the top of the range for height and weight among children his or her age, and small parents typically have a smaller child.

If your child is either substantially below or above the growth range for his or her age, there may be a problem. Growth disorders result from various factors, including nutritional disorders, hormonal disorders and chronic disease. If you suspect that your child has a growth disorder, discuss it with your child's health care provider. Depending on the physical findings, further studies — including blood tests and X-rays — may be necessary to determine the cause.

Treatment depends on the specific problem. An obese child may be placed on a diet and exercise plan, whereas one who is malnourished may need high-calorie supplements and even hospitalization. Hormone replacements may help children with growth disorders due to a hormone deficiency.

Nutritional disorders
Good nutrition contributes to normal growth. Malnutrition may result from insufficient food, an unbalanced diet, digestive problems, absorption problems or other medical conditions.

In the United States and other developed countries, malnutrition is uncommon. Severe cases of malnutrition may occur when a child has an associated chronic illness or disorder. Malnutrition can be the result of diseases such as cystic fibrosis or celiac disease, in which nutritional intake is normal but absorption of nutrients is not. The most common nutritional disorder in children in the United States is obesity.

Hormonal disorders
Sometimes, the pituitary or thyroid gland produces an insufficient or an excess amount of hormones, the result of which can be a growth disorder. Growth disorders are rare and they include conditions such as gigantism, dwarfism and hypothyroidism.

Chronic disease
Children with diseases such as congenital heart disease, chronic kidney failure or anemia may also have impaired growth.

Learning disorders

Children of normal or high intelligence can still have great difficulty in learning. These learning disabilities aren't disorders of seeing, hearing, emotions or overall mental capacity. Rather, they're often mental process disorders in acquiring or expressing knowledge — referred to as specific learning disorders or specific learning disabilities.

Learning disorders are more difficult to diagnose than are vision or hearing problems, and they often require consultation with specialists such as psychologists, developmental and behavioral pediatricians, or child psychiatrists. Disorders of mental processing may include problems with remembering, recognizing patterns, focusing attention, writing, speaking and interpreting written words.

Various causes have been cited for learning disorders. Some of them stem from birth injuries. More commonly, however, they occur in children with normal health and intelligence. In some cases, they may be genetic. In other cases, there's evidence of disordered brain function, although no evidence of brain damage can be found.

Frequently, the specific cause for a child's learning disorder is unknown. Some experts in the field believe that in such instances the disorder may be due to developmental delays or slowing of the maturation process. Boys are affected more frequently than are girls.

A learning disorder can lead to chronic academic failure and to

Stuttering

Stuttering typically begins between the ages of 2 and 5, while your child is mastering the basics of speech. In some children, stuttering first appears between ages 6 and 8, when school lessons include reading aloud and recitation, and often disappears by adolescence. Occasionally, older children develop the problem.

Two common characteristics of stuttering are repetition of sound, parts of words, whole words and phrases, and prolongation or stretching of sounds or syllables. Examples of repetition are *b-b-b-bath*, *da-da-daddy* and *base-base-baseball*. An example of prolongation is *c----at*.

The causes of stuttering are only partially understood. Certain factors may promote tension of the muscles involved with speech and lead to stuttering. Stress, fatigue or excitement may trigger stuttering. Stuttering can run in families. Stuttering commonly isn't linked to intelligence or any measurable brain abnormality.

Occasional stuttering is common among children. These episodes usually disappear as speech and language develop, and they don't require attention.

Seek professional evaluation if your child becomes apprehensive about speaking, struggles with speech, or begins to avoid sounds, words or speech altogether. A speech pathologist can help your child minimize his or her stuttering by reducing tension in his or her lips, tongue and jaw and monitoring his or her breathing and rate of speech.

As a parent, try not to interrupt your child, show impatience or finish your child's sentences. Build your child's self-confidence by reducing stressful speaking situations and making time to play and talk quietly together each day.

major social and emotional problems. Early diagnosis and treatment can often minimize these consequences.

With special education and tutoring, many children can overcome their problem and perform much closer to their potential. They can achieve most academic and occupational goals if the appropriate teaching methods and motivation are found.

If your child has a learning disorder, you may not become aware of it until learning problems are recognized in the third or fourth grade. Close and regular communication with teachers may help to identify an emerging learning problem earlier on.

A thorough evaluation is essential for determining the specific disorder and ways to improve your child's education as soon as possible. Language disorders, dyslexia and attention-deficit/hyperactivity disorder (ADHD) are examples of learning disorders.

Communication disorders

The first few years of life are a critical period in a child's speech and language development. Rapid progress typically continues through the preschool years as children build vocabulary and understanding of grammar. Occasional mispronunciations are normal up to about 7 years of age, as long as your child's conversational speech is understood readily.

Delayed development of certain communication skills may signal a language or speech disorder. Language disorders affect how sounds and language are processed in the brain. Speech disorders interfere with normal production of speech sounds and, though not considered learning disorders, affect a child's ability to communicate verbally. About 5 percent of children are identified with both speech and language disorders by the time they start first grade.

Signs and symptoms
- Failure to use speech sounds correctly
- Speech that's hard to understand or scrambled
- Slow speech development
- Stuttering

In a majority of children with speech and language disorders, the cause of the problem is unknown and no physical cause is found.

Types of speech disorders include difficulty in articulation, stuttered speech and voice problems. Articulation problems refer to substituting one letter for another and leaving off the beginning and ending of words. Stuttering is difficulty in getting the words out in a smooth flow. Voice problems include a hoarse or strained voice.

If your child has a language disorder, he or she may be normal physically, emotionally and intellectually but struggle with mentally processing spoken language. Receiving information and making sense of it may be difficult for him or her. Sentences may come out scrambled or with one word substituted for another. The correct ordering of sounds may be impaired. Your child might be unable to tell the difference between two sounds or might have problems focusing on one specific sound or focusing on conversation while ignoring background noise.

Communication disorders can also result from conditions such as cerebral palsy, a cleft palate or lip, hearing loss or deafness, intellectual disability, brain damage, or autism.

Diagnosis
If you suspect that your child has a communication disorder, talk to your child's teacher or health care provider. You may also need to seek help from a speech and language specialist. Most school systems offer these services. A speech pathologist will test your child's language and speech abilities. He or she may work with an

audiologist to check for hearing loss or deafness in your child. In some instances, a complete physical and neurological examination may be advised.

How serious are communication disorders?

With help from specialists — and from parents at home — many children with speech and language disorders are able to vastly improve their verbal communication, but that doesn't mean they won't experience frustration. The social penalty can be costly if your child is taunted or rejected by other children at school. Early diagnosis and treatment are desirable before frustration and low self-esteem become problems.

Treatment

Children with speech and language disorders generally require speech therapy. This usually entails weekly sessions with a speech professional. Your child's speech therapist can explain how you can help at home.

Dyslexia

Dyslexia is a specific learning disability that primarily affects a child's ability to read. It's the most common learning disability in children. However, not all children with dyslexia will qualify for special education services.

Dyslexia occurs in children with normal vision and normal intelligence. Children with dyslexia usually have normal speech, but they often have difficulty with reading and writing. The disorder is an impairment of the brain's ability to translate written images received from the eyes into meaningful language.

Common signs of dyslexia include difficulty associating letters on the printed page with their corresponding sounds and a reading ability that's much below the expected level. Although the key factor of this reading disability is unknown, evidence shows that it

Factors Affecting Learning

Your child's ability to learn depends on complex mental processes that make learning possible. But overall health, emotional comfort and motivation are other important factors. Factors that can interfere with your child's ability to learn include:

Illness

Illness can leave a child tired and listless. This can interfere with learning, especially if the illness is chronic.

Emotions

If a child is depressed, worried or concerned about problems at home, learning can suffer. Worrying or daydreaming in school distracts the child from schoolwork.

Motivation

Lack of motivation also can be an impediment to learning. Your child needs to be motivated to learn in order to make full use of his or her capacities.

may be associated with a malfunction of certain areas of the brain concerned with language.

A family history of language disorders is frequently found. Approximately 5 to 10 percent of school-age children have dyslexia, though some studies suggest it may affect up to 17 percent of children.

Dyslexia can be difficult to recognize before your child enters school, but some early clues may indicate a problem. If your child begins talking late, adds new words slowly and has difficulty rhyming, he or she may be at increased risk of dyslexia.

Children with dyslexia often have problems processing and understanding what they hear. They may have difficulty comprehending rapid instructions, following more than one command at a time or remembering the sequence of things. Reversals of letters (b for d) and a reversal of words (saw for was) are typical among children who have dyslexia. Reversals are also common for young children who don't have dyslexia. But with dyslexia they persist.

Dyslexia is characterized primarily by a delay in the age

at which a child begins to read. Most children are ready to learn this skill by age 6. Children with dyslexia often can't grasp the basics of reading in first or even second grade. Because a child with dyslexia has difficulty interpreting written language, reading is difficult.

The condition may also manifest itself by your child trying to read starting at the wrong end of the sentence, failing to see and hear similarities or differences in letters or words, and being unable to sound out the pronunciation of an unfamiliar word. Children with dyslexia usually have difficulty with their ability to write.

Diagnosis

Reading achievement that's significantly below that expected for a child's age is the key sign of dyslexia. A diagnosis is generally made based on a comprehensive evaluation of medical, cognitive, sensory processing (vision and hearing), educational and psychological factors.

A battery of specialized psychological tests may be performed. An expert may analyze the process

Hyperactivity

Hyperactivity, or extreme overactivity, isn't a diagnosis or a separate disorder. Rather, it's a behavior that often accompanies other symptoms of attention-deficit/hyperactivity disorder (ADHD).

Children vary in their level of physical activity. In general, young children are active. Some youngsters are naturally much more active than are others, and boys tend to be more active than girls. These variations in activity are normal.

However, a small percentage of children, more often boys than girls, are excessively active. Some seem to be in constant motion, and others are erratically active. These children aren't necessarily less coordinated or less intelligent than are other children. The difference lies in how organized or purposeful their activity is and if it can be stopped when appropriate or on request.

Hyperactive children tend to act without consideration for results, punishment or other people's reactions. They can't direct their activity, and it's often difficult for parents or teachers to do so.

Contrary to some opinions, sugar alone doesn't cause or increase hyperactivity.

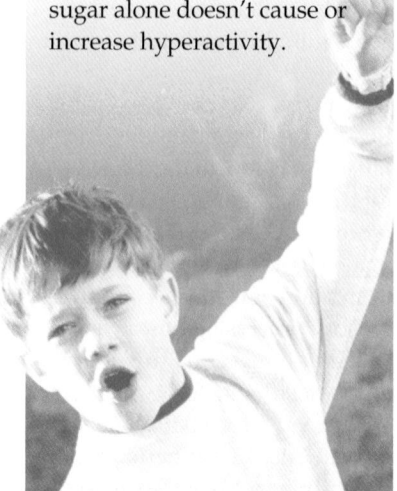

and quality of your child's reading skills. The results of these tests are used to plan treatment and track your child's progress.

Thorough vision, hearing and neurological examinations also may be necessary to verify that your child's poor reading ability isn't due to another disorder. Dyslexia varies in severity from relatively mild to severe.

How serious is dyslexia?

If you have a child with a reading disability, you may find that his or her inability to read doesn't affect achievement in other school subjects, such as arithmetic. However, because reading is a skill basic to most other school subjects, a child with dyslexia is at a great disadvantage in most classes.

If untreated, the disorder may result in low self-esteem, behavioral problems, delinquency, aggression, and withdrawal or alienation from friends, parents and teachers.

Treatment

Because there's no known way to correct the underlying brain malfunction, the primary form of treatment is generally remedial education. Psychological testing will help your child's teachers design a suitable remedial teaching program. Most important is frequent instruction by a reading specialist who uses both visual and phonic methods of teaching.

Techniques emphasizing many of the senses, including hearing, vision and touch, are used to improve reading. It's also important to provide emotional support and opportunities for achievement in areas other than reading.

If the reading disability is severe, your child may also benefit from several individual or small-group tutoring sessions each week. Be aware that progress is likely to be slow and laborious.

Children with milder forms eventually learn to read well enough to get through school and to be able to read newspapers.

Those with severe forms may always have difficulty reading and may need to learn ways to bypass their reading problems, such as by using tape-recorded textbooks.

Attention-deficit/hyperactivity disorder

Attention-deficit/hyperactivity disorder (ADHD) is another common learning disorder of childhood. Millions of children are affected by this condition. It typically begins in childhood and often continues into adolescence and adulthood.

The key signs and symptoms of ADHD are difficulty paying attention and concentrating (inattention), or difficulty staying still (hyperactivity) and controlling impulsive behavior (impulsivity), or a combination of those criteria. Boys are more likely to be hyperactive, whereas girls tend to be inattentive.

When this condition presents without hyperactivity, it is sometimes referred to as attention-deficit disorder (ADD).

As a result of this disability, your child may have problems with learning, following directions and remembering information. Your child's ability to learn depends on paying attention and remembering previous lessons and instructions.

Many sights, sounds, memories and other stimulating things compete for your child's attention. They can cause any child to have trouble paying attention, especially at a young age. However, most school-age children have the ability to focus their attention on a specific task and ignore distractions for a period of time. Among children with ADHD, this ability is underdeveloped.

ADHD may not noticeably affect your child's intelligence or early development. It may become apparent only later as your child has increasing difficulty with learning after the second or third grade, when sitting still in class and paying attention become increasingly important.

What causes ADHD remains a mystery; however, the disorder tends to run in families. It frequently occurs along with certain other conditions, including having a learning disorder or being a gifted learner.

Diagnosis
In making a diagnosis of ADHD, your doctor will likely want to observe your child's behavior and get a detailed history of early development. Early signs and symptoms may appear during infancy, including problems with feeding, sleeping and restlessness.

Physical and neurological exams may be recommended to identify any sensory or neurological disorders. Your child may also see specialists to partake in psychological and educational testing.

How serious is ADHD?
ADHD is a chronic problem that can continue through childhood and into adulthood. It has the potential to damage a child's self-esteem and confidence, generate rejection and ridicule by other children, and cause academic and social failure. Treatment can help a child with learning, behavior control, friendships, social interactions and self-esteem.

Treatment
Your child may need remedial education to help with learning. Some children with ADHD also have behavioral problems that require specialized counseling for the child and parents.

Treatment may focus on behavior modification techniques and restructuring home and school routines. Avoiding overstimulation and providing consistency can be effective for decreasing unacceptable behavior. Rewarding good behavior also is important.

Your child's doctor may prescribe medications to help focus your child's attention and reduce overactivity. Currently, stimulant drugs (psychostimulants) and the nonstimulant medication atomoxetine (Strattera) are the most commonly prescribed medications for treating ADHD. Stimulant medications include methylphenidate (Concerta, Ritalin, Daytrana), dextroamphetamine (Dexedrine) and dextroamphetamine-amphetamine (Adderall).

In a hyperactive child, these medications often can improve attention. When the medication is carefully prescribed and a health care provider is closely following the child's progress, the drug may be taken safely for as long as it's needed, even for years.

Some children experience side effects such as loss of appetite, nervousness, irritability and growth retardation. If your child experiences any of these signs or symptoms, discuss them with your child's health care provider.

Developmental disorders

Intellectual disability (formerly termed mental retardation) and autism are examples of developmental disorders in children. Although these conditions have no cures, resources are available to help parents and their children cope with them.

Intellectual disability
Intellectual disability can range from a mild slowness that makes school a struggle for the child to profound disability that requires the child have constant care or supervision.

If your child has an intellectual disability, he or she will be slow in acquiring motor skills and language. Your child will also lack the social skills and emotional maturity appropriate for his or her age.

Intellectual disability may be caused by inborn chromosomal or metabolic abnormalities such as Down syndrome or phenylketonuria (PKU). Other possible causes include prenatal German measles, toxoplasmosis and excessive alcohol use during pregnancy.

While a child with a learning disorder or an emotional immaturity due to a mental illness may be able to catch up to his or her peers through effort and treatment, intellectual disability is different from most other disorders. Children with an intellectual disability don't catch up with their peers in development, and their disorders generally can't be treated.

How serious is intellectual disability?
Intellectual disability is generally evident before age 18 and often many years earlier. Mild forms of disability may first become evident when your child begins school.

Children with mild disability are able to learn academic skills, but they do so more slowly than does the average child. Mild intellectual disability often isn't diagnosed until a child begins school because it's then that he or she is compared with large numbers of peers and developmental differences become more apparent. Children with mild forms of intellectual disability are often identified as being educationally mentally disabled.

Children with moderate intellectual disability may learn self-care skills such as dressing and using the toilet. They have limited ability to benefit from academic school programs but still profit greatly by attending school and may learn to perform certain simple jobs in a supervised setting.

Federal legislation guarantees an appropriate education to all developmentally disabled children in the United States. Community schools provide special education classes. Your child may spend part of the day in a class with other children with special needs and then attend a class or two with children who aren't disabled.

Children who are severely or profoundly disabled can learn

Taking Time for Yourself

Caring for a child with special needs can leave little time for the rest of the family. Even the most devoted parents need a break. However, because of your child's unique needs, you may be reluctant to leave him or her with a baby sitter.

Many communities recognize this problem and have opened respite centers where parents can temporarily leave a special needs child with a caregiver experienced in caring for such children. If this type of option is provided in your community, consider taking advantage of it.

minimal self-care skills such as using the toilet but require almost total supervision and care. These children often have limited communication skills.

Treatment

In the past, children with an intellectual disability were often institutionalized. Today, most of these children live at home or in group homes in their communities.

If your child is developmentally disabled, the goal of treatment is to help your child reach his or her potential, whatever that may be, and to enable him or her to cope as well as possible with limitations.

When a diagnosis of intellectual disability is made in infancy, you and your baby can enroll in an infant stimulation program or an early childhood intervention program. Such programs offer multisensory stimulation in an attempt to facilitate emotional, intellectual and physical development. They also help you to understand more about your child's strengths and weaknesses and offer you support during what is usually an emotionally difficult time.

Every child needs friends. Despite the mainstreaming of developmentally disabled children with other children in schools, classmates don't always accept these children as friends. Thus, you as a parent must often take it upon yourself to plan social and recreational activities for your child.

Organizations for developmentally disabled children offer various activities, including summer camps. Such programs help your child both to become more comfortable in social situations and to increase his or her independence. Working with a developmental disabilities case manager is essential to securing this help.

Autism

Autism is one of a group of developmental conditions called autism spectrum disorders that appear in early childhood — usually before age 3. Though symptoms and severity vary, autism disorders affect a child's ability to communicate and interact with others.

It's estimated that about 15 out of every 1,000 children in the United States have autism — and the number of diagnosed cases has been rising. This may be due to greater awareness of symptoms, better detection and reporting, and changing diagnostic criteria, as well as a possible real increase in the number of cases.

Children with autism generally have problems in three crucial areas of development — social interaction, language and behavior. But because the symptoms of autism vary greatly, two children with the same diagnosis may act quite differently and have strikingly different skills. In most cases, though, severe autism is marked by a complete inability to communicate or interact with other people.

Many children show signs of autism in early infancy. An autistic child may exhibit repetitive body movements, such as hand flicking, hand twisting, spinning or headbanging. He or she may be fascinated by parts of objects, such as the spinning wheels of a toy car. The child may become upset over even the slightest change in his or her environment and may be unreasonably insistent on established routines. Young children with autism also have a hard time sharing experiences with others. When read to, for example, they're unlikely to point at pictures in the book. This early-developing social skill is crucial to later language and social development.

Some children may develop normally for the first few months or years of life but then suddenly become withdrawn, aggressive or lose language skills they've already acquired. Signs of autism usually are seen by age 2.

In recent decades, controversy has persisted around a suggested (then debunked) link between autism and certain childhood vaccines, particularly the measles-mumps-rubella (MMR) vaccine and vaccines with thimerosal, a preservative that contains a small amount of mercury. Most children's vaccines have been free of thimerosal since 2001, and extensive studies have found no link between autism and vaccines.

As they mature, some children with autism become more engaged with others and show less marked disturbances in behavior. Some, usually those with the least severe problems, eventually may lead normal or near-normal lives. Others, however, continue to have great difficulty with language or social skills, and the adolescent years can mean a worsening of behavior problems.

There isn't a medical test to determine the disorder. Instead a specialist will look for certain behaviors and responses. Although autism has no cure, many therapies and interventions have been developed to treat its signs and symptoms. The most effective treatments use a combination of special education, behavioral therapy and medication.

Smoothing the Stubbornness

At a young age, children go through a period when *no* is their favorite word. It doesn't matter what you say to the child, most of the time it will be met by an emphatic no. "Do you want to stay in the bathtub?" you ask your young daughter. "No," she answers. "Well, then, do you want to get out of the bathtub?" "No."

Stubbornness and tantrums are normal parts of childhood development. Although it may seem as though your child is purposely trying to provoke you, he or she isn't. This is simply one step down the long road toward independence.

Getting through this sometimes difficult phase of development requires lots of patience and a good sense of humor. If you're the parent of a child in the thick of childhood stubbornness, remember that every parent goes through this and lives to laugh about it later.

The following tips may help make the road a little less bumpy:

- Don't take your child's negativism too seriously or too personally. Sometimes kids act stubborn when they are just being silly. Joining them in a sense of humor can make everything a little easier.
- Don't punish your child for saying no.
- Give your child choices: "Do you want to wear the red pants or the green pants?" Letting him or her choose will give your child a sense of freedom and control and make him or her more likely to cooperate. Be careful about asking a question with only one acceptable answer, such as a choice between staying up and going to bed.
- Give your child a transition time between activities. If, for example, it's time to leave the playground, give your child adequate time. "You can go down the slide three more times, and then we have to go home."
- Go easy on rules. Children this age aren't likely to follow a long list of house rules. Avoid arguing about unimportant things and decide which battles are really worth the struggle. Make sure that daily interactions with your child are weighted toward the positive, not the negative.
- Try to avoid saying no yourself. You want the child to see you as an agreeable person, someone he or she can imitate.
- Make sure all appropriate behavior is praised, no matter how insignificant it may be.

Personality and Behavior

The development of your child's personality is as important as his or her physical development. During the preschool years, issues may emerge that can affect the way your child behaves around you and others. His or her psychological and social development proceed at a rapid clip. Impressive changes take place in his or her ability to reason, learn, act in a moral fashion, follow rules intelligently, and interact with adults and other children. Many of these changes may seem surprising or even shocking to you as a parent. It helps to have some understanding of the normal course of events.

Normal changes

Keep in mind that a child's behavioral development doesn't adhere to a strict schedule. Every child is different and develops according to his or her own schedule. If you think there's a problem with your child's behavioral development, consult your child's doctor.

During your child's early years, seek your child's company. Discuss his or her interests and participate in activities, however mundane, together. The lines of communication that you keep open during these critical formative years may prove invaluable in later years as you help your child with behavior and personality issues.

Imagination

Preschoolers live part of their lives in a rich, imaginary world where anything is possible. Play during these early years often revolves around lots of pretending. Sometimes it's difficult for a child to know where pretending stops and reality starts.

For example, your 3-year-old may explain to you that he or she wasn't the one who broke your bottle of perfume but that it was a little green man with a yellow hat. Your child isn't lying, not in the true sense of the word. And you shouldn't punish your child or make him or her feel guilty for making up stories like this from time to time.

However, some children seem to live in their imaginations most of the day. If your child seems to be spending too much time with an imaginary friend whom he or

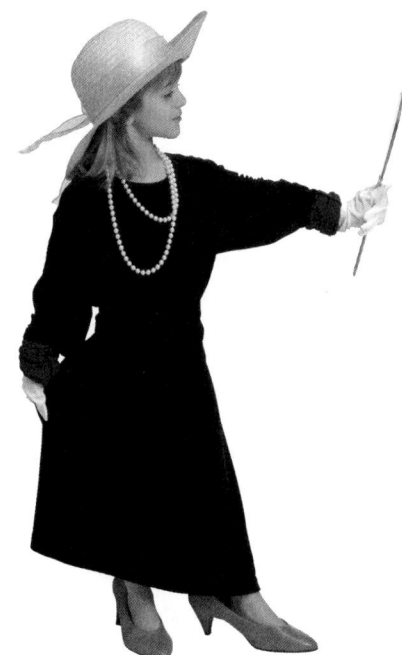

Thumb and Finger Sucking

All infants need to suck. Sucking on a thumb, finger or pacifier is common and helps soothe and calm most babies. By the time most children are 4, they've given up the practice, except when the issue has become a power struggle between parent and child or when it has become a deeply ingrained habit. Because thumb sucking during sleep is involuntary, it generally ceases when your child's sleep pattern matures.

Thumb or finger sucking in a preschool or school-age child isn't a serious problem. However, it makes your child appear babyish, which may subject him or her to ridicule from peers. Moreover, prolonged thumb or finger sucking can interfere with the normal alignment of the teeth, making orthodontic treatment necessary in later years.

If your child is younger than 4 and sucks his or her fingers or thumb, try to ignore or distract the child. Never punish, scold or pull your child's hand away from his or her mouth. These methods often make the problem worse.

Sometimes an older preschooler will suck his or her thumb as a way to "stay small." Remind your child often that you love him or her, and add that you are especially proud when he or she remembers not to suck his or her thumb.

she truly believes in, you might ask yourself if your child's real life is sufficiently interesting.

A child who lives in his or her own private dream world may need to spend more time with friends or may not be getting enough attention from his or her parents.

Increased independence
The increasing independence of your school-age child may stand in welcome contrast to the continual demands of your preschooler. Although it may be easy to allow your increasingly independent child to occupy himself or herself, an open and trusting relationship must be nurtured if it's to be maintained later during adolescence.

Social skills
During the preschool years, children tend not to conform. Social rules may be confusing to them. Behavior begins to change during the early school-age years. Children enjoy identifying with their peers and start understanding social situations. They often show a

rigid conformity that makes them embrace each new social norm that they come to comprehend. You may have noticed that your child relishes some strict compulsion, such as never stepping on a crack in the sidewalk. This is one form of the child's temporary infatuation with arbitrary rules.

Moral behavior
Up through the school-age years, children learn about moral behavior — how to distinguish between what's right and wrong. Your child must learn how to balance his or her needs and wants with the requirements of the family, school and society.

You can help your child develop a sense of duty, responsibility and realistic accomplishment. Encourage your child to assume a helpful role in the family. This may include assigning reasonable household chores such as setting the table. As your child accomplishes tasks you set, he or she will develop confidence in his or her abilities and a sense of responsibility regarding the tasks. This will

also reinforce that he or she is an important part of the family.

Setting an example of moral behavior is also important. In addition, it's a good idea to limit and monitor your child's TV watching and time online, to avoid or keep to a minimum his or her exposure to violence and inappropriate sexual behavior.

If you consistently specify what behavior you're rewarding or disciplining and explain why you're doing so, your child will be more likely to develop internal control of moral actions — a conscience. Less desirable are external controls, which influence behavior through fear of being caught or of displeasing parents.

Children who believe securely in their own worth tend to be more industrious, creative and successful. They're also better at resisting pressure to conform to their peers.

Peer pressure
Peers and siblings play important roles in the integration of your child into society. Children learn a great deal from their siblings and peers about competition and cooperation as well as about conformity and independence.

The influence of other children can rival or even exceed that of adults, partly because children play together as equals. It's easy for them to understand one another. Another child's perspective often provides an alternative to the prevailing wisdom that the child has been accustomed to hearing from his or her parents.

As children reach school age and become part of a peer group, new social traits become important to them, such as popularity and leadership. At this age, children are eager to be popular and don't want to be left out of the group.

Sibling relationships

Few things are as exasperating to parents as constant bickering among their children. These fights can make even easygoing parents wish they were raising an only child; still, fighting and competition between siblings is normal.

Problems between siblings include competition between a young toddler and a newborn, physical aggression, and incessant quarreling. Interestingly, in the moments your children aren't fighting, they may be the best of friends.

Sibling rivalry

A certain amount of rivalry between siblings is normal, and it can help them learn how to interact fairly with other people. You don't necessarily need to be concerned if your children compete, roughhouse and bicker with each other. Despite the friction between them, most older siblings do contribute greatly to the education, socialization and support of younger siblings. Frequently, overt rivalry gives way to closeness by the end of the school-age years.

Sometimes, though, the discord between siblings can be severe. If so, you may want to seek family counseling to identify how the trouble started and how it can be stopped. The underlying cause of sibling antagonism may be a family problem such as marital strain. Without realizing it, parents can cast a child in a role that enmeshes him or her in a conflict between the mother and father, and the other siblings react according to their sympathies.

The birth of a sibling also can make a school-age child feel that his or her place in the family has been upset. Compared with a preschooler, a school-age child is usually better equipped to control the jealousy of a newborn sibling.

It helps if you're sensitive to your child's needs and reserve some one-on-one time together.

Fighting

Children must be taught that they can't kick, punch or bite each other. When your children physically fight, separate them immediately. Send them to separate rooms for a few minutes to calm down.

Quarrels

Help children learn the skills to settle their own arguments. When they do argue, try to ignore it and stay out of the argument, even if it means you have to go into another room. If they bring their argument to you, help them clarify the problem — but let them find the solution. When children settle an argument, praise them. Avoid showing favoritism.

Sexuality

Your preschool child has a natural sexual curiosity that manifests itself in various ways. Through

?	**Question and Answer**

When is it a good time to talk with a child about the birds and the bees?

Your preschooler may be too young to understand how babies are made, but he or she isn't too young to learn about inappropriate touches. Explain that it's OK for your child to touch himself or herself in private but that it's not OK for others, even family or friends, to touch him or her that way except in special circumstances, such as during a doctor's examination.

A good time to begin talking about sex-related topics is when your child starts school. Pubertal changes generally begin at around age 11. Before your child reaches his or her early teens, your child should know about:

- The names and functions of male and female sex organs
- Puberty
- The menstrual cycle
- Sexual intercourse and pregnancy

the school-age years, your child will continue to define his or her sexuality. This process is a vital part of your child's larger task of discovering and deciding his or her identity. Answer questions about sex directly and simply. Use anatomically correct language.

A preschooler

It's normal for children to explore their bodies and to do what feels good. Self-stimulation is one way a child's natural sexual curiosity is manifested. Boys typically pull at their penises, and girls rub their external genitalia.

Occasional masturbation is normal and nothing to worry about. A child stimulates himself or herself simply because it feels good. Some children masturbate because they're unhappy or experiencing and reacting to some stressful circumstances.

If your young child masturbates, try not to get upset. Masturbation doesn't mean your child will grow up to be promiscuous or sexually deviant. It's not physically harmful, nor does it cause emotional problems, unless a parent overreacts and sends the message that sex is dirty and frightening.

Because it's difficult to stop a child from masturbating, it's best to simply accept it. However, you need to explain to your child that although it's all right to masturbate in the privacy of a bedroom or bathroom, other areas are off-limits. If your child suddenly starts masturbating in a social setting, try to distract him or her. If that fails, take your child aside and remind him or her that this is done only in the privacy of the bedroom or bathroom.

In addition to self-stimulation, many preschoolers are curious about their parents' bodies. A young child may want to touch a mother's breasts or a father's penis. Another child may be found half-undressed, playing doctor with the child next door. These behaviors are normal.

Avoid showing shock or anger. Instead, stress that some activities are private and, although it's OK for your child to touch himself or herself, it's not OK for others, even friends, to touch them that way except for an examination by a doctor or another health care provider. Then point out that no other adult may touch him or her in that way either.

Fears and phobias

As your child grows, he or she will inevitably have certain fears, which will change with age. Such fears are normal and may even be necessary for psychological development.

Fear refers to the perception of a threat, whether actual or just a possibility. Fear is necessary for survival. For example, fear of a barking, snarling dog is normal. Your child perceives a real threat, and it's correct to be frightened and to try to avoid the danger.

However, a child who continues to be terrified of the friendly, tail-wagging cocker spaniel who lives next door has an irrational fear or phobia.

Fears vary from child to child, but some appear more commonly in certain age groups. For example, some children are afraid of a bath. They're afraid of slipping under the water or of getting soap in their eyes. Preschoolers may be fearful of strangers. Separation from parents can be another common fear. As a child gets older, fears change and may revolve around the dark, monsters, being left alone or death.

If your child is going through a fearful time, try to be supportive and encouraging. Don't force your child to confront the object of the fear. For example, trying to make a child who's afraid of animals pet a dog will likely only complicate the situation.

Your reassurance in the form of a hug or kiss can be powerful medicine for a child who's afraid of the dark. A night light is often helpful.

Be creative in your quest for a solution. For instance, if your 3-year-old son is terrified that monsters are lurking in his dark room, initiate a nightly monster check. At bedtime every night, scour the room together in search of a monster. Once your son is reassured that no monsters are present, he'll likely go to bed and fall asleep. Within a few weeks, you'll no longer need to do the monster check.

This illustrates the years when magic seems real. You might also assign a stuffed bear the responsibility of staying awake all night to keep away monsters. In the morning, praise it for a job well done.

When your child conquers even a tiny part of his or her fear, make sure to praise him or her. Most fears resolve themselves in time. Those that don't or that hinder your child or family may require some counseling.

Preschool phobia

School phobia — avoidance of preschool or refusal to go to preschool — may be a way of responding to overwhelming stress and situations a child can't control. School phobia is often an anxiety disorder distinguished by anxiety and a cycle of physical symptoms that get worse instead of better.

If your child is fearful and unable to cope with a situation at school, he or she may experience symptoms such as a headache, stomachache, nausea, dizziness or hyperventilation. These are symptoms a child often has no conscious control over. Often, a child doesn't know exactly why he or she feels ill and finds it difficult to explain what's causing the discomfort.

Your child may be afraid of a preschool bully or being teased. Among younger children, the problem can often be resolved with patience and by providing emotional support for the child.

Common Concerns

As children age and move from one stage of growth and development to another, they'll experience various challenges and frustrations. Invariably these problems will pass, but proper coaching and reactions from parents can help.

Nutrition

Some days it may seem as if your preschooler doesn't eat enough to keep an ant alive, and other days you can't keep him or her away from food. Such is a preschooler's appetite. Unlike an infant, who triples his or her weight during the first year and eats well, a preschooler's rate of growth slows considerably, as does his or her appetite. Some preschoolers are reluctant to try new foods or expand their food repertoire beyond three or four old favorites. By the time your child is of school age, his or her habits are well on the way to being established.

A preschooler's diet

When your child is 2 years old, he or she should be eating a variety of foods. Daily recommendations include:

- **Dairy group (two servings or about 2 cups).** Milk, cheese and yogurt are excellent sources of calcium, which is necessary for building strong bones and teeth. Kids older than age 8 should get three servings a day.
- **Protein group (2 ounces).** This group includes beef, poultry, lamb, fish, pork, liver, eggs, dried peas and beans, and peanut butter. These foods are excellent sources of protein, which is necessary for the growth and repair of tissue cells.
- **Fruits (about 1 cup).** Aim for a total of at least 1 cup raw or cooked fruit, or ½ cup dried fruit. To obtain an adequate amount of vitamin C, be sure

that one or more servings are citrus fruit, berries, tomatoes or cantaloupe.

- **Vegetables (about 1 cup).** Aim for a variety of these nutrient powerhouses, such as 1 cup raw or cooked veggies or 2 cups leafy greens. Provide at least one serving of a green or yellow fruit or vegetable, which are excellent sources of vitamin A.
- **Grains (about 3 ounces).** This group includes whole-grain cereals, crackers, breads, rice and pasta.

Eating Well

Here are some tips for healthier eating for young children:

- *Reduce fat.* Use fat-free (skim) or low-fat (1 percent) milk. Instead of ice cream, serve ice milk, frozen low-fat yogurt or sherbet. Use ground beef with less than 15 percent fat and low-fat ham. Bake or broil rather than fry foods. Strain fried ground meat to reduce fat content.
- *Increase fiber.* Offer fresh fruits and vegetables regularly. Use whole-wheat flour when baking. Add low-fat granola, bran, rolled oats and corn-meal to quick breads.
- *Reduce sodium.* Remove the salt-shaker from the table. Reduce salt in recipes. Serve soups that are lower in sodium. Look for snacks that are low in sodium.
- *Reduce calories and sugar.* Use less sugar in recipes. Serve unsweetened fruit juice or fresh fruit whenever possible. Serve smaller portions of baked desserts.

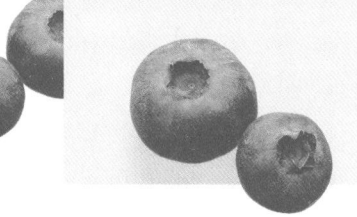

- **Other recommendations.** Limit fat and sugar in your child's diet. Your child should play actively every day. (Better yet, play actively together.)

These are the recommendations for a nutritionally balanced diet, but don't expect your preschooler to eat a completely balanced diet every day. When allowed to choose from a selection of nutritionally sound foods, most children tend to select diets that, over several days, offer the necessary balance. This may mean that one day your child might be eating a lot of peanut butter sandwiches, oranges and milk and the next day the menu is hamburgers, french fries and carrots.

Keep in mind that every child's energy needs are different. Your child isn't growing at the same rate he or she was as an infant, so it won't seem as if your child lives for the next meal. Your child doesn't need or want the quantities of food that he or she consumed with relish as an infant.

As your preschooler advances to the point where he or she can assume the same pattern of eating as that of older siblings or parents — a three-meal-a-day pattern — remember that snacking is acceptable. As parents, your role is to offer a variety of nutritious foods and to set a good example. Snacks are recommended for smaller preschoolers, who can't eat enough to satisfy their energy needs all at mealtimes.

Small amounts of a variety of foods eaten frequently over the course of the day as a snack are healthy and normal. However, uncontrolled snacking can diminish your child's appetite for meals.

Remember that a balanced diet may also include desserts and fats such as butter, margarine, mayonnaise and oils. Dietary fat and cholesterol are important for your infant's growth. However, after your child's second birthday, dietary fats should be consumed in moderation.

A school-age child's diet
The school-age years are a good time to continue the healthy eating habits initiated during the

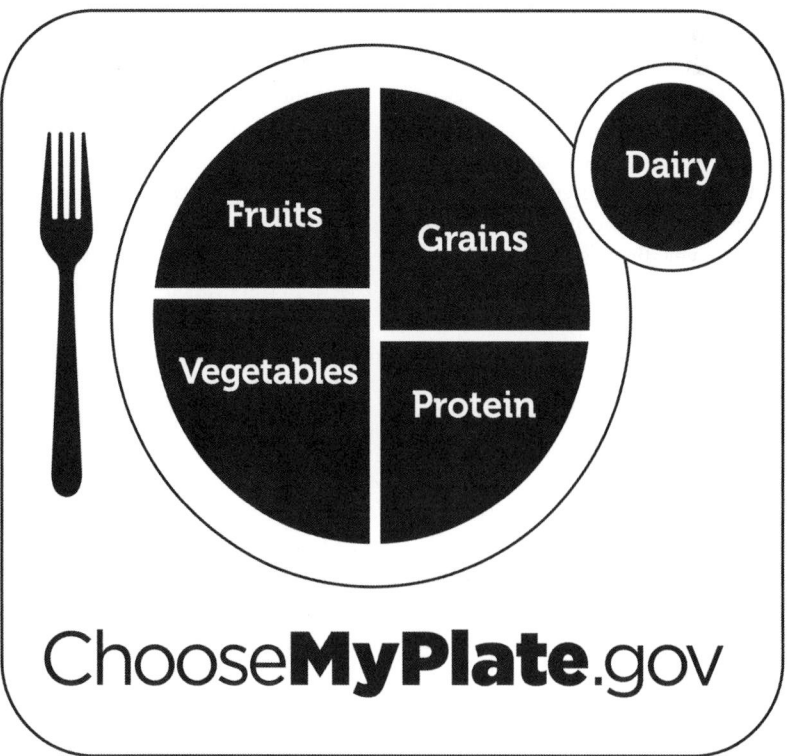

ChooseMyPlate.gov

Source: U.S. Department of Agriculture

10 Tips for Picky Eaters

If your child's nutrition is a sore topic in your household, you're not alone. Many parents are distressed by what their children eat — or don't eat. Until your child's food preferences mature, prevent mealtime battles one bite at a time.

1. *Young children tend to eat only when they're hungry.* If your child isn't hungry, don't force a meal or snack.
2. *Stay calm.* If your child senses that you're unhappy with his or her eating habits, it may become a battle of wills. Threats and punishments only reinforce the power struggle.
3. *Watch the clock.* Nix juice and snacks for at least one hour before meals. If your child comes to the table hungry, he or she may be more motivated to eat.
4. *Don't expect too much.* After age 2, slower growth often reduces a child's appetite.
5. *Limit liquid calories.* Low-fat or fat-free dairy products and 100 percent fruit juice can be important parts of a healthy diet — but if your child fills up on milk or juice, he or she may have no room for meals.
6. *Start small.* Offer several foods in small portions. Let your child choose what he or she eats.
7. *Don't force your child to clean his or her plate.* This may only ignite — or reinforce — a power struggle over food.
8. *Talk about things other than taste.* Discuss a food's color, shape, aroma and texture.
9. *Be patient with new foods.* Your child may need repeated exposure to a new food before he or she takes the first bite.
10. *Eat breakfast for dinner.* Who says cereal or pancakes are only for breakfast? The distinction between breakfast, lunch and dinner foods may be lost on your child.

preschool years. Equally important, promote regular physical activity to help maintain normal weight and physical fitness.

In general, the nutritional guidelines are similar for school-age children and adults. Have your school-age child eat a variety of foods that are lower in fat and higher in complex carbohydrates and fiber. At home, practice healthy-eating habits to guide what your child learns about food choices.

Although you may be setting a good example at home, your child will be receiving conflicting messages from television, other media and friends. These outside influences become even stronger as your child matures, but so does your child's ability to make his or her own choices.

Help your child learn that breakfast is an important meal. It's worth getting the whole family up early enough to enjoy this meal together. After school, your child may need a snack. The amount and type of this snack should be controlled so that it tides your child over until supper but doesn't dull his or her appetite for the meal. A good choice is a piece of fruit, a whole-grain muffin or some low-fat yogurt.

A nutritional problem in some preschool-age children in the United States is iron deficiency anemia. However, your child will get enough iron, zinc and other essential minerals if he or she eats lean meats, whole grains, dried beans, fruits and vegetables. If your child is involved in vigorous physical activity, he or she will need more calories.

If heart disease or high cholesterol runs in your family, discuss this with your child's doctor, who will decide if your child's blood cholesterol and triglycerides (lipids) should be measured. If the value is high, your child may need to follow a diet that controls dietary fat and cholesterol.

If your child's lipid values are normal, it's important not to over-do a low-fat diet. Your school-age child is still growing and needs a balanced diet and adequate calories to grow to his or her full potential. For this reason, you don't want to impose too many dietary restrictions on your child.

As in the preschool years, feed your child in response to hunger but not in response to boredom or inappropriate behavior. When your child feels restless, encourage him or her to go outside and play rather than give your child more food. And remember, the best way to teach your child about good nutrition is by setting a good example in your own eating habits. If you eat healthy, chances are your child will too.

Dental care

Some parents assume that a child has to be a certain age before dental hygiene becomes necessary. In fact, once your baby has a single tooth, you can begin a daily program of dental care.

Developing good habits early is key to preventive dental care. Encourage your child to brush his or her teeth every day. The technique might not be perfect, but it'll improve with time. Don't make teeth brushing a battle.

One by one, your child's permanent teeth will erupt during the school-age years. They replace the baby (primary) teeth at a rate of about four a year. Because perma-

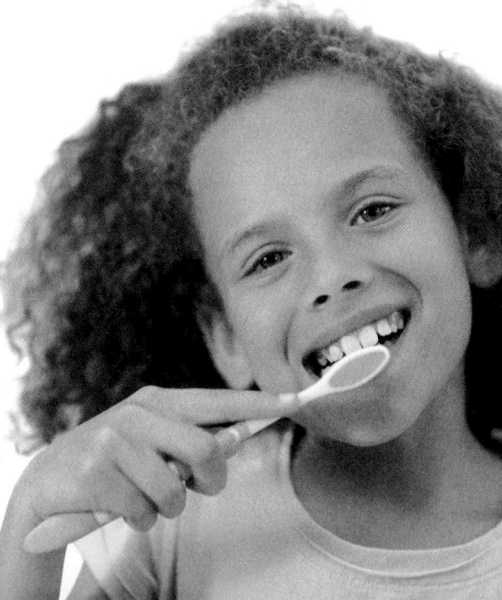

Obesity in Children

Obesity is more common during the first year of life, after age 5 or 6 and during adolescence than it is during the preschool years. Some medical disorders can cause obesity, but if your child is overweight, it's probably because he or she consumes more calories than necessary for growth and gets too little physical activity.

Not all children who are overweight are considered obese. Some children have larger than average body frames. These children tend to be stocky and look big, but they're not fat. A child is considered obese if he or she is more than 20 percent over what is considered his or her healthy weight.

Obesity is generally caused by a combination of factors. Heredity appears to play a role. If one or both parents are obese, their offspring are more likely to be overweight. In addition, overeating may be more common in households where family members are overweight than in households where family members aren't overweight. Lack of exercise also may be a factor. If your child is spending too many hours sitting in front of the television or computer, calories aren't being used and are turning to fat.

If your preschooler is obese, now is the time to do something, while you still have some control over what your child eats and how active he or she is. Once your child gets older and is more independent, modifying eating and exercise patterns is often much more difficult.

If you would like some assistance in developing a healthy diet for your child, consult your doctor or a dietitian. It's important to consider your child's nutritional needs and growth when making dietary changes. Don't use fad diets. They can be dangerous.

Of course, prevention is the best treatment. The time to be alert to obesity, especially if there's a family history of it, is when your child's eating and exercise habits are forming. Infant obesity has little correlation with adult obesity, but family eating habits may persist into adolescence and adulthood.

nent teeth need to last a lifetime, it's imperative to care for them well. Teach your child to brush his or her teeth after each meal. It's also a good time to demonstrate how to floss teeth.

Your child should begin to visit a dentist by age 1, or within six months of when the first tooth erupts. Schedule dental visits every six months or as your dentist recommends. When the permanent back teeth break through, your child's dentist may cover them with a brush-on sealant to protect them against tooth decay.

Fluoride

If your water doesn't contain fluoride, your child's doctor or dentist may prescribe a fluoride supplement. From the time your child is 6 months until he or she is 10 years old, fluoride is an important deterrent to tooth decay.

Fluoride helps make your child's tooth enamel cavity resistant. Typically, your child consumes fluoride either in drinking water or in a supplement.

Diet

You can do your part to decrease the risks of tooth decay by limiting your child's consumption of sugary and starchy foods and sugary beverages. It's virtually impossible to keep children away from sweets altogether, but try to get them to avoid those that stick to the teeth or linger in your child's mouth.

Offer healthy snacks as treats. Vegetables and fruits not only help minimize cavities but also are nutritionally better for your child.

A combination of measures that include water fluoridation, sealants, brushing and flossing, good nutrition, and regular dental visits can help prevent dental cavities.

Hand washing

Hand washing is the best way to prevent the spread of infectious diseases. Many ailments, from the common cold to serious diseases such as an intestinal infection or liver inflammation (hepatitis), may be spread from person to person.

Good hand washing habits are important for your entire family. It's important to wash your own hands regularly and to show your children how to wash their hands properly. Both hands, including the palms and between the fingers, should be washed thoroughly with soap or detergent and water. Remind your children to wash their hands after using the bathroom, whether at home or in school.

Although access to soap and water may not always be available, make an effort to find a place where you can wash your hands. Encourage your child to wash for as long as it takes to sing the alphabet song. For a description of proper hand washing technique, see page 452.

Hand washing is critical in the following situations:
- Before preparing or eating food
- After handling uncooked meat
- After blowing your nose, sneezing or coughing into your hand
- After changing a diaper
- After playing with a pet
- After handling garbage
- After handling money

Sleeping

One way to help maintain your child's health is to encourage good sleeping habits. Establish with

Children and Screen Time

Children in the United States spend a lot of time in front of screens. They spend about three hours each day watching television, recorded programs or DVDs or streaming video, playing video games, or doing other activities. Although television and online media can be educational and entertaining, healthier activities might be a better way to occupy your child's time. Children need to spend time socializing with their friends and family. Children need to be moving around and getting exercise. Too much time spent in front of the television, computer, tablet or cellphone can contribute to childhood obesity.

Parents often are concerned about TV and online programming, video content, and the messages from commercials. For example, children may watch programming that doesn't show the consequences of drinking alcohol, smoking or using other drugs. Commercials may advertise unhealthy foods targeted at children, such as candy, snacks, and sugary cereals and beverages.

One area of special concern is the depiction of violence and its effect on children. According to many studies, exposure to media violence can make children more aggressive, and it can desensitize them to the abuse of others. Media violence may set the cultural norm for what a child considers acceptable behavior.

The following suggestions may help parents create a safer media-viewing environment:

- *Set rules.* Establish limits on the amount and type of programming your child views.
- *Watch television with your child.* Discuss issues that may come up during a show. For example, if both of you see a violent scene, ask your child to think about the feelings of the victim.
- *Learn about TV and video game ratings.* A TV-Y rating is assigned to shows or games designed for children of all ages, and a TV-Y7 rating means that the show or game contains mild fantasy violence or comedic violence more appropriate for children age 7 and older. Video games are rated EC (early childhood) for children age 3 and older, E (everyone) for children age 6 and older, and T (teen) for users age 13 and older.
- *Use the v-chip.* The v-chip included in more recent TV models can be programmed to block inappropriate programs. An external v-chip box is available for televisions without the v-chip.

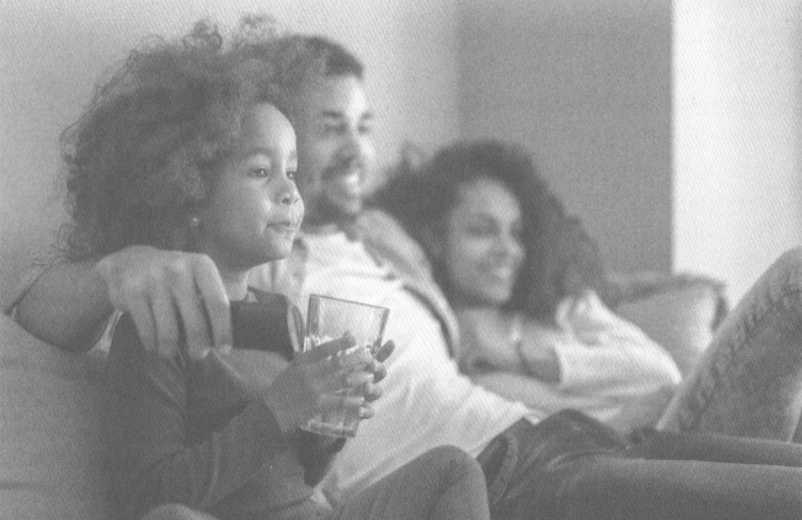

your child a regular sleep schedule with consistent wake and sleep times. An adequate amount of sleep gives your child energy and motivation. It can also enhance his or her learning and decrease behavioral problems.

Young children need plenty of sleep. Though sleep needs vary with each child, children between ages 2 and 5 generally require 10 to 12 hours of sleep to feel their best. This amount declines gradually to about nine hours by the time they reach their teens.

Sleep difficulties

Crying uncontrollably at bedtime, waking up frequently during the night, and getting out of bed and attempting to crawl in with mom and dad are common sleep problems among young children.

Sleep problems are a frequent complaint of parents. Whether the problem is temporary, intermittent or has been occurring for months, a child who's awake at night creates tired parents, not to mention a cranky child.

Causes of sleep difficulties vary, often depending on the age of your child. Common sleep problems that may interfere with your child's getting a good night's rest include:

- **Parental dependency.** If your child has always had problems sleeping through the night, you may have been too responsive to his or her night cries. Most infants awaken several times during the night but can put themselves back to sleep. If your child has learned that mom or dad will come rushing every time he or she cries, your child becomes dependent on a parent to get back to sleep. This can be a hard habit to break, especially with younger children.
- **Bed-wetting.** Bed-wetting (enuresis) is the most common reason children ages 3 to 15 wake up at night.
- **Nightmares.** Your child may have scary dreams that awaken him or her. These nightmares

may be in response to stress or trauma that occurs during waking hours. Calmly reassure your child if he or she awakes after a nightmare.

- **Night terrors.** Night terrors are a condition in which a sleeping child awakens screaming, with no recollection of a nightmare. Sometimes the child may scream and still be asleep and unresponsive to your actions. Emotional tension increases night terrors. They generally occur between ages 3 and 5, and they tend to run in families.
- **Sleepwalking.** Sleepwalking is a condition in which a child is partially awake with open eyes and a dazed expression. He or she may sit up in bed, walk, or do activities such as open doors, go to the bathroom or undress without being aware of what he or she is doing. If awakened, the child is often confused and disoriented. Sleepwalking tends to run in families and is most common in children ages 6 to 12. Gently guide your child back to bed without waking him or her. Keep doors and windows closed and locked and remove objects that your child could trip over.

Toilet training

The first question most parents ask is, "When is the right time to attempt toilet training?" That's not an easy question to answer. One child's readiness may be different from that of another. Some are toilet trained within 24 hours around age 2, and others still balk at the idea near their third birthday.

Unless a child appears extremely interested in being trained, most doctors usually advise waiting until your child is between 2 and 2½ years old. Most children continue to wear underwear-type absorbent pants at night for several months afterward.

The following are indications that your child may be ready for toilet training:

- Your child uses bathroom words such as *potty*, *pee pee* or *poo poo.*
- Your child watches others use the toilet.
- Your child indicates when he or she is wet or dirty and wants to be changed.
- Your child can briefly control his or her bowel and bladder.

How to train your child

You can go about toilet training in various ways. No matter which one you choose, try not to turn the bathroom into a battleground.

Many doctors suggest allowing the child to become trained according to his or her own free will. This means no coercion whatsoever. Ask your child if he or she wants to sit on the potty. If the answer is no, don't pressure him or her. If your child sits a minute but doesn't do anything, let him or her get off the potty when ready. If your child urinates or has a bowel movement, be free with your praise. And when the inevitable "accident" occurs, don't scold or shame your toddler.

Other methods use similar principles but require more parental involvement. For example, take your child to the potty chair at appropriate intervals and ask him or her to pee pee. If your child is reluctant to cooperate, try entertaining him or her with books or games while he or she is seated on the potty chair. If your child doesn't urinate within five minutes, take him or her off the potty chair and try again later. When your child does use the potty chair, offer praise.

Some children resist toilet training. The most common cause of resistance is parental pressure. The child may have been reminded too much to use the bathroom or been forced to sit for long periods on the potty chair.

In trying to train a resistant child, shift the responsibility to him or her. Tell your child that you're not going to remind him or her to go to the bathroom and that

Putting Your Child to Sleep

The following tips may prevent your child from developing sleep problems or help your child overcome sleep difficulties:

- Don't sleep in the same room as your child.
- Don't entertain your child at night.
- Don't let your child nap more than three hours a day.

If your child is having difficulty falling asleep at night or sleeping through the night, try the following steps. Although this approach may leave you wide awake for a while, it should improve the situation within about two weeks. Remember, each child's needs vary.

- Put your child to bed awake, read a book, say good night and leave the room despite protests.
- Give your child a transition object, such as a favorite blanket or stuffed toy. Put on a recording of soothing music.
- If your child begins crying, don't go into his or her room immediately. Wait 15 or 20 minutes before checking on him or her. When you do go in, stay in the room for less than a minute.
- Keep the light off and don't pick up your child. Simply reassure him or her that everything is all right and that it's time for sleep.

The first night that you begin using this method, your child may cry for an hour, but generally the crying time will decrease each night. Some children awaken terrified. If your child's cries sound fearful rather than simply angry, go to him or her immediately. After you reassure your child, you may have to sit there for a while. Don't play or talk.

Leaving the door open or using a night light also can work wonders. If you find your child crawling into bed with you at night, gently but firmly take him or her back to his or her bed. In the long run, this is better for you and your child.

193

he or she must decide when to go. Try to be patient, however difficult that may be.

Bed-wetting

"Mommy, Daddy, I wet my bed." Virtually every parent hears those words at one time or another, and many young children do on occasion have accidents during the night.

True bed-wetting (enuresis) is involuntary urination, mostly occurring at night, in a child age 5 or older. Usually, it doesn't indicate an emotional or physical problem. Children vary markedly in the age at which they're physiologically ready to stop wetting. Bed-wetting may be a problem if your child's bladder hasn't yet developed enough to hold urine through the night, or if your child hasn't learned how to recognize when his or her bladder is full, wake up and use the toilet.

If your child bed-wets and has never been totally dry for six months, the condition is known as primary enuresis. If your child starts wetting again after having been dry for at least a year, the condition is called secondary enuresis. This form of bed-wetting may develop temporarily in reaction to a stressful change in your child's development, such as the birth of a sibling or the first week of school.

Bed-wetting is much more common in boys than in girls, and it often runs in families. Your child may urinate during the first third of the night and remember nothing of the occurrence. Aside from wet pajamas, enuresis itself causes no direct impairment of your child's life, but a child who bed-wets is often afraid to attend sleepovers or go to camp.

Limiting your child's intake of liquids at bedtime is one way to make it easier for him or her to stay dry. Having your child urinate twice just a few minutes apart right before bedtime also may

help, as might getting him or her up to go to the bathroom at night. Behavior modification techniques are often effective in eliminating enuresis. You may want to use wall charts with gold stars awarded for cooperating with bedtime routines. Enuresis is involuntary, so avoid rewarding dry nights and punishing wet ones.

If your child is motivated to stop wetting, alarm devices attached to a pad that awakens your child when the pad gets wet may help. Your child's primary care provider may prescribe medication such as oxybutynin (Ditropan XL) if your child is older and the problem persists.

In the case of secondary enuresis, have your child examined to rule out any organic problems, such as urinary infection, seizure disorder or diabetes. Should the problem appear to be a reaction to stress, psychotherapy or family therapy may be helpful.

Although having to change bed linens repeatedly can be exasperating, try to express support for rather than anger toward your child. Doing so will not only help to enlist his or her cooperation but also prevent his or her losing self-esteem. Reward your child if he or she helps by getting into dry clothes and back to bed quickly.

Sun protection

Protect your child's skin from the sun's ultraviolet (UV) rays. A child who experiences a severe, blistering sunburn may have a greater risk of developing skin cancer as an adult. Practice sun safety:

- Buy sunscreen designed for children that has a sun protection factor (SPF) of at least 15. A sunscreen with an SPF of 30 or higher is even better.
- Use sunscreen even on cloudy days. Clouds block only a small portion of UV rays.
- Limit your child's time at the pool or beach.
- If possible, keep your child out of the sun when UV rays are

strongest. This is generally between 10 a.m. and 3 p.m.
- Dress your children in clothes made of tightly woven fabrics.

Insect repellents

When your child is outside, the following tips may help keep the insects away.

- Avoid using scented soaps or shampoos. Fragrances often attract insects.
- Avoid areas where insects may live, such as stagnant pools of water or gardens with blooming flowers.
- Don't dress your children in bright colors or flowery prints. They tend to attract insects. Wearing white can make it easier to find ticks.

When you're in an area that contains insects, use an insect repellent. The active ingredient in many insect repellent products is a chemical called DEET.

Although DEET is toxic if ingested or absorbed through the skin in large amounts, if used properly it doesn't present a health concern and it's effective in repelling potentially disease-carrying mosquitoes and ticks.

Make sure to follow these safety measures:

- Don't use repellents on infants and children younger than 2 months of age.
- Use insect repellents that contain no more than 30 percent DEET. Read the label before purchasing the repellent.
- Never apply insect repellent on children's hands because they're likely to put their hands in their mouths or rub their eyes.
- Apply insect repellent to clothing rather than directly on the skin.

Giving medicine

Many children resist taking medication. To sidestep such resistance, it helps to approach this task in a natural, matter-of-fact way. Explain that the medication needs to be taken and why. Apprehension on your part or the expectation of resistance can become a self-fulfilling prophecy.

It's generally best to avoid mixing medications with foods or drinks. If you do, make sure that the entire mixture is consumed. In addition, ask your pharmacist if the food or drink with which you mix the medication is compatible with the medication.

Don't try to get your child to take medication by promising a treat or, worse, telling him or her that the medication is candy. Children must learn to make a clear distinction between medicine and candy and to take all medications while supervised by an adult.

It's important to give your child his or her medications exactly as prescribed — in the correct dose and at the correct interval. When your child begins to show signs of improvement, don't stop giving the medication unless specifically instructed to do so. And don't use remnants of old prescriptions.

Tantrums and breath holding

Few children make it through their toddler and preschool years without demonstrating temper tantrums. This stubborn, oppositional and defiant behavior is a natural part of moving from total dependence to a taste of independence.

Nothing is more exasperating than when your child decides to throw a temper tantrum. Any parent who has been through one knows that it doesn't take much to drive some youngsters to uncontrollable kicking, screaming, headbanging and even breath holding.

Often, in fact, the temper tantrum has nothing to do with you, but is your child's response to frustration. When a child reaches this point, he or she is out of control and beyond reason. Generally, a temper tantrum, once started, has to run its course.

Giving in is not the answer. If, for example, your child has a tantrum because you deny him or her a second cookie, you'll be sending the wrong message if you suddenly reverse your decision. Once the tantrum starts, giving your child a timeout is most helpful. Leave the room and try to ignore what's going on. Even if your child holds his or her breath, don't worry because this generally isn't harmful. As for any headbanging, children hate pain as much as do adults. When things get too uncomfortable, they know it's time to quit.

When to return to your child is variable. Some parents find that their child finishes the tantrum on his or her own. Other children may need to be held for a moment before they can stop crying.

Although ignoring a tantrum is usually best, sometimes you must take other measures. Obviously, the child who decides to throw a tantrum in the middle of the supermarket can't be left there to kick and flail, nor should a child who is physically aggressive toward someone else or property be allowed to continue unchecked. Take the child to his or her room or separate your child from others until your child regains his or her composure.

Common Conditions

As many parents can attest, preschoolers do get sick with amazing frequency. Some months you seem to be caught in a revolving door between home and your child's clinic. No sooner is an ear infection cleared up than your child develops a cold. Before you know it, you're back.

Most parents are understandably concerned when their young child seems to fall prey to every virus that hits the block. In the back of your mind, you may wonder if something is wrong that's interfering with your child's ability to resist these infections.

Almost always such fears are groundless. If your child is active and gaining weight, there's probably nothing wrong with his or her health. It's a simple fact that young children are particularly susceptible to colds, ear infections and gastrointestinal viruses. Your child's immune system must be exposed to many viruses before it develops its own resistance.

School-age children gradually become less prone to common respiratory infections, such as colds. Most disorders of school-age children don't have serious consequences. At this age, children are extraordinarily resilient, and their young bodies easily recover from most common disorders.

Fever

A "core" temperature — oral or rectal — of more than 100.4 F is generally considered a fever. A fever is one of the body's ways of fighting infection.

Viral infections, strep throat and ear infections are the most common causes of fevers in children. More serious illnesses also can cause a fever, but fortunately they aren't common.

Although children tolerate most fevers quite well, high temperatures often provoke a great deal of anxiety for parents. If your child is responsive, continues to drink fluids and wants to play, there's probably nothing to worry about.

Contact your child's health care provider or go to the emergency department if the fever is accompanied by considerable listlessness, a severe headache, or a persistent stomachache or vomiting.

If you think your child will be more comfortable if you lower the fever, you can use children's acetaminophen (Tylenol, others) or ibuprofen (Advil, Motrin, others) to help reduce it. Extra fluids and minimal clothing also may help.

Don't use aspirin to reduce a fever in a child, unless specifically prescribed by your child's care provider. Aspirin use in children has been linked to Reye's syndrome, a potentially life-threatening illness.

Some medical experts believe that reducing a low-grade fever blunts the body's immune response and may possibly prolong some illnesses.

Vomiting

Vomiting may or may not be associated with diarrhea. If your child is vomiting, avoid feeding him or her solid foods for about eight hours. Your child may try to drink small amounts of clear liquids or suck on ice pops. If your child hasn't vomited for about eight hours, you can try foods such as soda crackers, white bread or chicken soup.

Seek medical care immediately if you see blood in vomit or note that your child has severe abdominal pain, has a swollen abdomen, is delirious or difficult to awaken, or exhibits signs of dehydration — no saliva or tears and absence of urination.

Diarrhea

Diarrhea is characterized by a change in one or more of the following stool patterns: frequency, volume or content. Diarrhea is a common gastrointestinal disturbance, usually caused by a virus. Less commonly, it is the result of a bacterial or parasitic infection.

Mild diarrhea is the passage of a few mushy stools. Moderate or severe diarrhea is indicated by an increased frequency of bowel movements and stools that are more watery and, possibly, greenish. Dehydration is the main danger. The body can lose large amounts of fluid in the stools.

If your child has diarrhea, take steps to avoid dehydration by increasing your child's fluid intake. Commercially available oral electrolyte replacement solutions, such as Pedialyte, provide excellent replacement of what the body loses with diarrhea. In addition, they help slow down the amount of fluid loss. Water, juice, ice pops, broth and sport drinks are good choices. Don't use diet soda or diet juices.

If your child isn't hungry, don't force food. If he or she wants to eat, offer a general diet and a lot of fluids. Foods that contain bulk — such as whole-grain cereal, fruits and vegetables — are good choices because they usually make the stool firmer. Diarrhea may last up to a week or a few weeks before bowel movements return to normal.

Some young children develop toddler's diarrhea. The child may have several days of loose stools that are foul smelling and runny. Some children are incredibly thirsty during this time.

Despite the diarrhea, a child with toddler's diarrhea usually is very active, appears healthy and doesn't have a fever. If the stool is tested for bacteria, it almost always is normal. This is because most cases of toddler's diarrhea are caused by viruses, such as the rotavirus.

It's unnecessary to call your health care provider every time your child has a bout of diarrhea unless any of the following signs or symptoms occur:
- Signs of dehydration — no wet diapers or urination for eight hours, tearless crying, no saliva in the mouth
- A bowel movement every hour for more than eight hours
- Blood, pus or mucus in the stool
- Severe abdominal pain or any abdominal pain lasting more than 12 hours
- Diarrhea that doesn't improve within 48 hours of dietary changes
- Mild diarrhea lasting more than a week

Constipation

Parents of young children are often overly concerned about their child's bowel movements. If your child doesn't have a daily bowel movement, you may incorrectly assume he or she is constipated. Although many people do have daily bowel movements, others may have a bowel movement only every second or third day.

The signs of constipation are the painful passage of stool, passage of a large, hard stool, an inability to pass stool even though the urge to defecate is strong, or going more than three days without having a bowel movement.

Constipation is often a result of not getting enough fiber or fluid in the diet. Constipation can also result from a child holding back passage of stool because it's inconvenient to go to the bathroom. Some children hold in the stool because a previous passage of a hard stool created a tear in the anal opening. It hurts when they try to have a bowel movement, so they try to avoid the pain.

Treatment for constipation generally involves eating lots of fruits and vegetables, foods high in fiber such as wheat breads, legumes and whole-grain cereals, and drinking water and other fluids. In addition, encourage your child to sit on the toilet at regular intervals, perhaps after breakfast or supper. If this doesn't resolve the constipation, talk to your child's doctor.

Colds

The common cold is one of the most frequent illnesses of childhood. Preschoolers have an average of five to eight colds each year.

If your child constantly has a congested head, is sneezing, and has a fever or sore throat, there are several possible causes. The most common cause of a constantly runny nose is simply a recurring cold.

Children older than 6 months often have recurring viral upper respiratory tract infections. A young child with a cold is generally sicker than are older children or adults with colds.

A fever may be an early sign of a cold. Irritability, restlessness and sneezing usually follow. Soon a clear liquid begins to drip from the nose, which gradually changes to a thick mucus that makes it difficult to breathe through the nose. The virus may irritate your child's throat and windpipe (trachea), causing a sore throat and cough. Other symptoms may include a headache, lack of appetite and muscle aches.

In general, there's little anyone can do to make your child better quickly. Usually, your child's temperature will return to normal in one to three days. Nose and throat symptoms often disappear within a week. However, the cough may persist for two to three weeks.

Cold medicines

Over-the-counter cold medications aren't recommended for children. The medicines won't cure a common cold or make it go away any sooner. In fact, cough and cold medicines haven't been proved effective at providing symptom relief for children. And there are serious risks to consider. For example, the sedating effects of antihistamines can be dangerous for kids already having trouble breathing. For young children, an accidental overdose of cough or cold medicine could be fatal.

The Food and Drug Administration (FDA) strongly encourages parents to avoid cough and cold medicines for children younger than 4 years of age, unless a health care professional has instructed you to use one.

If a cough or cold medicine seemed to work for your child in the past, chances are your child's signs and symptoms simply improved on their own — or the sedating effects of the medication made you think that your child was feeling better. Research shows that cough and cold medicines for kids are no more effective than a placebo.

Older children aren't as likely as younger children to experience side effects from cough and cold medicines, but side effects are still possible. Some cough and cold medicines may make kids sleepy, while others may have the opposite effect. Even then, remember that cough and cold medicines can't make a cold go away any sooner.

Experts from the FDA are studying the safety and effectiveness of cough and cold medicines for older children. In the meantime, if you choose to give cough or cold medicines to an older child, carefully follow the label directions.

What about antibiotics? Colds are caused by viruses, so antibiotics won't help. If your child uses antibiotics inappropriately, he or she could be at increased risk of getting sick with an antibiotic-resistant infection in the future.

An over-the-counter children's pain reliever — such as acetaminophen (Tylenol, others) or ibuprofen (Motrin, Advil, others) — can reduce a fever and ease the pain of a sore throat or headache. If you give your child a pain reliever, follow the dosing guidelines carefully. Don't give ibuprofen to a child younger than age 6 months, and don't give aspirin to anyone age 18 or younger. Aspirin has been associated with Reye's syndrome, a rare but potentially fatal illness.

You can do some things to make your child more comfortable:

- **Clear mucus from the nose.** If your child is too young to blow his or her nose, remove mucus from the nose using a soft, rubber suction bulb. If your child is managing OK with breathing and eating, there's really no need for nasal suction.
- **Use saline nose drops.** If your child's nose is stuffed, try administering over-the-counter saline nose drops 15 to 20 minutes before meals and at bedtime. For a young child, tilt his or her head back and place three drops in each nostril. After waiting about a minute, use a suction bulb to remove the loosened mucus. For an older child, put three drops in each nostril while he or she is lying faceup on the bed with his or her head over the side. After a moment, have your child blow his or her nose. This can be repeated several times in a row until the nose is cleared.
- **Use a humidifier or vaporizer.** If your child is congested or has a cough, use a cool-mist humidifier or vaporizer to moisten the air. It may help your child breathe easier. But make sure to keep the device clean to prevent the growth of bacteria and molds in it.

Ear infection

Middle ear infections (otitis media) are one of the most common

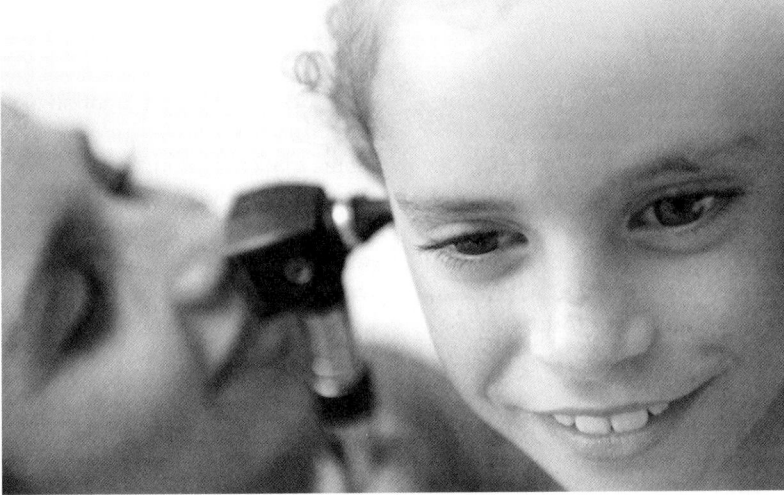

illnesses affecting young children. The majority of children will have at least one middle ear infection by age 3. Although ear infections recur in one-third of these children, most children stop having multiple ear infections by the time they reach school age.

Ear infections often follow a cold that leads to fluid buildup behind a child's eardrum. This trapped fluid is an ideal breeding ground for bacteria or viruses that cause infection. In addition to having an earache or a feeling of pressure in the ear, your child may become irritable, lose his or her appetite, develop a fever, and have trouble sleeping.

Most ear infections clear on their own without antibiotics. However, your child's health care provider may prescribe antibiotics if the infection is severe or if your child has recurrent ear infections.

If your child doesn't respond to antibiotics, your care provider may recommend surgically inserting a small drainage tube into the eardrum to help prevent fluid buildup. For more information on ear infections, see page 630.

Strep throat

Strep throat is a common infection and is caused by the bacterium *Streptococcus pyogenes* (group A beta-hemolytic streptococcus). Often, a person with strep was exposed to someone else with the illness in the preceding two to seven days.

Children ages 5 to 15 who are in a school classroom or some other group setting are most likely to get strep throat. The illness is generally spread by nasal or throat secretions. Less commonly, strep infection may be transmitted through food, milk or water contaminated with streptococci bacteria.

Common signs and symptoms of strep throat are a sore throat, red and swollen tonsils, swollen lymph glands in the front of the neck, a fever, headache, muscle aches, abdominal pain, and possibly vomiting.

Strep throat requires antibiotic treatment to prevent complications. For more information on strep throat, see page 449.

Croup

Croup is an inflammation of the voice box (larynx) and the airway just beneath it. Children with croup have a loud barking cough that may sound like the barking of a seal. Because of a narrowing of the airway, the voice becomes hoarse and breathing may become difficult.

Croup is caused by a virus and is usually preceded by symptoms similar to those of a cold. Symptoms of croup are usually worse at night and may last from five to seven days.

Children younger than 5 years are at greater risk of developing croup because their small airways are more susceptible to narrowing when swollen. Symptoms tend to be most pronounced in children younger than 3 years.

Most cases of croup aren't serious and can be treated at home. However, if your child has croup and develops stridor or other symptoms of airway distress, he or she should be seen for treatment. Stridor is a harsh, high-pitched sound made when a child breathes in after a bout of coughing.

For more information on croup, see page 450.

Pneumonia

Pneumonia refers to an infection or inflammation in the lungs. In young children it's often a passing illness that may remain undiagnosed and be regarded as a cold. Pneumonia can develop after a cold or the flu or on its own. It may result from a virus, a bacterium or another organism (see page 448).

A fever and a prominent cough are common warning signs. The cough may not produce phlegm

in children as it does in adults. Rapid and labored breathing or respiratory distress also are signs of pneumonia. Treatment varies depending on the cause.

Tonsillitis

Tonsillitis is an infection and inflammation of the tonsils. It's common in preschool and school-age children. If your child has tonsillitis, his or her tonsils may become red and swollen and you may notice small patches of white discharge on them.

Sometimes, the adenoids, located in the back and upper part of the throat, will be swollen too — although you can't see them. Other signs and symptoms may include a sore throat, difficulty swallowing, fatigue, a headache, fever, chills, and sore and enlarged glands in the jaw and neck.

Surgery to remove your child's tonsils and possibly adenoids is generally considered only if the tonsillitis interferes with breathing, is recurrent or doesn't respond to antibiotics (see page 653). Antibiotics treat tonsillitis that results from a bacterial infection.

Symptoms should disappear a few days after your child begins taking the medication. If the infection is resulting from a virus, no treatment is used aside from getting plenty of rest, drinking plenty of liquids and gargling with warm salt water to ease the symptoms.

Epiglottitis

Epiglottitis is an inflammation of the lid-like flaps of tissue and cartilage that cover your windpipe. It occurs among children between the ages of 2 and 5 but is very rare in populations with standard vaccinations. It is somewhat more common in boys than in girls.

Your child may have a sore throat, fever, difficulty swallowing and breathing, and hoarseness. Epiglottitis usually results from a bacterial infection and may respond to treatment with antibiotics.

Epiglottitis causes severe inflammation and serious breathing difficulties and can cause death. If you suspect that your child has epiglottitis, have him or her seen by a doctor immediately.

Sinusitis

Sinusitis is an infection of the lining of one or more of the sinuses. The sinuses are cavities in the bones around your nose. They're connected to your nasal cavities by small openings. Normally, air passes in and out of your sinuses, and mucus drains through these openings into your nose.

Sinusitis is relatively uncommon in young children but may occur in older school-age children. When a sinus cavity becomes infected, nasal membranes swell, causing nasal congestion or obstruction. Because the cavity can't drain, pus or mucus remains inside.

Sinus pain may result from the inflammation itself or from the pressure caused by built-up secretions in your sinus. For more on sinusitis, see page 649.

Rashes

Rashes can result from a variety of factors. Some of the most common include:

Chickenpox

Chickenpox (varicella) causes itchy red spots that quickly fill with a clear fluid to form blisters. The blisters eventually rupture and crust over. The initial rash tends to break out on the face, scalp, chest and back and may spread to the arms and legs (see the illustration on page 396).

Spots continue to appear over four to five days, often accompanied by a fever, runny nose or cough. Your child is contagious until the rash crusts. It usually takes a 10- to 21-day incubation period after exposure to chicken-

How Long Is My Child Contagious?

The following is a guide as to when a child who has had a contagious disease is no longer contagious:

Disease	No longer contagious
Chickenpox (varicella)	Generally after all sores are crusted, usually 7 days
Diarrhea	After stools form again
Head lice	After one treatment
Pink eye (conjunctivitis)	24 hours after treatment begins if bacterial, longer if viral
Strep throat	24 hours after treatment begins

pox before signs and symptoms appear. For most children, this period is 12 days.

Chickenpox occurs primarily in children, but adults who aren't immune can get it too. The incidence of chickenpox has declined drastically since the development of a chickenpox vaccine. The vaccine is given in two doses to children age 1 year or older and adults who haven't had the virus. For more information on chickenpox, see page 451. For more information on the chickenpox vaccine, see page 148.

Roseola

Roseola is a viral infection that typically affects children between ages 6 months and 3 years. It usually begins with a high fever lasting about three days. When the fever goes down, a rash appears on the trunk and neck lasting from a few hours to a few days.

The rash causes little discomfort and in most cases isn't serious. It disappears on its own without treatment, but acetaminophen

(Tylenol, others) and tepid sponge baths can help relieve discomfort and fever. Occasionally, young children experience convulsions caused by the high fever (febrile seizure). Contact a doctor immediately if this happens. For more information on roseola, see page 456.

Fifth disease

Fifth disease is a common, mild infection in children. It's caused by a virus called human parvovirus B19. Doctors often refer to the illness as parvovirus infection.

The primary symptom of fifth disease is the appearance of bright red, raised patches on both cheeks, resembling slap marks (see the illustration on page 396). A pink, lacy, slightly raised rash may also develop on the arms, trunk, thighs and buttocks. The rash may come and go for up to three weeks. Some children develop a slight fever and other mild, cold-like symptoms.

No specific treatment is recommended, but acetaminophen

Warning Signs of Serious Illness

The following signs and symptoms may suggest a serious illness. If your child has any of these, call your doctor or go to the emergency department:

- A fever higher than 100.4 F in infants (if infant is less than 2 months old, a fever is considered a medical emergency)
- A fever higher than 103 F in preschool-age children
- A fever without an obvious cause (a cold or the flu) that lasts longer than 24 hours
- A fever that lasts more than 72 hours
- Lethargy or no drinking of fluids
- A stiff or painful neck
- Such severe pain that he or she doesn't want to be touched
- A sudden inability to walk
- Breathing difficulty
- Difficulty being awakened
- A convulsion
- Pain in the groin
- Blue lips
- Profuse drooling
- Persistent vomiting
- Purple or deep red spots on the skin
- Painful urination or lack of urine output accompanied by other signs of serious illness
- Bloody stools or urine

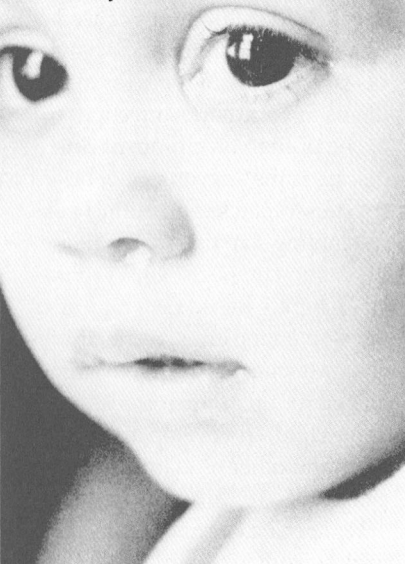

(Tylenol, others) may relieve the fever and discomfort. Pregnant women who suspect they've been exposed to the virus should contact their doctor because there's a chance the fetus could develop serious complications.

Measles (rubeola)

Measles (rubeola) typically begins with a fever, often as high as 104 F to 105 F, a cough, sneezing, a sore throat and red, watery eyes. A red, blotchy rash appears on the face and behind the ears and spreads to the trunk, arms and legs. The rash may begin as fine, red spots that increase in size.

Sometimes, small, white spots may appear on the inside lining of the cheek. The rash usually lasts about a week, during which time it typically spreads from the forehead to the legs.

Measles occurs primarily in children, but adults are susceptible too. A vaccine to prevent measles has significantly reduced the incidence of this disease. For more information on measles, see page 455.

Hand-foot-and-mouth disease

Hand-foot-and-mouth disease is a mild but highly contagious disease that primarily affects preschool children. Symptoms of this viral infection include blister-like lesions on the tongue, mouth, hands and feet.

Children in child care centers are especially susceptible to outbreaks because the illness is spread by person-to-person contact. Meticulous hand washing can help prevent spread of the disease.

This illness isn't related to foot-and-mouth disease, which is a highly infectious viral disease of ruminant animals.

Impetigo

Impetigo is a common skin infection caused by streptococcal or staphylococcal bacteria that penetrate the skin through a cut, scratch or insect bite. The infection starts as a red sore that blisters briefly, oozes for a few days and forms a sticky crust. It usually appears on the face and is more common among young children (see illustration on page 396).

The infection can easily spread to other people or other parts of your body just by scratching or touching the sores. Good hygiene can help prevent and limit the spread of impetigo. The sores and skin surrounding the infection should be kept clean. Trim your child's fingernails. If the infection spreads, your doctor may prescribe antibiotics to treat it.

Lice

Lice are tiny parasitic insects that cause intense itching. Head lice are often spread among children by direct contact, by shared combs and hairbrushes, or by clothing, such as coats and hats, that comes in contact with another child's clothes. Lice are commonly found on the scalp at the nape of the neck and over the ears. Small nits (eggs) that resemble tiny pussy willow buds attach to hair shafts.

Prescription and over-the-counter shampoos are available to remove lice. Read the directions carefully. Consult your health care provider before using these products on children younger than 2 months or if you're pregnant. Infected children should be kept home until after the first shampoo treatment. A mixture of vinegar and water may be useful in dislodging nits, which must be manually stripped from hair shafts to prevent recurrence.

To prevent the spread of lice or re-infestation, wash sheets, clothing and hats with hot, soapy water and dry them at high heat, which kills the lice. Soak combs and brushes in very hot, soapy water for at least five minutes.

Prevention of Diseases and Infestations

If you have a young child, you may have more colds and viral illnesses than your friends who don't have young children. Given the frequency with which young children contract these ailments and their high degree of contiguousness, this isn't a surprise. Infections that typically afflict families spread in various ways.

Respiratory infections such as colds most often spread through contact with secretions from the nose, mouth or eyes of an infected person. Toddlers are great at spreading colds because of their habit of touching and mouthing everything they come across.

Your child's sneeze can release potentially infectious agents into the air. Although colds are spread less commonly in this manner, the infectious particles contained in a sneeze or cough can travel up to 6 feet.

The sharing of combs, brushes and hats may contribute to the spread of ailments such as lice, ringworm and impetigo.

Although it's impossible to totally stop the spread of contagious disease and infestations within a family, you can take the following preventive steps:

- Wash your hands throughout the day and encourage your child to do likewise. This is particularly important before eating and after using the bathroom, blowing your nose or changing a diaper.
- Don't share combs, brushes and hats.
- Don't smoke around your child. Exposure to secondhand smoke increases both the frequency and the severity of your child's colds.
- After someone in your family has been ill, get him or her a new toothbrush and throw out the old one because it may contain bacteria that can cause reinfection.
- Use a disinfectant. Clean and disinfect bathrooms, the kitchen and diaper-changing areas frequently.
- Immunize your pets. It's likely your toddler and dog or cat will have frequent contact, so make sure your pet is immunized and wormed regularly.
- Cook foods thoroughly. To help prevent bacterial illness, cook eggs and meat thoroughly. And be sure that you carefully wash your hands and any object that comes into contact with uncooked food, particularly meat and eggs.

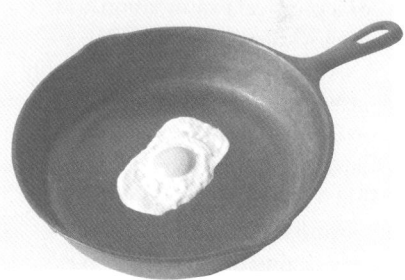

Vacuum carpets, mattresses, pillows, upholstered furniture and car seats. For more information on lice, see page 463.

Scabies

Scabies is a contagious skin disease caused by tiny mites that burrow under the skin. The mites are almost impossible to see without a magnifying glass, but they make a characteristic burrow that looks like a thin, irregular pencil mark (see the illustration on page 397).

The marks appear most often between the fingers, in the armpits, around the waist, along the insides of the wrists, on the back of the elbows, on the ankles and soles of the feet, around the breasts and genitals, and on the buttocks. Itching is usually worse at night.

Scabies can spread from person to person in a family, child care setting or schoolroom. Bathing and over-the-counter preparations aren't effective in removing scabies. Consult a medical provider for treatment.

Headaches

Headaches are more common during late childhood and early adolescence than during the preschool years. They rarely represent a serious problem. Usually, a headache is a sign that your child isn't getting enough fluids, food or sleep, or is experiencing stress. Headaches are also associated with many viral illnesses.

If your child frequently complains of headaches, even during times when he or she is otherwise well, consult a health care provider. Migraines may be the culprit, especially if there's a family history of migraines. In children, this type of headache often is accompanied by light sensitivity and sleepiness, so help your child rest in a quiet, dark room. Recovery often follows within a few hours of the onset of the headache.

Abdominal aches

Stomachaches are common in children. Typically, the pains are nothing more than the result of eating something that doesn't agree with the child or they're the beginning of a bout with a gastrointestinal virus.

Sometimes, a child may complain of intermittent stomachaches or abdominal pain. These symptoms may relate to stress or fear concerning a social situation or school issue. In many children, the symptoms gradually disappear, but others have recurrent bouts of pain over many years.

Consult with your child's doctor if your child refuses to participate in day-to-day activities because of a stomachache or if the stomachache is accompanied by blood in the stool or vomit, persistent vomiting or diarrhea, or weight loss.

Growing pains

Many school-age children, particularly during the later years of this period, experience severe, recurrent limb pain. These pains may come on at any time, but they seem to occur most frequently in the evening, particularly after a day of strenuous activity.

Usually, these pains are located in the thighs or calves, and last for an hour or two. The children are otherwise healthy, and the results of a physical examination and diagnostic tests are normal.

Although these pains probably aren't directly related to physical growth, the symptoms often are labeled growing pains. The pains have no known explanation and disappear over time without any lasting ill effects. The best treatment for growing pains is sympathy, understanding and the assurance that the symptoms don't represent a health problem.

To help alleviate some of the discomfort:
- Let your child use a warm (not hot) heating pad.
- Give recommended doses of children's acetaminophen (Tylenol, others) or ibuprofen (Advil, Motrin, others) for pain. Don't give aspirin unless advised by your medical provider to do so.
- Call your medical provider if the area becomes swollen, hot and tender, if your child develops a limp or an unexplained fever, or if the pain persists more than a week or two.

Genital infections and irritation in girls

Genital infections in girls (vulvovaginitis) can occur both before and after puberty. The usual cause is inadequate bathing and toilet habits. A young girl may not wash her genitals adequately. Or she may wipe herself from back to front after bowel movements and inadvertently transport bacteria that live harmlessly in the intestines to the vaginal and urinary openings, where they can colonize.

Yeast, parasites, bacteria and irritants found in soaps and other toiletries can cause genital infections. Yeast infections are more common in girls who have entered puberty, have diabetes or have been taking antibiotics.

Your daughter's health care provider may ask if she has had any vaginal discharge, itching or redness of the anus, vulva or vagina, or other infections. The doctor will likely examine the genital area and may take a sample of vaginal discharge to examine for bacteria, yeast and parasites.

Genital infections and irritation can often be prevented and treated by teaching your daughter about her genital area and showing her how to wipe from front to back. When she bathes, encourage her to wash her genital area and avoid taking bubble baths.

Your daughter's toilet paper and underpants should be white, not colored, because dyes can irritate the skin. Her underpants should also be all cotton and changed once a day. Discourage wearing clothing that increases moisture in the area, including attire such as tightfitting jeans and tights. Wearing a swimming suit for a prolonged period of time should be avoided.

For specific infections, treatment may involve taking oral antibiotics or applying a prescription cream to the genital area.

Urinary tract infection

Urinary tract infection occurs when bacteria enter the bladder via the channel leading from the bladder to the outside of the body (urethra). Under normal circumstances, these bacteria are rinsed out of the body during urination.

Urine itself has properties that inhibit the growth of bacteria. However, certain bacteria and anatomic abnormalities in the urinary system can increase the chance of a urinary tract infection.

Urinary tract infections are more common in girls than in boys. Usually, the infection is confined to the bladder, a condition called cystitis. Your child may feel as if she has to go to the bathroom constantly and may complain of pain with urination. The urine may be foul smelling.

A child who had been night trained and has a urinary tract infection may have episodes of bedwetting. Other signs and symptoms may include fever, vomiting and chills. In some cases, a child with a urinary tract infection has no signs or symptoms. Left untreated, the infection can lead to a more serious kidney infection.

Urinary tract infections in girls can result from improper wiping after going to the bathroom. Teach your child to wipe from front to back. In some cases, dyes in bubble baths may lead to a urinary tract infection. Other causes include genital abnormalities. Sometimes, urinary tract infections occur for no apparent reason.

Antibiotics are generally prescribed for a urinary tract infection. Some children who have recurrent urinary tract infections may need daily doses of an antibiotic for months or even years to keep their urine from becoming infected.

After an infection, X-rays may be taken to determine whether urine is flowing from inside the bladder back to the kidneys, a condition called refluxing. When an abnormality, such as reflux, is responsible for urinary tract infections, surgery may be considered if antibiotic treatment isn't sufficient to control the problem.

Special Concerns

If you have special concerns about some aspect of your child's health or development, discuss them with your child's doctor or another health care professional. The following information is presented as a starting point in your effort to understand how you can best help your child.

Some children may have vision or hearing problems, physical disabilities, orthopedic disorders, or sexual abnormalities. Others may exhibit signs of child abuse. Whatever their circumstances, every child in your care is counting on you to be informed and responsive to their needs.

Vision problems

The preschool years are crucial for the detection and successful treatment of many eye conditions. When detected in the preschool years, simple vision problems generally don't have an adverse effect on a child's learning. Sitting extremely close to the television or area of activity may be one indication of a vision problem. Others include squinting, eye rubbing, fatigue and headache.

Refraction abnormalities such as nearsightedness and farsightedness are the most common vision problems in children. A child with a refraction problem may seem to show a lack of interest in learning. A child who's farsighted may not want to look at books, and the one who is nearsighted may seem uninterested in activities more than a few feet away. These problems are usually easily corrected with prescription glasses.

Another condition that may be first noticed in early childhood is a misalignment of the eyes called strabismus (see page 602). Cross-eye is a type of strabismus. In some cases, one eye deviates only when your child is tired. In another form, both eyes deviate alternately.

The earlier the condition is discovered, the better the chances of improvement. If you feel your child's eyes may be misaligned, see your doctor. Early treatment can help prevent amblyopia, a condition in which the brain learns to ignore images from the weaker eye.

Hearing problems

In order to develop normal speech and language, a child must hear well. Even mild loss of hearing can interfere with your child's language development. The more severe the hearing loss, generally, the greater the learning problem.

In most states, a hearing screening is conducted at birth to identify possible hearing problems. If the child does not pass the test, a follow-up screening will be conducted in about a month. If hearing loss is suspected, the child will likely be referred to an audiologist for further testing.

Four types of hearing loss can occur in young children:

- **Conductive hearing loss.** It refers to an interference with the reception of sound from the external to the internal ear.
- **Sensorineural hearing loss.** It stems from abnormalities of the cochlear hair cells or the auditory nerve.
- **Mixed hearing loss.** It occurs when both conductive and sensorineural hearing loss are present.
- **Central auditory disorders.** They're the result of a dysfunction of the auditory center within the central nervous system.

Total deafness is often diagnosed within the first six months of life. If a child is partially deaf, however, the problem may not be detected until the child is 1 to 2 years old or older. At this point, your child may already have missed critical stages for language development and learning.

In the first three years of your child's life, look for the following warning signs that your child may have difficulty hearing:

- **1st year.** The child doesn't react to loud noises, doesn't imitate sounds or doesn't respond to his or her name.
- **2nd year.** The child doesn't play with his or her voice, doesn't imitate simple words, doesn't enjoy playing games, such as peekaboo or patty-cake, or isn't using two-word sentences to talk about or request things.
- **3rd year.** The child doesn't seem to understand "not now" and "no more" or can't follow simple directions.

The extent to which hearing loss influences your child's ability to learn depends on the severity of the loss, the range of frequencies affected, the age at which the loss occurs, how soon it's discovered and when treatment begins.

Some forms of hearing loss may be treated with medication. Others may require surgery, and still others may require a hearing aid. A hearing aid amplifies the hearing your child has and is considered the single most important tool toward allowing a hearing-impaired child to function normally. Techniques such as lip reading and sign language also may be beneficial, especially if the loss is more severe.

Orthopedic disorders

Beyond breaking a bone from time to time or pulling a muscle, most children don't have serious problems with their muscles, bones and joints. However, a wide range of growth patterns can occur in a preschool-age child. Flatfeet, intoeing, bowlegs and knock-knee are all stages through which most children pass during the normal pattern of leg and foot development.

For example, your infant's toes tend to bend inward and the feet appear flat because of the abundance of baby fat in the arch. As the child ages, the arches gradually become visible by the age of 5.

Likewise, legs are ordinarily slightly bowed from birth until about 2 years of age. Then your toddler's legs often overcorrect in the opposite direction, giving a knock-kneed appearance by age 3. Normally, legs straighten by 7 years of age.

Even when these variations continue through the school-age years, they seldom require treatment. Disease is rarely the cause.

Flatfeet

Your child's feet are flat if arches aren't apparent. There's no reason to be concerned about flatfeet in infants. Infants' baby fat always makes their feet look flat. However, if the arches don't become distinguished by age 5 years, your child may have flatfeet that are either flexible or fixed.

Flexible flatfeet look flat only when your child stands up. When he or she stands on tiptoe or the foot bears no weight, the arch is restored. Flexible flatfeet tend to run in families and are more common in Jewish and black people. The feet are mobile and painless and have excellent muscle strength.

Usually, flexible flatfeet don't require treatment. However, if the feet are extremely flat, your child's doctor may prescribe an arch support to be worn in his or her shoes. Although this won't correct the problem, it can prevent foot strain and make walking more comfortable.

Fixed or rigid flatfeet are cause for more concern because they may occur with congenital bone malformations. Your child's doctor will likely take X-rays to determine if this is the case. An operation may be appropriate if the condition isn't relieved by special footwear.

Intoeing

In children with intoeing, or pigeon toe, the toes turn inward. Most infants are born with intoeing as a holdover from their fetal position in the womb. They usually sleep with their toes pointed inward. Then, as they start to walk, their feet often turn inward to keep their balance and to make up for conditions such as flatfeet, bowlegs and knock-knee.

The condition usually resolves spontaneously by age 5. If it persists, your child's doctor may watch your child standing and walking and may also take X-rays. He or she will check for the presence of diseases that can cause intoeing, such as congenital bone malformations in which the bones of the thigh, shin, ankle or foot turn inward.

Medical providers have learned that without correction, the malformation generally resolves spontaneously. If the condition doesn't resolve itself, an operation may be necessary, but a doctor usually won't advise such a surgery before your child is at least 9 years old.

Knock-knee

When a child with knock-knee stands up, the knees touch each other but the ankles don't. Knock-knees are more common in girls than in boys, partly because their pelvis is wider. Knock-knee occurs more frequently in overweight children whose developing bones and joints are hard put to support their weight. Knock-knees also run in families.

A knock-kneed appearance can persist after age 4, but most children's legs straighten by age 7.

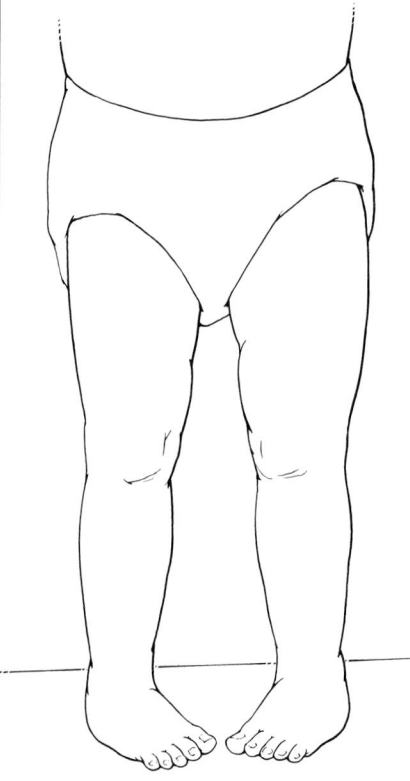

Newborns commonly arrive with intoeing, in which the toes turn inward. Most often the condition resolves itself by age 5.

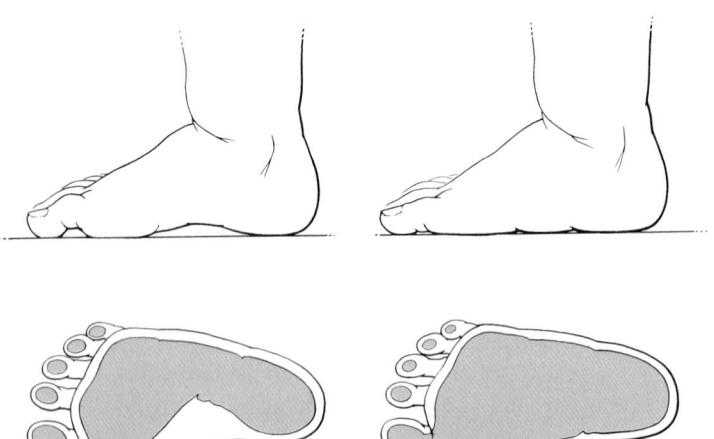

Flatfeet are feet that have little or no arch. Above at left (top and bottom) is a normal foot and footprint. If your child's foot and footprint more nearly resemble the illustrations at right, he or she has flatfeet.

If the legs don't straighten or if the condition develops after your child is of school age, your child's doctor may perform tests to rule out diseases of the knee joint that can cause knock-knees, such as juvenile rheumatoid arthritis, rickets and infections. An unrecognized injury or developmental problem can cause asymmetrical knock-knees.

Children with severe knock-knees often have flatfeet, because the weight falls on the inner edge of the foot and ankle. If your child is overweight, this condition may strain the feet and require an arch support to relieve foot fatigue and to prevent the inner border of the shoe from wearing.

A doctor may treat severe knock-knees with braces that are worn at night. Occasionally, an operation is needed, but not until the knees have had a chance to straighten on their own — after age 10 for girls and age 12 for boys — but before growth is complete. However, in most cases the legs tend to straighten as your child grows, so treatment is seldom required.

Bowlegs
Legs are considered to be bowed if, when the ankles touch each other, the unbent knees don't. Legs are normally bowed at birth because of the way the fetus's legs are folded over each other in the womb. Legs often stay bowed for up to two years. If bowed legs persist or worsen after age 3, they should be examined by your child's medical provider.

Sometimes, the legs merely appear bowed because of the distribution of the fat on your child's legs. When one leg is more bowed than is the other, it may be due to an injury or a growth problem. Persistently bowed legs usually straighten without treatment by age 8. A doctor may prescribe braces worn at night to help correct the disorder. Surgical correction is a possibility if other measures fail.

In rare cases, bowlegs are caused by disorders such as rickets or Blount's disease. In Blount's disease, the shinbone curves out below the knee and isn't securely inserted into the knee. Severe problems of the knee joint may develop.

This disease tends to occur more often in children who are overweight, short or who walked at an early age. It's more common in girls than in boys. An operation on the upper part of the shinbone can correct it.

Sexual abnormalities

The onset of puberty occurs in both boys and girls in the later

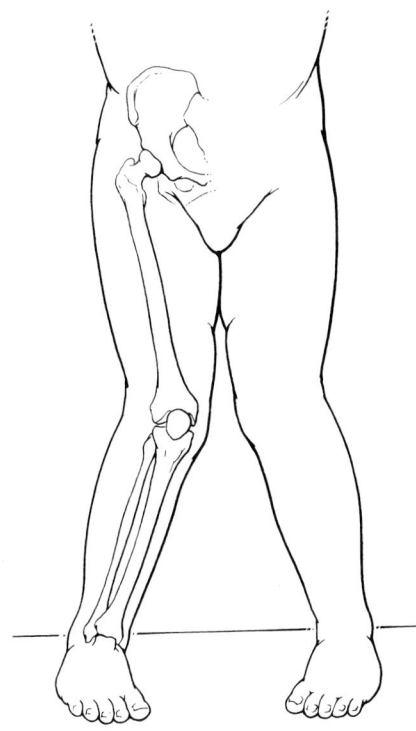

Knock-knees are the reverse of bowlegs. The knees are close together, but the ankles don't touch.

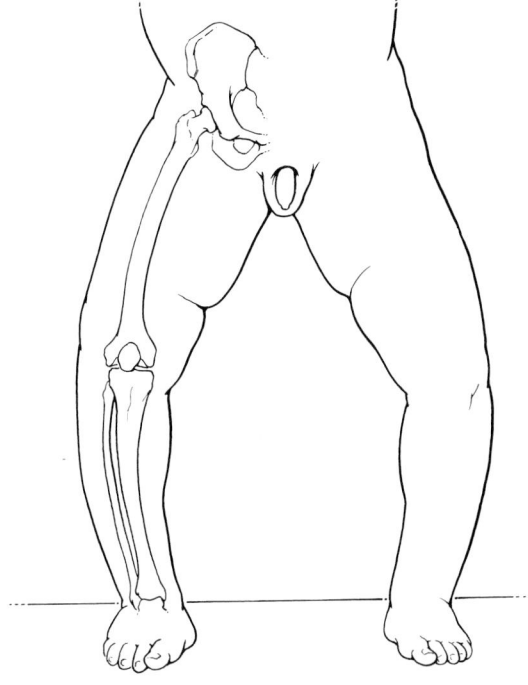

Most children are bowlegged as infants. If the legs are still bowed at age 3, consult your child's doctor.

stages of the grade-school years. In general, puberty is thought to be premature if it occurs before age 8 in girls and before age 9 in boys.

In girls, the first sign of puberty is generally the development of the breast bud (thelarche). The onset of menses (menarche) follows within several years. In boys, enlargement or growth of the testicles and penis is generally the first sign of puberty, to be followed by the appearance of pubic hair.

Several disorders concerning sexual development may occur during puberty, especially in girls:

Breast abnormalities
In girls, the development of the breast bud (thelarche) signals the onset of puberty. Breast development may be the only indication of puberty for six months or so. It's not unusual for one breast to develop first and remain larger for months.

When the breasts start budding in girls younger than 8 years, this sign of early sexual maturation is called premature thelarche. Most often, premature thelarche occurs between the ages of 1 and 3 years. If it's not followed by the other signs of sexual maturity, such as hair growth in the genital area, the girl's puberty is considered to be premature and incomplete.

The budded breasts often flatten within a year, but they may persist until the normal onset of puberty. The condition is harmless and seldom affects the girl's growth. Supportive counseling is usually all that's necessary to help a young girl cope with her temporary difference from other girls. Consult your health care provider for a full evaluation to differentiate premature thelarche from premature puberty.

Premature vaginal bleeding
Some girls may have bleeding from the vagina before the expected age of menstruation. Consult your daughter's doctor if this occurs.

A doctor will first want to ascertain the source of the bleeding. Often, the cause isn't the beginning of menstruation but another cause such as an inflammation of the genital and vaginal areas (vulvovaginitis), a genital tumor, trauma or a foreign body lodged in the vagina. In some cases, however, the cause is premature menstruation due to an early onset of puberty.

Premature adrenarche
Adrenarche refers to activity in the adrenal glands. Premature adrenarche occurs most often in girls between ages 5 and 8 years. It's often accompanied by rapid short-term growth. The armpits may sweat and grow hair. Pubic hair can develop (pubarche).

Your child's medical provider may perform tests to determine if your daughter has other abnormalities of the adrenal glands, which in rare cases can cause premature adrenarche.

Premature puberty
Premature (precocious) puberty occurs much more commonly in girls than in boys but is rare. If you're concerned about premature puberty in your child, consult his or her health care provider for a full evaluation.

Girls
In girls, premature puberty refers to the beginning of puberty before 8 years of age. The events of puberty may proceed as usual but start earlier than normal. In normal puberty (and usually in premature puberty), the breast buds appear first, then pubic hair appears and later menstruation begins, often with irregular cycles. Ovulation is uncommon but can occur.

Usually, no underlying cause can be determined. However, the condition is known to involve early maturation of one of the hormone-producing glands — the ovaries, pituitary or hypothala-

mus. Rarely, premature puberty results from a tumor of the brain or ovaries, so your child's doctor may initiate studies to rule out these possibilities. A doctor may also ask if your child has been exposed to or used any face creams or medications containing estrogens, which can also induce the disorder.

A potential long-term consequence of premature puberty is shorter height. It's usually associated with rapid short-term growth that stops earlier than normal.

Treatment for premature puberty may include psychological counseling for your child to help her deal with an appearance that's different from that of her peers. When puberty occurs very early, medication to change hormone balance may be considered to stop sexual development from progressing.

Premature puberty shouldn't be minimized. However, it's reassuring that by about age 10 most of the girl's peers will have caught up with her in sexual maturity, and she probably won't feel so different anymore.

If your daughter undergoes puberty prematurely, it's important not to respond to her based on her physical appearance or to deny her hugs. Keep treating her like the little girl she is and advise her teachers to do the same.

Boys
In boys, premature puberty refers to the beginning of puberty before age 9. If your child develops signs of advanced sexual development at an early age, see your medical provider. Signs generally include enlargement of the testicles and penis, appearance of pubic hair, deepening of the voice and accelerated growth.

Studies may be done to rule out a tumor of the brain and nervous system, adrenal gland, or testes. An identifiable cause of the premature puberty is found in about half the boys who experience it.

Sexual Abuse

Sexual abuse of children involves an adult or older child forcing or persuading a child to participate in a sexual act.

Young people need affection. Depriving a child of healthy physical contact, such as hugging, may cause significant problems in a youngster's psychological development. Young children often seek physical contact with adults, but their need for affection shouldn't be mistaken for adult sexuality. Some adults inappropriately respond to this behavior by exploiting children for their own sexual gratification.

Children often seek some sexual contact with their peers. This usually is normal curiosity and experimentation. However, if your child describes an experience in which he or she was touched in an inappropriate way by an older child or an adult, take it seriously and take appropriate measures to prevent it from happening again.

Signs and symptoms

Indications of possible sexual abuse in a child include:
• Provocative or promiscuous sexual behavior
• Withdrawal from friends, family or school activities
• Unusually hostile or aggressive behavior

Sometimes, a doctor may identify evidence of trauma to the genital area or the presence of sexually transmitted infections. However, the absence of all these signs and symptoms isn't necessarily proof that abuse didn't occur. In the vast majority of sexual abuse cases, there's no specific physical evidence of abuse.

How to respond

If you suspect that your child has been sexually abused, make sure that your child is safe from further harm. Take your child to his or her doctor or an emergency department at a hospital, preferably one that offers emergency and follow-up psychological support. The child will be checked and treated for any internal and external injuries, and the child may be tested for sexually transmitted diseases.

If the sexual abuse involved rape, handle it as a specific type of aggression against the child. This will help to minimize the sexual significance of the trauma and to prevent the child from experiencing lasting psychological effects. When you're in the presence of the child, it's best for you and the child's doctor not to dwell on the sexual nature of the assault. If you do, your child may become insecure and anxious, without clearly understanding what's going on.

Report the abuse to the proper authorities and have your child talk with a sensitive professional who's experienced at counseling victims of child abuse. This counseling is particularly important if the abuser was a family member or friend.

Don't keep the abuse a private or family matter. Most perpetrators are involved with several children. Seldom is the abuser a complete stranger to the child.

Child abuse

Children of all ages can be abused. There are many ways children can be abused. Physical harm by beating or sexual assault is the most obvious form of abuse, but children left hungry or in unsafe conditions or children who are emotionally abused with hurtful words are victims of child abuse as well.

Most often the abuser is related to the child and is involved in caring for the child. Parents who abuse their offspring come from all walks of life. Child abusers are of all races, faiths, economic strata and political beliefs.

Abusive parents often tend to be lonely, angry and unhappy people who often are under stress with which they can't cope. Many of them were physically abused as children. Still, there's never a valid excuse for child abuse.

In dealing with child abuse, protection of the child is the most important objective. The goal of treatment of the entire family is for the majority of families to remain intact and safe for the child, with the parents providing adequate care.

Abused children who are returned home without intervention run a significant risk of serious injury or even death.

Child abuse is a serious matter and everyone must help by reporting instances of suspected abuse or neglect. You can file a report by contacting professionals trained in dealing with suspected abuse.

Local social service agencies, law enforcement agencies or the child protective service office in your county can help. You may obtain further information and assistance by talking to doctors, counselors, clergy, school professionals or other professionals who deal with families having problems.

Parents who fear they have or may abuse their children are encouraged to contact these groups as well. In addition, many communities offer self-help groups such as Parents Anonymous.

Children with disabilities

The care of a child with a disability may require a combination of family support, social and academic adaptation, adjustments in the child's physical environment, and often, special medical care.

Permanent disabilities in children can include intellectual disability, physical deformities such as the absence of a limb, or sensory defects such as blindness or deafness.

Whatever a child's limitations, it doesn't take him or her long to realize that he or she is different. Helping your child develop a sense of self-worth and an ability to get along in the world despite his or her differences is fundamental to the successful rearing of your child.

You can achieve this, in part, by helping your child become as self-sufficient as possible and by creating an environment in which he or she can develop to his or her full potential.

Few things are as traumatic as the birth of a child with a major disability. Some parents initially try to deny the reality of the situation, especially if the disability isn't apparent to others. It's normal to feel guilt, anger and fear about your ability to cope with a disabled child, as well as anxiety over your child's future.

If your child's handicap is severe, you may need to consider placement in a supervised living service at an early age. It used to be common to place infants with severe intellectual disabilities in institutions. Today, doctors know that infants and young children do better developmentally if they have a consistent parent figure and are in a nurturing home environment.

Still, parents of children with disabilities often come to the realization that they alone can't care for their child. Thus, the child may enter a facility equipped for children with special needs. Even so, you may want to attempt home care before considering placing your child in an alternative environment.

Coping strategies

If you're attempting to rear a child with disabilities at home, you can use the following coping strategies to make your child as happy and well adjusted as possible.

Treat all of your children alike

Some parents relax household rules for a disabled child, which only makes the child feel different from the other children. Rules should apply equally to all of the children in the family. Like his or her siblings, your disabled child should have certain responsibilities and should be punished for breaking the rules, provided that he or she is capable of understanding them.

Be aware of your attitude

Children are amazingly deft at compensating for a defect. For example, a child born without one hand becomes very proficient with the other hand and, having known nothing else, doesn't miss the absent hand. However, if you're embarrassed about the deformity, your child will sense these feelings and probably become self-conscious.

Don't neglect your other children

The care of a child with special needs can be so time-consuming that it becomes easy to ignore other family members. Try to set aside time each week to be alone with each child. Honestly answer your other children's questions about their brother or sister.

Accept your child's individuality

All children have strengths and weaknesses. When your child with special needs accomplishes something, no matter how small, praise him or her.

Don't isolate your child

All children need friends. It's normal to want to protect your child from a contagious illness or the potential cruelty of some children, but don't do it at the expense of your child's socialization.

Schools now provide an education for all children within the community. Previously, children with special needs went to a separate school or were kept separate from regular classrooms. Today, most public schools by law must provide special classes for children with disabilities. And, in many cases, the children take classes with children in the mainstream student population. Mixing children with disabilities with the rest of the students can benefit everyone in the class.

Address special needs

A child's needs may range from a specially designed house and van to home care provided by a trained nurse or visits to a medical facility.

Accept help

Many community resources can help you meet the needs of your son or daughter. Some agencies offer financial help for qualifying parents who can't provide for their child's medical needs. Others offer services such as transportation, counseling, psychological evaluation, baby-sitting, child care and play activities.

Your child's health care provider can be an excellent source of information about available community resources, for your child and for you. Public health nurses and social workers also know of local resources and are often a very useful source of information and support.

In addition to supporting your child, don't be afraid to seek support for yourself. Parent support groups give parents a chance to express their common concerns and share information. In recent years, these groups have organized and become a force in influencing legislation that has expanded and improved opportunities for children with disabilities. ∎

Preteen and Teenage Years

Adolescence is the period of transition between puberty and adulthood. It's a time of physical, emotional, psychological, social and mental growth. Physical growth is especially apparent. Teenage boys and girls become taller and heavier, their body shape changes, and their facial features become more defined and mature.

Equally significant is their intellectual development, broadening to provide new insights and ability to understand more-complex matters. In addition, a teenager's psychological development helps integrate these changes into a better understanding of his or her physical and intellectual self.

Often, an individual's physical, intellectual and psychological developments occur at different rates and times. This can lead to anxiety, insecurity, conflict and other emotional hurdles. The tug of war between parent and child, involving the normal tension between the child's dependence on his or her parents and the need to be more independent, also begins to change in adolescence.

To ensure a good relationship between parents and teenagers, it's crucial for both generations to communicate with each other as openly as possible.

Growth and Development

Adolescence is the period of fastest growth and development except for the first year of life. Growth occurs unevenly, as periods of relatively slow change are interspersed with growth spurts.

Normal growth changes

Before around age 9, average height is similar for both sexes. By the age of 14 years, most boys have grown taller than have most girls. Girls tend to weigh less than boys until about age 9 and after age 14, but they're often heavier than boys are between those ages.

Toward the end of the grade school years, children begin to grow at a dramatic but highly variable rate. This preadolescent growth spurt is a part of puberty, a sequence of changes that transforms a child into a young adult. At the peak of the growth spurt, there's an increase in height of about 3 to 4 inches a year. Most boys grow faster than girls do. At the end of the growth spurt, adult height is nearly attained. If your child hasn't started an obvious increase in growth by age 15, consult your child's doctor.

Teenagers may feel insecure about being one of the shortest or tallest in the class. If your child is developing slower or faster than average, let him or her know there's nothing to worry about. Show your love and provide reassurance by neither minimizing nor overdramatizing your child's concerns.

Height is just one physical attribute that changes in puberty. Early on, fat collects on the buttocks and around the abdomen in both boys and girls. As development continues, boys accumulate mostly muscle and bone, and girls add more body fat, particularly over the hips and in the thighs and breasts. The result is that fat makes up about 10 to 12 percent more of total body weight in girls than in boys.

By the time of a girl's first menstrual period or the end of a boy's growth spurt, there's a distinct difference in contour between female and male bodies. The respective male and female sex hormones, along with family traits, account for most of the difference. These hormones are also responsible for secondary sex changes, which usually characterize puberty.

Sexual development

The first stages of puberty generally begin at ages 8 to 10 in girls and ages 9 to 12 in boys. The onset of puberty provides a good opportunity to educate your child about sexual development, whether or not you've already done so. You can help prepare your child for the cascade of changes that his or her body will go through during the next few years. The goal is for the child to welcome these changes without shame or anxiety that they're occurring too quickly or too slowly.

In the preteen years, children are most eager to conform. An obsession with "normality" coincides with the time when their bodies' development is diverging from that of their peers. Even children who are right in the middle of the spectrum of physical maturity often feel they're developing too rapidly or too slowly. You can help by reassuring your child that he or she fits well within the wide range of normal development.

Don't worry if your child's puberty starts a little earlier or later than that of his or her peers. This is rarely a medical problem. However, your child may feel awkward and self-conscious about diverging from the average schedule. Be sensitive to these feelings.

At the same time, reassure your child that he or she is fine. It may help to stress that every child, including your child and each of his or her peers, is traveling along the same road toward adulthood and that everyone takes a different amount of time to arrive.

Sexual changes in boys

The male body prepares for sexual maturity by producing more androgen hormones. Though these are commonly called male hormones, they're actually present in both sexes. These hormones, made mainly by the testes, cause the physical changes of puberty.

One of the first changes in boys is the appearance of sparse, lightly pigmented pubic hair on the skin surrounding the base of the penis. The scrotum also enlarges and darkens. These changes are likely to be well under way before growth reaches its peak. Your son shouldn't be worried if he happens to develop some breast tissue about this time. Only rarely is this change due to any medical or hormonal problem. The breast enlargement usually disappears within a few months. If it persists or is particularly concerning, see your child's doctor.

The penis is able to become erect from infancy. But it's usually not until about two years after the start of puberty and one year after the penis begins to lengthen that it becomes capable of ejaculating semen for the first time. This may occur during masturbation, spontaneously during a sexual fantasy or during a nocturnal ejaculation. Take this opportunity to talk about sexuality with your son, including information on sexual intercourse and contraception.

Later, hair begins to appear under the arms and on the face. As the voice box (larynx) enlarges, the Adam's apple becomes more prominent. The voice also starts to have a deeper tone. Occasionally, the higher, younger voice may still be heard fleetingly when the voice cracks.

Throughout this period of sexual maturation, which usually lasts four or five years, the testes continue to enlarge, and the penis gets longer and thicker. By the end of this period, the penis, testes and pubic hair have fully developed, and mustache and beard hair have started to appear.

Sexual changes in girls

Sexual changes in girls result from an increase in hormones made in the ovaries and adrenal glands. The first visible change in females is either the beginning of breast development (breast budding) or the appearance of sparse, lightly pigmented pubic hair. Girls shouldn't worry if one breast starts developing before the other.

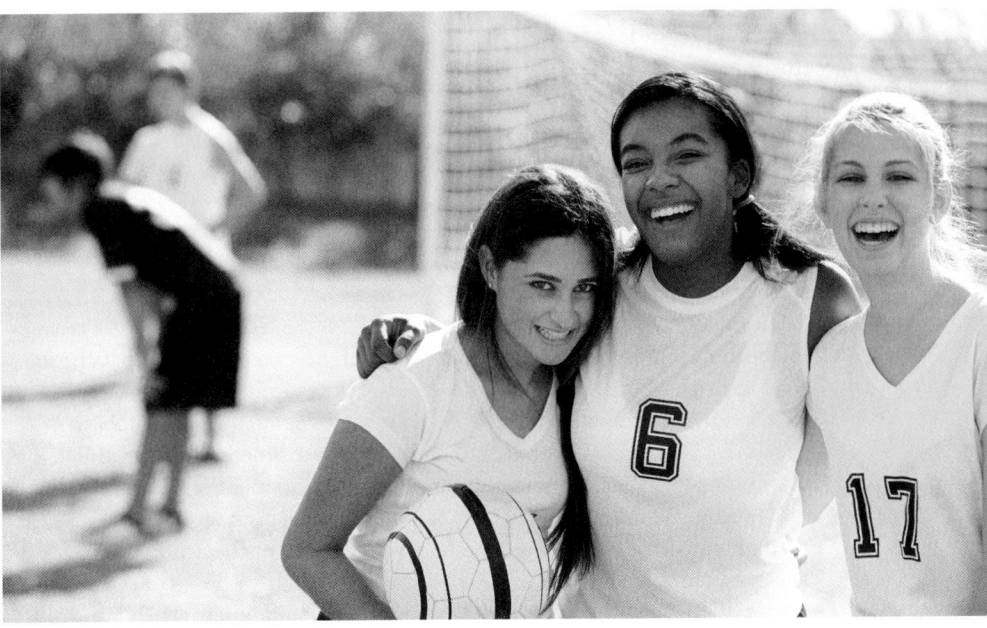

Even when the breasts have fully developed, they're rarely exactly equal in size.

About a year after the breasts begin to develop, the growth rate is likely to reach its peak. Within a year after the peak of a growth spurt, the menstrual period (menarche) may start. Take this opportunity to talk about sexuality with your daughter, including information on sexual intercourse and contraception.

There may be an intermittent increase in either white or yellow vaginal discharge during the months before the onset of menstruation. It's also normal for the first few menstrual periods to occur irregularly. Within about a year, menstruation should become more regular.

Physical changes include increasing height, breast growth, an increase in pubic and underarm hair, and deepening of the voice, though the voice doesn't change as much as that of a boy experiencing puberty. It usually takes four or five years from the onset of puberty to reach full body development.

There's a link between the timing of puberty and nutrition. Improvements in nutrition in recent decades are the principal explanation of why the onset of puberty occurs at younger ages in

successive generations of young females in industrialized nations, such as the United States. Environmental factors may play a role as well.

Puberty also tends to start earlier in girls who have more body fat and later in those who are thin. Children of parents who experienced puberty later may also experience later puberty and growth spurts.

Intellectual development

During adolescence, the thinking process undergoes a gradual transformation from childhood into adulthood. Until about age 12, learning primarily involves understanding the logic of concrete things, objects that can be seen and felt. The next step in intellectual development is abstract thinking.

Throughout adolescence, children become increasingly adept at dealing with intangible ideas, including concepts that involve the past and the future. Newfound abilities allow an adolescent's thoughts to take wing, traveling through time, including speculating about what he or she and the surrounding world might become.

Along the way, this increase in powers of thought may blur some boundaries. Teenagers may feel that they're at the center of the universe, with the ability to do anything and everything. They may assume that others are thinking about them — positively or negatively — more than they really are. This feeling of being on-stage can also make teenagers feel self-conscious, powerless or lost.

Ultimately, abstract reasoning becomes more mature and comprehensive. Your teenager is able to solve increasingly complex problems. Teenagers become able to think scientifically, conceiving of hypotheses and of ways to test them. In addition, teenagers can also think reflectively. For example, your teenager can frame an argument for a discussion or debate and make judgments about an argument's strengths and weaknesses.

Maturation in a teenager's intellectual development changes the way your teen thinks about the world and how he or she behaves in response to it. Teenagers are able to discern much more clearly how past actions have affected what's happening now. They also become capable of predicting more accurately what implications their current actions or those of others will have for the future.

At this same time, teenagers begin to appreciate the cause-and-effect relationship between destructive behaviors, such as drug and alcohol use, and poor health. The health benefits of good nutrition and regular physical activity also may begin to make sense.

For the first time, you may notice your teenager's interest in discussing various serious subjects with his or her friends, family, and teachers. Topics may involve love, morality, work, politics, religion and philosophy. Many teenagers spend a great deal of time wrestling with major questions, such as, "What's the purpose of life?"

Although a teenager will probably still be guided by parents, teachers and other adults, his or her decisions are made more inde-pendently. His or her decisions are also influenced by the thoughts and beliefs of peers.

Personality and Behavior

Much of an adolescent's psychosocial development involves coping with sexual development. Developing a distinct identity and becoming independent from parents also can be a struggle.

Adolescents basically go through three phases of psychosocial development: early, middle and late adolescence.

- **Early phase.** This phase starts at about age 13 or younger. In early adolescence, a teen's mental focus starts to shift from family to peers.
- **Middle phase.** The middle phase generally begins around ages 15 to 17. This phase may involve outright conflicts over independence.
- **Late phase.** The late phase extends from the middle phase to age 19, or well into the 20s or even 30s in some individuals. By the end of late adolescence, independence is virtually secured, parental advice can be taken or not, and body image and gender role definition are established.

The process of going through these stages can be challenging. The diverse aspects of physical, psychological and social development aren't synchronized. Teenagers may alternate between childish and adult behaviors.

The gradual changes of these years enable your teenager to develop a sense of who he or she is and to understand the nature of personal responsibility. Teenagers begin to understand that their actions and decisions have rewards or consequences. They begin to take an active role in making countless decisions about what to do and what not to do. Many times teenagers may prefer to seek the advice of an adult outside the family, such as a teacher or counselor.

Body image

Part of a teenager's maturation process is developing and accepting a realistic image of his or her body. If your teenager matures earlier or later than average — and many adolescents do — he or she may encounter trouble with peers and with his or her own body image. Difficulty with this image can manifest itself in eating disorders, particularly in girls. Peers and role models may influence your teenager's attitude toward his or her own body.

It's important to listen to what children say about their bodies and to observe their behavior. During maturation your teenager may:
- Feel uncomfortable with his or her physical self
- Be deeply concerned about whether his or her developing body is attractive
- Measure his or her body against that of his or her peers
- Fear that he or she is physically imperfect and develop anxiety

Some teens find it helpful to discuss these concerns with an understanding adult, whether it's a doctor, trusted teacher or parent.

Self-image

During adolescence, a teenager does a great deal of thinking about what kind of person he or she is and may become. He or she may muse on a career for later in life, naming career goals that are idealistic in early adolescence.

Later in adolescence, your teenager may set his or her sights more practically, considering careers that more immediately suit his or her abilities and interests. The merging of idle musings with practical planning is yet another part of the maturation process.

How do I offer reassurance to my teenagers who are struggling with their body images?

- Offer alternatives to our culture's beauty icons. Point out the number of successful people without "perfect" bodies.
- Focus on the numbers: There are billions of people in the world but fewer than 100 supermodels.
- Express affection for your children often. Tell them love doesn't depend on how tall they are or how much they weigh.

Increasing independence

In early adolescence, teenagers often start to experiment with new ways of behaving and dressing at home. At first a teen may seek some approval from family members before trying anything out on the outside world. As time goes by, your teenager may make a few tentative motions toward asserting his or her independence. Soon your teenager may become less interested in family activities and less willing to accept advice or criticism from family members. He or she may find more social comfort in a close relationship with a best friend of the same sex. As a parent, recognize that this is part of normal adolescent development.

As your teenager starts to break away from family influence, he or she may pay more attention to peers. For some time, the peer group may even dominate your teenager's thinking and behavior. At first, the peer group is likely to be restricted to members of the same sex. Then it usually shifts to a mixed group. A peer group may provide a teenager with a sense of social status and security.

In return, teenage cliques often demand conformity of behavior, attitudes and dress.

The struggle for independence is often most apparent in middle adolescence. Your teenager may start testing your controls and discipline. He or she may decide that your standards are unfair. A teenager may develop his or her own value system, or adopt that of his or her peer group, and challenge other authority figures.

Teenagers often delight in playing pranks and practical jokes. A teenager may also feel intense peer pressure to take risks that may pose dangers to himself or herself and others — for instance, experimenting with drugs, sex or vandalism. Some teenagers carry this activity even further into negative behavior. Rebellious acts taken too far can cause long-term trouble at home, at school and even with the law.

By late adolescence or early adulthood, teenagers often evolve another way of thinking about family. As a teenager becomes more comfortable with his or her own identity, he or she often starts to break free of the values of his or her peer group.

Achieving independence doesn't mean that your teenager cuts himself or herself off from others. Rather, your teenager has gained a foundation through education, family and community to allow him or her to start supporting himself or herself emotionally, socially and even financially. Part of this mature functioning is knowing when and how to use others for support. Your teenager may even be able to appreciate your values enough to seek your advice.

Parents often have a difficult time coping with the psychological changes in their adolescent children. But it's usually possible to achieve a delicate, ever-shifting balance between providing support and understanding while setting standards and limiting dangerous or harmful behavior.

When you disagree with what your teenager is doing, be firm without being harshly punitive. Respect your teenager's sincere efforts to achieve independence. Gradually, let go of the control that you've exerted over your teenager throughout childhood and trust your teen will be guided by the self-control that you've helped instill.

The challenge that parents face is to relinquish involvement gracefully rather than abdicate their role.

This increased independence will also be reflected in health-related visits. Your teen should have the opportunity to speak to the care provider independently. Generally, professionals in medicine, psychology and social work encourage teenagers to involve their parents in their psychosocial concerns. However, they won't reveal a teenager's confidences unless they perceive a serious danger to the teen or others.

Moral reasoning

Along with the psychosocial development of adolescence comes an evolution of standards. As teenagers move from childhood to adulthood, their moral standards may progress through more or less distinct phases. During each phase, a different type of moral reasoning predominates:

- **Influenced by self.** In early adolescence, children and young teens often evaluate situations in a self-centered or opportunistic manner. Judging if an action is moral may be based solely on whether the action will help or hurt them. The primary concern is avoiding punishment and gaining rewards for themselves.
- **Influenced by laws.** In middle adolescence, teenagers may become more motivated by conforming to legal standards. They start to realize that laws apply to everyone, including themselves. Accordingly, they may judge

actions based on whether the actions are legal or illegal — not only on whether there's a risk of punishment.

However, many adolescents go through a phase of rebelling, testing the limits of authority and sometimes even breaking the law. Some may be asking to be disciplined, to experience tangible proof of the reality of the law. Ultimately, most teenagers progress beyond this testing phase.

- **Influenced by others.** By late adolescence or early adulthood, teenagers start caring more about how their actions affect others. Their moral concerns may now extend to rules of human behavior beyond the letter of the law. Teenagers may follow standards based on broad ethical principles that in some cases may be even more restrictive than the law. They can recognize everyday examples of justice, equality, honesty, responsibility, cooperation and reciprocity — and their opposites.

Eventually, a teenager's standards evolve so that he or she becomes fully responsible for the morality of his or her actions. Ideally, teenagers develop their own detailed, individualized definitions of what society deems as right and wrong. They follow this internalized personal moral code relatively independent of the endorsement or disapproval of others. If they ever violate their principles, they feel guilty and experience self-condemnation.

The evolution of standards is intertwined with social interactions and intellectual development. Teenagers who participate in social activities have more opportunities to observe interactions. This experience may help them to form more-mature moral judgments. However, neither social nor intellectual maturity necessarily guarantees the development of high moral standards.

Parents can encourage their teenagers' development of standards by being role models and setting examples. Teenagers tend to develop more self-control and make more-mature moral judgments when their parents have followed a certain style of child rearing. This style includes the following:

- Consistently disciplining, with reasoning and explanation
- Discussing how others feel about actions taken
- Promoting democratic family discussions, in which even young children can have their input

Common Conditions and Concerns

Adolescence has the reputation of being the healthiest of times, but many teenagers have significant health problems. Some diseases are more likely to appear during the teenage years. Adolescence is often a good time to establish habits for preventive care and examinations.

Routine examinations

As your teenager matures, he or she likely will be ready to assume increased responsibility for his or her own health. Ideally, it's best if your teenager sees his or her doctor alone at each office visit. However, parental consent is required for a physician to treat a patient under 18 years old.

Routine examinations provide teenagers an opportunity to seek professional guidance regarding their health-related concerns. Privacy is important because your teenager's concerns may be different from what you have in mind. Your child's doctor may also use these medical visits to promote and discuss good health habits and healthy behaviors.

Trust should be a key part of the relationship between your child and his or her care provider. Still, many teenagers are reluctant to discuss health-related concerns, such as acne, contraception, depression, drugs, being overweight, sexual practices, sexually transmitted infections and getting along with parents and other adults. Providers understand this reluctance. Often, it takes time, privacy and special skill for a care provider to draw out the teenager's true concerns.

Although you may want to know everything that concerns your teenager, there are some health issues your child may not want to discuss with you. Continue to offer your support and let your child know that you're available to discuss any concerns that he or she has.

Checkups for teenagers offer an opportunity for early detection of chronic conditions that may pose health problems now or in adulthood. Let your teenager's doctor know about any diseases that run in the family. If your teenager has a chronic disease such as diabetes or asthma, a medical professional can teach him or her how to manage the condition.

Nutrition

Energy requirements and nutrient requirements increase during adolescence. But busy teenagers with full school schedules, extracurricular activities and part-time employment may be eating on the go and not getting enough calories and all the nutrients they need. Tight schedules may lead to skipping some meals, especially breakfast, or to eating more frequently. Many teenagers eat a great number of meals away from home, especially from fast-food restaurants and vending machines. This can lead to unhealthy eating habits. Overeating or restricting food consumption can make young people more vulnerable to eating disorders.

Greater independence from family and the desire to be accepted by peers often influence eating practices such as fad dieting, eating an unbalanced diet and indulging in alcohol. All of these factors put an adolescent at greater risk of inadequate nutrition. But this isn't true of all teens. Some families begin eating healthier because of the influence of their teens, who may follow vegetarian diets or other healthy-eating practices. Vegetarian diets can be nutritionally adequate — even for teens — if they're appropriately followed and steps are taken to ensure consumption of essential nutrients.

Parents have a crucial role in setting a good example and taking time to prepare and serve wholesome family meals. Get the entire family involved in meal planning and preparation. If family meals aren't possible because of different schedules, stock your kitchen with healthy, convenient snacks, such as fresh fruits and vegetables, yogurt, milk, and whole-grain bread.

Nutritional status doesn't depend on one specific food choice but rather on the sum of food choices over several days and weeks. Even fast foods and desserts can be included in a healthy diet if you regularly eat a variety of foods from the various food groups.

Iron

Ample iron is essential during adolescence because of the expanding volume of blood in the body and an increase in muscle mass that teens experience as they grow. Extra iron is needed during growth spurts because it's important for muscle development and healthy red blood cells. Teenage girls especially need additional iron because of iron loss during menstruation.

A lack of iron in the diet can cause iron deficiency anemia. Signs and symptoms include pale skin, fatigue, lightheadedness and poor appetite. Low iron without anemia can also contribute to fatigue and poor sleep quality.

To ensure an adequate supply of dietary iron, teenagers need to eat foods that contain iron on a regular basis. Foods that contain iron include meat, fish, poultry, eggs, legumes (peas and beans), potatoes and rice. Iron-fortified grain products are another alternative as are, if needed, multivitamins that contain iron.

Keep Up With Vaccinations

By the time they reach their teens, most boys and girls have completed their childhood immunizations. But they still may need a few vaccinations to boost immunity. For more information on these vaccinations, see page 148. For information on the HPV vaccine, see page 216.

Vaccine ▼ Age ▶	7-10 years	11-12 years	13-18 years
Influenza	Influenza (yearly)		
Tetanus, diphtheria, pertussis	Tdap	Tdap	Tdap
Human papillomavirus	HPV series	HPV (2 doses)	HPV series
Meningococcal (MenACWY)	MenACWY	MenACWY	MenACWY
Meningococcal (MenB)		MenB	
Pneumococcal	PPV		
Hepatitis A	HepA series		
Hepatitis B	HepB series		
Inactivated poliovirus	IPV series		
Measles, mumps, rubella (MMR)	MMR series		
Varicella	Varicella series		

Range of recommended ages

Catch-up immunization

Certain high-risk groups

Source: Advisory Committee on Immunization Practices, Centers for Disease Control and Prevention, 2017

Calcium

Calcium is important to the development of strong bones and teeth. Inadequate amounts of calcium in childhood may increase the risk of the bone-thinning disease osteoporosis common later in life.

Unfortunately, many children and adolescents don't get enough calcium in their diet. Only about 14 percent of teenage girls and less than half of teenage boys are meeting recommendations for calcium consumption. The American Academy of Pediatrics recommends that adolescents and teens consume at least 1,300 mg of calcium each day. One 8-ounce glass of milk provides 300 milligrams of calcium.

Dieting

Adolescents need certain nutrients and adequate calories to provide for their activity and growth. If they're not getting the nutrients they need, dieting may prevent teenagers from growing to their full height. Teenagers concerned about their weight should avoid skipping meals and focus on eating healthy meals, reducing excess snacking and increasing exercise.

If weight is a concern, consult your teen's doctor or a registered dietitian. In youth, it's important to establish healthy patterns of eating and exercise. Obese adolescents between ages 12 and 18 have an 80 percent chance of becoming obese adults. For more information on healthy eating, see Chapter 8, "Nutrition and Weight."

Exercise

Adolescents and young adults benefit greatly from a regular exercise routine. Regular exercise is good for overall health and helps control weight. Beginning good exercise habits as a teenager helps encourage healthy habits as an adult.

However, moderation is important. Excessive exercise can lead to injuries and, in females, menstrual abnormalities. Pain or swelling in the joints, a common complaint, is a sign of too much exercise or improper technique. Female athletes may experience discontinuation of menstrual periods (amenorrhea). When this occurs, a medical evaluation is important because the condition can increase a female's risk of bone thinning.

Injuries

Among adolescents, injury is a major public health problem.

Unintentional injuries are the leading cause of death among American teenagers.

Automobile accidents are the most common cause. About one-third of fatal accidents involving 16- and 17-year-old drivers occur during night hours, even though only about 11 percent of their driving is at night. Alcohol is often a factor, as is distracted driving. Seat belts could prevent many injuries and spare lives, but, unfortunately, adolescents often fail to buckle up.

HPV Vaccine for Adolescents and Teens

Human papillomavirus (HPV) is the name of a group of viruses that includes more than 100 different strains or types. More than 30 of these viruses are sexually transmitted through vaginal, anal or oral sex with someone who has the virus.

In many cases, HPV goes away on its own without causing health problems. But in some people, it can result in conditions such as genital warts and cancer.

Genital warts usually appear as a small bump or a group of bumps on the female or male genitals. Cancers associated with HPV include cervical cancer and others, such as cancer of the vulva, vagina, penis or anus. HPV is also a leading cause of oropharyngeal cancer, cancer that develops in the back of the throat, including the base of the tongue and tonsils.

Vaccine recommendation

The Centers for Disease Control and Prevention (CDC) recommends all girls and boys ages 11 or 12 get vaccinated for HPV, although some organizations recommend getting the vaccine as early as age 9 or 10 (see the chart on page 215).

In 2016, the CDC updated the HPV vaccine schedule to recommend that adolescents and teens ages 9 through 14 receive two doses of HPV vaccine at least six months apart, rather than the previously recommended three-dose schedule. Those who begin the vaccine series later, at ages 15 through 26, as well as individuals with weakened immune systems, should continue to receive three doses of the vaccine.

It's best for adolescents and teens to receive the vaccine before they have sexual contact and are exposed to HPV because once someone is infected with the virus the vaccine might not be as effective or might not work at all.

Three vaccines are currently available that protect against different forms of HPV. Gardasil, Gardasil 9 and Cervarix have been shown to protect against cervical cancer. Gardasil and Gardasil 9 also protect against genital warts.

For concerned parents, research has shown that receiving the vaccine at a young age isn't linked to an earlier start of sexual activity.

Athletic activities are leading causes of nonfatal injuries. Football is among the most hazardous. Knees and ankles are sites commonly injured, but head and neck injuries occur as well, despite advances in equipment and an increase in concussion awareness.

Although less hazardous, participation in sports such as soccer and basketball can lead to injury, especially among boys. For girls, gymnastics poses the highest risk. For both, even sports such as cross-country running, swimming and tennis carry some risk. You can help minimize your teen's risk of injury by ensuring that he or she wears protective equipment designed for each sport and gets appropriate physical conditioning.

Acne

Acne is a common problem and concern among teenagers. Three out of 4 teenagers have some acne. It can appear on the face, neck, chest, back, shoulders and scalp. Acne usually starts around puberty and significantly improves or resolves by the end of the teenage years, but it can affect adults too. Medical attention and treatment with prescription drugs may be beneficial if the acne is distressing, persistent or severe.

Usually, acne begins with an overproduction of oil (sebum) by the sebaceous gland of each hair follicle in the skin. Follicles then become plugged with oil and dead skin cells. When a follicle is plugged with white pus just

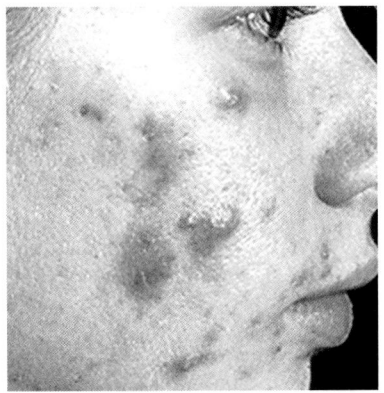

beneath the skin surface, it's called a whitehead. If this plug extends to the surface and is exposed to air, it turns black and is termed a blackhead. Pimples result from inflammation of follicles. This inflammation is usually caused by oil blocking the follicle and predisposing it to bacterial infection.

In both boys and girls, acne may be triggered by normal elevations of androgen hormones, which make the sebaceous glands produce extra oil. In girls, acne may worsen around the time of their menstrual periods. Psychological stress may also exacerbate acne.

For more information on acne, see page 1073.

Headaches

Recurrent headaches are common during late childhood and adolescence. They may be associated with a viral illness but rarely indicate a serious problem. Headaches may be related to factors such as stress, a reaction to a medicine or food, or a family history of migraines. If headaches occur frequently, come on suddenly without explanation, persist or get steadily worse, see your child's care provider. Also contact your child's provider if a headache follows a recent ear infection, toothache, strep throat or other infection.

Migraines usually occur for the first time in early adolescence, although they can also appear in young children. Migraines are repeated attacks of intense, throbbing head pain lasting at least an hour each episode. They're often accompanied by nausea, sensitivity to light and sometimes vomiting.

For more information on headaches, see page 516.

Painful menstruation

Many females experience some pain on the first or second day of their period. For some, though, the pain is so severe that it disrupts

normal daily activities. Painful menstruation (dysmenorrhea) is a common cause of teenage girls and adult women missing work and school. It's most common in adolescence. The problem often subsides by the mid-20s or after pregnancy.

There are two types of dysmenorrhea: primary and secondary. Primary dysmenorrhea is pain due to menstruation, when the muscles of the uterus contract and the uterus sheds its lining. Secondary dysmenorrhea is pain caused by an underlying gynecologic disorder, such as a fibroid tumor, sexually transmitted infection (STI) or endometriosis.

Signs and symptoms include general aching, pain in the lower abdomen possibly extending to the hips, lower back or thighs, nausea, vomiting, and diarrhea. Soaking in a warm tub or exercising may help relieve the pain. For many women, prescription or over-the-counter nonsteroidal anti-inflammatory drugs (NSAIDs), such as ibuprofen (Advil, Motrin IB, others) or naproxen sodium (Aleve, others), are effective. These medications work better if taken early, when the menstrual cycle is starting, rather than waiting until cramps become more intense. Birth control pills also may be beneficial.

For more information on painful periods, see page 1197.

Urinary tract infections

Urinary tract infections may result when bacteria normally found in the colon colonize and enter the bladder via the channel leading from the bladder to the outside of the body (urethra). In adolescents who haven't had a urinary tract infection as children, the onset of infection frequently coincides with the onset of sexual activity.

The most common urinary tract infection is cystitis, inflammation of the bladder. Cystitis usually results when traces of stool contaminate the urethra. It can be caused by sexual intercourse, which can irritate the urethra. Signs and symptoms include urination that's frequent, urgent and painful, foul-smelling urine, and, less commonly, a fever. If your adolescent has these signs and symptoms, he or she should be seen for treatment.

For more information on urinary tract infections, see page 909.

Infectious mononucleosis

Infectious mononucleosis is commonly referred to as mono or the kissing disease. Anyone can get mononucleosis, but its incidence is highest in teens and young adults.

The majority of cases of infectious mononucleosis are caused by the Epstein-Barr virus. Most adults have eventually been exposed to the Epstein-Barr virus and have built up antibodies. Although kissing can spread the virus, mono is more commonly spread by coughing, sneezing or sharing drinking glasses. It isn't highly contagious; however, it can cause prolonged illness. The condition typically results in complete recovery.

Initial infection in children between ages 4 and 15 usually results in only mild signs and symptoms such as a short-term fever and fatigue. In some instances, symptoms are minimal and the infection goes unrecognized. Later in adolescence and young adulthood, the virus may be a cause of a prolonged, exhausting illness.

Signs and symptoms include a fever that lasts several days, swollen glands, sore throat and fatigue. A blood test can indirectly check for evidence of the Epstein-Barr virus. Rest and plenty of fluids are the main treatments.

Most signs and symptoms ease within 10 days, but your teenager may still need another two to three weeks of rest before resuming routine activities — especially if his or her spleen is enlarged. He or she likely will need a couple of more months to feel completely back to normal.

For more information on infectious mononucleosis, see page 451.

Growth disorders

Many growth disorders are diagnosed in childhood, but certain growth disorders appear during the teenage years.

Scoliosis
Scoliosis is a sideways (lateral) curvature of the spine that makes the spine look like an S or a C. In most cases, the cause is unknown. The disorder can affect both boys and girls, but adolescent girls are more likely to have serious scoliosis that requires treatment.

The onset of scoliosis is gradual and usually painless. Screening for scoliosis is performed routinely at many schools. Some cases are too mild to need treatment. In other cases, special braces or surgery may be required. If untreated, scoliosis may cause permanent disability.

For more information on scoliosis, see page 953.

Osgood-Schlatter disease
Osgood-Schlatter disease is a painful inflammation below the kneecap, where the tendon attaches to the shinbone (tibia). It's common in young athletes, especially boys, during growth spurts.

This condition is caused by overuse, from repeated stress where the tendon of the kneecap inserts on the top of the shinbone. This repeated pulling on the tendon causes inflammation and pain, which is worsened by activity and relieved by rest.

Treatment involves resting and avoiding activities that place prolonged stress on the flexed knee. These include activities such as bicycle riding and playing basketball. Exercises to strengthen the quadriceps muscle also are advised. Anti-inflammatory medications, such as ibuprofen (Advil, Motrin IB, others), also may be helpful. When growth of the affected bone ends, the pain usually subsides on its own.

Teenage Sexuality

Parents often feel perplexed and even threatened by their teenager's emerging sexuality. If you're the parent of a teenager, it's best for everyone if you can come to terms with your child's sexuality, show your trust, and give him or her any help needed.

Your child may receive education about sex, family life and sexually transmitted infections (STIs) at school. STIs are also referred to as sexually transmitted diseases (STDs). But don't rely on the school to explain all of the complexities of sexual relationships that you want your child to understand. No matter how awkward it may be for you, you have a responsibility to inform your child about the facts of life.

As a parent, you are your child's primary sex educator. You may find it helpful to look through relevant materials before talking with your son or daughter. In addition, books that you and your child can read together are invaluable for opening up a discussion. Avoid overloading your child with too much information, but do answer all of his or her questions honestly.

If you don't know the answer to a particular question, tell your child that you'll look it up together. Sexual fantasies, masturbation, homosexuality, contraception, pregnancy and STIs are some topics your teenager may have questions about.

Emerging sexuality

Sexual feelings and fantasies normally increase during adolescence.

Your teenager may find it difficult to deal with such feelings, particularly if they seem to conflict with the attitudes that he or she has been taught about sex. Friendships with members of the same sex and the opposite sex will be influenced by these feelings and evolve during adolescence.

Friendships with the same sex

In early adolescence, your teenager's closest relationship outside the family is usually with a best friend. At first, your teenager may retreat from his or her emergence as a sexual being into the safety of friendships with members of the same sex.

At the same time, your teenager may be intrigued by sexual matters and may seek information about sex. Sometimes, the emergence of sexual feelings in early adolescence is expressed by telling dirty jokes.

When your teenager first becomes capable of sexual intercourse, he or she is probably years away from being emotionally prepared for this activity and its consequences.

Friendships in a peer group

In middle adolescence, your teenager starts feeling more aware of himself or herself as male or female. Your teenager may spend more time with a larger group of peers, a group within which a natural process of social experimentation occurs.

Your teenager may become more interested in forming relationships with members of the opposite sex, but the choice may be influenced by his or her peer group's acceptance. Dating may start, as well as some sexual experimentation.

Your teenager may feel strong pressure from his or her peers to lose his or her virginity. Some teenagers react to this pressure, and to their own curiosity, by starting to have sexual intercourse at a very young age.

Relationships with the opposite sex

By late adolescence, your teenager may become more secure about his or her sexual identity. Your teenager may be ready to establish an intimate relationship that demands a different type of sharing and commitment. Your teen may feel emotionally ready to have sexual intercourse with this person. But he or she is unlikely to be prepared to become a parent and should know about various methods to prevent pregnancy and to reduce the risk of sexually transmitted infections (STIs).

Sexual fantasies

Daydreaming is an important part of adolescence that can provide an outlet for expanding imaginations. Many daydreams have some sexual content. Your teenager may also have sexual fantasies at night. Sexual thoughts may be hypothetical experiences or memories of real-life experiences. It's normal to have sexual fantasies. Sexual fantasies may even be useful in the development of a teen's sexual identity because they allow exploration of sexual situations that would be inappropriate for the teen to act out.

Masturbation

Masturbation is self-stimulation of the genitals for sensual pleasure. Some teenagers feel guilty about masturbating because of old, unfounded myths, misinformation, cultural messages or plain embarrassment about it.

Your child may have started masturbation before adolescence. It provides a way for teenagers to release sexual tension, give themselves pleasure, savor sexual fantasies and even curb impulses to engage in inappropriate sexual activity with others. As long as your teenager doesn't masturbate publicly, there's nothing unusual,

Talking to Teens About Sex

Teaching your children about sex is most effective if you make it an ongoing discussion, beginning in the preschool and school-age years. During the teenage years, some new topics may come up.

- *Dating.* Your teenager may have questions such as: "When can I start dating?" or "How will I know if I'm ready to have sex?"
- *Abstinence.* Your teenager may be motivated to have sex because of peer pressure, curiosity or any number of other reasons. Tell your teenager that many teenagers decide to wait and that until he or she is ready, there are many other ways to be affectionate: intimate talks, holding hands while walking, listening to music and dancing together, kissing, touching, hugging.
- *Date rape.* Date rape happens when someone your teenager knows forces him or her into sexual activity. Teach your children that no always means no, and that only a clear "yes" means that touching or sexual activity is okay. Let your child know that avoiding alcohol and drugs helps make him or her less vulnerable to being involved in date rape either as a victim or perpetrator. In addition, discuss the danger of date-rape drugs with your teen.
- *Sexual orientation.* Many young people wonder at some point whether they're gay, lesbian or bisexual. Let your child know that it's normal to have crushes on members of the same sex and that just having these feelings doesn't mean he or she is homosexual or bisexual. Stress that if your teen is gay, lesbian or bisexual, you won't reject him or her.

harmful or unacceptable about the practice.

Homosexuality

Some teenagers seek out members of their own sex. Openly homosexual teenagers may face rejection by some of their peers, teachers and family members. Teenagers having difficulty adjusting to their sexual orientation, or to others' reactions to it, may find psychotherapy or counseling helpful.

Sexually active male homosexuals are at risk of contracting sexually transmitted infections (STIs), such as chlamydia, hepatitis B, gonorrhea, AIDS and syphilis. At even higher risk are those who've experimented with several sexual partners. Using a condom during sex can reduce, though not eliminate, the risk of getting infected.

Sexual activity

Teenagers who've had sexual intercourse at least once are considered sexually active. Many teenagers begin having sex in their mid- to late teens. Studies indicate around 40 percent of high school students have had intercourse. The average age of first intercourse for both girls and boys is about 17.

Male and female adolescents often have different reactions to their first experience of intercourse. Girls tend to say they felt scared, guilty, worried, embarrassed and curious. Boys, meanwhile, usually report feeling excited, satisfied, happy and mature.

A wide range of dating patterns is normal. Teenagers may not date at all in junior high or high school, or they may have one high school sweetheart. It's common to have two or three close emotional commitments as a teenager, one after the other. Typically, during the course of each relationship, neither partner dates others and, if sexual activity is part of the relationship, has no other sexual partners.

About 12 percent of all high school students have had four or more sexual partners. These individuals are at a higher risk of acquiring sexually transmitted infections (STIs).

Contraception

If your teenager is considering sexual intercourse, encourage some method of birth control. Both boys and girls should know what types are available.

Hormonal contraception options include the pill (oral contraceptives) and the vaginal contraceptive ring. Another type of birth control is the barrier method, including condoms or a diaphragm. Long-acting reversible contraceptives such as intrauterine devices (IUDs) are also safe and very effective in teens. The choice of methods may be affected by access and motivation to avoid pregnancy.

Each type of birth control has its advantages and disadvantages. Condoms provide the most protection from infection, compared with other forms of contraception. Condoms may not be as reliable in preventing pregnancy, though, so many people use both condoms and another method of birth control. The best way to protect against STIs and pregnancy is abstinence.

Make sure your teen is also aware of emergency contraception (the morning-after pill) in case of unprotected sex or possible failure of another method to prevent pregnancy.

For more information on preventing pregnancy, see page 1177. For more information on preventing pregnancy, see page 1177.

Teenage pregnancy

Teen births have steadily declined in recent years, but the United States still has one of the highest rates of teenage pregnancy of any Western industrialized nation.

Most teenage pregnancies are unplanned or unwanted. Poverty, lack of education about birth control, misinformation about birth control, lack of access to birth control, having a mother who became pregnant as a teen and denial of the risks of becoming pregnant are several factors that may contribute to the risk of teenage pregnancy.

Pregnancy Myths

Don't assume that your teenager knows everything about getting pregnant. Here are some common pregnancy myths:

Myth: You can't get pregnant the first time.
  Fact: It can take only one episode of sexual intercourse to become pregnant, even if it's your first time.

Myth: You can't get pregnant if the penis is pulled out before ejaculation.
  Fact: Fluid carrying sperm commonly leaks out of the penis before and after ejaculation.

Myth: You can't get pregnant during your period.
  Fact: Chances of pregnancy may be reduced during menstruation, but it's possible to get pregnant at any time.

Myth: You can't get pregnant if you douche.
  Fact: Flushing the vagina with water or another liquid doesn't prevent pregnancy.

Raising a child is a serious responsibility. Most teenagers aren't ready, emotionally or financially, to make the necessary commitment. Just as an adult father should participate in caring for and supporting his child, so too should a teenage father. But often a teenage mother ends up having to raise her child under difficult circumstances, without help from the child's father.

Sexually transmitted infections

More than 25 infections can be spread through sexual activity. Almost half the 20 million new cases of sexually transmitted infections (STIs) — also known as sexually transmitted diseases (STDs) — each year occur in people age 15 to 24. The highest reported rates of chlamydia, gonorrhea and human papillomavirus (HPV) all occur in this age group. Young women are more susceptible to STIs such as these than are young males, due to their anatomy.

Teenagers and young adults are at high risk of STIs because they're less likely to use condoms consistently, and they're more likely to have multiple partners and have a partner who's been sexually active with others. Further, adolescents' decision-making and communication skills are still developing and may not keep pace with their sexual activity.

Each type of STI is caused by a different infectious agent. The risk of catching a sexually transmitted infection increases with multiple sexual partners. Signs and symptoms don't accompany all STIs. When no signs or symptoms are present and if sexual partners aren't aware of an infection, the infection is more likely to be passed on.

Sexually active teens should see a doctor regularly to be tested and examined for common STIs.

Whenever one is diagnosed, it's important for all sexual partners to be examined and treated. In all cases, abstaining from sexual contact is important until the infection is successfully treated.

Many STIs can be treated and cured with medication. Antibiotics can kill the bacteria that cause some of them. Human immunodeficiency virus (HIV) is an exception. It causes AIDS, a life-threatening disease. Early treatment, however, can now keep people with HIV healthy for many years.

The longer treatment is delayed, the more difficult a sexually transmitted disease is to control and the greater the risk of complications. For instance, repeated bouts of pelvic inflammatory disease can leave a young woman incapable of getting pregnant.

Abstinence is the most effective way to avoid STIs. For teens who are sexually active, steps to minimize risk include using a condom and being selective about their sexual partners. Condoms are usually effective at blocking the spread of infectious agents, when used correctly. When a condom and contraceptive foam are used together, they offer added protection against pregnancy and the spread of STIs.

For more information on sexually transmitted infections, see Chapter 11, "Unhealthy Behaviors," and Chapter 16, "Infectious Diseases."

Special Concerns

Adolescence is often regarded as a turbulent phase, but studies

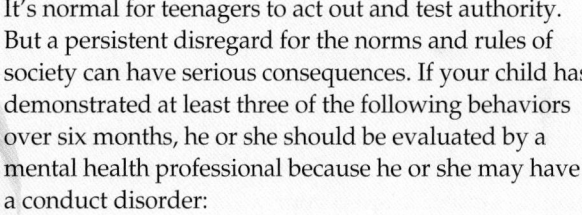

Conduct Disorders

It's normal for teenagers to act out and test authority. But a persistent disregard for the norms and rules of society can have serious consequences. If your child has demonstrated at least three of the following behaviors over six months, he or she should be evaluated by a mental health professional because he or she may have a conduct disorder:

- Stealing
- Constant lying
- Truancy
- Starting fires
- Breaking into homes, offices or cars
- Destroying others' property
- Displaying physical cruelty to animals or humans
- Forcing others into sexual activity
- Starting fights
- Using weapons in fights

Often children with a conduct disorder have underlying problems that have been overlooked or ignored, such as depression or attention-deficit/hyperactivity disorder (ADHD).

Appropriate treatment to help the adolescent realize and understand the effects of his or her behavior on others is important. Treatment may include behavior therapy and psychotherapy. Children with accompanying depression or ADHD may be treated with medications in addition to psychotherapy.

show that most teenagers don't go through the turmoil and rebellion often associated with this stage. For some adolescents, though, the teenage years can be very challenging.

Rebellious behavior

A child who previously has been obedient and calm may become moody, inconsistent, unpredictable and even rebellious in adolescence. Your adolescent may argue with you about a range of issues, large and small. They can include everything from what to wear and when to take out the garbage to when to come home at night and whether to engage in sexual activity.

A certain amount of teenage rebellion, risk taking and testing of authority is normal. It may be an essential stage in the adolescent's process of separating from parents and developing a personal identity. However, most teenagers don't rebel greatly.

Rebellion can be seen as part of the process by which adolescents define their identity. They may take an action merely to see what reactions it provokes in the people around them. This is why you shouldn't just give up on your rebellious teenager. Intervene when his or her behavior exceeds limits you have set. Eventually, a teenager will learn from the consequences of the behavior and work toward the establishment of his or her own boundaries.

Mild rebellion is common and even normal in early and middle adolescence. By late adolescence, most teenagers are on their way to developing a sense of perspective. They have become better able to delay gratification, compromise on conflicting demands and set limits.

If rebellious behavior becomes more self-destructive or lingers into late adolescence, consult your physician or a mental health professional. Family problems may be causing or worsening the rebel-

lion. Therapy involving the whole family may be helpful.

If your teenage child is rebellious, hold your ground. Keep stating your concerns and setting reasonable limits. Don't threaten punishments that you won't carry out. In most cases, with your firm handling, your teenager will outgrow this rebellious phase without any lasting damage.

Beliefs and behaviors usually change by the time a teen grows up and starts a family. Your child is likely to return to the viewpoints and standards learned from you during childhood. With this in mind, try to prevent rifts during your child's adolescence that will stand in the way of a later reunion.

As a parent, you remain the greatest influence on your teenager's beliefs and behavior. Even when your child appears to be disagreeing with everything you say, he or she needs you to hold and defend your own reasonable and consistent view of the world.

School problems

Problems in school can occur for a variety of reasons. While also evident in school-age children from kindergarten on, such problems can become more serious during the teenage years.

Learning disabilities
A learning disability can cause a teenager to perform poorly in school, regardless of intelligence. Though often diagnosed in the earlier school years, a learning disability sometimes doesn't come to light until a child has reached his or her teens.

Attention-deficit/hyperactivity disorder
Up to one-half of the children with attention-deficit/hyperactivity disorder (ADHD) continue to have symptoms as adolescents and adults. Behavior therapy together with medication, if needed, can help parents and teens to manage

symptoms. ADHD may cause additional frustration during the teenage years, when academic and social demands increase.

Failure to pay attention to details, excessive distractibility, inability to organize and impulsiveness can interfere with learning. Coping strategies such as using a daily planner for assignments, keeping a routine, and setting aside a quiet time and place to do homework may be helpful.

Participation in extracurricular activities such as sports, drama and debate teams can offer an outlet for excess energy and an opportunity to make friends. Keep in touch with your teen's teachers about how he or she is doing.

Chronic illness
If your teenager has had a chronic illness through childhood and adolescence, such as asthma or cystic fibrosis, he or she may need to miss school during acute episodes of the disease. Too often, these absences put your child at risk of school failure. Your child may need extra encouragement and support to make up the missed schoolwork. As parents, don't support frequent school absences for minor physical complaints. Work with your child's doctor, teachers and school nurse. Together, you can help minimize absences.

School phobia
Avoidance of school or refusal to attend school may be a way of responding to overwhelming stress and situations that an adolescent can't control. School phobia most often appears when a student first begins school. If the problem persists in an older child, evaluation and treatment by a mental health professional is often beneficial.

Truancy
Truancy may start with cutting an occasional class and then escalate into prolonged absences. Truancy can result from conflicts within the family, parental expectations that

are too high, lack of parental attention and peer pressure to drop out. Truants are often rebellious teenagers who are in trouble not only at school but also at home and elsewhere.

Sometimes, truancy can be reversed with an educational plan that emphasizes behavior management and involves the family, school and medical personnel. Individual and family psychotherapy also may help. If the teenager still doesn't attend school regularly, it may be possible to work out an educational alternative such as work-study and independent study programs.

School failure

School failure can result from truancy. It's difficult for your child to know what's going on in class if he or she doesn't attend. Some schools automatically drop students who've been absent more than a certain amount of time. A host of other problems can be involved in school failure. Future employment opportunities for high school dropouts are limited, so it's important to prevent school failure.

Depression

It was once thought that only adults got depressed, but researchers are finding that children and teenagers are prone to the same types of depression as adults. The incidence of major depression in children and teenagers peaks during adolescence. Unfortunately, depression in this age group often isn't recognized and treated. Below are some facts to consider:

- Depression may occur in an estimated 1 in 8 teenagers in the United States.
- If a child or teenager has an episode of depression, he or she has a greater than 50 percent chance of having another episode in the next five years.
- Suicide is the third-leading cause of death for 10- to 19-year-olds.

- About 18 percent of high school students have seriously considered attempting suicide in the past year.

Recognizing depression in teenagers can be challenging because its signs and symptoms may easily be attributed to a growing phase or hormonal changes. Many behaviors associated with depression in young people are common reactions in children and teenagers. For example, almost all teenagers argue with their parents or teachers or refuse to do chores from time to time. The criteria used to make a diagnosis of depression include the number, duration and severity of signs and symptoms.

Risk factors

During the teenage years, girls become twice as likely as boys to experience depression. A family history of depression also may be a risk factor. Other risk factors include the following:

- Experiencing significant stress
- Being the victim of abuse or neglect
- Experiencing the death of a parent or other loved one
- Breaking up with someone
- Having a chronic illness, such as diabetes
- Experiencing other trauma
- Having a behavioral disorder

Treatment

If you think your child may be depressed, arrange for him or her to see a doctor or mental health professional. Professional treatment can help your child regain hope that things can get better and that his or her problems will be overcome. Treatment may involve medication, psychotherapy or a combination of the two.

Although opinions differ on which form of treatment to use first, growing evidence shows that the best approach for most young people has been a combination of medication and a form of psychotherapy called cognitive behavioral therapy.

Suicide

Sometimes, depressed teenagers' lives become so painful that they feel they have nothing to live for. Most adolescents who attempt suicide are depressed. Other suicides may be motivated by triggers such as the breakup of a relationship, the death of a friend or family member, psychological problems within the family, chronic physical illness, drug abuse, or physical or sexual abuse.

There are many reasons why teenagers attempt suicide. Sometimes, they give no warning, and the attempt can't be predicted.

The rate of suicide among 10- to 24-year-olds in the United States has risen substantially since 1960. Teenage girls attempt suicide at a higher rate than boys. They more often ingest drugs, which may not be lethal. When teenage boys attempt suicide, they're more likely to use guns and be successful in killing themselves.

Because depressed adolescents often feel that their family doesn't understand them, make a special effort to bridge this communication gap. Your hopes and dreams for your child's happiness, strength and success shouldn't stand in the way of your accepting his or her revelations of depression.

Ask your child how he or she really feels — and then listen. Ask how long the mood lasts and how intense it is. You can help by offering your support and concern. You can also reassure your child that he or she won't feel this way forever. Most episodes of depression eventually end. A teenager who's experiencing deep depression for the first time may not recognize or believe it will end.

If your child confides that he or she has considered suicide, take it seriously and seek a psychiatric evaluation for him or her immediately. Even if you think you know with certainty that your child isn't really going to kill himself or herself, it's a cry for help that deserves to be heeded.

Medication

In the past, doctors were reluctant to prescribe antidepressants to children and teenagers because of the lack of evidence concerning the safety and effectiveness of these drugs on young people. However, studies have shown that antidepressants such as selective serotonin reuptake inhibitors (SSRIs) and newer related medications are safe and effective for use in children.

Commonly used SSRIs include fluoxetine (Prozac), citalopram (Celexa) and sertraline (Zoloft), among others.

Some studies suggest that a combined approach of medications and psychotherapy are more effective than either alone.

Generally, antidepressants are a first choice of treatment among providers when the child or teen:

- Has severe symptoms that likely won't respond well to psychotherapy
- Has psychosis or bipolar disorder
- Doesn't have immediate access to psychotherapy
- Has chronic depression or recurring episodes

Even after symptoms of depression have subsided, it's generally recommended that antidepressant medication continue to be taken for several months to help prevent a recurrence.

When it's time to stop taking the drug, your child's doctor likely will taper him or her off the medication over a period of weeks or months. If depression recurs — especially during the tapering period or shortly thereafter — it's usually necessary to resume the medication.

Psychotherapy

Certain types of short-term psychotherapy, especially cognitive behavioral therapy, have been shown to relieve symptoms of depression in children and teenagers. When a child or teenager is depressed, he or she often has distorted, negative views, which reinforce the depression. Cognitive behavioral therapy helps young people develop more-positive views of themselves, the world and their life situation.

Sometimes a therapist may recommend continuing psychotherapy for a period of time after depressive symptoms are gone. This may further enhance a child's or teenager's coping skills, decreasing chances of a relapse.

Recognizing and treating depression is important. Children and teenagers living with untreated depression may experience other problems. Family relationships can suffer, social development may be affected and school performance may decline. Depression may also lead to alcohol or drug abuse and an increased risk of suicide. Fortunately, if depression in teens is quickly identified and treated, its duration, severity and risk of complications can be reduced.

A Depression Checklist for Parents

The following checklist may help you gather information about your child's feelings, thinking, physical problems, behavior problems and suicide risk:

Feelings

Does your child demonstrate:
- Sadness
- Emptiness
- Hopelessness
- Guilt
- Worthlessness
- Lack of enjoyment in everyday pleasures

Thinking

Does your child have trouble:
- Concentrating
- Making decisions
- Completing schoolwork
- Maintaining grades
- Maintaining friendships

Physical problems

Does your child complain of:
- Headaches
- Stomachaches
- Lack of energy
- Sleeping problems — too much or too little
- Weight or appetite changes — gain or loss

Behavior problems

Is your child:
- Irritable
- Not wanting to go to school
- Wanting to be alone most of the time
- Having difficulty getting along with others
- Cutting classes or missing school
- Dropping out of sports, hobbies or other activities
- Drinking alcohol or using drugs

Suicide risk

Does your child talk or think about:
- Suicide
- Death
- Other morbid subjects

If your child experiences five or more of these signs or symptoms for at least two weeks, he or she may be experiencing depression or another mental illness. Note how long the signs and symptoms last and how often they occur. This information will help a doctor or therapist better understand your child's emotional state. Address suicide concerns without delay.

Eating disorders

Many teenagers are preoccupied with the way their bodies look. Some may occasionally go on a diet or change their eating habits to lose weight. If dieting becomes an obsession, it may be a sign indicating a potential eating disorder.

Eating disorders are more common during adolescence and early adulthood but can occur in childhood or midlife. Although eating disorders occur in both sexes, teenage girls and young women are more likely than teenage boys and young men to develop an eating disorder. Symptoms can result in serious medical complications and benefit from treatment by a multidisciplinary team of providers.

Anorexia nervosa

Anorexia nervosa is characterized by a significantly low body weight, fear of gaining weight (or persistent behavior to prevent weight gain) and a disturbance in perception of one's own body shape or weight. People with this disorder typically eat only small quantities of a few foods and may also exercise compulsively. Some routinely vomit, use laxatives or take other medications to control their weight.

One hallmark of anorexia nervosa is that someone with the disorder perceives his or her body as fat even if he or she is very thin. Often lacking body fat, girls with anorexia nervosa don't have much development of breasts, thighs or a waistline, and they maintain the appearance of younger children.

Signs and symptoms of anorexia include weight loss (sometimes severe), failure to maintain body weight at or above a minimally normal weight, menstrual changes or the absence of menstruation, and preoccupation with food intake, exercise and academic achievement.

For more information on anorexia nervosa, see page 1138.

Bulimia nervosa

Bulimia nervosa involves frequent uncontrolled eating (bingeing) and then throwing up (purging) or using other methods to avoid gaining weight. In addition, self-image is closely tied to one's weight and shape for those with bulimia. Unfortunately, this eating disorder doesn't always have clear outward signs. Individuals typically try to hide bingeing and purging episodes, and teenagers with bulimia may maintain their normal weight, lose weight or even gain weight.

Signs and symptoms of bulimia include an unhealthy focus on body shape and weight, uncontrollable eating behavior, and recurrent binge eating followed by efforts to prevent weight gain, such as self-induced vomiting, using laxatives or other medications, or excessive exercise.

For more information on bulimia nervosa, see page 1139.

Binge eating disorder

Frequent binge eating without subsequent behavior to prevent weight gain is now recognized as binge eating disorder. During binge episodes, people with this disorder feel a lack of control over eating. Episodes are different from routine overeating in that they include at least three of the following symptoms: eating very rapidly, eating until uncomfortably full, eating without physical hunger, bingeing alone due to shame and negative feelings following overeating.

Individuals with binge eating disorder may display depressive symptoms, fluctuations in weight and distress over their eating habits.

Other feeding or eating disorder

Sometimes an individual's eating pattern doesn't meet all the criteria for a specific disorder but may be considered disordered eating. Examples include less frequent binge eating or bingeing and purging, purging without binge eating, anorexic behavior with less severe weight loss, and excessive night eating.

Tobacco use

While numbers have declined, cigarettes continue to be the most commonly used form of tobacco, including among teenagers.

Online Safety

During the teenage years, parents generally allow their children to do more things on their own. Sexual predators may take advantage of this unsupervised time to befriend unsuspecting children. Through social media or other activities online, teenagers may innocently become friends with and be lured into meeting a sexual predator. Although the internet is a great tool for learning, make sure your children are aware of the potential dangers.

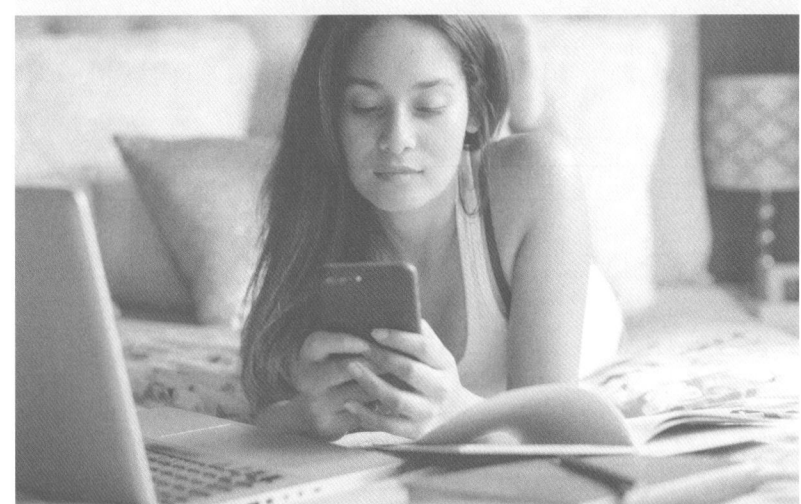

Several other forms of tobacco — including smokeless tobacco, e-cigarettes, cigars and cigarillos, hookahs or water pipes, and dissolvable tobacco — are available. All contain a variety of chemicals, including nicotine, and aren't safe alternatives to cigarettes.

Most teenagers recognize the health risks associated with smoking and tobacco use, but they overestimate their ability to stop once they start. About three-fourths of teenage smokers will still be smoking as adults. The earlier a child begins smoking, the greater the chance that he or she will become a heavy smoker as an adult.

Teenagers who smoke tobacco are also more likely to experiment with marijuana and other drugs.

Here are some strategies parents might try to keep their adolescent from smoking:

- **Set an example.** If you as a parent smoke, one of the best reasons to stop is for the sake of your children. Parents teach best by example.
- **Talk with your children.** Ask whether their friends smoke. The risk of your child smoking is much higher if his or her best friends smoke. Most teenagers smoke their first cigarette with a friend who already smokes.
- **Learn what your children think about smoking.** Ask them to read this information so that you can discuss it together.

- **Help your child explore ways to deal with peer pressure.** Use nonjudgmental questions and rehearse with them how they could handle tough situations.
- **Note the social repercussions.** Individuals who smoke often have bad breath, and smoking makes their hair and clothes smell. Smoking can also produce a chronic cough and makes skin wrinkle prematurely.

For more information on tobacco use, see page 310.

Alcohol use

Most young people try alcoholic beverages during their teenage years. Alcohol is widely available, and many adolescents drink excessively. Although it may take years for many adults to develop alcohol dependence, teenagers often become addicted within months. Alcohol use by itself or with other drugs can harm your child's normal growth and development and is associated with safety risks.

Alcohol use among teenagers increases dramatically during the 10th and 11th grades. Each year in the United States, binge drinking is responsible for 4,300 deaths among underage youth. Alcohol is also often implicated in other teenage deaths, including auto accidents, drownings, suicides and fires.

For young people, the likelihood of addiction depends on the influence of parents, peers and other role models, susceptibility to advertising, how early in life they begin to use alcohol, and genetic factors that may predispose them to addiction.

Look for these signs in your child:

- Loses interest in activities and hobbies
- Appears anxious or irritable
- Has difficulties in relationships with friends or joins a new crowd
- Receives lower grades in school

To prevent teenage alcohol use, set a good example regarding alcohol use. Talk to your children about alcohol use and discuss both the legal and medical consequences of drinking, especially drinking and driving.

For more information on alcohol use and alcoholism, see page 316.

Drug use and addiction

Just like an adult who may drink to feel more comfortable at a party, an adolescent may take a drug to relax and join the crowd. But drug use is a counterproductive strategy. Social interactions are more

Teens and Stress

All teens experience stress. In fact, teens may be more susceptible to stress overload because of the pressures faced on the road to becoming adults. Parents, school and work — and even friends — can add stress to everyday life.

While some stress is good and can motivate you to achieve your goals, if stressful situations pile up one after the other, your mind and body have no chance to recover.

Although you can't avoid stress completely, you can learn how to deal with it more effectively. For more information on stress, see Chapter 10, "Stress."

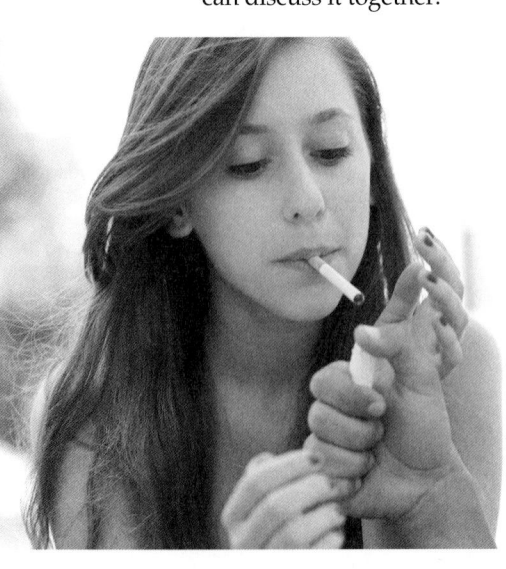

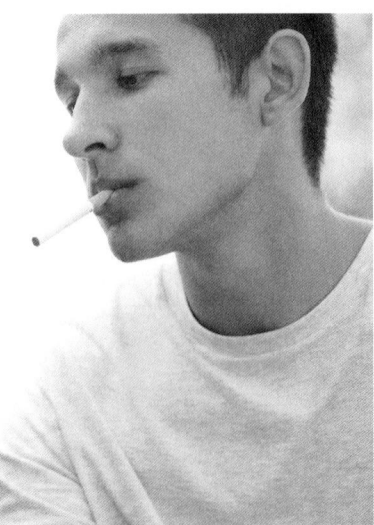

successful when one is really one's self, rather than some other personality induced by a drug. Drugged people often withdraw socially and may become depressed. Likewise, depressed adolescents may abuse more drugs in a vain effort to improve their mood.

For most adolescents, experimentation with drugs starts with alcohol or tobacco. Because alcohol and cigarettes are legal for adults, they're easily accessible to teenagers. The same is true for marijuana, now legalized for medical or recreational use in many states.

More than 70 percent of high school juniors and seniors in the United States have had one alcoholic drink, and more than 1 in 3 has smoked during their lifetime. Next may come smoking marijuana. Almost half the high school seniors in the United States have used marijuana in their lifetime. About 14 percent of high school seniors report trying other illegal drugs in the past year.

Peer pressure and learning problems at school may make teenagers more likely to abuse drugs. Conversely, drug abuse can dampen an adolescent's motivation to do well in school. Drugs can impair the learning process, causing memory loss and shortening the attention span. Teens who abuse drugs compromise their future outside of school too. They may get into legal trouble for abusing illicit drugs, selling them or stealing to get enough money to buy them.

Drugs can disrupt the process by which your teenager develops a secure identity. They can also mar judgment and self-control. They release inhibitions and can make it easier for your child to do things that he or she wouldn't normally consider doing, including sexual activity.

Most seriously, drug abuse raises the risk of death during adolescence. The leading killers of teenagers — accidents, murder and suicide — are more prevalent among drug abusers.

The most effective way to discourage your teenage child from abusing drugs is to gear your message to his or her level of intellectual and moral development. Particularly in early and middle adolescence, your child may be less impressed by the long-term health effects of these substances than by their immediate social consequences. Even more important than delivering an antidrug message is to set a good example. Addictive behavior often repeats itself in successive generations of a family. There may be a genetic component, but learning by the example of others also may play a role.

Helping to build your child's self-confidence can help him or her to resist peer pressure to use drugs and alcohol.

Inhalant use

Teens don't need to take drugs to get high. There are more than 1,000 types of inhalants that teens may abuse, including gasoline, paint thinners, aerosol sprays, nail polish remover and household cleaners.

Sniffing inhalants offers an inexpensive alternative to illicit drugs, and inhalants are readily available. Teens can also huff — soak rags in inhalants and press the rags to their mouth. Another option is bagging — inhaling fumes from chemicals poured into a plastic bag.

Inhalants may produce a quick, powerful high. Inhalant abuse can start in grade school and continue throughout adolescence. About 7 percent of American high school students report using inhalants at least once in their lives.

When children sniff, huff or bag, they may ingest a host of toxic chemicals — butane, propane, fluorocarbons, nitrites and more. Chronic abusers are at risk of weight loss, muscle weakness, lack of coordination and addiction.

? Question and Answer

How can I know if my teenager is using drugs?

These clues are only possible indications that your teenager is using drugs:
- *School.* Your child suddenly exhibits a dislike of school and looks for excuses to stay home. Contact school officials to see if your child's attendance record matches what you know about his or her attendance. A drastic fall in grades may be another sign.
- *Physical health.* Listlessness and apathy are possible indications of drug use.
- *Appearance.* Appearance is extremely important to adolescents. A warning sign of drug use can be a sudden lack of interest in clothing or appearance.
- *Personal behavior.* Teenagers enjoy privacy. However, be wary of exaggerated efforts to bar you from their bedrooms or keep you from knowing where they go with their friends.
- *Money.* Sudden requests for more money without a reasonable explanation for its use can be an indication of drug use. Some teens may also steal money or valuable objects from their parents.

Adolescents need to know that there's an open line of communication with their parents. Even in the face of your child's reluctance to share feelings, continue to express an interest in listening to your child talk about his or her experiences.

Other possible effects include damage to the brain, heart, kidneys and liver. Inhalant abuse can be deadly.

People who abuse inhalants often act like they're intoxicated with alcohol. Unfortunately, adults often fail to recognize inhalant abuse. Parents and care providers may be more concerned about adolescent use of alcohol, nicotine, marijuana and other illicit drugs. Preventing inhalant abuse starts with spotting clues to the problem.

Abusive Dating Relationships

It's estimated that between 10 and 25 percent of teens are involved in abusive dating relationships. The abuse may be verbal and emotional, with or without sexual abuse. Is your daughter or son at risk? Consider the warning signs:

- Increasingly distant from family and friends
- Unexplained injuries or an explanation that doesn't make sense
- Lost interest in school or dropping grades
- Moody or depressed
- Suddenly uninterested in her or his appearance
- Involved with someone who's verbally or physically abusive
- Involved with someone who demonstrates a violent temper
- Involved with someone who calls constantly and appears possessive

If you suspect abuse, talk with your child immediately. With the information you've gathered, get your daughter or son actively involved in developing a plan to end the abuse. If you have reason to believe that your child's partner is going to hurt her or him in a specific situation, take steps to protect her or him.

The Consumer Product Safety Commission suggests the following as possible signs of inhalant abuse:

- An unusual breath odor or chemical odor on clothing
- Slurred or disoriented speech
- Drunk or dazed appearance
- Signs of paint or other products on the face or fingers
- Red or runny eyes or nose
- Spots or sores around the mouth
- Sitting with a pen or marker near the nose
- Smelling clothing sleeves
- Hiding rags, clothes or empty containers of the potentially abused products in closets and other places

Tell your children about the risks and that even experimentation is dangerous. Make sure that your child's care provider, teachers, counselors and coaches know about inhalant abuse so that they can reinforce the danger of it and recognize potential signs of trouble. Open discussion can prevent a tragedy.

Sexual abuse

Sexual abuse can occur in adolescence as well as earlier in childhood. It can include a spectrum of unacceptable behavior from fondling to rape. Sexual abuse is any act of sexual contact forced on one person by another.

Rape usually involves force or the threat of force. However, rape also includes situations in which the victim is unable to give consent because of being drunk, drugged, mentally ill or developmentally disabled. Almost half the reported rape victims are adolescents. Most sexual abuse of teenagers involves girls, but the rate of assaults on boys may be increasing.

Sexual abuse can be devastating, hostile and dehumanizing. Sexual abuse often causes major psychological trauma that has lasting effects on the victim's self-worth and identity. This is especially true for adolescents, who are still figuring

out who they are, including their sexual identity. If rape is a teen's first sexual experience, future sexual relations may be difficult.

Following sexual abuse, the victim may go through rapid mood swings, feeling alternately degraded, angry, guilty and helpless. The victim may be plagued for a long time by fears, nightmares and disturbed sleep. The victim's relationships with peers and consensual sexual partners may suffer.

Counseling can help the victim and family to cope with long-term effects of sexual abuse. You may want to seek professional guidance from an established sexual abuse program or center. Some parents reject their children when they have become victims, while others overprotect them. You can help your child come to terms with the sexual abuse by neither denying nor overreacting to the abuse, and by reinforcing that the victim is never at fault.

The psychological ramifications of sexual abuse by a family member can be even more complex than those of abuse by a nonfamily member. Fearing that reporting these occurrences will disrupt the structure of the family, the victim may be too frightened to tell anyone about it. Thus, the abuse may occur repeatedly. The abusive relative may invoke family authority to keep the victim from reporting the abuse. As the abuse continues unreported, the victim may feel increasingly helpless, ashamed, guilty and even responsible.

Serious consequences can occur when adolescents don't have the opportunity to disclose the abuse. These individuals are at high risk of drug abuse, promiscuity, running away or even suicide. ■

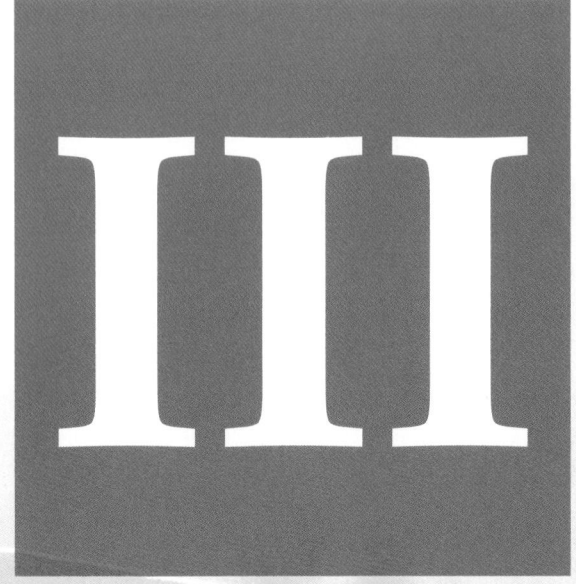

PART **THREE**

Healthy Adults

Vaccinations and Screenings

Prevention is crucial to good health. It's far better to prevent a disease than to treat it. One of the best ways to protect yourself and your family from disease is to get vaccinated. Vaccination, a method of immunization, is the best line of defense against diseases such as measles, mumps, rubella, tetanus, hepatitis, polio and many others. Vaccination stimulates your body's natural defense mechanisms to resist infectious disease, destroying the virus or bacterium before you become sick.

Thanks to vaccines, many infectious diseases that were once common in the United States are now rare or nonexistent. Children don't have to keep away from water fountains to avoid getting polio. Parents no longer have to fear that their children will die of or become disabled by diphtheria, whooping cough (pertussis) or measles. However, occasional outbreaks do happen.

Beginning in 20th century, widespread use of vaccinations has saved billions of lives worldwide. However, despite the availability of vaccines, many people remain underimmunized. One reason is that some people have concerns about the safety and risks of vaccines. These concerns are often the result of incorrect information.

How Vaccines Work

Every day, your body is threatened by bacteria, viruses and other germs. When a disease-causing microorganism enters your body, your immune system mounts a defense, producing proteins called antibodies to fight off the invader. The goal of your immune system is to neutralize or destroy the foreign invader, rendering it harmless and preventing you from getting sick.

Understanding immunity

Your body's immune system fights off foreign invaders and protects you from disease in the following two ways:

Post-exposure immunity
This type of immunity develops after you've been exposed to a certain organism. Your immune system puts into play a complex array of defenses to prevent you from getting sick again from the same type of virus or bacterium.

Exposure to a foreign invader, such as a virus, activates the production of certain white blood cells in your body called B cells (B lymphocytes). B cells produce plasma cells, which in turn produce a huge number of proteins known as antibodies that are designed to fight a specific invader. The antibodies circulate in your body's fluids, and the next time that invader enters your body, the antibodies recognize it and destroy it. Once your body produces a particular antibody, it can rapidly resume production of more if needed.

Other white blood cells called macrophages "process" all invaders. They confront foreign invaders, determine if they present a threat, and destroy them if necessary. If your body encounters a germ that it has never been exposed to before, information about the germ is relayed to white blood cells called helper T cells. These cells aid in the development of other infection-fighting cells, including memory T cells.

Once you've been exposed to a specific virus or bacterium, the next time you encounter it, antibodies and memory T cells react to the organism, attacking it before disease can develop.

Vaccine immunity
Vaccine immunity results from injection of a vaccine. The vaccine triggers your immune system's infection-fighting ability and memory without exposure to the

Vaccine Immunity

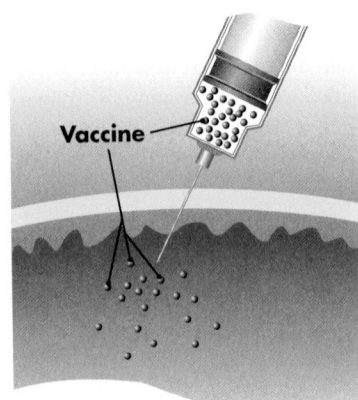
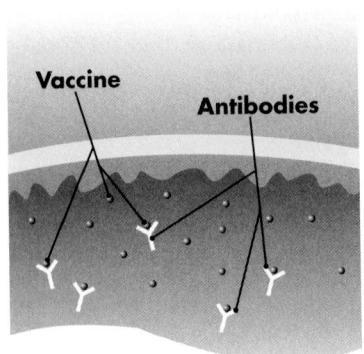
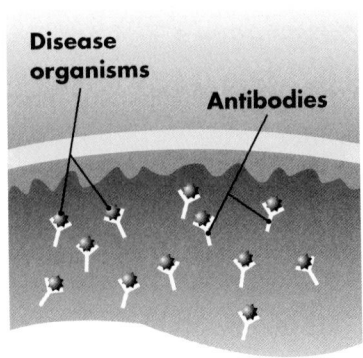

A vaccine with dead or harmless forms of a virus, bacterium or other organism is injected into an individual (left). The vaccine stimulates the immune system to produce antibodies against the organism (center). In any subsequent exposure to this germ, the antibodies attack and stop the infection (right).

actual disease. A vaccine contains a killed or weakened form or derivative of the infectious germ. When given to an individual who's healthy, the vaccine triggers an immune response. It makes your body think that it's being invaded by a specific organism, and your immune system goes to work to destroy the invader and prevent it from infecting you again.

If you're exposed to a disease for which you've been vaccinated, the invading germs are quickly met by antibodies prepared to destroy them. The immunity you develop after vaccination is similar to that acquired from natural infection. For most diseases, a vaccine is as good at creating immunity as the infection would be. And vaccines can be administered without the risk of the serious effects of disease.

Several doses of a vaccine may be needed for a full immune response. Some people fail to build immunity to the first doses of a vaccine but often respond to later doses. In addition, the immunity provided by some vaccines, such as tetanus and pertussis, isn't lifelong. Because the immune response may decrease over time, you may need another dose of a vaccine (booster) to restore or increase your immunity.

Types of vaccines

Vaccines are prepared in different ways. For each type of vaccine, the goal is the same — to stimulate an immune response without causing disease.

Weakened live
Some vaccines, such as those for measles, mumps, rubella and chickenpox (varicella), use live viruses that have been weakened (attenuated).

Killed or inactivated
Other vaccines use inactivated (killed) bacteria or viruses. The inactivated polio vaccine (IPV) is made this way.

Toxoid
Some types of bacteria cause disease by producing toxins that invade the bloodstream. Toxoid vaccines, such as those for diphtheria and tetanus, use bacterial toxins that have been rendered harmless.

Acellular and subunit
Acellular and subunit vaccines are made by using only part of the virus or bacterium. The hepatitis, *Haemophilus influenzae* type b (Hib) and injectable flu vaccines are made in this way.

Benefits of Vaccines

Because many vaccine-preventable diseases are now uncommon in the United States, some people wonder if it's necessary to keep up with immunizations. The answer is yes. Many infectious diseases that have virtually disappeared in the United States can reappear quickly. The germs that cause the diseases still exist and can be acquired by people who aren't protected by vaccination.

As travelers unknowingly carry disease from one country to another, a new outbreak in the United States may be only an airplane trip away. From a single entry point, an infectious disease can spread quickly among unprotected individuals.

The persistent threat of disease is just one reason public health officials recommend vaccinations. Vaccines provide a number of benefits to individuals, communities and the world population.

Safety

Many people have questions and concerns about vaccine safety. A common fear is that vaccines may trigger serious side effects or even cause disease.

In fact, vaccines are extremely safe. Before they can be used, they must meet strict safety standards set by the Food and Drug Administration (FDA). Meeting these standards requires a lengthy development process of up to 10 years followed by three phases of clinical trials.

Once vaccines are licensed and made available to the general public, the FDA and the Centers for Disease Control and Prevention (CDC) continue to monitor their safety. Furthermore, vaccines are subject to ongoing research, review and refinement by doctors, scientists and public health officials.

Your chances of being harmed by a disease are far greater than your chances of being harmed by a vaccine used to prevent disease.

Effectiveness

Vaccines are highly effective. Most childhood vaccines are effective in 85 to 99 percent or more of children who receive them. In some instances a vaccine provides only partial immunity. It doesn't prevent the disease, but it often lessens the duration of the illness and the severity of the symptoms.

A reduction in suffering and disability

In addition to being potentially fatal, many infectious diseases can cause permanent harm. Polio can cause paralysis. Meningitis can cause deafness. Measles can cause brain damage and death. Hepatitis can cause liver damage. Vaccines prevent these serious complications.

Take, for example, the *Haemophilus influenzae* type b (Hib) vaccine. Before the vaccine became available, this bacterium caused about 20,000 serious infections in American infants and children each year. Hib meningitis killed 600 children annually and left many survivors with deafness, seizures or mental disability. Immunization has reduced the incidence of Hib disease by almost 99 percent.

Protection of community health

Immunizing also protects the health of your community. In any community, you'll find a small number of people who shouldn't be vaccinated — for example, individuals who are allergic to an ingredient in a vaccine or who have a condition that precludes certain vaccinations. These people depend on others not passing disease on to them.

If 95 percent of the people in a community are immunized, unprotected individuals are much less likely to be exposed to the germ, so they have a smaller chance of becoming infected. This is called herd immunity.

Eradication of disease worldwide

Immunization protects more than one city, one country and one generation. Its benefits can extend across the world and into the future. The long-term goal of an immunization program is to completely eliminate a disease. At least in one instance, this goal has become a reality. The worldwide eradication of smallpox is a success story of modern medicine.

Smallpox was devastating to humankind for centuries. It spread in epidemics and killed as many as 30 percent of its victims. The disease caused severe headache, fever and a red, blistering rash that often left disfiguring scars on its survivors. Up to one-third of people with the disease were blinded from corneal infection.

At the end of the 18th century, Edward Jenner, an English physician, discovered that inoculating individuals with cowpox virus — a virus that's similar to smallpox but usually harmless — prevented them from getting smallpox. Campaigns were launched in the United States and in Europe to immunize people against smallpox. In 1967, the World Health Organization (WHO) launched a global campaign to eliminate smallpox. The last reported case occurred in 1977, signaling the end of one of the deadliest and most feared diseases in history. Smallpox vaccination is no longer required, but the United States has some vaccine in storage should the smallpox virus ever emerge again.

Side Effects of Vaccines

Although vaccines are considered very safe, like all drugs they aren't completely free of side effects. Most side effects are minor and temporary — such as a sore arm, a mild fever or swelling at the injection site. These effects typically go away on their own within a few hours to a couple of days. Serious side effects differ by vaccine and are rare. When any serious reactions are reported, they receive careful scrutiny from the Food and Drug Administration and the CDC. The risk of death from a vaccine is so slight that it can't accurately be determined.

Some vaccines have been blamed for chronic illnesses, such as autism or diabetes. But decades of vaccine use in the United States provides no credible evidence that vaccines cause chronic illness. Researchers have on occasion reported a link between vaccine use and chronic illness, but when other researchers have tried to duplicate those results — a test of good scientific research — they haven't been able to do so.

Weighing the risks and benefits

The consequences of acquiring a disease that can be prevented by immunization are far greater than the extremely rare risk of a serious side effect that may result from vaccine use.

Adult Vaccinations

Many adults believe that the need for immunization ends with childhood. They assume that the vaccines they received as children will protect them for the rest of their lives. This is partly true, but:
- Some adults were never vaccinated as children
- Immunity can decrease over time
- Newer vaccines weren't available when some adults were children
- Recommendations change as more scientific evidence becomes available
- With age you become more susceptible to infectious diseases, such as pneumonia and the flu
- Risk of a particular disease changes with factors such as

Vaccine Additives

In addition to the killed or weakened microorganisms that make up vaccines, small amounts of other substances may be added to enhance the immune response, prevent contamination, stabilize the vaccine against temperature variations and other conditions, and preserve its potency. Vaccines may also contain small amounts of materials used in the manufacturing process, such as gelatin.

One additive that has received much attention is a preservative called thimerosal, which is a derivative of mercury. Thimerosal has been used in medical products since the 1930s and in small amounts in some vaccines to prevent bacterial contamination. No evidence shows that children have been harmed by such mercury use in vaccines. Nonetheless childhood vaccines are now made without thimerosal or with only trace amounts.

occupation, travel, lifestyle and personal health

Each year people die of diseases that could have been prevented by routine adult vaccinations. Often the reason is lack of awareness that the shots are needed. Vaccines you may need depend on your health, medical history and risk of exposure to various illnesses.

Chickenpox (varicella)

Chickenpox (varicella) is a viral disease that spreads from person to person by inhaling infected respiratory droplets from the air or by physical contact with fluid from the chickenpox rash. The illness is much more serious in adults than in children.

Recommendation

If you've never had chickenpox or been vaccinated against the disease, consider getting the two-dose varicella immunization series. But don't get immunized if you've had a serious allergic reaction to gelatin or the antibiotic neomycin, both ingredients in the vaccine.

Flu (influenza)

Flu (influenza) is a highly contagious viral respiratory disease that spreads through the air. It's different from the common cold or the so-called stomach flu. It's a disease caused by one of two types of viruses — influenza A and B. Adults most at risk of developing serious complications from the flu are those age 65 and older, pregnant women and people with chronic medical conditions, such as asthma, diabetes and heart disease.

Recommendation

Vaccination is recommended for anyone who wants to avoid illness due to influenza. In particular, those who should receive a flu shot are children older than 6 months, adults age 50 and older (even though people age 65 and older are at higher risk), and individuals

at high risk. Because the influenza virus changes its structure slightly each year, you need to get immunized annually. In some years the vaccination is not as effective as in others. Still, vaccination is very important for prevention. Even if you get the flu, its severity and complications will be reduced. For more information on the influenza vaccine see page 237.

Haemophilus influenzae type b (Hib)

Haemophilus influenzae is a type of bacterium that causes illness mainly in infants and children, but it can cause infections in people of all ages. A vaccine is available that can prevent disease caused by *Haemophilus influenzae* type b (Hib), but not the other strains of the *Haemophilus influenzae* bacteria.

Recommendation

In addition to children, the Hib vaccine is recommended for adults with certain medical conditions who may be at increased risk of the disease and who haven't previously been vaccinated. This includes individuals who have sickle cell disease, leukemia or HIV infection, or who've had their spleen removed (splenectomy).

Hepatitis A

Hepatitis A is a liver disease caused by the hepatitis A virus. It's usually spread by eating or drinking contaminated food or water or by close personal contact.

Recommendation

The two-dose series of the hepatitis A vaccine is recommended for people who live in or will be traveling to places where the disease is prevalent, people who work in a lab conducting hepatitis research, and people who care for an individual adopted from a country where hepatitis A is common. This vaccination is also recommended for people who have chronic liver

Signs of a Severe Reaction

After vaccination, watch for any unusual conditions, such as a serious allergic reaction, high fever or behavior changes. Signs and symptoms of a serious allergic reaction include difficulty breathing, hoarseness or wheezing, hives, paleness, weakness, a fast heartbeat, dizziness, and swelling of the throat. If you think that you or your child may be experiencing a severe reaction, call your doctor or go to the emergency department immediately.

disease, have a clotting-factor disorder, use illegal drugs, or are male and have sex with other men.

A combination hepatitis A and B vaccine is available for adults who are at high risk of being exposed to both viruses. There's also an alternative rapid dosing schedule, which may be used if protection is needed more quickly than normal.

Hepatitis B

Hepatitis B is a viral liver disease spread by infected blood or body fluids, sexual contact, and prenatal exposure. The disease can result in liver damage or liver cancer.

Recommendation

The vaccination, which is administered in three doses, is recommended for the following groups:
- People whose sex partners have hepatitis B
- Sexually active individuals who aren't in a long-term monogamous relationship
- Men who have sexual contact with other men
- People who share needles, syringes or other drug-injection equipment
- People who have household contact with someone infected with the hepatitis B virus
- People in correctional facilities
- Victims of sexual assault or abuse

Recommended Adult Immunization Schedule

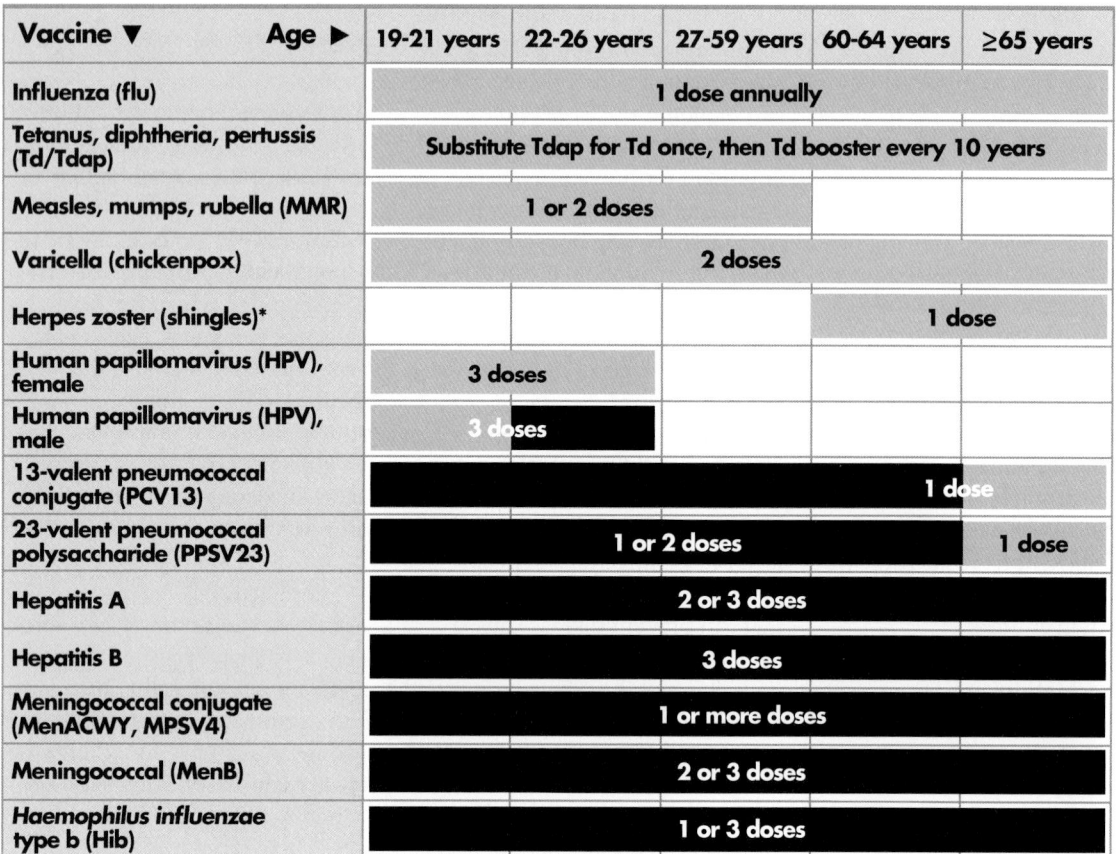

Vaccine ▼ Age ▶	19-21 years	22-26 years	27-59 years	60-64 years	≥65 years
Influenza (flu)	1 dose annually				
Tetanus, diphtheria, pertussis (Td/Tdap)	Substitute Tdap for Td once, then Td booster every 10 years				
Measles, mumps, rubella (MMR)	1 or 2 doses				
Varicella (chickenpox)	2 doses				
Herpes zoster (shingles)*				1 dose	
Human papillomavirus (HPV), female	3 doses				
Human papillomavirus (HPV), male	3 doses				
13-valent pneumococcal conjugate (PCV13)	1 dose				
23-valent pneumococcal polysaccharide (PPSV23)	1 or 2 doses				1 dose
Hepatitis A	2 or 3 doses				
Hepatitis B	3 doses				
Meningococcal conjugate (MenACWY, MPSV4)	1 or more doses				
Meningococcal (MenB)	2 or 3 doses				
Haemophilus influenzae type b (Hib)	1 or 3 doses				

Recommended for all adults

Recommended for certain high-risk groups

*Talk with your doctor about new shingles vaccination recommendations expected in 2018.
Source: Advisory Committee on Immunization Practices, Centers for Disease Control and Prevention, 2017

- Health care and public safety workers at risk of exposure to blood or body fluids
- Travelers to regions with increased rates of hepatitis B
- People with chronic liver disease, kidney disease, HIV infection or diabetes
- Anyone who wants to be protected from hepatitis B

A combination hepatitis A and B vaccine is available for adults who are at high risk of being exposed to both the hepatitis A and hepatitis B viruses. There's also an alternative rapid dosing schedule, which may be used if protection is needed more quickly than normal.

Human papillomavirus

Human papillomavirus (HPV) is the name for a group of viruses that includes more than 100 different strains or types. More than 30 of these viruses are sexually transmit-

ted and can infect the genital areas of men and women. HPV infection is a leading cause of cervical cancer.

Recommendation
The cervical cancer vaccine (Gardasil) is one of the first vaccines designed to prevent cancer. It blocks the most common cancer-causing types of HPV, in essence stopping the cancer before it can develop.

The vaccine is recommended for all girls and boys ages 11 or 12. It's also recommended for all women through age 26, all men through age 21 and the following through age 26, if they didn't get vaccinated when they were younger:
- Men who have sex with men, including young men who identify as gay or bisexual or who intend to have sex with men
- Individuals who are transgender
- Individuals with certain immunocompromising conditions, including HIV

Measles, mumps and rubella

Measles, mumps and German measles (rubella) are infectious viral diseases that can cause serious complications in adults. The viruses are spread from person to person through airborne droplets that are inhaled.

Recommendation
Anyone born after 1956 without documentation that he or she has had measles, mumps or rubella or the vaccines for those diseases should be immunized. One or two doses are recommended, especially for people in college, in the health care profession or traveling in a foreign country. The vaccination isn't recommended for people who are pregnant, have an impaired immune system, or recently received a blood transfusion or other blood products. Women

Flu (Influenza) Vaccines

A flu vaccination can keep you from getting the flu (influenza). And while the flu vaccine doesn't always provide total protection, it's still worth getting.

Influenza is a viral infection that sickens millions of people each year and can cause serious complications, especially in children and older adults.

The flu vaccine is generally offered between September and March, which is typically the flu season. Flu vaccines are designed to protect against strains of flu virus expected to be in circulation during the fall and winter. It takes up to two weeks to build immunity after a flu vaccine.

The Centers for Disease Control and Prevention (CDC) conducts studies each year to determine how well the flu vaccine protects against flu illness. While vaccine effectiveness can vary, recent studies show vaccine reduces the risk of flu illness by about 50 to 60 percent among the overall population during seasons when circulating flu viruses are like the vaccine viruses.

In some cases, people who receive the flu vaccine can still get the flu, but they may get a much less severe form of the illness and, most important, they'll have a decreased risk of flu-related complications — especially pneumonia, heart attack, stroke and death — to which older adults are especially vulnerable.

What are my options?
The flu vaccine comes in various forms:
- *A regular-dose shot.* A flu shot contains an inactivated vaccine made of killed virus. The shot is given in the arm. Because the viruses in the vaccine are killed (inactivated), the shot won't cause you to get the flu, but it will enable your body to develop the antibodies necessary to ward off influenza viruses. You may have a slight reaction to the shot, such as soreness at the injection site, mild muscle ache or fever. Reactions usually last one to two days and are more likely to occur in children who have never been exposed to the flu virus.
- *A high-dose shot.* Human immune defenses become weaker with age, which places older people at greater risk of severe illness from influenza. Also, aging decreases the body's ability to have a good immune response after getting influenza vaccine. An influenza vaccine is available that's designed specifically for people 65 years and older. A higher dose of antigen in the vaccine is supposed to give older people a better immune response and, therefore, better protection against flu.
- *A nasal spray.* The nasal spray vaccine, which is administered through your nose, consists of a low dose of live, but weakened, flu viruses. This type of vaccine was used primarily in young children. However, due to concerns about the effectiveness of the nasal spray vaccine, its use is under evaluation.

Why do I need to get vaccinated every year?
You need annual flu protection because the influenza virus changes from year to year. The flu vaccine you got last year wasn't designed to fight the virus strains in circulation this flu season. Influenza viruses mutate so quickly that they can render one season's vaccine ineffective by the next season.

Who should get the flu vaccine?
Everyone 6 months of age and older should get a flu vaccine every flu season.

Who shouldn't get the flu vaccine?
Don't get a flu shot if you:
- Have had an allergic reaction to the vaccine in the past.
- Are allergic to chicken eggs.
- Developed Guillain-Barré syndrome, a serious autoimmune disease affecting the nerves outside the brain and spinal cord, within six weeks of receiving the vaccine in the past.
- Have a moderate to severe acute illness. Wait until your symptoms improve before getting vaccinated.

Why do children need two doses of the flu vaccine?
Children younger than 9 years old require two doses of the flu vaccine if it's the first time they've been vaccinated for influenza. That's because children don't develop an adequate antibody level the first time they get the vaccine. Antibodies help fight the virus if it enters your child's system. If a flu vaccine shortage were to occur and your child couldn't get two doses of vaccine, one dose might still offer some protection.

should avoid pregnancy for 28 days after immunization.

Meningococcal disease

Meningococcal disease, caused by *Neisseria meningitidis* bacteria, can cause blood infection (septicemia) and meningitis, an infection of the brain and spinal cord coverings. Meningococcal disease can result in deafness, nervous system problems, seizures, strokes and death.

Recommendation
Vaccination for meningococcal disease is recommended for people considered at risk and travelers to countries where the disease is a concern. Because first-year college students, particularly those who live in dormitories, are at increased risk of getting the disease, they should consider getting vaccinated before starting college.

Three types of meningococcal vaccines are available:

- Meningococcal conjugate vaccines (Menactra, Menveo, MenHibrix)
- Meningococcal polysaccharide vaccine (Menomune)
- Serogroup B meningococcal vaccines (Bexsero, Trumenba)

Adolescents should be vaccinated with a meningococcal conjugate vaccine (Menactra or Menveo). Teens and young adults (16- through 23-year-olds) may be vaccinated with a serogroup B meningococcal vaccine. In certain situations, any of the three kinds of meningococcal vaccines may be recommended.

Serogroup B vaccines can't be interchanged, so check with the individual performing the vaccination to be sure you're receiving the same brand as your previous dose.

Pneumococcal disease

Pneumococcal disease is a serious bacterial infection that can cause pneumonia, bloodstream infections, ear infections, sinusitis and meningitis. The disease is most serious in older adults and individuals who are chronically ill.

Recommendation

Adults age 65 and older should receive two pneumococcal vaccines. The PCV13 vaccine is generally recommended first and the PPSV23 vaccine a year later. Some people may need PCV13 before age 65. Vaccination also is recommended for adults of any age who:

- Have a chronic medical condition, such as asthma, diabetes, or heart, lung or kidney disease
- Have an impaired immune system
- Have had their spleens removed
- Live in a nursing home or long-term care facility
- Have received an organ transplant
- Smoke tobacco

People who receive the vaccine at age 65 or later and who are generally healthy may need only one shot. Those who received their first shots before age 65 may need a booster shot. You can get a pneumococcal vaccination any time of the year,

Who Should Avoid Live Vaccines?

Weakened (attenuated) live vaccines usually are derived from the naturally occurring germ. They're made by passing the virus or bacterium through cell cultures over time until the germ's disease-causing ability has deteriorated. Attenuated live vaccines can infect people, but they typically don't cause disease. These vaccines include:
- Measles vaccine
- Mumps vaccine
- Rubella vaccine
- One type of influenza vaccine
- Chickenpox (varicella) vaccine
- Zoster vaccine

There's a very slight risk that attenuated live vaccines could cause disease if a person's immune system is weakened. For this reason, attenuated live vaccines aren't recommended for certain groups of people, including pregnant women and people with an impaired immune system. Women who get an attenuated live vaccine are advised to avoid pregnancy for up to three months afterward.

Check with your doctor before getting one of these vaccines if you:
- Have human immunodeficiency virus (HIV), AIDS or another disease that affects your immune system
- Are being treated with drugs that affect the immune system, such as steroids, for two weeks or longer
- Have cancer or are being treated for cancer
- Recently had a blood transfusion or received other blood products
- Have tuberculosis

but it's often convenient to get it when you receive your flu shot.

Shingles (herpes zoster)

Shingles is a painful localized skin rash often with blisters that's caused by the varicella-zoster virus, the same virus that causes chickenpox. Anyone who's had chickenpox can develop shingles because the varicella-zoster virus remains in the nerve cells of the body after the chickenpox infection clears. The virus can appear years later causing shingles.

Shingles is more common in older adults and in people with a weakened immune system.

Recommendation

The zoster vaccine can help prevent shingles in adults, even if they don't recall having had chickenpox. There are two vaccines — Zostavax and Shingrix. Shingrix is newer, more effective, and preferred by the CDC Advisory Committee on

Immunization Practices. At the time this book went to press, the Shingrix vaccine had received CDC approval but was awaiting official implementation.

The Shingrix vaccine is recommended for all adults age 50 and older, whether or not they've previously had shingles. People who received the Zostavax vaccine should also be vaccinated with Shingrix.

Tetanus and diphtheria

Tetanus is a bacterial infection that develops in contaminated wounds. Diphtheria is primarily a bacterial throat infection spread by breathing infected droplets from the air.

Recommendation

It's reasonable for adults to get a tetanus-diphtheria (Td) toxoid booster shot every 10 years. If you have a deep or dirty wound, you may need a booster shot if your last Td vaccination was more than five years ago. If you've never had a tetanus shot, you may need a three-dose series.

A newer vaccine called Tdap, which includes acellular pertussis (whooping cough), is recommended as a one-time booster shot and replaces one of the Td boosters. Whooping cough is a highly contagious respiratory infection that causes uncontrollable, strenuous coughing.

Preventive Screenings

Regular preventive screening exams and tests are the best method for catching potential problems in the early stages, when the odds for successful treatment are the greatest. Preventive screening exams are often performed during regular physical examinations.

Which preventive screening exams and tests are appropriate for you? Only you and your doctor can make that decision. However, there are some general guidelines for preventive exams.

Following is a list of exams and tests generally recommended for women and men without symptoms or risk factors for a particular medical condition.

If you have one or more risk factors for a disease, your doctor may order additional tests or perform certain tests more frequently.

Recommended screenings

These are the tests that you should undergo on a periodic basis. The following tests are for both men and women:

Blood cholesterol test
A blood cholesterol test is actually made up of several blood tests. A blood cholesterol test measures total cholesterol as well as low-density lipoprotein (LDL, or "bad") cholesterol, high-density lipoprotein (HDL, or "good") cholesterol and triglycerides, a type of blood fat.

LDL cholesterol deposits fatty substances on your artery walls. HDL cholesterol carries fatty deposits away from your arteries to your liver for disposal. Problems occur when your LDL cholesterol deposits too much of the fatty substances or when your HDL cholesterol carries away too little. This can lead to a buildup of fatty deposits (plaques) in your arteries, a condition called atherosclerosis.

What's the exam for?
It's to test the levels of cholesterol and triglycerides in your blood. Undesirable levels raise your risk of heart attack and stroke.

When and how often should you have it?
Have a baseline cholesterol evaluation at age 20, then have it checked every four to six years if the levels are within normal ranges. You may need to be screened earlier or more frequently if you have risk factors for heart disease or you have an abnormal blood cholesterol reading.

Blood pressure measurement
Blood pressure is determined by the amount of blood your heart pumps and the resistance to blood flow in your arteries. The test measures the peak pressure your heart generates when pumping blood out through your arteries (systolic blood pressure) and the amount of pressure in the arteries when your heart is at rest between beats (diastolic blood pressure).

What's the exam for?
It's for early detection of high blood pressure. In general, the more blood your heart pumps and the narrower your arteries, the harder your heart must work to pump the same amount of blood. The longer that high blood pressure goes undetected and untreated, the higher your risk of heart attack, stroke, heart failure and kidney damage.

When and how often should you have it?
You'll likely have your blood pressure measured when you see a doctor for any reason. Have this test done every three to five years if you're younger than age 40 and annually if you're age 40 or older or you have risk factors for high blood pressure.

Colon cancer screening
Colon cancer screening involves one or more tests to look for precancerous cells or signs of cancer in your colon. The screening may take one of several forms. Talk with your doctor about the goals and limitations of the following options:
- Stool tests
- Colonoscopy
- Sigmoidoscopy
- Stool DNA testing
- CT colonography

What's the exam for?
It's to detect cancer and precancerous growths (polyps) on the inside wall of the colon that may become cancerous. Many people skip colon cancer screening because of fear of embarrassment or discomfort. However, this screening could save your life by detecting growths before they turn cancerous or identifying cancer in its early stages when chances of curing the cancer are greatest.

When and how often should you have it?
For people at average risk, a colon cancer screening is recommended every five to 10 years, beginning after age 50. In low-risk individuals, stool DNA testing with Cologuard may be an acceptable alternative to other options. How often you should have a screening will depend on the test you receive, your doctor's recommendations and the results of the screening. If you're at high risk of colon cancer because of

family history or other factors, your doctor may recommend beginning screenings before age 50. For individuals who aren't at high risk of colon cancer, routine screenings can end at age 75. Depending on your health status, they may continue beyond age 75.

Dental checkup
During a dental checkup, your dentist examines your teeth and gums and checks for growths on your tongue, lips and soft tissues.

What's the exam for?
It's to detect cavities and diseases such as periodontal disease. Your doctor also looks for lesions and other abnormalities in your mouth that could indicate cancer.

When and how often should you have it?
Have your teeth checked twice a year or as your dentist recommends. Dental checkups should begin during childhood and continue throughout your adult life.

Eye exam
During an eye exam, an ophthalmologist or optometrist checks your vision and eye movement and looks for signs of disease.

What's the exam for?
It's to determine if you need corrective lenses and to identify if you may be at risk of diseases such as glaucoma, cataracts and age-related macular degeneration.

When and how often should you have it?
Adults with no risk factors for eye disease should have a baseline exam at age 40 and an eye exam every two to four years until age 54. At age 55 and after, have your eyes checked annually. You may need earlier and more frequent exams if you have risk factors for eye disease.

Fasting blood sugar test
This is a blood test that measures the level of sugar (glucose) in your blood after an eight-hour fast.

What's the exam for?
It's to check for high blood sugar levels, an indication of diabetes.

When and how often should you have it?
Have a baseline test by age 45. If the results are normal, have your blood sugar checked every three years. If you're at risk of diabetes because of family history or other factors, your doctor may recommend you be tested at a younger age and more frequently.

HIV screening
This involves a blood test.

What's the exam for?
It's to screen for human immunodeficiency virus (HIV), an infection that can lead to serious health problems. A positive test needs to be verified by a more specific blood test.

When and how often should you have it?
The U.S. Preventive Services Task Force recommends all people ages 15 to 65 be screened at least once for HIV. Those at increased risk should be tested more often.

Additional recommended screenings for women

Mammogram
In this screening examination, your breasts are compressed between plastic plates while a technologist takes X-rays of your breast tissue.

What's the exam for?
It's to detect cancer and precancerous changes in your breasts.

When and how often should you have it?
A baseline screening is generally recommended at age 40. Between ages 40 and 49, recommendations vary as to how often you should have a mammogram based on your risk factors. Talk to your doctor. After age 50, have the test every one to two years.

Pap test
In this test, your doctor inserts a plastic or metal speculum into your vagina. Then, using a soft brush, your doctor gently scrapes a few cells from your cervix, which are placed in a liquid-based medium for laboratory analysis.

What's the exam for?
It's to detect cancer and precancerous changes in your cervical tissue.

When and how often should you have it?
An initial Pap test should occur at age 21. Subsequent Pap tests are recommended every three years. If you're at high risk of cervical cancer or you have an abnormal test result, your doctor may recommend more frequent screening.

Women age 30 and older can consider Pap testing every five years if the procedure is combined with testing for human papillomavirus (HPV). HPV is a leading cause of cervical cancer.

Additional screenings women should consider

Women should consider having the health of their bones checked, especially after menopause.

Bone density test
A bone density test uses X-rays to measure how many grams of calcium and other bone minerals are packed into a segment of bone. Bones most commonly tested are in the spine, hip and forearm.

What's the exam for?
It's to detect osteoporosis, a disease involving loss of bone mass that can increase your risk of fractures.

When and how often should you have it?
Guidelines recommend all women

Recommended Age-Specific Tests for Women

Test	Ages 18-39	Ages 40-50	Older than 50
Breast cancer screening (mammogram)	Ask your doctor	Baseline at age 40, then ask your doctor	Every 1-2 years
Blood cholesterol test	Baseline by age 20, then every 4-6 years	Every 4-6 years	Every 4-6 years
Blood pressure measurement	Every 3-5 years	Annually	Annually
Cervical cancer screening (Pap test)	Every 3-5 years	Every 3-5 years	Every 3-5 years
Colon cancer screening	Ask your doctor	Ask your doctor	Usually every 5-10 years until age 75
Dental checkup	Every 6 months	Every 6 months	Every 6 months
Eye exam	Ask your doctor	Baseline at age 40, then every 2-4 years	Every 2-4 years to age 54, then annually
Fasting blood sugar test	Ask your doctor	Baseline by age 45, then every 3 years	Every 3 years
HIV screening	At least once between ages 15-65		

Other Tests Women Should Consider

Test	Ages 18-39	Ages 40-50	Older than 50
Bone density test	Ask your doctor	Ask your doctor	Baseline test at age 65
Chlamydia and gonorrhea screening	Ask your doctor	Ask your doctor	Ask your doctor
Clinical breast exam	Ask your doctor	Ask your doctor	Ask your doctor
Full-body skin exam	Ask your doctor	Ask your doctor	Ask your doctor
Hearing test	Ask your doctor	Ask your doctor	Baseline by age 60
Hepatitis B and C screening	Ask your doctor	Ask your doctor	Ask your doctor
Lung cancer screening	At least once between ages 55-80 in current or recent smokers		
Syphilis screening	Ask your doctor	Ask your doctor	Ask your doctor
Thyroid-stimulating hormone test	Ask your doctor	Ask your doctor	Ask your doctor
Tuberculosis screening	Ask your doctor	Ask your doctor	Ask your doctor

Recommended Age-Specific Tests for Men

Test	Ages 18-39	Ages 40-50	Older than 50
Blood cholesterol test	Baseline by age 20, then every 4-6 years	Every 4-6 years	Every 4-6 years
Blood pressure measurement	Every 3-5 years	Annually	Annually
Colon cancer screening	Ask your doctor	Ask your doctor	Usually every 5-10 years until age 75
Dental checkup	Every 6 months	Every 6 months	Every 6 months
Eye exam	Ask your doctor	Baseline at age 40, then every 2-4 years	Every 2-4 years to age 54, then annually
Fasting blood sugar test	Ask your doctor	Baseline by age 45, then every 3 years	Every 3 years
HIV screening	At least once between ages 15-65		

Other Tests Men Should Consider

Test	Ages 18-39	Ages 40-50	Older than 50
Bone density test	Ask your doctor	Ask your doctor	Baseline test at age 70
Full-body skin exam	Ask your doctor	Ask your doctor	Ask your doctor
Hearing test	Ask your doctor	Ask your doctor	Baseline by age 60
Hepatitis B and C screening	Ask your doctor	Ask your doctor	Ask your doctor
Lung cancer screening	At least once between ages 55-80 in current or recent smokers		
Prostate-specific antigen (PSA) test	Ask your doctor	Ask your doctor	Ask your doctor
Syphilis screening	Ask your doctor	Ask your doctor	Ask your doctor
Thyroid-stimulating hormone test	Ask your doctor	Ask your doctor	Ask your doctor
Tuberculosis screening	Ask your doctor	Ask your doctor	Ask your doctor
Ultrasound of abdominal aorta	Once between ages 65-75 in men who have ever smoked		

age 65 and older have a bone density test to screen for osteoporosis. Women at increased risk of bone fracture should have the test at an earlier age.

Clinical breast exam
This is a physical examination of the breasts and armpits performed by a doctor.

What's the exam for?
It's to detect cancer and precancerous changes in the breasts. Your doctor carefully examines your breasts, looking for lumps, color changes, skin irregularities and changes in your nipples. He or she then feels for swollen lymph nodes in the arm pits.

When and how often should you have it?
In women with no family history of breast cancer, many professional organizations don't recommend doctors perform a regular clinical breast exam. If you have a strong family history of breast cancer or other factors that place you at high risk, talk to your doctor about having a yearly clinical breast exam.

Chlamydia and gonorrhea screening
Chlamydia and gonorrhea screening is done either through a urine test or a swab from a woman's cervix. The sample is then analyzed in a laboratory.

What's the exam for?
Chlamydia and gonorrhea are common sexually transmitted infections. The infections are usually spread during unprotected sexual activity, but they can be passed from mother to child during childbirth.

When and how often should you have it?
Sexually active women age 24 and younger should be screened for both chlamydia and gonorrhea. Women older than age 24 at increased risk of these infections also should be screened.

Additional screenings men should consider

Men should consider having the health of their prostate glands checked, especially after age 50.

Digital rectal exam and prostate-specific antigen test
During a digital rectal exam, your doctor inserts a lubricated gloved finger into your rectum and feels the prostate gland for lumps or a variation in texture. These changes can raise suspicion for the presence of cancer.

The prostate-specific antigen (PSA) test is a blood test that measures the amount of a specific protein secreted by the prostate gland.

What's the exam for?
A digital rectal exam can detect noncancerous enlargement of the prostate gland (benign prostatic hyperplasia, or BPH), or it can detect suspicious nodules that may be associated with prostate cancer. Elevated results on a PSA test can indicate the possibility of prostate cancer. However, above normal PSA levels may stem from BPH or other noncancerous conditions as well.

When and how often should you have it?
After age 50, have a digital rectal exam annually.

Recommendations vary as to whether you should have a PSA test. Agencies such as the U.S. Preventive Task Force recommend against PSA screening, indicating that the harms of the test are greater than its potential benefit. But not all doctors and organizations agree with this recommendation.

Talk to your doctor about PSA screening — its potential benefits and drawbacks.

Bone density measurement
This test involves a specialized X-ray scan of your lower back and hip region.

What's the exam for?
It's to detect osteoporosis, a disease involving loss of bone mass that can increase your risk of bone fractures.

When and how often should you have it?
Guidelines recommend all men age 70 and older have a bone density test to screen for osteoporosis. Men at increased risk of bone fracture should have the test at an earlier age.

Ultrasound of abdominal aorta
This is an ultrasound examination of your abdomen.

What's the exam for?
It's used to detect weakening (ballooning) in the wall of the major artery that leads from the heart and runs through the abdomen (aorta). Weakness in a blood vessel wall puts you at high risk of an aneurysm — bulging of a blood vessel.

When and how often should you have it?
Men ages 65 and older who are current or former tobacco smokers are at highest risk of an abdominal aortic aneurysm. Men ages 65 to 75 who smoke or have smoked in the past should be screened for this condition. If you never smoked, talk to your doctor.

Screenings for women and men to consider

Ask your doctor which of these may be appropriate for you:

Full-body skin exam
Your doctor examines your skin from head to toe, looking for moles or other growths that are irregularly shaped, have varied colors, are asymmetric, or have grown or changed since the previous visit.

What's the exam for?
It's to check for skin cancer.

When and how often should you have it?

The American Academy of Dermatology encourages everyone to perform skin self-exams to check for signs of skin cancer and get a skin exam from a doctor during a routine physical. A dermatologist can make individual recommendations as to how often to have skin exams based on personal risk factors.

Hearing test

During a hearing test, a doctor checks how well you recognize speech and sound at various volumes and frequencies.

What's the exam for?

It's to screen for hearing loss.

When and how often should you have it?

A baseline test is recommended between ages 50 and 60. If you've been exposed to loud noises or suspect hearing loss, you may want to have a baseline test earlier.

Hepatitis screening

This is a blood test.

What's the exam for?

It's to screen for chronic hepatitis B or chronic hepatitis C. People with chronic hepatitis B or C are at greater risk of liver disease, including cancer.

When and how often should you have it?

If you're at high risk of becoming infected with hepatitis B or C (see pages 235 and 876), you should get screened for the illness. Your doctor may recommend the test if you have one or more risk factors.

Lung cancer screening

This exam is performed by taking a computerized tomography (CT) image of the lungs.

What's the exam for?

It's to detect cancer and precancerous changes in your lungs.

Gathering a Family History

In preparation for a physical examination, you might want to gather information about any childhood illnesses, accidents or operations.

It's important for your doctor to know about any genetic diseases in your family, such as Huntington's disease or sickle cell anemia. Parents can pass these ailments to their children, although not always to every child in each generation.

Similarly, many common diseases have apparent familial links. For example, if your father has heart disease, it doesn't necessarily mean that you'll also have heart disease. But your doctor should know about the history of this illness in your family so that he or she can watch for early signs and recommend preventive measures that may reduce other controllable risk factors.

To assemble a family history, make a list of any chronic diseases affecting your parents, grandparents, brothers, sisters, children, and even aunts and uncles. Keep track of whether the diseases are on your mother's or your father's side of the family. Such diseases include high blood pressure, diabetes, Alzheimer's disease, kidney disease, cardiovascular disease, and cancers of the breast, uterus, ovaries, colon and prostate. In addition, record any unusual diseases — even those that you don't believe are hereditary — and note if any immediate relatives died at a young age of an illness.

Provide this information to your primary care doctor to be included in your medical record.

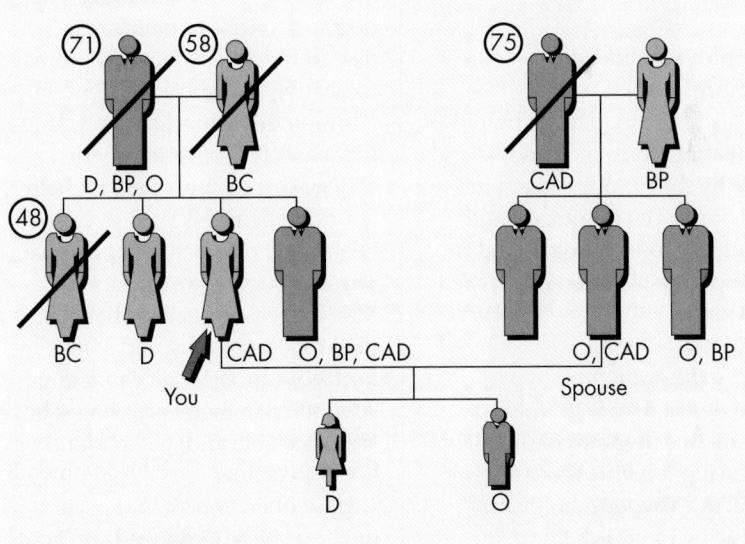

BC = Breast cancer
D = Diabetes
O = Obesity
CAD = Coronary artery disease
BP = High blood pressure

/ = Deceased
◯ = Age at death

Above is an example of a family tree that charts a family medical history.

When and how often should you have it?

Adults between the ages of 55 and 80 who are at high risk of lung cancer because they're current smokers or they've quit smoking within the past 15 years should be screened.

Syphilis screening

This also is a blood test.

What's the exam for?

Syphilis is caused by a spirochete bacterium. It's usually passed from person to person through sexual contact. It also can pass from mother to baby during pregnancy. The number of cases of syphilis has been increasing.

When and how often should you have it?

The U.S. Preventive Services Task Force recommends that all people who are at increased risk of syphilis (see page 474) be screened. Screening is also recommended for all pregnant women.

Thyroid-stimulating hormone test

This also is a blood test. Thyroid-stimulating hormone (TSH) is made by the pituitary gland in your brain. The pituitary gland stimulates your thyroid gland to produce its active hormone called thyroxine.

What's the exam for?

It's to detect if your thyroid is underactive (hypothyroidism), producing too little thyroxine, or overactive (hyperthyroidism), producing too much thyroxine.

When and how often should you have it?

There's no agreement among experts. Ask if you should be screened based on your personal health.

Tuberculosis (latent) screening

There are two types of screening tests for latent tuberculosis: a skin test and a blood test.

What's the exam for?

Tuberculosis is an infection caused by the bacterium *Mycobacterium tuberculosis* that most commonly affects the lungs. Active tuberculosis is highly contagious and is spread through the air. Latent tuberculosis is a dormant disease that produces no symptoms but can activate at any time.

When and how often should you have it?

Screening is recommended in all adults at increased risk of infection. This includes health care workers, people who work in high-risk settings such as correctional facilities, and people who come from countries where tuberculosis is common.

When to See a Doctor

Make an appointment to see your doctor if you have pain, shortness of breath or other symptoms indicating a medical problem. In addition, see your doctor on a regular basis for preventive care.

Regular preventive exams help your doctor assess your overall health and risk factors for disease. These checkups are important. Many diseases, such as diabetes, high blood pressure and some forms of cancer, don't cause any symptoms in their early stages but are detectable and, when found early, treatable.

How often you should get a medical checkup depends on your age, your health and your family medical history.

Finding a primary care doctor

A key step in preventive health and overall management of your health is developing an ongoing relationship with a primary care doctor who oversees all aspects of your medical care. Ideally, a primary care doctor is someone who knows you, your family health history, and the conditions under which you live and work that may impact your health.

This person treats problems as they arise and makes sure you receive basic screening tests to prevent disease or catch it early when it can most easily be treated. Your primary care doctor will refer you to a specialist when you need to see one for a complex or unusual medical problem. He or she also makes sure that one treatment you're receiving doesn't conflict with another. This is particularly important if you have long-term or multiple health problems that require consultations with various specialists.

A primary care doctor is usually a specialist in family medicine, internal medicine, obstetrics and gynecology, or pediatrics. A family medicine doctor has training in almost every aspect of medicine, including obstetrics and pediatrics. An internist is a doctor who specializes in the diagnosis and treatment of health problems that occur in adults. A pediatrician specializes in diseases of children and adolescents.

Increasingly, primary care is being provided by other trained and qualified individuals, such as physician assistants or nurse practitioners.

If you're looking for a primary care doctor, you can check with the American Medical Association (AMA) to get a list of doctors in your area. Also ask your friends, colleagues and neighbors for recommendations.

As you're researching potential primary care doctors, and during your first visit to his or her office, here are some questions that may help you decide if this individual is right for you and your family:
- Is the receptionist warm and friendly? Does this person answer your questions directly?
- What are the office hours?

- How much time does the doctor allot for appointments?
- Does the doctor accept your insurance plan?
- How and where would you get emergency care outside of normal office hours?
- What hospital does the doctor use?

Basic physical examination

A physical examination generally includes a discussion with your doctor about any current symptoms or concerns and your lifestyle habits. You also may review past health problems and your family health history, as well as undergo a head-to-toe examination.

What to expect
During the exam, anticipate that your doctor or a nurse will likely:
- Check your height, weight, blood pressure and heart rate
- Check the inside of your mouth
- Examine your eyes, ears, nose, neck (thyroid gland) and skin
- Feel for swollen lymph nodes in your neck, armpits and groin

- Listen for abnormal sounds from your heart, lungs or abdomen
- Feel for abnormalities or enlargements in your abdomen, especially your liver, spleen or kidneys
- Check your pulse in your neck, groin and feet
- Check reflexes

He or she also may perform certain screening tests depending on your age, your health and family history, and how long it's been since your last test.

Keep in mind that your doctor may not check everything. If you have specific concerns — for example, you're losing weight for no apparent reason or you've noticed that you're becoming increasingly short of breath — mention this to your doctor so that he or she can appropriately evaluate the problem.

When to have one
How often you need a complete physical examination depends on a variety of factors including your sex, age, health history and risk factors for specific conditions,

as well as your doctor's recommendations.

In the past, it was often recommended that you have a physical exam yearly. This often isn't necessary. A good rule of thumb would be to get a checkup at the following intervals. At your first checkup, you and your doctor can discuss what schedule fits your individual needs.
- Two times in your 20s
- Three times in your 30s
- Four times in your 40s
- Five times in your 50s
- Annually after age 60

When to See a Specialist

There may be times when your primary care provider may be uncertain about a diagnosis or about the best treatment for your problem. In this case, he or she may refer you to a specialist.

Seeing a doctor with specific training in a certain area may be necessary and to your benefit if:

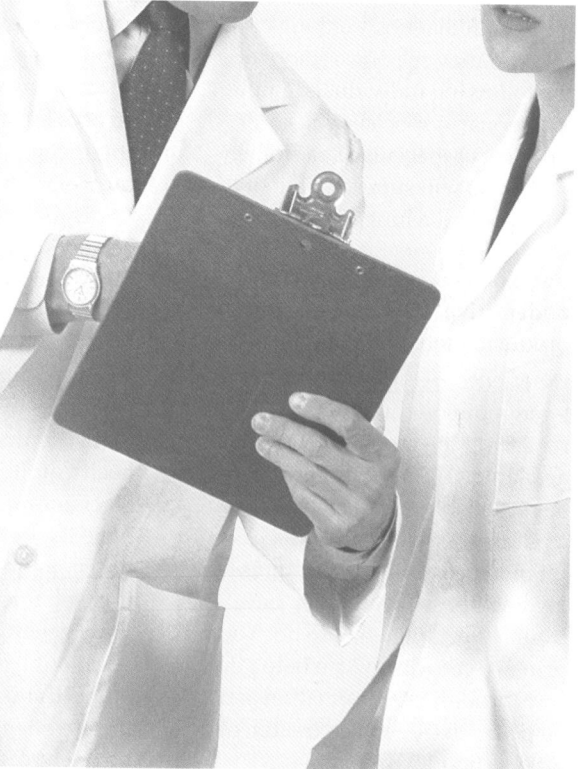

Second Opinions

There may come a time, especially if an illness develops, when you would like a second opinion before proceeding with a treatment recommended by your primary care doctor. In addition, some health insurance plans require a second opinion before agreeing to cover certain procedures.

Either you or your doctor can initiate the process of seeking a second opinion. A good personal physician should have no reservations about referring you to a specialist, when appropriate. Second opinions may also be useful when the diagnosis is unclear or when the choice of treatments isn't clear-cut.

A second opinion may also be in your best interest if:
- A condition for which you've received a diagnosis is serious
- The treatment your doctor advises is risky, experimental or controversial
- Major surgery appears necessary

If you'd like a second opinion to consider more options, tell your doctor so.

- You or your doctor would like a second opinion about your diagnosis or management options
- You have a rare disease or unusual manifestations of a common disease
- You need a special procedure or an operation
- You aren't responding to current therapy
- Your disease is progressing especially rapidly or new complications are developing

Your personal physician may refer you to a specialist that he or she works with frequently. Your doctor may contact the specialist, brief the specialist about your case and schedule an appointment for you. Or you can locate a specialist on your own.

Before you see a specialist, put together a list of questions that you want to ask that person. Be prepared that the specialist is likely to ask you about your medical history and he or she may repeat some of the tests you've already undergone. Nevertheless, have a copy of your medical records with you.

Often, areas of expertise overlap. For instance, if you've received a diagnosis of lung cancer, you may see one or more of the following individuals: a lung (pulmonary) specialist, a cancer (oncology) specialist, a radiotherapist who will supervise radiation therapy, and a lung (thoracic) surgeon.

Remember that medicine isn't an exact science. Different doctors — each highly qualified and experienced — may have different opinions and preferences regarding the therapies currently available. All the treatments may be reasonable, but each will have advantages and disadvantages.

Some people find this confusing and stressful, and they have trouble deciding what to do. Your primary care doctor can help you sort through the information and help you decide which treatment may be best for you.

Developing a Good Relationship

Better care and better health results when you actively participate in your health care and you work in partnership with your doctor and other medical professionals.

In this partnership, both you and your doctor each have important roles. Here are some suggestions to help the two of you work well together.

Expectations of your doctor

When you see a doctor, you likely have certain expectations regarding actions he or she should take or information that he or she should provide:

- **Reasonable access.** You should be able to make an appointment to see your doctor within a reasonable amount of time.
- **Time.** You should be allowed a reasonable length of time to ask questions and discuss concerns.
- **Timely appointments.** You should be able to see your doctor within a reasonable length of time once you arrive for your appointment. But realize that he or she may be called away on occasion to address medical emergencies.
- **Information.** You're entitled to as much information as you need regarding your illness.
- **Confidentiality.** Your condition and medical records are your and your doctor's business. For some conditions, such as certain infectious diseases, law requires that your doctor notify public health authorities.
- **Decision-making ability.** You have the right to participate in decisions about your care. This is called informed consent.
- **Emergency contacts.** Your doctor should give you information on how and where to go for care in case of an emergency, when he or she can't be reached.

Your responsibilities

You also have certain responsibilities. Your doctor expects that you:

- **Be on time for appointments.** If you must cancel, do so at least 24 hours in advance. This allows your doctor to see other people during that appointment time.
- **Be honest about the medications you take.** Let your doctor know of all of the medications you're taking, including over-the-counter medicines, vitamins and supplements. List them or bring in the medication bottles. This allows your doctor to review and assess what you're taking, to make sure certain medications aren't causing symptoms or interacting with one another.
- **Answer questions accurately and completely.** Having all of the information that you can provide helps your doctor better monitor your health, assess any health risks you may have and make the proper diagnosis, if one is needed.
- **Be informed.** If you have a disorder or illness, take time to learn about it, including treatment recommendations and steps that you can take to improve the prognosis.
- **Follow treatment recommendations.** When your doctor prescribes a medication or another type of treatment, do what he or she recommends.
- **Ask questions.** If you don't understand something, ask your doctor to clarify it for you until you do. Understand what your doctor and his or her staff are doing and why. To follow through on recommendations, you need to understand why a particular course of action is being prescribed.
- **Be proactive.** Contact your doctor if you experience any unexpected events or problems, or you feel that something isn't right. Don't wait for your signs and symptoms to become severe. ■

Nutrition and Weight

Whether you eat to live or live to eat, you no doubt take some interest in food. It's one of the great pleasures of life and a life-giving essential. Food is so important that from the beginning of recorded history, it has formed the basis for rituals in every society.

The food you eat is the source of energy and nutrition for your body. Getting enough food isn't a common problem for most Americans, but good nutrition can be a challenge. Many chronic diseases, including cardiovascular disease, diabetes, osteoporosis and cancer, are in part caused by eating too much of the wrong foods and not enough of the right ones.

According to the World Health Organization (WHO), unhealthy diets and physical inactivity contribute to millions of deaths worldwide each year. The number of people who are overweight or obese is high. Being overweight increases your risk of developing several diseases.

For these reasons, eating well and maintaining a healthy weight are crucial components of a healthy lifestyle. The decisions you make every day about selecting and preparing food affect how you feel and how well you'll live in the years ahead. To feel good, ward off disease and perform at a peak level, you should eat a nutritionally balanced diet.

Contrary to popular opinion, eating more healthfully doesn't have to require drastic changes in your diet. To eat well, you don't have to give up your favorite foods or spend a lot of time pouring over new recipes, scrutinizing labels and searching out exotic foods. For most people, a few small changes can make a big difference in their health.

This chapter provides an overview of the basics of good nutrition, as well as recommended dietary guidelines for all Americans. It looks at a number of healthy-eating plans and discusses the role of diet in preventing and managing certain diseases. By applying the principles outlined in this chapter to your daily eating habits, you should be able to maintain a healthy weight, keep your energy up and get the nutrients you need.

Nutrition Basics

No single food provides all of the nutrients that your body needs for good health. Eating a variety of foods ensures that you get the nutrients and other substances associated with good health.

A healthy diet is one that emphasizes vegetables, fruits, whole grains, heart-healthy fats such as nuts and olive oil, and lean sources of protein, including beans, fish, low-fat dairy products and lean meats. Such foods optimize nutrition and help promote a healthy weight. Simply by eating more plant-based foods — grains, fruits, vegetables and legumes — you can add more variety and health-enhancing nutrients to your diet.

Nutrition isn't the only reason to add variety. Choosing among many flavors, colors and textures in food also boosts your satisfaction and pleasure. If, for example, your fruit choice is limited to bananas, you're missing out on the sensual delights of other fruits — blackberries, kiwis and mangoes, to name a few.

Learning more about how your body uses the nutrients that different foods provide can help you better understand how eating patterns affect your health.

Key nutrients

Every day your body requires a certain amount of energy to function properly. Energy is provided by the major components in foods — carbohydrates, proteins and fats. Other compounds in food are needed in much smaller amounts. These include essential amino acids, fatty acids, minerals and vitamins. Each food component has a different function in the regulation, growth and repair of your body's cells.

Carbohydrates

Carbohydrates are your body's main energy source — the primary fuel for your cells. Carbohydrates are starches or sugars. Starches — found primarily in bread, rice, pasta, cereals, fruits and vegetables — are known as complex carbohydrates. Sugars — found in fruits, milk and foods made with sugar — are called simple carbohydrates. Digestion changes complex carbohydrates into simple sugars, the fuel your body uses.

Complex carbohydrates can be whole grain or refined. Whole-grain carbohydrates contain the endosperm (which is mostly starch), the bran (which contains fiber), and the germ (which contains nutrients and a small amount of healthy fat). Refined grains, such as white flour, contain only the endosperm and few nutrients. Whole grains are much healthier than refined grains.

For most people, about half of their daily calories should come from carbohydrates. Try to get most of them from whole-grain carbohydrates. Cane or beet sugar (sucrose) and high-fructose corn syrup make up a considerable portion of the average American diet. Unlike whole-grain carbohydrates and natural sugars found in milk and fruits, sucrose and high-fructose corn syrup contain no significant nutrients.

Fiber

Fiber is the part of plant foods that your body doesn't absorb. Two types of fiber are soluble and insoluble. Some foods are higher in soluble fiber. These include citrus fruits, strawberries, apples, legumes, oatmeal and oat bran. Soluble fiber may help lower blood cholesterol and blood sugar levels. It also absorbs water and provides bulk, helping to prevent constipation.

Insoluble fiber is found in wheat bran, whole-grain breads, pasta, cereals and many vegetables. Insoluble fiber also helps reduce constipation.

For men and women through age 50, 38 and 25 grams of fiber, respectively, is recommended. For men and women older than age 50, 30 and 21 grams, respectively, is recommended. Most Americans get less than half this amount.

Protein

Your body needs protein to make and maintain tissues, such as muscles and organs. Protein is composed of building blocks called amino acids. Your body naturally produces some — but not all — amino acids. Those that must be obtained from the foods you eat are called essential amino acids.

You can get protein from a variety of sources. Grains and vegetables supply small amounts. A plant-based diet that includes a wide variety of grains, legumes, vegetables, nuts and seeds can meet your daily protein needs. Meat, seafood, poultry, eggs, soy products and dairy products are the richest sources of protein. Studies suggest that for overall health, protein from plants is better than protein from animal sources.

The amount of protein people need depends on their weight. As an example, someone who weighs 176 pounds should get 64 grams of protein daily.

Fat

Fat is your most concentrated calorie source. Some fat in your diet is necessary for your body to function properly. But too much of the less healthy fat can have a negative effect on your health.

Fat comes in different forms. It's found in foods of animal origin, such as meat, poultry and fish, and in foods of vegetable origin, such as avocados and olives.

Chemists classify fat according to the molecular structure of its building blocks (fatty acids). Those that your body can't make are called essential, and must be supplied by the foods you eat. Other types of fatty acids are saturated and unsaturated. Unsaturated fat is further subdivided into mono-unsaturated, polyunsaturated and trans.

Many foods contain a mixture of fatty acids. For example, although olive oil is termed a monounsaturated fat, it also contains small amounts of both saturated and polyunsaturated fatty acids.

Dietary guidelines recommend saturated fat be limited to less than 10 percent of your daily calories.

Saturated fat

Saturated fat is usually solid or waxy at room temperature. It's less likely to turn rancid, which is why it's used in many processed foods that must withstand long storage times. Foods high in saturated fat include butter, cheese, whole milk, cream, chocolate, coconut oil, lard and solid short-enings. Meat — including beef, pork and lamb — can be high in fat, most of it saturated. In poultry, most of the fat is found in the skin.

Polyunsaturated fat

Polyunsaturated fat is usually liquid at room temperature and in the refrigerator. Foods high in this type of fat include vegetable oils, such as safflower, corn, sunflower, soy and cottonseed oils.

Monounsaturated fat

Monounsaturated fat is liquid at room temperature but begins to solidify in the refrigerator. Foods high in monounsaturated fat are olive, peanut and canola oils, avocados, and most nuts.

Trans fat

Trans fat generally comes from adding hydrogen to vegetable oil through a process called hydrogenation. This makes the fat more solid and less likely to spoil. Partially hydrogenated fat is a common ingredient in commercial baked goods and many other processed foods. Manufacturers are limiting their use, but check food labels. Most margarines

Fat and Blood Cholesterol

Different types of dietary fat have different effects on blood cholesterol. Your total blood cholesterol level can be divided into two major parts: low-density lipoprotein (LDL) cholesterol — commonly referred to as the "bad" cholesterol — and high-density lipoprotein (HDL) cholesterol — commonly referred to as the "good" cholesterol. LDL cholesterol is deposited in your arteries, narrowing them and increasing your risk of cardiovascular diseases, such as a heart attack. HDL cholesterol removes cholesterol deposits from your artery walls, reducing your risk of cardiovascular disease.

Saturated and trans fats raise LDL ("bad") cholesterol, while polyunsaturated and monounsaturated fats can lower LDL cholesterol. Trans fats have the additional disadvantage of lowering HDL ("good") cholesterol. Therefore, polyunsaturated and monounsaturated fats have the healthiest effect on blood cholesterol levels.

What this means is that in your daily diet you want to consume mainly monounsaturated fats, such as olive or canola oil, and polyunsaturated fat from vegetable oils. Avoid or limit saturated fats and trans fats. Most saturated fat comes from meat and dairy products and trans fat from processed foods.

and shortenings also are high in trans fat.

Water

Water seems so ordinary that you may forget how vital it is to health. Water plays an important role in nearly every major body function. It regulates body temperature, carries nutrients and oxygen to cells and removes wastes. Water also cushions joints and helps protect organs and tissues.

Most healthy adults can count on thirst for proper hydration. Some circumstances call for more water, such as when you're sweating on a hot day, exercising vigorously or breast-feeding. Young children and older adults may not sense thirst, so it's important they're offered water regularly.

The Institute of Medicine recommends roughly 13 cups of total fluid a day for men, and about 9 cups daily for women. You also may have heard the phrase, "Drink eight 8-ounce glasses of water a day." The "8 by 8" rule isn't that different from the Institute of Medicine's recommendations, and it's easy to remember.

You can meet part of your water requirement with fluids such as low-fat milk, unsweetened juice and soup.

To increase water consumption:
- Take frequent water breaks.
- Keep bottled water with you at work and when traveling.
- Drink a glass of water with your meals and snacks.
- Substitute sparkling water for alcoholic drinks at gatherings.

Vitamins

Vitamins play a role in many body functions. They enable your body to process proteins, carbohydrates and fat. Certain vitamins also help produce blood cells, hormones, genetic material and nervous system chemicals. Because your body is unable to synthesize adequate amounts of most vitamins, you need to get them from the foods you eat.

The 14 essential vitamins are divided into two categories: fat-soluble and water-soluble.

Fat-soluble

The fat-soluble vitamins are A, D, E and K. They're stored in body fat. Vitamins A and D are also stored in the liver, and reserve supplies may last as long as six months. Reserves of vitamin K, however, may be sufficient for only a few days, and the supply of vitamin E is somewhere in between. Because they're stored, excess amounts of vitamins A and D potentially can accumulate in your body and reach toxic levels.

Water-soluble

The water-soluble vitamins include C, choline, biotin and seven more B vitamins. They're stored in the body to a lesser extent than are fat-soluble vitamins.

Some people believe that water-soluble vitamins are harmless, even when taken in large amounts, but this isn't always true. Consuming excessive amounts of some water-soluble vitamins, including vitamins B-6, folic acid (B-9), niacin (B-3) and C, can have adverse effects.

Minerals

Your body also needs 16 minerals to function properly. Major minerals (macrominerals) include calcium, magnesium, phosphorus, potassium, sodium and chloride. Calcium, phosphorus and magnesium are important in the development and health of your bones and teeth. Sodium, potassium and chloride, known as electrolytes,

Vitamin D

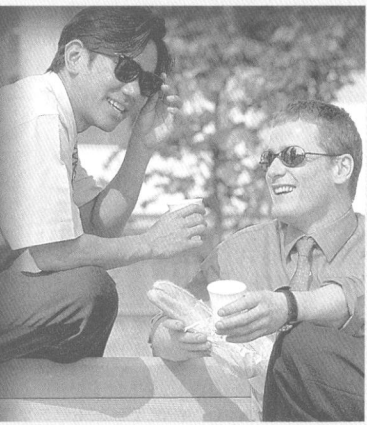

Calcium is essential for strong bones, but to enhance the amount of calcium that reaches your bones, you also need vitamin D.

Your body makes vitamin D from two sources — sunlight and food. Most of the vitamin D in your body results from sun exposure. When you're exposed to ultraviolet light rays, a chemical in your skin is converted into a form of vitamin D. Your liver and kidneys then change it into an active form that your body can use.

Egg yolks and fatty fish, such as herring, mackerel and salmon, naturally contain vitamin D. Several food products also are fortified with vitamin D, such as milk and some breakfast cereals.

Some people don't get enough vitamin D, either due to lack of exposure to sunlight or not eating foods that contain the vitamin. In addition, with age, the skin becomes less efficient at synthesizing vitamin D, and the body is less able to absorb it from food.

If you don't eat foods containing vitamin D or you rarely spend time outdoors, you might want to take a vitamin D supplement to meet your daily requirement. The recommended amount is 600 international units (IUs) daily through age 70 and 800 IUs for adults older than age 70. Some researchers and organizations suggest 1,500 to 2,000 IUs daily for optimal health. Talk to your doctor about the amount that's best for you.

Excessive sun exposure isn't healthy for your skin, but a little bit of sun — about 15 minutes a day — can be good for your bones.

Vitamin and Mineral Supplements

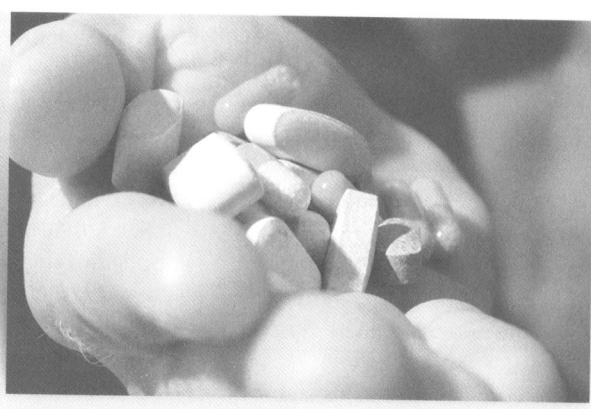

You can get your entire daily requirement of vitamin C by eating an orange — or by taking a vitamin C tablet. So which is better? In the vast majority of cases, the orange. The best way to get the vitamins and minerals you need is through food, not supplements.

Many American adults take vitamin supplements regularly. Some people regard them as essential food replacements. Others see them as harmless insurance. But supplements can't provide important elements found in food. And there's little evidence that multivitamins are beneficial to your health.

Before taking any supplement other than a standard multivitamin and mineral supplement, check with your doctor or a registered dietitian. It's also important that you not take more than the recommended amount. Many nutrients can be harmful if taken in large amounts.

Benefits of food

Whole foods provide a number of benefits that you can't find in a pill:

- *Whole foods are complex.* They contain a variety of the nutrients your body needs. An orange, for example, provides not only vitamin C but also beta carotene, calcium and other nutrients. Supplements contain only limited nutrients.
- *Whole foods provide fiber.* Fiber is important for digestion and may help prevent heart disease, diabetes and constipation.
- *Whole foods contain phytochemicals.* Fruits and vegetables contain substances called phytochemicals, such as lycopene or flavonoids. Phytochemicals are naturally occurring compounds that plants produce to protect themselves against bacteria, viruses or fungi. Unlike vitamins and minerals, phytochemicals aren't necessary to survive, but they may help protect against a variety of diseases, including cancer, heart disease, osteoporosis and diabetes.

Who needs supplements?

For most people, a healthy diet provides adequate vitamins and minerals. However, a vitamin or mineral supplement may be appropriate if:

- *You're age 50 or older.* As you get older, health problems may lead to a poor diet, making it difficult for you to get the vitamins and minerals you need. In addition, your body may not be able to absorb vitamins B-12 and D as well as it used to, making supplementation of these nutrients more necessary.
- *You're postmenopausal.* For some women, it can be difficult to obtain the recommended amounts of calcium and vitamin D without supplementation. Both calcium and vitamin D supplements have been shown to protect against osteoporosis. Some men also may benefit from vitamin D and calcium. A small proportion of older men develop osteoporosis.
- *You don't eat well.* If you don't eat the recommended daily servings of fruits and vegetables, taking a multivitamin supplement may be reasonable. However, your best course of action is to adopt better eating habits. There's no evidence a multivitamin can compensate for a poor diet.
- *You're on a very low-calorie diet.* If you eat fewer than 1,000 calories a day, you may benefit from a vitamin and mineral supplement.
- *You smoke.* Tobacco decreases the absorption of many vitamins and minerals, including vitamin B-6, vitamin B-12, vitamin C, folate and niacin.
- *You drink alcohol excessively.* Excessive alcohol use can impair digestion and absorption of thiamin, folate and vitamins A, D and B-12. Altered metabolism also affects minerals such as zinc, selenium, magnesium and phosphorus.
- *You're planning to become pregnant, are pregnant or are breast-feeding.* During these times, you need more of certain nutrients, especially folic acid — the synthetic form of folate. Folic acid helps prevent neural tube defects, such as spina bifida, in the fetus. Iron supplements taken during pregnancy can help prevent anemia in the mother.
- *You eat a special diet or have a chronic condition.* If your diet has limited variety because of intolerance or a food allergy, you may benefit from a vitamin and mineral supplement. If you're a vegan who eliminates all animal products from your diet, you may need additional vitamin B-12 and zinc. If you don't eat dairy products and don't get 15 minutes of sun exposure each day, you may need to supplement your diet with calcium and vitamin D.

Some medical conditions and certain medications can increase your need for nutrients while impairing your appetite or the way your body handles nutrients. In these cases, special supplements may be necessary.

help regulate the water and chemical balance in your body. Potassium is also important to muscle and your cells.

Your body needs smaller amounts of the remaining minerals, known as trace minerals (microminerals). These include iron, iodine, zinc, copper, fluoride, selenium and manganese, among others.

For young children, teenage girls and women of childbearing age, it's especially important to get adequate iron to allow for growth and development and prevent diseases such as iron deficiency anemia. Foods high in iron include:

- Shellfish, such as shrimp, clams, mussels and oysters
- Lean meats, especially beef, and organ meats, which are also high in cholesterol
- Dark turkey meat
- Sardines
- Spinach and other dark leafy greens
- Dried beans, peas and lentils
- Cereals with added iron
- Enriched and whole-grain breads

While many foods that contain iron are animal-based, the prevalence of iron deficiency isn't increased on a vegetarian diet.

Calories

A calorie is a measure of energy. When carbohydrates, protein, fat and alcohol are burned (metabolized) in the body, they produce energy, which is measured in a unit known as the kilocalorie. The kilocalorie — commonly referred to as calorie — is used to express both the energy provided by food and the energy your body needs to function.

People's energy needs vary considerably with their activity level, body size, sex and age. The average adult requires about 2,000 calories a day, but there's a wide range. An older, petite, sedentary woman may need only about 1,600 calories a day, and a young, physically active man may need 2,800 calories or more daily.

If you eat more food than your body can use or too many high-calorie foods, your body stores the extra energy as fatty tissue. If you eat less food than your body needs, you lose fatty tissue.

The term *empty calories* is often applied to sugar, alcohol and fat. They contribute energy (calories), but few, if any, essential nutrients, such as vitamins or minerals.

Consuming sugar and alcohol on occasion in small amounts is OK. The problem is, most people consume too much added sugar — more than is beneficial to their health. Too many calories from sugar, fat and alcohol can lead to weight gain.

Body composition

The phrase, "You are what you eat," is true. The same ingredients that make up foods — water, protein, fat and carbohydrates — are the primary components of the human body.

Water

Water is a major component of body tissues made of protein, such as muscles and organs, and of the body's carbohydrate stores. Water makes up about 40 percent of body weight for very obese people and about 70 percent of body weight for very lean individuals.

Protein

Tissues composed of protein — muscles and vital organs — function as the machinery of your body. These protein structures make up about 30 to 60 percent of body weight.

Carbohydrates

Carbohydrates are stored in the liver and muscles in the form of glycogen. Glycogen makes up about 1 to 5 percent of your body weight.

If you switch from a normal diet to a very low-calorie diet or a very low-carbohydrate diet, you may lose 3 or 4 pounds within a day or two. Such weight loss, however, comes from a reduction of glycogen containing water — not fat.

Fat

Unlike protein and carbohydrates, fat is an extremely concentrated form of reserve energy that contains little water. Among men at a healthy weight, 15 to 20 percent of their body weight is fat. In women, this figure is approximately 20 to 25 percent. In an extremely obese person, as much as 50 percent of body weight or more is fat.

Nutrition Professionals

If you feel that you need help in getting essential nutrients and developing a healthier diet, talk to a registered dietitian or a registered dietitian nutritionist. These individuals are registered with the Academy of Nutrition and Dietetics. A registered dietitian must earn an undergraduate degree in a four-year program in food science and nutrition at an accredited college or university, complete six to 12 months of training in practical aspects of dietetics, and pass a national examination. Registered dietitians also must complete at least 75 hours of professional education every five years.

Other professionals also may be helpful in dealing with nutrition-related questions. Some doctors have a particular interest in nutrition. Home economists are often a good source of information on meal planning.

Be aware that the term *nutritionist* is sometimes used by people who have no credible nutritional training and who may be selling dietary supplements or weight-loss schemes. Some of these people may even display a diploma or certificate that means very little.

Body fat primarily serves as a fuel reserve, but it also provides padding and insulation. Too much body fat, however, increases the risk of heart disease, diabetes, high blood pressure, stroke and various types of cancer.

A Healthy-Eating Plan

Eating well doesn't have to be complicated. Unless you need a special diet for a specific health problem, the best approach is to follow national dietary recommendations.

These recommendations have evolved over the years to keep pace with scientific knowledge as experts develop a better understanding of how diet influences general health and helps prevent disease.

National dietary recommendations incorporate the best judgment of nutrition professionals and are intended for healthy individuals older than age 2. Current guidelines recommend that you:

- Follow a healthy-eating plan throughout your lifetime
- Eat a variety of nutrient-dense foods
- Eat moderate portions
- Limit calories from added sugars and saturated fats
- Limit your sodium intake

A healthy-eating plan emphasizes vegetables, fruits, whole grains, low-fat dairy, and healthy proteins and oils.

Eat a plant-based diet

Adopting a diet that includes variety of vegetables, fruits, nuts, beans and grains — especially foods made from whole grains — is the basis of healthy eating. Fruits, vegetables, beans and grains are low in calories and fat and provide essential vitamins and minerals, fiber, and phytochemicals important for good health. Nuts contain some healthy fat and are loaded with nutrients.

Most people, including children, don't eat enough fruits and vegetables. Try to eat seven or more servings of fruits and vegetables each day — at least three servings of fruit and at least four servings of vegetables.

Fruits contain little or no fat and provide fiber, vitamins and minerals. In addition, fruits contain phytochemicals that can reduce your risk of cardiovascular disease and some cancers. Vegetables also contain vitamins, minerals, fiber and phytochemicals. They're low in calories and virtually fat-free.

All grains and foods made from grains — cereals, bread, rice and pasta — are high in complex carbohydrates and provide a variety of nutrients.

Aim for at least six servings of grains each day. Whenever possible, choose whole grains because they contain more fiber and other nutrients than do refined grains. Whole-grain foods differ in nutrient content, so eat foods made from a variety of them — such as whole-wheat bread, brown rice and oatmeal.

Beans are high in nutrients and fiber, and can help lower cholesterol. Nuts can reduce cholesterol and help prevent heart disease.

A plant-based diet that includes a variety of grains, legumes, nuts and seeds can meet your daily protein needs. Eat moderate amounts of foods high in protein. Most plant foods are naturally low in less healthy fats and they're cholesterol-free.

Healthy Additions

Here are some tips on easy ways to incorporate more fruits, vegetables and whole grains into your diet:

Fruits

- Keep a bowl of fruit on the kitchen counter or table for snacks.
- Add fresh or dried fruit to breakfast cereals.
- Replace the oil in foods to be baked with thick fruit purees such as applesauce or mashed bananas.
- Use fruit sauces as toppings on desserts and pancakes.
- Instead of drinking soda pop, use 100 percent fruit juice mixed with sparkling water.

Vegetables

- Keep ready-to-eat, raw vegetables handy in a clear container in the front of your refrigerator for snacks or meals on the go.
- Eat a variety of salad greens, including arugula, mixed baby lettuces, collards, kale, mustard greens, spinach and watercress.
- Stir-fry vegetables with a small portion of poultry, seafood or meat.
- Make soup with summer or fall vegetables.
- Top a baked potato with 1 cup of steamed vegetables.

Whole grains

- For breakfast, choose high-fiber cereals, such as bran flakes, shredded wheat and oatmeal.
- Substitute whole-wheat toast or multigrain muffins for bagels and pastries made with refined flour.
- Make sandwiches with whole-grain breads or rolls.
- Expand your grain repertoire with foods such as kasha, brown rice, wild rice, bulgur and wheat berries.
- Use rice or barley in soups, stews and casseroles.

Reduce saturated fat

Reducing saturated fat doesn't mean eliminating fat altogether. You want to select foods made from monounsaturated and poly-unsaturated fats, such as olive, canola and other vegetable oils.

Even though monounsaturated and polyunsaturated fats have some positive effects on blood, it's still important to consume them in moderation. Eating lots of fat of any type adds excess calories.

Aim for a total fat intake of no more than 25 to 35 percent of calories, with 10 percent or less from saturated fat. For example, if you consume 2,000 calories a day, your upper limit on total fat will be 55 to 78 grams, with 22 grams or less of saturated fat.

To reduce fat in your diet, eat fewer foods high in saturated fat. Limit meat and high-fat dairy products (butter, cheese and cream), as well as foods made from solid shortenings and palm and coconut oils.

Limit sugar and salt

Foods containing sugars added during processing or preparation generally provide calories but few vitamins and minerals. High-sugar foods also promote tooth decay. For these reasons, dietary guidelines recommend that you limit foods and beverages containing added sugars.

In the United States, a major source of added sugars is nondiet soft drinks. Other major sources include candies, cakes, cookies, fruit drinks and dairy desserts, such as ice cream. Don't let soft drinks or other sweets crowd out foods that you need to maintain good health.

Salt (sodium chloride) is the main source of sodium in foods. The recommended daily limit of sodium is 2,300 milligrams — found in about 1 teaspoon of table salt. Most Americans are unaware they consume much more than this.

Processed foods contain the most hidden sodium. They contribute about 75 percent of the average person's sodium intake. About 10 percent of sodium in your diet is added during food preparation or at the table. Only a small amount of sodium occurs naturally in foods.

People with high blood pressure, heart or kidney disease need to consume less than 2,300 milligrams.

To limit sodium, choose and prepare your foods carefully. Check labels on processed foods. Frozen dinners, soups, packaged mixes, cereals, cheese, salad dressings and sauces may be high in sodium. When preparing meals, flavor foods with herbs or spices instead of salt.

Limit alcohol

Alcoholic beverages supply calories but few nutrients. If you drink alcoholic beverages, do so in moderation — no more than one drink a day for women of all ages and men age 65 and older and two drinks a day for younger men.

One drink is defined as:
- 12 ounces of beer
- 5 ounces of wine
- 1.5 ounces of 80-proof distilled spirits

Consuming alcohol with meals will slow its absorption. Don't drink before or while driving.

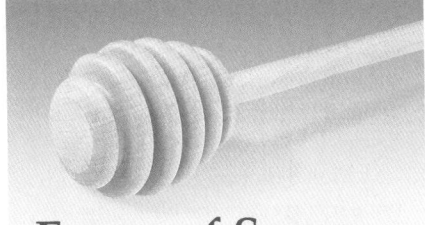

Forms of Sugar

Sugar travels under many disguises, depending on how it's formed and processed. A food is likely to be high in sugar if one of the following names appears first or second in the list of ingredients, or if several of these names are listed:
- Brown sugar
- Corn sweetener
- Corn syrup
- Dextrose
- Fructose
- Fruit juice concentrate
- Glucose
- High-fructose corn syrup
- Honey
- Invert sugar
- Lactose
- Maltose
- Malt syrup
- Molasses
- Raw sugar
- Sucrose
- Syrup
- Table sugar

Good Fat

One type of fat, called omega-3 fatty acids, may have a protective effect against heart disease. This type of fat can lower your triglyceride level in large amounts. Triglycerides are a type of blood fat. Omega-3 fatty acids may also lower blood pressure slightly.

Foods containing omega-3 fatty acids are part of a healthy diet, but the typical American diet has few of them. The best sources of omega-3 fatty acids are fatty, cold-water fish, such as salmon, mackerel, sardines, herring, bass, swordfish, tuna and trout. Other foods containing this type of fat include flaxseed, walnuts and soybean and canola oils. However, omega-3 fats from plant foods aren't utilized as well in the body.

Health experts recommend eating fish at least twice a week, unless you're pregnant or planning to become pregnant. Fish oil supplements generally aren't recommended.

Some individuals shouldn't drink any alcohol. This includes pregnant women and individuals with liver disease or other medical conditions sensitive to alcohol. In addition, people taking certain medications shouldn't consume alcohol.

Think variety and moderation

Eating a variety of foods provides you with a wider array of nutrients. Plus, it's fun to eat different foods and enjoy new flavors. Don't be afraid to try new foods and to experiment with new ways to prepare some of your favorites.

In general, plant-based foods are nutrient dense. Therefore, eating a variety of plant-based foods, such as vegetables, fruits, whole grains, beans and nuts, ensures that your body is benefiting from many different nutrients.

But keep the amounts you consume in check. With the trend toward larger food portions, many Americans have a distorted view of appropriate serving sizes. Knowing and controlling food portions also can help you maintain a healthier diet, whether or not you're trying to lose weight.

By avoiding large portions of certain foods, you're able to eat a wider variety of foods during a meal. The exceptions to this are vegetables and fruits, which most people don't get enough of.

Try these other suggestions for reducing food portions:
- Serve food on plates rather than put serving bowls on the table.
- Serve main dishes on a smaller plate.
- When eating out, ask for a take-home container. Save part of the meal for another time.
- Skip second servings.
- Don't feel as though you have to clean your plate.

For vegetables and fruits, you don't need to limit portions, just be careful about what you put on them, such as rich sauces.

Food Labels

Food labels can serve as an important guide to better nutrition. They have several parts, including the ingredients list and Nutrition Facts label. The Nutrition Facts label contains information pertaining to serving size, calories and daily values of various nutrients.

You can use the Nutrition Facts label to see if a food is a good source of a particular nutrient. Or you can compare labels to see, for example, which brand of frozen dinner is lower in saturated fat and sodium or which breakfast cereal contains more fiber.

Nutrition labeling is required for almost all foods. Voluntary information for commonly eaten raw fruits, vegetables and seafood also is available online and in most grocery stores. This information may be provided in a brochure, pamphlet, sign or poster.

Nutrition labeling is also voluntary for single-ingredient raw meat and poultry products. Ground beef and chicken parts, for example, aren't required to have a nutrition label. However, processed products such as corned beef, hot dogs and frozen entrees with meat must have nutrition labeling on each package.

Label components

Each food label contains information pertaining to:

Serving size
The serving size is based on the amount of the labeled food people normally eat and is listed in both household and metric measures. Check the serving size to see if the amount you normally eat is similar to the serving size on the label. If you eat more, then the number of calories and nutrients you get from that item will be higher. The number of servings per container also is listed so that you can calculate the calories and nutrients in the whole product.

Nutrition Facts

8 servings per container

Serving size   2/3 cup (55g)

Amount per serving	
Calories	**230**

	% Daily Value*
Total Fat 8g	**10%**
Saturated Fat 1g	**5%**
Trans Fat 0g	
Cholesterol 0mg	**0%**
Sodium 160mg	**7%**
Total Carbohydrate 37g	**13%**
Dietary Fiber 4g	**14%**
Total Sugars 12g	
Includes 10g Added Sugars	**20%**
Protein 3g	
Vitamin D 2mcg	10%
Calcium 260mg	20%
Iron 8mg	45%
Potassium 235mg	6%

* The % Daily Value (DV) tells you how much a nutrient in a serving of food contributes to a daily diet. 2,000 calories a day is used for general nutrition advice.

INGREDIENTS: ENRICHED FLOUR, (WHEAT FLOUR, CALCIUM GLUCONATE, REDUCED IRON, ASCORBIC ACID, RETINOIC ACID) GRAHAM FLOUR, ORGANIC CANE SUGAR, PARTIALLY HYDROGENATED COTTONSEED OIL, MOLASSES, LEAVENING (SODIUM BICARBONATE), SEA SALT, ARTIFICIAL FLAVOR

Calories and nutrients to limit
Nutrition labels include the number of calories in each serving. The limits for saturated fat, added sugars and other nutrients also are listed. Use this information to make sure that you aren't consuming too many calories or too much of those nutrients that you want to limit.

The figures shown on labels are based on a diet of 2,000 calories a day. Your calorie needs may be lower or higher based on your age, size and physical activity level.

Adults should consume less than 10 percent of their daily calories from saturated fat or added sugars. For a 2,000 calorie diet that equals 22 grams of saturated fat and 50 grams of sugar.

Consume as little trans fat as possible, and limit sodium to 2,300 milligrams daily.

Nutrients to increase

Certain nutrients you want to get more of. They include dietary fiber, vitamin D, calcium, iron and potassium. Most Americans don't get the recommended amount of these nutrients. Getting enough is important because it can decrease your risk of disease.

Daily Value

The Daily Value section tells you how much of the recommended daily amount of a nutrient one serving contains. The percentage is based on a diet of 2,000 calories a day. Use the figures listed to compare products and to tell which food is higher or lower in nutrients.

Nutrient claims

Some food labels also contain standardized claims, such as "low-fat" and "high in fiber." Claims involving nutrient content are defined and regulated by the Food and Drug Administration. The accompanying chart defines some of the common claims. In addition to claims such as "light" or "lean," sometimes health claims are made that link foods or food components with a reduced risk of certain chronic diseases.

Ingredients list

The ingredient list shows each ingredient in a food, listed by its common or usual name. On processed foods, ingredients are listed in order from the greatest amount to the least amount.

If, for example, sugar is listed as the first ingredient, it's present in a greater amount than any of the other ingredients. Be aware that an ingredient, such as sugar, may be listed with multiple names (see page 254).

Finding the Right Plan

There isn't one perfect plan for how to eat healthy. A healthy-eating plan can be created and implemented in many ways, taking into account your personal tastes and preferences.

People like different foods and they prepare food in different ways. Your culture, family background, religious and moral beliefs, and the cost and availability of food all affect your food choices.

While there may not be one perfect eating plan for everyone, as you've just read, healthy eating is based on certain general principles that apply to most people.

These principles are often portrayed in the shape of a pyramid — with the foods that should be eaten most forming the base — or a plate — with the healthiest foods taking up the greatest amount of space on your plate.

USDA MyPlate

The U.S. Department of Agriculture (USDA) uses a dinner plate, called MyPlate, to encourage people to make healthy food choices.

MyPlate offers ideas and tips to help you create a healthier eating style that meets your individual needs and preferences and improves your overall health.

MyPlate illustrates the five food groups that are building blocks for a healthy diet using a familiar

Nutrient Claims on Food Labels

Food term	What it means
Light or "lite"	*For fat:* If 50 percent or more of the calories are from fat, fat must be reduced by at least 50 percent *For calories:* If less than 50 percent of calories are from fat, calories must be reduced by 33 percent *For sodium:* Contains at least 50 percent less sodium than a comparable product
Reduced	Contains at least 25 percent less of a nutrient than a comparable product
Free	Contains negligible or insignificant amounts of the nutrient, such as fat, saturated fat, cholesterol, sodium, sugar or calories
Low	*For fat:* Contains 3 grams (g) or fewer *For saturated fat:* Contains 1 g or less *For sodium:* Contains 140 milligrams (mg) or fewer *For calories:* Contains 40 calories or fewer
High	Contains at least 20 percent of the recommended Daily Value for a nutrient, such as fiber or vitamin C, based on a 2,000-calories-a-day diet
Good source	Contains 10 to 19 percent of the recommended Daily Value for a nutrient, based on a 2,000-calorie-a day diet
Healthy	Must be low in fat, saturated fat and sodium and must provide at least 10 percent of the recommended Daily Value for vitamin A, vitamin C, calcium, iron, protein or fiber
Lean	Meat, poultry, seafood or game meat that has, per 3 ounces (oz.), less than 10 g of total fat, less than 4.5 g of saturated fat and less than 95 mg of cholesterol
Extra lean	Meat, poultry, seafood or game meat that has, per 3 oz., less than 5 g of total fat, less than 2 g of saturated fat and less than 95 mg of cholesterol

Source: U.S. Food and Drug Administration

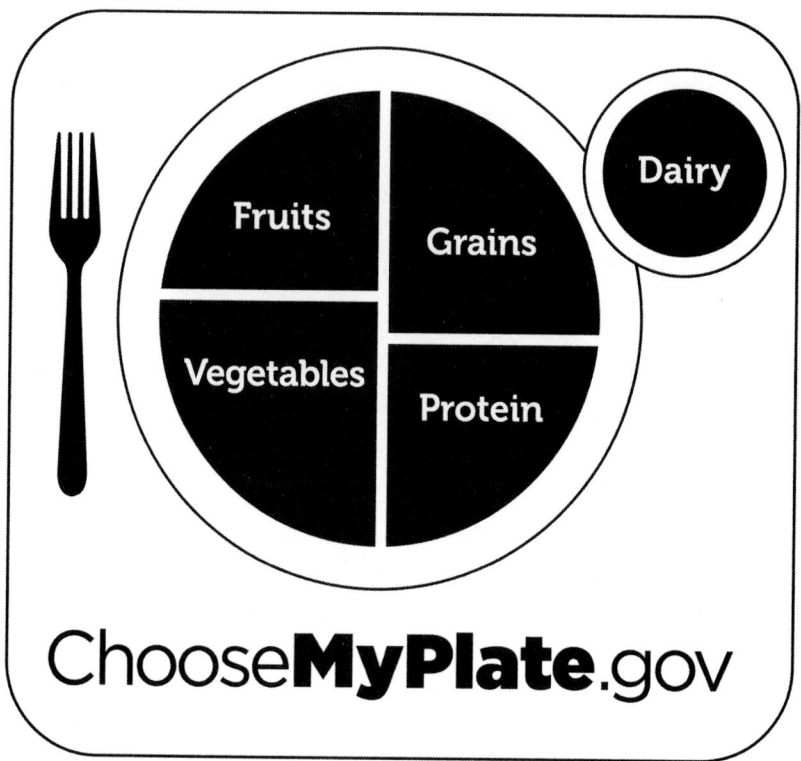

Source: USDA Center for Nutrition Policy and Promotion

How Much Should I Eat?

The 2015-2020 Dietary Guidelines recommends all Americans adopt an eating pattern that includes a variety of foods. But how much of each should you eat? Here are some good goals to aim for. These recommendations are based on diet of 2,000 calories a day.

Vegetables	2½ cups a day
Legumes (beans and peas)	1½ cups a week
Fruits	2 cups a day
Grains	6 ounces a day
Whole grains	≥ 3 ounces a day
Refined grains	≤ 3 ounces a day
Dairy	3 cups a day
Protein foods	5½ ounces a day
Seafood	8 ounces a week
Meats, poultry, eggs	26 ounces a week
Nuts, seeds, soy products	4 ounces a week
Oils	27 grams a day

Limit calories from added sugars, solid fats, added refined starches to 270 calories a day. That equates to 14 percent of your total calories.

Source: U.S. Department of Health and Human Services, 2015

image — a place setting. As you think about your meal and put food on your plate, try to replicate the MyPlate setting.

At each meal, vegetables and fruits should take up half of your plate. Grains should make up a quarter of your plate and protein the other quarter. Try to consume mostly whole grains, and vary your protein sources, including a variety of plant-based proteins in addition to seafood, poultry or meat. Make sure to include a serving of dairy with each meal and try to make it low fat or fat-free.

Many other eating plans are represented by food pyramids. These include the Mediterranean, Asian, Latin American and Vegetarian diet pyramids, just to name a few.

Mediterranean Diet Pyramid

Because the Mediterranean Diet Pyramid is based on a cultural eating pattern, it includes a more limited range of foods than does the USDA MyPlate.

The Mediterranean Diet Pyramid reflects traditional eating patterns in Greece, Crete and southern Italy. This eating style came into focus in the 1950s and 1960s, when studies showed that Greek men were the least likely to develop heart disease among men from seven countries that participated in the study, including the United States.

The Mediterranean eating plan emphasizes fresh fruits and vegetables, grains of all types and legumes such as beans, lentils and peas. Mediterranean dishes are also enhanced with olive oil, a monounsaturated fat that appears to help protect against heart disease. Wine, in moderation, is part of this pyramid, because red wine with meals is a Mediterranean tradition.

Asian Diet Pyramid

The Asian Diet Pyramid also reflects a cultural eating pattern.

It emphasizes grains, including rice, noodles, breads, millet and corn, as well as fruits, vegetables, legumes, nuts and seeds. As in the Mediterranean diet, fat in the Asian pyramid comes largely from vegetable oils high in unsaturated fat, such as peanut oil. The Asian Diet Pyramid contains limited dairy products, considering them optional and to be eaten only in low-fat forms.

The Asian and Mediterranean pyramids group plant-based proteins — soybeans, beans and nuts — separately from animal proteins found in meat, poultry, eggs and dairy products. Red meat is recommended infrequently — a few times a month or less — and poultry and eggs are recommended weekly.

Latin American Diet Pyramid

The Latin American Diet Pyramid is based on traditional healthy-eating patterns in Latin American regions, including Mexico, Central America and South America. The diet emphasizes food from plant sources, especially maize (corn) and potatoes, as well as fruits, vegetables, grains, beans, nuts and seeds.

In this diet, a variety of fruits and vegetables and whole grains are eaten at main meals. Fish, shellfish, plant oils (corn, soybean, olive), dairy products and poultry can be eaten once a day, and red meat, sweets and eggs are limited to once a week or less.

The pyramid places daily physical activity at the base to promote healthy weight, fitness and well-being.

Vegetarian Diet Pyramid

There are many vegetarian eating plans. At the very least, most vegetarian diets exclude red meat. Others omit all animal flesh, including chicken and fish. Some vegetarians don't eat eggs or milk products. The most strict vegetarians (vegans) eat only grains, legumes, fruits, vegetables, nuts and seeds, and products made from these foods.

If you don't eat any animal products, it can become more challenging to meet daily recommendations for essential amino acids from protein as well as requirements for calcium, iron, zinc and vitamins B-12 and D.

The Vegetarian Diet Pyramid can help in making good food choices. This pyramid specifies whole grains and puts them at the same level as fruits and vegetables, which are to be eaten at every meal. Daily choices include moderate amounts of nuts and seeds, egg whites, soy milk and dairy products, as well as plant oils.

Eggs and sweets are at the top of the pyramid and should be eaten once a week or less. The vegetarian pyramid also recommends at least six glasses of water each day. Water is also important to many other eating plans.

Sizing Up a Serving

Keep an eye on serving sizes as you prepare and eat meals. The number of servings that are appropriate for you depends on your age, sex and activity level.

For some foods, the number of recommended servings a day might seem high, but some of the serving sizes may be smaller than what you usually eat or what you see on food labels. For example, some people eat two slices of bread in a meal, which equals two servings. Serving sizes also differ. On food labels, one serving of cooked rice or pasta often is 1 cup, but on the USDA's MyPlate, one serving of these foods is only ½ cup.

If you follow the suggested number of servings in the recommended amounts, you'll help control your caloric intake.

Grains group
- ½ cup cooked cereal, rice or pasta
- 1 ounce (oz.) ready-to-eat cereal (check the label for the serving size)
- One slice whole-wheat bread
- ½ bagel, English muffin or hamburger bun

Vegetable group
- 2 cups raw leafy green vegetables
- 1 cup other vegetables, cooked or raw, or juice
- One medium potato

Fruit group
- One medium orange, apple, banana or pear
- 32 grapes
- ½ cup dried fruit
- 1 cup fruit juice

Milk, yogurt and cheese group
- 1 cup low-fat or fat-free milk or yogurt
- 1½ oz. natural cheese, such as cheddar
- 2 oz. processed cheese, such as American
- 2 cups low-fat or fat-free cottage cheese

Meat, poultry, fish, dry beans, eggs and nuts group
- 1 oz. cooked lean meat, fish or skinless poultry
- ¼ cup cooked legumes or dried beans
- One egg
- 1 tablespoon peanut butter
- 2 tablespoons seeds
- 12 almonds
- 7 walnut halves
- ¼ cup tofu

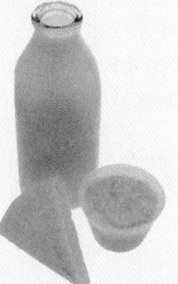

Mayo Clinic Healthy Weight Pyramid

Like other dietary plans, the Mayo Clinic Healthy Weight Pyramid — and its corresponding Healthy Dining Table — focus on vegetables, fruits and whole grains as the basis for a healthy diet. The emphasis is on nutritious foods that contain a small number of calories in a large amount of food.

In addition to helping you stay well, this pyramid is designed to help you lose weight. The Mayo Clinic Healthy Weight Pyramid and Healthy Dining Table are discussed in more detail on pages 270-271.

Food and Health

The relationship between diet and health is powerful. The food you eat can influence your health directly, or it can do so indirectly by way of the numbers on the scale. There's a definite link between obesity and poor health.

Not surprisingly, of the top 10 leading causes of death in the United States, more than half of them are related to being obese or to having an unhealthy diet.

An unhealthy diet lacks key nutrients or it includes generous amounts of animal-based foods or less healthy foods. As an example, consuming red or processed meat — meat that's been salted, smoked or cured — is associated with an increased risk of colorectal cancer, type 2 diabetes, cardiovascular disease and overall mortality. An unhealthy diet can also lead to obesity.

Some factors that affect your risk of disease are beyond your control, such as age and family history. But what you may not realize is how much you can control your disease risk. A healthy lifestyle that includes eating well can improve, or even eliminate, significant risk factors for several important chronic conditions. By following the dietary recommendations outlined in this chapter, you can reduce your risk of disease and improve the quality of your life.

Some chronic diseases, such as celiac disease, liver disease and kidney disease, require you to follow a specialized diet. For some of these conditions, dietary changes can be lifesaving. If you need to follow a special diet, it's important to work with a registered dietitian initially to develop an appropriate eating plan.

To help prevent diseases, it's not necessary that you follow a specialized diet, but it's important that you eat a healthy diet.

Coronary artery disease

High blood cholesterol can lead to accumulation of fatty deposits (plaques) in the arteries that feed your heart (coronary arteries), narrowing the arteries and increasing your risk of heart attack or stroke.

A diet low in saturated and trans fat can help reduce your blood cholesterol level and reduce your risk of coronary artery disease.

Heart-healthy foods that can help lower blood cholesterol or reduce heart disease risk include:

- A variety of vegetables and fruits
- Foods high in soluble fiber, such as legumes, oatmeal and apples
- Whole grains, such as whole-grain bread, oatmeal and brown rice
- Fish, especially salmon, mackerel and herring, rich in omega fat
- A variety of nuts
- Olive oil and foods containing plant sterols or stanols, such as spreads, dressings, juices and yogurt drinks

High blood pressure

Left untreated, high blood pressure can damage your arteries and increase your risk of stroke and heart disease. Limiting sodium and alcohol and maintaining a healthy weight can help prevent or reduce high blood pressure. In recent years, the role of diet in treating and preventing high blood pressure has drawn more attention.

Studies indicate that a diet rich in fruits, vegetables and low-fat dairy products can help lower your blood pressure. An eating guide based on these principles is called Dietary Approaches to Stop Hypertension, or the DASH diet.

The benefits of the DASH diet are improved even further by reducing sodium in your diet. Limiting sodium to less than 2,300 milligrams (mg) a day is generally recommended. The average American consumes about 3,400 mg of sodium a day.

For a detailed discussion of DASH, see page 711.

Cancer

Researchers continue to evaluate and clarify the role that diet and nutrition play in the development of cancer. Evidence suggests that about one-third of the cancer deaths in the United States each year may be related to weight or unhealthy habits associated with diet and exercise. Thus, your dietary choices, along with not smoking and getting regular physical activity, can help reduce your risk of cancer.

Maintaining a healthy weight through good eating habits is one of the most important things you can do to protect against cancer. Professional organizations dedicated to the prevention of cancer recommend that most of the foods you eat come from plant sources. In addition to fruits and vegetables, these include grains — especially whole grains — beans and other legumes.

Studies also suggest you limit your intake of red and processed meat, as well as energy-dense foods and sugary drinks that promote weight gain.

It's also a good idea to avoid processed foods in which a lot of salt is used in the preservation process. Salt-preserved foods are linked to cancer of the stomach. Avoiding or limiting alcohol also may reduce your risk of various cancers, including those cancers of the mouth, esophagus, pharynx, larynx, liver and breast. For more information, see Chapter 15.

Diabetes

Basic nutritional guidelines for people with diabetes are the same as those outlined earlier in this chapter, with greater emphasis on eating meals at regular times and on weight control. Most people with type 2 diabetes are overweight or obese.

The American Diabetes Association recommends that individuals with diabetes work with a registered dietitian to develop a meal plan based on food preferences, lifestyle and health concerns, such as blood cholesterol levels or weight management.

More than 90 percent of adults with diabetes have type 2 diabetes. Being overweight is the greatest risk factor for this form of diabetes. Eating plenty of whole grains, vegetables, fruits and legumes can make it easier to limit calories and lose weight. The fiber in these foods may also help lower your blood sugar.

Research has shown that weight loss resulting from a combination of a healthy diet and physical activity can be almost twice as effective as medication in preventing diabetes in people at risk.

If you have diabetes, you're at greater odds of developing cardiovascular disease, so it's important to limit saturated fat in your diet, and control blood cholesterol levels and other risk factors.

Simple carbohydrates, such as table sugar, honey, jelly, fruit juice and candy need to be planned into your diet. However, it's the total amount of carbohydrates

in your diet that affects glucose the most. For this reason, a Mediterranean diet that's slightly lower in carbohydrate consumption and higher in healthy fats from olive oil may offer some benefit, provided you take steps to control your daily calorie intake.

For more information on diabetes and nutrition, see Chapter 28, "Endocrine System."

Osteoporosis

About 1 in 4 women develops osteoporosis after menopause. For both women and men, risk increases with age. Osteoporosis results from a reduction in bone mass, causing your bones to become thin, fragile and prone to fracture.

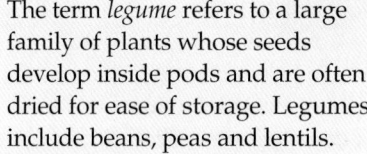

Love Those Legumes

The term *legume* refers to a large family of plants whose seeds develop inside pods and are often dried for ease of storage. Legumes include beans, peas and lentils.

Because legumes are high in protein, these plant foods make an excellent substitute for animal sources of protein.

Selecting legumes
Here are some common legumes to look for at your local supermarket:
• White or navy beans
• Lima beans
• Pinto and black beans
• Black-eyed peas
• Split peas
• Brown lentils
• Chickpeas (garbanzos)
Ethnic markets often have less common legumes. Indian markets, for example, usually offer a good selection of lentils, including red and green ones. Look for legumes of a uniform size that will cook evenly.

The recommended intake of calcium in women up to age 50 and men up to age 70 is 1,000 milligrams daily. For women older than age 50 and men older than age 70, the recommended amount is 1,200 milligrams daily. Adequate vitamin D also is important to preventing osteoporosis. See page 250 for more information on vitamin D.

In general, it's best to get as much calcium as you can from your diet (see the opposite page). Although vegetables and fruits aren't usually thought of in regard to osteoporosis risk, there's evidence they're beneficial in improving done density and lowering your risk of a fracture.

If you can't get the recommended amount from food,

Storing legumes
Store legumes at room temperature. After purchase, place them in tightly covered jars away from heat, light and moisture. They'll keep well for up to a year.

Cooking legumes
Carefully sort legumes before using them. Bags of legumes may include a few small stones or fibers that you'll want to remove before cooking.

Beans and other large dried legumes, such as chickpeas and black-eyed peas, require pre-soaking overnight or for about six to eight hours before cooking. This rehydrates them for more-even cooking. Split peas and lentils don't require pre-soaking. You can also purchase legumes that are precooked and canned.

To incorporate legumes into everyday meals:
• Feature beans, peas or lentils in soups, stews or casseroles.
• Add chickpeas or black beans to salads.
• Use pureed beans as the basis for dips and spreads.

supplements can help make up the difference. Discuss taking a dietary supplement with your doctor, particularly if you're past menopause.

Celiac disease

Celiac disease, also called celiac sprue or nontropical sprue, is a digestive disease caused by an intolerance to gluten, a protein found in wheat, barley and rye. For affected individuals, gluten triggers an immune system response that damages the small intestine and prevents absorption of some nutrients in food.

Lifelong avoidance of foods that contain gluten is the only treatment for celiac disease. Although it may sound simple, doing so can be challenging.

Products made from gluten-containing grains are staples of American and European diets. Wheat breads of all kinds contain gluten, as do most baked goods, cereals and pasta. In addition, many processed foods contain small amounts of emulsifiers, thickeners and other additives derived from these grains and must be avoided.

Rice, potatoes and corn don't contain gluten, and foods made from these ingredients are acceptable. Oats are naturally gluten-free, however, they're often grown and harvested along with wheat, barley and rye, creating the risk of cross-contamination. Plain meats, fish, poultry, eggs, dairy products, vegetables and fruits also don't contain gluten.

Even trace amounts of gluten can cause severe damage to the intestines. Strict diet compliance can control the disease and prevent life-threatening complications. Regular checkups with your doctor and a dietitian also are an important part of treatment.

Kidney stones

Kidney stones (renal calculi) are fairly common. A kidney stone is a mineralized deposit that forms on the inner surface of your kidney and may pass into the lower urinary tract.

In many cases, you can prevent kidney stones by making a few changes in your diet. The most important thing you can do to lower this risk is to drink lots of water. Drinking extra fluids dilutes urine, making it less likely that crystals will develop.

If you have a history of kidney stones, your doctor will probably recommend that you drink enough fluid to produce about 2½ quarts of urine each day. Although most liquids count, water is best. Lemonade also is a good choice. The citrate in lemonade helps prevent some stones from forming.

If you tend to form calcium stones in your kidneys, your doctor may recommend restricting foods rich in oxalates. Some common food sources include organ meats, beets, chocolate, coffee, rhubarb, cooked spinach, strawberries, tea and whole-wheat products.

With the exceptions of the foods just listed, a diet high in fruits and vegetables may decrease stone formation. Eating less animal protein, sodium and sugar, and decreasing consumption of vitamin C supplements also may help prevent stone formation.

Foods that contain calcium, such as dairy products, don't have to be restricted. However, calcium supplements may increase the risk of stone formation.

Kidney failure

Kidney (renal) failure may result from diseases such as diabetes, high blood pressure, kidney stones, infection, injury or exposure to toxins. The kidneys lose their ability to filter fluids and waste from blood, causing dangerous levels of these substances to accumulate in your body.

If you have acute kidney failure, you'll probably be placed on a diet high in carbohydrates and low in

Getting Adequate Calcium

Getting plenty of calcium in your diet is important for growth and maintenance of healthy bones and teeth throughout life. Adolescents and adults over age 50 have an especially high need for calcium. At younger ages, people are growing. At older ages, they begin to lose calcium from bone.

Sources of calcium include:

- *Milk or milk products.* Skim or low-fat milk, low-fat yogurt, and cheese are especially high in calcium. If you're lactose intolerant, try lactose-free or lactose-reduced milk. Lactaid and other lactose-reduction treatments are available as chewable tablets that you take with a meal that contains lactose.

- *Fish and vegetables.* Canned fish with soft bones included, such as salmon and sardines, is a good source of calcium. Dark leafy greens, such as collards and turnip greens, also contain calcium.

- *Calcium-enriched products.* These include breakfast cereal with added calcium, orange juice with added calcium, tofu made with calcium sulfate and soy milk with added calcium.

- *Calcium supplements.* Calcium carbonate and calcium citrate are two common types of calcium supplements. Avoid calcium supplements made from bone meal, dolomite or oyster shell. These products are often advertised as natural calcium, but they may contain toxic substances such as lead, mercury and arsenic.

protein, potassium and fluid to prevent excess fluids and wastes from accumulating in your blood while your kidneys heal. A sudden rise in potassium levels could impair your heart's function and may be life-threatening.

Chronic kidney failure has many nutritional implications. Eating a diet low in protein may ease symptoms of nausea, vomiting and lack of appetite. A modestly low-protein diet may also help slow progression of the disease and preserve kidney function. But too little protein isn't healthy either, so talk with your doctor or a dietitian.

You may need to curtail the amount of water you drink to reduce fluid accumulation. If your kidney disease is associated with high blood pressure, you may need to restrict salt in your diet as well as the amount of liquid that you drink. Your doctor may direct you to limit your consumption of foods high in potassium and phosphorus.

If you're receiving dialysis, you may need more protein, but need to restrict your intake of fluids, phosphorus, sodium and potassium.

Liver disease

Advanced liver disease can result in an increased amount of ammonia in your blood, retention of fluid in your abdomen (ascites) and fatigue. Several dietary measures can help relieve these problems. It's important that you work closely with your doctor and dietitian to develop an appropriate eating plan.

Some protein is broken down into ammonia, so your doctor may suggest that you avoid excessive protein. Instead of eating a whole day's worth of protein in one sitting, it's better to divide it into several smaller meals throughout the day. It's usually best to eat four to six smaller meals a day rather than two or three larger ones.

It's also important to make sure that you're getting adequate calories. If you have high blood pressure or fluid retention, you may need to limit your sodium intake.

Food Safety

Another important aspect of healthy eating is keeping the food you eat safe from foodborne illness caused by microorganisms such as bacteria, viruses and parasites.

Foodborne illness

Foodborne illness, often referred to as food poisoning, is a gastro-

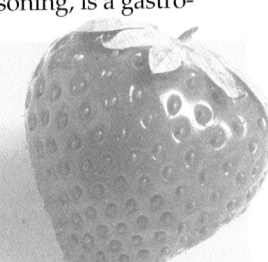

Antioxidants and Disease Prevention

Antioxidants are substances that protect your body's cells from the damaging effects of toxic molecules called free radicals. Free radicals may contribute to diseases, including cardiovascular and lung disease, cataracts and cancer. Important antioxidants include vitamins C, E and A (carotenoids), such as beta carotene. Other types of antioxidants, called flavonoids and polyphenols, are found in brewed tea (especially green tea), red wine and chocolate.

Despite the health benefits of vitamins C and E and beta carotene, current evidence doesn't support taking antioxidants in supplement form. Plus, there's good evidence that vitamin C and E supplements and beta carotene supplements taken by smokers and former smokers are associated with increased mortality. This is why nutrition experts recommend that you get antioxidants in your daily diet and not from supplements.

The following foods are good sources of antioxidants:

Vitamin C
- Green peppers and sweet red peppers
- Collards
- Broccoli
- Spinach
- Tomatoes
- Potatoes
- Strawberries
- Oranges and their juice
- Grapefruits and their juice

Vitamin E
- Vegetable oils and products made with them
- Wheat germ
- Nuts and seeds
- Fortified cereals

Vitamin A
Vitamin A (carotenoids) are found in deep yellow, dark green and red vegetables and fruits such as:
- Carrots
- Winter squash
- Sweet potatoes
- Spinach
- Broccoli
- Green peppers and sweet red peppers
- Tomatoes and tomato products
- Papaya
- Cantaloupe
- Mango
- Apricots
- Watermelon

intestinal infection caused by eating contaminated food. The food may contain harmful bacteria, toxins, parasites, viruses or chemical contaminants. Bacteria such as campylobacter, salmonella, *Escherichia coli* (*E. coli*) and listeria, and Norwalk-like viruses are among the most common causes of foodborne illness.

In most people, the discomforts of foodborne illness pass within a few hours. For some people, however, food poisoning may be life-threatening. This is especially true for infants, pregnant women, older adults, and people in poor health or with a weakened immune system.

Eating even a small portion of an unsafe food can make you sick. Common signs and symptoms are loss of appetite, nausea, vomiting, diarrhea and abdominal pain. They may appear within a half-hour of eating the food, or they may not develop for up to three weeks.

Many common foods can contain large numbers of bacteria. Perishable foods such as fresh fruits and vegetables, salads, eggs, meats, poultry, fish, shellfish and milk products are most susceptible to bacterial contamination. Seafood also is a leading cause of foodborne illness.

Preventing foodborne illness

Food and water supplies in the United States are generally safe and are subject to inspection and regulation. But it's impossible to keep the entire food supply completely free of potentially dangerous bacteria. For this reason, you're the final line of defense against food hazards.

How do you make sure that the food you eat is safe? These tips can help prevent foodborne illness:

Wash your hands, utensils and food surfaces often
Wash your hands with warm,

Chocolate: A Healthy Food?

Healthy chocolate sounds like a dream come true, but chocolate hasn't gained the status of health food quite yet. Still, chocolate's reputation is on the rise, as a growing number of studies suggest that it can be a heart-healthy choice.

Chocolate and its main ingredient, cocoa, appear to reduce risk factors for heart disease. Flavonols in cocoa beans have antioxidant effects that reduce cell damage implicated in heart disease. Flavonols — which are more prevalent in dark chocolate than in milk chocolate — also help lower blood pressure and improve vascular function.

In addition, some research has linked chocolate consumption to reduced risks of diabetes, stroke and heart attack. However, more research is needed to confirm these results.

In the meantime, if you want to add chocolate to your diet, do so in moderation, and choose dark chocolate over milk chocolate.

Most commercial chocolate has ingredients that add fat, sugar and calories. And too much can contribute to weight gain, a risk factor for high blood pressure, heart disease and diabetes. Milk chocolate contains saturated fat, and it isn't as healthy as dark chocolate.

Cocoa itself, however, is low in both sugar and fat while offering potential health benefits. If you enjoy the flavor of chocolate, consider adding some plain cocoa to your low-fat glass of milk or morning bowl of oats.

soapy water before and after handling or preparing food, especially raw meat, poultry, fish, shellfish and eggs. Then use hot, soapy water to wash the utensils, cutting board and other surfaces you used.

You can wash an acrylic cutting board in your dishwasher. Disinfect a wooden cutting board with a solution of 2 teaspoons of household bleach mixed with 1 quart of water. Wash the board after applying the bleach. Replace cutting boards when they become worn or have hard-to-clean grooves.

In addition, wash your hands after using the toilet, changing diapers or playing with pets.

Keep raw foods separate from ready-to-eat foods
When shopping, preparing food or storing food, keep raw meat, poultry, eggs, fish and shellfish away from other foods. This prevents cross-contamination from one food to another. Store raw foods in containers in the refrigerator so that the juices don't drip onto other foods.

Cook foods to a safe temperature
Uncooked and undercooked animal foods are potentially unsafe. The best way to tell if meat, poultry or egg dishes are cooked to a safe temperature is to use a food thermometer. Cook fish and shellfish until the outside is opaque. Fish should flake easily with a fork.

Heat sauces, soups and gravies to a boil. If you marinate meat or poultry, don't serve the unused marinade. Make sure to reheat leftovers thoroughly. Also, don't consume raw or partially cooked eggs, unpasteurized milk products or unpasteurized juices.

Refrigerate perishable foods promptly
Refrigerate or freeze perishable foods within two hours of purchasing or preparing them. If the temperature is above 85 F,

Coffee, Caffeine and Your Health

As you probably realize when you stumble into the kitchen for that first cup of morning java, coffee is a stimulant because of the caffeine it contains. However, coffee also contains hundreds of other compounds, including antioxidants, that may be beneficial for health.

Coffee intake has been associated with a slightly reduced risk of type 2 diabetes, liver disease, liver cancer, Parkinson's disease and depression, and it's associated with improved mood. It's not the health effects that should limit your intake, but rather the side effects, which some people are more susceptible to. Coffee can predispose you to insomnia, heart palpitations, gastroesophageal reflux disease (heartburn) and urinary symptoms.

If you experience these side effects, you may want to cut down on your consumption. Other foods and drinks also contain caffeine. If you're concerned about your caffeine intake, ask your doctor for advice.

Approximate Caffeine Content

	Milligrams of caffeine
Coffee drinks	
Brewed, 8 oz.	95-190
Brewed, decaf, 8 oz.	2-5
Espresso, 1 oz.	47-64
Espresso, decaf, 1 oz.	0
Instant, 8 oz.	63
Instant, decaf, 8 oz.	2
Latte or mocha, 8 oz.	63-126
Teas	
Black, brewed, 8 oz.	25-48
Black, brewed, decaf, 8 oz.	2-5
Chai latte, regular or iced, 8 oz.	25-48
Green, brewed, 8 oz.	25-29
Ready-to-drink, bottled, 8 oz.	5-40
Soft drinks	
Citrus (most brands), 12 oz.	0
Citrus, yellow or green, 12 oz.	48-64
Cola, 12 oz.	24-46
Root beer (most brands), 12 oz.	0
Energy drinks	
Energy drink, 8 oz.	27-164
Energy shot, 1 oz.	40-100

refrigerate them within an hour. Freeze fresh meat, poultry, fish and shellfish that can't be used in a few days. Thaw meat, poultry, fish or shellfish in the refrigerator, microwave or in cold water that's changed every 30 minutes.

Follow safety instructions
Read the label on food products and follow the safety instructions, such as "Keep refrigerated," "Refrigerate after opening," "Safe-handling suggestions" and "Cook thoroughly."

Serve foods safely
Keep hot foods hot — 140 F or above — and cold foods cold — 40 F or below. Harmful bacteria can grow rapidly in the danger zone between these temperatures.

Avoid letting food sit out on the table after meals. When serving large quantities of food, bring out small batches at a time. Throw out any leftovers that have been at room temperature more than two hours or have been in hot weather more than an hour.

Pay attention to leftovers
Many leftovers can be kept for three to four days in the refrigerator. After that, the risk of food poisoning increases. If you don't think that you'll be able to eat the leftovers within four days, freeze them immediately.

When in doubt, throw it out
If you're unsure if a food has been prepared, served or stored safely, it's best to discard it. Food that's been left at room temperature too long may contain bacteria that can't be destroyed by cooking. Don't taste food that you're unsure about. Discard foods that are moldy. Hard cheese can be an exception.

Ensuring safe drinking water

America's drinking water is among the safest in the world, and most people don't have to worry about the quality of their water. But water-treatment equipment sometimes can break down, or other unforeseen problems can occur.

Even though water may look, smell and taste pure, it still can contain substances that can make you ill.

Here are some general precautions to keep in mind regarding water safety:

- Don't drink water of unknown safety. Water from streams or lakes should be considered contaminated. Carry your own bottled water or place the contaminated water through a purifying device before drinking it.
- If your water supply comes from a private well or groundwater source, such as a lake or stream, have your water tested annually or anytime that you notice a change in color or odor.

Recommended Safe-Cooking Temperatures

145 F	Steaks, roasts and fish
160 F	Ground beef, pork and egg dishes
165 F	Chicken breasts and whole poultry

PREVENTION TIP

Foodborne illness is especially serious for pregnant women, young children, older adults and people with weakened immune systems. Individuals at high risk should take extra precautions by avoiding the following foods:

- Unpasteurized juices and ciders
- Unpasteurized milk and milk products
- Soft cheeses — such as feta, brie and Camembert — blue-veined cheese and unpasteurized cheese
- Raw sprouts (alfalfa and bean)
- Raw or rare meat and poultry
- Raw fish and shellfish
- Raw eggs and egg products
- Pâtés

Note: Deli and luncheon meats and hot dogs may harbor the bacteria listeria monocytogenes even if they've been properly refrigerated. They should be reheated to steaming before eating them.

Fish and Sushi

Fish is an important part of a healthy diet. It's a lean source of protein, and it contains heart-healthy omega-3 fatty acids. Eating fish regularly may protect you against coronary artery disease and some cancers.

But you also need to be careful about your fish choices. In some locations, sushi is a popular way to prepare fish. Sushi refers to a Japanese dish of small cakes of cold rice flavored with vinegar, sugar and salt, typically garnished with raw fish, other types of seafood and vegetables. Rarely, fish may harbor parasites that can cause gastrointestinal disease or reactions ranging from hives to shock.

Some fish may also contain environmental toxins, particularly polychlorinated biphenyls (PCBs) and methyl mercury. Heed the guidelines from your state's Department of Natural Resources or your local health department about consumption of freshwater fish.

Here are some guidelines when eating fish:

- Only eat sushi fish that was fresh frozen. Freezing raw fish can kill the parasites. If you're pregnant, don't eat raw fish.
- If you're breast-feeding, pregnant or planning to become pregnant, avoid shark, swordfish, king mackerel and tilefish. In addition, avoid serving these fish to children. The fish contain the highest levels of mercury, which may harm an unborn baby's developing nervous system. Currently, it's recommended that you limit other varieties of fish to no more than 12 ounces of cooked fish a week. Choose shellfish or smaller, younger fish, such as perch or stream trout.
- At the market, look for fresh fish with clear eyes that bulge slightly, firm and shiny flesh that springs back when pressed, bright pink or red gills, no slime, and no discoloration. The fish shouldn't have a strong fishy smell.
- Remove visible fat and skin before cooking. Broil the fish on a rack or grill so that the fat drips away.
- Vary the fish you eat to limit exposure to possible contaminants.
- Cook fish and seafood thoroughly and wash your hands, cutting boards and utensils with soap and water after coming in contact with fish.

Weight Loss

Obesity is a major health problem in the United States. Two-thirds of the adult population is overweight, and 1 in 3 adults is considered obese. Childhood obesity also is at an all-time high.

With the easy availability of calorie-dense foods, the bombardment by commercial messages urging you to eat, and the prevalence of sedentary work and leisure activities, it's easy to pack on pounds.

After a certain point, body fat can interfere with your health. The more your weight increases, the more problems you'll face in staying healthy and living longer. Excess weight can lead to a variety of health problems, including diabetes, high blood pressure and unhealthy cholesterol levels.

Improving your health over the long term is the most important reason for reaching and maintaining a healthy weight. Along with that, you'll likely feel better physically, feel better about yourself and have more energy.

Losing weight is challenging. There's no quick, easy fix. But despite the challenges, you aren't doomed to be overweight.

The pages that follow include strategies for losing weight gradually by changing your eating and activity habits. These long-term changes in your lifestyle can lead to successful weight loss and better health.

Is Your Weight Healthy?

For a moment, put aside thoughts of weight and dieting and looking thin — think about what it means to simply be healthy. If you take steps to maintain good health, you can enjoy a more active, energetic, higher quality of life and reduce your risk of many diseases.

In addition, you likely can avoid aging prematurely.

A combination of three measurements — body mass index (BMI), waist measurement and medical history — can give you an idea of whether it would be beneficial to you to lose a few pounds. Even a small reduction in weight can reduce your risk of many diseases.

Body mass index

The first step in determining if your weight is healthy is to determine your body mass index (BMI). Weigh yourself and have your height measured. Then determine your BMI by using the chart on the next page.

BMI considers weight in relation to height. The BMI ranges shown are for adults. They're not exact ranges of healthy and unhealthy weights, but they show that health risks increase with a higher body mass index. BMI doesn't consider your individual makeup and factors such as being big boned or more muscular, but it's an improvement over traditional height and weight tables.

A BMI of 18.5 to 24.9 is desirable. If your BMI falls within this range, there's generally little health advantage to your losing weight. A BMI of 25 to 29.9 suggests that you're overweight. If you have a BMI of 30 or more, you're considered obese.

The further your BMI is above the healthy range, the higher your weight-related health risks. If your BMI is 25 or more, losing weight may improve your health and reduce your risk of weight-related diseases. If your BMI falls below 18.5, you're probably underweight. Ask your doctor to assess your weight and health.

Waist circumference

Your waist circumference measurement indicates where most of your fat is located. People who carry most of their weight around their waists are often referred to as apples. Those who carry most of their weight below their waists — in their thighs, hips and buttocks — are known as pears.

Generally, it's better to have a pear shape than an apple shape. Extra weight around your waist puts you at higher risk of heart disease, diabetes and some cancers. How body fat is distributed begins with genetics, but it's also influenced by your environment.

To measure your waist, find the highest point on each of your hips and measure horizontally across your abdomen above the two points.

- For women, a waist measurement of 35 inches or more is associated with higher health risks.
- For men, a waist measurement of 40 inches or more is associated with higher health risks.

Despite these specific cutoffs, the message to keep in mind is the smaller the waist measurement, the lower the health risks.

Excess abdominal fat may place you at greater risk of health problems, even if your BMI is about right. If your BMI is 25 or higher and your waist circumference exceeds healthy guidelines, the risk is even greater.

Medical history

Your medical history provides additional information about your health, based on your weight.

If you answer yes to any of the following questions, you're likely to benefit from weight loss if you're overweight (BMI 25 to 29.9) or obese (BMI 30 or higher):

- Do you have high blood pressure, diabetes, heart disease, sleep apnea, osteoarthritis or abnormal blood fats (cholesterol and triglycerides)?
- Have you gained at least 10 pounds as an adult?
- Do you smoke cigarettes, overeat, have more than two

alcoholic drinks a day or lead an inactive lifestyle?

Assessing your weight

If your BMI is 25 or greater, your waist circumference equals or exceeds the healthy guidelines, or if you answered yes to at least one of the medical history questions, you're likely to benefit from losing weight. Discuss your weight with your doctor during your next checkup.

If your weight falls into the obese category, even losing just a few pounds may improve your health. A modest reduction in weight — 3 to 10 percent of your total weight — can improve many health conditions associated with excess weight. These include diabetes, high blood pressure, high cholesterol and sleep apnea.

If your extra weight is mostly around your waist, taking just 2 inches off your waist may reduce your blood pressure and lower your risk of many diseases.

Your Weight and Your Health

Obesity is a chronic disease that develops from the interaction between genes and the environment. Researchers' understanding of how and why people become obese is incomplete, but it involves a combination of factors.

Risk factors for becoming overweight

Weight is largely determined by how you balance your intake of calories with the energy you burn in everyday activities. If you consume more calories than you burn, you gain weight. Overeating and lack of physical activity are the main causes of being overweight. But many other factors contribute to this condition.

Genetics
Genes play a part in how your body balances calories and energy.

Body Mass Index (BMI)

	Healthy		Overweight					Obese				
BMI	19	24*	25	26	27	28	29	30	35	40	45	50

Height						Weight in pounds						
4'10"	91	115	119	124	129	134	138	143	167	191	215	239
4'11"	94	119	124	128	133	138	143	148	173	198	222	247
5'0"	97	123	128	133	138	143	148	153	179	204	230	255
5'1"	100	127	132	137	143	148	153	158	185	211	238	264
5'2"	104	131	136	142	147	153	158	164	191	218	246	273
5'3"	107	135	141	146	152	158	163	169	197	225	254	282
5'4"	110	140	145	151	157	163	169	174	204	232	262	291
5'5"	114	144	150	156	162	168	174	180	210	240	270	300
5'6"	118	148	155	161	167	173	179	186	216	247	278	309
5'7"	121	153	159	166	172	178	185	191	223	255	287	319
5'8"	125	158	164	171	177	184	190	197	230	262	295	328
5'9"	128	162	169	176	182	189	196	203	236	270	304	338
5'10"	132	167	174	181	188	195	202	209	243	278	313	348
5'11"	136	172	179	186	193	200	208	215	250	286	322	358
6'0"	140	177	184	191	199	206	213	221	258	294	331	368
6'1"	144	182	189	197	204	212	219	227	265	302	340	378
6'2"	148	186	194	202	210	218	225	233	272	311	350	389
6'3"	152	192	200	208	216	224	232	240	279	319	359	399
6'4"	156	197	205	213	221	230	238	246	287	328	369	410

*Asians with a BMI of 23 or higher may have an increased risk of health problems.
Based on Circulation, 2014;129(suppl 2):S102; NHLBI Obesity Expert Panel, 2013.

If one or both of your parents are overweight, your chances of being overweight increase by 25 to 30 percent. Your genes also affect the amount of body fat you store and how that fat is distributed. But your genetic makeup doesn't guarantee that you'll be overweight.

Diet
Large portion sizes and regular consumption of high-calorie foods contribute to weight gain. Foods high in sugar — such as candy, desserts and soft drinks — are dense in calories. Loading up on these foods promotes weight gain.

Another dietary factor that can contribute to increased weight is eating out regularly at restaurants.

Inactivity
Sedentary people are more likely to gain weight because they burn fewer calories through physical activity.

Psychological factors
Some people overeat to cope with problems, such as stress, anxiety or depression.

Sex
Men have more muscle and less fat than do women. Because muscle burns a greater number of calories than does fat, men expend up to 20 percent more calories than do women, even at rest. For women, achieving and maintaining a healthy weight may be a tougher challenge.

Age
As you get older, you gradually lose muscle, and fat accounts for a greater percentage of your weight. Less muscle mass leads to a decrease in the rate at which your body uses calories. The result is a reduction in calorie needs. Activity also tends to decline with age.

As you get older, if you don't reduce the number of calories you consume, you'll likely gain weight. Weight generally increases until you reach your 60s and then it tends to level off.

Pregnancy
After each pregnancy, women tend to gain an average of 4 to 6 pounds over their pre-pregnancy weight.

Medications
Side effects of some medications — such as corticosteroids and tricyclic antidepressants, insulin and other hormones — may lead to weight gain.

Quitting smoking
Some people gain weight after quitting smoking. This may be partially due to nicotine's ability to raise the rate at which your body burns calories (metabolic rate). When smokers quit, they tend to eat more because their senses of taste and smell improve.

Medical problems
Endocrine and metabolic disorders contribute to only a small percentage of cases of obesity. Less than 1 percent of all cases of obesity can be traced to a medical cause, such as low thyroid function or other hormonal imbalances. A low metabolic rate is rarely a cause of obesity.

Health effects of being overweight

Regardless of how a person becomes overweight, the condition can ultimately affect your health and your quality of life. Overweight and obese people are more likely to develop a number of potentially serious health problems.

Studies show that your risk of certain diseases and disorders increases as your body mass index increases. In addition, your overall risk of dying increases the more obese you are.

High blood pressure
When you have excess body fat, you tend to retain sodium. Extra sodium causes your body to hold on to more water. This increases the volume of your blood, and eventually the pressure inside your arteries builds up. The excessive force makes your heart work harder.

Excess weight is associated with altered nervous system activity and metabolic and vascular abnormalities that also increase blood pressure.

Abnormal blood fats
Obesity is associated with reduced levels of high-density lipoprotein (HDL, or "good") cholesterol and with high levels of a type of blood fat known as triglycerides.

Over time, these blood substances can contribute to the buildup of fatty deposits in arteries, particularly those in your heart. This condition is called atherosclerosis, and it puts you at risk of coronary artery disease and stroke.

Diabetes
Obesity is a leading cause of type 2 diabetes. Excess fat makes your body resistant to insulin, the hormone that helps transport sugar (glucose) from your blood into individual cells. If your body is resistant to insulin, the sugar remains in your blood. Your cells can't get the glucose they need for energy, and your blood glucose rises.

Metabolic syndrome
The combination of too much weight around your abdomen (abdominal obesity), high blood pressure, elevated blood sugar (glucose), abnormal blood fats (cholesterol and triglycerides) and other abnormalities is called metabolic syndrome.

Coronary artery disease
If you're overweight, you may be at increased risk of coronary artery disease, largely related to metabolic syndrome. However, there's also an increased risk from obesity itself.

Aging and Body Fat

Your body composition changes as you age. Muscle mass decreases slowly after ages 30 to 35 and more rapidly after age 55. Translated into what your scale may be telling you, if you weigh 10 pounds more at age 65 than you did at 30, you may actually be carrying 15 to 20 pounds more fat.

The distribution of fat also changes with age. As you get older, body fat tends to shift from the face, arms, legs and neck to the trunk and abdomen — hence the appearance of the spare tire or love handles.

For women, menopause can play a role in midlife body changes. During the years leading up to menopause, you begin to produce less estrogen, a process that's associated with weight shifting to your middle. And, because of changes in physical activity, metabolic rate and possibly diet, women often gain weight or have more trouble staying at the same weight during and after menopause.

An excellent way to deal with age-related weight change is to exercise. Aerobic exercise helps you burn calories, and strength-training exercises increase muscle mass and strengthen bones. See Chapter 9, "Fitness," for detailed information about aerobic exercise and strength training.

Coronary artery disease typically results from the buildup of fatty deposits (plaques) in the arteries that feed your heart. Over time, these deposits can narrow your heart's arteries, and complete blockage can lead to a heart attack.

Stroke

The accumulation of deposits (plaques) in arteries that feed the brain can lead to a stroke. When an artery leading to your brain becomes narrowed, a blood clot can form in the artery, interrupting blood flow to your brain. The result is an ischemic stroke. Being overweight or obese increases risk of an ischemic stroke, even in the absence of high blood pressure and diabetes.

Osteoarthritis

This joint disorder most often affects the knees, hips and lower back. Excess weight puts extra pressure on these joints and wears away the cartilage that protects them, resulting in joint pain and stiffness.

Sleep apnea

Obstructive sleep apnea is a serious condition that causes you to stop breathing for short periods during sleep. The upper airway becomes blocked intermittently during sleep, resulting in lower blood oxygen levels and subsequent drowsiness during the day. Sleep apnea can also contribute to high blood pressure and heart failure.

Most people with sleep apnea are overweight. The more overweight an individual is, the more severe his or her sleep apnea tends to be. Obesity is associated with other sleep problems, including snoring.

Cancer

Many types of cancer are associated with being overweight. In women, these include cancers of the breast, uterus, colon and gallbladder. Overweight men have a higher risk of colon and prostate cancers.

Gallstones

Gallstones are more common in people who are overweight, although it's not clear how being overweight results in gallstones.

Physical discomfort

As fat accumulates, it crowds the space occupied by your organs. Some obese people have trouble moving around because of their obesity, and some have trouble getting up from the ground.

Social and emotional consequences

In a country that tends to equate thinness with beauty, intelligence and success, overweight adults may experience psychological stress, reduced income and discrimination.

Benefits of modest weight loss

The good news is that you don't have to lose a lot of weight to enjoy health benefits. A modest reduction of just 3 to 10 percent of your body weight can lower your blood pressure, reduce your risk of cardiovascular disease and stroke, improve control of diabetes, improve symptoms of osteoarthritis and sleep apnea, and lower your risk of cancer.

The amount of weight you need to lose to improve your health may actually be much less than what you envision you need to lose to be thin or achieve an "ideal" appearance.

The first goals in dealing with being overweight are to take steps to lose some weight and to maintain the weight loss. For example, if you weigh 200 pounds and are obese by BMI standards, start by trying to lose 10 pounds — that's 5 percent of your weight. Talk to your doctor about setting realistic weight-loss goals to improve your health.

How to Lose Weight

If you've struggled with your weight, you likely know that both losing weight and keeping it off can be very difficult. Many diets promote temporary weight loss, but they may also encourage unhealthy eating habits, and their long-term effects are often minimal.

Healthy weight loss is weight loss that's slow and steady over the long term. The first couple of weeks weight loss may be more rapid, but after that aim to lose no more than 1 to 2 pounds a week.

A good weight-loss plan has three components — a healthy diet, regular physical activity and changes to your lifestyle that you can sustain for life.

Eat a healthy diet

What you eat and how much you eat play key roles in managing your weight. Eating a healthy diet means learning to enjoy a variety of healthy foods.

There's not one best diet that will help you easily shed pounds. To lose weight and keep it off you need to decrease the number of calories you consume each day. You want to choose a diet that's healthy and that will work for you, based on your preferences and lifestyle.

Decreasing calories, however, doesn't mean decreasing the taste or satisfaction of the food you eat or increasing preparation time. You can lower your calorie intake by eating foods that are tasty, healthy and practical.

Select the right mix of foods

To help guide your daily food choices, Mayo Clinic doctors and nutrition experts developed the Mayo Clinic Healthy Weight Pyramid and Mayo Clinic Healthy Dining Table.

The pyramid and dining table are tools that can help you improve your health while reducing your weight. They illustrate the types and amounts of food you need to eat every day from each of five key food groups.

The triangular shape of the pyramid shows you where to focus when selecting foods that can help promote healthy weight. The dining table helps you to visualize what your meals should look like on your plate. It shows approximately how your servings should be divided at each meal.

Mayo Clinic Healthy Weight Pyramid

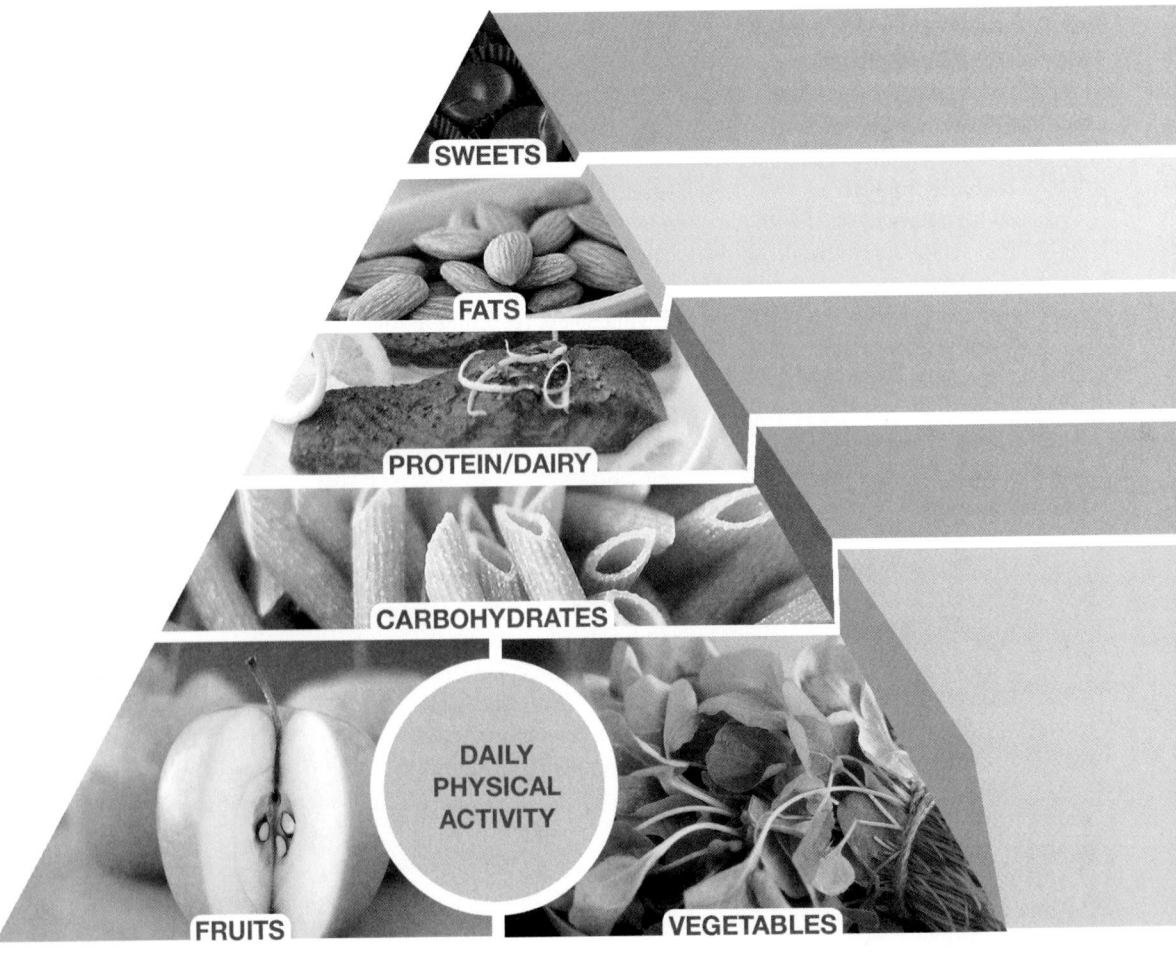

The most important foods — vegetables and fruits — form the foundation of the pyramid. That's because vegetables and fruits are lower in energy density — they provide few calories for their bulk. If you eat foods with low energy density, you can eat more food but consume fewer calories.

Fruits and vegetables are low in energy density because they're composed mainly of water and fiber. Water provides weight and volume to help you feel full and has no calories. Fiber provides bulk, so you feel full sooner. Fiber also takes longer to digest, making you feel full longer.

The Mayo Clinic Healthy Weight Pyramid and Healthy Dining Table provide all of the nutrients you need for good health. Unlimited fresh or frozen fruits and vegetables make it high in vitamins, minerals, fiber and plant nutrients called phytochemicals. The diet is low in fat, saturated fat, cholesterol and sodium, and it provides adequate protein and calcium.

Vegetables

Vegetables are low in calories and virtually fat-free while providing a variety of vitamins, minerals and, in most cases, fiber. In addition, vegetables contain phytochemicals, substances that can reduce your risk of cardiovascular disease and cancer. Some vegetables belong within the carbohydrates group instead of the vegetable group because they're high in starch, contain more calories than typical vegetables and function more like a carbohydrate in your body. These include corn, potatoes, sweet potatoes and winter squash.

Fruits

Along with few calories and little or no fat, fruit also contains vitamins, minerals, fiber and phytochemicals. Fresh and frozen fruits are best because they're bulkier and lower in energy density than are canned fruits, fruit juices and dried fruits. Foods and beverages that are lower in energy density have fewer calories relative to their volume.

Carbohydrates

Carbohydrates include grain products such as cereal, bread, rice and pasta. These foods provide a variety of nutrients and are generally low in fat and calories.

Mayo Clinic Healthy Dining Table

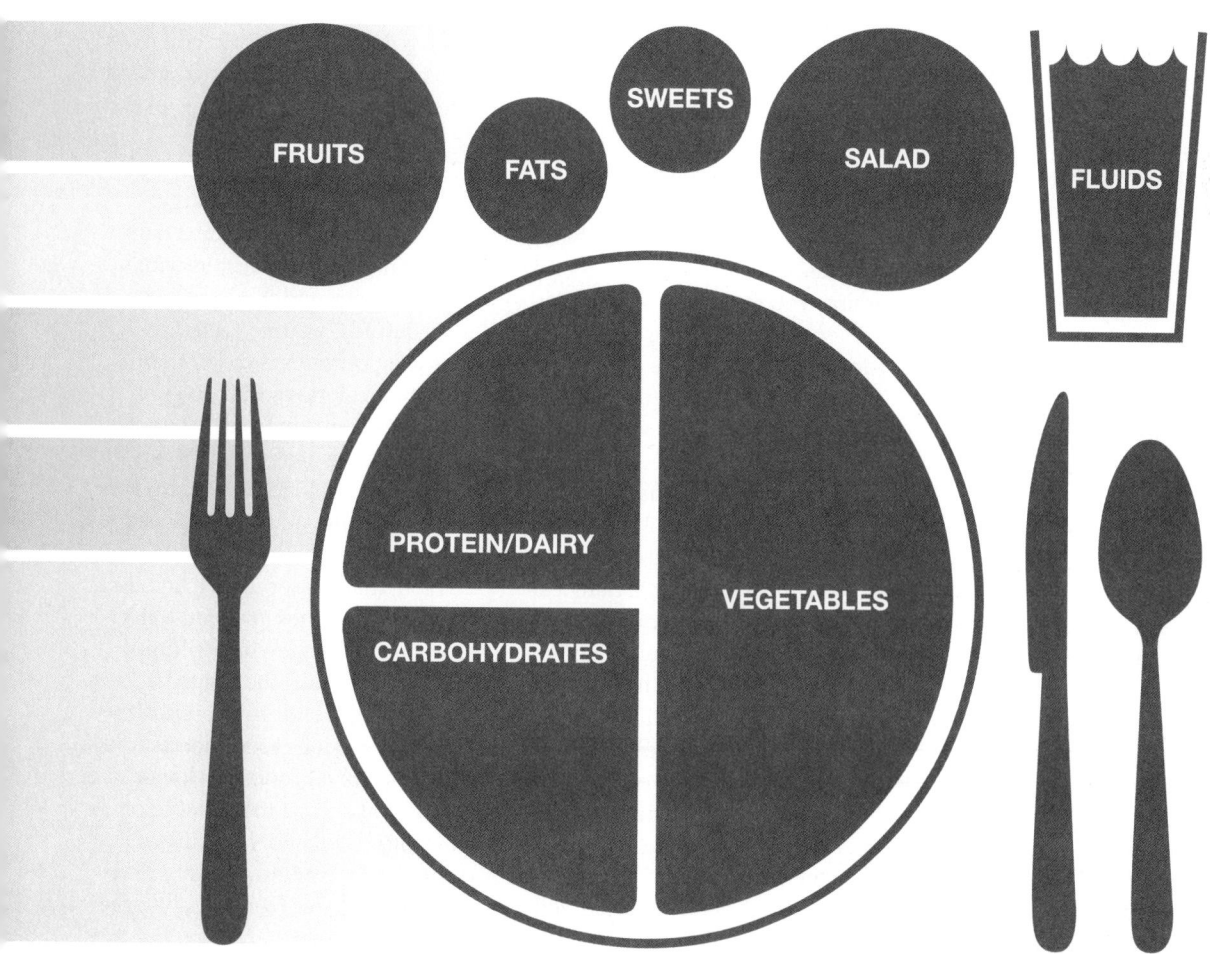

Calorie Targets

On the chart below, find your current weight and the calorie target associated with that weight. This is a good place to start. You can adjust the target based on your personal goals and how quickly you want to lose weight. If you feel exceptionally hungry all of the time, consider moving up to the next calorie level. If you want to move down a level, don't drop below the lowest level listed.

Weight in pounds	Starting calorie target			
Women	**1,200**	**1,400**	**1,600**	**1,800**
250 or less	✔			
251 to 300		✔		
301 or more			✔	
Men	**1,200**	**1,400**	**1,600**	**1,800**
250 or less		✔		
251 to 300			✔	
301 or more				✔

It's often other ingredients added to grain products or creamy sauces served with them that add calories and fat.

The best grains are whole grains because they're higher in fiber, vitamins and minerals. Choose brown rice, whole-grain pasta, and breads made from whole-wheat or whole-grain flour.

Protein and Dairy

The foods in the protein and dairy group usually provide most of the protein in your diet. Because many animal-based protein sources are high in saturated fat, the Mayo Clinic Healthy Weight Pyramid emphasizes healthy sources of protein, such as beans, peas and lentils; fish; and low-fat or fat-free dairy products. Dairy products are good sources of calcium, and milk is fortified with vitamin D.

Fats

Because gram for gram fat has more than twice the calories of carbohydrates and protein, reducing the fat in your diet is an important way to cut calories if you're trying to lose weight. Prepare foods with little or no oil or other fats. When using fats, choose healthy unsaturated fats, such as olive or canola oil. Nuts are also a good source of healthy fat.

Sweets

This group includes candies, desserts and other processed sweets. You can eat sweets in amounts that average 75 calories a day. Once you get used to a diet that emphasizes fruits, vegetables and grains, you may not miss sweets.

Identify your calorie target

To lose weight, your goal is to consume fewer calories than you burn. The number of calories you need each day depends on several factors, including your age and your activity level. See chart above to determine your initial daily calorie target based on your weight.

Over time, your calorie needs may change based on health risks, how much weight you lose, and your goals and preferences. Calories can be adjusted to the next higher level if you've reached your target weight and your goal now is maintenance.

Cutting calories to below 1,200 a day if you're a woman or 1,400 a day if you're a man usually doesn't provide enough food to keep you to satisfied long term. Eating below these calorie levels also makes it difficult for you to get some of the nutrients you need for good health.

Determine your servings goals

Using your daily calorie target, look at the chart on the next page to determine how many servings from the pyramid food groups you should consume each day. Tracking servings is easier than counting calories and it gives a "close-enough" measurement of calorie intake. It also provides a guide to what kind of foods to eat, ensuring that you get a balanced diet.

Note that the servings listed for the carbohydrates, protein/dairy and fats groups are upper limits. Try not to exceed the limits.

Vegetables and fruits are different. The serving recommendations for these food groups are lower limits. Eat at least the number of servings listed and you can eat more if you want to. When you're hungry, feel free to snack on vegetables and fruits.

Serving Recommendations

The number of servings to choose from each food group depends on your daily calorie target. The following chart lists the number of servings recommended for various calorie levels:

| Food group | Starting calorie targets | | | |
	1,200	1,400	1,600	1,800
	Recommended number of daily servings			
Vegetables	4 or more	4 or more	5 or more	5 or more
Fruits	3 or more	4 or more	5 or more	5 or more
Carbohydrates	4	5	6	7
Protein/Dairy	3	4	5	6
Fats	3	3	3	4

Check product labels to learn how much of the food is considered a serving and how many calories and grams of fat are in the food. Many items sold as single portions actually provide two or more servings.

Learn serving sizes

Don't be worried by how many servings of some foods you should eat each day, such as four servings of vegetables. It's easy to confuse servings with portions.

A serving is an exact amount of food, compared with a portion, which is the amount you put on your plate. A serving may be smaller than you think, and a portion may contain several servings. One of the reasons more people today are overweight is that portion sizes have increased, especially in restaurants.

On page 274 is a chart that offers visual cues to help you gauge Mayo Clinic Healthy Weight Servings for the various food groups. The cues will get you "close enough" to actual serving sizes. Keep these cues in mind as you plan your meals and place food on your plate.

Be physically active

Studies show that people who want to optimize weight loss — and keep it off — must do more than transform their eating habits. They need to make physical activity and exercise a part of their daily routine. To stay fit and maintain a healthy weight, you need to keep active.

The goal of exercise to promote weight loss is to burn calories, but it has many other benefits as well. Physical activity promotes loss of body fat and development of muscle. Muscle uses more calories than fat does. So the more muscle mass your body has, the more calories it'll burn, even when you're at rest.

The best way to lose body fat is to sit less and move more. Compared with five decades ago, people today move less. At work, if you sit for hours at your desk, you're burning an average of 130 fewer calories a day. Most people are less active at home as well, where it's all too tempting to sit in front of the TV or computer for the evening.

All of that inactivity adds up. It's not good for your health and it leads to weight gain.

Find ways to move more during the day and try to build steady aerobic exercise into your daily routine — activities that increase your breathing and heart rate, such as walking, bicycling, jogging and swimming.

Remember, any extra movement helps burn calories. Activities such as mowing the lawn, cleaning the house, taking the stairs instead of the elevator at work or walking the dog, also can help with weight management.

Your goal should be at least 30 minutes of moderate to vigorous physical activity on most or all days of the week. Start slowly and gradually build up your time and intensity level and stick to it.

If you're obese — particularly if you're unfit and you have health problems — check with your doctor before starting an exercise program.

For more information about developing an exercise program, see Chapter 9, "Fitness."

Adopt a positive attitude

Anyone who has tried to lose weight knows that it's more challenging than it sounds. To make lasting changes, you need to address your habits, emotions,

Quick guide to serving sizes

Vegetables	Calories	Visual cue
1 cup broccoli	25	1 baseball
2 cups raw, leafy greens	25	2 baseballs

Fruits	Calories	Visual cue
½ cup sliced fruit	60	Tennis ball
1 small apple or medium orange	60	Tennis ball

Carbohydrates	Calories	Visual cue
½ cup pasta or dried cereal	70	Hockey puck
½ bagel	70	Hockey puck
1 slice whole-grain bread	70	Hockey puck
½ medium baked potato	70	Hockey puck

Protein/Dairy	Calories	Visual cue
3 ounces of fish	110	Deck of cards
2-2½ ounces of meat	110	⅔ deck of cards
1½-2 ounces of hard cheese	110	⅓ deck of cards

Fats	Calories	Visual cue
1½ teaspoons peanut butter	45	2 dice
1 teaspoon butter or margarine	45	1 die

needs, thinking and the behaviors that made you overweight in the first place.

Part of being successful is to plan how you'll incorporate changes into your lifestyle. This takes time and effort. A variety of tools are effective in helping change attitudes and behaviors:

Make a commitment
Focus on all of the good things about losing weight, such as having more energy and improving your health. Then look at the negatives, such as finding the time to exercise. Look for creative solutions to overcome the negatives and then commit yourself to losing weight.

Set small, realistic goals
Remember that you're in this for the long haul. You're making lifestyle changes, and the goals you write down are your first steps in that direction. Anything you undertake too intensely or too vigorously will quickly become uncomfortable, and you're more likely to give it up. Don't set a weight goal that's unrealistic.

Focus on the positive
Rather than dwelling on what you can't eat, focus on what you can. Discover new tastes and activities.

Know your habits
To become aware of your eating behaviors, ask yourself if you tend to eat when you're bored, angry, tired, anxious or depressed. Assess your eating style and shopping and cooking techniques. Were you taught to always clean your plate? Do you eat fast? Do you eat while watching TV? See if any patterns emerge.

Eating Out

According to the U.S. Department of Commerce, Americans spend more money at restaurants these days than they do at grocery stores. That isn't good for your health or your waistline! You're less likely to make healthy choices when you eat out than when you eat at home. But that doesn't mean that you can't eat out on occasion. You just need to play it smart.

When dining out, the rules you use at home still apply. And remember, eating out includes more than just restaurants. No matter if you're in the coffee shop, buying food at a convenience store, or attending an office potluck or catered event, you're still eating out! As always, selecting the right foods is key.

Plan ahead

When it comes to eating out, being prepared can make all the difference. Set yourself up for success before you even step out the door.

- *Consider your options.* If you don't have a lot of time, it may seem easiest to go to a fast-food restaurant, but remember there are other options. You can stop at a convenience store and pick up some fruit, a prepackaged salad or a small sandwich. If you have time for a more relaxed meal, stop at a restaurant that has low-calorie options and plenty of fruits and vegetables on the menu.

- *Go online.* Review the menus at restaurants you're considering. When you get to the restaurant it may be hard to study what's available. When you're online, you can check out which restaurants have offerings that fit with your meal plan. You can even look up nutrition information at some restaurant chains. If the calories are posted, consider a meal that provides about 500 to 600 calories. Also check to see if they have healthy side dishes.

- *Have a snack first.* If you're meeting friends for a late dinner, eat something an hour or two before you leave. That way, you won't show up famished and be tempted to order more food than you need. You'll also be less likely to fill up on the chips and salsa or bread rolls that sit at the table before your meal arrives.

- *Don't eat on the go.* Even if your day is packed, take a few minutes to sit down and eat. If you're eating while you're driving, you're more likely to eat too much too quickly and make unhealthy food choices. (It's hard to eat a salad when you're hands are on the wheel!) The end result: You feel guilty and frustrated afterward.

Eating at fast-food restaurants

Fast-food restaurants are everywhere, and they're popular. Among other things, they offer a meal in a hurry when you don't have much time. But eating at fast-food restaurants on a regular basis isn't a good idea. Perhaps the biggest reasons why are because fast food is often loaded with calories and the portions are often very large. This doesn't mean an occasional stop at a fast-food restaurant is out of the question. Just be smart in what you eat.

Fortunately, making healthy choices at fast-food and other chain restaurants is now easier. The Food and Drug Administration has established new regulations for nutrition labeling in chain restaurants. All fast-food and sit-down restaurant chains with at least 20 locations are required to provide nutrition information about the foods they serve on their menus or menu boards. These regulations also apply to drive-thru windows, and to foods sold in bakeries and coffee shops, and many vending machines.

Have a plan

Work out a strategy to gradually change your habits and any attitudes that may have undermined past efforts to lose weight. If possible, write it down and place it in a location where you can see it.

Avoid your food triggers

Store food out of sight and don't keep junk food around. Practice substituting healthy food for unhealthy food. Distract yourself from your desire to eat with something positive, like calling a friend or going for a walk.

Plan ahead for unusual circumstances

Think of effective strategies for keeping your commitment while at work, on vacation, at parties and during the holidays. For example, envision yourself at a party taking a small portion of a few items or taking only fresh fruits and vegetables. Mentally rehearse this plan.

Keep a record

Studies show that keeping a food record helps with weight loss. In addition to keeping track of the food servings you eat, you might want to keep track of the amount of time you're physically active each day. Some people track other important health parameters, such as their blood pressure or blood sugar (glucose) levels.

Draw on support from others

Ultimately, only you can help yourself lose weight, and you have to take responsibility for your own behavior. But that doesn't mean that you have to do everything alone. Ask for support from your spouse, partner, family or friends.

Action Guide to Weight-Loss Barriers

To lose weight — and maintain a healthy weight — you need to identify your barriers to weight loss and find solutions. Check all the barriers that apply to you.

Barriers	Possible solutions
❑ I tried to lose weight before, but it didn't work. So I don't have a lot of confidence that it'll work this time.	• Set realistic expectations. • Focus on behavioral changes rather than numbers of pounds. • Make small changes to your lifestyle so that you don't give up. • When you have a setback, start fresh the next day. • Write down previous obstacles and strategies for dealing with them. • Identify what will motivate you to be successful.
❑ My family doesn't like to try new things, and it's too much work to make two different meals.	• Take it slow. Make a few small changes each week. • Keep fruit in a location where it's visible and easy to grab. • Prepare a favorite dish using a different cooking method, such as baking chicken instead of frying. • Ask family members which healthy foods they'd like to try. Give them several options so that they might be more willing to experiment.
❑ I don't like vegetables and fruits.	• Find a few that you do like and eat them more often. • Try vegetables that you've never had. Add them to your favorite soups or replace some of the meat in casseroles or pizzas with vegetables. • Include fresh fruit with your cereal, and stir fruit into low-fat yogurt or low-fat cottage cheese.
❑ I can't resist certain foods that I shouldn't eat, such as potato chips and other junk foods.	• Avoid keeping junk food at home. • If you can't resist the urge, buy only a small amount, such as a single serving. Have it with your meal. • Eat healthy foods first, so you won't be so hungry when you eat your favorites. • Try healthier versions, such as baked rather than regular chips.
❑ I eat when I'm stressed, depressed or bored.	• Instead of high-fat, high-calorie "comfort foods," keep healthy foods in your house. • Try to distract yourself from eating by calling a friend, running an errand or going for a walk. • Try to think positively. For example, write down what you want to achieve with weight loss.
❑ I don't have time to make healthy meals.	• Keep it simple. For example, serve a fresh salad with fat-free dressing, a whole-grain roll and a piece of fruit. • Stop at a deli or grocery store and buy a healthy sandwich, soup or entree that's low in calories and fat.
❑ When eating out, I like to eat my favorite foods — not something healthy.	• Eat only half of your favorite foods and save the other half for the next day. (But if you dine out often, make healthy eating routine.) • If you know that you'll be eating extra calories, increase your exercise for the day.
❑ I don't like to exercise.	• Remember that physical activity — anything that gets you moving — burns calories, too. • Choose activities that you enjoy and include variety. • Exercise with a friend or a group so that you can socialize. • Take a class or buy an exercise video if you need structure.

It may be helpful to talk to a weight-loss specialist or others trying to lose weight who can help you think of food and exercise in a new light. Group programs such as Weight Watchers, Take Off Pounds Sensibly (TOPS) or Overeaters Anonymous can support your efforts, giving you eating plans and reinforcement from others on the same path.

Don't give up

No matter how prepared you are, you'll occasionally overeat or eat foods that you're trying to avoid. Rather than letting a setback derail your efforts, accept that the setback happened and get back on track. Don't expect to be perfect — no one is. And never give up.

Set SMART goals

Your ability to reach your weight goals is closely tied to how realistic your expectations are. Goals that are too unrealistic or too long term just set you up for frustration and disappointment.

You want to set goals that are SMART: specific, measurable, attainable, relevant and time-limited.

- **Specific.** State exactly what you want to achieve, how you're going to do it, and why you want to achieve it.
- **Measurable.** Track your progress. For example, whether your goal is to walk for 30 minutes a day or jog 3 miles a day, track this in an exercise log. If your goal is to eat more servings of vegetables and fruits, track the number of servings you eat each day in a food record or food diary.
- **Attainable.** Set a goal that's realistic and that you have sufficient time and resources to achieve. If anything, err on the side of starting off too easily.
- **Relevant.** Set a goal that's important and that means something to you. It doesn't have to be huge and lofty to be relevant.

- **Time-limited.** It's helpful to plan a series of smaller goals that build on each other instead of one major long-term goal. Setting and achieving short-term goals helps keep you motivated.

Deal with obstacles

There's no greater reward for your efforts than to step on the scale and see that you've lost weight. But what happens when the indicator on the scale doesn't change from week to week, even if you're eating a healthy, low-calorie diet and exercising regularly? Or you see results the first few weeks then you hit a plateau?

Before you get discouraged, understand that long-term results don't always show up right away. It's normal to hit plateaus, and if you do hit one, don't give up!

To help you get past the plateau, try one of these tips:
- Review your food and activity records. Make sure you haven't loosened the rules, letting yourself get by with more calories or less exercise.
- Focus on three- to four-week trends in weight loss instead of daily fluctuations.
- Reassess your program. Is it possible you've accomplished about as much as you can with the goals you've set? Maybe you need to adjust your goals.

For more on common weight-loss obstacles and how to deal with them, see the opposite page.

When You Need Extra Help

It's best to lose weight by adopting a healthy diet and getting regular physical activity. Some people, though, have physical limitations that keep them from exercising. Others need extra help reducing their calorie intake.

In such cases, medications or surgery may help.

Medications

If you have serious health problems because of your weight — and lifestyle changes haven't resulted in significant weight loss — prescription weight-loss drugs may be an option. You should know, though, that prescription weight-loss drugs don't replace the need to make healthy changes in your eating habits and your activity level.

Are you a candidate?
Prescription weight-loss drugs are generally reserved for people who haven't been able to lose

Willpower vs. Self-Control

Some people think that they can achieve a healthy weight if they exert enough willpower. But that just sets you up to fail when your willpower cracks. Try focusing on self-control rather than willpower. Self-control is, "Ice cream is my problem food, so I'm not going to keep it in the house." Willpower is, "I'm going to keep buying ice cream, but I won't eat it." Self-control means planning for success ahead of time.

If you like sweets, consider finding a way to occasionally fit them into your diet without destroying your overall eating plan. You may be surprised to discover that just knowing it's all right to allow yourself a treat now and then can make it easier to say no.

weight through diet and exercise, and who have health problems because of their weight. They're not for people who want to lose just a few pounds for cosmetic reasons.

Your doctor may consider weight-loss drugs if you haven't been able to lose weight through diet and exercise and you meet one of the following:

- Your body mass index (BMI) is greater than 30.
- Your BMI is greater than 27 and you have a serious medical problem related to obesity, such as diabetes or high blood pressure.

Before selecting a medication for you, your doctor will consider your health history, any potential interaction of weight-loss drugs with other medications you're taking and the possible side effects of the medications being considered. Some weight-loss drugs can produce serious side effects and their use needs to be monitored.

How well do they work?

When combined with a low-calorie diet and regular exercise, weight-loss drugs produce an average weight loss of 5 to 10 percent of total body weight within a year, which is a typical weight-loss goal. Diet and exercise are responsible for part of this weight loss, and the medications are responsible for part as well.

Losing 5 to 10 percent of your total weight may not seem like much, but even modest weight loss can improve your health.

Keep in mind, however, that these medications may not work for everyone. And when you stop taking the medications, you're likely to regain much or all of the weight you lost if you don't change your unhealthy habits.

Factors to consider

If you meet the criteria for prescription weight-loss drugs, you'll want to evaluate the potential benefits of the drugs against

their possible risks. Cost also is a consideration. Not all health insurance plans cover prescription weight-loss drugs. In addition, adverse effects are common with many weight-loss drugs, which may make it difficult to stick with treatment.

While taking the medications, you'll still want to make every effort to exercise, change your eating habits and adjust any other lifestyle factors that may have contributed to your excess weight.

Weight-loss drugs aren't the easy answer to weight loss, but they may be a useful tool to help you make the dietary and lifestyle changes. Keeping off the pounds that you lose is an ongoing concern. Many people, despite their efforts, eventually regain the weight they've lost.

Surgery

Generally, weight-loss surgery is reserved for people who are severely overweight and who have health problems as a result.

Before you consider surgery, make sure that you've made every effort to exercise, change your eating habits and address any lifestyle factors that may have contributed to your weight gain.

If you do have surgery, its success will depend in part on your commitment to carefully follow the guidelines given to you about food choices and exercise.

Weight-loss (bariatric) surgery helps you lose weight and lowers your risk of medical problems associated with obesity. Bariatric surgery contributes to weight loss in two main ways:

- **Restriction.** Surgery is used to physically limit the amount of food the stomach can hold, which limits the number of calories you can eat.
- **Malabsorption.** Surgery is used to shorten or bypass part of the small intestine, which reduces the amount of calories and nutrients the body absorbs.

Are you a candidate?

In general, weight-loss surgery may be an option if:

- Your body mass index (BMI) is 40 or higher (extreme obesity).
- Your BMI is 35 to 39.9 (obesity) and you have a serious weight-related health problem, such as type 2 diabetes, high blood pressure or severe sleep apnea. In some cases, you may qualify for certain types of weight-loss surgery if your BMI is 30 to 34 and you have serious weight-related health problems.

You likely will go through an extensive screening process to see if you qualify. When conducting an evaluation for gastric bypass surgery, the health team considers:

- **Your nutrition and weight history.** The team reviews your weight trends, diet attempts, eating habits, exercise regimen, stress level, time constraints, motivation and other factors.
- **Your medical condition.** Some health problems, such as blood clots, liver disease, heart problems, kidney stones and nutritional deficiencies, increase the risks associated with having surgery or may be worsened by surgery. The team evaluates what medications you take, how much alcohol you drink and whether you smoke. You'll also undergo a physical exam and laboratory testing. The results of these tests and exams may help determine eligibility for weight-loss surgery.
- **Your psychological status.** Certain mental health conditions may contribute to obesity or make it more difficult for you to maintain the health benefits of gastric bypass surgery. These may include binge-eating disorder, substance use disorder, depression, anxiety disorders and issues related to childhood sexual abuse. These may not prevent you from having gastric bypass surgery, but your doctors may want to postpone surgery to ensure that any con-

Weight-Loss Drugs

This chart shows some prescription weight-loss drugs, how they work and their possible side effects.

Drug	How it works	Possible side effects
Benzphetamine hydrochloride	Decreases appetite, increases feeling of fullness	Increased blood pressure and heart rate, nervousness, insomnia, dry mouth, constipation
Diethylpropion (Tenuate)	Decreases appetite, increases feeling of fullness	Headache, increased blood pressure and heart rate, nervousness, insomnia, dry mouth, constipation
Lorcaserin (Belviq)	Decreases appetite, increases feeling of fullness	Headache, nausea, dry mouth, dizziness, fatigue, constipation
Naltrexone and bupropion extended-release (Contrave)	Decreases appetite, increases feeling of fullness	Nausea, constipation, headache, vomiting, dizziness
Phendimetrazine	Decreases appetite, increases feeling of fullness	Increased blood pressure and heart rate, nervousness, insomnia, dry mouth, constipation
Phentermine (Adipex-P)	Decreases appetite, increases feeling of fullness	Headache, increased blood pressure and heart rate, nervousness, insomnia, dry mouth, constipation
Orlistat (Xenical)	Blocks absorption of fat	Decreased absorption of fat-soluble vitamins, oily spotting, intestinal cramps, gas with discharge, diarrhea, fecal urgency and incontinence
Phentermine and topiramate extended-release (Qsymia)	Decreases appetite, increases feeling of fullness	Insomnia, dry mouth, dizziness, constipation, pins and needles feeling, changes in sense of taste or smell
Liraglutide (Saxenda)	Slows gastric emptying, increases feeling of fullness	Nausea, vomiting, pancreatitis

dition is appropriately treated and managed.
- **Your motivation.** The team will also assess your willingness and ability to follow through with recommendations and carry out prescribed changes in your diet and exercise routine.
- **Your age.** Although there's no specific age limit for gastric bypass surgery, the risks increase as you get older. The surgery remains controversial in people under age 18.

Types
Four common types of weight-loss surgery are:
- Roux-en-Y gastric bypass
- Laparoscopic adjustable gastric banding
- Sleeve gastrectomy
- Biliopancreatic diversion with duodenal switch

Roux-en-Y gastric bypass
In this procedure, a surgeon creates a small pouch at the top of the stomach. The pouch is the only part of the stomach that receives food. This greatly limits the amount that you can comfortably eat and drink at one time.

The small intestine is then cut a short distance below the main stomach and connected to the new pouch. Food flows directly from the pouch into this part of the intestine. The main part of the stomach, however, continues to make digestive juices. The portion of the intestine still attached to the main stomach is reattached farther down. This allows the digestive juices to flow to the small intestine. Because food now bypasses a portion of the small intestine, fewer nutrients and calories are absorbed.

Laparoscopic adjustable gastric banding

In the laparoscopic adjustable gastric banding procedure, a band containing an inflatable balloon is placed around the upper part of the stomach and it's fixed in place. This creates a small stomach pouch above the band with a very narrow opening to the rest of the stomach.

A port is then placed under the skin of the abdomen. A tube connects the port to the band. By injecting or removing fluid through the port, the balloon can be inflated or deflated to adjust the size of the band.

Gastric banding works by restricting the amount of food that your stomach can hold, so that you feel full sooner. Unlike some other weight-loss surgeries, it doesn't reduce the absorption of calories and nutrients.

Sleeve gastrectomy

In a sleeve gastrectomy, part of the stomach is separated and removed from the body. The remaining section of the stomach is formed into a tubelike structure. This smaller stomach cannot hold as much food. It also produces less of the appetite-regulating hormone ghrelin, which may lessen your desire to eat. However, sleeve gastrectomy doesn't affect the absorption of calories and nutrients in the intestines.

Biliopancreatic diversion with duodenal switch

As with sleeve gastrectomy, this procedure begins with a surgeon removing a large part of the stomach. The valve that releases food to the small intestine is left, along with the first part of the small intestine, called the duodenum. The surgeon then closes off the middle section of the intestine and attaches the last part directly to the duodenum. This is the duodenal switch.

The separated section of the intestine isn't removed from the body. Instead, it's reattached to the end of the intestine, allowing bile and pancreatic digestive juices to flow into this part of the intestine. This is the biliopancreatic diversion.

As a result of these changes, food bypasses most of the small intestine, limiting the absorption of calories and nutrients. This, together with the smaller size of the stomach, leads to weight loss.

Results

When used appropriately, weight-loss surgery can result in dramatic improvements in weight and health. In the first one to two years after this operation, many people lose up to 50 to 60 percent of their excess weight. Generally, individuals who follow dietary and exercise recommendations are able to keep most of that weight off long term.

However, weight-loss surgery does have side effects. Vitamin deficiencies can develop if you can't take the recommended supplements. Rapid weight loss can result in fatigue, dry skin and temporary hair loss. A hernia or weakness, which may require surgical repair, can develop at the site of your incision.

In addition, if you eat too much or too fast, you may experience nausea, vomiting, sweating and shakiness, called dumping syndrome. Over time, you'll be able to increase your food intake.

Keep in mind that surgery for weight reduction isn't a miracle procedure. Though you can expect to lose weight and it's possible to keep it off, you still need to eat healthy foods and remain physically active. ■

Fitness

Modern society seems to conspire against physical activity. With modern phones, computers, TVs and countless labor-saving devices, it's easy to get through each day with little physical exertion. Yet our bodies are designed to move. And it's important that they do.

Regular physical activity results in a number of health benefits. Adding more physical activity to your day doesn't mean that you have to become a marathon runner or head to the gym each morning. Simple modifications to your lifestyle can go a long way toward improving your health.

For many years the common belief was that you had to exercise vigorously if you wanted to become physically fit and improve your health. Vigorous exercise has its benefits, but studies show that even light activity is good for your health — and it's definitely better than doing nothing at all.

Moderate physical activity performed on a regular basis gives you most of the health benefits of more vigorous exercise, according to the Centers for Disease Control and Prevention and the National Institutes of Health.

Fitness Pays

The decision to become more active is an investment in yourself, your family and your future. For a modest time investment, the rewards are enormous.

Along with eating well, physical activity is the key to improving your overall health and preventing illness. People who are physically active can often perform at a level comparable with that of an inactive person who's 10 to 20 years younger.

Regular physical activity can help you control your weight, improve your coordination and balance, reduce muscle aches and pains, and avoid insomnia. It may also prevent, delay or control the following diseases and conditions, among others:

High blood pressure

Physical activity is critical to efforts to prevent or control high blood pressure. Activity challenges your heart, which is a muscle. With exercise your heart becomes stronger and can pump more blood with less effort. The result is less pressure on your arteries.

Abnormal blood fats

Daily physical activity can reduce your low-density lipoprotein (LDL) cholesterol level and increase your high-density lipoprotein (HDL) cholesterol level. LDL cholesterol is commonly referred to as the "bad" cholesterol, and HDL cholesterol as the "good" cholesterol. Regular activity also helps reduce triglycerides, another type of blood fat (lipid).

Diabetes

Physical activity lowers the amount of a sugar (glucose) in your blood. Diabetes is characterized by blood sugar levels that are too high. If you have or are at risk of diabetes, daily activity combined with a healthy diet can help keep your glucose levels under control.

Coronary artery disease and stroke

Coronary artery disease is damage to the arteries that supply blood to your heart. The damage typically results from narrowing of the arteries (atherosclerosis), which may stem from a variety of factors, including high blood pressure, diabetes, smoking or high cholesterol. Complete blockage of the arteries can cause a heart attack.

Physical activity helps prevent coronary artery disease — and reduces your risk of having a heart attack — by helping you achieve and maintain a healthy weight, controlling diabetes, and lowering cholesterol and blood pressure.

Physical activity also helps reduce your risk of stroke by preventing or slowing the narrowing

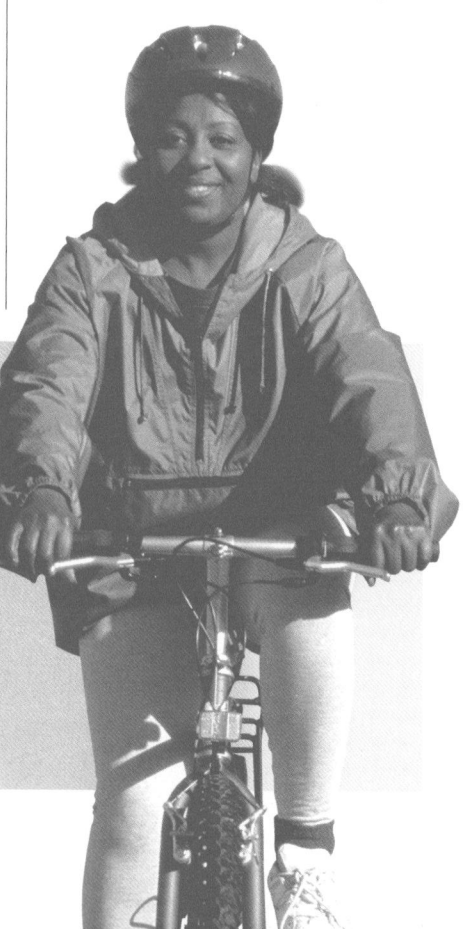

Physical Activity vs. Exercise

The terms *physical activity* and *exercise* are often used synonymously, but there is a difference between the two. Physical activity refers to any body movement that burns calories, such as mowing the lawn, walking up stairs, making the bed or walking your dog. Exercise is a more structured form of physical activity. It involves a series of repetitive movements designed to strengthen or develop some part of the body or to improve your heart and lung capacity. Exercise includes walking, swimming, bicycling and many other activities.

Both physical activity and exercise are valuable to your health. The important thing is to keep moving, whether or not the activity is structured.

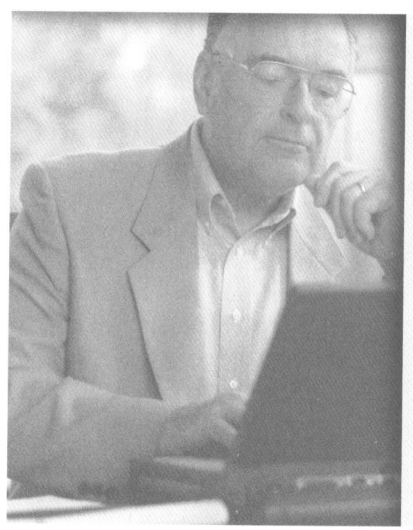

Avoid 'Sitting Disease'

Compared to just five decades ago, people today move less. At work, where many of us sit at our desks for hours, we're burning an average of 130 fewer calories a day. We're less active at home as well, where it's all too tempting to park ourselves in front of the television or computer.

All of that inactivity adds up. Prolonged periods of sitting are associated with an increased risk of health problems such as diabetes, heart disease, some cancers and depression — not to mention weight gain and obesity.

Unfortunately, regular exercise doesn't seem to overcome the health effects of too much sitting. As an example, people who sit for eight hours or more a day have an increased risk of heart disease even if they exercise an hour daily.

To stay healthy and happy, sit less and move more throughout the day!

---

of the arteries that supply blood to the brain. Blockage of these arteries can cause a stroke.

Osteoporosis

Women and men who perform strength training and weight-bearing activities, such as walking, have a better chance of avoiding osteoporosis, a bone-thinning disease. Osteoporosis is more common in women than in men.

Arthritis

If you have arthritis, appropriate exercises to maximize the range of motion and strength of muscles surrounding your joints may reduce pain and injury. Low impact aerobic activity won't flare joint pain, but it will improve your energy level and help you control your weight, which is important because excess weight places unnecessary stress on your joints.

Cancer

Staying active may reduce your risk of some cancers, including cancers of the colon, rectum, prostate, breast, kidney and lining of the uterus (endometrium). Activity may reduce cancer risk by helping prevent obesity, a risk factor for many types of cancer.

Regular physical activity reduces cancer risk in other ways, too. For example, it may cut your risk of colorectal cancer by stimulating movement through your bowel and reducing the time your colon is exposed to harmful substances that may cause cancer.

And for breast and prostate cancer, regular physical activity may act on hormone levels in a way that reduces your risk.

Depression and anxiety

Studies indicate that aerobic exercise and strength training help relieve symptoms of depression. When you exercise, your body releases chemicals called endorphins, which are your body's natural painkillers. Endorphins also help relieve stress and anxiety.

Everyday Fitness

For many people, not enough activity simply may be a matter of time. You know that activity is good for you, but you just can't seem to set aside time in your day to be active. You're not alone. Despite the proven benefits of physical activity — and the risks of inactivity — most American adults don't get the recommended amount of physical activity. Medical and fitness organizations generally recommend partaking in at least 30 minutes of light to moderate physical activity most, if not all, days of the week.

Never Too Old

If you haven't exercised before, it's never too late to incorporate more physical activity into your life. Studies show that beginning an activity program anytime in your 70s and 80s reduces the risk of dying over the next several years. Not surprisingly, people who were more active at age 78 were twice as likely to be functioning independently when they were 85. Studies have also found that people older than 85 who walk at least three times a week have significantly less risk of heart disease than those who are sedentary.

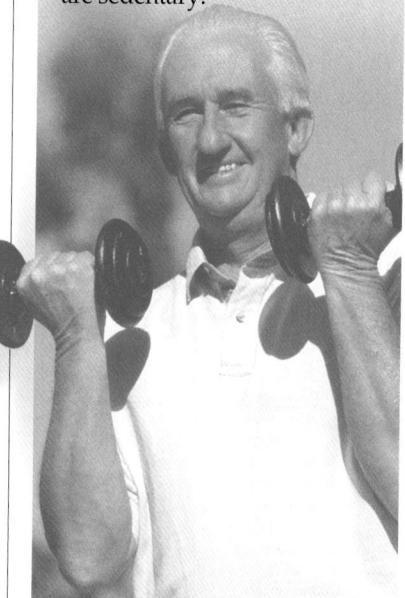

On the Move

Here are some suggestions for incorporating more activity into your everyday life:

- Instead of sitting and talking with a friend, go for a walk together.
- Walk around while talking on your cellphone.
- Walk or bike to a nearby store instead of driving.
- Listen to music and dance your way through housecleaning.
- Use a push lawn mower instead of a motorized or riding mower.
- Wash your car by hand instead of using the automatic carwash.
- Rake leaves, prune bushes and spend time in the garden.
- Play with your kids instead of watching them play.
- When watching television, pedal a stationary bike, walk on a treadmill, stretch or lift free weights.
- Hide your remote control and get up to change the channel.
- Park farther away from work or the shopping mall.
- Avoid drive-throughs. Park the car and walk in.
- Climb the stairs instead of using the elevator.
- Do stretching exercises at your desk.
- Take a break from what you're doing and walk around.

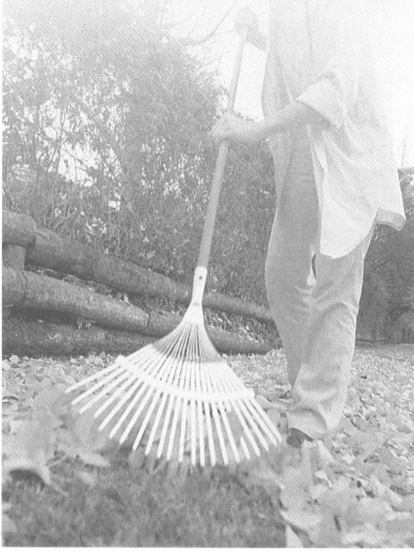

If you have trouble carving 30 minutes out of your day for a specific activity, such as taking a walk or going for a bicycle ride, try another approach. Incorporate more physical activity into the things you already do. This lifestyle activity approach is like "snacking" on exercise. Do a smidgen of activity in the morning. Have two or three more servings later in the day, and perhaps one in the evening. Over the course of the day, five or 10 minutes of activity here and there add up.

The key to your success is attitude. You have to want to get out of your sedentary habits and embrace new, more-active ones.

So how do you get your exercise servings? There are many ways. You might park your car at the far end of the parking lot every time you go to the store. You could make it a habit to take the stairs instead of the elevator. If your job involves a lot of sitting, think about small movements you can attach to simple tasks. On the phone a lot? Walk while you're talking. Check emails often? Stand up when you're reading them or stretch whenever you hit "send."

The point is, every move counts — and the more, the better.

As you get started, make sure to pick activities that you like to do. If you enjoy what you're doing, you're more likely to stick with it. Make a date to go dancing every Friday. Invite a friend to join you on your walks. Go bike riding with your grandchildren.

And when you want to enjoy some downtime, look for ways to incorporate some physical activity into that time. For instance, you might stretch or walk slowly on a treadmill while watching your favorite TV program.

Doing something is better than nothing, and consistency is more important than intensity. It's the total amount of activity that counts, not great exhibits of endurance. Think of physical activity as an ongoing part of your day.

Family Fitness

A great way to integrate fitness into your daily life is to make it a family affair. Family exercise builds healthy bodies — and healthy families. Look for fun, creative activities that provide an opportunity for the whole family to get up and moving. That might be going to the zoo, biking together or going bowling.

Some children get enough exercise just by being kids, but many don't. Today's children are increasingly out of shape compared with those of previous generations. Approximately 1 in 5 school-age children in the United States is obese — a number that has more than tripled since the 1970s.

Many factors contribute to the increase in childhood obesity. The biggest culprit is television, followed closely by video games, cellphones, computers and other mobile devices. Spending time in front of a screen encourages a sedentary lifestyle. To make matters worse, increasingly fewer school-age children are in physical education courses, meaning that fewer kids get exercise at school.

Studies show that active children are healthier, stronger, more flexible, and have greater endurance and lung capacity. In addition, they perform better in school, are more mentally alert, sleep better, are sick less often and bounce back more quickly when they do catch a bug.

Equally important, children who exercise regularly are more likely to grow up to be fit, lean adults, with better posture and sleep habits.

Teaching healthy habits

Parents play a key role in their children's attitudes toward physical activity. As a parent you help them make good decisions about nutrition and exercise.

When your family does active things together, you teach your

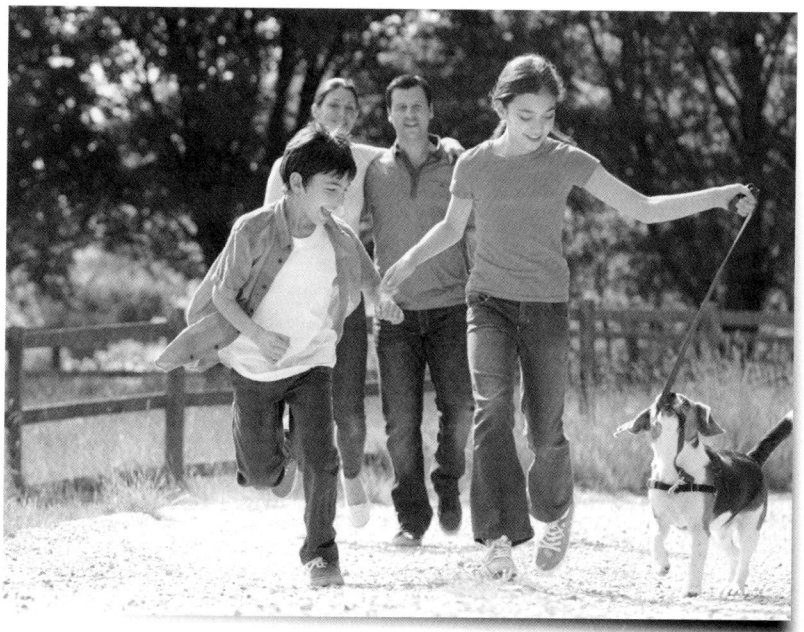

kids healthy habits that can last a lifetime. Research shows that children are much more likely to be active when both parents exercise.

Exercising together also provides good family time. The sheer pleasure of doing something fun together eases conflicts, tensions and pressures. Family fun time breaks up the routine of seeing one another only at the breakfast table before everyone dashes off their own separate ways. Structured family activities also help control disruptive behavior.

The earlier you start adding fitness to your family routine, the more readily your kids will accept it as a normal part of family life. A child who grows up taking after-dinner walks with mom or dad accepts the walks as family routine.

Getting the ball rolling

How can you nurture an active child? How do you get a 3-year-old interested in exercise? And what about your 12-year-old, who's embarrassed to be seen with you? Getting kids of any age to be active doesn't have to be a tough sell. Consider the following steps:

Limit television, computer time and video games

Many studies have found a direct relationship between childhood obesity and hours of television watching. As hours of viewing increase, so does weight.

Sitting in front of a computer or playing video games is just as sedentary. Set a limit on these activities, such as one to two hours a day or 10 TV programs a week. Don't let your child have a television in his or her bedroom.

Plan a family activity three times a week

A family activity could be a trip to the playground, a driveway game of basketball, a bike ride or just a family stretch time. Spur-of-the-moment activities can be fun, but if you set aside a certain time of the day or week when your family can be together, you're more likely to accomplish your goal. Plan for at least three family activities a week.

Emphasize activity, not exercise

Your family activity doesn't have to be a structured exercise program — the object is just to get the kids moving. Free-play activities such as hide-and-seek, tag or jump-rope can be great for burning calories and improving fitness.

Making Exercise Fun

Be creative when choosing activities. Every family is different. Do whatever gets your kids pumped. Start with the ideas below, then add some of your own.

- Don't just go for a walk. Take the kids on an adventurous treasure hunt.
- Don't just run. Run like a gorilla. Fly like a bee. Walk like a spider. Hop like a bunny. Stretch like a cat.

- Play fast-moving games such as tag, Simon Says or kickball.
- Build a fort.
- See who can pull the most weeds in the vegetable garden or who can collect the most litter in the neighborhood.
- Plot the mileage of each family hiking and biking trip on a map of the United States to see how far your outings would have taken you if you had traveled in one direction.
- Plan family vacations around hiking, skiing, snorkeling or camping. Take along a ball for rest stops.

- Organize neighborhood volleyball or baseball games or sledding or skating parties.

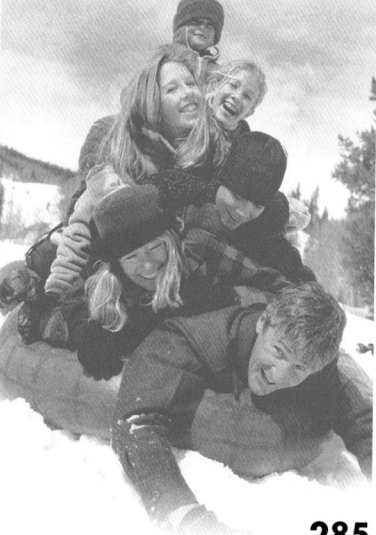

Make your activity fun and varied. A lot of kids' games involve exercise by nature.

Do things your children enjoy

Engage your children in physical activities related to their interests and abilities. For example, if a child is artistic, go on a nature hike to collect leaves and rocks that he or she can use in a collage. If a child likes to climb, head for the nearest neighborhood jungle gym or climbing wall. If a child likes to read, walk to the neighborhood library.

Promote physical education

If you're concerned about the lack of physical education opportunities at your child's school, work with your local parent organization, school board or school administrators to improve the offerings in your district. If your child is in child care, make sure the program offers plenty of physical activity each day.

Participating in sports

Sports offer many benefits. On the physical side, participants experience improved fitness, coordination and weight control. Sports also offer meaningful lessons in social and psychological development, such as interacting with others, following directions, and dealing with setbacks and defeat. Children who participate in sports tend to have a better body image and better self-esteem.

To help your child find the right sport, expose him or her to a variety of athletic activities. Let him or her try team sports such as softball or soccer, as well as sports that offer an opportunity for more individual participation, such as tennis, running or golf.

If your child shows interest in a sport, consider the time commitment, cost, characteristics of the sport and your child's physical maturity level. You can help by being positive and encouraging.

Emphasize effort and improvement over winning or personal performance. And keep the sport in perspective. It's important to be supportive, but don't become overly invested in whether your child wins or loses.

And if your kids show no interest whatsoever in sports, don't worry. A healthy lifestyle doesn't have to include organized sports. What's more important is that your children be involved in some form of physical activity.

A Personal Fitness Program

Daily activity is good, but for maximum health benefits, a structured fitness program is best. The program doesn't need to be strenuous, but the activity needs to be regular and it should be moderately challenging.

A fitness program takes time to show results. Don't expect to whip yourself into shape overnight. By gradually increasing the duration and intensity of your activity, you can improve your overall fitness in eight to 12 weeks.

Identify your goals

Tailor your fitness program to your needs, abilities, schedule and other personal factors. Develop a routine that works for you and your lifestyle. If your program is so difficult you're rarely able to do it, or your workout is so long that you can't fit it into your schedule more than once or twice a week, you probably won't stick with it.

What do you want to gain from your program? Be specific. Are you 55 and concerned about warding off a heart attack? Are you 75 and want to enjoy more recreational activities and prolong your independence? Do you want to lose weight? Relieve your stress? Lower your blood pressure? Maybe you just want to feel better.

Keep your expectations realistic. If you have short, thick legs, your fitness program isn't going to give you a ballet dancer's body. What you can expect is an increased level of fitness and more energy.

Plan your activities

An optimal fitness program incorporates activities designed to meet four basic goals: improved aerobic capacity, strength, flexibility and stability. Each activity session should begin with a warm-up period and end with a cool-down and stretching.

Aerobic exercises

Aerobic means "with oxygen," as opposed to *anaerobic*, meaning "without oxygen." Aerobic activities involve continuous motion as you repeatedly use your muscles. Aerobic activities increase your breathing and heart rate, improving your cardiovascular fitness — the health of your heart, lungs and circulatory system. Anaerobic exercises work muscle groups, but they don't provide as much cardiovascular benefit. Weightlifting is an example of anaerobic exercise.

From a health standpoint, aerobic exercise is about as close as you can get to a "magic potion." Besides making your heart work more efficiently, aerobic exercise can help you lose weight, ease stress, boost your immune system and reduce your risk of disease. Aerobic exercise also improves your stamina and muscle health, making it easier for you to do everyday tasks such as household chores and climbing stairs.

Moderate-paced walking, bicycling, running, cross-country skiing and swimming are examples of aerobic exercises.

Strength exercises

Strength exercises (resistance or strength training) build your muscle strength and endurance, which in turn can improve your posture, balance and coordination. To increase strength, an exercise must involve resistance to muscle contractions. In other words, your muscles have to push or pull against some force, such as when you lift weights.

In general, people who aren't active lose about 10 percent of their lean muscle mass each decade after age 30. Strength training can help slow and prevent or even reverse this process. Because strength exercises also strengthen bones, the exercises protect against the bone-thinning effect of osteoporosis. In addition, these exercises support your joints, cut your risk of injury and increase your metabolism, which helps keep your weight in check.

Two ways to build muscle mass are working out with free weights (dumbbells or barbells) and using weight machines. Workouts with free weights simulate moves made in everyday life. Newer weight machines also permit more natural body movements than do older machines, and they emphasize body stabilization during exercise.

Core Exercises (abdominal and back muscles)

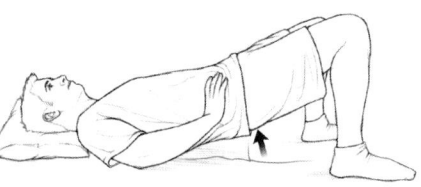

Lie on a firm surface with your feet flat, about shoulder-width apart. Raise your buttocks off the mat, keeping a level line from your knees to your hips. Keep your shoulders, head and neck relaxed and on the surface. Hold the position until you're fatigued and can no longer keep your knees and hips in a straight line. Relax and repeat.

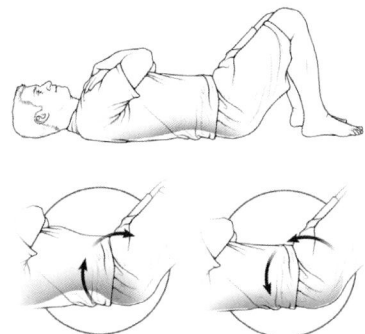

Lie on a firm surface with your knees bent. Flatten the small of your back against the surface and concentrate on tightening your abdominal muscles. Relax and repeat.

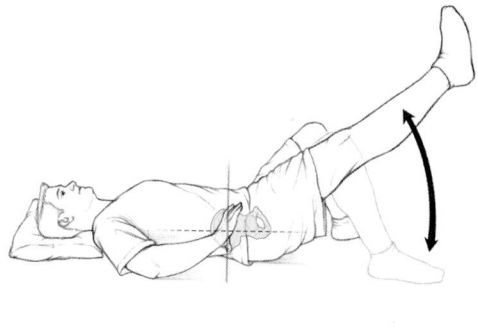

Lie on a firm surface. Bend your left knee and keep your right knee straight. Hold your abdominal muscles tight and slowly raise and lower your right leg. Relax and repeat. Reverse legs.

Back Exercises

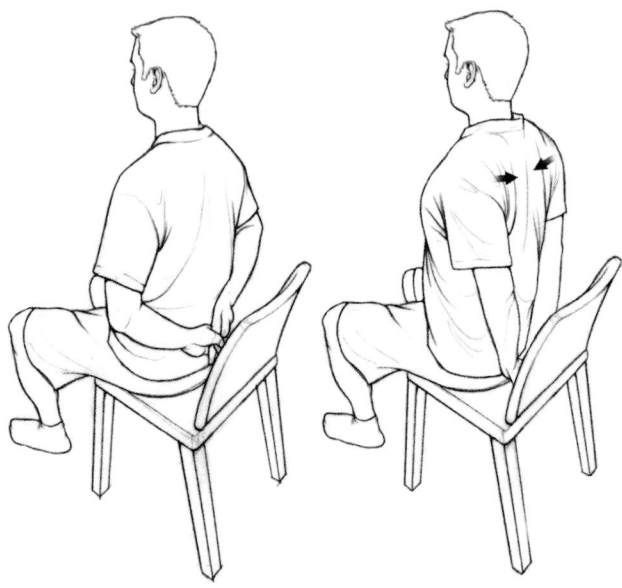

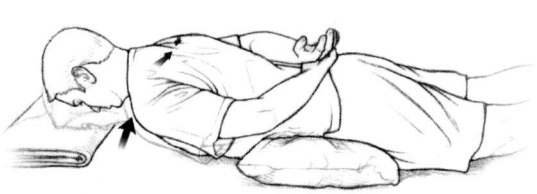

Sit upright in a chair. Put your hands on your hips or behind your back and pull your shoulder blades together. Relax and repeat.

Lie facedown over a large pillow. Position the pillow under your navel to keep your spine in a neutral position. Place your hands behind your hips. Pulling your shoulder blades together, raise your head and chest. Keep your neck relaxed. Return to the starting position and repeat.

Chest and Arm Exercises

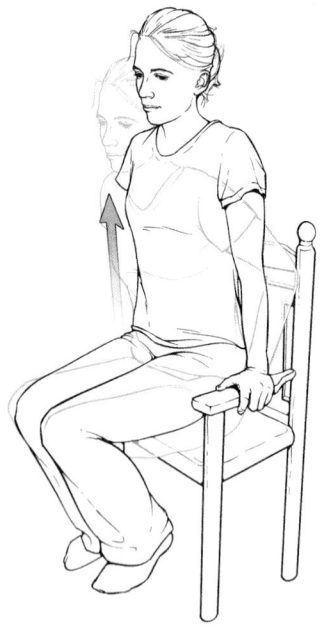

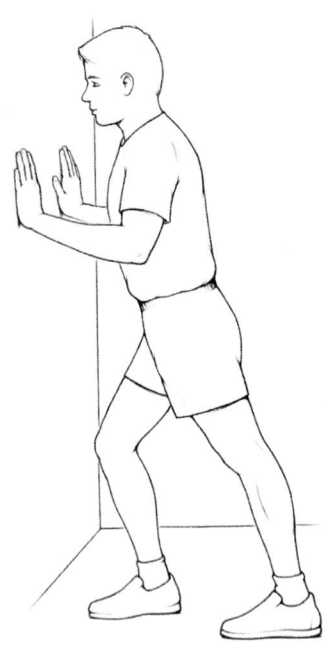

Sit in a sturdy chair that has arms, with your feet firmly on the floor. Place your hands on the arms. Push your body up off the surface of the chair using your arms only, not your feet. Relax and repeat.

Stand facing a wall, far enough away from it so that you can place your palms on the wall with your elbows slightly bent. Keeping your heels flat on the floor, slowly bend your elbows and lean toward the wall, supporting your weight with your arms. Straighten your arms and return to a standing position. Repeat. As you build strength, try standing farther from the wall.

Leg Exercises

Stand with your feet flat on the floor, slightly more than shoulder-width apart. Keeping your back straight and looking straight ahead, slowly lower your hips downward and backward as you bend your knees to between 30 and 60 degrees. Pause for a moment and return to your starting position. Repeat. To maintain balance, lightly hold on to a table or countertop.

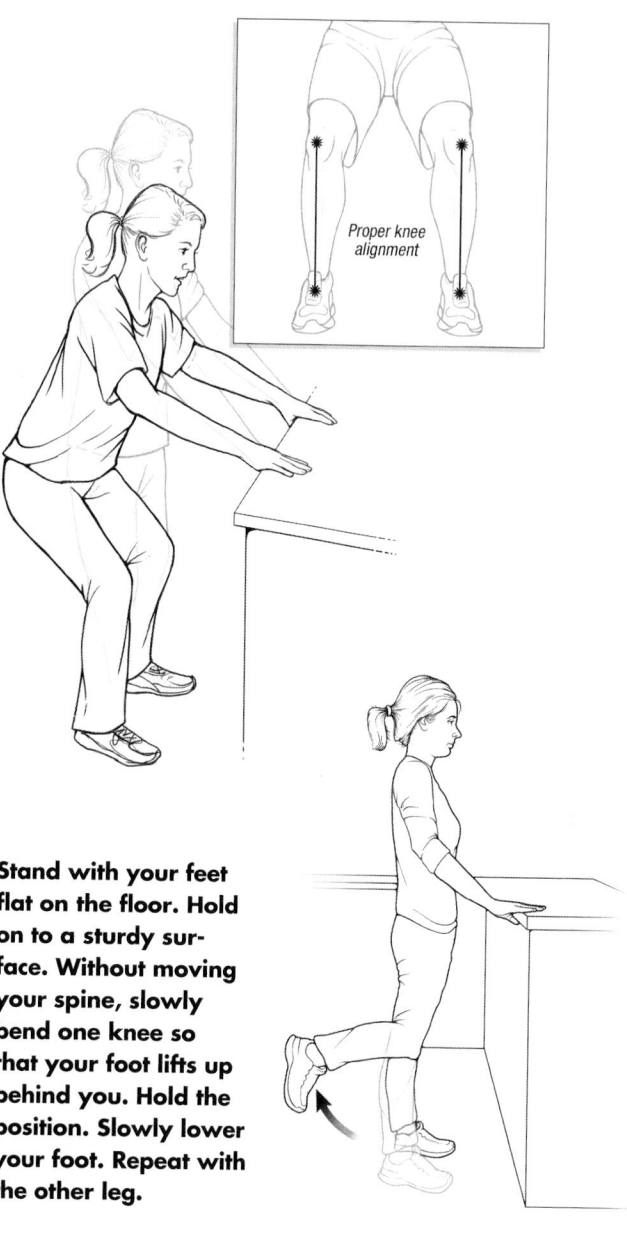

Proper knee alignment

Stand with your feet flat on the floor. Hold on to the back of a sturdy surface. Slowly raise your heels and stand on tiptoe. Hold the position for a few seconds. Then slowly lower your heels and repeat.

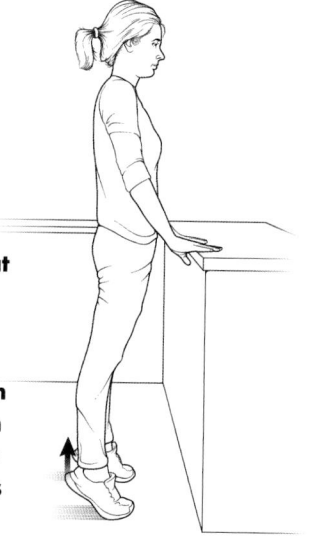

Stand with your feet flat on the floor. Hold on to a sturdy surface. Without moving your spine, slowly bend one knee so that your foot lifts up behind you. Hold the position. Slowly lower your foot. Repeat with the other leg.

Stability Exercises

Stand with the heel of your left foot touching the toes of your right foot. Focus on an object in front of you to maintain your balance. Hold this position for 30 seconds. Repeat with your right foot in front of your left foot. If you're unsteady, place your fingertips on a wall to balance yourself.

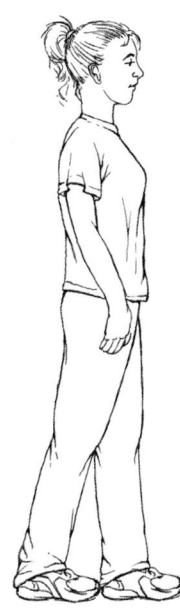

Stand shoulder-width apart. Lift one leg slightly off the floor. Hold for five seconds and relax. Repeat at least five times then switch legs. If you're unsteady, place your fingertips on a wall to balance yourself.

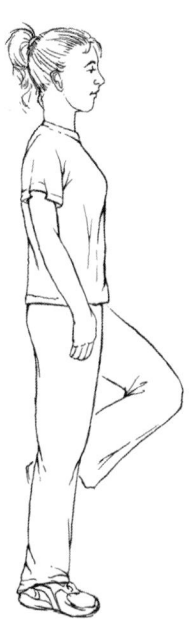

But free weights and machines aren't the only ways to gain strength. You also can use resistance bands, your own body weight or the resistance of water to challenge your muscles.

You want to lift a weight or use some type of resistance that tires (fatigues) your muscles after 12 to 15 repetitions (reps). Many studies show that you can achieve most of the benefits of strength training by working muscle groups for a single set of repetitions. It isn't necessary to repeat the same exercise over and over to gain benefit. But make sure to use proper technique and form when performing any resistance exercise.

If you're concerned that strength training may not be good for you, talk to your doctor, a physical therapist or a certified athletic trainer. No matter what your physical condition, there are usually ways to modify exercise to enable you to train safely and effectively.

The exercises shown on pages 287-290 are designed to strengthen various muscle groups. Include some or all of them in your fitness routine at least twice a week. If you're out of shape, begin with five repetitions each and build to 12 to 15 repetitions.

Calf Stretch

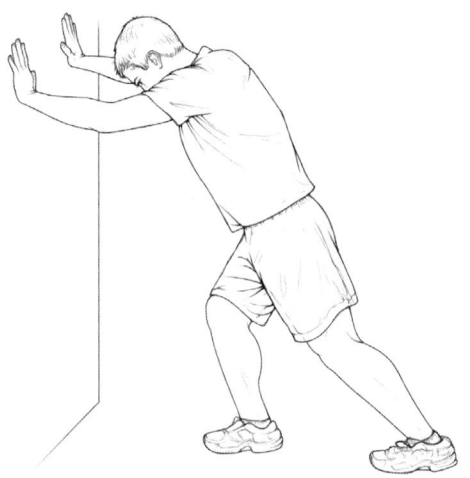

Stand at arm's-length from the wall. Place one leg forward with the knee bent. Keep your other leg back with the knee straight and heel down. Keeping your back straight and your heels on the ground, move your hips toward the wall until you feel a stretch in the calf of your extended leg. Relax. Repeat with the other leg.

Upper Thigh Stretch

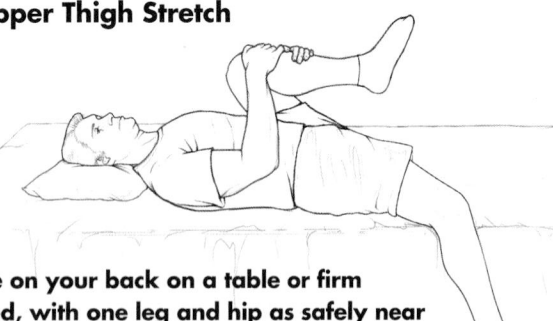

Lie on your back on a table or firm bed, with one leg and hip as safely near the edge as possible. Grasp the knee of the other leg with both hands and pull it toward your chest until your lower back flattens against the table. If you have knee problems, pull from the back of your thigh. Then relax your straight leg so that it hangs over the edge. Relax. Repeat with the other leg.

Lower Back Stretch

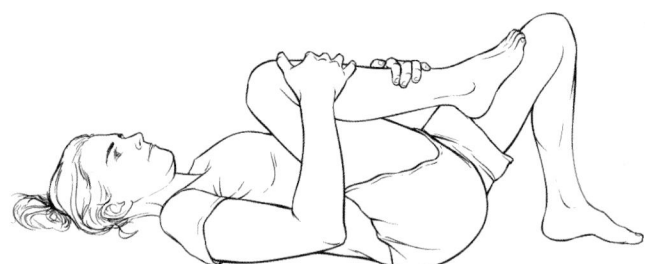

Lie on a firm surface with your knees bent and feet flat. Pull your right knee toward your shoulder with both hands. If you have knee problems, pull from the back of your thigh. Relax. Repeat with your other leg.

Chest Stretch

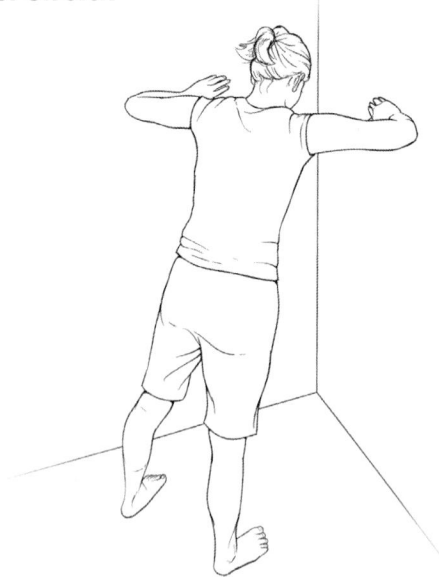

Stand with your feet shoulder-width apart, arm's length from a room corner. Place one hand on each wall at shoulder level. Bend your elbows and let your chest move toward the corner until you feel a gentle stretch in your chest muscles. Hold for 5 to 10 seconds. Return to starting position and repeat.

Stability exercises

Stability exercises help you maintain good balance, reducing your risk of falling and injury. Do stability exercises at least once a day most days of the week. If you have balance problems, talk to your doctor before starting the exercises.

Stretching and flexibility exercises

Regular, careful stretching can help you limber up, feel younger and reduce your risk of injury. Stretching exercises get the blood flowing, literally warming up your muscles and getting them ready to work out. At the end of a period of physical activity, it's good to stretch your muscles. It helps them cool down and retain their flexibility.

Flexibility is a "use it or lose it" function. To prevent your muscles from shortening and tightening, you need to regularly flex your muscles and move your joints through their full range of motion.

Basic stretches to improve your flexibility focus on the body's major muscle groups, including your calf muscles, thigh muscles, lower back muscles, and neck and shoulder muscles.

Never bounce when you are stretching and flexing your muscles, and stretch only until you feel a noticeable pull — not pain. Try to do at least three repetitions of the exercises shown on page 290.

Common Types of Exercise

The choices are endless when it comes to physical activity. No single form of exercise or piece of equipment is best. Select an activity or activities that fit your personality and lifestyle. Do you like to exercise alone or in a group? Do you like to be outdoors or to stay inside?

In the following pages, you'll read about some of the most common physical activities. These are just starting points for a world of physical activity.

Walking

A brisk walk is a simple and cost-free means of improving your physical fitness. It requires no special skills, equipment, lessons or other participants. If you've been inactive and are a bit out of shape, a walking program could be just the challenge you need.

Walking, like other forms of aerobic exercise, can help increase the efficiency of your heart and lungs, allowing you to do more work with less effort. It can improve muscle tone and help shape muscles in your legs, hips, buttocks and abdomen.

Walking can also be a valuable part of a weight-loss program. On

Features of a Walking Shoe

Achilles notch. Reduces stress on the Achilles tendon.

Ankle collar. Cushions the ankle and ensures proper fit.

Upper. Holds the shoe on your foot and is made of leather, mesh or synthetic material. Mesh allows better ventilation and is lighter weight.

Insole. Cushions and supports your foot and arch. Removable insoles can be laundered or taken out to dry.

Midsole. Provides comfort, cushioning and shock absorption.

Outsole. Makes contact with the ground. Grooves and treads help maintain traction.

Toe box. Provides space for the toes. A roomy and round toe box helps prevent calluses.

Gel pad. Cushions and reduces impact when your foot strikes the ground.

Roll bar. Stabilizes your foot if it tends to roll inward when striking the ground.

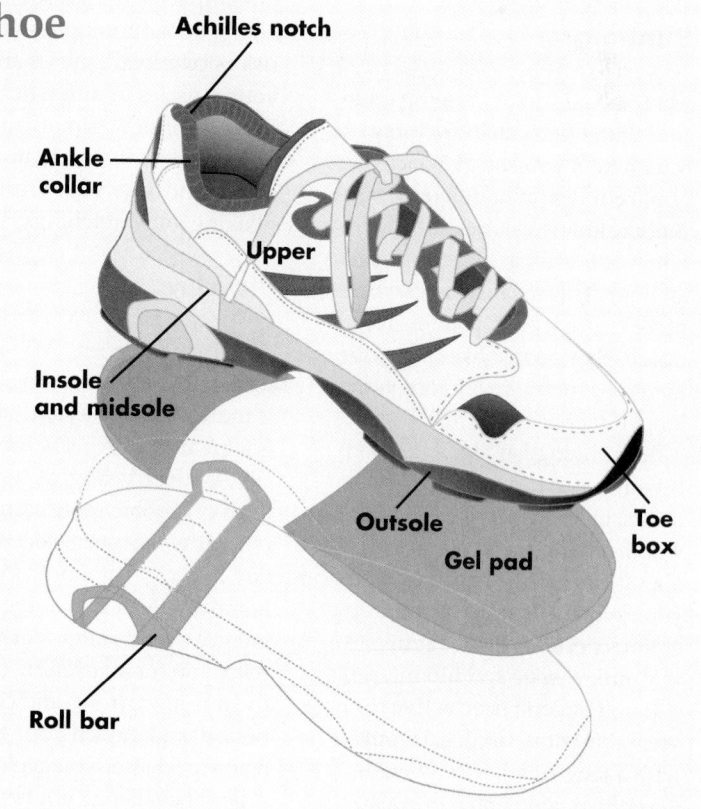

average, a brisk one-hour walk burns about 250 to 350 calories, depending on your weight and level of fitness.

Regular walking can help prevent some age-related diseases. Walking increases bone density and may lower the risk of osteoporosis and lessen the pain of arthritis. Walking improves balance and coordination, so walkers are less prone to injury from falls.

Walking can also be a tonic for the mind. It can help you unwind at the end of a busy day or after a difficult task. Get your spouse or a friend to join you, and it's a chance to connect with others.

Start out slowly and increase the duration and pace of your workout over a period of four to six weeks. Begin by walking on flat ground. When that becomes too easy, look for gentle hills to increase the intensity of your workout. Many people find that it helps to establish a routine, such as walking at the same time each day. Vary your route to keep it interesting.

Running

Many people enjoy running and find that it fits well into a busy schedule. If you run at a pace of about 8 miles an hour, you'll burn twice as many calories as you do when you walk at a pace of 4 miles an hour. This means you can be more efficient with your exercise time. Other people like the excitement of running in 5-kilometer, or longer, races.

But running isn't for everybody. If you have a heart or lung condition, talk to your doctor about whether running is appropriate for you. It can also be hard on some of your joints. The impact from repetitious pounding can aggravate foot, ankle, knee and hip injuries.

If you haven't been active for several months, don't start out with a long run. Begin by walking. When you're able to walk 2 miles in 30 minutes comfortably,

A Walking Program

The following chart outlines how to gradually increase the pace and intensity of your walking program.

Week of program	Distance in miles	Time in minutes per mile
1-2	1-2	15-30
3-4	2-2½	13-25
5-6	2½-3	13-20
7-8	3-4	13-20
9-10	4-5	13-20

you may be ready to try alternating jogging and walking. Run at a comfortable pace — slowly enough that you can carry on a conversation without gasping for breath. Over time you can gradually increase the intensity of your workout.

To minimize the risk of injury and muscle and joint discomfort, run on alternate days and don't run more than three or four times a week. Alternating running with low-impact activities such as biking or swimming lessens the risk of overload injuries and works your muscles in different ways. Remember to warm up and cool down. Allow five to 10 minutes before and after your workout for walking and stretching.

Bicycling

As the saying goes, "You never forget how to ride a bicycle." This is more or less true, and bicycling is a great way to get aerobic exercise. With bicycling, as with any form of aerobic exercise, schedule regular workouts. Select a time of day to cycle that works for you. For example, if managing stress is a goal, a ride after work may relax you for an evening at home. Include a warm-up and cool-down period, and stretch your muscles before and after you cycle.

Don't challenge yourself by setting the gears to make ped-

aling hard, producing a strain resembling that of a hard run. This doesn't work your heart and lungs effectively and puts excessive strain on your knees. Pedaling more rapidly at all times — even while going downhill — helps make your ride an aerobic activity. A pedaling rate of 80 to 100 revolutions a minute is generally ideal. Cycle computers can help you keep track of this, plus speed, distance and elapsed time.

Make sure that you have the right bike to suit your needs. Some bikes are designed for smooth surfaces and high speeds, and others are suitable for rough terrain. Touring bicycles (racing or road bikes) are lightweight and have narrow tires, low-slung handlebars and about 18 to 21 gear settings. Mountain bicycles are designed for off-road riding. They have sturdier frames and wider tires with more tread. The handlebars are more upright, and the riding posture is more erect.

Hybrid bicycles are a cross between mountain and racing bicycles. The riding posture is more upright, and the tire width is midway between road and mountain bike tires. Hybrid bikes often have 21 speeds. Those with shock absorbers built into the front wheel struts and seat posts provide added comfort on uneven surfaces.

Make sure the bike fits you well. When you're seated on a

bicycle with your foot on the pedal lowest to the ground, your leg should be not quite fully extended. You should be able to reach the handlebars, work the brakes and shift gears while keeping your eyes on the road. When straddling a racing bicycle with your feet on the ground, there should be 1 to 3 inches of clearance between you and the crossbar. For a mountain or hybrid bicycle, the clearance should be 3 to 6 inches.

Always wear a helmet for protection from serious head injury should you fall or be in an accident.

Exercise machines

Each type of exercise machine has something unique to offer. Some machines exercise your lower body only, and others build upper body strength or aerobic capacity. The following devices can build both strength and aerobic capacity:

Stationary cycle

A stationary cycle builds leg strength and cardiovascular capacity and is an excellent choice for both beginning and serious exercisers. Some cycles have moving handlebars that provide an upper body workout as well. If you have knee problems, be sure the cycle's resistance can be adjusted to a low setting and that your seat height is set appropriately.

If you have low back problems, you might want to use a recumbent cycle, in which you sit in a chairlike seat with pedals in front of you rather than below the seat.

Rowing machine

A rowing machine offers a good aerobic workout by putting your entire body in action. It helps strengthen your back, shoulders, stomach, legs and arms. Proper technique is important to avoid back strain.

Treadmill

A treadmill helps build leg strength and aerobic capacity.

How Many Calories Does It Burn?

The chart below shows approximately how many calories you burn while performing various activities for one hour. Calorie expenditure varies widely depending on the exercise, intensity level and individual. For example, a trained athlete may exercise with greater economy of motion and expend less energy.

Activity	Average calories used in 1 hour	
	160-lb. person	240-lb. person
Aerobics		
low impact	365	545
water	402	600
Basketball game	584	872
Bicycling		
< 10 mph, leisure	292	436
Bowling	219	327
Dancing, ballroom	219	327
Elliptical trainer		
moderate effort	365	545
Golfing		
carrying clubs	314	469
Hiking	438	654
Ice skating	511	763
Jogging		
5 mph	606	905
Racquetball, casual	511	763
Resistance training	365	545
Rowing, stationary	438	654
Running		
8 mph	861	1,286
Skiing		
cross-country	496	741
downhill	314	469
Softball or baseball	365	545
Stair treadmill	657	981
Swimming laps		
moderate or light	423	632
Tennis, singles	584	872
Volleyball	292	436
Walking		
2 mph	204	305
3.5 mph	314	469
Yoga, hatha	183	273

Based on from Ainsworth BE, et al., *Medicine and Science in Sports and Exercise*, 2011;43:8.

Shopping for Exercise Equipment

Most health clubs and many workplaces have exercise machines. Or you can purchase exercise equipment to use at home. Before buying home fitness equipment, carefully consider your situation. If you've made physical activity a habit, then the investment is probably worth it. If you're still exploring various activities and haven't established a routine, you may want to wait before buying equipment.

In general, you get what you pay for when you purchase an exercise machine. The low-priced models may be unstable, uncomfortable and even unsafe. Look at the warranty — it's usually one sign of quality. Make sure the equipment is solidly built, with no exposed cables or chains. Look for a machine that operates smoothly and is comfortable to use. A comfortable seat is critical for cycles and rowing machines. Before buying a machine, try out various types at a dealer or fitness center.

Most treadmills offer an adjustable degree of incline to simulate walking or running up hills. You can adjust speed for walking or running. Higher horsepower models generally run more smoothly and are more durable.

Stair climber

A stair climber helps tone and strengthen your hips, buttocks, thighs, hamstrings, calves and lower back and provides an effective aerobic workout. Compared with running, a stair climber causes less impact stress on your ankles and knees. However, the device can aggravate certain knee problems.

A stair climber may consist of a moving flight of stairs (such as walking up a down escalator) or independent steps that move up and down at various rates or heights.

Cross-country ski machine

A cross-country ski machine offers a good overall workout, but some people find it hard to master. It requires some practice in learning to move your arms and legs in opposing directions.

Elliptical trainer

An elliptical trainer provides a total upper and lower body workout and aerobic conditioning. The device is similar to a cross-country ski machine, but the leg-and-arm action is elliptical — up and down in an oval shape — rather than back and forth. It can be easier to master than the cross-country ski machine.

Swimming and water workouts

Water exercise is as close as you can get to a zero-impact aerobic workout. Water's buoyancy supports your weight and significantly reduces stress on your joints, bones and muscles. Water pressure also helps reduce swelling. Swimming or water exercises are a good choice if you have arthritis or an injury or disability that prevents you from doing other forms of exercise, are recovering from illness or surgery, or are pregnant or overweight.

For individuals who run or walk regularly, swimming is a good cross-training activity. Indoor swimming is also a good option for bad-weather days. You can also do strengthening exercises in water. Water provides resistance as you move through it. Walking in water works the leg and abdominal muscles. While in the water, you can use barbells, weighted boots, paddles and webbed gloves if you want extra resistance.

Even if you fear deep water or don't like to swim, you can try a water workout in the shallow end of the pool. Simply walking in shallow water provides significant aerobic benefits. Most water aerobic classes are taught in the shallow end of the pool. Such classes often are offered by organizations such as health clubs, YMCAs, YWCAs and medical centers.

Resistance training

Resistance training, also referred to as strength training or weight-lifting, builds the strength and endurance of your muscles. Resistance training reduces body fat and increases lean muscle mass.

Increased lean muscle mass provides you with a bigger "engine" to burn calories. Because muscle tissue burns more calories than does fat tissue, the more muscle mass you have, the more calories you burn, even at rest.

Resistance training involves working your muscles against some form of resistance This is typically done with free weights, weight machines or resistance bands. You can also exercise using the weight of your own body as the resistance, as happens with exercises such as pushups, lunges and squats.

Regardless of the method you choose, begin slowly. For example, start with a weight that you can lift comfortably 12 times in a row. If you start with too much resistance or too many repetitions, you may damage muscles and joints. A single set of 12 to 15 repetitions can help you gain strength just as effectively as doing multiple sets.

It's best to start with conservative amounts of resistance to minimize the risk of injury. Before each session, take a five- to 10-minute walk to warm up your muscles.

In general, three workouts a week will build muscle, and two a week will maintain the strength you've gained. Typically, increases in strength are noticeable after four to six weeks of training. Improvement in muscle shape and size takes longer.

When beginning a resistance program, it's also good to get advice and instruction from a qualified instructor, such as a physical therapist, athletic trainer or fitness specialist. Many gyms and health clubs have such an adviser on staff. This person can help you design a program that fits your fitness level, abilities and goals yet is varied enough to keep you interested. Correct technique also is very important.

Vigorous Exercise

If you're looking for more-vigorous exercise, high-intensity interval training is an excellent, time-efficient way to improve fitness.

However, you should see your doctor to make sure that it's safe to perform vigorous exercise before you get started, especially if you haven't been involved in regular exercise. Your doctor may recommend that you have an exercise stress test before beginning a vigorous exercise program.

Interval training

High-intensity interval training begins with a three- to five-minute warm-up period and ends with a three- to five-minute cool-down period. In between, you alternate between short periods of intense physical activity and recovery periods.

Periods of intense activity are usually performed for about 30 seconds. They're followed by periods of recovery, which typically last two to four minutes in duration. During the periods of intense activity you want to "go as hard as you can," and during the periods of recovery you want to take it easy and catch your breath.

An example might be cycling very hard for 30 seconds, backing off and spinning more easily for two to three minutes, and then cycling very hard again for 30 seconds. Repeat the cycle three or four times, or as many cycles as you feel you're capable of doing.

During the periods of intense activity, your exertion level should be at approximately 85 to 90 percent of your target heart rate, or 17 to 18 on the Borg Rating of Perceived Exertion Scale (see page 298). During recovery periods, aim for approximately 65 percent of your target heart rate, or approximately 12 to 13 on the Borg scale. A common mistake is not slowing down enough during the slow periods to let your heart and body recover.

If you don't have a lot of time to exercise, interval training is one way to get an effective workout in a short period. Three to four cycles of intense activity and recovery take only about 15 to 20 minutes.

In addition, research suggests that interval training may offer as

Calculating Your Target Heart Rate

To get the best results from aerobic exercise, it's recommended that you exercise at approximately 50 to 85 percent of your maximum heart rate.

A mathematical formula known as the Karvonen Formula can help you determine your target heart rate (HR) so that you know at what level of intensity you should be exercising. The formula uses your maximum and resting heart rates, combined with the recommended 50 to 85 percent intensity level, to determine your target heart rate.

$$((\text{max HR} - \text{resting HR}) \times \% \text{ intensity}) + \text{resting HR}$$

You can get a rough determination of your maximum heart rate by subtracting your age from the number 220. To determine your resting heart rate, take your pulse while you're resting, counting the number of beats in one minute.

So, here's how the formula would look for a 50-year-old individual with a maximum heart rate of 170 (220 - 50 = 170) and a resting heart rate of 70 beats per minute.

    50% intensity: ((170 - 70) x .50) + 70 = 120
    85% intensity: ((170 - 70) x .85) + 70 = 155

This person's target heart rate would be 120 to 155 beats per minute. To get the most benefit from his or her workout, this is the level of exertion this person should try and achieve while exercising.

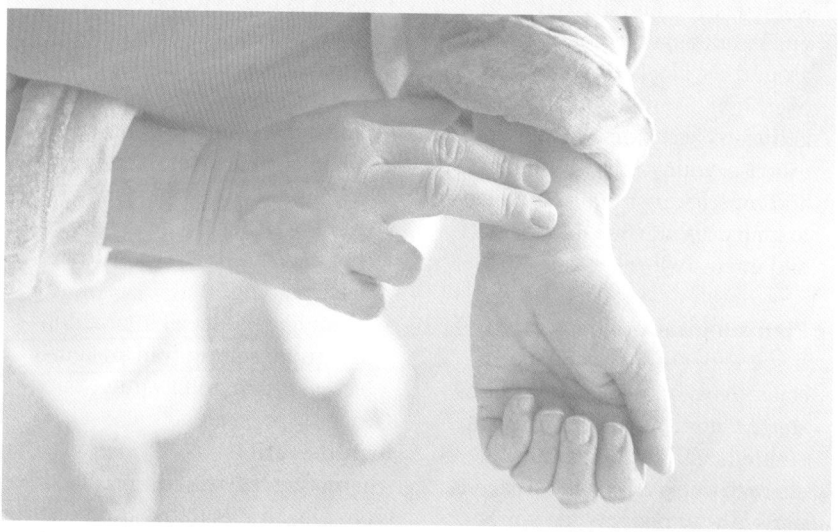

good or greater health and fitness benefits as classic moderate intensity exercise. This is even true for individuals with health conditions such as heart disease, type 2 diabetes or obesity.

Try to incorporate high-intensity interval training into your exercise program two to three days a week. If possible, work with a trained instructor, such as an exercise specialist. This person can help you develop a training schedule and can help you determine which activities to perform during high-intensity and recovery periods. Low-impact activities, such as cycling, using an elliptical trainer or swimming, work best for individuals with arthritis or joint problems.

Getting and Keeping Going

Once you've come up with some reasonable goals and developed a workable exercise plan, the next — and perhaps the biggest — challenge is to do it! Starting a fitness program takes initiative. Sticking with it takes commitment. Here are some tips to help you get and stay on track:

Begin gradually
Rome wasn't built in a day, and you're not going to zip from strolls around the block to a marathon overnight. Don't overdo it. If your body isn't accustomed to vigorous exercise, your joints, ligaments and muscles are more vulnerable to injury. Establish a suitable pace and intensity level.

Plan a logical progression
If you're out of shape or have unstable joints from injury or arthritis, start by improving your muscle strength and flexibility. Build strength by exercising the weakest parts of your body. When you're

ready to add aerobic exercise, start at a comfortable level, such as walking slowly for five to 10 minutes. Gradually increase the duration and speed each time you exercise.

Schedule exercise appointments
A written plan might encourage you to stay on track, and an exercise diary or log helps chart your progress. Schedule an exercise appointment just as you would a golf game or meeting. An exercise log is also helpful in establishing the habit of physical activity. Try to exercise at least 30 minutes most, if not all, days of the week.

Once you've been at it awhile, a typical session might include a five-minute warmup, 30 minutes of aerobic activity, and five to 10 minutes to cool down and stretch. And every two or three days, include 10 to 20 minutes of strength exercises. At first this may seem quite time-consuming. But once you're in the habit, it won't seem like a strain on your schedule. You may even look forward to the break from work and other obligations. And remember, you don't have to do your activities all at one time. A good night of dancing is an exercise session all in itself.

Make it fun
Boredom is a major reason people quit exercising. To keep exercise interesting and combat boredom:
- Listen to music while exercising. Music makes you daydream, which makes time pass more quickly.
- Watch television, read or listen to books on tape while using a treadmill.
- Exercise with a friend. You can chat and encourage each other to keep going.
- If you like the social interaction of a group setting, join an aerobics class or a golf league.

Include variety
Alternating between different types of activities (cross-training)

reduces your chance of injury from overusing a specific muscle or joint. You might walk one day, bicycle the next and swim later in the week. Doing different types of exercise also reduces boredom.

Don't be afraid to try a new sport. There are many physical activities that you might enjoy. How about taking tennis or cross-country skiing lessons? Or check out activities such as tai chi or yoga.

Find an exercise buddy
Knowing that someone is waiting for you to show up at the park or the gym is a powerful incentive and can keep you accountable. Working out with a friend, co-worker or family member can bring a new level of motivation to your workouts. Plus, it's nice to have someone to visit with.

Be flexible and forgiving
If you're traveling or too busy on a certain day to do your full workout, it's OK to adapt your exercise program to accommodate your schedule. If you have a cold or the flu, it's better for your body to take a few days off. If you fall off your fitness program for some reason, don't lose hope. It happens to everyone. Just get going again and gradually return to your previous fitness level.

Set goals
Reaching a goal gives you encouragement. Start with simple, realistic goals, such as walking three or four days a week. You're more likely to quit in frustration if you bite off more than you can chew.

Once you've been exercising for a while, consider increasing your goals. For example, your new goal might be to walk for 30 minutes six days a week, to complete a 5-kilometer run or to bicycle 10 miles. Change your goals to keep things interesting and to advance to the next level of fitness.

Track your progress
Keep a record of your progress.

Be Aware of Warning Signs

If you experience any of the following signs or symptoms during exercise, stop and consult your doctor:

- Chest pain or tightness
- Dizziness or faintness
- Pain in an arm or your jaw
- Severe shortness of breath
- Bursts of very rapid or slow heart rate
- An irregular heartbeat
- Excessive fatigue
- Severe joint or muscle pain

Muscle soreness during exercise is common, especially if you're new to physical activity. If you're exercising at a moderate level of intensity, your breathing will be faster, and you'll feel like you're working, but you shouldn't be exhausted or feel pain.

Pain during exercise sends a different signal — it can be a warning sign of impending injury.

An exercise log helps you see what you've accomplished and helps determine your goals for the future. There's no right or wrong way to track your progress. What matters is that you pick a method you find easy to use and that works for you.

Common tracking tools include smartphone apps, wearable devices, computer-based logs, and old-fashioned pen and paper.

Reward yourself

When you reach a goal, treat yourself. If a gold star doesn't do the trick, buy yourself a new CD or go out for the evening. Equally important, work on developing internal rewards that come from feelings of accomplishment, self-esteem and control of your own behavior. Savor the good feelings that being active gives you.

Preventing Injury

Most injuries that occur during physical activity result from the "terrible toos" — too much, too hard, too fast, too soon, too long.

For example, a novice runner who attempts and struggles to complete five miles the first day out is bound to feel aches and pains. And a couch potato who comes to life for the annual company softball game is an excellent candidate for a sprain or some other painful injury.

Warm up

Warming up prepares your body for exercise and helps you avoid muscle stiffness, soreness and injury. Muscles that have been inactive are "cool." One way to warm them up is to start off with a low-intensity aerobic exercise, such as a slow to moderate walk. This gradually increases your heart rate (pulse), body temperature and blood flow to your muscles.

Another way to warm up is to slowly and gently stretch your muscles. This increases flexibility and helps maximize the range of motion around your joints. To avoid a pulled muscle that can result from stretching, it's often best to walk for at least three to five minutes before stretching. If you only have time to stretch once during an exercise session, it's best to do it right afterward, when your muscles are warmer and more elastic. See page 290 for examples of warm-up and cool-down stretches.

Exercise at the appropriate intensity

The intensity of a workout refers to how hard you work when you exercise. Moderate intensity exercise improves your cardiovascular fitness. But your workout shouldn't be too strenuous. Going full tilt doesn't provide many additional fitness benefits and may put you at increased risk of muscle or joint soreness or injury.

The following three measurements and tests can help you gauge whether you're exercising at the right intensity level to achieve cardiovascular fitness:

Talk test

The first method, the talk test, is the simplest. While you're exercising, you should be able to carry on a short conversation without being short of breath. If you can't do this, you're probably pushing too hard and need to slow your pace.

Heart rate

The more intense your aerobic exercise, the higher your heart rate (pulse) will be. When you exercise as hard as you can, your heart beats at its maximum rate. Most people should exercise at a level that puts their heart rate at 50 to 85 percent of their maximum. This is called the target heart rate (see page 295).

To determine if you're within your target range, take your pulse while you're exercising. Place two fingers on the inside edge of your wrist, press gently and feel for your pulse. Count your pulse for one minute or for 10 seconds and multiply the number you get by six.

Some medications, such as beta blockers, slow the heart rate and may invalidate the use of the target heart rate. To gauge the intensity of a workout, individuals on these medications need to rely more on their perceived exertion rather than on an actual heart rate.

Borg perceived exertion scale

Another way to gauge the intensity of your exercise is to use the Borg Rating of Perceived Exertion Scale. Perceived exertion is the total amount of physical effort you experience during a physical activity, taking into account all sensations of exertion, physical stress and fatigue.

For an activity to produce significant health benefits, you need to exert a moderate to somewhat hard effort — a 13 to 14 on the Borg perceived exertion scale.

Drink plenty of water

Water helps maintain a normal body temperature, and it cools working muscles. To help replenish lost fluids, drink water before and after your activity. Don't rely on thirst to tell you when you need a drink. During exercise your thirst mechanism is suppressed.

Use pain relievers with caution

If you're taking pain relievers, masking your pain may make it easier to overexert and damage your muscles, ligaments or tendons without realizing it. In addition, fluid loss with longer duration exercise may amplify the side effects of anti-inflammatory medications.

Cool down

Immediately after your aerobic exercise, allow your heart rate to gradually return to normal by spending three to five minutes in a low-intensity activity, such as slow walking. This also helps prevent blood from pooling in your legs, which may cause dizziness.

Stretching after exercise also is important. It helps keep your muscles limber and prevents muscle soreness and stiffness. You can use the same stretching exercises you used to warm up.

Take precautions in hot weather

When exercising in the heat, it's important to take precautions to avoid heat stress (see page 67). On hot days, more blood circulates through your skin to dispel heat. As a result, less blood is available for your muscles, so your heart rate during exercise will be higher than on cool days. To compensate, decrease the intensity of your exercise to keep your heart rate within your target range (see page 295).

Borg Perceived Exertion Scale

20	Maximal exertion
19	Extremely hard
18	
17	Very hard
16	
15	Hard
14	
13	Somewhat hard
12	
11	Light
10	
9	Very light
8	
7	Extremely light
6	No exertion at all

© Borg G. Borg Rating of Perceived Exertion Scale. 1998.

On hot days, exercise outside early in the morning or later in the evening, when it's cooler. If possible, do your exercise in the shade, indoors or in a pool. Drink water before and after exercising. If you plan to exercise for more than 30 minutes, stop and drink water every 15 to 20 minutes.

Proper attire is also important. Wear lightweight, loosefitting clothes made of fabrics that breathe and that wick moisture away from your body. White fabrics reflect sunlight and are cooler on sunny days. A light-colored hat or cap also will help.

Take precautions in cold weather

In extremely cold, windy weather, exposed skin can freeze in a short time (frostbite). If you exercise in extreme cold, protect exposed skin as much as possible. As with warm-weather exercising, make sure you drink plenty of fluids. Your body needs water in cold weather, too.

Dress for the conditions. Dressing in layers is the best strategy for cold weather. This provides added insulation and allows you to add or shed layers as appropriate. High-tech, lightweight fabrics keep you warmer and drier and are more resistant to wind and water than are old-fashioned cotton sweats.

In extremely cold or windy conditions, wear a soft scarf or cold-air mask over your mouth and nose. In addition, try to breathe through your nose because your nose warms, filters and humidifies the air before it enters your lungs.

Polypropylene glove liners can help keep your hands drier and warmer inside your gloves or mittens. In addition, be sure to wear a hat — most heat loss is through the head.

Treat an injury

Mild muscle soreness is common after exercise, but pain sends a different signal. If you sprain an ankle or twist a knee, don't ignore it and just hope that it will get better. See a doctor and follow his or her recommendations. Allow the injury time to heal.

Activity and Chronic Illness

There was a time when people with certain chronic medical conditions were told to avoid physical activity for fear it would make their conditions worse. But research has shown that physical activity actually can improve the health of many people with chronic illnesses.

Some chronic conditions, such as arthritis, asthma, diabetes and cardiovascular disease, can't be cured. However, many can be effectively managed with healthy lifestyle choices, medications and other treatments.

If you have a chronic condition, talk to your doctor about a physical activity program that's appropriate for you.

Arthritis

Although pain and stiffness may discourage you from being active, the only way to keep your joints functioning their best is to move them and strengthen the muscles that support them. Exercising can also help control your weight, reduce pain and injury, and improve your energy level and ability to accomplish daily tasks.

Any movement, no matter how little, can help. Take part in low-impact activities that place less stress on your joints. Water exercises such as swimming and walking in a pool are ideal because water's buoyancy takes the weight off your joints.

Other low-impact activities include biking and cross-country skiing. Strengthening exercises are important, too. If you can't lift weights, try more-gentle forms of resistance training, such as strength exercises you do while seated in a chair or standing against a wall.

As with all physical activity, start out slowly and gradually increase the amount of time and the intensity level. Take breaks when you feel you need to.

Asthma

Exercise is a common trigger of asthmatic symptoms, a condition called exercise-induced asthma. You're more prone to exercise-induced asthma if you have asthma due to allergies. Signs and symptoms of exercise-induced asthma include coughing, wheezing, chest tightness and shortness of breath.

Just because you have asthma doesn't mean you can't exercise. In fact, it's best if you're active. Regular exercise strengthens your heart and lungs and helps you lose weight so that you can breathe more easily.

Here are some tips for exercising with asthma:
- To help prevent symptoms, inhale a fast-acting bronchodilator

medication 15 to 30 minutes before exercising.
- Before beginning vigorous activity, warm up for five to 10 minutes with light activity and stretching, to help open your airways.
- Choose an activity that is less likely to trigger asthma symptoms. Swimming is a good choice. Some sports, such as distance running, soccer and basketball, are more likely to trigger symptoms.
- Choose activities that involve short or intermittent periods of exercise, such as golf, volleyball or softball.
- Be aware that cold-weather activities, such as skiing or ice hockey, are more likely to cause wheezing. If you do exercise in cold weather, wear a face mask to warm the air you breathe. Don't exercise in subzero temperatures.
- Try to exercise in an environment that doesn't aggravate your condition. For instance, if there's a high pollen count, exercise indoors.

Diabetes

Exercise can help you manage your diabetes by lowering your blood sugar and increasing insulin efficiency. It also helps prevent or delay the development of complications that can result from diabetes, such as high blood pressure and coronary artery disease. In addition, exercise helps control weight, an important factor for many people with type 2 diabetes.

Try to exercise at least 30 minutes a day most days of the week. Aerobic activities are generally best. Plan your activities to fit your mealtimes and medication dose, and check your blood sugar before and after exercising. If it's below 100 milligrams per deciliter (mg/dL), you may need to eat a snack before you exercise to avoid low blood sugar. You shouldn't

exercise if your blood sugar level is above 300 mg/dL.

If you've lost some of the feeling in your feet due to diabetic neuropathy, talk to your doctor about appropriate forms of exercise. You may want to avoid high-impact exercises such as running. Swimming or bicycling may be better choices.

High blood pressure

Physical activity is critical to controlling high blood pressure. Regular activity makes your heart stronger, so it doesn't have to work as hard to pump blood. Exercise also helps promote weight loss. Increased weight can contribute to high blood pressure.

Regular physical activity can lower your blood pressure by about the same amount as many blood pressure medications — 5 to 10 millimeters of mercury. This change may be enough to prevent you from having to take medication. If you're already taking medication, exercise can help your medication work more effectively.

Consistency is more important than intensity. Try to get at least 30 minutes of moderately intense activity most, if not all, days of the week. Aerobic activity has the greatest effect on blood pressure.

Coronary artery disease

If you have coronary artery disease, exercise is important. Regular exercise can help prevent a heart attack by reducing pressure on damaged arteries and reducing buildup of cholesterol-containing plaques. When plaques form in an artery, they narrow the passageway for blood flow and can lead to formation of a blood clot.

If you've had a heart attack, regular exercise helps reduce the risk of a second heart attack. Many people worry that they'll have a heart attack during exercise. The chances of that happening are small. Most heart attacks occur during rest, not activity. To minimize health risks and maximize exercise benefits:

- **See your doctor.** Before you begin a regular exercise program, have a physical examination and talk with your doctor about the best way to get started.
- **Exercise regularly.** Cardiovascular risk increases if you alternate intense workouts with weeks or months of inactivity.
- **Warm up and cool down.** This reduces stress on your heart and risk of muscle strain.
- **Wait two to three hours after a large meal before exercising.** Digestion increases blood flow to your digestive system and away from your heart.
- **Listen to your body.** If you experience heart palpitations, lightheadedness, or pain in your chest, jaw or arm, stop and seek immediate medical attention.

Osteoporosis

Regular exercise helps maintain, and may even increase, bone density. It also strengthens muscles. Strengthening your muscles and bones helps improve your balance, which can reduce the risk of falls and, therefore, fractures associated with osteoporosis.

Because of the varying degrees of osteoporosis and the risk of fracture, ask your doctor or a physical therapist for advice on exercises that are safe and appropriate for you. Walking is often an ideal weight-bearing activity because you can do it anywhere with minimal risk of injury.

Strength training may include use of free weights, weight machines, resistance bands or water exercises. These exercises strengthen muscles and bones and help slow bone mineral loss. Core exercises help strengthen back and abdominal muscles.

Avoid high-impact exercises that place excessive stress on your bones, such as running. Also avoid rowing machines, which require deep forward bending that could contribute to the development of a compression fracture in a vertebra.

Chronic pain

A common misconception is that exercise increases pain. Not so — exercise can help reduce it. When you're inactive, you become deconditioned — you lose muscle tone and strength, and your cardiovascular system works less efficiently. Regular physical activity builds stronger muscles, bones and joints, which can help reduce pain.

In addition, during physical activity your body releases chemicals called endorphins. Endorphins are natural pain-relieving chemicals that can block pain signals from reaching your brain. The more endorphins you produce on your own, the less you need to rely on external forms of pain management, such as medications.

Endorphins also help alleviate anxiety and depression, conditions that can make pain more difficult to control.

Your fitness program should be tailored to your specific condition. Talk with your doctor or a physical therapist about activities that may be beneficial for you. ■

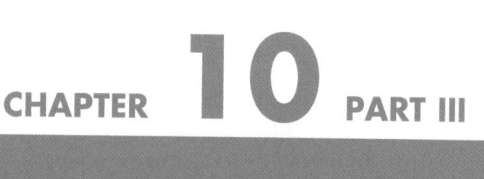

Stress

Constant time pressures, a heavy workload, a demanding family life, aging parents — these situations and countless others can lead to a high level of stress. Stress is something that most people know well and experience often. It's unavoidable. Stress comes from events that you consider to be positive — a job promotion, vacation or marriage — as well as from negative events — the loss of a job, a divorce or financial problems. In short, stress is a normal part of everyday life.

Understanding Stress

Stress results from both your response to an event and the event itself. It's how you react physically and emotionally to certain situations and circumstances that causes you to feel pressure, or stress.

Long days — both at home and at work — too little sleep and information overload are among the leading sources of stress. However, situations that create stress are as unique as you are. Your personality, your genetic makeup and your past experiences — your overall ability to cope — influence how you deal with stressful situations. Standing in line at the store or getting a parking ticket may not bother you, but another person may find them extremely stressful.

Whatever the cause of your stress, the thing to remember is that when perceived demands exceed your ability to cope, it creates stress, and stress can produce symptoms and lead to illness.

Stress can be short term (acute) or long term (chronic), and the effects of stress can accumulate over time. Acute stress commonly is a reaction to an immediate or perceived threat. In such cases, you respond with an alarm reaction that readies your body for an emergency. Chronic stress is often related to situations that aren't short-lived, such as relationship problems, loneliness or 24/7 access to work.

When you experience stress — especially severe stress — a physical response occurs to meet the energy demands of the situation. After the threat passes, your body begins to relax again.

You may be able to handle an occasional stressful event, but when stressful situations occur regularly, the effects multiply and compound over time. Developing effective coping strategies to help you manage stress can be a lifesaver.

Stress and Health

Many of the physical reactions that accompany stress can damage your long-term health by contributing to both emotional and physical illness. Stress may be a factor in many illnesses, from anxiety to heart disease.

Stress may aggravate an existing health problem, such as asthma or a gastrointestinal condition. Or, it may trigger a new illness if you're already at risk of that particular condition.

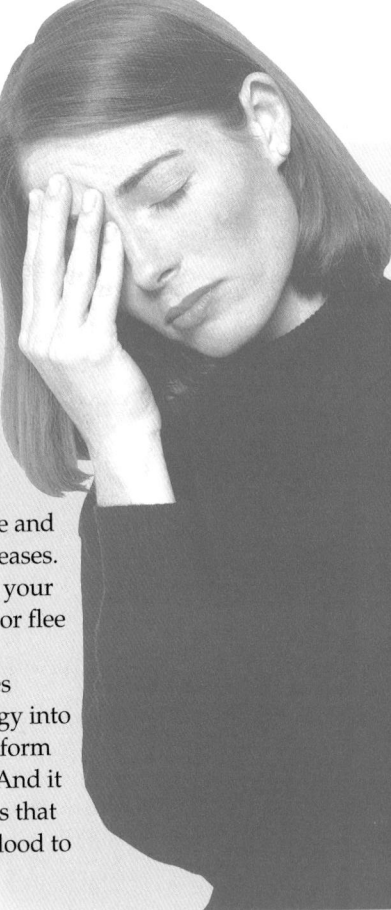

The Fight-or-Flight Response

Your brain comes hard-wired with an alarm system for your protection. When you perceive danger or experience fear — for instance, an angry-looking dog barks at you during your morning run — a tiny region at the base of your brain called the hypothalamus sets off an alarm system in your body known as your fight-or-flight response.

The same type of reaction occurs when you encounter stressful situations — such as having to speak before a large audience or take an important exam. Your body responds to the situation similar to a physical threat.

During the fight-or-flight response, your pituitary gland, which is located at the base of your brain, secretes hormones that regulate many body processes, kicking into action a number of physical responses. Through a combination of nerve and hormone signals, your internal alarm system prompts your adrenal glands, located atop your kidneys, to release a surge of hormones, including the hormones adrenaline (epinephrine) and cortisol. Immediately, your heart starts to beat faster, your muscles tense and your blood pressure increases. These responses prepare your body to fight the danger or flee the situation.

Your body also releases potential sources of energy into your bloodstream in the form of blood sugars and fat. And it secretes certain chemicals that make it easier for your blood to clot in case of an injury.

Suppresses the immune system

The hormone cortisol produced during the stress response may suppress your immune system, increasing your susceptibility to infectious disease. Studies suggest the risk of bacterial infections such as tuberculosis and group A streptococcal disease increases during stress. Stress may also make you prone to upper respiratory viral infections such as a cold or the flu.

Increases the risk of cardiovascular disease

During acute stress your heart beats quickly, which makes you more susceptible to heart rhythm irregularities and a type of chest pain called angina. If you're a "hot reactor" experiencing an "amygdala hijack," acute stress may add to your risk of a heart attack. Hot reactors exhibit extreme increases in heart rate and blood pressure in response to stress. These surges may injure your coronary arteries and heart. Increased blood clotting from persistent stress can put you at risk of a heart attack or stroke.

Worsens other illnesses

Other relationships between illness and stress aren't as clear-cut. However, stress may worsen your symptoms if you have any of the following conditions:

Asthma
A stressful situation can make your airways overreactive, precipitating an asthma attack.

Gastrointestinal problems
Stress may trigger or worsen symptoms associated with some gastrointestinal conditions, such as irritable bowel syndrome or nonulcer dyspepsia.

Chronic pain
Stress can heighten your body's pain response, making chronic pain associated with conditions such as arthritis, fibromyalgia or a back injury more difficult to manage.

Mental health disorders
Stress may trigger depression in people prone to the disorder. It may also worsen symptoms of other mental health disorders, such as anxiety or substance abuse

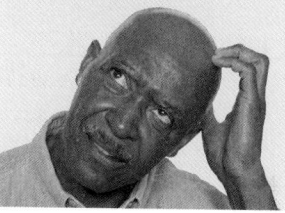
Your nervous system also moves into action by causing the pupils in your eyes to dilate so that you can see better if the lighting is poor and by tensing your facial muscles, possibly to make you look more menacing. Perspiration increases to keep your body cool, and respiration accelerates to increase oxygen in your blood. All of these changes prepare your body for an emergency, real or perceived.

The amygdala, located in the front portion of the temporal lobe, is the brain's stress center. It helps fuel certain emotions, including fear. It controls how you react when you perceive a potential threat, and it regulates the fight-or-flight response.

When you're facing a physical danger, you can release your stress through physical activity, such as running away from the threat. When the danger is mental, you don't have an avenue to get rid of your stress energy and it accumulates.

When you become angry, you may stop thinking logically and have difficulty controlling your behaviors. It's not uncommon for people to overreact when they experience overwhelming emotional responses from too much stress. This is known as an amygdala hijack. During periods of extreme or constant stress, people may do or say things that they later regret.

Your body's stress response system is usually self-limiting. Once a perceived threat has passed, your body is meant to return to a normal, relaxed state, with hormone levels returning to normal. As adrenaline and cortisol levels drop, your heart rate and blood pressure reach their baseline levels, and other systems resume their regular activities.

However, when stressors are always present and you constantly feel under attack, that fight-or-flight response stays turned on. Long-term activation of your stress response system — and the subsequent overexposure to cortisol and other stress hormones that this causes — can disrupt almost all of your body's processes. This puts you at increased risk of numerous and varied health problems. And this is why ongoing, uncontrolled stress is bad for your health.

Recognizing Stress

You may not recognize that you're under stress. Indications that your body and brain are feeling pressured may be associated with certain symptoms — headache, muscle tension, fatigue, insomnia, upset stomach or digestive changes. A nervous habit such as nail biting may reappear. Instead of recognizing these as signs of stress, you may interpret them as an illness.

Stress may also become apparent through psychological changes. The most common change is increased irritability with people close to you. You may also feel more cynical, pessimistic or resentful. Many people with stress report a sense of being victimized, misunderstood or unappreciated. Things you once enjoyed may now seem burdensome.

Some people become anxious, reclusive, or prone to crying or laughing. Others engage in unhealthy behaviors, such as smoking or drinking too much alcohol. The changes may be so gradual that you or those around you don't recognize them until your health or relationships change.

Coping With Stress

You can manage stress in many different ways. You may talk about your problems with others, listen to soothing music, or sit in a warm bathtub or hot tub at the end of the day. Exercise, relaxation activities and being in nature also are great stress reducers.

Most of the time you may do pretty well in getting through life's crises. For times when you probably could do better, below are some strategies to help you out.

Signs and Symptoms of Stress

Physical	Psychological	Behavioral
Headache	Anxiety	Overeating or loss of appetite
Grinding teeth	Irritability	Impatience
Tight, dry throat	Feeling of impending doom	Being argumentative
Clenched jaws	Depression	Procrastination
Chest pain	Slowed thinking	Increased use of alcohol or drugs
Shortness of breath	Racing thoughts	Increased tobacco use
Pounding heart	Feeling of helplessness	Withdrawal or isolation
High blood pressure	Feeling of hopelessness	Neglecting responsibilities
Muscle aches	Feeling of worthlessness	Poor job performance
Indigestion	Feeling of lack of direction	Burnout
Constipation or diarrhea	Feeling of insecurity	Poor personal hygiene
Increased perspiration	Sadness	Biting nails or chewing on pencils
Cold, sweaty hands	Defensiveness	Consuming more caffeine
Fatigue	Anger	Being less physically active
Insomnia	Hypersensitivity	Change in close relationships
Frequent illness	Apathy	Change in religious practices

Identify your stressors

The first step in learning to manage your stress is to identify what's causing it. Not everyone responds to events the same way.

For instance, a so-called workaholic may be thought by others to be working too much, when in fact that person feels more in control when taking on extra challenges at work. For this person, work itself may be a form of stress management, and the unstructured time of a vacation or "relaxation" at home may actually be a greater source of stress.

Your stress may be linked to external factors, such as:
• Work
• Family
• Community
• Environment
• Unpredictable events

Stress can also come from internal factors, such as:
• Unrealistic or high expectations
• Perfectionism
• Worry
• Negative attitudes and feelings
• Irresponsible behavior
• Poor health and health habits

Once you identify the sources of your stress, you might not be able to avoid them, but you'll at least know what's causing your symptoms. That in itself may be a benefit by making you feel more in control.

Practice tolerance

As a part of your overall strategy to better manage stress, try to become more tolerant — of yourself and of situations over which you have no control. You need to understand and accept that changes are constant. Some of them you can control and others you can't. Understand that some things will continue to occur, like it or not.

Interpersonal Conflicts

Often life's hurdles revolve around dealing with interpersonal conflicts. The three most typical types of interpersonal conflicts are marital conflicts, family conflicts and job-related conflicts.

Marital conflicts

Often, couples enter into a relationship with unrealistic expectations. An overly romantic view of marriage fosters this tendency. Instead of realizing that they're marrying ordinary human beings with strengths and weaknesses, some people tend to idealize their mates and expect nothing less than perfection.

Over the course of a marriage, couples typically face a series of predictable transitions. Adjustments to having children, changing jobs and losing parents, as well as changing sexual needs, all present challenges. If their marriages are to flourish, couples must communicate and resolve inevitable conflicts effectively.

A licensed marriage counselor often can bring troublesome issues to light and foster communication so that a couple can recognize and deal with stress in the marriage.

Family conflicts

A family is a complex network of relationships. Each member has a different relationship with each other member in the family. These differences may be a reflection of age, birth order, sex, personality type or a combination of several such factors. Each of these relationships, in turn, affects the rest of the family unit.

Difficulties within a family are often brought to the surface when one member is showing signs of a problem — for example, trouble in school or excessive use of alcohol. These occasions may reveal a pattern of behavior that everyone is contributing to, such as spending too little time with one another, and that everyone in the family needs to help change. Licensed family therapists often help identify specific problems that all family members can work on.

Job-related conflicts

Interpersonal conflicts in the workplace present a multitude of issues. Competition can develop among co-workers. Conflict may stem from an individual's desire for power and control, a perception of disrespect, workplace changes, or differences in work habits.

These problems often result from a lack of proper communication among co-workers and between management and employees. Employee assistance programs (EAPs) can be a valuable resource for stress due to work-related conflict.

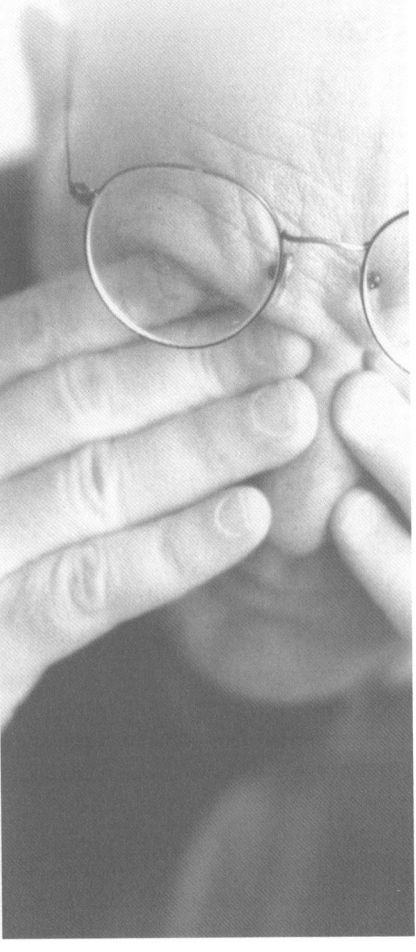

Getting Professional Help

You don't need to handle all of your problems alone. Help from a licensed mental health professional, such as a psychiatrist, psychologist or counselor, may be what you need to better handle stress. Many people believe that seeking outside help is a sign of weakness, which adds to their sense of inadequacy, hopelessness or anger. To the contrary, it takes strength to realize that you need professional help and good judgment to seek it. If you need assistance finding someone who can help you, ask your doctor, local health organization or employer for recommendations.

With professional guidance, you may be able to determine if what you're feeling is stress or an illness. If you're experiencing symptoms that affect your ability to work, enjoy positive relationships or find pleasure in life, they may be a signal of something more than stress.

If you're like most people, you're more understanding of other people's distress than of your own. You may think that you should always feel happy or you should always be able to cope. As long as you believe this, you're bound to be disappointed. The reality is, you'll always experience some stress — a certain level of stress is normal.

Learn to manage anger

For many people, anger management is an important technique for reducing stress. Anger can significantly increase and prolong stress if you remain angry for an extended period. Anger can even trigger a heart attack. Learning to manage anger is a lot like learning to manage stress. Here are some suggestions to help you get started:

Identify your anger triggers
Once you know what sets you off, plan ahead for how you'll avoid becoming angry when you're in such a situation.

Identify signs and symptoms of emerging anger
What do you do when you start to get angry? Do you clench your teeth? Do your shoulders begin to tense up? Do you feel your heart begin to beat faster? Does your face flush? Read these signs and symptoms like a caution light — a warning that you're getting angry.

Respond to your symptoms
When you find yourself becoming angry, take a short timeout. Count to 10, take a few deep breaths, look out a window — anything to buy time so that your brain can catch up with your emotions and you can think before you act.

Take time to cool down
Before you confront a person or situation that has made you angry, find a way to release some of your emotional energy. Go for a walk, clean the house, or call a friend. Don't hit the send button on that angry email you just wrote.

Don't bottle up your anger
If your anger stems from what someone said or did, talk to that person in an assertive, not aggressive, manner. Don't verbally attack the person with accusations. Deal only with this episode and approach it from the perspective of how you feel instead of what the person did.

Find release valves
Look for creative ways to release the energy produced by your anger. These might include exercise, listening to music, painting, dancing or writing in your journal.

Seek advice
If you find yourself becoming angry often, confide in people who care about you, such as family members or close friends. Ask them to help you brainstorm possible coping solutions or find a medical professional who can help you.

Practice positive thinking

Positive self-talk is another effective way to cope with stress. Self-talk is the endless stream of thoughts that run through your head every day.

These automatic thoughts can be positive or negative. Some are based on logic and reason. Others may be misconceptions you formulate from lack of adequate information. The goal of positive self-talk is to weed out the misconceptions and challenge them with rational and positive thoughts. Studies indicate that a positive, hopeful attitude can help manage stress, but a negative attitude can aggravate it.

Positive self-talk is simple, but it takes time and practice. Throughout the day, stop and evaluate what you're thinking. Are you focusing only on the worst-case scenarios? Find a way to replace negative thoughts with positive ones. A reasonable rule about self-talk is this: Don't say to yourself anything you wouldn't say to someone else.

Develop an action plan

Once you've identified your stressors, it's time to address them. Some stressors are under your control; others aren't. Concentrate on events that you can change. For example, if your busy day is a source of stress, ask yourself if it's because you tend to squeeze too many things into your day or because you aren't organized. Here are some tips that may help:

Plan your day
Planning can help you feel more in control. Keep a schedule of your daily activities so that you're not faced with conflicts or last-minute rushes to get to an appointment or activity on time.

Managing Your Time

Often, stress is a result of too much to do and too little time. Or it may stem from procrastination. Setting priorities and practicing some simple time management skills may go a long way toward depressurizing your day, for example:

1. Put all of your tasks onto a master list. Include everything you have to do, large and small. Mark key dates and deadlines for big projects on your calendar.
2. Each day, list five to 10 items that you want to accomplish that day.
3. Divide your daily list into three levels — A, B and C:
   - *A* items are the two or three tasks that you must do. These tasks are both important and urgent and probably will take the most energy. Do them first or when your energy level is the highest.
   - *B* items are important but not urgent. These activities will help you move toward your long-range goals.
   - *C* items are routine stuff, but things that you must do today. Can you delegate any of these?

If you're still having problems getting the right things done, analyze how you spend your time for several days. You may be wasting time on things that aren't on your list, such as time on the internet or on social media.

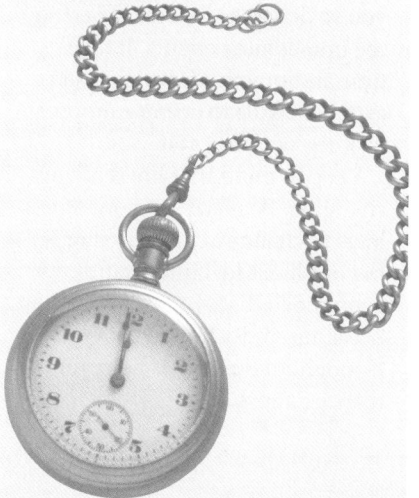

Simplify your life

Prioritize, plan and pace yourself. Simplify your life by cutting out some activities or delegating tasks. Keep your house, car and personal belongings in working order to prevent untimely, expensive and stressful repairs.

Get organized

Organize your home and work space so that you don't have to spend time looking for things you've misplaced.

Take occasional breaks

Periodically during the day, take time to relax, stretch or walk.

Get adequate sleep, stay physically active and eat well

A healthy body helps promote good mental health. Sleep helps you tackle problems with renewed vigor. Physical activity helps burn off stress-related tension. A healthy diet provides you with energy to handle daily stress.

Discuss your concerns

Talking with a trusted friend helps relieve stress and may put events in perspective. At times, just venting can be helpful.

Remember what's important

Concentrate on the things of most importance to you.

Get away

Take a break from your normal routine and take part in enjoyable activities — alone, with friends or family, or with a group.

Enjoy a good laugh

It's healthy to spend time with people who take themselves lightly or have a sense of humor. Laughter helps reduce or relieve tension.

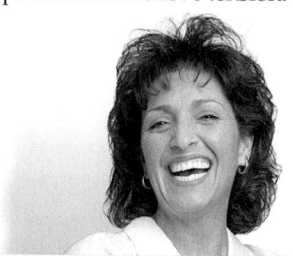

Turning Negatives Into Positives

Here are some examples of typical negative thoughts or mental messages and how you can give them a positive twist:

Negative thought	Positive thought
I've never done it before.	It's an opportunity to learn something new.
It's too complicated.	Let's break it into smaller, manageable tasks.
I don't have the necessary skills.	Let me think of what resources are available that I can use.
There's not enough time.	Let's re-evaluate some priorities.
There's no way it'll work.	Let's be positive and test this out.
I don't have the expertise.	I'll find people who can help me.
It's not perfect.	There's always room for improvement, but I did well.
It's too radical a change.	Let's give it a shot.

Practice relaxation techniques

Relaxation is more than watching television or taking a break from work. True relaxation is positive and satisfying — a feeling of peace of mind. As you learn to relax, you want to seek out activities that give you pleasure or satisfy you, such as physical activity, art, music or some other hobby.

Try to devote at least 60 minutes to these relaxing activities every day. You don't have to do the activities all at once. You can reach your 60 minutes by breaking up the activities into several 10-minute blocks throughout the day.

There are many techniques that can lessen the discomfort and duration of stress. See Chapter 38, "Integrative Medicine," for more information on different ways to relax and reduce stress.

To get you started, here are three techniques you might try — relaxed breathing, progressive muscle relaxation and visualization. The techniques are fairly easy to learn, and you can use them almost anywhere, during times when you feel stress getting the better of you.

Relaxed breathing
This form of relaxation focuses on deep, relaxed breathing. Rehearse it throughout the day so that it becomes natural, and you can apply it when you feel stressed.
1. Lie on a bed or couch or sit comfortably in a chair.
2. Place your feet slightly apart and rest your hands on your abdomen or in your lap.
3. Slowly inhale while counting to four, allowing your abdomen to rise about 1 inch — you should feel the movement with your hand. Don't pull up your shoulders or move your chest.
4. As you breathe in, imagine the air flowing into all parts of your body.
5. Pause one or two seconds after inhaling.
6. Slowly exhale and count to four. As you exhale, your abdomen will slowly fall.
7. As air flows out, imagine your tension also flowing out.
8. Pause one or two seconds after exhaling.
9. Repeat five to 10 times.

If it's difficult to make your breathing regular, take a slightly deeper breath, hold it for a second or two and let it out slowly through pursed lips for about 10 seconds. Repeat this once or twice. Practice relaxed breathing whenever you're waiting in line or at a stoplight.

Progressive muscle relaxation
Progressive muscle relaxation is a technique that involves relaxing a series of muscles one at a time.
1. Sit or lie in a comfortable position and close your eyes. Allow your jaw to drop and your eyelids to relax, but don't squeeze your eyelids shut.
2. Mentally scan your body, starting with your toes and working slowly up through your legs, buttocks, torso, arms, hands, fingers, neck and head. Focus on each part individually.
3. Tighten the muscles in one area of your body, hold them for a count of five, and then relax them. Imagine the tension melting away from your muscles as you relax. Then move on to the next area.

Visualization
Also known as guided imagery, visualization involves lying quietly and picturing yourself in a pleasant and peaceful setting — a location you truly enjoy.
1. Allow thoughts to flow through your mind, but don't focus on any of them. Tell yourself that you're relaxed and calm, that your hands are heavy and warm — or cool if you're hot — and that your heart is beating calmly.
2. Breathe slowly, regularly and deeply.
3. Once you're relaxed, imagine yourself in a favorite place or in a spot of beauty and stillness.
4. After five or 10 minutes, rouse yourself gradually.

With practice, you'll be able to imagine your favorite place or a spot of great beauty and stillness and trigger the relaxation response in your body.

An added benefit of stress management is that it promotes resiliency — the ability to bounce back and grow from life's experiences. Studies indicate that people who are more resilient to life's challenges tend to be healthier and happier.

How to succeed

No matter what steps you take to manage stress, two simple reminders can help you be successful: practice and be patient.

Practice
The steps you're taking may be new to you. In fact, at first you may feel uncomfortable doing them. Work on your coping skills daily, and be open to trying new techniques. You want to get to the point that you can use them anytime and anywhere.

When you're practicing relaxation techniques, get comfortable — loosen tight clothing and remove your shoes and belt if needed.

Be patient
Don't worry about how well you're doing, and don't expect to see immediate benefits. It takes time and practice for stress management skills to become automatic. Keep working at it.

Keep in mind that life is always changing. Be ready for your stress level to change at various stages in your life. Most importantly, continue to discover and practice stress-reduction techniques throughout the day to help you manage stress. ■

Unhealthy Behaviors

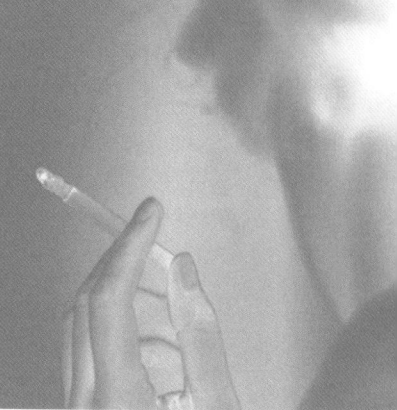

Your health in later life depends as much on your lifestyle choices as on your genes. And the sooner you adopt healthy habits, the greater is your chance of living to a ripe old age.

What are your health trouble spots — activities or habits that increase your risk of disease? For some people, the answer may be inactivity and an unhealthy diet. For others, trouble spots may be activities that have a more direct negative impact on health. These activities — commonly referred to as unhealthy behaviors — include tobacco, excessive alcohol, drug use and unsafe sex.

If you aren't involved in any of these activities, don't start. If you are, it's not too late to change. Addressing risky behaviors can add years to your life.

Tobacco Use Disorder

Smoking is the single largest preventable cause of premature death and disability in the United States. Yet approximately 36 million Americans smoke — that's about 15 percent of the adult population. Among high school teens, about 8 percent smoke cigarettes. If smoking continues at the current rate among youth in this country, more than 5 million of today's Americans younger than 18 will die early from a smoking-related illness.

Doctors frequently see people whose serious medical conditions are related to smoking. Medical care for smoking-related illnesses in the United States costs billions of dollars annually. The indirect costs of smoking are equally astounding. Fires started by cigarettes cause significant property damage. Higher insurance premiums and taxes needed to fund disability benefits for people who are ill as a result of smoking also are part of the cost.

Consider these facts:
- Cigarette smoking is responsible for about 1 in 5 deaths in the United States.
- Cigarette smoking is responsible for more than 480,000 deaths annually, including deaths from secondhand smoke.
- The life expectancy for smokers is at least 10 years shorter than it is for nonsmokers.

Smoking and disease

The popularity of the cigarette is a 20th-century phenomenon. The number of cigarette smokers skyrocketed in the early 1900s following the introduction of new mass production technology combined with highly effective advertising campaigns. Before long, reports of a connection between smoking and the incidence of diseases such as lung cancer began to appear.

Today, tobacco use is recognized as a major risk factor in many diseases. This should come as no surprise. Cigarette smoke contains more than 7,000 chemicals, including at least 70 known to cause cancer in humans and animals.

The delicate tissues of your mouth, throat and voice box (larynx) are affected by repeated exposure to cigarette smoke. After the smoke passes through your mouth, your lungs retain 70 to 90 percent of the compounds you inhale.

Just a few puffs on a cigarette reduce the effectiveness of the cilia inside your bronchial tubes. Cilia are tiny, hair-like bodies that normally work like brooms to sweep foreign particles out of your lungs. Smoking just one cigarette can slow the sweeping actions of the cilia for almost an hour, allowing unwanted substances to stay in your lungs.

A smoker experiences airway inflammation with mucus-secreting glands producing larger than normal volumes of sputum. Regular smoking virtually paralyzes the cilia, leaving your lungs exposed to billions of tiny particles from cigarette smoke. With the cilia largely inactive, tar from the cigarette smoke begins to build up and damage lung tissues. When cooled inside your lungs, the tar forms a brown sticky layer on the lining of breathing passages. This layer contains the tar and other chemicals that can cause cancer.

Cancer
Smoking is a major risk factor for cancers of the mouth, larynx, pharynx, esophagus, lung, stomach, pancreas, kidney, urinary bladder and cervix.

Here are some other sobering statistics:
- About one-third of cancer deaths in American men and one-quarter in American women are smoking-related.
- Lung cancer is the leading cause of cancer deaths in American men and women. The risk of death from cigarette smoking continues to increase among women, and is now nearly identical to that of men.
- Smoking cigarettes kills more Americans than alcohol, car accidents, HIV, guns and illegal drugs combined.

Chronic obstructive pulmonary disease
Smoking is a major cause of chronic lung diseases such as chronic obstructive pulmonary disease (COPD). This disease includes lung disorders such as emphysema and chronic bronchitis.

As many as 8 out of 10 COPD deaths are related to cigarette smoking. In addition to paralyzing or destroying the cilia in your lungs, tobacco smoke irrevocably damages or destroys the tiny air sacs (alveoli) in your lungs in which carbon dioxide is exchanged for oxygen. When these air sacs are injured, your body is less able to transport adequate levels of oxygen to your vital organs. Eventually, as you struggle for each breath, COPD often becomes fatal.

Attention Women Smokers

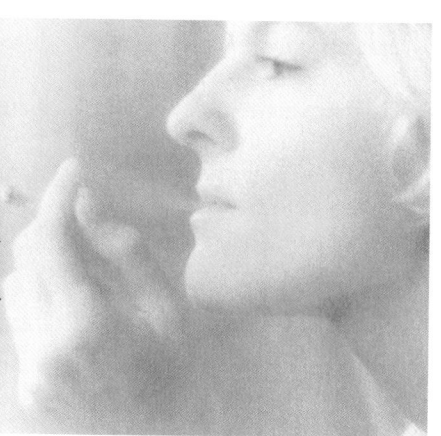

Women who smoke have additional risks to consider:
- Female smokers older than age 35 who use birth control pills are at high risk of heart attacks, strokes and blood clots in the legs.
- Female smokers have an increased risk of developing osteoporosis, a disease that makes bones brittle.
- Women who smoke during pregnancy are more likely to have a miscarriage or stillbirth, or a baby with a low birth weight. Studies also show a direct relationship between smoking during pregnancy and risk of sudden infant death syndrome.

Cardiovascular disease

Cardiovascular disease includes conditions such as high blood pressure, coronary artery disease and stroke. The single most important health effect of smoking may be its role in developing cardiovascular disease.

Nicotine in tobacco smoke acts on your adrenal glands, causing them to secrete hormones that temporarily increase your blood pressure and your heart rate. The carbon monoxide from tobacco smoke binds to hemoglobin in your blood, taking the place of valuable oxygen and reducing the amount of oxygen available to your tissues and organs.

Carbon monoxide may have a direct effect on the heart muscle itself, on your blood vessels and perhaps even on the clotting of your blood. Smoking may increase the clumping (clotting) action of certain blood cells (platelets), and it decreases the ability of the arteries to dilate when they need to do so. The mechanism is complex, but smoking is also a contributing factor to the accumulation of cholesterol in arteries (atherosclerosis). In addition, smoking raises your triglyceride level and lowers the "good" (high-density lipoprotein, or HDL) cholesterol in your blood. All of this increases your risk of cardiovascular disease. Smoking contributes to other circulatory problems as well.

Here are some statistics about tobacco use and the risks to your heart:

- Smoking causes 1 in 3 deaths from cardiovascular disease.
- A smoker is at least two times more likely to die of a heart attack than is a nonsmoker, and the risk is even higher for heavier smokers.
- A smoker who has had a heart attack and continues to smoke is much more likely to have a second heart attack than is a person who stops smoking.

Why smokers smoke

Increased knowledge of the hazards of smoking, along with increased smoking restrictions or bans, has had a deterring effect on smokers. More than 40 million Americans identify themselves as former smokers. The number of men who smoke has declined substantially, from one-half of the adult men in 1965 to about 17 percent today. Among women, there's been a slower decline. As a result, the numbers of male and female smokers are now about equal.

The reasons people start smoking or refuse to quit are rarely simple. Some smokers report that their cigarettes offer them a surge of energy, especially to wake them up in the morning or keep them awake at other times. Nicotine acts as a stimulant with an adrenaline-like effect. Your heart rate and blood pressure increase while you're smoking.

Some smokers note that cigarettes calm them down when they're under stress. In addition, a cigarette gives them something to do with their hands if they're nervous or even gives them a sense of security.

Nicotine in tobacco is an addictive drug that leads to an addictive response. The degree of addiction depends to some degree on how much and how long the smoker has smoked. The addiction most smokers experience is both psychological and physical. For some, regular use of cigarettes in many life situations has convinced them that they can't cope with life without smoking.

Nicotine can be as addictive as alcohol, heroin or cocaine. The central element of addiction is loss of control. Nicotine controls your behavior by making you feel good, so you want to use it more. You may want to quit, but you can't or won't, even when you know tobacco is harmful to your health.

You may be dependent on or addicted to nicotine if you experience one or more of the following characteristics:
- You have a cigarette within 30 minutes of the time you wake up in the morning.
- You've made a serious but unsuccessful attempt to stop or reduce the amount of tobacco you use.
- Your attempts to stop have led to withdrawal symptoms, such as craving tobacco or feelings of anxiety, irritability, frustration or anger. Other signs and symptoms include trouble

concentrating or sleeping, and an increase in appetite with possible weight gain.

- You continue to use tobacco even when you have a serious health problem, such as heart or lung disease, that you know is made worse by tobacco use.
- You develop a "tolerance" for tobacco. You may notice that a certain number of cigarettes daily produces less effect than it used to and that you need to smoke more to achieve a desired effect.

Teenage smoking

Most cigarette smokers start early in life. Among smokers born since 1935, more than 80 percent started smoking before age 21, and more than half started before age 18. Presently in the United States, each day an estimated 2,100 youth and young adults who've been occasional smokers become daily cigarette smokers. Even though smoking has generally declined since the mid-1960s, an increasing number of teenagers smoke. This group continues to be a major target for advertising by the tobacco industry.

It's been well-documented that a high percentage of teenagers who smoke come from families in which one or both parents smoke. Cigarette smoking among teenagers also seems to be connected to peer pressure. Surveys suggest a common predictor of whether a boy or girl smokes is having friends who smoke.

While most teenagers are aware that smoking is harmful to their health, most also indicate that they don't plan to smoke for a lifetime. The majority of teen smokers say they plan to quit within a few years. Interestingly, most teens who took up smoking had been adamantly against smoking in their younger years. Parents who continue to smoke with no visible ill effects can have a substantial influence. In such sit-uations teenagers' concerns about smoking diminish, and many take up smoking.

Cigarette alternatives

Contrary to popular belief, using other types of tobacco products or cigarette alternatives endangers your health just as much as smoking regular cigarettes.

E-cigarettes
In the past five years e-cigarettes have become popular among smokers, but adolescent users have increased significantly. An e-cigarette is a battery-operated module that contains an atomizing device and a reservoir for nico-tine. When you inhale, air passes through the atomizing device, pro-ducing heat that results in aerosol-ization of the nicotine mixture.

This process results in a nic-otine vapor that you inhale. Vaping is the term used for inhaling the e-cigarette vapor. There are 27 different nicotine strengths across more than 400 brands.

The highest use of e-cigarettes is among current smokers, fol-lowed by ex-smokers and then nonsmokers. A recent survey found that more than 13 percent of high school students had exper-imented with e-cigarettes.

There are very few reliable stud-ies that have looked at the health risks of these products. Although there have been claims that e-ciga-rettes are a substitute for smoking and may aid in smoking cessation, there's inadequate data or research to substantiate this claim. E-ciga-rettes have not received Food and Drug Administration approval as a smoking-cessation product.

Cigars
According to some figures, a little more than 8 percent of U.S. males smoke cigars. Unlike cigarettes, cigars vary in size and appearance. And whereas cigarettes are made from blends of tobacco, cigars are made primarily of a single tobac-co. Like cigarette smoking, the health risks from cigar smoking increase with the number of cigars a person smokes each day.

Although many cigar smokers don't fully inhale smoke into their lungs, they're still exposed to smoke in their oral cavity, as well as to the secondhand smoke in the smoking environment. Cigar smoke contains as many poison-ous chemicals as cigarette smoke, putting cigar smokers at the same risk of smoking-related illnesses. Plus, a single large cigar can con-tain more than ½ ounce of tobacco — as much as an entire pack of cigarettes. One cigar also contains 100 to 200 milligrams of nicotine, while a cigarettes averages only about 8 milligrams.

Cigar smokers and cigarette smokers have similar risk levels of cancers of the mouth, throat and esophagus. And cigar smokers are still four to 10 times more likely to die of cancers of the lung and larynx than are nonsmokers.

Pipes
Studies on the risks of lung or heart disease in people who smoke only a pipe compared with people who smoke only cigarettes or cigars are limited. However, pipe smoking is associated with cancers of the lip, mouth and lung, and it clearly increases the level of carbon monoxide in your blood. There's enough evidence avail-able on the dangers of pipe use to recommend that you become a nonsmoker.

Spit tobacco and snuff
Spit tobacco (chewing tobacco) is usually sold in loose leaf form or compressed in a plug. Users gen-erally place spit tobacco between their cheek and gum and keep it there for several hours. Nicotine is absorbed into the bloodstream through the cheek lining. Snuff is powdered tobacco. A small amount is placed between the lower lip and the gum.

In recent years, there's been an increase in the use of spit tobacco and snuff. Approximately 3 percent of the U.S. population uses spit tobacco, primarily white males. Spit tobacco and snuff have been thought to be a safe alternative to cigarette smoking. But they're not safe at all. Studies show that smokeless tobacco can produce a high level of nicotine in the blood. The consequence of regular use is long-term nicotine dependence and addiction and associated health risks.

Health risks include cancers of the oral cavity and throat, particularly where tobacco is held in the mouth. Frequently, a white, leathery patch forms at the place in your mouth where you hold tobacco. This condition, called leukoplakia, is precancerous.

Spit tobacco and snuff can cause swollen, bleeding gums and lead to the loss of teeth. They can also cause an increased heart rate, higher blood pressure and even an irregular heartbeat. The bottom line is, no smoke is safe smoke, and no tobacco use is safe.

Secondhand smoke

More than 41,000 Americans die each year of exposure to second-hand (passive) smoke. As a result, most states have enacted laws limiting smoking in public places.

Since 1964, more than 2½ million nonsmoking adults have died from exposure to secondhand smoke. Each year, secondhand smoke causes approximately 7,330 deaths from lung cancer and 33,950 deaths from heart disease. Secondhand smoke contains more than 7,000 chemicals, 70 of which can cause cancer.

Inhaling secondhand smoke causes your heart to beat faster, your blood pressure to increase and the level of carbon monoxide in your blood to rise. Side-stream smoke from a burning cigarette contains twice as much tar and nicotine as does inhaled smoke, three times more of a cancer caus-

ing compound called 3,4-benz-pyrene, five times more carbon monoxide and possibly 50 times more ammonia.

- More than 24 million (about 37 percent) of U.S. children have been exposed to secondhand smoke.
- Secondhand smoke is especially harmful to young children. It's responsible for between 150,000 and 300,000 lower respiratory tract infections in infants and children under 18 months of age. It also causes 430 sudden infant death syndrome (SIDS) deaths in the U.S. annually.
- Secondhand smoke exposure may cause a buildup of fluid in the middle ear, resulting in close to 800,000 doctor's office visits per year, as well as more than 200,000 asthma flare-ups among children each year.

How to stop smoking

Most smokers understand that tobacco use is hazardous to their health. What many beginning smokers fail to understand, however, is that smoking also is an addiction. It involves chemicals that affect human emotions and behavior.

Because nicotine is an addictive drug, quitting smoking can be very difficult. In fact, most people fail in their first attempt. If you don't succeed the first time, don't stop trying.

Develop a stop plan

Becoming smoke-free is a result of planning and commitment, not luck. It helps to develop a stop plan that combines various strategies, or plans of action, for:

Coping With a Lapse

A lapse usually occurs when an ex-smoker is placed in a situation in which he or she would have smoked in the past but currently lacks a plan to cope without a cigarette or is unable to resist when someone offers one.

Lapses happen. It may be one puff or it may be days of smoking. The thing to remember is a lapse doesn't mean failure. And it doesn't mean you should stop trying to quit. Millions of ex-smokers experienced lapses before they were finally able to maintain a smoke-free lifestyle.

Here are some tips for how to get back on track so that a lapse doesn't become a return to regular smoking:

Stop what you're doing
Stop smoking and throw away all of your cigarettes, lighters and ashtrays. Take a break or go for a walk and give yourself time to think. Call a friend or professional to help you get back on track.

Assess and learn
If you're kicking yourself for having a cigarette, stop. Take this opportunity to catch your breath, assess what happened and make a new plan. By looking at what happened, you can learn about the risks you faced and modify your approach to quitting.

Get back on track
Return to being smoke-free. Review your stop-smoking plan and figure out where you can strengthen and improve.

If your lapse occurred over several days, you may want to use nicotine replacement products to manage renewed signs of withdrawal. Follow your original plan regarding how much and how often to use this medication. If you have questions, consult your doctor.

- Coping with symptoms of nicotine withdrawal
- Surviving urges to smoke
- Gaining social support and guidance, when necessary

Don't expect to find a ready-made stop plan that you simply adopt as your own. No one plan works for everybody. Build a stop plan you feel comfortable with and that fits your lifestyle. Choose various techniques and tools that you feel suit your needs. These become your strategies to stop smoking.

Generally, stop plans combine several strategies. Studies show that using more than one strategy increases your chance of becoming smoke-free. Experiment with and adapt strategies to achieve a combination that you feel comfortable with.

For the first week, keep it simple and be flexible. If you're using your stop plan but feel something isn't working, revise your plan.

You may experience physical withdrawal symptoms for up to 10 days. When these symptoms begin to lessen, you may still have an impulse to smoke at those times you usually would light up, such as after a meal or when getting behind the wheel of your car.

For some ex-smokers, periodic urges to smoke may come and go for months to years. However, the intensity and duration of these urges invariably grow smaller with the passage of time.

Stop strategies

Your doctor is a valuable resource as you work to become smoke-free. Following are some important strategies to help you quit smoking.

Self-help

The self-help method involves working on your own to quit smoking. You may want to use health resources to plan and maintain your efforts, which may include publications and internet sites sponsored by national health organizations such as the American Cancer Society or the American Lung Association. The knowledge you gain can help you handle cravings and avoid high-risk situations to smoke. In addition, there are several apps you can download to your phone or other mobile device to help you monitor your progress and offer advice.

Medication

Medication helps ease the withdrawal symptoms of nicotine addiction until the worst effects are over. It also allows you to focus on other concerns, such as changing behaviors that lead to smoking. Remember, though, that any medication you decide to use is only an aid. You still need to be psychologically ready to quit. You

Medications to Help You Quit

Many treatments, including nicotine replacement therapy and non-nicotine medications, have been approved as safe and effective in treating nicotine dependence. The best time to start using nicotine replacement medication is on the date you've set to stop smoking. Using more than one medication may help you get better results.

Here are some of the nicotine replacement and non-nicotine options currently available:

Nicotine replacement therapy

Nicotine replacement therapy gives you nicotine without tobacco and the harmful chemicals in tobacco smoke. Nicotine replacement products help relieve withdrawal symptoms and cravings.

The following nicotine replacement products are available over-the-counter:

- **Nicotine patch (NicoDerm CQ, Habitrol, others).** The patch delivers nicotine through your skin and into your bloodstream. You wear a new patch each day. You typically use the patch for eight weeks or longer. If you haven't been able to stop smoking completely after two weeks of wearing the patch, ask your doctor about adjusting the dose or adding another nicotine replacement product. Common side effects include skin irritation, insomnia and vivid dreams.
- **Nicotine gum (Nicorette, others).** This gum delivers nicotine to your blood through the lining of your mouth. Nicotine gum is often recommended to curb cravings. Chew the gum for a few times until you feel a mild tingling or peppery taste, then park the gum between your cheek and gumline for several minutes. This chewing and parking allows nicotine to be gradually absorbed in your bloodstream. Mouth irritation is a common side effect. Other side effects are often a result of overly vigorous chewing that releases nicotine too quickly. These include heartburn, nausea and hiccups.
- **Nicotine lozenge (Commit, Nicorette mini lozenge, others).** This lozenge dissolves in your mouth and, like nicotine gum, delivers nicotine through the lining of your mouth. Place the lozenge in your mouth between your gumline and cheek or under your tongue and allow it to dissolve. You'll start with one lozenge every one to two hours and gradually increase the time between lozenges. Avoid drinking anything right before or right after the lozenge.

and your doctor can decide which medication is right for you.

Two basic types of medication are used: non-nicotine medications designed to reduce nicotine cravings and nicotine replacement products. Nicotine replacement products deliver nicotine to your brain via the bloodstream without smoking. As your nicotine dependence weakens, you gradually decrease the use of the medications (see "Medications to Help You Quit").

Counseling, support groups and other programs

Combining medications with behavioral counseling provides the best chance for establishing long-term smoking abstinence.

Medications help you cope by reducing withdrawal symptoms including tobacco craving, while behavioral treatments help you develop the skills you need to avoid tobacco over the long run. The more time you spend with a counselor, the better your treatment results will be.

Several types of counseling and support can help with stopping smoking:

- **Telephone counseling.** No matter where you live, you can take advantage of phone counseling to help you give up tobacco. Every state in the U.S. has a telephone quit line, and some have more than one. To find the options in your state, call 800-QUIT-NOW (800-784-8669).
- **Individual or group counseling program.** Your doctor may recommend local support groups or a treatment program where counseling is provided by a tobacco treatment specialist. Counseling helps you learn techniques for preparing to stop smoking and provides support for you during the process.

Many hospitals, health care plans, health care providers and employers offer treatment programs or have tobacco treatment specialists who are certified to provide treatment for nicotine dependence. Nicotine Anonymous groups are available in many locations to provide support for smokers trying to quit. Some medical centers provide residential treatment programs — the most intensive treatment available.

- **Internet-based programs.** Several websites offer support and strategies for people who want to stop smoking. BecomeAnEX is free and provides information and techniques as well as blogs, community forums, ask the expert and many other features. Text messaging services, including personalized reminders about a quit-smoking plan, also may prove helpful.

Side effects include mouth irritation as well as nicotine-related effects such as heartburn, nausea and hiccups.

These nicotine replacement products are available by prescription:

- **Nicotine nasal spray (Nicotrol NS).** The nicotine in this product, sprayed directly into each nostril, is absorbed through your nasal membranes into your blood vessels. The nasal spray delivers nicotine a bit quicker than gum, lozenges or the patch, but not as rapidly as smoking a cigarette. It's usually prescribed for three-month periods for up to six months. Nasal and throat irritation, runny nose, sneezing and coughing are common side effects.
- **Nicotine inhaler (Nicotrol).** This device is shaped something like a cigarette holder. You puff on it, and it delivers nicotine vapor into your mouth. You absorb the nicotine through the lining in your mouth, where it then enters your bloodstream. Common side effects are mouth and throat irritation and occasional coughing.

Non-nicotine medications

Medications that don't contain nicotine and are available by prescription include:

- **Bupropion (Zyban).** The antidepressant drug bupropion increases levels of dopamine and norepinephrine, brain chemicals that are also boosted by nicotine. Typically your doctor will advise you to start bupropion one week before you stop smoking. Bupropion has the advantage of helping to minimize weight gain after you quit smoking. Common side effects include insomnia, agitation, headache and dry mouth. If you have a history of seizures or serious head trauma, such as a skull fracture, you shouldn't take this drug.
- **Varenicline (Chantix).** This medication acts on the brain's nicotine receptors, decreasing withdrawal symptoms and reducing the feelings of pleasure you get from smoking. Typically your doctor will advise you to start varenicline one week before you stop smoking. Common side effects include nausea, headache, insomnia and vivid dreams. Rarely, varenicline has been associated with serious psychiatric symptoms, such as depressed mood and suicidal thoughts.
- **Nortriptyline (Pamelor).** This medication may be prescribed if other medications haven't helped. This tricyclic antidepressant acts by increasing the levels of the brain neurotransmitter norepinephrine. Common side effects may include dry mouth, drowsiness, dizziness and constipation.

What to expect when you stop

Immediately after quitting, you may feel more hungry, tired and short-tempered than usual. You may have strong cravings for a cigarette and find it difficult to concentrate and maintain your focus. You may also have trouble sleeping and experience a temporary increase in coughing.

Nicotine withdrawal symptoms are the result of your body's clearing itself of the nicotine. Most of the nicotine will be gone within three days, but your body's desire for it may continue much longer.

Increased hunger and improvement in your senses of taste and smell may indirectly result in modest weight gain. Quitting doesn't mean that you'll automatically gain weight, however. Some people lose weight after quitting smoking.

Here are some tips to guard against a major weight gain:

- Drink a glass of water before every meal.
- Eat more slowly so that you don't have second helpings.
- Leave the table as soon as you're finished eating.
- If you miss having something in your mouth, chew sugarless gum or snack on foods such as carrots, pickles or celery.
- Find things to keep your hands busy that don't involve food. Try gardening or another hobby.
- Do other things when the urge to eat strikes.
- Exercise daily. This is one of the most important practices you can adopt. Exercise stimulates your body's endorphin and dopamine levels, creating a stimulation similar to that of nicotine.

These suggestions are by no means complete, nor are they suitable for everyone. Find out what works for you. Also see Chapter 8 on "Nutrition and Weight."

When you get tense, find ways to relax. Take a walk or a shower, or soak in the bathtub. Breathe deeply and slowly, as if you're inhaling a cigarette. Repeat this several times.

The benefits of quitting

Within a few days of quitting smoking, you'll begin to notice some changes in your body. Your senses of smell and taste may improve. You may notice an improvement in your stamina. You may breathe easier, and your smoker's cough will begin to disappear, although you may experience increased cough and sputum production for a while as the hair-like structures (cilia) lining your airways attempt to expel tobacco tars and chemicals from your lungs.

Even more lasting and important benefits of quitting smoking begin almost immediately. Within 12 to 24 hours, the levels of carbon monoxide and nicotine in your system will decrease significantly. The effects of smoking on bronchitis will begin to reverse from the very first day you quit. Although the effects of emphysema are irreversible, breathing is made easier, and progression of the disease is slowed.

By the end of your first nonsmoking year, your risk of a heart attack will decrease by half, and by five years it'll be almost the same as that of individuals who have never smoked. Quitting smoking decreases your chances of esophageal or pancreatic cancer. Within seven years, your risk of bladder cancer will drop to that of a nonsmoker. And after 10 to 15 years of not smoking, your statistical risk of getting cancer of the lung, larynx or mouth will approach that of people who've never smoked.

Just as importantly, by stopping smoking you've taken control of a very important part of your life. You'll feel better about yourself. In addition, those around you will benefit from not inhaling smoke from your cigarettes. And you'll set the right example for your children and grandchildren.

Alcohol Use Disorder

Many people who choose to drink alcohol are able to limit their consumption to amounts that cause no harmful health or social consequences. Millions of others, though, drink alcohol excessively and suffer adverse consequences.

According to the 2015 National Survey on Drug Use and Health, more than 15 million U.S. adults ages 18 and older have alcohol use disorder. The disorder also affects more than 600,000 adolescents ages 12 to 17.

Problem drinking, once referred to as alcohol abuse or alcoholism, is now known as alcohol use disorder, or AUD. Alcohol use disorder causes major social, economic and public health problems. In the United States alone, the cost of excessive alcohol consumption is estimated at $233 billion annually. This number includes lost productivity expenses, health care expenses, criminal justice expenses and motor vehicle crash expenses.

It's important to keep in mind that alcohol use disorder is a disease. It's also a leading killer in the United States. If traffic fatalities and death certificate diagnoses related to alcohol use were included in disease-related statistics, alcohol use disorder would be recognized as the nation's No. 1 killer.

Controversy persists over what levels of drinking are problematic or unhealthful. The importance of distinguishing between mild alcohol use disorder and more severe disease is chiefly related to treatment approaches.

What is alcohol use disorder?

Alcohol use disorder is a pattern of alcohol use with a spectrum of severity that includes problems controlling your drinking, being preoccupied with alcohol, continuing to use alcohol even when it causes problems, having to drink more to get the same effect, or having withdrawal symptoms when you rapidly decrease or stop drinking.

Unhealthy alcohol use includes consumption that puts your health or safety at risk or causes other alcohol-related problems. It also includes binge drinking — a pattern of drinking in which a male consumes five or more drinks within two hours or a female consumes at least four drinks within two hours.

People who misuse alcohol continue its use despite knowing that their consumption is causing problems — physical, psychological or social — to themselves and their family and friends.

Alcohol use disorder isn't limited to adults. Teenagers can develop drinking problems in just months. Alcohol consumption among high school students appears to be decreasing, but misuse is still a significant issue.

What is alcoholism?

Alcoholism is a moderate to severe form of alcohol use disorder. It's a chronic, progressive and sometimes fatal disease that involves a preoccupation with alcohol and impaired control over its use.

A person experiencing alcoholism continues to misuse alcohol despite serious adverse health, personal, work-related and financial consequences. Genetic, psychological and social factors all contribute to alcoholism.

Signs and symptoms
Signs and symptoms of more-severe alcohol use disorder include:
- Being unable to limit the amount of alcohol you drink
- Wanting to cut down on how much you drink or making unsuccessful attempts to do so
- Spending a lot of time drinking, getting alcohol or recovering from alcohol use
- Feeling a strong craving or urge to drink alcohol

- Failing to fulfill major obligations at work, school or home due to repeated alcohol use
- Continuing to drink alcohol even though you know it's causing physical, social or interpersonal problems
- Giving up or reducing social and work activities and hobbies
- Using alcohol in situations where it's not safe, such as when driving or swimming
- Developing a tolerance to alcohol so you need more to feel its effect or you have a reduced effect from the same amount
- Experiencing withdrawal symptoms — such as nausea, sweating and shaking — when you don't drink, or drinking to avoid these symptoms

Causes
Genetic, psychological, social and environmental factors can impact how drinking alcohol affects your body and behavior. Theories suggest that for certain people drinking has a different and stronger impact that can lead to alcohol use disorder.

In addition, social and cultural factors can contribute to the addiction process. The glamorous way that the advertising industry and the entertainment media portray alcohol use sends messages that it's OK to drink excessively.

Over time, drinking too much alcohol may change the normal function of the areas of your brain associated with the experience of pleasure, judgment and the ability to exercise control over your behavior. This may result in craving alcohol to try to restore good feelings or reduce negative ones.

Alcohol Myths

There has never been a shortage of myths about alcoholism.

Myth: *Older adults don't become alcoholics.*
Fact: More free time, social events and life losses can lead to increased drinking and problem drinking in older adults.

Myth: *A drink can warm you up.*
Fact: Alcohol dilates your blood vessels and may give you a sensation of warmth, but only temporarily. Increased heat loss through your skin actually decreases your body temperature when you drink alcohol. Consequently, the risk of serious, even fatal, low body temperature (hypothermia) is increased if you drink alcohol in a cold environment.

Myth: *When drunk, you reveal your true personality.*
Fact: Alcohol may permit traits to surface that you suppress when sober, and excessive drinking can distort your personality. But your true personality is revealed when you're sober.

Myth: *Strong black coffee can help you sober up.*
Fact: Coffee neither increases the rate at which your liver processes alcohol nor changes your blood alcohol levels. The initial lift that coffee provides may lead you to believe that you're reasonably alert and sober when, in fact, you're not.

Risk factors

Continued alcohol use over time can produce a physical dependence on alcohol. However, drinking by itself is just one of the risk factors that contribute to alcohol use disorder. Others include:

- **Age.** People who begin drinking at an early age — in their teens or earlier — are at a higher risk of alcohol use disorder.
- **Family history.** The risk of alcohol use disorder is higher for people who have a parent or other close relative who has problems with alcohol. This may be influenced by genetic factors.
- **Mental health disorders.** It's common for people with a mental health disorder such as anxiety, depression, schizophrenia or bipolar disorder to have problems with alcohol or other substances.
- **Social and cultural factors.** Having a partner or close friends who drink regularly could increase your risk of alcohol use disorder. For young people, the influence of parents, peers and other role models can impact risk.

How alcohol affects your body

Alcohols are a group of compounds, many of which are ingredients in perfumes, extracts, tinctures, paints and other products. Alcohols are essential to many manufacturing processes.

The form of alcohol in the beverage you drink is ethyl alcohol (ethanol), a colorless liquid that in its pure, undiluted form has a biting or burning taste. It's produced by the fermentation of sugars that occur naturally in grains, such as barley, and in fruits, such as grapes.

When you drink alcohol, it depresses your central nervous system by acting as a sedative or tranquilizer. In some people, the initial reaction may be stimulation, but as drinking continues, sedative effects occur. By depressing the controlling centers of your brain, alcohol relaxes you and reduces your inhibitions. The more you drink, the more sedated you become.

Initially, alcohol affects areas of thought, emotion and judgment. Eventually, alcohol can impair your speech and muscle coordination and produce sleep. Taken in large enough quantities, alcohol can be lethal. It can cause a life-threatening coma by severely depressing vital centers of your brain.

The principal site for alcohol absorption is your small intestine, although very small amounts are absorbed in your mouth and esophagus and only slightly more is absorbed in your stomach. The rate at which the alcohol is absorbed depends on whether you've recently eaten. If your stomach is empty, alcohol is usually quickly absorbed. Food in your stomach or small intestines, especially solid and fatty foods, slows the emptying of your stomach and the absorption of the alcohol into your bloodstream.

Once alcohol has been absorbed, it's quickly transported throughout your body to wherever there's water, including inside individual cells. This distribution accounts for the intoxicating effects of alcohol. Taking a drink on a full stomach spreads the metabolism of that drink over a longer period of time and results in a lower concentration of alcohol in your blood.

Nearly all of the alcohol is burned as fuel for your body, although small amounts are lost in your urine and from the lungs. It's the alcohol in the air you exhale that's measured in breath tests to determine the amount of alcohol in your body. The level of alcohol in your exhalations closely reflects the concentration of alcohol in your blood.

Alcohol dilates the blood vessels nearest your skin to produce an initial feeling of warmth, although this is only temporary. Your pulse rate increases, and you produce more urine because of increased fluid intake and the action of the alcohol on your kidneys. Alcohol also stimulates your stomach to secrete acid.

Your body uses alcohol just as it uses other food, metabolizing it in the liver to produce heat and energy. The food value of alcohol is limited because it provides no vitamins, minerals or proteins. People with severe alcohol use disorder often have deficiencies in nutrients. Doctors once thought that liver damage common among people who misuse alcohol, such as fatty liver and cirrhosis, was related to the effect of alcohol on nutritional status. Today, it's known that the toxic effect of alcohol can harm the liver directly.

Alcohol intoxication

How much food you've eaten and how recently you've eaten aren't the only factors that affect how you respond to alcohol. Your sex, age, size and body fat also play important roles. Drinking equal amounts of alcohol may have a greater effect on a woman than on a man. Women generally are smaller and have a higher percentage of body fat than do men. They may also metabolize alcohol less efficiently than do men. Older adults also are more susceptible to the effects of alcohol than are younger people.

The intoxicating effects of alcohol relate to the concentration of alcohol, which in turn reflects levels present in your blood and brain. Most states define legal intoxication as a blood alcohol concentration of at least 0.08 or 0.10 percent. Even at concentrations much lower than the legal limit, many people lose some coordination and reaction time.

Health effects of excessive alcohol use

Drinking excessive amounts of alcohol produces several harmful effects on your brain and nervous system. Excessive use of alcohol can also damage your liver, pancreas and cardiovascular system and cause other illnesses.

Brain and nervous system disorders

People who misuse alcohol, as well as occasional or first-time drinkers, may forget all or part of what occurred during the time they were drinking. This temporary loss of memory is referred to as a blackout. Some excessive drinkers have problems with short-term memory that may persist for several weeks after they have stopped drinking.

Excessive alcohol use can leave you exhausted in the morning, even after a full night's sleep. This morning fatigue is caused by the sedating effect of alcohol that interferes with your brain's ability to produce an adequate amount of deep, dreaming sleep, called rapid eye movement (REM) sleep.

Individuals who are deficient in nutrients, particularly thiamin, may be affected by a neurological disorder called Wernicke-Korsakoff syndrome. This condition consists of two separate disorders — Wernicke's syndrome and Korsakoff's syndrome. They often occur together in people who misuse alcohol.

The first symptom of Wernicke's syndrome is often weakness and paralysis of your eye muscles, which may result in double vision. Later on you may not be able to stand or walk without help. Korsakoff's syndrome involves severe amnesia, particularly loss of recent memory. If you have both syndromes, you may experience episodes in which you forget your identity, become disoriented and have hallucinations.

Gastrointestinal disorders

Alcohol can irritate the mucous lining of your stomach and produce gastritis. This also may cause severe retching and vomiting that can tear the upper part of your stomach and the lower part of your esophagus. These tears, called Mallory-Weiss tears, can bleed.

Persistent drinking can interfere with the absorption of the B vitamins, particularly folate and thiamin, as well as other nutrients. Most of these problems will improve if you stop drinking.

Other alcohol-induced problems, such as liver damage, hepatitis and dilated veins of the esophagus (esophageal varices), may require immediate medical attention. Damage caused by alcohol-induced cirrhosis of the liver tends to be progressive. When alcohol reaches your liver, enzymes metabolize it. A healthy liver can process alcohol at a rate of about 50 calories an hour. This is equivalent to about 1 ounce of 40 percent alcohol in about an hour. If your liver becomes overwhelmed by larger amounts of alcohol, the alcohol will remain in your blood until your liver can process it. In people with alcohol use disorder, acute and chronic inflammation of the pancreas (pancreatitis) may develop.

Cardiovascular system disorders

A drink of alcohol temporarily reduces blood pressure. But if you consume alcohol excessively, it can increase your blood pressure. Similarly, although some reports indicate that moderate daily drinking may prevent one type of heart trouble, the harmful effects of excessive use of alcohol clearly outweigh any potential benefits.

One or two alcoholic drinks a day, or up to 1 ounce of ethyl alcohol, may reduce your risk of coronary artery disease. This protective effect may be due, in part, to changes in blood fats. People who regularly consume alcohol have increased levels of high-density lipoprotein (HDL) cholesterol. This "good" cholesterol may inhibit narrowing of the arteries (atherosclerosis).

However, a condition called alcoholic cardiomyopathy can develop in people who use alcohol excessively. This disease injures and destroys the heart muscle and

Are You at Risk?

Some disorders have manifestations that make a diagnosis easy. Alcohol use disorder, however, often defies easy classification because its characteristics vary greatly from one person who misuses alcohol to the next.

To cope with this difficulty, Mayo Clinic developed the Self-Administered Alcoholism Screening Test (SAAST). Based in part on the Michigan Alcohol Screening Test, the SAAST consists of 37 questions. In use since 1972, the test can identify 95 percent of individuals ill enough to be hospitalized.

The test aims to identify behavior patterns, medical signs and symptoms, and consequences associated with misuse of alcohol. Here's a sample of questions:

1. Do you have a drink now and then?
2. Do you feel you're a normal drinker (that is, you drink no more than average)?
3. Have you ever awakened the morning after drinking the previous evening and found that you couldn't remember a part of the previous evening?
4. Do close relatives ever worry or complain about your drinking?
5. Can you stop drinking without a struggle after one or two drinks?
6. Do you ever feel guilty about your drinking?
7. Do friends or relatives think you're a normal drinker?
8. Are you always able to stop drinking when you want to?
9. Have you ever attended a meeting of Alcoholics Anonymous (A.A.) because of your drinking?
10. Have you gotten into physical fights when drinking?

If your responses match four or more of those listed below, you may be at risk of alcoholism:
1. yes 2. no 3. yes 4. yes 5. no 6. yes 7. no 8. no 9. yes 10. yes

produces signs and symptoms that range from an irregular heartbeat (arrhythmia) to heart failure.

Sexual disorders

Alcohol misuse can cause erectile dysfunction (impotence) in men. In women, it can disrupt menstruation.

Cancer

Individuals who drink excessive amounts of alcohol have a higher rate of cancer than that of the general population, especially cancer of the voice box (larynx), esophagus, stomach and pancreas.

Diabetes complications

Alcohol prevents the release of sugar (glucose) from your liver and increases the risk of low blood sugar (hypoglycemia). This is dangerous if you have diabetes and are taking insulin to control your blood sugar level.

Recognizing alcohol use disorder

How can you tell if you, a friend or a family member is having a problem with alcohol? Alcohol use disorder knows no social or economic bounds. Many people who misuse alcohol are highly regarded and pass for years among friends and associates as healthy and normally functioning people. Alcohol use disorder strikes young and old, men and women, rich and poor, and people of all races.

The American Medical Association has recognized alcoholism as an illness for more than 50 years, yet many people still believe that a person who misuses alcohol is someone who has disgraced himself or herself because of personal weakness.

Because of a lingering social stigma, many people who misuse alcohol see themselves as weak and bad people. Some may rationalize the problems that are brought on by their illness, such as a broken marriage or a lost job, as the consequence of bad luck or something

caused by others. This burden of shame and blame is one of the greatest stumbling blocks to seeking help and achieving recovery.

Alcohol use disorder is a treatable disease. A step toward recognizing if you or someone you know may have a drinking problem is to evaluate the drinking patterns. Indications of alcohol misuse include:

Denial

Believing that your problems are caused by factors other than drinking, even when the consequences of drinking behaviors are clearly evident, is a sign of alcoholism. Rather than admitting the problem, an alcoholic often becomes defensive, gets angry, blames others and continues to drink without seeking help.

Increased tolerance

Tolerance to the effects of alcohol is an early sign of alcohol dependence. The need to drink more than the usual amount of alcohol to feel its effects is evidence of increased tolerance. Alcoholics may appear sober even after consuming more alcohol than would intoxicate moderate drinkers.

But beware. No matter how much tolerance you seem to develop, your liver is still unable to metabolize pure alcohol at a rate faster than approximately 1 ounce of 40 percent liquor an hour. Using tolerance as a measure of how much to drink is unsafe.

Withdrawals and delirium tremens

If your body is dependent on alcohol and you suddenly stop drinking, you're likely to experience physical and psychological withdrawal symptoms. Signs and symptoms include:
- Hand tremors
- An increase in pulse, blood pressure and body temperature
- Nausea, diarrhea and other gastrointestinal discomfort
- Insomnia

These signs or symptoms often last three to seven days, although some may last for weeks. With delirium tremens (DTs), more-dangerous withdrawal signs and symptoms can occur:
- Delirium
- Confusion
- Aggression
- Vivid hallucinations
- Severe tremors
- Paranoid ideas
- Seizures

These signs and symptoms often last three to five days, sometimes longer, and usually require urgent medical evaluation and treatment in a hospital setting.

Your doctor can help you deal with withdrawal symptoms. For some individuals who want to stop drinking, a hospital-based detoxification program can be helpful and may be necessary.

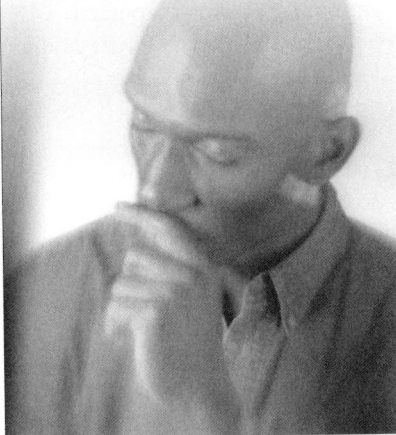

Treating alcohol use disorder

Most people with alcohol problems who enter treatment do so reluctantly, usually under pressure from their family, employers or friends. In some cases, health or legal problems motivate them to seek help. Such pressure to seek treatment is often necessary because many people who have a drinking problem use denial, enabling them to believe they don't need help.

Acknowledging the problem
People who misuse alcohol often build a protective shell by developing strategies, both conscious and unconscious, to avoid being confronted. Denial may be so profound that an individual may genuinely not recognize the extent of his or her problem. One of the first goals of treatment is to penetrate personal defenses that have developed over the years.

Blaming the person with an alcohol problem for the illness only feeds that person's feeling that no one understands him or her. It's important to understand that a person who misuses alcohol is someone who has been made ill by a disease.

Motivational enhancement
Motivational enhancement approaches address the concerns of the individual with an alcohol problem in a nonconfrontational manner. A friend, family member or medical professional works with the individual to find ways to make the changes the person seeks. This approach may include goal setting, behavior change techniques, use of self-help manuals and counseling.

Intervention
The pre-treatment phase is crucial for family members, friends, employers and other people concerned about someone who has a drinking problem. Chances of recovery increase if the person who has a drinking problem can be confronted with the seriousness of the negative consequences of his or her drinking.

There are different ways to approach intervention. Seeking the help of a professional knowledgeable about alcoholism and alcohol misuse can result in sparing family members, including the person with a drinking problem, years of suffering and destruction of relationships. An employer or respected authority figure also may be appropriate. Sometimes, the best person to intervene is someone recovering from the disease.

There's no ideal time or place for a confrontation. However, don't confront an individual with an alcohol problem when the person is drunk or drinking. Pick a time when he or she is sober or in the process of getting sober.

In a kind but candid way, share facts and feelings, neither of which the individual can deny. Facts about the person's drinking may include DUIs, marital conflicts or problems at work. An example of shared feelings may include a statement such as, "I was sad when you missed my birthday party because you were intoxicated."

Don't try to bail the person out of trouble or offer another chance. An escape from the consequences of drinking is usually interpreted as permission to drink again.

Addressing the needs of family members
Drinking problems usually impair family and workplace relationships. If a family is unaware of the true nature of alcohol misuse and the need for treatment for someone who has a drinking problem, it continues to become increasingly distraught and traumatized.

Families may experience psychological, marital, parental, economic, physical and spiritual problems as the disease of alcoholism progresses. By directing their

Alcoholics Anonymous and Al-Anon

The Fellowship of Alcoholics Anonymous was formed in 1935. As a self-help group, Alcoholics Anonymous (A.A.) offers a sober peer group as an effective model of how you can achieve total abstinence.

The A.A. program is built around the Twelve Steps, which are straightforward suggestions for men and women who choose to lead sober lives. The Twelve Steps aren't requirements for membership but rather are guides for people who choose to live their lives sober. As guides to recovery, the Twelve Steps help individuals who misuse alcohol accept their powerlessness over alcohol. They also stress the necessity for honesty about the past and present.

Recovery in A.A. is based on accepting the unique experience of each person. Through listening and sharing stories, members learn that they're not alone. There are no fees for membership, only a willingness to remain sober.

In the mid-1950s, family members of individuals who misuse alcohol formed a complementary self-help group called Al-Anon. This group is designed for people who are affected by someone else's alcoholism. In sharing their stories, Al-Anon members gain a greater understanding of how the disease affects the entire family. Al-Anon also accepts the Twelve Steps of A.A. as the principles by which participants are to conduct their lives. It emphasizes how members need to learn detachment and forgiveness if they too are to be free of the disease.

In many communities, Alateen groups are available to provide support for teenage children of individuals who misuse alcohol.

Pregnancy and Alcohol Use

Some women believe that small amounts of alcohol don't hurt their unborn child. The truth is, there's no amount of alcohol that's safe to consume during pregnancy. If you drink alcohol during pregnancy, you place your baby at risk of fetal alcohol syndrome.

Fetal alcohol syndrome is a condition that results from alcohol exposure during the mother's pregnancy. The Centers for Disease Control and Prevention estimates that for every 1,000 births .2 to 1.5 infants are born with fetal alcohol syndrome. Some studies suggest the prevalence of the condition is higher. Fetal alcohol syndrome causes brain damage and growth problems that are irreversible.

The more you drink while pregnant, the greater the risk to your unborn baby. However, any amount of alcohol puts your baby at risk. The severity of fetal alcohol syndrome symptoms varies, with some children experiencing problems to a far greater degree than others. Signs and symptoms of fetal alcohol syndrome may include any mix of physical defects, intellectual or cognitive disabilities, and problems functioning and coping with daily life. These consequences are collectively called fetal alcohol spectrum disorders.

Physical defects may include:
- Distinctive facial features, including small eyes, an exceptionally thin upper lip, a short, upturned nose, and a smooth skin surface between the nose and upper lip
- Deformities of joints, limbs and fingers
- Slow physical growth before and after birth
- Vision difficulties or hearing problems
- Small head circumference and brain size
- Heart defects and problems with kidneys and bones
- Brain and central nervous system problems

Problems with the brain and central nervous system may include:
- Poor coordination or balance
- Intellectual disability, learning disorders and delayed development
- Trouble with attention and with processing information
- Difficulty with reasoning and problem-solving
- Difficulty identifying consequences of choices
- Poor judgment skills
- Jitteriness or hyperactivity
- Rapidly changing moods

Problems functioning, coping and interacting with others may include:
- Difficulty in school
- Trouble getting along with others
- Poor social skills
- Trouble adapting to change or switching from one task to another
- Problems with behavior and impulse control
- Problems staying on task
- Difficulty planning or working toward a goal

There's no cure or specific treatment for fetal alcohol syndrome. The physical defects and mental deficiencies typically persist for a lifetime. However, early intervention services may help reduce some of the effects of fetal alcohol syndrome and may prevent some secondary disabilities.

attention toward the individual with the alcohol problem, families may neglect these other issues. Families commonly use denial to cope as readily as the person who has the drinking problem. It often becomes the family's major defense mechanism in attempting to deal with the unending series of crises that present themselves.

Family members often respond to the havoc in their lives with anger, sarcasm, emotional outbursts or depression. Although blame is understandable, it's counterproductive in dealing with alcohol use disorder. With professional guidance, family members can learn how to avoid enabling and rescuing the alcoholic. Instead, they need to react constructively and establish a climate for positive responses.

Countless problem drinkers are recovering today simply because their families chose to start the process of recovery, often by entering treatment programs for family members, such as Al-Anon (see page 321).

Treatment programs

A wide range of treatments is available to help with alcohol problems. Treatment is tailored to the individual and may involve evaluation, brief intervention, counseling, an outpatient program, a residential program or an inpatient program.

The first step in treatment is to determine whether you have an alcohol use disorder. If you haven't lost control over your use of alcohol, your treatment may involve reducing your drinking. If you're dependent on alcohol, cutting back is ineffective and inappropriate. Abstinence must be a part of your treatment goal.

Mild alcohol use disorder
For people who aren't physically dependent on alcohol but still experience the adverse effects of drinking, the goal of treatment is

the prevention of more-serious disease through a screening procedure or brief interventions.

Screening

Two major types of screening are used. One is designed for people who seek medical care for problems unrelated to alcohol use or those who participate in random alcohol testing programs. It's also used for drivers who are stopped at random to test of their breath for the presence of alcohol.

The other type of screening program involves people who've been identified as possibly having a drinking problem. Hospital-based programs screen people admitted for traumatic injuries. Court-mandated programs screen adolescents or adults arrested for violent crimes or drivers who have positive results on a breath or blood alcohol test. Employee assistance programs screen employees with impaired performance.

Brief interventions

Brief interventions usually involve specialists who establish a specific treatment plan with an individual identified as having an alcohol problem. These interventions may include many components:
- Direct feedback
- Contracting and goal setting
- Behavior modification
- Use of written material such as self-help manuals
- Counseling
- Follow-up care extending over multiple visits to a treatment center

Moderate to severe alcohol use disorder (alcoholism)

Treatment for alcoholism typically takes place in an outpatient setting with services for all stages of recovery. However, residential or inpatient care is still the most appropriate treatment if you have other serious medical or psychiatric problems or if you're living in an environment that won't support your recovery.

The most common residential alcoholism treatment programs in the United States are based on an approach that includes abstinence, individual and group therapy, participation in Alcoholics Anonymous (A.A.), educational lectures, activity therapy, and use of recovering lay counselors and multiprofessional staff. Many outpatient services include these same components.

Here's what you might expect from a typical treatment program:

Detoxification and withdrawal

If you arrive at the facility intoxicated or are a heavy, chronic drinker, treatment may begin with a program of detoxification that may take three to seven days. You may be given medications to prevent delirium tremens (DTs) or other withdrawal symptoms. Then you enter either a residential treatment program or outpatient treatment program, depending on your needs.

Acceptance of the illness

Effective treatment is impossible unless you accept that you have a problem with alcohol. This is one of the most important steps to recovery.

Medical assessment and treatment

Medical problems often associated with alcoholism are high blood pressure, diabetes, and liver and heart disease. A doctor may review your health status and take steps to treat any complications.

Abstinence

Most treatment programs for alcoholism require abstinence from alcohol and drugs.

Recovery

Education about alcoholism, the damage it does to the body, the problems it causes and the experience of recovery is a critical part of treatment. During this phase, most programs include daily classes, group therapy, individual coun-

seling, recreational therapy and an introduction to the principles of A.A. or other self-help organizations. Psychological support and additional medical care also may be provided, if needed.

Some of the trained staff involved in recovery programs may be recovering from alcohol misuse themselves and able to share their experiences and serve as role models.

Psychological support and psychiatric treatment

A psychologist or psychiatrist may provide an assessment and assist with individual counseling and support. Sometimes, emotional symptoms of alcoholism may mimic mental health disorders, or an alcoholic may have an accompanying psychiatric illness. If you have a mental health disorder, such as significant depression or anxiety, this condition also needs to be treated to facilitate recovery.

Medication

Medications can be used in combination with other therapies to treat alcoholism. Some medications help you to achieve abstinence and increase long-term recovery. Others reduce the desire to drink and the craving for alcohol.
- **Oral medications.** A drug called disulfiram (Antabuse) may help to prevent you from drinking, although it won't cure alcohol use disorder or remove the compulsion to drink. If you drink alcohol, the drug produces a physical reaction that may include flushing, nausea, vomiting and headaches. Naltrexone, a drug that blocks the good feelings alcohol causes, may prevent heavy drinking and reduce the urge to drink. Acamprosate (Campral) may help you combat alcohol cravings once you stop drinking. Unlike disulfiram, naltrexone and acamprosate don't make you feel sick after taking a drink.
- **Injected medication.** Vivitrol, a version of the drug naltrexone,

is injected once a month by a health care professional. Although similar medication can be taken in pill form, the injectable version of the drug may be easier for people recovering from alcohol use disorder to use consistently.

Continuing support
Aftercare programs available through treatment centers, A.A. and other self-help organizations can help recovering from alcohol misuse abstain from alcohol, manage relapses and cope with lifestyle changes.

Substance Use Disorders

Misuse of addicting drugs is an increasing public health issue in this country. Substance use disorder doesn't involve only those substances considered illicit. It occurs if you take any drug inappropriately — for purposes other than for what it's intended or in a manner or quantity other than directed. Nicotine and alcohol, discussed earlier, also are addicting substances.

Most of the millions of people who take prescription medications don't abuse them. However, many misuse them, sometimes out of ignorance and carelessness.

People misuse drugs — prescription or illicit — for various reasons. Mind-altering psychedelics produce effects that alter the way you experience reality. Stimulants such as amphetamines give a temporary sensation of increased energy and lifted spirits. Painkillers (analgesics) reduce the sensation of pain and induce drowsiness. And sedative drugs create a feeling of relaxation. To achieve such effects is a frequent motivation for misuse.

Drugs to which you can become addicted include:

- **Cannabis compounds.** These compounds are found in marijuana and hashish. Cannabis is now legal in some states, and it may be used in many individuals with limited consequences. However, like alcohol, it's also addictive and can cause health, psychological and social consequences.
- **Hallucinogens.** These include lysergic acid diethylamide (LSD) and phencyclidine (PCP).
- **Designer drugs.** Designer drugs include synthetic compounds such as Ecstasy, which has both amphetamine-like and hallucinogenic effects.
- **Opiates and opioids.** These include narcotic painkillers produced naturally from opium or made synthetically. They include heroin and the prescription medications morphine, codeine and methadone.
- **Central nervous system depressants.** These include barbiturates and benzodiazepines. Benzodiazepines include prescription tranquilizers such as diazepam (Valium), alprazolam (Xanax), lorazepam (Ativan), clonazepam (Klonopin) and chlordiazepoxide (Librium).
- **Central nervous system stimulants.** These include amphetamines and cocaine.
- **Inhalants.** Some people become addicted to substances found in glue, paint and solvents.

Medications

Millions of Americans abuse prescription and nonprescription medications, sometimes with tragic results. Hospital emergency departments report that approximately the same percentage of drug emergencies are due to misuse of legal medications as to misuse of illicit drugs. The abuse of prescription drugs is widespread. Many people are able to maintain a dependence on prescription medications by obtaining prescriptions from multiple doctors.

You can misuse over-the-counter drugs as well. Aspirin, cough medicines, laxatives, diet pills, nasal sprays and numerous other medications can be abused if taken in higher doses or more frequently than recommended.

Addiction to tranquilizers
Numerous emergency department visits each year are related to misuse of tranquilizers, and every year thousands of people enter drug treatment centers for the same reason.

Tranquilizers such as diazepam (Valium), alprazolam (Xanax) and lorazepam (Ativan) — all part of a family of drugs named benzodiazepines — are typically prescribed for a limited time to help alleviate nervousness or tension caused by the stress of everyday life or associated with an emotional disorder. Sleeping aids such as flurazepam and temazepam (Restoril) also are part of this family. Problems arise when people use the drugs too long, too often or at too high a dosage.

Another issue related to the abuse of benzodiazepines is the mistaken belief that they're not addicting. When they first became available, many people used them instead of barbiturates, another family of sedatives, which carry a higher risk for overdosage and toxicity. However, benzodiazepines have been found to have strong addictive potential. In fact,

Pregnancy and Drug Abuse

Many drugs pass through the placenta and reach the fetus. The first trimester of pregnancy generally is the stage at which the fetus is most sensitive to drugs in the mother's body.

Many women who smoke marijuana during their pregnancy deliver premature babies or babies who have a low birth weight. Women who use tranquilizers and amphetamines while pregnant may have a baby born with congenital malformations. Taking barbiturates, opiates and cocaine while pregnant may cause fetal addiction.

If you use marijuana when breast-feeding, the drug may pass through your breast milk to your baby.

virtually all of the medications in the benzodiazepine group can cause physical and psychological addiction if used at a high dosage or over a prolonged time.

Addiction to painkillers (opioids)

The ideal painkiller (analgesic) would be one that furnishes sufficient pain relief, produces a minimum of side effects, acts promptly, prevents development of increased tolerance and is non-addicting. Unfortunately, there is no such ideal painkiller.

The strongest painkillers are opiates and opioids. Opiates are narcotic drugs derived from the opium plant. Opioids are synthetic narcotic substances with the same properties. They include the medications oxycodone (OxyContin, Roxicodone) and those containing hydrocodone (Norco, Zohydro ER).

Opioids and opiates (narcotics) generally are prescribed to relieve severe pain. The medications are often are obtained illegally. Given in low doses over short periods, narcotics aren't addictive, but in large doses taken over time, they're highly addictive.

Side effects, especially when taken in high doses, include decreased respiration, a drop in blood pressure, dizziness, nausea, sweating, general weakness and a depressed sex drive.

Oxycodone (OxyContin), a prescription pain reliever, has become a popular street drug with a high market value. Its effects are more intense when the long-acting tablets are chewed.

Opioid abuse has become a serious public health issue. According to the Department of Health and Human Services, it's estimated that more than 12 million Americans misuse prescription opioids, and each year more than 30,000 people die from overdosing on the prescription drugs.

In addition to relieving pain, opioids activate reward regions in the brain causing the euphoria — or high — that underlies their potential for misuse and addiction.

Chemically, these medications are very similar to heroin, which was originally synthesized from morphine as a pharmaceutical in the late 19th century. As a result of the opioid epidemic, there's also been an increase in heroin use. Heroin provides the same physical effects, but it's much cheaper. Approximately 13,000 people die an-

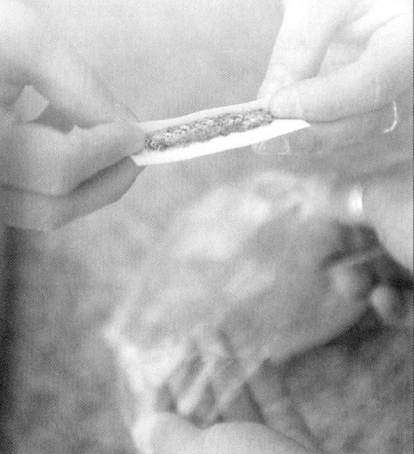

nually from overdosing on heroin, and the numbers are increasing.

Drug overdose, driven largely by the opioid epidemic and its consequences, is now the leading cause of unintentional injury death in the United States.

Illicit drugs

The term *street drugs* is often used to describe illicit drugs because the drugs often are sold on the street. Many people abuse illicit drugs by using them "recreationally" in an attempt to relax, experience euphoria, enhance sexual activity or heighten the senses. Some athletes use street drugs to try to improve their athletic performance.

Whatever their intended use, illicit drugs can be extremely hazardous to your health not only because of their nature but also because of the unknown potency of the drug and risk of contamination with other dangerous substances. Most of these drugs are highly addictive.

Marijuana

Marijuana is still often referred to as an illicit drug, but its use is now legal in some states.

The hemp plant *(Cannabis sativa)*, from which marijuana is derived, contains more than 400 chemicals, including tetrahydrocannabinol (THC). The THC is what causes marijuana's effect on mood and is probably responsible for the hunger that many people experience after using marijuana.

The amount of THC varies from plant to plant and from cigarette to cigarette. Hashish, a more powerful derivative drug prepared from the resin of the hemp plant, contains far greater concentrations of psychoactive THC.

If you smoke marijuana, THC is quickly absorbed from your lungs into your bloodstream and rapidly distributed to most tissues and organs of your body. To eliminate THC, your liver converts the substance into waste products (metabolites). The rate at which

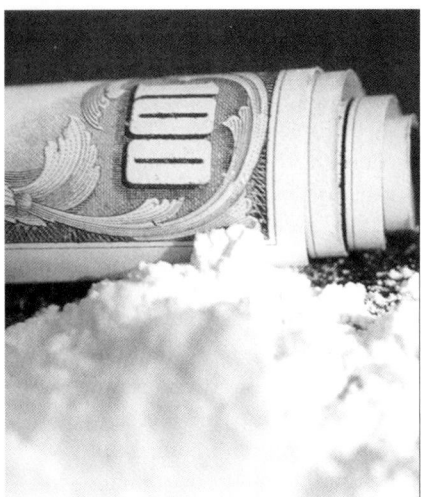

they're cleared from your body is slower than that of many other psychoactive drugs.

The effects of marijuana are almost immediate. Your heart rate increases by as much as 50 percent, depending on the potency of the marijuana. People with a poor blood supply to the heart may have chest pains. High doses of marijuana may produce many of the same behavioral effects as severe alcohol intoxication. Although the high may subside, many of the negative effects may linger for up to six hours after you smoke marijuana. These include difficulty in performing functions that require concentration, rapid reactions and physical coordination.

Chronic marijuana smokers show evidence of decreased lung capacity and chronic bronchial irritation. Because chronic marijuana smoking may impair your body's immune system, your lungs may be more susceptible to aspergillus and other infectious agents. Marijuana may negatively affect your reproductive system, including temporary loss of fertility in both men and women. Some studies have suggested that there may be a significant relationship between use of marijuana during pregnancy and premature birth.

Although often misunderstood and misrepresented to the public, marijuana may lead to addiction. Regular use often results in the same type of misuse described for other substances.

Cocaine and crack

Cocaine was once referred to as the champagne of drugs, in part because it was an expensive drug preferred by the wealthy. Today, it's one of the most widely used illicit drugs in this country. Cocaine is popular with drug users because it leads to a sense of euphoria.

Signs and symptoms of cocaine use include dilation of the pupils, increased heart rate and breathing, and a slight rise in body temperature. These effects are mostly of short duration. They reach their peak about 15 to 20 minutes after you inhale the drug through your nose (snort it) in the form of a powder and last about an hour.

Unwanted effects of cocaine use disorder include a persistent restlessness, anxiety and sleeplessness. Another problem associated with inhaling cocaine is a mildly stuffy or runny nose. Long-term use can cause ulcers on the mucous membranes of your nose and even a hole (perforation) in your nasal septum. In addition, people who chronically abuse cocaine may develop paranoid hallucinations, called cocaine psychosis, which may involve the senses of smell, taste, touch or sight.

Crack's name comes from the sound of burning "rocks" of cocaine. It produces an intense high in a matter of seconds. A profound low may follow, leaving the chronic user desperate for more.

Cocaine can overwork your heart, forcing it to beat too fast and too powerfully. As your heart tires, it becomes susceptible to irregularities in its rhythm that can be life-threatening. Cocaine can also induce coronary artery spasm, a sudden narrowing of the arteries leading to your heart. This can cause a blood clot to form, which could cause a heart attack or sudden death.

Injecting cocaine with shared needles increases the risk of exposure to human immunodeficiency virus (HIV), infectious hepatitis and other diseases.

Hallucinogens

Hallucinogenic drugs were widely used in the 1960s and early 1970s. The popularity of such drugs diminished during the next 20 years, but some observers report a renewed interest in the use of hallucinogens. The most common hallucinogens used today are lysergic acid diethylamide (LSD) and phencyclidine (PCP).

LSD

Hallucinogens were popular because they produced a vivid perception of changes in sensation, depth perception, passage of time and body image. Some users reported experiencing a mixing of the senses. Under the influence of LSD, one could seemingly hear colors or see sounds.

LSD can also cause powerful negative experiences, referred to as bad trips, in which the user has an overwhelming sense of fear, perhaps of being abandoned or dying. In some instances, abusers have had no comprehension of their limitations and have died because they tried to fly out of windows or walk on water.

Another effect of hallucinogenic drugs is the production of sustained altered mental states that can last eight hours or more. Flashbacks also may occur days or weeks after the conclusion of the initial trip, in which the user reexperiences previous effects even though he or she hasn't ingested any more of the drug.

LSD and similar drugs increase heart rate and blood pressure, dilate the pupils, and cause sleeplessness, tremors and loss of appetite. Heavy, long-term use of hallucinogens can cause impaired memory, an abbreviated attention span and difficulty with abstract thinking.

PCP

This powerful hallucinogen, sometimes referred to as angel dust, is less commonly used today. PCP taken in very small doses by humans causes a loss of inhibition and induces a state of general euphoria. Other effects include increased heart rate and breathing, sweating, flushing of the skin, and increased body temperature. It may also cause some unsteadiness.

What makes the drug especially dangerous is its unpredictability. Almost any dose may result in destructive, violent behavior. When users have turned violent or acted in bizarre ways, they've been known to lose all control. PCP has been known to induce a toxic psychosis that resembles schizophrenia.

Club drugs

Club drugs tend to be used by teenagers and young adults at bars, nightclubs, concerts and parties. Club drugs include the drugs GHB, Rohypnol, ketamine and MDMA (Ecstasy).

- GHB (gamma-hydroxybutyrate) is a depressant approved for use in the treatment of narcolepsy, a disorder that causes daytime sleep attacks.
- Rohypnol is a benzodiazepine chemically similar to prescription sedatives such as Valium and Xanax.
- Ketamine is a hallucinogen that causes the user to feel detached from reality.
- MDMA (3,4-methylenedioxymethamphetamine) is a synthetic drug that alters mood and awareness of surrounding objects and conditions. Known as Ecstasy, it's chemically similar to both stimulants and hallucinogens, producing feelings of increased energy, pleasure, emotional warmth, and distorted sensory and time perception.

GHB and Rohypnol are available in odorless, colorless and tasteless forms and may be combined with alcohol and other beverages. Both are also known as "date rape," "drug rape," "acquaintance rape," or "drug-assisted" assault drugs due to their ability to sedate and incapacitate unsuspecting victims.

Methamphetamine

Misuse of methamphetamine, a potent and highly addictive stimulant, remains an extremely serious problem in the United States. Methamphetamine (meth) comes in many forms and can be smoked, injected, ingested orally or snorted. Users may feel an intense sensation (rush) or a long-lasting high, depending on how it's taken.

Most of the pleasurable effects of methamphetamine are believed to result from the release of very high levels of the neurotransmitter dopamine. Dopamine is involved in motivation, the experience of pleasure, and motor function, and is a common mechanism of action for most drugs of abuse. The elevated release of dopamine produced by methamphetamine is also thought to contribute to the drug's damaging effects on nerve terminals in the brain.

Methamphetamine, even in small doses, can increase wakefulness and physical activity and decrease appetite. Methamphetamine can also cause a variety of cardiovascular problems, including rapid heart rate, irregular heartbeat and increased blood pressure. Hyperthermia (elevated body temperature) and convulsions may occur with a methamphetamine overdose, and if not treated immediately, can result in death.

Beyond its devastating effects on individual health, methamphetamine abuse threatens whole communities, causing new waves of crime, unemployment, child neglect or abuse, and other social problems.

Sports and school performance drugs

When you exercise, your nervous system is stimulated naturally. This stimulation boosts the production of hormones, including adrenaline (epinephrine). These hormones increase the amount of blood your heart pumps, resulting in increased blood to your muscles, the release of sugar (glucose) from the liver and the release of fatty acids from body fat to fuel your muscles. These effects are important to anyone who's exercising.

To further improve their athletic performance, some athletes turn to drugs. The abuse of anabolic steroids and other drugs by athletes is often front-page news, involving professional and amateur athletes in a wide range of sports.

An elevated level of awareness of the problem has led to more drug testing of athletes. In addition to putting an athlete's future in jeopardy, sports performance drugs cause health risks.

Anabolic steroids

A group of drugs used by some athletes are androgenic-anabolic steroids. Because these drugs are closely related chemically to natural male hormones, anabolic steroids mimic the effects of the male sex hormone testosterone. They increase the buildup of muscle tissue.

Anabolic steroids have several legitimate medical uses. They may be used to treat skeletal and growth disorders and certain types of anemia, as well as to offset the negative effects of irradiation and chemotherapy. But when the drugs are used over a prolonged period, serious side effects can result. An overload of anabolic steroids can lead to jaundice and liver failure.

Another potential liver problem is peliosis hepatitis. In this condition the liver develops blood-filled cysts that can rupture. Liver failure can result. There's also the potential for formation of liver tumors. In addition, anabolic steroids may increase blood pressure and decrease levels of high-density lipoprotein (HDL) cholesterol — the "good" cholesterol. Studies suggest that anabolic steroids may also cause heart damage.

Anabolic steroids can lead to a reduction in sperm production, a decrease in the size of the testicles and a reduction in the amount of sex hormones produced, resulting in a diminished sex drive. In female athletes the drugs may reduce production of the female sex hormones estrogen and progesterone, inhibit development of eggs and ovulation, reduce breast size, and disrupt the menstrual cycle.

All of these changes are reversible when use of anabolic steroids is discontinued. However, female athletes sometimes find that male secondary sex characteristics, such as an increase in facial hair or a deepening of the voice, persist after they stop using anabolic steroids.

Sympathomimetic amines

Some professional and world-class athletes have admitted using sympathomimetic amines, a class of stimulant drugs that mimic the natural effects of a stimulated sympathetic nervous system. The drugs can increase alertness and physical endurance and delay the onset of fatigue.

This class of drugs includes ephedrine and its derivative pseudoephedrine, which are often used as decongestants in cold and hay fever preparations. Ephedrine is also an ingredient in many asthma medications.

Stimulant drugs

Stimulant medications including amphetamines (Adderall) and methylphenidate (Ritalin, Concerta) are often prescribed to treat children, adolescents or adults diagnosed with attention-deficit/hyperactivity disorder (ADHD). These medications have a calming and "focusing" effect.

The drugs are often abused, however. They're taken in higher quantities or in a different manner than prescribed, or taken by those without a prescription.

A growing number of teenagers and young adults are taking prescription stimulants to boost their study performance in an

Getting High off Inhalants

Some people inhale substances that give them a high. A common prescription inhalant is called amyl nitrite, or "poppers." The drug relaxes smooth muscle in small blood vessels, causing them to expand and lower blood pressure. It's usually prescribed for treating angina pectoris. However, people inhale amyl nitrite because it produces an intense and immediate high and seems to intensify sexual orgasm.

Amyl nitrite isn't physically addictive, but users often suffer headaches, dizziness, an accelerated heart rate, nasal irritation and coughing spells.

More often people inhale substances that don't require a prescription, including a category of volatile inhalants that contain butyl nitrite and isobutyl nitrite sold as room deodorizers. Butyl nitrite is thought to intensify a sexual experience.

Other inhalants that people use include:
- Solvents
- Glue
- Paint
- Nitrous oxide

The physical risks from inhaling these substances range from an irregular heartbeat (cardiac arrhythmia) to liver and kidney impairment. Children and teens may experience permanent cognitive impairment. The products are also highly toxic.

effort to improve their grades in school, and there's a widespread belief that the drugs can improve a person's ability to learn (cognitive enhancement).

While prescription stimulants do promote wakefulness, studies indicate they don't enhance learning or thinking ability when taken by people who don't have ADHD.

Stimulants can increase blood pressure, heart rate, and body temperature and decrease sleep and appetite. When abused, they can lead to malnutrition and its consequences. Repeated abuse of stimulants can lead to feelings of hostility and paranoia. At high doses, they can result in serious cardiovascular complications. Addiction to stimulants is also a very real consideration for anyone taking them without medical supervision.

How to recognize substance use disorders

Substance use disorder occurs if you take any drug other than as directed — whether for a different reason or in another manner or quantity. Such misuse may lead to an addiction. Substance use disorders can cause health problems that range from physical to psychological, mild to severe, and reversible to permanent — or even fatal.

Compulsive use of a drug, or loss of control over its use, suggests addiction. The state of addiction includes both psychological dependence and physical dependence, causing a need to take the drug again.

Psychological dependence occurs when the desire or need for a drug evolves into a preoccupation with it. The individual needs the drug to feel better. A person who misuses drugs may develop a tolerance, so he or she needs more and more of the substance to achieve the desired effects.

Physical dependence occurs when withdrawal symptoms appear shortly after discontinuing use of the drug. They may be severe and possibly life-threatening, sometimes requiring immediate medical attention. Examples of these signs and symptoms include agitation, tremors, anxiety, insomnia, depression, convulsions and hallucinations.

Recognizing early signs and symptoms of addiction can be difficult. They vary from drug to drug and person to person. However, people who are addicted to one or more drugs usually exhibit changes in their behavior that may gradually affect personal relationships and work performance. Their behavior may be erratic and their mood unpredictable, alternating between periods of exhilaration or agitation and exhaustion or lethargy. Irritability is another sign. Some addicted individuals no longer sleep well, and others may crash and sleep for long periods. They may lose interest in eating or experience unexplained weight loss.

Other possible clues to substance abuse disorder are bloodshot eyes, dilated pupils, and a dazed or expressionless appearance. Individuals abusing hallucinogens may appear distracted and have to be spoken to several times before responding, or they may gaze at an object without reason for long periods. Some drugs may produce excessive sweating or flushed skin. An unexplained rash or an irritated nostril or runny nose may be a sign that someone has been using an opiate.

However, many people with a substance use disorder appear normal, even to close friends.

Treating substance use disorders

Treatment for addiction typically involves steps to help the person withdraw from using the drug, followed by counseling and self-help groups to help him or her resist the urge to use the drug again.

Withdrawal therapy
The goal of withdrawal therapy (detoxification) is for the person to stop taking the addictive drug as quickly and safely as possible. Detoxification may involve gradually reducing the dose of the drug or temporarily substituting other substances with less severe side effects. For some people it may be safe to undergo withdrawal therapy on an outpatient basis. Other people may require placement in a hospital or residential treatment center.

Withdrawal from different types of drugs often produces different side effects and requires different approaches.

Depressants
Withdrawal from depressants (sedative medications and alcohol) may be dangerous without professional monitoring. Minor side effects of withdrawal may include restlessness, anxiety, sleep problems, rapid heartbeat, high blood pressure, low-grade fever and sweating. More-serious signs and symptoms include hallucinations, whole-body tremors, seizures, profuse sweating and vomiting. The most serious stage of withdrawal may include delirium and is potentially life-threatening. Withdrawal therapy may involve gradually scaling back the amount of the drug you've been using. It can take that long for your body to adjust to low doses of the medication and then get used to taking none at all.

Stimulants
Side effects of withdrawal from stimulant drugs typically include depression, excessive sleepiness, fatigue, headaches, irritability and an inability to concentrate. In some cases, signs and symptoms may include suicide attempts, paranoia and impaired contact with reality (acute psychosis). There are no approved drugs used for treating stimulant withdrawal. Treatment during withdrawal is usually limited to emotional support from your family, friends and doctor. Your doctor may recommend medications to treat paranoid psychosis or depression.

Opioids
Opioid tapering involves gradually decreasing the dose of medication until it's no longer used. Other medications — such as clonidine (Catapres), a drug mainly used for high blood pressure — can be used to help manage opioid withdrawal symptoms during this process. Buprenorphine, buprenorphine with naloxone (Suboxone) or methadone may be used by doctors under specific, legally regulated and monitored conditions to ease symptoms of withdrawal from opioid painkillers. Vivitrol, a version of the drug naltrexone, given by injection once a month by a doctor may help people stay off opioids early in their recovery.

Continuing treatment
After detoxification, therapies such as counseling, treatment programs and self-help group meetings can help you stay off drugs.

Counseling
Individual or family counseling with a psychiatrist, psychologist or addiction counselor may help you resist the temptation to resume using addictive drugs. Behavioral therapy can help you develop ways to cope with your drug cravings, strategies to avoid drugs and prevent relapse, and ideas on how to deal with a relapse, if it occurs. Counseling may involve discussions related to your job, legal problems, or relationships with family and friends. Family members also may receive counseling to help them develop better communication skills and be more supportive.

Treatment programs
Treatment programs involve both pharmacologic and psychosocial treatment interventions. They generally include educational sessions and individual, group and family counseling. They're available in various settings — outpatient, residential and inpatient.

Self-help programs
Narcotics Anonymous is a self-help program that uses the 12-step program first developed by Alcoholics Anonymous. Self-help groups exist for people addicted to drugs such as cocaine, sedatives and narcotics. The message is that addiction is a chronic disorder with a danger of relapse and that ongoing maintenance treatment — which may include medications, counseling and attending self-help group meetings — is necessary to prevent a relapse. Your doctor or another medical professional can help you locate a self-help group.

Unsafe Sex

Sexually transmitted infections (STIs) are on the increase in the United States. To avoid them, it's important that you understand what puts you and your family and friends at risk. Most STIs — also known as sexually transmitted diseases (STDs) — are treatable, but some, such as AIDS, have no cure.

If you suspect that you may have a sexually transmitted infection, see your doctor right away. The sooner you get tested and begin treatment — if necessary — the less chance of serious complications developing.

Preventing sexually transmitted infections

Sexually transmitted infections include chlamydial infections, gonorrhea, genital herpes, venereal warts, syphilis and the human immunodeficiency virus (HIV), which causes AIDS. Many can be acquired during a single sexual encounter. Although HIV can also result from shared use of contaminated needles or, rarely, a blood transfusion, its main mode of transmission is sexual contact.

None of these infections is spread through casual contact such as handshaking, sitting on a toilet seat or living in the same house with an infected person. The microorganisms that cause STIs, including HIV, all die quickly once they're outside the body.

Entering into a monogamous relationship
The only sure way of preventing a sexually transmitted infection is through sexual abstinence or a mutually monogamous relationship with an uninfected person. If you or your partner has several sexual partners — either heterosexual or homosexual — you'll be at high risk of contracting an STI.

Using condoms
Use of a condom during sexual intercourse doesn't eliminate the risk of acquiring or transmitting a sexual infection, but it can significantly reduce the risk. The key is correct and consistent condom use.

Condoms are available in various thicknesses, colors and shapes. They may be lubricated or unlubricated, have a plain end or a reservoir end, and have a smooth, ribbed or corrugated texture. Condoms sometimes are made of animal membrane, but pores in this type of natural material may allow HIV to pass through. Latex condoms are recommended instead. When purchasing condoms, look for packages that mention STI protection and check the expiration date on the package.

To be effective, a condom must be undamaged, applied to the erect penis before any genital contact and kept snugly in place until it's removed on completion of sexual activity. Extra lubrication — even with lubricated condoms — can help prevent a condom from breaking. Use only water-based lubricants. Oil-based lubricants can cause a condom to break down.

After intercourse of any kind, the proper way to remove the condom is to hold on to it tightly at the rim and pull out slowly while the penis is still hard, to prevent spillage.

Female condoms also can help reduce the risk of contracting a sexually transmitted infection. Female condoms give women more control over their personal health. Most forms of female-directed contraception, such as the pill or diaphragm, don't protect against STIs. However, studies indicate that use of a spermicide decreases the frequency of gonorrhea and chlamydial infections. Using a spermicide in conjunction with a diaphragm also may help kill bacteria.

Avoiding certain sexual practices
Various sexual practices carry different degrees of risk of contracting a sexually transmitted infection. Receptive (passive) anal intercourse is the riskiest behavior for acquiring HIV because it may damage the anal and rectal membranes and allow the virus to enter the bloodstream. The passive partner is at much higher risk of contracting HIV than is the active partner, although gonorrhea and syphilis can be acquired from infection in the passive partner's rectum. Most studies have focused on male homosexuals, but heterosexual anal sex involves similar risks.

Heterosexual vaginal intercourse, particularly with multiple partners, also carries a risk of contracting HIV. The virus is believed to be more easily transmitted from the man to the woman than vice versa. This type of sex is how most other STIs are transmitted or acquired.

Oral sex is another possible means of transmission of HIV, gonorrhea, herpes, syphilis and other STIs. Accepting the penis in the mouth (fellatio) with ejaculation and swallowing of semen is the most common cause of throat gonorrhea. Oral contact with the clitoris and vaginal opening is a frequent method of transmission of the herpes virus.

Common sexually transmitted infections

Sexually transmitted infections result from bacteria, viruses and other organisms transmitted through sexual contact. For more information on the specific infections and their treatment, see Chapter 16, "Infectious Diseases."

Gonorrhea

Gonorrhea is an infection caused by a sexually transmitted bacterium (*Neisseria gonorrhoeae*) that can infect both males and females. Gonorrhea most often affects the urethra, rectum or throat. In females, gonorrhea can also infect the cervix.

Gonorrhea is most commonly spread during sex. But babies can be infected during childbirth if their mothers are infected. In babies, gonorrhea most commonly affects the eyes.

Gonorrhea is a common infection that, in many cases, causes no symptoms. You may not even know that you're infected. When symptoms do appear, gonorrhea infection can affect multiple sites in your body, but it commonly appears in the genital tract.

Signs and symptoms of gonorrhea infection in men include:
- Painful urination
- Pus-like discharge from the tip of the penis
- Pain or swelling in one testicle
Signs and symptoms of gonorrhea infection in women include:
- Increased vaginal discharge
- Painful urination
- Vaginal bleeding between periods, such as after vaginal intercourse
- Painful intercourse
- Abdominal or pelvic pain
Adults with gonorrhea are treated with antibiotics. Due to emerging strains of drug-resistant *Neisseria gonorrhoeae*, the Centers for Disease Control and Prevention recommends that uncomplicated gonorrhea be treated only with the antibiotic Ceftriaxone — given as an injection — in combination with either azithromycin (Zithromax, Zmax) or doxycycline (Monodox, Vibramycin, others) — two antibiotics that are taken orally.

Some research indicates that oral gemifloxacin (Factive) or injectable gentamicin, combined with oral azithromycin, can successfully treat gonorrhea. This treatment may be helpful in treating people who are allergic to cephalosporin antibiotics, such as ceftriaxone.

Your partner also should undergo testing and treatment for gonorrhea, even if he or she has no signs or symptoms. Even if you've been treated for gonorrhea, you can be reinfected if your partner isn't treated.

Babies born to mothers with gonorrhea receive a medication in their eyes soon after birth to prevent infection. If an eye infection develops, babies can be treated with antibiotics.

Chlamydia

Chlamydia trachomatis is a common sexually transmitted infection caused by the bacterium *Chlamydia trachomatis*. This bacterium affects both men and women and occurs in all age groups, though it's most prevalent among young women.

You may not know you have chlamydia because many people never develop the signs or symptoms. When signs or symptoms do occur, they usually start one to two weeks after exposure to chlamydia. Often, they're mild and passing, making them easy to overlook. Signs and symptoms may include:
- Painful urination
- Lower abdominal pain
- Vaginal discharge in women
- Discharge from the penis in men
- Painful sexual intercourse in women
- Bleeding between periods and after sex in women
- Testicular pain in men
Chlamydia can also infect the rectum. You may experience rectal pain, discharge or bleeding, or not have any signs or symptoms. It's also possible to acquire chlamydial eye infections (conjunctivitis) through contact with infected secretions.

Chlamydia is treated with antibiotics. You may receive a one-time dose, or you may need to take the medication daily or multiple times a day for five to 10 days.

In most cases, the infection resolves within one to two weeks. During that time, you should abstain from sex. Your sexual partner or partners also need treatment even if they have no signs or symptoms. Otherwise, the infection can be passed back and forth between sexual partners.

Having chlamydia or having been treated for it in the past provides no immunity against reinfection in the future.

Syphilis

Syphilis is an infection caused by the bacterium *Treponema pallidum* that's usually spread by sexual contact. The disease starts as a painless sore — typically on your genitals, rectum or mouth. Syphilis spreads from person to person via skin or mucous membrane contact with these sores.

After the initial infection, the syphilis bacteria can lie dormant in your body for decades before becoming active again. Early syphilis can be cured, sometimes with a single injection of penicillin. Without treatment, syphilis can severely damage several organs and can be life-threatening, or be passed from mother to an unborn child.

Syphilis develops in stages, and symptoms vary with each stage. But the stages may overlap, and symptoms don't always occur in the same order:
- **Primary syphilis.** The first sign of syphilis is a small sore (chancre) that appears at the spot where the bacteria entered your body. It usually develops about three weeks after exposure. The chancre is usually painless and may be hidden within the vagina or rectum. It will heal on its own within three to six weeks.

- **Secondary syphilis.** Within a few weeks of the original chancre healing, you may experience a rash that begins on your trunk and eventually covers your entire body. It may be accompanied by wart-like sores in the mouth or genital area. Some people also experience hair loss, muscle aches, a fever, sore throat and swollen lymph nodes. These signs and symptoms may disappear within a few weeks or repeatedly come and go.
- **Latent syphilis.** If you aren't treated for syphilis, the disease moves from the secondary to the latent (hidden) stage, when you have no symptoms. The latent stage can last for years. Signs and symptoms may never return, or the disease may progress to the tertiary stage.
- **Tertiary (late) syphilis.** About 15 to 30 percent of people with syphilis who don't get treatment will develop complications of late syphilis. In the late stages, the disease may damage your brain, nerves, eyes, heart, blood vessels, liver, bones and joints.
- **Congenital syphilis.** Babies born to women with syphilis can become infected through the placenta or during birth. Most have no symptoms, although some experience a rash on the palms of their hands and the soles of their feet. Later symptoms may include deafness, teeth deformities and collapse of the bridge of the nose.

When treated in its early stages, syphilis is easy to cure. The antibiotic penicillin is the preferred treatment. A single injection can stop the disease from progressing if you've been infected for less than a year. If you've had syphilis for longer than a year, you may need additional doses. If you're allergic to penicillin, your doctor will suggest another antibiotic.

Even if you're treated for syphilis during your pregnancy, your newborn child should also receive antibiotic treatment.

Genital herpes

Genital herpes is a common sexually transmitted infection caused by the herpes simplex virus (HSV). Sexual contact is the primary way that the virus spreads. After the initial infection, the virus lies dormant in your body and can reactivate several times a year.

Genital herpes may cause pain, itching and sores in your genital area, or you may have no signs or symptoms. When present, symptoms may begin about two to 12 days after exposure to the virus. In addition to pain and itching, you may experience:

- **Small red bumps or tiny white blisters.** These may appear a few days to a few weeks after infection.
- **Ulcers.** They form when blisters rupture and ooze or bleed. Ulcers may make it painful to urinate.
- **Scabs.** Skin will crust over and form scabs as ulcers heal.

You can spread the infection by touching a sore and then rubbing or scratching another area of your body, including your eyes. During an initial outbreak, you may have flu-like signs and symptoms such as swollen lymph nodes in your groin, a headache, muscle aches and a fever.

Signs and symptoms may recur, off and on, for years. Some people experience numerous episodes each year. For others, the outbreaks are less frequent as time passes.

There's no cure for genital herpes. Treatment with antiviral medications such as acyclovir (Zovirax), famciclovir and valacyclovir (Valtrex) may help sores heal sooner, lessen the severity and duration of symptoms during outbreaks, reduce the frequency of recurrence, and minimize the chance of transmitting the virus to another person.

Your doctor may recommend that you take the medicine only when you have symptoms of an outbreak or that you take a certain medication daily, even when you have no signs of an outbreak.

Genital warts

Genital warts are one of the most common types of sexually transmitted infections. Many sexually active people will become infected with the virus that causes genital warts, at some point during their lives.

Like warts that appear elsewhere on your body, genital warts are caused by the human papillomavirus (HPV). Some strains of genital HPV can cause genital warts, while others can cause cancer. Vaccines can help protect against certain strains of genital HPV.

In many cases, the warts are too small to be visible. Sometimes, though, the warts may multiply into large clusters. If your warts aren't causing discomfort, you may not need treatment. If your symptoms include itching, burning and pain, or if visible warts are causing you emotional distress, your doctor can help clear an outbreak with medications or surgery. However, the lesions are likely to come back after treatment.

HIV and AIDS

AIDS is a chronic, life-threatening condition caused by the human immunodeficiency virus (HIV). By damaging or destroying the cells of your immune system, HIV interferes with your body's ability to effectively fight off viruses, bacteria and fungi that cause disease. This makes you more susceptible to many infections your body would normally resist.

HIV is most commonly spread by sexual contact with an infected partner. Untreated women with HIV can also pass the infection to their babies during pregnancy, delivery or later through their breast milk.

Symptoms vary depending on the phase of the infection. For more information on HIV and AIDS, see page 476. ■

Healthy Travel

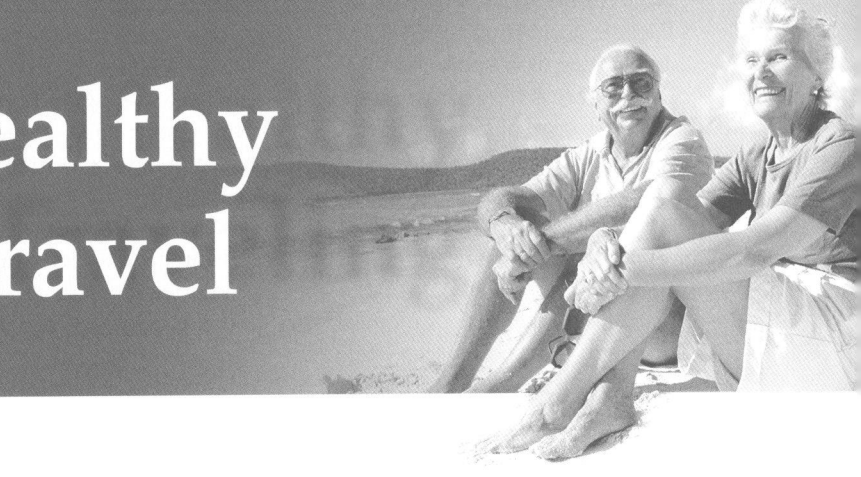

Each year, millions of Americans travel within the United States and abroad. Packing appropriate clothes and getting a passport and visa in order are activities that most travelers take for granted. Equally important, but often overlooked, is making sure you're properly vaccinated before traveling abroad, especially if you're traveling to a developing country. Also anticipate and plan for minor medical problems that could occur while traveling. It's not uncommon for people to experience some type of illness or injury while traveling that may need medical attention or require hospitalization.

Pre-travel Planning

If you're traveling, especially if you're going to a foreign country, it's important not to wait until the last minute to make all of your preparations. If you have a medical condition or if you may need vaccinations, it's especially important to see a doctor early. Follow these tips for a smoother trip:

Prepare early
As soon as you know your travel destinations, contact your doctor to see if you'll need any vaccinations. Some vaccinations are given in a series that you need to start several weeks to months before you leave. If you're planning to stay in a developing country for longer than one to three months, you may need to start your vaccinations six months before your departure.

If you have underlying health conditions such as heart disease or diabetes, or you're disabled, discuss with your doctor problems that you might anticipate and recommendations for dealing with them. If you take medication, make sure that you take enough with you.

Talk to your doctor or pharmacist about advance filling of your prescriptions. Also talk to your doctor about what medications or medical supplies you should carry with you. All of this can be discussed with your primary doctor or with a travel medicine doctor.

Inquire about nearby medical facilities
Your travel guide or a travel medicine doctor may be able to supply you with information on hospitals near the destinations at which you'll be staying. The U.S. Embassy or Consulate in the country you'll travel to also may be able to provide you with a list of hospitals and English-speaking doctors.

Another reference for a list of medical facilities in the country to which you'll be traveling is the organization International Association for Medical Assistance to Travellers (IAMAT).

See your dentist
Don't let the excruciating pain of a toothache spoil your trip as you fly in a pressurized airplane cabin or bite into an unfamiliar delicacy. Have any needed dental work done before you leave.

Be aware of health precautions at your destination
High altitudes or severe air pollution, often a problem in large, foreign cities, can be a health risk for some individuals with chronic health conditions. Talk to your doctor about how to avoid or handle these situations.

Consider travel protection insurance
If you need medical care, many foreign doctors and hospitals won't bill your American insurance company directly. Rather, they'll require cash in advance or at least verification of your ability to pay for their services. You'll need to seek reimbursement when you return home.

Medicare doesn't pay for foreign medical services. Some travel protection plans offer an immediate hospital deposit, emergency travel

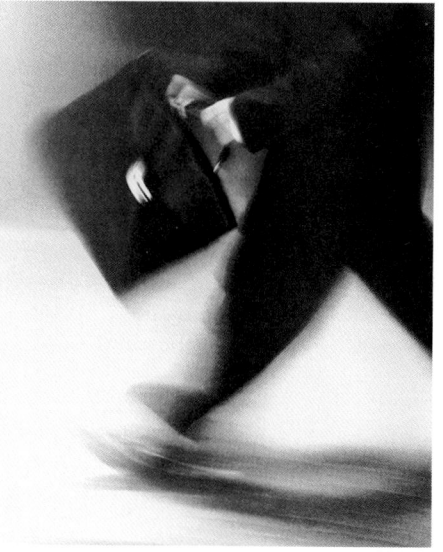

Travel Clinics

During the last decade, many travel clinics have been established across the United States. Services at travel clinics vary widely. Some offer vaccinations and informational handouts. Others offer comprehensive overviews on infectious diseases and other hazards you may encounter on a particular itinerary and detailed advice on how to minimize your risk of these illnesses. Some travel clinics are staffed with doctors trained in diagnosing and managing illness acquired while traveling in other countries.

In general, it's useful to see a travel medicine physician before any foreign travel, but especially for prolonged travel — four weeks or more — to any country and before travel to Asia, Africa or Latin America. If you have a medical condition, it's particularly important that you see someone before you travel.

arrangements and, if necessary, emergency air evacuation. Ask your travel agent or insurance agent for detailed information.

Vaccinations

Many countries have vaccination requirements that travelers must fulfill before entering. These are listed in the booklet updated regularly by the Centers for Disease Control and Prevention (CDC) called *Health Information for International Travel*. It's also known as the *CDC Yellow Book*.

You can also ask your doctor, your local travel clinic, state health department, or the consulate or embassy of the country you plan to visit about required immunizations.

Every adult and child should have up-to-date immunity against tetanus, polio, measles, mumps and rubella. Other immunizations you may need depend on the country you're visiting and perhaps the region of that country. If a vaccine isn't available for a disease or isn't recommended, take precautions.

Generally, you're more likely to be exposed to an infectious disease in a rural area than in an urban one, particularly in less-developed countries. Water supply systems and sanitary conditions may not be up to date in rural areas.

Diseases for which you may need to be vaccinated include:

Hepatitis A

Vaccination for hepatitis A is recommended for all travelers to any area of the world where sanitation is poor. Hepatitis A is generally contracted from contaminated food or water or from contact with someone who's infected.

Hepatitis B

Get vaccinated for hepatitis B if you plan to travel for more than a

A Medical Kit

When traveling abroad, it's a wise idea to take with you a list of past or present major illnesses, in addition to medications that you take and first-aid supplies.

Medications

Make sure you have an ample supply of medications that you or anyone in your family takes regularly. Prescriptions should be up to date. Keep prescription medications in their original pharmacy containers with the labels intact. This can help you avoid problems if security or customs officials check for illicit drugs.

Transport your medications and first-aid kit in your carry-on luggage, in case your checked luggage is missing on arrival. An extra supply of essential medications kept in your checked luggage also is a good idea in case you stay longer than you anticipated or you lose your carry-on baggage. Be sure to include any special medications your doctor recommends, such as for motion sickness if that's a problem for you.

Taking a simple first-aid kit with you is a sensible precaution. Supplies might include alcohol wipes, antiseptic cream, adhesive and gauze bandages, aspirin or acetaminophen, a thermometer, elastic wrap for sprains, insect repellent, sunscreen, lip balm, an antacid, a mild laxative, and a decongestant. Also include sunglasses and a second pair of prescription glasses or contact lenses with more wetting and cleaning solutions than you would ordinarily use.

Medical records

In case of illness or an emergency, the doctor you consult on your trip will need to know something about your medical history. Carry a brief medical report in your wallet or a location where it's easily accessible. Make sure

other members of your family or traveling group know where it is so that they can quickly and easily provide relevant information to any medical professional who may need it.

The medical information should include the following:

- Your name, address, telephone number, Social Security number and person to notify in case of an emergency.
- Your health status, including any chronic diseases you have or any allergies to medications, food or insects.
- Recent test results of any abnormalities for comparison in an emergency.
- A list of your medications and eyeglass or contact lens prescription for easier replacement. For medications, include the generic and brand names (if any) and the doses and frequency at which you take them. Also include typewritten copies of your prescriptions in case you lose your medication and need to have it refilled during your trip.
- Your immunization record, including dates you received your vaccines. Some countries require certificates of vaccination against diseases such as yellow fever.
- The name, address and telephone number of your primary care doctor.

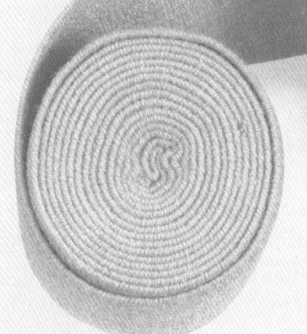

month to an area where hepatitis B is prevalent, such as Southeast Asia, Africa, the Middle East, some islands in the Pacific, Haiti or the Dominican Republic, or if you're at high risk of the disease. Individuals at increased risk include people who handle blood or blood products, men who have sex with men, intravenous drug users, or people who stay more than six months in a developing country.

Flu (influenza)

Individuals at high risk of serious illness from the flu (influenza) should be vaccinated before leaving the country. This includes children, adults over age 50 and individuals with a chronic illness. High-risk individuals should receive the influenza vaccine in the spring or summer months if traveling to the Southern Hemisphere, during the fall or winter months if traveling to countries in the Northern Hemisphere, or anytime if traveling to the tropics.

Japanese encephalitis

Talk with your doctor about a vaccine for Japanese encephalitis if you're traveling to areas of Southeast Asia or the Indian subcontinent, especially if you'll be traveling in rural areas or you're staying longer than four weeks. This vaccination series involves two shots given 28 days apart, and it should be completed at least seven days before you depart, in case side effects from the vaccination need attention.

Measles

You may need to be vaccinated for measles before going abroad if you haven't already had two doses. If you were born before 1957, you're more than likely immune to measles and may not need the vaccine. In some situations, a blood test can be done to check your immunity to measles.

Meningitis

If you're traveling to regions such as sub-Saharan Africa where a certain type of meningitis — meningococcal meningitis — is prevalent, get the meningococcal vaccine. It's required before entry into Saudi Arabia for travelers going to Mecca during the annual hajj pilgrimage.

Pneumonia

Travelers at increased risk of contracting pneumonia include adults older than age 65, as well as individuals with compromised immune systems and those with chronic illnesses such as diabetes or liver disease.

There are two different pneumococcal vaccines that are recommended for all adults age 65 and older and for those with immune problems. For adults younger than age 65 with a chronic illness such as diabetes, only one vaccine may be needed.

If you had your first shot before age 65, you may need a five-year booster shot. If you've had your spleen removed or you have another chronic illness that puts you at increased risk of pneumonia, you may need a repeat dose.

Polio

For people who've had their childhood polio immunizations, a booster shot of the inactivated vaccine may be recommended for travel to certain areas such as Pakistan, Afghanistan and some countries in Africa.

Rabies

If you plan to stay for more than a month in areas where rabies is common or where you're likely to have extensive exposure to animals, you may want to acquire immunity to the disease before leaving by obtaining the rabies vaccine series.

Tetanus and diphtheria

A booster dose of adult tetanus-diphtheria (Td) toxoid is recommended every 10 years. Every child and adult should have up-to-date immunity at all times. If you have a contaminated wound and it's been more than five years since you last received a tetanus booster, get a booster dose. You may also receive the booster in combination with the whooping cough (pertussis) vaccine — what's known as the tetanus, diphtheria and pertussis (Tdap) vaccine.

Typhoid

If you're traveling to a country where typhoid is prevalent, your doctor may suggest that you receive a weakened live oral vaccine or an injectable vaccine. The oral vaccine is generally effective for up to five years, and the injectable vaccine is effective for two years.

In the United States, both the oral and the injectable vaccines are available. If you live in a country where typhoid is prevalent for an extended period of time, the vaccine should be repeated every five or two years, respectively, as long as you remain there.

Yellow fever

If you're traveling to certain areas of Africa and South America where yellow fever is widespread, get the live virus vaccine. This vaccine is available only at certain yellow fever vaccination centers. It's also not given to people who have a significantly weakened immune system. You may need to repeat the vaccination.

Precautions

Most travel precautions are based on common sense. They include protecting yourself from insect bites and sunburns, and being responsible for your own safety. Following are precautions you should review prior to foreign travel.

Accident prevention and safety

The most common reason travelers require hospitalization is accidents. Car accidents are very common. Always use seat belts and child safety seats. Avoid forms of transportation that you don't feel are safe.

Always be aware of your surroundings and avoid being alone. Try not to draw attention to yourself and don't wear or carry expensive items. Have the telephone number for the U.S. Embassy in that country with you. The U.S. Embassy can be very helpful when there are problems or you need advice regarding a serious matter.

Food and water precautions

Ordinary traveler's diarrhea and more-serious foodborne illnesses, such as cholera and typhoid, can be prevented by following strict food and water precautions. All water and other drinks should be bottled or boiled. Bottled water and other drinks should be sealed and purchased from a reliable source. Avoid ice cubes.

Ideally, food should be freshly prepared, well-cooked and served steaming hot. Food that's steaming hot has been cooked to a high enough temperature to kill any bacteria. Fruits can be made safer by peeling them. However, bacteria can get into thinner-skinned fruit. A fruit with a thick skin, such as a banana, should be safe if you peel it yourself. Dairy products should be avoided unless you're certain they're pasteurized. Eat at restaurants with a reputation for cleanliness and food safety and avoid food from street vendors.

Frequent hand washing and use of an alcohol-based hand sanitizer can decrease the likelihood of diarrhea and many other infections.

Insect precautions

Many illnesses are transmitted by insects. Avoiding insect bites is your best protection against illness. Wear long-sleeved clothing, tuck your pants into your socks and cover up your skin as much as possible. Stay in dwellings with screens on exterior doors and windows or sleep under an insecticide-treated insect net.

A 20 to 50 percent concentration of a DEET-containing insect repellent should be applied to clothing and exposed skin. The repellent shouldn't be applied to children younger than 2 months old. Don't apply it to children's hands because they may touch their mouthes or eyes. The repellent shouldn't be used over open wounds or irritated skin. Sunscreen should be used, and reapplied every four to six hours when DEET is reapplied.

Permethrin is an insecticide that can be applied to clothing, shoes, tents and mosquito nets. Permethrin-treated clothing is effective for up to five to six washes. DEET should still be used.

Malaria prevention

Malaria is transmitted by mosquitoes that bite at night. There's no vaccine against malaria, but effective preventive medications are available. In most countries of the world where malaria exists, resistance has developed to the medication chloroquine. Depending on the malaria endemic to the area you'll be traveling to, your doctor may prescribe chloroquine or another antimalarial medication, such as mefloquine, doxycycline or a combination pill of atovaquone and proguanil.

Start taking this medication just before you arrive in the malarial area and continue to take it during your travel and for the recommended period of time after leaving the area. Discuss with your doctor possible adverse reactions to the medication. Your doctor will want to review your past and current medical history for any indications that you shouldn't take the medication.

Because malaria infection often mimics a flu-like illness or other viral diseases, be wary if you develop an illness with fever within 12 months of traveling to a malaria-prone area. Tell your doctor about your trip. A blood test can determine if you have the disease.

Zika prevention

Zika is a virus spread mostly by the bite of an infected aedes species mosquito. These mosquitoes bite primarily during the day.

Zika infection during pregnancy can cause serious birth defects including microcephaly, which results in incomplete brain development. Doctors have also found other problems in pregnancies and among fetuses and infants infected with the Zika virus before birth. If you're pregnant or there's a chance of pregnancy in the near future, avoid travel to areas with risk of Zika. In addition, if you have a partner who lives in or has traveled to an area with risk of Zika, use condoms or don't have sex during your pregnancy.

The CDC has issued guidance for travel, prevention, testing, and preconception counseling related to risks for pregnant women and couples considering conception in areas of active Zika virus transmission. For more information on Zika, visit the CDC website and see page 468.

Other precautions

Depending on the location you are traveling to, keep these precautions in mind.

Rabies prevention

Although there's a vaccine that's helpful in preventing rabies, most people visiting countries where rabies is present aren't immunized prior to travel. Travelers should avoid contact with mammals because of the risk of getting bitten.

Any bite or scratch should be taken seriously. The wound should be washed thoroughly with soap and water, and you should seek immediate medical attention. Travelers who haven't been vaccinated should receive immediate rabies treatment if there's any question that the mammal could have rabies.

Sunburn prevention

The risk of sunburn increases the closer you are to the earth's equator and the higher the altitude. Also be aware that some medications, including medications to prevent malaria, can significantly increase the risk of sunburn.

Wear a sunscreen with a sun protection factor (SPF) of 30 or above. If you expect to be in sunlight for lengthy periods, take other steps to protect yourself. Wear a hat and a shirt with long sleeves, and avoid shorts. Several clothing manufacturers market items designed to provide protection from the sun while you're outdoors.

Swimming precautions

Swimming in lakes and rivers in developing countries should be avoided because of risk of infection. The water may be contaminated by animal urine, bacteria, viruses and parasites. When swimming in the ocean, wear watershoes and be aware of jellyfish, sea coral and anemones, which can cause painful and toxic allergic reactions. Before swimming in unfamiliar water, ask about currents that can overpower swimmers and cause drowning.

Common Ailments of Travelers

Traveling can cause a variety of illnesses. Most often, the illness is related to a chronic condition. For example, individuals with circulatory problems are at increased risk of formation of a blood clot in a leg if confined to a tight space and unable to move for a considerable period, such as on a long airplane trip. A few conditions, though, tend to be fairly common during travel.

Altitude sickness

Signs and symptoms

- Headache
- Shortness of breath with mild exertion
- Fatigue
- Nausea
- Disturbed sleep
- Loss of appetite

Emergency signs and symptoms

- Severe breathing difficulty

Altitude sickness may occur when people who live in a low altitude make a trip to an altitude of more than 8,000 feet. It usually develops several hours after arriving at a high altitude. Skiers, hikers or others who travel to mountain slopes from lower elevations are often affected, especially if they fly into the high-elevation area.

How serious is altitude sickness?

Many people experience mild to moderate symptoms that generally resolve as the individual becomes adjusted to the change in altitude. However, symptoms can persist for several days. Rarely, some people experience a more severe form of altitude sickness that can produce severe breathing distress or severe brain illness. This is a medical emergency that can be fatal if not treated.

Treatment

Increasing intake of fluids and carbohydrates can help minimize the effects of mild altitude sickness. Rest is also helpful. For serious altitude sickness, get the affected person to a lower altitude and, if possible, provide him or her with oxygen.

Prevention

To avoid altitude sickness:

- **Allow time to adjust.** Rest a day after arriving to help you get used to the altitude.
- **Ascend slowly.** If possible, begin at an altitude below 6,000 feet.
- **Take it easy.** Slow down if you're out of breath or tired.
- **Limit ascent.** Don't climb more than 3,000 feet a day or 1,000 feet if you're at 12,000 feet or above.
- **Sleep safely.** Avoid increasing your sleeping altitude by more than 1,000 feet a night after reaching an altitude of 10,000 feet.
- **Avoid cigarettes and alcohol.** They worsen symptoms.
- **Consider medication.** Ask your doctor about acetazolamide or other prescription medications that may prevent or lessen symptoms.

Move Around

During a long trip, take time to stretch and walk. Extended sitting can put you at risk of a potentially fatal condition in which a blood clot forms in your leg, breaks loose and blocks an artery in your lung (pulmonary embolism).

Support hose also can help prevent clots or swelling of your feet and ankles during lengthy airline flights or train, bus or car trips. But avoid socks or stockings with tight elastic tops that constrict your legs and interfere with blood circulation.

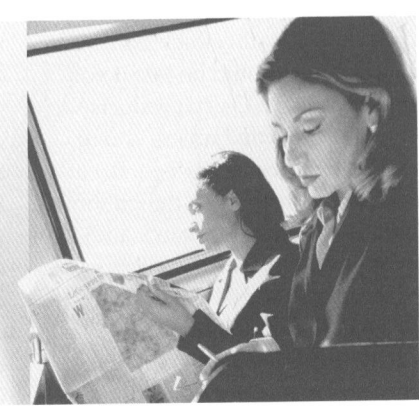

Jet lag

Signs and symptoms
- Fatigue, drowsiness
- Irritability
- Difficulty sleeping
- Loss of mental acuity
- Minor coordination problems

If you've ever traveled by air across several time zones, you're probably familiar with what it's like to experience jet lag — that dragged-out, out-of-sync feeling that can affect your pattern of eating, working, relaxing and sleeping. Jet lag results from the readjustment you demand of your body when traveling across time zones.

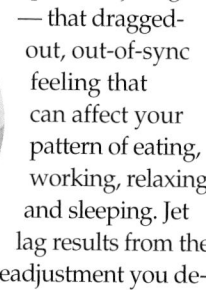

How serious is jet lag?
Flying eastward — thus resetting your body clock forward — is often more difficult than flying westward and adding hours to your day. Flying north or south doesn't produce jet lag. Most people's bodies adjust at the rate of about an hour a day. If you pass through four time zones, for example, that means that your body may require about four days to resynchronize its usual rhythms.

Prevention
To prevent jet lag or reduce its effects:

Reset your body clock
Begin resetting your body's clock a few days in advance of your departure by adopting a sleep-wake pattern similar to the day-night cycle at your destination. Or set your watch to the time of your destination while on the airplane so you start thinking in terms of the new time.

Another strategy is to try to schedule your arrival at your destination at roughly your usual bedtime, according to the clocks in the time zone to which you're flying. Or try sleeping on the plane and plan to arrive at the hour you usually start your day. If it's daytime when you arrive, stay in the sun as much as possible. This can help you immediately begin to orient your body to the new time schedule.

Getting added sleep before departure also may reduce jet lag. Alternatively, if you have an important event or meeting at your destination, get there two or three days in advance. That way, you won't be disadvantaged by jet lag.

Drink plenty of fluids and eat lightly
Drink extra liquids during your flight to avoid dehydration, but limit beverages with alcohol and caffeine. They increase dehydration and may disrupt your sleep.

Limit your intake of salty or fatty food. If you have a special diet, be sure to follow it. Many airlines offer special meals, but you'll need to make arrangements in advance.

Adjust your medication schedule
If you're on a regimen of medications, you may have to make adjustments as to when you take them to account for changes in time zones. Check with your doctor before leaving. If you have diabetes and are taking long-acting insulin, you may have to switch to regular insulin until you adjust to your new time change, food and activities. However, be sure to discuss the time change with your doctor.

Motion sickness

Signs and symptoms
- Restlessness that may progress to a cold sweat
- Dizziness
- Nausea and vomiting

Any type of transportation can produce motion sickness. You may experience motion sickness in a plane, on a boat, on a train or in a car.

Motion sickness results from increased activity of inner structures that control balance. The increased activity is often brought on by the motion of a vehicle. As soon as the motion stops, symptoms generally begin to improve.

How serious is motion sickness?
The illness isn't serious, but it can ruin a vacation. Some people find that the more they travel, the more their body adjusts to being in motion.

Prevention
If you're susceptible to motion sickness, try the following:
- In a ship, request a cabin in the middle, near the waterline.
- On a plane, ask for a seat over the front edge of a wing.
- On a train, sit near a window and face forward.
- In an automobile, drive, or sit in the front passenger's seat.
- Keep your head still, rested against a chair back.
- Sleep or lie down.
- If you're on a boat, breathe plenty of fresh air.
- Avoid spicy foods and alcohol and don't overeat.
- Don't read.

Take an over-the-counter antihistamine such as meclizine or dimenhydrinate (Bonine, Dramamine Less Drowsy, others) before you feel sick, unless your doctor advises otherwise. Expect some drowsiness as a side effect of the medication.

Ask your doctor about the scopolamine patch (Transderm-Scop) used to treat motion sickness. You need a prescription for this product. You place the dime-sized patch behind your ear before you experience symptoms of motion sickness. One patch works for up to three days.

Traveler's diarrhea

Signs and symptoms
- Diarrhea
- Abdominal cramps

Traveler's diarrhea, turista, Montezuma's revenge and Tut's tummy are familiar names for this common ailment of travelers. A trip to a foreign country by no means guarantees a bout with gastrointestinal discomfort. But if you travel to a country where the climate, social conditions, or sanitary standards and practices are different from yours at home — particularly in developing nations — risk of traveler's diarrhea may be high.

Traveler's diarrhea may be attributed to a number of causes, including consuming food and drink that you're unaccustomed to, a difference in living habits, and a change in the balance of bacteria that naturally live in your bowel. Usually, the problem is related to inadequate sanitation. Contaminated food and water may contain bacteria, viruses or parasites that cause diarrhea and abdominal cramps.

How serious is traveler's diarrhea?

Traveler's diarrhea most often begins abruptly while traveling or shortly after you return home. Usually, it's mild and subsides in three or four days, but you may not feel well for several more days. Sometimes, traveler's diarrhea can be more troublesome. If it's caused by organisms other than common bacteria, symptoms may be more severe, long lasting and difficult to overcome. Medication may then be needed to rid your body of the organism.

Treatment

If you do get traveler's diarrhea, drink plenty of safe liquids to replace lost fluids, salts and minerals. It's important not to get dehydrated. Orange, apple or other fruit juices are good for replacing lost potassium, but remember to avoid juices diluted with tap water. Broth, sweetened tea and soft drinks also are good for keeping up your strength. The most

Replacing Lost Fluids

If you experience severe weakness after a bout of traveler's diarrhea, your body may have lost an excessive amount of fluids and minerals. If medical help is unavailable, prepare the following solution to help correct the problem. Mix $\frac{1}{2}$ teaspoon of table salt (sodium chloride), $\frac{1}{2}$ teaspoon of baking soda (sodium bicarbonate) and 4 tablespoons of table sugar (sucrose) in 1 liter of safe drinking water. If carbonated or bottled water isn't available, tap water boiled for three minutes or more is a suitable substitute. Drink the mixture over the course of the day, as a supplement to a clear liquid diet.

important treatment for traveler's diarrhea is fluids.

As soon as you feel like eating again, start with fat-free, soft foods to avoid irritating your intestinal tract. Bananas are a good source of potassium and can help slow diarrhea. Bland cereals, rice, gelatin, jellied consomme, simple puddings and soft-cooked eggs are other possibilities.

Some immunosuppressed travelers take antibiotics as a preventive measure. Public health experts discourage this for travelers with normal immune systems. For healthy travelers, it's recommended that you carry antibiotics to take only in the event of serious diarrhea.

For mild to moderate diarrhea, medications such as loperamide (Imodium A-D) often ease cramps and diarrhea, and drugs containing diphenoxylate (Lomotil, Lonox) can be taken orally. Most people experience prompt relief. Such medications shouldn't be taken if you have a fever or bloody diarrhea.

The medication bismuth subsalicylate (Pepto-Bismol, Kaopectate) can decrease the frequency of your stools and shorten the duration of your illness. However, it isn't recommended for children, pregnant women or people who are allergic to aspirin.

Prevention

To reduce your risk of traveler's diarrhea when traveling to a foreign country, talk to your doctor about preventive medications.

No vaccines offer protection against traveler's diarrhea. You might consider taking bismuth subsalicylate (Pepto-Bismol, Kaopectate) tablets throughout your trip as a preventive measure. Doing so can decrease your risk of diarrhea. However, the medication isn't recommended for children, pregnant women or people who are allergic to aspirin.

Bismuth subsalicylate can interfere with the absorption of other medications, so take it a few hours before or after your medications. It can also turn your stools a dark charcoal color, so don't be alarmed if this occurs. Talk with your doctor about use of bismuth subsalicylate. ■

End-of-Life Issues

One of life's few guarantees is that, someday, it will end. End-of-life planning isn't just about how you will die but how you will live until that time. It also involves the many decisions that need to be made about the care you receive at the end of your life and decisions your family will deal with after your death. Making these decisions when you're healthy and sharing them with your family and health care providers will help to ensure that the care you receive aligns with the care you want. This type of planning also helps to prevent disputes among loved ones.

Estate Planning

Whether you have a complex network of assets or you live simply, estate planning allows you to choose the individuals and organizations that you would like to benefit from your life of hard work. When you die, your assets are distributed. If you leave no indication of how you want your assets divided, state law decides for you.

Now is the time to set up a formal plan to make your wishes known. With these issues settled, you're free to enjoy your final years without the stress of worrying about how your assets will be distributed after your death.

Assessing your estate

Before you begin to make plans for your estate, you need to take an inventory of what it entails. Your estate includes everything you own that conceivably has some value. Major items in your estate may include:
- A home
- Additional real estate
- Ownership interest in a business

- Life insurance
- Investments
- Retirement accounts
- Savings accounts
- Vehicles
- Other personal property

Drafting a will

The simplest way to ensure that your heirs get what you want them to have is to prepare a will. About half of all Americans, however, don't have wills in effect when they die. In these cases, a probate judge decides who gets what from an individual's estate. If you don't have any heirs and you don't leave a will, your state government may claim your money and property.

An attorney can be helpful in making sure your wishes are carried out. With an attorney you can draw up a will that describes your estate, names your beneficiaries and details what they're to receive and when they should receive it. You may make any other special provisions you wish and name a manager of your estate (personal representative).

It isn't necessary, however, to involve an attorney. You can use a pre-made will in which all you need to do is fill in the necessary information.

Most wills go through probate court to some degree or another. The smaller your estate, the simpler that process is apt to be. Probate rarely takes longer than a year.

Preparing a living trust

Another way to pass on your estate to your heirs is to create what's called a revocable living trust. A living trust is a legal document created by a lawyer. It describes how you would like your estate distributed after you

die and names a trustee to execute your wishes.

The benefit of a living trust is that it allows your assets to be passed along to beneficiaries without going through the process of probate. In addition, you have the option of specifying how your property should be handled in the event that you become incapacitated.

Seeking estate counseling

No matter if your estate is small and simple or large and complex, it's often helpful to enlist the aid of an experienced attorney, certified public accountant, financial planner or other appropriate professional. Estate laws change frequently and are usually complicated. Someone with experience in financial and estate matters can help ensure that your heirs aren't left with a larger tax liability than necessary.

Long-Term Care Insurance

Long-term care insurance provides financial protection if you're unable to care for yourself because of a chronic illness, disability or cognitive impairment, such as Alzheimer's disease.

If you should need long-term care, it's often very expensive and it generally isn't covered by Medicare or it involves substantial copayments. In addition, individuals who receive long-term care often must spend most all of their personal assets before receiving long-term care benefits. This can be a hardship to the surviving spouse.

Long-term care insurance is designed to help pay the cost of continued medical care, protecting your savings. This type of insurance generally covers a wide variety of services, from the cost of home health care to monthly nursing home payments.

However, long-term care insurance can be expensive, especially if you wait until you're older to purchase it. Buying the insurance when you're younger — such as in your 50s or 60s — can prevent the insurance from being too expensive. However, if you purchase it too young you may pay many years of unnecessary premiums.

Also keep in mind that long-term care insurance isn't for everyone. This type of insurance probably isn't the right choice if you have a limited income and few assets. Nor do you need it if you've saved enough money to pay for long-term care, though you might still want to buy it to protect your assets.

Most people purchase long-term care insurance for peace of mind. Keep in mind, though, that many people never end up in nursing homes, and of those that do, the majority are there for only a short period of time.

When thinking about long-term care insurance, consider all the pros and cons, and make certain you understand exactly what the insurance covers and for how long. Long-term care insurance can be complicated. Therefore, it's a good idea to talk to an expert before you buy.

Funeral Costs

A traditional funeral and burial can cost thousands of dollars. For this reason, more Americans are setting aside money to cover future funeral expenses. Or they're entering into contracts with funeral homes and prepaying for funeral packages. Either approach will relieve some of the stress on loved ones when you die.

If you decide to purchase a funeral package — whether it's simply a cemetery plot or an entire package that includes a casket or cremation and the funeral service

— it's a good idea to shop around. If possible, call or visit at least two funeral homes and cemeteries. The Federal Trade Commission's "Funeral Rule" requires funeral homes, though not cemeteries, to disclose their prices by telephone. Many will mail you their price lists.

If you're buying a package, be sure to get prices for the casket, the outer burial container — which is often required by cemeteries to prevent the ground from sinking — and the funeral home's general services, which may include:

- An initial consultation
- Copies of death certificates — you may need more than a dozen to settle matters such as insurance claims, social security issues and pension benefits
- Transportation of the body to the funeral home and burial site
- Preparation of the body for burial
- Use of the facilities for visitation or a memorial ceremony
- Other options, such as flowers, music or preparing obituary notices

An increasing number of people are choosing cremation over burial. Cremation can be less costly, especially if the remains are transported across state lines. However, there are costs and options associated with cremation as well. The body must be cremated in a container,

although not necessarily a casket. And many families choose to purchase a memorial spot for the urn containing the remains. Some cemeteries allow burial of the urn in a traditional plot, and others have urn gardens. Ask about the various options and costs.

Advance Directives

As people age, medical care can become increasingly complex. While advances in modern medicine can extend the length of a person's life, this life prolongation may not be accompanied by improvements in quality of life. Many people are just as concerned with how well they'll live as they are about how long they'll live.

It's important to have regular, honest conversations with your doctor about your hopes and worries concerning the types of medical care you wish to receive in your later years, and how that care does or does not fit with your goals, preferences and values for how you want to live.

You have the right to determine how you want to live your life, even when dealing with a serious

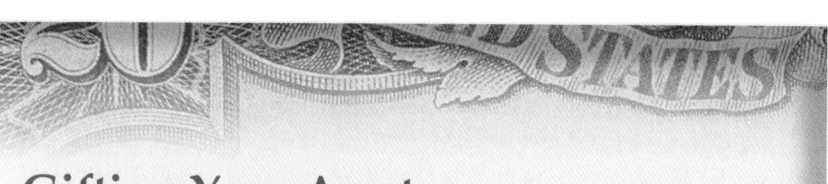

Gifting Your Assets

One way to ensure that your heirs and your favorite charities or organizations get as much of your estate as possible is to gradually begin passing on your assets to them while you are alive.

There are several approaches that you can take — including cash gifts, an irrevocable trust, a revocable living trust, a charitable remainder unitrust or annuity trust, or a charitable lead trust — to divide and disperse your assets.

Rules and regulations regarding these types of financial arrangements change, so make sure to visit with a professional to determine which route would be best for you. Also make sure that you save enough money for yourself so that you can live comfortably during your retirement.

illness. Many doctors are uncomfortable initiating conversations about end-of-life care or care during a serious illness. Therefore, you may need to approach such a conversation with your doctor and let him or her know your wishes.

Advance directives are a set of guidelines that can help guide your medical providers and your family to help them make the best decisions regarding your care in case you aren't able to communicate your wishes.

Advance directives shouldn't be viewed as a list of procedures or types of care that you may or may not want, but a way to communicate how you wish to live your life. It's beneficial to think about medical care at the end of your life and those aspects of your care that are very important to you — that you want to make sure do or do not happen.

Most advanced directives allow you to appoint someone who can make medical decisions for you if you lose the capacity to make those decisions yourself. It's critical to have open and honest conversations with this person (and an alternate individual if possible) about your preferences regarding your quality of life and what you value at the end of life.

If you're over age 18 and are being admitted to a hospital, nursing home, hospice or home health care agency that receives Medicare funds, the institution is required by federal law to ask whether you have an advance directive. That information is documented in your record. The institution must also give you written information about your right, under state law, to accept or reject medical treatment. Whether or not you have an advance directive, federal law requires the institution to provide all individuals the same treatment options.

If you want to prepare an advance directive, your doctor or hospital staff can give you the necessary form and provide resources explaining the relevant state laws. You can also contact an attorney.

One of the most useful aspects of advance directives is that they provide an opportunity for individuals to discuss important matters with their family members before a life-threatening event. And if you ever do become seriously ill or injured and unable to communicate, this document can help relieve some of the anguish of family who would otherwise have to guess what medical treatment you would want.

Types of directives

The most common types of advance directives are living wills and durable powers of attorney for health care. The combination of a durable power of attorney for health care and a living will provides maximum personal participation in the face of many medical situations that require difficult decisions.

A living will

Living wills are usually written in general language because no one can anticipate all possible circumstances that may surround a death. Living wills may follow a standard format or be specific. For example, your living will might prohibit heroic procedures, but your doctor has to make certain distinctions: Is the use of a respirator a heroic measure? What about a blood transfusion?

As new technologies develop and yesterday's heroic treatments become routine, the problem becomes increasingly complicated. For doctors, one of the biggest challenges is keeping patients and family members informed of ever-changing life-sustaining technologies, and the personal impact of these treatments. It's a well-informed individual who's most likely to make thoughtful decisions about medical treatment.

To draft a living will, it's useful, but not essential, to get help from an attorney. More importantly, talk to family members. With a living will, family members aren't expected to make difficult decisions, but they will be carrying out your wishes, so make sure they understand your thinking.

It's also important to realize that all living wills have limitations because few people can predict their manner of death. You might consider stating your wish that extraordinary technological procedures be used if they will preserve useful life but not if they will only prolong the dying process.

A living will by itself carries only moral force in stating your preferences. To give legal authority to living wills, most states have passed statutes, often called natural death acts. In these states, the statutes interpret the extent of the authority and the legal force of the living will. The statutes aren't

Health Care Services and Facilities

Near the end of life, there may come a time when it makes sense to get some extra help with day-to-day tasks. Or you may need extra help while you recover from an illness. There are several ways to receive this help, and it makes sense to think now about what you might want if someday you should need some assistance.

Options include:
- Home health care
- Assisted living
- Elder care
- Nursing homes

uniform among states. To ensure that your living will conforms to your state's requirements and will be followed, be familiar with the appropriate laws in your state before you prepare your living will, or let an attorney or health care professional trained in these matters help you.

Once you've created a living will, review it periodically with your doctor. Medical technology and your views and wishes may change. You have the option of revoking your living will and other advance directives at any time.

A durable power of attorney for health care

In addition to a living will, you may want to consider a document creating a durable power of attorney for health care. This document identifies the person you've selected to make health-related decisions for you should you become unable or unwilling to do so, giving this person legal authority to act on your behalf. Usually, the person is a spouse, partner, family member or trusted friend.

This person, also called a proxy, helps ensure that your wishes aren't misinterpreted or ignored. And, unlike a living will, your proxy can respond specifically to the unique questions that your condition may create. When selecting someone to serve as your proxy, choose a person you trust and are comfortable with. He or she should fully understand your medical care philosophy and wishes and agree to serve in representing them. It also may be helpful, but not necessary, if this person lives close to you.

You need to be careful not to confuse a durable power of attorney for health care with a financial power of attorney. A financial power of attorney, also called a statutory short form power of attorney, allows a person you authorize to manage your money and property if you aren't able to do so.

What to address

It's impossible to predict exactly what issues will need to be addressed as you approach death. Therefore, it's not always clear what to include in an advance directive. However, the following health care scenarios are common and provide a guideline for discussions:

Discontinuing or withholding lifesaving treatment

Terminal illness may reach a point at which further treatment may only prolong the process of dying. At this point, you and your family, with help from your doctor and perhaps a religious adviser, may decide in advance not to attempt cardiopulmonary resuscitation (CPR) in the event you stop breathing or your heart stops beating. You and your family may also decide to stop further treatment except to ease pain and provide comfort.

Decisions that involve highly sensitive ethical matters often bring out differences of opinion among family members. For example, removing life-support systems may not present a dilemma for someone who sees the choice only in terms of death with dignity. For another relative, removing life-support systems may violate deep beliefs about the preservation of life.

The best course of action isn't always obvious. This is why it's critical to communicate your feelings about what you judge to be useful in life to those you entrust with decisions about your care.

Artificial feeding

In addition to the use of CPR and ventilators to breathe, questions regarding use of other life-sustaining measures, such as nutritional support, may arise in the care of a person with a terminal illness.

Artificial feeding involves providing artificial nutrition in a manner other than normal eating — usually by inserting into the stomach a tube that allows liquids to go directly into it. Several difficult questions arise in these situations: Is such feeding permanent? What will be the quality of life of the person? If feeding is discontinued, will the person experience thirst and hunger? Your caregiver can help answer these questions.

Many difficult decisions can arise with a terminal illness. In making such decisions, unique factors must be weighed. Although there are few rules, each person has his or her own framework of moral and ethical principles limited by legal boundaries that need to be considered.

Helpful Organizations

As you go about your day-to-day activities, it's difficult to think about the end of your life. It also can be difficult to discuss matters relating to your or a loved one's death and dying. However, there are organizations designed to help people with end-of-life issues.

For example, the Center for Practical Bioethics, an independent organization, has developed a workbook with questions to consider, answer and discuss with family members. Its program, called Caring Conversations, is designed to help individuals and families share meaningful conversations while making practical end-of-life decisions.

The workbook covers everything from reflecting on your personal relationships and religious beliefs to more specific, practical issues, such as whether you would want to refuse food, water or any other life-sustaining services. The resource guide also goes over an advance directive and information on how to create one.

'Do Not Resuscitate' Orders

The directive "Do not resuscitate" (DNR) means that cardiopulmonary resuscitation (CPR) is not to be performed when a person's heart stops or he or she stops breathing. CPR is rarely appropriate for a person with a terminal, irreversible illness when death is expected at any time. The initials *DNR* are usually prominently displayed on the charts of people in hospitals or nursing homes when it has been decided that CPR is not to be used. The decision to place *DNR* on the chart is made by the individual who is ill and his or her doctor. If the individual isn't competent or able to communicate, relatives, a doctor or someone who's been designated to make medical decisions for the person may make the decision. Sometimes, a request for a DNR order is part of a living will.

It's best not to make the decision whether to use CPR in an emergency situation, if possible. It's better to make the decision in advance and have everyone who might be involved aware of it. Placing *DNR* on your chart doesn't imply that any lesser quality of care will be given. Rather, it's to consider if attempting CPR or proceeding with intubation corresponds with your wishes. You're still given optimal treatment for other conditions. For example, your doctor would still ask if you wanted antibiotics should an infection develop.

Organ Donation

Every year tens of thousands of people await organ transplants. Some are waiting for a donated cornea to help them see again. For others, the transplant is a matter of life and death, such as the donation of a heart or liver. Unfortunately, each year the number of organ donations fills only a fraction of the need.

The United Network for Organ Sharing (UNOS), the organization charged with organizing the sharing of organs, believes that the better people understand the donation process, the more willing they'll be to become a donor.

Who can donate?

First off, anyone can donate organs. There's no upper age limit. Older adults are often evaluated as donors. In addition, a medical illness doesn't necessarily mean that you can't donate your organs. At the time of death, the appropriate medical professionals will determine whether your organs are usable. What about your religion? Donation is acceptable to and even lauded by most religions.

Organ transplantation is less common at hospitals outside major medical centers. However, all hospitals are required by law to inform the relatives of an individual who has died and is a potential donor about UNOS, which was established in 1984 by the National Organ Transplant Act. UNOS maintains an extensive computer network of individuals in need of donated organs.

The donation procedure

Some people have concerns about the donation procedure. They worry about disfigurement or if their care will be affected by their decision to donate.

Donation doesn't disfigure the body. Needed organs are removed surgically, in an operation similar to a gallbladder or appendix removal. When a person has stated a desire to be an organ donor after death, the procedure takes place only after all efforts to save the individual have been exhausted and death has been legally declared. The medical professionals who retrieve organs for transplantation aren't the same doctors who provide care for an ill person.

Organs that can be taken from one individual and transplanted into another include the heart, kidneys, pancreas, lungs, liver, intestines and eyes. Tissues that can be donated include skin, bone, heart valves and tendons.

Who receives the organs or tissues?

One myth that's difficult to dispel is that wealthy or famous people move to the top of the recipient list when they need a transplant. In reality, the organ allocation and distribution system is blind to wealth or social status.

The length of time it takes to receive a transplant is governed by many factors, including blood type, length of time on the waiting list, severity of illness and other medical criteria.

UNOS doesn't consider factors such as race, sex, age, income or celebrity status when determining who receives an organ.

Becoming a donor

If you wish to be an organ donor, you can indicate that in an advance directive. In some states you can also make a notation on your driver's license indicating your preference. However, even if you take both of these steps, it's also crucial to discuss this issue with your family so that they are aware of your wishes.

Organ removal must happen shortly after death, and often family members don't have much time to make a decision on whether to donate a loved one's organs. Knowing the person's preference ahead of time can make the decision less difficult.

Terminal Illness

Death is quite different from the process of dying. Death is an endpoint when life ceases. But dying is the final part of the life process. Dying can be intense and shaped by the individual's history of illness, his or her response to stress, the nature of the illness, and his or her interactions with others during the process. Cultural influences and belief systems also play a role.

For many dying people, life's experiences still have significant meaning and importance. Understanding the process of dying can often help terminally ill individuals and their families and friends cope during this difficult time.

The paths to death are as varied as the lives preceding it. Sometimes, death comes suddenly and without warning. Other times, people live with impending death as part of life. With a terminal illness, the dying person, the attending doctor, and a circle of family and friends are given time to prepare for death. They can discuss important issues, such as how various medical procedures (artificial nutrition or invasive procedures) may or may not help the dying individual achieve comfort during the dying process.

During a terminal illness, a dying person can often make clear his or her choices regarding an autopsy, organ donation, funeral arrangements — including burial or cremation — and legal matters. The reality of dying can be frightening to many people, but with support and encouragement, terminally ill individuals and their families can come to experience the remarkable possibilities that exist during this time in life.

Families, too, have to cope with complicated and painful emotional reactions when someone they love is terminally ill. Everyone copes in his or her own way. In some instances, the bereaved may choose to ignore or deny their loved one's inevitable death and avoid any talk of it, even with the dying person.

Although dying can be traumatic for everyone involved, it's also a time to come to terms with the ending of a life. Dying can be an occasion filled with moments of grateful remembrance and hope-filled meaning.

Discussing death

Most dying people can and should be told of their impending death. Unless a specific cultural tradition requires that the dying person not be told, people with a terminal illness generally want to be informed honestly of their situation. In most cases, a properly informed person is fortified, not undermined. In addition, this may give the dying person an opportunity to tell and see others, put affairs in order, and leave memories, such as a journal.

That doesn't mean it's easy news to give or to digest. Dying people often fear abandonment, humiliation and loneliness at the end of life. Some also fear dying in a hospital or on a machine. Others worry about becoming a burden to loved ones. And some believe that their personal relationships will suffer during this time and that they won't be treated as normal human beings. These concerns are often reinforced if the dying person is deprived of an opportunity to talk about feelings of fear and wonder when faced with death.

A person who's terminally ill may find it easier to talk to someone other than a relative. Most hospitals have a supportive care program with trained staff members who can make it easier to get through this difficult time. In some instances, a social worker or a hospital chaplain can help a dying individual and family members talk about their attitudes toward death.

A dying person and his or her family members often need to discuss practical matters as well. It's helpful to understand the estimated length of the dying process, if it's known. Will it be days, weeks or months? This allows family members to adjust work schedules or consider taking time off. The 1993 Family and Medical Leave Act permits most employees up to 12 weeks of unpaid leave for such a purpose.

The process of dying

Pain, both physical and emotional, is generally a dying person's principal fear. Fortunately, various methods of pain management make it possible to provide relief, with minimal side effects to compromise the comfort and dignity of dying.

Most large hospitals have teams trained in providing relief of pain and other symptoms of serious illness. Called palliative care teams, these teams have expertise in managing symptoms and improving quality of life for individuals and their families during a serious illness or the dying process.

Medications can successfully control most physical pain. Other therapies, such as biofeedback and relaxation therapy, also may be of benefit. These approaches alone may not relieve all of the pain, particularly the profound psychological pain that some people experience when dying.

Common reactions to impending death

When someone is told that he or she has a terminal illness, it's not uncommon for the person to feel a wide range of emotions — shock, anger, denial, depression. A dying individual may feel resentful toward anyone and everyone and robbed of the rest of his or her life. He or she may ask, "Why me?"

Some people attempt to negotiate or postpone the inevitable. There may be an element of bargaining with God or fate.

Often the desired "deal" involves a period of time without pain and discomfort.

Others experience a peaceful acceptance of the importance and value of each day, for however long that may be. With this acceptance comes the ability to explore options and opportunities that present themselves at the end of life and to provide input into decisions that need to be made. This level of acceptance may come after having grappled with various and often-conflicting emotions and experiences. For some, this might come more easily and even automatically.

Chaplains

Hospital and hospice chaplains are often invaluable resources to individuals and families facing death. Chaplains can be from any faith tradition, but when they're ministering in a hospital setting, they're trained to be sensitive to an individual's personal religious beliefs.

In most hospitals, chaplains are unit based, which means that they work with all of the patients and family members in a particular area of the hospital or hospice organization, regardless of a person's religious background.

Sometimes, a chaplain helps put dying individuals in touch with members of their own faith. Other times a chaplain becomes integrally involved in an individual's care, working with doctors, nurses, therapists and social workers. A chaplain becomes familiar with medical procedures and recurring concerns and questions of people in a particular unit.

The hospital environment can create feelings of dependence and helplessness. A person in the hospital may feel alienated from family and friends. He or she may be unwilling to share feelings of guilt or anxiety. A chaplain can help facilitate communication among family members and between a patient and his or her medical staff. In addition, a chaplain often helps terminally ill individuals and family and friends with coping mechanisms to assist them during this difficult time.

Chaplains are trained in dealing with important decisions such as maintaining or discontinuing life-sustaining measures and organ donation.

Perhaps the most important role of a chaplain is to provide comfort in the traditional role of offering individuals and their families a chance to share in the formal rituals of their faith community and to search for answers to difficult questions regarding suffering and dying.

For people with specific cultural or religious convictions related to medical care, a chaplain can serve as a mediator between faith and scientific communities.

Hospice Care

Until the 20th century, most people spent their last days at home, comforted and cared for by family and loved ones. That tradition faded as hospitals became widespread. But recently, renewed interest in this time-honored philosophy has given rise to the field of hospice care.

Hospice care is a program focused on comfort. It's available to individuals with terminal illness. Hospices are based on the philosophy that people near the end of life should be as comfortable as possible and in the setting they prefer. For many people, a hospital — with its busy atmosphere, numerous interruptions and focus on getting better — isn't where they prefer to spend their final days. By definition, hospice care is for people with six months or less to live.

Hospice addresses the two biggest fears that most dying people have — the fear of pain and other debilitating symptoms, and the fear of being alone. Although 80 percent of hospice care is provided at home or in nursing homes, hospice is available wherever an individual may reside, including assisted living facilities. Residential hospices, in which a dying individual can come to the hospice facility to spend his or her last days, also are available in some communities.

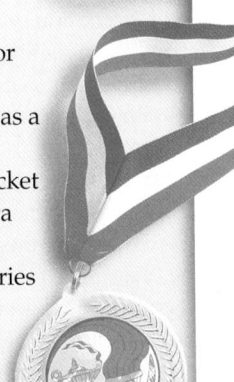

Creating a Memory Box

During a terminal illness, a dying person or family members may want to create a memory box. Gathering items with special meaning and writing down thoughts and wishes can be good ways to create special memories for family members. The box will be treasured for a lifetime, especially by young children of a dying parent.

Find a nice box and consider adding some of the following items:
- Favorite family pictures
- Special trinkets, books, knickknacks or medals
- A distinctive article of clothing, such as a favorite shirt, hat or scarf
- Beloved personal items, such as a pocket watch, reading glasses or a harmonica
- A journal in which everyone writes down his or her thoughts and memories
- An audio or video recording of the individual
- Letters written by the dying individual to family members

By choosing to receive hospice care, a terminally ill person accepts that death is near, and the treatment reflects that. Efforts to prolong life are cut back or stopped, and the emphasis shifts from finding a cure to maximizing the quality of life remaining. Although many people receiving hospice care have cancer, hospice is available to anyone of any age with any type of terminal illness.

Increasing popularity

In 1974, only one hospice program existed in the entire United States. Today, there are more than 4,000. The majority of hospice programs are run by nonprofit, independent organizations. Many are affiliated with hospitals, nursing homes or home health care agencies. Some programs are operated by for-profit organizations.

Hospice programs help individuals and family members meet the physical, emotional, social and spiritual challenges of a terminal illness. Hospice also offers bereavement services that tend to the needs of grieving family members and friends.

What distinguishes hospice is the nature of the care: The goal is to affirm life yet accept death as a normal part of the life process.

Cost

The cost of hospice care varies greatly depending on the length and type of care necessary and an individual's insurance coverage. Medicare — and in some states Medicaid — and most private insurance plans, including managed care organizations, cover hospice care. Coverage may be with benefits beyond standard plans. Medicare and Medicaid provide a package of services that includes professional services, medications related to the terminal illness, and supplies and equipment needed for management of symptoms at the end of life.

Family involvement

The core of hospice is an integrated and cooperative effort by family, friends, and a team of professional and volunteer caregivers to meet a dying person's needs. In some situations, family members or friends are able to provide most or almost all of the care, with support and instruction from the hospice team. Other times, the hospice team plays a more active role.

Normally, a physician trained in hospice medicine leads the hospice team. He or she will work with the primary care physician who has been overseeing your loved one's medical care. A nurse typically coordinates the day-to-day care. Chaplains and social workers are available to counsel individuals and families and to make sure emotional, spiritual and social needs are being addressed. Trained volunteers perform a wide variety of tasks as needed, such as providing companionship, doing light housekeeping, preparing meals and running errands.

Palliative Care

Modern-day palliative care grew out of the hospice movement, and it shares many of the same goals. The main difference between palliative care and hospice care is time.

Hospice care is for people with six months or less to live. Palliative care provides the greatest benefit when it's integrated early in the care of an individual with a serious illness. In fact, the current standard of care for all individuals diagnosed with incurable cancer is to integrate palliative care at the moment of diagnosis.

In practice, the two are quite similar. Both seek to include the active participation of family and friends in end-of-life care. The palliative care team encourages, and even may facilitate, open communication among family members and between the family and the medical team. This includes frank discussions of treatment options and disease progression. Emphasis is also placed on attending to the emotional, spiritual and psychological needs of family and friends. Like hospice care, palliative care involves not only doctors but also social workers and nurses.

Research shows that palliative care has a number of benefits:

- Less time in the hospital
- More time at home among friends and family
- Higher likelihood of dying at a place of one's own choosing
- Increased satisfaction with medical care
- Better symptom control, including acute and chronic pain
- Reduction in the cost of care

The National Hospice and Palliative Care Organization can provide information on hospice care available in your region.

Approaching Death

New technologies have forced a new definition of death. Today, doctors can keep people alive in circumstances that would have been impossible in the past. Most states recognize that a person is legally dead when he or she has experienced irreversible cessation of circulation and respiration or irreversible cessation and function of the entire brain, including the brainstem, which controls breathing.

Only a few years ago, anyone who had lost consciousness, was unable to breathe and had no heartbeat was considered dead. Now, in some instances, life-support systems can revive an individual not breathing and with no heartbeat and, in part, continue to support or replace some of these necessary functions. In addition, doctors often are able to maintain heart or lung function even when the brain ceases to function.

The remarkable ability to sustain life brings with it certain ethical, legal and medical concerns, discussed earlier in this chapter.

The moment of death

Caretakers' actions and attitudes, especially those of loved ones, can have a strong influence on the dying experience. For example, dying people frequently request that they not be left alone. They may fear not only the moment of death with its uncertainties but also abandonment. Offering consolation and reassurance at these moments may be difficult but necessary.

Many dying people are also comforted by their faith traditions and by having members of their faith community with them in their final moments.

Usually, there are signs that the moment of death is near. The dying person may become fidgety or restless and have irregular breathing. In such circumstances a doctor may provide medications or oxygen to make the person more comfortable. In some cases, the dying person's breathing can be eased if he or she is placed in a sitting position or allowed to lie on one side with a pillow under the head.

Even though the dying person may not be able to communicate, he or she often can hear much of what's being said. Despite any sense of powerlessness you may feel, your very presence can be all of the comfort a dying person seeks. Simply hold the person's hand or give him or her a hug. Physical contact is often soothing. If you don't know what to say, remember that silence can be golden.

The formalities of death

Death is a legal event that calls for several formalities.

The death certificate

Before a burial or cremation can take place, a medical death certificate must be obtained that shows the cause of death and formally registers the death. A death certificate is signed by a licensed physician. If a doctor has examined or treated a dying individual regularly or shortly before death, he or she generally isn't obliged to examine the body before signing the certificate. Sometimes, a medical examiner or coroner, rather than a physician, states the cause of death and signs the certificate.

In some instances, an autopsy may be ordered, or it may be requested by the family. An autopsy provides more information about a person's illness. It may be required by law if the death resulted from an accident, is unexpected and unexplained, or is the result of a suspected homicide or suicide. After such matters are resolved, the family usually works with a funeral home on any final arrangements.

Funeral arrangements

If a loved one has died, a funeral director can be helpful in making virtually all of your decisions concerning funeral and burial arrangements. However, people who knew they were dying may have made these decisions with their family while they were still able to do so.

The funeral director will come to the deceased's home, hospital or nursing home to remove the body and take it to the funeral home. Later, members of the family meet with the funeral director to discuss funeral arrangements. Federal law requires that funeral homes provide consumers with itemized price lists of products and services to ensure that people pay for only what they want or need.

Family members should make it quite clear how elaborate or simple they want the funeral to be and how the details are to be handled. Because these are emotionally dif-

ficult times, you may want to seek help in making these decisions from someone who isn't personally involved, such as a member of the clergy, a close friend or an attorney.

Funeral decisions include the type and location of the funeral service and whether the remains are to be buried, cremated or both.

Funeral ceremonies can be held at the funeral home or a place of worship or both. If your family has a religious affiliation, the funeral director can contact your clergy member or recommend a member of the clergy or an appropriate authority. Fees and terms of payment are made with the funeral director at the time funeral arrangements are made. Usually, payment isn't required in advance, but these expenses become the first legal obligation of the estate of the deceased.

The estate

After the funeral, a probate judge may need to designate the executor or personal representative of the estate. This is often a member of the family, family attorney or close friend. The executor is responsible for the financial affairs of the deceased, which may include the funeral expenses.

After all payments are made, any remaining assets are distributed according to the deceased's will or the laws of the state in which the person lived. Procedures may vary from state to state. Some terminally ill people like to provide guidance to their families regarding estate and funeral matters to lessen the sense of burden that family members may feel.

The autopsy decision

Autopsy comes from Greek words meaning "to see with one's own eyes." An autopsy is a detailed examination of a deceased person's body to determine the cause of death. An autopsy is performed by a medical doctor who specializes in the nature of disease (pathologist). He or she then reports the findings to the attending doctor. On request, the doctor discusses the findings with the family.

In the 1940s, an autopsy was performed after about half the hospital deaths. Now less than 10 percent of people who die are autopsied. One reason for the decline is that modern diagnostic measures performed on terminally ill individuals often make it clear what's causing them to die.

Although their use has declined, autopsies play an important role in medical science, and can provide useful information for surviving family members and doctors.

Hereditary disorders
An autopsy may reveal conditions that could affect children and siblings. For example, if polycystic kidney disease is found, close relatives of childbearing age may want genetic counseling to determine if they're at risk of passing on the disease to their children. An autopsy can also confirm some illnesses that have been diagnosed based on behavior alone, such as Alzheimer's disease.

Emotional security
Family members often feel that they could have done something to prevent the death of a loved one. In the case of a fatal heart attack, they might berate themselves for not insisting that their loved one take it easier. An autopsy may reveal that the person had a pre-existing heart condition that could have taken his or her life at any time — regardless of whether the person "took it easy."

Insurance settlements
Establishing the cause of death can help resolve disputes that may affect the benefits that survivors receive. For example, if a person with a heart problem dies from a fall, insurance benefits may vary depending on whether the death was accidental or the result of heart disease.

Benefits to medical science
Much of what researchers and doctors know about diseases, including statistical information, was discovered or confirmed through autopsies. Advances in medical knowledge depend in part on the study of human tissue removed at autopsy. Pathological observations reveal a great deal about human disease.

For example, such data helped to confirm the association between cigarette smoking and lung cancer. Autopsies also helped doctors discover the nature and character of conditions such as hyperparathyroidism and viral hepatitis. And they revealed the effects of toxic chemicals and other industrial hazards on body organs.

Quality assurance
Doctors often use autopsy data to assess their accuracy in diagnosis and treatment. Autopsy findings also can help assess the overall quality of care in a hospital and community.

Vital statistics
Causes of death keep changing. Deaths from infectious diseases are less common today than years ago, but degenerative illnesses are taking a greater toll. Public health officials use information from autopsies to monitor such trends. Death statistics influence government spending for health care, the enactment of safety standards and the design of medical equipment.

Emerging illness
Early medical understanding of illness such as AIDS, Legionnaires' disease and toxic shock syndrome all came from autopsy studies.

Bereavement

Humans experience many losses throughout life. The longer people live, the more losses they suffer. Bereavement is the natural response to a loss. Bereavement usually refers to feelings after the loss of a loved one — usually through death, but also after the dissolution of a relationship.

The death of a loved one is never easy to accept, and a sudden loss can be especially distressing. However, a long, terminal illness before a death can be emotionally, physically and financially draining.

To protect yourself from grief-related illness, take care of your own health. Monitor any medical problems you had before the loss, and seek professional help if new symptoms develop. Your ability to adapt to the stress of a death can influence your overall health. Severe or prolonged grief that disrupts daily routines or lifestyles can contribute to illnesses such as depression and alcoholism.

Although cultural norms for mourning determine behavior to some degree, there's no single right way to grieve. Nor is there a fixed timetable. Some people seem to return to normal emotions and activities within a month, but for others bereavement is measured in years rather than weeks or months.

People cope with their grief in different ways. Some people grieve openly, others privately. And it's not always evident that someone is grieving. During your bereavement, don't be afraid to seek help from clergy, friends and counselors. And remember that it's entirely appropriate — and essential for both your mental and physical health — to express your emotions. Healthy mourning is the process that helps you accept your loss so that you can go on with your life. Suppressing your emotions through excess activity, work, alcohol or drugs can prolong the mourning process.

Arranging for an autopsy

Autopsies are often required by state or local law when death results from an accident, is unexpected or unexplained, or is a suspected homicide or suicide. Otherwise, autopsies require the permission of the next of kin.

When you sign an autopsy consent form, you can authorize a limited autopsy, which restricts the procedure to specific parts of the body, or a more thorough autopsy. A disadvantage of a limited autopsy is that it limits the amount of useful information the procedure provides and may leave some questions unanswered. Consent forms generally permit removal of internal organs and tissue.

There are many misconceptions about autopsy and tissue removal. In many cases, families are reluctant to permit an autopsy, believing that the procedure is degrading or that the deceased has "suffered enough." Another common misconception about autopsy is that it will disfigure the body. The truth is, an autopsy that's performed properly won't disfigure the body. At an open casket funeral service, observers won't be able to tell if an autopsy was performed. Autopsies don't interfere with embalming of the body, and the procedure doesn't need to delay the funeral.

In most instances, when you grant permission for an elective autopsy, the bill will be paid by the hospital. Medicare won't pay for the procedure. However, if the death occurs outside a hospital and family members request an autopsy, they usually must pay for it.

A dying individual who would like an autopsy performed after his or her death should make a provision for it in his or her advance directive and notify loved ones of the provision. This can help to spare loved ones the burden of having to make this decision during a time of grief. ■

Visual Guide: Anatomy and Common Disorders

Bones and Joints

There are approximately 206 bones in your body. All of them are alive and continually changing, providing mobility, support and protection for your body. Some bones contain marrow, a soft core that manufactures blood cells. Ends of bone that meet at a joint are cushioned with a layer of cartilage, which absorbs shock or weight involved in movement. Ligaments bind the joint together, connecting bone to bone.

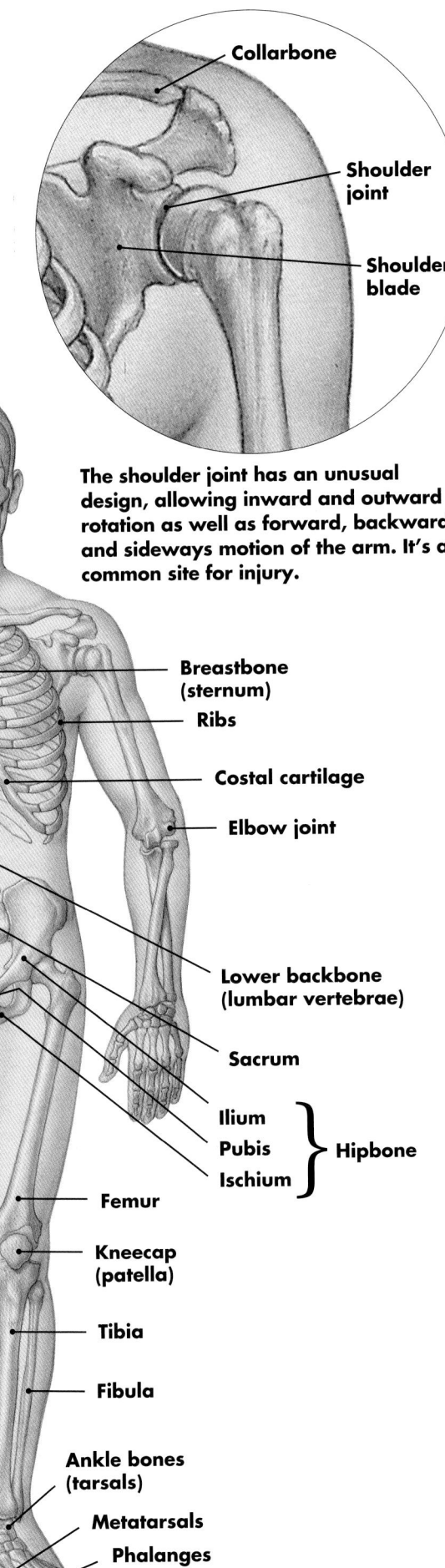

Collarbone

Shoulder joint

Shoulder blade

The shoulder joint has an unusual design, allowing inward and outward rotation as well as forward, backward and sideways motion of the arm. It's a common site for injury.

Skull

Cervical vertebrae

Collarbone (clavicle)

Shoulder joint

Shoulder blade (scapula)

Humerus

Radius

Ulna

Wrist bones (carpals)

Metacarpals

Phalanges

Breastbone (sternum)

Ribs

Costal cartilage

Elbow joint

Lower backbone (lumbar vertebrae)

Sacrum

Ilium

Pubis } **Hipbone**

Ischium

Femur

Kneecap

Tibia

The knee joint has a hinge design, allowing bending (flexion) and straightening (extension) of the leg. It is also a common location for injury.

Femur

Kneecap (patella)

Tibia

Fibula

Ankle bones (tarsals)

Metatarsals

Phalanges

Your skull and vertebrae protect your brain and spinal cord. A column of bones called vertebrae makes up the spine. In between the vertebrae are spongy structures called disks. The vertebrae and disks are held together by a network of ligaments.

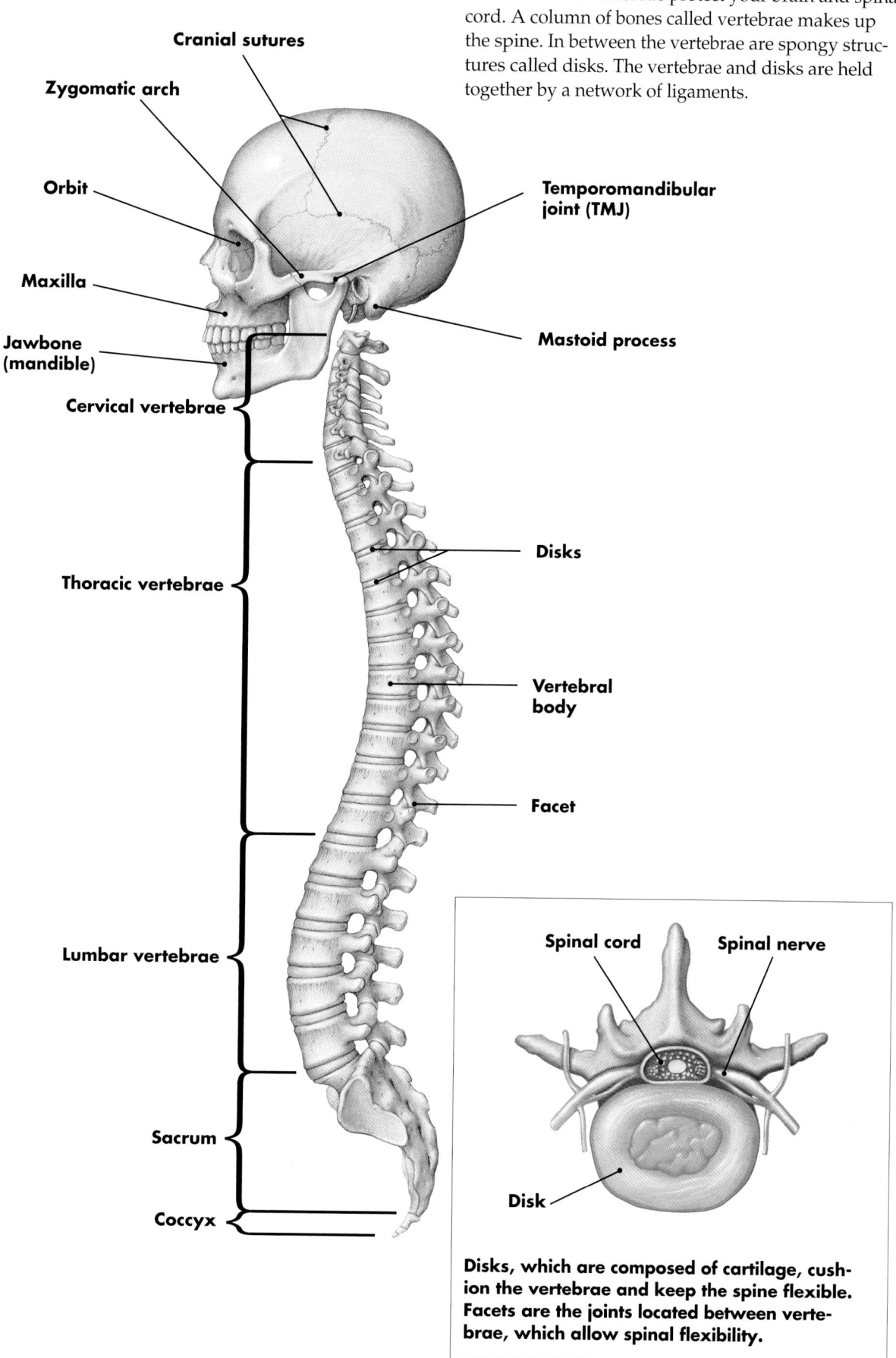

Cranial sutures

Zygomatic arch

Orbit

Maxilla

Jawbone (mandible)

Cervical vertebrae

Thoracic vertebrae

Lumbar vertebrae

Sacrum

Coccyx

Temporomandibular joint (TMJ)

Mastoid process

Disks

Vertebral body

Facet

Spinal cord

Spinal nerve

Disk

Disks, which are composed of cartilage, cushion the vertebrae and keep the spine flexible. Facets are the joints located between vertebrae, which allow spinal flexibility.

Anatomy and Common Disorders **355**

Muscles

The superficial and deep muscles of the musculoskeletal system contract to produce movement at the joints. Virtually all of these muscles are paired. For example, contraction of the biceps muscles causes the forearm to flex, whereas contraction of the opposing triceps muscles causes the forearm to extend. Many muscles are connected to bones by tendons.

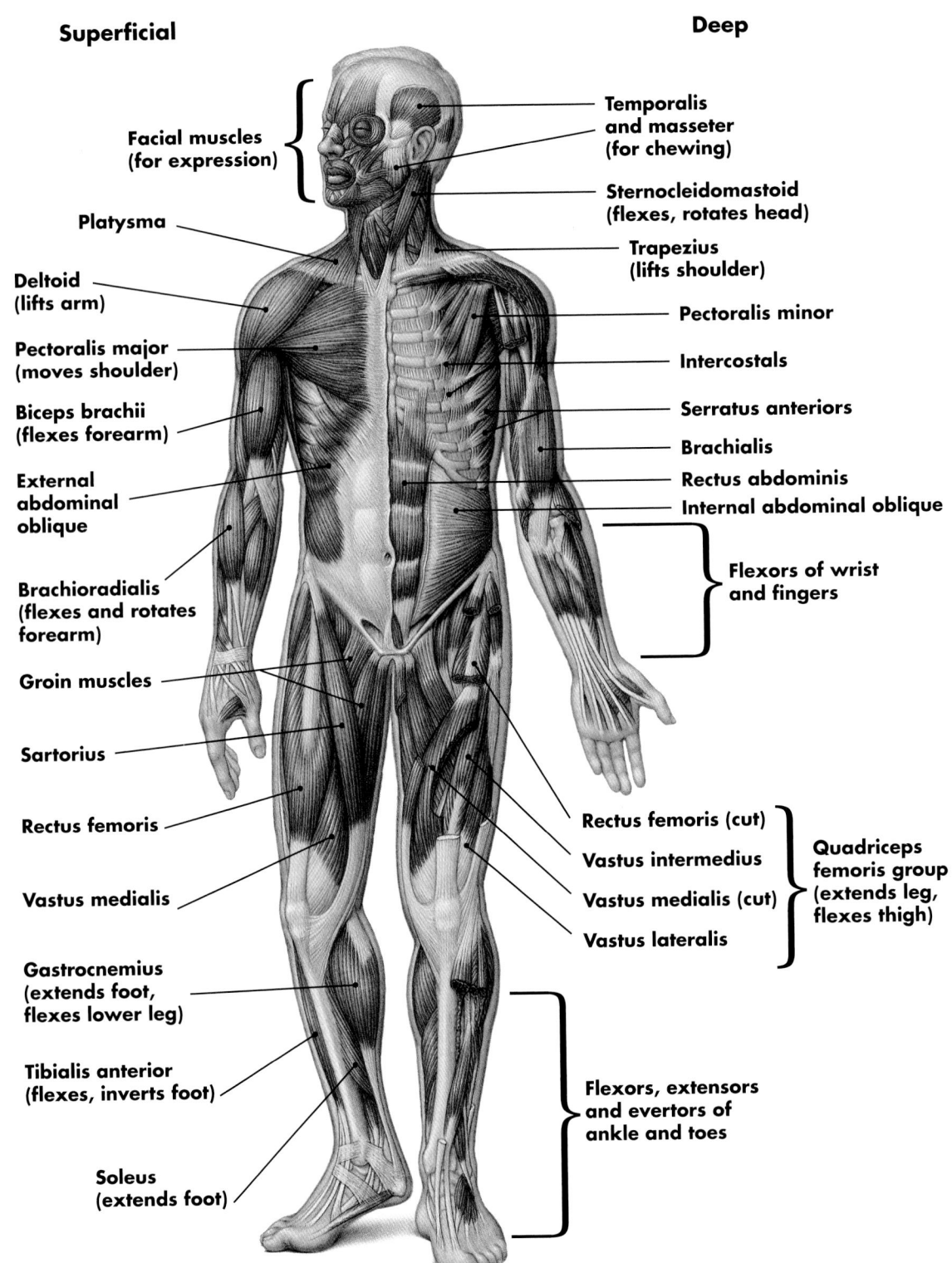

Superficial

Deep

Facial muscles (for expression)

Platysma

Deltoid (lifts arm)

Pectoralis major (moves shoulder)

Biceps brachii (flexes forearm)

External abdominal oblique

Brachioradialis (flexes and rotates forearm)

Groin muscles

Sartorius

Rectus femoris

Vastus medialis

Gastrocnemius (extends foot, flexes lower leg)

Tibialis anterior (flexes, inverts foot)

Soleus (extends foot)

Temporalis and masseter (for chewing)

Sternocleidomastoid (flexes, rotates head)

Trapezius (lifts shoulder)

Pectoralis minor

Intercostals

Serratus anteriors

Brachialis

Rectus abdominis

Internal abdominal oblique

Flexors of wrist and fingers

Rectus femoris (cut)

Vastus intermedius

Vastus medialis (cut)

Vastus lateralis

Quadriceps femoris group (extends leg, flexes thigh)

Flexors, extensors and evertors of ankle and toes

Superficial   **Deep**

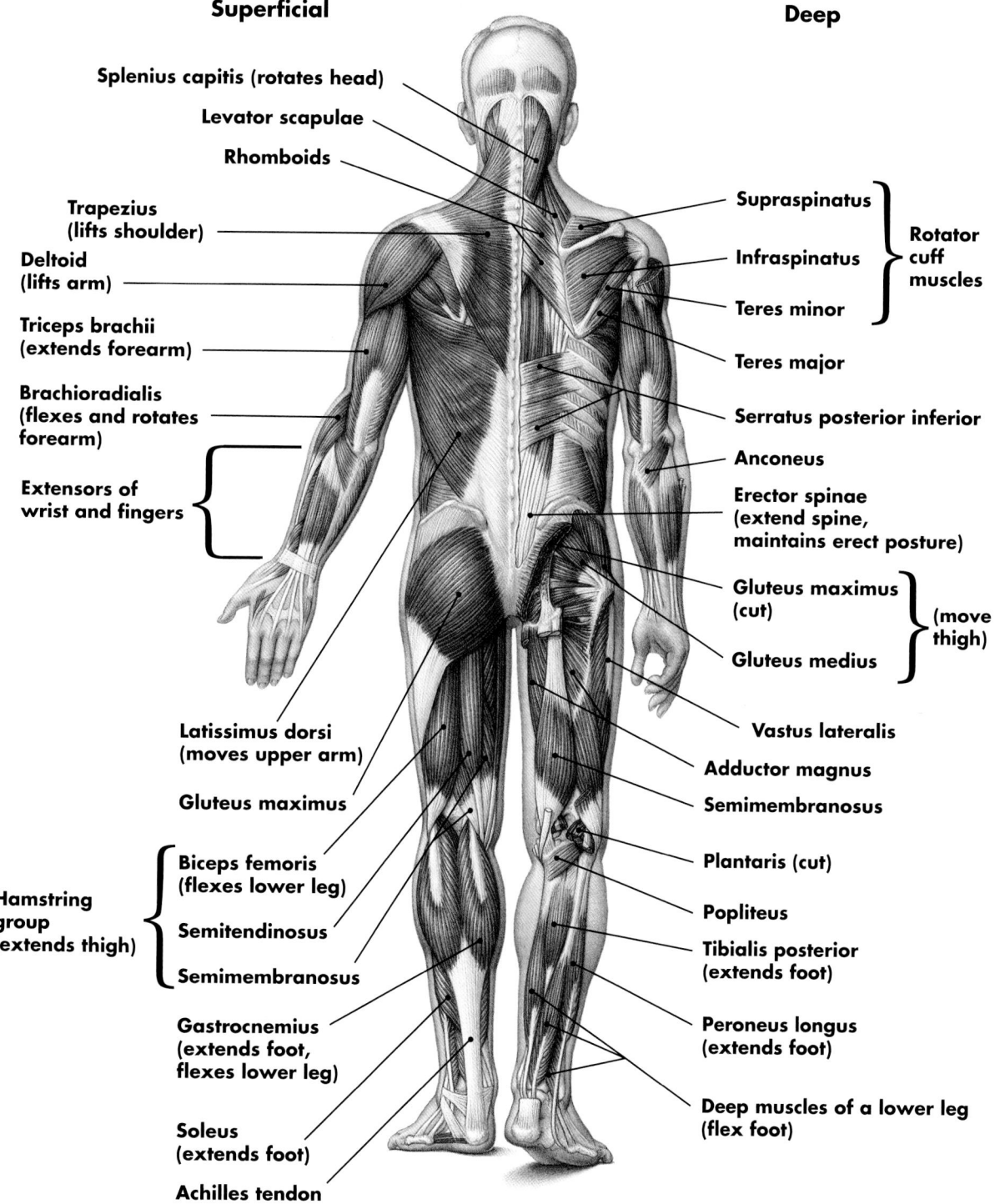

Splenius capitis (rotates head)

Levator scapulae

Rhomboids

Trapezius
(lifts shoulder)

Deltoid
(lifts arm)

Triceps brachii
(extends forearm)

Brachioradialis
(flexes and rotates
forearm)

Extensors of
wrist and fingers

Latissimus dorsi
(moves upper arm)

Gluteus maximus

Hamstring
group
(extends thigh)

Biceps femoris
(flexes lower leg)

Semitendinosus

Semimembranosus

Gastrocnemius
(extends foot,
flexes lower leg)

Soleus
(extends foot)

Achilles tendon

Supraspinatus

Infraspinatus   Rotator
                    cuff
                    muscles
Teres minor

Teres major

Serratus posterior inferior

Anconeus

Erector spinae
(extend spine,
maintains erect posture)

Gluteus maximus
(cut)   (move
                        thigh)
Gluteus medius

Vastus lateralis

Adductor magnus

Semimembranosus

Plantaris (cut)

Popliteus

Tibialis posterior
(extends foot)

Peroneus longus
(extends foot)

Deep muscles of a lower leg
(flex foot)

Organs

Protected by skin and bones, the body's internal organs function day and night, serving the body's needs. The insets on the right show how the body's internal organs appear on computerized tomography (CT) scans.

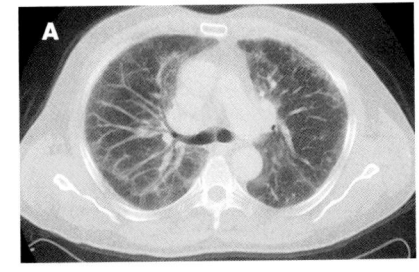

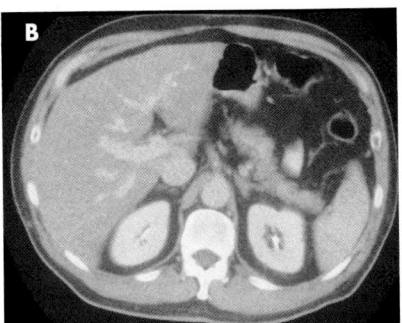

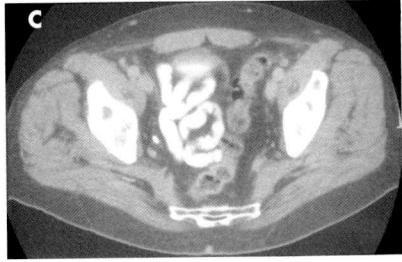

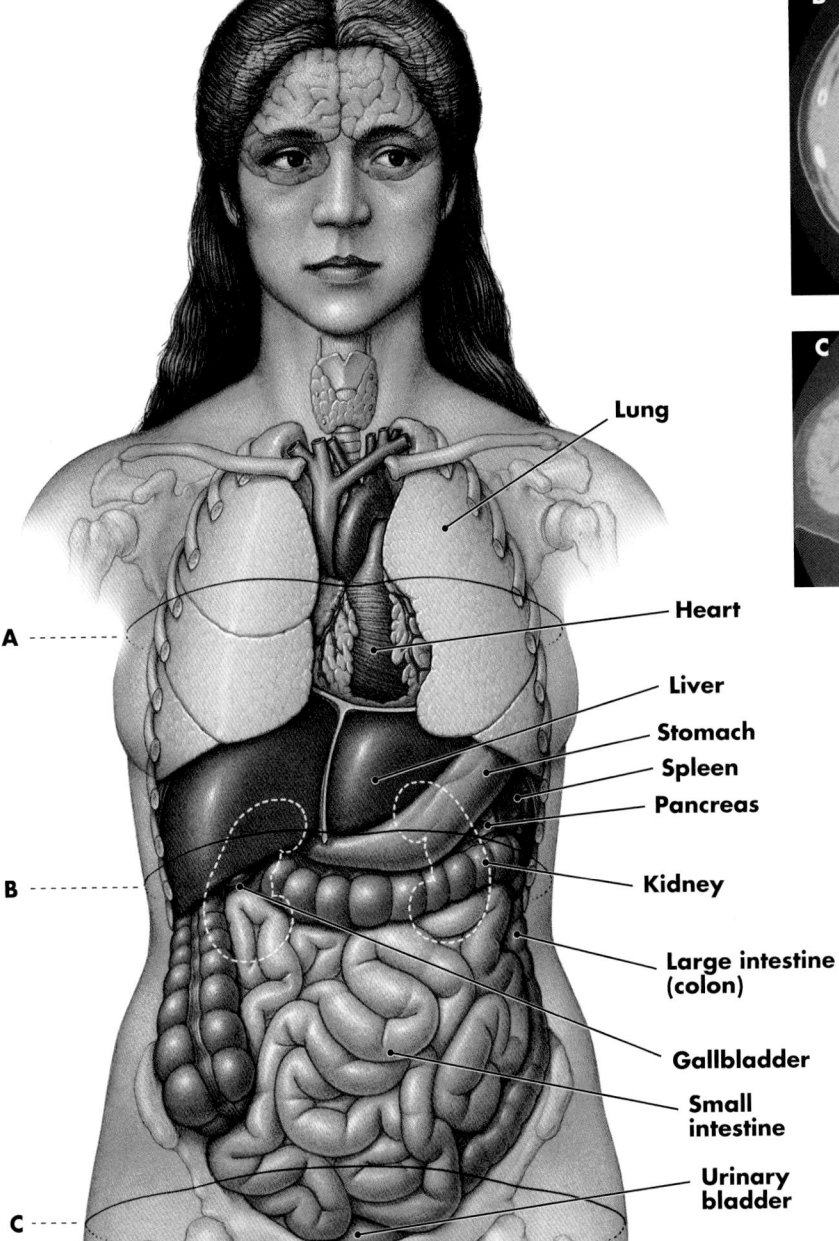

Lung

Heart

Liver

Stomach

Spleen

Pancreas

Kidney

Large intestine (colon)

Gallbladder

Small intestine

Urinary bladder

A

B

C

Digestive System

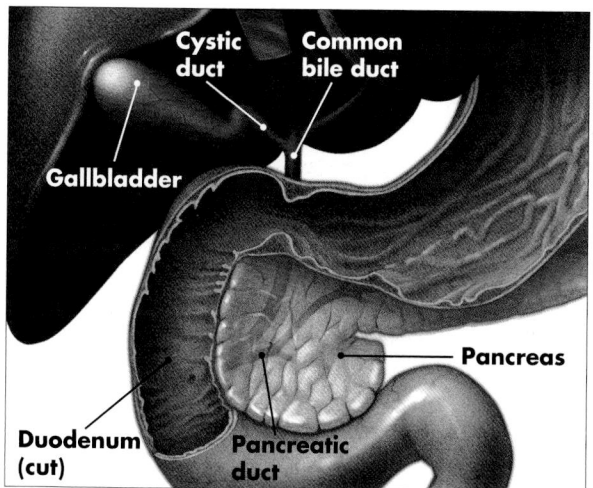

Cystic duct

Common bile duct

Gallbladder

Pancreas

Duodenum (cut)

Pancreatic duct

Digestion begins when food enters the mouth. Food is broken down by chewing and salivary gland enzymes. Once swallowed, wavelike muscular contractions (peristalsis) move the food through the digestive tract. Food nutrients are absorbed and waste products eliminated.

The small intestine is the body's main digestive organ. Digestive juices are released into the upper portion of the small intestine (duodenum) from the pancreas, liver and gallbladder by way of a system of tiny ducts.

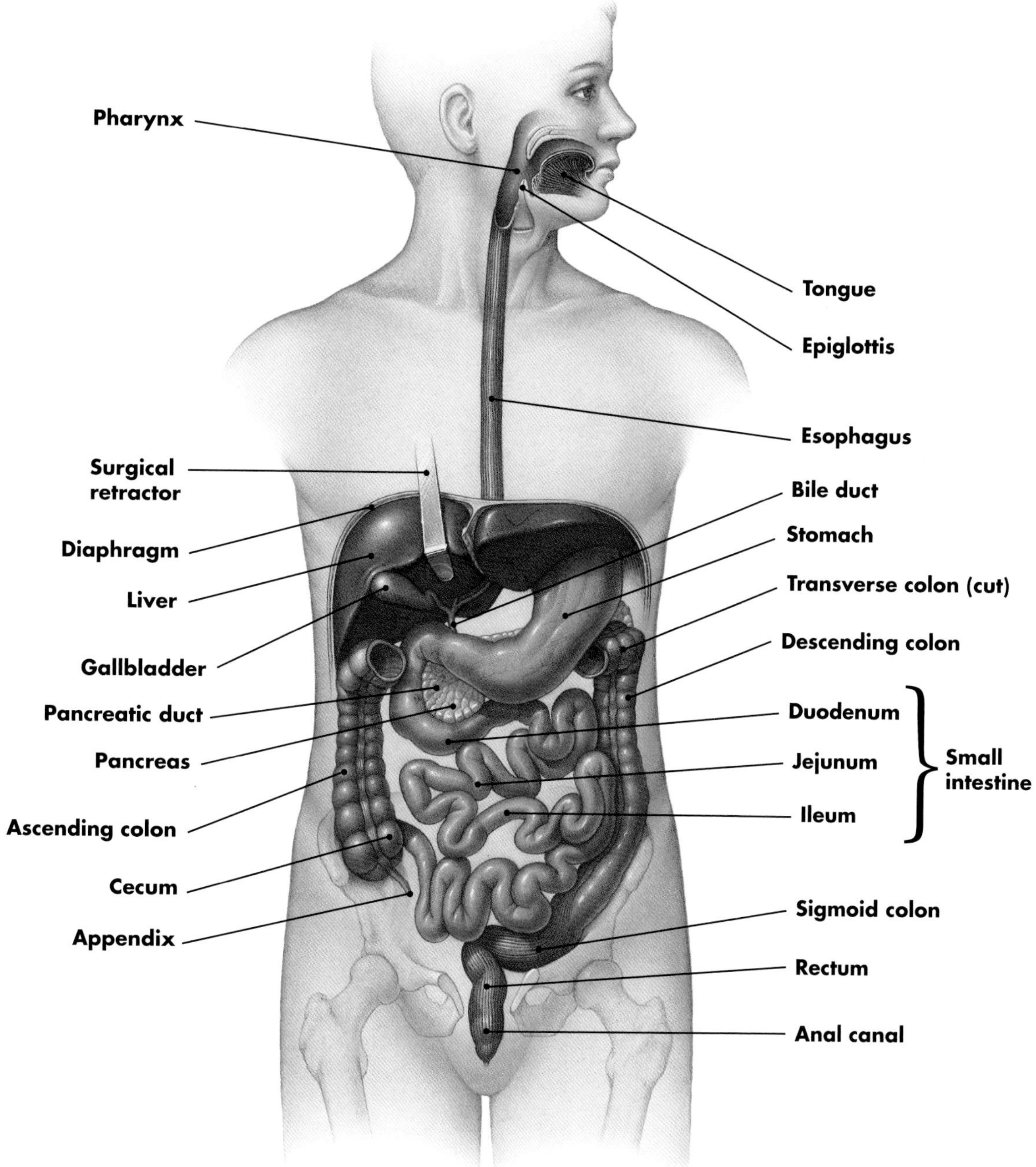

Pharynx

Tongue

Epiglottis

Esophagus

Surgical retractor

Diaphragm

Liver

Gallbladder

Pancreatic duct

Pancreas

Ascending colon

Cecum

Appendix

Bile duct

Stomach

Transverse colon (cut)

Descending colon

Duodenum

Jejunum — **Small intestine**

Ileum

Sigmoid colon

Rectum

Anal canal

Heart and Blood Vessels

The heart and blood vessels supply body tissues with life-sustaining oxygen and nutrients. The heart pumps blood into the arteries (red). The major arteries that emerge from the heart are the aorta and pulmonary arteries. Veins (blue) return blood to the heart. The large veins that enter the heart are the superior vena cava, inferior vena cava and the pulmonary veins.

The coronary arteries supply nourishing blood to the heart muscle itself. Coronary arteries emerge from the aorta and extend over the surface of the heart. Blood returns from the heart muscle through coronary veins.

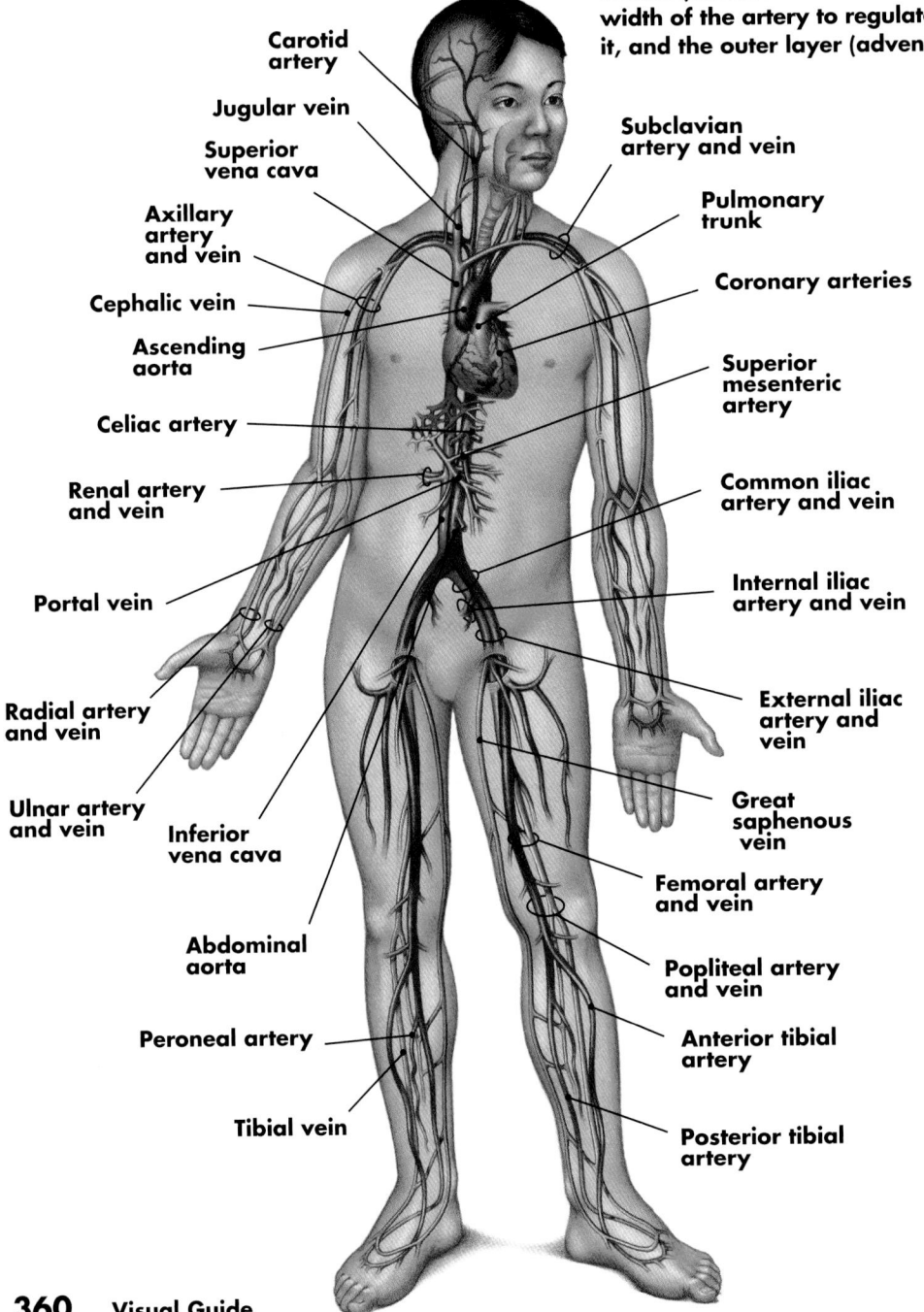

Adventitia (outer layer)

Tunica media vasorum (muscle layer)

Endothelium (inner lining)

The artery wall consists of three layers: the smooth inner lining (endothelium), the middle layer of muscle (tunica media vasorum) that controls the width of the artery to regulate blood flow through it, and the outer layer (adventitia).

Carotid artery

Jugular vein

Superior vena cava

Axillary artery and vein

Cephalic vein

Ascending aorta

Celiac artery

Renal artery and vein

Portal vein

Radial artery and vein

Ulnar artery and vein

Inferior vena cava

Abdominal aorta

Peroneal artery

Tibial vein

Subclavian artery and vein

Pulmonary trunk

Coronary arteries

Superior mesenteric artery

Common iliac artery and vein

Internal iliac artery and vein

External iliac artery and vein

Great saphenous vein

Femoral artery and vein

Popliteal artery and vein

Anterior tibial artery

Posterior tibial artery

Contraction (Systole)

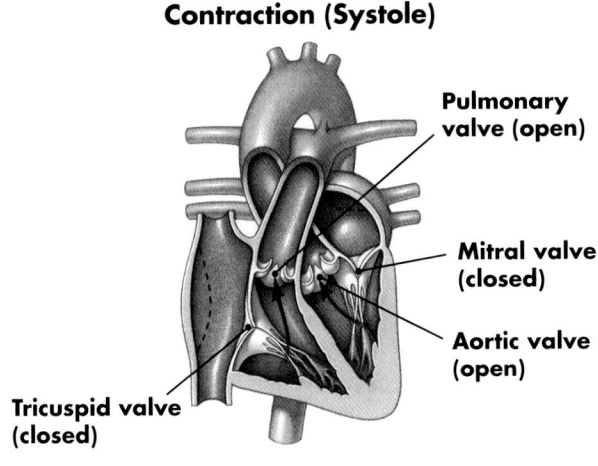

Pulmonary valve (open)

Mitral valve (closed)

Aortic valve (open)

Tricuspid valve (closed)

Relaxation (Diastole)

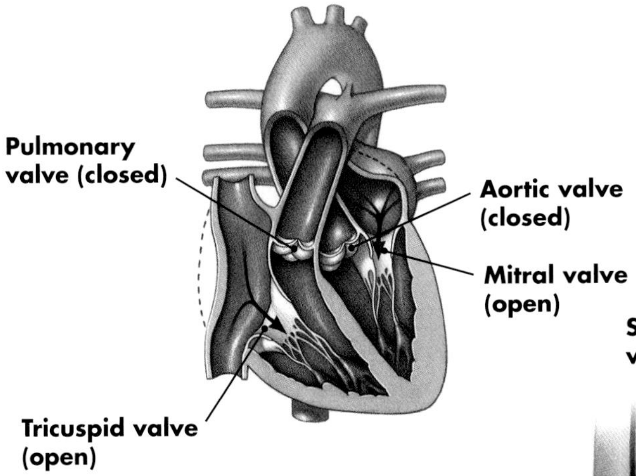

Pulmonary valve (closed)

Aortic valve (closed)

Mitral valve (open)

Tricuspid valve (open)

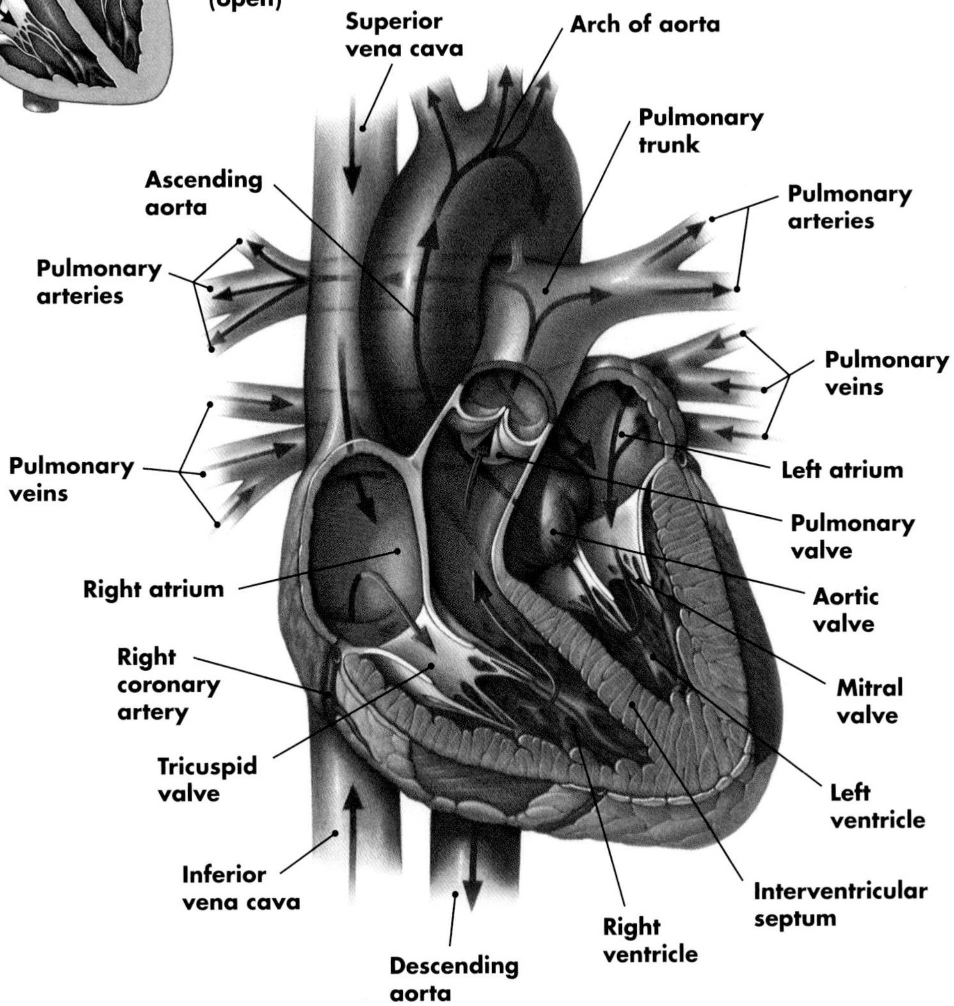

The heart has four chambers connected by valves. Blood from the veins flows through the superior and inferior vena cava into the right atrium, and then through the tricuspid valve into the right ventricle. The right ventricle pumps blood through the pulmonary valve and into the lungs via the pulmonary arteries. Re-oxygenated blood from the lungs enters the left atrium via the pulmonary veins and flows through the mitral valve into the left ventricle. The left ventricle pumps the blood through the aorta for delivery to body tissues.

Valves keep blood flowing through the heart in one direction. As the ventricles relax (diastole), pressure within them decreases. The mitral and tricuspid valves are forced open, allowing blood to flow from the atria into the ventricles. The aortic and pulmonary valves are closed to prevent the return of blood pumped out on the previous beat. During contraction (systole), pressure pushes the aortic and pulmonary valves open, and the mitral and tricuspid valves are forced shut.

Superior vena cava

Arch of aorta

Pulmonary trunk

Ascending aorta

Pulmonary arteries

Pulmonary arteries

Pulmonary veins

Pulmonary veins

Left atrium

Pulmonary valve

Right atrium

Aortic valve

Right coronary artery

Mitral valve

Tricuspid valve

Left ventricle

Inferior vena cava

Interventricular septum

Descending aorta

Right ventricle

Anatomy and Common Disorders   **361**

Lungs

The lungs supply oxygen to blood and remove carbon dioxide from it. This exchange takes place in tiny air sacs called alveoli. Oxygen passes from the air in the alveoli into the blood. The oxygenated blood flows through tiny capillaries surrounding the alveoli into the pulmonary veins. The pulmonary arteries carry the blood to the lungs. Pulmonary veins return the blood to the heart.

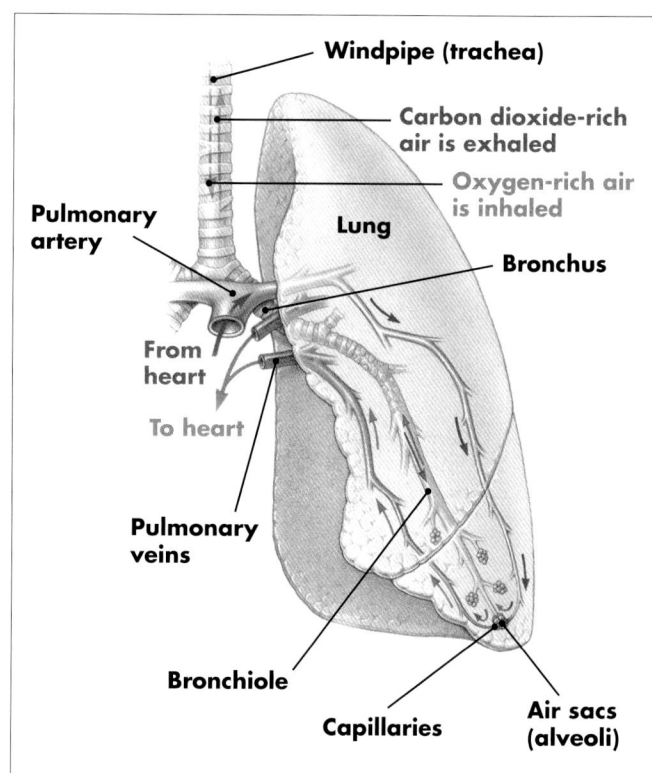

Windpipe (trachea)

Carbon dioxide-rich air is exhaled

Oxygen-rich air is inhaled

Pulmonary artery

Lung

Bronchus

From heart

To heart

Pulmonary veins

Bronchiole

Capillaries

Air sacs (alveoli)

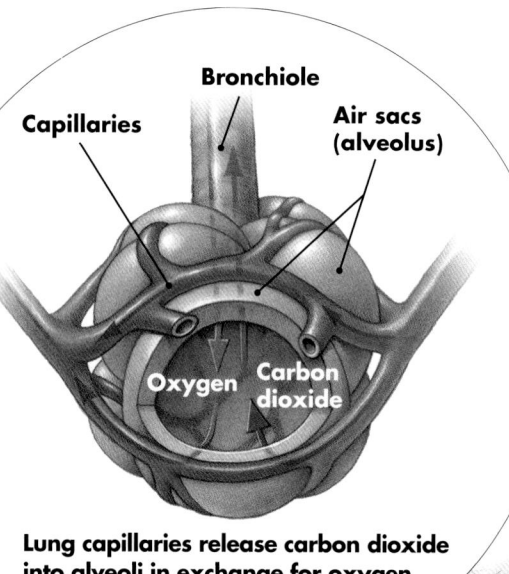

Bronchiole

Capillaries

Air sacs (alveolus)

Oxygen

Carbon dioxide

Lung capillaries release carbon dioxide into alveoli in exchange for oxygen.

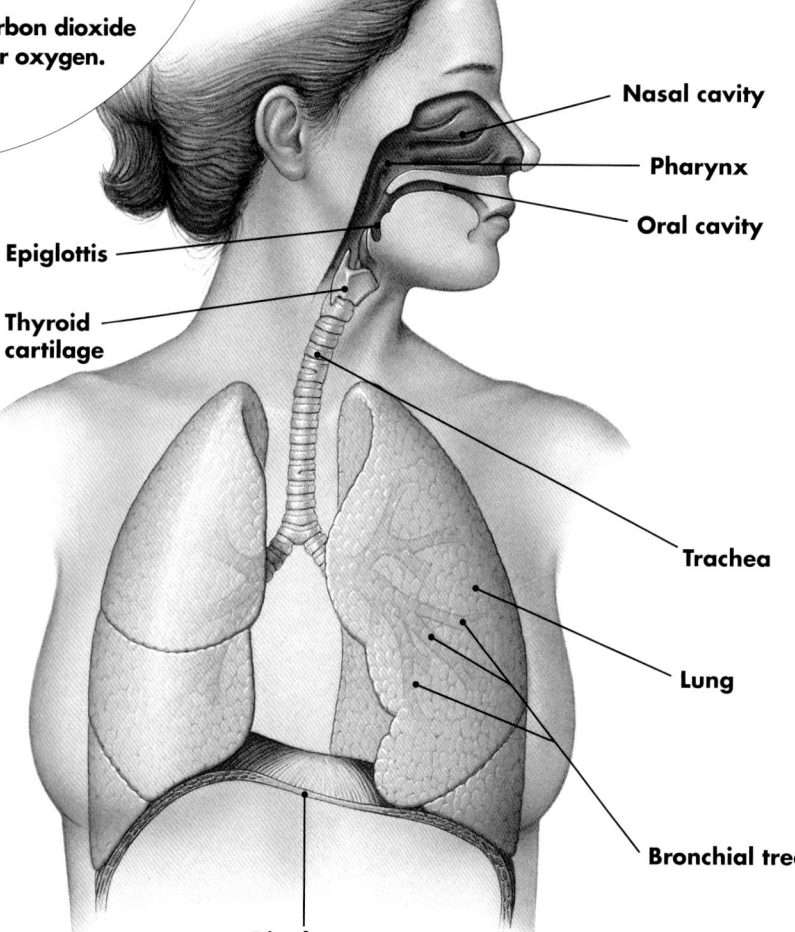

Nasal cavity

Pharynx

Oral cavity

Epiglottis

Thyroid cartilage

Trachea

Lung

Bronchial tree

Diaphragm

Endocrine Glands

The endocrine glands control many body activities as well as the response of body systems to usual and stressful events. The glands secrete hormones into the bloodstream. These chemical messengers deliver instructions to organs and tissues.

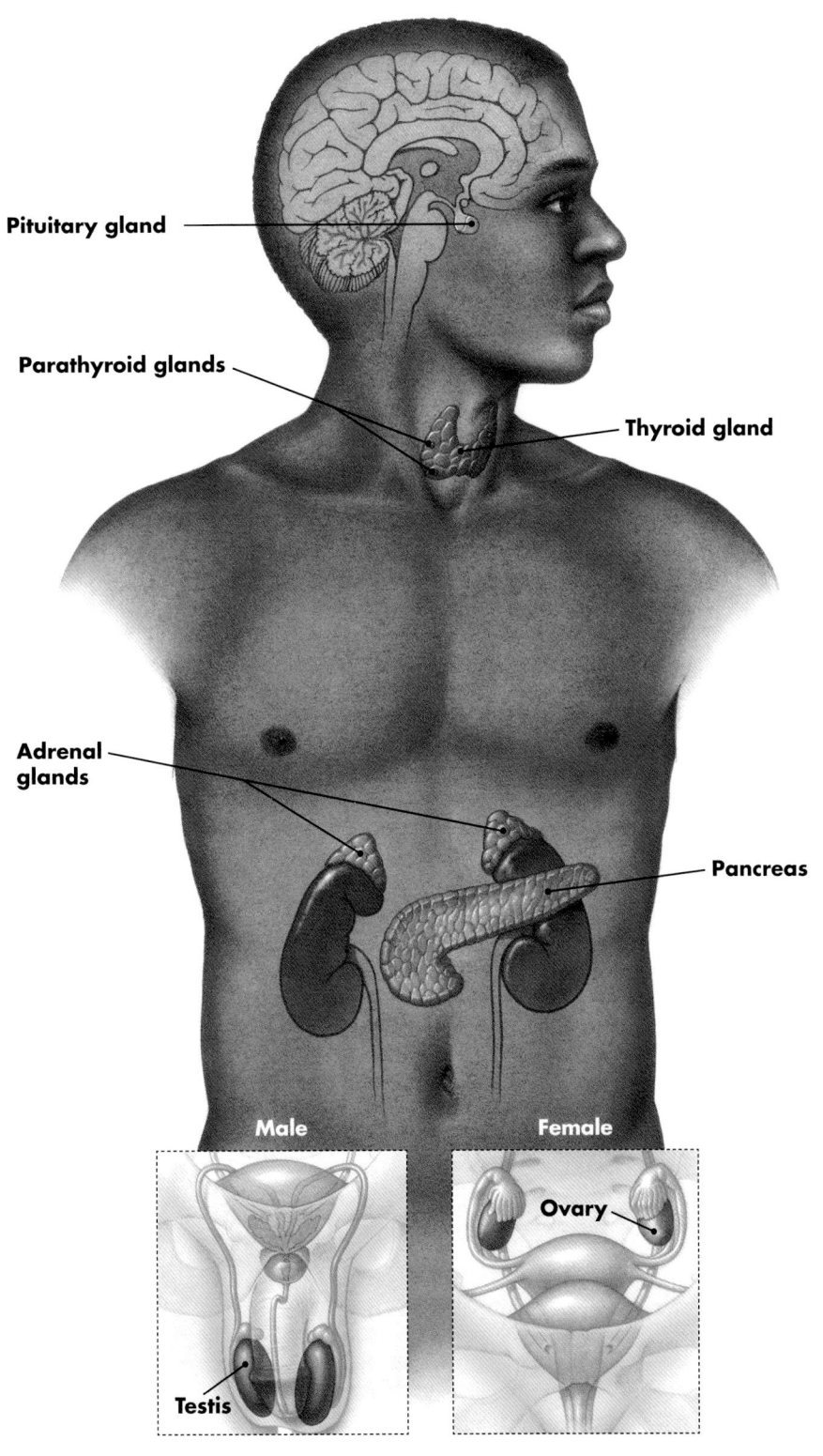

Pituitary gland

Parathyroid glands

Thyroid gland

Adrenal glands

Pancreas

Male

Female

Ovary

Testis

Breast and Female Reproductive Organs

The female breast produces milk to feed infants. Each breast has between 15 and 20 sections (lobes). Each lobe is made up of many smaller structures (lobules) that end in tiny bulbs that can produce milk. The lobes, lobules and bulbs are linked by a network of thin tubes (ducts). Ducts carry milk from the bulbs to the dark area of skin in the center of the breast (areola), where it's expressed from the nipple.

Female reproductive organs include the ovaries, which release an egg at ovulation, the fallopian tubes, where an egg may meet with the sperm, and the uterus, where the fertilized egg implants itself and grows into a fetus. The reproductive organs are located near the bladder and the urethra.

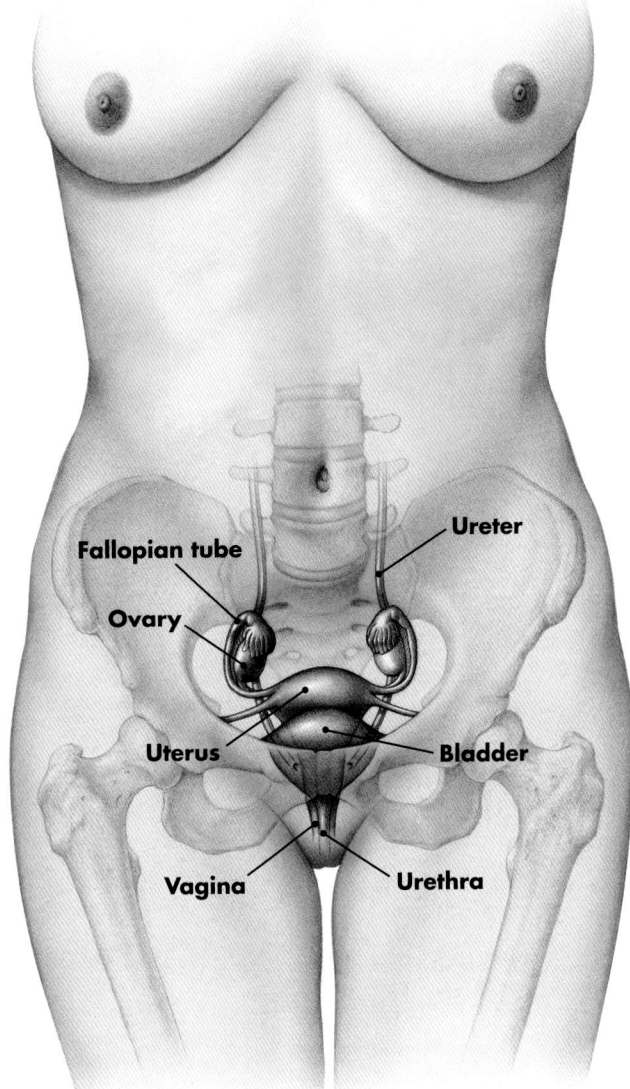

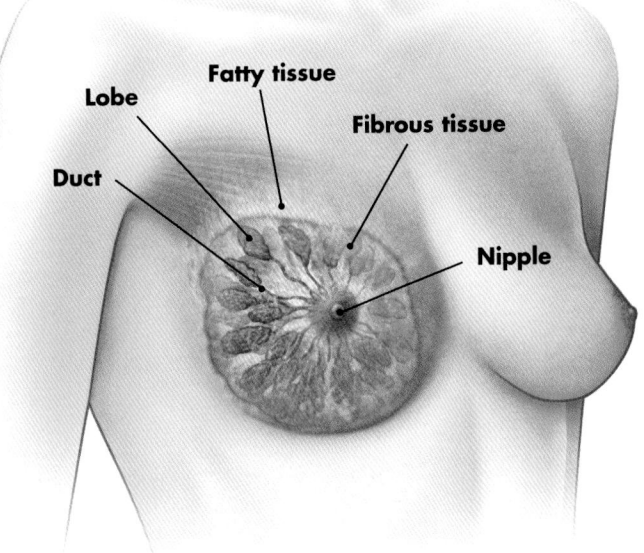

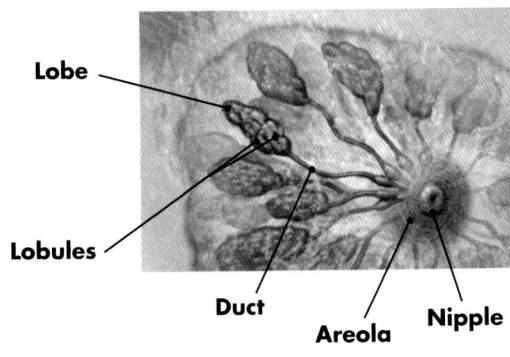

Male Reproductive Organs and Urinary Tract

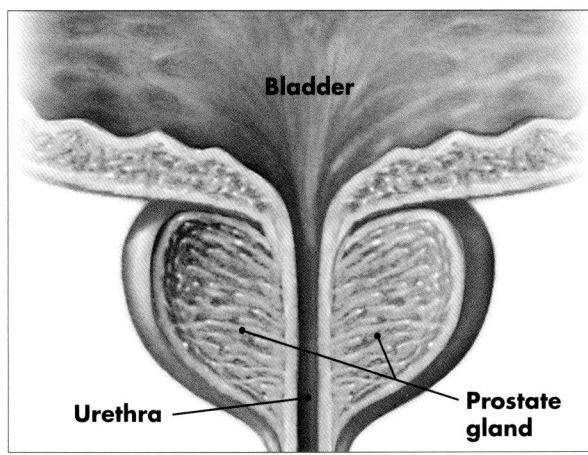

Bladder

Urethra

Prostate gland

The primary function of the prostate gland is to produce most of the fluid in semen. Tiny ducts within the prostate convey the fluid to the urethra, where it mixes with sperm. About the size of a walnut, the prostate gland is located just below the bladder, and it surrounds the top portion of the urethra.

Male reproductive organs include the testicles, where sperm are produced, the epididymides and vasa deferentia, which transport sperm into the seminal vesicles and prostate gland. Fluids from the seminal vesicles and prostate gland are mixed with the sperm and ejaculated as semen through the urethra.

In men, the urethra serves both the reproductive and urinary systems — transporting both semen and urine. The urinary tract includes the kidneys, ureters, bladder and urethra. In both men and women, the kidneys cleanse blood of excess fluid and waste products as they manufacture urine, which is passed to the bladder by way of the ureters. The bladder stores urine and expels it through the urethra.

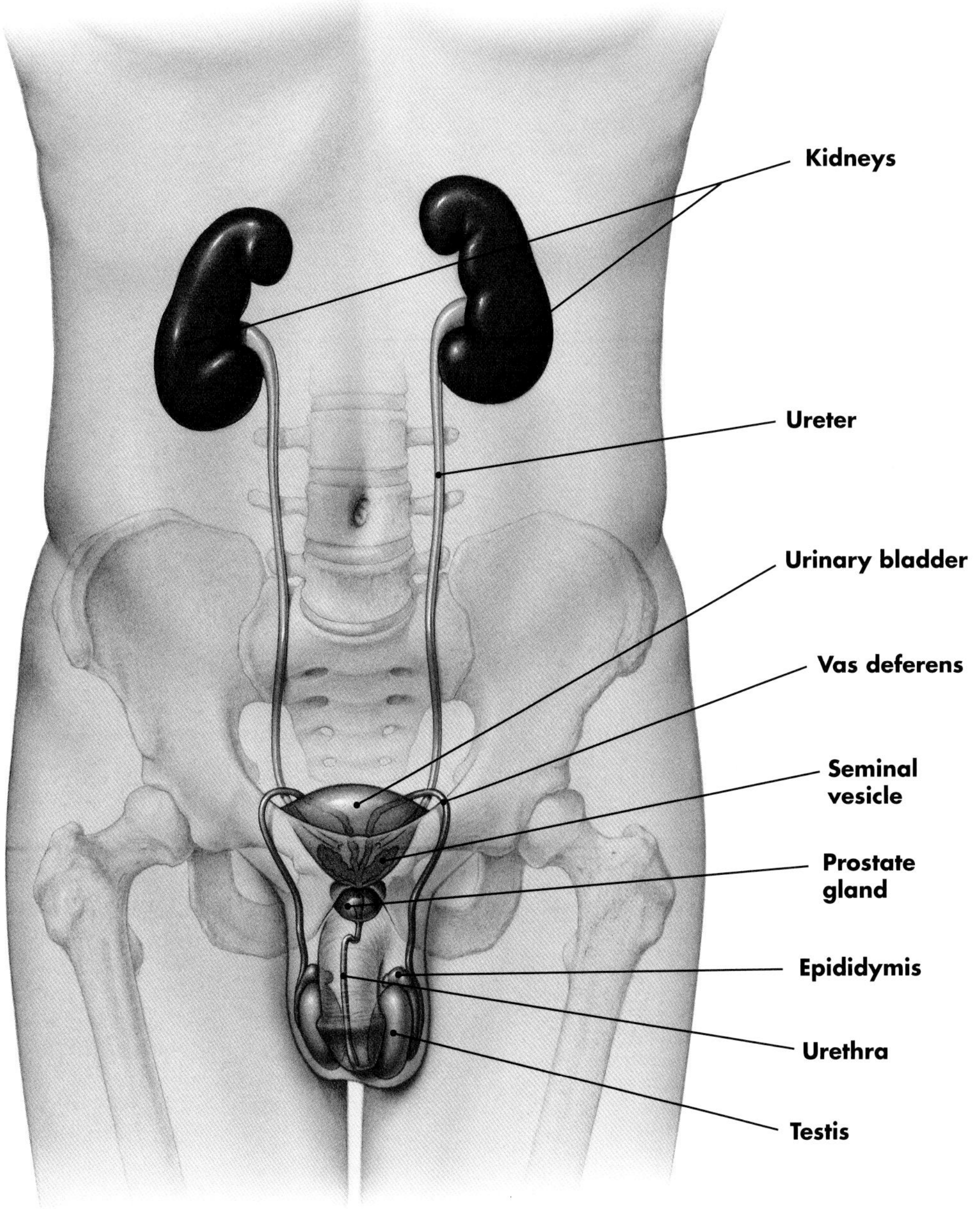

Kidneys

Ureter

Urinary bladder

Vas deferens

Seminal vesicle

Prostate gland

Epididymis

Urethra

Testis

Brain

The brain controls virtually all of the body's activities, from basic instincts of survival to intellectual analysis and creative thought. It organizes and shapes emotions and monitors and directs body functions and physical actions. The basic structures of the brain include the brainstem; the cerebellum, responsible for balance and movement; and the cerebrum, the largest structure of the human brain and perhaps the most recognizable, due to its heavily folded appearance. The cerebrum (see opposite page) is divided into two hemispheres. Each hemisphere is composed of four lobes — frontal, parietal, temporal and occipital — each of which directs different activities.

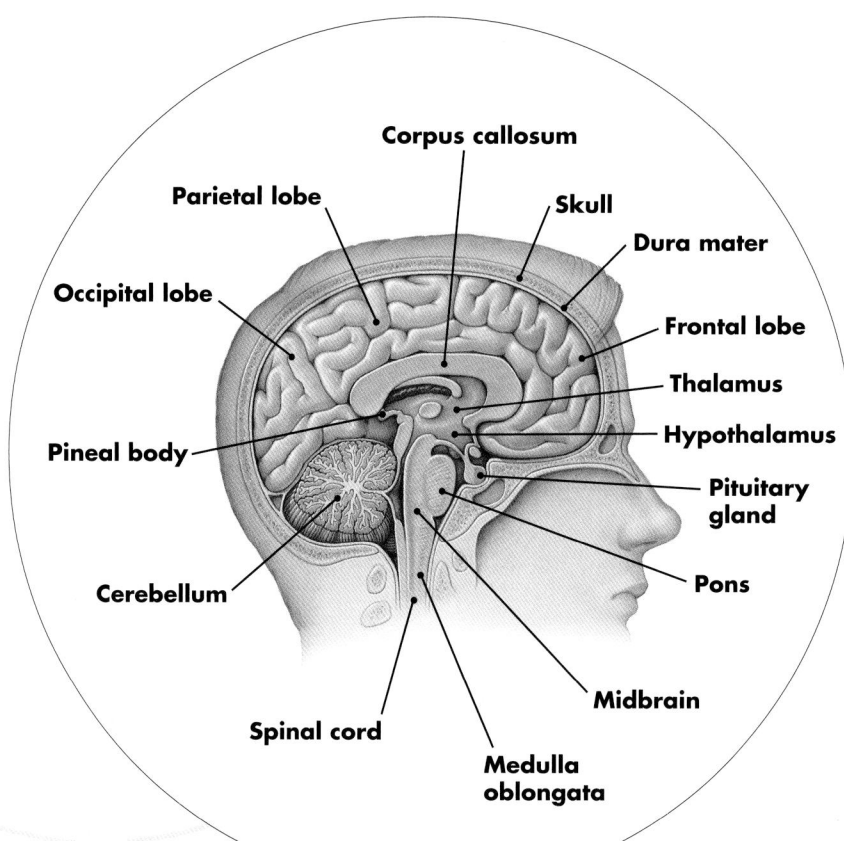

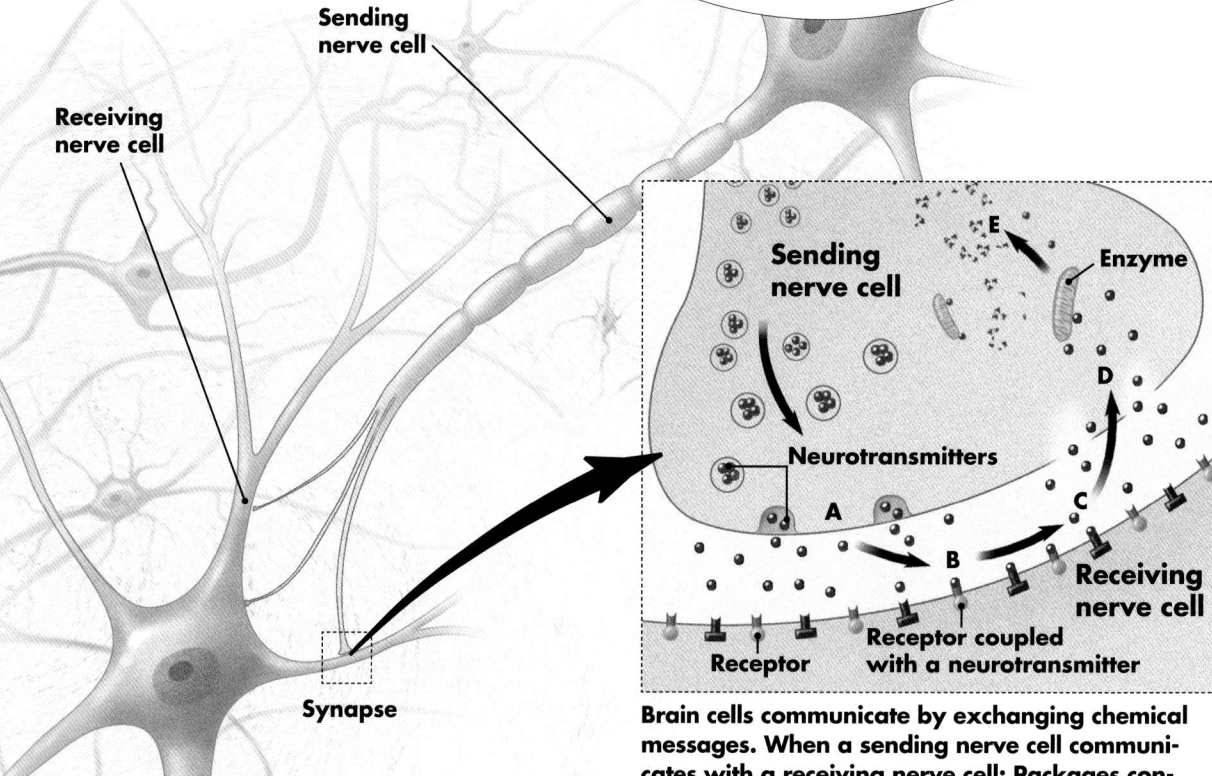

Brain cells communicate by exchanging chemical messages. When a sending nerve cell communicates with a receiving nerve cell: Packages containing chemical messengers (neurotransmitters) are released into a gap (synapse) between the two cells (A). The neurotransmitters bind with receptors on receiving nerve cells (B). Once communication is complete, the neurotransmitters return to the synapse (C). The neurotransmitters re-enter the sending nerve cell (D). The neurotransmitters are repackaged for future use or broken down by enzymes (E).

Nervous System

The human body communicates by its nervous system, which is composed of the brain, spinal cord and peripheral nerves. Peripheral nerves receive messages from various body parts and the outside world. These messages are transmitted to the spinal cord and passed on to the brain, which interprets and responds to the messages. The spinal cord continuously transmits messages back and forth between the brain and the outermost regions of the body.

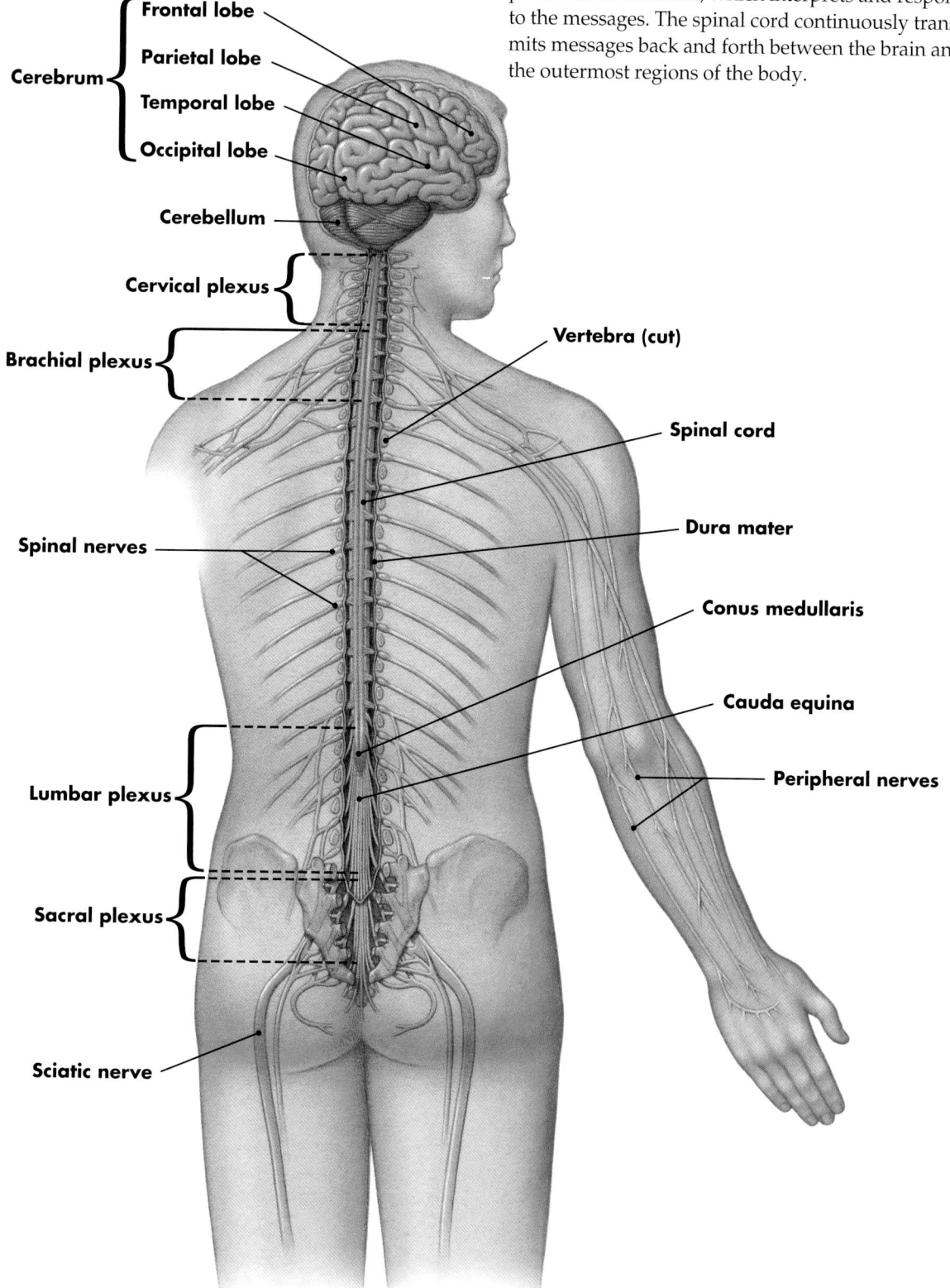

Cerebrum
Frontal lobe
Parietal lobe
Temporal lobe
Occipital lobe

Cerebellum

Cervical plexus

Brachial plexus

Spinal nerves

Lumbar plexus

Sacral plexus

Sciatic nerve

Vertebra (cut)

Spinal cord

Dura mater

Conus medullaris

Cauda equina

Peripheral nerves

Eyes and Ears

An image passes through the pupil at the front of the eye and onto the lens, located behind the pupil. The lens projects the inverted image onto the retina, located at the back of the eye. The retina, which is composed of light-sensitive cells, converts the image into electrical impulses that are delivered to the brain by way of the optic nerve.

The two main functions of the ears are hearing and balance. The eardrum transmits sound by means of tiny connective bones (hammer, anvil, stirrup) to the inner ear. There, sound is transmitted as electrical impulses to the brain via the auditory nerve. The inner ear also contains the semicircular canals of the vestibular labyrinth, structures essential to balance.

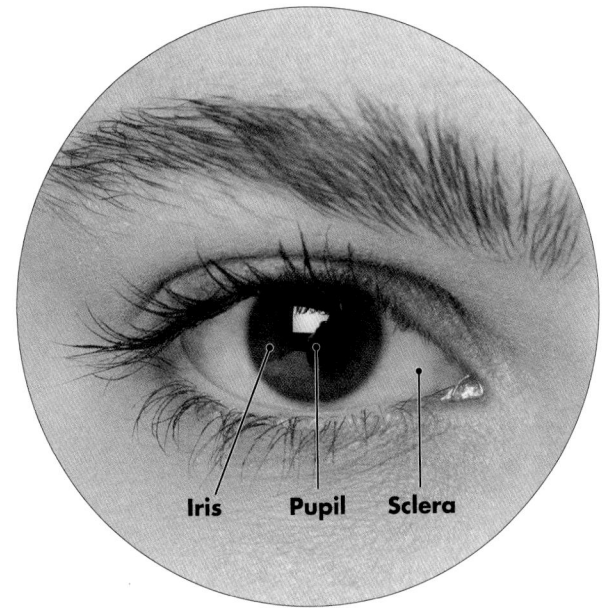

Iris   Pupil   Sclera

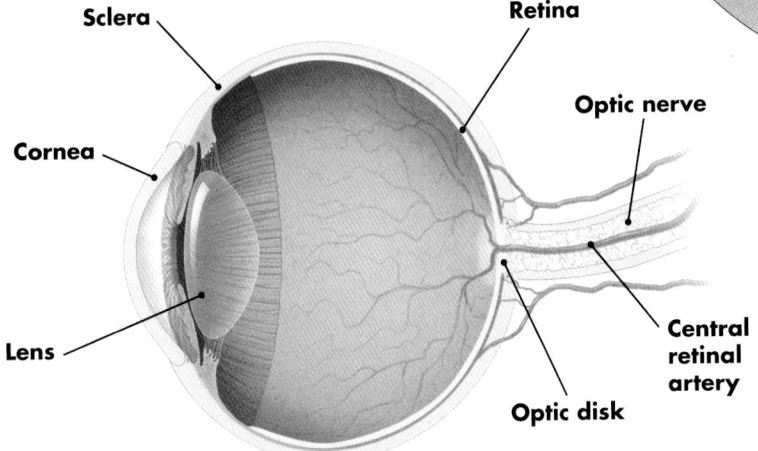

Sclera

Retina

Optic nerve

Cornea

Central retinal artery

Lens

Optic disk

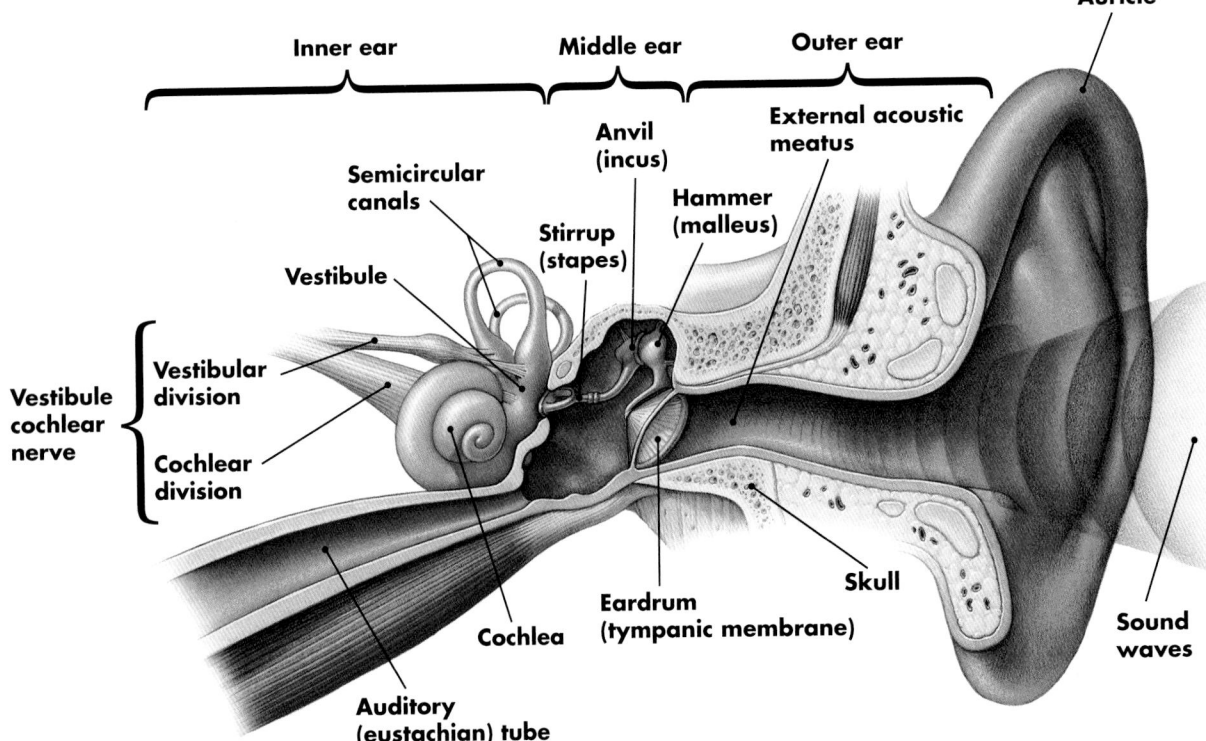

Inner ear   Middle ear   Outer ear

Auricle

Anvil (incus)

External acoustic meatus

Semicircular canals

Stirrup (stapes)

Hammer (malleus)

Vestibule

Vestibule cochlear nerve

Vestibular division

Cochlear division

Skull

Cochlea

Eardrum (tympanic membrane)

Sound waves

Auditory (eustachian) tube

Nasal and Oral Cavities

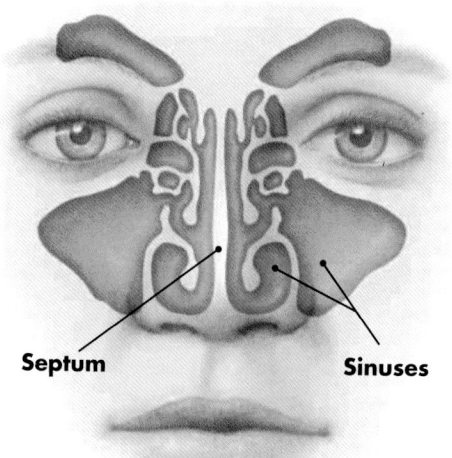

Septum   **Sinuses**

The nose is divided into two identical passages called nostrils, which are separated by a partition (septum) of cartilage and bone. The nasal passages also open into the sinuses, tiny air-filled cavities in the skull. The adenoids are an aggregation of lymphatic tissue located behind the nasal passages.

The oral cavity is composed of the mouth and teeth. Many important acts, such as speaking and singing, use the teeth and mouth to shape sounds. The teeth and mouth are also responsible for the first phase of digestion.

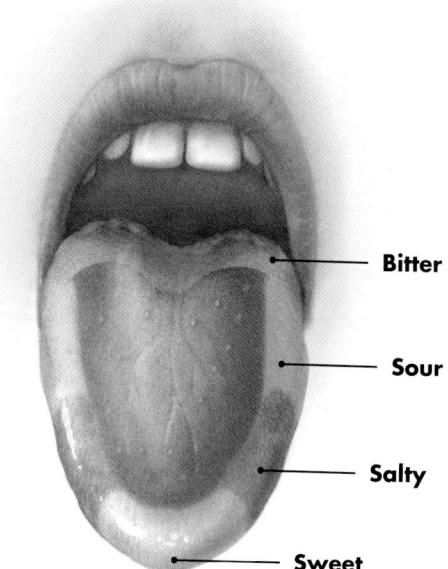

Bitter

Sour

Salty

Sweet

Working in conjunction with your sense of smell, your taste buds can distinguish sweet, salty, sour and bitter flavors.

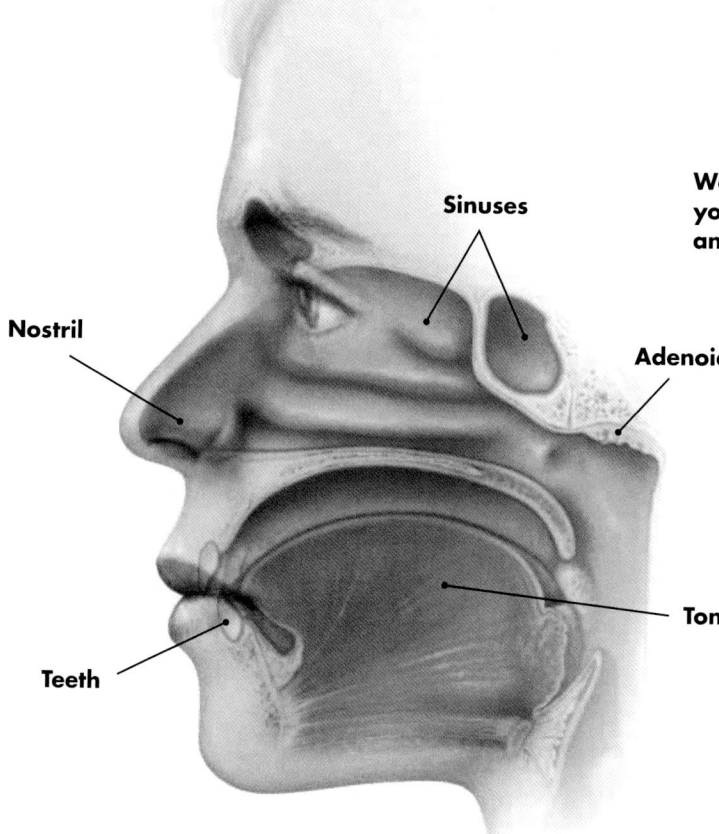

Nostril

Sinuses

Adenoids

Tongue

Teeth

Skin

Skin keeps out invaders, helps control body temperature and protects vital internal organs. The adult human body has 2 square yards of skin. One square inch of skin contains millions of cells and includes structures such as oil glands, hair roots (follicles) and sweat glands. Specialized nerve endings in skin sense heat, cold and pain.

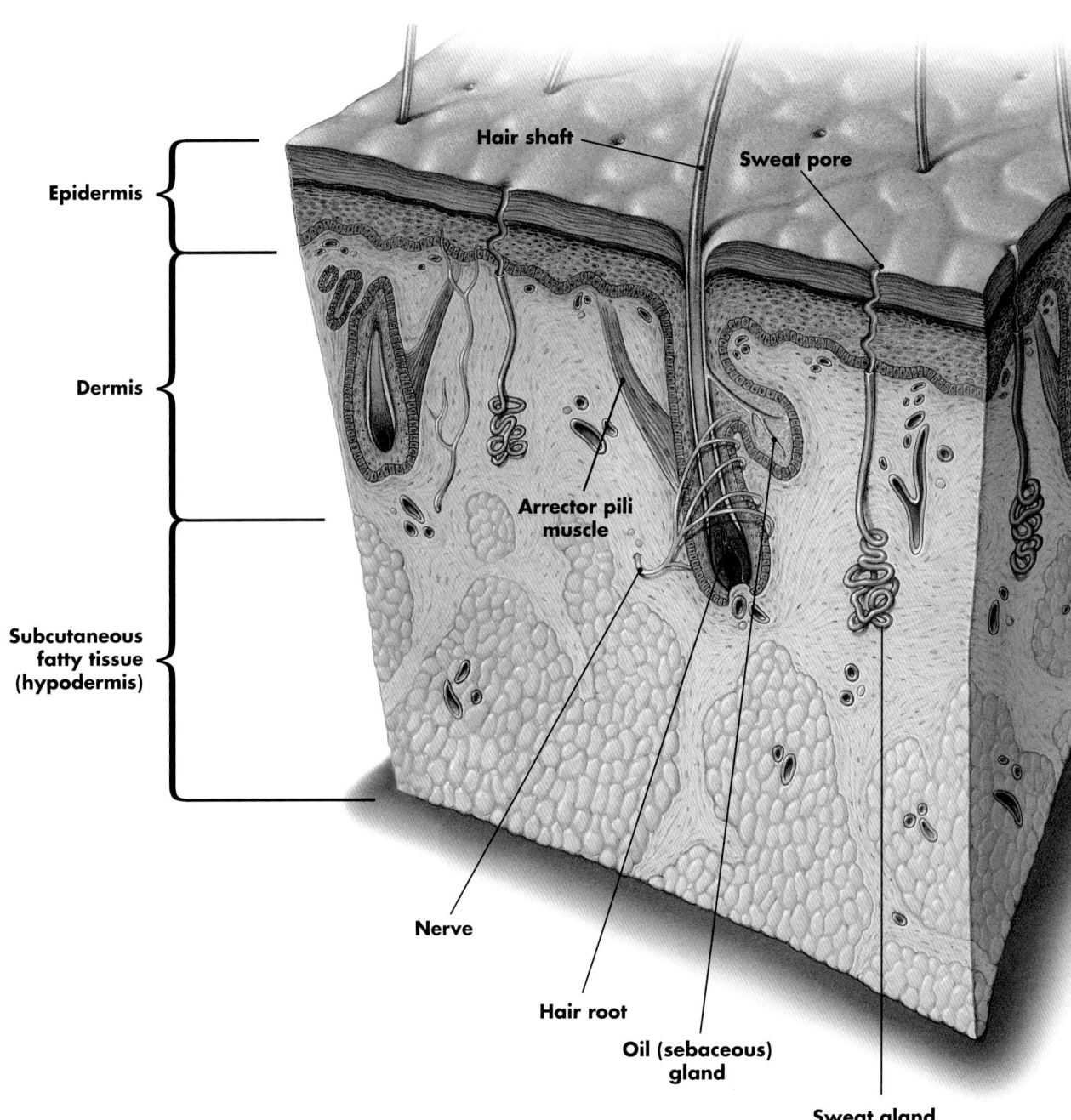

Epidermis

Dermis

Subcutaneous fatty tissue (hypodermis)

Hair shaft

Sweat pore

Arrector pili muscle

Nerve

Hair root

Oil (sebaceous) gland

Sweat gland

Immune System

The immune system is a complex array of organs, cells and molecules distributed throughout the body, responsible for protecting the body from harmful invaders (antigens), such as germs, viruses and other foreign substances. Each part of the immune system contributes to the growth, development or activation of lymphocytes, specialized white blood cells that play a major role in the body's immune response. White blood cells originate in bone marrow. Some migrate to the thymus gland and develop into specialized types of immune cells. Some white blood cells from bone marrow and the thymus gland gather in lymph nodes and other immune organs, including the spleen, tonsils, adenoids and appendix. Other cells circulate throughout blood and lymphatic vessels.

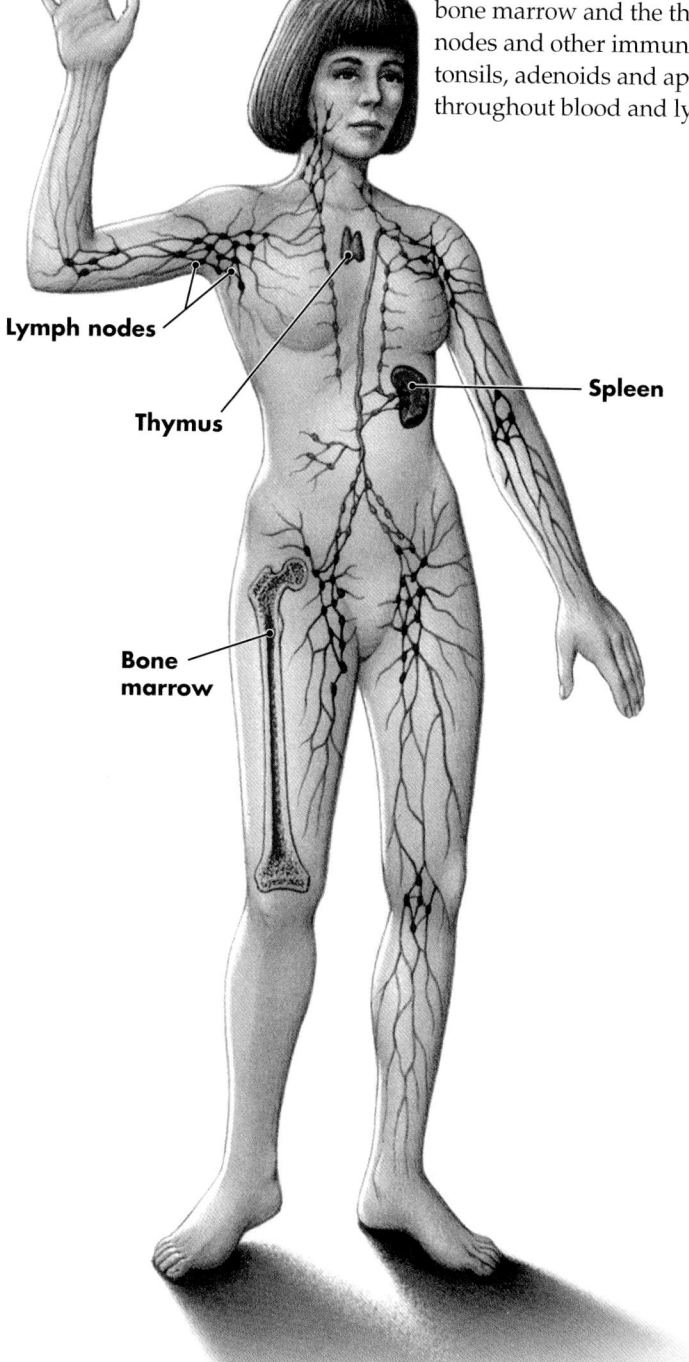

Lymph nodes

Thymus

Spleen

Bone marrow

Genes

1. Your body is made up of cells, about 100 trillion of them. Different kinds of cells — for example, skin, muscle, bone and blood — perform different functions. Each cell has a control center called the nucleus.

2. Within the nucleus of each cell are 23 pairs of structures called chromosomes. Half of a person's chromosomes are inherited from the mother and the other half, from the father.

3. Each chromosome contains strands that resemble a twisted ladder. The strands, called deoxyribonucleic acid (DNA), are held together by chemical "rungs."

4. Chromosomes are made up of genes. Each gene is composed of sequences of thousands of pairs of the chemicals adenine (A) and thymine (T), and the chemicals cytosine (C) and guanine (G). The precise sequence of these chemical pairs in the gene directs the cell to produce another chemical, usually a protein, which has a specific task to do. This is how each gene tells each cell in your body precisely how to act — controlling your features and growth, and influencing or directly affecting the function of your organs.

DNA strand

Chromosome

Cell

Gene

1

2

3

4

A
T

C
G

Nucleus

Spinal Disorders

Many types of spinal disorders cause back pain. Back pain generally isn't life-threatening, but the pain can make you miserable.

Pain radiating from your back down your buttock to your lower leg, called sciatica (see left), may be associated with inflammation or compression of the roots of the sciatic nerve.

Sciatic nerve

Pinched nerve

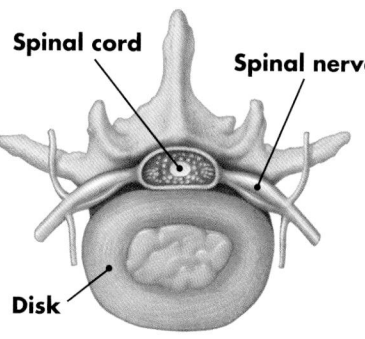

Normal Disk

Spinal cord

Spinal nerve

Disk

Herniated Disk

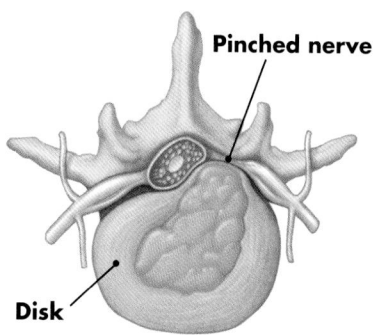

Pinched nerve

Disk

A slipped (herniated) disk places pressure on a spinal nerve, causing pain and, sometimes, loss of sensation or paralysis.

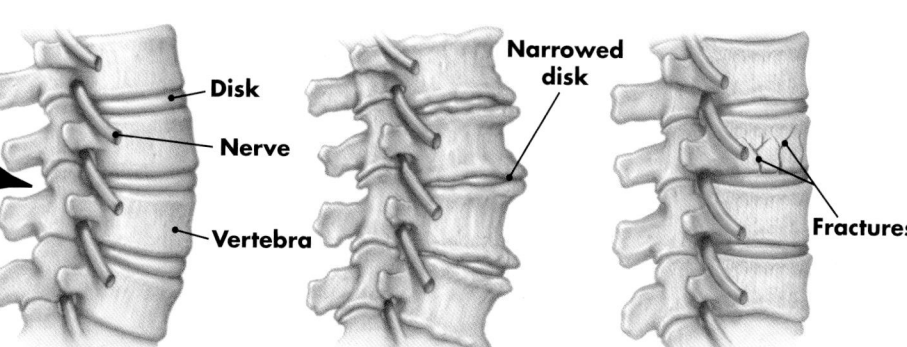

Normal Spine

Disk

Nerve

Vertebra

Osteoarthritis

Narrowed disk

Osteoporosis

Fractures

Elastic structures called disks cushion vertebrae in a normal spine, keeping it flexible. In osteoarthritis, disks may narrow and spurs form. Pain and stiffness may occur where bone surfaces rub together. With osteoporosis, vertebrae may become compressed and fractured due to bone weakness.

Joint Disorders

Pain and stiffness in a joint often result from osteo-arthritis. This common form of arthritis affects nearly all adults older than age 60. Joint replacement surgery can help restore near-normal, pain-free joint movement. Many joints, including the hip, knee, shoulder, elbow, wrist and even finger joints, can be replaced.

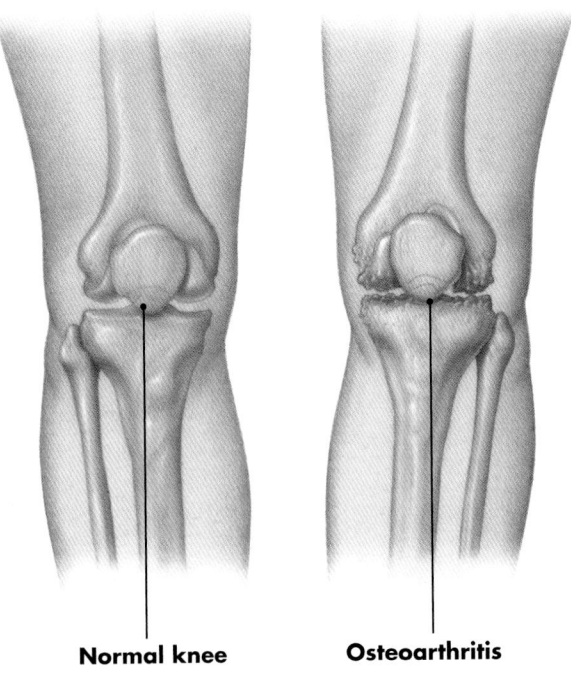

Normal knee   **Osteoarthritis**

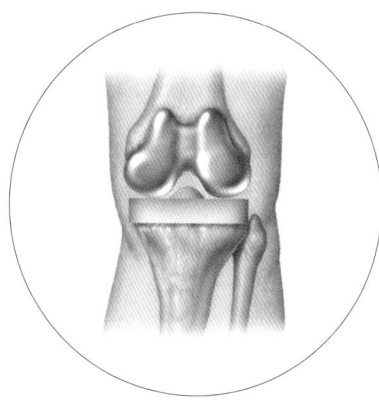

At left, a normal knee joint and a knee damaged by osteoarthritis. The inset above shows a knee repaired by total knee replacement.

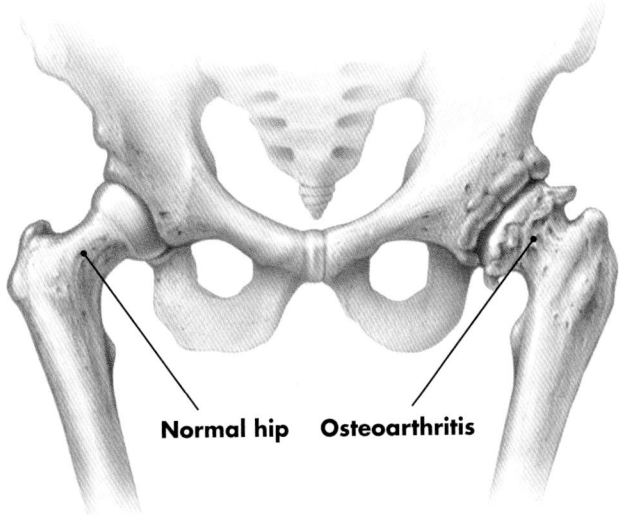

Normal hip   Osteoarthritis

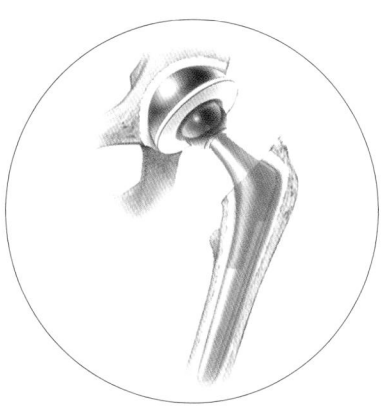

At left, a hip showing a normal joint and a joint that has been damaged by osteoarthritis. The inset above shows how an implant can replace a damaged joint.

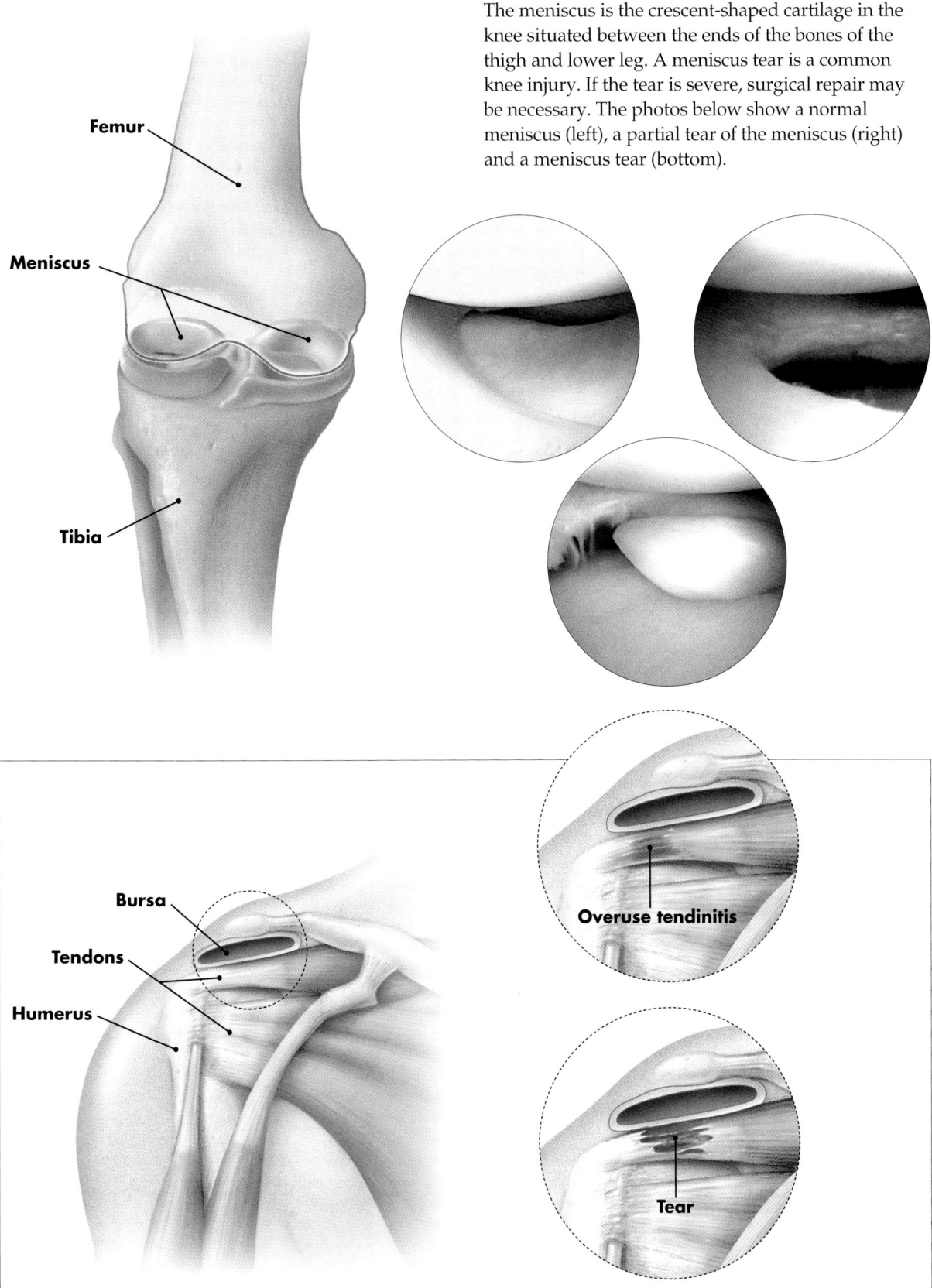

The meniscus is the crescent-shaped cartilage in the knee situated between the ends of the bones of the thigh and lower leg. A meniscus tear is a common knee injury. If the tear is severe, surgical repair may be necessary. The photos below show a normal meniscus (left), a partial tear of the meniscus (right) and a meniscus tear (bottom).

Femur

Meniscus

Tibia

Bursa

Tendons

Humerus

Overuse tendinitis

Tear

The rotator cuff is made up of muscles and tendons that attach the upper arm bone to the shoulder blade. Typical rotator cuff injuries involve inflammation of the tendons (tendinitis) or one or more tears in the tendons.

Breast Disorders

All breast lumps need to be taken seriously and investigated promptly. However, the vast majority of lumps are noncancerous (benign) and may be associated with the female menstrual cycle.

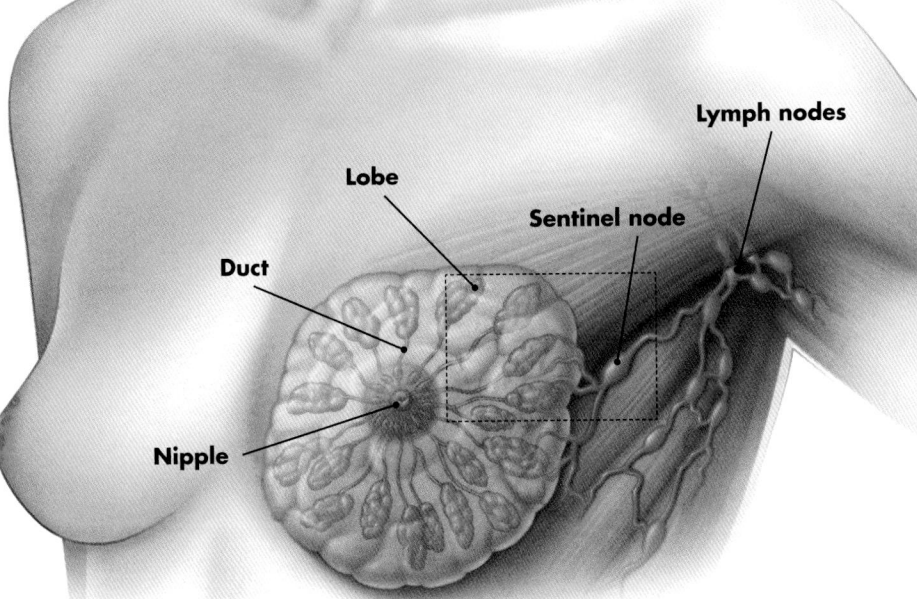

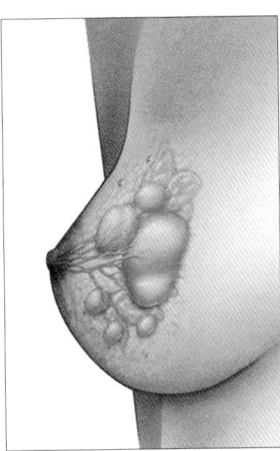

A breast cyst (see above) is a fluid-filled sac that tends to enlarge near the end of the female menstrual cycle, when the body is retaining more fluid. Some cysts are tiny, but others can be as large as an egg.

The sentinel node is the first lymph node into which a tumor drains. By finding the sentinel node before surgery, doctors can remove the node for study during surgery. If the sentinel node is free of cancer, it's unlikely the cancer has spread.

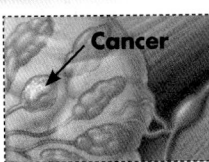

Early breast cancer is confined to the duct.

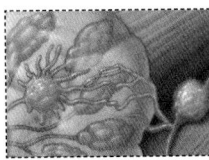

Invasive breast cancer has spread from a duct into adjacent breast tissue and the nearby sentinel node.

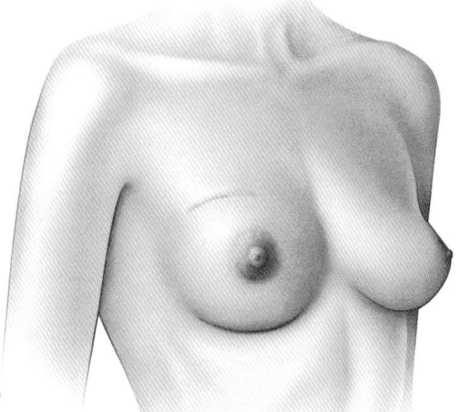

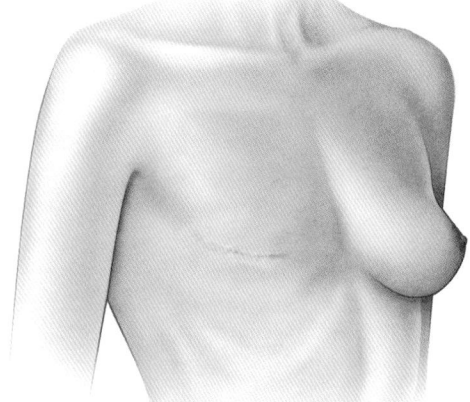

During a lumpectomy, the tumor is removed along with some of the lymph nodes. During a modified radical mastectomy, the breast is removed, and possibly some underarm lymph nodes. Chest muscles are left intact.

Prostate Disorders

Benign prostatic hyperplasia (BPH) is a noncancerous enlargement of the prostate gland that's common in older men. Your prostate gland may enlarge and gradually compress your urethra, slowing the flow of urine.

A more serious disorder is prostate cancer. Prostate cancers grow within the gland. The tumor may not produce any signs and symptoms.

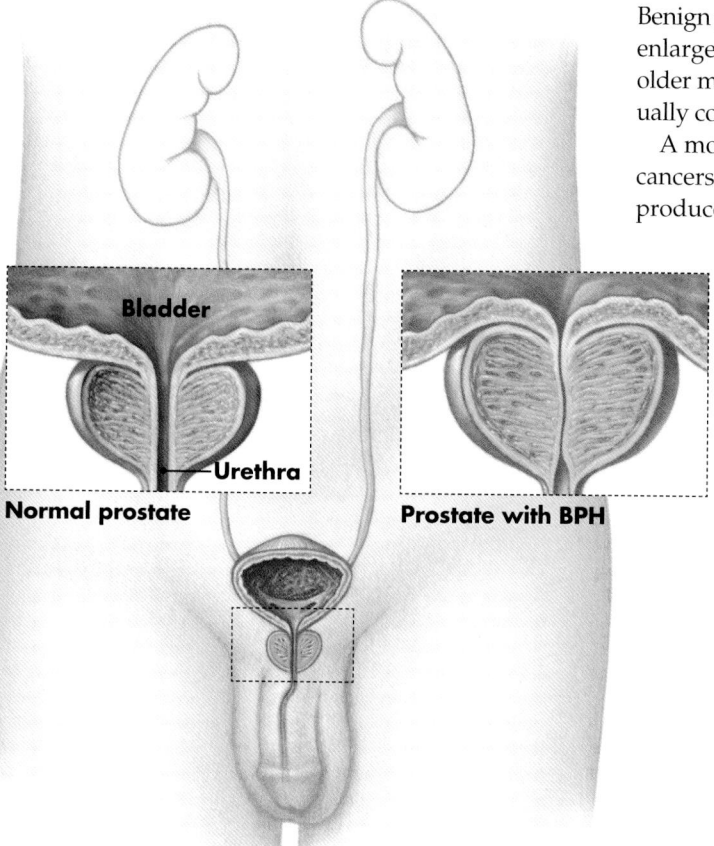

Bladder

Urethra

Normal prostate

Prostate with BPH

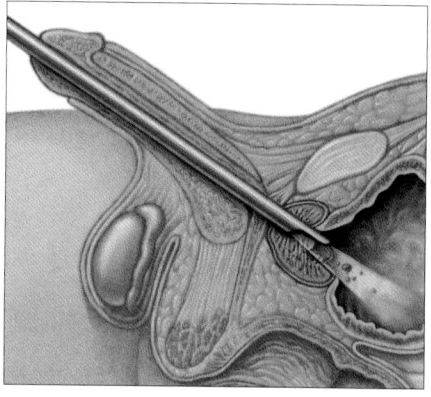

For BPH, a surgeon can reduce the size of the prostate gland with a procedure called transurethral resection of the prostate (TURP). Other procedures also may be used.

Staging and grading prostate cancer. When a biopsy confirms the presence of cancer, the cancer is staged to determine how far it has spread, with stage I being the most confined and stage IV the most widespread. The cancer is also graded to determine whether it's a slow- or fast-growing form. The most common grading scale runs from I to V, with I being the least aggressive form of cancer.

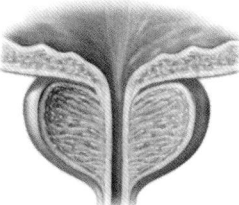

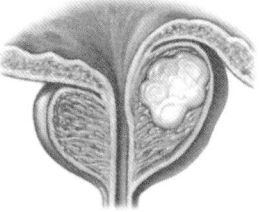

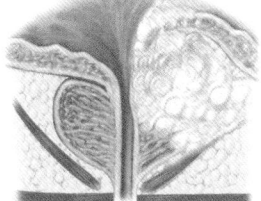

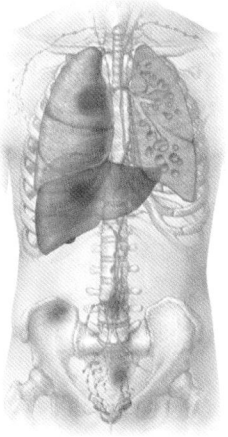

Stage I. Very early cancer that's confined to microscopic particles that can't be felt on examination.

Stage II. Cancer that can be felt but is confined to the prostate.

Stage III. Cancer that has spread beyond the prostate to seminal vesicles or adjacent bladder tissue.

Stage IV. Advanced cancer that has spread to lymph nodes, bones, lungs or other organs.

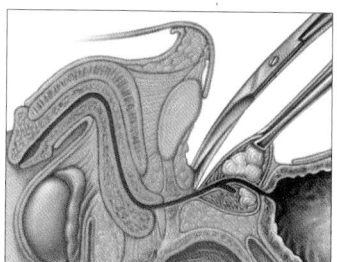

For prostate cancer, removal of the prostate gland (radical prostatectomy) is a common treatment option. Other procedures also may be used.

Heart Disorders

Coronary artery disease is a common cause of heart disease. In this condition, fatty deposits (plaques) accumulate on the interior walls of the arteries in your heart. This narrowing reduces blood flow and can cause chest pain (angina) or lead to a heart attack (see opposite page). A common procedure to widen arteries and restore circulation is balloon angioplasty followed by placement of a stent (see below).

An alternative to opening blocked arteries is coronary bypass surgery (see right). Bypass surgery involves rerouting blood around blockage sites. Bypasses can be surgically constructed out of veins taken from a leg or from arteries arising near the collarbone. A double bypass operation routes blood around blockages in two vessels.

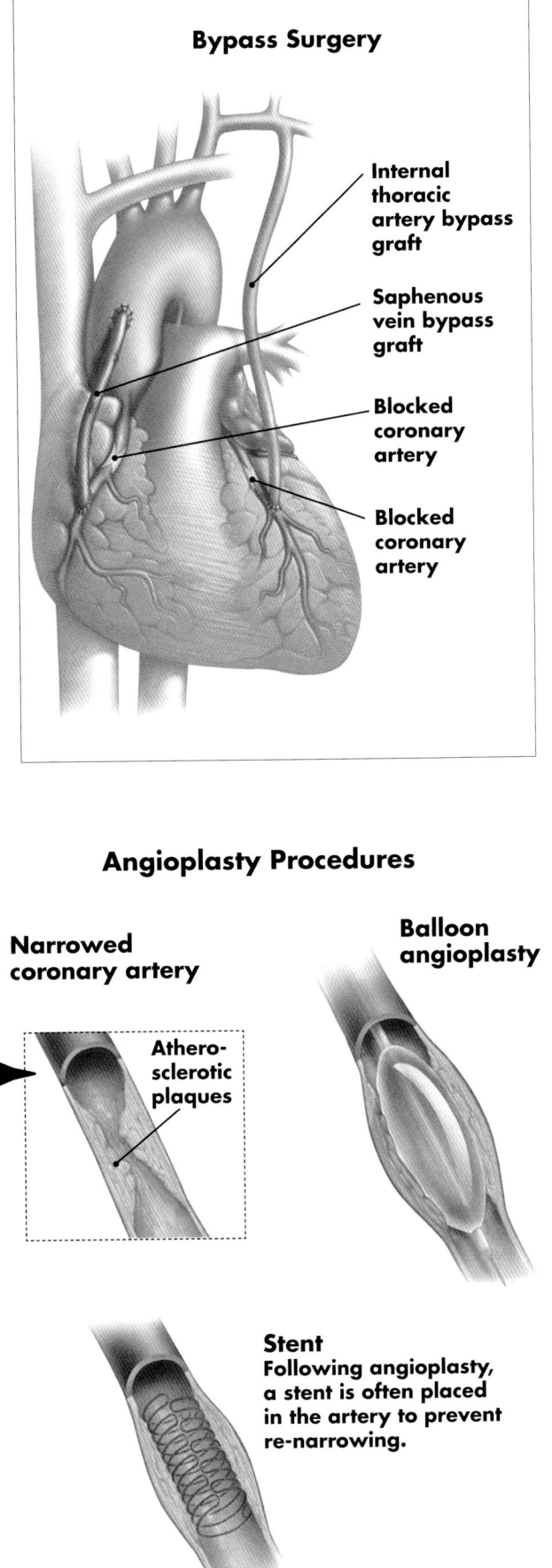

Bypass Surgery

Internal thoracic artery bypass graft

Saphenous vein bypass graft

Blocked coronary artery

Blocked coronary artery

Angioplasty Procedures

Narrowed coronary artery

Athero-sclerotic plaques

Balloon angioplasty

Stent
Following angioplasty, a stent is often placed in the artery to prevent re-narrowing.

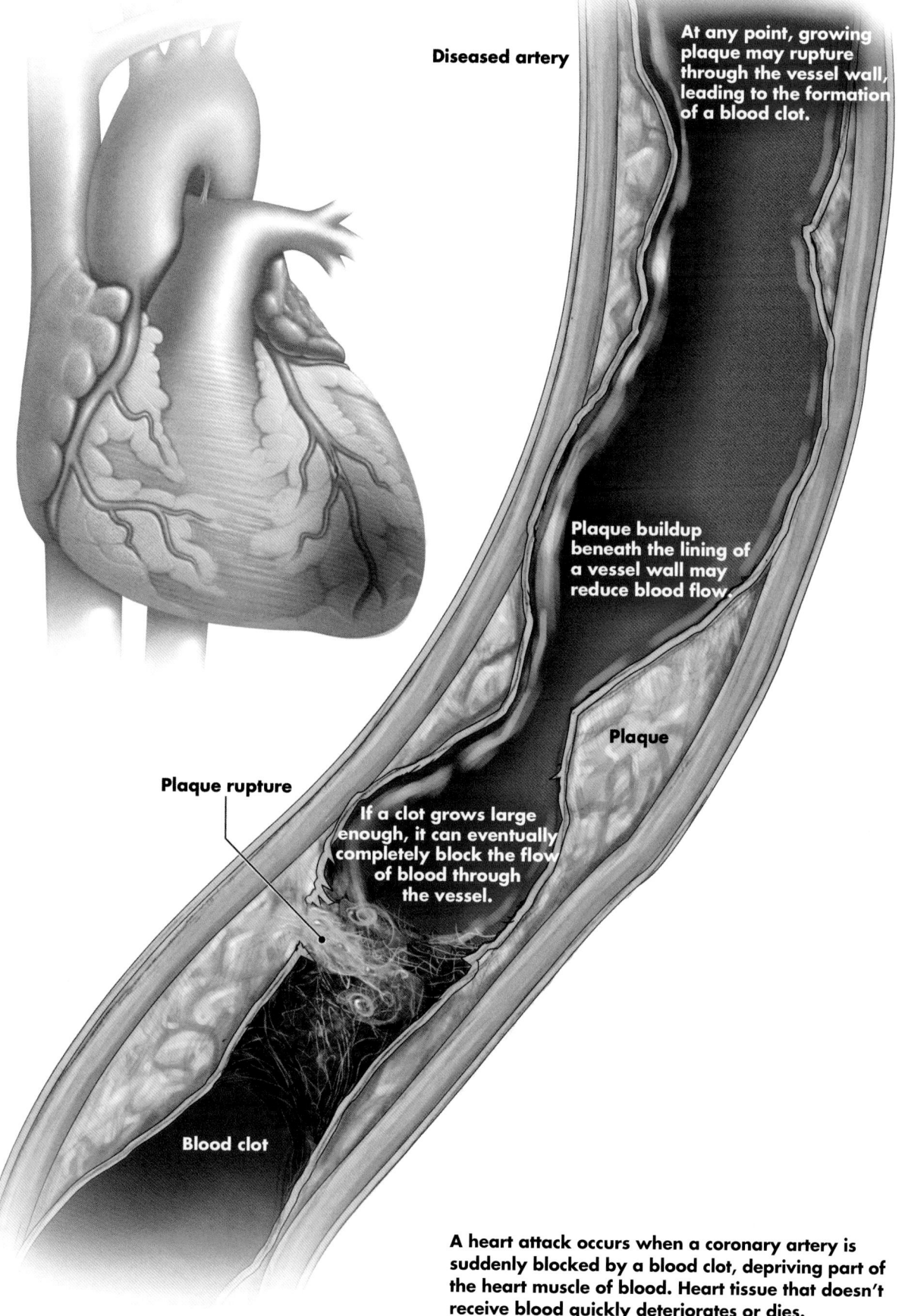

Diseased artery

At any point, growing plaque may rupture through the vessel wall, leading to the formation of a blood clot.

Plaque buildup beneath the lining of a vessel wall may reduce blood flow.

Plaque

Plaque rupture

If a clot grows large enough, it can eventually completely block the flow of blood through the vessel.

Blood clot

A heart attack occurs when a coronary artery is suddenly blocked by a blood clot, depriving part of the heart muscle of blood. Heart tissue that doesn't receive blood quickly deteriorates or dies.

Heart valve disease can cause heart valves to narrow, restricting blood flow through them (valve stenosis). Valves also may not close properly, allowing blood to flow backward (valve regurgitation).

If a damaged valve cannot be repaired, it may need to be replaced (see below). After removing the valve, a surgeon replaces it with a mechanical valve or a biological tissue valve made from animal or human heart tissue.

Mitral valve regurgitation　　**Aortic valve stenosis**　　**Mitral valve stenosis**　　**Aortic valve regurgitation**

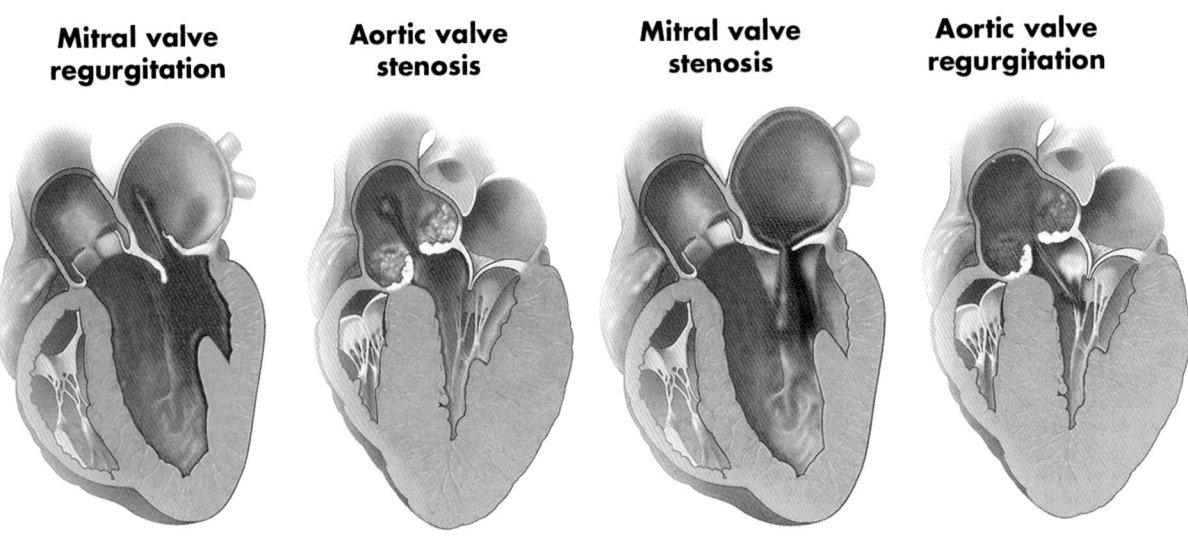

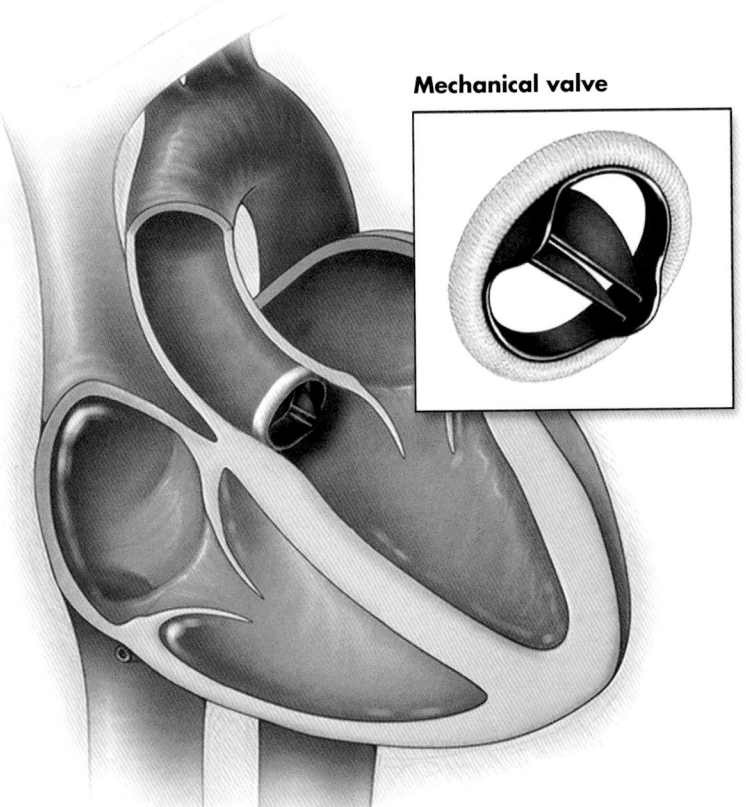

Mechanical valve

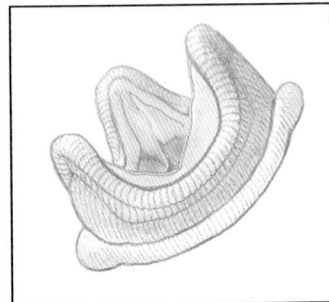

Biological tissue valve

Blood Disorders

There are many blood disorders, each caused by a malfunction of a certain blood component. Anemias are caused by too few red blood cells and leukemias by too many white blood cells. Bleeding disorders are often caused by defects in platelets or clotting factors.

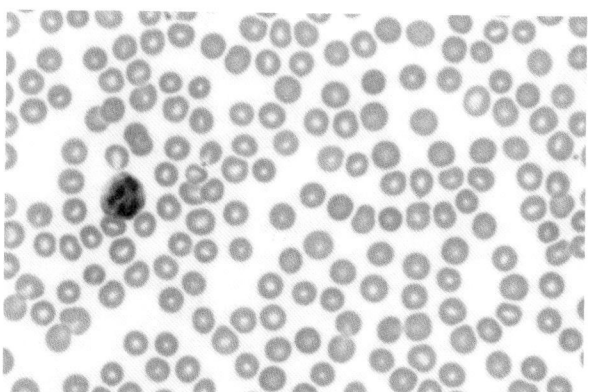 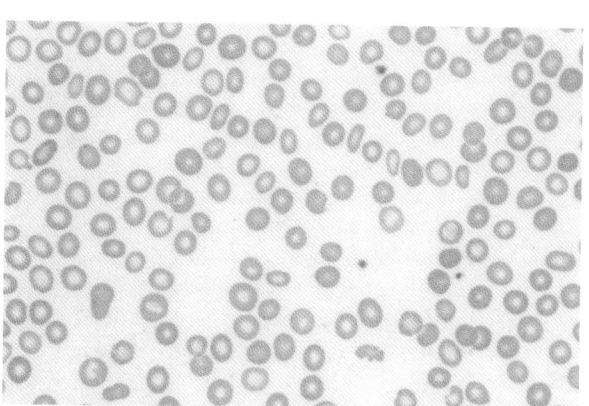

On the left is a normal blood smear. On the right is a blood smear showing iron deficiency anemia. The cells are smaller, and the white area in the middle of the cells is larger (increased central pallor).

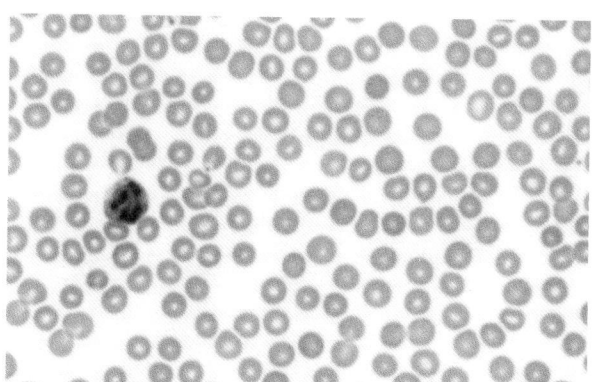 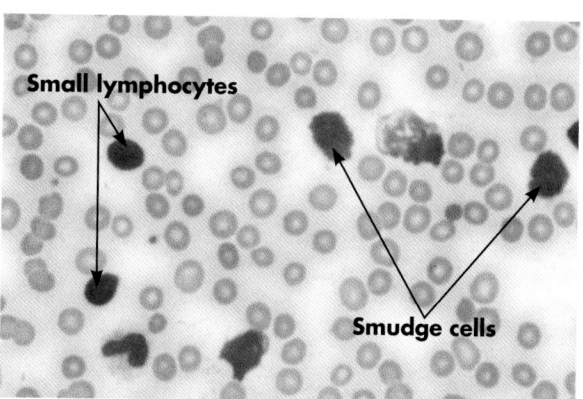

Small lymphocytes

Smudge cells

On the left is a normal blood smear. On the right is a blood smear showing chronic lymphocytic leukemia. There's an increased number of small lymphocytes and some smudge cells.

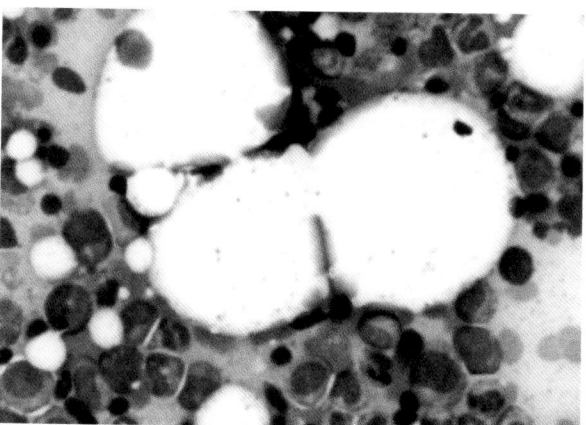 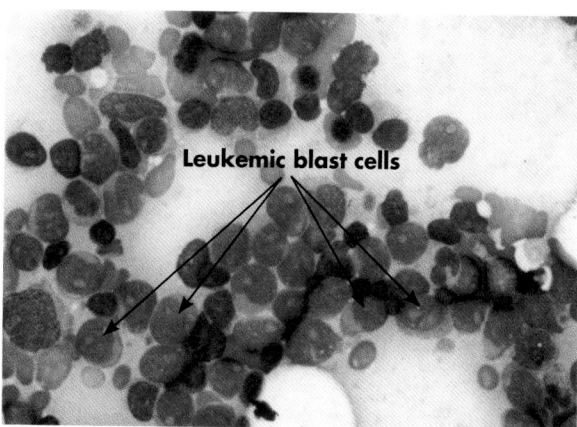

Leukemic blast cells

On the left is a slide of normal bone marrow showing a variety of cells. On the right is a slide showing acute leukemia, a primary cancer of bone marrow. Most of the cells on the slide to the right are leukemic blast cells.

Lung Disorders

Common chronic lung disorders that restrict the flow of air out of the bronchial passages include chronic bronchitis, emphysema and asthma. Another lung disorder, lung cancer, is a leading cause of cancer deaths in the United States.

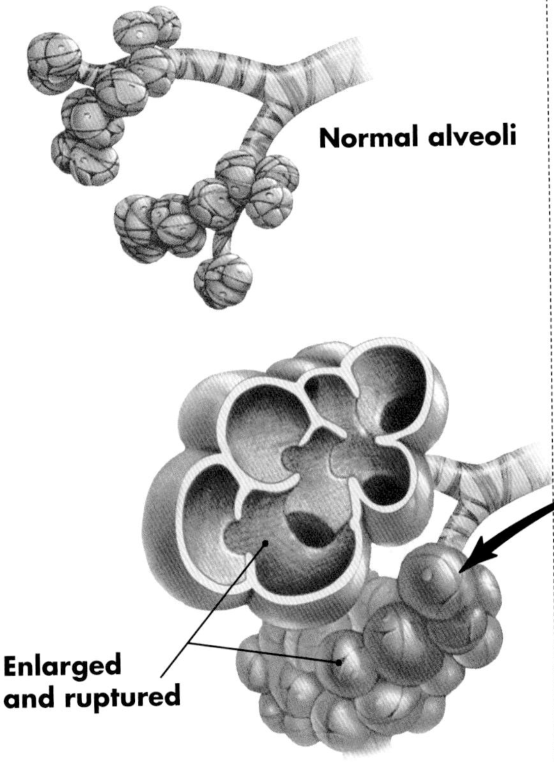

Normal alveoli

Lung

Trachea

Bronchus

Normal bronchial tube

Bronchitis

Enlarged and ruptured

In emphysema, air sac (alveolar) walls are damaged by inflammation. Alveoli can lose their natural elasticity, become overstretched and rupture.

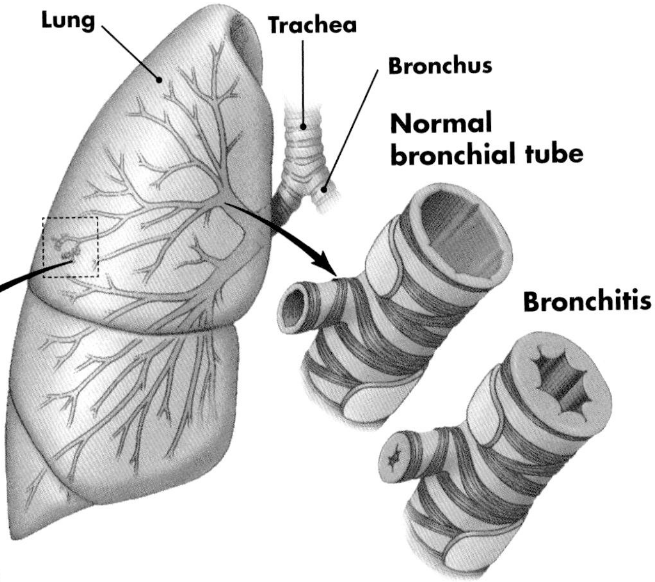

Chronic bronchitis is a chronic inflammation and thickening of the walls of the bronchial tubes, which narrows them.

Lung Cancer

Surgery to treat lung cancer involves removing the cancer and a portion of surrounding lung tissue. The most common surgery is lobectomy.

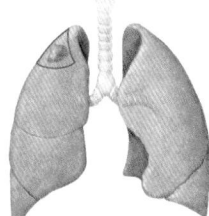

Wedge resection is removal of a small portion of a lobe.

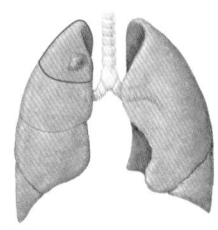

Segment resection is removal of a larger portion of a lobe.

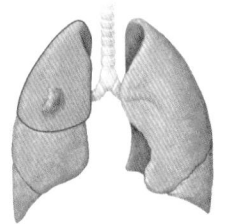

Lobectomy is removal of an entire lobe.

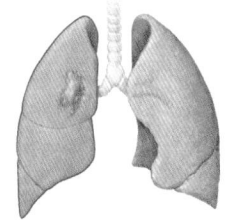

Pneumonectomy is removal of an entire lung.

Normal lungs

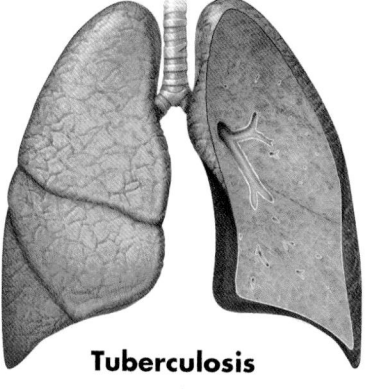

Tuberculosis

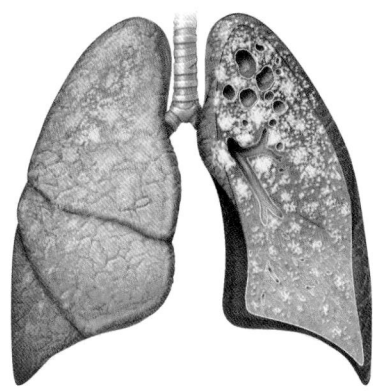

Tuberculosis (TB) is an infectious disease caused by bacteria that most commonly attacks the lungs. In some individuals the disease remains inactive (latent); in others it becomes active (TB disease).

In asthma, lung airways become inflamed and swollen. Muscles surrounding the airways tighten and constrict, and membranes in airway linings secrete excess mucus.

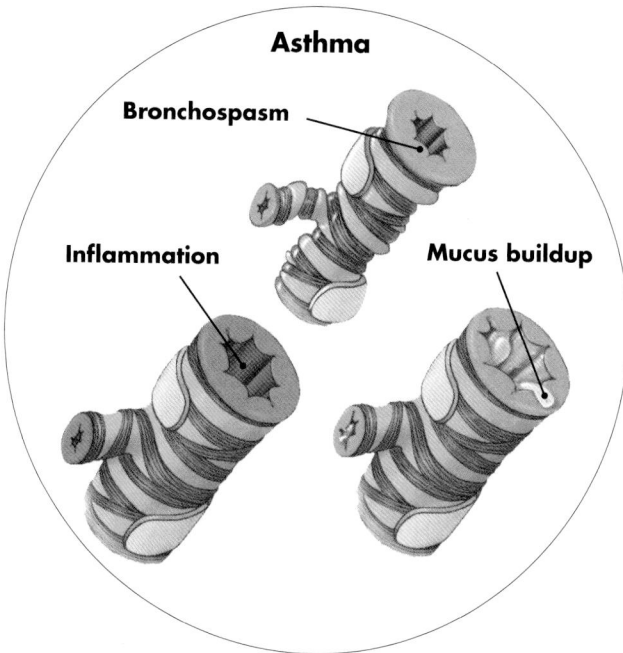

Asthma

Bronchospasm

Inflammation

Mucus buildup

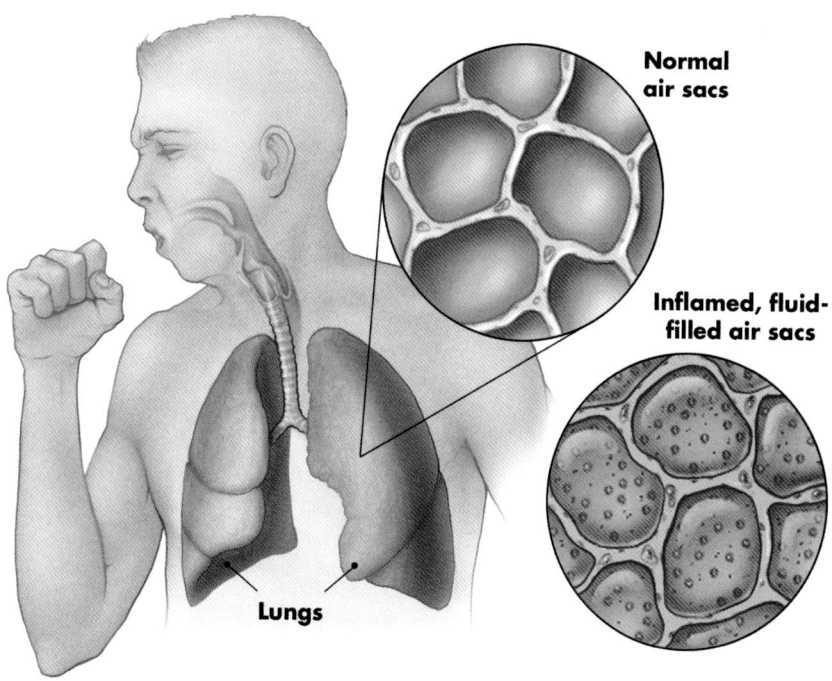

Normal air sacs

Inflamed, fluid-filled air sacs

Lungs

Pneumonia is an inflammatory condition of the lungs primarily affecting the microscopic air sacs. The sacs become inflamed, and they may fill with fluid or pus.

Gastrointestinal Disorders

The digestive system is composed of a complex network of organs that convey and convert food into energy the body needs. There are many disorders that can affect this intricate system.

Gallstones (shown below) are made up of various components of bile and form in the gallbladder. If the stones leave the gallbladder, they can become lodged in ducts and cause problems.

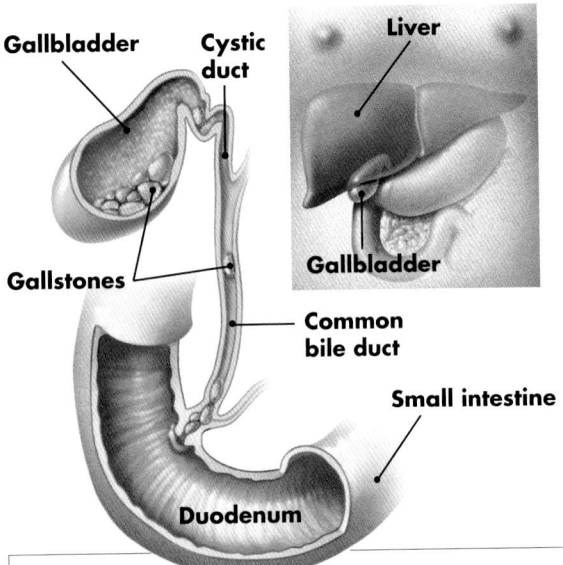

Gallbladder **Cystic duct** **Liver** **Gallbladder** **Gallstones** **Common bile duct** **Small intestine** **Duodenum**

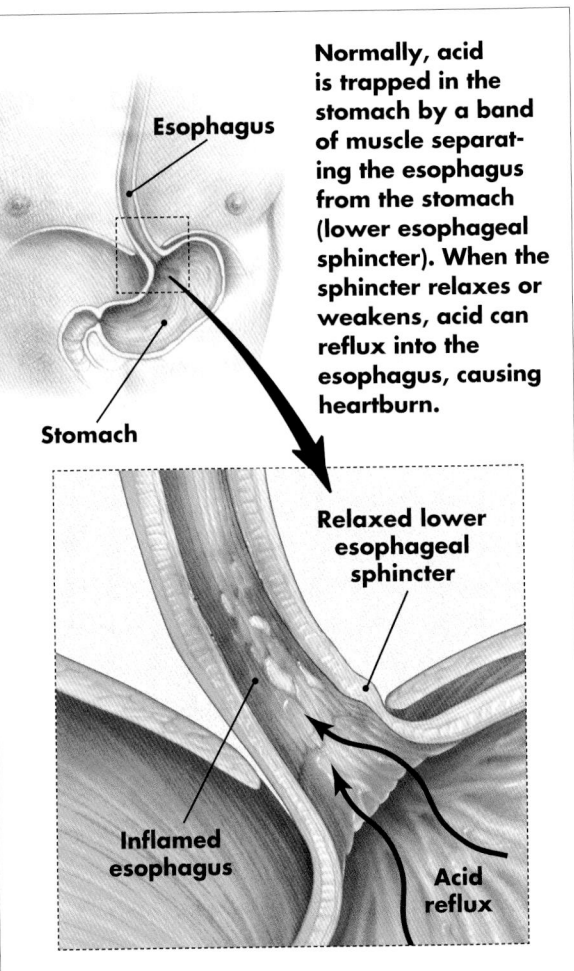

Normally, acid is trapped in the stomach by a band of muscle separating the esophagus from the stomach (lower esophageal sphincter). When the sphincter relaxes or weakens, acid can reflux into the esophagus, causing heartburn.

Esophagus **Stomach** **Relaxed lower esophageal sphincter** **Inflamed esophagus** **Acid reflux**

Stage 0. The cancer is in its earliest stage. It hasn't grown beyond the inner layer (mucosa) of the colon or rectum.

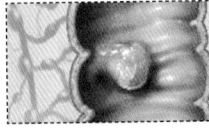

Stage I. The cancer has grown through the mucosa but hasn't spread outside the colon wall.

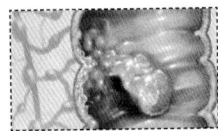

Stage II. The cancer has grown through the wall of the colon or rectum but hasn't spread to nearby lymph nodes.

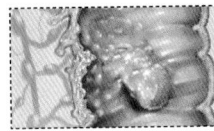

Stage III. The cancer has spread to nearby lymph nodes but hasn't spread to other parts of the body.

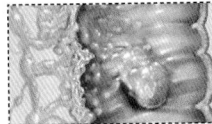

Stage IV. The cancer is advanced and has spread to distant organs, such as the liver or lungs, or the lining of the abdominal cavity.

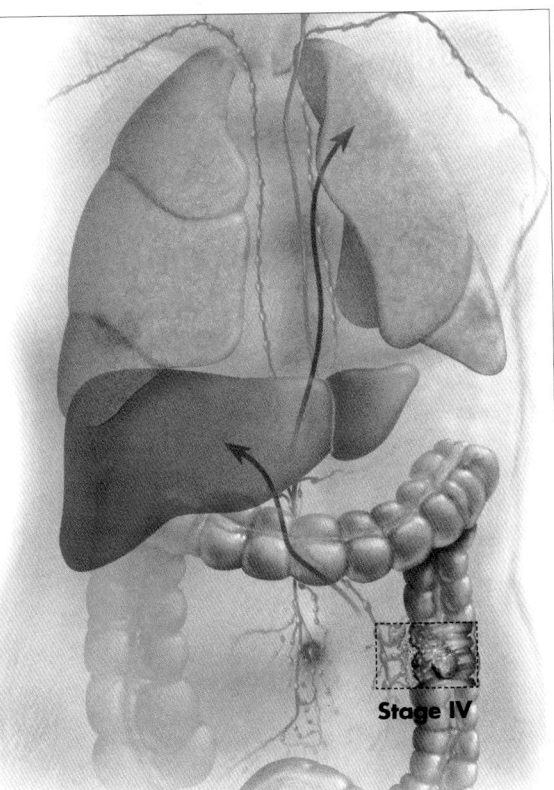

Stage IV

Unlike some other cancers, the size of the cancerous tumor isn't a major factor in determining the outcome of colorectal cancer. Of greater importance is how far the cancer has spread.

A hernia occurs when an organ pushes through an opening in the muscle or tissue that holds the organ in place. Types of hernias include hiatal, umbilical and inguinal.

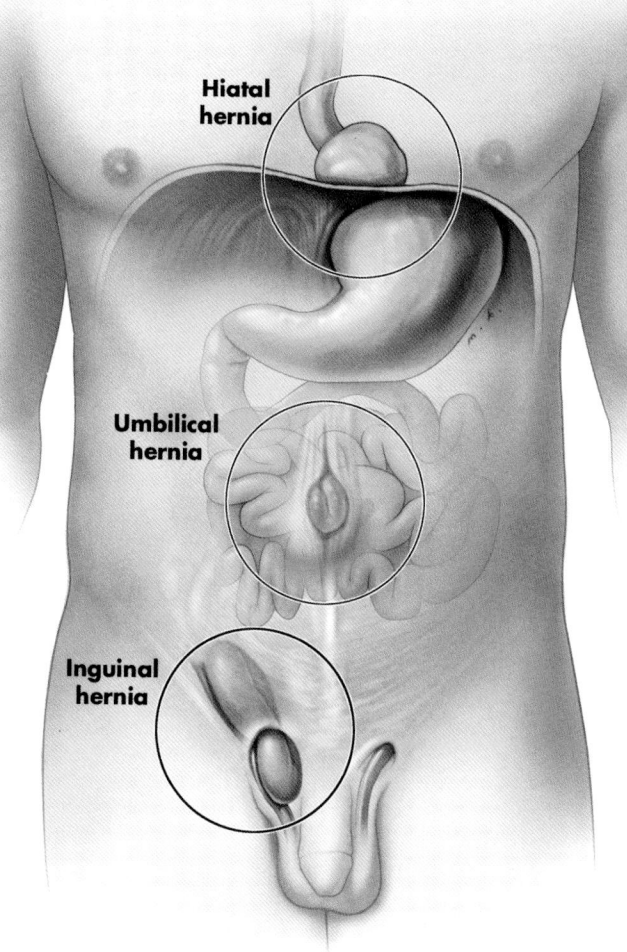

Hiatal hernia

Umbilical hernia

Inguinal hernia

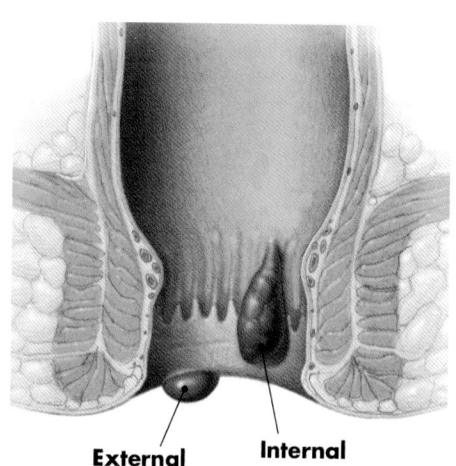

External　**Internal**

Hemorrhoids are swollen and inflamed veins in the anus and rectum. Hemorrhoids may be located inside the rectum (internal hemorrhoids), or they may develop under the skin around the anus (external hemorrhoids).

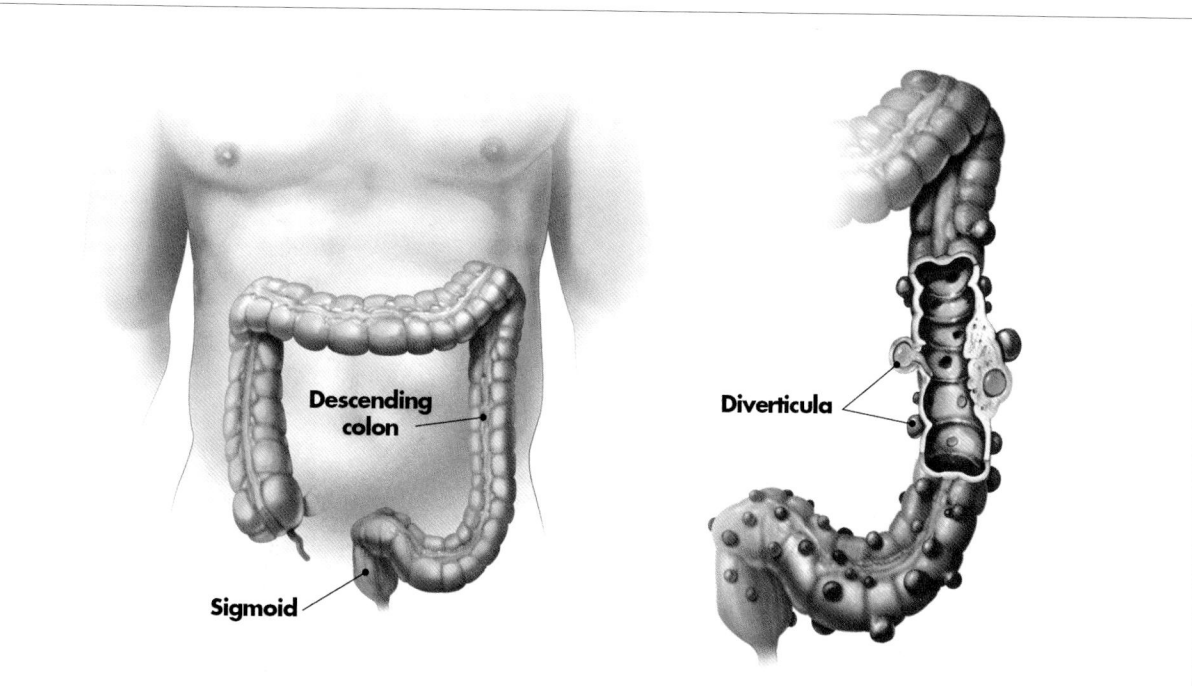

Descending colon

Diverticula

Sigmoid

Diverticulosis occurs when small, bulging pouches (diverticula) develop in the digestive tract. When one or more of these pouches becomes inflamed or infected, the condition is called diverticulitis.

Anatomy and Common Disorders **385**

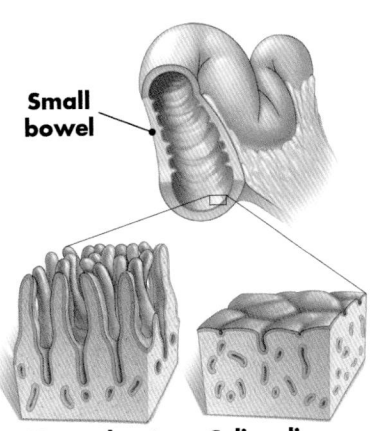

Small bowel

Normal gut   **Celiac disease**

The small intestine is lined with tiny hairlike projections called villi, which absorb vitamins, minerals and other nutrients from food. Celiac disease damages the villi, leaving the body unable to absorb nutrients necessary for health and growth.

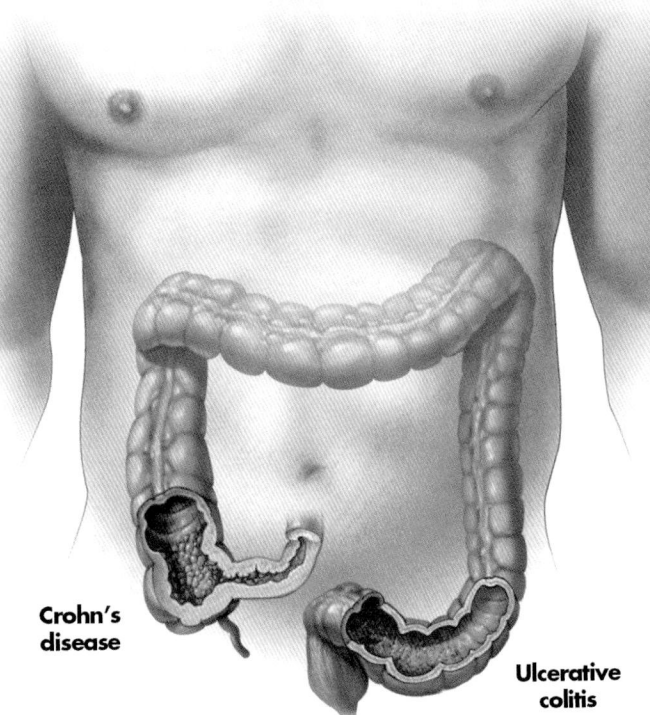

Crohn's disease

Ulcerative colitis

In ulcerative colitis, the lining of the large intestine (colon) becomes inflamed and develops open sores (ulcers). Crohn's disease can affect any part of the gastrointestinal tract, and it may spread deeper to all layers of tissue.

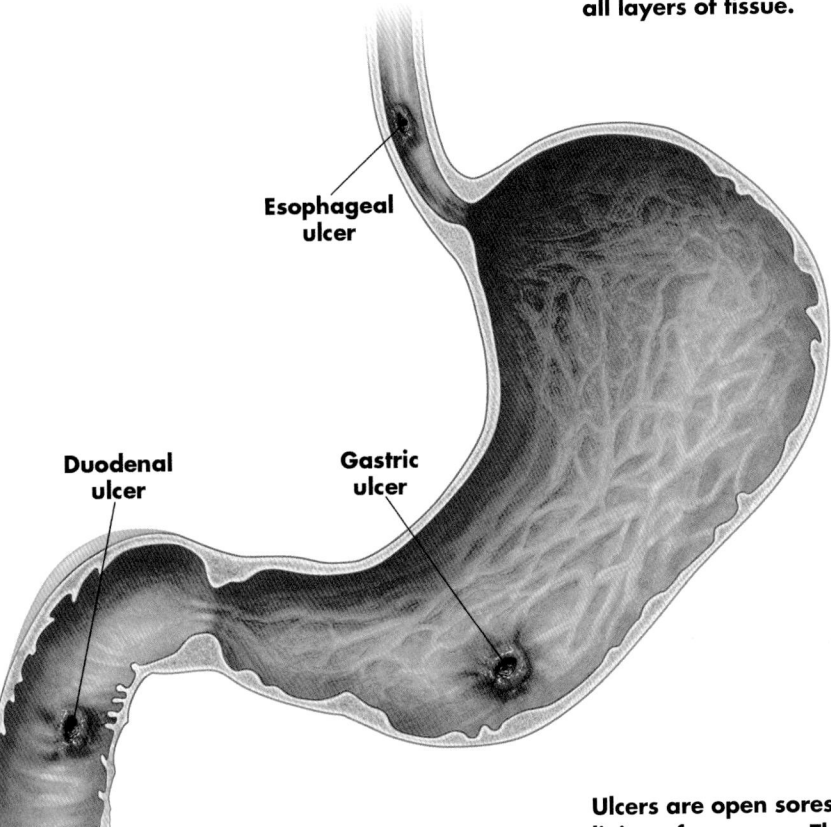

Esophageal ulcer

Duodenal ulcer

Gastric ulcer

Ulcers are open sores that develop in the inner lining of an organ. The most common are peptic ulcers, which may form in the esophagus (esophageal ulcer), the stomach (gastric ulcer) or the upper portion of the small intestine (duodenal ulcer).

Brain Disorders

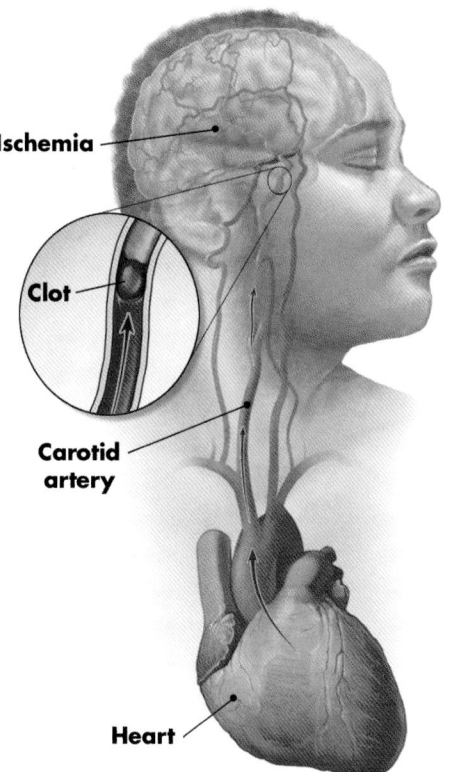

Trauma or disease can lead to a brain disorder. A violent blow to the head and neck or the upper body can result in a concussion, in which the brain slides back and forth forcefully against the inner walls of the skull. Sometimes, a brain injury can rupture a blood vessel within the brain and cause blood to collect within the skull. This condition is known as an intra-cranial hematoma (see below).

Common diseases to affect the brain include stroke and Alzheimer's disease.

(see below)

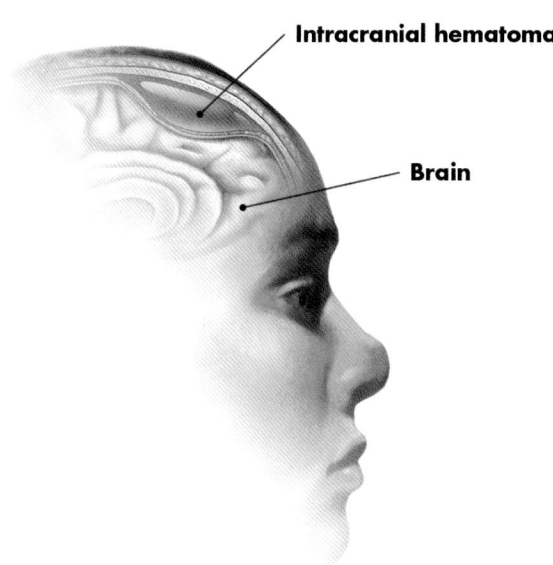

The most common type of stroke, an ischemic stroke, results when a blood clot lodges in a brain artery, disrupting blood flow. The clot may form in a carotid artery in the neck or elsewhere in the body, such as the heart, and travel through the bloodstream to the brain.

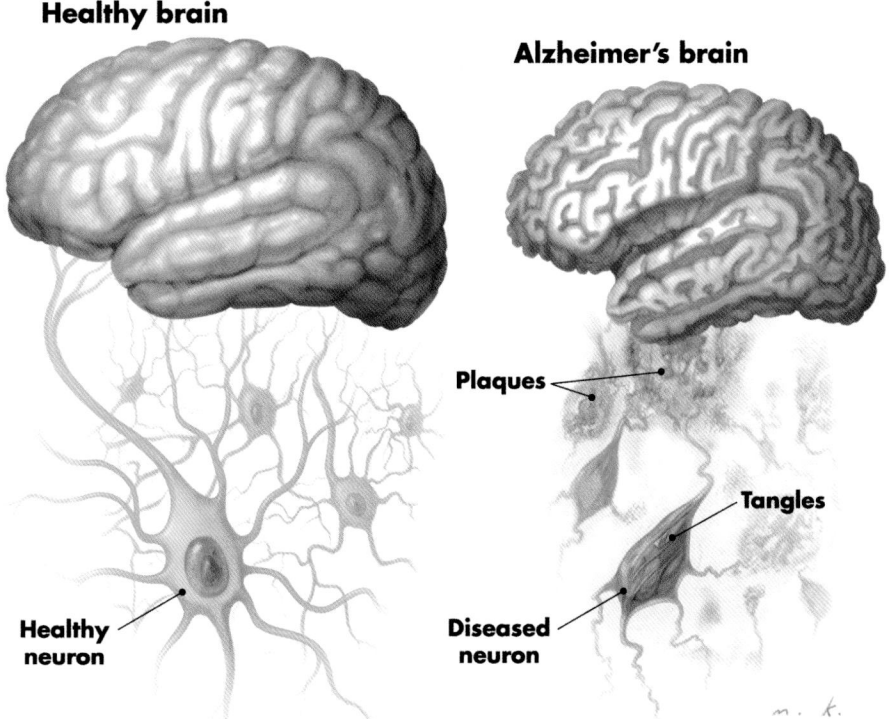

Alzheimer's disease is associated with plaques and tangles that destroy brain cells. Plaques are clumps of a protein called beta-amyloid that damage brain cells in several ways. Tangles result from abnormal twisting of a protein called tau that prevents the transportation of nutrients.

VISUAL GUIDE

Ear, Nose and Throat Disorders

Several conditions can affect the ears, nose and throat. An ear infection (see below), results when swelling, inflammation and mucus block the tiny eustachian tubes that drain fluid from the ears. Fluid accumulates and serves as a breeding ground for viruses and bacteria. When the cavities around the nasal passages (sinuses) become inflamed and swollen, mucus may accumulate in the cavities. This is known as sinusitis (see bottom left).

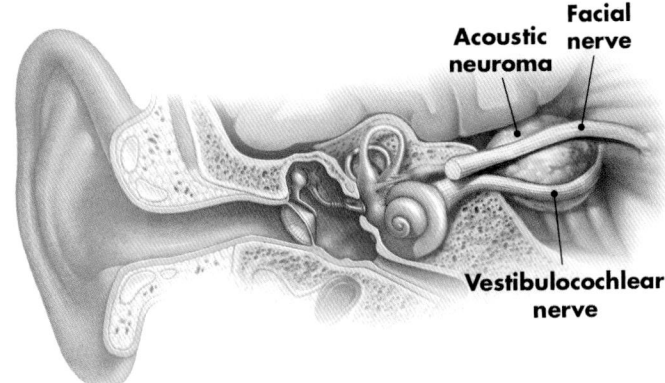

Acoustic neuroma
Facial nerve
Vestibulocochlear nerve

An acoustic neuroma is a benign tumor that develops on the auditory (cochlear) nerves leading from your inner ear to the brain. Pressure on the nerves from the tumor may cause hearing loss or imbalance.

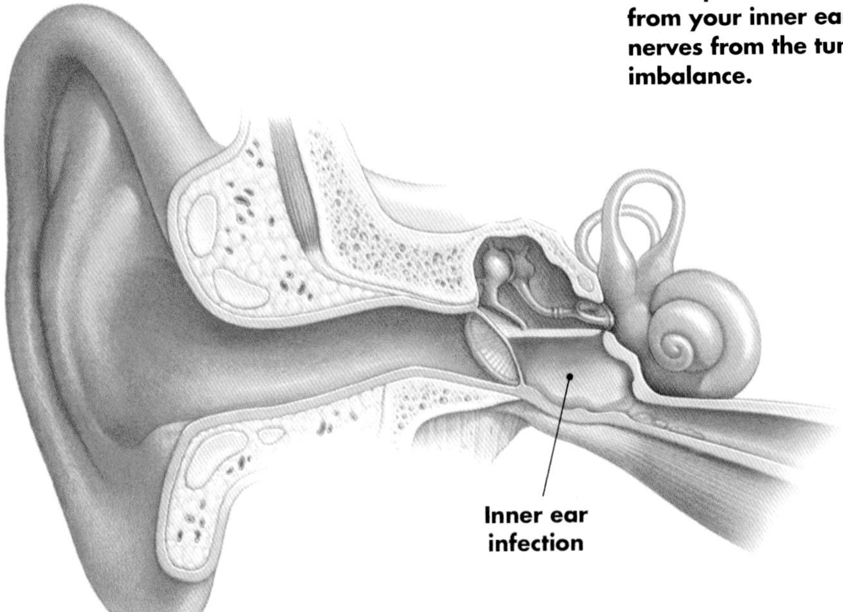

Inner ear infection

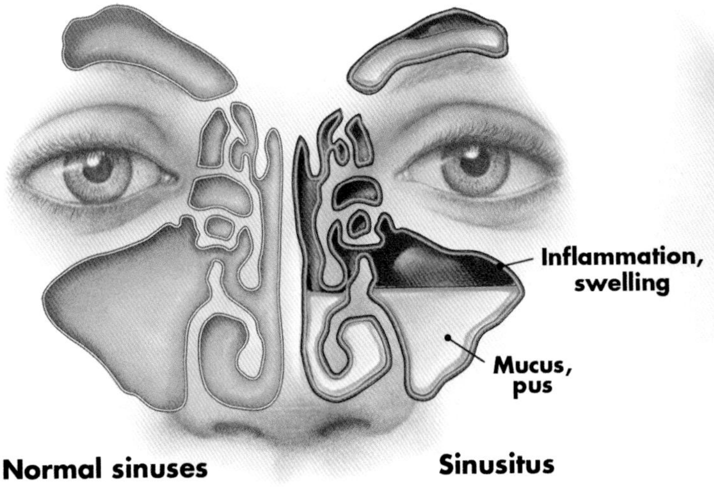

Polyps

Inflammation, swelling

Mucus, pus

Normal sinuses

Sinusitus

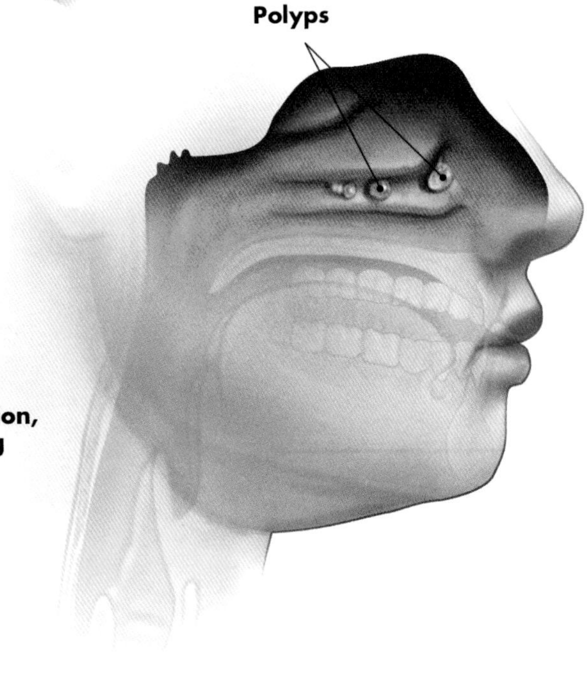

Nasal polyps are noncancerous growths that hang down like teardrops or grapes. Larger polyps or groups of polyps can block nasal passages, interfering with breathing.

Kidney and Urinary Disorders

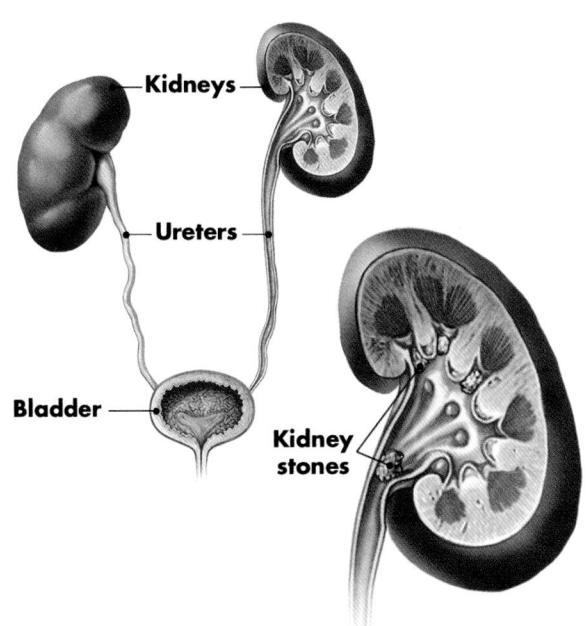

Kidney stones are hard deposits of minerals and salts that form in the kidneys (see left). As the stones move into the ureters — the thin tubes that allow urine to pass from the kidneys to the bladder — signs and symptoms, including severe pain, can result.

Bladder cancer (see middle left) develops when cells that line the inside of the bladder begin to grow abnormally, forming a tumor.

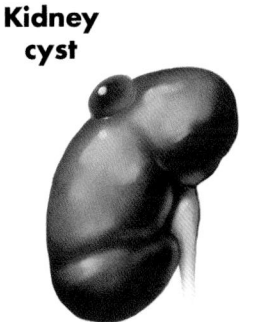

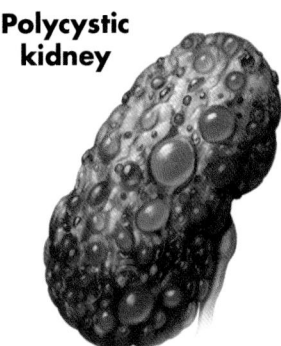

A kidney cyst is a fluid-filled pouch that typically grows on the surface of the kidney. Some cysts may develop inside. Simple kidney cysts rarely cause complications. With polycystic kidney disease, an inherited disorder, clusters of cysts develop within the kidneys, causing the kidneys to enlarge and lose function over time.

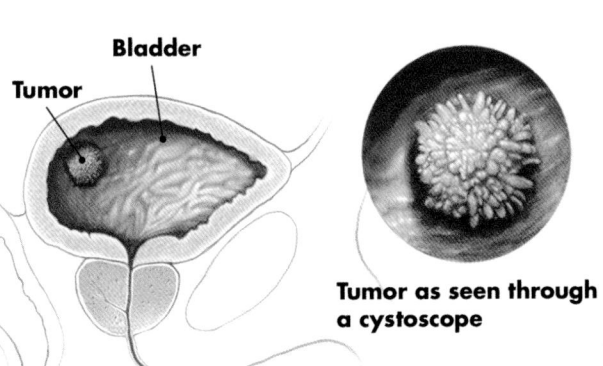

Tumor as seen through a cystoscope

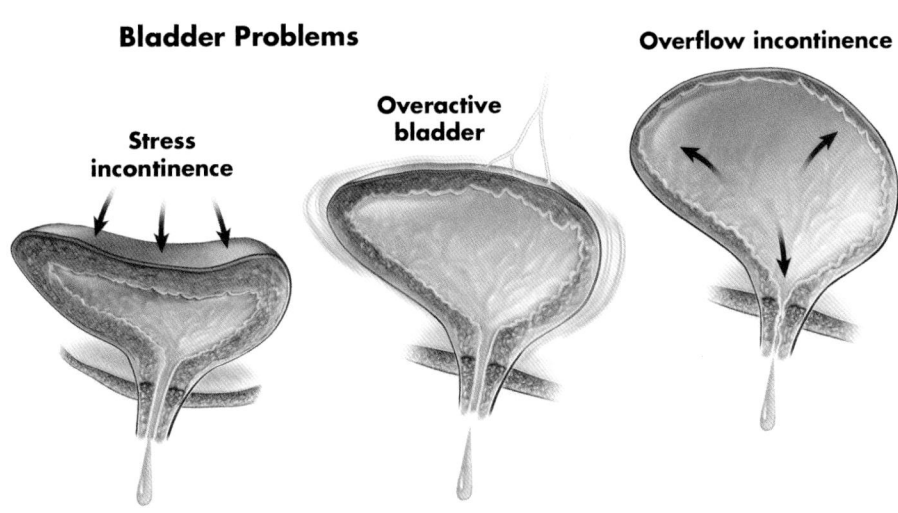

With stress incontinence (left) urine leaks when pressure is exerted on the bladder, such as from coughing, sneezing or laughing. With an overactive bladder (center), the bladder muscle contracts too often, signaling to the brain the need to urinate. Overflow incontinence (right) stems from the inability to completely empty the bladder, causing urine to accumulate and leak.

Liver Disorders

Liver disorders may be inherited (genetic) or be caused by a variety of factors that damage the liver, such as viruses and alcohol use.

Liver cysts, also called hepatic cysts (see below), are fluid-filled cavities in the liver. They generally don't cause signs or symptoms, but some can become large enough to produce discomfort.

Nonalcoholic fatty liver disease (see bottom illustration) includes a range of liver conditions affecting people who drink little to no alcohol. The main characteristic is too much fat stored in liver cells.

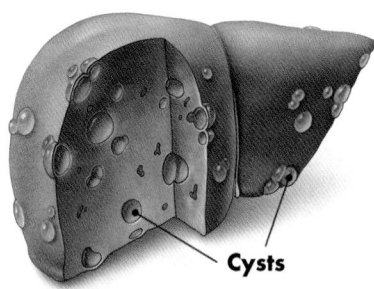

Cysts

Normal liver

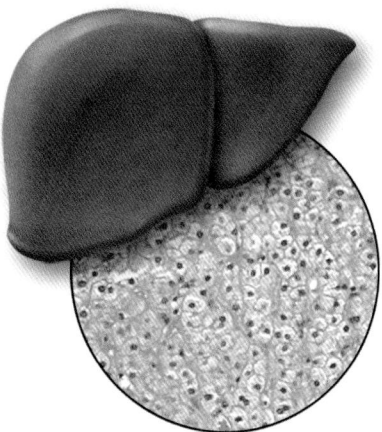

Fatty liver

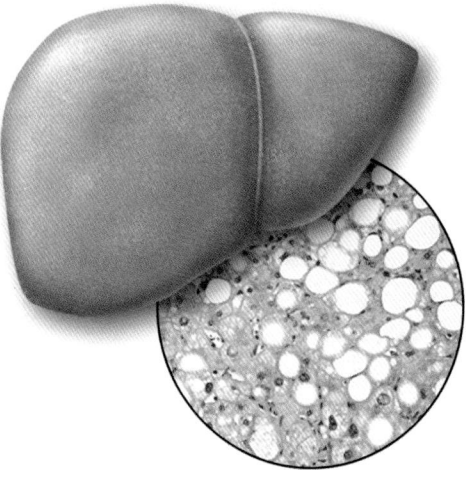

Normal

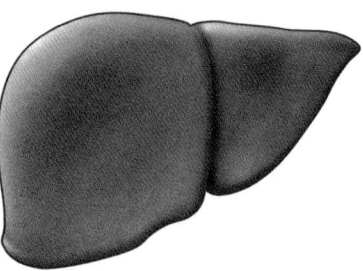

Chronic hepatitis

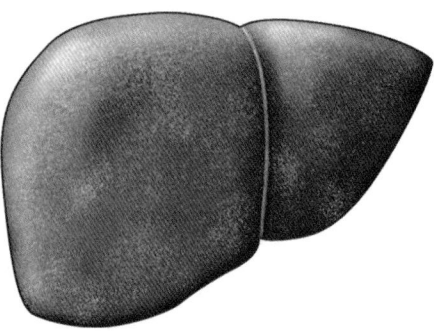

Cirrhosis

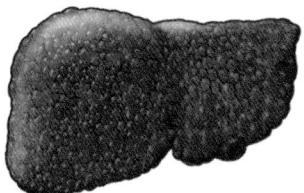

Cancer

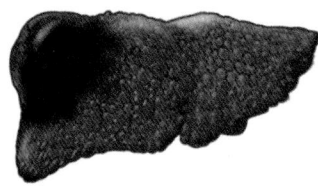

A normal liver is about the size of a football. Chronic hepatitis causes the liver to inflame and enlarge due to infection or other causes. Inflammation that continues over many years can lead to scarring (cirrhosis) of the liver. Cirrhosis also can result from chronic alcohol use. Hepatocellular carcinoma is the most common form of cancer that originates in the liver as a primary cancer. It occurs most often in people who have cirrhosis of the liver.

Eye Disorders

The delicate structures of the eye often change with age, making it more difficult to see. Aging also increases the risk of serious eye disorders.

Although certain vision problems may be an unavoidable, natural part of aging, others can be prevented. Even those that are unavoidable can often be slowed or stopped through early detection and treatment.

Some of the most common eye disorders include cataracts, glaucoma, macular degeneration and diabetic retinopathy.

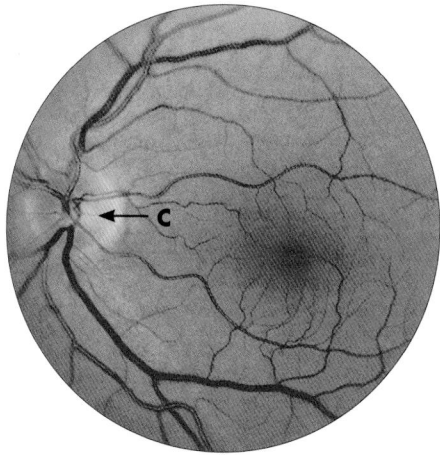

A cataract occurs when the lens of the eye becomes cloudy, giving the pupil a white appearance.

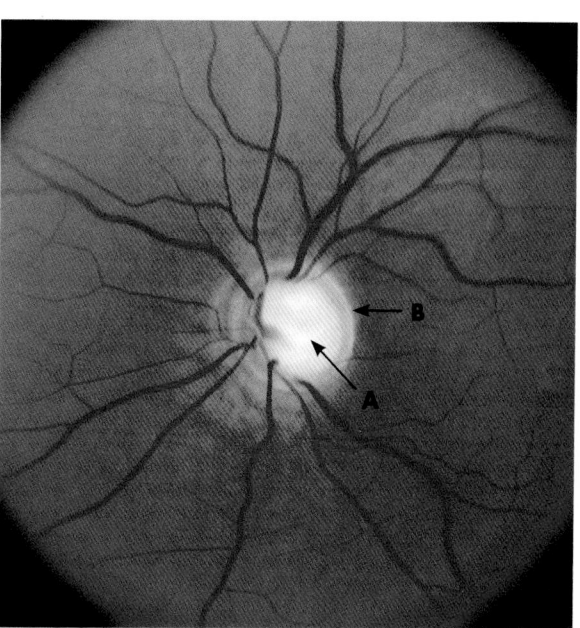

The photo on the right shows an optic nerve that's damaged by advanced glaucoma. This is evident from the evacuation (cupping) at the center of the optic disk (A). Only a narrow rim of optic nerve tissue remains (B). In comparison, the optic disk of a healthy eye (above) has more even and reddish coloration (C).

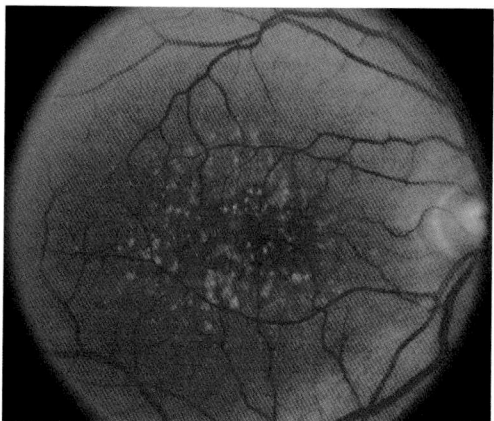

The hallmark of early-stage dry macular degeneration is the appearance of waste deposits (drusen) in and around the macula. Drusen have the appearance of yellow spots.

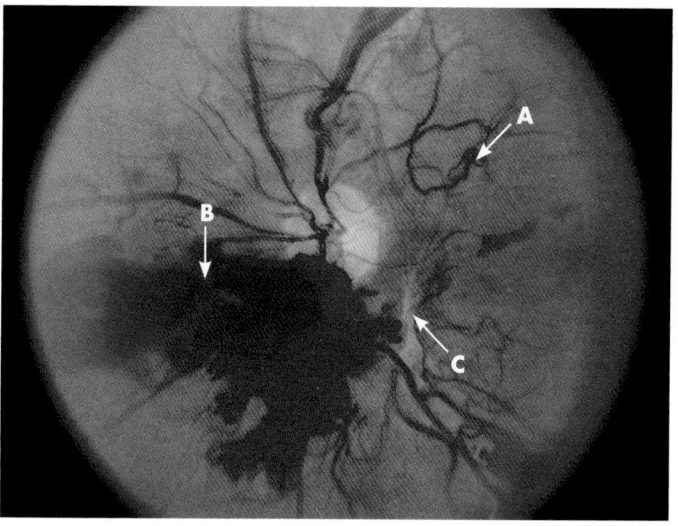

In late-stage proliferative diabetic retinopathy, abnormal blood vessels grow on the optic nerve and the retina and into the vitreous cavity (A). These blood vessels break, causing bleeding (B) and the formation of scar tissue (C).

Skin Disorders

The color and texture of your skin can reveal a great deal about the health of your skin and your health in general. Sometimes the first clue to illness is revealed by a rash or welts. At other times, the skin disorder itself is the only abnormality.

Psoriasis and Dermatitis

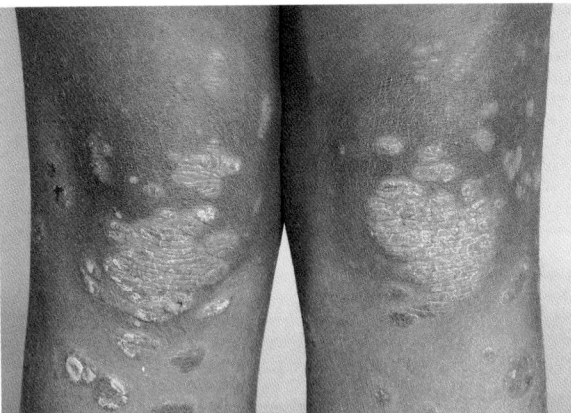

Psoriasis. Areas of skin are covered with dry, red patches with silvery scales. Lesions may itch.

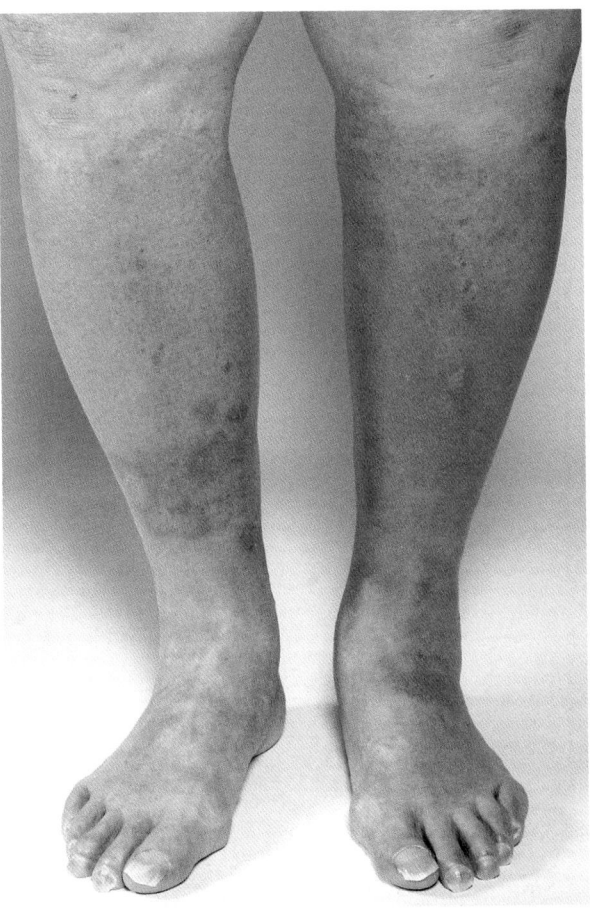

Stasis dermatitis. Thickening, redness and itching of the skin of the lower legs and ankles, often associated with varicose veins.

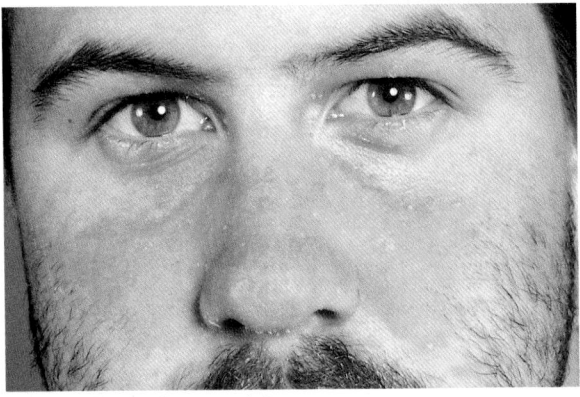

Seborrheic dermatitis. Greasy-appearing, scaly, itchy areas on the sides of the nose, between the eyebrows, behind the ears or on the scalp.

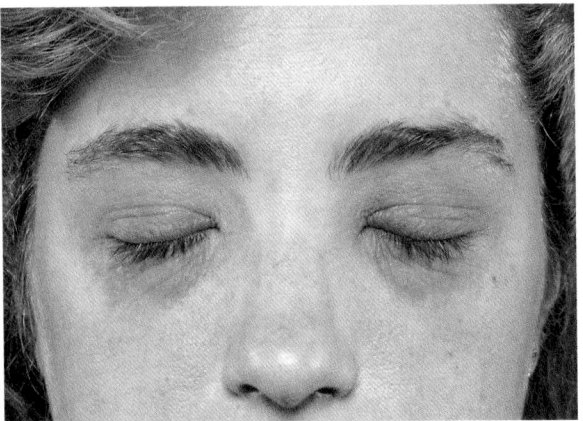

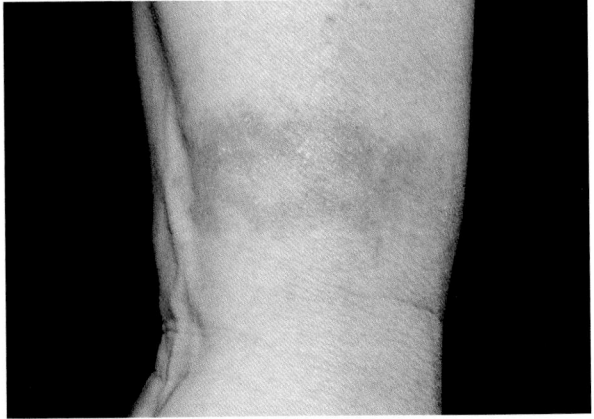

Contact dermatitis. Skin redness and itching resulting from direct contact with a plant, chemical or other substance, such as makeup (left) or a bracelet made from nickel (right).

Pigmentary Disorders

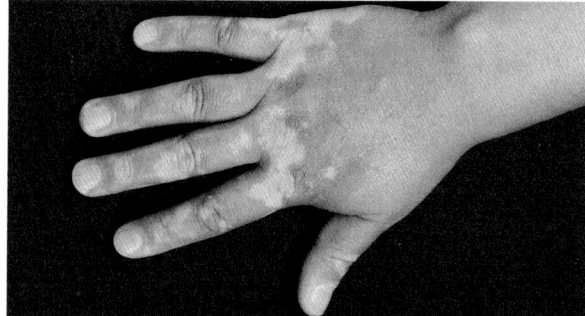

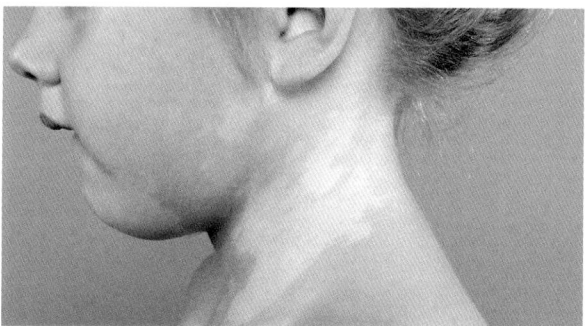

Vitiligo. The development of patches of white or depigmented skin.

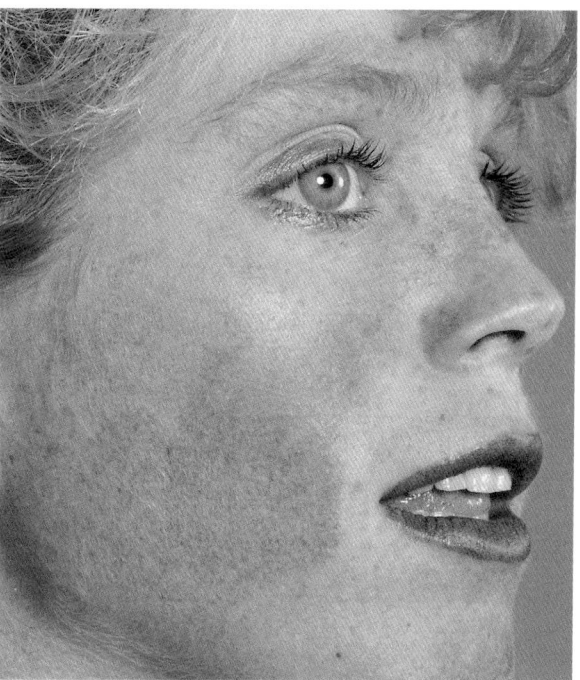

Melasma. Patches of darker skin, most commonly found on the face. Results from excessive melanin in the skin. The condition is common during pregnancy.

Aging Skin

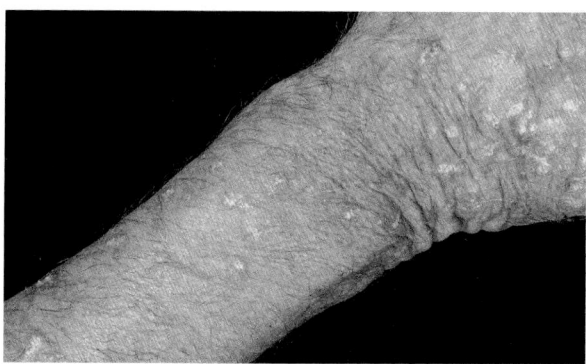

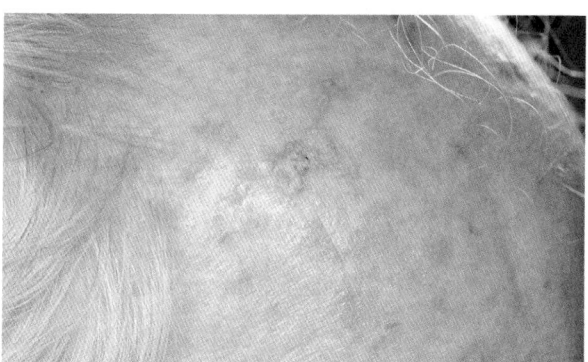

Actinic (solar) keratoses. Gritty, scaly, gray to dark pink patches on face, scalp and back of hands. The patches have a sandpaper surface. They may be precancerous.

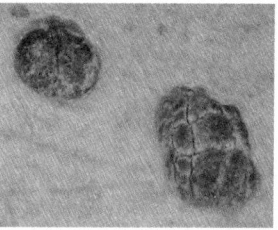
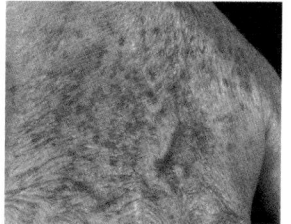
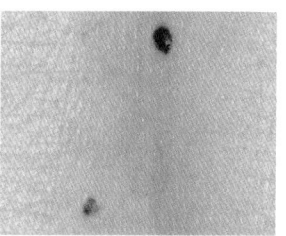
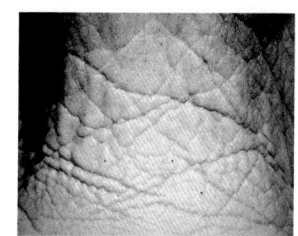

Seborrheic keratoses (upper left). Oval lesions with a waxy, scaly, slightly elevated appearance.

Solar lentigines (upper right). Flat patches of increased pigmentation that range from freckle sized to a few inches across. Also called liver spots.

Cherry angiomas (bottom left). Characterized by small, smooth, cherry-red bumps on skin. Range in size from a pinhead to ¼-inch across.

Sun-damaged skin (bottom right). Coarse wrinkles, sagging folds, dryness or leathery toughness.

Skin Cancer

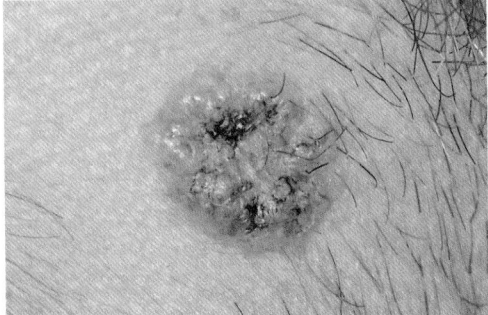

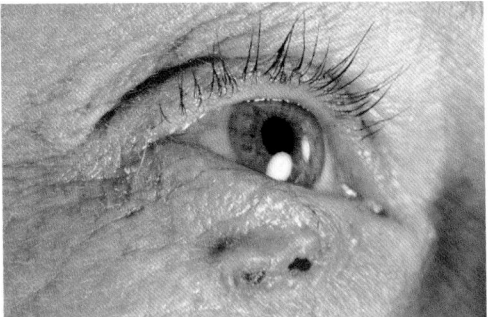

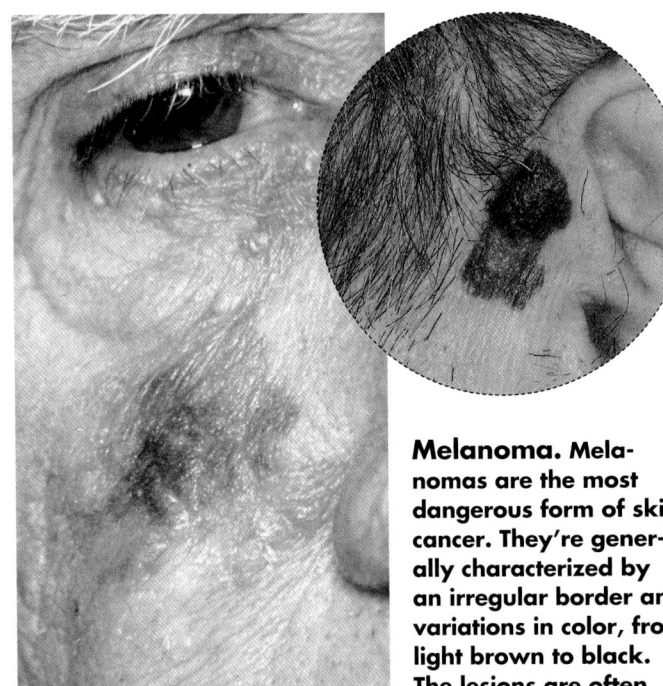

Basal cell cancer. The most common malignant skin tumor. Characterized by a pearly or waxy bump commonly found on the face, ears or neck. Or it may be a flat, flesh-colored or brown scar-like lesion.

Melanoma. Melanomas are the most dangerous form of skin cancer. They're generally characterized by an irregular border and variations in color, from light brown to black. The lesions are often firm and dome shaped.

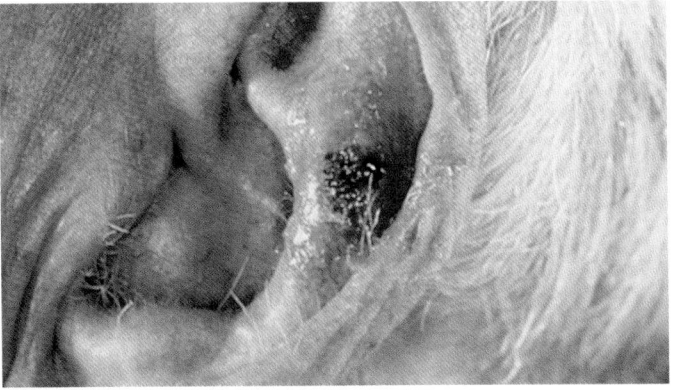

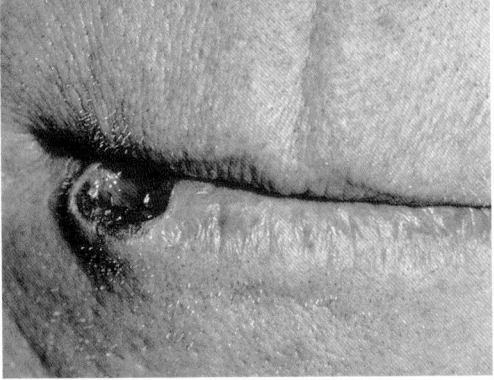

Squamous cell cancer. This skin cancer typically appears in areas exposed to sun. The lesion is generally firm, red, nodular or flat and has a scaly, crusted or ulcerated surface.

Noncancerous (Benign) Growths

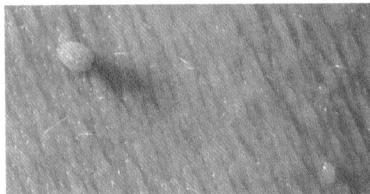

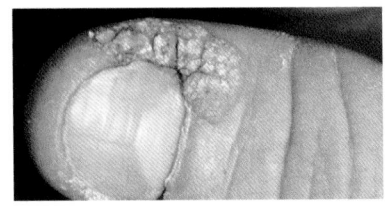

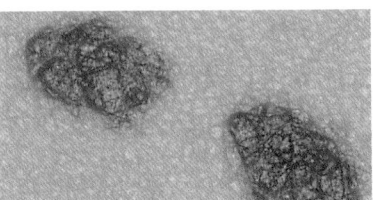

Skin tag. Tiny, soft growth attached to a narrow stalk. Often skin colored but may be darker.

Warts. Caused by a virus that stimulates rapid reproduction of skin cells. Most commonly occur on hands or feet.

Moles. Accumulations of pigment cells. May stay smooth or become raised or wrinkled, and may contain hair.

Acne

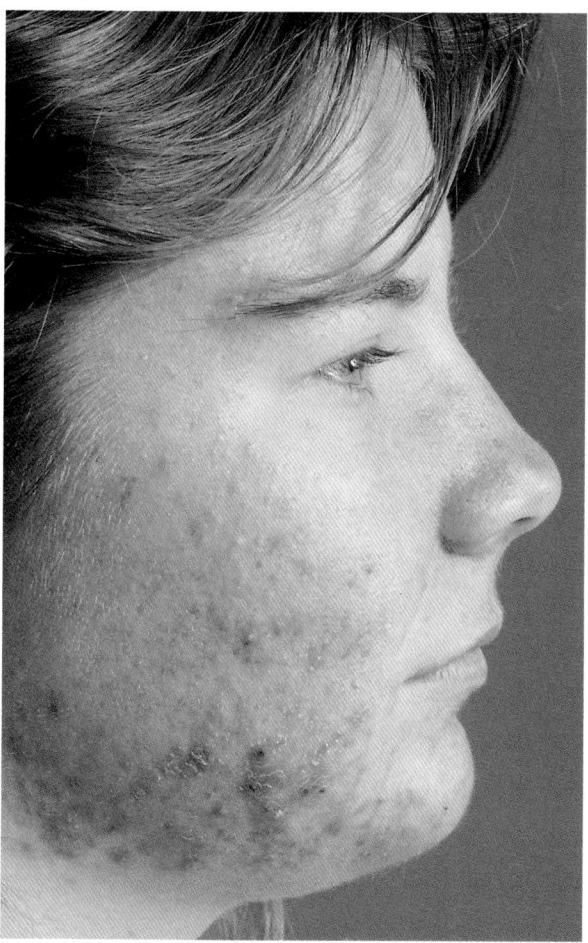

Common acne. Clogging of hair pores (follicles) in skin, causing the development of whiteheads or blackheads on the face, neck, shoulders or back.

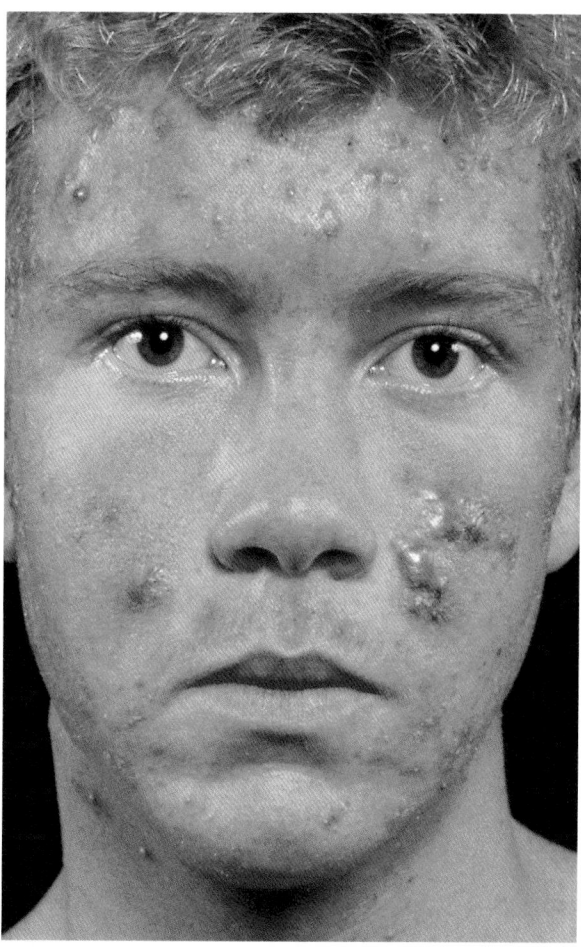

Cystic acne. Most severe form of acne. Clogged pores cause boil-like infections (cysts) in the skin.

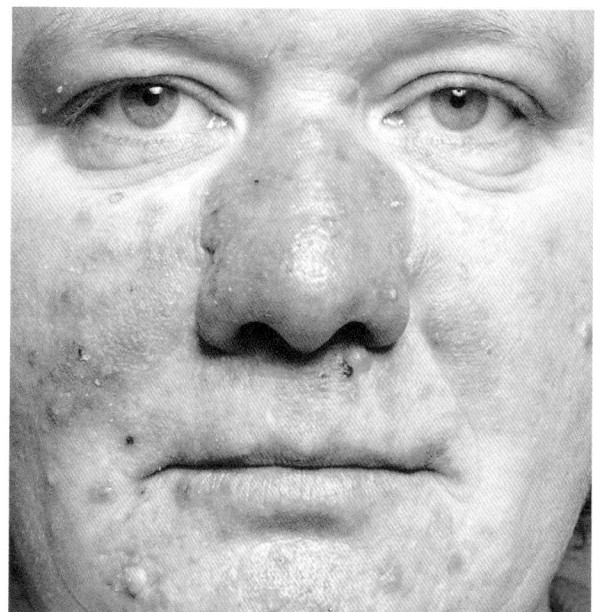

Acne rosacea. Chronic inflammation of the central face with pustules in the reddened area. Occurs most often in adults.

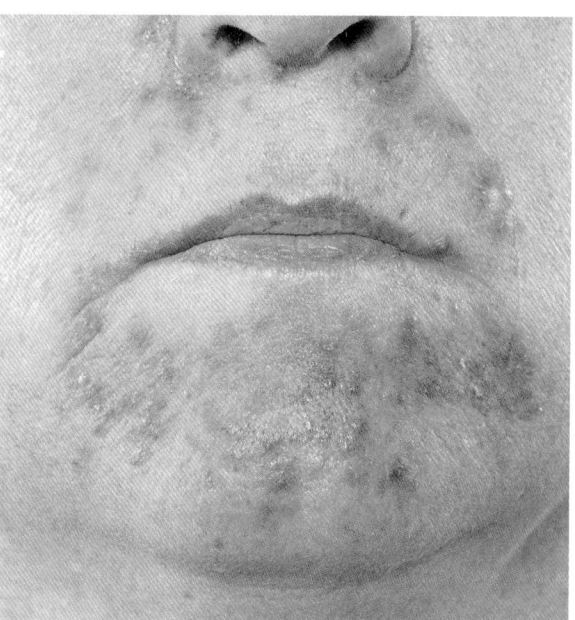

Perioral dermatitis. Red, often bumpy, rash around the mouth and chin. An area of normal skin usually separates the edge of the lips from the rash.

Childhood Diseases

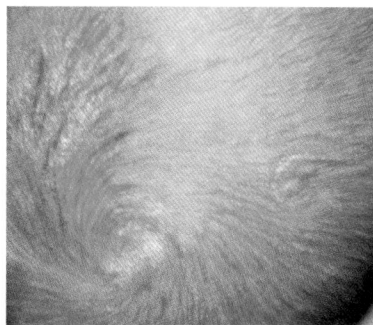

Cradle cap (infantile seborrheic dermatitis). Dry, scaly patches. Yellow crust may form over the patches.

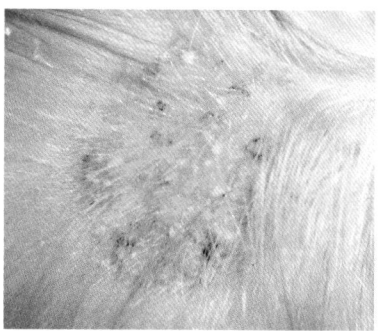

Scalp ringworm (tinea capitis). A fungal infection that causes an itchy, red, circular patch on the scalp.

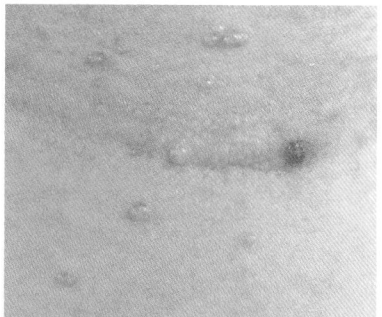

Molluscum contagiosum. Tiny pearl-like projections with a white, cheesy core.

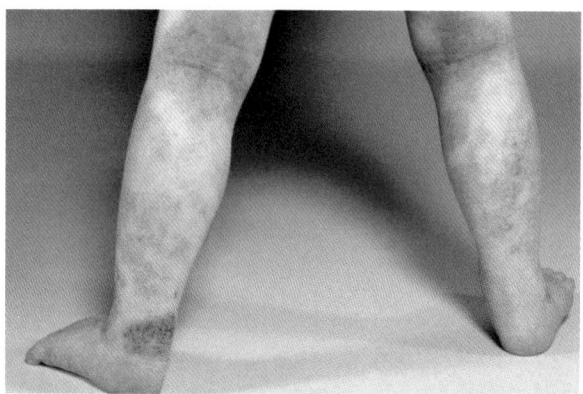

Infantile eczema. Rough, red, patchy rash usually associated with extremely dry skin.

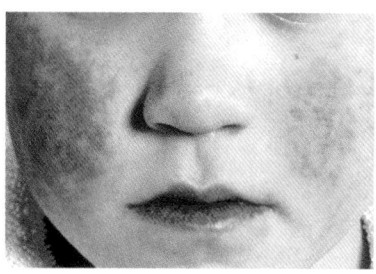

Fifth disease. A viral infection that causes a red rash on the cheeks, appearing as if the cheeks have been slapped.

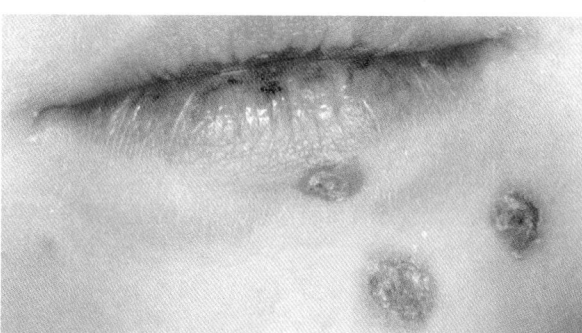

Impetigo. Bacterial infection that starts with a red sore, blisters briefly, oozes and forms a thick crust.

Keratoses pilaris. Dead skin cells plug hair follicle openings, causing small, pointed pimples.

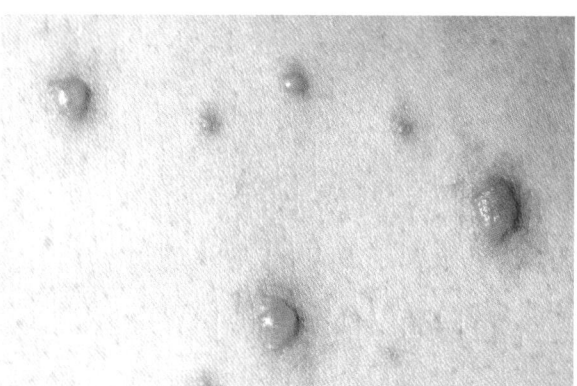

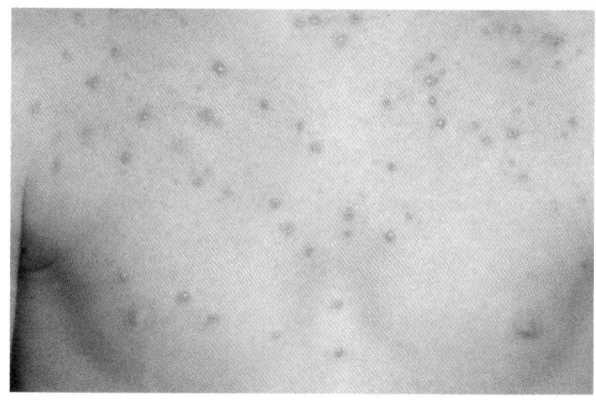

Chickenpox (varicella). Itchy, red rash that breaks out (erupts) on the face, scalp, chest, back, and arms and legs. Spots fill with clear fluid, rupture and then crust over.

Infestations and Bites

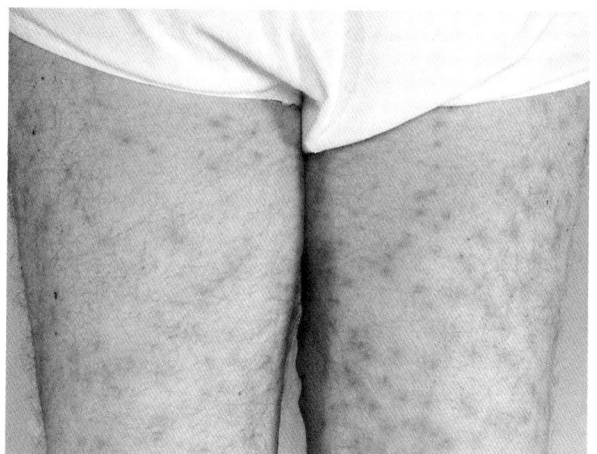

Swimmer's itch. Sandpaper-like rash caused by parasitic infestation. Develops after swimming in fresh water. Most noticeable beneath swimsuit.

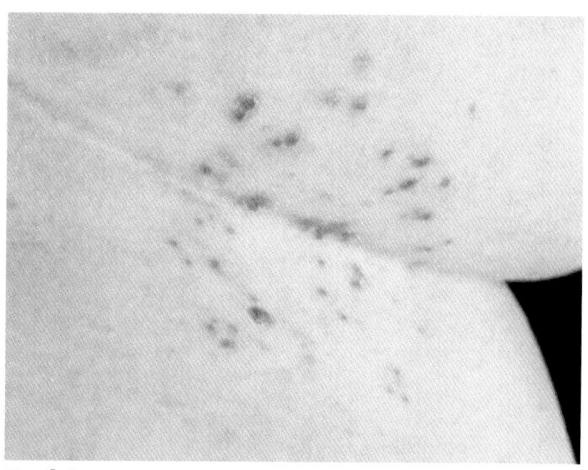

Scabies. Lesions where tiny mites burrow in the skin. Itching is often severe.

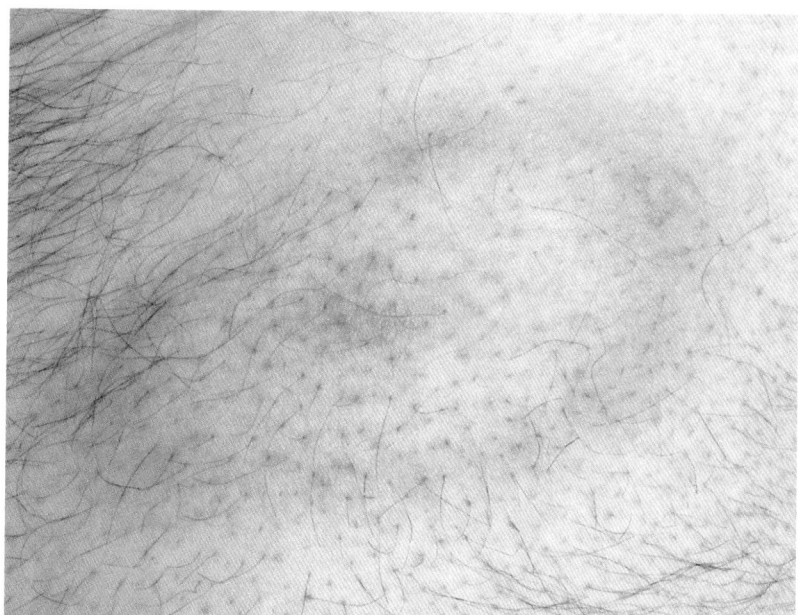

Lyme disease. Red rash that usually occurs at the site of a tick bite. Central portion clears as the rash spreads outward.

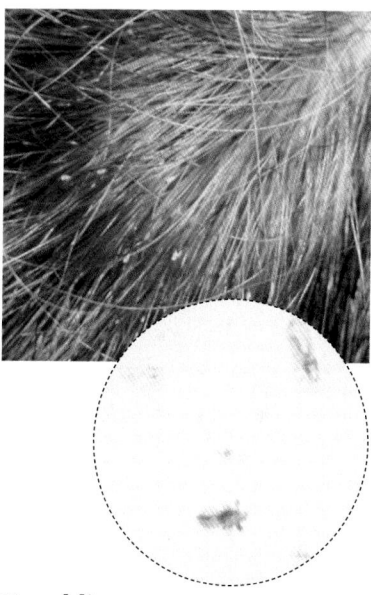

Head lice. Tiny insects found on the scalp. Small nits (eggs) resembling tiny pussy willow buds are found on hair shafts.

Hives

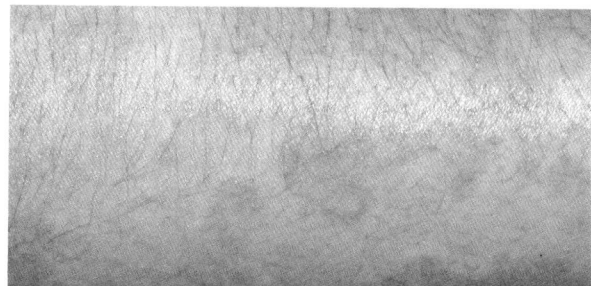

Hives (urticaria). Characterized by raised, red, itchy welts of various sizes on the surface of the skin.

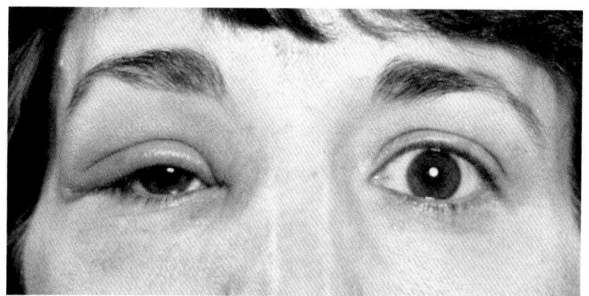

Angioedema. Large welts develop below the surface of the skin, particularly on the eyes and lips, but also on the hands, on the feet and in the throat.

Fungal Infections

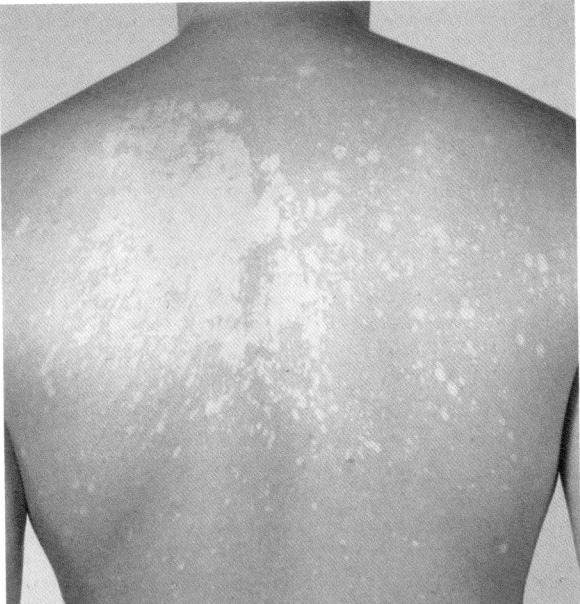

Tinea versicolor. Characterized by small, scaly, pale patches on the upper body and neck or face.

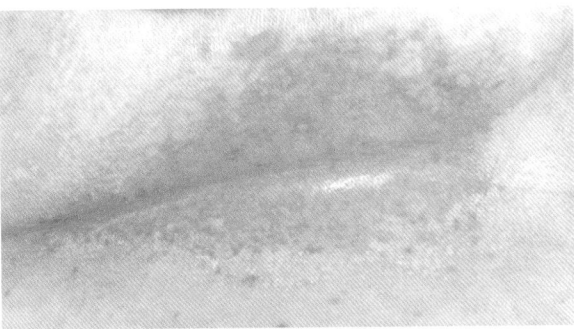

Intertrigo. Red, moist patches rimmed with small, red bumps found under the breasts, in armpits, in groin or buttock folds, or between fingers or toes.

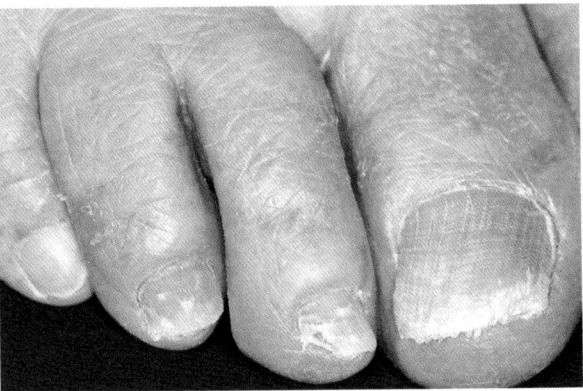

Onychomycosis. Fungal infection in the toenails or fingernails. Nails become discolored, pitted and may thicken.

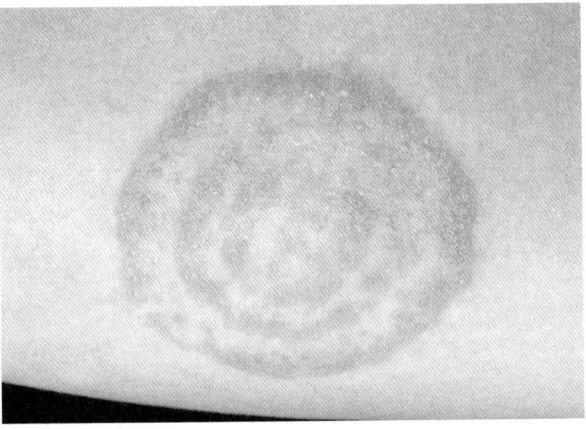

Ringworm (tinea corporis). Itchy, red, scaly, slightly raised expanding rings on the trunk, face, groin or thigh.

Other Infections

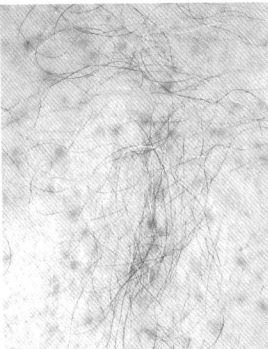

Folliculitis. Infection of hair follicles caused by bacteria or fungi.

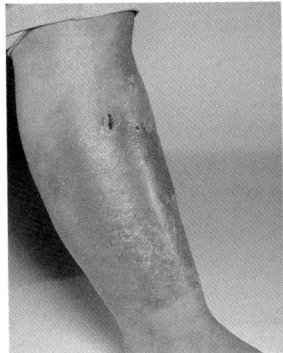

Cellulitis. Generally caused by bacterial infection. Characterized by hot, red, swollen and painful skin.

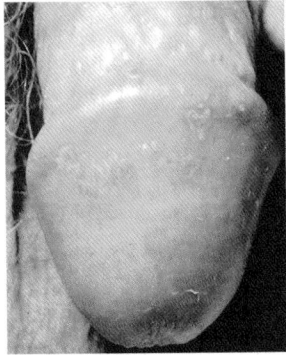

Genital herpes. Lesions characterized by blisters or open sores (ulcers). Often accompanied by burning or tingling sensation or pain.

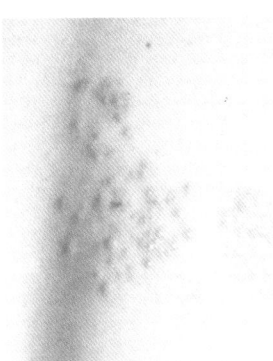

Shingles (herpes zoster). A red rash with small fluid-filled blisters, often extending out from the spine along a nerve pathway.

Hair Disorders

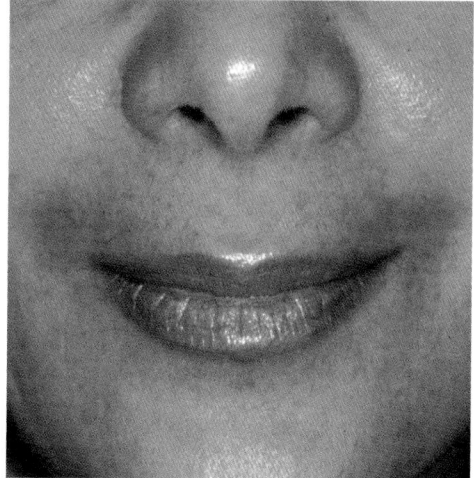

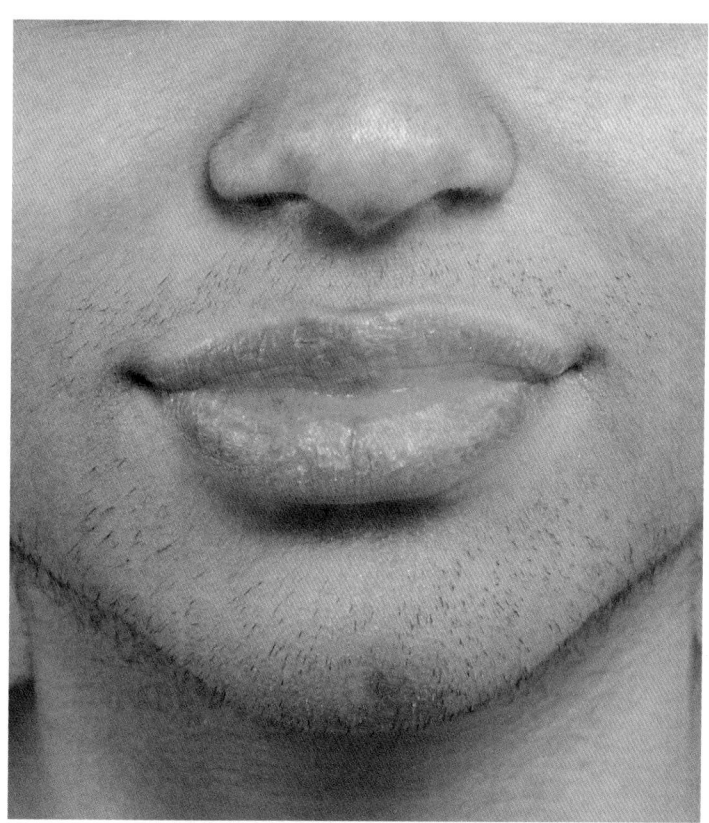

Hirsutism. Excess hair. Most often noticeable around the mouth and on the chin and neck of women.

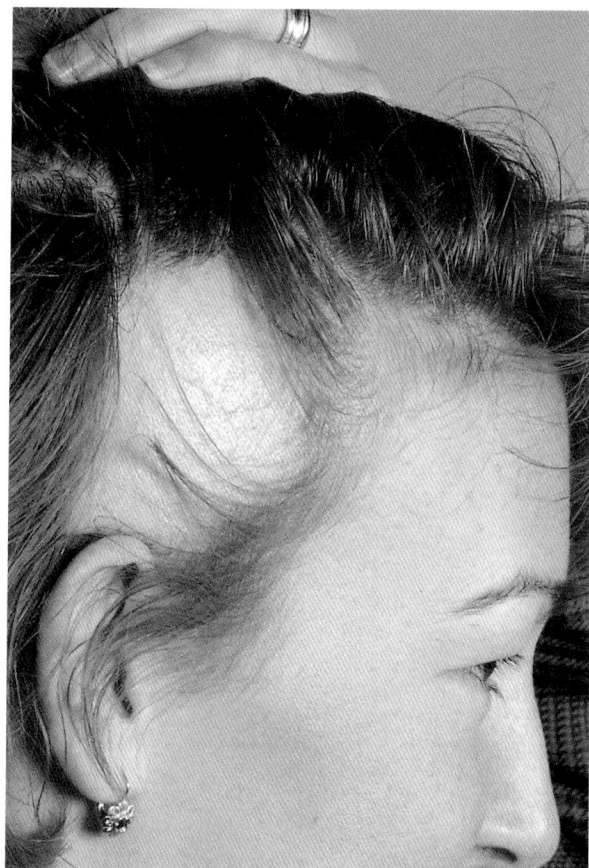

Alopecia areata. Hair loss that often starts with circular bald patches, which may overlap.

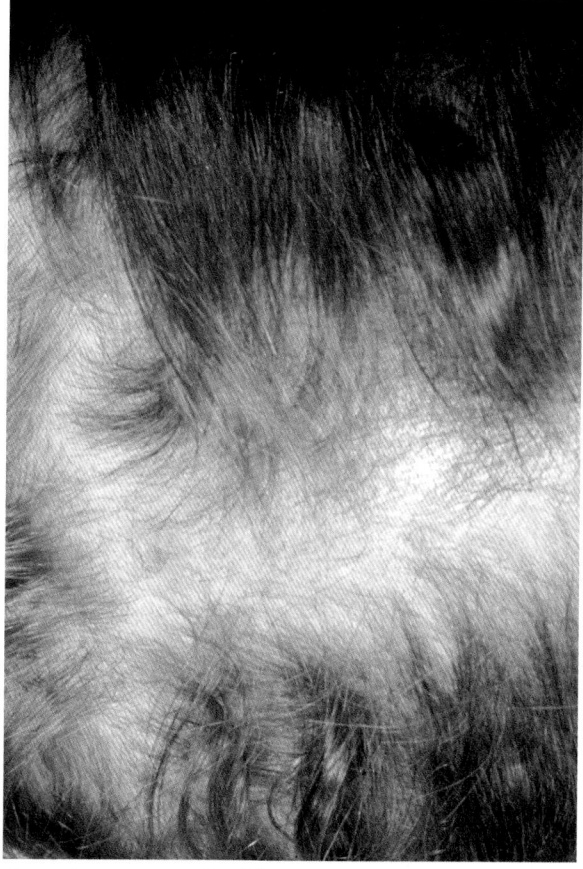

Female-pattern baldness. Generally, thinning of the hair all over the head, especially on the crown.

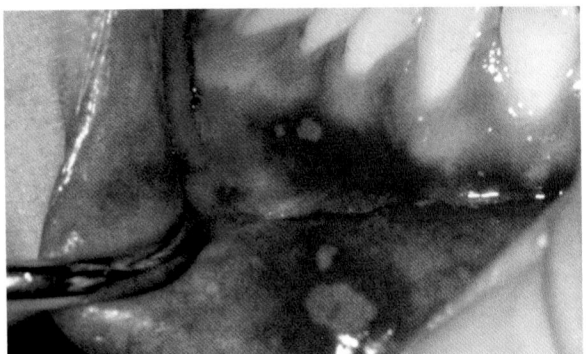

Canker sore. Occurs inside the oral cavity. A painful sore with a white or yellow center and a red border.

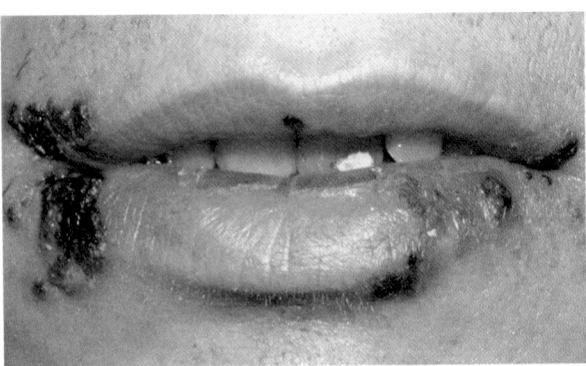

Cold sore (herpes simplex). Small, fluid-filled blisters on a raised, red, painful area. Blisters break and ooze. Yellow crust forms that sloughs off.

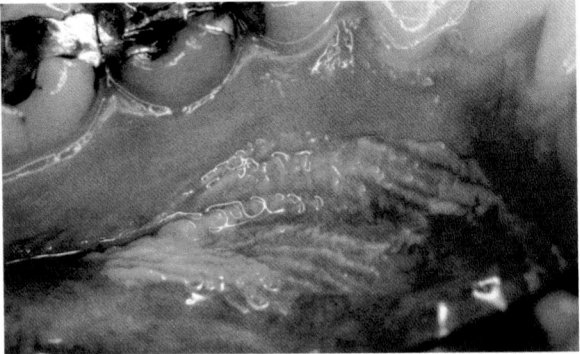

Leukoplakia. Thickened, hardened white patch on the cheek or tongue. May be a precancerous lesion.

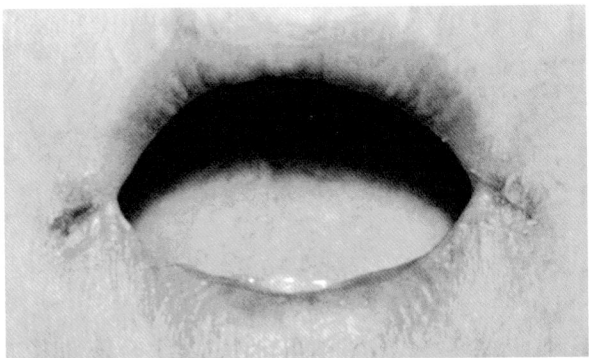

Cheilitis. Corners of the mouth become irritated, red and cracked. Fungus can grow in the corners of the mouth, keeping them inflamed and sore.

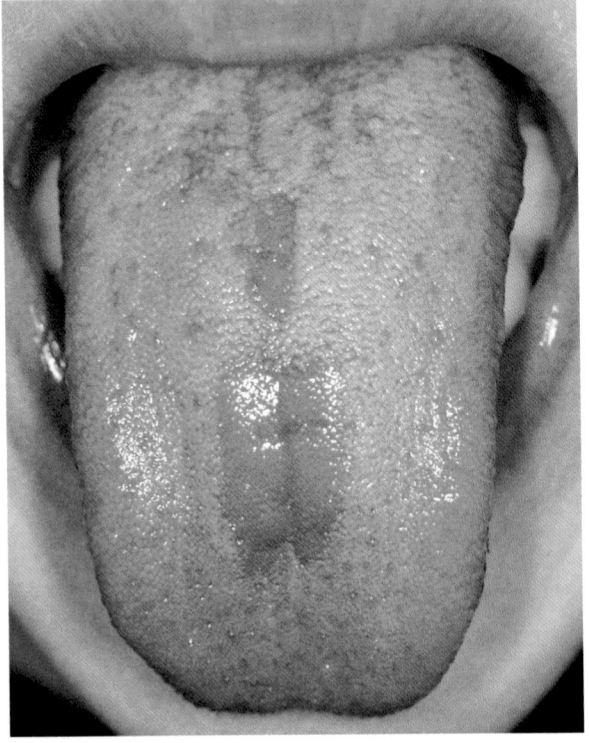

Geographic tongue. Patches with an absence of papillae, making the tongue appear smooth and bright red in the patches.

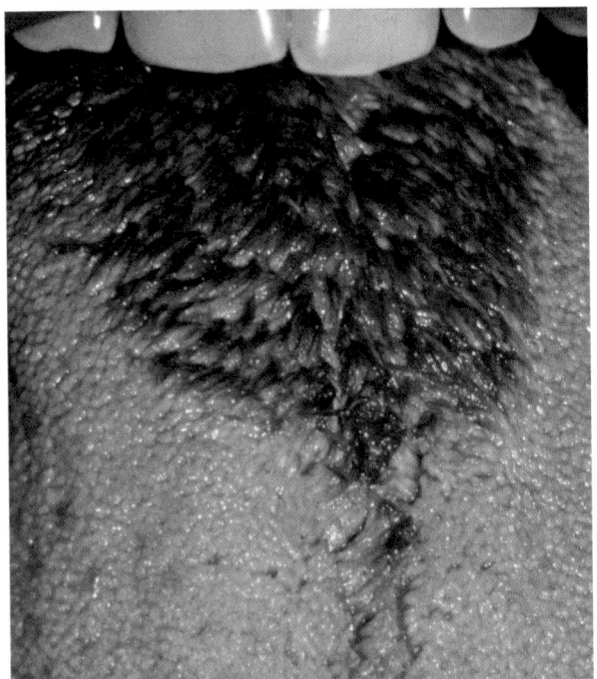

Black hairy tongue. Hairlike projections that grow on the tongue, giving it a hairy appearance.

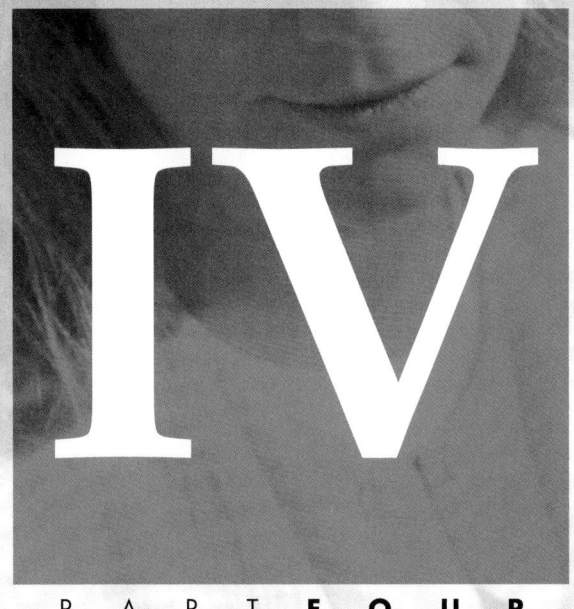

Diseases and Disorders

Genetics and Disease

Let's say you want to make a cake. If you don't know the ingredients and instructions by heart, you'll probably start off by finding a recipe. It should contain a detailed list of the ingredients that you'll need and directions on how to put them together so that the end result is a cake that's good to eat.

In much the same way, there's a recipe that makes you a living, breathing human being, entirely different from any other person on the planet. A complete version of this recipe is contained in virtually every cell in your body. Passed along to you from your parents, the recipe is coded into a long, twisted molecule of a chemical called deoxyribonucleic acid (DNA).

DNA is tightly packed into a set of structures — called chromosomes — within the nucleus of your cells. Within your chromosomes, DNA is arranged into segments called genes. Each one of your genes contains specific instructions for making a particular protein — a molecular structure that can do any number of jobs, from making up your skin and hair to acting as a hormone or enzyme and controlling chemical reactions in your cells. Just as ingredients such as flour, water and eggs come together to produce a cake, when these proteins are put together, they result in a human body.

When a cell divides, each gene must be copied so that the two resulting cells each has a complete set of genes. Mistakes in this copying process can and do occur. Most of the time, these mistakes are harmless and easily repaired, but sometimes they can cause disease and premature death. Genetics — the study of genes and diseases that genetic anomalies may cause — is a rapidly advancing medical field that's receiving a lot of attention.

Scientists have mapped out a rough draft of the specific components that make up the genes — approximately 20,000 of them —

typically present in a human being. The hope is that by studying and understanding the role of each of these genes, doctors and scientists will gain a better understanding of why and how things go wrong to cause illness.

In order to gain better insights into how genetics and disease are intertwined, it's helpful to understand some basic information about genes and chromosomes, inheritance patterns, and how living beings progress from a single cell to a fully formed adult. It's also useful to learn how some diseases may be passed on from one generation to the next, how genes and environment can work together to produce illnesses, and how the study of genes may lead

The Human Genome Project

The Human Genome Project has been one of the most ambitious projects ever undertaken by science. The international research effort, coordinated by the Department of Energy and the National Institutes of Health, took 13 years to complete, resulting in a literal map of all of the genes contained in the human genome. Project goals were to:

- Identify the approximately 20,000 genes in human DNA
- Determine the sequences of the 3 billion chemical base pairs in egg and sperm gamete cells (haploid genome)
- Store the information in databases
- Improve tools for data analysis
- Transfer related technologies to the private sector
- Address the ethical, legal and social issues that may arise from the project

The project was completed in 2003, but additional work followed to close gaps in information and reduce ambiguities.

to better treatment and, perhaps, even the cure or prevention of some diseases.

The Basics of Genetics

Your body is made up of trillions of microscopic cells. A typical human cell is about one-tenth the diameter of a human hair. Your cells are categorized into approximately 200 different types. For example, skin, muscle, bone and blood cells all perform different functions: making your skin soft, your muscles flexible, your bones solid and your blood fluid. Each cell's

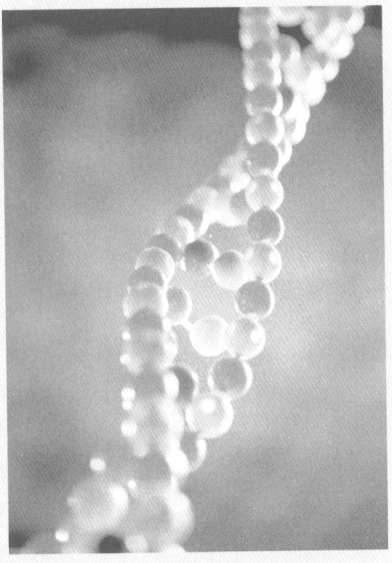

The map details the sequence of the 6 billion base pairs (nucleotides) that make up the 6 feet of DNA contained in the human genome of each cell. The genome map also shows genetic landmarks along each of the 23 pairs of chromosomes, including the locations of genes that are known to mutate and cause disease and other genes that are known to repair DNA.

Although the project is technically finished, analyses of the data will continue for many years.

function is largely determined by which of its approximately 20,000 genes are activated.

Chromosomes, genes and DNA

Each cell, except for mature red blood cells, has a control center called the nucleus. The nucleus houses your DNA, contained in two sets of 23 chromosomes, for a total of 46 chromosomes. One set comes from your mother, the other from your father. Two of these 46 chromosomes — called X and Y — are the sex chromosomes, which determine whether you are male or female. Females have a pair of X chromosomes. Males have an X chromosome and a Y chromosome. All other chromosomes are called autosomes.

The only cells that don't contain two sets of chromosomes are the egg and sperm. Known as your reproductive cells, each contains only one set of chromosomes. When an egg cell and sperm cell join together to form a zygote, the zygote contains the complete 46 chromosomes. This is how you get one set of 23 chromosomes from each parent.

The DNA contained in your chromosomes is a double-stranded structure composed of sugar and phosphate molecules that are joined together by paired chemicals called nucleotide bases. Four types of nucleotide bases are found in DNA: adenine (A), thymine (T), cytosine (C) and guanine (G). Adenine always pairs up with thymine, and cytosine always pairs up with guanine. The end result, known as the double helix, resembles a long, twisted ladder.

Cell proteins

One of the most important functions of genes is to produce proteins. Just as many kinds of genes control your traits, many kinds of proteins play various roles in your body. Some function as structural components, others as enzymes that control chemical reactions within your body. Other proteins help convert food from your diet into energy. Proteins are vital to the development and maintenance of your body. In fact, the two main components of your body are water and protein.

Amino acids are the basic building blocks of proteins. There are a total of 20 different amino acids, and they come together in various combinations to form different proteins. Proteins can be simple structures, made up of only a few amino acids, or complex, made of several chains of amino acids.

Some genes continuously produce proteins for basic cell metabolism, and other genes are "switched on" (activated) only when their protein-coding information is needed. In fact, some genes in a particular cell may be permanently "switched off." In other words, not all genes are activated in a cell at any given time.

When a cell needs a specific protein, it initiates a process called transcription. Transcription uses the blueprint provided by DNA to produce ribonucleic acid (RNA). First, an enzyme called RNA polymerase makes an exact copy of a gene's DNA. This copy, called

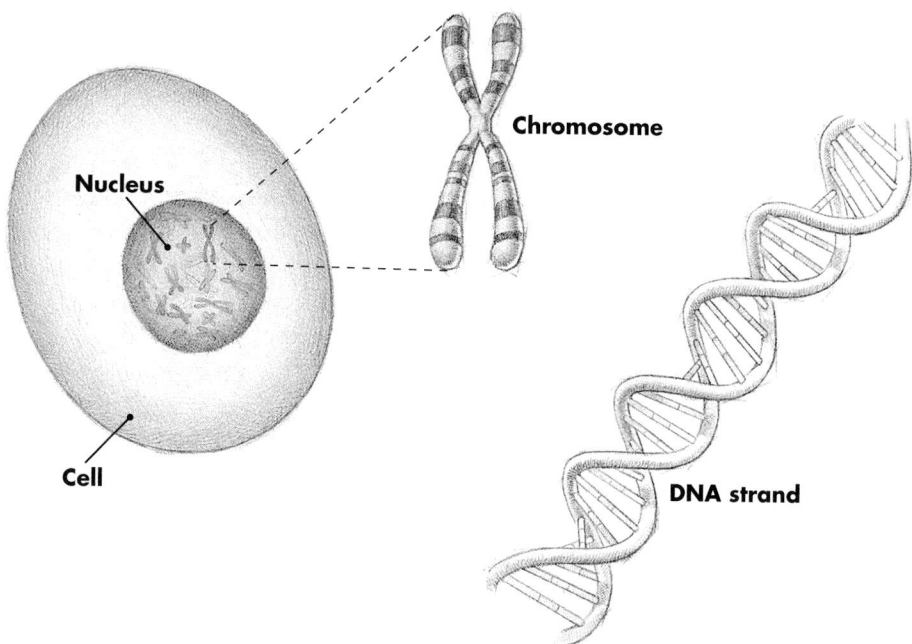

Nucleus

Cell

Chromosome

DNA strand

Virtually every cell in your body has a nucleus that contains 46 chromosomes (23 pairs) — half coming from each parent. Each chromosome consists of spirals of deoxyribonucleic acid (DNA), divided into units called genes. Your genes control the traits you inherit from your parents and can pass on to your children.

messenger RNA (mRNA), then travels outside of the nucleus to the outer part of the cell, where it links up with an enzyme called a ribosome. The ribosome translates the mRNA into protein by creating a corresponding chain of amino acids. This amino acid chain folds into a unique shape, forming a protein that's ready to function.

Controlling cell function

Throughout your lifetime, your body is in the business of generating new cells. During growth and development before adulthood, your cells are particularly busy dividing and specializing — developing your brain, increasing your height and creating a fully functional immune system, among many other things.

The exact way in which your cells are able to selectively activate or deactivate parts of the genome remains a mystery, but your health depends on it. For example, it's believed that cancer results, in part, from the failure of a growth-control gene to switch off properly or failure of a tumor-suppressing gene to turn on, resulting in uncontrolled growth of cells.

In order to know what to do and when to do it, each new cell requires a complete set of your genetic material (genome). When a cell divides, its DNA is replicated so the newly formed cells have a complete copy of the genome. Sperm and egg cells undergo yet another division process, resulting in four cells with half the original amount of genetic material. This prepares the sperm and egg cells for a potential union. When a sperm and egg unite, the new structure (zygote) has 46 chromosomes in 23 pairs. This is how the number of chromosomes and genes remains the same from one generation to the next.

Genes and inheritance

The genes you inherit from your parents are expressed in a variety of ways, but are perhaps most discernible in your physical characteristics, such as the shape of your ears, your eye color and your body type. Genes can also influence the risk of disease, such as heart disease or type 2 diabetes.

Gene versions (alleles) can be either dominant or recessive. The effects of a dominant allele take precedence over the effects of a recessive allele. In general, for a recessive allele to express itself, it must be paired with a similar recessive allele.

Variations in genes (polymorphisms) occur on a regular basis and can influence the way genes are expressed. Rarely does a single allele control one specific trait. Most of the time, traits are governed by the interplay of a variety of genes.

Genetic Disorders

Understanding how DNA normally functions can help you understand how genetic information might go awry. The topic of genetics and disease is frequently reported in the news, with many reports speculating on how a particular disease may be related to genetic makeup. Understandably, some of the most frequent questions that people now ask their doctors relate to whether a disease can be inherited.

Genetic disorders can stem from an abnormality (mutation) in your DNA that's significant enough to alter the function of a specific protein or other gene product. This abnormality can involve an entire chromosome or a single gene.

Chromosome abnormalities

Chromosome abnormalities typically consist of an extra or a missing chromosome. An example is Down syndrome, a condition caused by the presence of extra genetic material from chromosome 21. Most of the time, an entire extra copy of chromosome 21 is present (trisomy 21). Chromosome anomalies such as trisomy 21 may

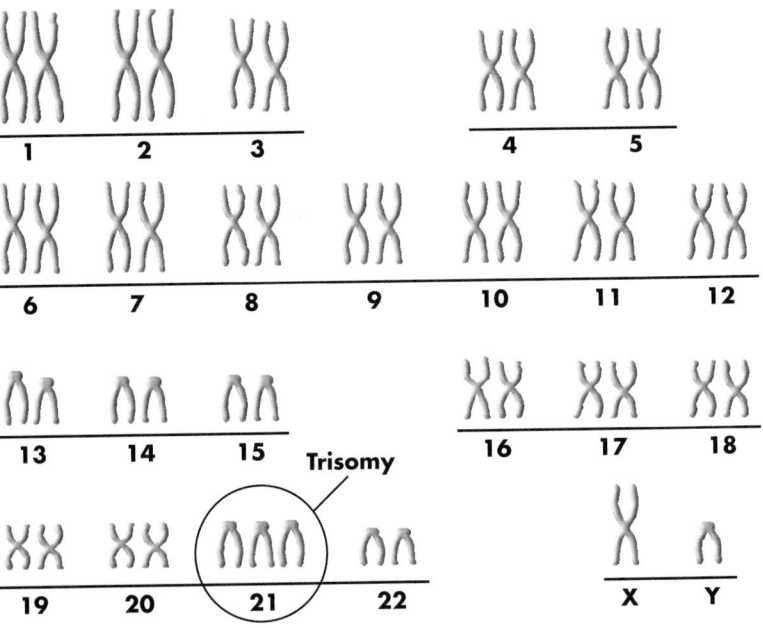

Down syndrome occurs when one of the reproductive cells from the parents that combine at fertilization contains extra material from chromosome 21. Individuals with Down syndrome usually have three copies of chromosome 21 (trisomy 21) instead of two copies.

cause intellectual disability and other birth defects.

Gene abnormalities

Diseases may also result from abnormalities within a single gene or gene pair, often referred to as a gene mutation. A common example of a single gene disorder is cystic fibrosis. About 30,000 people in the United States have this disorder. It results from abnormalities in the gene known as the cystic fibrosis transmembrane regulator. Cystic fibrosis is a recessive disorder, so an affected person must have two mutated copies of the gene.

Some diseases called multifactorial conditions likely require the presence of one or more genetic mutations and specific environmental factors. For example, scientists have discovered some people who develop cancer have both a genetic predisposition to the disease as well as a history of exposure to environmental toxins.

Breast cancer is an example. Defects in one of several genes — especially BRCA1 or BRCA2 — put you at greater risk of developing breast cancer. Usually, these genes help prevent cancer by making proteins that keep cells from growing abnormally. If these genes have a mutation, they're less effective at blocking unwanted cell growth.

In addition, factors such as excess body weight and long-term exposure to estrogen may increase your risk of breast cancer. Similarly, a combination of a genetic defect and smoking may increase your risk of the disease.

Alzheimer's: Is It in Your Genes?

Researchers have identified several genes associated with Alzheimer's disease. But genetic risk factors are just one part of the Alzheimer's story. Most people with Alzheimer's disease have no family history of the disorder.

The most common variety of Alzheimer's usually begins after the age of 65 — what's called late-onset disease. The most common gene associated with late-onset Alzheimer's is called apolipoprotein E (APOE). It has three forms:
- APOE e2 is the least common. It appears to reduce the risk of Alzheimer's.
- APOE e4 is a bit more common and may increase the risk of Alzheimer's.
- APOE e3 is the most common. It doesn't seem to affect the risk of Alzheimer's.

Because you inherit one APOE gene from your mother and another from your father, you may have two different types of APOE genes — for example, one APOE e3 gene and one APOE e4 gene. Having at least one APOE e4 gene increases your risk of developing Alzheimer's. If you have two APOE e4 genes, your risk is even higher. But not everyone who has an APOE e4 gene — or even two APOE e4 genes — develops Alzheimer's. And the disease occurs in people who have no APOE e4 gene. This indicates other factors are involved in the development of Alzheimer's disease.

Studies also show a link between late-onset Alzheimer's and a gene known as sortilin-related receptor L (SORL1). This is the first gene, other than APOE, to be linked to the most common form of Alzheimer's. Some variations of SORL1 appear to increase the production of amyloid-beta fragments, which form structures in the brain called amyloid plaques. These plaques are one of the hallmarks of Alzheimer's disease.

With early-onset disease, which is less common, scientists have identified three genes that cause this form of Alzheimer's. If you inherit one of these mutated genes from either parent, you almost certainly will experience Alzheimer's symptoms before the age of 65. The genes involved are: amyloid precursor protein (APP), presenilin 1 (PSEN1) and presenilin 2 (PSEN2).

Pathogenic variants in these genes cause the production of excessive amounts of a toxic protein fragment called amyloid-beta peptide. As these fragments accumulate in the brain, neurons begin to die, causing Alzheimer's disease. However, at least half the people who have early-onset Alzheimer's disease don't have any of these three gene mutations. That suggests that this aggressive form of Alzheimer's disease is linked to other genetic mutations that haven't been identified yet.

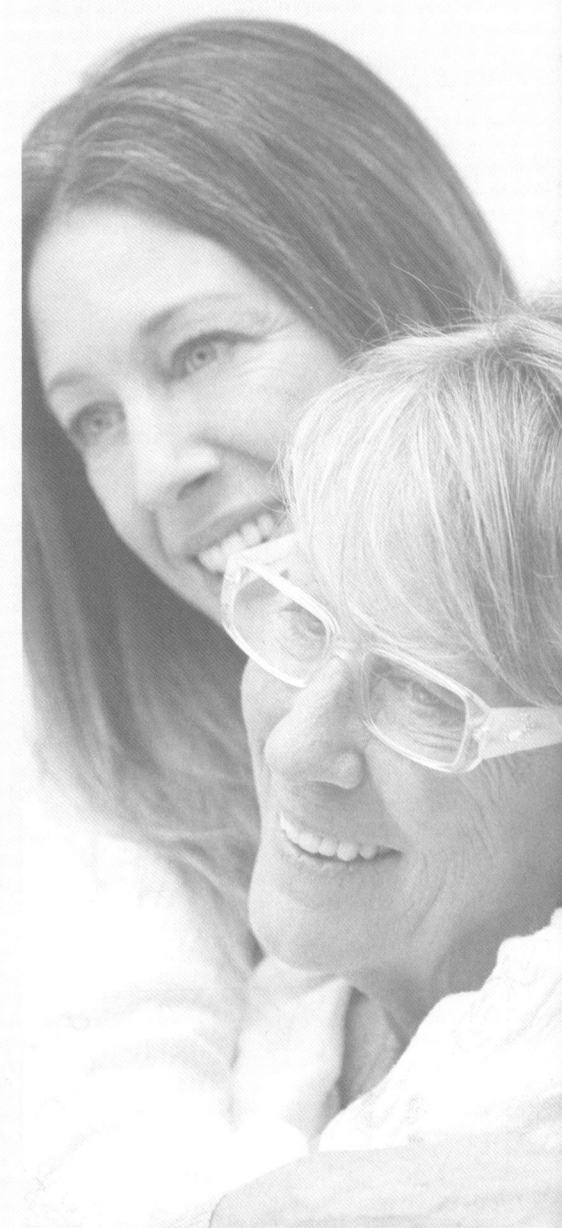

Genes mutate in several ways:

- **Substitution.** When DNA is copied, one nucleotide base may be substituted for another (such as C for T), resulting in a different sequence than the original. When a ribosome reads the DNA to gather the appropriate amino acids for the desired protein, one of the amino acids will be wrong.
- **Deletion or insertion.** Sometimes a nucleotide base is dropped or ignored as the DNA is being read. Other times an extra base is added to the sequence. The result is a different amino acid chain.
- **Expansion.** A portion of the DNA strand may contain additional information, disrupting the normal gene.

Each of these alterations results in a change in protein function, which may alter your body's chemistry and result in disease.

Acquired and inherited mutations

If a genetic mutation occurs during a person's lifetime, it's called an acquired mutation. For example, skin cancer is most often caused by damage to skin cell DNA from ultraviolet B (UVB) radiation given off by the sun or by special lights used for tanning. An acquired mutation is typically present in just one or a few cells.

A gene mutation is termed inherited if it's present in reproductive cells or occurs at the time of fertilization and is thus present at birth. Like other inherited traits, the mutation may reside in a dominant or recessive gene, or it may be located on a sex chromosome. An inherited gene mutation is present in every cell of the body.

Autosomal dominant mutations

If you inherit a dominant gene mutation for a disease, you usually develop that condition because the dominant gene takes precedence over the recessive gene it's paired with. In addition, each of your children will have a 50 percent chance of inheriting the mutation and have an increased risk of developing the disease.

An example of an autosomal dominant disorder is familial hypercholesterolemia, a condition marked by very high levels of blood cholesterol.

Autosomal recessive mutations

An autosomal recessive genetic disorder requires inheritance of a recessive gene from each parent in order for the disease to develop. If you inherit only one such recessive gene, the normal gene on the other allele still functions normally, and you won't develop the disorder. But you still are a carrier of the gene mutation and can pass it on to your children.

If you have children with someone who's also a carrier, each child has a 25 percent chance of inheriting both recessive gene mutations and developing the associated disease. It's relatively rare for two people to be carriers for the same mutated recessive gene.

When both genes of a pair are required to cause a particular condition, this is called autosomal recessive disorder. Cystic fibrosis

Autosomal Dominant Gene Mutations

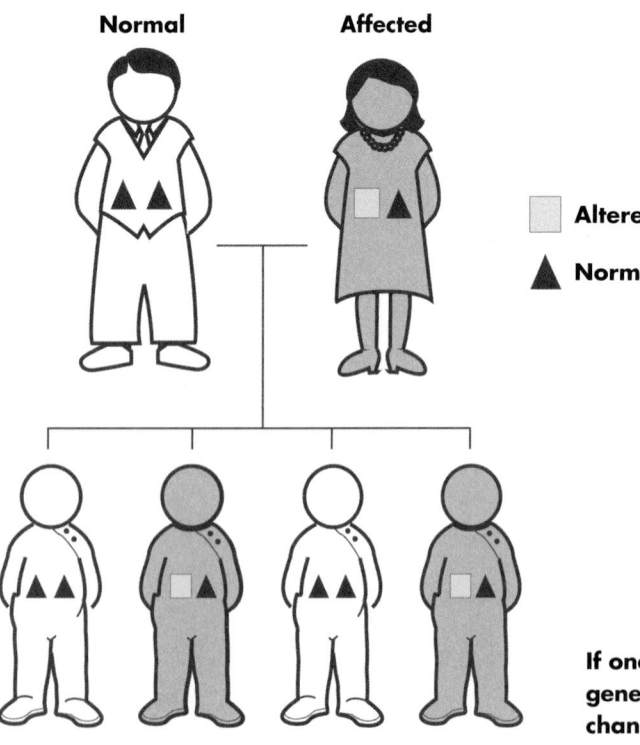

Normal   **Affected**

■ **Altered gene dominates**

▲ **Normal gene**

Normal   **Affected**   **Normal**   **Affected**

If one parent carries an altered (mutated) dominant gene, such as the gene for Huntington's disease, the chance is 50 percent the couple's child, regardless of sex, will be born with the altered gene.

Autosomal Recessive Gene Mutations

Unaffected carrier   **Unaffected carrier**

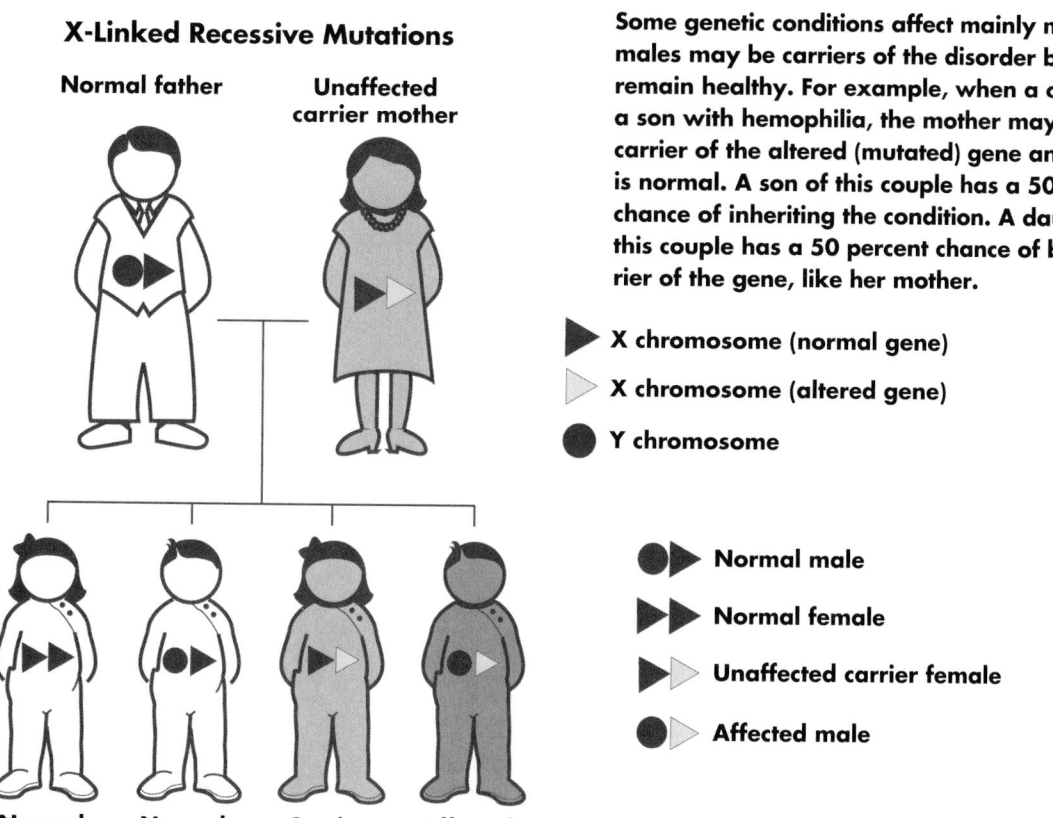

■ Normal gene

△ Altered gene

Normal   Unaffected carrier   Unaffected carrier   Affected

A recessive disorder, such as cystic fibrosis, can occur even if neither parent has the disorder. If both parents are carriers of an altered (mutated) recessive gene, their offspring may be affected. The chance is 1 in 4 that their child, regardless of its sex, may be born with cystic fibrosis, 2 in 4 that it may be a healthy, unaffected carrier and 1 in 4 that it may neither carry the gene nor have the disease.

X-Linked Recessive Mutations

Normal father   **Unaffected carrier mother**

Some genetic conditions affect mainly males. Females may be carriers of the disorder but usually remain healthy. For example, when a couple has a son with hemophilia, the mother may be the carrier of the altered (mutated) gene and the father is normal. A son of this couple has a 50 percent chance of inheriting the condition. A daughter of this couple has a 50 percent chance of being a carrier of the gene, like her mother.

▶ X chromosome (normal gene)

▷ X chromosome (altered gene)

● Y chromosome

Normal daughter   Normal son   Carrier daughter   Affected son

●▶ Normal male

▶▶ Normal female

▶▷ Unaffected carrier female

●▷ Affected male

is an autosomal recessive disorder that results from an abnormality in the copy of the cystic fibrosis gene inherited from each parent. Another example is the blood disorder sickle cell anemia.

Reproductive chromosome mutations

Some mutations that cause disease are found only on the X chromosome. These are called X-linked disorders. Men are more likely to develop these disorders because they have only one X chromosome. (The other male reproductive chromosome is the Y chromosome.) Women have two X chromosomes, and the normal X chromosome functions sufficiently so that no disease develops. Thus, women are more likely to remain unaffected, even if they carry the mutation, than they are to develop the related disorder.

A father with the disease will pass the mutation on to his daughters, who will usually be unaffected because they'll have one normal X chromosome from their mother that will function normally so no disease develops. Hemophilia is an example of an X-linked disorder.

These patterns of disease inheritance may seem fairly straightforward, but in real life things are much more complicated. People express genes in a number of ways and may express a disease differently as well. This is why two people who have cystic fibrosis may not have the same symptoms or experience the same degree of disease severity. With multifactorial conditions, the influence of a person's individual genome and personal life experience can be even more pronounced. Thus, multifactorial disorders can vary significantly from one person to the next. So even though scientists are coming to a better understanding of genetic disorders and inheritance patterns, many more contributing factors have yet to be explored.

Cancer Family Syndromes

Cancer family syndromes are often inherited in an autosomal dominant fashion. This means that if a parent has the condition, each child has a 50 percent chance of inheriting the mutated gene.

Lynch syndrome is one example. It's a rare inherited condition that increases your risk of colon and other cancers. Also known as hereditary nonpolyposis colorectal cancer (HNPCC), Lynch syndrome is believed responsible for about 2 to 10 percent of all colon cancers. Endometrial, urethral, pancreatic and ovarian cancers also occur with increased frequency in families with the disorder.

When an individual inherits a mutation in a gene responsible for Lynch syndrome, the lifetime risk that he or she will develop colon cancer can be as high as 80 percent. While the mutations that cause many familial cancers act in a dominant fashion, they may have reduced penetrance, meaning they don't always cause disease.

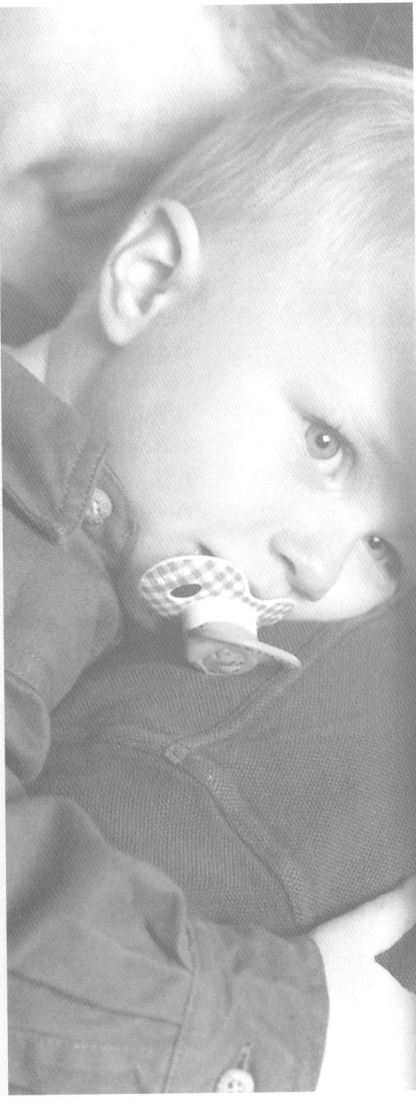

Genetic Testing

A variety of genetic tests may help guide your medical care. But keep in mind that genetic testing is complicated, and it may raise more questions than it answers.

Genetic testing can't tell, for example, if you'll definitely develop breast cancer or when you'll start to notice symptoms of Alzheimer's disease. But genetic testing can determine your risk of certain diseases, and it may help alleviate anxiety. If you learn you have a below-average likelihood of developing a frightening disease, testing can prevent needless worrying.

? Question and Answer

How helpful is genetic testing?

Genetic testing isn't always 100 percent predictive. Even when a genetic test reveals that a person has the gene for a particular disorder, the following may remain uncertain:

- Whether the disorder will actually appear
- When symptoms may begin
- Which symptoms will occur first
- How severe the condition will be
- How the condition will progress over time

Damaged DNA

An organism's complete DNA sequence is its genome. The human genome contains approximately 20,000 genes, each holding the molecular recipe for a gene product — a protein produced by a cell. Genes with missing, duplicated or misplaced nucleotides may function improperly. They may not produce any of the needed protein, or they may produce the protein but in an ineffective amount or form. The result is known as a single-gene disorder.

When you undergo a genetic test, it's this damaged DNA — genes with missing, duplicated or misplaced nucleotides — that the test looks for.

Single-gene disorders account for only a small proportion of medical conditions. About 1.5 percent of your DNA is made up of genes that code for proteins. Researchers have begun studying what the remaining 98 percent of "noncoding DNA" does. The answers are slowly beginning to emerge.

Types of genetic testing

Genetic tests are used to determine if a person may have a genetic mutation that causes a disease or increases susceptibility to a disease. The tests also may be used to identify carriers of a genetic mutation or to confirm a suspected disorder.

Until recently, genetic testing was available only from a handful of laboratories affiliated with genetics departments at major medical centers. Your doctor might have referred you to a medical genetics department for genetic counseling and testing if you had a family history of a specific genetic disorder, if you were having repeated miscarriages, or if you had an increased likelihood of having a baby with a genetic or chromosomal disorder.

Today, many labs offer thousands of different genetic tests.

Finding Diseases That Run in Families

With some genetic disorders, the exact mutation isn't known, but the general location of the mutated gene on the chromosome is known. In such cases, scientists begin by studying families in which multiple members across several generations have developed the condition. By comparing DNA samples from relatives who have the disease with samples from relatives without the disease, researchers can identify genetic markers that are consistently inherited by people with the disease. These markers are usually located in the vicinity of the mutated gene or genes. This process of DNA comparison is called linkage analysis.

Doctors can now send samples of their patients' blood, saliva or tissue to a commercial or academic genetics laboratory for a number of different tests. It's even possible to order some types of genetic tests on your own. However, it's best to work with a genetic specialist to make sure the test is ordered and interpreted properly.

Diagnostic testing

Many genetic disorders, such as some forms of polycystic kidney disease and iron overload (hemochromatosis), appear in adolescence or later. If you have signs and symptoms of an adult-onset genetic disorder, genetic testing may confirm the diagnosis. In the case of cystic fibrosis, genetic testing is able to detect most disease causing the genetic mutation. Thus, the DNA test can confirm the diagnosis of cystic fibrosis in a person with clinical symptoms.

Sometimes, though, a gene mutation is found and it's unclear if it's causing a disease. This type of change is called a variant of uncertain significance (VUS). And for many genetic disorders, the gene alterations responsible for the disease haven't yet been identified.

When might diagnostic testing be used? Couples having difficulty conceiving may undergo genetic testing for disorders that cause infertility. If a hereditary cancer syndrome runs in your family, you can be tested for the genetic

variations associated with the syndrome. If the results show that your likelihood of eventually developing hereditary cancer is high, you may want to have appropriate cancer-screening tests more often than generally recommended and starting at an earlier age. This can help detect the cancer at its earliest stage. Genetic testing may also affect your options for medical treatment of hereditary cancer syndromes.

Carrier testing

Couples with family histories of single-gene disorders may undergo genetic testing and genetic counseling before starting a family. In these circumstances, genetic testing determines whether either parent also carries a copy of the altered gene and is, as a result, at risk of passing the mutation on to a child. Among the most common of these disorders are sickle cell anemia and cystic fibrosis.

Prenatal genetic testing

Doctors are able to diagnose chromosomal abnormalities, such as Down syndrome, by doing prenatal genetic testing on fetal cells, which are obtained through diagnostic tests such as amniocentesis. Genetic testing is also an option when other prenatal screening tests suggest a genetic disorder, or when one or both parents have a family history of a single-gene disorder.

Newer technology such as cell-free DNA testing, also known as noninvasive prenatal screening (NIPS), allows screening for genetic disorders by way of blood tests as early as nine weeks, holding great promise for the future.

Preimplantation genetic testing

Couples conceiving through in vitro fertilization may benefit from genetic testing of the embryo before it's implanted in the female uterus. Preimplantation genetic tests can detect some of the same conditions as prenatal tests.

Newborn genetic screening

Some babies are born with gene abnormalities that cause specific diseases. With relatively inexpensive technology, virtually all newborns in the United States are now screened for several genetic conditions, many that can be treated early in life to improve outcomes. The number of conditions being screened for continues to expand every year.

Whole exome/genome sequencing

Another type of genetic testing detects DNA variations at the single nucleotide level across the genome. There are a number of names for this technology including next-generation sequencing and massively parallel sequencing.

The whole-exome sequencing (WES) test is for identifying disease-causing DNA variants within the 1 to 2 percent of the genome that encodes for proteins (exons) or regions that flank exons known as splice junctions.

It's predicted that whole-genome sequencing, which looks at all DNA rather than just protein-coding DNA, will replace other forms of sequencing as the cost of sequencing and knowledge of noncoding DNA continues to improve. Sometimes, though, it may be best to look at a small number of genes rather than the entire genome.

It's important to remember that large parts of the human genome still cannot be interpreted. However, this is likely to change as more testing is done and more knowledge is gained.

Pharmacogenetics

Pharmacogenetics is the study of gene-drug interactions, specifically looking at how genetics influences an individual's response to medication.

The overall goals of pharmacogenetics are to select and administer the appropriate drug at the right dose, to reduce drug therapy failures, to limit side effects and to improve medical care. Pharmacogenomic testing is now widely available.

Privacy and genetic testing

The Genetic Information Non-discrimination Act (GINA) of 2008 prohibits health insurers from requesting, requiring or using genetic information to make decisions about your eligibility for health insurance, health insurance premiums, contributing amounts or terms of coverage. Under GINA, employment discrimination based on genetic risk also is illegal. However, the act does not cover other types insurance related to your health.

When you apply for life, long-term care or disability insurance, you may have to disclose your complete medical history, including results of genetic tests, or risk losing your benefits if anything you omit comes to light.

Genetic test results kept in your medical record may be available to your current insurer without your disclosure.

Regardless of the type of genetic testing that you're considering, make sure to talk with your doctor or a genetics professional about all the advantages and disadvantages of obtaining personal genetic information.

Genetic Counseling

Medical geneticists and genetic counselors are often called upon to help individuals understand inherited diseases and disorders. A medical geneticist is a doctor who has completed additional training in medical genetics. Look for an individual who is board certified in medical genetics. Genetic counselors have a master's degree in genetic counseling.

In the past, people were most often sent to a medical geneticist for evaluation of a rare disorder caused by a single-gene abnormality. Now doctors and scientists realize that many complex and common disorders are due in part to genetic factors.

For instance, a congenital abnormality of one of the major organ systems, such as a congenital heart defect, is often due in part to genetic factors and may prompt genetic evaluation.

If a person has multiple congenital anomalies, a genetic component is often involved. Sometimes, a person has a family history of a known inheritable disorder, such as cystic fibrosis, sickle cell anemia or hemophilia.

Benefits of counseling

If you're considering genetic testing for yourself or your child, there are many issues to think about. Speaking with a medical geneticist or a genetic counselor can help you sort them out.

These health care professionals are specially trained to deal with the complex issues surrounding genetic testing. They can offer valuable information before you make your decision. Should you choose to go ahead with the testing, they can help you interpret the results and provide support in the weeks and months ahead. Some issues to think about include:

- Are there treatments available for the genetic disorder under consideration?
- What impact might the test results have on your relationships with your partner, family, children and friends? For some people, relationships improve after genetic testing. For others, they become more complicated.
- Will the test results cause others to think less of you?
- Results of a genetic test sometimes can give unexpected information. For example, revealing nonpaternity — that a father isn't the biological father.
- Who will give you emotional support through the process?
- How will you react if your test results are uncertain?
- What are your plans and hopes for having children?
- What's the cost of the test, and who will pay?
- Do you want your insurance company to know the results?
- Can the results be used to discriminate against you, or will they be regarded as a pre-existing condition?
- Will the results become a part of your medical record?
- Would you like to be tested at this time, or would postponing the testing be better?

Family health history

If you're referred to a medical geneticist for evaluation, it's helpful to put together your family health history — also called a family pedigree or family health tree — before the appointment.

For instance, in the case of a family history of cancer, it's helpful to know the type of cancer each affected family member had and the person's age at diagnosis. Also provide information about unaffected family members because it can be helpful in interpreting the family pedigree and in creating a risk assessment.

The more information you provide about the health conditions in your family, the better a medical geneticist can help you. He or she analyzes the family pedigree in order to determine the inheritance pattern of a disorder in the family. The analysis often helps the geneticist develop a screening or treatment plan for individuals in your family who may be at risk of or have the disorder.

Creating a family pedigree

You can create a family health history by gathering information about the health of first- and second-degree relatives. First-degree relatives are your parents, sisters, brothers and children. Second-degree relatives include aunts, uncles, grandparents and grandchildren.

For each family member, record his or her relationship, sex, year of birth, illnesses and age at diagnosis, and other significant lifestyle factors (when known), such as tobacco and alcohol use or obesity. If any family members have died, note the age at death and cause of death. Other things you might want to include are:

Family background or ethnicity
The ethnic background of a family can be important. For instance, if a family is of Northern European background, the risk of family members being carriers of a cystic fibrosis gene mutation is increased. Likewise, among black people, the risk of family members being carriers of sickle cell anemia is increased. Remember that a carrier of a genetic disorder doesn't have the condition.

Intermarriage
When taking a family history, pay attention to the possibility that a couple may have been blood relatives. This increases the risk of certain disorders in their children.

History of birthing difficulty
A history of previous miscarriages or stillborn or neonatal deaths may be relevant.

Environmental exposures
Illnesses can also be influenced by exposure to factors such as illicit drugs, prescription medications, radiation and toxic chemicals.

Gene Therapy and Editing

Gene therapy and editing involves altering the genes inside your body's cells to stop disease. Genes contain your DNA — the code that controls much of your body's form and function. Your cells use the information from your genes to manufacture proteins that do the work in your body, from making you grow taller to regulating your body systems. Throughout your life, your genes turn on and off as needed to control cell activity.

Genes that don't work properly can cause disease. Gene therapy replaces a faulty gene or adds a new gene in an attempt to cure disease or make changes within your body so that it's better able to combat disease. Gene therapy holds promise for treating a wide range of diseases, including cancer, cystic fibrosis, heart disease, diabetes, hemophilia and AIDS.

Researchers are still learning about how gene therapy works and the best way to administer gene therapy.

Why it's done

Gene therapy is used to correct defective genes in order to cure a disease or to help the body better fight disease. Researchers are investigating several ways to do this, including:
- **Replacing missing or mutated genes.** This is currently the most common gene therapy approach. Some cells become diseased because certain genes have been permanently turned off. Other cells may be missing certain genes. Researchers hope that

replacing missing or defective genes can help treat certain diseases. For instance, a common tumor suppressor gene called p53 normally prevents tumor growth in your body. Several types of cancer have been linked to a missing or inactive p53 gene. If doctors could replace p53 where it's missing, that might trigger the cancer cells to die.

- **Changing the regulation of a gene.** Mutated genes that cause disease could be turned off so that they no longer promote disease, or healthy genes that help prevent disease could be turned on so that they can inhibit the disease.
- **Making diseased cells more evident to the immune system.** Sometimes, the body's immune system doesn't attack diseased cells because it doesn't recognize them as intruders. Using gene therapy, doctors could potentially infuse mutated cells with genes that make them more recognizable to your immune system. Or enhancements could be made to immune cells to make it easier for them to recognize mutated cells.

Risks

Gene therapy poses a number of risks. First, the way the genes are delivered can be problematic. A gene can't be inserted directly into your cells; it has to be delivered using a carrier, called a vector. The most common gene therapy vectors are viruses because they can recognize certain cells and carry genetic material into the cells' genes.

Researchers are trying to take advantage of this unique capability by removing the original disease-causing genes from the viruses and replacing them with the genes needed to stop disease, and then inserting the altered viruses into a person's diseased cells, where they can deliver their genetic material.

This technique presents the following risks:

- **Immune response.** Your body's immune system may see the newly introduced viruses as intruders and attack them. This may cause inflammation, toxicity and, in severe cases, organ failure.
- **Viral spread.** Because viruses can affect more than one type of cells, it's possible that the viral vectors may infect cells beyond just those containing mutated or missing genes. If this happens, healthy cells may be damaged, causing other illness or diseases.
- **Reversion of the virus to its original form.** It's possible that once introduced into the body, the viruses may recover their original ability to cause disease.

Another risk of gene therapy is that the new DNA introduced into your body may affect your reproductive cells — egg cells in women and sperm cells in men. This could result in genetic changes that could affect any children you have after treatment.

Gene therapy clinical trials underway in the U.S. are closely monitored by the Food and Drug Administration (FDA) and the National Institutes of Health (NIH) to ensure the safety of those who participate in the studies.

What you can expect

The most common way to receive gene therapy is to participate in a clinical trial. Clinical trials help doctors determine whether a gene therapy approach is safe for people. They also demonstrate the effects of gene therapy on the body. For instance, doctors may analyze samples of cells from people in a clinical trial to look for signs the makeup of the diseased cells is changing. They might also look to see how the immune system reacts to the gene therapy.

In addition to viruses, other vectors used to carry altered genes into your body's cells may include:

- **Stem cells.** Stem cells are the raw material cells of your body — cells from which all other cells in your body with specialized functions are created. For gene therapy, stem cells can be altered in a laboratory to accept new genes that can help fight disease.
- **Liposomes.** These fatty particles have the ability to carry the new, therapeutic genes to the target cells and pass the genes into your cells' DNA.

Obstacles

Although the promise of gene therapy is exciting, many issues need to be resolved before it becomes a standard form of medical practice. In addition to developing effective methods of delivery, scientists face other hurdles.

Unknown genetic effects
Little is known about the activity of specific genes at different times in different cells. If new genes are introduced, will they express themselves long enough and at high enough levels to accomplish their mission? In addition, could

Editing DNA

A new technology called CRISPR that allows researchers to edit DNA may have a wide range of potential applications. Compared with previous methods, it's faster, cheaper and easier to manipulate DNA sequences.

CRISPR works when a piece of RNA (guide RNA) is guided to an enzyme called Cas9. Within the enzyme, the RNA acts like a molecular scissors and cuts DNA at a specific location. A specific sequence embedded in the guide RNA is then used to repair the DNA sequence.

Human trials have been approved, and the outcomes will be watched closely by the scientific community.

Stem Cell Research

Stem cells and their potential for curing disease are popular topics.

What are stem cells?

Stem cells are master cells of the body — cells from which all other cells with specialized functions are created. Under the right conditions in the body or a laboratory, stem cells divide to form more cells, called daughter cells. These daughter cells either become new stem cells (self-renewal) or become specialized cells (differentiation) with a more specific function, such as blood cells, brain cells, heart muscle or bone. Stem cells are unique — no other cell in the body has the ability to self-renew or to differentiate.

Where do stem cells come from?

Researchers have discovered several sources of stem cells:

- *Embryonic stem cells.* These stem cells come from embryos that are 4 to 5 days old. These are pluripotent stem cells, meaning they can divide into more stem cells or they can specialize and become any type of cell in the body. Because of this versatility, embryonic stem cells have the highest potential for use to regenerate or repair diseased tissue and organs in people.
- *Adult stem cells.* These stem cells are found in small numbers in most adult tissues, such as bone marrow. Adult stem cells are also found in children and in placentas and umbilical cords. Until recently, it was felt that adult stem cells could only create similar types of cells. However, emerging evidence suggests that adult stem cells may be more versatile than previously thought and able to create unrelated types of cells.
- *Adult cells altered to have properties of embryonic stem cells.* Researchers have reported being able to transform regular adult cells into stem cells in laboratory studies. By altering the genes in the adult cells, researchers were able to reprogram the cells to act similarly to embryonic stem cells, and thus become induced pluripotent stems cells acting similarly to embryonic stem cells.
- *Amniotic fluid stem cells.* Stem cells are also located in amniotic fluid. Amniotic fluid fills the sac that surrounds and protects a developing fetus in the uterus. Researchers have used amniotic fluid to identify stem cells that could develop into several other types of cells. More study of amniotic fluid stem cells is needed to understand their potential.

Why is there a controversy about using embryonic stem cells?

Embryonic stem cells are obtained from early-stage embryos — a group of cells that forms when a female egg is fertilized with a male sperm. Extracting stem cells from the embryos destroys the embryos. This raises important ethical questions.

Have stem cells already been used to treat diseases?

Yes. Stem cell transplants, also known as bone marrow transplants, have been performed in the United States since the late 1960s. Bone marrow transplants use adult stem cells.

Adult stem cells also are being tested in other applications, including a number of degenerative diseases, such as heart failure. Stem cells from umbilical cord blood have been successfully used in clinical trials to treat rare genetic diseases.

What does the future hold for stem cell therapy?

Researchers say the field has promise. Stem cell transplants using induced pluripotent cells continue to be refined and improved. And researchers are discovering that these cells may be able to treat a wider variety of diseases than once thought.

Regenerative medicine is a growing field, and researchers are enthusiastic about the potential for regenerative medicine treatments.

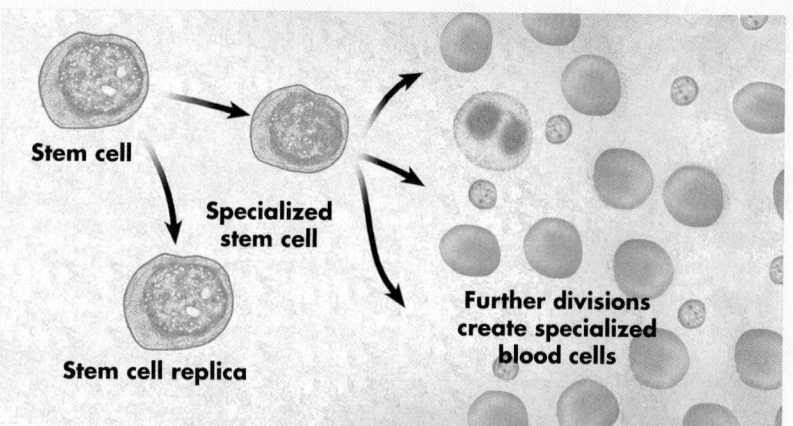

Stem cell

Specialized stem cell

Stem cell replica

Further divisions create specialized blood cells

When a stem cell divides, it creates a stem cell that's specialized — a cell that can create cells that perform specific functions, such as blood cells. It also creates an exact replica of itself.

the new genes alter more than the intended cells, or could they over-express themselves, producing so much of the new protein that it becomes harmful?

Ethical issues

There are concerns regarding the short- and long-term consequences of manipulating the human genome. Gene therapy focuses on delivering corrective genes to diseased cells. It doesn't involve altering the genome in reproductive cells, which would permanently change the genetic characteristics of future generations.

Manipulating genetic information in reproductive (germ) cells is called germline therapy. Presumably germline therapy could be used to correct defective genes so that a family could be free of a disease, such as hemophilia. But might it also be used to enhance genetic traits, such as intelligence or athletic ability?

Germline therapy isn't approved by the National Institutes of Health, but its potential exists, and this is what many people are concerned about. The U.S. branch of the Human Genome Project has set aside a specific portion of its budget to study the ethical, legal and social issues surrounding the project with the goal of being better prepared for other complex issues that may arise in the future.

Results

Some clinical trials have recorded small successes for a few participants, but several significant barriers stand in the way of gene therapy becoming a reliable form of treatment. They include developing reliable vectors, consistently ensuring safety, targeting the correct cells and preventing genetic changes from being passed on from parents to children.

Still, gene therapy remains a very active area of research. ■

What's Cloning?

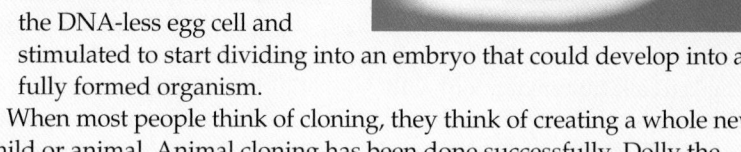

Cloning involves taking a single organism's genetic material and using it to create a genetically identical organism, without the use of sexual reproduction. This process basically has three steps:

1. First, an egg cell is obtained from a donor, and its nucleus (genetic material) is removed.
2. Next, any cell other than an egg or sperm cell (somatic cell) is taken from the organism that's to be cloned.
3. The somatic cell is fused with the DNA-less egg cell and stimulated to start dividing into an embryo that could develop into a fully formed organism.

When most people think of cloning, they think of creating a whole new child or animal. Animal cloning has been done successfully. Dolly the sheep is the most famous example. After Dolly was cloned in Scotland in 1997, other animals also were successfully cloned. But the subject of most debate is human cloning. There are actually two types of human cloning: reproductive cloning and therapeutic cloning.

Human reproductive cloning is the attempt to create a new person who is genetically identical to the person who donated his or her DNA. After an embryo is cloned in a laboratory, it would be implanted in the uterus of the surrogate mother who donated the egg cell. A host of ethical and legal issues surround this topic. To date, no human has been successfully cloned. In fact, cloned human embryos have yet to reach a stage beyond a few cells.

Many scientists are opposed to reproductive cloning because of the dangers involved, as illustrated by animal cloning. For every 100 animal cloning attempts, only three, at the most, produce actual offspring, and even then survival beyond birth is improbable. If cloned human babies survive birth, it's likely that many of them would have severe birth defects, malfunction of various body systems and premature death. Not many people want to pay this sort of price for the ability to create a human clone, regardless of how they feel about its moral aspects.

Another form of human cloning that particularly interests scientists is therapeutic cloning. Therapeutic cloning is a technique to create versatile stem cells independent of fertilized eggs. In this technique, the nucleus, which contains the genetic material, is removed from the unfertilized egg. The nucleus is also removed from the somatic cell of a donor. This donor nucleus is then injected into the egg to replace the nucleus that was removed — a process called nuclear transfer. The egg is allowed to divide, and it soon creates a line of stem cells identical to the donor's — in essence, a clone. Some researchers believe that stem cells derived from therapeutic cloning may offer benefits over those derived from fertilized eggs because they're less likely to be rejected once transplanted back into the donor.

Cloning is a hotly debated topic. On one side, many people see it as a major technological and medical advance toward the treatment of incurable diseases. Those on the other side regard it as an irresponsible use of human life.

Cancer

Many people have a fear of cancer, perhaps because they view it as an incurable disease. But the truth is that although cancer remains a serious illness, it's no longer the inevitable death sentence it once was. Instead, it's increasingly becoming a tale of survivorship.

As the cancer death rate continues to decline, millions of people are alive today, having survived cancer. Well over 15 million living Americans have a history of cancer. In the United States, 3.5 million women are breast cancer survivors, and 3.3 million men are prostate cancer survivors.

But the battle against this disease isn't over. Annually, cancer (excluding nonmelanoma skin cancer) is diagnosed in almost 1.6 million Americans. In the United States, cancer causes almost 600,000 deaths each year — approximately 1 in every 4 to 5 deaths is cancer related.

There are at least 200 different kinds of cancer. Some cancers affect just one organ, and others are more generalized. But the basic characteristic of all cancers is the same — uncontrolled growth and spread of abnormal (malignant) cells.

Why cancer develops in some people but not in others isn't fully known. But medical professionals are gaining knowledge about what factors may contribute to the development of cancer. These factors include some that can be controlled or eliminated, such as certain dietary habits and use of tobacco.

Researchers know also that most cancers develop slowly. You may not detect evidence of the disease for five to 40 years after you've been exposed to a cancer-causing agent. Cancer of the lung, for example, may not appear until 25 years or more after sustained exposure to tobacco smoke. This long delay between exposure and development of the disease may partly explain why so many people ignore the warnings associated with smoking.

This chapter provides an overview of cancer: what it is, how it develops, and how it's detected and treated. It also offers some guidelines on potential ways to prevent cancer, as well as what to do when you have cancer. Other chapters in this book offer more-detailed information on specific types of cancer. Cancers are generally named according to the body system or organ where the cancer started.

The following list shows you where to find more-specific information on some of the more common cancer types:

New Cases of Cancer and Cancer Deaths by Site and Sex — 2017

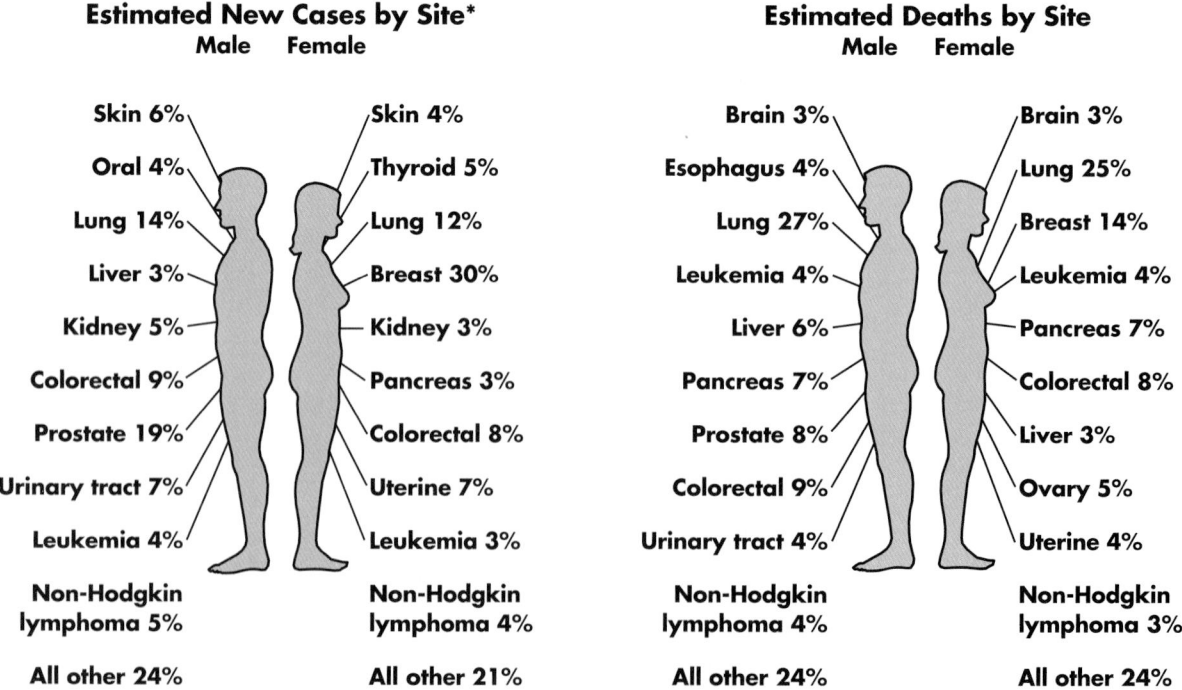

Estimated New Cases by Site*
Male   Female

Male	Female
Skin 6%	Skin 4%
Oral 4%	Thyroid 5%
Lung 14%	Lung 12%
Liver 3%	Breast 30%
Kidney 5%	Kidney 3%
Colorectal 9%	Pancreas 3%
Prostate 19%	Colorectal 8%
Urinary tract 7%	Uterine 7%
Leukemia 4%	Leukemia 3%
Non-Hodgkin lymphoma 5%	Non-Hodgkin lymphoma 4%
All other 24%	All other 21%

Estimated Deaths by Site
Male   Female

Male	Female
Brain 3%	Brain 3%
Esophagus 4%	Lung 25%
Lung 27%	Breast 14%
Leukemia 4%	Leukemia 4%
Liver 6%	Pancreas 7%
Pancreas 7%	Colorectal 8%
Prostate 8%	Liver 3%
Colorectal 9%	Ovary 5%
Urinary tract 4%	Uterine 4%
Non-Hodgkin lymphoma 4%	Non-Hodgkin lymphoma 3%
All other 24%	All other 24%

*Excluding basal and squamous cell skin cancers and *in situ* carcinomas, except urinary bladder.
Source: American Cancer Society, Surveillance Research, 2017

What Is Cancer?

Your body is made up of trillions of individual cells. It grows and develops as a result of increases in the numbers of new cells that become different types of tissue.

New cells are created through a process of cell division called mitosis. Cells acquire various specialized functions through an accompanying process called cell differentiation.

In the early developmental years of your life, cells divide rapidly in order to bring your body and all of its organs to full growth and maturity. Once you reach adulthood, most of your cells switch into maintenance mode, dividing only to replace cells that are injured or dead. Normal cellular function and, in turn, the overall health of your body depend largely on the delicate balance between normal cell growth and normal cell death.

Unlike normal cells, cancer cells either lack the controls that switch off growth or they lose their ability to undergo natural cell death. They divide without restraint, crowding out neighboring cells. In addition, they affect the function and growth of normal cells, invading and destroying normal tissues.

Uncontrolled cells can grow into a mass called a tumor that can invade and destroy nearby normal tissue. Cancer cells can also spread to other parts of the body via the bloodstream or lymphatic system in a process called metastasis.

Not all cells that exhibit rapid or uncontrolled growth patterns are cancer cells. Cells may accumulate as benign tumors, which often don't damage surrounding tissues. Benign tumors grow only locally and typically aren't life-threatening unless they're in a confined space, such as the skull.

Cancer cells, on the other hand, have the ability to spread beyond their place of origin and, if not detected early, can be life-threatening. Cancer can develop in several forms.

Carcinomas

Cancers that originate on external or internal body surfaces, such as skin and colon cancers, are called carcinomas. These are the most common types in the United States.

Sarcomas

Sarcomas develop in the body's supportive tissues, such as bones and muscles.

Lymphomas

Lymphomas originate in the lymph nodes and immune system.

Leukemias

Leukemias originate in blood-forming cells of bone marrow and are evident in the bloodstream.

Damaged DNA

What goes wrong to produce cancer cells? This is a basic question scientists are still attempting to answer. Although they have yet to understand the exact processes by which all cells grow, divide, communicate and differentiate, they have learned much about what goes on within a cell to activate or alter a normal cell to become cancerous.

Your body contains approximately 100 trillion cells. In the core (nucleus) of each cell reside 23 pairs (46 total) of structures called chromosomes — half of them inherited from each parent. Each chromosome is composed of long, double-stranded sequences of a material called deoxyribonucleic acid (DNA), arranged as a double helix.

Normal Cells

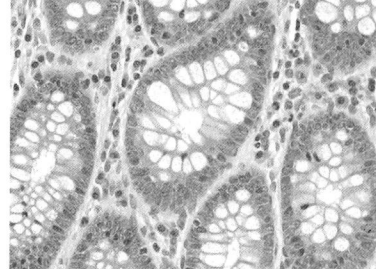

This slide shows normal tissue cells. The cells are oval shaped, with all of the cells looking similar. They're very well-organized into a single layer of cells.

Cancer Cells

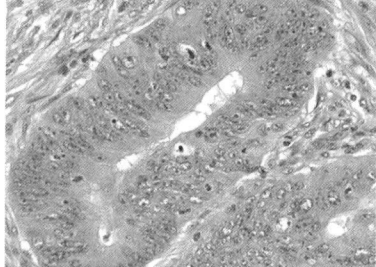

This slide shows cancer cells. Cancer cells are stacked up and highly disorganized. They also look very different from each other.

Benign Tumor Cells

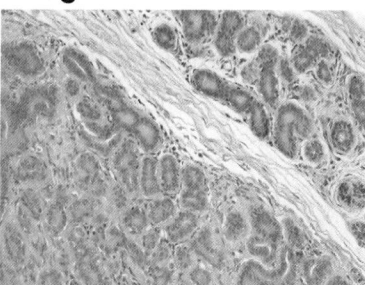

This slide shows a benign tumor (fibroadenoma). Unlike cancer cells, these cells remain well-formed. Benign tumors also don't invade normal surrounding tissue.

Each chromosome is made up of smaller units called genes. Each gene consists of a specific section of DNA. A set of instructions encoded within the DNA determines almost everything about you, from the color of your eyes to your susceptibility to different diseases.

The code used in these instructions is composed of four chemical components: adenine (A), thymine (T), guanine (G) and cytosine (C). Different sequences of these molecules within a gene are translated or expressed as different proteins, substances that make up practically every part of your body and play a role in most of your body's activities (see Chapter 14, "Genetics and Disease"). Each cell contains about 20,000 genes, forming a complete recipe for a human being.

Not all genes are active all of the time. Cells selectively switch on certain genes in response to stress, injury, infections, hormones, growth factors and many other external stimuli. Some genes act as control (regulatory) genes. Some control genes can cause other genes to manufacture their protein continuously, such as an enzyme required for cells to transform nutrients into energy. Others can adjust a gene's production in response to a particular need of the body, such as for the production of insulin, which is a hormone needed to control blood sugar levels. Still others can regulate cell division and differentiation.

When the genetic programming of a normal cell is disrupted or mutated, serious harm may result in the form of disease. Genes that

Advances in Cancer Research

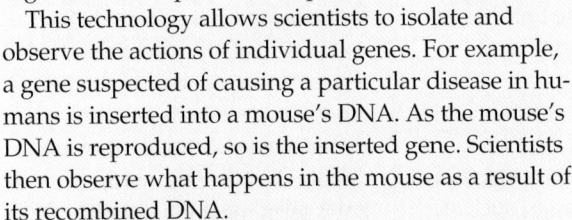

During the past three decades, great strides have been made in understanding how genes are activated and inactivated. This progress is due in great part to the development of recombinant DNA technology, a laboratory procedure that allows the genetic information contained in the DNA of a particular organism to be spliced (manipulated).

This technology allows scientists to isolate and observe the actions of individual genes. For example, a gene suspected of causing a particular disease in humans is inserted into a mouse's DNA. As the mouse's DNA is reproduced, so is the inserted gene. Scientists then observe what happens in the mouse as a result of its recombined DNA.

Recombinant DNA technology has made it possible for scientists to show that multiple mechanisms (agents) may be involved in activating cancer-causing genes (oncogenes). Altered chromosomes have long been suspected of playing a role in the origin of tumors. Research on a family of tumor-producing viruses (retroviruses) led investigators to specific genes associated with cancer in humans and to the exploration of whether chromosome rearrangement may be one way that proto-oncogenes, the precursors to oncogenes, are activated.

Such discoveries were possible partly because of the development of polymerase chain reaction (PCR) — a laboratory technique by which a small fragment of DNA can be quickly reproduced millions of times, making it easier to study. PCR led to the identification of the first genetic marker for cystic fibrosis and is now aiding scientists in the search for specific cancer genes.

Investigators have also discovered a set of genes that actually plays a protective role against cancer development, particularly in inherited cancers. Known as tumor-suppressing genes, these genes act to prevent the unregulated growth of cancer cells and the cancer-inducing effect of activated oncogenes. If one of these tumor-suppressing genes is absent or its protein product is unable to work properly, the cancer-producing action of an oncogene may not be completely suppressed and a tumor may develop.

Researchers continue to investigate how transformed or mutated cells are able to bypass the body's immune response. Remember, since cancer cells originate as normal cells, they are not foreign, so your immune system doesn't recognize them as foreign. However, cancer cells can produce things that alter immune recognition.

Improved understanding of the differences between normal and cancer cells has led to the development of "targeted therapies." These are medications that specifically target abnormalities within cancer cells that cause the cells to grow rapidly. By blocking or altering the abnormal signals, cancers often regress or stop growing. These drugs tend to produce different side effects from those of traditional chemotherapy, and they may be combined with other treatments.

A major roadblock that remains is finding a way to safely deliver immune system antibodies or anti-cancer drugs to the site of the cancer. One approach is monoclonal antibodies, artificial agents designed to attach themselves to cancer cells and deliver drugs or radiation with great precision. The potential of these immunological "bullets" in locating and treating cancer is an exciting prospect (see page 426).

Strategies to conquer cancers are progressing. The oncogene hypothesis, discovery of tumor-suppressing genes and application of targeted therapies are a few advances under study. The future holds promise for applying such new information to the diagnosis, treatment and, ultimately, prevention of cancer.

have the potential for initiating cancer are known as oncogenes. Normally, these genes perform useful functions, such as regulating cell division and tissue repair. But when an oncogene's DNA is disrupted or damaged, these functions may be altered, and oncogenes can become cancer-causing genes (the root word *oncos* comes from the Greek word for "mass," or "tumor"). Oncogenes convert normal cells into cancer cells when the genes are "turned on" or overproduced.

Damage to DNA can result from a variety of environmental factors, including chemicals, radiation, tobacco use and viruses. Damage can also occur because of factors inside your body, such as immune and metabolic disorders, and inherited genetic mutations. Some factors are avoidable; others are not.

Very few cancers are directly inherited. The majority of people who develop cancer have no family history of the disease. Scientists have, however, identified many of the controllable factors that increase a person's chances of getting cancer (see page 437). Most researchers believe that a complex mix of such factors, acting together or in a sequence of events, promotes cancer cell growth.

Diagnosing Cancer

Along with prevention, one of the best approaches to fighting cancer is an early diagnosis. In most cases the earlier a cancer is detected, the greater the chances are that it can be treated before it spreads to other tissues or organs. With the cancer-screening procedures available today, many cancers can be detected early enough to be cured.

The first step is generally to identify the type of cancer you have, so your doctor can plan an appropriate treatment regimen.

While each type of cancer has a tendency to grow and spread in certain patterns, every cancer is unique in every individual. Doctors can anticipate how each cancer is likely to behave to some extent, but growth and spread varies from person to person.

If your doctor suspects that cancer may be present because of signs or symptoms or the results of a cancer-screening procedure, a biopsy may be done. A biopsy involves taking a sample of the affected tissue for microscopic examination. Tissue samples may be removed surgically or with a needle. A biopsy can help determine if a tumor is benign or malignant. Biopsies are also used as screening tools to check for cellular abnormalities (precancerous changes) that often occur before cancer development.

Grading

The microscopic examination of a tissue sample may provide clues about the way a tumor will behave or respond to treatment. The more normal the cells appear and the fewer the number of dividing cells, the more likely the cancer will be slow growing. Based on the sample's cellular appearance, a grade is assigned to the tumor. A lower grade generally indicates fewer cellular abnormalities. Higher grades indicate more abnormalities.

Staging

If a tumor is benign, your doctor may advise its removal to avoid the possibility of it becoming cancerous. If the tumor is cancerous, your doctor will want to determine if or how far the cancer has spread, a process called staging.

Staging is accomplished through a number of steps. It begins with a thorough history and physical examination and is followed by diagnostic tests, which might include a computerized tomography

(CT) scan or magnetic resonance imaging (MRI), bone scans, X-rays, blood tests, or other laboratory procedures. Staging is different for each type of cancer.

Information obtained from these tests is used to help classify the stage of the cancer. There are different ways of assigning malignant tumor classifications. The most common method is the TNM staging system. This system evaluates three components — the primary tumor (T), regional nodes (N) and metastasis (M) — by answering the following key questions:

- T — How big is the tumor, and has the cancer spread locally?
- N — Have cancer cells spread to nearby lymph nodes?
- M — Has the cancer spread (metastasized) to other, distant areas of the body?

Numbers are assigned to each of these categories, indicating the degree to which the tumor has grown or spread. Once the TNM classifications have been determined, your doctor can determine the stage of your cancer. Like cancer grades, a lower number indicates that the cancer is still in its early stages, and a higher number means it's more advanced.

If cancer cells are present in a particular location but haven't invaded nearby tissues, the stage can also be described as *in situ* — a Latin term meaning "in place." This is a very early stage of cancer development and generally carries a very good prognosis. If the cancer has invaded nearby tissues, then it's called invasive. If the cancer has traveled to a different part of the body, it's known as metastatic.

In addition to grade and spread, new staging systems in development also take into account biological data such as the presence of gene mutations and the overexpression of certain cancer markers.

Estimating a survival rate

Doctors often use statistics to help them estimate a prognosis, which is a prediction of the course and outcome of the disease and the likelihood of recovery. A common statistic used is the five-year survival rate. This rate is based on people who've survived the cancer for a period of five years, whether the cancer is receding (in remission), cured or under treatment. This statistic provides a rough estimate of how an average person may do with a specific type of cancer. Your situation may be different.

Evaluating the results

All of these diagnostic tools — laboratory tests, imaging scans, grading and staging classifications — can help guide you and your doctor toward the treatment best suited to your cancer. The diagnosis and staging of your cancer may require several days or weeks.

Specific Cancers

A number of tests are helpful in screening for cancer. They vary in complexity and cost. Most of the widely used tests are designed to discover the more common forms of cancer in people at high risk and for whom an early diagnosis may allow more-effective treatment and better chances of survival.

Because everyone is different, the screening methods you and your doctor choose should address your specific circumstances and the type of cancer for which you're at risk. Safety also is important. The test shouldn't pose a health threat.

Screening tests for cancer don't have the same preventive value in all cases and for all cancer types. With lung cancer, for example, tests often don't identify the disease early enough to make a significant difference in survival rates. Other cancers, such as cervical cancer, are more easily detectable in their early stages.

The tests and procedures described here are recommended by the American Cancer Society (ACS). Routine cancer screening should be stopped when age or other medical conditions make living another 10 years unlikely.

Breast cancer

Warning signs. An abnormality on a mammogram, any lump or thickening in the breast, bleeding, or discharge from the nipple
Risk factors. In addition to being female, breast cancer is associated with:
- Being older than age 50
- Having never given birth
- Having your first child after age 30
- Having never breast-fed
- Being more than 40 percent over your ideal weight
- Reaching sexual maturity early or having late menopause
- Having dense breast tissue on a routine mammogram
- Using hormone therapy for more than five years after menopause
- Having a family history of premenopausal breast cancer, cancer in both breasts or ovarian cancer
Checkup guidelines. It's recommended that women become familiar with their breasts (see page 802) and that women ages 20 to 39 with a strong family history of breast cancer have their breasts examined yearly by a doctor.

There's disagreement within the medical profession about the age at which women should begin having regular mammograms.

Most medical experts agree that women younger than 35 who aren't in a high-risk category don't need mammograms and that women older than 50 should have them every one to two years.

If you're in your 40s, talk with your doctor about how often you should have a mammogram, based on your risk factors, personal preferences and your understanding about the benefits and limitations of mammography.

Women with a family history of breast cancer should have regular mammograms beginning five to 10 years before the age the youngest first-degree with breast cancer received her diagnosis.

Cervical cancer

Warning signs. Abnormal vaginal bleeding
Risk factors. Cervical cancer is associated with:
- Genital herpes or genital wart infections
- Onset of sexual activity shortly after reaching puberty
- Many sexual partners
- Tobacco use
Checkup guidelines. If you're a female who's sexually active or older than age 18, it's recommended you have a Pap test that includes a test for human papillomavirus (HPV) and a pelvic examination annually. After three or more consecutive normal annual examinations, your doctor may decide the Pap test can be performed less frequently.

The HPV vaccine recommended for all girls and boys before the onset of sexual activity can prevent cervical cancer.

Colorectal cancer

Warning signs. Rectal bleeding or a change in bowel habits
Risk factors. Colorectal cancer is associated with:
- A history of colorectal polyps
- A family history of colorectal cancer or inflammatory bowel disease
- A family history of hereditary nonpolyposis colorectal cancer (HNPCC) or familial polyposis
- African-American people
- Tobacco use
- Physical inactivity
- A high-fat or low-fiber diet or both
- A diet low in fruits and vegetables
- Obesity
- Excessive alcohol consumption
Checkup guidelines. If you're age 50 or older and at average risk of colorectal cancer, it's recommended that you have one or more of the following screening procedures:

- A fecal occult blood test annually
- A barium enema and flexible sigmoidoscopy every five years
- A colonoscopy every 10 years

A digital rectal exam should be done at the same time as a barium enema or colonoscopy.

Collecting a stool sample that's tested for abnormal cells associated with colorectal cancer (Cologuard test) may be an option for some.

If you're at an increased risk, your doctor may request more-frequent screening.

Endometrial cancer

Warning signs. Abnormal vaginal bleeding

Risk factors. Endometrial cancer is associated with:
- A history of infertility or failure to ovulate
- Late onset of menopause or prolonged estrogen therapy or tamoxifen use after menopause
- Obesity
- Diabetes
- Gallbladder disease
- High blood pressure
- Hereditary nonpolyposis colo-rectal cancer (HNPCC)
- The drug tamoxifen for treat-ment of breast cancer

Checkup guidelines. Most endo-metrial cancer is detected early due to postmenopausal bleeding. If you're a woman with a person-al or family history of HNPCC, consider an annual endometrial biopsy beginning at age 35.

Lung cancer

Warning signs. A persistent cough, coughing up blood, bron-chitis, chest pain and recurrent pneumonia in the same location

Risk factors. Lung cancer is asso-ciated with:
- Tobacco use
- Exposure to secondhand smoke
- Exposure to environmental pollutants such as asbestos and arsenic
- Exposure to radon and radiation
- Tuberculosis

Checkup guidelines. If you're older than age 40, consider having a baseline chest X-ray. Subsequent chest X-rays may be done at the discretion of your doctor. Low-dose helical (spiral) computerized tomography (CT) scans and molecular markers in sputum are being studied for possible use in early lung cancer detection, and the results are controversial.

Oral cancer

Warning signs. A change of color, a lump or thickening inside your mouth, or a sore that fails to heal

Risk factors. Oral cancer is associ-ated with:
- Being male and age 40 or older
- Use of chewing tobacco
- Heavy use of smoking tobacco
- Excessive alcohol consumption
- Human papillomavirus (HPV)

Checkup guidelines. See a doctor or dentist if you have a sore in your mouth that doesn't heal or if you notice a lump inside your mouth.

Prostate cancer

Warning signs. Often none. Some men experience difficulty urinat-ing. Blood in urine or persistent pain in the lower back, pelvis or upper thighs.

Risk factors. Prostate cancer oc-curs most often in men who:
- Are older than age 65
- Are black
- Have a family history of the disease
- Are obese

Checkup guidelines. Men older than age 40 should have a digi-tal rectal examination during an annual physical. At age 50 — or earlier if you're black or have a family history of prostate cancer — discuss with your doctor the benefits of having a prostate-specific antigen (PSA) blood test.

The accuracy of the PSA test is frequently debated. Some health experts view it as a needless and expensive procedure. Mayo Clinic urologists agree the test isn't ideal, but they support its use because it's the best screening tool available for identifying prostate cancer. No study has shown the test to decrease the risk of dying of prostate cancer.

Mayo Clinic urologists recom-mend a yearly PSA test beginning at age 50. After age 75, Mayo urol-ogists believe a yearly digital exam to be sufficient, although some organizations recommend lifelong screening. For more on the PSA test, see page 1249.

Skin cancer

Warning signs. Skin cancer can present itself in many ways:
- A lesion with an irregular border
- A firm bump, nodule or lesion — from pearl colored to black — anywhere on the skin
- Dark lesions on the palms, the soles of your feet, or the tips of your fingers or toes
- A shiny, waxy, pearl-colored bump on your face, ear or neck
- A firm, red nodule or a flat lesion with a scaly or crusted surface
- A change in a mole
- A sore that fails to heal

Risk factors. Skin cancer is associ-ated with:
- Fair skin
- Blue eyes
- Red hair
- Severe sunburns during childhood
- A family history of birthmarks or moles
- Exposure to coal, tar, creosote, arsenic compounds or radium

Checkup guidelines. If you have a skin lesion that fits the warning signs, see your doctor.

Testicular cancer

Warning signs. Any lump on the testicle, a change in its size or a sensation of fullness

Risk factors. Testicular cancer strikes younger men and is less common after age 40. A known risk factor for this cancer is unde-scended testicles — one or both — at birth.

Checkup guidelines. Beginning in their late teens, men should examine their testicles monthly (see page 1245).

Throat cancer

Warning signs. Hoarseness
Risk factors. Heavy smoking, particularly when coupled with excessive alcohol use
Checkup guidelines. Have an annual throat examination if you're a heavy smoker or in case of unexplained hoarseness or a change in the character of your voice lasting more than a few weeks.

Urinary tract and bladder cancer

Warning signs. Blood in urine, back pain, loss of weight and appetite, fever, and anemia
Risk factors. Urinary tract and bladder cancer is associated with:

- Being male and age 50 or older
- Tobacco use
- A history of chronic urinary tract infections
- Obesity
- Work around certain chemicals, such as dyes or petrochemicals

Checkup guidelines. Have a routine urinalysis during an annual physical examination to check for blood in your urine (hematuria), the most common warning sign.

Treating Cancer

More than ever before, many cancers can be successfully treated. The probability of a complete cure or extended survival is continuously improving due to growing knowledge and understanding of cancer. As a result, new therapies that selectively kill cancer cells are steadily being developed. These therapies are not only more effective but also safer. In addition, management of cancer pain and other symptoms has improved to the point that most people with cancer can live and work comfortably while undergoing treatment.

Treatment regimens for cancer are based on the health needs of the individual being treated and the type of cancer he or she has. But the basic therapeutic options available to most people with cancer are similar. Why one form of treatment is more appropriate than another for a given person depends on a variety of factors, including the diagnosis, the stage of the disease, the individual's age, sex and general health, and his or her individual preferences. In women, menopausal status also can be a factor in treatment decisions.

During the diagnostic phase, your doctor is usually able to determine if a localized form of treatment, such as surgery or radiation therapy, can treat your cancer or if a total body (systemic) form of treatment, such as chemotherapy, is necessary because cancer cells have spread to other body parts.

Surgery

Surgery has long been the foundation of cancer treatment. The goal of any operation can vary — it may be to determine whether a growth is malignant, to remove a cancerous growth from the body or to learn if malignant cells have spread to other body parts. Sometimes, surgery is directed primarily toward relief of a symptom, for example, removing a growth that's obstructing the bile ducts. At other times, when it's not possible to remove all of the cancerous growth, a surgeon may remove as much as possible (debulking procedure) in order to make chemotherapy or radiation more effective.

Surgery is most successful if the cancer is contained in one location (localized). Sometimes, however, cancer cells spread from the site where the cancer first appeared (primary tumor) and travel by way of the bloodstream or the lymphatic system to other sites in the body to form secondary tumors (metastases). If cells spread before the primary growth is taken out, cancer may recur at other locations, even after the primary tumor has been fully removed.

Metastatic tumors are still named based on the location

Cancer Clusters in Populations

Data collected by public health officials sometimes show an increase in the frequency of occurrence of a certain type of cancer or group of cancers in a region or community. This increase is often referred to as a cancer cluster.

Further study usually finds that such clusters are explained by the laws of chance or by changes in medical referral patterns. Sometimes, though, the increase is traced to an environmental factor.

The laws of chance tell us that most communities or groups of people of similar age and background will have about the same frequency of various diseases. They also suggest that from time to time there will be an unusual concentration of one disease or another within certain groups of people.

This statistical phenomenon might be compared to dealing a hand of cards. Usually, the cards in a hand will be fairly evenly distributed among the four suits, but you can also expect that now and then you'll be dealt a hand composed almost entirely of one suit. Mathematicians can even calculate the odds of such an event occurring.

It's important to separate cancer clusters that are merely random from those related to environmental factors. Scientific proof that a cancer cluster is a consequence of exposure to potentially toxic substances depends on careful evaluation.

where the cancer started. For example, breast cancer that has spread to the lungs is called breast cancer metastasis, not lung cancer.

If the cancer is widespread, an operation is rarely able to cure it. Occasionally, a single metastatic tumor appears after removal of the primary cancer and, in some cases, the surgical removal of this single lesion can result in a complete recovery. This situation may be experienced by people with cancer of the colon or testicles, among others. Metastatic tumors, in most of these circumstances, are located in the lung, liver or brain.

Radiation therapy

Radiation is another option for destroying cancer cells. Radiation therapy — also referred to as radiotherapy, X-ray therapy, cobalt treatment or irradiation — may be one part of a treatment regimen or the only form of treatment. Radiation affects only the cancer cells located within the area of the body (field) receiving the radiation.

Proton therapy is a type of radiation therapy that uses energy from positively charged particles called protons to treat tumors.

Radiation is sometimes used before surgery to shrink a cancerous tumor, after surgery to destroy any remaining cancer cells, in combination with anti-cancer drugs or alone. Radiation is particularly effective on certain types of localized cancers, such as malignant tumors of the lymph nodes or vocal cords.

Radiation, like surgery, usually isn't curative if the cancer cells have spread throughout the body or outside the field of radiation. However, it may still be used even if a complete recovery isn't probable because it can shrink tumors to decrease signs and symptoms the cancer is producing, such as pressure, pain or bleeding.

Generally, radiation produces less physical disfigurement than does radical surgery, but it may

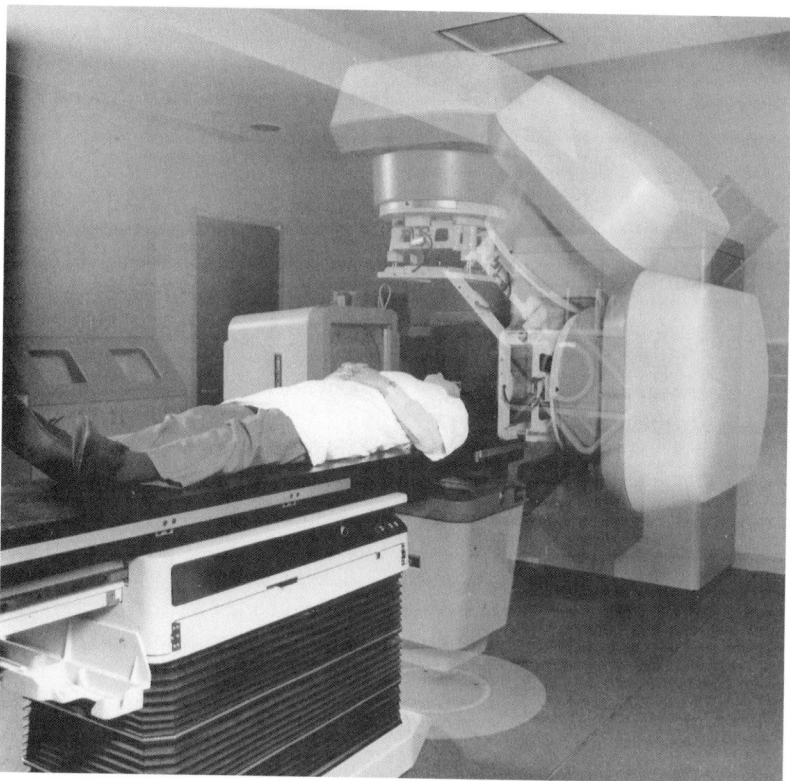

Radiation therapy can effectively destroy cancer cells. During treatment this radiation source slowly rotates to deliver radiation more effectively.

produce some troublesome side effects, such as irritated or thickened skin, difficulty swallowing, dry mouth, nausea, diarrhea, hair loss, and loss of energy. How serious and extensive these side effects become depends on where and how much radiation is used.

Chemotherapy

Chemotherapy is the systemic use of medication to treat cancer. The medication is generally administered by injection or intravenously, but is also available in topical form or may be taken as a pill. For some types of cancer, such as Hodgkin lymphoma, leukemia and testicular cancer, chemotherapy may produce a cure even when the cancer is widespread.

Chemotherapy is frequently administered after an operation has removed the cancer, even when there's no clear sign of the cancer having spread. This is referred to as adjuvant chemotherapy. For some cancers, especially breast and colorectal, adjuvant

chemotherapy has been shown to decrease the chance the cancer will return. And people with cancer who receive this therapy generally live longer than do those who don't have the treatment.

Chemotherapy may also be given before an operation to shrink the cancer and make the operation easier or more successful. This is called neoadjuvant chemotherapy and is used in cancers of the head, neck, breast and bladder. In instances in which the cancer isn't curable, chemotherapy may relieve symptoms and enhance quality of life. This is known as palliative treatment.

Chemotherapy may involve the use of more than one medication. Combination chemotherapy consists of giving a group of drugs that work together to kill more cancer cells. The downside of anti-cancer medications is that they often affect normal tissue cells as well as cancer cells.

Normal cells most likely to be affected are those that divide rapidly, such as those found in bone marrow, the lining of the gastrointestinal tract, the reproductive system and hair follicles. After treatment is complete, these cells usually recover.

Side effects vary depending on the medications used. They include hair loss, mouth sores, difficulty swallowing, dry mouth, nausea, vomiting, diarrhea, bleeding and infection.

Less common problems include damage to the heart, liver, lungs, kidneys or nerves. Nerve damage may result in numbness or tingling of the hands or feet. Often, the side effects disappear once the treatment is complete. Experts are working to reduce and even eliminate these side effects.

Immunotherapy

Your body's immune system acts as a surveillance system to guard against what it interprets to be foreign substances. For example, when your immune system detects harmful bacteria or a virus in your body, it responds by mobilizing certain cells and producing specific proteins (antibodies) that attack and destroy the invaders. Your immune system also views cancer cells as foreign invaders but often is prevented from attacking them.

Immunotherapy is a type of cancer treatment that helps your immune system fight cancer. Other names for the technique include biological therapy, biotherapy and biologic response modifier therapy. Immunotherapy may be prescribed alone or in combination with other cancer treatments.

One variation of immunotherapy is to administer substances that stimulate the immune system — nonspecific immunomodulating agents. Two such agents are used in conjunction with surgery for bladder cancer and surgery for advanced colon cancer.

Another variation is to produce specific immune system proteins (cytokines) in the laboratory and then use them in treatment.

Called biologic response modifiers (BRMs), they account for the majority of immunotherapeutic agents currently being used or studied. BRMs include:

Interferons

Interferons are cytokines that occur naturally in your body. There are several types. The type most commonly used in cancer treatment is interferon-alfa. Interferons may directly inhibit cancer cells, or they may stimulate other immune system cells to help in the battle.

Interferons are used for a number of cancers, including hairy cell leukemia, melanoma, chronic myeloid leukemia and AIDS-related Kaposi's sarcoma. They're also being studied for use in the treatment of metastatic kidney cancer and non-Hodgkin lymphoma.

Interleukins

Like interferons, interleukins are a type of cytokine. Interleukin-2, the most widely studied interleukin, works by interfering with cancer growth pathways. It has been approved for the treatment of metastatic kidney cancer and metastatic melanoma and is being studied as a treatment for several other cancers.

Monoclonal antibodies

Monoclonal antibodies are designed and produced in a laboratory to target specific types of cancer. By attaching themselves to tumor cells, they can either react with that tumor cell or be used to deliver anti-cancer medications or radiation.

Examples of monoclonal antibodies approved by the Food and Drug Administration are rituximab (Rituxan) for the treatment of B-cell non-Hodgkin lymphoma and trastuzumab (Herceptin) for the treatment of breast cancer. Additional monoclonal antibodies are being studied for use in other cancers, including other lymphomas, leukemias, brain tumors, and cancers of the lung, colon, rectum and prostate.

Checkpoint inhibitors

Certain cancers can block your immune system's ability to recognize and attack cancer cells. New immune treatments known as checkpoint inhibitors are designed to remove this blockage so that your immune system can mount its natural defenses to attack the cancer. The drugs block "checkpoint proteins" called PD-1 and PD-L1 that prevent your immune cells from taking action.

Checkpoint inhibitors are approved to treat melanoma, certain lung cancers and bladder cancer. They include the drugs pembrolizumab (Keytruda), nivolumab (Opdivo), atezolizumab (Tecentriq) and avelumab (Bavencio).

Vaccines

Researchers are working on vaccines that can help your immune system recognize cancer cells. Unlike infectious disease vaccines, which are given to prevent a disease, cancer vaccines are given only after a tumor develops. The vaccine is intended to help your body reject the tumor and prevent the cancer from recurring. These remain experimental.

Side effects

Side effects of BRMs may include a rash or swelling at the site of injection, flu-like symptoms and fatigue. Some may cause allergic reactions. Muscle aches and fever may occur after a cancer vaccine.

Side effects of checkpoint inhibitors include fatigue, cough, nausea, loss of appetite, skin rash and itching. These drugs can cause serious, even life-threatening, problems in the lungs, intestines, liver, kidneys and hormone-producing glands.

Because they can be severe at times, talk with your doctor about the possible side effects of your particular treatment.

As researchers learn more about how the immune system recognizes and attacks malignant cells, their studies may lead to more-effective immunotherapy techniques.

Hyperthermia therapy

Hyperthermia therapy involves exposing body tissue to high temperatures — up to 106 F — damaging the cells. This therapy can be performed in a small area, for example, on a limb or an organ, with the use of a small probe. It can be very effective at relieving local symptoms such as pain.

Cryotherapy

Cryotherapy is the opposite of hyperthermia therapy. It uses extreme cold to destroy cancer cells. Cryotherapy consists of the application of liquid nitrogen to a tumor. It's used most often to treat early-stage skin cancers and precancerous skin conditions, as well as cancer of the retina (retinoblastoma). Researchers are studying cryotherapy as a possible treatment for some internal cancers, such as those affecting the prostate and the liver. For these cancers, liquid nitrogen reaches the tumor through a device called a cryoprobe.

Stem cell transplantation

Stem cell transplantation is used to replace cells within bone marrow that have been destroyed by radiation or chemotherapy. During the procedure, you receive a supply of stem cells — immature cells that haven't yet differentiated into the various types of blood cells. You may receive your own stem cells (autologous transplant), stem cells from an identical twin if you have one (syngeneic transplant), or stem cells from a sibling or a parent or even an unrelated donor (allogeneic transplant).

Knowing that you'll have a supply of healthy stem cells available to you allows your doctor to use higher doses of chemotherapy or radiation therapy. Stem cell transplantation is used most often as a treatment for leukemia and lymphoma.

Targeted therapies

Targeted therapy is a type of cancer treatment that targets the changes in cancer cells that help them grow, divide and spread. As researchers learn more about cellular changes that drive cancer, they're better able to design promising therapies that target these changes or block their effects.

A primary goal of targeted therapy is to fight cancer cells with more precision and potentially fewer side effects.

The Food and Drug Administration has approved numerous targeted therapies and many more are being studied in clinical trials. Similar to newer immunotherapy drugs, these medications can be expensive. Also, in some cases, the benefits may only be temporary. Here are some examples of targeted therapies and how they work:

Bevacizumab
All tumors require new blood vessel development to supply oxygen and nutrients to their cells so that they can grow. The formation of new blood vessels is called angiogenesis. The drug bevacizumab (Avastin) is designed to stop new blood vessels from forming and has been approved for use in lung, colon, breast, brain, cervical fallopian tube and kidney cancers.

Imatinib
The drug imatinib (Gleevec) is used to treat certain forms of blood cancer (leukemia), as well as bone marrow disorders, skin cancer, and certain tumors of the stomach and digestive system. Leukemia results from a genetic mutation that allows a blood cell enzyme to be switched on permanently. Imatinib works by inhibiting the enzyme, thereby interfering with the abnormal growth of white blood cells.

Rituximab
Your immune system produces antibodies to fight germs, but sometimes things go wrong, and instead it produces harmful antibodies called autoantibodies that attack healthy tissue and cells. Autoantibodies are produced by immune cells called B cells.

The drug rituximab (Rituxan) decreases the number of B cells by targeting those that have a specific marker on their cell surface. It attaches to B cells, causing them to commit cellular suicide, a process called apoptosis.

Rituximab is approved to treat non-Hodgkin lymphoma and certain leukemias.

Erlotinib
The drug erlotinib (Tarceva) is used to treat non-small cell lung cancer and pancreatic cancer that has spread to other parts of the body (metastasized). The medication is thought to interfere with the activity of a specific protein called epidermal growth factor receptor (EGFR). Some cancer cells need this protein to help them grow and divide.

Coping With Side Effects

Sometimes the side effects of cancer treatment are temporarily more distressing than the cancer itself. Both radiation therapy and chemotherapy have common side effects that include fatigue, nausea, hair loss, skin problems, mouth and throat difficulties, diarrhea, and constipation. Immunotherapy also can cause fatigue.

Although scientists have made strides in modifying the severity of such problems, including effective anti-nausea medications, you'll likely experience some side effects during your treatment.

Many people continue to work or go to school — though perhaps on a less demanding schedule — and carry on daily activities while receiving cancer treatment. You can do things to reduce side effects and improve your quality of life during this period.

Hair loss

Certain chemotherapy drugs and radiation therapy to the head can cause hair loss (alopecia). The hair tends to come out in clumps, most often during washing or brushing.

Your doctor can tell you in advance if hair loss is a likely side effect of your treatment. If you know hair loss is likely, you may wish to purchase a wig or hair piece before the treatment begins so that you can match your natural hair color and texture. Some people choose to wear turbans or scarves. Others have their hair cut short before it begins to fall out so that the process of losing their hair isn't quite as overwhelming.

Several treatments have been investigated as possible ways to prevent hair loss, but none has been absolutely effective. One treatment is called scalp hypothermia. During your chemotherapy infusions, ice packs or similar devices are placed on your head to slow blood flow to your scalp. This way, chemotherapy drugs are less likely to have an effect on your hair.

Studies of scalp hypothermia have found it works somewhat in the majority of people who have tried it. However, the procedure also causes a small risk of cancer recurring in your scalp, as this area doesn't receive the same dose of chemotherapy as the rest of your body. People undergoing scalp hypothermia report feeling uncomfortably cold and having headaches.

Fatigue

People frequently feel more tired during cancer treatment. The level of fatigue can vary — you may feel a mild lack of energy, or you may feel completely wiped out. Your fatigue also may last for several months until your treatment ends.

There are many different causes for fatigue from cancer treatment. Some may be treatable. For example, cancer treatment can cause anemia. Medications that stimulate your body to produce new blood cells can be used to reverse this. Blood transfusions also may help in some situations.

Regardless of your level of fatigue, pay attention to it. Try to get a good night's sleep and rest as needed throughout the day. Routine exercise is beneficial to help you maintain energy, but let others help you do things too. It's also important to eat well and drink plenty of fluids. The herbal supplement ginseng also has been shown to help decrease fatigue in people undergoing cancer therapy.

Nausea

Anti-nausea medications help prevent or decrease nausea and vomiting in many people undergoing cancer treatment. Newer anti-nausea medications have made cancer therapy much more tolerable. Other things you can do to help prevent nausea include:

- Eat bland foods such as toast, crackers and ice pops.
- Drink small amounts of clear liquids frequently.
- Eat cold foods because hot foods can have a more pungent odor.

Cancer Centers

Choosing doctors and a hospital to treat your cancer can be stressful. Sometimes the process seems automatic. Your family doctor may refer you to a cancer specialist (oncologist) within the same practice or at an associated medical facility. Sometimes you're faced with many options. Before making a decision, ask for advice from your personal physician or another doctor with whom you feel comfortable and have confidence. Also check with your insurance company to make sure it covers treatment at the center you are considering. Don't forget to factor in hotel costs, meal expenses and time away from work if you need to travel.

Many larger medical centers are equipped to treat cancer cases that don't require a high degree of specialization. But if you need complicated or experimental treatment or if the doctors at your local hospital are inexperienced in treating your specific type of cancer, you might want to visit a specialized cancer center.

Usually, a hospital connected to or affiliated with a medical school offers a broad range of treatment options because these institutions often draw prominent clinicians, researchers and educators to their medical facilities. Teaching hospitals — those that train doctors but don't necessarily have a direct medical school affiliation — also often are good facilities.

Teaching hospitals and hospitals associated with medical schools often conduct clinical trials in which they investigate potential new cancer treatments. If you're offered a chance to enter one of these trials, make sure that you fully understand the possible risks and benefits. Although clinical trials are clearly experimental, the therapies under investigation often include some of the most promising treatments.

The National Cancer Institute has designated more than 60 medical centers throughout the United States as comprehensive cancer centers. These centers provide leadership in cancer research and education and develop programs involving scientists and doctors from many fields. Comprehensive cancer centers generally offer the most extensive range of cancer treatment found in the United States. To find out more about these centers, see the National Cancer Institute.

- Eat foods that you like.
- Eat smaller meals.

Mouth and throat disorders

It's important to maintain good oral hygiene during cancer treatment because gum disease, mouth sores and mouth dryness can result from chemotherapy or radiation. Radiation therapy to the chest or throat area also can cause gagging, coughing or swallowing problems. Do the following:
- Brush your teeth and gums after every meal.
- Rinse your mouth often with warm salt water.
- Avoid mouthwashes with alcohol.
- Eat soft foods, such as ice cream, mashed potatoes or yogurt.
- Keep your lips moist with lip balm or petroleum jelly.
- Avoid spicy or acidic foods, such as tomatoes and citrus fruits.
- Carry a water bottle with you and sip throughout the day.

Diarrhea

Cancer treatment can affect the cells that line your intestines, causing diarrhea. The following steps can help limit diarrhea:
- Drink plenty of mild, clear liquids, such as water, ginger ale, weak tea or sports drinks. Diarrhea can cause dehydration.
- Eat smaller meals throughout the day.
- Eat low-fiber foods, such as white rice, noodles or chicken.
- Eat foods rich in potassium, a vital nutrient that's lost during diarrhea. Foods with plenty of potassium include bananas, oranges, potatoes and apricots.
- Avoid beverages containing alcohol or caffeine, sweets, dairy products, and extremely hot or cold foods because these can make diarrhea worse.

If you have diarrhea for more than 24 hours, or if it's associated with abdominal pain or cramping, talk to your doctor.

Constipation

Certain medications, physical weakness, lack of activity, or a diet low in fiber and liquids can cause constipation. If you experience constipation for more than one or two days, your doctor may prescribe a stool softener or laxative. Try taking these steps too:

Integrative Therapies

When cancer is diagnosed, many people look beyond standard medical practices to help fight the cancer or cope with its side effects. Although some nontraditional therapies may be helpful, others may be harmful, especially if they're used in place of proven treatments.

Complementing standard care

When complementary therapies for cancer are used in conjunction with standard medical treatments, it's known as integrative medicine. These therapies won't cure your cancer, but they may enhance your quality of life by reducing stress, lessening side effects of treatment and improving your general sense of well-being. In addition, because most integrative therapies are self-managed, they can give you a sense of control over your situation.

The types of integrative therapies that may accompany cancer treatment are many and varied:
- Meditation
- Acupuncture or acupressure
- Therapeutic massage
- Music, movement and art therapy
- Prayer and other spiritual practices
- Yoga
- Tai chi
- Hypnosis

To improve your sense of well-being, you don't necessarily have to enroll in an organized program. Taking the time to relax and enjoy the small things in life is a complementary therapy in and of itself.

In place of standard care

Some people explore nontraditional therapies in an effort to replace more-standard treatment. However, the safety and effectiveness of many nontraditional therapies hasn't been tested, and some therapies may even be harmful. Beware of alternative therapies that haven't been documented for safety and effectiveness. Also, do your homework when it comes to herbal supplements. People often think of herbal supplements as "all natural," but that doesn't mean they're safe. Supplements aren't regulated in the same manner as foods and drugs and may contain contaminants.

A good rule of thumb in terms of integrative therapies is to first discuss them with your doctor and avoid any treatment that promises a cure, encourages you to give up conventional therapies or requires you to travel to another country. See Chapter 38, "Integrative Medicine," for more information.

- Increase the amount of high-fiber foods in your diet, such as whole-grain breads, raw fruits and vegetables, or dried fruits.
- Drink plenty of liquids.
- Get regular exercise.
- Avoid foods that commonly cause constipation, such as chocolate, cheese and eggs.

Appetite and weight changes

Eating a balanced diet can help you better tolerate the side effects of chemotherapy, radiation or surgery. Good nutrition also enhances your immune function and sense of well-being.

Difficult problems often associated with cancer are weight loss and malnutrition. Many factors can contribute to weight loss. Cancer or its treatment can decrease appetite and food intake or interfere with your body's consumption, digestion and absorption of food. In addition, many people experience appetite and weight changes even before a diagnosis of cancer is made.

Often a person with cancer who experiences severe weight loss simply can't eat. Some people also are unable to taste their food, and it's not uncommon to feel full after eating only a few bites.

Radiation therapy, chemotherapy or surgery may also cause nausea, changes in your sense of taste or smell, a sore mouth, diarrhea, anorexia, or difficulty swallowing, which can increase nutritional issues.

You can take many simple, constructive steps to improve your appetite during cancer treatment to prevent weight loss (see page 434). If these steps don't help, talk to your doctor about medications that may help stimulate your appetite. The medication megestrol (Megace), taken several times each day, has been shown to increase appetite and weight in individuals with cancer. However, you may only be gaining fat and water weight. People taking the drug generally don't gain any muscle tissue or become stronger.

Studies also indicate that good nutrition can improve a person's chance of undergoing successful treatment, if the cancer is found early and has a good chance of being cured. There's no evidence that decreased or excessive amounts of any specific nutrient has a beneficial role in the treatment of cancer. Your doctor or a registered dietitian can provide advice on how to maintain adequate nutrition.

Skin problems

Dry skin can be a side effect of radiation therapy or chemotherapy. To reduce the effects of dry skin:
- Avoid hot baths.
- When you do take a bath, add bath oil to the water.
- Don't bathe more than once daily.
- Apply moisturizers and lotions while your skin is still moist.
- Avoid skin products that contain alcohol.

Pain

Cancer doesn't always cause pain, but pain is the most feared symptom associated with cancer. More than half the people with cancer don't experience significant pain. Some, though, have severe pain. In general, the more advanced the cancer, the greater the likelihood of periods of severe pain.

Causes
Cancer pain may be dull, aching, sharp, constant, intermittent, mild, moderate or severe. The pain may stem from the destruction of healthy tissues around the primary tumor or other areas in the body where the cancer has spread. Or, it may result from pressure on nerves, bones or other organs as the cancer continues to grow. Cancer also can cause pain by secreting substances that directly stimulate nerves and cause pain without tissue destruction. Treating the cancer can help alleviate this type of pain.

In addition, cancer treatments can be a source of pain. Surgery may be painful. Radiation therapy may cause skin reactions or scars that are painful. Chemotherapy may result in mouth sores, diarrhea or damaged nerves. Emotional responses to the cancer, such as anxiety, depression or feelings of hopelessness, can make the pain seem worse.

Treatments
Pain relief can be obtained in many ways, and most people with cancer don't have to deal with severe pain. One of the components of cancer treatment is to decrease pain with as few side effects as possible.

Cancer treatments
The ideal way to treat cancer pain, when possible, is to remove the source of pain through surgery, chemotherapy or radiation therapy.

Medications
Pain medications (analgesics) are another option. Many drugs are used to treat cancer pain, but most fall into two categories: nonopioids and opioids.
- **Nonopioids.** Nonopioids include acetaminophen and nonsteroidal anti-inflammatory drugs (NSAIDs). NSAIDs are also helpful if inflammation is responsible for some of the pain. Antidepressants and anti-seizure medications and steroids are other nonopioid agents that may help control cancer pain.
- **Opioids.** Opioids, such as morphine and codeine and derivatives, are powerful pain-killers most often prescribed for moderate to severe pain. People with cancer often worry that using opioids will lead to addiction. It's true that people who use opioids for purposes other than pain control may become addicted to them. But when taken for pain and under

proper direction, opioids rarely cause addiction. If an opioid is needed to relieve severe pain for a long time, the comfort it provides often outweighs the risk of addiction.

A common side effect of opioids is constipation, which can be treated with appropriate measures prescribed by your doctor. Other side effects include confusion, lethargy and sleepiness. They usually occur when first taking the medication and often go away with regular use.

Occasionally, tranquilizers (sedatives) are used in combination with analgesics. Tranquilizers provide no pain relief, but they may help you tolerate the discomfort and can be an integral part of treatment. Tranquilizers or large doses of opioids can cause confusion or delirium. This can limit their usefulness.

Most pain medications can be taken orally. Others are given by injection or intravenously through a needle inserted into a vein in your arm. Some pain medications are available in patch form. For some people with cancer, this is a convenient and effective way of providing durable pain relief.

Other therapies

Beyond medications, other options for treating pain include:

- **Nerve blocks.** Nerve pathways that carry pain impulses to the brain are blocked either by injection of substances into or around nerve fibers or by surgery. For people who can't tolerate the side effects of pain medications, they can be helpful. Nerve blocks are frequently used for pancreatic cancer and some other types of cancer.
- **Behavior modification therapies.** These therapies help decrease anxiety and can build confidence in your ability to cope with pain. Behavior modification therapies include hypnosis, biofeedback, relaxation exercises and massage.

Childhood Cancer

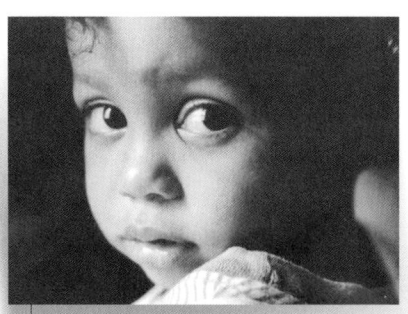

More than 15,000 new cases of childhood cancer are diagnosed each year in the United States, making cancer a rare condition among children. In addition, modern treatment now makes prolonged survival and recovery not only possible but likely with many childhood cancers — more than 80 percent of all children with cancer in America now survive.

Still, cancer remains responsible for more deaths than any other disease in school-age and preschool children. Only accidents claim more lives in these age groups.

The most common childhood cancer is leukemia. It accounts for a third of childhood cancers. With new treatments, the outlook for children with this disease has brightened considerably. Another type of cancer seen in children is a malignant brain tumor. Less common cancers that occur in children include a tumor of the kidney (Wilms' tumor), a nervous system cancer (neuroblastoma), cancer of the eye (retinoblastoma) and bone cancer (osteosarcoma). The causes of these cancers remain largely unknown.

It's important to choose carefully when deciding where to have your child treated for cancer. Seek out a medical center with a team that specializes in childhood cancer. This team often includes pediatric oncologists, pediatric surgeons and pediatric nurses. In addition to physical care for your child, the center and its staff should provide emotional support for the entire family.

Dealing with your child's cancer

Having a child with cancer is very stressful for even the strongest of families. The best approach is to be honest with your child about his or her disease and to be support-

ive. Both you and your child's health care team should prepare your child for the experiences involved in his or her treatment. Reassure your child that everybody is trying to make him or her better. Ask doctors and nurses to help answer your child's questions.

The goal of pediatric cancer treatment is not only to get rid of the cancer but also to help your child continue to function at an age-appropriate level — developmentally, psychologically and emotionally.

Although it's important to support and console your child, it's also critical to maintain as much normalcy as possible in his or her life. Keeping schedules, rules, family activities and previous expectations in place conveys a message that you trust your child's ability to cope with this difficulty. It also suggests that, as a parent, you'll help him or her prepare for a long future.

While your child is receiving cancer treatment, communicate closely with school personnel to establish behavioral and academic expectations that are as realistic as possible. Most schools are able to provide individualized instruction if required during periods of intense treatment. In addition, they often have school re-entry programs for children who have been out for a period of time.

It's also important to take care of yourself and one another. Siblings can be very supportive of their ill brother or sister but must know that their own special place in the family is secure.

Economic stress isn't unusual for families with a seriously ill child. Financial burdens not only include the cost of treatment but also may involve the costs of travel, lodging and child care. Incomes also may be affected by disrupted work schedules.

Many pediatric cancer centers are staffed with child life specialists, mental health professionals, social workers and clergy who are trained to help families with difficult emotions and situations. In spite of the difficulties, many families develop closer, more supportive and trusting relationships as a result.

Living With Cancer

A diagnosis of cancer can truly change your life. The disease can dominate your thoughts and actions and affect your daily routine, your relationships with others and your view of life.

But these effects don't all have to be negative. Armed with the advice of health professionals and the insights of others who have dealt with cancer, you can learn to cope with cancer's impact. Life with and after cancer not only is possible but also can be lived fully.

Survivorship care plan

As you make the transition from cancer treatment to cancer survivorship, the National Cancer Institute (NCI) recommends that you work with your health care team to develop a survivorship care plan, a blueprint that can help you navigate the ebbs and flows of post-treatment life.

In addition to helping your doctor prescribe follow-up cancer screenings and monitor for late effects of cancer treatment, you will feel reassured that the appropriate steps are being taken to monitor your health.

Survivorship plans can vary, but these are the basic elements that the NCI recommends you include in your plan:

- Your cancer type, treatments received and their potential consequences
- Specific information about the type of follow-up care you should receive and how often
- Recommendations regarding preventive practices and how to maintain health and well-being
- Information on legal protections regarding employment and access to health insurance
- The availability of psychosocial services in the community

Rehabilitation

Rehabilitation is an important component of cancer treatment. Whatever form your rehabilitation happens to take, the goal is always the same — to restore your life to as normal as possible.

This might mean developing an exercise program, learning to use a prosthesis after an amputation or even retraining for a job. Depending on your needs, you may work with a number of health care professionals, including physical therapists, occupational therapists and social workers.

Don't be discouraged if at first you find the process difficult. Progress may come slowly, and the effort may be intense. If you have problems, discuss them with your therapist, a doctor who specializes in physical rehabilitation (physiatrist) or another doctor.

Follow-up visits

Going in for checkups is one thing many people with cancer fear. Several days before each visit, you may start worrying, afraid that your doctor will find something terribly wrong. And once you get to the doctor's office, the sights, sounds and smells may bring back memories you'd prefer to forget.

This is natural. But try to balance these negative associations with positive ones. Keep in mind that the medical treatment you've received, and continue to receive, is good. It's helping you stay alive.

Before a follow-up exam, write down any questions you may have and bring them with you so that you can ask your doctor for answers and advice.

At first, these questions may include some of the following:

- Will my checkups always be the same?
- What are some signs or symptoms that the cancer has returned or progressed?
- What changes might I experience that are OK, that aren't warning signs?
- If I feel pain what should I do?
- What's the best way for me to get in touch with you if I have questions or concerns?

Emotional issues

Cancer generally produces a roller coaster of emotions. What's important is that you recognize and accept your emotions and find healthy ways to deal with them.

When you were first diagnosed, you might have experienced a variety of emotions including disbelief, fear and anger. Some of these emotions may continue after treatment. Other emotions common in cancer survivors include:

Anxiety
If you experience side effects from your treatment, such as hair loss or skin reactions, you may feel embarrassed, worry what others will think and lose your self-confidence. This can make you anxious. You might also withdraw from others and from social and business gatherings.

These feelings can be especially difficult if you've always been a self-confident, outgoing and active person.

Emptiness
If you've had surgery to remove part of your body, you may feel a void that's hard to describe.

Women often feel less feminine after a hysterectomy or surgery to remove a breast. It's not uncommon for men to feel less masculine after prostate removal.

Depression

Depression is common among people with any serious illness, including cancer. You may grow sad and discouraged over what has happened. You may be pessimistic about your future. Such feelings may last only a short time, or they may linger for weeks or months.

Depression that lingers can interfere with your ability to manage your life. It can precipitate a downward spiral that makes you more and more miserable. Because you're depressed, you don't feel motivated to cope with your daily problems. When the problems become worse, so does your depression. To find out the common warning signs of depression, see page 1124.

If you think you may be depressed, talk to your doctor or a

Cancer Coping Strategies

You may not be able to get rid of distressing feelings, but you can find positive ways to deal with them so that they don't take over your life. The following strategies can help you cope with the difficulties of cancer:

Be prepared

Ask your doctor questions and read about your specific type of cancer and its potential side effects. The fewer the surprises, the more quickly you'll adapt.

Maintain a routine

Don't let the cancer or side effects of treatment dominate your day. Try to follow at least some of the routine and lifestyle you had before learning of your cancer. Go back to work, take a trip, or visit your children or grandchildren. You need activities that give you a sense of purpose, fulfillment and meaning. But realize that initially you may have some limitations. Start slowly and gradually build up your level of endurance.

Set reasonable goals

Having goals helps you feel in control and can give you a sense of purpose. But don't choose goals you can't possibly reach. You may not be able to work a 40-hour week, for example, but you may be able to work at least part time. In fact, many people find that continuing to work can be helpful.

Get plenty of exercise

Exercise helps to fight depression and relieve tension and aggression. Recent data suggest improved outcomes and survival for people who are able to maintain an exercise program during cancer treatment.

Enjoy some humor and laughter

Find ways to help lighten your day with laughter, whether by spending time with someone who makes you laugh or watching a funny movie. Laughter helps distract your attention from your health problems. It's also a kind of analgesic — that is, it promotes the release of chemicals that help fight pain and reduce depression.

Try not to wallow in sad feelings

Seek diversions and plan at least two or three enjoyable experiences a week. These might include a new hobby, playing golf or going to a movie. Make it something you enjoy and look forward to.

Take time for yourself

Eating well, relaxing and getting enough rest can help combat the stress and fatigue of cancer. Plan ahead for the downtimes, when you may need to rest more or limit what you do.

Look for ways to compensate

If you have trouble eating, for example, reserve mealtimes for when you're at home and plan outings that don't revolve around food. If you frequently need to use the bathroom, sit in the back of the movie theater or the meeting room so that you'll feel less conspicuous if you need to leave.

Open up to a friend, family member or counselor

Sometimes it helps to talk with someone about your feelings and fears. Your mind and body aren't separate. The better you feel emotionally, the better able you are to physically cope with your illness.

Don't avoid sexual contact

People with cancer sometimes feel as if they're no longer adequate as sexual beings. Don't fall for this feeling. You can express your sexuality in many ways. Touching, holding, hugging and caressing may become far more important to you and your partner. In fact, the closeness you develop through these actions can produce greater sexual intimacy than you've ever had before.

Look for the positive

Cancer doesn't have to be all negative. Good can come out of it. Confrontation with cancer may lead you to grow emotionally and spiritually, to identify what really matters to you, to settle long-standing disputes, and to spend more time with people who are important to you.

therapist. With treatment, which may involve counseling or taking antidepressant medications or both, the majority of people affected by depression show significant signs of improvement.

Regaining your strength

Fatigue is a common side effect of cancer and treatment. Your body is dealing with a number of physical challenges, and the effort involved in coping with them is often exhausting and stressful. Fatigue can be a frustrating obstacle when you're struggling to keep a normal schedule and maintain a good quality of life.

To help reduce fatigue, consider taking the following steps:

Tell your doctor
Don't hide or ignore your fatigue. Tell your doctor about it because it may have a treatable physical cause, such as anemia.

Rest
Don't fight fatigue. If you find that you need to take short naps during the day, take them.

Go easy on yourself
Take one day at a time and try not to overdo it. But don't sit back and do nothing, either. Inactivity also produces fatigue.

Delegate
You may need to ask others to do tasks that traditionally you've done, such as cutting the grass or shoveling snow.

Practice relaxation techniques
Wrestling with heavy emotions, such as anxiety and fear, can contribute to your fatigue. Talk with your doctor, nurse or counselor about stress-reduction techniques and which ones might work best for you.

Try to get a good night's sleep
Establishing a nightly relaxation routine, such as reading a book or taking a warm bath, may make it easier to fall asleep. Avoiding caffeine, getting some exercise during the day and keeping your bedroom at a comfortable temperature also can be helpful sleep inducers.

Exercise
One of the most helpful ways to fight cancer-related fatigue is to get regular exercise. Research hasn't found any harmful effects from moderate exercise among people with cancer. In fact, studies show that people with cancer who exercise experience less fatigue than those who don't exercise.

It's best to start slowly and build gradually. Depending on your fitness and comfort level, you may want to start with a 10-minute walk around the block. Or you many find that you can exercise for 20 minutes (or longer) right away.

Your goal should be at least 30 minutes of aerobic activity five days a week or more. Be careful not to overdo it. If you try to do too much too quickly, you may become discouraged and stop exercising altogether. On the other hand, if you were a regular at the gym before you developed cancer, you may have to lower the intensity of your workouts for a while.

Eating better to feel better

A nutritious diet provides the fuel that lets your body maintain its strength and operate at its best. That's why a nutritious diet is especially important if you have cancer. If you don't eat enough food or the right kinds of food, your body resorts to using stored nutrients. This weakens your natural defenses against infection, a major threat for people with cancer. In addition, the better you eat, the more able you may be to handle treatment, such as radiation therapy, which in turn improves the chances of destroying your cancer.

When you have cancer, what you should eat and how often you should eat may be different from when you're healthy. Normally, nutrition recommendations stress eating plenty of fruits, vegetables and grains and cutting back on fat, sugar and salt. But if you're having difficulty maintaining your weight because of your cancer or your cancer treatment, proper nutrition involves eating more high-calorie foods to promote strength and energy and eating more foods that are high in protein. Protein helps repair body tissues.

The following steps can help add more calories and protein to your diet:

- **Emphasize dairy products.** Foods such as milk, cream and cheese are good sources of calories and protein.
- **Eat plenty of peanut butter.** Spread it on toast, fruit slices, crackers or celery. Peanut butter is high in calories and protein.
- **Choose breaded or fried meat.** Beef, poultry and fish prepared this way contain more calories. Meat is also a good source of protein.
- **Add high-calorie toppings.** Top your hot cereal with brown sugar, honey or cream. Top your pie, cake, pudding and gelatin with ice cream or whipping cream. Top fruit with sugar or cream.
- **Drink high-calorie beverages.** Good choices include milk, fruit juice, lemonade, fruit-flavored drinks, malts, floats, soft drinks, cocoa and eggnog. Water, black coffee and tea have no calories.
- **Stock up on nutritional drinks.** These products, available as a liquid or powder, are sold under brand names such as Ensure, Boost and Carnation Breakfast Essentials. The drinks are high in both calories and protein, and they contain extra vitamins and minerals.

If you don't feel like eating, nutritional drinks can be used as snacks or as meal substitutes. Some people find nutritional products difficult to drink because they don't care for the flavor or texture. If this is true for you, you may want to try this recipe: Combine one can of a liquid drink with a piece of fruit or scoop of ice cream or both. Blend the mixture in a blender and serve it over ice.

Stimulating your appetite

A loss of appetite is common when you're ill or recovering from an illness. The nausea, vomiting, depression and fatigue that often accompany cancer can make food unappealing.

Try the following suggestions to improve your diet and stimulate your appetite:

- **Eat whenever you're hungry.** If your appetite and taste buds seem in disarray, eating smaller meals throughout the day may work better for you than trying to eat three big meals. Taking just a few bites of healthy foods or a few sips of a nutritious drink every hour or so also can help a lot.
- **Prepare and freeze meals ahead of time.** This way you won't have to cook when you don't feel like it.
- **Choose foods that look and smell good.** Cancer treatment can alter your sense of taste and smell. If red meat is unappetizing, try other sources of protein: chicken, fish or dairy products. Most people with cancer find that soups and soft foods, such as pasta or mashed potatoes, are the easiest to eat and digest. If your favorite foods suddenly don't look appetizing anymore, don't force yourself to eat them.
- **Enhance the flavor.** Food may taste bland to you. Try small amounts of seasoning or marinate meat and vegetables.
- **Drink less with meals.** Although you should aim to drink 6 to 8 cups of fluids daily, limit beverages at mealtimes because they can make you feel full and keep you from eating adequate amounts of food. Drink beverages after your meals.
- **Change the atmosphere.** Eating in a different setting may stimulate your appetite. Invite a friend to join you, play music, light some candles, or watch a video or TV program.

If you're still having trouble eating a few weeks after your treatment, contact your doctor. He or she may want you to talk with a registered dietitian. Some dietitians specialize in assisting people with cancer and can help devise a customized eating plan that meets your individual needs.

Getting back to work

Work is an important part of life, providing personal fulfillment, income or enjoyment. If you have cancer, work can also be rehabilitative and uplifting, especially if you're treated as a valuable team member. Many people with cancer find getting back to work helps them regain a sense of normalcy and control over their lives.

If you're an employee, having cancer doesn't mean that your career is ruined or that you'll never again pull your weight at work. In fact, 8 of 10 employees with cancer return to their jobs. And surveys show that employees who have had cancer are just as productive

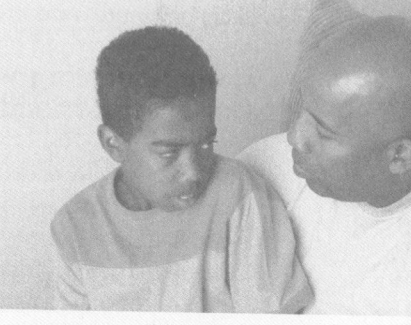

Telling Your Children You Have Cancer

If you've received a diagnosis of cancer and have children, the prospect of telling them about your cancer can be overwhelming. It helps to come to grips with the diagnosis yourself before communicating it to them. But at some point, your children must be told. Remember, too, that children, particularly younger children, don't understand cancer in the same way that adults do, so often they don't experience the shock, anxiety or fear that parents expect them to. Here are some suggestions as to how you might explain your cancer:

- Be honest about your diagnosis, what you're going through, and what your children can expect at various stages of your disease and treatment.
- Encourage your children to ask questions, share their feelings, and help out around the home or with your care.
- Reassure your children that nothing they did or thought caused your cancer, that it's not contagious, and that they'll continue to be loved and cared for no matter what happens to you.
- Enable your children to carry on as normal a schedule as possible — and assure them that it's OK to do so.
- Alert your children's teachers, counselors and child care providers of your situation.
- If you need it, ask for help from doctors, nurses, social workers, counselors, support groups, psychologists and psychiatrists.
- Continue to discipline your children as you normally would.
- Give answers that are truthful yet hopeful. Children can sense when something is wrong and might imagine the worst.
- Don't put too much responsibility on your children. It's reasonable for them to help, but they shouldn't become adults in the home.
- If possible, avoid sending your children away to a friend or relative. Being sent away can cause feelings of abandonment.

as other workers, and no more likely to take sick days.

At first, you may need to make a few adjustments, such as working fewer hours. But eventually you should be able to resume your regular schedule and activities. Before you return to work:

- Talk with your doctor about how much you should work. It's often best to ease back into your work schedule.
- Talk with your supervisor about adjusting your hours or duties when you first return.
- Consider how you'll respond to co-workers who may have questions about your cancer and how you're doing. Practicing what you're going to say ahead of time can make the interchange more comfortable.

Communicating with family and friends

Cancer has a way of stifling communication when you need it the most. Family members may find it difficult to come to grips with your illness, so they aren't able to talk with you about important issues. And well-meaning friends — not knowing what to say or do, and not wanting to upset you — may steer clear of conversations about your health.

Here are some ways you can make it easier for family and friends to give you needed support:

Give it time
You may want to talk about important issues related to your illness before some of your family and friends are ready. Interpret their body language, such as whether they make eye contact. If they aren't ready to talk, give them a little more time to adjust.

In the same way, if some of your loved ones are ready to talk before you are, acknowledge their feelings but say that you're not ready to talk yet.

Not all families are open and sharing. Sometimes it's easier to open up to someone outside your immediate circle of family and friends, such as a counselor or someone else who has experienced cancer.

Reach out to family and friends
Reach out to the people you care about. You may think it should be the other way around. And with some of your closest family and friends, it will be. They'll come to you. But try to remember people you knew who were ill and how difficult it was for you to think of what to say or do to help them.

Think of ways to put family and friends at ease. Ask a busy friend what projects he or she has going. Invite a friend who's not a great talker to help you with a chore, such as cleaning out the garage. For friends who have plenty of their own problems, ask how things are going.

Accept help
Don't be afraid to ask for help either. Many times your family and friends are waiting for clues as to how they can help. When they say,

"Let me know how I can help," respond positively to the offer. Give some suggestions as to what they can do. Most family and friends are grateful to have a chance to show you, in tangible ways, that they care.

Joining a support group

Not everyone with cancer needs a support group. Having family and friends may be all of the support that you need. But some people find it helpful to have people they can turn to outside of their immediate circles.

In general, support groups fall into two main categories: those led by health care professionals, such as a psychologist or nurse, and those led by group members. Some are more educational and structured and may include discussions on new treatments. Others emphasize emotional support and shared experiences.

In addition, the internet offers online virtual support groups in which you can communicate with others by way of chat groups. But be careful about the reliability of information about therapy or treatment that you may find online. Talk with your doctor to make sure it's accurate and, more importantly, not harmful.

If you think that you would like to join a support group, check with a member of your health care team or community health services. A variety of volunteer support groups exist that can help you during this transition in your life.

Hospice Care

The word *hospice* comes from the Latin word for "guest." It's the root that forms the words *hospital*, *hospitality* and *hostel*.

In the Middle Ages, a hospice was a way station for travelers. Today *hospice* has another meaning. Hospice offers a coordinated, interdisciplinary program of care and services for people who are terminally ill and their families. The program may be in a medical center, a person's home or in a separate facility dedicated to hospice care.

Hospice care neither hastens nor postpones death. Rather, hospice programs emphasize quality of life, with the focus on the management of side effects and psychosocial counseling instead of on treatment of the disease.

The goals of hospice programs are to allow people to adequately prepare for death and to live their last days in as much comfort as possible.

For more information on hospice care, see page 348.

Preventing Cancer

Scientists and doctors don't understand many of the reasons why people develop cancer, but there's still a lot that you can do to help decrease your risk of getting it. Smoking causes just under 30 percent of cancer deaths. Evidence suggests that another third of cancer deaths may be due to dietary factors. Obesity also plays a role in cancer development.

If Americans applied to their daily lives everything that's known about cancer prevention, cancer rates might be reduced significantly.

Cancer prevention can take the form of a few key decisions in your everyday life. No matter what your age, it's never too late to set a course that could help you avoid cancer down the road. Here are some strategies to get you started on a healthier lifestyle.

Tobacco

If you smoke, you likely find it to be an enjoyable habit. Perhaps you smoke to calm your nerves or to curb your appetite. People smoke for a number of reasons. Combine that with the addictive nature of nicotine, and the prospect of quitting becomes fairly unappealing and often difficult.

But there's no two ways around it. Not using tobacco, or deciding to stop using it — whether it's cigarettes, chewing tobacco, pipes or cigars — is one of the most important health decisions you can make.

You may have heard it a hundred times, but it's true. Tobacco use can be fatal. If you smoke cigarettes, you're inhaling air that contains more than 40 substances that can cause cells to become cancerous (carcinogens). Tar in cigarette smoke also forms a sticky brown layer on the lining of your lungs and air passageways. This layer traps the carcinogens you inhale when you smoke, enhancing cancer development.

Smoking is responsible for the vast majority of lung cancer cases. It also increases your risk of cancer of the esophagus, larynx, mouth, bladder and kidneys. In addition, tobacco use is linked to emphysema, bronchitis, cardiovascular disease and stroke. Chewing (spit) tobacco isn't harmless, either. Evidence suggests chewing tobacco increases your risk of oral cancer.

Diet

Your diet is another important risk factor for cancer. Although

Quitters Do Win

Tobacco users who quit, regardless of their age, live longer than do those who continue to use tobacco. By quitting, you can reduce your chances of getting lung cancer by more than half, as well as reduce your risk of other types of cancers and diseases.

A number of aids are available to help you break nicotine's grip. They include the following products and medications:

Nicotine patch
Now available over-the-counter, the nicotine patch is placed on your skin, where it gradually releases nicotine into your body. This helps battle nicotine addiction by reducing nicotine cravings when you cut back or stop smoking. Eventually you taper off using the patch.

Nicotine gum and lozenges
When you chew the gum, it releases nicotine into your body. The lining of your mouth absorbs the nicotine. After you get the initial burst of effect from the nicotine, you can "park" the gum alongside your cheek until you have another nicotine craving. Nicotine lozenges are tablets that contain a small amount of nicotine. You place a lozenge between your gumline and cheek and suck it slowly, allowing it to dissolve. These products are often used in combination with other quit-smoking products.

Nicotine inhaler
The nicotine inhaler, available by prescription, is a device that gives you a small dose of nicotine. When you puff on the inhaler, nicotine vapor is released from a cartridge inside the device. The nicotine enters your bloodstream as it's absorbed through the lining of your mouth and throat.

Nicotine nasal spray
Your nose is another way to get nicotine into your body. A nicotine nasal spray, available by prescription, is absorbed by the lining of your nose.

Non-nicotine medication
Bupropion (Zyban) is an antidepressant medication that's been proved to help people combat nicotine addiction. Unlike nicotine replacement therapy, bupropion doesn't contain nicotine. It's thought to decrease tobacco cravings and withdrawal symptoms by increasing the levels of certain brain chemicals.

Varenicline (Chantix) is a prescription medication that can help reduce cravings for tobacco and control nicotine withdrawal symptoms. It also blocks nicotine receptors in your brain, which decreases the pleasurable effects of smoking.

It can take several days for both medications to reach effective levels in your blood. People often start the medication just before they quit smoking.

Reducing Your Risks

Here's how your health improves after stopping smoking:

Immediately	The air around you is no longer dangerous to children and other adults.
20 minutes	Your blood pressure drops to normal.
	Your pulse rate drops to normal.
	The temperature in your hands and feet increases to normal.
8 hours	The carbon monoxide level in your blood drops to normal.
	The oxygen level in your blood increases to normal.
24 hours	Your chance of having a heart attack decreases.
48 hours	Your senses of smell and taste improve.
2 to 12 weeks	Your circulation improves.
	Your breathing improves.
	Walking becomes easier.
1 to 9 months	Your coughing and sinus congestion decrease.
	Your shortness of breath decreases.
	Your overall energy increases.
	The ability of your lungs to self-clean and reduce infection increases.
1 year	For men, the risk of premature heart disease is half that of a male smoker.
5 years	Your risk of stroke is comparable to that of a nonsmoker.
10 years	Your life expectancy is comparable to that of a nonsmoker.
	Your risk of dying of lung cancer is about half that of a smoker.
	Your risk of cancers of the mouth, throat, esophagus, bladder, kidney and pancreas decreases.
15 years	All other factors being equal, your risk of heart disease is comparable to that of a nonsmoker.
Before age 50	Your risk of dying in the next 15 years has decreased by 50 percent compared with that of people who continue to smoke after age 50.

making healthy food selections can't guarantee you won't get cancer, it can help reduce your risk. The American Cancer Society recommends the following dietary guidelines:

Eat plant-based foods

Whether it's cauliflower or cranberries, eating more fruits and vegetables may play a role in preventing a variety of cancers. The same is true of foods made from whole grains, such as breads and cereals.

Plant foods contain more than 100 vitamins, minerals, fibers and other beneficial substances. Fruits, vegetables and whole grains are excellent sources of fiber, which may help reduce your risk of colorectal cancer. Green and dark yellow vegetables, soybean products, and vegetables such as broccoli and cauliflower may play a role in reducing your risk of cancer of the colon, rectum and stomach.

Most Americans eat far fewer plant-based foods than they should. To stay healthy and help reduce your risk of cancer, try to eat at least four servings of vegetables and three servings

PREVENTION TIP

There are no miracle foods for cancer prevention. Eat as if your diet were an investment. Just as you would diversify your portfolio, diversify your diet. Eating a variety of foods provides a variety of nutrients that promote health.

? Question and Answer

Can eating more soy foods reduce my risk of cancer?

Some studies suggest that substances in soy may cause changes at the cellular level that hinder cancer cell development and growth. In addition, some kinds of cancer occur far less often in cultures where soy is a food staple, such as many of those in Asia. Although soy hasn't been proved to help prevent cancer, it's an excellent source of protein and a good alternative to meat in your diet.

of fruit daily. And when eating carbohydrates, choose whole-grain products instead of those made from processed (refined) grains.

Limit high-fat foods

Studies suggest that people with high-fat diets that include a lot of high-fat meats are at increased risk of cancer of the prostate, colon, rectum, uterus and breast.

Try to reduce the percentage of fat in your diet to less than 30 percent of the calories you consume each day. Eat foods with little or no saturated fat and avoid trans fats. Monounsaturated and polyunsaturated fats found in nuts, avocados and olive and vegetable oils are the healthiest.

Physical activity

Regular physical activity plays a key role in helping you stay healthy and control your weight. When you're at a healthy weight, you lower your risk of many kinds of cancer.

But despite the benefits of exercise, many people avoid it. The majority of older adults — the age group with the highest risk of cancer — are inactive.

One reason may be that many people believe that exercise must be strenuous, even painful, to be beneficial. The truth is, the frequency and duration of physical activity are more important than the activity's intensity.

Experts recommend that you get 30 to 60 minutes of physical activity most days of the week. That may sound daunting, but those 30 minutes can include activities such as a brisk walk, raking the yard and dancing. And you can perform the activities in 10-minute segments.

Obesity

Studies suggest that obesity is a risk factor for a number of cancers, including cancers of the endometrium, colon and rectum, uterus,

pancreas, kidney, and in post-menopausal women, breast.

The links between body weight and cancer are complex and aren't fully understood. Excess weight may affect cancer risk through a number of mechanisms. Obesity may influence your immune system function and the development of inflammation. It may affect the levels of certain hormones, such as insulin and estrogen. It may modify substances that regulate cell growth.

Maintaining a healthy weight can reduce your risk of several cancers. The best way to lose weight is with regular physical activity and a healthy diet.

Alcohol

Your risk of cancer increases with the amount of alcohol you consume and the length of time you've been consuming alcohol on a regular basis. Even a moderate amount of alcohol — one drink a day for women and men over age 65 and two drinks a day for all other men — may increase your cancer risk.

This is particularly true if you smoke. Using both alcohol and tobacco significantly increases your risk of cancer of the mouth, esophagus and larynx.

Skin protection

Skin cancer is one of the most common forms of cancer, and one of the most preventable. Although repeated exposure to X-rays or contact with certain chemicals can play a role in this disease, sun exposure is by far the most common cause of skin cancer. Approximately 90 percent of skin cancer occurs on parts of the body that usually aren't covered with clothing — your face, hands, forearms and ears.

Cancer signals

Knowing your risk of cancer and being aware of changes in your body can help you prevent cancer or help your doctor detect it early, increasing your chances of a full recovery.

One way to assess your cancer risk is to find out if your family has a history of cancer. If so, find out what type of cancer and at what age the person with cancer received a diagnosis. In general, the more frequent and earlier that cancer occurs in your relatives, the more likely you're at risk. But just because someone in your family had cancer doesn't mean you'll get it. Remember, only 5 to 10 percent of cancer cases run in families.

While doing your research, if you see a pattern of cancer that occurred at an early age, you may wish to schedule a visit with your doctor. He or she can help you decide your next step, which may include seeing a medical geneticist. Genetic testing can help determine if you may have inherited an increased risk of some types of cancer. For more information on genetic testing, see Chapter 14, "Genetics and Disease."

You also need to stay alert to changes in your body that could signal cancer. If you notice warning signs, talk to your doctor. While it's important to know some of the general signs and symptoms of cancer, keep in mind that having any of these doesn't mean that you have cancer. Many other conditions cause similar signs and symptoms.

If you have any of the following and they persist or get worse, see a doctor:

- Unexplained weight loss
- Unexplained fever
- Fatigue
- Unexplained pain
- A recent change in a wart or mole or any new skin change
- Thickening or a lump in a breast or elsewhere in your body
- Changes in bowel habits or bladder function
- A sore that doesn't heal
- White patches inside your mouth or white spots on your tongue
- Unusual bleeding or discharge
- Indigestion or difficulty swallowing
- A nagging cough or hoarseness

Other symptoms

The signs and symptoms listed above are the more common ones seen with cancer, but there are many others. If you notice any major changes in the way your body works or the way you feel —especially if it lasts for a long time or it gets worse — let a doctor know. If it has nothing to do with cancer, your doctor can determine the cause and, if needed, treat it. If it is cancer, you'll give yourself the chance to have it treated early, when treatment works best.

Regular checkups

You and your doctor should discuss which cancer screening tests are best for you, based on your age, occupation, lifestyle, family history and personal preferences.

Between doctor visits, examine yourself at home for changes that may signal some kinds of cancer, including cancers of the breast, skin and testicles. If you aren't familiar with when and how to do such self-exams, ask your doctor during your next visit. If you already perform self-exams, your doctor can help you determine if you're doing them correctly. ■

Infectious Diseases

Understanding Your Immune System

Keeping infectious micro-organisms out of your body and destroying any that get in are the missions of your immune system.

Not that long ago, scientists had only fragments of information about how the variety of cells that make up your immune system interact to help protect you against disease. But through research advances, scientists now believe that more than 100 million types of immune cells exist. For each virus or bacterium, there seems to be an immune cell that's specifically designed to hunt it down and destroy it.

However, viruses and bacteria are cunning adversaries, constantly seeking new ways to breach your immune system's defenses. In addition, some antibiotics long used to treat infections are becoming less effective.

Your immune system is a complex array of organs, cells and molecules distributed throughout your body. Each part of the system contributes to the growth or action of lymphocytes, sophisticated white blood cells that play a major role in your body's immune response.

White blood cells originate in bone marrow. Some then migrate to your thymus gland, where they develop into specialized types of immune cells. Some of these cells from bone marrow and the thymus gather in lymph nodes and other organs involved in immunity, including your spleen, tonsils, adenoids, appendix and small intestine. Other white blood cells circulate throughout your blood and lymphatic vessels. Lymphatic vessels transport lymph, a colorless fluid that can carry microorganisms and dead cells from distant infections into lymph nodes, where they're eliminated. Lymph vessels also transport white blood cells to sites of infection.

Immune army 'soldier' cells

The key to your immune response is a remarkable arsenal of white blood cells. The main "soldiers" include macrophages, lymphocytes, neutrophils and phagocytes.

Macrophages
Macrophages are "scavenger" white blood cells located within tissues. Their role is to engulf and digest worn-out cells and other debris and foreign invaders (anti-

Your Immune Armament

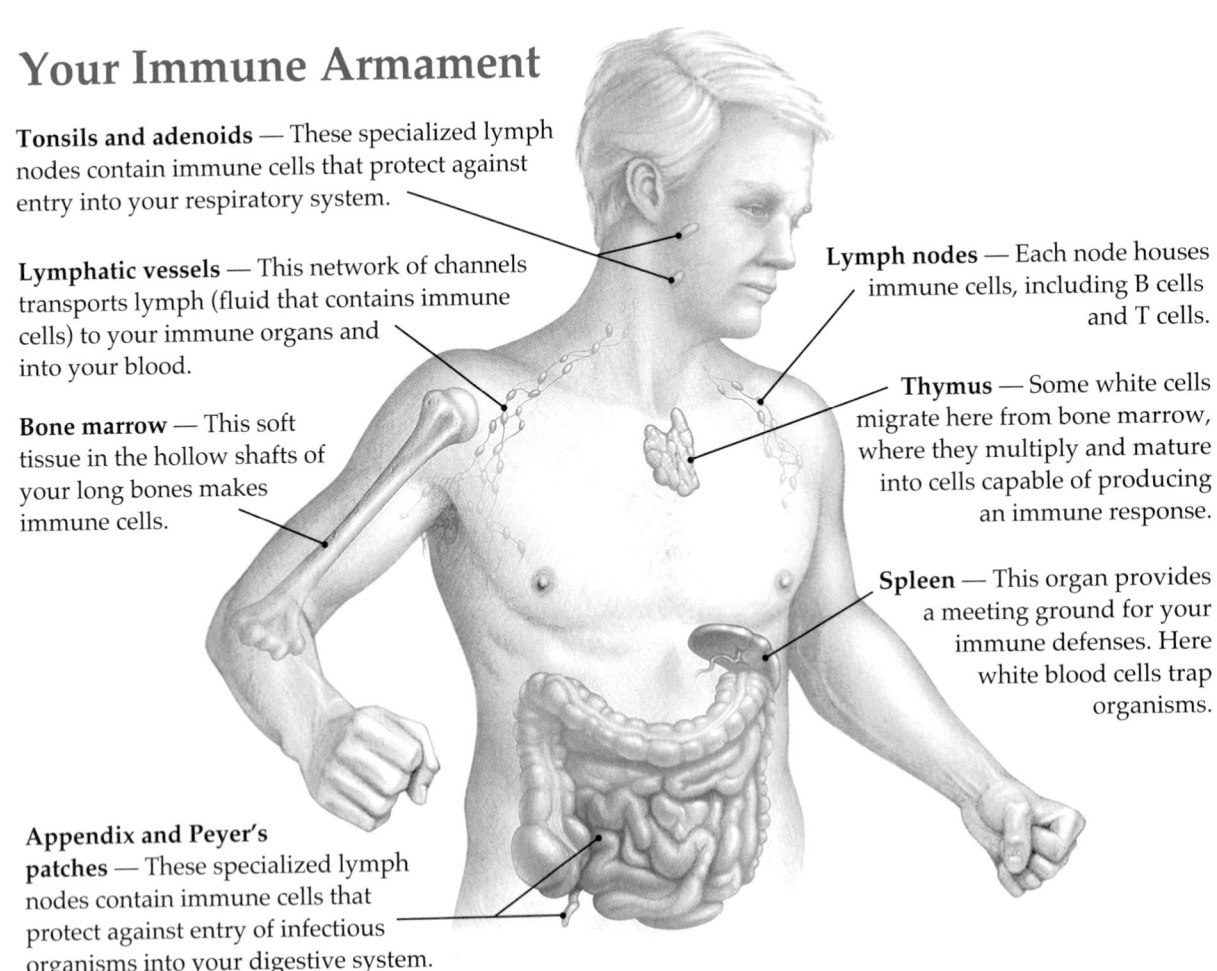

Tonsils and adenoids — These specialized lymph nodes contain immune cells that protect against entry into your respiratory system.

Lymphatic vessels — This network of channels transports lymph (fluid that contains immune cells) to your immune organs and into your blood.

Bone marrow — This soft tissue in the hollow shafts of your long bones makes immune cells.

Appendix and Peyer's patches — These specialized lymph nodes contain immune cells that protect against entry of infectious organisms into your digestive system.

Lymph nodes — Each node houses immune cells, including B cells and T cells.

Thymus — Some white cells migrate here from bone marrow, where they multiply and mature into cells capable of producing an immune response.

Spleen — This organ provides a meeting ground for your immune defenses. Here white blood cells trap organisms.

gens), such as germs. Macrophages also stimulate other immune cells to respond to the invaders.

Lymphocytes

Lymphocytes include white blood cells known as natural killer cells and T cells and B cells. Natural killer cells help defend host cells against tumors and virally infected cells. B cells work chiefly by producing antibodies, substances that attach themselves to and destroy antigens. Each antibody is designed to attack a specific antigen. T cells coordinate immune defenses and seek out organisms in cells. They may secrete potent chemicals, which are particularly good at attacking cancerous cells or cells infected by viruses.

Neutrophils

Some white blood cells are chemical killers called neutrophils, eosinophils and basophils. These cells also ingest unwanted microorganisms and release powerful chemicals that help destroy such microorganisms.

Phagocytes

Phagocytes are another type of white blood cell. The main function of these "eater" cells is to gobble up anything unwanted, from a speck of dust or pollen to a virus. The macrophage is a specific type of phagocyte that helps carry out the immune response.

Lines of defense

As foreign invaders attempt to invade your body, they're confronted by increasingly sophisticated layers of protective defenses.

Physical barriers

Your skin effectively shields your body from invaders, whether they're harmful or not. Your respiratory system also helps keep out microorganisms. Defenses include trapping irritants in nasal hairs and mucus, carrying the mucus upward and outward on tiny hair-like projections lining the respiratory tract (cilia), and coughing and sneezing.

Your skin and the mucous membranes lining your respiratory and gastrointestinal tracts also contain macrophages and antibodies. Fluids such as saliva, sweat and tears contain destructive enzymes. Stomach acids also play a role, killing most microorganisms ingested in food or water.

General defenses

Invaders that slip through physical barriers are met by scavenger cells circulating in your blood and lymphatic vessels. One general defense mechanism is the inflammatory response. It halts disease-causing microorganisms early in their invasion and confines them to a localized area. Immune cells cause small blood vessels near the invasion site to widen (dilate), causing redness and warmth. Swelling occurs when blood vessels leak fluid into surrounding tissue. Nearby lymph nodes then trap the microorganisms and trigger production of more immune cells that kill the organisms and limit the infection.

Complement defenses

Complement defenses involve a complex series of circulating proteins that complement the work of antibodies. When a complement protein comes in contact with an invading organism, each component of the complement system is activated. The result is a protein complex that attaches to the organism's surface and destroys it by puncturing its cell membrane.

Antibody defenses

Unwanted microorganisms that pass through the front-line defenses confront even more sophisticated defenses. When a T cell identifies and presents an antigen, B cells produce antibodies that attach themselves to the antigen, neutralizing it or rendering it harmless. Antibodies are specific: Each is effective against only the antigen that led to its creation.

Cellular defenses

T cells concentrate on trickier assignments, such as finding microorganisms hidden within cells. For help in finding the foe, macrophages act as undercover agents, moving among cells, checking for foreign substances.

Building resistance

When you're born, your immune system is relatively weak; however, you possess many of the benefits of your mother's immunity. Your immune system becomes stronger as you mature and are exposed to infectious agents and receive vaccinations. This is known as post-exposure immunity.

Each time you're exposed to a foreign invader, your immune system creates T and B memory cells specific to the invading organism. After you recover, your immune system stores a few of the memory cells. The next time you come into contact with that same type of organism, the memory cells rapidly multiply to stop the infection.

Vaccines work in a similar manner. When you're vaccinated, a killed portion of a weakened virus or bacterium is injected into your body. Although the injected organism isn't strong enough to make you sick, it still stimulates an immune response. Memory cells are formed, providing immunity against the disease for years or even a lifetime.

The Enemy

Substances that can invade your body live everywhere — in the air, on food and plants, on and in animals, in the soil and water, and on virtually every other surface. They range from microscopic organisms to larger parasites. The vast majority of these organisms don't produce disease because they're kept under control by your immune system. But if that system becomes weakened or you encounter an organism to which you haven't built up resistance, illness can result. Many types of organisms cause infectious disease.

Bacteria

Bacteria are single-cell organisms that are visible only under a microscope. They appear as short rods (bacilli) or round cells (cocci), are self-sufficient and multiply by subdivision.

When infectious bacteria gain entry to your body, they increase in number and potentially produce powerful chemicals, called toxins, that damage specific cells

Infectious Agents

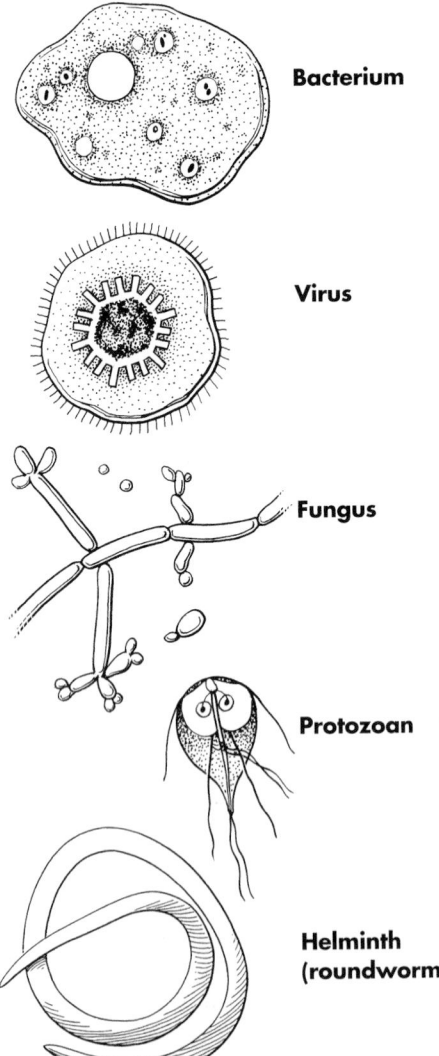

Bacterium

Virus

Fungus

Protozoan

Helminth (roundworm)

in the tissue they've invaded, causing you to become ill.

A few of the more-common groups of disease-causing bacteria include staphylococcus, escherichia (the principal species of which is the well-known *E. coli*), streptococcus, chlamydia, haemophilus, gonococcus and rickettsia.

Not all bacteria are harmful. Some bacteria that reside in the body — such as those in the mouth and intestinal tract — are actually of benefit.

Viruses

In its simplest form, a virus is a capsule that contains genetic material. But it isn't able to reproduce on its own. When a virus invades your body, it enters some of your cells and takes them over by instructing the host cells to manufacture the parts it needs to multiply. In the process, the host cells are eventually destroyed. Polio, AIDS and the common cold are viral illnesses.

Fungi

Molds, yeasts and mushrooms all are types of fungi. Obviously, mushrooms aren't infectious, but certain yeasts and molds can be. These single-cell organisms are slightly larger than bacteria. Candida is one example of a yeast that causes infection. It can produce thrush — an infection of the mouth and throat — in infants, in people taking antibiotics and in people with impaired immunity. It's also responsible for most types of infection-induced diaper rash.

Protozoans

Protozoans are single-cell organisms that can live within you as a parasite. Many protozoans reside in the intestinal tract and are harmless. Others may cause disease. Often, these organisms spend part of their life cycle outside of humans or other hosts, living in food, soil, water or insects. The

diseases malaria and giardiasis are caused by protozoan parasites.

Helminths

Helminths are among the larger parasites. The word *helminth* comes from the Greek word for "worm." If this parasite or its eggs enter your body, they take up residence in your intestinal tract, lungs, liver, skin or brain, where they live off the nutrients in your body. The most common helminths are tapeworms and roundworms.

Treating Infections

Medication can fight many of the infections that your immune system may not be equipped to handle. Most bacterial infections can be treated with antibiotics, substances produced by microorganisms that destroy other bacteria. Some antibiotics are produced from synthetic antibacterial agents.

Unfortunately, antibiotics have no effect on viruses. A few medications have been developed that help control viral infections, but these drugs usually don't cure the infections. However, the development of vaccines that can prevent certain viral infections has led to the eradication of a number of deadly diseases, including smallpox and polio. Some vaccines are also effective against bacterial infections, such as tetanus and diphtheria.

Parasitic infestations caused by protozoans and helminths often can be successfully treated with appropriate medications. Antifungal medications exist to treat infections such as athlete's foot, jock itch and ringworm.

Antibiotics

Before penicillin was discovered, very few medications were available to combat bacterial infections.

Antibiotic Resistance

When bacteria are exposed to an antibiotic, they can develop a resistance or tolerance to that antibiotic. This may happen quickly or slowly.

Because of this, some antibiotics have become less useful today than they were in the past. Newer antibiotics are constantly being developed. However, it's likely that they too will become less effective in future years.

To help prevent antibiotic resistance, it's important to take antibiotics only when they're needed. If you take an antibiotic unnecessarily — such as for the common cold, which is caused by a virus and not bacteria — you increase your chances of developing drug-resistant bacteria. Such resistance makes future treatment more difficult.

Now antibiotics are common, and new antibiotic medications are continuously being developed.

Specificity

Each antibiotic works against specific types of bacteria. Some destroy only one or two kinds of bacteria. Others affect many. When your doctor suspects that you have an infectious disease, he or she may take samples of your blood, pus, urine, stool or sputum to grow (culture) the offending organism in a laboratory. This is done to identify the organism and determine how resistant or susceptible that particular strain is to antibiotics. It usually takes at least 24 hours to get the results of these tests. Therefore, depending on the diagnosis, your doctor may first prescribe an antibiotic that attacks a broad array of bacteria (a broad-spectrum antibiotic) and then, depending on the test results, change your prescription to a more specific antibiotic.

Topical vs. oral

For certain localized infections, such as of the eye or skin, antibiotics may be applied on the surface (topically) as a solution or ointment. In most cases, though, antibiotics are taken orally or administered intravenously or as an injection into muscle. Antibiotics are given intravenously or intramuscularly if the infection is serious or if the drug isn't properly absorbed when taken orally.

Types

Once absorbed into your bloodstream, the antibiotic circulates rapidly throughout your whole body. It takes only about a minute for your heart to circulate all of the blood in your body. However, the antibiotic acts only where it encounters particular bacteria. Depending on the type of antibiotic and the dosage, the medication works either by killing the bacteria or preventing it from multiplying.

Antibiotics such as penicillins and cephalosporins kill bacteria by interfering with their ability to form cell walls. This ultimately causes their death. Most other antibacterial agents, including tetracyclines, sulfonamides, aminoglycosides (gentamicin, streptomycin) and macrolides (erythromycin), interfere with the proteins and chemicals the bacteria need to multiply and survive. This allows your body's immune system to take control of and eliminate the bacteria.

Common Infectious Diseases

A wide range of diseases can challenge your immune system. Some seem to occur rather frequently, others once in a lifetime, if at all.

In the following pages, we discuss several of the most common infectious diseases. Some are also discussed in other chapters, especially those that affect predominantly only one organ or body system. The following list shows you where to find more information on such diseases:

- Gastrointestinal infections, see page 834.
- Heart infections, see pages 746-752.
- Respiratory infections, see page 763.
- Skin infections, see page 1092.
- Urinary tract infections, see page 909.

Colds

Signs and symptoms

- A runny or stuffy nose
- Itchy or sore throat
- Cough
- Congestion
- Mild headache or body aches
- Sneezing
- Watery eyes
- Low-grade fever
- Mild fatigue

Everyone experiences a cold now and then. Colds are most common during childhood. Children usually experience their first cold during their first year of life and are especially susceptible to them until about age 6, when their immunity seems to be established. Adults tend to be less vulnerable to colds, but statistics suggest that on average each person gets three or four colds a year.

The common cold is a viral infection of your upper respiratory tract. Because more than 200 different viruses cause a common cold, symptoms can vary greatly. These viruses include the rhinoviruses, those most often associated with the common cold, which primarily affect the nose and throat.

A cold virus usually enters your body through your mouth. The virus can spread through droplets in the air when someone who is sick coughs, sneezes or talks. But it also spreads by hand-to-hand contact by someone who has a cold or by using shared objects, such as towels, utensils, toys or telephones. Touch your eyes, nose or mouth after such contact or exposure and you're likely to "catch" a cold.

Myths and popular wisdom about catching colds abound: If you get wet in a rainstorm or go out with wet hair, you'll surely catch one. If you're exposed to cold air, you'll come down with a cold. Fatigue and lack of sleep can cause colds. But none of these has been proved in clinical studies to increase your risk of getting a cold.

Colds, though, do have a seasonal pattern. More people have colds during fall, winter and spring than during summer.

Diagnosis

Signs and symptoms of a cold include a runny nose, nasal and head congestion, coughing, sneezing, hoarseness, and watery eyes.

Symptoms usually develop within a day or two after exposure and may be signaled at first by an itching or sore throat, increasing nasal congestion, and mild body aches or a headache. A watery, runny nose is often the first major sign. After a while the discharge becomes thick and turns yellowish green.

An otherwise healthy person has no need to see a doctor for a cold. However, if it lasts more than two weeks, see your doctor to make sure that a secondary bacterial infection of the lungs, larynx, trachea, sinuses or ear hasn't set in. If you have a history of any such infections, consult your doctor without delay.

How serious is a cold?

Colds are general nuisances that for the most part must just be waited out. Occasionally, a more serious secondary bacterial respiratory infection, such as pneumonia, can follow a cold and require medical treatment.

Treatment

There's no cure for the common cold. Antibiotics are of no use against cold viruses. Over-the-counter cold preparations won't cure a common cold or make it go away any sooner. They may ease your symptoms, but be aware of side effects.

- **Pain relievers.** For a fever, sore throat and headache, many people turn to acetaminophen (Tylenol, others) or other mild pain relievers. Keep in mind that acetaminophen can cause liver damage, especially if taken frequently or in larger than recommended doses. Be especially careful when giving acetaminophen to children because the dosing guidelines can be confusing. For instance, the infant-drop formulation is much more concentrated than the syrup commonly used in older children. Never give aspirin to children. It's been associated with Reye's syndrome — a rare but potentially fatal illness.

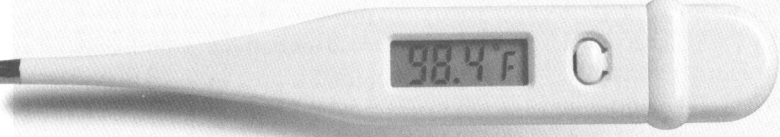

Temperature and Thermometers

Normally, your body temperature shows a definite pattern: low in the morning, gradually increasing during the day, and reaching its maximum during late afternoon or evening. Ordinarily, body temperature varies by 1 to 2 degrees Fahrenheit over the course of the day but usually doesn't exceed 99.9 F.

Thus, the mark at 98.6 F on your thermometer is only a general guide. A reading slightly above 98.6 F isn't abnormal and doesn't automatically signal illness. An increased body temperature usually isn't considered dangerous until it goes above 105 F.

What's a fever?

Ordinarily, your body controls its temperature to be within a range of 97 F in the morning to 99 F in the evening. When a fever is present, the mechanisms that control body temperature are set a few degrees higher. This increase in temperature is usually triggered by an immune system response to a foreign invader. When the cause of the fever disappears, or if you take medication to reduce the fever, the set-point returns to the normal range.

Taking your temperature

There are several ways to take your temperature. Older oral and rectal thermometers were essentially glass tubes containing a column of mercury. As the mercury expands in response to the heat from your body, it moves up the column. These types of thermometers pose a risk of mercury contamination and have been replaced by nonmercury thermometers.

Other types of thermometers include electronic thermometers and temperature strip thermometers. These are generally safer, although they may be slightly less accurate than the older, mercury-containing thermometers.

When taking someone's temperature, follow the instructions that came with the thermometer. In adults and children age 7 or older, you usually take the temperature orally by inserting the bulb end of the thermometer under the tongue and having the person close his or her mouth. After about a minute, you can remove the thermometer and read it. Some newer thermometers may be even faster and often work by gently inserting the end of the device into the ear canal.

- **Decongestant nasal sprays.** Adults shouldn't use decongestant drops or sprays for more than a few days because prolonged use can cause chronic inflammation of mucous membranes. And children shouldn't use decongestant drops or sprays at all. There's little evidence that they work in young children, and they may cause side effects.
- **Cough syrups.** The American College of Chest Physicians strongly discourages the use of these medications because they're not effective at treating the underlying cause of a cough due to a cold. Some contain ingredients that may alleviate coughing, but the amounts are too small to do much good and may actually be harmful for children.

The college recommends against using nonprescription cough syrups or cold medicines for anyone younger than age 14. The Food and Drug Administration strongly recommends against giving cough and cold medicines to children younger than age 2.

Under an agreement announced by manufacturers in 2008, several brands of nonprescription cold and cough medications began carrying a warning that these products should not be used in children under age 4. For young children, an accidental overdose could be fatal. A cough associated with a cold usually last less than two to three weeks. If a cough lingers longer than that, see your doctor.

PREVENTION TIP

The primary way to prevent the flu (influenza) is with a flu shot (influenza vaccine), given each fall. Because influenza can lead to complications, the flu shot is strongly recommended for people at increased risk of acquiring the disease. For more information on the flu shot, see page 237.

Flu (influenza)

Signs and symptoms
- Fever over 101 F (38 C) in adults, often higher in children
- Chills and sweats
- Headache
- Dry cough
- Muscle aches and pains
- Fatigue and weakness
- Loss of appetite
- Nasal congestion
- Diarrhea and vomiting in children

Influenza is a viral infection that attacks the respiratory system, including your nose, throat, bronchial tubes and lungs. Influenza, commonly called the flu, is not the same as the stomach viruses that cause diarrhea and vomiting.

Anyone can get the flu, but young children, older adults, people with weakened immune systems and those with chronic illnesses are especially vulnerable.

According to the Centers for Disease Control and Prevention, from 10,000 to 50,000 people in the United States die each year of complications of influenza and hundreds of thousands of people are hospitalized.

Flu viruses travel through the air in droplets when someone with the infection coughs, sneezes or talks. You can inhale the droplets directly or you can pick up the germs from an object, such as a telephone or doorknob, and then transfer them to your eyes, nose or mouth.

There are three types (strains): A, B and C. Type A usually is responsible for the large flu outbreaks. Types B and C generally aren't as widespread. Type B causes smaller, more localized outbreaks. Type C is the least common and usually causes only a mild illness.

Type C is a fairly stable virus, but types A and B are constantly changing and new strains appear regularly. Once you've had the flu, you develop antibodies to the strain that caused it, but the antibodies won't protect you from new strains.

Diagnosis
The flu usually has a sudden onset. Signs and symptoms are similar to those of the common cold but tend to be much more severe.

Influenza typically develops one to four days after coming into contact with the virus. The fever may last three to five days, although it can last as long as a week.

Diagnosing the flu with complete certainty requires a lab culture. What makes the diagnosis difficult is that influenza is similar to many other illnesses.

If your doctor suspects the flu, he or she may be able to isolate the virus from throat washings or may do a blood test to look for antibodies to the virus. These tests are mainly of value to public health officials, who can better advise the public if they know the character and extent of the disease circulating in a community.

How serious is the flu?
Isolated cases of the flu generally resolve without complications. However, flu epidemics still are responsible for thousands of deaths each year.

The illness can result in complications such as bronchitis, pneumonia and worsening of existing chronic diseases, such as heart disease or asthma.

Complications are more common in older adults and in individuals with weakened immune systems or chronic medical disorders.

Treatment
Usually, you need nothing more than lots of bed rest and plenty of fluids to treat the flu. But in some cases — such as individuals with a suppressed immune system or pregnant women — a doctor may prescribe an antiviral medication such as oseltamivir (Tamiflu) or zanamivir (Relenza).

These drugs are members of a class of antiviral agents called neuraminidase inhibitors. They treat both influenza A and B and work by deactivating an enzyme the virus needs to grow and spread. If taken soon after you notice symptoms, they may shorten your illness by a day or so. Oseltamivir is an oral medication, but zanamivir is inhaled through a device similar to an asthma inhaler and shouldn't be used by anyone with respiratory conditions, such as asthma and lung disease.

Both medications can cause side effects, including lightheadedness, nausea, vomiting, loss of appetite and trouble breathing. They can also lead to the development of antiviral-resistant viruses.

The Food and Drug Administration (FDA) has required the maker of Tamiflu to include a warning that people with the flu, particularly children, may be at increased risk of self-injury and confusion after taking Tamiflu. The FDA recommends that individuals with the flu who take Tamiflu be closely monitored for signs of unusual behavior. Discuss possible side effects with your doctor before starting any antiviral medication.

Pneumonia

Signs and symptoms
- Shaking chills
- High fever
- Sweating
- Shortness of breath
- Chest pain
- Cough that produces thick, greenish or yellow phlegm

Pneumonia is an inflammation of the tissues of your lungs caused by an infection with bacteria, viruses, fungi or other organisms. When you have pneumonia, air sacs in your lungs become inflamed and filled with fluid. This causes difficulty breathing that characterizes many types of pneumonia.

There are many kinds of pneumonia ranging in seriousness from mild to life-threatening. Because it often mimics a cold or the flu, pneumonia can be difficult to spot. You may not realize that you have a more serious condition. Pneumonia is a particular concern for older adults and people with chronic illnesses or impaired immune sys-

tems, but it can also strike young, healthy individuals.

Pneumonia is sometimes classified according to its cause.

Community-acquired pneumonia
Community-acquired pneumonia is acquired in the course of daily life — at school, work or the gym, for instance.

Hospital-acquired pneumonia
This type of pneumonia is acquired in the hospital or long-term care facility, and it tends to produce more-severe illness. The microorganisms that cause this type of pneumonia tend to be more resistant to antibiotics. A common predisposing factor to this type of pneumonia is gastroesophageal reflux, when contents from your stomach back up into your upper esophagus and are aspirated into the trachea and then the airways.

Aspiration pneumonia
This type of pneumonia occurs when foreign matter is inhaled (aspirated) into your lungs — most often when the contents of your stomach enter your lungs after you vomit. This can happen when

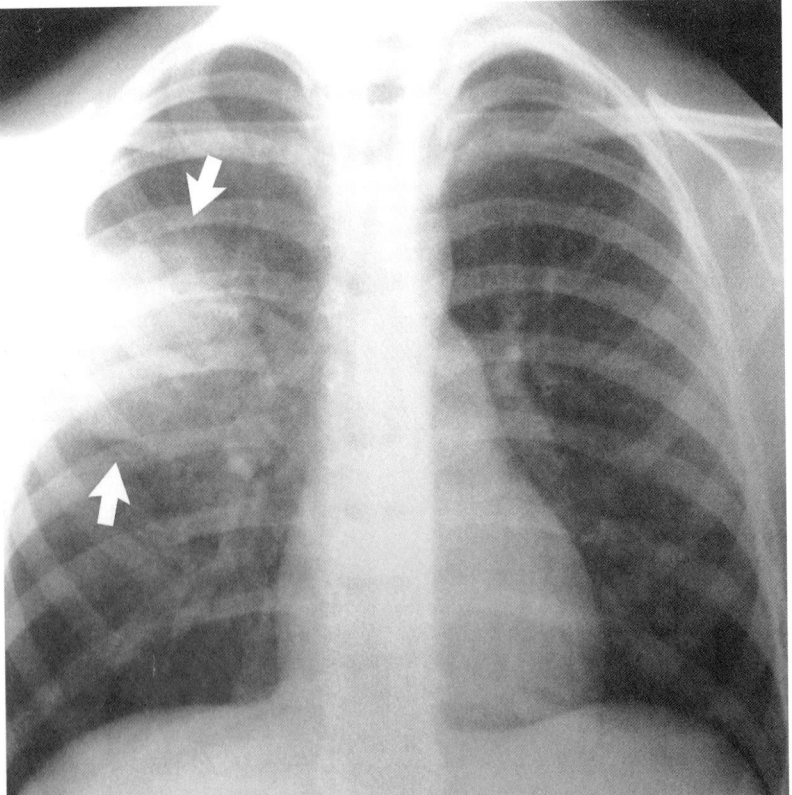

This chest X-ray reveals pneumonia in the upper lobe of the lung (see arrows).

a brain injury or other condition affects your normal gag reflex. Another common cause of aspiration pneumonia is consuming too much alcohol. This happens when the inebriated person passes out, and then vomits due to the effects of alcohol on the stomach.

Pneumonia caused by opportunistic organisms

Pneumonia is more likely to strike people with impaired immune systems. Organisms that aren't harmful in healthy people can be extremely dangerous in people with diseases such as AIDS, sickle cell anemia and other conditions that impair the immune system. Medications that suppress your immune system, such as corticosteroids or certain types of chemotherapy for cancer, also increase your risk of opportunistic infections.

Emerging pathogens

Outbreaks of the bird flu (H5N1 influenza) virus and severe acute respiratory syndrome (SARS) have caused serious, sometimes deadly pneumonia infections.

Diagnosis

Using a stethoscope, your doctor may detect distortions in the sounds of your breathing that suggest the presence of infection. Chest X-rays can help identify the location and extent of the infection. You may have blood tests to check your white cell count, or to look for the presence of viruses, bacteria or other organisms. A sample of your sputum may be tested (cultured) to help identify the infecting agent.

How serious is pneumonia?

Pneumonia is common. Every year approximately 50,000 Americans die of pneumonia. The seriousness of this disorder depends largely on the cause of the illness and your overall health.

A healthy person generally has sufficient defense mechanisms to be able to resist or control the invading organism. Among individuals whose defense mechanisms are impaired, fighting the condition is more difficult. Proper medical care, adequate rest and careful monitoring are essential.

Treatment

Pneumonia treatments vary, depending on the severity of your symptoms and the type of pneumonia you have.

- **Bacterial.** Doctors usually treat bacterial pneumonia with antibiotics. Although you may start to feel better shortly after beginning your medication, be sure to complete your entire course of antibiotics. Stopping medication too soon may cause your pneumonia to return. It also helps create strains of bacteria that are resistant to antibiotics — an increasingly serious problem in the United States.
- **Viral.** Antibiotics aren't effective against most viral forms of pneumonia. And although a few viral pneumonias may be treated with antiviral medications, the recommended treatment is generally the same as for the flu — rest and plenty of fluids.
- **Fungal.** If your pneumonia is caused by a fungus, you'll likely be treated with antifungal medication.
- **Mycoplasma.** Mycoplasma pneumonias are treated with antibiotics. Even so, recovery may not be immediate. In some cases fatigue may continue long after the infection itself has cleared.

In addition to these treatments, your doctor may recommend over-the-counter medications to reduce a fever, treat your aches and pains, and soothe the cough associated with pneumonia. You don't want to suppress your cough completely, though, since coughing helps clear your lungs. If you must use a cough suppressant, use the lowest dose that helps you get some rest.

Hospitalization and treatment with oxygen and intravenous

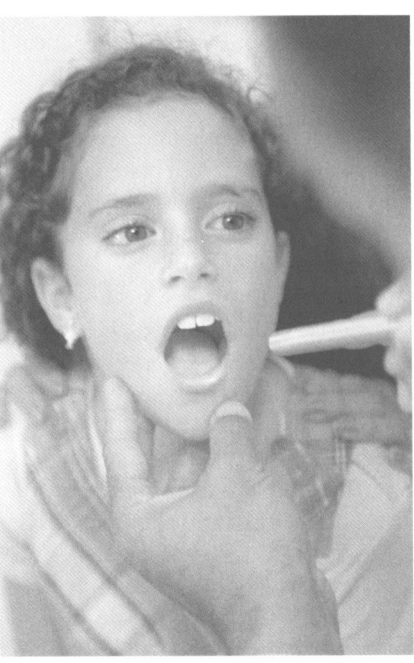

antibiotics are often necessary for severe pneumonia.

Strep throat

Signs and symptoms

- A sore throat
- Difficulty swallowing
- Red, swollen tonsils
- Tiny red spots on the soft or hard palate of your mouth
- Swollen, tender lymph glands
- Fever
- Headache
- Rash
- Stomachache

Strep throat is a bacterial infection that can make your throat feel sore and scratchy. It's caused by the bacterium *Streptococcus pyogenes* (group A beta-hemolytic streptococcus). The bacteria spread through airborne droplets or direct contact, such as touching a contaminated doorknob or other surface.

Strep throat is most common between the ages of 5 and 15, but it affects people of all ages. Some people are carriers of strep, which means they can pass the bacteria on to others, but the bacteria don't make them sick.

Diagnosis

It's important to identify strep because if left untreated it may lead to serious complications, such as kidney infection or rheumatic fever. Your doctor will likely do a throat test for strep infection. He or she is likely to use one or more of the following tests to check for the presence of bacteria, including streptococcal bacteria:

- **Throat culture.** For this test, a sterile swab is rubbed over the back of the throat and tonsils to get a sample of the secretions. It's not a painful procedure, but it may cause brief gagging. The sample is then cultured in a laboratory for the presence of bacteria, but results may take as long as two days.
- **Rapid antigen test.** Because of the waiting period for a throat culture, your doctor may also order a rapid antigen test on the swab sample. This test can detect strep bacteria in minutes by looking for foreign substances (antigens) in the throat. If you or your child tests positive for strep bacteria, antibiotic treatment can begin right away. But rapid strep tests have a downside. They may miss some strep throat infections. For this reason, many doctors still use throat cultures, especially if the results of the rapid test are negative.
- **Rapid DNA test.** Rapid tests use DNA technology to detect strep throat in a day or less from a throat swab. These tests are as accurate as throat cultures, and the results are available sooner.

How serious is strep throat?

Although strep throat usually isn't dangerous, without treatment it could lead to serious complications.

Treatment

Treatment for strep throat generally includes:

- **Antibiotics.** If you or your child has strep throat, your doctor will likely prescribe an oral antibiotic such as penicillin, amoxicillin (Amoxil), azithromycin (Zithromax), clarithromycin (Biaxin), clindamycin (Cleocin) or a cephalosporin (Keflex). Penicillin may be given by injection in some cases — such as if a young child is having a hard time swallowing or is vomiting from strep throat. These antibiotics reduce the duration and severity of symptoms, as well as the risk of complications and the likelihood the infection will spread to others.

  Be sure to finish the entire course of medicine. Stopping medication early may lead to recurrences and serious complications.
- **Pain relievers.** In addition to antibiotics, your doctor may suggest ibuprofen (Advil, Motrin IB, others) or acetaminophen (Tylenol, others) to relieve throat pain and reduce a fever. Because of the risk of Reye's syndrome, a potentially life-threatening illness, don't give aspirin to infants or children. Be careful with acetaminophen, too. In large doses, it can cause liver problems. Read and follow label directions.
- **Surgery.** For individuals with recurrent strep throat, removal of the tonsils and adenoids may be necessary.

Croup

Signs and symptoms
- Harsh, barking cough
- Difficulty breathing
- Fever
- Hoarse voice

Emergency signs and symptoms
- Noisy, high-pitched sounds when inhaling (stridor)
- Drooling or difficulty swallowing
- Agitated or extremely irritable
- Struggles to breathe
- Blue or grayish skin
- High fever

Croup — marked by a harsh, barking cough — results from a viral infection that causes swelling around the vocal cords (larynx) and windpipe (trachea). Rarely, croup may be caused by a bacterial infection. Because children have small airways to begin with, those younger than age 5 are most susceptible to having more symptoms with croup.

Croup typically lasts three to four days. During that time, it may go from mild to severe several times. Your child will probably be more comfortable sitting up than lying down. Usually, the condition worsens at night and improves in the morning.

How serious is croup?

Most cases of croup are mild. Rarely, the airway swells enough to interfere with breathing.

Treatment

Because croup is usually caused by a virus, antibiotics aren't helpful. Antibiotics work against bacteria, not viruses.

Warm, moist air may relieve some of the airway swelling and ease the cough. Run hot water in your shower for 10 minutes with the bathroom door closed. Once the room looks like a steam bath, take your child into the bathroom for at least 10 minutes. Another method of creating increased humidity is to use a vaporizer in the child's room. Have the child put his or her face in the mist and breathe deeply through the mouth. A wet washcloth placed loosely over the nose and mouth also may help relieve symptoms.

Encourage your child to drink clear, warm fluids, which may help loosen thickened secretions. A child with croup is often agitated and crying, which makes breathing more difficult, so try to both reassure and distract him or her.

During the illness it's a good idea to sleep in the same room with your child so that you'll be alert to any worsening of his or her condition. Don't let anyone smoke in the house because smoke will worsen the symptoms.

If symptoms persist for more than a few days or become severe, contact your child's doctor. Occasionally, croup may cause

Aspirin and Children

Aspirin is effective for treating a wide range of symptoms and disorders in adults. It's generally thought of as mild and harmless, but in certain cases, it can be dangerous, particularly when given to children. Aspirin use is related to a serious childhood condition called Reye's syndrome (see page 543). You shouldn't give aspirin to your child for any reason unless it's prescribed by a doctor.

Instead, try acetaminophen, which can help relieve minor aches and pains. It's available over-the-counter in generic form or under the brand name Tylenol.

Acetaminophen comes in several forms, including liquid and tablet. Each form has a different strength, so read labels and follow directions carefully, paying particular attention to dosage instructions for age or weight.

complete airway obstruction. To guard against this, be alert for emergency signs and symptoms and seek urgent medical attention if they occur.

Chickenpox (varicella)

Signs and symptoms
- A red, itchy rash
- Fever
- Abdominal pain or loss of appetite
- Mild headache
- Unease and discomfort (malaise)
- Dry cough

Chickenpox, also known as varicella, occurs primarily in children, although adults can contract the disease if they haven't had it already or haven't been immunized.

Chickenpox, which is caused by the varicella-zoster virus, is spread by inhaling infected respiratory droplets or by direct contact with the fluid from a blister when it ruptures. The virus is highly contagious and it spreads quickly. In people who've had chickenpox, the virus can reactivate later in life and cause shingles (see page 1097).

Diagnosis
The most recognized symptom of chickenpox is the itchy, red rash and small blisters that break out on the face, scalp, chest, back and, to a lesser extent, arms and legs (see the illustration on page 396). The rash usually appears about two weeks after exposure to the virus.

The spots turn into blisters, which quickly fill with a clear fluid and then rupture and turn crusty. They gradually slough off in one to two weeks. The rash continues to break out for about five days, so blisters at various stages of development may be present at the same time. A fever and malaise, often mild in children and more severe in adults, also develop.

How serious is chickenpox?
In children, chickenpox is often a mild disease, but in adults it can be more serious and may lead to pneumonia. In people with suppressed immune systems, the disease can be very serious. Although uncommon, inflammation of the brain (encephalitis) may occur, but recovery usually is complete.

If a pregnant woman contracts chickenpox during the first or second trimester, there's a small risk the child will be born with a congenital deformity. If a pregnant woman contracts the disease within a week before delivery, there's a high risk of a serious, life-threatening infection in her newborn.

Chickenpox seldom lasts for more than two weeks, from the appearance of the first blisters to the disappearance of the last ones. A secondary bacterial infection of the ruptured blisters may cause a fever and skin scarring.

Treatment
In otherwise healthy children, chickenpox typically requires no medical treatment. Keep the skin moist with frequent baths or, once the fever has subsided, showers. Cool, wet compresses also may help to relieve itching.

For people who have a high risk of complications from chickenpox, doctors sometimes prescribe medications to shorten the duration of the infection and to help reduce the risk of complications.

If you or your child falls into a high-risk group, your doctor may suggest an antiviral drug such as acyclovir (Zovirax) or another drug called immune globulin intravenous (IGIV), which may lessen the severity of the disease if given within 24 hours after the rash first appears. Other antiviral drugs, such as valacyclovir (Valtrex) and famciclovir, also may lessen the severity of the disease, but are approved for use only in adults.

In some cases, a doctor may recommend getting the chickenpox vaccine after exposure to the virus. This may prevent the disease or lessen its severity.

Prevention
A vaccine to prevent chickenpox is recommended for:
- Young children, with the first vaccine between 12 and 15 months, and the second between ages 4 and 6
- Unvaccinated older children
- Adults who haven't had chickenpox and have never been immunized against the disease

The vaccine isn't approved for pregnant women, people with weakened immunity, or people who are allergic to gelatin or the antibiotic neomycin.

A separate vaccine is recommended for adults age 60 and older to help prevent shingles (see page 1098).

Infectious mononucleosis

Signs and symptoms
- Fatigue and weakness
- A sore throat

- Fever
- Swollen lymph nodes in neck and armpits
- Swollen tonsils
- Headache

Infectious mononucleosis (mono) is usually caused by the Epstein-Barr virus. This infection most often occurs in adolescents and young adults. It's transmitted through saliva. You may be exposed through a cough or sneeze, kissing, or sharing a glass or utensil with someone who has mono.

Diagnosis

Your doctor may suspect mononucleosis based on your signs and symptoms and a physical examination. He or she will be looking for signs such as swollen lymph nodes, tonsils, liver or spleen. You may also receive blood tests.

- **Antibody tests.** If there's a need for additional confirmation, a monospot test may be done to check your blood for antibodies to the Epstein-Barr virus. This screening test gives results within a day, but it may not detect the infection during the first week of the illness. A different antibody blood test

requires a longer result time, but can detect the disease within the first week of symptoms.

- **White blood cell count.** Your doctor may use other blood tests to look for an elevated number of white blood cells (lymphocytes) or abnormal-looking lymphocytes. These blood tests won't confirm mononucleosis, but they may suggest it as a possibility.

How serious is infectious mononucleosis?

Mononucleosis isn't a serious disease, except in rare cases in which the spleen becomes severely enlarged and ruptures or when other vital organs, such as your liver or heart, are infected. Seek urgent medical care if you experience sudden sharp pains in the upper left side of your abdomen. This could mean a rapidly enlarging or ruptured spleen. In case of a rupture, emergency surgery may be required to control the bleeding.

In most cases, the fever, swollen lymph nodes and enlargement of the spleen improve after 10 days. However, the disease may cause prolonged fatigue and weakness. It may take two to three months before you feel completely normal.

Treatment

There's no specific therapy available to treat infectious mononucleosis. Antibiotics don't work against viral infections such as mono. Treatment involves bed rest and adequate fluid intake.

Medications

Occasionally, a streptococcal (strep) infection accompanies mononucleosis. You may also develop a sinus infection or infection of your tonsils (tonsillitis). You may need an antibiotic to treat these accompanying bacterial infections.

To ease some of your symptoms, such as severe swelling of your throat and tonsils, your doctor may prescribe a corticosteroid medication such as prednisone.

Self-care

Rest is an important part of treatment. Drinking plenty of fluids helps to relieve the fever and sore throat and keeps you from becoming dehydrated. For a sore throat, try gargling warm, salty water several times a day. Acetaminophen (Tylenol, others) or ibuprofen (Advil, Motrin IB, others) can help relieve pain or a fever.

Don't expect to return to your normal routine for a while. Your doctor may ask you to avoid contact sports for several months if your spleen is enlarged.

Gastrointestinal infections

Signs and symptoms

- Watery diarrhea
- Nausea and vomiting
- Fever
- Abdominal cramps
- Occasional muscle aches and headache

Emergency signs and symptoms

- Profuse diarrhea, to the point of causing lightheadedness
- Bloody diarrhea

Bacteria, viruses, fungi and parasites can cause gastrointestinal infections. These infections are most commonly contracted by drinking contaminated water, eating unwashed raw fruits or vegetables, or eating meat or fish that hasn't been cooked properly.

A common viral infection of the gastrointestinal tract is rotavirus. This infection occurs mainly in infants between the ages of 6 and 24 months. Other types of gastrointestinal infections include norovirus, *Campylobacter jejuni*, *Escherichia coli* (*E. coli*), *Staphylococcus aureus*, *Clostridium difficile* (*C. difficile*) and salmonella.

Diagnosis

Most gastrointestinal infections take a day or two to cause signs or symptoms, depending on the incubation period of the infectious agent. Diarrhea is the most common symptom. If the lining

---

PREVENTION TIP

Proper hand washing is the best way to prevent many infections. That's why it's important to wash your own hands regularly and to show your children how to wash their hands properly.

The Centers for Disease Control and Prevention recommends taking the following steps:

- Use soap and running water.
- Rub your hands vigorously as you wash them.
- Wash all surfaces, including backs of hands, wrists, between fingers and under fingernails.
- Rinse well and leave the water running until after drying hands.
- Dry hands with a single-use towel.
- Turn off the faucet using a paper towel.

Escherichia Coli O157:H7

In 1982, 47 people in two states became sick with bloody, watery diarrhea, abdominal pain and severe cramps. Public health officials were stumped. It appeared obvious that it was a gastrointestinal infection of some sort, but how could so many people, across two states, become sick at the same time with similar signs and symptoms? What was the cause of such an outbreak?

After three months of investigation, medical experts found the answer. All of the individuals affected had eaten hamburger from the same stock at a national fast-food restaurant. The infectious culprit in the meat was a strain of the bacterium we now know as *Escherichia coli* O157:H7. *E. coli* O157:H7 adheres to the intestinal wall after being ingested. Once established, it produces a toxin that can cause bloody diarrhea.

Today, in the United States, *E. coli* infections cause about 265,000 illnesses and about 100 deaths annually. In addition to O157:H7, other forms of the *E. coli* bacteria also can cause infections.

As a result of *E. coli* outbreaks, the Department of Agriculture has changed its regulations on meat handling. It now requires safe-handling labels on raw meat and poultry products and has instituted monitoring programs to test random beef samples. Meat processing plants are required to take steps to prevent contamination from pathogens and other hazards.

Transmission

The bacterium can live in the intestines of healthy cattle and is found on some cattle farms. Eating meat that hasn't been cooked enough, particularly ground beef, is the most common way of acquiring an *E. coli* infection. The bacterium has also been found in unpasteurized milk and juice, and in produce such as lettuce and alfalfa sprouts.

In addition, you can become infected through contact with contaminated stool. This is particularly apt to occur with young children who are still being toilet trained or still learning how to properly wash their hands. Families and people at child care centers with infected children are at increased risk of developing the illness.

Treatment

Within a day to two weeks of exposure to the bacterium, you may experience watery diarrhea and abdominal cramps. In most people, this eventually progresses to bloody diarrhea. Generally, the symptoms resolve within one to nine days.

For mild diarrhea, drink plenty of fluids to avoid dehydration. This is especially important for children. As you begin to feel better, you might try eating semisolid foods and low-fat fibers, such as soda crackers and toast.

Diarrhea is your body's way of attempting to get rid of the offending organism. For this reason, health experts generally don't recommend anti-diarrheal medications, as they may contribute to keeping the bacteria from being eliminated.

In a small percentage of people infected with *E. coli*, particularly the very young and the very old, a serious complication called hemolytic uremic syndrome (HUS) may occur. HUS destroys red blood cells and causes kidney failure (see page 893). It requires intensive care and may lead to further kidney complications and possibly the need for kidney dialysis later in life. In a few cases, it may be fatal.

Prevention

According to food safety experts, the best way to prevent such an infection is to use common sense. Avoid having raw meat come into contact with other foods. Cook your meat until it's done. For hamburger, meat should reach at least 160 F, and for steaks and roasts, between 145 and 170 F.

In addition, properly wash hands, foods and cooking utensils that have come in contact with raw meat. Keep meat and produce separate while in the refrigerator and while cooking. Wash vegetables and fruits thoroughly, especially if they'll be eaten raw. Don't drink unpasteurized milk or fruit juices.

Practicing proper hand-washing techniques, and teaching them to your children, can go a long way toward preventing a host of infectious diseases.

---

of the intestine is damaged, stool may be bloody.

Vomiting also is common. In some cases, a fever, loss of appetite, abdominal cramps, nausea and weight loss occur. Diarrhea and vomiting that begin within several hours of eating may suggest food poisoning from a preformed toxin, rather than a toxin that's released after the bacteria have lodged in your intestine. To determine the cause, your doctor may take blood or stool samples to be grown (cultured) and analyzed in a laboratory.

How serious are gastrointestinal infections?

In the United States, gastrointestinal infections generally aren't serious, although they can be fatal in small children, the elderly and people with impaired immune systems. In developing countries, where sanitation levels may be poor and health care inadequate, diarrheal diseases are among the top causes of sickness and death.

The loss of fluids brought on by diarrhea can cause dehydration, a serious problem in older adults and young children. For this reason, it's important to drink plenty of liquids. Avoid alcohol, caffeine and milk products.

If your child exhibits signs of dehydration — dry mouth, pale skin, sunken eyes, decreased urination — talk to your doctor. Other reasons to contact your doctor include severe or prolonged diarrhea or vomiting, either a high fever or a sudden drop in body temperature, changed levels of consciousness, severe abdominal pain, or bloody stools.

Treatment

For the most part, gastrointestinal infections get better within a few days and complete recovery occurs without treatment. During your illness stay hydrated with nonalcoholic, noncaffeinated fluids. Water and sports drinks, which contain sodium, potassium and other nutrients, are generally best. If you're severely dehydrated, you may need an intravenous electrolyte solution.

Most intestinal infections don't require antibiotics. Some infections, however — such as diarrhea caused by *E. coli* O157:H7 or *C. difficile* — may lead to serious complications. In addition to severe diarrhea, other signs and symptoms may include nausea, vomiting and abdominal pain.

Prevention

Good hygiene is key in the prevention of gastrointestinal infections. Frequent hand washing is one of the most effective ways of getting rid of germs. In addition, wash any surfaces, cookware and utensils that have been in contact with raw meat — especially poultry — with hot, soapy water.

Make sure all meat is thoroughly cooked before you eat it. If you're in a foreign country, avoid local drinking water and ice cubes, unsanitary eating establishments, and raw fruits and vegetables, unless you peel them yourself.

Other Infections

Many other infectious diseases occur less often than the illnesses described so far, but they can cause very serious illness. Immunizations now make it possible to avoid many — but not all — of these.

Tetanus

Signs and symptoms
- Stiffness of the jaw, neck and other muscles
- Spasms of the jaw and neck muscles
- Irritability
- Painful convulsions
- Fever

Tetanus, also known as lockjaw, is caused by the bacterium *Clostridium tetani*, whose spores are found in soil. If the spores enter a deep wound with low oxygen content, they germinate and produce a toxin (tetanospasmin) that interferes with nerves that control your muscles. The incubation period from the time of the injury until symptoms appear is usually eight to 12 days.

Some people with tetanus experience only pain and tingling at the wound site and some spasms in nearby muscles, but most develop a stiff jaw and neck, difficulty swallowing and irritability.

Staph Infections

Staph infections are caused by staphylococcus bacteria, types of germs commonly found on the skin or in the nose of even healthy individuals. Most of the time, these bacteria cause no problems or result in relatively minor skin infections. But staph infections can become serious if the bacteria invade deeper into your body, entering your bloodstream, joints, bones, lungs or heart. Signs and symptoms of staph infections vary widely, depending on the location and severity of the infection.

A variety of factors — including the status of your immune system to the types of sports you play — can increase your risk of developing staph infections. People with weaker immune systems, either from a disease or medications that suppress the immune system, are more likely to develop a staph infection. Staph bacteria can spread easily through cuts, abrasions and skin-to-skin contact. The bacteria may spread in locker rooms through shared razors, towels, uniforms or equipment. Staph infections are also more common in individuals who are hospitalized or have recently been in a hospital.

Treatment usually involves antibiotics, and for some skin infections drainage of the infected area. However, some staph infections no longer respond to common antibiotics. The emergence of antibiotic-resistant strains of staph bacteria — often described as methicillin-resistant *Staphylococcus aureus* (MRSA) strains — has led to the use of IV antibiotics, with the potential for more side effects.

Most MRSA infections occur in people who've been in hospitals or other health care settings, such as nursing homes. This type is known as health care-associated MRSA (HA-MRSA). Another type of MRSA infection occurs among healthy people in the wider community. This form is called community-associated MRSA (CA-MRSA). It often starts as swollen, painful red bumps that might resemble pimples or spider bites or a painful skin boil.

Spasms of the jaw or facial muscles often follow, progressing to spasms and rigidity of the neck, abdominal and back muscles. Finally, painful convulsions caused by minor stimuli affect the respiratory muscles so that the individual is unable to breathe.

Diagnosis

Laboratory tests generally aren't helpful for diagnosing tetanus. A diagnosis is generally based on signs and symptoms and a physical examination.

How serious is tetanus?

In most cases of tetanus, the illness is severe, and there's a risk of death despite treatment. Death may result from constriction of airways, pneumonia or instability in the autonomic nervous system. The autonomic nervous system is the part of your nervous system that controls your heart muscles, other involuntary muscles and glands. Tetanus is especially serious in small children and older adults.

Treatment

Treatment may consist of certain medications and supportive care.

Medications

You may receive:

- **Antitoxin.** Your doctor may give you a tetanus antitoxin, such as tetanus immune globulin (TIG). However, the antitoxin can neutralize only toxin that hasn't yet combined with nerve tissue.
- **Antibiotics.** Your doctor may give you antibiotics, either orally or by injection, to fight tetanus bacteria.
- **Vaccine.** You'll need a tetanus vaccine in order to prevent future tetanus infection.

Supportive therapies

Tetanus infection often requires a long period of treatment in an intensive care setting. You may need drugs to sedate you and to paralyze your muscles, and that may result in shallow breathing

that needs to be supported temporarily by a ventilator.

People who've had tetanus often recover completely. However, some people have lasting effects, such as brain damage from a lack of oxygen when muscle spasms in the throat cut off the airway.

Prevention

Immunization is vital for everyone. The tetanus vaccine is usually initially given to children as part of the diphtheria, tetanus and pertussis (DTaP) vaccine. You should receive a booster shot every 10 years, or at the time of a major injury if it's been more than five years since your last booster. Booster shots are generally part of the tetanus, diphtheria and pertussis (Tdap) vaccine. Vaccination is also recommended for pregnant women to ensure transfer of maternal antibodies to the baby.

Measles (rubeola)

Signs and symptoms

- Fever
- Dry cough
- Runny nose
- Inflamed eyes
- Sensitivity to light
- Tiny white spots on the lining of the cheek
- A rash

Measles (rubeola) is primarily a respiratory infection caused by a highly contagious virus. The virus is transmitted by inhalation of infected droplets in the air, such as from a sneeze. Measles is most contagious before its rash appears, making it difficult to avoid the disease. The rash — a red, blotchy rash that appears on the face and behind the ears — begins about four days after onset of symptoms. It spreads to the chest and back and, finally, to the arms and legs.

Diagnosis

A diagnosis is typically made on the basis of the characteristic rash and the small, white spots on the lining of the cheek.

How serious is measles?

Typically, a measles infection lasts 10 days to two weeks and you recover completely. In a small number of cases, pneumonia or other bacterial infections develop during the course of the illness, or complications such as encephalitis arise immediately after appearance of the rash. Encephalitis can cause convulsions and brain damage.

Treatment

Acetaminophen (Tylenol, others) can help relieve fever, and a sedative cough medicine may help relieve coughing. A person with measles should remain isolated until a week after the rash disappears, and he or she should stay in bed until the fever disappears. Severe symptoms may require additional treatment.

Prevention

The measles vaccine is effective and is usually given as a combined measles-mumps-rubella (MMR) inoculation. Doctors recommend that the MMR vaccine be given to children between 12 and 15 months of age, and again between 4 and 6 years of age.

German measles (rubella)

Signs and symptoms

- Mild fever
- Headache
- Stuffy or runny nose
- Inflamed, red eyes
- Enlarged lymph nodes
- Fine, pink rash

German measles (rubella) is only moderately infectious. It's caused by a different virus than measles (rubeola). The disease is transmitted by inhalation of droplets in the air carrying the virus. Symptoms of this disease are usually mild and sometimes hardly noticeable. A fine, pink rash may appear on the face and trunk and then the arms and legs. The rash usually disappears in three to five days. Sometimes, a rash doesn't occur.

Diagnosis

A diagnosis is usually made on symptoms. Your doctor may take a blood sample to check for antibodies to the virus.

How serious is German measles?

In itself, German measles is a mild infection. However, if a woman has rubella when she's pregnant, the consequences for her unborn child may be severe. The child may have one or more problems, including growth retardation, cataracts, rashes, deafness, congenital heart defects and defects of other organs.

Treatment

The standard treatment for rubella is to let the infection run its course. Taking acetaminophen (Tylenol, others) may help to relieve symptoms. If you're exposed to rubella while you're pregnant, contact your doctor promptly.

Prevention

A vaccine can protect against the disease. It's usually part of the combined measles-mumps-rubella (MMR) vaccination. Doctors recommend that the MMR vaccine be given to children between 12 and 15 months of age, and again between 4 and 6 years of age.

Roseola

Signs and symptoms

- Fever
- Rash made up of small pink spots or patches
- Swollen lymph nodes
- Fatigue

Roseola is a mild infection most often caused by the human herpes virus 6. The viral infection usually affects children by age 2. It rarely develops in adults. The infection typically isn't serious, but sometimes complications occur. The primary sign of roseola is a sudden, high fever. As the fever goes down, a rash appears on the trunk and neck that lasts a few hours to a few days.

Fever of Unknown Origin

A fever is the most common reaction to an infection. But a fever doesn't always signify that you have an infection. A fever can also be a sign of a noninfectious disease or result from a medication. Sometimes, the cause is not apparent. If you have recurrent temperatures greater than 100.5 F for more than three weeks and there's no obvious cause, even after extensive evaluation, the diagnosis may be "fever of unknown origin." However, with persistence, a cause can usually be identified.

Some of the tests that your doctor may use to try to identify the cause of an unknown fever include blood tests, X-ray examinations, computerized tomography (CT) scans and biopsies of the arteries, lymph nodes, bone marrow, liver or muscles.

Diagnosis

Roseola is usually diagnosed by its signs and symptoms and can be confirmed by a blood test to check for antibodies to the virus.

Treatment

Treatment consists of acetaminophen (Tylenol, others) or ibuprofen (Advil, Motrin IB, others) and applying cool sponges or washcloths to lower the fever. Some doctors may prescribe the antiviral medication ganciclovir to treat the infection in people with weakened immunity.

Whooping cough (pertussis)

Signs and symptoms

- A hacking cough, often followed by explosive coughs that end in a high-pitched whoop
- A runny nose and sneezing
- Nasal congestion
- Mild fever
- Unease and discomfort (malaise)
- Fatigue from coughing

Emergency signs and symptoms

- Difficulty breathing
- Blue lips

Whooping cough — known medically as pertussis — gets its name from the Latin word for intensive cough. It's a highly contagious respiratory tract infection marked by a severe, hacking cough that's followed by a high-pitched intake of breath that sounds like a "whoop."

The condition is caused by the *Bordetella pertussis* bacterium. Once in your airways, the bacteria multiply and produce toxins that interfere with your respiratory tract's ability to sweep away germs. Thick mucus accumulates inside your airways, causing uncontrollable coughing. The bacteria also cause inflammation of the airways. This narrowing leaves you gasping for air — sucking in air with a high-pitched "whoop" — after a fit of coughing.

The incidence of whooping cough has been increasing, primarily among children too young to have completed the full course of vaccinations and teenagers whose immunity has faded.

Diagnosis

Diagnosing whooping cough in its early stages can be difficult because symptoms resemble those of a cold. Once the characteristic cough sets in, a diagnosis may be made on symptoms. Medical tests may be needed to confirm the diagnosis.

- **A nose or throat culture and test.** Your doctor takes a nose or throat swab or suction sample. The sample is then sent to a lab and tested for whooping cough bacteria.
- **Blood tests.** A blood sample may be drawn and sent to a lab to check for a high white blood cell count. White blood cells help the body fight infections,

such as whooping cough. A high white cell count typically indicates the presence of an infection or inflammation. This is a general test and not specific for whooping cough, however.

- **A chest X-ray.** Your doctor may order an X-ray to check for fluid in your lungs, which can occur when pneumonia complicates whooping cough and other respiratory infections.

How serious is whooping cough?

With proper care, most people recover from the illness without incident. However, it can lead to pneumonia and damage the lungs. In very severe cases, lack of oxygen (asphyxia) may lead to brain damage. If a person's lips turn blue, this means that he or she is having severe difficulty breathing and needs emergency care.

Treatment

Treatment for whooping cough varies, depending on your age and the severity of signs and symptoms.

When whooping cough is diagnosed early in older children, teenagers and adults, doctors usually prescribe bed rest along with an antibiotic such as azithromycin or erythromycin. Although antibi-

otics won't cure whooping cough, they can shorten the duration of the illness and they shorten the period in which the disease is communicable.

If the illness has progressed to the point of severe coughing spells, antibiotics aren't as effective but may still be used. Unfortunately, not much is available in the way of symptom relief. Over-the-counter cough medicines have little effect on whooping cough. A case of whooping cough usually resolves in six weeks but may last longer.

Almost all infants with whooping cough who are younger than 3 months, as well as many older babies, are admitted to the hospital to decrease the risk of serious complications. Most babies treated for whooping cough overcome the condition without lasting effects, but the risk of complications exists until the infection clears.

In the hospital, your child is likely to receive intravenous (IV) antibiotics to treat the infection and perhaps corticosteroid medications, which help reduce inflammation in the airways. Sometimes a child's airway may also be suctioned to remove mucus that's blocking it. In some cases, prescription sedatives may be given to help your child rest.

Prevention

Vaccination for whooping cough is generally given as part of the diphtheria, tetanus and pertussis combination vaccine (DTaP) administered during childhood. Because immunity from the pertussis vaccine tends to wane by age 11, and because of the increase of whooping cough in adolescents and teens, doctors recommend a booster shot at age 11 or 12. This is the tetanus, diphtheria and pertussis vaccine, or Tdap.

Adults who didn't get the Tdap vaccine as an adolescent should get one dose of this vaccine. Once they have had this dose, a Td booster should be given every 10 years. All pregnant women also should be vaccinated.

Mumps

Signs and symptoms

- Swollen, painful salivary glands that cause the cheeks to puff out
- Pain with chewing or swallowing
- Fever
- Weakness and fatigue

Mumps is a viral infection that primarily affects the parotid glands — one of three pairs of salivary glands, located below and in front of your ears. The medical term for the illness is *epidemic parotitis*.

Mumps was common until the mumps vaccine was licensed in the 1960s. Since then, the number of cases has dropped dramatically.

Diagnosis

The primary — and best known — sign is swollen, painful parotid salivary glands, causing puffing of the cheeks. About a quarter of teenage boys and adult men who contract mumps experience inflammation of the testicles (orchitis).

Your doctor can confirm a diagnosis of mumps by identifying the mumps virus in your saliva or by finding an increase in mumps antibodies in your blood. However, this testing is rarely necessary.

Smallpox

The eradication of smallpox is a success story of modern medicine. Small- pox was once a highly infectious viral disease that would spread in epidemics, causing death in up to 40 percent of its victims. The disease caused severe headaches, a fever and a red, blistering rash that often left scars. At the end of the 18th century, Edward Jenner, an English physician, discovered that inoculation with cowpox virus, which is usually harmless, prevented smallpox. Campaigns were launched in the United States and Europe to inoculate people against smallpox. However, as late as 1967, when the World Health Organization launched a global campaign to eliminate this disease, outbreaks still occurred regularly in many countries.

After 10 years of effort, this international campaign was successful and the disease was eradicated. Smallpox vaccination is no longer necessary, and in 1972 routine vaccination in the United States stopped.

The potential use of smallpox as a biological weapon has renewed interest in the disease, spurring the manufacture of the vaccine. Vaccination would only be reinstituted as a defense against biological warfare.

How serious is mumps?

Mumps makes you uncomfortable, but it's usually not a serious disease and rarely lasts more than two weeks. Encephalitis, an uncommon but serious complication of the illness, can cause neurological symptoms. Rarely, it can be fatal. Swelling of the testicles (orchitis) is uncomfortable and occasionally causes male infertility.

Treatment

There's no specific treatment for mumps. Your doctor may advise bed rest until the fever disappears. Isolation to prevent the spread of the disease is sometimes appropriate. For most of the complications that may arise, treatment depends on the symptoms.

Prevention

The vaccine against mumps is safe and effective. It's usually given as a combined measles-mumps-rubella (MMR) inoculation. The first dose is given to children between ages 12 and 15 months. A second dose is given between ages 4 and 6 years. Since the recommendation for a second dose of the mumps vaccine didn't begin until the late 1980s or early 1990s, many young adults may not have received their second dose and should have one now.

Rabies

Signs and symptoms

- Fever
- Headache
- Unease and discomfort (malaise)
- Insomnia and anxiety
- Hallucinations and agitation
- Salivation
- Convulsions and paralysis

Rabies is a serious viral disease that affects your central nervous system. It results from a virus belonging to the rhabdoviridae family that affects the brain. The virus is typically transmitted to humans by way of saliva from infected animals — often, but not always, through a bite.

The incubation period from the time of exposure until symptoms appear is one to three months. There have been rare cases in which rabies didn't occur for more than six months after exposure.

Diagnosis

If you've been bitten or had contact with an animal that may have rabies, it's essential to capture the animal. Once a potentially rabid animal is captured, it may be confined for observation. Another option is for health officials to conduct tests of the animal's brain tissue to determine whether it has rabies. Testing can be done quickly, but only after the animal is dead.

If you have signs and symptoms of rabies, a number of tests using blood, saliva, spinal fluid or skin tissue may be required to identify or rule out rabies infection.

How serious is rabies?

Quick action is important. If you think you may have been exposed to an animal with rabies, thoroughly wash the wound or area of exposure with soap and water. This is one of the most effective methods to decrease the chance of infection. Then immediately call your doctor or go to the emergency department. Once the earliest signs and symptoms appear, death almost always follows. Most rabies deaths occur because the person didn't seek immediate medical care.

Treatment

If your doctor determines that you likely were exposed to rabies, treatment will begin at once. The sooner the treatment begins, the greater your chance of recovery.

In the United States, treatment consists of one dose of rabies immune globulin and five doses of the rabies vaccine over a 28-day period. You're given the immune globulin by injection around the site of the bite, and you receive the injections of the vaccine into your upper arm muscle.

Immune globulins are disease-fighting proteins that provide you with temporary antibodies. The rabies vaccine helps your body start producing its own antibodies, which are longer lasting than the ones contained in the immune globulin. The vaccine isn't painful, but you might have a mild physical reaction, such as swelling or redness at the injection site.

Scarlet fever

Signs and symptoms

- Red rash that feels like sandpaper
- Red lines in folds of skin around the groin, armpits, elbows, knees and neck
- Red and bumpy appearance of the tongue
- Fever, often with chills
- Very sore and red throat
- Swollen lymph nodes in the neck
- Headache

Scarlet fever was once a common, serious childhood illness but is now rare. The most common source of scarlet fever is a specific type of streptococcal bacteria infection that produces strep throat. However, the strain of bacteria causing scarlet fever also releases toxins that produce a rash, red lines and red tongue. Infrequently, scarlet fever stems from bacterial infections affecting other organs.

Diagnosis

Diagnosis generally involves a physical examination to look for characteristic signs and symptoms. If your doctor suspects strep as the cause of the illness, he or she will also swab the back of the throat to collect material that may harbor strep bacteria. Tests for the strep bacterium are important because other conditions can cause the signs and symptoms of scarlet fever, and these illnesses may require different treatments.

Your doctor may order one or more of the following tests:

- **Throat culture.** The sample from the throat is examined in a laboratory test in which the bacteria can thrive. Although this is a very reliable test, the results may take as long as two days.

- **Rapid antigen test.** Sometimes called a rapid strep test, it can detect foreign proteins (antigens) associated with strep bacteria infection. This test can be completed during a visit to your doctor's office. If a rapid antigen test is negative, your doctor will probably order a throat culture to ensure an accurate diagnosis.
- **Rapid DNA test.** This test uses DNA technology to detect strep bacteria from a throat swab within a day. The test is at least as accurate as a throat culture, and the results are available sooner.

How serious is scarlet fever?
Scarlet fever was once considered a serious childhood illness, but antibiotic treatments have made it less threatening. Scarlet fever rarely results in serious complications.

Treatment
The standard treatment for scarlet fever is an antibiotic that's usually given for a minimum of 10 days. Bed rest and drinking plenty of liquids also are important. After 24 hours on an antibiotic an individual is no longer contagious.

Typhoid fever

Signs and symptoms
- Fever
- Headache
- Weakness and fatigue
- A sore throat
- Rash
- Diarrhea or constipation

Emergency signs and symptoms
- Become delirious
- Lie motionless and exhausted with your eyes half-closed (typhoid state)

Typhoid fever is caused by the *Salmonella typhi* bacterium. It's rare in industrialized countries, but in developing countries with poor sanitary conditions and unsafe water supplies epidemics still occur.

The disease is acquired by consuming contaminated food or fluids or through close contact with someone who's infected. The bacteria penetrate the wall of the small intestine and cause inflammation of the lymph nodes and spleen.

Chronic carriers also are possible sources of the disease. A chronic carrier is someone who carries typhoid bacteria in his or her intestinal tract for years but has no symptoms.

Diagnosis
Your doctor is likely to suspect typhoid fever based on your symptoms and your travel history. The diagnosis is usually confirmed by identifying the *S. typhi* bacteria in a sample of your blood, urine, feces or bone marrow.

How serious is typhoid fever?
Untreated, typhoid fever is very serious. Even when treated, a few people don't survive the disease's complications. Older adults and people with chronic illnesses are especially vulnerable. In children, the disease usually is milder. A few people become chronic carriers.

Treatment
Antibiotics are available to treat typhoid fever. The choice depends on the strain of the bacteria. Other treatment steps include drinking fluids to avoid dehydration and eating a high-calorie diet to supply your body with the nutrients it may lose during the illness. At times, administration of fluids through a vein (intravenously) is necessary. Because the bacteria are present in the stool and urine, proper hand washing is important.

Prevention
Currently, two types of typhoid vaccines are available — an oral form and an injected form. The oral vaccine is given as four capsules, taken one a day every other day. Protection lasts five years. The injectable vaccine lasts two to three years and is given in a single dose.

Neither is 100 percent effective, and both require repeat vaccinations. People who plan to live or to travel in an area where the disease is prevalent or who may have been exposed during an epidemic outbreak should be immunized.

Diphtheria

Signs and symptoms
- A sore throat and hoarseness
- Painful swallowing
- Swollen glands
- A thick gray membrane covering the throat and tonsils
- Difficulty breathing
- Fever and chills
- Unease and discomfort (malaise)

Diphtheria is an acute infection caused by a toxin produced by the bacterium *Corynebacterium diphtheriae*. It usually attacks the upper respiratory tract. Infection occurs by inhalation of airborne droplets exhaled by a person with the disease or by a carrier who has no symptoms.

A second type of diphtheria can affect the skin. A wound infected with diphtheria is typically red, painful and swollen. It may also have patches of a sticky, gray material. In rare cases, diphtheria affects the eye.

Diagnosis
A doctor may suspect diphtheria in someone who has a sore throat with a gray membrane covering the throat and tonsils. He or she will confirm the diagnosis by taking a sample of the membrane from the throat with a swab and having the sample grown (cultured) in a laboratory. Doctors can also take a sample from an infected wound and have it cultured.

How serious is diphtheria?
With proper treatment and no complications, the prognosis is good. However, the gray diphtheria membrane in the upper airway can be dangerous because it may obstruct breathing. In addition, the disease may cause a serious heart

infection called myocarditis. Sometimes, the bacteria affect the cranial nerves, causing nasal-sounding speech, regurgitation of food and an inability to swallow. This is seldom fatal, unless paralysis of respiratory muscles develops.

Treatment

The disease is treated immediately and aggressively with these medications:

- **An antitoxin.** The antitoxin neutralizes the diphtheria toxin already circulating in your body. The antitoxin is injected into a vein (intravenously) or into a muscle (intramuscular injection). But first, doctors may perform skin allergy tests to make sure that the infected person doesn't have an allergy to the antitoxin. People who are allergic must first be desensitized to the antitoxin. Doctors accomplish this by initially giving small doses of the antitoxin and then gradually increasing the dosage.
- **Antibiotics.** Diphtheria is also treated with antibiotics, such as penicillin or erythromycin. Antibiotics help kill bacteria in the body, clearing up infections. Antibiotics also reduce the length of time that a person with diphtheria is contagious.

People who have diphtheria often need to be in the hospital for treatment. They may be isolated in an intensive care unit because the disease can spread easily to anyone not immunized against the disease. Doctors may remove some of the thick, gray covering in the throat if it's obstructing breathing.

Prevention

The diphtheria vaccine can prevent the disease. The vaccine is usually combined with vaccines for tetanus and whooping cough (pertussis). The three-in-one vaccine is known as the diphtheria, tetanus and pertussis vaccine, or DTaP vaccine.

The DTaP vaccine is one of the childhood immunizations that doctors in the United States recommend begin during infancy. The vaccine consists of a series of five shots, typically administered in the arm or thigh, and is given to children beginning at 2 months and ending at 4 to 6 years.

The diphtheria vaccine is very effective at preventing diphtheria. Rarely, the vaccine causes serious complications in a child, such as an allergic reaction (hives or a rash develops within minutes of the injection), seizures or shock — complications that are treatable.

After the initial series of immunizations in childhood, booster shots of the diphtheria vaccine are needed to help you maintain immunity. That's because immunity to diphtheria fades with time.

The first booster shot is needed around age 12, and then every 10 years after that — especially if you travel to an area where diphtheria is common. A booster shot of the diphtheria vaccine is given in combination with a booster shot of the tetanus and pertussis vaccines, and is known as Tdap.

Wound infections

Signs and symptoms

- Swelling and redness
- Hot, inflamed skin around a wound
- Drainage of pus
- Elevated temperature
- Decrease in blood pressure
- Rapid heartbeat

After an injury causes a break in the skin or after an operation, wound infections may occur. These can range from minor to severe, depending on the cause of the infection, whether the organism produces toxins, and how quickly the infection is identified and treated. Some severe wound infections include:

Necrotizing subcutaneous infection

This infection is caused by bacteria that infect tissue through wounds. Primary symptoms are swelling, discoloration and death (necrosis) of the surrounding tissue. The skin around the wound becomes hot, inflamed, tender and red. If the infection worsens, the skin becomes discolored and gangrene may develop. Some necrotizing infections have been referred to as "flesh-eating bacteria" infections.

To determine the correct antibiotic to treat the infection, your doctor will take a sample of pus from the wound for culture to identify the bacteria present.

Your doctor may also have to thoroughly open the wound (debride) so that all infected tissue can be removed. One operation usually isn't sufficient to remove all the dead tissue. Additional operations frequently are necessary. If the infection involves an arm or leg, amputation may even be necessary.

Gas gangrene

Gangrene is defined as death of infected tissue. Gas gangrene results when a wound becomes infected by a certain type of bacteria, called clostridium, which produces several toxins.

The infection causes sudden pain and swelling around the wound, a moderate increase in temperature, a decrease in blood pressure, and a rapid heartbeat.

Skin around the wound becomes pale due to fluid that builds up under it. A watery, foul-smelling, brownish-red fluid is released later. The tissue changes from pale to dusky to highly discolored as the infection worsens. Left untreated, stupor, delirium, a coma and death can result.

Treatment requires surgical removal of infected tissue and removal of surrounding tissues, along with administration of antibiotics.

Cutaneous abscess

A cutaneous abscess is a raised, swollen collection of pus, usually due to bacteria such as staphylococci. Sometimes the lymph glands in the area become swollen, and you may have a fever.

Treatment consists of opening the infected area, cleaning and irrigating the wound with saline, and packing it with gauze for 24 to 48 hours to absorb the pus and discharge. Application of heat and, if possible, elevating the affected area, may help relieve the inflammation. Your doctor may recommend antibiotics, in addition to drainage of recurrent abscesses.

A particular strain of resistant staphylococci bacteria has become resistant to commonly used antibiotics.

Anthrax

Signs and symptoms

The signs and symptoms of anthrax vary according to type:

- A raised, itchy bump that develops into an open sore with a black center
- Nausea and vomiting
- Loss of appetite
- Fever
- Abdominal pain
- Bloody diarrhea
- A sore throat
- Muscle aches
- Chest discomfort and difficulty breathing

An anthrax infection is caused by the bacterium *Bacillus anthracis*. The disease usually affects livestock, but it can also occur in humans. Anthrax was once common in areas where livestock was raised, but animal vaccination programs have greatly reduced the natural occurrence of the disease among animals and humans.

Anthrax has renewed importance because of its use as a biological weapon. The anthrax bacillus is highly lethal. However, it isn't contagious. There are no reports of the disease spreading from one person to another.

Refined anthrax spores form a fine, white dust. Crude preparations have a sand-colored tint and are clumpier. There are three forms of the infection — skin (cu-

taneous) anthrax, gastrointestinal anthrax, which is contracted from eating infected meat, and inhalation anthrax, the deadliest form.

Skin (cutaneous) anthrax

Skin anthrax occurs when a cut, blister or other skin wound comes into contact with anthrax spores. The infection usually becomes apparent within seven to 12 days of the exposure. It begins as a raised, sometimes itchy bump. Within a day or two, it develops into an open sore with a black center. This is the mildest form of the disease.

Gastrointestinal anthrax

Gastrointestinal anthrax results when a person eats undercooked meat from an infected animal. It causes sores (ulcers) within the intestines.

Initial signs and symptoms generally show up a day to a week after eating contaminated meat. They may include nausea and vomiting, fever, and loss of appetite, followed by abdominal pain and bloody diarrhea. This form can be fatal.

Inhalation anthrax

Inhalation anthrax occurs if enough anthrax spores are inhaled. Once inhaled, the spores can take anywhere from a day to two months to become active.

Initial signs and symptoms are similar to those of the flu or a cold and may include a sore throat, fever, fatigue, muscle aches and chest discomfort. These may last a few hours or a few days. Within three days of onset, the disease progresses, producing a high fever and breathing problems. This type of anthrax destroys lung tissue and may spread to the brain, causing meningitis. It's fatal in the majority of cases, even with appropriate treatment.

Diagnosis

Tests to detect the presence of anthrax bacteria include a skin biopsy, sputum tests and blood tests. A rapid anthrax test allows doctors to

diagnose anthrax in blood samples in less than an hour. To confirm evidence of inhalation anthrax, a chest X-ray may be taken. An endoscopy and stool samples can be used for diagnosing intestinal anthrax, and a spinal tap may be done to check for anthrax meningitis.

How serious is anthrax?

Cutaneous anthrax is rarely fatal. Gastrointestinal anthrax can be fatal without appropriate treatment. Inhalation anthrax is dangerous because its early symptoms are often difficult to distinguish from the flu or a common cold. Once the disease has spread, inhalation anthrax is often lethal.

Treatment

All three forms of anthrax are treated with antibiotics. The medications work by killing the anthrax bacteria. However, antibiotics may fail in inhalation anthrax once symptoms become severe because the bacteria may already have released large amounts of toxin that aren't affected by antibiotics.

Prevention

An anthrax vaccine for humans was approved by the Food and Drug Administration in 1970, but it's currently unavailable to the public, and the supply is limited. The vaccine is presently recommended for military personnel and people who work with anthrax or who live or travel in areas of high exposure. Scientists are working to produce a new vaccine that may require fewer doses and be available in larger quantities.

Hantavirus

Signs and symptoms
Early
- Fatigue
- Fever and chills
- Muscle aches, especially the thighs, hips and back
- Rattling sounds in your lungs (rales)
- Fast breathing

- Fast heartbeat
- Headaches and dizziness

Late
- Coughing
- Shortness of breath
- Fluid in your lungs
- Respiratory shock or failure

The first prominent outbreak of hantavirus pulmonary syndrome (HPS) in the United States occurred in 1993, in the Four Corners area — where the borders of Utah, Colorado, New Mexico and Arizona meet. Other cases likely occurred before then but weren't recognized as such.

The hantavirus is a distant cousin of the Ebola virus and can cause respiratory failure in infected people. Humans become infected by breathing air infected with hantaviruses that are shed in rodent urine and droppings. This may happen when a person is cleaning out sheds, barns, attics or other areas infested by infected rodents, and contaminated dust is kicked up into the air.

Hantavirus is most common during the spring and summer months. Like many infections, the early signs and symptoms of HPS are similar to those of the flu (influenza) — a fever, fatigue and muscle aches, especially around the thighs, hips, back and sometimes shoulders. About half the infected individuals also have headaches, dizziness, chills and abdominal problems, such as nausea, vomiting, diarrhea and abdominal pain.

Symptoms may appear to improve, but within one to two days coughing and shortness of breath occur as the lungs fill with fluid. Breathing difficulty may be subtle at first but rapidly gets worse. Internal bleeding develops, followed by respiratory failure.

Diagnosis
Blood tests are the main method for diagnosing hantavirus pulmonary syndrome. The tests analyze blood samples for the presence of certain antibodies your body produces as a defense against the virus. Your doctor may order further tests to rule out other conditions.

How serious is hantavirus?
HPS is a serious infection that usually requires hospitalization and intensive therapy. Among diagnosed cases, the death rate has been more than 50 percent. If you have a history of contact with rodents and subsequently experience abrupt, flu-like symptoms or have difficulty breathing, see your doctor immediately. Tell your doctor of your contact with rodents so that he or she may know to look for the hantavirus as a possible cause of your illness. When treated early in the disease process, chances of recovery are better.

Treatment
There's currently no effective treatment for HPS. Oxygen therapy is given to help with severe breathing distress. People who are severely ill may be given a breathing tube and ventilator to provide respiratory support. In extremely severe cases, people may be hooked up to a machine that removes carbon dioxide from the blood and adds oxygen to it.

Prevention
To prevent HPS infection, avoid contact with rodent feces, urine and nests. If you're cleaning out a barn or shed or area that may contain rodents, take special precautions, such as wearing a respirator and neutralizing rodent droppings or urine with disinfectants before sweeping or vacuuming.

Variant Creutzfeldt-Jakob (mad cow) disease

Signs and symptoms
- Personality changes
- Anxiety
- Depression
- Memory loss
- Impaired muscle coordination
- Blurred vision
- Speech impairment

Creutzfeldt-Jakob disease (CJD), related to mad cow disease, is a degenerative brain disorder that eventually leads to dementia. The disease captured public attention in the 1990s when individuals in the United Kingdom developed a form of the disease called variant CJD after eating meat from cattle suspected of having bovine spongiform encephalopathy (BSE), the medical term for mad cow disease. Variant CJD causes a rapidly progressive loss of memory, thinking and reasoning skills (dementia), as well as personality changes and problems with muscular coordination.

So far, no cases of BSE or variant CJD have been confirmed in the United States. Public health officials and regulators began monitoring the food industry in the United States after BSE first appeared in the United Kingdom. British authorities eventually traced the outbreak to meat-and-bone meal, a type of feed made from remnants of slaughtered animals. In 1997, the Food and Drug Administration banned the use of this type of feed to protect the food supply from contamination by imported feeds. Regular inspection of cattle in the United States hasn't found any cases of BSE.

Diagnosis
CJD can be diagnosed with 100 percent accuracy only with a brain biopsy or autopsy, when examination of the brain reveals characteristics of the disease, such as buildup of certain proteins called prions. But doctors often can make an accurate diagnosis based on your medical and personal history, a neurological exam, and certain diagnostic tests.

Treatment
No effective treatment exists for Creutzfeldt-Jakob disease and any of its variants. A number of drugs have been tested — including steroids, antibiotics and antiviral agents — and have not shown

Insect and Mite Infestations

Small insects can sometimes attach themselves to your skin and feed on your blood. Some insects do transmit viruses or bacteria that can cause serious illness in humans.

Lice

Signs and symptoms
- Intense itching
- Lice on the scalp, body, clothing, pubic hair or other body hair
- Nits (eggs) on hair shafts
- Small, red bumps on the scalp, neck and shoulders

Lice are tiny, wingless, parasitic insects that feed on your blood. Lice are easily spread — especially by schoolchildren — through close personal contact and by sharing belongings.

Several types of lice exist:
- **Head lice.** These lice develop on your scalp. They're easiest to see at the nape of your neck and over your ears.
- **Body lice.** These lice spend most of their time in the seams and folds of your clothing.
- **Pubic lice.** Commonly called crabs, these lice occur on the skin and hair of your pubic area and on eyelashes.

You can get lice by coming into contact with lice or their eggs. Eggs hatch in about one week. Methods of transmission include head-to-head contact, sharing items such as brushes, clothing or blankets, storing infected clothing in closets, lockers or side by side on hooks, sharing a bed or furniture with an infected person, and through sexual contact.

The first sign of lice is intense itching of the affected area. People with body lice may develop hives or abrasions from scratching. Head lice are easiest to detect at the nape of the neck and over the ears. Small nits that resemble tiny brown buds can be found on the hair shafts (see the illustration on page 397). Body lice are difficult to find on the body because they burrow into the skin, but they usually can be detected in the seams of underwear. Pubic lice are found on the skin and hair of the pubic area.

Diagnosis
Lice are generally diagnosed based on symptoms and identifying the insects.

Treatment
Lice can be treated with medications and some self-care.

Head lice
Over-the-counter lotions or shampoos specifically designed to kill head lice (Nix, Rid, others) are usually the first line of defense. After shampooing your hair or your child's hair, treat it with vinegar. Grasp a lock of hair with a cloth soaked in vinegar and strip the hair downward to remove any remaining eggs (nits). Repeat until you have treated all of the hair this way. You can also remove the nits with a tweezers or fine comb. Repeat this process every three to four days for two weeks to make sure all of the eggs are gone.

In some geographical locations, head lice have grown resistant to the ingredients in over-the-counter products. If nonprescription products don't kill the lice, your doctor

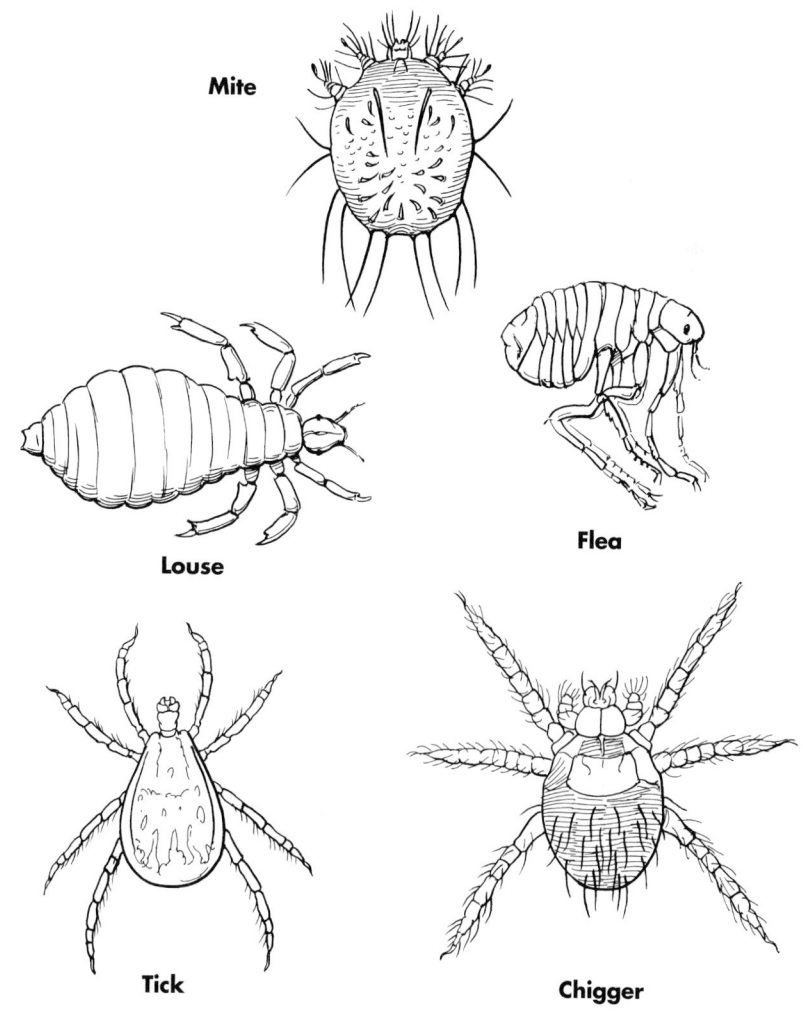

Mite

Louse

Flea

Tick

Chigger

can prescribe a stronger shampoo or lotion. Prescription treatments for head lice include the products malathion (Ovide), benzyl alcohol lotion (Ulesfia), ivermectin lotion (Sklice) and spinosad topical suspension (Natroba).

These products are applied to the scalp and hair for a set period of time and then rinsed off. Some are single-dose treatments, while others require repeat treatment.

Side effects may include redness or irritation of the skin and eyes. Malathion is flammable, so keep it away from heat sources such as hair dryers, curling irons or cigarettes.

Lindane is a prescription shampoo that's sometimes prescribed when other measures fail. Due to increasing resistance of lice to this medication and to potential neurological effects, it's no longer a first-line treatment for head lice.

Whether you use an over-the-counter or prescription shampoo to kill lice, much of the treatment involves steps you can take at home. These include making sure all the nits are removed and that all clothing, bedding, personal items and furniture are decontaminated. Washable items should be washed in hot, soapy water and dried at high heat for at least 20 minutes. Unwashable items should be sealed in an airtight bag for two weeks. In most cases, killing lice on your body isn't difficult. The challenge is getting rid of all the nits and avoiding contact with other lice at home or school.

Body lice

If you have body lice, you don't need treatment, yourself. However, you must take the same self-care measures, such as treating clothing and other items, as you would for head lice.

Pubic lice

Pubic lice can be treated with the same nonprescription and prescription treatments used for head lice. Your sexual partner should be examined and treated if infected.

Scabies

Signs and symptoms
- Severe itching that's often worse at night
- Thin, irregular marks, or burrows, on your skin

Scabies infection is caused by a tiny mite called *Sarcoptes scabiei*. It makes a characteristic burrow that looks like a thin, irregular pencil mark (see the illustration on page 397). Intense itching occurs in places where the mite has burrowed — generally in the folds of your skin, such as between fingers, in armpits, around the neck, around the waist, on the inner elbow, around the breasts and in the male genital area.

The eggs mature in 21 days and the new mites work their way to the surface of your skin, where they mature and then spread to other areas of your body or other people. Scabies is contagious and can spread quickly through close physical contact. It often infests an entire family.

Diagnosis

Your doctor will look for a burrow mark and remove the mite located at the end of one to confirm the diagnosis. Although not serious, scabies are very annoying.

Treatment

Scabies treatment involves eliminating the infestation with medications. Several creams and lotions are available. You usually apply the medication over all your body, from your neck down, and leave the medication on for at least eight hours. Prescription medications commonly prescribed are permethrin (Elimite) and crotamiton (Eurax). Although these medications kill the mites promptly, you may find that the itching doesn't stop entirely for several weeks.

Doctors sometimes prescribe oral medications for people with altered immune systems or for people who don't respond to the prescription lotions and creams.

Because scabies spreads so easily, your doctor may recommend that all family members and other close contacts receive treatment, even if they show no signs of scabies infestation.

Fleas

Signs and symptoms
- A localized rash
- Severe itching

Fleas are small insects that suck blood from dogs, cats, humans and other animals. By using their tremendous jumping ability, they often spread from family pets to their owners. Eggs laid in bedding hatch and remain there to feed off animals or humans.

Fleabites cause intense itching. Clusters of bites can be seen around the waist, along the ankles, in the armpits, and in the crooks of elbows and knees. Hives may develop in people who are especially sensitive to flea saliva.

Diagnosis

The surest way to diagnose flea infestation is by identifying the tiny insects themselves. In the United States, having fleas isn't serious, and you normally don't need to see your doctor if you have them. However, they're annoying and should be eliminated to relieve symptoms.

Treatment

Calamine lotion may help to relieve the itching, but the problem will continue until the fleas are eliminated. Persistent treatment of animals and their living areas is necessary. Once fleas are established, getting rid of them is difficult, and just putting a flea collar on your pet isn't sufficient.

Various flea insecticides are available. Spray one of these on your pet's bedding, as well as on your own, if you suspect that fleas have established there. Furniture and carpeting also should be sprayed. Home foggers help eliminate the insects. However, be careful to remove other pets, such as birds and fish, because they're very sensitive to these insecticides. If you have a heavy infestation of fleas, or other treatments aren't effective, you may have to call a professional exterminator.

Chiggers

Signs and symptoms
- Intense itching
- Pimple-like bumps or hives

Chiggers, also known as redbugs or harvest mites, are the larvae of a type of mite. In North America, they're located primarily in the South, but can be found elsewhere.

Chiggers live in areas of tall grass or brush and on the edges of woods. Farmers, hunters, hikers and others who spend a lot of time in the woods are most likely to become infested.

The larvae prefer warm, moist places and usually take up residence around your waist, on your ankles, in the crooks of your elbows and armpits, in the groin area, and wherever clothing is tight.

These small, red insects attach themselves to the skin and insert a feeding tube to reach a source of blood. This causes small, red pimples and sometimes hives. Several hours after they've inserted their feeding tube, you'll experience intense itching at the site. Chiggers feed in the same spot for up to four days and then drop off.

Diagnosis
The best way to diagnose an infestation of chiggers is by identifying the mites. They can be found in the center of pimples that have not yet been scratched. In the United States, chiggers don't cause any diseases but are annoying because of the intense itching.

Treatment
The aim of treatment is to relieve the itching. Your doctor may prescribe an antihistamine. Corticosteroid creams or lotions also can be applied directly to the pimples.

Ticks

Signs and symptoms
- Itching
- A tick embedded in your skin
- A small lump surrounded by a red circle

Ticks are small, flat insects that feed on blood. They live in tall grasses, brush and wooded areas and attach to animals or people passing by.

Diagnosis
After walking through areas that might contain ticks, check to see if any have attached themselves to your skin or clothing. They can lodge anywhere on your body but are often found in hair, around the ankles and in the genital area. Once embedded, they can cause a small, hard, itchy lump surrounded by a red halo.

How serious is a tick bite?
A tick bite can be serious because ticks may be carriers of many illnesses, including Lyme disease and Rocky Mountain spotted fever. A condition called tick paralysis can occur after a tick has fed on a person for several days. The condition can resemble poliomyelitis, a viral disease that affects your spinal cord. Tick paralysis can be very serious; however, if the tick is removed, the symptoms usually disappear.

Treatment
Don't detach a tick from a pet with your bare hands because infection may result. Don't scratch a tick bite. The body may break off, leaving the head embedded in your skin. Treatment consists of gently — slowly and steadily — removing the tick using a tweezers. Place the tweezers as close to the head of the insect as possible (see page 59).

Lyme disease

Signs and symptoms
- A characteristic red rash at the site of a tick bite
- Headache
- Chills and fever
- Body aches
- Joint pain and swelling
- Temporary paralysis

In the United States, Lyme disease is caused by the bacterium *Borrelia burgdorferi*. Named after a large outbreak among children in Lyme, Connecticut, the illness is transmitted by the deer tick. From May to October, this tick is found throughout the United States, especially on the East and West coasts and in Wisconsin and Minnesota. The ticks are brown and about the size of a head of a pin, making them difficult to spot.

Other *Borrelia* species can cause Lyme disease in Western Europe.

Only a minority of deer tick bites lead to Lyme disease. To get

Deer tick

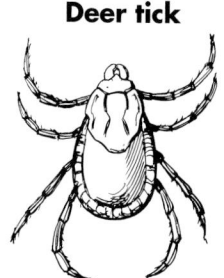

Actual size

Wood tick

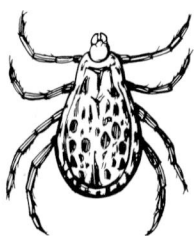

Actual size

The deer tick and wood tick are two common ticks.

Tick-Transmitted Diseases

Although tick bites are usually harmless, they can at times pass on infectious organisms that cause serious illness. In addition to Lyme disease and Rocky Mountain spotted fever, ticks can transmit other less familiar diseases. The following diseases have a number of signs and symptoms in common, including chills, headaches, a fever, profuse sweating, muscle aches, nausea and weight loss. Antibiotics are generally the recommended treatment.

Human anaplasmosis

Signs and symptoms of human anaplasmosis generally develop about a week after the bite. In addition to the common tick-bite symptoms, diarrhea, an altered mental state, rash and other problems also may develop later. In some cases, the condition can be fatal.

Human ehrlichiosis

Ehrlichiosis is a bacterial disease that's spread by infected ticks. It causes flu-like symptoms that generally appear within a week or two of the tick bite. Most infections are mild or without symptoms, but some can be severe and life-threatening. If treated quickly with antibiotics, ehrlichiosis generally improves within a few days.

Human babesiosis

Human babesiosis is carried by the same tick that carries Lyme disease. It can be very severe in people with no spleen. The infectious agent's incubation period can last weeks to months.

Tularemia

Tularemia can be acquired from tick bites or from eating improperly cooked meat or drinking contaminated water. Among reported cases in the United States, the death rate is less than 2 percent. It can be treated with intravenous (IV) antibiotics.

the disease, you must be bitten by an infected tick. The longer the tick remains attached to your skin, the greater your risk of getting the disease.

If you know you've been bitten and you experience signs or symptoms of the disease, contact your doctor immediately.

Diagnosis

Lyme disease is difficult to diagnose because it mimics several other diseases. A characteristic target-shaped red rash usually occurs at the site of the tick bite (see the illustration on page 397), followed by flu-like symptoms.

Sometimes, the bite may go entirely unnoticed. A few weeks to months later, the person who was bitten may experience facial paralysis, joint inflammation, various neurological symptoms and sometimes heart palpitations and heart block, a condition where impulses are improperly conducted within the heart.

Your doctor may perform a blood test to check for antibodies to the organism. However, the test isn't always conclusive. In the earliest stages of the disease, the test often doesn't produce positive results. In the case of an inflamed and swollen joint, fluid may be drawn from the joint for analysis.

Many people who have unexplained symptoms such as fatigue, malaise and trouble concentrating believe they have Lyme disease. However, in most cases Lyme disease isn't the cause.

How serious is Lyme disease?

If detected in its early stages, the disease can be treated with medication. If not treated early, complications involving the joints, heart, and central and peripheral nervous system can occur.

Treatment

Treatment may include:

Oral antibiotics

Oral antibiotics are the standard treatment for early-stage Lyme disease. These usually include doxycycline for adults and children older than age 8, or amoxicillin or cefuroxime axetil for younger children and pregnant or breast-feeding women. The drugs often clear the infection and prevent complications. A 14- to 21-day course of antibiotics is usually recommended, but some studies suggest that courses lasting 10 to 14 days are equally effective. In some cases, longer treatment has been linked to serious complications.

Intravenous antibiotics

If the disease has progressed, your doctor may recommend treatment with an intravenous antibiotic for 14 to 28 days. This is effective in eliminating infection, although it may take some time to recover from your symptoms. Intravenous antibiotics can cause various side effects, including gallstones and mild to severe diarrhea.

Prevention

When walking in wooded or grassy areas, wear shoes, light-colored

Beware of Bismacine

The Food and Drug Administration (FDA) warns consumers and health care providers to avoid bismacine, an injectable compound prescribed by some alternative medicine practitioners to treat Lyme disease.

Bismacine, also known as chromacine, contains high levels of the metal bismuth. Although bismuth is safely used in some oral medications for stomach ulcers, it's not approved for use in injectable form or as a treatment for Lyme disease. Bismacine can cause bismuth poisoning, which may lead to heart and kidney failure.

clothing, long pants tucked into your socks and long-sleeved shirts. Apply tick repellents containing 20 to 50 percent DEET to your skin or clothing.

Check yourself and your pets often for ticks. If you find any, remove them by using a tweezers. Grasp the tick close to the head and pull directly outward. Don't yank or crush the tick. Pull carefully and steadily. If the tick has been attached for less than 24 hours, infection usually doesn't follow, but it's a good idea to see your doctor.

Rocky Mountain spotted fever

Signs and symptoms
- High fever and chills
- Severe headache
- Widespread aches and pains
- Restlessness
- Fatigue
- Loss of appetite
- A rash of red spots or blotches

Rocky Mountain spotted fever is a bacterial infection caused by the organism *Rickettsia rickettsii*. It's transmitted to humans by tick bites. The illness is named after the Rocky Mountain region, where it was first identified.

In the western United States, Rocky Mountain spotted fever is transmitted by the wood tick. In the eastern United States, where the disease is most common, it's transmitted by the American dog tick. In the southern United States and Central and South America, the disease is transmitted by other types of ticks.

In the United States, Rocky Mountain spotted fever occurs primarily during the late spring and early summer, when the ticks are most active, and during warm weather when people tend to spend more time outdoors.

The illness begins with flu-like symptoms. Between the second and sixth days, a red rash appears on your wrists and ankles. The rash spreads up your arms and legs to your chest.

Diagnosis
Your doctor may attempt to establish a diagnosis of the condition by doing a blood test or examining a specimen (biopsy) of the rash to search for the presence of the *Rickettsia rickettsii* organism.

How serious is Rocky Mountain spotted fever?
A mild case of Rocky Mountain spotted fever that's treated promptly causes few problems. Even without treatment, mild cases may disappear after two weeks. In a small percentage of infected people, the disease can be serious or even fatal, especially in older adults.

Treatment
Treatment for Rocky Mountain spotted fever involves careful removal of the tick from your skin and antibiotic medication, such as doxycycline or tetracycline, to eliminate the infection.

Prevention
When walking in wooded or grassy areas, wear shoes, light-colored clothing, long pants tucked into your socks and long-sleeved shirts. Apply tick repellents containing 20 to 50 percent DEET to your skin or clothing. Check yourself and your pets often for ticks. If you find any, remove them with a tweezers.

West Nile virus

Signs and symptoms
- Skin rash
- Headache
- Fever
- Nausea
- Diarrhea and vomiting
- Muscle aches

Emergency signs and symptoms
- High fever
- Severe headaches
- Stiff neck
- Disorientation and confusion
- Tremors or muscle jerking
- A coma

West Nile virus is transmitted by mosquitoes. If you become infected, you may not experience any signs or symptoms or you may experience only mild signs or symptoms. However, some people, particularly those with suppressed immune systems, can develop life-threatening illness that includes inflammation of the brain (encephalitis) and membranes surrounding the brain and spinal cord (meningitis).

West Nile virus made its first appearance in the United States in 1999, when an outbreak occurred in and around New York City. An epidemic of the virus resulted in severe illness in 59 people and seven deaths. The virus was first identified in Uganda in 1937.

Mosquitoes transmit the virus to humans. The main reservoirs for the virus are wild birds. It's of particular concern that the migratory patterns of birds have led to the spread of the virus to new locations. Since the outbreak in New York, the virus has been detected in several states.

Infection with the virus occurs primarily when the weather is mild and mosquito populations are active. It takes five to 15 days from the time of infection before symptoms of the illness appear.

Diagnosis
West Nile virus can be confirmed by rising levels of antibodies to the virus in your blood, or from a positive culture of West Nile virus drawn from a blood sample. Finding West Nile virus genetic material in body fluids also confirms an infection.

How serious is West Nile virus?
Anyone bitten by an infected mosquito is at risk of acquiring the virus, although the chance of developing a West Nile virus-related illness after being bitten is very small.

In most cases, people who become infected recover fully. The risk of severe infection is greater for people over age 50 or who have weakened immune systems.

Treatment

There's no specific treatment for West Nile virus and no vaccine is currently available, although steps are being taken in this direction. Many people recover without treatment. However, severe cases may require hospitalization.

Scientists are investigating interferon therapy — a type of immune cell therapy — as a treatment for encephalitis caused by West Nile virus. Some research shows those who receive the therapy recover better than those who don't, but more study is needed.

Prevention

To prevent a West Nile virus infection, take precautions against exposure to mosquitoes. This includes wearing pants and long-sleeved shirts and using insect repellent. Mosquitoes are most active between dusk and dawn.

Zika virus

Signs and symptoms
- Mild fever
- Rash
- Joint or muscle pain
- Headache
- Red eyes (conjunctivitis)

Zika virus disease is a mosquito-borne viral infection that primarily occurs in tropical and subtropical areas of the world. Most people infected with Zika virus have no signs and symptoms, while others report mild symptoms and a general feeling of discomfort. When symptoms do occur, they usually begin two to seven days after being bitten by an infected mosquito. Most people recover fully, with symptoms resolving in about a week.

Zika virus is transmitted primarily through the bite of an infected Aedes species mosquito. It was first identified in the Zika Valley in Africa in 1947. Outbreaks have since been reported worldwide. When a mosquito bites a person infected with Zika virus, the virus enters the mosquito. When the infected mosquito bites another person, the virus enters that person's bloodstream. Spread of the virus through sexual contact and blood transfusion also have been reported.

Factors that put you at greater risk of developing Zika virus disease include:
- **Travel to outbreak areas.** Being in tropical and subtropical areas increases your risk of exposure to the virus that causes Zika virus disease. Because the mosquito that carries Zika virus is found worldwide, it's likely that outbreaks will continue to spread to new regions.
- **Having unprotected sex.** Isolated cases of sexually transmitted Zika virus have been reported. If a man has traveled to an area of active Zika virus transmission, abstinence from sexual activity or condom use during all sexual contact with a pregnant sex partner is advised.

Diagnosis

See your doctor if you think you or a family member may have Zika virus, especially if you've recently traveled to an area where there's an ongoing outbreak. The Centers for Disease Control and Prevention (CDC) has blood tests to look for Zika virus or similar diseases such as dengue or chikungunya viruses, which are spread by the same type of mosquitoes.

Talk to your doctor about which tests for Zika virus or similar diseases are available in your area.

How serious is Zika virus?

Zika virus infections during pregnancy have been linked to miscarriage and can cause microcephaly, a potentially fatal congenital brain condition. Zika virus may also cause other neurological disorders such as Guillain-Barre syndrome.

A pregnant woman with no symptoms of Zika virus infection who recently traveled to an area with active Zika virus transmission may be offered testing two to 12 weeks after her return. A doctor may also perform an ultrasound to detect microcephaly or other abnormalities of the brain or offer to take a sample of amniotic fluid using a hollow needle inserted into the uterus (amniocentesis) to screen for Zika virus.

Treatment

No specific antiviral treatment for Zika virus disease exists. Treatment is aimed at relieving symptoms with rest, fluids and nonprescription medications to relieve joint pain and fever.

Prevention

All blood donations are not screened for Zika virus. Researchers also are working on a Zika virus vaccine; to date, none exists.

The best prevention is to avoid mosquito bites. The Centers for Disease Control and Prevention (CDC) recommends pregnant women avoid traveling to areas where there's an outbreak of Zika virus. If you're trying to become pregnant, talk to your doctor about upcoming travel plans.

If you have a male partner who lives in or has traveled to an area where there's an outbreak of Zika virus, the CDC recommends abstaining from sex or using a condom if you're pregnant or trying to become pregnant.

If you live in or must travel to areas where Zika virus exists, follow these tips:
- **Stay in air-conditioned or well-screened housing.** The mosquitoes that carry the Zika virus are most active from dawn to dusk, but they can also bite at night.
- **Wear protective clothing.** When you go into mosquito-infested areas, wear a long-sleeved shirt, long pants, socks and shoes.
- **Use mosquito repellent.** Permethrin can be applied to your clothing, shoes, camping gear and bed netting. You also can buy clothing made with permethrin already in it. Use a repellent containing a 20 to 50 percent concentration of DEET.

Parasitic Infestations

Parasites range from microscopic, single-celled organisms called protozoans to larger worms called helminths. Protozoans often spend part of their life cycle outside of humans, living in food, soil, water or insects. The protozoan that causes malaria is an example. Some protozoans are commonly present in your body but are kept under control by your immune system.

Tapeworms and roundworms are the most common types of helminths. If they enter your body, they may take up residence in your intestinal tract, lungs, liver, skin or brain, where they live off nutrients available at those sites.

Malaria

Signs and symptoms

- Moderate to severe shaking chills
- High fever
- Sweating as body temperature falls
- Feelings of unease and discomfort
- Headache
- Nausea and vomiting

Malaria is caused by a parasite that's transmitted by mosquitoes. Malaria may also be transmitted through contaminated blood transfusions and by the sharing of contaminated needles. The disease is found primarily in the rural areas of tropical and subtropical countries. It's one of the leading infectious killers in the world, particularly of children.

The female mosquito becomes infected with the malarial parasite when it bites a human who has malaria and ingests blood containing the protozoa. After developing in the mosquito, the parasite is then transmitted to other humans by subsequent bites of the mosquito. In humans, the parasite migrates to the liver. Later it enters the bloodstream and infects red blood cells. The parasites multiply in the cells and, 48 to 72 hours later, depending on the species, cause the red blood cells to rupture, releasing a new generation of parasites.

Symptoms of malaria relate closely to the parasite's life cycle. After an incubation period anywhere from eight days to eight months, chills and fever begin, lasting 15 minutes to an hour, which correspond to the rupture of the red blood cells. A headache, vomiting and nausea also may occur. A fever remains high for several hours, and then sweating begins as body temperature falls. The cycle may recur every 48 to 72 hours, depending on the species of protozoan.

Diagnosis

After noting your symptoms and travel history, your doctor will likely obtain a sample of your blood for microscopic observation. Two to three blood samples taken at six- to 12-hour intervals can usually confirm the presence of the parasite and its type.

How serious is malaria?

Left untreated, some forms of malaria can be fatal. Approximately 150 to 300 million cases of malaria occur worldwide each year, and approximately 430,000 people die of this disease annually. In the United States, about 1,500 to 2,000 cases are reported each year, primarily among people returning from mosquito-prone areas.

Treatment

Doctors can often treat malaria effectively with one or more of the following medications:

- Chloroquine
- Quinine sulfate (Qualaquin)
- Hydroxychloroquine (Plaquenil)
- Combination of sulfadoxine and pyrimethamine
- Mefloquine
- Combination of atovaquone and proguanil (Malarone)
- Doxycycline (Doryx, Vibramycin)
- **Artemisinin-derived medications.** These antimalarial medications are derived from artemisinin, a sweet wormwood extract.
- **Halofantrine.** Doctors sometimes will use halofantrine to treat malaria, although it's not marketed in the United States. If you've been taking mefloquine for prevention of malaria or if you have heart problems, don't take halofantrine because it can be dangerous and possibly fatal.
- **Primaquine.** This drug may be given to fight the dormant liver form of the parasite and prevent relapses. However, the Centers for Disease Control and Prevention (CDC) has warned against taking primaquine if you're pregnant or have an enzyme deficiency called glucose-6-phosphate dehydrogenase (G6PD).

Which drug you take and the length of treatment depend on the type of malaria, where you were infected, your age and how sick you were when treatment began.

Prevention

There is no vaccine yet for malaria. However, many drugs are effective preventive medications. Consult with a travel medicine expert to find out if you need one of these medicines and which one.

Possible reactions to mefloquine include nausea, dizziness, insomnia and vivid dreams. People with epilepsy or other seizure disorders shouldn't take mefloquine. Children under age 8 should avoid doxycycline, as it can permanently stain their teeth. Malarone shouldn't be taken by people with severe kidney impairment. Some drugs that prevent malaria may cause miscarriage or stillbirth in pregnant women.

Take precautions in malaria-prone areas. Sleep under permethrin-treated mosquito netting, stay in buildings with screens on doors and windows, and stay indoors during times when the mosquitoes feed. Wear mosquito repellent containing 20 to 50 percent DEET.

Tapeworm

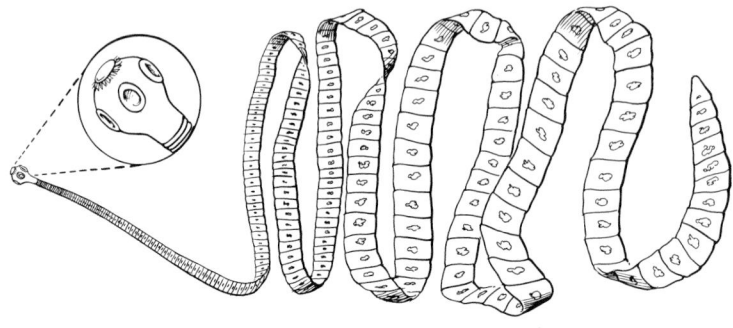

The largest species of tapeworm can grow up to 75 feet long.

Tapeworms

Signs and symptoms
- Segments of adult tapeworm in stool
- Nausea
- Loss of appetite
- Weakness
- Abdominal pain
- Diarrhea
- Weight loss

Tapeworm infection usually occurs when you eat food or drink water that's contaminated with tapeworm eggs or larvae. The parasites are generally ingested through food, water or soil that's contaminated with human or animal feces.

Tapeworms occur in humans in one of two forms. If ingested as eggs, they might develop into larvae that migrate out of the intestines and form cysts in other tissues, such as the lungs or liver. These cysts can cause serious problems. If ingested as larvae, they typically develop into adult tapeworms in the intestines and cause few or no symptoms.

Adult tapeworms can measure up to 50 feet long and can survive as long as 20 years. Some tapeworms attach themselves to the walls of the intestine, where they can cause irritation or mild inflammation, while others pass through your stool and exit your body.

In humans, tapeworm infection is most commonly caused by one of several tapeworm species: the pork tapeworm, the beef tapeworm, the dwarf tapeworm and the fish tapeworm.

Factors that increase your risk of tapeworm infection include poor hygiene, improper disposal of human and animal feces, frequent travel to developing countries, and eating raw or undercooked meats.

Tapeworms usually cause few symptoms. When symptoms do occur they generally include fatigue, loss of appetite, weight loss, vomiting and irritability — especially in children. In severe cases, nausea, diarrhea and abdominal pain may be present.

Diagnosis
Tapeworms are usually discovered when eggs are found in the stool or worm segments are found in the stool, bedding or clothing. A doctor generally makes the diagnosis by obtaining eggs or segments and having them examined in a laboratory. The lab might need two or three samples over a period of time to detect the parasite, since eggs and tapeworm segments are released irregularly in stool.

Your doctor may also test your blood for antibodies your body may have produced to fight the tapeworm infection.

How serious is a tapeworm infestation?
Usually, the presence of tapeworms in the intestines isn't a serious situation. But some types of tapeworms can penetrate the intestinal wall and spread to various internal organs. The resulting condition may become very serious.

Treatment
The most common treatment for tapeworm infection involves oral medications that are toxic to the tapeworm. These drugs include praziquantel (Biltricide) or albendazole (Albenza), as well as niclosamide, although this drug is not available in the United States. The medication prescribed depends on the species of organism and site of infection involved.

The medications are poorly absorbed by your digestive tract and generally work by dissolving or attacking the adult tapeworm. Be aware that these drugs target the adult tapeworm, not the eggs, so take care to avoid reinfecting yourself. Always wash your hands after using the toilet and before eating.

Treatment should render your stool free of tapeworm eggs, larvae or proglottids. The success rate is very good in people who receive appropriate treatment.

In cases in which the tapeworm infection has migrated to tissues outside your intestine, your doctor may prescribe an anti-inflammatory steroid to reduce any swelling caused by the development of cysts.

Surgery may be required to remove cysts that have developed in your liver, lungs or other organs, and organ transplantation may be your last resort in some cases.

Trichinosis

Signs and symptoms
- Diarrhea and cramps
- Malaise

- Fever
- Muscle pain and tenderness
- Facial swelling

Trichinosis is a type of round-worm infection. Roundworms are parasites that use a host body to stay alive and reproduce.

Trichinosis occurs primarily among meat-eating animals. People get trichinosis when they eat infected meat — such as pork, bear, horse or walrus — that's undercooked. Some cases have been linked to eating beef that was mixed with infected pork or ground in a grinder previously used for contaminated pork.

In the United States, trichinosis was most commonly found in hog-producing regions. However, due to increased regulation of pork feed and products, pigs are now a less common source of infection. Bear meat has now become the most common source of trichinosis in the United States.

Two to 12 days after eating infected meat, you may experience diarrhea, abdominal cramps and malaise lasting from one to seven days, although some people experience no symptoms. When the muscles are invaded by the larvae, muscle pain and tenderness, fever, swelling of the face, and weakness may develop and last about six weeks.

Diagnosis
In addition to your symptoms, your doctor may use blood tests and a sample of muscle tissue (muscle biopsy) to confirm the diagnosis.

How serious is trichinosis?
Except in severe cases, trichinosis usually isn't serious and often gets better on its own.

Treatment
Trichinosis often gets better on its own. More-severe infections may respond to medication.
- **Anti-parasite medication.** Anti-parasite (anti-helminthic) medication is the first line of treatment against trichinosis. If the trichinella parasite is discovered early, in the intestinal phase, albendazole (Albenza) or mebendazole can be effective in eliminating the intestinal worms and larvae. You may have mild gastrointestinal side effects during the course of treatment, and you may need to take repeat doses to get rid of the infestation completely.
- **Pain relievers.** After muscle invasion, pain relievers may be given for muscle aches. Eventually, the larvae cysts in your muscles tend to calcify, resulting in destruction of the larvae and the end of muscle aches and fatigue.
- **Corticosteroids.** Some cases of trichinosis cause allergic reactions when the parasite enters muscle tissue or when dead or dying larvae release chemicals in your muscle tissue. Your doctor may prescribe a corticosteroid to control inflammation during larval migration.

Pinworms

Signs and symptoms
- Itching of the anal or vaginal area
- Insomnia, irritability and restlessness
- Vague gastrointestinal symptoms

Pinworm infection is the most common type of roundworm infection in the United States. Inside your body, the pinworm's microscopic eggs hatch and grow into adults, measuring about 0.2 to 0.4 inches. The worms mature in your intestine and then travel through your digestive tract to lay eggs in the anal area. The primary symptom is severe itching around the anus, particularly at night.

You acquire a pinworm infection by ingesting pinworm eggs from contaminated food, drink or hands. After the eggs are swallowed, they hatch in the small intestine and migrate to the large intestine. The entire cycle takes three to four weeks,

Pinworm

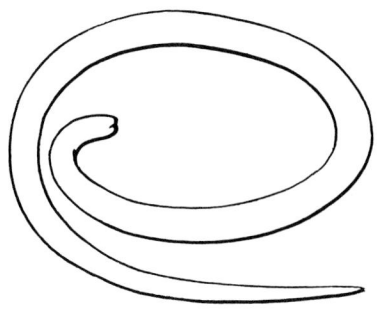

Pinworms are very small. The actual size of a pinworm is about 3/8 inch long.

and the eggs are contagious for up to two to three weeks. Pinworms occur more frequently in children than in adults.

Many pinworm infections cause no symptoms or only mild digestive problems. But if you're infected with hundreds of worms, more-serious symptoms and complications can occur.

Diagnosis
Pinworms are diagnosed by identifying eggs taken from the skin around the anal area. The most reliable method is to apply a short piece of cellophane tape to the area. A doctor may press a piece of clear plastic tape against the skin around the anus and examine the tape under a microscope for pinworms.

Because the parasite typically lays eggs at night, you may want to do the tape test yourself first thing in the morning before defecating or bathing. Take the tape sample to your doctor.

How serious is pinworm infestation?
A pinworm infestation is annoying, but it isn't serious. It's easily treated, but reinfection is common.

Treatment
If you have symptoms, you may need an anti-parasite medication. The most commonly used for pinworms is albendazole (Albenza).

Ascaris lumbricoides

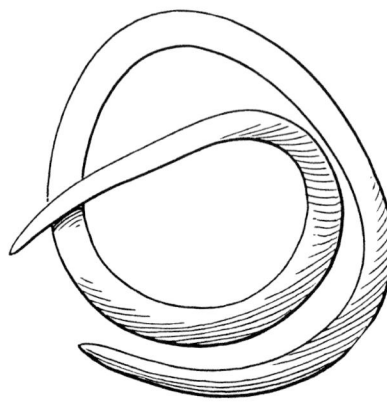

***Ascaris lumbricoides* is the largest of the roundworms, ranging in length from 6 to 16 inches.**

These medications work by killing the adult worms as well as the larvae and eggs to prevent reinfection. You may have mild gastrointestinal side effects during the course of treatment, and you may need to take multiple doses to get rid of the pinworms completely.

If anal or vaginal itching is severe or interfering with your sleep, your doctor may prescribe a soothing ointment or cream to use until the pinworms are gone.

Pinworm reinfection is common, so your doctor may remind you to avoid scratching the anal area, keep your fingernails clean, clean toilet seats twice a day, thoroughly launder any potentially infected clothing or sheets, and wash your hands thoroughly after defecating.

Strongyloidosis

Signs and symptoms
- Small, possibly itchy, skin lesions
- Diarrhea, sometimes alternating with constipation
- Abdominal pain
- Gas (flatulence)

Strongyloidosis is caused by the small worm *Strongyloides stercoralis*. Also known as threadworm, it's found in many tropical and subtropical areas. Strongyloidosis sometimes occurs in temperate areas, including the United States. It's common in overcrowded, unsanitary conditions.

The first sign of a strongyloidosis infestation is the appearance of small, red and sometimes itchy lesions caused by the larvae entering the skin. The larvae travel through the bloodstream to the lungs, where they rise to the throat and are swallowed. They then inhabit the intestine, causing gastrointestinal symptoms. In severe cases, diarrhea is accompanied by blood and mucus.

Diagnosis
Making a diagnosis can be difficult because of the wide variety of symptoms. Finding larvae in stool or fluid from the small intestine confirms the diagnosis.

How serious is strongyloidosis?
Unless the infection is severe, most people recover completely once the worms are eliminated.

Treatment
Strongyloides infection is treated with anti-parasite (anti-helminthic) medication, medications used to treat worm infections.

Ascariasis

Signs and symptoms
- Persistent cough
- Shortness of breath
- Wheezing
- Vague abdominal pain
- Nausea and vomiting
- Diarrhea or bloody stools

Ascariasis is a type of roundworm infection. Eggs of the ascaris roundworm are microscopic, but adult worms can reach lengths up to 16 inches.

The highest rates of ascariasis infection occur in places where sanitation and hygiene are poor. The ascaris parasite can be transmitted when infected human feces are mixed with soil. The eggs infect their hosts when humans eat contaminated vegetables or fruit grown in that soil.

After migrating to the lungs, the larvae rise to the mouth and are swallowed. Eventually, they take up residence in the small intestine, where they develop into an adult form that lives for up to two years.

Diagnosis
If you notice anything resembling a worm when you cough or vomit, keep it and let your doctor examine it. Other tests, such as stool tests, blood tests and imaging tests, also can help your doctor identify the parasite.

How serious is ascariasis?
Ascariasis generally isn't a serious condition and sometimes may get better without treatment. Heavy infestations can cause severe symptoms.

Treatment
Anti-parasite (anti-helminthic) medications are the first line of treatment against ascariasis. The most common are mebendazole and albendazole (Albenza). They work by killing the adult worms. You may have mild gastrointestinal side effects during treatment.

Although the medications are generally effective at killing adult worms, you may need to take multiple doses to get rid of the infestation completely or if you become reinfected.

In cases of heavy infestation, surgery may be necessary to repair damage the worms have caused and to remove worms. Intestinal obstruction or perforation, bile duct obstruction and appendicitis are complications that may require surgery.

Hookworms

Signs and symptoms
- A dry cough
- Difficulty breathing
- A low-grade fever
- Weakness and fatigue
- Loss of appetite
- Diarrhea
- Ulcer-like abdominal pain

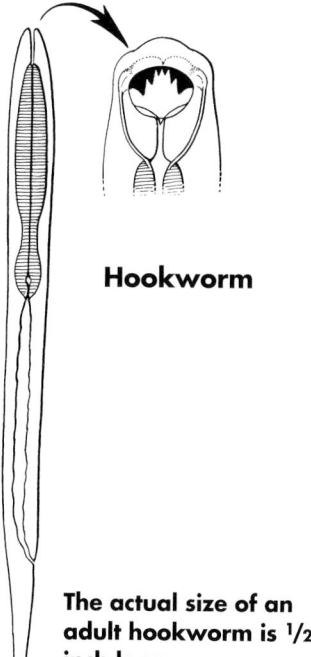

Hookworm

The actual size of an adult hookworm is ¹/₂ inch long.

- Pallor
- Blood-tinged sputum

Hookworm infections are widespread in tropical and subtropical areas. The larvae live in damp soil and can penetrate the skin between the toes, enter the bloodstream and proceed to the lungs.

From the lungs, the larvae go to the throat, are swallowed and attach to the lining of the small intestine, where they develop into half-inch-long adult worms. The disease may affect anyone, but children are particularly susceptible to severe infestations.

At the spot where the hookworms enter the skin, the larvae cause an itchy rash called ground itch. When in the lungs, they provoke a dry cough, wheezing, difficulty breathing, a low-grade fever and sputum tinged with blood. Two weeks after entering the skin, they reach the intestines.

Diagnosis

You may experience no symptoms, but in people with serious infestations or without adequate iron intake, the worms can cause a loss of appetite, bloody diarrhea, abdominal pain, weakness and fa-

tigue, pallor, and anemia. Finding microscopic hookworm eggs in the feces confirms the diagnosis.

How serious is hookworm infestation?

Because hookworms don't reproduce in humans, they die and disappear in one to five years, depending on the species. People with mild or severe cases usually recover completely with proper treatment.

Treatment

If you have no intestinal symptoms, treatment for hookworms is unnecessary. The worms eventually will be passed out of your system. If you have a heavy infestation, an anti-parasitic medication is necessary. Several types of prescription medications are available. However, certain drugs shouldn't be used by pregnant women. If you're pregnant, be sure to tell your doctor. A diet high in protein, vitamins and iron supplements will prevent malnutrition and anemia until the infestation is eradicated.

Sexually Transmitted Infections

Several bacterial and viral infections are sexually transmitted infections (STIs) — also known as sexually transmitted diseases. They can be transmitted by sexual contact. Gonorrhea, chlamydia and syphilis are bacterial infections. Herpes and venereal warts are viral infections. Other infections also can be sexually transmitted.

Gonorrhea

Signs and symptoms
- Thick, pus-like discharge from the urethra or rectum
- Painful urination
- Abdominal or pelvic pain
- Anal itching
- Sore throat

Gonorrhea is a sexually transmitted bacterium that can infect men and women. It can affect the urethra, rectum and throat of both men and women. In women, gonorrhea can also infect the cervix.

Most people contact gonorrhea during sex. But pregnant women with gonorrhea can also pass the bacterium to their babies. In babies, gonorrhea most commonly affects the eyes.

The Centers for Disease Control and Prevention reports about 400,000 people contract gonorrhea each year in the United States. Many don't know they have it. About half of infected women don't experience symptoms at all, which increases the risk of spreading the disease. Homosexual men also may not have symptoms, especially when the infection affects the pharynx or rectum.

Men may experience a tingling sensation in the tube that carries urine from the bladder (urethra). A few hours later, urination becomes painful and a milky discharge is noted. As the infection progresses, urethral pain becomes more pronounced and large amounts of creamy, pus-like discharge are produced.

In women, the infection usually affects the cervix and other reproductive organs as well as the urethra. You may develop frequent, urgent and painful urination, and a pus-like discharge from the vagina or urethra. The symptoms are often so mild that many women don't realize they have the infection.

In both sexes, rectal gonorrhea may result from anal intercourse with an infected person or from the infection spreading to the rectum from the genital area. It may cause discomfort in the anal area and rectal discharge. Oral sex can produce pharyngeal gonorrhea, resulting in a sore throat and painful swallowing. Again, many people have no symptoms.

Diagnosis

To confirm a diagnosis of gonorrhea, your doctor will likely take specimens of the discharge or infected tissue for laboratory examination. This must be done before antibiotics are taken. The symptoms of gonorrhea are similar to those of a number of other STIs, so it's important to know exactly what's causing them.

How serious is gonorrhea?

Gonorrhea is an acute infection that can become chronic if not treated. In men, gonorrhea may lead to epididymitis (see page 1242). In women, it can spread to the uterus and fallopian tubes, causing pelvic inflammatory disease (PID), which can cause scarring and infertility.

Gonorrhea can also spread through the bloodstream to cause infection in other parts of the body. A fever, rash, joint pain and stiffness are possible. These complications can cause permanent joint damage. If treated appropriately, gonorrheal infections usually can be cured. However, some strains of gonococci are resistant to many antibiotics.

Treatment

If you have gonorrhea, it's important that you abstain from sexual contact until your infection is completely eliminated. Your doctor will prescribe antibiotics to treat the infection. You may receive the treatment as an injection or as a tablet taken by mouth. Because some forms of the disease have become drug resistant, a combination of antibiotics may be needed.

Your partner should also undergo testing and treatment, even if he or she has no symptoms. Your partner will likely receive the same treatment as you do. You can be reinfected with gonorrhea if your partner isn't treated.

Babies born to mothers with gonorrhea receive a medication to their eyes soon after birth to prevent infection. If an infection does develop, babies can be treated with antibiotics.

Chlamydia

Signs and symptoms

- Painful urination
- Lower abdominal pain
- Vaginal discharge in women
- Discharge from the penis in men
- Painful sexual intercourse in women
- Testicular pain in men

Chlamydia is a bacterial infection of the genital tract that spreads easily through sexual contact. It's one of the most common sexually transmitted diseases in the United States. Each year, approximately 1.5 million Americans are infected with chlamydia.

In men, chlamydial infection may cause a burning sensation during urination and a discharge from the urethra. Symptoms may appear one to three weeks after exposure. Women may have no symptoms, or they may experience burning urination, a thin vaginal discharge or lower abdominal pain. Many must rely on having their sexual partners inform them that they have the disease.

Diagnosis

Diagnosing can be difficult because symptoms may be slight or nonexistent. When they are present, they're similar to those of gonorrhea.

Tests for chlamydial infection involve identifying the bacteria in secretions from the cervix (in women) or from urethral or seminal fluid (in men). A urine sample also may indicate this infection.

How serious is chlamydia?

In men, chlamydial infections can cause epididymitis (see page 1242) and inflammation of the urethra. In women, they can cause urethral infection and inflammation of the cervix and other pelvic organs. If you engage in anal sex with an infected partner, the organism may cause inflammation of the rectum. In a newborn, conjunctivitis or pneumonia may occur during the first two weeks after birth.

Treatment

Doctors treat chlamydia with prescription antibiotics such as azithromycin (Zithromax), doxycycline or erythromycin. Your doctor usually prescribes these antibiotics as pills to be swallowed. You may be asked to take your medication in a one-time dose, or you may receive a prescription medication to be taken daily or multiple times a day for five to 10 days.

In most cases, the infection resolves within one to two weeks. During that time you should abstain from sex. Your sexual partner or partners also need treatment even though they may not have signs or symptoms. Otherwise, the infection can be passed back and forth. It's possible to be reinfected with chlamydia.

Syphilis

Signs and symptoms

Primary
- Painless sores on the genitals, rectum, tongue or lips
- Enlarged lymph nodes in the groin

Secondary
- A rash over any area of the body, but especially on the palms of the hands and soles of the feet
- Fever
- Fatigue
- Soreness and aching
- Swollen lymph glands

Tertiary
- Jerky or uncoordinated muscle movements
- Paralysis
- Gradual blindness
- Dementia

Syphilis is a bacterial infection usually spread by sexual contact. Syphilis rates in the United States have been rising in recent years. According to the Centers for Disease Control and Prevention, nearly two-thirds of new infections occur in men who have sex with men.

The organism gains entrance to the body through minor cuts or abrasions in the skin or mucous membranes. The disease can also be transmitted by infected blood and from a mother to her unborn child during pregnancy (congenital syphilis).

Syphilis develops in stages and symptoms vary with each stage. In some cases, signs or symptoms don't develop for many years after infection, or they disappear for a considerable period of time. This is known as the latent, or hidden, stage.

Diagnosis

Syphilis can be diagnosed with a blood test identifying antibodies to the bacteria in your blood, or by testing a sample of fluid from sores. Your doctor may scrape a small sample of cells from a sore to be analyzed in a laboratory. In the disease's later stage, examination of your spinal fluid may be necessary to determine whether the nervous system is involved.

How serious is syphilis?

Syphilis can be cured if it's diagnosed early and the infection is treated appropriately. If not treated, the disease can be fatal. If a woman contracts the disease while she's pregnant, it can be transmitted to her unborn child, causing deformities or death of the child.

Treatment

When diagnosed and treated early, the disease is easy to cure. Penicillin is highly effective in treating syphilis. If you're sensitive to penicillin, your doctor may prescribe another type of antibiotic or desensitize you to penicillin. The first day you receive treatment you may experience a reaction that includes a fever, chills, nausea, body aches and a headache. This reaction usually doesn't last more than a day.

Genital herpes

Signs and symptoms

- Small, red bumps, blisters or open sores in the genital area
- Pain or itching in the genital area

Genital herpes is a highly contagious infection caused by the herpes simplex virus (HSV).

There are two types — oral and genital. That which affects the mouth and lips, causing a cold sore, generally stems from herpes simplex virus type 1 (HSV-1). That which affects the genital area is typically caused by herpes simplex virus type 2 (HSV-2).

Genital herpes may be transmitted by vaginal, oral or anal sex. The virus enters the body through tiny cuts in the skin or mucous membranes. It can infect the eyes by contact with a contaminated finger. It affects both men and women.

Signs and symptoms tend to come and go, and they may recur for years. Some people experience numerous episodes each year. For many people, though, the outbreaks become less frequent as time passes. Various factors may trigger outbreaks, including stress, menstruation, illness, surgery or certain medications. Some people with mild disease don't experience any signs and symptoms.

Diagnosis

A doctor usually can diagnose genital herpes by taking a tissue scraping or culture of the blisters for examination in a laboratory. A blood test also can detect a herpes infection. Examination for other sexually related diseases, including HIV, is important. Another sexually transmitted disease may be present in addition to herpes.

How serious is genital herpes?

Other illnesses may be due to herpes, including injury to the cornea of the eye and meningitis. It can also cause severe illness in infants. The rate of herpes infection in newborns is increasing as the rate of genital herpes in women increases.

Treatment

There's no cure for genital herpes. Treatment includes oral prescription antiviral medications, including acyclovir (Zovirax), famciclovir and valacyclovir (Valtrex), to help heal the sores sooner and reduce the frequency of relapses. If taken daily, these medications may also reduce the chance you'll infect your partner with the herpes virus.

Genital warts

Signs and symptoms

- Wart-like growths on the genitals
- Itching or discomfort in the genital area
- Bleeding with intercourse

Genital warts, also called venereal warts, are one of the most common sexually transmitted diseases. They may develop in both men and women and are caused by the human papillomavirus (HPV). The warts may look like small, flesh-colored bumps or have a cauliflower-like appearance. In addition to appearing on the genitals, these warts can also appear in the mouth or throat of someone who's had oral sexual contact with an infected person.

Genital warts may develop from three weeks to three months after exposure to the virus. Sometimes they're so small they can't be seen with the naked eye.

Diagnosis

Because it can be difficult to detect genital warts, your doctor may apply an acetic acid solution to your genitals to whiten any warts. Then, he or she may view them through a special microscope called a colposcope.

For women, it's important to have regular pelvic exams and Pap tests, which can help detect vaginal and cervical changes caused by genital warts or the early signs of cervical cancer — a possible complication of HPV infection.

Have an initial Pap test within three years of having sex or at age 21, whichever comes first. If you've had genital warts, you may need to have a Pap test every three to six months, depending on the severity of your condition.

How serious are genital warts?
Cervical cancer has been closely linked with HPV infection. Certain types of HPV also are associated with cancers of the vulva, anus and penis.

Treatment
Your doctor can help you clear an outbreak of warts with medications or surgical treatments. The underlying virus is never completely eliminated, however, and genital warts may reappear even after treatment.

Medications
Genital warts treatments that can be applied directly to your skin include:

- **Imiquimod (Aldara).** This cream appears to boost your immune system's ability to fight genital warts. Avoid sexual contact while the cream is on your skin. It may weaken condoms and diaphragms and may irritate your partner's skin.
- **Podofilox (Condylox).** Podofilox works by destroying genital wart tissue. Your doctor may want to administer the first application, and will recommend precautionary steps to prevent the medication from irritating surrounding skin. Never apply podofilox internally. Additionally, this medication isn't recommended for use during pregnancy.
- **Trichloroacetic acid (TCA).** This chemical treatment burns off genital warts. TCA must always be applied by a doctor.

Surgery
Surgery may be necessary to remove larger warts, warts that don't

respond to medications, or — if you're pregnant — warts that your baby may be exposed to during delivery.

Surgical options include:

- **Freezing with liquid nitrogen (cryotherapy).** Freezing works by causing a blister to form around your wart. As your skin heals, the lesions slough off, allowing new skin to appear. You may need repeated cryotherapy treatments.
- **Electrocautery.** This procedure uses an electrical current to burn off warts.
- **Surgical excision.** Your doctor may use special tools to cut off warts. You'll need local anesthesia for this treatment.
- **Laser treatments.** This approach, which uses an intense beam of light, can be expensive and is usually reserved for very extensive and tough-to-treat warts.

Prevention
While it won't completely prevent genital warts or cervical cancer, a vaccine known as Gardasil offers protection from the most dangerous types of HPV.

The national Advisory Committee on Immunization Practices recommends routine vaccination for all children ages 11 or 12. The vaccine is most effective if given before adolescents become sexually active.

The vaccine is also recommended for young women through age 26 and young men through age 21 who have not been vaccinated. In addition, the following individuals should receive the vaccine if they have not been previously vaccinated:

- Young men who have sex with men, including young men who identify as gay or bisexual or who intend to have sex with men through age 26
- Young adults who are transgender through age 26
- Young adults with certain immunocompromising conditions (including HIV) through age 26

HIV and AIDS

Acquired immunodeficiency syndrome (AIDS) is a chronic condition affecting the immune system. It's caused by the human immunodeficiency virus (HIV). This virus, which causes a progressive weakening of the immune system, has reached global epidemic proportions. HIV affects an estimated 36.7 million people worldwide.

By damaging or destroying the cells of your immune system, HIV interferes with your body's ability to effectively fight off viruses, bacteria and fungi that cause disease. This weakening also makes you more susceptible to infections that your body would normally resist, such as some types of pneumonia, meningitis and cancer.

Infection with the virus is known as an HIV infection. The term *AIDS* denotes the late stages of HIV infection.

HIV and the immune system

When your immune system is healthy, specialized white blood cells (lymphocytes) and antibodies help to resist germs to keep you free from disease. When most unwanted organisms enter your body, they're attacked and destroyed. This response is coordinated by a type of lymphocyte known as a helper T cell.

When HIV enters your body, it can't live on its own. It must take over another living (host) cell to survive. HIV enters helper T cells by attaching to a protein on the surface of the cells called CD4 — thus the name CD4 cells for helper T cells. Once inside the CD4 cells, the virus inserts its own genetic material into the cells and uses them to make copies of itself.

When the newly formed viruses burst out of the host cells, they find other cells to attack. In the meantime, the old host cells die. The cycle repeats itself again and again.

In the process, more than 10 billion new HIV particles can be produced every day. Your immune system tries to overcome this massive infection by producing antibodies and forming more helper T cells (CD4 cells), turning out as many as 2 billion new cells daily.

Ultimately, the virus wins the race. The number of new cells your body can produce gradually decreases, and you develop a severe immune deficiency. Your body is no longer able to effectively fight off infection.

How do you get HIV?

You can be infected with HIV in the following ways:

Sexual activity
You may become infected if you have vaginal, anal or oral sex with an infected partner and his or her blood, semen or vaginal secretions enter your body. You can also become infected from shared sexual devices if they're not washed or covered with a condom. The virus is present in the semen or vaginal secretions of someone who's infected. It enters your body through small tears that can develop in your rectum or vagina during sexual activity.

If you already have another sexually transmitted disease, you're at greater risk of contracting HIV. Women who use the spermicide nonoxynol 9 are at higher risk of acquiring HIV infection. The spermicide irritates the lining of your vagina and may cause tears that allow the virus into your body.

Infected blood
In some instances, the virus may be transmitted through blood and blood products — including whole blood, packed red cells, fresh-frozen plasma and platelets — that you receive in blood or blood-product transfusions.

Since 1985, American hospitals and blood banks have screened the blood supply for HIV antibodies. This testing, along with improvements in donor screening and recruitment practices, has substantially reduced the risk of acquiring HIV through transfusions.

Needle sharing
HIV is easily transmitted through needles and syringes contaminated with infected blood. That's why sharing intravenous drug paraphernalia puts you at high risk of HIV, as well as infectious diseases such as hepatitis. Your risk is increased if you inject illicit drugs frequently or also engage in high-risk sexual behavior. Avoiding the use of injected illicit drugs is the most reliable way to prevent infection.

Accidental needle sticks
Transmission of the virus between HIV-infected people and health care workers through needle sticks and cuts is low. More than 99 percent of needle sticks or cut exposures don't lead to infection.

Transmission from mother to child
Untreated pregnant women infected with HIV can pass the infection to their babies. Among women who receive treatment for their HIV infection during pregnancy, the risk to their babies decreases by as much as two-thirds.

Other routes
In very rare cases, the virus may be transmitted through organ or tissue transplants or unsterilized dental or surgical equipment.

Signs and symptoms

The signs and symptoms of HIV and AIDS vary, depending on the phase of the infection.

Early infection
When first infected with HIV, you may have no signs or symptoms

Human immunodeficiency virus (HIV) belongs to a family of viruses called retroviruses. These viruses carry their genetic information on single-stranded ribonucleic acid (RNA). Once inside a host cell, HIV uses an enzyme called reverse transcriptase to convert its RNA into double-stranded deoxyribonucleic acid (DNA). The viral DNA enters the nucleus and is inserted into the host cell's DNA. After this, HIV is able to reproduce (replicate) itself. When the cell bursts, the replicated viruses are released.

at all, although it's more common to develop a brief flu-like illness for two to four weeks. Signs and symptoms may include:

- Fever
- Headache
- Sore throat
- Swollen lymph glands
- Rash

Even if you don't have symptoms, you're still able to transmit the virus to others.

Later infection

During the last phase of HIV infection — which occurs approximately 10 or more years after initial infection — more-serious signs and symptoms may begin to appear, and the infection may then meet the official definition of AIDS. To meet the definition you must have:

- The presence of HIV infection
- An opportunistic infection — an infection that occurs when your immune system is impaired, such as pneumonia
- A CD4 lymphocyte count of 200 or less — a normal count ranges from 800 to 1,200

By this time, your immune system has been severely damaged. Signs and symptoms of late HIV infection may include:

- Soaking night sweats
- Shaking chills or fevers higher than 100 F (38 C) for several weeks
- Dry cough and shortness of breath
- Chronic diarrhea
- Persistent white spots or unusual lesions on your tongue or in your mouth
- Headaches
- Blurred and distorted vision
- Weight loss
- Persistent, unexplained fatigue
- Swelling of lymph nodes for more than three months

Testing and diagnosis

HIV is diagnosed by testing your blood or oral mucus for the presence of antibodies to the virus.

The Centers for Disease Control and Prevention (CDC) encourages voluntary HIV testing as a routine part of medical care for all adolescents and adults ages 13 to 64. Although the CDC says that everyone should be tested at least once, yearly testing is recommended only for people at high risk of infection.

Unfortunately, HIV tests aren't accurate immediately after infection because it takes time for you to develop these antibodies — usually about 12 weeks. In rare cases, it can take up to six months for an HIV test to become positive.

ELISA and Western blot tests

For years, the only available test for HIV was the enzyme-linked immunosorbent assay (ELISA) test that looked for antibodies to the virus in a sample of your blood. If this test was positive — meaning you had antibodies to HIV — the same test was repeated. If the repeat test was also positive for HIV antibodies, you'd have another confirming blood test called the Western blot test, which checks for the presence of HIV proteins. The Western blot test was important because you may have non-HIV antibodies that cause a false-positive result on the ELISA test. Combining the two types of tests helped ensure that the results were accurate, and you'd receive a diagnosis of HIV only if all three tests were positive. The downside is that it can take up to two weeks to get the results of the ELISA and Western blot tests, a period of time that can take an emotional toll.

Rapid tests

Today, several rapid tests can give highly accurate information within as little as 20 minutes. These tests look for antibodies to the virus using a sample of your blood or fluids collected on a treated pad that's rubbed on your upper and lower gums. The oral test is almost as sensitive as the blood test and eliminates the need for drawing

blood. A positive reaction on a rapid test requires a confirming blood test. And because the tests are relatively new and were originally approved for use only in certified laboratories, they may not be available everywhere.

Home tests

The Food and Drug Administration (FDA) has approved HIV test kits for home use. These tests are as accurate as a clinical test, and all positive results are automatically retested.

Unlike a home pregnancy test, you don't evaluate the test yourself. Instead, you mail in a drop of your blood, then call a toll-free number to receive your results within a few days. This approach ensures your privacy and anonymity — you're identified only by a code number that comes with your kit. The greatest disadvantage is that you're not offered the counseling that you typically receive in a clinic or doctor's office, although you're given referrals for medical and social services.

Additional testing

If you receive a diagnosis of HIV or AIDS, your doctor will use a test to help predict the probable progression of your disease. This test measures the amount of virus in your blood (viral load).

Studies have shown that people with higher viral loads generally fare more poorly than do those with a lower viral load. Viral load tests are also used to decide when to start and when to change your treatment.

Complications

HIV infection weakens your immune system, making you highly susceptible to a large number of bacteria, viruses, fungi and parasites. You may also be more vulnerable to certain types of cancers. Treatment with antiretroviral drugs can markedly decrease the risk of these conditions.

Bacterial infections
These may include:

Bacterial pneumonia
Dozens of types of bacteria can cause bacterial pneumonia, which may develop on its own or after you've had an upper respiratory infection such as a cold or the flu.

Mycobacterium avium complex
This infection is caused by a group of mycobacteria referred to by a single name — MAC. The mycobacteria normally cause an infection of the respiratory tract. But if you have advanced HIV infection and your CD4 lymphocyte count is less than 50, you're more likely to develop a systemic infection that can affect almost any internal organ, including your bone marrow, liver or spleen.

Tuberculosis (TB)
In resource-poor nations, TB is the most common opportunistic infection associated with HIV and a leading cause of death among people living with AIDS. Millions of people are currently infected with both HIV and tuberculosis, and many experts consider the two diseases twin epidemics. TB increases the rate at which the AIDS virus replicates. What's more, TB often strikes people with HIV years before other problems associated with HIV develop.

Salmonellosis
You contract this bacterial infection from contaminated food or water. Although anyone exposed to salmonella bacteria can become sick, salmonellosis is far more common in people who are HIV-positive.

Bacillary angiomatosis
This infection, caused by the *Bartonella henselae* bacterium, first appears as purplish to bright red skin patches. It often resembles Kaposi's sarcoma, but it can cause disease in other parts of your body, including your liver and spleen.

How HIV Is *Not* Transmitted

There are many myths regarding human immunodeficiency virus (HIV) transmission. You *can't* become infected through ordinary contact, such as hugging, dancing or shaking hands, with someone who has HIV or AIDS. And you *can't* be infected in any of the following ways:

- Coming into contact with the sweat or tears of someone with HIV or AIDS.
- Sharing food, utensils, towels, bedding, a swimming pool, a telephone or a toilet seat with someone who has the virus.
- Being bitten by bedbugs or mosquitoes.
- Kissing someone who's HIV-positive or who has AIDS. There's no evidence that the virus is transmitted through kissing. Although HIV is sometimes found in the saliva of people with the virus, it occurs in low concentrations. In addition, natural inhibitory substances in saliva help prevent the virus from being transmitted.
- Donating blood. Donation centers use new, sterilized needles for each person donating blood. They also employ screening methods to test donated blood for disease-causing agents.

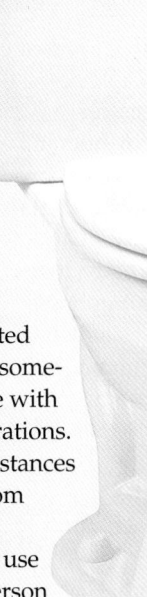

Viral infections
These may include:

Cytomegalovirus (CMV)
This common herpes virus is transmitted in body fluids such as saliva, blood, urine, semen and breast milk. But a healthy immune system inactivates the virus, and it remains dormant in your body. If your immune system weakens, the virus resurfaces, causing damage to your eyes, digestive tract, lungs or other organs.

Viral hepatitis
Viral hepatitis is a viral infection of the liver. There are several types but the most common are hepatitis A, B and C. Hepatitis B and C can lead to persistent or chronic infection and put you at risk of long-term complications such as cirrhosis or liver cancer. If you're HIV-positive and also have hepatitis, you may be more likely to develop liver toxicity from your medications.

Herpes simplex virus (HSV)
HSV, which usually causes genital herpes, may be transmitted during unprotected anal or vaginal sex. If you have HIV, your skin infection is likely to be more severe than it would be in people who don't have HIV, and the sores may take longer to heal.

Human papillomavirus (HPV)

If you're HIV-positive, you're especially susceptible to infection with HPV and more prone to recurrent infections. HPV infection is especially serious because it significantly increases a woman's risk of cervical cancer. And infection with both HPV and HIV increases a woman's risk even further — cervical cancer seems to occur more often and more aggressively in women who are HIV-positive.

Progressive multifocal leukoencephalopathy

PML is an extremely serious brain infection caused by human polyomavirus and JC polymavirus. Signs and symptoms vary and may include speech problems, weakness on one side of the body, loss of vision in one eye, or numbness in an arm or leg. PML usually occurs only when your immune system has been severely damaged.

Fungal infections

These may include:

Candidiasis

Candidiasis is a common HIV-related infection. It produces inflammation and a thick white coating on the mucous membranes of your mouth, tongue (thrush), esophagus (Candida esophagitis) or vagina.

Cryptococcal meningitis

Meningitis is an inflammation of the membranes and fluid surrounding your brain and spinal cord (meninges). Cryptococcal meningitis is a common central nervous system infection associated with HIV, caused by a fungus that's present in soil. Once you've had cryptococcal meningitis, you'll need to be on long-term medication to prevent a recurrence.

Pneumocystis jiroveci pneumonia (PJP)

Anti-retroviral drugs have helped reduce the number of cases of PJP, but it remains one of the most common opportunistic infections affecting people with AIDS in the United States. PJP attacks the lungs, making it difficult to breathe.

Parasitic infections

These may include:

Toxoplasmosis

This potentially deadly infection is caused by *Toxoplasma gondii*, a parasite spread primarily by cats. Humans generally contract toxoplasmosis by touching their mouths with their hands after changing cat litter or by eating raw or undercooked meat, especially pork, lamb and venison. For people with AIDS, toxoplasmosis may lead to encephalitis, a brain infection.

Cryptosporidiosis

This infection is caused by an intestinal parasite that's commonly found in animals. You contract cryptosporidiosis when you ingest contaminated food or water. The parasite grows in your intestines and bile ducts, leading to severe, chronic diarrhea in people with AIDS.

Cancers

These may include:

Kaposi's sarcoma

Kaposi's sarcoma is a tumor of the blood vessel walls. Although rare in people not infected with HIV, it's common in HIV-positive people. Kaposi's sarcoma usually appears as pink, red or purple lesions on the skin and mouth. In people with darker skin, the lesions may look dark brown or black. As with most opportunistic infections associated with AIDS, the use of anti-retrovirals has reduced the incidence of this cancer and has even reduced the lesions in people already affected.

Non-Hodgkin lymphoma

This cancer originates in lymphocytes, a type of white blood cell. Lymphocytes are concentrated in your bone marrow, lymph nodes, spleen, digestive tract and skin. Although lymphomas can start in other organs, they usually begin in your lymph nodes.

Other complications

These may include:

Wasting syndrome

Aggressive treatment regimens have reduced the number of cases of wasting syndrome, but it does still affect many people with AIDS. It's defined as a loss of at least 10 percent of body weight and is often accompanied by diarrhea, chronic weakness and a fever.

Neurological complications

Although AIDS doesn't appear to infect the nerve cells, it can still cause neurological symptoms such as confusion, forgetfulness, changes in behavior, depression, anxiety and trouble walking. One of the most common neurological complications is AIDS dementia complex, which leads to behavioral changes and diminished mental functioning.

Treatment

When HIV was first identified in the early 1980s, there were few drugs to treat the virus and the opportunistic infections associated with it. Since then, a number of medications have been developed to treat both HIV/AIDS and opportunistic infections.

For many people, including children, these treatments have extended and improved their quality of life. Scientists at the National Institutes of Health estimate that since 1989, anti-retroviral medications have provided HIV-positive Americans with years of extended life.

But none of these drugs can cure HIV/AIDS, many have side effects that can be severe, and most are expensive. What's more, after several years on AIDS drugs, some people develop resistance to the drugs and no longer respond to treatment. Newer drugs are being researched and developed to help this group of people.

Treatment guidelines

According to current guidelines, treatment should focus on achieving the maximum suppression of symptoms for as long as possible. This aggressive approach is known as highly active anti-retroviral therapy (HAART). The aim of HAART is to reduce the amount of virus in your blood to very low or even nondetectable levels, although this doesn't mean the virus is gone. Achieving nondetectable levels is usually accomplished with a combination of three or more drugs.

Treatment guidelines also emphasize the importance of quality of life. Thus the goal of AIDS treatment is to find the strongest possible regimen that is also simple and has the fewest side effects. If you have HIV/AIDS, it's important that you take an active role in treatment decisions. You and your doctor should discuss the risks and benefits of all therapies so that you can make an informed decision about what will likely be a complex and long-term treatment.

Anti-retroviral drugs

Anti-retroviral drugs inhibit the growth and replication of HIV at various stages of its life cycle. Seven classes of these drugs are available:

Nucleoside analogue reverse transcriptase inhibitors (NRTIs)
NRTIs were the first anti-retroviral drugs to be developed. They inhibit the replication of an HIV enzyme called reverse transcriptase. They include zidovudine (Retrovir), lamivudine (Epivir), didanosine (Videx), stavudine (Zerit) and abacavir (Ziagen). The drug emtricitabine (Emtriva), which is used in combination with at least two other AIDS medica-

tions, treats both HIV and hepatitis B.

A major side effect of zidovudine is bone marrow suppression, which causes a decrease in the number of red and white blood cells. A small percentage of people treated with abacavir experience hypersensitivity reactions such as a rash, fever, fatigue, nausea, vomiting, diarrhea and abdominal pain. Symptoms usually appear within the first six weeks of treatment and generally disappear when the drug is discontinued. If you've had a hypersensitivity reaction to abacavir, avoid taking the drug again. Side effects of emtricitabine include skin discoloration.

Protease inhibitors (PIs)
PIs interrupt HIV replication at a later stage in its life cycle by interfering with an enzyme known as HIV protease. This causes HIV particles in your body to become structurally disorganized and non-infectious. Among these drugs are saquinavir (Invirase), ritonavir (Norvir), indinavir (Crixivan), nelfinavir (Viracept), amprenavir, lopinavir/ritonavir (Kaletra), atazanavir (Reyataz) and tipranavir (Aptivus). Darunavir (Prezista) is intended for people who haven't responded to treatment with other drugs. Darunavir is used with ritonavir and other anti-HIV medications. Protease inhibitors are usually prescribed with other medications, to help avoid drug resistance.

The most common side effects of protease inhibitors include nausea, diarrhea and other digestive tract problems. PIs can also cause a significant number of side effects when they interact with certain other medications. That's because all PIs, to one degree or another, affect an enzyme system in your liver that is responsible for metabolizing a large number of drugs. Newer side effects have also appeared with the continuing and widespread use of protease inhibitors. These include elevated

triglyceride levels and problems with sugar metabolism that may sometimes progress to diabetes.

There may also be abnormalities in the way fat is metabolized and deposited in your body. Some people lose much of their total body fat. Others gain excess fat on the back between their shoulders (buffalo hump) or in the stomach (protease paunch). No one knows exactly why these abnormalities occur. In fact, it's not even certain whether these problems are a direct result of treatment with protease inhibitors or due to some other cause that has yet to be identified. Similar metabolic abnormalities have occurred in people on anti-retroviral therapy that doesn't include PIs. Although these body changes can be distressing, the possibility that they may occur should not stop you from getting treatment for HIV or AIDS.

Non-nucleoside reverse transcriptase inhibitors (NNRTIs)
These drugs bind directly to the enzyme reverse transcriptase. NNRTIs that are approved for clinical use include nevirapine (Viramune), delavirdine (Rescriptor), efavirenz (Sustiva) and etravirine (Intelence) and rilpivirine. A major side effect of all NNRTIs is a rash. In addition, people taking efavirenz may have side effects such as abnormal and worsening of underlying mood disorders.

Nucleotide reverse transcriptase inhibitors (NtRTIs)
NtRTIs work much like nucleoside analogues: They interfere with the replication of reverse transcriptase and prevent the virus from inserting its genetic material into cells. But NtRTIs act more quickly than NRTIs do. The only approved drug in this class, tenofovir (Viread), inhibits both HIV and hepatitis B and appears to be effective in people who are resistant to NRTIs. The most common side effects of tenofovir, when used in combination with other anti-

retrovirals, are nausea, vomiting, diarrhea and gas. As with all reverse transcriptase inhibitors, the possibility of severe, and even fatal, liver damage exists.

Fusion inhibitors
One of the most alarming developments in the AIDS epidemic is the emergence of drug-resistant strains of HIV. Worldwide, a majority of people receiving treatment for HIV are resistant to at least one drug, and many don't respond to a typical three-drug combination. A drug called enfuvirtide (Fuzeon) is the first in a class of drugs called fusion inhibitors. It appears to suppress resistant strains of HIV. Fusion inhibitors stop the virus from replicating by preventing its membrane from fusing with the membrane surrounding healthy cells.

Fuzeon is used in combination with other HIV drugs for people who have advanced infection and who have developed resistance to other drugs. Doctors administer Fuzeon by injection.

Integrase inhibitors
These drugs are aimed at treating individuals who become resistant to other treatments. Drugs in this class include raltegravir (Isentress), dolutegravir (Tivicay) and elvitegravir. They're intended to be used in combination with other anti-retroviral drugs rather than alone. This is the first class of drugs that blocks replication of the HIV integrase enzyme, which keeps HIV DNA from inserting itself into human DNA. Common side effects include diarrhea, nausea, headaches and fevers.

Chemokine co-receptor inhibitors
Chemokine co-receptor inhibitors (Ccr5 antagonists) make up a new class of drugs used to treat a particular type of HIV infection called CCR5-tropic HIV-1. The only drug in this class — maraviroc (Selzentry) — is for treatment of Ccr5-tropic HIV-1 in adults.

Maraviroc is the first drug that targets a human protein rather than components of the HIV virus itself.

Maraviroc is used in combination with other anti-retroviral drugs for the treatment of adults with Ccr5-tropic HIV-1 who have elevated levels of HIV (high viral load) in their blood despite treatment with other HIV medications. Maraviroc reduces viral load by preventing HIV from entering uninfected white blood cells. It does this by blocking Ccr5, a major route of entry into the cells. Ccr5 is a protein found on the surface of some immune cells, and maraviroc blocks the Ccr5 co-receptor from accepting HIV.

During two large clinical trials, approximately twice as many people with Ccr5-tropic HIV-1 infection who received maraviroc had undetectable viral loads after 24 weeks as did those who received more-standard therapy.

Side effects of maraviroc may include liver and cardiovascular problems, as well as a cough, fever, upper respiratory tract infections, a rash and abdominal pain.

Prevention

There's no vaccine for HIV infection and no cure for AIDS. But it's possible to protect yourself and others from infection. That means educating yourself about HIV and avoiding any behavior that allows HIV-infected fluids into your body. ■

Allergies and Asthma

Allergies occur when your immune system reacts to a foreign substance — such as pollen, bee venom or pet dander — or to a food that doesn't cause a reaction in most people.

Most foods, drinks or substances that you come in contact with don't trigger an immune response. Occasionally, though, your immune system goes astray and reacts — or rather overreacts — to an harmless invader. It perceives the substance as harmful and launches an attack against it.

Nasal allergies, which generally include mild to moderate symptoms such as sneezing, itchy eyes and a runny nose, are common, affecting an estimated 50 million Americans. And up to 2 percent of the population may be at risk of anaphylaxis, a more serious condition often accompanied by hives, swelling and wheezing, that can sometimes cause death.

Asthma is a lung condition that often coincides with allergies. While many people experience mild symptoms, for some the condition can be severe and even fatal.

Because of the high frequency of allergies and asthma and their potential for serious complications, these conditions are a concern for many individuals.

Allergic Reactions

To fully understand allergies and asthma, it's important to know how your body's immune system works. The main players in the majority of allergic reactions are white blood cells known as lymphocytes (B cells).

Lymphocytes are manufactured in bone marrow. Some migrate to your thymus, where they develop into specialized types of immune cells (T cells). Some migrate from bone marrow and the thymus to your lymph nodes and other organs, including your spleen, tonsils, adenoids, appendix and small intestine. Other lymphocytes circulate throughout your body in blood and lymphatic vessels.

The role of lymphocytes is to seek out and destroy harmful foreign invaders that enter your body. In people with allergies, lymphocytes perceive harmless substances such as pollen, dust mites and dander as harmful and launch an attack against them. These innocent substances are known as allergens.

When an allergen enters your body, it meets up with an antigen-presenting cell. Allergens, a type of antigen, are processed by the antigen-presenting cell, and with the help of T cells they stimulate the development of B cells. Both T and B cells are lymphocytes, types of white blood cells. Upon stimulation, B cells develop into plasma cells, which may produce a large number of substances called antibodies that identify a specific allergen. The antibodies, composed of a special kind of protein called immunoglobulin (Ig), attach themselves to certain cells, such as basophils or mast cells. The IgE antibody is most often involved in allergic responses. As more allergens enter your body, they attached to the antibodies, triggering basophils and mast cells to release powerful chemicals including histamine. This causes a range of allergic signs and symptoms, including sneezing, coughing and itching.

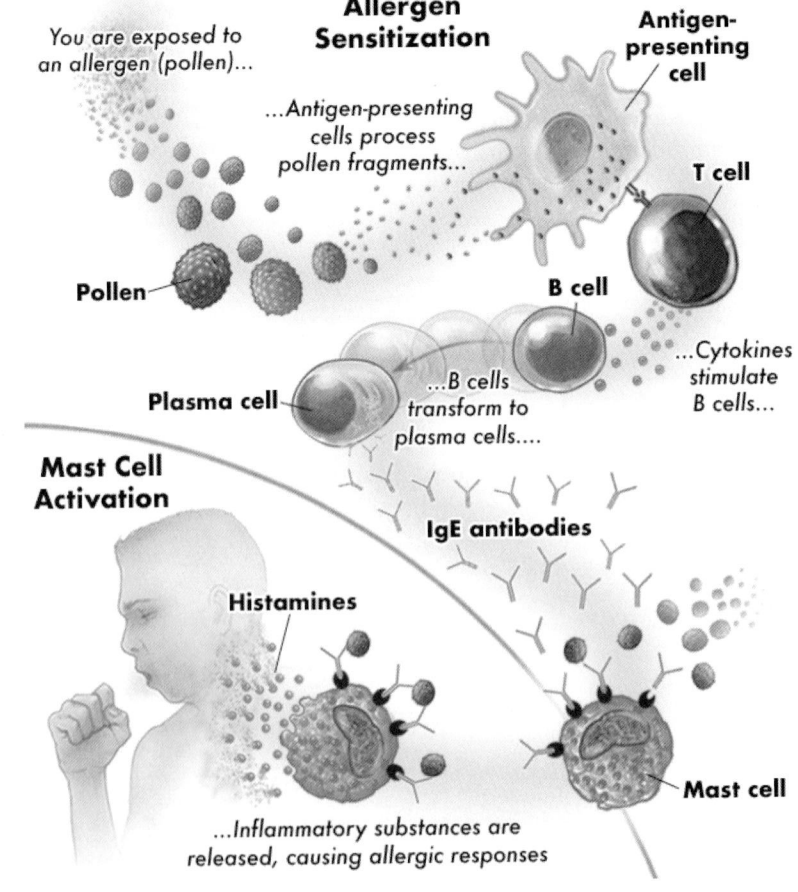

You are exposed to an allergen (pollen)...

Allergen Sensitization

...Antigen-presenting cells process pollen fragments...

Antigen-presenting cell

T cell

Pollen

B cell

Plasma cell

...B cells transform to plasma cells....

...Cytokines stimulate B cells...

Mast Cell Activation

IgE antibodies

Histamines

...Inflammatory substances are released, causing allergic responses

Mast cell

When allergens enter your body, certain lymphocytes combat them by releasing a variety of chemicals. One of these is called histamine, which acts as an irritating stimulant. Often other white blood cells respond to allergens by releasing powerful chemicals intended to destroy them.

These immune responses result in a host of signs and symptoms that vary in severity. When histamine and other chemicals are released in the lungs, the lining of lung air passages becomes inflamed, causing it to swell and narrow and secrete mucus. This leads to wheezing, coughing and, sometimes, shortness of breath.

When these chemicals are released in nasal cavities, they cause a runny nose, teary eyes, and itching in the nose, throat, roof of the mouth and eyes. Histamine in the skin produces hives and other rashes. When the chemicals are activated in the digestive system, abdominal cramps and diarrhea may result.

Occasionally, the entire body experiences a serious allergic response known as anaphylactic shock (anaphylaxis). In severe cases, blood vessels may dilate and air passageways narrow, causing a drop in blood pressure, difficulty breathing, and other signs and symptoms. Unconsciousness or death may result (see page 507).

Each allergen stimulates its own specific set of antibodies. For this reason, a person may be sensitive to ragweed but not to mold allergens. It is, however, fairly common for a person who's allergic to specific substances, such as pollens, to be allergic to other substances that may share structural similarities with the pollen.

Allergic reaction triggers

A surprising number of substances found outdoors, indoors or in foods can trigger an allergic reaction. You may be allergic to substances present in certain medications, parts of plants (such as pollen), dust mites in household dust, animal dander, molds, fungi or insect venom released during a sting, such as a bee sting. Some people are also sensitive to chemical changes that occur in the body in response to exercise or to exposure to heat or cold.

Paths of exposure

Different allergens have different routes of entry into the body.

Inhalation
Inhalation is a common way to be exposed to allergens. Millions of people have hay fever (allergic rhinitis) due to sensitivity to certain plant pollens. Spring, summer and fall are the pollen-producing seasons.

Because pollen is easily airborne, during these seasons exposure is inevitable. As part of their reproductive cycle, molds also release particles that travel in the air. When inhaled, these particles can trigger an allergic reaction.

A similar reaction can occur when a sensitive person inhales animal dander or dust mites, which are common in household dust. Substances in the air such as smoke, fumes, mists and baby powder also can irritate inflamed airways.

The reaction to an inhaled allergen typically is characterized by signs and symptoms such as a drippy nose, a cough and itchy, teary eyes. An inhaled allergen can also trigger asthma symptoms.

Wheezing associated with asthma can occur when airways in the lungs become inflamed and swollen. Other asthma symptoms include a feeling of tightness in the chest, a cough and the production of thick mucus.

Contact
Exposure to plant allergens such as the resins of poison ivy, poison oak and poison sumac occurs when you come into contact with the resin. You can get poison

PREVENTION TIP

The best way to prevent allergies is to avoid the allergen, which can be fairly easy in the case of something such as poison ivy or penicillin. It's more difficult to avoid pollens, molds and dust because they're airborne and present even in the best-kept homes.

When indoors, you can minimize exposure to pollens and outdoor molds by keeping your doors and windows closed and the humidity low. When needed, use an air conditioning system equipped with good filters. Discard all moldy or mildewed items from your home.

If you're allergic to dust, keep your house and work environment as dust-free as possible. This means vacuuming, dusting and damp mopping frequently. Avoid decorating with items that trap dust, such as bed ruffles and curtains.

ivy by accidentally brushing against the plant's leaves while walking in a wooded area, while gardening or even by touching clothing that has had resin deposited on it. The allergic reaction usually occurs on your skin wherever contact was made.

Other contact reactions can occur from prolonged exposure to certain metals, such as nickel and chromium. People who are sensitive to components in cosmetics can develop rashes after exposure to the components. Health care workers may become allergic to latex after repeated exposure to gloves and other latex-containing products.

Absorption
Certain foods and medications that are absorbed into the body by

Common Myths

Allergies often appear to be mysterious in origin and unpredictable in response. At times they can also be difficult to treat. So it's not surprising that misconceptions and myths regarding allergies abound.

Myth: Allergies are all in your head

Fact: For most people, allergies are a real medical condition. However, allergy symptoms may be aggravated by stress or emotions. Although stress and emotions don't cause allergies, they can exaggerate your body's response to the allergens. Scientists don't fully understand the relationship between allergic responses and emotions.

Myth: Moving to Arizona will cure allergies

Fact: For years people bothered by seasonal allergies to pollens and molds thought that if they moved to the desert Southwest, where the foliage and climate are different from other regions, their allergies would disappear. Although the desert is lacking in maple trees and ragweed, it does have other pollen-producing plants, such as sagebrush and cottonwood, ash and olive trees. People who are sensitive to some pollens and molds often find that in a new environment they eventually develop sensitivities to new allergens. For example, people sensitive to ragweed may become sensitive to sagebrush pollen.

Myth: Short-haired pets don't cause allergies

Fact: The length of an animal's fur doesn't determine its allergic potential. In fact, the fur itself isn't the culprit. The cause is the dander, the scales of skin that are constantly shed by all animals with hair or feathers. In addition, saliva and urine may trigger a sensitivity. If you have allergies to furry pets, potential pets may include fish and reptiles.

Myth: You won't get poison ivy unless you touch the plant

Fact: It's true that the plant resin responsible for a sensitivity to poison ivy, poison oak and poison sumac must actually touch your skin to cause a reaction. But that resin may first touch your clothing and then later be transferred to your skin quite easily while you're handling that clothing. This may explain why people who haven't touched the plants have reactions. These resins can even be carried in smoke if the plants are burned.

Myth: Most people outgrow hay fever

Fact: Many people believe that hay fever is a childhood disorder that you outgrow by the time you reach adulthood. On the contrary, hay fever can develop at any life stage, and you can recover from it at any point in your life.

Myth: No one ever dies of allergies

Fact: Although it's true that many allergies are merely an inconvenience, some allergic reactions can be serious. People who are highly sensitive to allergens can experience life-threatening shock (anaphylaxis) after being stung by a certain insect, being injected with a certain drug or eating a certain food. Asthma attacks also can be fatal. Severe reactions must be taken seriously and treated promptly and properly.

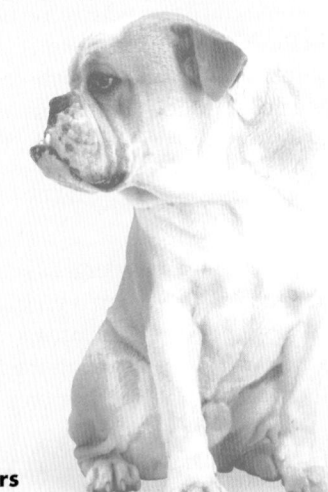

way of digestion or injection can cause an allergic response in some people. The foods most likely to produce reactions include peanuts and other legumes, tree nuts, and fish and shellfish.

Almost any medicine has the potential to cause an allergic reaction. The most common offenders by far are penicillin and its relatives, followed by other antibiotics. Some people are sensitive to aspirin and to intravenous contrast agents used in some X-ray tests.

Stings

Some allergens find their way into people by way of stings. For most people, venom from the sting of a bee, wasp or yellow jacket causes a reaction that's locally uncomfortable for a couple of hours. But in people who are sensitive to these allergens, such a sting can trigger a whole-body (systemic) reaction and could potentially be serious or fatal without immediate treatment.

Other sensitivities

In rare cases, people are sensitive to heat, cold, pressure, light, sun rays or exercise. They may experience responses such as rashes or hives. These responses generally don't involve the antibodies responsible for most allergic reactions.

Diagnosing Allergies

To determine if you have an allergy, your doctor may ask you a series of questions about your symptoms, your family's medical history, any past medical problems, past or current emotional or relationship problems, and your lifestyle, including work, eating and recreation habits. You can also expect questions about possible exposure to allergens. This interview is one of the most important sources of information in making a diagnosis.

For example, because the tendency to develop allergies is inherited, it's important for your doctor to know whether your parents have or had allergies. People who have allergies frequently have a close relative with allergies — although the types of allergies may not be the same. You're less likely to inherit a sensitivity to a specific agent than you are the general tendency to develop sensitivities.

Testing for allergens

When being evaluated for allergies, you may undergo one or more tests to see if your body responds when exposed to certain allergens.

Skin test

The skin test is the most commonly used test, and it can be administered in several ways. Generally, a small amount of a purified allergen extract is pricked or injected into the skin on your arm or upper back. If you're allergic to the allergen, you usually develop a raised bump (hive) at the test location on your skin.

Several allergens are generally tested at the same time to eliminate possible allergens and because people are often sensitive to several substances.

Skin tests aren't foolproof. You may test positive and yet not respond to the allergen in daily life, and a negative result doesn't rule out sensitivity to that allergen. Or, if too much allergen is placed on the skin, you may get a positive reaction even if you aren't allergic to the substance. Therefore, skin tests must be conducted carefully and interpreted cautiously.

Skin tests are particularly useful for respiratory allergies, insect sting allergies, latex allergy and penicillin allergy.

Allergy blood test

The in vitro allergen-specific immunoglobulin E (IgE) antibody test, formerly known as the radioallergosorbent test (RAST),

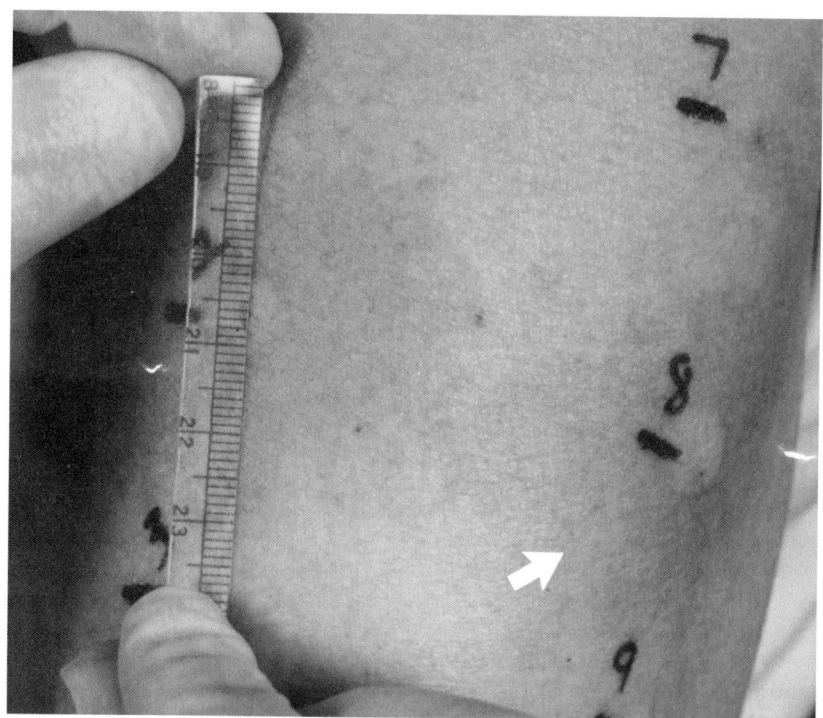

An area of red and swollen skin (see arrow) resulting from a skin test indicates that this person is allergic to the allergen introduced beneath the skin surface.

is a blood test that's useful for diagnosing sensitivity to inhaled allergens, such as pollen. It measures the amounts of specific IgE antibodies in your blood. In contrast to skin tests, this test may be more convenient, and it doesn't pose any risks because all of the testing is done on a blood sample in a test tube (in vitro). In addition, any antihistamine drugs you're taking won't affect the test.

The downside to the in vitro allergen-specific IgE antibody test is that it may not be as sensitive as are skin tests. The test may also be more expensive than are skin tests.

Treating Allergies

Several strategies are effective for treating allergies. The best approach is simply to avoid exposure to the allergic substance, but that may not always be possible. Medications and allergy shots are other options.

Avoidance

Avoiding a known allergen is fairly simple in the case of an allergy to penicillin or poison ivy. Avoidance isn't so simple for people allergic to such things as pollen and dust mites. Pollen is constantly in the air during certain months of the year, and even the best-kept homes contain dust. For tips on reducing exposure to these and other inhalant allergens, see pages 490-493.

Medications

There are a number of over-the-counter and prescription medications available that help relieve allergy symptoms. They include pills, liquids, nasal sprays and eyedrops. Many people get the best relief from a combination of allergy medications. You may need to try several medications to identify what works best for you.

Over-the-counter medications may be enough to relieve your symptoms, or you may need a prescription medication.

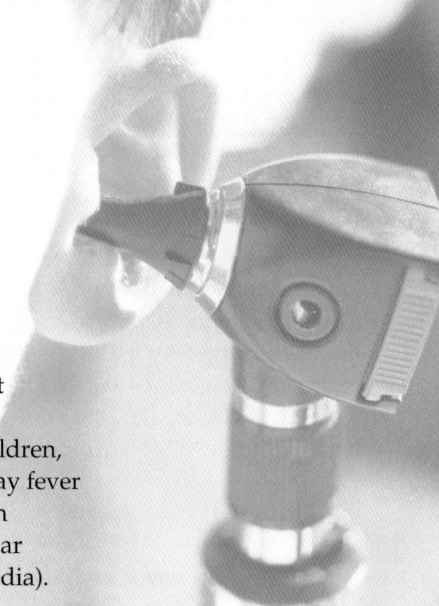

Allergies Often Associated With Other Conditions

Allergies often occur together with another health condition. If you have allergies, you also may be bothered by one of these diseases or disorders:

- *Asthma.* Allergies and asthma often occur together. In fact, allergic asthma is the most common type of asthma in the United States. If you experience signs and symptoms such as difficulty breathing, shortness of breath, a tight feeling in the chest, coughing and wheezing, you may have asthma.
- *Eczema.* Also called dermatitis, this condition causes swollen, red or itchy skin.
- *Sinusitis.* Prolonged sinus congestion due to hay fever may increase your susceptibility to sinusitis — an infection or inflammation of the membrane that lines the sinuses.
- *Ear infection.* In children, allergies such as hay fever often are a factor in recurrent middle ear infection (otitis media).

If your child has allergies, talk with your doctor about the best treatment. Some medications are approved for use in children, while others are only approved for adults. With over-the-counter medications, be sure to read the labels carefully.

Nasal corticosteroids

These nasal sprays help prevent and treat the inflammation caused by allergies. For many people they're the most effective medications, and they're often the first medication prescribed. Examples include fluticasone (Flonase Allergy Relief, others), mometasone (Nasonex), beclomethasone (Beconase AQ, QNASL), triamcinolone (Nasacort Allergy 24HR, others) budesonide (Rhinocort Aqua) and ciclesonide (Omnaris, Zetonna).

Although these medications can start to work after a few days of treatment, you may not notice any improvement until after you've used them for a week or so. Nasal corticosteroids are generally considered a safe long-term treatment for most people. Side effects can include an unpleasant smell or taste and nose irritation.

Oral corticosteroids

Corticosteroid medications in pill form, such as prednisone, are sometimes used to relieve severe allergy symptoms. Because long-term use can cause serious side effects such as cataracts, osteoporosis and muscle weakness, they're usually prescribed only for short periods of time.

Antihistamines

These oral medications and nasal sprays can help with itching, sneezing and a runny nose, but have less effect on congestion. They work by blocking histamine, an inflammatory chemical released by your immune system during an allergic reaction.

Older over-the-counter antihistamines such as diphenhydramine (Benadryl) and clemastine (Tavist-1) work as well as newer ones, but can make you drowsy. Newer oral antihistamines are less likely to make you drowsy.

Over-the-counter examples include loratadine (Claritin, Alavert), cetirizine (Zyrtec, others) and fexofenadine (Allegra, others). The prescription antihistamine nasal sprays azelastine (Astelin) and olopatadine (Patanase) start to relieve symptoms within minutes of use. Side effects include a bad taste in the mouth right after use.

Decongestants

These medications are available in over-the-counter and prescription liquids, tablets and nasal sprays. Over-the-counter oral decongestants include Sudafed and Drixoral Cold and Allergy. Nasal sprays include phenylephrine (Neo-Synephrine) and oxymetazoline (Afrin).

Because oral decongestants can raise blood pressure, avoid them if you have high blood pressure (hypertension). Oral decongestants can also worsen the symptoms of prostate enlargement, making urination more difficult. They may also cause insomnia and glaucoma.

Nasal decongestants shouldn't be used long term because they can worsen the congestion.

Cromolyn sodium

This medication, available as an over-the-counter nasal spray, must be used several times a day. It helps prevent allergy symptoms by stabilizing the cells that release histamine. Cromolyn sodium doesn't have serious side effects.

Leukotriene modifiers

Montelukast (Singulair) is a prescription tablet taken to block the action of leukotrienes — immune system chemicals that cause allergy symptoms such as excess mucus production. It's proved effective in treating asthma and also in treating hay fever. Possible side effects include headaches. In rare cases, aggressive behavior has been reported with montelukast. Less common side effects include abdominal pain and a cough.

Medication Side Effects

Antihistamines can be very useful in treating allergy symptoms, but side effects need to be considered. Antihistamines can cause drowsiness, dryness of the nose and mouth, and blurred vision. One study reported that diphenhydramine, an antihistamine in some over-the-counter allergy and cold remedies (Benadryl, Chlor-Trimeton), can cause more

driving impairment than can being legally drunk. Nonsedating antihistamines such as fexofenadine (Allegra) and loratadine (Claritin) tend to cause much less drowsiness. Cetirizine (Zyrtec) is less sedating than are older antihistamines such as diphenhydramine.

You may want to avoid driving a car or operating heavy machinery when you're taking an older over-the-counter antihistamine. Even if you don't feel drowsy, your driving may be impaired as long as the drug is in your system. Also avoid alcohol, which speeds the

absorption of some antihistamines and intensifies the drowsiness.

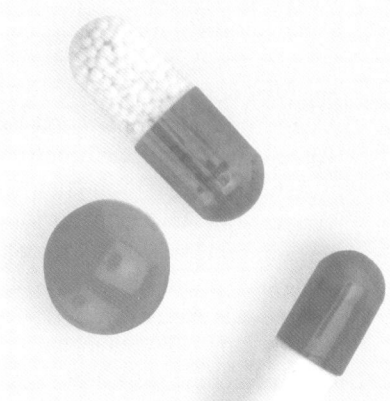

This medication is often used when nasal sprays can't be tolerated or for mild asthma.

Another leukotriene modifier zileuton (Zyflo) may have a special role in treating aspirin-induced asthma. Liver function monitoring is required every two to three months the first year and periodically thereafter. Neuropsychiatric events have been reported in some people taking the medication.

Nasal atropine

Available in a prescription nasal spray, ipratropium bromide (Atrovent) helps relieve a severe runny nose by preventing the glands in your nose from producing excess fluid. It's not effective for treating congestion, sneezing or postnasal drip. Mild side effects include nasal dryness, nosebleeds and a sore throat. Rarely, it can cause blurred vision, dizziness and difficult urination. The drug isn't recommended for people with glaucoma or men with an enlarged prostate.

Other treatments

In addition to medications, your doctor may recommend other treatments to relieve allergy symptoms.

Allergy shots

Certain allergies may be treated with what's commonly referred to as allergy shots, also known as

immunotherapy. It involves injecting very small amounts of known offending allergens under the skin in the upper arm. The intent is to decrease your immune system's reaction to the allergens by helping your body learn to accept them as harmless substances.

This treatment requires regular injections, often weekly, of increasing doses of the allergens until a maintenance dose is established. Then, injections of the maintenance dose are given monthly for three to five years or longer.

Severe reactions to immunotherapy are rare but can occur. As a precaution, your doctor will likely recommend that you stay in a waiting room for around 30 minutes after you receive an injection. Most, but not all, serious reactions occur within 30 minutes.

Allergy shots may provide hay fever relief that continues even after the shots are discontinued. They may be especially effective if you're allergic to insect stings, cat dander, dust mites or pollen produced by trees, grass and weeds. In children, immunotherapy may help prevent the development of asthma.

Oral allergy tablets

Another form of immunotherapy approved by the Food and Drug Administration to treat grass pollens and ragweed involves use of oral tablets. Side effects

I have respiratory allergies and asthma. I'll be traveling to an area with many plants and trees. What should I do?

See your doctor for a pre-trip evaluation and advice. Make sure your allergies and asthma — particularly your asthma — are well-controlled before you leave.

Ask your doctor for a contingency plan in case you have an attack on your trip. Your doctor may recommend that you take along emergency medications such as antihistamines, bronchodilators or corticosteroids. You might take a peak flow or another special asthma breath meter with you to monitor your peak flow rates. This can help guide adjustments to your asthma medication. In addition:

- Pack all of your medications in your carry-on luggage so that you have them in case you need them en route or if your luggage doesn't arrive on time. Be sure to pack more medication than the minimum you'll need. Store medications in their original containers. The containers provide instructions on dosages and refills and identify the drugs for customs officials when needed.
- Smoke can irritate asthma, so if you're traveling abroad, you may want to book a nonsmoking flight. If this isn't possible, ask for seats far away from the smoking section. Commercial flights within the United States are smoke-free.
- If you cross several time zones, allow for time differences so that you maintain your medication dosage schedule.
- Find out ahead of time if and how your health insurance plan handles medical care abroad, in case you should need medical treatment.

---

may include itching of the mouth and oral swelling. Serious reactions including anaphylaxis and severe throat swelling have been reported.

Nasal lavage

To help with irritating nasal symptoms, your doctor may recommend that you rinse your nose with salt water to help relieve congestion. Use an over-the-counter nasal saline spray or prepare your own saltwater solution using 1/4 teaspoon of salt mixed with 2 cups of warm water. It's important that you use good hygiene with this process, using distilled or boiled water and frequently changing or cleaning the rinse bottles.

Epinephrine

The most severe allergic reaction is anaphylaxis, which can cause blood vessels to dilate and air passages in the lungs to constrict. This reaction can cause severe wheezing, low blood pressure, unconsciousness and, in some instances, even death. Treatment for anaphylaxis involves an injection of epinephrine (adrenaline). Epinephrine quickly opens narrowed airways and constricts blood vessels to restore normal blood pressure.

Respiratory Allergies

Allergies of the respiratory tract often produce signs and symptoms that are similar to those of a cold: a congested head and chest, stuffy or runny nose, coughing, sneezing, and wheezing. In fact, allergies and colds are often confused. Some allergy symptoms typically last far longer than do those of a cold. Others may appear and disappear briefly, which is also uncharacteristic of the common cold.

For some people, allergy symptoms appear during a pollen season. For others, the symptoms manifest primarily at home from dust mite or mold exposure. Still others experience symptoms only during certain events, such as when visiting a home occupied by a cat or dog.

Hay fever (allergic rhinitis)

Signs and symptoms
- Stuffy or runny nose
- Frequent sneezing
- Watery or itchy eyes
- Cough

- Itchy nose, roof of mouth or throat
- Sinus pressure and facial pain
- Swollen, blue-colored skin under the eyes
- Decreased sense of taste and smell

Hay fever, also called allergic rhinitis, causes cold-like signs and symptoms such as a runny nose, congestion, sneezing and sinus pressure. It's one of the most common allergic conditions, affecting about 8 percent of American adults.

Unlike a cold, however, hay fever isn't caused by a virus — it's caused by an allergic response to indoor or outdoor airborne allergens, such as pollen, dust mites or pet dander. Some people have hay fever year-round. For others, it gets worse at certain times of the year, usually in the spring, summer or fall. This allergen sensitivity is thought to be partly an inherited trait that affects the ability of your immune system to deal with potential invaders.

For some people hay fever symptoms are a minor, temporary nuisance. But if your symptoms are more persistent, they can make you miserable and affect your performance at work, school or leisure activities. Finding the right hay fever treatment probably

That Pesky Pollen

Wherever plants grow, pollen is in the air at some time of the year. Trees, both deciduous and evergreen, produce pollen in spring. Grasses and most flowers produce their pollen during summer months. Late-blooming plants such as ragweed produce pollen in early fall. In warm climates with long growing seasons, pollen may be present in the air for 10 months of the year. In climates with shorter growing seasons, the pollen is present for less time.

Ragweed, a roadside plant, heads the list of hay fever-causing plants east of the Rocky Mountains. Other plant pollens that produce allergy symptoms include sagebrush, tumbleweed, pigweed, spiny amaranth, burning bush and English plantain.

Grasses that cause troublesome pollens include rye, timothy, redtop, Bermuda, orchard, sweet vernal and bluegrass. Most trees, including maple, oak, ash, birch, poplar, elm, pecan, juniper and cottonwood, produce pollens that can trigger hay fever.

Pollens that are carried by insects from one plant to another tend to be larger grains that are relatively harmless. Those carried by the wind are lighter and smaller and can cause hay fever. The amount of pollen in the air depends on the weather. Hot, dry breezes stir up pollen, whereas dampness washes the pollen to the ground.

Most pollen particles are so small that they can be carried by the air into a house through doors and screens. It doesn't take much pollen to produce an allergic reaction — as little as 20 particles per cubic yard. Many plants can produce up to a million such particles.

The most effective way to avoid pollen is to stay indoors, especially when pollen counts are high. Keep doors and windows closed. Air conditioning also is helpful.

won't completely eliminate your symptoms — but for most people, it makes a big difference.

During a process called sensitization, your immune system mistakenly identifies a harmless airborne substance as something harmful. Your immune system then starts producing allergy-causing antibodies. The next time you come in contact with the substance, these antibodies recognize it and signal your immune system to release chemicals such as histamine. These chemicals cause a reaction that leads to the irritating signs and symptoms of hay fever.

A hay fever attack generally lasts about 15 to 20 minutes and may recur several times a day. For people with severe hay fever, the condition can be continuous and disrupt their lives. For those with minor symptoms, the illness is only an annoyance.

Seasonal hay fever triggers include tree, grass and weed pollens and spores from fungi and molds. Year-round hay fever triggers often include dust mites or cockroaches, Asian beetles, dander from pets or mice, and spores from indoor or outdoor fungi or molds.

Diagnosis

To help in identifying the cause of your hay fever, your doctor may ask you a series of questions regarding the severity of your symptoms, when you first noticed them and if they seem to get worse at any particular time. You may be asked to keep a diary to determine accurately when your allergic reactions occur most frequently.

Your doctor may recommend tests such as skin prick tests or a blood test to determine which pollens may trigger your symptoms (see page 487).

Treatment

For mild hay fever, nonprescription oral antihistamines and decongestants are often effective (see page 488). Some over-the-counter antihistamines can produce drowsiness and dryness of the throat and mouth, causing as much discomfort as that of the hay fever. Nonsedating antihistamines such as loratadine (Claritin) and fexofenadine (Allegra) have less tendency to cause drowsiness.

Avoid regular use of over-the-counter decongestant nasal sprays. These sprays should only be used twice a day for a maximum of three to four days. Although they relieve symptoms at first, they can make the problem worse. If used too often or for too long, they cause your nose to become increasingly congested, and more frequent doses are needed to clear it. The only way to resolve the problem is to stop using the spray and wait for the congestion to subside. This may take a month or two.

Your doctor may also recommend a corticosteroid nasal spray. You may need to use the product for one or two weeks before you experience benefits. Cromolyn sodium may be used prior to allergen exposure to prevent symptoms. If you're bothered by watery or itchy eyes, your doctor may recommend an eye-drop such as ketorolac (Acular) or olopatadine (Patanol, Pataday, Pazeo), azelastine (Optivar), epinastine (Elestat), or lodoxamide (Alomide).

The closest thing to a cure for hay fever are allergy shots or tablets (immunotherapy) to desensitize your immune system to allergens (see "Allergy shots," page 489). Many people who undergo this therapy lose their sensitivity to a particular allergen, usually within two years. But it isn't appropriate for all individuals.

Animal dander, mold and dust allergies

Signs and symptoms
- Stuffy, runny nose
- Frequent sneezing

- Itchy eyes, nose, roof of mouth or throat
- Coughing
- Wheezing

Not all respiratory allergies are caused by pollen. Identical allergic reactions can occur because of sensitivity to molds, animal dander and the microscopic mites that live in house dust. For some people, mold, dust or animal allergies are an inconvenience, producing mild symptoms that last only a few weeks each year. Others experience more-severe, and sometimes year-round, symptoms.

Animal dander

Some people are allergic to the dander of animals and birds. The fur and feathers themselves are not the cause of year-round irritation. It's the scales shed from the skin that cause the allergy, along with the pet's saliva and urine. The only way to eliminate the problem is to avoid the source. This means not keeping pets. If you're sensitive to the tiny amounts of dander found in wool, avoid products made mostly of wool. Don't buy furniture or rugs that contain animal hair.

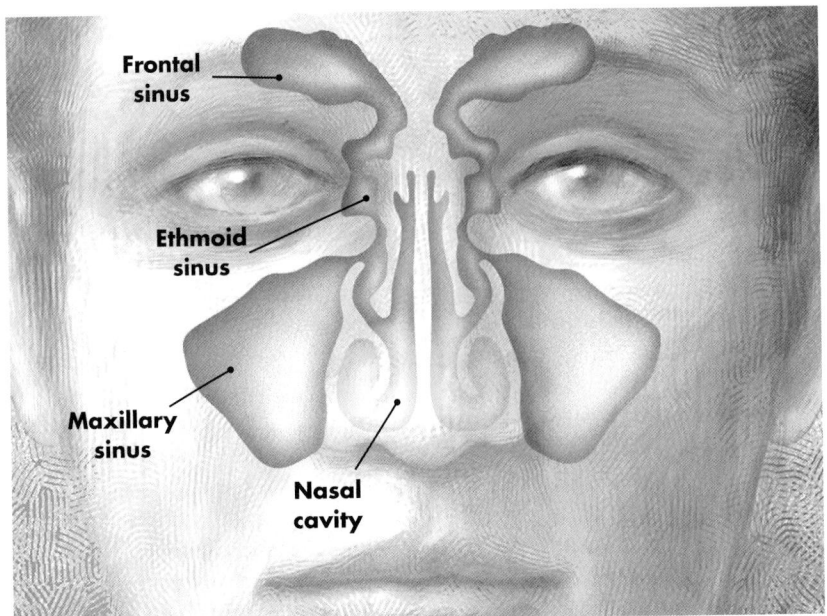

Sinuses are hollow spaces within the bones of your face. They produce mucus, which normally drains through sinus openings into your nose. If drainage is blocked, a sinus infection can result.

Molds

People with many allergies are often sensitive to the spores of common molds carried in the air. Mold allergy symptoms vary from person to person, and range from mild to severe. Some people have year-round symptoms and for others symptoms flare up only during certain times of the year.

Outdoor molds produce spores mostly in the summer and early fall, although in warm climates mold spores can be present all year. They live in the soil and on compost or damp vegetation. People who are susceptible to mold spores react most noticeably when they're mowing grass, harvesting crops, raking leaves or walking

Coping With Pet Allergies

A pet allergy occurs when your immune system reacts to certain animal proteins. The linings of your nasal passages become inflamed, causing sneezing, a runny nose, and other signs and symptoms.

Any animal with fur can be a source of a pet allergy, but pet allergies are most commonly associated with cats, dogs, rodents and horses. If you have a pet allergy, the best strategy is to avoid or reduce exposure to the animal as much as possible. If you're allergic to the pet in your home, take these steps:

- *Keep the pet out.* If your pet can live comfortably outside, this will greatly help reduce your allergy symptoms. However, this option isn't appropriate in certain climates.
- *Wash your pet once a week.* Have a family member or friend do this for you. Bathing can reduce the amount of your pet's airborne allergens by close to 90 percent.
- *Establish a pet-free zone.* Make certain rooms in your house, such as your bedroom, off-limits to your pet.

- *Avoid carpets and upholstered furniture.* It's difficult to remove pet allergens from upholstery. If possible, replace carpeting, particularly in your bedroom. Mop and vacuum floors frequently.
- *Use a high-efficiency particulate air (HEPA) filter.* This type of air filter that attaches to your furnace and air conditioning system, and some vacuums, can reduce airborne pet allergens.
- *Increase ventilation.* This will help decrease allergen levels.

If you or someone in your home has asthma triggered by a pet allergy, find your pet a new home. Continued exposure to pet allergens may lead to narrowing of the airways, increasing your risk of an attack.

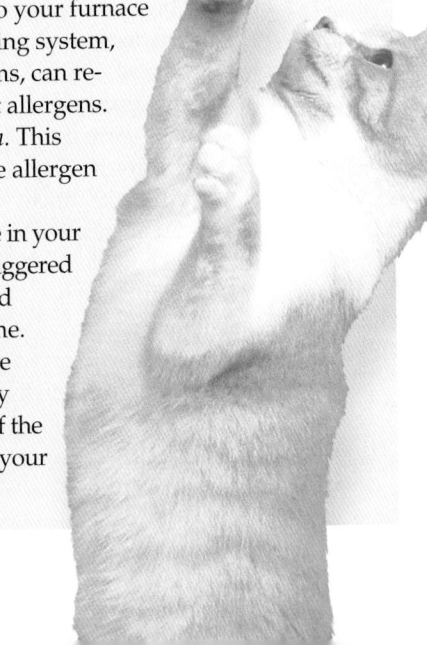

through tall grass and plants — activities that cause the spores to become airborne.

Indoor molds shed spores all year long, producing constant problems for people who are sensitive to them. Molds thrive indoors in damp locations, such as basements and bathrooms, and in upholstered furniture, bed linens, rugs, wood, books and wallpaper.

To reduce mold spores, keep doors and windows closed as much as possible and, when needed, use air conditioning in your home, car or office. Dry out a damp basement by using a dehumidifier. Be sure to clean the dehumidifier regularly so that molds and other growths don't develop inside it. Clean bathroom and basement walls with disinfectants.

Dust

House dust harbors all kinds of substances, including pollen, mold spores and animal dander. However, the primary cause of an allergic reaction to dust is microscopic mites. Dust mites, relatives of the spider, are too small to see without a microscope. They eat skin cells people shed and thrive in damp, warm environments.

If you have a dust mite allergy, your body generates an allergy-causing antibody to a protein found in dust mite debris. In other words, it mistakenly views the protein as something that could harm you.

The best way to deal with dust mites is to keep your home as dust-free as possible and the humidity low. This means mopping and dusting often. Wash throw rugs and furniture covers weekly. If you're the one with the allergy, if possible, have someone else do the cleaning or wear a dust mask.

Avoid dust trappers such as bed ruffles, canopy beds, bunk beds, carpeting, curtains, Venetian blinds and upholstered furniture. Enclose pillows, mattresses and box springs in allergen-proof coverings.

A central heating and air conditioning system that filters the air is a big help. You may also want to use a dehumidifier.

Miscellaneous irritants

Dozens of other inhaled substances can irritate the nose or bronchial tubes. These substances include:
- Industrial smoke and fumes
- Tobacco smoke
- Face and baby powder
- Powdered soaps and detergents

People who are sensitive to respiratory allergens are more likely to be sensitive to such irritants. If you seem to be bothered by these substances, try to avoid them as much as possible.

Diagnosis

To determine the cause of your symptoms, your doctor may ask you questions to determine how severe the reaction is, how often it occurs, whether it's year-round or seasonal, and the situations in which it generally occurs.

Your doctor may recommend tests such as skin prick tests or a blood test to confirm your allergy triggers (see page 487).

How serious are these allergies?

The cold-like symptoms of this type of allergy are inconvenient and annoying, but they're generally not a serious health threat.

Treatment

The most effective treatment for an allergy to molds, dust and animal dander is avoidance. This may be easier said than done because some allergens, particularly mold spores, are wind-borne just like pollen. With pollen, staying indoors in an air-conditioned atmosphere is often the most useful preventive measure.

When the allergen is house dust or animal dander, you can take steps to decrease your exposure. In addition, medications such as antihistamines and corticosteroids can help alleviate symptoms (see page 488). Some people also

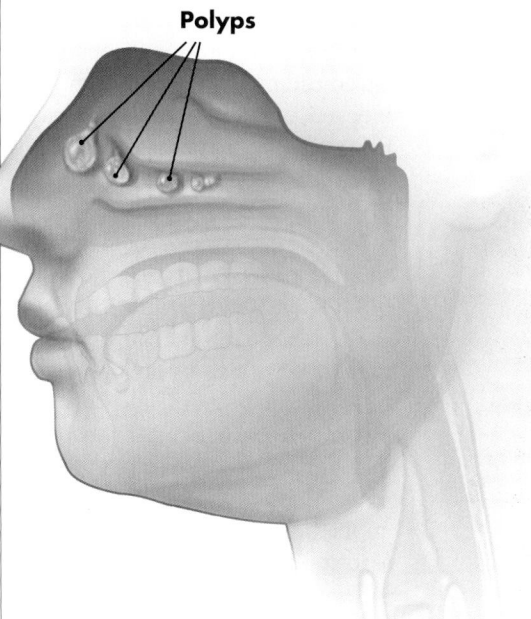

Polyps

Pearl-like lumps in the lining of the nasal passage are called nasal polyps. If they cause breathing difficulty or recurrent sinus infections, these polyps can be removed surgically.

receive immunotherapy to help desensitize their immune systems to the allergens (see page 489).

Chronic sinusitis and nasal polyps

Signs and symptoms
- Pain around your eyes or cheeks
- Tenderness of your sinuses to pressure or touch
- Difficulty breathing through your nose
- Drainage of thick, yellow or greenish discharge from the nose or down the back of the throat
- Reduced sense of taste and smell

Your sinuses are hollow spaces within the bones of your face, behind and above your eyes and nose. They help humidify and warm the air you breathe, aid your sense of smell, and improve the sound of your voice. They also secrete mucus, which cleans and moisturizes your nasal passages.

Inside your sinuses, tiny hair-like projections called cilia constantly sweep mucus out of your sinuses and into your nose and throat. Your sinuses drain into your nose through small openings called ostia. When ostia become blocked, mucus accumulates in sinus cavities. Microorganisms such as viruses and bacteria can multiply and cause an infection. An infection produces swelling, which can decrease sinus drainage.

Sometimes, respiratory allergies can lead to an infection or inflammation of your sinus cavities, causing pain and difficulty breathing through your nose. If you've had sinusitis for three months or longer and it doesn't respond to antibiotics, you may have chronic sinusitis.

Chronic sinusitis is different from acute sinusitis caused by a bacterial infection, which typically responds to treatment within a few weeks. Chronic sinusitis is also associated with nasal polyps — small, benign tissue growths within nasal passages that hinder breathing.

Causes

Allergies to such elements as pollen, animal dander and dust mites can cause a stuffy nose, leading to chronic sinusitis. With seasonal allergies, symptoms tend to occur during distinct seasons. With non-seasonal allergies, symptoms persist throughout the year or recur.

A nasal passage abnormality, such as a deviated septum, also increases your risk of chronic sinusitis. So do nasal polyps. Nasal polyps occur when the mucous membrane that lines the inside of the nose swells and protrudes into the nasal passage, reducing sinus drainage. These polyps may appear singly or in clusters, making breathing difficult and interfering with your sense of taste and smell.

Nasal polyps are caused by an overproduction of fluid in the mucous membrane, sometimes as a result of hay fever or some other nasal allergy.

Chronic sinusitis, nasal polyps and asthma are commonly associated with sensitivity to aspirin or nonsteroidal anti-inflammatory drugs (NSAIDs). This combination is called aspirin-exacerbated respiratory disease (AERD).

Diagnosis

People often have several episodes of severe but acute sinus infections (sinusitis) before developing chronic sinusitis. If you've had sinusitis a number of times and the condition doesn't respond to treatments such as nasal sprays, decongestants and antibiotics, you might have chronic sinusitis.

To look for the cause of your symptoms, your doctor may use a tool to hold your nose open and apply medication that constricts blood vessels in your nasal passages. This makes it easier to see inside your nasal passages. This visual inspection can also help rule out physical conditions that trigger sinusitis, such as nasal polyps or other abnormalities.

Several tests may be used to screen for chronic sinusitis:

- **Nasal endoscopy.** A thin, flexible tube (endoscope) with a fiber-optic light inserted through your nose allows your doctor to visually inspect the inside of your sinuses.
- **Imaging studies.** Images taken using computerized tomography (CT) or magnetic resonance imaging (MRI) can show details of your sinuses and nasal area. These may identify a deep inflammation or physical obstruction that's difficult to detect using an endoscope.
- **An allergy test.** If your doctor suspects that the condition may be triggered by allergies, an allergy skin test may be recommended. A skin test is safe and quick and can help pinpoint the allergen that's responsible for your nasal flare-ups.

Treatment

Your doctor may recommend treatments to help relieve sinusitis symptoms. These include:

- **Saline.** You squirt or spray a saline solution into your nose several times a day to rinse your nasal passages.
- **Nasal corticosteroids.** These nasal sprays help prevent and treat inflammation. Examples include fluticasone (Flonase Allergy Relief, others), budesonide (Rhinocort Aqua), triamcinolone (Nasacort Allergy 24HR, others), mometasone (Nasonex), beclomethasone (Beconase AQ), flunisolide and ciclesonide (Zetonna, Omnaris).
- **Oral or injected corticosteroids.** Because these medications can cause serious side effects, they're rarely used to relieve inflammation from severe sinusitis. Examples include prednisone and methylprednisolone.
- **Decongestants.** These medications are available over-the-counter and by prescription. Over-the-counter oral decongestants include Sudafed and Drixoral Cold and Allergy. Nasal sprays include phenylephrine (Neo-Synephrine) and oxymetazoline (Afrin). Nasal decongestants should be taken for only a few days at most; otherwise they can cause more-severe congestion (rebound congestion).
- **Antibiotics.** Most often chronic sinusitis isn't caused by bacteria, so antibiotics won't help. But in some cases, a bacterium may be responsible, in which case an antibiotic may be prescribed.
- **Allergy shots.** If allergies are contributing to your sinusitis, allergy shots (immunotherapy) that help reduce the body's reaction to specific allergens may help treat the condition.
- **Surgery.** In cases that continue to resist treatment or medication, endoscopic sinus surgery may be an option. For this procedure, the doctor uses an endoscope, a thin tube with an attached light, to explore your sinus passages. Then, depending on the source of obstruction, the doctor may use various tools to remove tissue or shave away a polyp that's causing nasal blockage.

Asthma

Asthma occurs when the airways in your lungs (bronchial tubes) become inflamed and constricted. The muscles of the bronchial walls tighten, and your airways produce extra mucus that blocks your airways. Signs and symptoms of asthma range from minor wheezing to life-threatening asthma attacks.

An estimated 24 million Americans have asthma. Of these about 6 million are children. Asthma is the leading cause of chronic illness in children.

Signs and symptoms
- Wheezing
- Difficulty breathing
- Tightness in the chest
- Coughing

Emergency signs and symptoms
- Extreme difficulty breathing
- Bluish lips and nails
- Severe breathlessness
- Increased pulse rate
- Severe coughing

Some people with asthma have persistent symptoms. For others, symptoms are intermittent. Fortunately, asthma is a treatable disease. With professional help, asthma attacks can be controlled and are seldom disabling or life-threatening.

In recent years scientists have gained a better understanding of asthma's causes. New drugs have been developed to replace older medications, and greater emphasis is now being given to managing the condition.

Risk factors

A growing number of people are diagnosed with asthma each year. However, it isn't clear why numbers are increasing. Several factors are thought to increase the chances of developing asthma. These include:
- A family history of asthma
- Frequent respiratory infections as a child

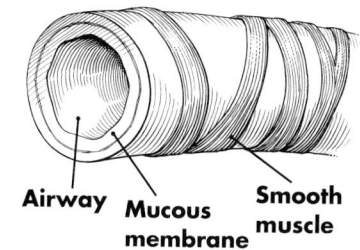

Normal airways in your lungs

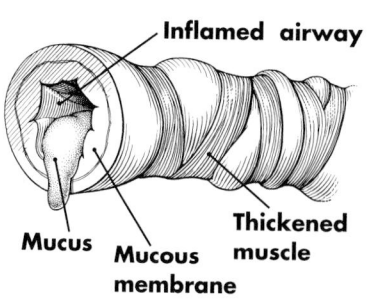

In asthma, airways in your lungs are inflamed and swollen.

- Exposure to secondhand smoke
- Living in an urban area, especially if there's a lot of air pollution
- Exposure to occupational triggers, such as chemicals used in farming and manufacturing
- Low birth weight
- Being overweight

For people under age 30, asthma is typically triggered by allergies. Among individuals age 30 and older with asthma, approximately 40 to 70 percent also have respiratory allergies.

For individuals in whom allergies aren't a factor, asthma may be related to an irritant or a medical condition. In most cases, asthma is the result of a combination of environmental and genetic (inherited) causes.

Diagnosis

Diagnosing asthma can be difficult. Signs and symptoms can range from mild to severe and are often similar to those of other conditions, including emphysema, early congestive heart failure or vocal cord problems. In children, it can be hard to differentiate asthma from wheezy bronchitis, pneumonia or reactive airway disease.

In order to rule out other possible conditions, your doctor likely will do a physical exam and ask you questions about your signs and symptoms and any other health problems. You may also be given lung (pulmonary) function tests to determine how

much air moves in and out as you breathe.

Tests used to measure lung function include:
- **Spirometry.** This test measures the narrowing of your bronchial tubes by checking how much air you can exhale after a deep breath, and how fast you can breathe out.
- **Meters.** Peak flow and home FEV-1 meters are simple devices that can be used at home to help detect subtle respiratory changes before you notice symptoms (see page 499). If the readings are lower than usual, it's a sign your asthma may be about to flare up. Your doctor will give you instructions on how to track and deal with low readings.

Lung function tests generally are done before and after using a bronchodilator to open your airways. If your lung function improves with

PREVENTION TIP

If you have asthma, you're more likely to be bothered by stomach acid backing up (refluxing) into your esophagus, a condition called gastroesophageal reflux disease (GERD). In some cases, GERD may actually cause asthma symptoms. To help prevent GERD, don't eat or drink for several hours before going to bed. You may also find it helpful to elevate the head of your bed. See page 818 for more information about GERD.

use of a bronchodilator, it's likely that you have asthma.

Other tests to diagnose asthma include:

- **Methacholine bronchial challenge.** If you have asthma, inhaling a known asthma trigger called methacholine will cause mild constriction of your airways. A positive methacholine test supports a diagnosis of asthma. This test may be used if your initial lung function test is normal.
- **Nitric oxide test.** This test is sometimes used to diagnose and monitor asthma. It measures the amount of a gas called nitric oxide you have in your breath. If your airways are inflamed — a sign of asthma — you may have higher than normal levels of nitric oxide. This test isn't as widely available as other lung studies.

Based on the results of your tests, your doctor may classify your asthma as mild intermittent, mild persistent, moderate persistent or severe persistent. It's not uncommon for asthma severity to change over time.

Asthma Medications

Medications used to treat asthma include long-term control medications, quick-relief (rescue) medications and medications to treat allergies. The right medication for you depends on your age and symptoms, and what seems to work best to keep your asthma under control.

Long-term control medications

In most cases, these medications need to be taken every day. Types of long-term control medications include:

- **Inhaled corticosteroids.** Inhaled corticosteroids include the drugs fluticasone (Flovent Diskus, Flovent HFA), budesonide (Pulmicort Flexhaler), flunisolide, beclomethasone (Qvar), fluticasone furoate (Arnuity Ellipta), mometasone furoate (Asmanex Twisthaler, Asmanex HFA) and ciclesonide (Alvesco). These medications reduce airway inflammation and are the most commonly used long-term asth-

Occupational Asthma

Some people regularly experience wheezing, coughing or shortness of breath at work. When they leave work, their signs and symptoms improve.

This is commonly referred to as occupational asthma. It's caused by inhaling dust, vapors, gases or fumes particular to the workplace. These substances can irritate your respiratory system.

Occupational asthma generally develops in one of two ways:

Direct response to an irritant
Asthmatic symptoms occur immediately following exposure to substances such as ammonia, hydrochloric acid, sulfur dioxide or environmental smoke. This is especially common in people who already have asthma.

Long-term sensitization
Continued exposure — sometimes over months or years — causes an allergic response. Symptoms develop more gradually. An example is a veterinarian who after regular exposure to animals develops an allergy to one or more of them.

Common irritants

It's estimated that occupational asthma may account for up to 15 percent of all asthma cases in the United States. An estimated 11 million workers in a wide range of industries and occupations are thought to be exposed to at least one of numerous substances known to cause occupational asthma.

More than 300 workplace substances have been identified as possible causes of occupational asthma, and the list keeps growing. These substances generally fall into one of these categories:

- Chemicals such as anhydrides, diisocyanates and acids that are used in the manufacture of paints, varnishes, adhesives, laminates and soldering fluxes (resin used in soldering)
- Enzymes used in detergents, flour conditioners, some pharmaceuticals and meat tenderizers
- Proteins found in animal dander, hair, scales, fur, saliva and body wastes
- Flour and grain dust
- Proteins found in rye, barley, oats, rice and soy
- Products used during seafood and egg processing
- Chlorine gas, sulfur dioxide, hydrochloric acid and smoke

If your asthma is severe and there's a strong connection between your illness and your job, your doctor might recommend that you eliminate any exposure to irritants or other substances that can cause asthma. This might mean that you can't work in the same location, at the same job or in the same industry.

Changing jobs is a difficult decision with many potential consequences, and such a recommendation is never made without careful consideration. Working with your doctor, you can arrive at the best decision for your overall health.

ma medication. Unlike oral corticosteroids, these medications are considered relatively low risk for long-term corticosteroid side effects. You may need to use the medications for several days to weeks before they reach their maximum benefit.

- **Long-acting beta-2 agonists.** These include salmeterol (Serevent Diskus) and formoterol. These inhaled medications, called long-acting bronchodilators, mainly open lung airways. This type of medication should be used in combination with an inhaled corticosteroid that's being used regularly.
- **Leukotriene modifiers.** These medications — montelukast (Singulair), zafirlukast (Accolate) and zileuton (Zyflo CR) — work by opening airways, reducing inflammation and decreasing mucus production.

Quick-relief medications

Also called rescue medications, you use quick-relief medications for rapid, short-term relief of symptoms during an asthma attack, or before exercise, if your doctor recommends it. Only use these medications as often as your doctor advises you to. Using rescue inhalers too often is a clue to poorly controlled asthma. Your doctor may need to increase your long-term control medications or take other action to prevent a potentially serious asthma flare.

Types of quick-relief medications include:

- **Short-acting beta-2 agonists.** These inhaled medications, such as albuterol, are called bronchodilators. They ease breathing by temporarily relaxing airway muscles. They act within minutes, and their effects last four to six hours.
- **Ipratropium (Atrovent).** Your doctor might prescribe this inhaled medication for immediate symptom relief. Like other bronchodilators, ipratropium

relaxes the airways, making it easier to breathe. Ipratropium is mostly used for emphysema and chronic bronchitis.

- **Oral and intravenous corticosteroids.** These drugs are used to treat acute asthma attacks or very severe asthma. Examples include prednisone and methylprednisolone. The medications relieve airway inflammation. They may cause serious side effects when used long term, so they're only used for severe symptoms.

Medications for allergy-induced asthma

The purpose of these medications is to decrease your body's sensitivity to a particular allergen or prevent your immune system from reacting to allergens. Depending on what you're allergic to and the severity of your allergy symptoms, a variety of drugs may be prescribed. For more information on allergy treatments, see page 487.

Combination therapy

If one drug isn't keeping your asthma in check, your options generally are to increase the strength (dose) of that medication or to take an additional medication of a different type.

A number of studies indicate that adding another medication is often the most effective therapy. Combining two different medications may reduce the risk of potential side effects from taking a high dose of one drug, such as an inhaled corticosteroid. In addition, the different drugs treat asthma in

Future Therapies

Asthma is likely the result of a combination of genetic and environmental factors. Researchers have discovered several genes associated with airway inflammation and constriction. These discoveries may lead to new therapeutic approaches to the prevention and treatment of asthma. As their understanding of asthma evolves, scientists are developing many new classes of drugs that interrupt the asthma process at key points.

different ways. For example, one drug may control inflammation to prevent attacks, while another may help keep airways open.

Some combination drug products are now available on the market, such as Advair Diskus, an inhaler that combines the corticosteroid fluticasone and the bronchodilator salmeterol; Symbicort, an inhaler that combines the medications budesonide and formoterol; Dulera, which combines the medications mometasone furoate and formoterol; and Breo Ellipta, a combination of fluticasone furoate and vilanterol. Asthma medications can be prescribed in a number of combinations. An inhaled corticosteroid often is one component.

The right combination depends on the severity of your asthma and your treatment goals. For instance, you may prefer a pill instead of an inhaler. Perhaps you experience greater problems at night or during a favorite activity. Maybe you've experienced certain side effects with one drug but not with another. By discussing these issues with your doctor, the two of you can select the treatment program that controls your symptoms and works best for you.

Other medications

Asthma can be difficult to control despite regular use of high-dose inhalers. Rarely, a doctor may prescribe a steroid administered by mouth or injection. For severe asthma that doesn't respond to high-dose preventive inhalers, a doctor may prescribe a biologic agent to help control symptoms.

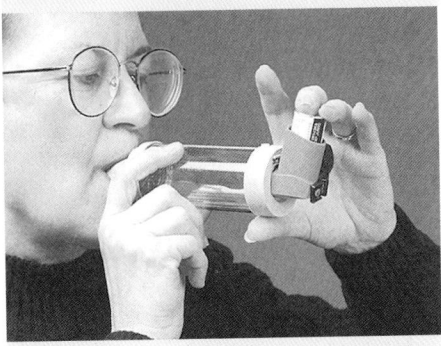

To use a metered dose inhaler:

1. Shake the inhaler well, perhaps five or six times.
2. Attach a spacer to the nozzle end of the inhaler. A spacer is a 4- to 8-inch-long plastic tube that helps to distribute the medication evenly in the bronchial tubes. Releasing your medication into the chamber gives you time to inhale more slowly. It decreases the amount of medication that's deposited on the back of the throat and increases the amount that reaches the lungs.
3. Hold your head erect and sit up straight. Breathe in and out normally once, then stop for a moment. Don't try to push all of the air from your lungs.
4. Close your mouth around the end of the spacer.
5. Squeeze the inhaler once as you breathe in slowly, like you're sipping hot soup. Keep inhaling even after finishing the squeeze. Continue inhaling for a total of five to seven seconds.
6. After inhaling, remove the spacer from your mouth and hold your breath for 10 seconds. Then exhale through your nose.
7. If you've been directed to take two doses at a time, breathe normally four or five times and repeat steps 1 through 6.
8. Gargle with water or brush your teeth after using an inhaled corticosteroid. Spit out the water. This reduces the amount of drug that's swallowed and absorbed into the body by way of the stomach. It also reduces side effects such as mouth and throat irritation and oral yeast infections (thrush).

Asthma Inhalers

Inhalers have transformed asthma treatment. They enable people with asthma to deliver medication directly to their lungs almost anytime, anyplace. During the past several decades, a variety of inhalers have been developed to relieve or prevent asthma symptoms. The most common device used to deliver inhaled medication is a metered dose inhaler.

There's one catch, however. Metered dose inhalers help only when you know how to use them. It takes a certain amount of coordination and skill to use a metered dose inhaler properly. Many surveys have shown that most people who use a metered dose inhaler — maybe up to two-thirds — use it improperly. But studies also show that with careful and repeated instruction, more than 90 percent of people who use inhalers can learn to do so correctly.

Carefully follow the instructions that come with your inhaler and ask your health care provider for a demonstration. Try using the inhaler in front of this person and ask for feedback. Then practice at home in front of a mirror.

Types of inhalers

Inhalers are hand-held, portable devices that deliver medication directly to the lungs. A variety of inhalers are available, but basically they fall into two categories — metered dose and dry powder.

Metered dose inhalers
Metered dose inhalers use a chemical propellant to force a measured dose of medication out of the inhaler. The inhaler includes a pressurized canister with measured doses of medication inside. The medication is released either by squeezing the canister or by inhaling. You may find it easier to use a hand-actuated inhaler with a spacer — a short tube that attaches to the inhaler. The idea is to inject the medication into the incoming air and slowly breathe this mixture into your lungs.

Dry powder inhalers
Dry powder inhalers are breath-activated. The medication is released when you suddenly inhale from the device. A dry powder inhaler requires you to place your lips on the mouthpiece and inhale more rapidly than with a traditional metered dose inhaler. Some people find dry powder inhalers easier to use than the conventional pressurized metered dose inhalers because hand-lung coordination isn't required. Spacers shouldn't be used with dry powder inhalers.

Who should use an inhaler?

Both children and adults can use inhalers. Generally children age 6 and older can be trained to use an inhaler properly, and some children as young as age 4 may be able to use the device. Parents should supervise their children's use of all medications.

For people who are unable to use an inhaler, a nebulizer is often recommended. Nebulizers are most commonly used by infants, young children and people who are seriously ill. The device includes a compressor-driven pump that converts the medication into a mist that's inhaled.

Inhaler pros and cons

The benefits of inhalers are that they're convenient to carry and use, and they can provide immediate relief. But they need to be used properly to be effective. Noncompliance is a problem for many people with asthma who use metered dose inhalers to manage their disease — either they forget to take the medication, or they use the inhaler incorrectly.

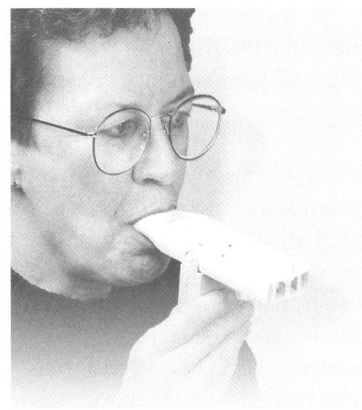

To use a peak flow meter, follow these steps:
1. Connect the mouthpiece to the peak flow meter.
2. Push the indicator to the bottom of the scale.
3. Take a deep breath and blow as hard and fast as possible — like you're blowing out a candle 6 feet away — with your lips tight around the mouthpiece.
4. Note the reading of the indicator. This is your peak flow rate.
5. Slide the indicator back to the bottom of the scale and repeat the test two more times.
6. Record the highest reading of the three tests.

This can lead to the second problem: People with asthma can rely too much on short-acting bronchodilator inhalers.

These fast-acting medications usually relieve symptoms quickly. But they're no substitute for the long-term medications that keep asthma under control. Most people with controlled asthma use fast-acting inhalers twice a week or less. If you use a fast-acting inhaler more than twice a week your asthma may not be well-controlled. Overuse of a bronchodilator can also put you at risk of toxic drug levels, which can cause an irregular heartbeat, especially if you have a heart condition.

Managing Asthma

In addition to medication, self-care is very important in controlling asthma. The best way to overcome anxiety that can accompany asthma is to take steps to reduce your risk of an attack. Try to avoid or limit activities that make your asthma worse.

- **Monitor your breathing.** You may learn to recognize warning signs of an impending attack, such as slight coughing, wheezing or shortness of breath. But because your lung function may decrease before you notice any signs or symptoms, regularly measure your peak airflow with a peak flow meter.

- **Identify and treat attacks early.** If you act quickly, you're less likely to experience a severe attack. When your peak flow measurements decrease and alert you to an impending attack, take your medication as instructed and stop any activity that may have triggered the attack. If your symptoms don't improve, get medical help.
- **Don't let up on your medication program.** Just because your asthma seems to be improving, don't stop your medication. Your doctor can help you step-down your medications when appropriate.
- **Identify and avoid triggers.** A number of outdoor allergens and irritants — ranging from pollen and mold to cold air and air pollution — can trigger asthma attacks. Find out what causes or worsens your asthma, and take steps to avoid those triggers. Also understand that most flares of asthma occur after a common cold.

Here are some simple strategies that may help:
- **Use your air conditioner.** Air conditioning helps reduce the amount of airborne pollen from trees, grasses and weeds that finds its way indoors. Air conditioning also lowers indoor humidity and can reduce your exposure to dust mites.
- **Maintain optimal humidity.** Keep humidity low in your home and office. If you live in a damp climate, talk to your doctor about using a dehumidifier.

- **Keep indoor air clean.** Have your air conditioner and furnace checked once a year. Change the filters in your furnace and air conditioner according to the manufacturer's instructions. Consider installing a small-particle filter in your ventilation system. If you use a room humidifier, change the water daily.
- **Decontaminate your decor.** Minimize dust by replacing certain items in your bedroom. For example, encase pillows, mattresses and box springs in dust-proof covers. Remove carpeting and install hardwood or linoleum flooring. Use washable curtains and blinds.
- **Clean regularly.** Clean your home at least once a week. If you're likely to stir up dust, wear a mask or have someone else do the cleaning.
- **Prevent mold spores.** Clean damp areas in the bath, kitchen and around the house to keep mold spores from developing. Get rid of moldy leaves or damp firewood in the yard.
- **Reduce pet dander.** If you're allergic to dander, avoid pets with fur or feathers. Having pets regularly bathed or groomed also may reduce the amount of dander in your surroundings.
- **If it's cold out, cover your face.** If your asthma is worsened by cold, dry air, wearing a face mask can help.
- **Get regular exercise.** Exercise strengthens your heart and lungs, which helps relieve asthma symptoms.

Children and Asthma

More than 6 million people under age 18 in the United States have asthma. With effective treatment, many children with asthma can enjoy a full range of activities, including exercise and sports. In many cases, their symptoms decrease during their adult years.

To reduce asthma episodes, have a treatment plan in place and know the signs of a possible attack.

Follow a treatment plan
Work with your child's doctor to develop a treatment plan. The two overall objectives are to:
- Minimize the frequency and severity of asthmatic episodes
- Control the condition to allow for a normal quality of life

Your child's treatment plan may include several strategies:
- Medications
- Avoidance of asthma triggers
- Daily use of a peak flow meter
- Allergy shots

Be supportive
Attitudes can be especially important. Children with asthma may emphasize what they can't do. Help them focus on what they can do — and how they can help keep their asthma under control. Be encouraging and supportive.

Be prepared for an attack
An asthma attack can be an anxious time for you and your child. That's exactly why you need to prepare for how to handle the situation. Your doctor can help you put together a written contingency plan that outlines what to do in an asthma attack. This plan will help you avoid panic when an attack does occur.

Copies of the plan should be kept in places where they're accessible at a moment's notice. Be sure that your child and everyone who cares for him or her — such as grandparents, a babysitter and schoolteachers — knows where the plan is kept. Also keep copies of the plan in your wallet or purse, the car, and your child's backpack in case an asthma attack occurs away from home.

Although every child's plan will be different, it should contain the phone number of your child's doctor and this basic information:
- **Warning signs.** Symptoms and peak flow meter readings that often are a precursor to an attack.
- **How to manage an attack at home.** Medications that should be used during an asthma attack — also where they're located and how to use them.
- **Indications of a serious attack.** Information needed to evaluate if your child needs medical care. List criteria for determining how much difficulty your child is having breathing. Note what level of medication use indicates a serious attack. List instructions for using medications that are designed specifically for treating a serious asthma attack.
- **What to do in an emergency.** Warning signs of a life-threatening asthma attack, emergency phone numbers and the location of the nearest hospital.

If you're in doubt about the seriousness of your child's symptoms, it's better to be safe than sorry. Call your child's doctor or take your child in for evaluation at your local clinic or emergency department, if needed. Successful treatment of asthma attacks depends on recognizing symptoms and acting early.

Work with school personnel
Every parent of a child with asthma faces the dilemma of how

Exercise-Induced Asthma

If you cough, wheeze or feel out of breath during or after exercise, you may have exercise-induced asthma. Exercise-induced asthma occurs when the main air passages of your lungs, the bronchial tubes, become inflamed, causing tightening and narrowing of the bronchial walls.

If you have exercise-induced asthma, physical exertion may be the only thing that triggers your symptoms. Or exercise may just be one of several things that trigger an asthma attack. Factors that can worsen exercise-induced asthma include cold weather, dry air, air pollution such as smoke or smog, high pollen counts, having a respiratory infection such as a cold, and being out of shape.

The good news is exercise-induced asthma doesn't have to limit your athletic goals. Proper treatment can help keep symptoms under control — and help you exercise as much as you want. Because exercise-induced asthma has the same symptoms and results as involved in regular asthma, standard asthma medications can control it (see page 496).

To prevent or reduce symptoms, make a habit of warming up and cooling down for at least 15 minutes before and after exercise. Avoid exercising outdoors in extremely cold temperatures or when pollen levels are high. If you have to exercise in the cold, wear a face mask. Using a short-acting bronchodilator 15 minutes before exercise may help you prevent symptoms.

If you feel mild symptoms coming on during a workout, try continuing your activity. Your symptoms may remain mild. Otherwise, if your doctor has prescribed an inhaler with a short-acting bronchodilator, pause and inhale two puffs. You should breathe more easily within a few minutes. If you don't, stop exercising.

Children and Corticosteroids

For several years, the Food and Drug Administration has required drug manufacturers to add language on the labels of corticosteroids stating that they may reduce the rate of growth in some children. Does this mean that it's not safe for a child to take inhaled or intranasal corticosteroids?

Inhaled and intranasal corticosteroids are, by expert consensus, still the best and most effective medications for asthma. Most doctors appropriately continue to recommend these products for many, if not most, people with asthma.

Inhaled corticosteroid use may reduce growth rates in some children. It's not possible to predict accurately which children will be affected. Studies don't reveal conclusively whether the slowed growth rate is permanent or whether affected children "catch up" later.

Asthma is a chronic disease that can be debilitating and even life-threatening. For children with asthma, the benefits of inhaled corticosteroids largely outweigh the risk of a potential reduction in growth.

To reduce possible side effects, it's important to use inhaled or intranasal corticosteroids with care. Here are some important things to remember if your child is taking these medications:

- Carefully follow the instructions.
- Together with your child's doctor, determine over time the lowest dose of inhaled or intranasal corticosteroids that will manage your child's allergies or asthma.
- Discuss other options with your child's doctor. Other medications for allergies and asthma do exist. But they also have possible side effects and may not offer the same benefits as inhaled or intranasal corticosteroids.
- Talk to your child's doctor before discontinuing inhaled or intranasal corticosteroids. Stopping the medication suddenly without careful follow-up could seriously impair your child's health.
- Be sure your doctor monitors your child's growth.

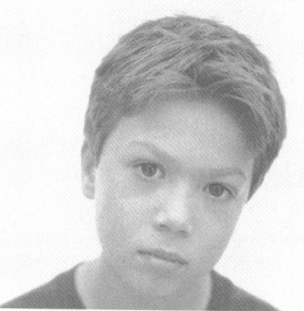

to help the child control his or her asthma at school. Create a feedback system to detect how well your child is managing asthma during the school day.

Share your child's treatment plan
Share your child's treatment plan with all of the adults who regularly interact with him or her:
- Homeroom teacher
- School nurse
- Specialists, such as music, art and physical education teachers
- Classroom aides
- Counselors
- Coaches

Meet with your child's teachers and other school personnel early in the school year. Describe any medications that your child takes, how those medications are administered and possible side effects. Explain how your child can manage an asthma episode.

Set up a medication location
This may help your child so he or she doesn't feel self-conscious about taking medication at school.

Make arrangements for your child to take his or her daily medication with minimal disruption.

Monitor your child's learning
Ask your child's teachers to contact you if your child has difficulty paying attention or following instructions, and follow up promptly on any decline in grades. It's possible that asthma symptoms or medications might be playing a role.

Meet with the physical education teacher
Flexibility is key in physical education. Ask your doctor to write a letter to your child's physical education teacher. This letter may include guidelines for appropriate levels of exercise. Have the doctor explain your child's asthma management plan.

Assess the results
Observe your child's symptoms and overall health and well-being. If you notice any change, consult your doctor.

Skin Allergies

Most Americans experience skin reactions at some time during their lives. The most common sensitivity is to plants such as poison ivy, poison oak or poison sumac. In people who are susceptible to these plants, contact with the irritants of the plants produces an itchy rash that may blister. Many other substances also can produce skin allergies.

Contact dermatitis

Signs and symptoms
- Red rash or bumps
- Itching, which may be severe
- Dry, red patches, which may resemble a burn

Contact dermatitis is an inflammation of the skin that results from direct contact with certain substances, such as chemicals, soap, cosmetics, jewelry or weeds. The resulting red rash isn't contagious, but it can be very uncomfortable.

Latex Allergy

Allergic reactions to latex — a substance found in many medical and consumer products — are common. Latex is a natural rubber product derived from the milky sap of the rubber tree. It may be found in examination and surgical gloves, intravenous and respiratory supplies, and many other medical and dental products. Consumer products containing latex include condoms, diaphragms, rubber gloves, balloons and tires.

Reactions to latex allergy can take two forms. One is a skin rash (contact dermatitis). It's often seen in people who wear latex gloves, and it resembles the skin rash of poison ivy. This type of allergic response generally isn't a reaction to the latex but to the chemical additives used in the manufacture of latex products. The second type of reaction is a classic allergy reaction, and it can be more serious. In this case, the allergens are proteins in the latex itself. Signs and symptoms include hives, hay fever, a runny nose and those associated with occupational asthma (see page 496).

The best way to avoid latex allergy reactions is to avoid latex or reduce your exposure as much as possible. If you think that you may have a latex allergy, visit an allergist to find out. A medical history and allergy tests can determine your sensitivity to latex.

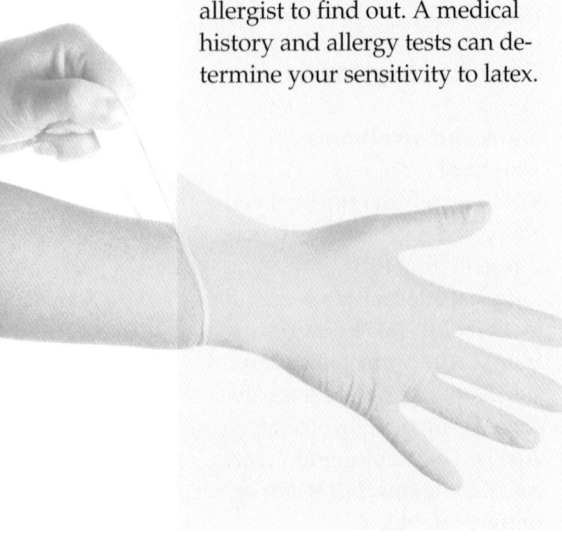

Based on the cause, contact dermatitis falls into two categories: irritant contact dermatitis and allergic contact dermatitis. Irritant contact dermatitis is the more common of the two.

- **Irritant contact dermatitis.** This type of dermatitis results from repeated contact with a substance, such as soap, cosmetics or skin products, including deodorant, that irritates the skin. The exposure produces red, dry itchy patches, usually on the hands, fingers and face. Some substances, such as bleach or strong acids, can cause irritant contact dermatitis after just one exposure. These substances typically remove oil and the protective barriers from the skin.

- **Allergic contact dermatitis.** This type of dermatitis is caused by a reaction to substances called allergens. The resulting reaction is your body's response to the sensitive agent. Allergic contact dermatitis produces a red rash, bumps and sometimes blisters when severe.

Common allergens include rubber or latex, metals such as nickel, costume jewelry (nickel), perfume, cosmetics, hair dyes and weeds, including poison ivy. It may take several years for an allergy to develop. Once an allergy has developed to a specific substance, however, it remains for life. Exposure to even a small amount of the allergen will reliably result in skin eruption. This usually occurs within 48 hours of contact, but time may vary.

Diagnosis

Your doctor may diagnose contact dermatitis after talking to you about your signs and symptoms and examining your skin. If the cause of your rash isn't apparent or if your rash recurs often, your doctor may recommend a patch test (contact delayed hypersensitivity allergy test).

During a patch test, small quantities of potential allergens are applied to small patches, which are then placed on your skin to check for a reaction. The patches remain on your skin for two days before being evaluated by your doctor.

If you're allergic to a particular substance being tested, you'll develop a raised bump or a reaction limited to the skin just beneath the patch.

How serious is contact dermatitis?
Contact dermatitis is irritating. It causes pain and discomfort, and the blisters it produces can become infected. But while it may be temporarily debilitating, it has no lasting effects.

Treatment
Contact dermatitis treatment consists primarily of identifying what's causing your irritation and then taking steps to avoid it. If this is done, it may take two to four weeks for the rash and irritation to clear up.

In mild to moderate cases, self-care measures, such as using creams containing hydrocortisone or applying wet dressings, can help relieve redness and itching. In severe cases, oral corticosteroids and antihistamines may be necessary to reduce the inflammation and relieve the intense itching.

Prevention
Avoidance is the best way to prevent contact dermatitis. Allergens in household agents aren't always easy to detect, but harmful plants are. Learn to recognize offending plants and avoid them or wear protective clothing.

If you're allergic to a chemical such as formaldehyde, take steps to avoid exposure to it. For example, wash all new permanent-press clothing several times before wearing it. In the case of nickel sensitivity, make sure to wear solid (not plated) gold and sterling silver jewelry.

Leaves of Three, Let Them Be

The phrase, "Leaves of three, let them be," is familiar to many people, and with good reason. Certain three-leaved plants — especially poison ivy and poison oak — are the most common cause of contact dermatitis.

Poison sumac, which has many leaves, is a common offender as well. Four of every 5 Americans become sensitive to these plants to some degree. The problem-causing substance is the same for each plant, an oily resin called urushiol.

A reaction to urushiol occurs when a sensitive person comes in contact with the resin by brushing against the plant or something, such as clothing or pet fur, that has brushed against it.

It takes only a tiny amount of urushiol to cause a reaction, but direct contact is essential. The resin can be spread by accidentally rubbing it onto other areas of the skin before all of the resin is washed off.

If you come in contact with a poisonous plant, washing off the harmful resin with soap within five to 10 minutes after exposure can help avert an episode of contact dermatitis. Don't try to remove the resin by taking a bath, because this can spread the resin to other parts of your body.

Carefully remove and wash clothing, jewelry, shoes and shoelaces that may have come in contact with the resin.

Poison Ivy

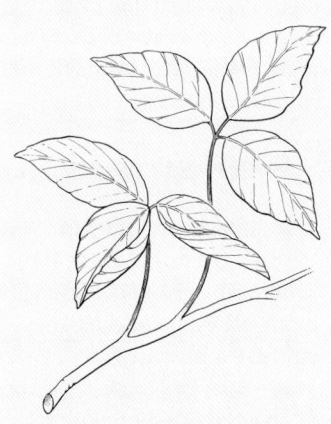

Poison Oak

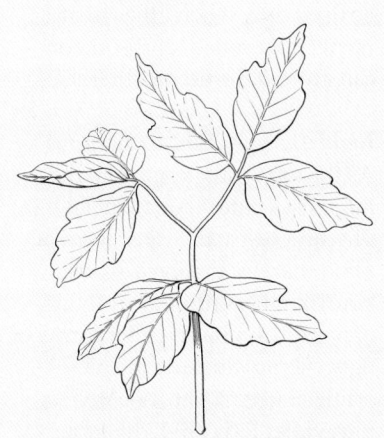

Poison Sumac

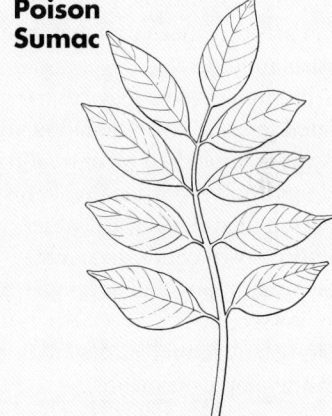

Poison ivy can be a low-growing plant, bush or vine. Its elliptical leaves grow in groups of three on a stem. Poison oak can grow as a low plant or bush. Its leaves, which resemble oak leaves, also grow three to a stem. Poison sumac may be a bush or tree. It has two rows of leaflets on each stem and a leaflet at the tip. The smooth edges of its leaves distinguish it from its harmless sumac relatives.

Eczema

Signs and symptoms
- Red to brownish-gray colored patches
- Itching, which may be severe
- Small, raised bumps
- Thickened, cracked or scaly skin

Eczema, also known as atopic dermatitis, is an itchy eruption of the skin. It's a long-lasting (chronic) condition that may be accompanied by asthma or hay fever. Eczema is most often seen in infants and children, but it can continue into adulthood or first appear later in life. When it occurs in infants, it's called infantile eczema.

Although eczema may affect virtually any area, it classically involves skin on the arms and behind the knees, as well as the face, neck, and upper chest. It can also affect the skin around your eyes, including your eyelids.

Eczema tends to flare periodically and then subside for a period of time, even up to several years. The exact cause of eczema isn't known, but it may result from a malfunction in the body's immune system. Eczema often occurs along with allergies and frequently runs in families in which other family members have asthma or hay fever.

Factors that may worsen signs and symptoms include hot baths or showers, sweating, stress, rapid changes in temperature, low humidity, and cigarette smoke.

Diagnosis
There is no laboratory test or skin test that diagnoses eczema. Instead, the condition typically is diagnosed based on an examination of your skin and a review of your medical history. Your doctor will likely ask questions about your signs and symptoms and whether you or any family members have asthma, hay fever or other allergies.

Children often outgrow their eczema by about age 6, although among some individuals, improvement doesn't occur until puberty or adulthood.

How serious is eczema?

Eczema is irritating, but for most people it's a passing problem. Some people have severe eczema.

Treatment

Treatments for eczema aim to reduce inflammation, relieve itching and prevent future flare-ups. Over-the-counter (nonprescription) anti-itch creams, along with other self-care measures, may help control mild disease.

Although eczema may be related to allergies, eliminating allergens is rarely helpful in treating the condition. Occasionally, items that trap dust — such as feather pillows, down comforters, mattresses, carpeting and drapes — can worsen the condition. Allergy shots usually aren't successful in treating atopic dermatitis.

Medications

Your doctor may recommend prescription corticosteroid creams or ointments to ease scaling and relieve itching. Regular use of nonprescription skin treatments for eczema may prevent the progression to other treatment.

Some low-potency corticosteroid creams are available without a prescription, but always talk to your doctor before using any topical corticosteroid. Side effects of long-term or repeated use can include skin irritation or discoloration, thinning of the skin, infections, and stretch marks on the skin.

If itching is severe, oral antihistamines may help. Diphenhydramine (Benadryl, others) can make you very sleepy and may be helpful at bedtime.

If these steps don't help, your doctor may prescribe a short course of oral corticosteroids, such as prednisone, to reduce inflam-

mation and to control symptoms. These medications are effective but can't be used long term because of potentially serious side effects.

A class of medications called immunomodulators, such as tacrolimus (Protopic) and pimecrolimus (Elidel), may help maintain normal skin texture and reduce flares of atopic dermatitis. This prescription-only medication is approved for children over the age of 2 and for adults. Due to possible concerns about the effect of these medications on the immune system when used for prolonged periods of time, the Food and Drug Administration recommends they be used only when other treatments have failed, or if someone can't tolerate other treatments.

Light therapy (phototherapy)

As the name suggests, this treatment uses natural or artificial light. The simplest and easiest form of phototherapy involves exposing your skin to controlled amounts of natural sunlight. Other forms of light therapy include the use of artificial ultraviolet A (UVA) or ultraviolet B (UVB) light either alone or in combination with medications.

Though effective, long-term light therapy has many harmful effects, including premature skin aging and an increased risk of skin cancer. For these reasons, it's important to consult your doctor before using light exposure as treatment for eczema. Your doctor can advise you on possible advantages and disadvantages of light exposure in your specific situation.

Infantile eczema

Treatment for infantile eczema includes identifying and avoiding skin irritations, avoiding extreme temperatures, and using bath oils, lotions, creams or ointments to lubricate your baby's skin.

See your baby's doctor if these measures don't improve the rash or if the rash looks infected. Your

baby may need a prescription medication to control the symptoms or to treat the infection. Your doctor may recommend an oral antihistamine to help lessen the itch and to cause drowsiness, which may be helpful for nighttime itching and discomfort.

Prevention

Avoiding dry skin may be one factor in helping prevent future bouts of eczema. These tips can help you minimize drying effects on your skin:

- **Bathe less frequently.** Most people who are prone to atopic dermatitis don't need to bathe daily. Try going a day or two without a shower or bath. When you do bathe, limit yourself to 15 minutes, and use warm,

? Question and Answer

I've heard conflicting reports on home humidifiers. Should someone with allergies and asthma use a humidifier?

It's a good question with a complicated answer. On one hand, high indoor humidity can promote mold and dust mites — both of which can trigger asthma and allergy symptoms. In addition, humidifiers can be a source of airborne bacteria and fungi. On the other hand, low indoor humidity can aggravate eczema, along with nasal dryness and coughing — especially in people who have a cold or croup.

The best advice is to use humidifiers cautiously. Keep indoor humidity no higher than 50 percent. Clean the humidifier regularly according to instructions. You might consider limiting humidifier use to times when someone is sick or has a symptom flare-up.

rather than hot, water. Using a bath oil also may be helpful.

- **Use only certain soaps or synthetic detergents.** Choose mild soaps that clean without excessively removing natural oils. Deodorant and antibacterial soaps may be more drying to your skin. Use soap only on your face, underarms, genital areas, hands and feet. Use clear water elsewhere.
- **Dry yourself carefully.** Brush your skin rapidly with the palms of your hands, or gently pat your skin dry with a towel after bathing.
- **Moisturize your skin.** Moisturizers provide a seal over your skin to keep water from escaping. Thicker moisturizers work best, such as over-the-counter brands Cetaphil, Vanicream or Eucerin. You may also want to use cosmetics that contain moisturizers. If your skin is extremely dry, you may want to apply an oil, such as baby oil, while your skin is still moist. Oil has more staying power than moisturizers do and prevents the evaporation of water from the surface of your skin.
- **Use a humidifier.** Hot, dry indoor air can parch sensitive skin and worsen itching and flaking. A portable home humidifier or one attached to your furnace adds moisture to the air inside your home. Portable humidifiers come in many varieties. Choose one that meets your budget and any special needs. And be sure to keep your humidifier clean to ward off bacteria and fungi.
- **Wear cool, smooth-textured cotton clothing.** Avoid clothing that's rough, tight, scratchy or made from wool. These types of clothing can irritate eczema and intensify the itching. Also, wear appropriate clothing in hot weather or during exercise to prevent excessive sweating. Sweating can exacerbate symptoms.

Hives and angioedema

Signs and symptoms
Hives
- Raised, red, itchy welts of various sizes that appear and disappear at random on the surface of the skin
- Formation of welts where the skin is scratched (dermatographism)

Angioedema
- Large welts below the surface of the skin, particularly around the eyes and lips but also on the hands and feet and in the throat

As many as 1 in 5 people experiences hives or angioedema at one time or another. Often, the exact cause for the outbreak can't be determined. The medical name for hives is *urticaria*, from the Latin word *urtica*, for "nettle." Hives usually occur in batches rather than singly, and may last a few minutes to one or two days. Hives occur on the surface of the skin. Angioedema is a similar swelling that occurs deeper in the skin.

Hives and angioedema are thought to result from the release of histamine and other chemicals. The cause of the release is unknown, although a range of substances have been found to cause hives, including foods, pollen, animal dander, drugs, latex, insect venom, infections, illness, cold, heat, light and emotional distress. As with many allergies, heredity may play a role in the development of hives and angioedema.

Foods that may cause hives in sensitive people include shellfish, fish and nuts. Penicillin and aspirin also are known culprits. Some people experience hives from emotional stress, exercise, sunlight or temperature extremes.

Diagnosis
The primary sign of hives and angioedema is a swelling of the skin in the form of red welts. With hives, the welts are on the surface of the skin and are often very itchy.

In the case of angioedema, the welts are deeper and appear primarily around the eyes and mouth, making them appear swollen. Welts may occur on the hands and feet, although less frequently.

To help determine the cause of your condition, your doctor may ask you to create a detailed diary indicating exposure to possible triggers. Hives and angioedema may be triggered by many different things.

How serious are hives and angioedema?
Hives and angioedema are generally harmless. They leave no lasting marks and sometimes cause few symptoms. But when angioedema affects the throat or tongue, it can obstruct the air passage and be life-threatening or fatal.

In addition, hereditary angioedema, a rare form of the condition, is more troublesome and can be especially dangerous. It results from a blood protein disorder involving your immune system response. The symptoms of this disorder include nonitchy swelling, possibly with painful abdominal cramping and diarrhea.

Treatment
The standard treatment for hives and angioedema is an antihistamine. For more acute or severe swelling, other drugs may be used, such as an injection of epinephrine. Occasionally, doctors prescribe a corticosteroid medication. To prevent hives and angioedema, avoid substances known to trigger an allergic response.

Reactions to heat, cold or light

Signs and symptoms
- Rash
- Welts such as hives that appear as a result of exposure to heat, cold, sun or rubbing

Emergency signs and symptoms
Emergency signs and symptoms can occur as a result of immersion in cold water. They include:

Feel Like You're Allergic to Almost Everything?

For most people allergic reactions stem from sensitivities to specific agents, such as pollen or peanuts. Some people, though, feel as if they're allergic to almost everything around them. Strong fragrances, exhaust fumes, new carpet, cigarette smoke, solvents, plastics, formaldehyde and pesticides are among the irritants people cite as causing an array of symptoms.

These individuals may experience dizziness, impaired concentration, headaches, joint pain, fatigue, memory loss and heat intolerance. The condition is known by several names, including multiple chemical sensitivity, total allergy syndrome and idiopathic environmental intolerances — the term recommended by the World Health Organization.

Allergies aren't the cause of such symptoms. Several theories as to a cause have been proposed, but none has been proved. Some people suggest the symptoms may be related to an immune deficiency. Others believe they may be due to immunologic hypersensitivity, overstimulation of the olfactory (smell) area of the brain, damaged tissues, stress, depression or an anxiety disorder. About half the people with idiopathic environmental intolerances also have depression or anxiety. It's uncertain whether these cause the condition or are merely associated with it.

People with idiopathic environmental intolerances sometimes become frustrated when doctors can't find a physical cause for their symptoms, and they often consult other health care providers in search of an explanation for their illness. Some take drastic measures that are expensive and disruptive to their lives. These may include quitting a job to move to the mountains, living in a home free of synthetic materials or eating only organic foods. Despite such measures, rarely are the symptoms relieved permanently.

The most effective treatment tends to be a multifaceted approach that includes controlling — not curing — the symptoms and treating other associated conditions, such as depression or anxiety.

- Muscle cramping
- Vomiting
- Fainting

One of the most puzzling allergy-like reactions is that to physical stimuli, such as pressure, heat, cold, light and sunlight. People who have this type of response often have very sensitive skin. Sometimes, just rubbing a blunt object on the skin produces swelling within a few minutes.

Diagnosis

Signs and symptoms include tiny hives that may result in response to vigorous exercise, a hot shower, emotional stress or a rewarming of body parts that have been exposed to cold air. Swelling of the hands and feet may occur in response to pressure. In testing for heat and cold reactions, your doctor may apply cold and hot objects to your skin to see if a reaction occurs.

Treatment

The best method for treating hypersensitivity to heat and cold is to avoid temperature extremes whenever possible.

You can prevent sun-induced hives by avoiding sun exposure or using sunscreens. This is especially important if you're taking certain medications, such as antibiotics, antihistamines, diuretics, antifungal agents, tranquilizers or hypoglycemics, which may make your skin more sun sensitive.

Food, Drug and Insect Sting Allergies

Allergies to foods, drugs and insect stings are thought to result from an antibody response to allergens.

Signs and symptoms may range from a simple rash to a more severe reaction involving the gastrointestinal tract, respiratory tract or cardiovascular system. Signs and symptoms often appear soon after a food is eaten, a drug is administered or an insect sting occurs.

Food allergies

Signs and symptoms
- Hives, eczema or swelling beneath the skin
- Swelling of the lips, eyes, face, tongue and throat
- Nasal congestion
- Asthma

Emergency signs and symptoms
- Severe symptoms of the reactions listed above
- Abdominal pain, diarrhea, nausea or vomiting
- Fainting
- Anaphylactic shock

Few things are more distressing than a reaction to food because food represents something that nourishes and comforts. Many Americans believe they're allergic to specific foods, but in actuality most are bothered by food intolerances (see page 508). Only a small percent of Americans have true food allergies.

You can develop food allergies at any age, but children are much more likely to have a food allergy than are adults. Foods associated with allergies in children include milk, eggs, soy, peanuts, wheat, fish, shellfish and tree nuts, such as cashews, almonds and Brazil nuts. Chocolate, long thought to be allergenic, seldom causes allergy.

Fortunately, many children outgrow allergies to milk, eggs and wheat by about age 6. Allergies to nuts and shellfish are more likely to be lifelong.

Diagnosis

Most food allergies provoke an almost immediate reaction. If you eat something and within a few minutes your tongue and lips are swollen, it's fairly easy to suspect the cause. It's unusual for a food to cause a reaction that begins more than two hours after eating.

Your doctor may take several steps to determine if you have a true food allergy. You'll need to review your symptoms and when they occurred, and you may be asked to keep a detailed diary of everything you eat and drink for several weeks, as well as any medications you take. Various tests may help determine specific allergens.

Skin test

In this test, a small amount of a food extract is pricked into your skin. Negative skin tests are helpful in excluding a food allergy, but positive skin tests are less accurate.

One approach is the double-blind challenge test. In this test, you're given suspected foods in disguised form so that neither you nor the individual dispensing the food knows what food is being administered. These results are more conclusive, but this test can be difficult and is time-consuming.

Immunoassays

These tests involve examining a blood sample for immunoglobulin E (IgE) antibodies specific to certain foods.

How serious are food allergies?

For most people, food allergies are merely a nuisance, but for a few they can be life-threatening. Responses vary from minor sniffles and a cough to life-threatening anaphylactic shock.

Treatment

The only truly effective treatment for a food allergy is to avoid the food causing the problem. For some people this isn't a problem. For people allergic to foods or food ingredients common in the average diet, such as nuts or shellfish, it can mean having a very restricted diet.

Emergency treatment, including an immediate injection of

Anaphylactic Shock

Anaphylactic shock, also called anaphylaxis, is the most severe and frightening allergic response. Luckily, it's also the most infrequent, although each year several hundred Americans die of this reaction.

This allergic overresponse is often sudden, beginning seconds or minutes after an offending allergen is encountered.

Signs and symptoms

- Flushing of skin and intense itching
- Swelling of the lips and tongue
- Constriction of airways, including a swollen throat, resulting in breathing difficulty
- Shock associated with a severe decrease in blood pressure
- Rapid pulse
- Generalized hives, or hives and welts below the skin surface (angioedema)
- Nausea, vomiting or diarrhea
- Dizziness

The anaphylactic reaction is systemic, meaning that it's not limited to the site of exposure. Constriction of air passageways in the bronchial tract or throat or both is common in an anaphylactic reaction.

The constriction may be accompanied by shock — a situation in which there can be a sudden decrease in blood pressure that causes a rapid pulse as well as weakness, paleness, mental confusion and unconsciousness. An anaphylactic reaction requires immediate medical treatment. It can cause death if it's not treated quickly.

A person who experiences only a mild reaction may have a severe reaction with a subsequent exposure. A person may also become hypersensitive at any time, no matter whether he or she was previously sensitized.

Causes

Many allergens can cause this type of response. Anaphylaxis can occur after certain insect stings or intravenous injection of certain drugs. Certain foods such as peanuts, tree nuts and shellfish also can cause fatal reactions. Only rarely do pollens cause the anaphylactic response. Some people have anaphylactic reactions for which no cause can be found.

Treatment

The standard treatment for anaphylaxis is injection of adrenaline (epinephrine) as soon as possible. It opens airways and improves blood circulation.

Cardiopulmonary resuscitation (CPR) and an emergency tracheotomy — an incision creating an opening in the windpipe through the neck — sometimes have to be performed as lifesaving measures.

If you observe someone experiencing an allergic reaction with signs of anaphylaxis, summon emergency medical personnel immediately. Check to see if the person is carrying auto-injectable epinephrine (Epi-Pen, Auvi-Q, AdrenaClick) to counter the effects of an allergic attack. If you're trained in CPR, perform the procedure if the person isn't breathing or has no pulse.

epinephrine, is necessary when anaphylaxis develops. If you have a food allergy, talk to your doctor about carrying such medication for emergency use.

Drug allergies

Signs and symptoms
- Rash
- Hives
- Generalized itching
- Wheezing and difficulty breathing

Emergency signs and symptoms
- Obstruction of the throat due to swelling
- Severe asthma
- Anaphylactic shock

Almost any drug can cause an adverse reaction that may range from irritating to life-threatening. Some reactions are true allergic responses — antibodies are mobilized against the offending drug and histamine is released. Nonallergic reactions also can occur.

Penicillin and its relatives are responsible for many drug allergy reactions, including mild rashes, hives or even anaphylactic shock. Most reactions are minor rashes.

Other drugs that cause allergic reactions include sulfas, barbiturates, anticonvulsants, insulin and local anesthetics. In addition, contrast dyes injected into blood vessels to outline major organs in X-ray studies may cause an allergic reaction.

Diagnosis
A rash is the most common allergic reaction to drugs. Penicillin and its relatives can cause a rash, similar to hives, and another reaction known as serum sickness. This reaction, which can take up to three weeks to develop, is characterized by a fever, aching joints, swelling of the lymph glands and a rash. In some cases, these medications, as well as the drugs streptomycin, insulin and tetracycline, can cause anaphylactic shock.

Sensitivity to penicillin drugs can be diagnosed with a skin test.

Allergy vs. Intolerance

Food allergies and food intolerance are often thought to be the same thing, but they're not. In a true allergic reaction, the body releases histamine and other substances that produce the gastrointestinal, respiratory and skin symptoms associated with food allergies. Only a small percentage of the population has true food allergies.

Food intolerance can produce allergy-like symptoms, but the chemistry is quite different, as no histamine is released. In addition, if you have a food intolerance, you can usually eat a small amount of the problem food without a reaction. By contrast, if you have a true food allergy, even a tiny amount of the food may trigger an immediate allergic reaction.

One of the tricky aspects of diagnosing a food intolerance is that some people are sensitive not to the food but to a substance or ingredient used in the preparation of it. This is particularly true of foods containing lactose, wheat, monosodium glutamate (MSG), sulfites, salicylates and possibly tartrazine.

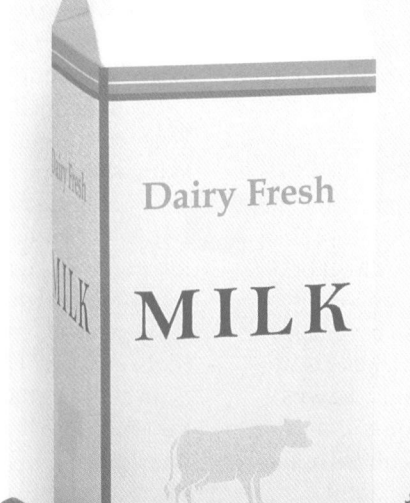

Causes of food intolerance include emotional and physical stress, irritable bowel syndrome, and the absence of an enzyme needed to digest a specific food, causing incomplete digestion (malabsorption). Intolerance disorders include:

Lactose intolerance
As most people grow older, they're less able to tolerate lactose, a sugar found in milk and some other dairy products. Even in infancy 1 to 3 percent of all babies are lactose intolerant. For more information on this condition, see page 840.

Wheat and vegetable intolerance
Intolerance to gluten, found primarily in wheat products, most commonly occurs in young children, who may or may not outgrow their sensitivity. Vegetables to which some people are intolerant include broccoli and peas, which produce intestinal gas, and mushrooms, which produce indigestion and diarrhea.

MSG intolerance
MSG, a commonly used flavor enhancer, may cause flushing, a headache and numbness around the mouth in people who are sensitive to it. Because many Chinese restaurants use MSG, this type of intolerance is sometimes called Chinese restaurant syndrome. MSG is also found in some seasoning mixtures and prepared foods.

Sulfite intolerance
Sulfites are present in various foods and beverages, particularly wine, beer, fresh and dehydrated fruits, seafood, dehydrated soups, maraschino cherries, and some soft drinks. The sulfites help sanitize and preserve foods. Only a few people are sensitive to sulfites.

Skin tests to detect sensitivity to other medications are limited. However, depending on the need for a medication and the specific history of a prior reaction, an allergist may discuss select testing, a drug challenge or drug desensitization.

How serious is a drug allergy?

Severe reactions such as anaphylaxis or acute asthma can be life-threatening. But such reactions are rare. Most reactions are limited to rashes and hives, but this doesn't mean that they can be ignored.

Treatment

The most common drug allergy reactions — a rash, itching and hives — are treated with antihistamines or, occasionally, corticosteroid drugs. Asthma reactions are treated with bronchodilators and corticosteroids. Anaphylaxis is treated with epinephrine injections.

In some cases, sensitivity to penicillin can be reduced with treatment so that the person can tolerate the drug. Small amounts of the drug are given in slowly increasing amounts. Sometimes, antihistamines and corticosteroids are given before and with the penicillin doses to lessen the allergic reaction.

Prevention

If you know that you're allergic to certain drugs, avoid them. This means alerting your doctor of your drug sensitivities.

People sensitive to aspirin should avoid all aspirin-containing drugs. Wearing a medical alert necklace or bracelet at all times can alert medical personnel to your allergy in case of an emergency.

Insect sting allergies

Signs and symptoms
- Hives
- Itchy eyes
- Constricted feeling of the throat and chest

Nonallergic Drug Reactions

Many drugs can cause adverse reactions that mimic the symptoms of an allergy, but the reactions aren't the result of an immune system response, as are true allergies. Almost 1 million Americans, primarily adults, have reactions to the common drug aspirin. The reaction can include hives, welts (angioedema) and anaphylaxis. About 10 percent of people with asthma are sensitive to aspirin. In these individuals, aspirin can cause asthma to worsen. Reactions can also occur with other nonsteroidal anti-inflammatory drugs, such as ibuprofen (Advil, Motrin IB, others).

Angiotensin-converting enzyme (ACE) inhibitors — a class of drugs that relax blood vessels and are used to reduce blood pressure or treat congestive heart failure — sometimes cause a cough and swelling (angioedema) that occur in a different manner than the typical IgE allergy response. Opiates such as morphine and codeine can cause reactions that mimic allergic anaphylaxis.

Some antibiotics, such as erythromycin, can cause stomach upset or diarrhea, and the antibiotic ampicillin may cause a rash that develops differently than the typical allergy response.

Emergency signs and symptoms
- Swelling of the throat that causes difficulty breathing
- Coughing or wheezing
- Severe hives
- Abdominal cramps, nausea and vomiting
- Decrease in blood pressure that may result in unconsciousness

For most people, the sting of a bee or wasp is a temporary irritation. The area may swell and itch or sting for several hours, but then it returns to normal.

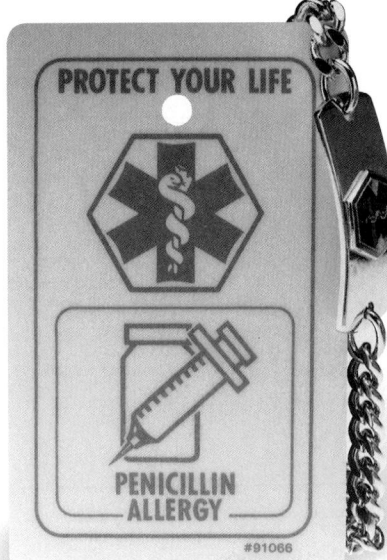

If you have a drug allergy, carry appropriate identification, such as a drug alert necklace or bracelet, at all times.

For a small percentage of people, however, such stings cause serious symptoms. These people are extremely sensitive to some insect venoms, particularly that of bees, wasps, hornets, yellow jackets and fire ants. An allergy-causing immunoglobulin antibody response occurs, releasing histamine into the body.

Diagnosis

Symptoms of an insect sting allergy usually appear within a few minutes after the sting occurs. In addition to pain and an intense itch around the site of the sting, a mild reaction might include hives and itchy eyes. Extremely sensitive people may have more-serious signs and symptoms such as severe hives and anaphylactic shock (see page 507).

Severe reactions to insect stings can happen within two or three minutes. Generally, the sooner the reaction begins, the more severe it will be.

To confirm an allergic response to a certain insect, your doctor may perform allergy blood tests and skin tests several weeks after the incident. Your doctor may also screen for a rare mast cell disorder called mastocytosis, which occurs in approximately 1 to 2 percent of individuals with an anaphylactic reaction to stings.

How serious are insect sting allergies?
Reactions to insect stings range from mild to life-threatening.

Treatment
In the case of severe reactions, an injection of epinephrine is administered and emergency care may be required. Corticosteroids, which act over a longer period of time than does adrenaline, are often prescribed to reduce hives and other swelling. If the person stops breathing, cardiopulmonary resuscitation (CPR) may be needed. Rarely, if the throat is constricted enough to block an air passageway, a tracheotomy might be performed. A tube is inserted into the throat to allow for the flow of air.

When the reaction is less severe, you can minimize the effects by keeping the venom as localized as possible. Remove the stinger if it's present and place a cold pack on the wound to limit swelling and reduce itching.

Prevention
Once an insect sting allergy is confirmed by testing, immunotherapy may be used to increase your tolerance to the offending venom. Injections of small amounts of the venom will be administered every week until you can tolerate the amount of venom in a sting. From then on, you receive maintenance injections every four to six weeks, usually for a three- to five-year period.

It's also important to avoid exposure to the insect as much as possible. For example, when you're outside, avoid wearing clothing with flowery prints or bright colors, which are attractive to certain insects. Don't use sweet perfumes or scented soaps, body lotions and cosmetics. Wear shoes and long-sleeved shirts as much as possible. And try to stay away from places where stinging insects are found, such as orchards, flower gardens, and fields or lawns containing clover. If you feel in danger of being stung, stay calm. Move away from the insect slowly and without sudden movement. Panicky flailing only agitates insects, increasing the risk of a sting.

People who are extremely sensitive to insect stings can safeguard themselves by carrying auto-injectable epinephrine (Epi-Pen, Auvi-Q, AdrenaClick). Wearing a medical alert bracelet or necklace or carrying a medical identification card will provide helpful information in case of an emergency. ■

Brain and Nerves

You might think of your brain as the chief executive organ in your body. It shapes and controls all of your thoughts and emotions and virtually all of your bodily functions and physical actions. Together with your spinal cord, it makes up your central nervous system.

The peripheral nervous system extends from your spinal cord and branches out to the tips of your fingers and toes. Sensory nerves are continuously gathering information from both inside and outside your body, busily sending messages to your brain.

Your brain receives hundreds of impulses from this network of nerves. While it interprets the messages, it sends information to different parts of the brain for memory storage. It then shoots back instructions that determine the appropriate response of your fingers, legs, mouth or other body part. By processing, sorting, filing and responding to incoming information, your brain gives meaning to the world around you. The individual manner in which your brain does this makes you the unique person you are.

cerebellum, cerebrum and limbic system. The brainstem, located at the base of the brain, is responsible for regulating some of your most basic survival functions, such as breathing and heart rate. The cerebellum, which sits at the back of the brainstem, controls movements such as brushing your teeth and riding a bike. The cerebrum, resting on top of the brainstem, is the largest part of the human brain and the most easily recognized. It's responsible for all of your intellectual activities — your ability to think, reason, remember, imagine and plan for the future.

The limbic system, located in the deeper regions of the brain and responsible for emotions, is composed of the following structures:

- **Hypothalamus.** It controls body functions and urges — such as eating, sleeping and sexual behavior — and regulates body temperature.
- **Thalamus.** It acts as an information relay center, sorting and sending messages to and from various parts of the brain.
- **Amygdala.** It governs emotions such as anger and fear and triggers your response to danger,

whether it be confronting the situation or fleeing it, a reaction commonly called the fight-or-flight response.
- **Hippocampus.** It plays an important role in forming and retrieving your memories, sending them to be stored in appropriate sections of the cerebrum or cerebellum, and recalling them when necessary.

The cerebrum is divided into left and right hemispheres. Putting your two fists together in front of you can give you a rough picture of what your cerebrum looks like. Each hemisphere is subdivided into four lobes that control different activities. The frontal lobes in each hemisphere, located directly behind your forehead, govern such activities as speech production, abstract thought and voluntary movement. Behind the frontal lobes are the parietal lobes, which receive sensory information such as pain, taste and touch. Situated under the frontal and parietal lobes are the temporal lobes, areas that help you hear and interpret sounds and that are responsible for memory. The temporal lobe of the dominant half of your brain

Structures of the Brain

Your brain is made up of many structures that have specific functions. In a healthy brain, these parts work together in an efficient yet incredibly complex fashion. Although scientists are still discovering basic information about the workings of the brain, they know much more about it now than they did even 10 years ago. Advances in science and technology have provided so many new insights into this vital part of the human body that the U.S. Congress labeled the 1990s as the Decade of the Brain.

Some of the brain's basic structures include the brainstem,

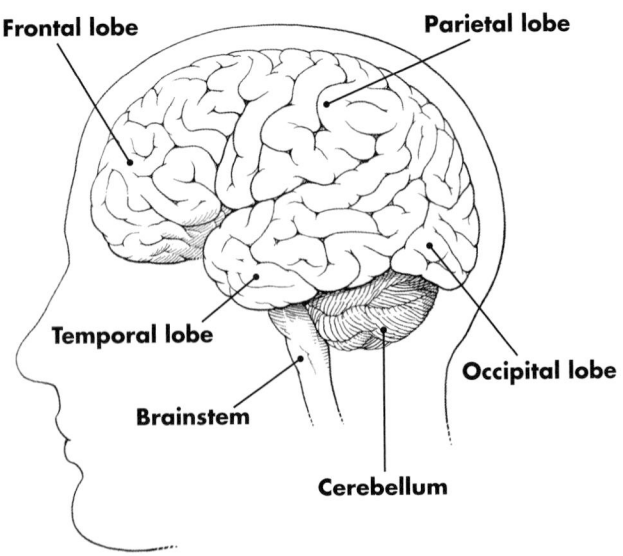

The outer cerebrum is composed of the frontal, parietal, occipital and temporal lobes. Other major areas of your brain include the brainstem and cerebellum.

— usually the left — plays a major role in language function. At the back of the brain are the occipital lobes, responsible for your vision.

Covering your cerebrum is a layer of tissue less than a quarter-inch thick. Grayish-brown and wrinkled in appearance, this layer is the cerebral cortex — commonly called the gray matter. The cerebral cortex is where most information processing in your brain takes place. All of the grooves, bulges and folds in the cortex allow a greater surface area to fit inside the skull, thus increasing the amount of information that can be processed. The human brain has more wrinkles than any other animal brain.

In addition, there are structures under the cortex called the basal ganglia. They play a critical role in relaying messages between different areas of the brain. Some disorders, such as Parkinson's disease, involve abnormalities in the basal ganglia.

Your brain and spinal cord are encased in bone. The brain is protected by the skull, and the spinal cord is protected by the vertebrae. The brain and spinal cord are sheathed in three layers of membranes (meninges): the outermost layer is called the dura mater, the middle layer the arachnoid and the innermost layer the pia mater. These layers provide cushioning for the brain and spinal cord. In addition, a liquid called cerebrospinal fluid, located between the arachnoid and pia mater, further protects your brain and spinal cord from injury.

Structures of the Nervous System

Peripheral nerves run from the spinal cord to all other parts of your body. Parts of the peripheral nervous system are named for the four spinal regions from which they branch: neck (cervical), chest (thoracic), lower back (lumbar) and pelvis (sacral). The spinal cord acts as a central communication network to transmit signals back and forth between your brain and the farthest reaches of your peripheral nervous system.

Your autonomic nervous system distributes nerves to smooth muscles in blood vessels (vascular) and internal organs (visceral), to exocrine and endocrine glands, and to function-controlling cells of internal organs. This intricate system controls unconscious but vital activities such as distribution of blood flow, regulation of blood pressure, heartbeat, sweating and body temperature. Connections between autonomic and other brain functions occur in the brainstem and hypothalamus.

Cranial nerves are those nerves connected directly to your brain. They exit from the brain to control muscles in your face, eyes, tongue, ears and throat. They also convey sensations from these parts back to the brain.

Your arteries, which carry oxygen and nutrients from your lungs and heart, are critical to the functioning of your brain. Despite its small size and weight, your brain uses 20 percent of the heart's output of blood and 20 percent of the oxygen consumed by your body at rest. Blood is brought to the brain by the paired vertebral and carotid arteries, which extend up through

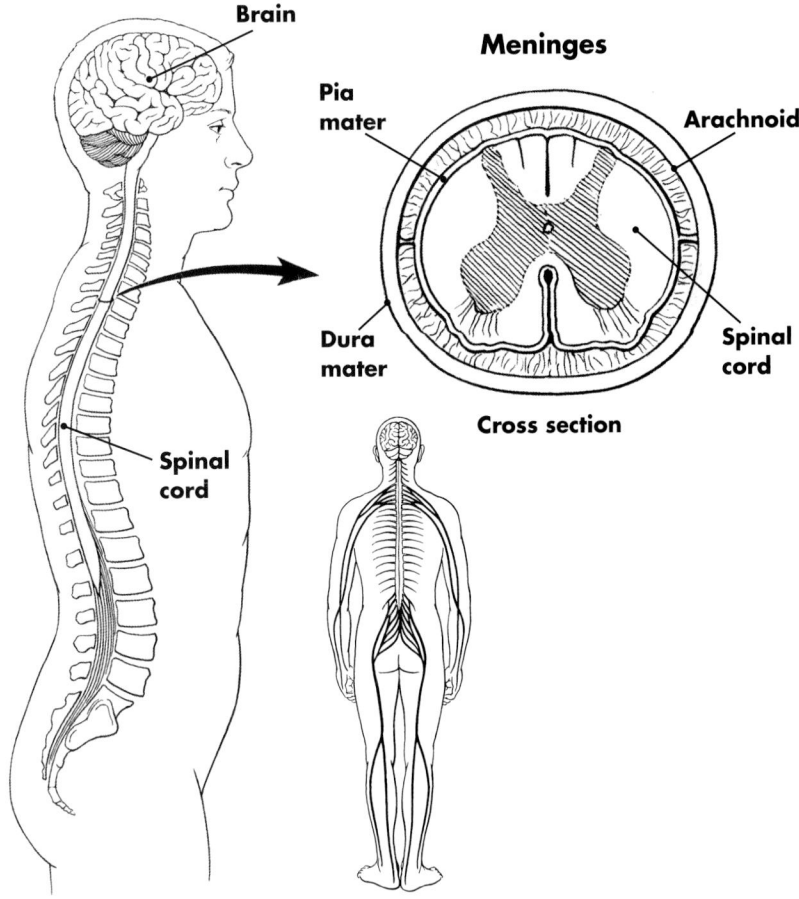

Your central nervous system, composed of your brain and spinal cord, is protected by your skull and vertebrae and by three layers of membranes — dura mater, arachnoid and pia mater — collectively known as meninges. Your peripheral nervous system (lower right) extends from your spinal cord to all other parts of your body.

your neck from your aorta. These large arteries then divide into smaller ones to distribute blood to various regions of your brain.

A Healthy Brain at Work

The basic unit of your brain and nervous system is a nerve cell called a neuron. Neurons allow different parts of your body to communicate. They do so by generating electric impulses — messages — and relaying them near and far, to and from your brain and the rest of your body. Surrounding the neurons are glial cells that act as bodyguards — protecting, nourishing and supporting neurons. The human brain contains about 12 billion neurons and 50 billion glial cells.

Each neuron is made up of a cell body, which contains a nucleus and several other structures essential to the neuron's functioning. Extending from the cell body are branches called dendrites, which receive incoming messages from other nerve cells. Also extending from the cell body is a larger branch called an axon. Axons carry outgoing signals from the cell body to other cells, such as a nearby neuron or a muscle cell. Interconnected with each other, neurons are able to provide efficient, lightning-fast communication.

Covering some axons is a white fatty substance called myelin. Myelin helps insulate the axons and speeds the transmission of impulses.

A neuron communicates with other nerve cells or body cells through electric impulses. In order to send an impulse, the neuron must be stimulated by something, whether it be a prick on your finger, a funny scene in a movie or an incoming impulse from an adjoining neuron. The message is then passed from one neuron to the next.

Within a neuron, the impulse travels through the cell body to the tip of the axon where there are tiny sacs containing neurotransmitters, chemicals that act as data messengers. The arrival of an electric impulse signals the release of the neurotransmitters into the synapse, the tiny gap between two nerve cells. In the synapse, neurotransmitters bind to receptors on a receiving cell. This allows the impulse to enter the receiving cell and pass on to that cell's axon. Once the neurotransmitters have done their job, they're released back into the synapse and return to their cell of origin, where some of them may be reused (see the illustration on page 366). This process is repeated from neuron to neuron as the impulse travels to its destination.

Neurons maintain their health by converting nutrients found in circulating blood, such as glucose and oxygen, into energy by a process called metabolism. Neurons are constantly renovating and repairing themselves so that they can continue to function properly.

When things go wrong

Like a finely tuned machine, your brain and nervous system depend on a harmonious balance among all of their parts for efficient opera-

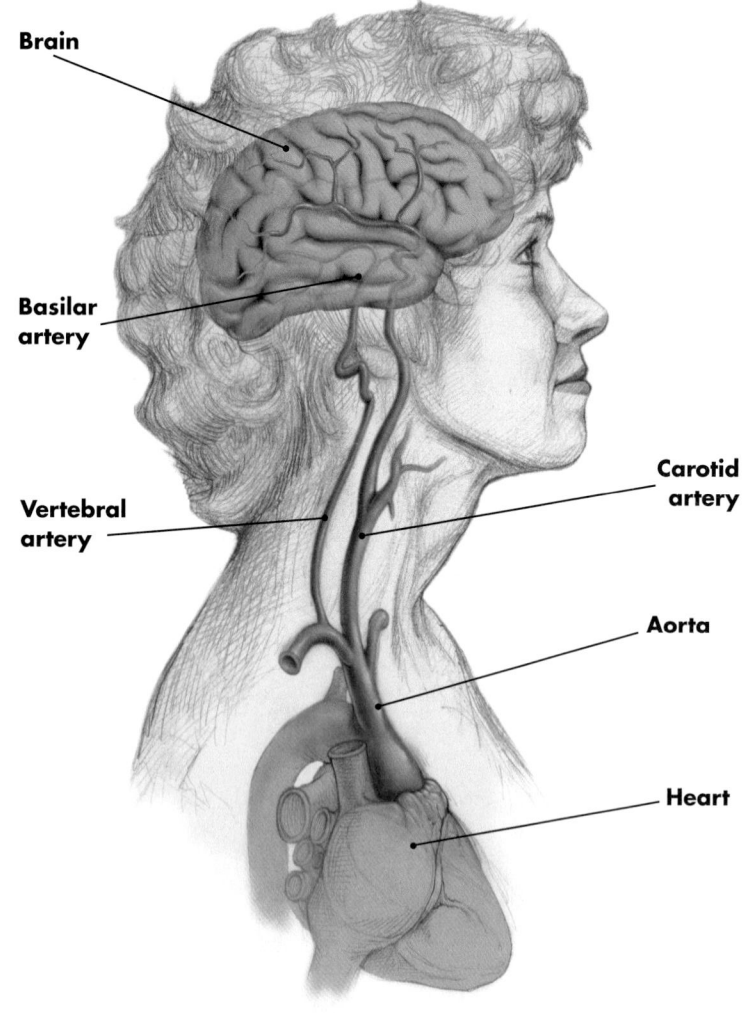

Brain

Basilar artery

Vertebral artery

Carotid artery

Aorta

Heart

Your brain needs a constant supply of oxygen and nutrients from blood delivered through several key arteries.

tion. Your brain and nervous system are vulnerable to a wide variety of injuries.

Interruption of the blood supply to the brain causes strokes. Degeneration of nerve cells causes illnesses such as Alzheimer's disease, amyotrophic lateral sclerosis and Parkinson's disease. An inflammatory reaction of the brain to an infection can cause meningitis and encephalitis. A head injury or brain tumor may cause structural damage. Problems in mental processing and learning are called cognitive disorders and can result from a variety of conditions affecting special brain functions. Seizures are caused by abnormal firing of nerve cells.

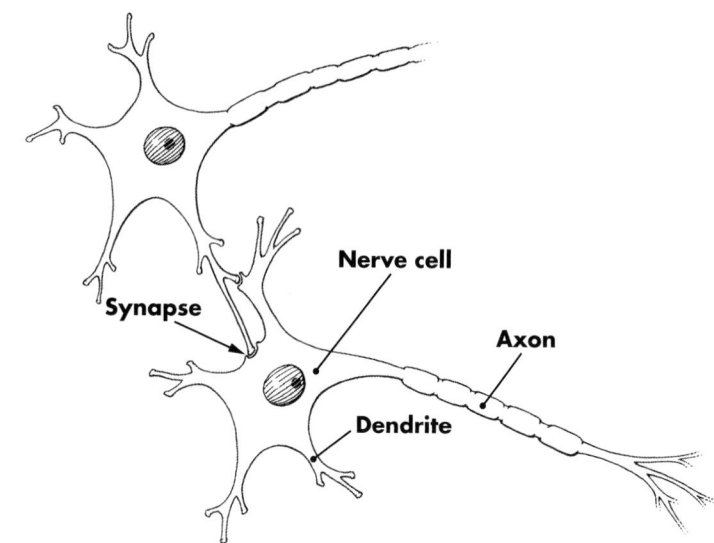

The nerve cell (neuron) is the basic unit of the brain and nervous system. It consists of the cell body, a major branching fiber (axon), and numerous smaller branching fibers (dendrites). Every nerve cell is linked to adjacent nerve cells at contact points called synapses.

A Neurological Examination

The most important element in the diagnosis of a nervous system disorder is a description of your signs and symptoms and how they developed. Headaches, blurred vision or tingling sensations, for example, can be caused by many disorders. To determine what condition you might have, your doctor will likely ask detailed questions about your signs and symptoms and then conduct a neurological examination.

A neurological examination systematically tests how well the various parts of your nervous system are functioning. Many abnormalities that you may not notice can be detected with simple tests done in your doctor's office.

Tendon reflexes
Your tendon reflexes are tested to evaluate motor and sensory nerve functions, spinal cord connections and peripheral nerve conditions. For example, your doctor may stimulate your reflexes by tapping your knee or ankle lightly with a special rubber-tipped hammer.

Babinski's reflex
Light stroking of the underside of your foot may produce a certain type of involuntary movement of your big toe, which can suggest an abnormality in the nerve tracts that originate in the brain or spinal cord.

Muscle strength
Weakness of a muscle or group of muscles can be a manifestation of a neurological disorder. Your doctor may test the strength of various muscles as part of your exam.

Muscle tone
A doctor moves your arm or leg to assess the ease and range of movement. Increased tone (spasticity or rigidity) or decreased tone (flaccidity) can indicate particular problems in the nerves that control different muscle groups.

Cranial nerve exam
There are 12 pairs of cranial nerves located at the base of the brain. Some bring information from the sense organs, others control muscles, and others are connected to glands and organs. To ensure the nerves are functioning properly, a variety of tests — from vision to tongue movements — are done.

Sensory function
Sensory tests are important in a neurological examination because sensations such as pain, heat, touch and vibration travel through your peripheral nerves to your central nervous system. Your doctor evaluates these functions by asking what you feel when your skin is touched lightly by a pinprick, a hot or cold object, a cotton ball, or a tuning fork.

Nervous system disorders can also affect your eyes and senses of taste, smell and hearing. Eye testing is particularly useful. The size of your pupils, a difference between the sizes of the pupils, range of eye movement, gaze and field of vision are often useful for diagnosing disturbances that may include the nerves that control your vision.

Gait, posture, coordination and balance
To evaluate these abilities, your doctor may ask you to stand, walk or move your body in a particular way to reveal possible abnormalities.

Mental status
Your doctor may also ask you questions that help determine whether your thinking, judgment or memory is impaired.

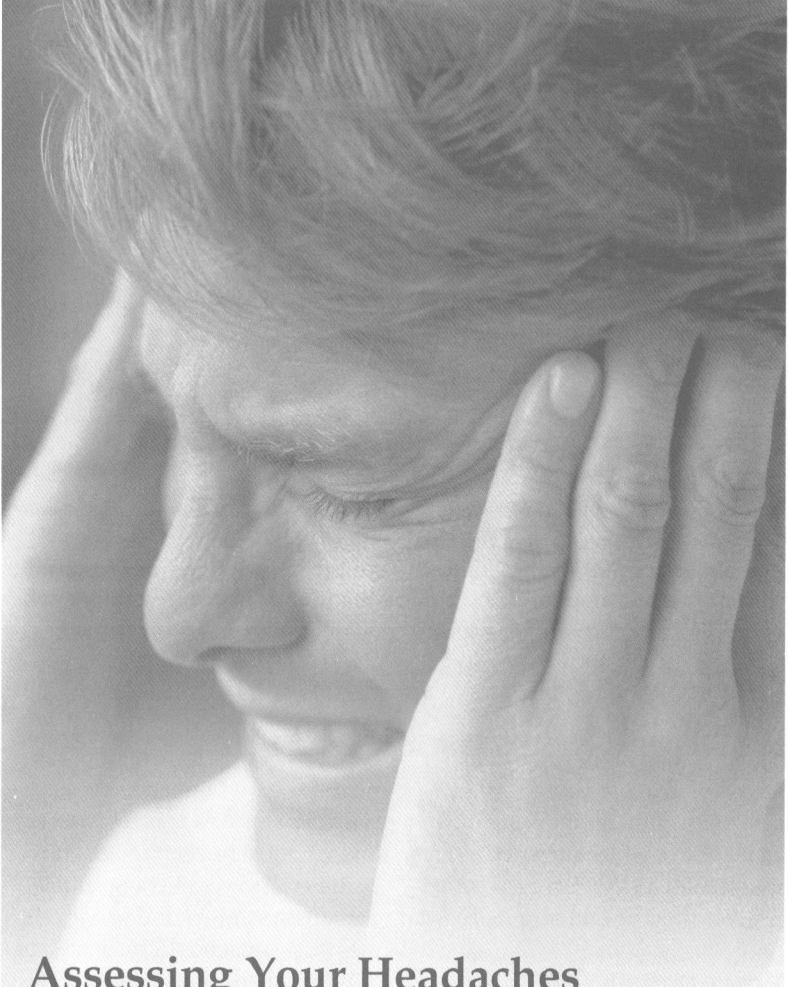

Neurologists and neurosurgeons are the medical specialists who treat brain and nervous system disorders. Diagnosis can be difficult because signs and symptoms can be numerous and diverse. Difficulties may also be encountered in distinguishing between neurological and psychiatric disease. A careful assessment of the character and pattern of signs and symptoms over time, in addition to laboratory tests, are sometimes necessary to reach an accurate diagnosis.

Headaches

Almost everyone experiences a headache at one time or another. Headaches are among the most common medical complaints. Headaches have many causes, and the site, severity and frequency with which they occur vary greatly. About 95 percent of all headaches are primary headaches, meaning that they aren't caused by an underlying disease or tumor. Sometimes, a headache may result from a serious medical problem, but this is uncommon.

What causes head pain?

Although your brain tissue can't ache, there's evidence that certain pathways within the brainstem and other portions of the brain may contribute to the production of various types of headaches. In fact, pain can't occur in most of your skull and a large portion of your brain membranes. Observations made during surgery indicate that only certain structures in your head are pain sensitive. These structures include skin and tissues lying just beneath it on the outside of your skull — muscles, arteries, the skull coating, eyes, ears and nasal and sinus cavities. Pain-sensitive structures inside your skull include arteries, venous sinuses and their tributary veins, parts of the outer membrane at

Assessing Your Headaches

To help assess your pain, your doctor may ask several questions about your headaches, such as:
- Do certain things trigger your headaches?
- How frequently do your headaches occur?
- Do they occur at regular intervals, and if so, at what time of day or night?
- Where do you experience the first pain?
- What does the pain feel like — pressure, throbbing, stabbing?
- Do your headaches begin slowly or rapidly? How soon does the pain peak?
- How long do your headaches typically last?
- Do other signs and symptoms precede your headache?
- Do other signs and symptoms accompany your headache?
- What relieves your headaches?
- Is there a history of headaches in your family?
- How do you respond to headache medication?
- Do your headaches affect your ability to work or participate in other activities?
- What thoughts do you have about your headaches?
- Why are you seeking help now?

If you have frequent headaches, it may be useful to keep a headache diary, including answers to the questions listed above. Such a journal may help you and your doctor identify headache triggers to avoid in the future.

the base of the brain, and certain cranial and cervical nerves.

Cranial or cervical nerves send pain sensations from these parts of your head to your central nervous system. Dental and jaw pain, for example, are conveyed by the cranial nerves. Your cervical nerves also convey messages about pain in your neck and at the base of your head.

Outside of your skull, pain may result from inflammation or tension in muscles, inflammation of scalp arteries, or inflammation in your sinuses, ears or gums. Inside your skull, enlargement or contraction of arteries, inflammation of brain membranes, or pressure from a tumor or hemorrhage can produce a headache.

Although the exact nature of headache pain is unclear, research suggests that headaches may occur as a result of changes in the levels of brain chemicals (neurotransmitters), such as serotonin and noradrenaline. An imbalance in the levels of these neurotransmitters may lead to inflammation of scalp arteries and subsequent irritation of pain-sensitive structures. This causes pain impulses to travel along the trigeminal nerve, a major pain pathway, into the brain. The level of endorphins, natural painkillers produced by your brain and spinal cord, also may be disrupted, causing pain.

Your headache might feel dull, throbbing (pulsatile) or sharp. Precise description of your pain can be helpful in diagnosing what type of headache you have. Primary headaches are generally classified into three categories: tension-type, migraine and cluster.

Tension-type headaches usually produce a dull pain, knot or pressure in your forehead, scalp or the back of the neck. Migraines are associated with moderate to severe pain, often, but not always, on one side of your head. They may be accompanied by nausea and sensitivity to lights and sound. Cluster headaches are characterized by a steady, severe pain in and around one eye or on one side of the head and tend to occur in episodes.

If you have a headache more days than not, you may be experiencing chronic daily headaches. An estimated 3 to 5 percent of adults worldwide experience chronic daily headaches. Many people with chronic daily headaches are actually experiencing a rebound effect from taking pain medication too frequently.

Headaches can be triggered by any number of things. Headaches, especially migraines, occur in some women just before or during a menstrual period. Such headaches are likely related to hormonal fluctuations. Headaches from high

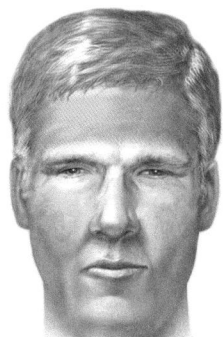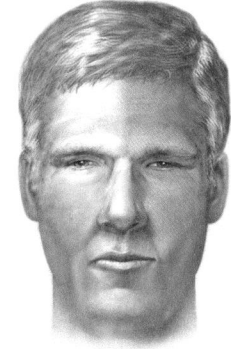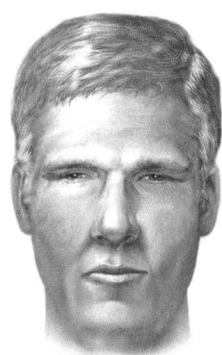

The three most common types of headaches cause different types of pain. The pain of a tension headache is usually a dull, squeezing pain that may involve the forehead, scalp, temples or back of the neck. A migraine usually occurs on only one side of the head. Cluster headaches occur on one side of the head or as a stabbing sensation in an eye.

When a Headache Spells Trouble

Headaches that signal a serious medical condition are uncommon, but a headache can accompany conditions such as a cerebral hemorrhage, brain tumor or weakened blood vessel (aneurysm).

If you have one or more of the following headache warning signs, seek urgent care:

- Abrupt, severe headache, often like a thunderclap
- Headache with fever, stiff neck, rash, mental confusion, seizures, double vision, weakness, numbness or speaking difficulties
- Headache after a head injury, even if it's a minor fall or bump, especially if it's associated with a seizure, weakness, drowsiness, nausea or vomiting
- Chronic, progressive headache that worsens after coughing, exertion, straining or a sudden movement
- New headache pattern after age 55

A rare headache-related condition that almost always begins after age 50 is temporal arteritis, an inflammation of arteries in your scalp, brain and eyes. It's treatable, but if ignored, it can lead to blindness or, rarely, stroke.

You generally don't need to be concerned by an occasional headache. Most everyone experiences them, and they're usually related to common conditions such as stress, allergies or overuse of alcohol. If, however, your headache appears with other signs and symptoms or you have one that you might call the worst ever, seek medical help.

Effects of Too Much Medication

If you find yourself taking pain relievers for headaches three or more times a week on a regular basis, you may be experiencing a rebound effect. In other words, your medication may actually be contributing to your head pain, a condition known as medication overuse headaches.

Although scientists aren't sure why this happens, they think that overuse of pain medications may short-circuit your brain's pain control system. When your pain reliever wears off, your headache returns, at times even stronger than before. The most common over-the-counter medications that cause this are ibuprofen (Advil, Motrin IB, others), acetaminophen (Tylenol, others) and combination medications that include caffeine. Overuse headaches also can result from prescription headache medications.

Signs and symptoms

Medication overuse headaches are typically continuous throughout the day but not necessarily severe. You may notice increasing pain at certain times, especially when your pain reliever begins to wear off, such as at night. Nausea, anxiety, restlessness, irritability, difficulty concentrating and depression may accompany rebound headaches.

Breaking the cycle

To break the rebound cycle, you'll need to wean yourself off your pain medications. Start by making an appointment with your doctor or a headache specialist.

Depending on what you've been taking, you may be advised to temporarily stop all pain medication. Doing so will likely mean increased headaches for the next week to 10 days. But most people who successfully stop pain relievers experience significant pain relief within two weeks.

Once you've broken the cycle, you can work with your doctor to develop a headache management plan. Often, daily preventive therapy is available. Avoiding or minimizing certain headache triggers, caffeine, stress or irregular eating patterns, is critical. In addition, your doctor may prescribe a specific medication to treat your headaches, matching it with the type of headache to which you're prone.

Alternative pain management

Instead of pain medication, try some of the following techniques. They may be just as effective as medication, without the side effects:

- *Rest in a quiet, dark room.* Place a cold towel on your forehead and compress your temples. Ice also may help.
- *Take a hot shower or warm bath to relax.* Massage your scalp, face, neck and shoulder muscles.
- *Learn stress-relief techniques.* These include relaxed breathing, yoga and meditation.

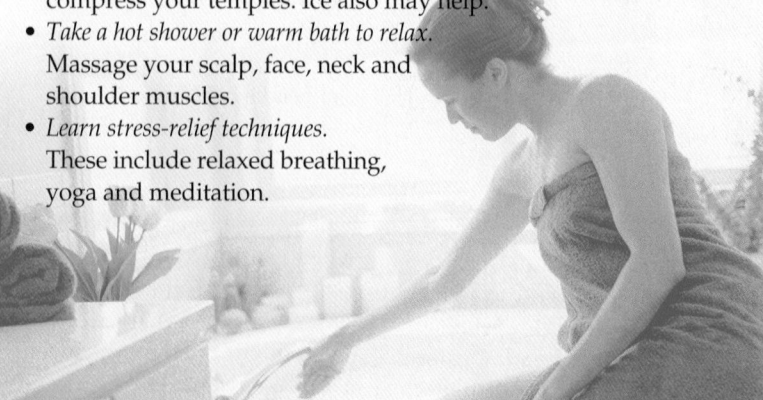

blood pressure tend to occur on awakening in the morning, but this type is uncommon. Morning headaches are often caused by untreated sleep apnea.

A headache that results from an infection in your nasal cavity can be particularly painful when you bend over. It's usually accompanied by other signs and symptoms of infection, such as a fever. Eyestrain headaches may occur after long periods of reading or driving a car at night. Headaches also result from overexertion and dehydration.

Making a diagnosis

Diagnosis of a headache is generally based on a medical history and examination. If your headache is of recent onset, occurs in abrupt attacks, is triggered by exertion, and is often present in the morning and accompanied by vomiting or is associated with other signs and symptoms, such as vision loss, weakness on one side, seizure or speech impairment, further testing may be required.

Testing may include a computerized tomography (CT) scan or magnetic resonance imaging (MRI) of your head to look for any structural abnormalities and to examine your sinuses, facial bones, and neck tissue and bones. X-rays of the upper spine may be needed if your headaches began after a head or neck injury.

In rare cases, a doctor may need additional tests to establish a diagnosis.

Tension headaches

Signs and symptoms

- Dull, aching head pain
- Tightness or pressure across your forehead or on the sides and back of your head
- Tenderness on your scalp, neck and shoulder muscles

A tension headache — or tension-type headache as it's medically known — is the most common type of headache, and yet its causes aren't well-understood. A tension headache is generally a diffuse, mild to moderate pain that many people describe as feeling as if there's a tight band around their heads.

A tension headache can last from 30 minutes to an entire week. You may experience these headaches only occasionally, or nearly all the time. If your headaches occur 15 or more days a month for at least three months, they're considered chronic. If you have headaches that occur fewer than 15 times a month, your headaches are considered episodic. However, people with frequent episodic headaches are at a higher risk of developing chronic headaches.

Researchers suspect that tension headaches may result from changes among certain brain chemicals — serotonin, endorphins and numerous other chemicals — that help nerves communicate. It's not clear why the chemical levels fluctuate, but the process is thought to activate pain pathways to the brain and interfere with the brain's ability to suppress the pain. It's likely other factors also contribute to tension headaches. Potential triggers may include stress, depression, anxiety, poor posture, working in awkward positions, jaw clenching and poor sleep.

Diagnosis

Your doctor will likely ask you questions or have you undergo tests to exclude other possible sources of your pain. Tests may include vision tests and a computerized tomography (CT) scan or magnetic resonance imaging (MRI).

Your doctor may look for evidence of anxiety or depression. You may be asked if stress at work or at home might be associated with worsening of the headaches.

How serious are tension headaches?

These headaches don't lead to more-serious disorders. They may,
however, be a sign that you're stressed, anxious or depressed.

Treatment

Most people with tension headaches don't seek medical advice because they've been able to manage the discomfort with over-the-counter (OTC) pain relievers. Be aware that using OTC pain relievers more than two to three days a week can cause medication overuse headaches (see page 518).

Medications

A variety of medications, both OTC and prescription, can stop or reduce the pain of an existing headache attack, including:

- **Analgesics.** Analgesics are pain relievers. A class of analgesics known as nonsteroidal anti-inflammatory drugs (NSAIDs) are usually the first line of treatment for reducing headache pain. NSAIDs include the OTC drugs ibuprofen (Advil, Motrin IB, others) and naproxen sodium (Aleve). Prescription NSAIDs include naproxen (Naprelan, Naprosyn), indomethacin (Indocin, Tivorbex) and ketoro-

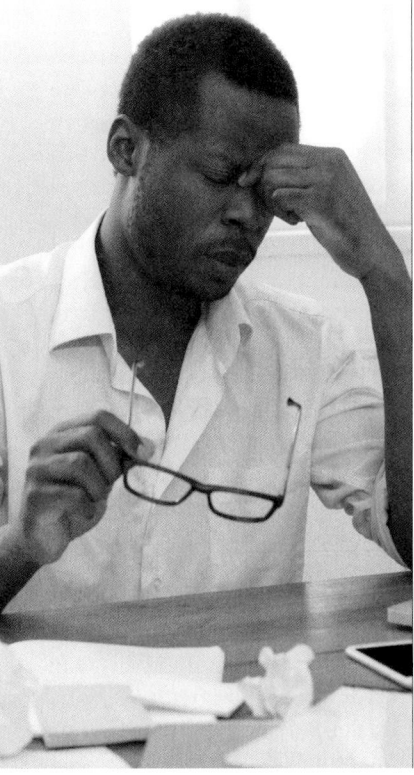

lac. Acetaminophen (Tylenol, others) and aspirin also are analgesics.

- **Combination medications.** Aspirin or acetaminophen or both are often combined with caffeine or a sedative drug into a single medication. For example, Excedrin combines aspirin, acetaminophen and caffeine. Combination drugs may be more effective than pure analgesics for pain relief but carry a higher risk of a medication overuse headache. Although many combination drugs are available OTC, analgesic-sedative combinations are obtained only by prescription because they may be addictive and can lead to chronic daily headaches. Use them only with careful monitoring by your doctor.

- **Other medications.** For people who experience both migraines and episodic tension headaches, a triptan can effectively relieve the pain of both headaches. Opiates (narcotics) are rarely used because of their side effects and potential for dependency and medication overuse.

Pain medications don't cure headaches; they relieve the symptoms temporarily. Over time, painkillers and other medications may lose their effectiveness or they might even cause headaches. To avoid the development of medication overuse headaches, don't use over-the-counter pain relievers for more than nine days a month. Also remember that most medications have side effects.

Preventive medications

Certain medications taken at regular intervals may reduce the frequency and severity of attacks. Your doctor may prescribe these if you have frequent headaches or tension headaches that aren't relieved by acute medication and nondrug therapy such as stress management. Your doctor may also recommend preventive medication if your headache pain becomes disabling or causes you to overuse pain relievers.

Doctors may prescribe antidepressants to prevent tension headache, especially the chronic form. They work to stabilize the levels of brain chemicals such as serotonin, which may be involved in the development of a headache. You don't have to have depression in order to use these drugs.

Preventive medications may include:

- **Tricyclic antidepressants.** Tricyclic antidepressants, including amitriptyline and nortriptyline (Pamelor), are the most commonly used medications to prevent tension headaches. They're effective against both the episodic and chronic forms. Side effects of these medications may include weight gain, drowsiness and dry mouth.
- **Other medications.** Other medications that may prevent tension headaches include anticonvulsants, such as topiramate (Topamax, Qudexy XR, others) and gabapentin (Neurontin, Gralise, others), and muscle relaxants, such as tizanidine (Zanaflex).

Preventive medications may require several weeks or more to build up in your nervous system before they take effect. Also be aware that overusing caffeine or painkillers for acute relief may reduce the effect of a preventive drug. If your headaches are under control, you may be able to gradually reduce the dose of medication over time.

Self-care
Tension-type headaches usually respond well to relaxation techniques, such as massage, hot showers, warm baths, biofeedback and meditation. Adequate exercise and rest also can be helpful. Sometimes, physical therapy is recommended.

Keeping a headache diary might help you to identify what may be triggering your headaches, so that you can take steps to avoid the triggers.

Migraine attacks

Signs and symptoms
- Moderate to severe head pain, which may be confined to one side of the head or affect both sides
- Nausea and vomiting
- Sensitivity to light and sound
- Fatigue, dizziness, difficulty concentrating
- Sparkling, rainbowlike colors or blank spots in your field of vision (aura)
- Tingling on one side of the body

A migraine can begin anytime with intense, throbbing pain on one side of your head that may gradually spread. Migraine attacks are often associated with nausea and, sometimes, vomiting. Sensitivity to lights, sounds and smells is common.

An attack typically reaches the peak of severity in minutes to an hour or two and can last for hours to up to three days, unless treated. Sleep generally improves signs and symptoms, but you may be listless after waking up. The frequency of attacks can range from daily to occasional.

Migraine is a brain sensation and pain processing disease that's often inherited. Researchers have demonstrated that migraines are caused by functional changes in the trigeminal nerve system, a major pain pathway in your nervous system, and by imbalances in brain chemicals, including serotonin, which plays a regulatory role for pain messages going through this pathway.

During a migraine, serotonin levels drop. Researchers believe this causes the trigeminal nerve to release substances called neuropeptides, which travel to your brain's outer covering (meninges). There they cause blood vessels to become dilated and inflamed. The result is headache pain.

It's likely that individuals with migraine are born with a tendency to develop the condition. Common migraine triggers include:

- **Hormonal changes.** Although the exact relationship between hormones and headaches isn't clear, fluctuations in estrogen levels seem to trigger headaches in many women with known migraines. Women with a history of migraines often report headaches immediately before or during their periods, and this corresponds to a major drop in estrogen. Others have an increased tendency to develop migraines during pregnancy or menopause. Hormonal medications, such as contraceptives and hormone replacement therapy, also may worsen migraines.
- **Foods.** Certain foods appear to trigger headaches in some people. Common offenders include alcohol, especially beer and red wine; aged cheeses; chocolate; fermented, pickled or marinated foods; aspartame; overuse of caffeine; monosodium glutamate — a key ingredient in some Asian foods; certain seasonings; and many canned and processed foods. Skipping meals or fasting also can trigger migraines.
- **Stress.** A difficult week at work followed by relaxation may lead to a weekend migraine. Stress at work or home also can instigate migraines.
- **Sensory stimuli.** Bright lights and sun glare can produce head pain. So can unusual smells — including pleasant scents, such as perfume and flowers, and unpleasant odors, such as paint thinner and secondhand smoke.
- **Changes in wake-sleep pattern.** Either missing sleep or getting too much sleep may serve as a trigger for migraine attacks in some individuals.
- **Physical factors.** Intense physical exertion, including sexual activity, may provoke migraines.
- **Changes in the environment.** A change of weather, season, altitude, barometric pressure or time zone can prompt a migraine.
- **Medications.** Certain medications can aggravate migraines.

Types

Migraine attacks have several clinical patterns:

Migraine with aura

About 10 percent of people with migraine regularly get a neurological warning about five to 20 minutes before their headache begins. This warning, called an aura, may include sparkling flashes of colored light, dazzling zigzag lines, slowly spreading blind spots and dizziness. You may also have a feeling of numbness on one side of your body. Less commonly, symptoms include a slowly spreading weakness or numbness of your face or a hand or leg, tingling and numbness in your lips, or difficulty talking or writing. Rarely, these symptoms persist longer than an hour.

Migraine without aura

This type is most common. It begins gradually with no characteristic warning symptoms. Hours before the headache, you may be elated, full of energy, thirsty, hungry for sweets, drowsy, experience yawning, or be irritable or depressed. These are sometimes referred to as premonitory symptoms. The headache usually builds to full intensity over several minutes or longer.

Others

Less common types of migraine attacks include:

- **Migraine aura without headache.** This form occurs most commonly in older adults.
- **Status migrainosus.** This is a migraine that persists longer than 72 hours.
- **Migrainous infarction.** This term describes a stroke that is induced by a migraine.

Migraine attacks may begin in childhood, adolescence or early adulthood. In more than half of all cases, there's a family history of migraines. Women are three times more likely to have migraines than are men.

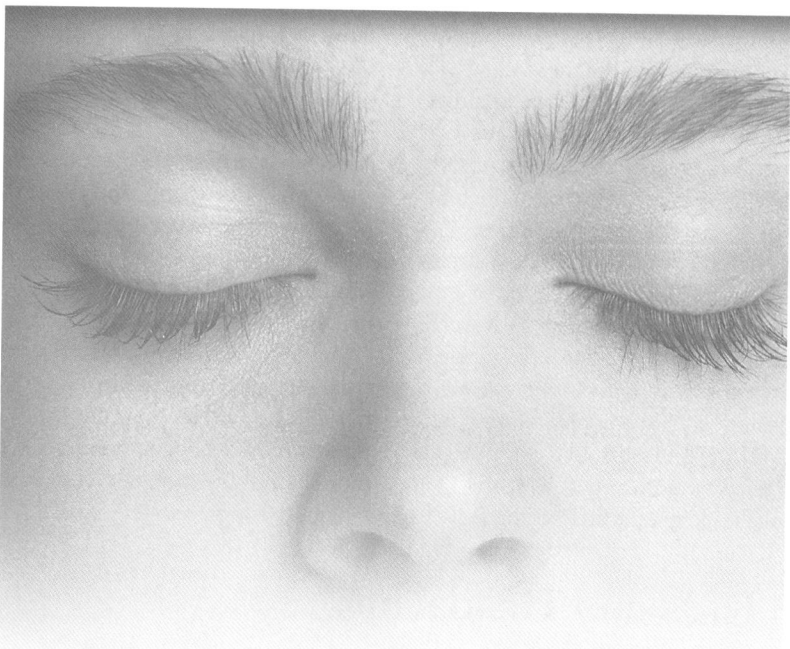

Muscle Relaxation

People sometimes develop habitual muscle responses to stress — a tension habit. Muscle relaxation techniques can reduce pain from muscle tension. These techniques have been useful in disorders such as tension headaches, temporomandibular joint (TMJ) syndrome and backaches.

Practiced relaxation techniques are successful stress relievers for many individuals. If you feel anxious, try the following relaxation strategy:

1. Sit in a comfortable chair or lie down. Close your eyes. Begin to breathe slowly and deeply. Keep breathing deeply and rhythmically for a number of minutes. As you breathe in, let your abdomen and chest expand with air. Contract them as you breathe out. In between, hold your breath for a few seconds. After some practice, a few breaths taken this way can calm you down during stressful situations.

2. Tense the muscles of your toes and press down your feet. Hold them taut. Feel the tension in your toes and feet. Notice where the tightness is. Keep the muscles tight and concentrate on the tension for about 20 seconds. Then relax your toes and feet. Feel the tension leave your muscles. Feel them become more and more relaxed, more and more heavy. Feel the warmth circulate through them as the tension drains away. Say the words *calm* and *relax* silently to yourself. When your feet and toes feel limp, go through the same procedure with another set of nearby muscles, moving very slowly up your body with one group of muscles at a time: your ankles and lower legs, your thighs, your pelvis and buttocks, your abdomen, your fists, your arms, and your shoulders.

3. Press your head into the cushion or pillow and tense the muscles in your neck. Clench your jaws. Frown and squint your eyes. Then relax. As you relax each section of your neck and head, keep saying *calm* and *relax*. Breathe deeply and fully.

For more information on ways to reduce stress, see Chapter 10, "Stress."

Diagnosis

People may self-diagnose their headaches as tension-type or sinus headaches (migraines can cause nasal congestion and runny nose), but most people who see a doctor for headaches have migraines.

If you have characteristic warning signs or a family history of migraines, your doctor may have little difficulty making a diagnosis. In some cases, a doctor may request tests such as a spinal tap (see page 542), vision tests and a computerized tomography (CT) scan or magnetic resonance imaging (MRI).

How serious are migraine attacks?

Migraines are a chronic disorder without a cure that can significantly affect your quality of life and ability to function. The headaches aren't life-threatening, and there's no proof that they lead to other disorders. With treatment you should be able to reduce the number and severity of attacks.

Sometimes, complications result from efforts to control the pain. If you take over-the-counter or prescription headache medications more than three times a week, you may be setting yourself up for a complication known as medication overuse headache (see page 518). Although these drugs can provide temporary relief, your body gets used to them over time. The result is that your headaches may become worse or more frequent, requiring more pain medication, which traps you in a vicious cycle.

In addition, aspirin or nonsteroidal anti-inflammatory drugs (NSAIDs), such as ibuprofen (Advil, Motrin IB, others), may cause side effects such as stomach pain, bleeding and ulcers, especially if taken in large doses a long time.

Kids and Headaches

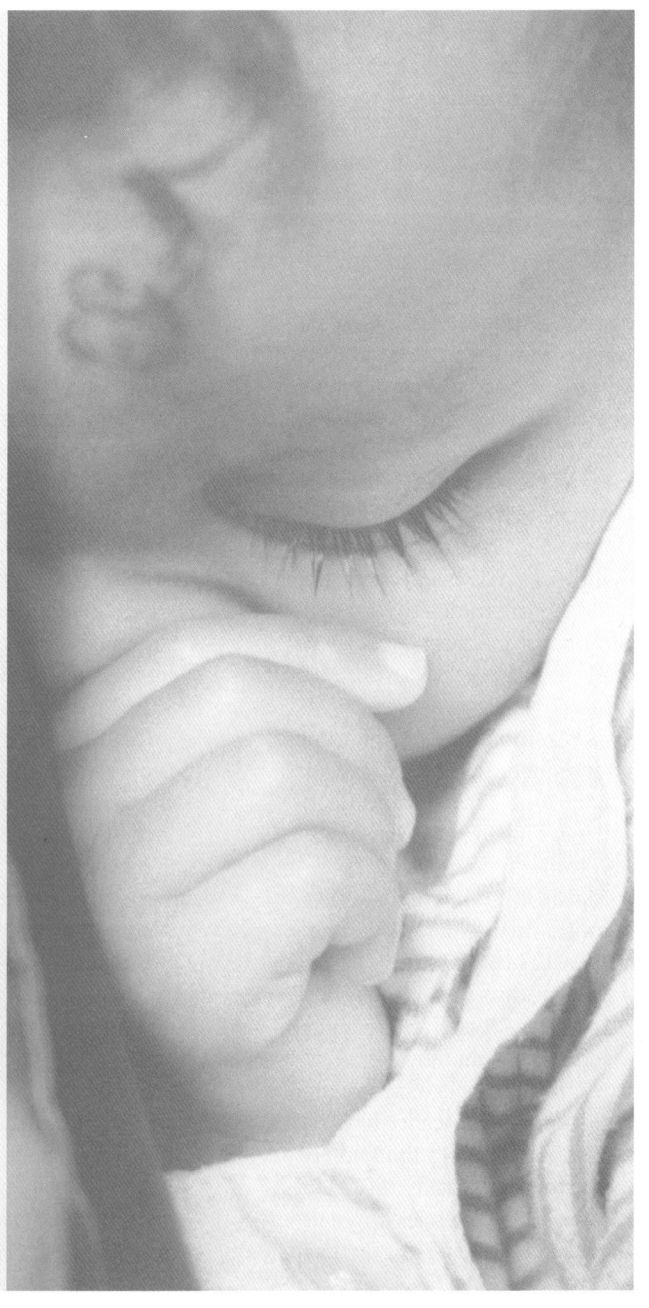

Headaches are one of the top reasons older children miss school. Recurrent headaches are common during late childhood and adolescence, although they're rarely due to a serious problem. Headaches are associated with many viral illnesses. However, if your child frequently complains of a headache, even during times when he or she is otherwise well, consult your doctor.

A headache may indicate stress related to school, friends or family. It may be a reaction to a medication, particularly a decongestant.

If you think it's a tension-type headache, help your child find ways to relax and avoid unnecessary stress. If headaches occur frequently, help your child keep a headache diary. Use acetaminophen (Tylenol, others) or ibuprofen (Advil, Motrin IB, others) sparingly and briefly to avoid missing serious problems that the pain reliever may be masking.

Don't give aspirin to children under age 16 unless instructed to do so by a doctor. Aspirin use in children is associated with Reye's syndrome, a rare and potentially life-threatening condition.

Migraines also may occur in children and are often accompanied by vomiting, light sensitivity and sleepiness. Recovery typically follows within a few hours.

If your child's headache persists, comes on suddenly without explanation or gets steadily worse, call your doctor. Also seek medical help with a headache that follows a recent ear infection, a toothache, strep throat or other infections.

Be sure to tell your doctor if there's any family history of migraines. That information could help lead to a diagnosis.

Treatment

A variety of drugs have been specifically designed to treat migraines. In addition, some drugs commonly used to treat other conditions also may help relieve or prevent migraines. Medications used to combat migraines fall into two broad categories:

- **Pain-relieving medications.** Also known as acute or abortive treatment, these types of medications are taken during migraine attacks and are designed to stop symptoms that have already begun.
- **Preventive medications.** These types of drugs are taken regularly, often on a daily basis, to reduce the severity or frequency of migraines.

Choosing a strategy to manage your migraines depends on the frequency and severity of your headaches, the degree of disability your headaches cause, and your other medical conditions.

Some medications aren't recommended if you're pregnant or breast-feeding. Some aren't used for children. Your doctor can help find the right medication for you.

Pain-relieving medications

For best results, take pain-relieving medications as soon as you experience signs or symptoms of a migraine. It may help if you rest or sleep in a dark room after taking them:

- **Combinations and nonsteroidal anti-inflammatory drugs (NSAIDs).** Drugs marketed specifically for migraine, such as the combination of acetaminophen, aspirin and caffeine (Excedrin Migraine), may ease moderate migraines. NSAIDs, such as ibuprofen (Advil, Motrin IB, others), may help relieve mild migraines. If over-the-counter medications don't help, your doctor may suggest a stronger, prescription-only version of the same drug. If taken too often or for long periods of time, NSAIDs can lead to ulcers, gastrointestinal bleeding and rebound headaches.
- **Triptans.** For many people with moderate to severe migraine attacks, triptans are the drug of choice. They're effective in relieving the pain, nausea and sensitivity to light and sound associated with migraines. Sumatriptan (Imitrex) was the first drug specifically developed to treat migraines. Related medications include rizatriptan (Maxalt), naratriptan (Amerge), zolmitriptan (Zomig), almotriptan (Axert), frovatriptan (Frova) and eletriptan (Relpax). Side effects of triptans include nausea, dizziness, muscle weakness and, rarely, stroke and heart attack. Studies indicate a single-tablet combination of sumatriptan and naproxen sodium relieves migraine symptoms more effectively than either individual medication.
- **Ergots.** Ergotamine (Ergomar) has been in use for more than 60 years and was a common prescription for migraine before newer medications were introduced. Dihydroergotamine is an ergot derivative that is more effective and has fewer side effects than ergotamine.
- **Anti-nausea medications.** Since migraine attacks are often accompanied by nausea with or without vomiting, medication to treat these symptoms is appropriate. Frequently prescribed medications include metoclopramide (oral) or prochlorperazine (oral or rectal suppository). There's some evidence these drugs can help relieve migraine pain as well.
- **Butalbital combinations.** Medications that combine the sedative butalbital with aspirin or acetaminophen are sometimes used to treat migraine attacks. Some combinations also include caffeine or codeine. These medications, however, have a high risk of rebound headaches and withdrawal symptoms and accordingly should be used infrequently.
- **Opiates.** Medications containing narcotics, particularly codeine, may be used to treat migraine pain when people can't take triptans or ergots. These drugs are habit-forming and are prescribed only as a last resort.

Preventive medications

Preventive medications can reduce the frequency, severity and length of migraines and may increase the effectiveness of symptom-relieving medicines used during migraine attacks. Your doctor may recommend that you take preventive medications daily, or only when a predictable trigger, such as menstruation, is approaching.

In most cases, preventive medications don't eliminate headaches completely, and some can have serious side effects.

- **Cardiovascular drugs.** Beta blockers — which are commonly used to treat high blood pressure and coronary artery disease — can reduce the frequency and severity of migraines. These drugs are considered among first line treatment agents. Calcium channel blockers, another class of cardiovascular drugs, especially verapamil (Calan), also may be helpful. In addition, the antihypertensive medications lisinopril (Prinivil, Zestril) and candesartan (Atacand) are useful migraine-prevention medications. Researchers don't understand exactly why all of these cardiovascular drugs prevent migraines. Side effects can include dizziness, drowsiness or lightheadedness.
- **Antidepressants.** Certain antidepressants are good at helping prevent all types of headaches, including migraines. Most effective are tricyclic antidepressants, such as amitriptyline, nortriptyline (Pamelor) and protriptyline (Vivactil). These medications are considered among first line treatment agents and may

reduce migraines by affecting the level of serotonin and other brain chemicals. You don't have to have depression to benefit from these drugs. Newer antidepressants, however, generally aren't as effective for migraine prevention.

- **Anti-seizure drugs.** Although the reason is unclear, some anti-seizure drugs, such as divalproex (Depakote) and topiramate (Topamax, Qudexy XR, others), which are used to treat epilepsy and bipolar disease, seem to prevent migraines. Gabapentin (Neurontin, Gralise, others), another anti-seizure medication, is considered a second line treatment agent. In high doses, however, these anti-seizure drugs may cause side effects, such as nausea and vomiting, diarrhea, cramps, hair loss and dizziness.
- **Cyproheptadine.** This antihistamine specifically affects serotonin activity. Doctors sometimes give it to children as a preventive measure.
- **Botulinum toxin type A (Botox).** Some people receiving Botox injections for their facial wrinkles have noted improvement of their headaches. The mechanism by which Botox might prevent migraines is unclear, although the drug may cause changes in your nervous system that modify your tendency to develop migraines. Botox has been shown to be safe and effective. It's only approved for people who experience chronic migraines — who have headaches more than half the days in a month for at least three months.

Self-care

If you know that certain foods trigger a migraine, avoid them. For some people, maintaining a regular sleep schedule helps reduce or prevent migraines.

Aerobic exercise — about 30 minutes on most days — reduces tension and can prevent migraines

in some people. Be sure to warm up slowly because sudden, intense exercise can actually trigger a headache. Relaxation techniques also can be helpful.

If you think your migraines may be related to medications, such as birth control pills or hormone replacement therapy, consider discontinuing their use. These medications contain the hormone estrogen, which can trigger or contribute to headaches and increase the risk of stroke in individuals with migraine aura. Talk to your doctor about other options or dosage changes.

If you have frequent headaches, keep a diary to see what triggers your attacks. Note the time a headache began, what you ate during the preceding 24 hours, how you felt and what you were doing when the headache started, any unusual stress, how long the headache lasted, and what made it stop.

Cluster headaches

Signs and symptoms
- Excruciating pain, generally located in or around the eye, but may radiate to other areas of the face, head, neck and shoulders
- One-sided pain
- Restlessness
- Excessive tearing
- Redness in the eye of the affected side
- Stuffy or runny nasal passage in the nostril on the affected side of your face
- Sweaty, pale skin (pallor) on the face
- Swelling around the eye on the affected side of your face
- Reduced pupil size
- Drooping eyelid

A cluster headache is one of the most painful types of headache. A striking feature of cluster headache is that the attacks occur in cyclical patterns or clusters, giving the condition its name.

Bouts of frequent attacks — known as cluster periods — may

last from weeks to months, usually followed by remission periods when the headache attacks stop completely. The pattern varies from one person to another, but most people have one or two cluster periods a year. During remission, no headaches occur for months, and sometimes even years.

During a cluster period:
- Headaches typically occur every day, sometimes several times daily.
- A single attack may last from 15 minutes to three hours.
- The attacks often happen at the same time each day.
- The majority of attacks occur between 9 p.m. and 9 a.m.

The pain usually ends as suddenly as it begins, with rapidly decreasing intensity. After attacks, most people are completely free from pain but exhausted.

The exact cause of cluster headaches is unknown, but abnormalities in the hypothalamus likely play a role. Cluster attacks typically occur with clocklike regularity during a 24-hour day, and the cycle of cluster periods often follows the seasons of the year.

These patterns suggest that the body's biological clock is involved. In humans, the biological clock is located in the hypothalamus, which lies deep in the center of your brain. Abnormalities of the hypothalamus may explain the timing and cyclical nature of cluster headaches. Studies have detected increased activity in the hypothalamus during the course of a cluster headache.

Other factors that may be involved include:
- **Hormones.** People with cluster headaches have abnormal levels of certain hormones, such as melatonin and cortisol, during cluster periods.
- **Neurotransmitters.** Changes in the levels of some of the chemicals that carry impulses in the brain (neurotransmitters), such as serotonin, may play a role in cluster headaches.

Unlike migraines and tension headaches, cluster headaches generally aren't associated with triggers such as foods, hormonal changes or stress, except of alcohol use.

Diagnosis

If your signs and symptoms are typical of cluster headaches, your doctor may have little difficulty in diagnosing the condition. Still, you may need tests to exclude other problems that can cause similar pain, such as an aneurysm of an artery in your head, a tumor made up of newly formed blood vessels, sinusitis or glaucoma.

How serious are cluster headaches?

Cluster headaches are a chronic problem. There's no known cure and little understanding of the periodic pattern of attacks. The pain during an attack can be debilitating, but there's no permanent physical harm, and the condition doesn't lead to other disorders.

Treatment

There's no cure for cluster headaches. The goal of treatment is to help decrease the severity of pain and shorten the headache period.

Because the pain of a cluster headache comes on suddenly and may subside within a short time, over-the-counter pain relievers such as aspirin or ibuprofen (Advil, Motrin IB, others) aren't effective. The headache is usually gone before the drug starts working. Fortunately, other types of acute medication can provide some pain relief. Treatment of cluster headache is focused more on prevention, with more medication options available to choose from.

Acute treatments

Fast-acting treatments available from your doctor include:

- **Oxygen.** Briefly inhaling 100 percent oxygen through a mask provides dramatic relief for most who use it. The effects of this safe, inexpensive procedure can be felt within 15 minutes. The major drawback is the need to carry an oxygen cylinder and regulator with you, which can make the treatment inconvenient. Small, portable units are available, but some people still find them impractical. Sometimes, oxygen may only delay rather than stop the attack, and pain may return.
- **Triptans.** The injectable form of sumatriptan (Imitrex), which is commonly used to treat migraines, also is an effective acute treatment for cluster headaches. Some people may benefit from using sumatriptan in nasal spray form, but for most people this isn't as effective as an injection. Sumatriptan isn't recommended if you have uncontrolled high blood pressure or ischemic heart disease. Another triptan medication, zolmitriptan (Zomig), can be taken in nasal spray form for relief of cluster headaches. This medication may be an option if you can't tolerate other forms of fast-acting treatments.
- **Dihydroergotamine.** This medication derivative is available in intravenous, injectable and inhaler forms. Dihydroergotamine (D.H.E. 45, Migranal) is an effective pain reliever for some people with cluster headaches. If administered intravenously, you have to go to a hospital or doctor's office to have an intravenous (IV) line placed in a vein. The inhaler form of the drug works more slowly.
- **Octreotide (Sandostatin).** This drug, an injectable synthetic version of the brain hormone somatostatin, is an effective treatment for cluster headaches and is safe if you have high blood pressure and ischemic heart disease.
- **Local anesthetics.** The numbing effect of local anesthetics, such as lidocaine, may be effective against cluster headache pain when used in the form of nasal drops.

Preventive medicines

Whenever a cluster period starts, you'll likely take both a long-term medication and a short-term medication. After your headaches are under control, you may discontinue use of the short-term medication but continue with the long-term drug.

- **Corticosteroids.** Corticosteroids, such as prednisone, are fast-acting preventive medications. Your doctor may prescribe corticosteroids if your cluster headache condition has only recently started or if you have a pattern of brief cluster periods and long remissions. Serious side effects make them inappropriate for long-term use.
- **Ergotamine.** Ergotamine (Ergomar, others), available as a tablet that you place under your tongue or available as a rectal suppository, can be taken before bed to prevent nighttime attacks. Ergot medications are effective, but can't be combined with triptans.
- **Nerve block.** Injecting a numbing agent (anesthetic) and corticosteroid into the area around the occipital nerve, located at the back of your head, can prevent pain messages from traveling along that nerve pathway. An occipital nerve block can be useful for temporary relief until long-term preventive medications take effect.
- **Calcium channel blockers.** The calcium channel blocking agent verapamil (Calan, Verelan, others) is often the first choice for preventing cluster headaches. Sometime after your cluster period ends, the use of this medication is gradually tapered and discontinued under your doctor's direction. Occasionally, longer term use is needed to manage chronic cluster headache.
- **Lithium carbonate.** Lithium (Lithobid), used to treat bipolar disorder, also is effective in preventing chronic cluster headaches. Side effects include tremor,

increased urination and diarrhea. Your doctor can adjust the dosage to minimize side effects.

Other preventive medications used for cluster headaches include anti-seizure medications such as divalproex (Depakote) and topiramate (Topamax, Qudexy XR, others).

Newer treatments

As scientists learn more about the causes of cluster headaches, they're able to develop more-selective treatments for the condition. One development that shows promise is the use of a device to stimulate the occipital nerve, which influences the trigeminal nerve. Researchers are testing a stimulator — a pacemaker-sized device that sends impulses via electrodes — that is implanted over the occipital nerve. Several small studies, including one by Mayo Clinic researchers, of implanted occipital nerve stimulators found that the devices reduced chronic headache pain in some people, and the devices were well-tolerated and appeared to be very safe.

Similar research is underway using an implanted stimulator in the hypothalamus, the area of the brain associated with the timing of cluster periods. Deep brain stimulation of the hypothalamus may provide relief for people with severe, chronic cluster headaches.

Prevention

To help avoid a cluster attack during a cluster cycle:

- **Stick to a regular sleep schedule.** Cluster periods may begin when there are changes in your normal sleep schedule.
- **Avoid alcohol.** Alcohol almost always triggers a headache during a cluster period.
- **Avoid tobacco products.** Nicotine may trigger a headache during a cluster period.
- **Avoid nitrates.** Nitrates, found in smoked and processed foods, may trigger a headache.

Seizures

Brain cells communicate with each other through electric signals. Seizures occur when there's a sudden change in these signals, causing them to become disorganized. During a seizure, some brain cells send abnormal signals, which stop other cells from working properly. Abnormal signals may cause temporary changes in sensation, behavior, movement or consciousness.

Seizures can occur as a result of a disease, accident that affects the brain, or for no clear reason. If you have a single episode, it doesn't necessarily indicate that you have epilepsy. When seizures recur spontaneously, the condition is called epilepsy. Seizure disorder is a broader term that includes both a single seizure and epilepsy.

Seizure disorders aren't mental disorders, although mental health can influence control of seizures. They also don't cause psychiatric problems or mental retardation, even though people with epilepsy may also have those conditions. In some people, hereditary or environmental factors may contribute to repeated seizures.

Grand mal seizure

Signs and symptoms

Grand mal seizures have two stages.

- **Tonic phase.** Loss of consciousness occurs, and the muscles suddenly contract and cause the person to fall down. A period of rigidity follows.
- **Clonic phase.** The muscles go into rhythmic contractions, alternately flexing and relaxing. Convulsions usually last for less than two minutes.

When to See a Doctor

Seek medical evaluation as soon as possible after your first grand mal seizure. If your medical evaluation shows that you have epilepsy, you don't need to seek medical help each time you have a seizure. But do seek prompt medical advice if any of the following conditions are present:

- The seizure lasts longer than five minutes.
- Recovery from the seizure is slow.
- A second seizure follows immediately.
- You're pregnant.
- Signs of injury or illness are present.
- Your seizures become more frequent.
- There's a change in the way you feel during and after the seizures.
- You have changed your seizure medication or started taking other medicines.

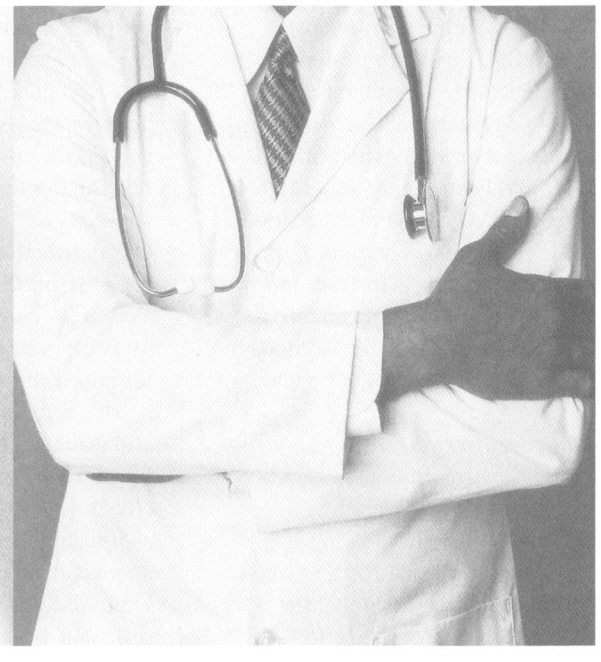

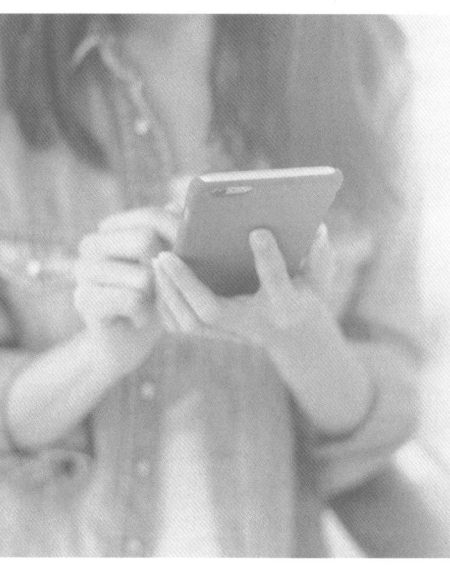

What to Do When Someone Has a Seizure

If you come across someone having a seizure, promptly call for medical help and follow these instructions:

- Gently roll the person onto one side and put something soft under his or her head.
- Loosen tight neckwear on the person.
- Don't try to put your fingers or anything else in the person's mouth. The tongue can't be swallowed.
- Don't try to restrain the person.
- Look for a medical alert bracelet on the person. It should state who to contact in an emergency and what medications he or she uses. Allergies to medications may be noted.

A grand mal seizure — also known as a tonic-clonic seizure — features a loss of consciousness and violent muscle contractions. It's the type of seizure most people picture when they think about seizures in general. Loss of consciousness occurs, which may be accompanied by falling. The seizure ends with a few minutes to a few hours of deep, relaxed sleep before consciousness returns with no memory of the seizure. Headache and drowsiness or confusion may follow a grand mal seizure.

Grand mal seizure is caused by abnormal electrical activity throughout the brain, so signs and symptoms typically involve the entire body. In some cases, this type of seizure is triggered by other health problems, such as extremely low blood sugar or kidney failure. But most grand mal seizures are related to epilepsy.

Sometimes, seizures run in families. In fact, a number of genes have been linked to certain seizure syndromes. Other causes of recurring seizures include scar tissue from prior brain disease or injury, a brain infection, tumor, abscess or hemorrhage, or alcohol or drug withdrawal. Rarely, seizures are life-threatening and can lead to death.

Diagnosis

A grand mal seizure is easily recognized, but the cause may be difficult to diagnose. Your doctor will want a detailed medical history. After a physical examination, you may need a test called electroencephalography (EEG), which records the electrical activity of your brain cells.

Other diagnostic tests may include magnetic resonance imaging (MRI) and blood tests. An MRI may help reveal seizures caused by scarring or by a tumor in a specific part of the brain.

How serious is a grand mal seizure?

The seriousness of a grand mal seizure depends on what caused it. Therefore, it's important to see a doctor when a grand mal seizure has occurred.

When a seizure results from a condition such as low blood sugar and the condition is corrected, seizure disorder isn't serious. In some cases, though, a seizure may be due to a serious medical disorder such as a brain tumor or brain infection.

A seizure that produces loss of awareness or loss of control can be dangerous if you're driving a motor vehicle or operating certain types of equipment. Therefore, many states have driving restrictions that are related to how well your seizures are controlled. Seizures can also result in injuries due to falling.

Treatment

Sometimes, treatment isn't started until you've experienced at least two seizures. In some cases, treatment begins after a single seizure if the risks appear to warrant it. Not everyone who has one seizure will have another one. The most common type of one-time seizure is the grand mal variety.

Medication

A number of medications are used to treat of epilepsy and seizures. Most are taken by mouth. Many people with epilepsy are able to prevent seizures by taking only one drug, but others require more than one.

Several standard anti-seizure drugs have been in use for decades. Anti-seizure drugs, which became available in the late 1990s, are generally no more effective in controlling seizures than the old standbys. But some recently developed drugs may have fewer side effects.

Finding the right medication and dosage can be complex. Your doctor likely will first prescribe a single drug at a relatively low dosage, and may increase the dosage gradually until your seizures are well-controlled. If you've tried two or more single-drug regimens without success, your doctor may recommend trying a combination of two drugs.

Anti-seizure medications have some side effects, which can include mild fatigue, dizziness and weight gain. More severe side effects include mood disruption, skin rashes, loss of coordination, speech problems and extreme fatigue.

If anti-seizure medications don't provide satisfactory results, your doctor may suggest other treatment options — such as vagus nerve stimulation, a ketogenic diet or brain surgery.

Vagus nerve stimulation
A device called a vagus nerve stimulator is implanted into your chest under the collarbone. Wires from the stimulator are attached to the vagus nerve in your neck (see page 531). The device turns on and off according to an adjustable program, and can be activated by the use of a magnet. This stimulation can inhibit seizures in some people. The exact mechanism by which this occurs is unclear.

Ketogenic diet
This treatment consists of a strict low-carbohydrate diet that leads to an increase in ketones, which may result in a reduction in seizures. To follow a ketogenic diet, you need a dietitian to assist you, and you need to perform regular urine tests at home to monitor your ketone levels. Even a tiny intake of sugar can significantly reduce the effectiveness of this treatment. In children with severe epilepsy, a third of those on the diet gain control over their seizures, and another third have fewer seizures. For the remainder, the diet has no effect. This approach has not been widely studied in adults.

Surgery
Individuals with tumors or scar tissue in the brain may benefit from surgery to remove the abnormality. People with uncontrolled seizures should see a specialist to determine if they may benefit from advanced nonmedication therapies, such as surgery.

Absence seizure

Signs and symptoms
- Brief staring spells with loss of awareness
- Eyelid fluttering
- Lip smacking
- Chewing
- Hand movements

An absence seizure — also known as a petit mal seizure — involves a brief, sudden lapse of conscious activity. Occurring most often in children, an absence seizure may look like the person is merely staring into space for a few seconds.

Compared with other types of epileptic seizures, petit mal seizures are very mild. But that doesn't mean they can't be dangerous.

Absence seizures last only a few seconds. Full recovery is almost instantaneous. Afterward, there's no confusion, and no memory of the incident.

Absence seizures may occur for weeks or months before an adult notices them, because they're so brief. A noticeable decline in a child's learning ability may be the first sign of this disorder. Teachers also may comment about a child's inability to pay attention.

In most cases, no underlying cause can be found. Some children simply seem to have a genetic predisposition to them. Sometimes flashing lights or hyperventilation can trigger an absence seizure.

Diagnosis
Electroencephalography (EEG), which measures brain wave activity, is generally used to look for signs of a distinctive brain electric pattern associated with absence seizures. In some instances, a doctor may also order blood tests or a computerized tomography (CT) scan or magnetic resonance imaging (MRI) to check for other possible causes of the seizures.

How serious are absence seizures?
Most children with absence seizures have significantly fewer or no seizures when they take medication. Up to 70 percent of children stop having them by late adolescence. At this age, most teens may be able to discontinue their medication under their doctor's supervision.

Treatment
Many medications can effectively reduce or eliminate the number of petit mal seizures. Finding the right medication and dosage can be complex, requiring a period of trial and error. Taking the medications on a regular schedule is crucial to maintaining the proper drug levels in the blood.

The most effective medications include ethosuximide (Zarontin), valproic acid (Depakene) and lamotrigine (Lamictal). Most children can discontinue anti-seizure medications, under a doctor's supervision, once they have been seizure-free for two years.

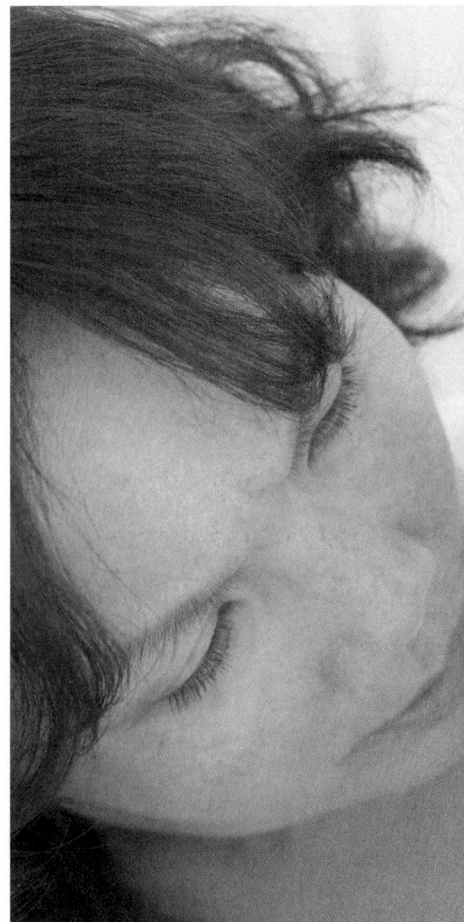

Febrile seizure

Signs and symptoms

- A brief episode of loss of consciousness and convulsions during a fever

A febrile seizure is a convulsion that occurs in young children caused by a sudden spike in body temperature, often from an infection. Watching your child experience a febrile seizure can be alarming, but it generally lasts only a few minutes.

Fortunately, febrile seizures aren't as dangerous as they may look. A seizure triggered by a sudden fever is usually harmless and typically doesn't indicate a long-term or ongoing problem.

Febrile seizures are classified as simple or complex:

- **Simple febrile seizures.** These are the most common. They last from a few seconds to 10 minutes and stop on their own. After the seizure, your child may cry, act confused or be quite sleepy.
- **Complex febrile seizures.** A complex febrile seizure lasts longer than 15 minutes, occurs more than once within 24 hours or is confined to one side of your child's body.

The fevers that trigger febrile seizures are caused by an infection in your child's body, such as a middle ear infection or roseola — a viral infection that causes swollen lymph nodes, usually in the neck, and a rash.

The risk of febrile seizures also increases after some common childhood immunizations. In the past, febrile seizures occasionally occurred the day a child received the diphtheria, tetanus and whole-cell pertussis (DTP) vaccination. However, this vaccine has been replaced by a newer version, commonly called DTaP. Now, febrile seizures may occur eight to 14 days after a measles-mumps-rubella (MMR) vaccination. The seizure is caused by the fever that may accompany the vaccination — not by the vaccination itself.

Diagnosis

If your child has a convulsion while a fever is present, seek medical attention immediately. Your child's doctor likely will perform a physical examination on your child. An electroencephalography (EEG) test to check brain wave activity may be performed. If the test shows no sign of an abnormality, the diagnosis is usually a febrile seizure.

How serious is a febrile seizure?

Although a febrile seizure may be alarming to you as a parent, it's usually harmless to your child and generally doesn't lead to a long-term or ongoing problem. Still, a febrile seizure always warrants medical attention to determine the cause of the fever.

Treatment

Don't try to give your child fever medications during a seizure, and don't place your child in a cooling tub of water. It's much more practical, more comfortable — and safer — for your child to remain lying on the carpet or a bed.

Most febrile seizures stop on their own within a couple of minutes. If your child has a febrile seizure that lasts more than five minutes — or if your child has repeated seizures — call for emergency medical attention.

In rare cases, the seizure may continue until your child arrives at the emergency department. If this happens, a doctor may order medication to stop the seizure.

If the seizure is prolonged or accompanied by a serious infection or if the source of the infection can't be determined, your doctor may want your child to stay in the hospital for further observation. A hospital stay generally isn't necessary for an uncomplicated seizure.

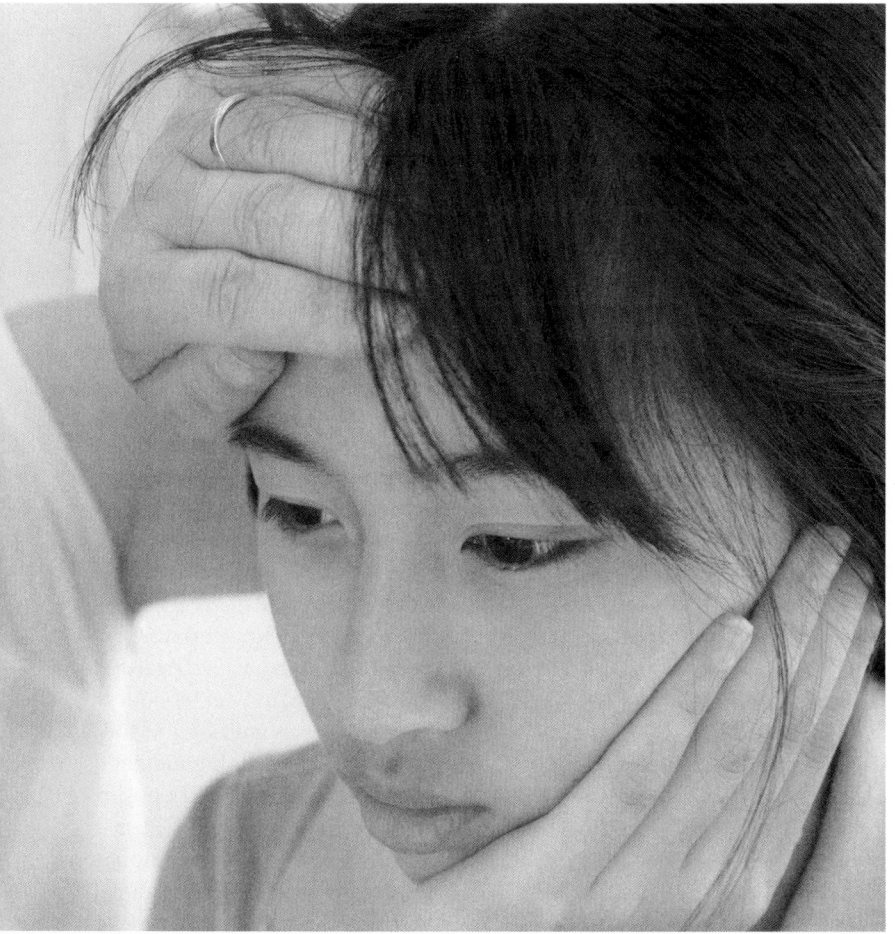

Anti-seizure Medications

Medication can control or greatly reduce the number of seizures for many people with a seizure disorder. Drug selection and dosage require close medical supervision and testing. You may have side effects such as drowsiness, upset stomach and a rash.

In some cases, medication can be discontinued after several years without seizures, but this must be done gradually and under the supervision of your doctor. If your seizures are due to an underlying condition, such as an infection or stroke, your doctor may decide that your anti-seizure medication can be eliminated after the underlying cause has been treated and is under control.

Commonly prescribed anti-seizure (anticonvulsant) medications include:

- Carbamazepine (Carbatrol, Tegretol)
- Clonazepam (Klonopin)
- Ethosuximide (Zarontin)
- Phenytoin (Dilantin)

- Primidone (Mysoline)
- Valproic acid (Depakene)
- Divalproex (Depakote)

In the past decade, newer anti-seizure medications have been developed, including the following:

- Gabapentin (Neurontin, Gralise, others)
- Felbamate (Felbatol)
- Lamotrigine (Lamictal)
- Topiramate (Topamax)
- Tiagabine (Gabitril)
- Oxcarbazepine (Trileptal)
- Levetiracetam (Keppra)
- Zonisamide (Zonegran)
- Lacosamide (Vimpat)

For prolonged or cluster seizures, your doctor may prescribe a sedative, such as diazepam (Diastat, Valium) or lorazepam (Ativan). For a child with a type of epilepsy called infantile spasms, or for severe seizures that don't respond to commonly used medications, a steroid drug called adrenocorticotropic hormone (ACTH) may be prescribed and given as an injection.

Many seizure medications can increase the risk of birth defects. If you're considering becoming pregnant, talk to your doctor about your seizure disorder and your medications.

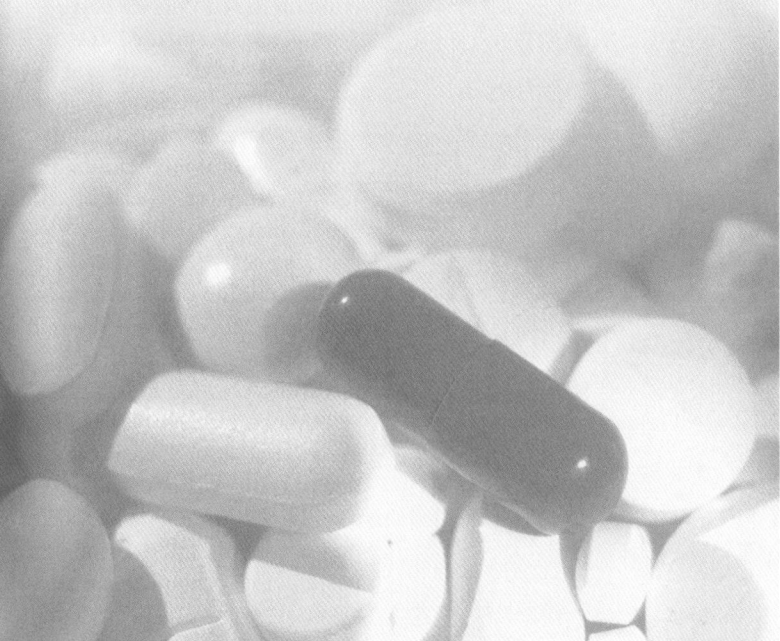

Complex partial seizure

Signs and symptoms

- A sudden sense of unprovoked fear
- A deja vu experience
- The sudden occurrence of a strange odor or taste
- A rising sensation in the abdomen
- Loss of awareness of your surroundings
- Staring
- A simple, repetitive act, such as lip smacking or repeated swallowing

These seizures most often originate in the temporal lobe, the part of your brain that extends from your temple to just behind your ear. Complex partial seizures are frequently preceded by a peculiar sensation (aura) that's followed by a brief loss of awareness or contact with surroundings. The physical component can be a simple repetitive act such as lip smacking, repeated swallowing or picking at clothes.

During normal waking and sleeping, your brain cells produce varying electrical activity. If the electrical activity from these cells becomes abnormally synchronized, a convulsion or seizure may occur.

Complex partial seizures may occur as a result of traumatic injury, infections, lack of oxygen, blood vessel malformations in the brain, stroke, brain tumors or genetic syndromes.

Diagnosis

In making a diagnosis, your doctor will want to know your medical history and that of your family. Diagnostic tests usually include electroencephalography (EEG) to check for abnormal electrical activity in the brain, and blood tests to detect any chemical imbalances. Imaging tests, including magnetic resonance imaging (MRI), positron emission tomography (PET) or single-photon emission computerized tomography (SPECT), may be performed to check for any structural abnormalities of the brain that may be the cause of seizures.

How serious are complex partial seizures?

The seizures themselves generally aren't life-threatening, but they can cause injuries associated with falling. A seizure that produces loss of awareness or control can be dangerous if you're driving a car, swimming, working at heights or operating certain types of equipment. In some cases, seizure disorders may require restrictions of physical activities. Still, limitations are often temporary, and many people with a seizure disorder are able to live an active life.

Treatment

The goal of seizure treatment is to eliminate or reduce seizures, minimize the side effects of treatment and allow you to live a normal, healthy life. This may involve the use of medications, surgery or, in some cases, a treatment called vagus nerve stimulation.

Medication

Most of the medications used to control seizures are taken by mouth. Several standard anti-seizure drugs have been in use for decades. Newer anti-seizure drugs, most of which became available in the late 1990s, are generally no more effective in controlling seizures than are the older standbys. There are some recently developed drugs, however, that may have fewer side effects.

Common side effects with all anti-seizure medications may include fatigue and dizziness. More than half of people who have complex partial seizures continue to have seizures despite taking anti-seizure drugs.

Surgery

Surgery for complex partial seizures has the highest success rate of all epilepsy surgery. At least 75 percent of these procedures result in a cure. Some studies place the

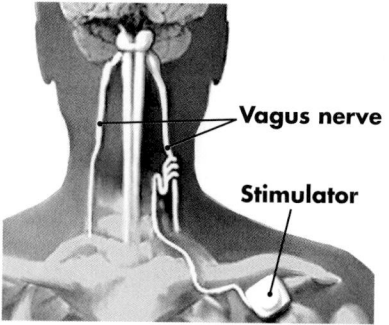

A vagus nerve stimulator delivers tiny, intermittent electric pulses to the vagus nerve. In some people, the pulses inhibit seizures.

success rate at over 90 percent. These high success rates are due to the nature of the seizures, which typically are linked to a defect or scar in the brain. Removing the defect or scar stops the seizures. However, surgery is rarely an option if your seizures originate from a region of the brain that contains vital brain functions.

During the procedure, your surgeon makes an incision in your scalp and removes a piece of the skull bone. He or she then cuts into or removes the area of the brain that's causing the seizures.

Although many people continue to need some medication to help prevent seizures after surgery, you may be able to take fewer drugs and reduce your dosages. In some cases, epilepsy surgery can cause complications, such as permanently altering your cognitive abilities.

Vagus nerve stimulation

A device called a vagus nerve stimulator may be an option if medications are ineffective or they cause serious side effects. In the procedure, a stimulator is implanted into your chest under the collarbone. Wires from the stimulator are carefully threaded underneath the skin and attached to the vagus nerve in your neck. The stimulator delivers tiny electric impulses to the vagus nerve. The impulses help inhibit seizures in some people. The device turns on and off according to an adjustable program.

Stroke and Vascular Disorders

Two major artery systems extend through your neck to carry blood to your brain. An interruption of blood flow in one of these systems — even for a few seconds — usually produces a dramatic effect on your brain's functions. Depending on what areas of your brain are affected, you can have vision or speech difficulties, paralysis in part of your body, or loss of consciousness. If this interruption continues for more than a few minutes, brain cells in the affected area may die, causing permanent impairment or death. Two conditions that can affect blood supply to brain cells are reduced blood flow (ischemia) and bleeding (hemorrhage).

Transient ischemic attack

Signs and symptoms
- Sudden onset of weakness or numbness of the face, arm or leg, often on one side of the body
- Sudden lack of coordination of the limbs
- Sudden vision loss or double vision
- Sudden difficulty speaking or understanding others
- Sudden severe dizziness, loss of balance or difficulty walking

A transient ischemic attack (TIA) is like a stroke, producing similar symptoms, but usually lasting only a few minutes and causing no permanent damage. Often called a ministroke, a transient ischemic attack may be a warning. About 1 in 3 people who have a transient ischemic attack eventually has a stroke, with about half occurring within a year after the transient ischemic attack.

Most TIAs are due to atherosclerosis, a condition where cholesterol-containing fatty deposits (plaques) form inside arteries.

Emergency Treatment

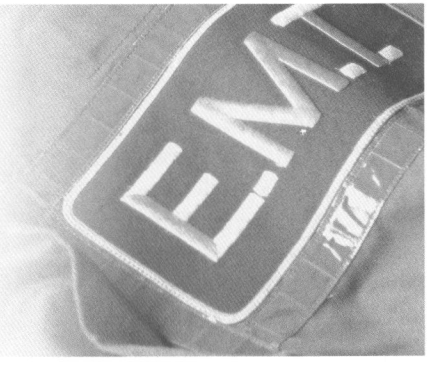

While waiting for emergency help to arrive, carefully watch the person suspected of having a stroke. If breathing ceases, cardiopulmonary resuscitation (CPR) is necessary.

If the person is having difficulty breathing, position the person's head and shoulders on a pillow. If vomiting occurs, turn the person's head to the side so that he or she doesn't choke on the vomit.

Don't let the person eat or drink anything.

The plaques narrow the pathway of blood through the artery and decrease flow. A blood clot (thrombus) can form on an injured plaque. A plaque fragment or a small piece of clot forming in the heart can break off and lodge in a smaller artery. When the clot or fragment temporarily blocks blood flow at a distant site in the brain, the result is a TIA.

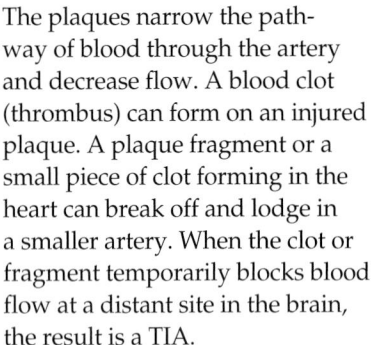

Various factors can increase your risk of a TIA. Risk factors that you can change or control include high blood pressure, tobacco use, diabetes and abnormal blood cholesterol levels. Certain cardiovascular diseases also can make you more prone to a TIA, including congestive heart failure, a previous heart attack, heart valve disease or valve replacement, and an irregular heart rhythm (atrial fibrillation).

Black people are at greater risk of a TIA than are white people, partly because of their higher prevalence of high blood pressure and diabetes. Risk is also greater if one of your parents or siblings has had a TIA or stroke.

Diagnosis

The most significant feature of a TIA is the speed with which it comes and goes. Rapid onset, brief duration and then a return to normal is the usual sequence. Recurrent episodes of similar signs and symptoms also are significant.

A detailed description of your signs and symptoms can help in the diagnosis of a TIA. Weakness in only one arm or leg, for example, may point to a disturbance in a branch of the internal carotid artery, whereas weakness in both arms or legs suggests disturbances in blood flow through the vertebral arteries or basilar artery.

Other information that your doctor may obtain to assist in a diagnosis includes your eye pressure, blood pressure and the noise (bruit) heard over the neck with a stethoscope when blood flow in various arteries is impaired.

You may also undergo various tests to gather additional information and provide images of brain arteries for evaluation. These may include a computerized tomography (CT) scan or magnetic resonance imaging (MRI), cerebral arteriography, magnetic resonance angiography (MRA), carotid ultrasonography, or transesophageal echocardiography to check for blood clots in a heart chamber.

How serious is a transient ischemic attack?

You should regard a TIA as an emergency because of the risk that a stroke may follow. Approximately one-third of people with TIAs later have a stroke, a third have more TIAs, and a third have no further brain-related signs or symptoms.

Treatment

Once your doctor has determined the cause of your transient ischemic attack, the goal of treatment is to correct the abnormality and prevent a stroke. Your doctor may prescribe medication to reduce the tendency for blood to clot or may recommend surgery or a balloon procedure (angioplasty).

Medications

Doctors use several medications to decrease the likelihood of a stroke after a transient ischemic attack. The medication selected depends on the location, cause, severity and type of TIA. Two frequently prescribed types of drugs are:

- **Anti-platelet drugs.** These medications make your platelets, one of the circulating blood cell types, less likely to stick together. When blood vessels are injured, sticky platelets begin to form clots, a process completed by clotting proteins in blood plasma. The most frequently used anti-platelet medication is aspirin. Aspirin is also the least expensive treatment with the fewest potential side effects. An alternative to aspirin is the anti-platelet drug clopidogrel (Plavix). Some studies indicate that aspirin is most effective in combination with another anti-platelet drug. Your doctor may consider prescribing Aggrenox, a combination of low-dose aspirin and the anti-platelet drug dipyridamole, to reduce blood clotting. The way dipyridamole works is slightly different from aspirin.
- **Anticoagulants.** These drugs include warfarin (Coumadin, Jantoven) and newer anticoagulants such as dabigatran (Pradaxa), rivaroxaban (Xarelto), apixaban (Eliquis) and edoxaban (Savaysa). Anticoagulants affect clotting-system proteins instead of platelet function. Anticoagulant drugs require careful selection and monitoring.

Are You at Risk?

Many risk factors for stroke are the same as those for a heart attack. These include:

- *Family history.* Your risk of stroke is greater if one of your parents or a brother or sister has had a stroke or TIA.
- *Age.* Your risk of stroke increases as you get older. It doubles each decade past age 35.
- *Sex.* Men are at greater risk of ischemic stroke than are pre-menopausal women. Men and women have similar risks of intracerebral hemorrhage, but women are more likely to have subarachnoid hemorrhage.
- *Race.* Black people are more likely to have strokes than are white people. The increase is partly due to greater risk of high blood pressure and diabetes.
- *High blood pressure.* High blood pressure increases your risk of both ischemic and hemorrhagic stroke. It can weaken and damage blood vessels in and around the brain, leaving them vulnerable to hemorrhage and atherosclerosis. Excessive dietary salt, lack of exercise and excess weight contribute to high blood pressure.
- *Cardiovascular disease.* Several other heart and blood vessel conditions can increase your risk of a stroke: congestive heart failure, a heart attack, aortic heart valve disease, or valve replacement and an irregular heart rhythm (atrial fibrillation). With these conditions, your heart doesn't pump blood efficiently or it beats irregularly. This can lead to formation of blood clots (thrombosis) in a chamber of the heart or on a diseased valve. About 15 to 20 percent of all ischemic strokes occur in people who have atrial fibrillation.
- *Tobacco use.* If you smoke, your risk of a stroke may be two or three times greater than if you don't. Smoking contributes to the formation of fatty deposits (plaques) in your arteries. Nicotine makes your heart work harder, increasing your heart rate and blood pressure. The carbon monoxide in cigarette smoke replaces oxygen in your blood, decreasing the amount of oxygen delivered to the walls of your arteries and tissues, including tissues in your brain. The combination of smoking and using oral contraceptives greatly increases your risk of stroke.
- *Diabetes.* Diabetes doubles your risk of a stroke. It increases the severity of atherosclerosis and interferes with normal breakdown of fibrin, a protein in your blood that binds clots together.
- *Undesirable blood cholesterol levels.* High levels of low-density lipoprotein (LDL or "bad") cholesterol and low levels of high-density lipoprotein (HDL or "good") cholesterol increase your risk of narrowed or blocked arteries, including those leading from your heart to your brain (carotid and vertebral arteries).
- *Previous transient ischemic attack (TIA) or stroke.* If you've had a TIA, your risk of a stroke increases significantly. The more frequent the TIAs, the greater your risk. If you've already had a stroke and you're over age 45, your risk of having another increases by about 10 to 20 times.
- *Elevated homocysteine level.* This amino acid occurs naturally in your blood. Studies indicate people with elevated levels of homocysteine may have a higher risk of heart and blood vessel damage.
- *Sedentary lifestyle.* Lack of physical activity on a regular basis increases the risk of stroke.

Decreasing your risk of stroke involves many of the same lifestyle changes as those for decreasing your risk of cardiovascular disease, such as quitting smoking, limiting fat and cholesterol in your diet, exercising regularly, controlling blood pressure and diabetes, and managing stress.

It may not be easy to change an old habit, or to start a new one such as daily exercise. But doing so may help protect you from the most common cause of serious, long-term disability and the third most common cause of death in the United States — stroke.

Talk to your doctor about your stroke risk factors and the treatments, medications and resources that may be available to help you reduce your risk.

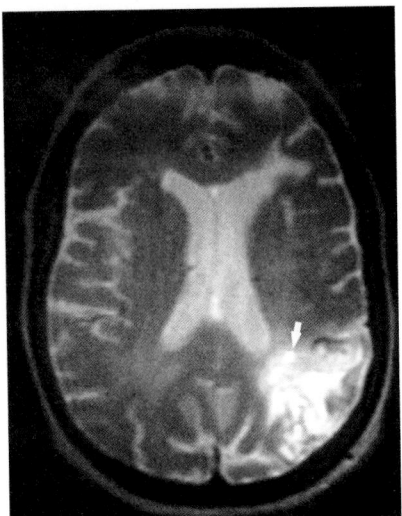

The arrow reveals an area of brain tissue affected by a stroke, as shown on magnetic resonance imaging (MRI).

Surgery and angioplasty (stenting)
If you've had a TIA or stroke and have a moderately or severely narrowed neck (carotid) artery, your doctor may suggest carotid endarterectomy. This surgery clears carotid arteries of fatty deposits (atherosclerotic plaques) before another TIA or stroke can occur. An incision is made to open the artery, the plaques are removed, and the artery is closed.

In selected cases, a procedure called carotid angioplasty, or stenting, is an option. This procedure involves using a balloonlike device to open a clogged artery and placing a small wire tube (stent) into the artery to keep it open.

Some people have carotid artery damage not caused by a TIA or stroke. Medication may be prescribed to lower the risk of stroke. Surgery or the placement of a stent may benefit certain individuals.

Stroke

Signs and symptoms
- Sudden onset of weakness or numbness of the face, arm or leg, often on one side of the body
- Sudden lack of coordination of the limbs
- Sudden vision loss or double vision

- Sudden difficulty speaking or understanding others
- Sudden severe dizziness, loss of balance or difficulty walking
- Sudden severe headache accompanied by other symptoms

A stroke occurs when the blood supply to a part of your brain is interrupted or severely reduced, depriving brain tissue of oxygen and nutrients. Within a few minutes, brain cells begin to die.

Just as for a heart attack, every minute counts. The longer a stroke goes untreated, the greater the damage. Success of treatment depends in part on how soon care is given.

Almost 800,000 Americans have a stroke each year. About 1 in 6 die of the injury. Warning signs may be temporary. Even symptoms lasting only a short time may indicate an impending stroke. It's important to take them seriously.

Types
Strokes are characterized by the location and type of disturbance. The two basic types are ischemic stroke and hemorrhagic stroke.

Ischemic stroke
More than 80 percent of strokes are ischemic strokes. They occur when the arteries to your brain are narrowed or blocked, causing severely reduced blood flow (ischemia). This deprives your brain cells of oxygen and nutrients, and cells may begin to die within minutes. The most common ischemic strokes are:
- **Thrombotic stroke.** This type occurs when a blood clot (thrombus) forms in one of the arteries that supply blood to your brain. A clot usually forms in areas

damaged by atherosclerosis — a disease in which the arteries are clogged by fatty deposits (plaques). Atherosclerosis can occur within one of the two carotid arteries of your neck that carry blood to your brain, as well as in other neck or brain arteries.
- **Embolic stroke.** An embolic stroke occurs when a blood clot or other particle forms in a blood vessel away from your brain — commonly in your heart — and is swept through your bloodstream to lodge in narrower brain arteries. This type of blood clot is called an embolus. It's often caused by irregular beating in the heart's two upper chambers (atrial fibrillation), which can lead to poor blood flow and the formation of a blood clot.

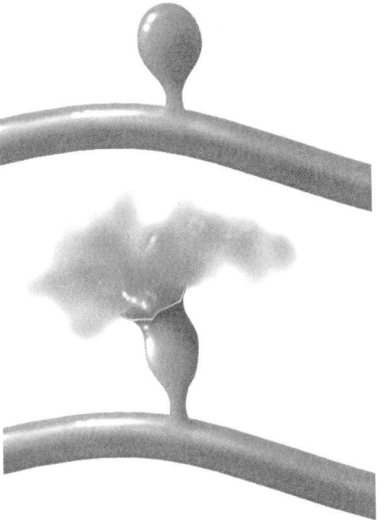

An aneurysm is a ballooning of an artery from a weak area in its wall. Over time, the wall stretches and becomes thin enough to rupture.

Hemorrhagic stroke

Hemorrhage is the medical term for bleeding. Hemorrhagic stroke occurs when a blood vessel in your brain leaks or ruptures. Hemorrhages can result from a number of conditions that affect your blood vessels, including uncontrolled high blood pressure (hypertension) and weak spots in your blood vessel walls (aneurysms). A less common cause of hemorrhage is the rupture of an arteriovenous malformation (AVM) — an abnormal tangle of thin-walled blood vessels, present at birth. There are two types of hemorrhagic stroke:

- **Intracerebral hemorrhage.** In this type of stroke, a blood vessel in the brain bursts and spills into the surrounding brain tissue, damaging cells. Brain cells beyond the leak are deprived of blood and also are damaged. High blood pressure is the most common cause of this type of hemorrhagic stroke. Over time, high blood pressure can cause small arteries inside your brain to become brittle and susceptible to cracking and rupture.
- **Subarachnoid hemorrhage.** In this type of stroke, bleeding

Carotid Endarterectomy

Endarterectomy is a surgical procedure that removes cholesterol-containing fatty deposits (plaques) from inside a blood vessel. Plaques can reduce the flow of blood through an artery or break off and travel to, and lodge in, the brain. Plaque formation (atherosclerosis) is common. It frequently occurs in the neck arteries to the brain, particularly in the carotid artery where it branches.

Plaque formation at this junction is a common cause of transient ischemic attack (TIA) or ischemic stroke. Carotid endarterectomy is usually done after one or more TIAs to prevent their recurrence or a subsequent stroke. Occasionally, carotid endarterectomy is performed during the first few hours of an evolving ischemic stroke.

Carotid endarterectomy is also effective in reducing the risk of stroke in people who have severe narrowing of the carotid artery but haven't yet experienced symptoms.

Benefits vs. risks

Although it has a high success rate, the procedure has risks. Your doctor will discuss them with you and determine whether to recommend the procedure for you. In addition to the severity and location of the narrowing, your doctor will consider other factors before recommending this operation, such as whether you have high blood pressure or other forms of cardiovascular disease. Unstable coronary artery disease may make the risk of this operation too great.

In individuals for whom the risks of the surgery may be too high, nonsurgical therapy is considered. This generally includes medication to prevent blood clotting.

The procedure

The procedure begins with an incision in the neck to expose the carotid branching site (bifurcation). Clamps are inserted to stop blood flow. The artery is opened to remove the plaques. Closure of the artery may require a patch of synthetic material. Restoring blood flow through the artery must be done carefully to prevent clots from entering the blood flow.

Complications, including stroke, can arise during this operation. To minimize the risk of stroke during surgery, brain activity is monitored by a test called electroencephalography. It allows the surgeon to determine if circulation to the brain is adequate while the carotid artery is clamped for repair. If not, steps can be taken to improve blood flow. Sometimes, the person undergoing surgery is kept awake to allow cooperation with surgical staff.

As with any surgical procedure, the success rate of carotid endarterectomy depends on the expertise of the doctor and surgical team. Blockage may recur, but that's uncommon. In properly selected individuals, the operation usually eliminates risk of further transient ischemic attacks (TIAs) and reduces the chance of a stroke.

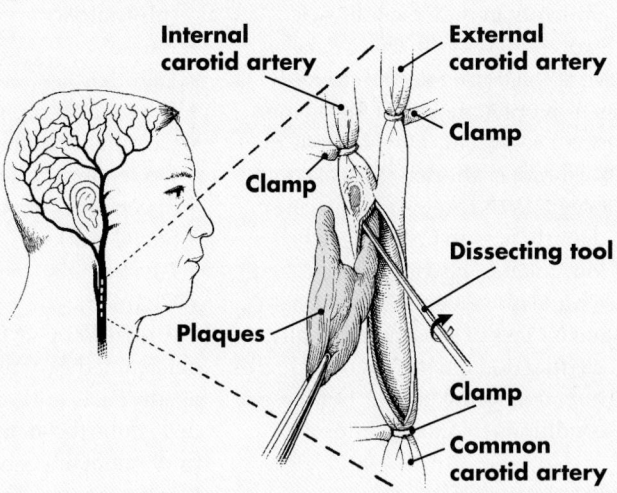

Internal carotid artery

External carotid artery

Clamp

Clamp

Dissecting tool

Plaques

Clamp

Common carotid artery

If blood flow to the brain is blocked by an obstruction in the carotid artery, a surgical procedure called an endarterectomy may be done. Clamps are placed on the artery to stop blood flow while fatty deposits (plaques) inside the artery are removed with a dissecting tool.

Stroke Rehabilitation

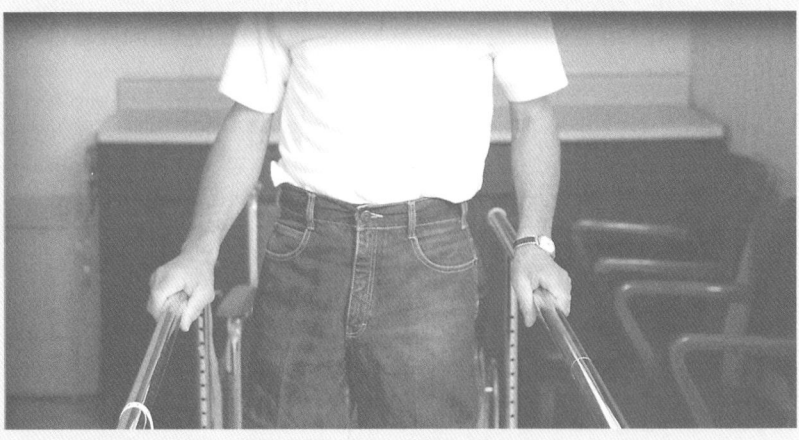

More than 6 million Americans are stroke survivors. Some have only minor disabilities, and well over half of all stroke survivors regain their independence. Other stroke survivors require extended care, some because of permanent mental or physical disabilities and others because they lack home care.

Following a stroke, rehabilitation is crucial for morale and a return to maximal function. Recovery and rehabilitation depend on the area of the brain involved and the amount of tissue damaged. Stroke may affect you physically, psychologically and cognitively.

Physically
Harm to the right side of the brain may impair sensation and movement on the left side of the body. Damage to brain tissue on the left side may affect movement on the right side and may also cause speech and language disorders.

Language disorders may include difficulty in understanding or expressing words. This can be very frustrating for the stroke survivor. Some loss of vision may occur regardless of which side of the brain is affected. A stroke that occurs in the brainstem can cause disturbances in breathing, swallowing, balance, hearing, and eye and tongue movements. You may also have a loss of sensation. Initially, bladder and bowel function are disturbed in many people, but these conditions frequently improve.

Psychologically
Depression is a common response to stroke. Affected individuals may feel helpless, frustrated and uninterested in activities they once enjoyed. Diminished sex drive, mood changes and thoughts of suicide aren't unusual.

Cognitively
The way in which a person learns, remembers, interacts with others or interprets everyday events may be affected. These side effects may be due in part to changes in the production of brain chemicals. Antidepressant medications may be prescribed.

Stroke rehab team

A stroke rehabilitation team can help you get started on your way to recovery. The team may include some or all of the following people:
• Rehabilitation physician (physiatrist)
• Nurse
• Dietitian
• Physical therapist
• Occupational therapist
• Recreational therapist
• Speech therapist
• Social worker
• Psychologist
• Chaplain

The makeup of the team is determined by your particular needs. Early and repeated tests to determine the status of your improvement are used to design your rehab program. Therapy is focused on maximizing your capabilities, such as getting you back to work or improving mobility at home and in the community. Many stroke survivors regain partial use of affected limbs, especially with the help of rehabilitation professionals.

Recovery

Some individuals recover satisfactorily without specific rehabilitation therapy. Others require it. In some, the damage is so severe that intensive rehabilitation is impractical. Among individuals in whom rehabilitation may not be possible, the goal of treatment and care is to prevent complicating muscle contractures, skin ulcers, pneumonia, malnutrition, bowel and bladder dysfunction, social isolation, and depression. The most important and effective help over the long term may come from family and friends, and it requires patience and persistence.

A supportive home environment has a beneficial effect on rehabilitation. Regardless of age, stroke survivors who can go home to a healthy spouse or other companion are more likely to become independent and productive. In case of severe damage, the home environment can reduce risk of further complications. Encouragement is important.

Various adaptive devices and architectural modifications such as ramps, hand bars on the tub and toilet, and bath benches or shower chairs can help facilitate independence and safety. Contact your doctor, local rehabilitation professionals or independent living center for information and assistance.

starts in a large artery on or near the surface of the brain and spills into the space between the surfaces of your brain and your skull. This type of hemorrhage is often signaled by a sudden, severe "thunderclap" headache. This type of stroke is commonly caused by the rupture of an aneurysm, which can develop with age or be genetically inherited. After the hemorrhage, the blood vessels in your brain may widen and narrow erratically (vasospasm), causing brain cell damage by further limiting blood flow to parts of your brain.

Diagnosis

A diagnosis of stroke doesn't depend on any single symptom, but on a rapid development of symptoms. The presence of specific symptoms that correspond to specific arterial areas within the brain is further evidence of stroke. However, even with a completed stroke, early care may decrease the amount of damage.

Other possible causes of your signs and symptoms, such as a tumor, need to be excluded. One or more of the following diagnostic tests may be used to evaluate your blood vessels: carotid ultrasonography, cerebral arteriography, computerized tomography (CT), magnetic resonance imaging (MRI) and magnetic resonance angiography (MRA).

How serious is stroke?

Stroke is a very serious illness that warrants prompt medical attention. The range of treatments for early stroke is expanding, so it's critical that you arrive at the emergency room as soon as possible. If available, see a stroke specialist.

After any kind of stroke, an area of dead brain tissue (cerebral infarct) may remain. Recovery depends on whether other nerve tissue can assume the function of that area. A series of strokes can lead to a long-term (chronic) brain disorder called vascular dementia.

Stroke most frequently results from chronic conditions such as high blood pressure, atherosclerosis and heart disease. If you have one or more of these disorders, see a doctor regularly.

Treatment for ischemic stroke

Prompt medical treatment for stroke is important. Treatment depends on the type of stroke. For an ischemic stroke, doctors must quickly restore blood flow to your brain.

Medications

Therapy with clot-busting drugs must start within 3 to 4½ hours. Quick treatment not only improves your chances of survival, but may also reduce the amount of complications resulting from the stroke. You may be given:
- **Tissue plasminogen activator.** Some people who are having a stroke can benefit from an injection of tissue plasminogen activator (TPA). TPA is the best-proven immediate treatment after a stroke to reduce the likelihood of having another stroke. It is a potent clot-busting drug that helps some people who have had stroke recover more fully. However, it's best if the drug be administered within a 3- to 4½-hour window of the stroke occurring, and it can only be given in situations in which doctors are certain that giving TPA will not worsen bleeding in the brain. TPA cannot be given to people who are having a hemorrhagic stroke.
- **Aspirin.** In an emergency room, you may be given aspirin. The dose may vary, but if you already take a daily aspirin for its blood-thinning effect, you may want to make a note of that in your purse or wallet on an emergency medical card so that the doctors will know if you've already had some aspirin. Do not take aspirin before you go to the hospital. If you are having a hemorrhagic stroke, taking aspirin could worsen the bleeding.

Other blood-thinning drugs, such as warfarin (Coumadin, Jantoven), also may be given, but they aren't as commonly used as aspirin.

Surgical and other procedures

Your doctor may recommend a procedure to open up an artery that's moderately to severely narrowed by the accumulation of plaques. This may include:
- **Intra-arterial TPA.** To treat a large acute stroke, doctors may insert a long, thin tube (catheter) through an artery in your groin and thread it to your brain to deliver TPA directly to the area where the stroke is occurring. The time window is somewhat longer than for intravenous TPA but is still limited.
- **Mechanical thrombectomy.** For a large clot, doctors may use a catheter to maneuver a tiny device into your brain to break up or grab and remove the clot.
- **Carotid endarterectomy.** In this procedure, a surgeon removes plaques that block the carotid arteries that run up both sides of your neck to your brain. The blocked artery is opened, the plaques are removed and your surgeon closes the artery. The procedure may reduce your risk of ischemic stroke. However, in addition to the usual risks associated with any surgery, a carotid endarterectomy can trigger a stroke or heart attack by releasing a blood clot or fatty debris. Surgeons now place filters (distal protection devices) at strategic points in your bloodstream to "catch" any material that may break free during the procedure.
- **Angioplasty and stents.** Angioplasty can widen the inside of an artery leading to your brain, usually the carotid artery. In this procedure, a balloon-tipped catheter is maneuvered into the obstructed area of your artery. The balloon is inflated, compressing the plaques against your artery walls. A metallic mesh tube (stent) is usually left

in the artery to prevent recurrent narrowing. Angioplasty and stenting of carotid arteries may be an appropriate stroke prevention option for some people who've had a stroke or transient ischemic attack (TIA) but can't undergo surgery. Intracranial stenting is similar to stenting the carotid arteries. Using a small incision in the groin, doctors thread a catheter through the arteries and into the brain. Sometimes they use angioplasty to widen the affected area first; in other cases, angioplasty is not used before stent placement.

Treatment for hemorrhagic stroke

Surgery may be used to treat a hemorrhagic stroke or prevent another one. The most common procedures — aneurysm clipping and arteriovenous malformation (AVM) removal — carry some risks. Your doctor may recommend one of these procedures if you're at high risk of spontaneous aneurysm or AVM rupture:

- **Aneurysm clipping.** A tiny clamp is placed at the base of the aneurysm, isolating it from the circulation of the artery to which it's attached. This can keep the aneurysm from bursting, or it can prevent re-bleeding of an aneurysm that has recently hemorrhaged. The clip will stay in place permanently.
- **Coiling (aneurysm embolization).** In an embolization procedure, a catheter is maneuvered into the aneurysm. A tiny coil is pushed through the catheter and positioned inside the aneurysm. The coil fills the aneurysm, causing clotting, and sealing the aneurysm off from connecting arteries.
- **Surgical AVM removal.** It's not always possible to remove an AVM if it's too large or if it's located deep within the brain. Surgical removal of a smaller AVM from a more accessible portion of the brain, though, can eliminate the risk of rupture, lowering the overall risk of hemorrhagic stroke.

Intracranial hematoma

Signs and symptoms

- Headache
- Nausea and vomiting
- Drowsiness
- Dizziness
- Confusion
- Slurred speech or inability to speak
- Pupils of unequal size
- Weakness in limbs on one side of your body

Emergency signs and symptoms
- Lethargy
- Seizures
- Unconsciousness

Although head injuries can be minor, an intracranial hematoma is a serious and possibly life-threatening condition that often requires immediate treatment.

Your brain floats within your skull, surrounded by fluid that cushions it from the bounces of everyday movement. But the fluid may not be able to absorb the force of a sudden blow or a quick stop. In these situations, your brain may slide forcefully against the inner wall of your skull and become bruised.

An intracranial hematoma occurs when a blood vessel ruptures within your brain or between your skull and your brain. The collec-

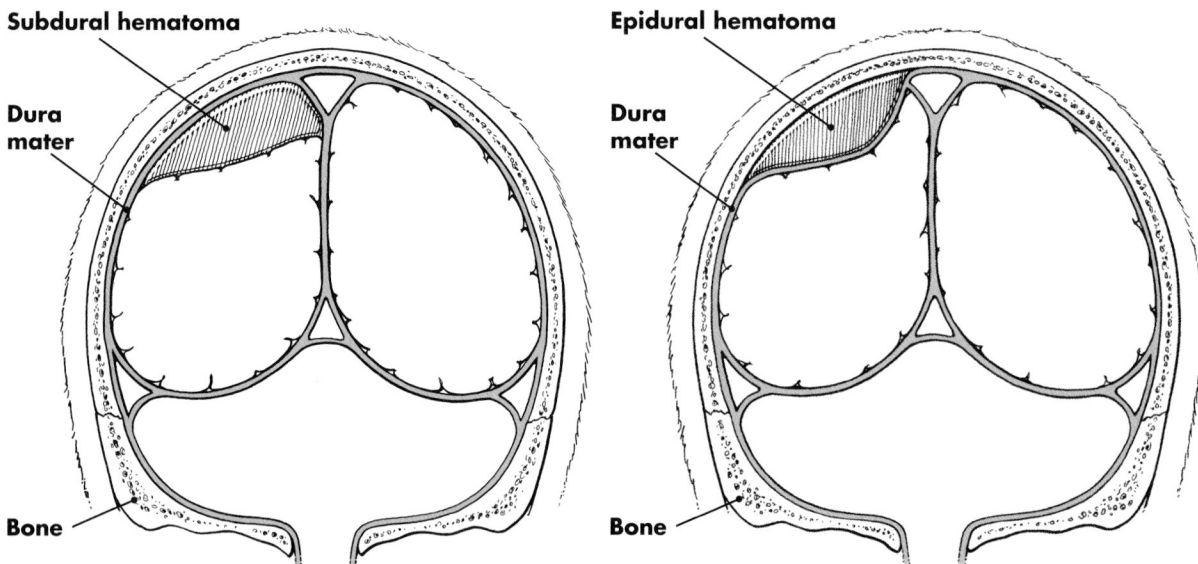

When an injury results in bleeding between the brain and the outer membrane of the brain (dura mater), blood may accumulate, producing a mass called a subdural hematoma (left). When bleeding occurs between the dura mater and the skull, the accumulation is termed epidural hematoma (right). Both can put pressure on the brain.

tion of blood (hematoma) compresses your brain tissue.

The cause of intracranial bleeding (hemorrhage) is an injury to the head, often as a result of an automobile or motorcycle accident or a seemingly trivial event, such as bumping your head. Mild head trauma is more likely to cause a hematoma in older adults. There may be no open wound, bruise or other outward sign.

A hematoma may occur as a subdural hematoma, an epidural hematoma or an intraparenchymal hematoma.

Subdural hematoma

This occurs when blood vessels — usually veins — rupture between your brain and the outermost of the three membrane layers that cover your brain (dura mater). The leaking blood forms a hematoma that compresses the brain tissue. If the hematoma keeps growing, a progressive decline in consciousness occurs, possibly resulting in death.

There are three types of subdural hematomas:

- **Acute.** This type is the most serious and potentially life-threatening. It's generally caused by a severe head injury, and signs and symptoms usually appear immediately.
- **Subacute.** In subacute subdural hematoma, signs and symptoms take longer to appear, generally several hours.
- **Chronic.** Less severe head injuries may cause a chronic subdural hematoma. Bleeding from chronic subdural hematoma may be much slower, and symptoms may take days, or even months, to appear.

All three types require medical attention as soon as signs and symptoms are apparent, or permanent brain damage may result. The risk of subdural hematoma is greater for people who use aspirin or anticoagulants daily, who are alcoholics, or who are either very young or very old.

Epidural hematoma

Also called an extradural hematoma, this type occurs when a blood vessel — usually an artery — ruptures between the outer surface of the dura mater and the skull. The blood vessel usually is damaged by a skull fracture. Blood then leaks between the dura mater and the skull to form a mass that compresses the brain tissue.

The risk of dying of an epidural hematoma is substantial unless prompt treatment occurs. Some people with this type of injury may remain conscious, but most become drowsy or comatose from the moment of trauma.

Epidural hematomas are more common in children and teenagers. They are often the result of motorcycle, automobile or other traumatic accidents.

Intraparenchymal hematoma

This type of hematoma, also known as intracerebral hematoma, occurs when blood pools in the brain. After head trauma, there may be multiple severe intraparenchymal hematomas.

The trauma that causes intraparenchymal hematomas is often responsible for what are called white matter shear injuries. These injuries occur after a trauma literally tears axons in the brain's white matter. Axons are the connections that carry messages (electrical impulses) from the neurons in the brain to the rest of the body. When this connection is sheared, serious brain damage can result because the neurons can no longer communicate.

Intraparenchymal hematoma can also result from blood vessel disorders, long-term hypertension, neurological conditions, brain tumors, liver disease, use of blood thinners and certain autoimmune diseases.

Diagnosis

Chronic subdural hemorrhage can be difficult to diagnose. Progressive loss of consciousness following a head injury, however, generally should be presumed to be caused by a hemorrhage inside the head until proved otherwise. The best method to define the position and size of the hematoma is a computerized tomography (CT) scan, if there's time to perform it. In some cases, magnetic resonance imaging (MRI) may be used instead. Sometimes, immediate surgery is necessary, leaving no time to perform tests.

How serious is an intracranial hematoma?

Intracranial bleeding (hemorrhaging) can be fatal without immediate treatment.

Some forms have less risk, but still require medical attention as soon as signs and symptoms are apparent, or permanent brain damage may result. Risk of serious complications is greater for people who use aspirin and anticoagulant medications on a daily basis.

Treatment

Hematoma treatment often requires surgery. The type of surgery depends on the characteristics of your hematoma. Options include:

- **Perforation.** If the blood is localized and isn't clotting excessively, a doctor may create a hole in the skull (perforation) and then remove the liquid by suction.
- **Craniotomy.** Large hematomas may require the opening of a section of skull (craniotomy) to remove the blood.

Some subdural hematomas don't need to be removed because they're small and produce no signs or symptoms.

Doctors may use medications, such as corticosteroids and diuretics, to control brain swelling (edema) after a head injury.

A significant period of recovery may be required after an intracranial hemorrhage. In adults, most recovery occurs within the first six months, but smaller adjustments may be made over two years.

Infections

Infections can attack your central nervous system in several ways. They may result from a direct invasion of your nervous system by a virus, bacterium or fungus. A minor condition, such as an ear infection or the measles, can lead to central nervous system involvement. You can also become infected from tick or animal bites or mosquito-borne agents.

Infections vary in seriousness. They may result in several days in bed, months of sickness with residual mental and physical impairment, or even death.

Meningitis

Signs and symptoms
- Fever
- Severe headache
- Vomiting
- Confusion
- Seizures
- Progressive lethargy
- Drowsiness
- In infants, bulging in the soft spot of the skull
- Stiff neck

Advanced signs and symptoms
- Stupor
- Coma
- Convulsions

Meningitis is an infection and inflammation of the membranes (meninges) and fluid surrounding your brain and spinal cord (cerebrospinal fluid). It's most often caused by a bacterial or viral infection. Of the two, bacterial meningitis is usually much more serious.

Meningitis usually strikes suddenly, with a high fever, severe headache and vomiting. Most cases of meningitis occur in children under age 5, but the disease is increasing in frequency among people between ages 15 and 24. Older adults also tend to have increased incidence of meningitis.

Some types of meningitis are contagious. You may be exposed to the bacteria when someone with the infection coughs or sneezes.

The bacteria can spread through kissing or sharing eating utensils or a toothbrush. You're also at increased risk if you live or work with someone with the disease.

The infection often starts as a respiratory illness. An infection of the heart valves, bones or some other organ can spread to the meninges via the bloodstream. Infection can also occur by direct invasion of bacteria already localized near your central nervous system, for example, from an infected ear, sinus, nose or tooth.

Types
Meningitis most often results from a bacterial or viral infection. Less commonly, a fungal infection may cause meningitis.

Bacterial
The *Streptococcus pneumoniae* (pneumococcus) bacterium is the most common cause of meningitis

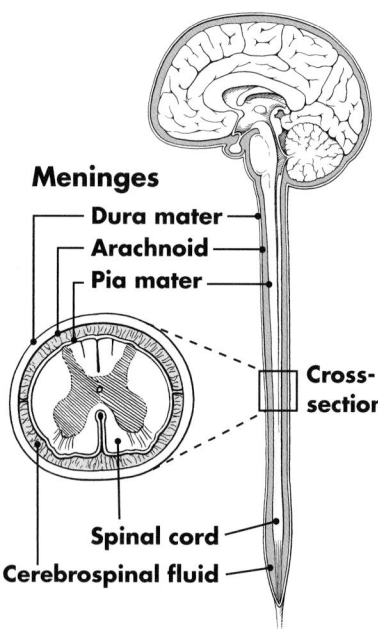

Meninges
- **Dura mater**
- **Arachnoid**
- **Pia mater**

Cross-section

Spinal cord
Cerebrospinal fluid

Like the brain, the spinal cord is protected by several layers of membranes (meninges): dura mater, arachnoid and pia mater. Cerebrospinal fluid (shown in blue) surrounds the brain and spinal cord. Meningitis affects the meninges and cerebrospinal fluid.

in adults and children. It most often occurs when the bacterium enters your bloodstream and migrates to your brain and spinal cord. You may also have this type of bacterium in your lungs, where it can cause pneumonia. Pneumococcal meningitis can also follow an ear infection or head injury.

The bacterial strain meningococcus may cause local epidemics within relatively confined environments, such as universities, boarding schools or military bases. It produces a purplish rash in about half of cases. Other bacterial strains that cause sporadic cases of meningitis include *Haemophilus influenzae* type b and staphylococcus.

Less frequent causes for acute bacterial meningitis include an epidural abscess and medical procedures such as a spinal tap (lumbar puncture). Alcoholism, diabetes, AIDS and immunosuppressant medications taken after organ transplantation may make you more vulnerable to meningitis.

Viral
Viral (aseptic) meningitis is most commonly caused by certain viruses but also can be a reaction to certain medications or chemicals that aren't normally present in cerebrospinal fluid. This form of meningitis causes many of the same signs and symptoms as does a bacterial infection.

Fungal
Fungal meningitis is relatively uncommon. Cryptococcal meningitis is a fungal form of the disease that affects people with immune deficiencies, such as AIDS. It's life-threatening if not treated with an antifungal medication.

Chronic
Ongoing (chronic) forms of meningitis occur when slow-growing organisms invade the membranes and fluid surrounding your brain. Human immunodeficiency virus (HIV), tuberculosis, fungal infec-

tions, malignant cancer cells or syphilis may cause chronic meningitis. Signs and symptoms often evolve over a period of weeks.

Diagnosis

Signs and symptoms of meningitis may not develop early in the course of the infection. If you experience signs and symptoms consistent with meningitis, your doctor will likely examine your head, ears and skin — especially along the spine — for evidence of infection. You may have X-rays taken of your chest, skull and sinuses. A computerized tomography (CT) scan may be done to determine if there's an abscess. A definitive diagnosis, however, will likely require analysis of your cerebrospinal fluid, obtained by a spinal tap. One of the main laboratory signs of meningitis is an increased white blood cell count in the fluid. Some of the fluid can be cultured to determine the type of organisms present.

How serious is meningitis?

Acute bacterial meningitis is a medical emergency. The longer you have the disease without treatment, the greater your risk of permanent neurological damage, such as hearing loss, brain damage, loss of memory or death. Meningitis is most dangerous to infants and older adults. In infants, a bulging in the soft spot of the skull (fontanel) and a stiff neck are key signs.

Meningococcal meningitis may be rapidly fatal if not treated promptly with an appropriate antibiotic. Viral meningitis is usually mild and often resolves on its own in one to two weeks.

Treatment

Treatment is dependent on the type of meningitis you have.

Bacterial meningitis

Acute bacterial meningitis requires prompt treatment with intravenous antibiotics to ensure recovery and reduce the risk of complications. The antibiotic or combination of antibiotics that your doctor may choose depends on the type of bacteria causing the infection. Often, analyzing a sample of cerebrospinal fluid can help identify the bacteria. If you or your child has bacterial meningitis, your doctor may recommend a broad-spectrum antibiotic until he or she can determine the exact cause of the meningitis.

If you or your child has bacterial meningitis, your doctor may recommend treatments for brain swelling, shock, convulsions or dehydration. Infected sinuses or mastoids — the bones behind the outer ear that connect to the middle ear — may need to be drained. Any fluid that has accumulated between the brain and the membranes that surround it also may need to be drained or surgically removed.

Viral meningitis

Antibiotics can't cure viral meningitis, and most cases improve on their own in a week or two without therapy. Treatment of mild cases of viral meningitis is usually with bed rest, plenty of fluids and over-the-counter pain medications to help reduce fever and relieve body aches. If the cause of your meningitis is the herpes virus, your doctor may also recommend an antiviral medication aimed at this virus.

Prevention

Some forms of bacterial meningitis are preventable with the following vaccinations:

- *Haemophilus influenzae* **type b (Hib) vaccine.** Children in the United States routinely receive this vaccine as part of the recommended schedule of vaccines, starting at about 2 months of age. The vaccine is also recommended for some adults, including those who have sickle cell disease or AIDS and those who don't have a spleen.

- **Pneumococcal conjugate vaccine.** This vaccine is also part of the regular immunization schedule for children younger than 2 years in the United States. In addition, it's recommended for children between the ages of 2 and 5 who are at high risk of pneumococcal disease, including children who have chronic heart or lung disease or cancer.

- **Pneumococcal polysaccharide vaccine.** Older children and adults who need protection from pneumococcal bacteria may receive this vaccine. The Centers for Disease Control and Prevention (CDC) recommends the pneumococcal polysaccharide vaccine for all adults older than 65 and younger adults and children who have weak immune systems, chronic illnesses such as heart disease, diabetes or sickle cell anemia, and those who don't have a spleen.

- **Meningococcal conjugate vaccine.** The CDC recommends that a single dose of meningococcal conjugate vaccine be given to children ages 11 to 12 or to any children ages 11 to 18 who haven't yet been vaccinated. However, this vaccine can be given to younger children who are at high risk of bacterial meningitis or who have been exposed to someone with the disease. It's approved for use in children as young as 2 years old.

Epidural abscess

Epidural abscess is an uncommon condition whose symptoms are similar to meningitis. The condition is usually due to a bacterial infection that causes pus to form between the outermost brain membrane (dura mater) and the bones of the spine or skull. Sometimes, it invades the bone surface inside the skull or vertebrae. It can also penetrate membrane layers to become a subdural abscess, a brain abscess or meningitis.

Epidural and similar abscesses are now relatively rare because antibiotics can control many infections in their early stages. The greatest risk is from chronic sinus or ear infections.

Encephalitis

Signs and symptoms
- Drowsiness
- Confusion and disorientation
- Seizures
- Sudden fever
- Severe headache
- Nausea and vomiting
- Tremor
- Occasionally, a stiff neck

Advanced signs and symptoms
- Altered levels of consciousness

Encephalitis is a rare but severe inflammatory disease of the brain that's usually caused by a viral infection. Encephalitis sometimes occurs due to a direct viral invasion of your central nervous system.

Another form is secondary (post-infectious) encephalitis, which follows or accompanies a viral illness such as measles, chickenpox, German measles (rubella) or mumps. It may be an overreaction of the immune system to a foreign substance.

Secondary encephalitis arises from within your body, but the

A Spinal Tap

A spinal tap (lumbar puncture) is used to measure pressure in your cerebrospinal fluid and to remove some of the fluid for laboratory analysis. This procedure is also used to inject spinal anesthetics, some medications and substances for diagnostic imaging.

The procedure
A local anesthetic is used at the puncture site. A thin, hollow needle is then inserted between two vertebrae in your lower back (lumbar region), through the spinal membrane (dura) and into the spinal canal. The vertebrae must be spread apart slightly to provide access, so you'll be asked to lie on your side with your knees drawn up to your chest and both arms clasped around your knees. This position flexes the back and spreads the vertebrae. Some conditions require the puncture to be made between two cervical vertebrae in your neck rather than the lower back.

Once the needle is in place, fluid pressure is measured, a small amount of fluid is withdrawn, and the pressure is measured again. If a drug or substance is being injected, its volume will equal the volume of the fluid that's withdrawn. The procedure usually takes about 30 minutes if only cerebrospinal fluid is being extracted, but more time may be required for an injection. After the procedure, the puncture site is covered with a bandage.

You may have a feeling of pressure during the procedure. Afterward, you may have a headache due to a decrease in cerebrospinal fluid pressure, especially if there is a persistent leak of fluid into tissues. Lying down usually alleviates the headache, and it usually goes away as the pressure returns to normal in a few days.

Uses
A sample of cerebrospinal fluid can aid in the diagnosis of various diseases. These include multiple sclerosis, Reye's syndrome, Guillain-Barré syndrome, infections of the central nervous system, certain kinds of tumors and subarachnoid hemorrhage. A cerebrospinal fluid sample can be tested for protein, sugar, red and white blood cells, and cancerous (malignant) cells. The fluid can also be cultured to identify bacterial, viral or fungal organisms.

A spinal tap may also be used for injecting dye (contrast material) or radioactive substances into cerebrospinal fluid when needed to make diagnostic images of the fluid's flow, a procedure called myelography. Occasionally, a spinal tap is used to inject medications such as antibiotics and chemotherapy drugs.

Risks
Some risks accompany lumbar puncture, although they're fewer now than they once were. Greater care is used to prevent infection, and the procedure is used more selectively. The availability of improved imaging procedures has reduced the need for a spinal tap in many conditions.

You're at increased risk of complications from a spinal tap if you have a blood-clotting disorder or increased spinal fluid pressure, which can lead to compression of the brainstem after a sample of cerebrospinal fluid is removed.

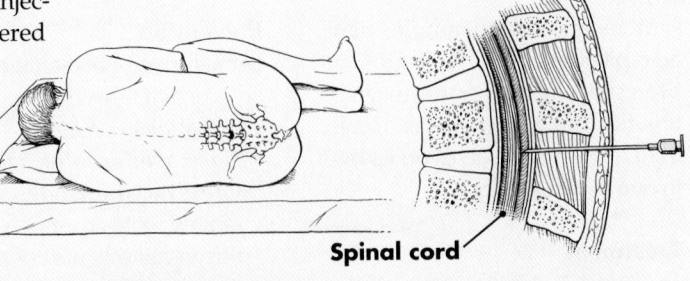

Spinal cord

In a spinal tap (lumbar puncture), you lie on your side, knees pulled to your chest, while a needle is inserted into an anesthetized site between two vertebrae and a small amount of cerebrospinal fluid is extracted for laboratory testing.

primary viral form results from the environment around you. Viral encephalitis can occur sporadically at any time of the year or as an epidemic. The most common sporadic form is herpes simplex encephalitis. It can start as a minor illness with headache and fever. This is followed by neurological signs and symptoms, which may include difficulty in talking, weakness, confusion, unconsciousness or repeated seizures.

Epidemic varieties are commonly caused by mosquito-borne viruses and occur during the summer months. The major types of mosquito-borne encephalitis in the United States are eastern equine encephalitis, western equine encephalitis, St. Louis encephalitis, La Crosse encephalitis and, more recently, West Nile encephalitis, caused by the West Nile virus.

Diagnosis

The onset of neurological signs and symptoms can be variable. You may be severely ill within 24 hours after initial signs and symptoms, or a week may pass before neurological involvement is apparent. In the case of secondary viral encephalitis, the disease may develop seven to 30 days after onset of the initiating viral infection.

Encephalitis usually is diagnosed by analyzing your cerebrospinal fluid, removed by a spinal tap (lumbar puncture). Analysis of the fluid reveals an increased white blood cell count, which signals that your body is fighting infection, and absence of bacteria, which helps rule out acute bacterial meningitis. When hemorrhages are part of the illness, your cerebrospinal fluid may be slightly bloody. Electroencephalography, magnetic resonance imaging (MRI) or a computerized tomography (CT) scan can help establish the diagnosis.

A diagnosis of herpes simplex encephalitis can be difficult. Recent advances using sensitive DNA methods have allowed detection of the virus in spinal fluid. If results are negative, and if signs and symptoms warrant, a brain biopsy may be necessary.

How serious is encephalitis?

The course of viral encephalitis is variable. It may be of short duration and leave no lasting effects, or it may strike with great severity and leave significant impairment. This can include loss of memory, the inability to speak coherently, lack of muscle coordination, paralysis, or hearing or vision defects.

The most severe (acute) phase of the illness may last from a few days to a week. The duration of the fever may be four to 14 days. Resolution is sometimes gradual, other times abrupt. Resultant neurological defects may continue to resolve over weeks or months. Even severely ill individuals can have a complete recovery.

Treatment

Because viruses that cause encephalitis don't respond to antibiotics, treatment generally consists of rest, nourishment and sufficient fluid intake to let your natural defenses fight the virus. Early on, irritability is common. For those who experience mental impairment, physical and speech therapies may be necessary.

In the case of herpes simplex encephalitis, antiviral agents such as acyclovir (Zovirax) have been used with success in early stages. For some people, anti-seizure medication may be needed.

Prevention

Even though viral encephalitis is rare, a good way to prevent secondary encephalitis is to make sure that you and your children are immunized against viral infections that may lead to encephalitis — chickenpox, measles, mumps and German measles (rubella).

Reye's syndrome

Signs and symptoms
- Persistent nausea and vomiting after a viral infection

Emergency signs and symptoms
- Drowsiness
- Stupor
- Loss of consciousness or coma
- Delirium, seizures or convulsions

AIDS and the Nervous System

AIDS is caused by the human immunodeficiency virus (HIV) and may lead to various nervous system diseases. HIV may directly infect your central nervous system and cause progressive degeneration of nerve cells. The virus also suppresses your immune system. HIV can infect any component of the nervous system, including the outer covering of the brain (meninges), the brain, spinal cord or peripheral nerves.

Approximately one-third of individuals with AIDS develop nervous system diseases, including viral, fungal or bacterial infections that cause meningitis, encephalitis or myelitis. Other diseases of the nervous system that occur in association with AIDS include parasitic cysts in the brain, abnormal growth of lymphoid tumors in the nervous system and a progressive form of dementia. Peripheral nerve disease also can be associated with AIDS.

Some AIDS-related diseases of the nervous system are treatable, but the effectiveness of standard treatments, such as antibiotic therapy for bacterial infections, is limited by the immunodeficiency. Treatment often requires lifelong therapy.

Triple-drug treatment of the HIV infection has lessened the frequency of opportunistic infections in the brain. Research on treatment is very active, and new medications are being tested.

Reye's syndrome is a relatively rare but serious illness that can follow a viral infection in children. Reye's syndrome affects the blood, liver and brain. Characteristics of the syndrome include high levels of ammonia and acidity and low levels of sugar in blood, fat deposits and swelling in the liver, and brain swelling that may cause loss of consciousness, delirium or seizures.

Reye's syndrome was first identified as a distinct disease in 1963. In the United States, the number of cases peaked in 1980 and have since decreased sharply. Today, only a few cases are reported each year. Many people assume that the decline is the result of the warnings against children taking aspirin, which is associated with the syndrome, but that may be only part of the reason.

Although aspirin use may trigger it in children, the specific cause for Reye's syndrome is unknown. The condition occurs almost exclusively in children between ages 2 and 16, following a viral infection

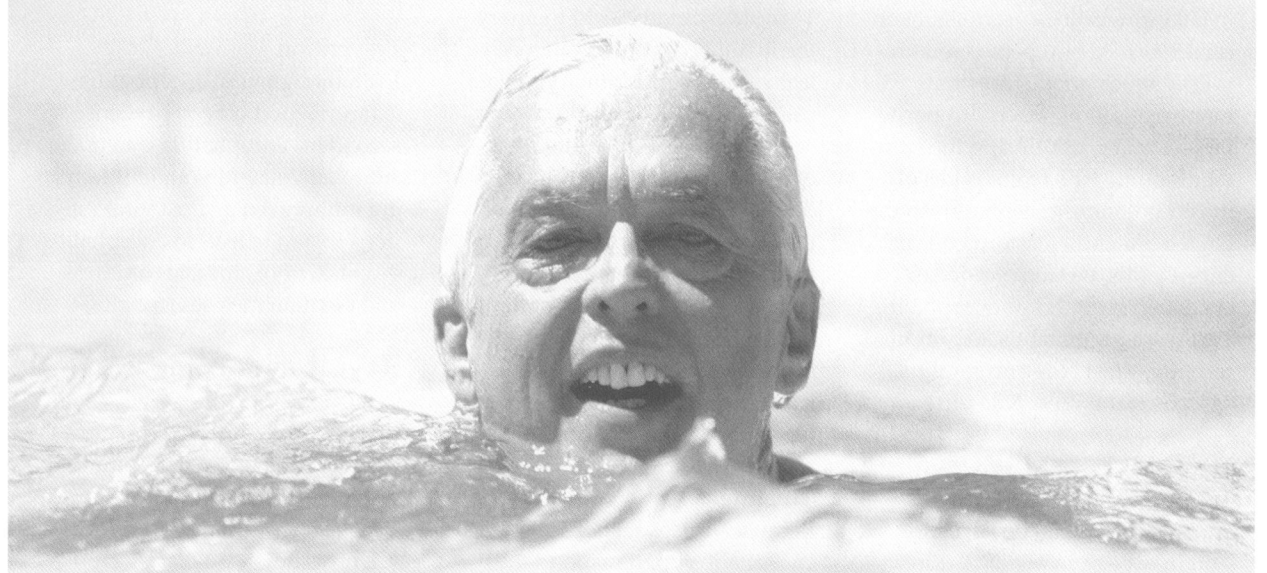

Post-Polio Syndrome

Late effects of polio, which some doctors call post-polio syndrome, can resemble arthritis, tendinitis or amyotrophic lateral sclerosis (ALS). Weakness usually develops in muscles that were involved during the earlier polio attack. Joint pain and flu-like aching of the muscles are common. The syndrome affects about 25 percent of polio survivors.

Scientists aren't sure of the exact cause of post-polio syndrome. It appears to not be a reactivation of a long-dormant virus or a new infection. Because most individuals with post-polio syndrome are in their 30s or 40s, it can't be attributed to aging either.

Current research focuses on nerve cells in the spinal cord. Normally, these cells deteriorate over time, but other cells compensate for their loss. Polio survivors, however, lost some of their nerve cells during their initial illness. People who recovered and then led physically active lives may have unknowingly overworked their remaining spinal nerve cells. Overuse of undamaged muscles in an effort to compensate for those that have been damaged can lead to pain and weakness after many years.

To confirm the diagnosis of post-polio syndrome, doctors generally look for these criteria:

- *Previous exposure to polio.* The syndrome usually occurs in people who were age 10 or older at the initial attack of polio and whose symptoms were often severe.
- *Long interval period.* The onset of late effects varies widely but typically begins about 30 years after the initial infection.
- *Gradual onset.* Weakness can develop quickly over a few months but may be imperceptible until it interferes with daily activities. You may awaken refreshed but feel exhausted by midday, tiring after activities that once were no problem.

It's difficult to forecast the course of symptoms. Fortunately, the progressive weakness in post-polio syndrome commonly is mild.

Although there's no specific treatment for the syndrome, see your doctor if you're a polio survivor experiencing new muscle weakness or pain. Medications, including aspirin and other nonsteroidal anti-inflammatory drugs (NSAIDs), may relieve some signs and symptoms. An occupational or physical therapist can analyze the ways that you move during work or leisure and suggest ways to reduce muscle fatigue. Try swimming or water aerobics and avoid overuse of your muscles.

Your attitude also plays an important part in your adjustment. Many communities are developing support groups for polio survivors that offer counseling, self-help tips and practical advice.

such as chickenpox or influenza or even an ordinary upper respiratory infection. Some researchers believe Reye's syndrome may be an underlying metabolic condition unmasked by a viral illness. Signs and symptoms often start a week after the viral infection.

Diagnosis
Your doctor may request blood tests, but a liver biopsy is the definitive diagnostic test. Cerebrospinal fluid may be obtained by a spinal tap (lumbar puncture) to exclude other diseases with similar signs and symptoms, such as meningitis or encephalitis.

Your doctor may also evaluate the possibility that your child has one of the rare, inherited metabolic disorders that can mimic the signs and symptoms of Reye's syndrome. The key to diagnosing or excluding these unusual conditions is obtaining blood and urine samples during the acute phase of the illness and having them analyzed in a qualified biochemical genetics laboratory. Many of these metabolic conditions are termed mitochondrial diseases because the problems arise from the part of body cells called the mitochondria.

How serious is Reye's syndrome?
Although its severity varies greatly, Reye's syndrome can be a severe, life-threatening disorder. Emergency treatment is required. The chances for your child's survival depend on how far the disease has progressed, how soon treatment is started and how quickly body chemistry is stabilized.

The fatality rate was once more than 40 percent, but with earlier diagnosis and better treatment, it has decreased to about 10 percent. Most children recover completely in two to three months, but in a few cases brain damage persists.

Treatment
Medications are given, usually intravenously, and vital signs are monitored. Your child's low blood sugar level is treated by giving glucose; blood chemistry values are corrected with electrolyte solutions containing sodium, potassium and chloride; and acidity is treated with counteracting basic solutions. Small amounts of insulin may be given to increase glucose metabolism.

Brain swelling is generally controlled with a corticosteroid (dexamethasone) that reduces inflammation, and a diuretic (mannitol) may be given to increase fluid loss through urination. Other medications may include purgatives, vitamin K-1 and an oral nonabsorbable antibiotic (neomycin).

Monitoring of the pressure inside your child's skull may be used to guide the effectiveness of therapy. Other common procedures include the insertion of a tube into your child's airway to aid breathing.

Prevention
The occurrence of Reye's syndrome is reduced by avoiding the use of aspirin (acetylsalicylic acid) in children younger than age 16 during a viral illness. Aspirin isn't recommended for children younger than age 12 with any illness.

Keep in mind that other common medications, including Alka-Seltzer and Pepto-Bismol, contain salicylates and should be avoided by children.

Structural Disorders

The nerve tissue in your brain is delicate and easily torn, bruised or damaged by pressure. Under ordinary circumstances, your skull and spinal membranes (meninges) provide protection for your brain. But upon sudden or severe impact, such as in a motor vehicle or industrial accident, the skull and membranes may prove to be inadequate. Structural damage to your brain from an accident can range from a mild concussion to permanent disability or even death.

Other structural problems described in this section include a disruption in the balance of cerebrospinal fluid in your brain (hydrocephalus) and the development of tumors inside your head.

Concussion

Signs and symptoms
- Brief loss of consciousness or memory after a head injury
- Headache
- Faintness
- Nausea or vomiting
- Slightly blurred vision
- Difficulty concentrating
- Loss of smell or taste

Emergency signs and symptoms
- Persistent confusion or delirium
- Persistent drowsiness
- Progressive lethargy
- Difference in size of eye pupils
- Speech disturbance
- Partial paralysis
- Stupor
- Coma

Concussions range in significance from minor to major, but they all share one common factor — they temporarily interfere with the way your brain works. They can affect memory, judgment, reflexes, speech, balance and coordination.

Your brain has the consistency of gelatin. It's cushioned from everyday jolts and bumps by the cerebrospinal fluid that it floats in, inside your skull. A violent blow to your head can cause your brain to slide forcefully against the inner wall of your skull. Even the sudden stop of a car crash can bounce your brain off the inside of your skull. This can result in bleeding in or around your brain and the tearing of nerve fibers.

Usually caused by a blow to the head, concussions don't always involve a loss of consciousness. In fact, most people who have concussions never black out. Some people have had concussions and not even realized it.

Concussions are common, particularly if you play a contact sport such as football. But every concussion, no matter how mild, injures your brain. This injury needs time and rest to heal properly.

While most concussions get better on their own, some blows to the head can cause more-serious injuries. Seek immediate medical advice if you experience signs and symptoms.

Diagnosis

Diagnosing a concussion is usually straightforward. If a blow to your head has knocked you out or left you dazed, you've had a concussion. It's more difficult, however, to determine whether the blow has caused potentially serious bleeding or swelling in your skull. Signs and symptoms of these injuries may not appear until hours or days after the injury.

After your doctor asks detailed questions about your accident, he or she may perform a neurological exam. This evaluation includes checking your memory, vision, hearing, balance, coordination and reflexes.

Brain imaging also may be done. A computerized tomography (CT) scan is the standard test to assess post-concussion damage.

How serious is a concussion?

A concussion is often a minor, temporary injury without permanent brain damage. Accidental head injuries, however, can cause death or brain damage in some cases, and any head injury is potentially serious. Thus, any traumatic injury to your head should be medically evaluated.

Treatment

If there are no complications, a concussion generally requires little or no treatment. Your doctor may prescribe acetaminophen or a stronger pain medication to relieve your headache. Aspirin should be avoided because it can contribute to bleeding. Rest and relaxation with limitation of activities requiring concentration or vigorous movement will usually facilitate recovery within a few days.

Athletes, such as football players or boxers, who've had a concussion should have a medical evaluation before returning to their sports.

Other traumatic brain injury

Signs and symptoms
- Headache

Emergency signs and symptoms
- Persistent confusion, drowsiness or delirium
- Speech disturbance
- Difficulty breathing
- Difference in size of eye pupils
- Partial paralysis
- Seizures or convulsions
- Stupor
- Coma

Traumatic brain injury may result from a blow to the head or from an object that penetrates the skull, such as a bullet or piece of industrial equipment. Traffic accidents, falls, industrial accidents and physical assaults are the major causes of such injuries.

An estimated 1.7 million cases of traumatic brain injury occur in the United States annually. These injuries range from mild concussions to severe brain damage. About 3 percent of these injuries end in death. Most head injuries are mild.

Moderate to severe brain injuries can be associated with a skull fracture, torn membranes or nerve tissue, and bruises or hemorrhaging within your brain. You may experience brain swelling or leaking of cerebrospinal fluid. Subdural or epidural (extradural) hemorrhage also is possible. Symptoms may not appear for several days after an accident.

Diagnosis

Get prompt medical evaluation for any head injury that causes even a brief loss of consciousness or persistent symptoms.

Your doctor may recommend hospitalization for observation, testing and treatment if you show any indications of possible brain injury. Diagnostic tests such as a computerized tomography (CT) scan or magnetic resonance imaging (MRI) may be necessary to observe the structure of your brain.

How serious is a traumatic brain injury?

The severity and effects of a head injury depend on the extent of damage and which area of the brain was most affected. Previous injuries and diseases as well as your overall state of health can play a role in potential complications. Most people with moderate head injuries recover in weeks to months, although some disability may persist. Severe injuries can be fatal or permanently disabling despite the best medical and surgical treatment.

Treatment

Emergency treatment is required for people who have entered a coma. A comatose state usually is indicative of severe brain injury. Brain swelling, which can cause death, may require treatment with medications such as corticosteroids and, possibly, surgery. Surgery may also be done to remove bone fragments, blood clots or damaged tissue, or to insert a shunt to control the pressure inside the brain.

Hydrocephalus

Signs and symptoms
- In newborns, abnormal enlargement of the head
- Mental decline
- Slow and restricted body and eye movements
- Urinary incontinence

Hydrocephalus — *hydro* meaning "water" and *cephalus* meaning "head" — is a condition in which excess fluid accumulates in the brain. Although hydrocephalus is often referred to as water on the brain, the "water" is actually cerebrospinal fluid — a clear fluid surrounding the brain and spinal cord.

Normally, this fluid is produced in the brain, flows through the four ventricles of the brain, exits into closed spaces (cisterns) that serve as reservoirs at the base of the brain, cleanses the surfaces of the brain and spinal cord, and is then absorbed into the bloodstream. The balance between production and absorption of cerebrospinal fluid is critical.

Usually, the fluid is almost completely absorbed into the bloodstream as it circulates. However, some circumstances prevent or disturb the production or absorption of cerebrospinal fluid or inhibit its normal flow. When this balance is disturbed, hydrocephalus results.

Hydrocephalus may be present at birth (congenital) or acquired. Congenital hydrocephalus can be due to a blockage in the brain's cerebrospinal fluid circulation system or to an inability to reabsorb the fluid. The resulting pressure expands the loosely connected sutures in the skull so that in a newborn or young child, the head is enlarged abnormally in all directions, especially in the frontal area.

Your infant's symptoms may be mild, and the progression might stop but then reappear in later childhood. The skull becomes firmly closed by age 5 years, so subsequent symptoms don't include further appreciable head enlargement.

Congenital or childhood hydrocephalus due to a blockage in the circulation of cerebrospinal fluid in the brain may be caused by various congenital malformations of the brain, a fetal infection, birth injury or tumor. Hydrocephalus due to problems of reabsorption can result from brain malformation, an infection such as bacterial menin-

gitis, subarachnoid hemorrhage, or spinal cord defects such as syringomyelia or myelomeningocele.

In adults, a variation of hydrocephalus may occur in which cerebrospinal fluid pressure is normal but reabsorption of cerebrospinal fluid is defective. Symptoms may arise slowly after meningitis, head injury or subarachnoid hemorrhage, or they may develop for no known reason.

Hydrocephalus is relatively uncommon, occurring in approximately 1 in 1,000 children. In adults, normal-pressure hydrocephalus is also uncommon and occurs most frequently among older adults with an unexplained decline in gait and cognitive function that may be accompanied by urinary incontinence.

Diagnosis

Your child's head may be measured at birth. If the circumference of the head exceeds a certain size, your doctor may measure the head frequently during the first weeks of life. If the soft spot (fontanel) on your infant's head is still open, an ultrasound of the head can distinguish between a normal large head (macrocephaly) and hydrocephalus. If the results of the ultrasound are abnormal, your infant will need further evaluation.

In later childhood and adulthood, signs and symptoms such as mental decline and slowed body movements may lead to further testing. In all cases, a diagnosis generally requires a computerized tomography (CT) scan or magnet-

ic resonance imaging (MRI) and an examination and culture of cerebrospinal fluid obtained by a spinal tap (see page 542).

How serious is hydrocephalus?

The severity of this condition depends on the child's age at onset and whether the disease is progressive. If the condition is well-advanced at birth, major brain damage and physical handicaps are often inevitable. Death usually occurs early from an underlying infection. In less severe cases, with proper treatment, 40 percent of affected individuals have a nearly normal life span and intelligence.

Treatment

The goal of treatment is to re-establish the balance between cerebrospinal fluid production and reabsorption. In young children with a slowly progressive condition, the drug acetazolamide (Diamox) sometimes diminishes cerebrospinal fluid production. When the imbalance is due to a reabsorption problem, treatment may consist of repeated spinal taps to relieve pressure.

An operation to implant a flexible tube (shunt) is effective in many children and adults. A shunt is placed to circumvent the blockage or to divert excess cerebrospinal fluid into the bloodstream or abdominal cavity, where it's reabsorbed. A successful shunt procedure will allow an infant's head size to become normal and will relieve signs and symptoms in older children and adults. Shunt

---

? **Question and Answer**

What's a meningioma?

A meningioma is a noncancerous brain tumor that originates in the cells of the outer covering of the brain (meninges). Treatment usually is surgical removal of the tumor. If the tumor is located in an area that isn't very accessible, complete removal may be difficult or impossible. Sometimes, functions of the brain already affected by pressure from the meningioma may be permanently damaged. A small tumor not causing symptoms may be monitored with imaging.

tubes may require replacement as a child grows. Successful shunts usually are maintained for life, but shunt infections are a serious complication.

Brain tumor

Signs and symptoms
- Headaches that become more frequent and severe, usually accompanied by other symptoms
- Unexplained nausea or vomiting
- Weakness and lethargy
- Personality or behavior changes
- Double vision
- Recent incoordination or clumsiness of an extremity
- Speech difficulties
- Change in gait or walking ability

Emergency signs and symptoms
- Vision, sight or speech difficulty
- Seizures
- Stupor

A brain tumor is a mass or growth of abnormal cells in your brain. Many different types of brain tumors exist. Some brain tumors are noncancerous (benign), and some brain tumors are cancerous (malignant). Brain tumors can begin in your brain (primary brain tumors), or cancer can begin in other parts of your body and spread to your brain (secondary, or metastatic brain tumors).

Primary brain tumors originate in the brain or close to it, such as in the brain-covering membranes (meninges), cranial nerves, pituitary gland or pineal gland. Primary brain tumors begin when normal cells acquire errors (mutations) in their DNA. These mutations allow cells to grow and divide at increased rates and to continue living when healthy cells would die. The result is a mass of abnormal cells, which forms a tumor.

Primary brain tumors are much less common than are secondary brain tumors, in which cancer begins elsewhere and spreads to the brain. Many different types of primary brain tumors exist.

Secondary (metastatic) brain tumors are tumors that result from cancer that starts elsewhere in your body and then spreads (metastasizes) to your brain. In some cases you may have a history of cancer when a brain tumor is discovered. In other cases, a brain tumor is the first sign of cancer that began elsewhere in your body.

A brain tumor, primary or secondary, can directly compress or invade brain tissue, damaging or destroying areas responsible for sight, movement, balance, speech, hearing, memory or behavior. Pressure from a brain tumor can also cause surrounding brain tissue to swell, leading to an increase in pressure and symptoms.

Though doctors aren't sure what causes the genetic mutations that can lead to primary brain tumors, they've identified factors that may increase your risk of a brain tumor:

- **Your race.** Brain tumors occur more frequently in whites than they do in others. One exception is meningioma, which occurs most frequently in blacks.
- **Your age.** Your risk of a brain tumor increases as you age. The majority of brain tumors occur in people 45 and older. However, a brain tumor can occur at any age. Certain types of brain tumors, such as medulloblastomas, occur almost exclusively in children.
- **Exposure to radiation.** People who've been exposed to a type of radiation called ionizing radiation have an increased risk of brain tumor. Examples of ionizing radiation include radiation therapy used to treat cancer and radiation exposure caused by atomic bombs. More common forms of radiation, such as electromagnetic fields from power lines and radiofrequency radiation from cellphones and microwave ovens, haven't been conclusively linked to brain tumors.
- **Chemical exposure on the job.** People working in certain industries have an increased

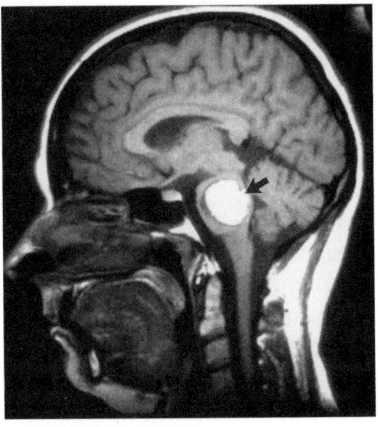

Magnetic resonance imaging (MRI) shows a tumor in the brainstem (see arrow).

risk of brain tumors, possibly because of the chemicals they're exposed to on the job. Studies don't always agree, but there is some evidence of an increased risk of brain tumor in certain industries, including agricultural, electrical, health care and oil refineries.
- **Family history of brain tumors.** A small portion of brain tumors occur in people with a family history of brain tumors or a family history of genetic syndromes that increase the risk of brain tumors.

Diagnosis
Diagnosis of brain tumor usually involves several steps. A thorough physical and neurological examination might lead to suspicion of a brain tumor. Depending on the results of that exam, your doctor may request a computerized tomography (CT) scan or magnetic resonance imaging (MRI) of the head to obtain detailed images of the brain.

Tests that evaluate other areas of the body may be needed to search for a tumor that may spread to the brain. Other tests, such as magnetic resonance spectroscopy (MRS), single-photon emission computerized tomography (SPECT) or positron emission tomography (PET) scanning, can help doctors gauge brain activity by observing brain chemistry and blood flow.

A biopsy, which involves removing a piece of the tumor so that it can be examined under a microscope, may be needed to identify the type of brain tumor.

How serious is a brain tumor?

Benign tumors are frequently curable, although sometimes their location makes total removal impossible. If a tumor infiltrates the brain so that tumor tissue can't be totally removed, recurrence after surgery is likely. Both benign and malignant tumors can produce profound and irreversible neurological impairment. Most malignant brain tumors — primary or secondary — are not curable.

Brain tumors may block the flow of cerebrospinal fluid in the brain, leading to the buildup of fluid in and around the brain and increased pressure on the structure of the brain. This is a serious complication known as hydrocephalus. The fluid may require drainage to relieve pressure and reduce the risk of further brain injury.

Treatment

Treatment for a brain tumor depends on the type, size and location of the tumor, as well as your overall health and your preferences.

Surgery

If the brain tumor is located in a place that makes it accessible for an operation, your surgeon will work to remove as much of the brain tumor as possible.

In some cases, tumors are small and easy to separate from surrounding brain tissue, which makes complete surgical removal possible. In other cases, tumors are located near sensitive areas in your brain, making surgery risky. In these situations your doctor may try to remove as much of the tumor as is safe. Even removing a portion of the brain tumor may help reduce signs and symptoms you experience. In some cases only a small biopsy is taken to confirm the diagnosis.

Surgery to remove a brain tumor carries risks, such as infection and bleeding. Other risks may depend on the part of your brain where your tumor is located. For instance, surgery on a tumor near nerves that connect to your eyes may carry a risk of vision loss.

Radiation therapy

Radiation therapy uses beams of high-energy particles, such as X-rays, to kill tumor cells. Radiation therapy can come from a machine outside your body (external beam radiation), or in very rare cases, radiation can be placed inside your body close to your brain tumor (brachytherapy).

External beam radiation can focus just on the area of your brain where the tumor is located, or it can be applied to your entire brain (whole-brain radiation). Whole-brain radiation may be used after surgery to kill tumor cells that might have been left behind. It may also be an option if you have several brain tumors that can't be removed through surgery. Whole-brain radiation is often used in situations where cancer has metastasized to the brain.

Radiosurgery

Stereotactic radiosurgery is not a form of surgery in the traditional sense. Instead, radiosurgery uses multiple beams of radiation to give a highly focused form of radiation treatment to kill the tumor cells in a very small area. Each beam of radiation isn't particularly powerful, but the point where all the beams meet — at the brain tumor — receives a very large dose of radiation to kill the tumor cells.

Radiosurgery may be an option if your brain tumor can't be removed with traditional surgery. Radiosurgery is typically done in one treatment, and in most cases you can go home the same day.

Chemotherapy

Chemotherapy uses drugs to kill tumor cells. Chemotherapy drugs can be taken orally or injected into a vein (intravenously) so that they travel throughout your body. Chemotherapy drugs can also be administered into your spinal column, so treatment affects only your central nervous system.

Another type of chemotherapy can be placed during surgery. When removing all or part of the brain tumor, your surgeon may place one or more disk-shaped wafers in the void left by the tumor. These wafers slowly release a chemotherapy drug over the next several days.

Targeted drug therapy

Targeted drug treatments focus on specific abnormalities present within cancer cells. By blocking these abnormalities, targeted drug treatments can cause cancer cells to die. Many targeted drug therapies are still undergoing careful study in clinical trials.

One targeted drug therapy used to treat brain tumors is the drug bevacizumab (Avastin) that's administered through a vein (intravenously). The medication stops the formation of new blood vessels, cutting off the blood supply to the tumor and killing tumor cells.

Neuroblastoma

Signs and symptoms

- An abdominal mass, perhaps accompanied by liver enlargement
- Bone pain, if a tumor has spread to bone
- Respiratory distress, if a tumor has spread to the chest
- Pallor
- High blood pressure
- Diarrhea

A neuroblastoma is a cancerous tumor made up of neuroblasts, embryonic cells from which nerve tissue is formed.

Neuroblastomas can originate in nerve tissue in the neck, chest or pelvis, but they occur most often in the abdomen, generally near the adrenal gland. The disease then may spread to the liver, bone marrow and bones.

Unlike most tumors, a neuroblastoma has a high rate of decreasing in size without treatment (spontaneous regression). Neuroblastomas occur mostly in children, and most cases are diagnosed by the time a child is age 5. The disease may be present at birth but usually isn't detected until later.

Diagnosis

The site and extent of a suspected tumor determine what diagnostic tests will be needed. If there's an abdominal mass, a computerized tomography (CT) scan or magnetic resonance imaging (MRI) may be done. A bone scan or bone marrow biopsy — in which a tissue sample is removed for laboratory study — may indicate whether the cancer has spread to bone.

How serious is a neuroblastoma?

The prognosis of this disease depends in large part on the age of the child and how advanced the disease is. Spontaneous regression is more common in very young infants. The older the child and the more widespread the disease, the more likely it is that the cancer won't respond to treatment.

Treatment

Your child's doctor will select a treatment plan based on several factors that affect your child's prognosis. These factors include your child's age, the stage of the cancer, the type of cells involved in the cancer, and whether there are any abnormalities in the chromosomes and genes.

Using this information, your child's doctor will categorize the cancer as low risk, intermediate risk or high risk. The treatment or combination of treatments that your child receives for neuroblastoma will depend on the risk category.

Surgery

A surgeon may attempt to remove cancer cells. In children with low-risk neuroblastoma, surgery to remove the tumor may be the only treatment needed. Whether the tumor can be completely removed depends on its location and its size. Tumors that are attached to nearby vital organs — such as the lungs or the spinal cord — may be too risky to remove.

In intermediate-risk and high-risk neuroblastoma, surgeons may try to remove as much of the tumor as possible. Other treatments, such as chemotherapy and radiation, may then be used to kill remaining cancer cells.

Chemotherapy

Chemotherapy uses chemicals to destroy cancer cells. Chemotherapy targets rapidly growing cells in the body, including cancer cells. Unfortunately, chemotherapy also damages healthy cells that grow quickly, such as cells in the hair follicles and in the gastrointestinal system, which can cause side effects.

Children with low-risk neuroblastoma that can't be removed surgically may receive low doses of chemotherapy. Sometimes chemotherapy is administered before surgery (neoadjuvant chemotherapy) to shrink the tumor to a size that's more easily removed. In other cases, chemotherapy may be the only treatment.

Children with intermediate-risk neuroblastoma often receive a combination of moderate-intensity chemotherapy drugs. Chemotherapy is often given before surgery to improve the chances that the entire tumor can be removed.

Children with high-risk neuroblastoma usually receive high doses of chemotherapy drugs to shrink the tumor and to kill any cancer cells that have spread elsewhere in the body. Chemotherapy is usually used before surgery and before bone marrow stem cell transplant.

Radiation therapy

Radiation therapy uses high doses of energy particles to destroy cancer cells. Radiation therapy primarily affects the area where it's aimed. Your child's radiation therapy team tries to protect the healthy cells near the cancer, but some healthy cells may be damaged by the radiation. What side effects your child experiences depends on where the radiation is directed.

Children with low-risk or intermediate-risk neuroblastoma may receive radiation therapy if surgery and chemotherapy haven't been helpful. Children with high-risk neuroblastoma may receive radiation therapy after chemotherapy and surgery, to prevent cancer from recurring.

Stem cell transplant

Children with high-risk neuroblastoma may receive a transplant using their own blood stem cells (autologous stem cell transplant). The bone marrow makes stem cells, which mature and develop into the red and white cells and platelets that make up the blood.

Your child undergoes a procedure that filters and collects stem cells from his or her blood. High doses of chemotherapy are used to kill any remaining cancer cells in your child's body. After chemotherapy is complete, your child's stem cells are injected back into your child's body, where they can form new, healthy blood cells.

Bell's palsy

Signs and symptoms
- Sagging muscles and weakness on one side of the face
- An inability to close one eye

Bell's palsy (facial palsy) causes a weakness or paralysis of the muscles that control expression on one side of your face. The condition results from damage to the facial nerve, which runs beneath the ear to the facial muscles of the same side.

The cause of the disorder is unknown, and its development isn't well-understood. The prevalent theory is that the facial nerve becomes swollen, perhaps by a viral infection, such as shingles (herpes zoster). The nerve has no room to expand within the bony channel it runs through. Bell's palsy results from nerve injury due to restriction or compression.

Complete paralysis on one side of your face leaves you looking expressionless because you have no movement of the muscles from the forehead to below the mouth on the paralyzed side. The corner of your mouth may droop, and you may have difficulty retaining saliva on that side of your mouth. When you move the muscles of the unaffected side, the face is distorted. The eye on your affected side may close only partially if at all, so tears may leak from that eye.

Some people complain of pain behind the ear, in the jaw or on the entire side of the face. You may feel that the unaffected side seems twisted or contracted, and you may experience changes in salivation and sense of taste, heightened sensitivity to sound, or difficulty in speaking or eating.

Bell's palsy can occur at any age, but it's most common between ages 30 and 60. Sometimes, it's associated with an infection of the middle ear. Cases associated with blisters or rash in the ear on the same side as the facial palsy are usually do to a viral infection. If both sides of the face are simultaneously involved, a disorder such as Lyme disease or sarcoidosis may be the cause.

Diagnosis

Your doctor may make a preliminary diagnosis by looking at your face and asking you to try to move your facial muscles. Other conditions, such as a stroke, also can cause one-sided facial paralysis, so careful evaluation is needed to exclude these disorders. Bell's palsy usually affects all of the muscles on one side of the face equally, including the forehead muscles. Strokes usually don't cause paralysis of the forehead muscles on the affected side.

Your doctor may also arrange for you to be tested by electromyography. This test measures a muscle's electrical activity in response to stimulation, to determine the severity of nerve damage.

How serious is Bell's palsy?

Bell's palsy is usually a temporary problem. In 80 percent of cases, recovery begins within two to three weeks and is complete within a few months. A mild case may be noticeable only when you smile. Improvement of the paralysis by the end of the first week suggests a favorable outcome.

Recovery is variable, and electromyography may be helpful in determining the prognosis. If the damage to the facial nerve is unusually severe, the fibers may be irreversibly damaged. A complication can arise from misdirected regrowth of nerve fibers. The misdirected fibers can cause unintended contraction of some muscles during facial movement.

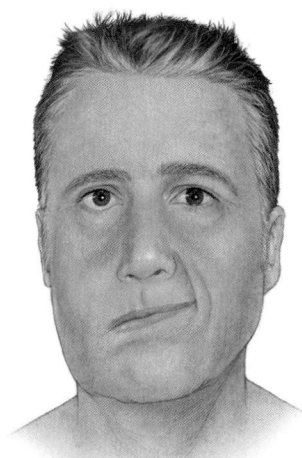

Bell's palsy may cause the corner of your mouth to droop, and you may have trouble retaining saliva on that side of your mouth. The condition may also make it difficult to close the eye on the affected side of your face.

Treatment

Most people with Bell's palsy recover fully — with or without treatment. Your doctor may suggest medications or physical therapy to help speed your recovery. Surgery is rarely an option for Bell's palsy.

Medications

Study results have been mixed regarding the effectiveness of two types of drugs commonly used to treat Bell's palsy — corticosteroids and antiviral medications.

Corticosteroids, such as prednisone, are powerful anti-inflammatory agents. If they can reduce the swelling of the facial nerve, the nerve will fit more comfortably within the bony corridor that surrounds it. It's best if corticosteroids are started within three days of the onset of signs and symptoms.

If Bell's palsy is triggered by a virus, then an antiviral drug — such as acyclovir or valacyclovir — may stop the progression of the viral infection. Most people do not require antiviral medication.

Physical therapy and basic care

Paralyzed muscles can shrink and shorten, causing permanent contractures. Massaging and exercising your facial muscles may help prevent this from occurring. Moist heat may help relieve pain. Place a warm washcloth on your face several times a day. Using lubricating eyedrops during the day and an eye ointment at night will help keep your eye moist. Wear glasses, goggles during the day and an eye patch at night to protect your eye from getting poked or scratched.

Surgery

One way to relieve the pressure on the facial nerve is to surgically open the bony passage through which it passes. This decompression surgery is controversial and rarely recommended. In some cases, however, plastic surgery may be needed to make your face look and work better.

Degenerative Disorders

Your brain, spinal cord and peripheral nerves form an intricate system consisting of billions of nerve cells. These cells are complex transmitters that carry electric and chemical signals to make your muscles move and to relay information throughout your nervous system.

If a few scattered cells die or malfunction, you likely won't notice any change because surrounding cells will carry the transmissions. When there's progressive deterioration in any part of your nervous system, you eventually lose some ability to function. This loss can be related to mental ability, muscular movement, and muscular control and coordination.

Degenerative disorders may be disabling and, in most cases, there's no known cure. Nonetheless, research is progressing rapidly. Scientists have discovered and learned more about the brain and its disorders in the last decade than in the previous 50 years. The hope is that increased understanding will lead to new methods of treatment and prevention.

Alzheimer's disease

Signs and symptoms
- A gradual loss of memory for recent events and an inability to learn new information
- A progressive tendency to repeat oneself, misplace objects, become confused and get lost
- A gradual disintegration of personality and judgment
- Increasing irritability, anxiety, depression, confusion and restlessness

Alzheimer's disease is the most common cause of dementia — the loss of intellectual and social abilities severe enough to interfere with daily functioning. In Alzheimer's disease, healthy brain tissue degenerates, causing a steady decline in memory and mental abilities.

Alzheimer's disease is not a part of normal aging, but the risk of the disorder increases with age. An estimated 5.5 million Americans in the United States have Alzheimer's disease. Of that number, approximately 5.3 million are age 65 and older. About 200,000 Americans below age 65 have early-onset Alzheimer's disease.

Dementia

A number of disorders that cause progressive deterioration in any part of your nervous system (neurodegenerative disorders) produce a collection of signs and symptoms (syndrome) called dementia.

Dementia is characterized by a progressive decline in intellectual and social abilities to a degree that interferes with daily functioning. Signs and symptoms vary from individual to individual, depending on a person's genetic makeup, lifestyle, cultural background and personal life experiences. Some of the more general characteristics of dementia include a reduction in or loss of memory, reasoning, judgment and language. Personality changes and abnormal behavior also may occur as dementia progresses. Eventually, people with dementia may lose the ability to perform even the most basic of tasks, such as speaking or eating.

Such signs and symptoms can be evidence of Alzheimer's disease, vascular dementia or other brain disorders known to cause dementia. In the past, people referred to dementia as senility and considered it to be an inevitable part of aging. Today, we know that dementia isn't a normal part of the aging process but is caused by an underlying disease affecting the brain.

If you notice such manifestations in yourself or a loved one, don't brush it off as simply "getting old." An early diagnosis is important because prompt treatment may affect the course of the disease.

Brain disorders that cause dementia

Diseases of the brain that can cause dementia include:

Alzheimer's disease
Alzheimer's disease is the most common cause of dementia. Changes in the brain of people with Alzheimer's disease include a loss of nerve cells in the areas vital to memory and other mental functions. Individuals with Alzheimer's disease also have lowered levels of brain chemicals that carry messages back and forth between nerve cells. The first sign of Alzheimer's disease may be worsening forgetfulness. As the disease progresses, it affects your language, reasoning, understanding, reading and writing. Eventually, you may become anxious or aggressive.

Vascular dementia
Vascular dementia results either from narrowing and blockage of the arteries that supply blood to the brain or from strokes that result from an interruption of blood flow within the brain. The onset of symptoms is often abrupt, but sometimes the disease progresses slowly, making it difficult to distinguish it from Alzheimer's disease. It's common to experience problems with thinking, language, walking, bladder control and vision.

Parkinson's disease
Many people with Parkinson's disease develop dementia late in the disease. Conversely, some people with Alzheimer's develop physical signs and symptoms similar to those in Parkinson's disease, such

Everyone has occasional lapses in memory. But Alzheimer's disease — a progressive, degenerative brain disease — goes beyond simple forgetfulness. It may start with slight memory loss and confusion, but it gradually worsens and leads to severe, irreversible mental impairment that destroys a person's ability to remember, reason, learn and plan for the future.

The course of the disease and how rapidly changes occur varies from person to person. For some, the progression from simple forgetfulness to severe dementia takes five to eight years. For others, it can take a decade or longer.

No one factor appears to cause Alzheimer's disease. Instead, scientists believe the disease may result from a combination of genetic, lifestyle and environmental factors that trigger the onset of symptoms.

Interestingly, the same factors that put you at risk of heart disease may also increase the likelihood that you'll develop Alzheimer's disease. Examples include high blood pressure, high cholesterol and poorly controlled diabetes. And keeping your body fit isn't your only concern — you've got to exercise your mind as well. Some studies suggest that remaining mentally active throughout your life, especially in your later years, reduces the risk of Alzheimer's disease.

Studies have found an association between less education and the risk of Alzheimer's. But the precise reason why this occurs is unknown. Some researchers theorize that the more you use your brain, the more synapses you create, which provides a greater reserve as you age. But it may simply be harder to detect Alzheimer's in people who exercise their minds frequently or who have more education.

Your risk of developing Alzheimer's also appears to be slightly higher if a first-degree relative — a parent, sister or brother — has the disease. Although the genetic mechanisms of Alzheimer's among families remain largely unexplained, researchers have identified several genetic mutations that greatly increase risk in some families.

While the causes of Alzheimer's aren't clearly understood, its effect on brain tissue is evident. Alzheimer's disease damages and kills brain cells. Two types of brain cell

as stiffness of the limbs, shaking at rest (tremor), speech impairment and a shuffling gait.

Lewy body dementia
Lewy bodies are protein deposits found in deteriorating nerve cells. They often appear in damaged regions deep within the brain of people with Parkinson's disease. When widespread throughout the brain, Lewy bodies cause signs and symptoms similar to those of Alzheimer's disease.

Lewy body dementia can affect your dreams, speed of thinking, memory, language, judgment and reasoning. It can also cause you to hallucinate and lose your sense of direction, which may result in a tendency to get lost.

Huntington's disease
Huntington's disease stems from an inherited disorder within the brain that leads to abnormal involuntary movements called chorea, and later dementia. As the disorder progresses, you experience personality changes and a decline in intellect, memory, speech and judgment. Dementia may develop in the later stages of the disease.

Creutzfeldt-Jakob disease
Dementia that sometimes occurs in young or middle-aged people may be caused by Creutzfeldt-Jakob disease. This rare and fatal brain disorder is thought to be caused by prions, infectious agents that can transform normal protein molecules into transmissible, deadly ones.

The earliest signs and symptoms of the disease may be memory impairment and behavior changes. The disease progresses rapidly with mental deterioration, muscle jerks (involuntary movements), weakness in the limbs, blindness and eventually coma. Bovine spongiform encephalopathy, commonly known as mad cow disease, is believed to be a prion disorder.

Frontotemporal dementia
Frontotemporal dementia is an uncommon brain disorder characterized by disturbances in behavior, personality and eventually memory. The disease is relentless in its progression and may ultimately include language impairment, erratic behavior and dementia.

Disorders that mimic dementia

Some conditions produce signs and symptoms similar to those of dementia, particularly in older adults. Two conditions sometimes mistaken for dementia are depression and delirium.

Depression can cause difficulty in remembering, thinking clearly and concentrating. Sometimes, depression occurs in conjunction with dementia. In these cases, the deterioration of emotions and intellect can be more extreme.

Delirium is an acute state of temporary mental confusion. It tends to be most common in older adults who have lung or heart disease, infections, poor nutrition, medication interactions or hormone disorders. A person who exhibits sudden disorientation, loss in mental skills, or loss of consciousness is likely to have delirium rather than dementia.

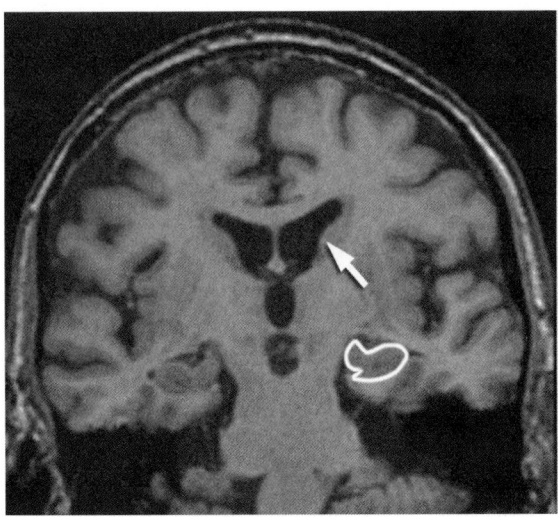
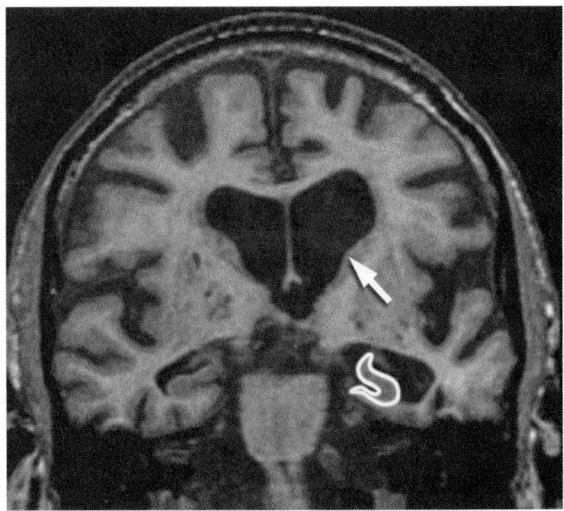

Magnetic resonance imaging (MRI) of the brain shows a person without Alzheimer's disease (left) and a person in the moderate stage of the disease (right). Signs of Alzheimer's disease include noticeable shrinkage of the hippocampus (circled in white) and enlarged interior cavities of the brain that have filled with cerebrospinal fluid (see arrows).

Mild Cognitive Impairment

Mayo Clinic researchers have identified a state of memory loss called mild cognitive impairment that may one day come to be known as pre-Alzheimer's.

This memory loss falls somewhere between that associated with normal aging and that common in early Alzheimer's disease. People with mild cognitive impairment may experience forgetfulness beyond what's typical for their ages, but not have full symptoms of Alzheimer's or dementia.

Identification of this category of memory loss could help doctors more accurately diagnose and advise their patients. It could also alert individuals to an increased risk of developing Alzheimer's disease.

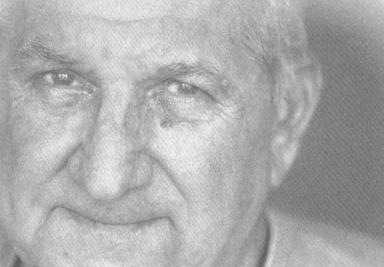

(neuron) damage are common in people who have Alzheimer's:

- **Plaques.** Clumps of a normally harmless protein called beta-amyloid may interfere with communication between brain cells. Although the ultimate cause of neuron death in Alzheimer's isn't known, evidence suggests abnormal processing of beta-amyloid protein may be the culprit.
- **Tangles.** The internal support structure for brain cells depends on the normal functioning of a protein called tau. In people with Alzheimer's, threads of tau protein undergo alterations that cause them to become twisted. Many researchers believe this may seriously damage neurons, causing them to die.

Diagnosis

Doctors can clinically diagnose 90 percent of Alzheimer's cases, but the disease can only be identified with complete accuracy after death, when examination of the brain reveals plaques and tangles.

While it is possible for researchers to identify individuals likely to develop Alzheimer's disease before memory loss develops, it's unlikely such tests will be routinely used until a treatment for Alzheimer's has been found.

To help distinguish Alzheimer's disease from other causes of memory loss, doctors typically rely on the following types of tests.

Lab tests
Blood tests may be done to help doctors rule out other potential causes of the dementia, such as thyroid disorders or vitamin deficiencies.

Neuropsychological testing
Sometimes doctors undertake a more extensive assessment of thinking and memory skills. This type of testing, which can take several hours to complete, is especially helpful in trying to detect Alzheimer's and other dementias at an early stage.

Brain scans
By looking at images of the brain, doctors may be able to pinpoint visible abnormalities — such as clots, bleeding or tumors — that may be causing signs and symptoms.

- **Magnetic resonance imaging (MRI).** An MRI machine uses radio waves and a strong magnetic field to produce detailed images of your brain. You lie on a narrow table that slides into the tube-shaped MRI machine, which makes loud banging noises during scans. The entire procedure can take an hour or more. MRIs are painless, but some people feel claustrophobic in the machine.

- **Computerized tomography (CT).** For a CT scan, you lie on a narrow table that slides into a small chamber. X-rays pass through your body from various angles, and a computer uses this information to create cross-sectional images, or slices, of your brain. The test is painless and takes about 20 minutes.
- **Positron emission tomography (PET).** During a PET scan, you're injected with a low-level radioactive material, which binds to chemicals that travel to the brain. You lie on a table while an overhead scanner tracks the radioactive material. This helps show which parts of your brain aren't functioning properly. The test can be particularly useful in distinguishing between different types of dementia.

How serious is Alzheimer's disease?
Alzheimer's disease isn't an acute condition, and it rarely requires emergency treatment. Abrupt changes in mental status are usually due to other diseases, which may require an immediate evaluation.

Alzheimer's disease, however, is ultimately fatal. Individuals with the disease may become bedridden and unable to care for themselves. They often die of pneumonia or other infections because of the disability. People with Alzheimer's may become disoriented, increasing their risk of falls, which can cause serious fractures or head injuries.

Treatment
Presently, there's no cure for Alzheimer's disease. Doctors sometimes prescribe drugs to improve signs and symptoms that often accompany Alzheimer's, including sleeplessness, wandering, anxiety, agitation and depression.

In some studies, two varieties of medications have been shown to slow the cognitive decline associated with Alzheimer's. They are:
- **Cholinesterase inhibitors.** This group of medications — which includes donepezil (Aricept), rivastigmine (Exelon) and galantamine (Razadyne) — works by improving the levels of neurotransmitters in the brain. But cholinesterase inhibitors don't work for everyone. As many as half the people who take these

Alzheimer's Warning Signs

When people forget something, they often joke that they're developing Alzheimer's disease. But having Alzheimer's isn't the same as having an occasional memory lapse or failing to immediately remember someone's name. Alzheimer's is a condition that becomes progressively worse. Most people with Alzheimer's share certain characteristics. These may include:

Increasing and persistent forgetfulness
At its onset, Alzheimer's disease is marked by periods of forgetfulness, especially of recent events or simple directions. But what begins as mild forgetfulness persists and increases. People with Alzheimer's may repeat things and forget conversations or appointments. They routinely misplace things, often putting them in illogical locations. They frequently forget names, and may even forget the names of family members and everyday objects such as a comb or watch.

Problems with abstract thinking
People with Alzheimer's disease may initially have trouble balancing their checkbook, a problem that progresses to trouble understanding and recognizing numbers.

Difficulty finding the right word
It may be a challenge for individuals with Alzheimer's to find the right words to express their thoughts or even to follow conversations. Eventually, reading and writing also are affected.

Disorientation
People with Alzheimer's disease may lose track of time and dates. They may get lost in familiar surroundings. They may even wander from home and get lost.

Loss of judgment
Solving everyday problems, such as knowing what to do if food on the stove is burning, becomes increasingly difficult. Alzheimer's is characterized by difficulty doing things that require planning, decision-making and judgment.

Difficulty performing familiar tasks
Once-routine tasks that require sequential steps, such as cooking, become a struggle as the disease progresses. People with Alzheimer's may forget how to do the most basic things, such as brushing their teeth.

Personality changes
Individuals with Alzheimer's may exhibit mood swings. They may express distrust in others, show increased stubbornness and withdraw socially. Early on, this may be a response to the frustration they feel as they notice uncontrollable changes in their memory. Depression often coexists with Alzheimer's disease. Restlessness also is a common sign. As the disease progresses, individuals may become anxious or aggressive and behave inappropriately.

What's cognition?

Cognition comes from the Latin word *cognoscere*, meaning "to know." Thus, your cognitive skills are the ones that enable you to know things. This includes your powers of awareness, intuition and memory, combined with your ability to perceive, reason and make judgments. Cognitive impairment is the loss of these powers.

drugs show no improvement. Other people choose to stop taking the drugs because of the side effects, which include diarrhea, nausea and vomiting. There's a common myth that these medications can slow Alzheimer's disease itself, but they don't.

- **Memantine (Namenda).** The first drug approved to treat moderate to severe stages of Alzheimer's, memantine protects brain cells from damage caused by the chemical messenger glutamate. It sometimes is used in combination with a cholinesterase inhibitor. Memantine's most common side

effect is dizziness, although it also appears to increase agitation and delusional behavior in some people.

Caregiving
Education is very important for caregivers. Learning more about the disease process and techniques for dealing with problems can be beneficial to family and friends of the person with Alzheimer's disease.

An individual with Alzheimer's disease should be encouraged to continue his or her daily routines, physical activities, and social interactions as much as possible.

Tests for Dementia

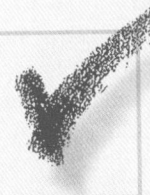

One of the purposes of testing for dementia is to help identify a possible treatable cause. Therefore, an accurate diagnosis is important.

Evaluation of a person with dementia typically begins with a detailed history, followed by physical and neurological evaluations. Depending on the results, laboratory tests are selected. Neuropsychological testing can provide additional information about a person's cognitive abilities, including memory, judgment, reasoning and planning skills. Some of the things a doctor typically evaluates include:

Mental status
A mental status assessment is often included in the neurological exam. This test assesses various mental functions, such as memory, attention, language and perception skills. A doctor or clinical psychologist may ask questions to assess several mental processes. These questions may include an evaluation of:
- *Insight into symptoms.* What do you think your problem is?
- *Orientation.* What's the date, month and year? Where are you now?
- *Memory.* Memorize a list of words and repeat them later.
- *Recall.* Remember information learned at a previous time.
- *Abstract reasoning.* Explain a proverb.
- *Attention.* Recite the months of the year forward and backward.
- *Thought content.* What are your fears and concerns?

- *Language.* Name objects and demonstrate an ability to read, write and comprehend the spoken word.
- *General knowledge.* Who's the president? How many weeks are there in a year?

Memory
Memory tests may be used to evaluate a person's ability to learn verbal and nonverbal information and to recall items from the remote past. The ability to construct objects by drawing also may be assessed, and the person may be asked to recall these drawings at a later time.

Cognitive skills
Cognitive function may be assessed by formal neuropsychological testing. This examination uses standardized tests of intelligence, memory, language and prior academic achievements. Typically, an individual's performance score is compared with scores obtained from other people of the same age and education level. These tests help determine if changes in mental status performance are within the normal range of aging or if an underlying disease may be involved. For example, depression may interfere with some attention and memory tasks in a manner somewhat similar to that found in Alzheimer's disease.

Several laboratory tests may be performed to identify a disease that may be causing the signs and symptoms. These tests include a computerized tomography (CT) scan or magnetic resonance imaging (MRI), electrocardiography, a chest X-ray, blood chemistry and urine tests, and drug screening. Additional neurological tests that may help in the diagnosis include electroencephalography, spinal tap (lumbar puncture) and radioisotope studies.

Proper nutrition and fluid intake are critical, but special diets and supplements are usually unnecessary. Exercise is important, and your doctor may recommend physical therapy. Travel with a supportive companion may be possible if arrangements aren't overly complicated.

Whenever possible, avoid dramatic changes, such as moving to a new location, rearranging the furniture and disrupting established routines. Also avoid dangerous equipment or materials in the living environment, and monitor carefully the person's ability to drive.

Use notes as reminders of activities and a calendar listing routine tasks and directions for daily activities. A medical alert bracelet may be helpful in case the person becomes disoriented and wanders into an unfamiliar setting.

Alzheimer's disease can be a difficult disorder to deal with, but concern and compassion on the part of the individuals providing care can make a major difference.

Vascular dementia

Signs and symptoms
- Problems with language and memory
- Confusion and agitation
- Walking disturbances
- Loss of bowel or bladder control
- Personality and mood changes

Emergency signs and symptoms
- An abrupt change in mental state

Vascular dementia is an umbrella term that describes impairments in cognitive function caused by problems in the blood vessels that feed the brain. Individuals who develop vascular dementia often have experienced a stroke or several strokes.

In some cases, a blood vessel may be completely blocked, causing a stroke. Some strokes result in dementia while others don't. It depends on the severity of the stroke and the portion of the brain that's affected. Vascular dementia also

can occur when blood vessels in the brain narrow, reducing blood flow to those sections of the brain. Risk of the condition increases dramatically with age.

Vascular dementia symptoms often begin suddenly and may worsen in a stepwise fashion, following a series of strokes or mini-strokes. But some forms of vascular dementia develop gradually and can easily be confused with Alzheimer's disease. One difference is that memory loss is one of the first symptoms of Alzheimer's. In vascular dementia, memory problems typically occur much later in the disease process.

Alzheimer's disease and vascular dementia often occur together. In fact, some scientists believe that it's more common for these two disorders to occur together than apart.

Diagnosis
Diagnosing vascular dementia requires fulfilling certain criteria and eliminating other possible causes of dementia that might be treatable, such as normal-pressure hydrocephalus, vitamin deficiencies or hypothyroidism.

This is generally accomplished through a series of tests, including physical and neurological examinations, neuropsychological testing, brain imaging and various laboratory tests. A history of high blood pressure, transient ischemic attacks (TIAs) or stroke may be an indication that the dementia is vascular in origin.

How serious is vascular dementia?
Vascular dementia is a disorder that becomes progressively worse. There may be periods where signs

Dementia and Communication

People with dementia often have problems using language and understanding others. Common changes in the ability to communicate include repetition and the use of inaccurate and socially inappropriate words that may reflect jealousy, paranoia or impulsiveness. Here are some tips to help communicate with someone who has dementia:
- Approach the person from the front, identify yourself and address the person by name.
- Speak slowly and clearly in a gentle, relaxed tone.
- Use short, simple and familiar words. Repeat when necessary, using the same words.
- Use one-step commands and requests.
- Ask one question at a time, preferably those that can be answered with a yes or no. Give the person extra time to respond.
- Offer encouragement when the person has difficulty expressing thoughts and feelings.
- Don't interrupt, criticize, correct or argue. Be patient and flexible.
- Avoid pronouns. Identify people by name.
- Avoid negative statements and quizzing, such as, "You know who that is, don't you?"
- Let the person know you're listening and trying to understand.
- Maintain eye contact to show interest.
- Don't talk to others about the person as if he or she weren't there.
- Use nonverbal communication, such as pointing and touching, when appropriate.
- Provide appropriate touch. This is perhaps the greatest form of communication in the later stages of dementia. Offering hugs, applying hand lotion and giving back rubs can be wonderful ways of communicating care and acceptance.

and symptoms improve, followed by further decline. Death may result from a stroke or complications such as pneumonia or infection.

Treatment

There is no cure for vascular dementia, and no drugs have been approved by the Food and Drug Administration to treat it. However, medications designed to treat the symptoms of Alzheimer's disease also appear to help people with vascular dementia. In addition, medications may be prescribed to reduce the risk of a stroke.

Cholinesterase inhibitors — such as donepezil (Aricept), galantamine (Razadyne) and rivastigmine (Exelon) — are Alzheimer's drugs that work by boosting levels of a chemical messenger involved in memory and judgment. Side effects can include nausea, vomiting and diarrhea.

Another Alzheimer's drug, called memantine (Namenda), also has been shown to provide a modest benefit in people who have vascular dementia. Memantine works by regulating a chemical messenger involved in information processing, storage and retrieval. Side effects can include headache, constipation, confusion and dizziness.

Doctors sometimes prescribe both types of drugs, memantine and one of the cholinesterase inhibitors.

Parkinson's disease

Signs and symptoms

- Shaking (tremor) at rest
- Masking (reduction) of facial expression and blinking
- Slowness of movements
- A shuffling gait with short steps
- Stiffness or rigidity of limbs
- A slow, soft, monotone voice
- Difficulty in maintaining balance
- A stooped posture
- Dementia

Parkinson's disease was first described by James Parkinson in England in 1817. It's a progressive degeneration of nerve cells (neurons) in parts of the brain that control muscle movements.

This particular group of neurons, called the substantia nigra, releases a chemical called dopamine. Dopamine is important for transmitting signals from the substantia nigra to another part of the brain called the corpus striatum. These signals help your muscles make smooth, controlled movements. In Parkinson's disease, the substantia nigra is damaged or destroyed, resulting in impairment of walking, arm movement and facial expression.

Parkinson's disease manifests itself in various ways. It may be evident only on one side or both sides of the body. Blinking, smiling and swinging your arms when you walk all are unconscious acts that are part of human behavior. In Parkinson's disease, these acts tend to be lost. Many develop a fixed staring, expression and unblinking eyes — the so-called masked face of the disease. And instead of gesturing while talking, some people lack animation when they speak.

People with Parkinson's disease may gradually develop a slow, shuffling walk with an unsteady gait, stooped posture and a tendency to fall. In the later stages of the disease, their muscles may freeze up, making it hard to initiate normal movement. This is especially distressing because it can make performing the simplest tasks difficult and time-consuming. Even the functioning of the digestive tract may slow down, causing problems with swallowing, digestion and elimination. In fact, constipation is often a major problem for people with Parkinson's disease.

Tremors often start with a slight shaking in one finger that later may spread to the whole arm. Sometimes, tremors in the hand cause a back-and-forth rubbing of

Use It or Lose It?

Studies suggest that maintaining mental fitness may delay the onset of dementia.

One study focused on a large group of nuns reported to have low rates of Alzheimer's disease, even though their average age was 85 and many were in their 90s. Many of the nuns had advanced academic degrees and led intellectually challenging lives into old age.

Some researchers believe that lifelong learning may promote the growth of additional connections between neurons (synapses) and delay the onset of dementia. Other researchers argue that advanced education gives a person more experience with the types of memory and thinking skills used in tests to measure dementia. This advanced level of education simply may help some people "cover" their condition longer.

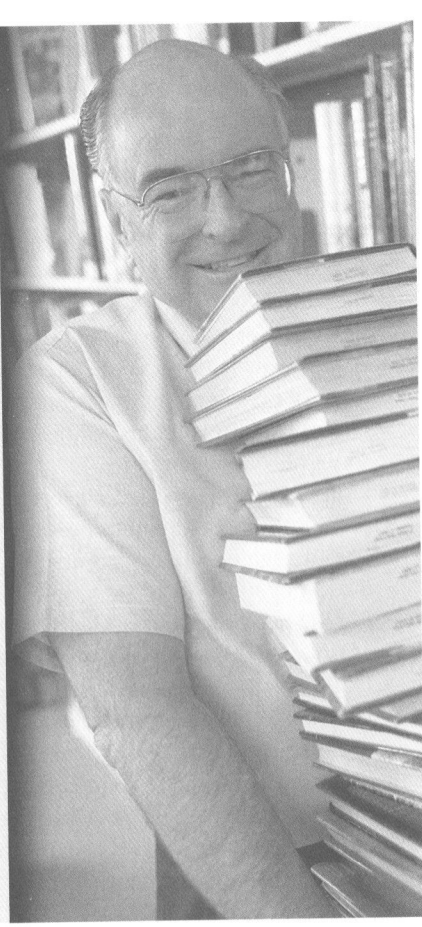

the thumb and forefinger known as pill-rolling. A person with Parkinson's may also develop tremors in the head, lips or feet. These signs and symptoms may occur on one or both sides of the body and may be more noticeable under stress. Although tremors can be very distressing, they're usually not disabling and often disappear during sleep and during movement.

Muscle stiffness (rigidity) often occurs in the limbs and neck. When stiffness is severe, it limits the size of movements. For example, the handwriting of people with Parkinson's disease often becomes extremely small. In addition, many people with Parkinson's disease have trouble speaking, and their voice may become a soft monotone.

During the later stages of the disease, up to one-third of people with Parkinson's disease develop dementia, with the loss of intellectual and social abilities.

Although much research has been done on Parkinson's disease, researchers still aren't certain about what sets this chain of events in motion. Some theorize that genetic mutations or environmental toxins — or a combination of both — may play a role in Parkinson's disease.

Studies indicate that people who have a first-degree relative, such as a parent or sibling, with Parkinson's are at greater risk of developing the condition themselves, suggesting a genetic connection. Other studies have linked the disease to exposure to herbicides and pesticides.

Diagnosis

A diagnosis of Parkinson's disease is based on your medical history and a neurological examination. As part of your medical history, your doctor will want to know about any medications you take and whether you have a family history of Parkinson's. The neurological examination includes

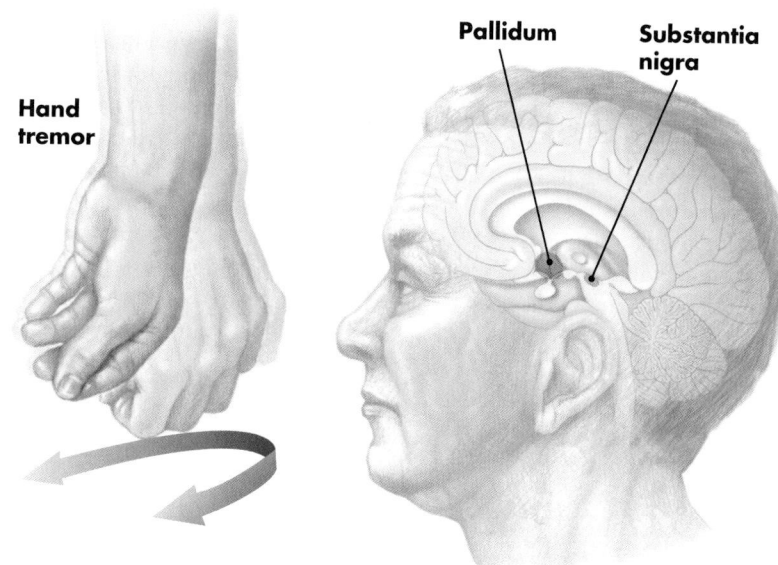

Movement problems associated with Parkinson's disease, such as tremor, are caused primarily by inadequate levels of the brain chemical dopamine, which transmits messages from the substantia nigra to other parts of the brain. One treatment involves surgically destroying tissue in the part of the brain called the pallidum.

an evaluation of your walking and coordination, as well as some simple hand tasks.

A diagnosis of Parkinson's is most likely if you have:
- At least two of the three cardinal Parkinson's symptoms — tremor, slowing of motion and muscle rigidity
- Onset of symptoms on only one side of the body
- Symptoms that aren't explained by medication use, stroke or other causes
- Tremor that's more pronounced at rest, for example, when your hands are resting in your lap
- A strong response to levodopa, a Parkinson's drug

How serious is Parkinson's disease?

Parkinson's disease tends to be progressive — its signs and symptoms gradually worsen. The time involved in this process varies greatly. You may have years of active living after developing this disease. For others, the progression is more rapid. During the later stages of the disease, many

individuals need assistance. In its most severe form, the disease can leave you incapacitated by rigidity and tremor, although this occurs in only a small minority of cases.

Treatment

Your initial response to Parkinson's treatment can be dramatic. Over time, however, the benefits of drugs frequently diminish or become less consistent, although symptoms can usually still be fairly well-controlled. Your doctor may recommend lifestyle changes, such as physical therapy, a healthy diet and exercise, in addition to medications. In some cases, surgery may be helpful.

Medications
Medications can help manage problems with walking, movement and tremor by increasing the brain's supply of dopamine. Taking dopamine itself is not helpful, because it is unable to enter your brain.
- **Levodopa.** The most effective Parkinson's drug is levodopa, a substance that occurs naturally in the body. When taken by

mouth in pill form, it passes into the brain and is converted to dopamine. Levodopa is combined with carbidopa to create the combination drug Sinemet. The carbidopa protects levodopa from premature conversion to dopamine outside the brain; in doing that, it also prevents nausea. Levodopa side effects include confusion, delusions and hallucinations, as well as involuntary movements called dyskinesia. These resolve with dose reduction, but sometimes at the expense of reduced parkinsonism control.

As the disease progresses, the benefit from levodopa may become less stable, with a tendency to wax and wane ("wearing off"). This often requires medication adjustments. A newer extended release form of carbidopa-levodopa called Rytary may provide a more sustained effect.

- **Carbidopa-levodopa infusion.** The Food and Drug Administration recently approved a drug called Duopa. This medication is made up of carbidopa and levodopa. However, it's administered through a feeding tube that delivers the medication in a gel form directly to the small intestine.

  Duopa is for select people with more advanced Parkinson's who still respond to carbidopa-levodopa, but who have a lot of fluctuations in their response. Because Duopa is continually infused, blood levels of the two drugs remain constant.

  Placement of the tube requires a small surgical procedure. Risks associated with having the tube include the tube falling out or infections at the infusion site.

- **Dopamine agonists.** Unlike levodopa, these drugs aren't changed into dopamine. Instead, they mimic the effects of dopamine in the brain and cause neurons to react as if dopamine is present. They're not nearly as effective in treating Parkinson's symptoms. However, they last longer and are often used to smooth the sometimes off-and-on effect of levodopa.

  Pill forms of dopamine agonists include pramipexole (Mirapex) and ropinirole (Requip). Rotigotine (Neupro) is a skin patch. A short-acting injectable dopamine agonist, apomorphine (Apokyn), is used for quick relief.

  The side effects of dopamine agonists include those of carbidopa-levodopa, although they're less likely to cause involuntary movements. However, they are substantially more likely to cause hallucinations, sleepiness or swelling. These medications may also increase your risk of compulsive behaviors such as hypersexuality, compulsive gambling and compulsive overeating. If you are taking these medications and start behaving in a way that's out of character for you, talk to your doctor.

- **MAO inhibitors.** These types of drugs, including selegiline (Eldepryl, Zelapar) and rasagiline (Azilect), help prevent the breakdown of both naturally occurring dopamine and dopamine formed from levodopa. They do this by inhibiting the activity of the enzyme monoamine oxidase B — the enzyme that metabolizes dopamine in the brain. Side effects are rare but can include serious interactions with other medications, including drugs to treat depression and certain narcotics.

- **Catechol O-methyltransferase (COMT) inhibitors.** These drugs prolong the effect of carbidopa-levodopa therapy by blocking an enzyme that breaks down levodopa. Entacapone (Comtan) doesn't cause liver problems and is now combined with carbidopa and levodopa in a medication called Stalevo.

- **Anticholinergics.** These drugs have been used for many years to help control the tremor associated with Parkinson's disease. A number of anticholinergic drugs, such as trihexyphenidyl and benztropine (Cogentin), are available. However, their modest benefits may be offset by side effects such as confusion and hallucinations, particularly in people over the age of 70. Other side effects include dry mouth, nausea, urine retention — especially in men with an enlarged prostate — and severe constipation.

- **Antivirals.** Doctors may prescribe amantadine alone to provide short-term relief of mild, early-stage Parkinson's disease. It also may be added to carbidopa-levodopa therapy for people in the later stages of Parkinson's disease, especially if they have problems with involuntary movements (dyskinesia) induced by carbidopa-levodopa. Side effects include swollen ankles and a purple mottling of the skin.

Physical therapy
Exercise is important for general health, but especially for maintaining function in Parkinson's disease. Physical therapy may be advisable and can help improve mobility, range of motion and muscle tone. Although specific exercises can't stop the progress of the disease, improving muscle strength can help you feel more confident and capable. A physical therapist can also work with you to improve your gait and balance. A speech therapist or speech pathologist can improve problems with speaking and swallowing.

Surgery
Deep brain stimulation is the most common surgical procedure to treat Parkinson's disease. It involves implanting an electrode deep within the parts of your brain that control movement. The amount of stimulation delivered by the electrode is controlled by a

pacemaker-like device placed under the skin in your upper chest. A wire that travels under your skin connects the device, called a pulse generator, to the electrode.

Deep brain stimulation is most often used for people who have advanced Parkinson's disease who have unstable medication (levodopa) responses. It can stabilize medication fluctuations and reduce or eliminate involuntary movements (dyskinesias). Tremor is especially responsive to this therapy. Deep brain stimulation doesn't help dementia and may make it worse.

Like any other brain surgery, this procedure has risks — such as brain hemorrhage or stroke-like problems. Infection also may occur, requiring parts of the device to be replaced. In addition, the unit's battery beneath the skin of the chest wall must be surgically replaced every few years. Deep brain stimulation isn't beneficial for people who don't respond to carbidopa-levodopa.

Essential tremor

Signs and symptoms
- Rhythmic, alternating movement of your hands, head, tongue or voice box (larynx)
- Hand tremor that worsens with use

Essential tremor is a common movement disorder. Almost half of all cases run in families, appearing from adolescence to later in life. It most commonly begins in middle to late life and progresses slowly. Over time, the tremor may affect your hands, head or voice. Voluntary movements, such as holding a coffee cup or a fork, usually make the tremor worse. This is in contrast to Parkinson's disease, in which the tremor tends to decrease with such movement.

The tremor usually stops when you're at rest. Jerky movements begin when you start a voluntary action, such as eating or writing. Essential tremor can make coordinated movements, such as

touching your nose, difficult. Signs and symptoms may increase the more active you are. Fatigue or stress can make the tremor worse. The tremor disappears when you're asleep.

Diagnosis
Diagnosing essential tremor generally involves ruling out other conditions that can result in hand, head or voice tremors. Your doctor will likely ask about your medical history and perform a physical and neurological exam. You may be asked to write, drink from a glass or hold a piece of paper.

You may also undergo blood, urine and neurological tests to check for other causes, including thyroid disease, drug side effects and other neurological disorders, such as Parkinson's disease.

How serious is essential tremor?
Essential tremor isn't life-threatening and usually is only a mild nuisance. But if it becomes disruptive, treatment is available to keep it under control.

Treatment
Some people with essential tremor may not require treatment if their symptoms are mild. But if your essential tremor is making it difficult to work or perform daily activities, you may want to discuss treatment options with your doctor.

Medications
They include:
- **Beta blockers.** Used to treat high blood pressure, beta blockers — such as propranolol (Inderal), atenolol (Tenormin), metoprolol (Lopressor) and nadolol (Corgard) — help relieve tremors in some people. They may not be an option if you also have asthma, diabetes or some heart problems.
- **Anti-seizure medications.** Epilepsy drugs — including primidone (Mysoline), gabapentin (Neurontin, Horizant) and topiramate (Topamax, Trokendi XR) — may be effective in people who don't respond to beta blockers. The main side effects are drowsiness and flu-like symptoms, which usually disappear within a short time.
- **Tranquilizers.** Doctors sometimes use drugs such as diazepam (Valium, Diastat) and alprazolam (Xanax) to treat people whose tremors are made much worse by tension or anxiety. Side effects can include confusion and memory loss. Additionally, these medications should be used with caution because they can be habit-forming.
- **Botulinum toxin type A (Botox) injections.** You're probably familiar with Botox as a treatment for facial wrinkles, but it can also be useful in treating some types of tremors, especially of the head and voice. Botox

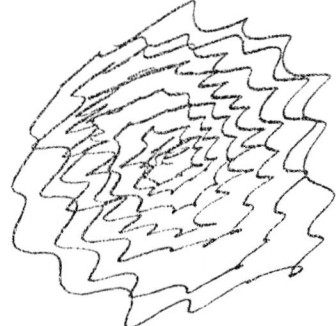 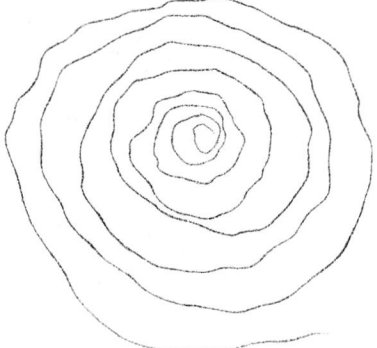

One test used to evaluate essential tremor involves having you draw a spiral. The spiral on the left was drawn by a hand affected by essential tremor. The spiral on the right was drawn by an unaffected hand.

injections can improve problems for up to three months at a time. If used to treat hand tremors, it may cause finger weakness.

Therapy
Physical therapy exercises can sometimes reduce tremor and improve coordination and muscle control. Occupational therapists may suggest some of the following adaptive devices to reduce the effect of your tremors on your daily activities: heavier plates, glasses and utensils, wrist weights, and wider writing implements.

Surgery
Surgery may be an option for people whose tremors are severely disabling and who don't respond to medications.

The most common procedure is called deep brain stimulation. It involves inserting a long, thin electrical probe into your thalamus — the portion of your brain responsible for causing your tremors. A wire from the probe is tunneled under your skin to your chest, where a pacemaker-like device has been inserted. This device transmits painless electrical pulses to interrupt signals from your thalamus that may be causing your tremors.

Tic disorders

Signs and symptoms
- Habitual, repetitive movements or twitches of the face and body
Tics are semivoluntary mannerisms that usually develop in childhood. Grimaces, eye or mouth twitches, head turning, and shoulder shrugging are examples of common tics. Adolescents sometimes have such tics, which resolve as they get older.

A condition called Tourette syndrome is characterized by more prominent tics that develop in youth and include vocalizations such as sniffing, grunting and compulsive swearing. It's four times more frequent in boys than in girls and may run in families.

The tics of Tourette syndrome aren't exactly involuntary, but compulsive or urgent, like the urge to scratch an itch. Sometimes, they can be suppressed, but ultimately the tics are expressed. The cause of this condition is not known but may be associated with abnormal metabolism of certain brain chemicals.

Diagnosis
A history and physical examination can help your doctor determine if you have a tic disorder, as well as its type and severity. Tests to exclude other disorders also may be necessary.

How serious are tic disorders?
Tic disorders typically are more frustrating than serious. Emotional stress can aggravate signs and symptoms and focus inordinate attention on the disorder.

Some conditions that may accompany Tourette syndrome include obsessive-compulsive disorder, autism, anger control problems and poor social skills. People with Tourette may experience periods free of signs and symptoms. Signs and symptoms often decrease with time and, in some cases, may even disappear.

Treatment
Treatment options include:
- **Medications.** Some medications can be used to help control or minimize tics. These may include certain antipsychotic medications, antidepressants, stimulant medications and central adrenergic inhibitors. But none of the drugs will completely eliminate the symptoms, and the side effects may outweigh any benefits gained.
- **Psychotherapy.** Psychotherapy can be helpful for two reasons. It can help with accompanying problems, such as attention-deficit/hyperactivity disorder (ADHD), obsessions, depression and anxiety. Therapy can also help people cope emotionally.

- **Deep brain stimulation.** For debilitating tics that don't respond to other treatment, research suggests that deep brain stimulation (DBS) may be effective. DBS consists of implanting a battery-operated medical device (neurostimulator) in the brain to deliver electrical stimulation to targeted areas that control movement.

Multiple sclerosis

Signs and symptoms
- Numbness, weakness or paralysis in one or more limbs
- Brief pain, tingling or electric shock sensations
- Impaired vision with pain during movement in one eye
- Tremor, lack of coordination or unsteady gait
- Double vision or rapid, involuntary eye movement
- Fatigue
- Dizziness
- Exacerbations and remissions of signs and symptoms
Multiple sclerosis (MS) is a potentially debilitating disease in which your body's immune system eats away at the protective sheath that covers your nerves. This interferes with the communication between your brain and the rest of your body. Ultimately, this may result in deterioration of the nerves themselves, a process that's not reversible.

Symptoms vary widely, depending on the amount of damage and which particular nerves are affected. People with severe cases of multiple sclerosis may lose the ability to walk or speak. Multiple sclerosis can be difficult to diagnose early in the course of the disease, because symptoms often come and go — sometimes disappearing for months.

Multiple sclerosis is an autoimmune disease, where the body's immune system attacks its own tissues. In multiple sclerosis, this process destroys myelin — the fatty substance that coats and

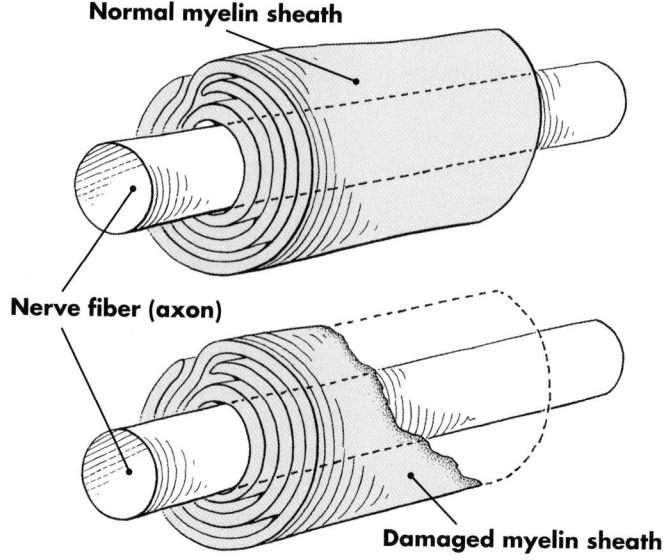

Normal myelin sheath

Nerve fiber (axon)

Damaged myelin sheath

Your nerve fibers are protected by an insulating sheath (myelin). In multiple sclerosis, the sheath is damaged.

protects nerve fibers in the brain and spinal cord. Myelin can be compared to the insulation on electrical wires. When myelin is damaged, the messages that travel along that nerve may be slowed or blocked.

Doctors and researchers aren't sure exactly why multiple sclerosis occurs in some people and not others. A combination of factors, ranging from genetics to childhood infections, may play a role.

The disease generally occurs in episodes (attacks) that last weeks or months and are separated by periods in which signs and symptoms improve or disappear (remission). Disability may persist, and the signs and symptoms may increase in severity.

Although multiple sclerosis can occur at any age, it most often begins in people between the ages of 20 and 40. Women are more likely to develop multiple sclerosis than are men. Your risk of MS is greater if a relative has the disease. The disease is not, however, passed on reliably from one generation to the next like other genetic diseases. White people of Northern European descent, especially those of Scandinavian heritage, are more susceptible to multiple sclerosis.

Diagnosis

There are no specific tests for multiple sclerosis. Ultimately, the diagnosis relies on ruling out other conditions that might produce similar symptoms. Your doctor may base a multiple sclerosis diagnosis on the following:

Blood tests
Analysis of your blood can help rule out some infectious or inflammatory diseases that have symptoms similar to multiple sclerosis.

Spinal tap (lumbar puncture)
In this procedure, a doctor removes a small sample of cerebrospinal fluid from within your spinal canal for laboratory analysis. This sample can show abnormalities associated with multiple sclerosis, such as abnormal levels of white blood cells or proteins. This procedure can also help rule out viral infections and other conditions that can cause neurological symptoms similar to those of multiple sclerosis.

Magnetic resonance imaging (MRI)
MRI can reveal lesions, indicative of the myelin loss caused by multiple sclerosis, on your brain and spinal cord. However, these types

of lesions can also be caused by other conditions, such as lupus or Lyme disease, so the presence of these lesions isn't definitive proof that you have multiple sclerosis.

You may also receive an intravenous dye that may help highlight "active" lesions. This helps doctors know whether your disease is in an active phase, even if no symptoms are present. Newer MRI techniques can provide even greater detail about the degree of nerve fiber injury or permanent myelin loss and recovery.

Evoked potential test
This test measures the electrical signals sent by your brain in response to stimuli. An evoked potential test may use visual stimuli or electrical stimuli, in which short electrical impulses are applied to your legs or arms.

How serious is multiple sclerosis?

The course of MS varies widely. The average life expectancy after onset of the disease has increased in the past few decades as a result of better medical care, particularly in dealing with complications of the disease. Most people with MS are ambulatory, and many are employed even after having MS for 20 years. It's very uncommon to be permanently disabled within weeks or months of initial signs and symptoms of MS.

Treatment

There is no cure for multiple sclerosis. Treatment typically focuses on combating the autoimmune response and managing the symptoms. Some people have such mild symptoms that no treatment is necessary.

Medications
Drugs that are commonly used for multiple sclerosis include:
• **Corticosteroids.** They are the most common treatment for multiple sclerosis. Intravenous corticosteroids reduce the

inflammation that spikes during a relapse.

- **Interferons.** These medications — such as Betaseron, Avonex and Rebif — appear to slow the rate at which multiple sclerosis symptoms worsen over time. But interferons can cause serious liver damage.
- **Glatiramer (Copaxone).** Doctors believe that glatiramer works by blocking your immune system's attack on myelin. You must inject this drug subcutaneously once daily. Side effects may include flushing and shortness of breath after injection.
- **Natalizumab (Tysabri).** This drug is designed to work by interfering with the movement of potentially damaging immune cells from your bloodstream to your brain and spinal cord. Tysabri is generally reserved for people who see no results from or can't tolerate other types of treatments. This is because Tysabri increases the risk of progressive multifocal leukoencephalopathy (PML) — a brain infection that's usually fatal. Testing can identify individuals who may be at high risk of PML.
- **Mitoxantrone.** This immunosuppressant drug can be harmful to the heart, so it's usually used only in people who have advanced multiple sclerosis.
- **Oral immunomodulatory therapies.** Individuals with active relaxing remitting multiple sclerosis may be candidates for new oral medications that lower the chances of relapses. These medications include fingolimod (Gilenya), dimethyl fumarate (Tecfidera) and teriflunomide (Aubagio). All of these medications require monitoring.

Therapies
A physical or occupational therapist can teach you stretching and strengthening exercises, and show you how to use devices that make it easier to perform daily tasks.

Procedures
Plasma exchange (plasmapheresis) looks a little like dialysis, as it mechanically separates your blood cells from your plasma, the liquid part of your blood. Plasma exchange is sometimes used to help combat severe symptoms of multiple sclerosis relapses, especially in people who are not responding to intravenous steroids.

Amyotrophic lateral sclerosis (ALS)

Signs and symptoms
- Slow loss of strength and coordination in one or more limbs
- Muscle twitches or cramps
- An increasingly stiff and clumsy gait
- Difficulty swallowing, speaking or breathing

Amyotrophic lateral sclerosis (ALS) is a progressive degeneration of the nerve cells in the brain and spinal cord that control your voluntary muscles. It's commonly called Lou Gehrig's disease after the New York Yankees baseball player who died of ALS in 1939.

The affected nerve cells shrink and disappear with no other signs of abnormality. Muscles then waste away because the nerves that stimulated them are gone.

In the United States, ALS occurs in 3.9 of 100,000 people. In 5 to 10 percent of those cases, the disease is inherited. The vast majority of the time, doctors don't know why ALS occurs in some people and not in others. The disease isn't contagious.

The onset of the disease is often gradual. Generally, there's increasing weakness in one limb, especially a hand. Later, other limbs may be affected. This may be accompanied by muscle twitching and cramping. Additional muscles become affected as ALS progresses, and complete paralysis may result. The disease eventually affects semivoluntary muscles, such as the ones used for chewing, swallowing, speaking and breathing.

Diagnosis
The disease is often well-advanced before people seek medical attention. In these instances, a doctor may be able to make a diagnosis based on signs and symptoms. Electromyography to test for nerve damage may be required. Other tests may include a nerve conduction study or magnetic resonance image (MRI). In a nerve conduction study, electrodes are attached to your skin above the nerve or muscle to be studied. A small shock is passed through the nerve to measure the strength and speed of nerve signals.

How serious is amyotrophic lateral sclerosis?
ALS is a chronic degenerative disorder that becomes progressively worse. Most people with ALS die of respiratory failure due to paralysis of the muscles used in breathing. Sometimes, people with ALS stop breathing because they inhale (aspirate) food and oral secretions into the lungs.

Generally, death occurs within two to 10 years after receiving a diagnosis. Only 1 in 5 people with the disease live longer than five years.

Treatment
There's no cure for ALS. Individualized therapy is useful for maintaining muscle function and general health during the disease's early stages. ALS doesn't affect your mind, and several years of productive and enjoyable life may be possible. The complications of aspiration of food and saliva inhaled into the windpipe (trachea) can be avoided by insertion of a tube through the wall of the abdomen and into the stomach through which liquid feedings can be given.

The Food and Drug Administration has approved the medication riluzole (Rilutek) for the treatment of ALS. It may slow the progression of the disease slightly in some people.

Huntington's disease

Signs and symptoms

- A wide, swinging gait
- Hesitant or slurred speech
- Involuntary, jerky movements in arms, neck, trunk and face
- Clumsiness or problems with balance
- Personality changes, such as moodiness and paranoia
- Intellectual deterioration, including memory loss and inattention

Huntington's disease, also known as Huntington's chorea, is a progressive degenerative brain disease that causes certain nerve cells to waste away. As a result, emotions, motor skills and mental skills are typically affected. The disorder was first identified in 1872 by American physician George Huntington.

Huntington's disease is an inherited condition caused by a single abnormal gene. Doctors refer to the illness as an autosomal dominant disorder because only one copy of the defective gene, inherited from either parent, is necessary to produce the disease. If one parent has the single faulty gene, the chance that an offspring will have the defect is 50 percent. Because signs and symptoms typically first appear in middle age, some parents may not know they carry the gene until they've already had children and possibly passed on the trait.

If your child doesn't inherit the faulty gene, he or she won't develop Huntington's disease and can't pass it on to the next generation. Everyone who has the gene eventually develops Huntington's disease, if he or she lives long enough.

In 2006, researchers discovered that the protein expressed by the Huntington's gene interacts with another protein to disturb the way that cholesterol accumulates in the brain. Cholesterol is essential for healthy brain cells and the network among those brain cells — but the cholesterol needs to be in proper levels and in the proper locations. When the network of brain cells is disrupted, motor skills, cognitive skills and speech can be affected.

Signs and symptoms usually appear between the ages of 30 and 50. Individuals who develop the disease at a younger age often have a more severe condition, but the disease is rare in children. Approximately 30,000 people in the United States have Huntington's disease.

Progression of the disease is slow. Personality changes, from moodiness to paranoia, may occur first. Involuntary facial movements such as grimacing may be mild initially. Other signs and symptoms, including severe chorea and mental impairment (dementia), appear as the disease progresses.

Diagnosis

To determine if you may have Huntington's disease, your doctor will likely perform a physical examination and obtain your medical history and that of your family. Your doctor may also ask about any recent emotional or intellectual changes that you may have experienced.

A computerized tomography (CT) scan or magnetic resonance imaging (MRI) may show any changes to your brain's structure. Your doctor may suggest a blood test to determine whether you carry the defective gene.

How serious is Huntington's disease?

After onset of the disease, signs and symptoms will progress in severity until death occurs. Although signs and symptoms vary from person to person, vital functions such as swallowing, eating, speaking and walking usually deteriorate over time. Death generally occurs as a result of complications of the disease, such as an infection or a fall.

Treatment

No satisfactory treatment is available to stop or reverse Huntington's disease, but some approaches can control signs and symptoms.

Medications

Tranquilizers such as clonazepam (Klonopin) and antipsychotic drugs such as haloperidol (Haldol) and clozapine (Clozaril) can help control movements, violent outbursts and hallucinations. While these medications can be helpful, a common side effect is sedation, and in some cases, these medications may cause additional stiffness and rigidity.

Various medications, including fluoxetine (Prozac), sertraline (Zoloft) and nortriptyline (Pamelor), can help control depression and the obsessive-compulsive rituals that some people with Huntington's disease develop. Medications such as lithium (Lithobid) can help control extreme emotions and mood swings.

Speech therapy

Huntington's disease can impair your speech, affecting your ability to express complex thoughts. You may find that speech therapy helps. Remind friends, family members and caregivers that if you don't speak, it doesn't necessarily mean that you don't understand what's going on. Ask people to continue talking to you and keep your environment as normal as possible.

Physical and occupational therapy

Physical therapy can help keep muscles stronger and more flexible, which helps maintain balance and may lessen the risk of falling. Occupational therapy can help make your home safer and give you strategies for coping with memory and concentration problems. Later in the disease, occupational therapy can assist you with eating, dressing and hygiene challenges.

Friedreich's ataxia

Signs and symptoms

- Difficulty in maintaining balance while walking or standing
- Abnormal speech rhythm or articulation
- Weakness in limbs
- A tremor of the hands or arms
- Deformed spine or feet
- Paralysis, particularly of the legs

Friedreich's ataxia was named in 1863 for German physician Nikolaus Friedreich, who first described the condition. Ataxia is the medical term for coordination problems, such as clumsiness or difficulty maintaining balance. Ataxia can be caused by many different conditions.

Friedreich's ataxia, a rare, inherited disease, is due to nerve fiber degeneration in areas of the spinal cord, peripheral nerves or cerebellum caused by a faulty gene. Normally, nerve fibers are encased in a sheath of a fatty substance called myelin, which enables smooth conduction of electric impulses between cells. In Friedreich's ataxia, nerve fibers lose some of their myelin sheath, and the spinal cord becomes thinner.

Signs and symptoms of the disease typically begin between the ages of 5 and 15, although they sometimes appear in adulthood. The condition affects about 1 in 50,000 people in the United States. In addition to problems with coordination and speech, many people develop curvature of the spine (scoliosis) and deformities in their feet. This often occurs as muscles weaken.

Friedreich's ataxia is an autosomal recessive disorder. You must inherit the abnormal gene from both parents in order to develop the condition. You may also be a carrier of the gene, without ever developing signs and symptoms, if you inherit it from only one parent. If there's a history of the disorder in your family, you may wish to speak with a genetic counselor before beginning a family.

Torticollis

Torticollis, sometimes called wryneck, is an intermittent or continuous spasm of the large muscles of the neck. It's a form of dystonia — sudden, involuntary contractions of a muscle or group of muscles. The condition may be inherited or acquired after damage to the neck muscle, or it may develop for no apparent reason.

The spasm is usually more prominent on one side than the other. This may cause permanent turning or tilting of the head. Stress or anxiety may make signs and symptoms worse.

Application of heat and massage may ease head and neck pain. Stretching exercises and a neck brace may improve spasms. Injections of botulinum toxin type A (Botox) to relax the muscles may provide relief, although repeat injections are usually required. In severe cases, surgery may be an option.

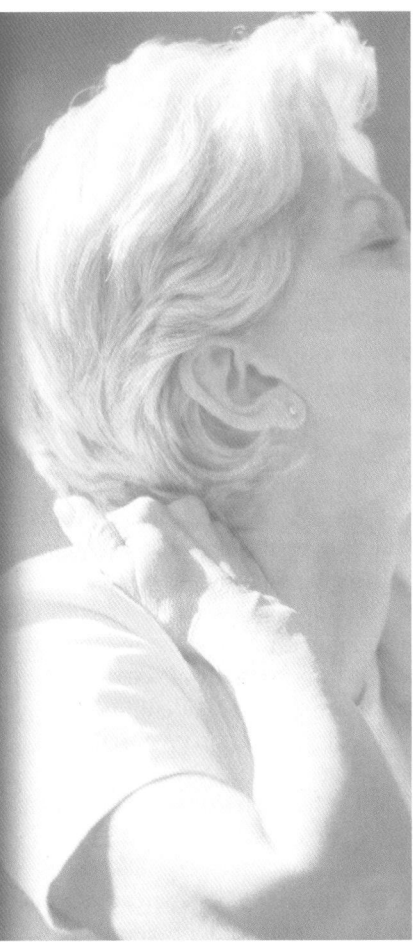

Mutation of the gene responsible for the disease causes reduced production of a protein called frataxin. Research suggests that a lack of frataxin leaves nerve cells vulnerable to oxidative stress, a condition caused by molecules called free radicals. Free radicals normally assist in your body's processing of fuel for energy, but too many of them can be damaging.

Diagnosis

Diagnosis of this disorder is based on family history and neurological findings including tests such as an electromyogram, which measures electrical activity in muscle cells, or an electrocardiogram (ECG). Tests to exclude other disorders may include a computerized tomography (CT) scan or magnetic resonance imaging (MRI) of the brain and spinal cord, and a spinal tap (lumbar puncture) with analysis of cerebrospinal fluid. Genetic testing can confirm the diagnosis.

How serious is Friedreich's ataxia?

Although signs and symptoms vary from person to person, most people with this disease eventually need a wheelchair to get around. Complications include various forms of cardiovascular disease, such as enlargement of the heart, heart failure, impairment of the conduction of electric impulses within the heart (heart block) and abnormal heart rhythms (tachycardia). Diabetes also may develop. Survival beyond early adulthood is rare. Death is frequently caused by a heart condition.

Treatment

No specific treatment is available for Friedreich's ataxia. Continued physical activity is recommended for general health, and physical therapy is often helpful.

Treatment of heart problems and diabetes can help maintain quality of life for a longer time.

Physical Therapy for Neurological Problems

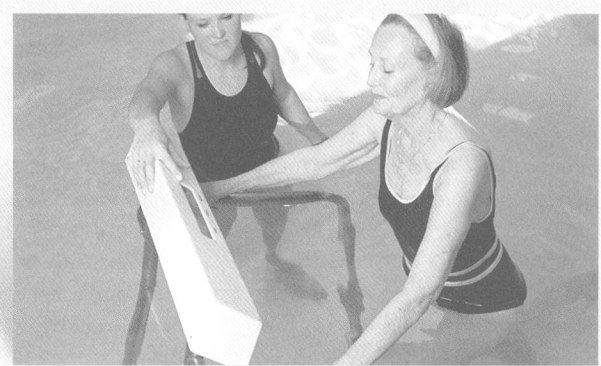

Physical therapy is used to achieve maximal potential in people with disabilities, including those resulting from neurological diseases and disorders. Physical therapy treatments can be valuable in helping relieve pain, improve strength and mobility, and perform essential tasks to maintain independence.

Before you begin a program of physical therapy, have a complete medical examination with diagnostic, functional and psychological testing, as determined by your doctor. A physical therapist generally consults closely with your doctor to plan a program that will work for you. The therapist and your doctor will also re-evaluate the therapy frequently as you make progress.

Your physical therapy program may address problems related to joint mobility, muscle strength, coordination, heart and lung capacity, posture, and ability to change position, walk, communicate, follow directions and perform other daily activities.

Physical therapists are trained and licensed in the use of a variety of therapies that may help relieve signs and symptoms of disease. Some of the therapies they may use include:

Exercise

Exercise is the most varied and widely used of all physical therapy techniques. Your exercise routine will be designed to overcome the manifestations of your disorder as much as possible, whether it be to increase the degree of joint mobility or to retrain your muscles to contract and relax in useful coordination with other muscles.

Exercises may be simple or complex. They may be performed actively by you alone or with the help of your therapist or passively as your physical therapist moves your arm or leg through a range of motions. Active exercises are necessary to improve your muscle function, but passive exercises are helpful when you have muscle contractures or need to relearn certain movements. Resistance exercises can improve muscle strength.

Various types of equipment may be used, including an exercise table or mat, a stationary bicycle, walking aids, a wheelchair, practice stairs, curbs, ramps, parallel bars, and pulleys and weights.

Hot and cold treatment

Heat can stimulate circulation, relax tense muscles and relieve pain. It can be applied with warm-water compresses, infrared lamps, short-wave radiation, ultrasound, hot paraffin wax or warm baths. In some cases, cold treatment with ice packs or cold-water soaking may be necessary. Alternating hot-and-cold water immersion of the hands or feet is used in certain circumstances.

Whirlpool baths

Whirlpool baths can ease pain from muscle spasms and help guide or strengthen your movements because the water partially supports you but provides resistance to your motion.

Massage

Massage therapy can improve circulation, help you relax, relieve local pain or muscle spasms, and reduce swelling. It can be done by trained therapists with special equipment or by family members trained in proper techniques.

Electricity

Electric currents of very low strength applied through your skin can stimulate superficial muscles and make them contract. This helps to produce response in paralyzed or weakened muscles. Certain medications can even be administered through your skin by means of a low-voltage electrical apparatus. Portable electric current devices called transcutaneous electrical nerve stimulation (TENS) units are sometimes used to control chronic pain (see page 1309).

Assistive devices

Your therapy may include learning how to use assistive devices for walking, such as a cane, brace or walker, or a mobility aid such as a wheelchair or motorized scooter. You may also receive training in use of devices that can make it easier to fasten buttons, hold a fork, dial a telephone or drive a car.

Other therapies

In addition to your doctor and physical therapist, you may meet with an occupational therapist to help you regain the ability to perform routine daily tasks such as grooming and dressing or develop alternative methods of compensating for lost function.

Orthopedic problems may be improved through surgery or the use of a brace.

It's hoped that identifying the genetic cause of the disorder will eventually lead to effective methods for a prevention or cure.

Myasthenia gravis

Signs and symptoms
- Facial muscle weakness, including drooping eyelids
- Difficulty breathing, talking, chewing or swallowing
- Double vision
- Muscle weakness in the arms or legs

Emergency signs and symptoms
- Increasing difficulty breathing or swallowing

Myasthenia gravis is a chronic disorder characterized by weakness and rapid fatigue of your voluntary muscles. Muscle weakness develops gradually and may affect any of the muscles that you control voluntarily. It commonly affects muscles of the face, eyes, arms and legs, and those involved in chewing, swallowing and breathing.

The more a muscle action is repeated, the worse the weakness becomes. In myasthenia gravis, good days alternate with bad. Remissions may occur and can last for months. In rare cases, breathing or swallowing problems worsen, requiring emergency medical care.

Myasthenia gravis is an autoimmune disease, which means that antibodies normally formed to fight infection instead attack normal tissue. When your nervous system is functioning normally, the chemical acetylcholine transmits nerve impulses to muscles. At specialized areas of your muscles, called neuromuscular junctions, receptor sites receive these impulses and signal your muscles to contract, allowing you to, for example, raise a spoon to your mouth.

In myasthenia gravis, there's a breakdown in communication between your nerves and muscles.

For unknown reasons, myasthenia gravis causes your immune system to produce antibodies that block or destroy many of your receptor sites. With fewer receptor sites, your muscles receive fewer nerve signals, causing weakness.

The thymus gland, a part of your immune system located in the upper chest beneath the breastbone, may trigger or maintain the production of these antibodies. Larger in infancy, the thymus gradually shrinks in healthy adults. However, some people with myasthenia gravis have an abnormally large thymus gland. A small percentage of those with the disease develop tumors of the thymus.

Myasthenia gravis is rare and develops most frequently in women between the ages of 20 and 40 and men older than age 60.

Diagnosis
A key symptom that may alert your doctor to the possibility of myasthenia gravis is muscle weakness that improves with rest. Tests to confirm the diagnosis may include a neurological examination, electromyography and a blood analysis for the presence of certain antibodies.

How serious is myasthenia gravis?
There's no cure for myasthenia gravis, but treatment can often lead to a remission. In a crisis phase of the illness, affected individuals become so weak that they need help breathing or swallowing, but this rarely persists beyond a few weeks. With proper treatment, most people with the condition can lead productive lives.

Treatment
Plan activities to take advantage of your energy peaks, and schedule daily rest periods. To relieve double vision, wear an eye patch. Because stress can worsen your condition, try to avoid situations that may provoke anxiety.

Medication
A drug called pyridostigmine (Mestinon, Regonol) is often prescribed to improve signal transmission between your nerves and muscles. Arrange to eat meals about 30 minutes after taking the medication to minimize chewing and swallowing difficulty. Medications that suppress or alter your immune system also may be prescribed. Examples include prednisone, azathioprine (Imuran, Azasan), cyclosporine (Sandimmune), mycophenolate (CellCept) and intravenous immunoglobulin.

Other therapies
Plasmapheresis is a treatment in which the plasma component in your blood is removed and discarded because it contains antibodies that may contribute to your disease. Other fluids to replace your plasma are mixed with your blood cells and returned to your body. This treatment may reduce the immune response and improve muscle strength temporarily, usually during a crisis.

Surgery
In some cases, removal of the thymus gland may be recommended. This can lead to permanent improvement in signs and symptoms. This procedure is used mainly in young individuals because the thymus gland shrinks with advancing age. As with any type of surgery, there are associated risks.

Spinal Cord and Peripheral Nerve Disorders

Your peripheral nervous system runs from your spinal cord to all other parts of your body. It's the network of nerves that you use to initiate movements and perceive sensations. Damage to your spine or peripheral nerves can interfere with communication between your brain and other areas of your body.

Damage to your peripheral nerves or spine can result in numbness or abnormal sensations and an inability to move your muscles. The seriousness of these disorders may range from temporary numbness to permanent paralysis.

Spinal cord injury

Emergency signs and symptoms
• Weakness, incoordination or paralysis in a part of the body after an accident
• Numbness or loss of sensation
• Loss of bladder or bowel control
Most spinal cord injuries are the result of traffic or industrial accidents, falls, gunshot wounds and recreational or athletic injuries. Sometimes, a relatively minor injury can produce severe damage if you have a predisposing condition, such as rheumatoid arthritis.

Your spinal cord is composed of long nerve fibers leading to and from your brain. The nerve fibers of the spinal cord feed into nerve roots that emerge between the vertebrae and organize into peripheral nerves that extend to your skin and muscles.

If the spinal cord is injured, the nerve fibers passing through the injured area can be affected. Part or all of your corresponding muscles and nerves below that injury site may be impaired.

Spinal injuries occur most frequently in the lower back (lumbar) and neck (cervical) areas. A lumbar injury can affect leg, bowel and bladder control and sexual function. A neck injury may affect breathing as well as movements of your upper and lower limbs. Injury to one side of the spinal cord typically impairs the muscles on the same side and some sensations on the same and opposite sides of your body.

Injury may result from your spinal cord being stretched, com-

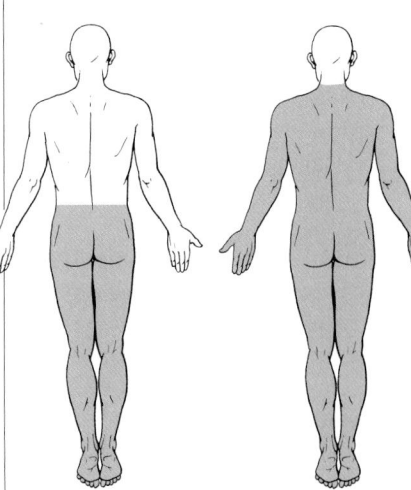

Paralysis of the lower body is called paraplegia. Paralysis below the neck is called quadriplegia.

pressed, pushed sideways or cut. It could also result from bleeding or the accidental insertion of a fragment of bone or metal into your spinal cord. Striking your chin on the steering wheel during a traffic accident, for example, may stretch your spinal cord and cause injury. A bullet or knife wound can sever the cord.

Often, injury to the spinal cord in the neck area results from a sharp bending of the neck during contact while playing football, from a shallow-water dive or from a motor vehicle accident. Injury to the lower spine, another common result of car and motorcycle accidents, may result in a crushing injury of the spinal cord.

Bleeding within the spinal cord can cause some permanent loss of sensation and muscle weakness. Bleeding around the spinal cord may compress it and result in weakness or loss of sensation in your limbs and trunk.

Compression may also occur from fluid accumulations and swelling in your spinal cord. The resulting paralysis may continue for several days and then improve dramatically when the swelling subsides or the accumulated fluid is removed surgically, although some impairment may persist.

Most cuts and other severe forms of trauma to the spinal cord cause permanent disability or paralysis because nerve fibers seldom regenerate. Paralysis below the neck can involve all four extremities, a condition called quadriplegia, or only the legs and lower body, resulting in paraplegia.

Diagnosis
Numbness or paralysis may occur immediately after a spinal cord injury or develop gradually as bleeding or swelling occurs in or around the spinal cord. Urgent medical attention is required to minimize long-term effects of such trauma.

After a physical and neurological examination, other diagnostic

Rehabilitation in Paraplegia and Quadriplegia

An accident that results in paralysis is a life-changing event, whether you've lost movement in your legs and lower body (paraplegia) or all four extremities (quadriplegia). Recovery from such an event takes time, but many people who are paralyzed move on to lead productive and fulfilling lives. The will to live is amazingly strong in humans, and the creativity with which many affected people lead their lives is infinite.

Initial recovery

In the early stages of paraplegia or quadriplegia, your doctor will treat the injury or disease that caused the loss of function. He or she will also watch for possible dangers such as stool or urine retention, respiratory or cardiovascular difficulty, stomach or intestinal ulcers, skin problems, muscle contractures, and formation of deep vein blood clots (thrombosis) in the extremities.

After the initial injury or disease stabilizes, attention will be given to problems that may arise from immobilization, such as deconditioning, muscle contractures, bedsores, urinary infection and blood clots. Early care will likely include changing your position frequently, range-of-motion exercises for paralyzed limbs, help with your bladder and bowel functions, applications of skin lotion and use of soft bed coverings or flotation mattresses. Hospitalization can last from several days to several weeks, depending on the cause and extent of the paralysis and the progress of your therapy.

Rehabilitation team

During this time, a rehabilitation team will work with you to improve your remaining muscle strength and to give you the greatest possible mobility and independence for living a full and active life. Your team may include a physiatrist, physical therapist, occupational therapist, rehabilitation nurse, rehabilitation psychologist, social worker and recreation therapist.

Rehabilitation therapy

Rehabilitation therapy may include exercise and various therapeutic methods, such as whirlpool baths and massage, to relieve pain and relax your muscles. You may receive training on day-to-day tasks and on the devices you'll need to assist you, such as a wheelchair or equipment that can make it easier to fasten buttons or use a telephone. This therapy may require several months in a rehabilitation facility.

Transitioning home

The rehabilitation team may smooth your transition to living at home by means of short-term leaves from the hospital. Such visits can acquaint you with support services in your community. Your doctor will continue to monitor your health and help you, with the assistance of your family or friends, adapt to a lifestyle that's healthy and as independent as possible.

Rehabilitation professionals can help you select needed equipment and modifications in your home. The goal is optimal independence and efficiency at minimal cost. Your rehab team can also help you address transportation needs.

Your part

Your mental state is extremely important. Sudden disability can be followed by depression. Many people with a disability learn to counter their depression by vigorous rehabilitative activity. It's essential for you to find or rediscover interesting things to do for yourself as well as with others. Don't hesitate to seek out support groups and peer counselors to help you.

---

tests may be needed. These usually include X-rays, a computerized tomography (CT) scan or magnetic resonance imaging (MRI). Occasionally, a spinal tap (lumbar puncture) is necessary.

How serious is a spinal cord injury?

The immediate effect of a spinal cord injury is often paralysis or loss of sensation in part of your body. This can be fatal if a neck injury has paralyzed breathing. The time between injury and treatment is a critical factor that can determine the extent of your recovery.

Recovery of movement or sensation within the first week is usually followed by eventual recovery of most or all functions. Any impairment remaining after six months probably will be permanent. If your bladder control is lost, your risk of recurring urinary tract infections increases. You also become susceptible to injury of any part of your body that has impaired sensation.

Treatment

Treatment consists of emergency care, hospitalization while the injuries heal and rehabilitation.

Medication

Corticosteroid medications may be prescribed to help reduce swelling that may be compressing your spinal cord. In case of urinary tract infections that may result, antibiotics may be required to treat the infection.

Surgery

Surgical procedures may be necessary to remove fragments of bone or foreign objects, to fix fractured vertebrae by fusing the bone or inserting metal pins, or to decompress the spinal cord.

Other therapies

Traction may reduce some dislocations of your spine and immobilize the back during healing. Sometimes, traction is accomplished by placing metal braces, attached to weights or a body harness, into the skull to hold it in place.

Bed rest is the primary treatment. Further neurological assessment is used to check for signs that reflexes and sensations are returning. Injuries usually heal in two to four months. Then a doctor can often estimate how much disability will remain.

Your doctor may recommend physical therapy to benefit from remaining muscle function and strength or to learn how to move with mechanical assistance.

Spinal tumor

Signs and symptoms
- Steadily increasing back pain
- Muscle weakness in the limbs
- Numbness or cold sensations

Emergency signs and symptoms
- Loss of bowel or bladder control
- Progressive loss of lower limb strength or sensation

A spinal tumor is a growth that develops within your spinal canal or within the bones of your spine. It may be cancerous or noncancerous. The cause is often unknown, although noncancerous tumors can be present from birth (congenital) or hereditary.

There are two main types of tumors that may affect the spinal cord. Intramedullary tumors begin in the cells within the spinal cord it-self. Extramedullary tumors develop within the supporting network of cells around the spinal cord.

Sometimes, tumors of the spine start elsewhere in your body, usually a lung or breast, and move through your bloodstream (metastasize) to the spinal area.

Signs and symptoms generally appear when the growing tumor presses against the spinal cord. Back pain and muscle weakness become progressively worse, and cold sensations may be felt in the legs, fingers or hands. Loss of bowel and bladder control and muscle spasms sometimes occur. Early treatment of a spinal tumor is important, so have your signs and symptoms evaluated by a doctor as soon as possible.

Diagnosis

Similar signs and symptoms can result from other spinal disorders, so an accurate diagnosis is important. If a spinal cord tumor is suspected, your doctor may request diagnostic tests, which may include X-rays, a computerized tomography (CT) scan or magnetic resonance imaging (MRI).

How serious is a spinal tumor?

If you're diagnosed with a spinal tumor, proceed with treatment as quickly as possible to minimize risk of permanent impairment. Early diagnosis and treatment provide a higher success rate, although neurological signs and symptoms may continue after initial treatments.

Treatment

Corticosteroids, such as dexamethasone, are used to reduce spinal cord swelling. Surgical removal is usually successful for isolated tumors located outside the spinal cord. Other tumors may not be completely removable, and radiation therapy may be necessary. Physical therapy programs are often needed to help with rehabilitation after completion of surgical or radiation therapy.

Cervical spondylosis

Signs and symptoms
- Pain or stiffness in the neck
- Pain, numbness, or pins-and-needles sensation in the shoulder or arm
- A burning sensation or clumsiness in fingers
- Bladder control problems
- Numbness or weakness in the legs or arms
- Imbalance or stiffness of the legs

Cervical spondylosis is a general term for age-related wear and tear affecting the joints in your neck. Also known as cervical osteoarthritis, this condition usually appears in men and women older than 40 and progresses with age.

As you age, the bones and cartilage that make up your backbone and neck gradually deteriorate. Your body attempts to fix the damage, but repairs may result in growth of new bone along the sides of the existing bone, which produces prominent lumps or bone spurs. These changes, which are characteristic of cervical spondylosis, eventually occur in everyone's spine. Still, many people with signs of cervical spondylosis on X-rays manage to escape the associated symptoms, which include pain, stiffness and muscle spasms.

At the other extreme, cervical spondylosis may compress one or more of the spinal nerves branching out of the cervical vertebrae — a condition called cervical radiculopathy. Bone spurs and other irregularities caused by cervical spondylosis also may reduce the diameter of the canal that houses the spinal cord, resulting in cervical myelopathy. Cervical radiculopathy and cervical myelopathy can lead to permanent disability. Fortunately, most adults with cervical spondylosis — nearly 90 percent — will not lose nerve function, even temporarily.

Diagnosis

A stiff neck is the key symptom, and it may not be very painful. If your signs and symptoms become troublesome, your doctor may request a neck X-ray, a computerized tomography (CT) scan or magnetic resonance imaging (MRI) to assess how much the spurs interfere with your nerve roots and spinal cord and if there's a need for surgery.

How serious is cervical spondylosis?

The signs and symptoms of cervical spondylosis are often mild and may not require medical treatment. Your discomfort may be long term or it may occur only under certain circumstances, such as sleeping in the wrong position or turning your head suddenly.

In limited cases when there's pressure on the spinal cord or nerve roots, cervical spondylosis can cause permanent disability.

Treatment

Mild cases of cervical spondylosis may respond to:
- Wearing a neck brace (cervical collar) during the day to help limit neck motion and reduce nerve irritation.
- Taking nonsteroidal anti-inflammatory drugs such as ibuprofen (Advil, Motrin IB, others) for pain relief.
- Doing exercises prescribed by a physical therapist to strengthen neck muscles and stretch the neck and shoulders. Low-impact aerobic exercise, such as walking or water aerobics, also may help.

For more-severe cases, treatment may include:
- Taking muscle relaxants, such as methocarbamol (Robaxin) or cyclobenzaprine, particularly if neck muscle spasms occur.
- Injecting corticosteroid medications into the joints between the vertebrae (facet joints). The injection combines corticosteroid medication with a local anesthetic to reduce pain and inflammation.

Surgery

If conservative treatment fails or if your neurological signs and symptoms, such as weakness in your arms or legs, are getting worse, you may need surgery.

The procedure your surgeon recommends may depend on your underlying condition, such as the presence of bone spurs or spinal stenosis.

The most common surgical options include:
- **Frontal approach (anterior).** Your surgeon makes an incision in the front of your neck and moves aside the windpipe (trachea) and swallowing tube (esophagus) to expose the cervical spine. Your surgeon can then remove a herniated disk or bone spurs, depending on the underlying problem. Sometimes, with disk removal, a surgeon will fill the gap with a graft of bone or other implant.

  With the anterior approach, your surgeon can relieve pressure on your spinal cord from bone or from multiple disk protrusions by removing two disks and the bone between them (corpectomy). Then, to support your head and neck, your surgeon reconstructs the area with bone from your body or a bone bank or with an implant made of metal combined with bone.
- **Back approach (posterior).** Your surgeon may opt to remove or rearrange bone from the back of your neck, especially if several portions of the channel that houses the cord have narrowed. The operation, called a laminectomy, removes the back part of the bone over the spinal canal through an incision in the back of your neck. Laminoplasty, an alternative to laminectomy, involves cutting and moving pieces of vertebrae to make more room for the spinal cord. Although laminoplasty takes longer, it is less likely to leave the neck unstable.

Peripheral neuropathy

Signs and symptoms
- Gradual onset of numbness and tingling in your feet or hands, which may spread upward into your legs and arms
- Burning pain
- Sharp, jabbing or electric-like pain
- Extreme sensitivity to touch, even light touch
- Lack of coordination
- Muscle weakness or paralysis if motor nerves are affected
- Bowel or bladder problems if autonomic nerves are affected

Peripheral neuropathy, in its most common form, causes pain and numbness in your hands and feet. The pain typically is described as tingling or burning, while the loss of sensation often is compared to the feeling of wearing a thin stocking or glove.

Peripheral neuropathy can result from such problems as traumatic injuries, infections, metabolic problems and exposure to toxins. One of the most common causes of the disorder is diabetes.

Your nervous system is divided into two broad categories. Your central nervous system consists of your brain and spinal cord. All the other nerves in your body are part of your peripheral nervous system, which includes:
- Sensory nerves to receive feelings such as heat, pain or touch
- Motor nerves that control how your muscles move
- Autonomic nerves that control such automatic functions as blood pressure, heart rate, digestion and bladder function

Most commonly, peripheral neuropathy begins in the longest nerves — the ones that reach to your toes. Specific symptoms vary, depending on which types of nerves are affected.

Signs and symptoms of peripheral neuropathy usually progress over many months, but in certain cases, such as Guillain-Barré syndrome, the onset may be abrupt.

A tingling sensation (paresthesia) usually begins in your toes or the balls of your feet and spreads upward. Occasionally, it begins in your hands and extends up your arms. Numbness may proceed in the same way. Your skin may become sensitive, and even the lightest touch can be painful. In some peripheral neuropathies, weakness may come before or may be more noticeable than the sensory signs and symptoms.

Diagnosis

Peripheral neuropathy has many potential causes. For that reason it can be difficult to diagnose. To help in the diagnosis, your doctor will likely take a full medical history and perform a physical and neurological exam that may include checking your tendon reflexes, your muscle strength and tone, your ability to feel certain sensations, and your posture and coordination. Often the disorder is inherited, so it's important to let your doctor know if immediate family members have similar symptoms.

Your doctor may also request blood tests to check your level of vitamin B-12, a urinalysis, thyroid function tests and, often, electromyography — a test that measures the electrical discharges produced in your muscles. As a part of this test, you'll be asked to have a nerve conduction study, which measures how quickly your nerves carry electrical signals. A nerve conduction study is often used to diagnose carpal tunnel syndrome and other peripheral nerve disorders.

Your doctor may recommend a nerve biopsy, a procedure in which a small portion of a nerve is removed and examined for abnormalities. But even a nerve biopsy may not always reveal what's damaging your nerves.

How serious is peripheral neuropathy?

In contrast to the nerves in your central nervous system, peripheral nerves may regenerate with proper care. In some disorders, recovery occurs, but signs and symptoms may recur if the cause isn't eliminated.

Damage to the nerves in your feet increase the risk of pressure-related injuries and, along with poor circulation, can lead to skin ulcers and even gangrene.

Treatment

The first goal of treatment is to manage the condition causing your neuropathy. If the underlying cause is corrected, the neuropathy often improves on its own. The second goal of treatment is to relieve the painful symptoms. Many types of medications can be used to relieve the pain of peripheral neuropathy.

- **Pain relievers.** Mild symptoms may be relieved by over-the-counter pain medications. For more-severe symptoms, your doctor may recommend prescription painkillers. Drugs containing opiates, such as codeine, can lead to dependence, constipation or sedation, so these drugs are prescribed only when other treatments fail.
- **Anti-seizure medications.** Drugs such as gabapentin (Neurontin, Horizant), pregabalin (Lyrica), carbamazepine (Tegretol, Carbatrol) and phenytoin (Dilantin, Phenytek) were originally developed to treat epilepsy. However, doctors also prescribe them for nerve pain. Side effects may include drowsiness and dizziness.
- **Lidocaine patch.** It contains the topical anesthetic lidocaine. You apply it to the area where your pain is most severe, and you can use up to three patches a day to relieve pain. This treatment has almost no side effects except, for some people, a rash at the site of the patch.
- **Antidepressants.** Tricyclic antidepressant medications, such as amitriptyline and nortriptyline (Pamelor), were originally developed to treat depression. However, they have been found to help relieve pain by interfering with chemical processes in your brain and spinal cord that cause you to feel pain. The selective serotonin and norepinephrine reuptake inhibitor duloxetine (Cymbalta) also has proved effective for peripheral neuropathy caused by diabetes.

Guillain-Barré syndrome

Signs and symptoms
- Numbness and tingling beginning in the fingers or toes
- Muscle weakness
- Difficulty with eye movement, facial movement, speaking, chewing or swallowing
- Severe pain in the lower back
- Difficulty with bladder control or intestinal functions

Emergency signs and symptoms
- Widespread tingling and numbness
- Difficulty breathing

Guillain-Barré syndrome is an uncommon inflammatory disorder in which your body's immune system attacks your nerves, typically causing severe weakness and numbness that usually starts in your extremities and quickly worsens over hours to days. Eventually your whole body can become paralyzed, even the muscles used for breathing.

The exact cause of Guillain-Barré syndrome is still unknown. In a number of the cases, an infection affecting either the lungs or the digestive tract precedes the disorder. But scientists don't know why such an infection can lead to Guillain-Barré syndrome for some people and not for others.

The most common triggering factor for Guillain-Barré syndrome appears to be infection with campylobacter, a type of bacteria commonly found in undercooked food, especially poultry. Guillain-Barré may also be triggered by surgery and, in very rare cases, influenza immunizations. Many cases appear to occur without any identifiable triggers.

In Guillain-Barré syndrome, your immune system — which usually only attacks foreign material and invading organisms — begins attacking the nerves that carry signals between your body and your brain. Specifically, the nerves' protective covering (myelin sheath) is damaged and this interferes with the signaling process, causing weakness, numbness or paralysis.

Diagnosis

A diagnosis of Guillain-Barré syndrome is generally based on signs and symptoms, a physical examination and diagnostic tests, including an analysis of cerebrospinal fluid obtained by a spinal tap (see page 542).

How serious is Guillain-Barré syndrome?

In its most severe form, Guillain-Barré syndrome is a medical emergency that requires hospitalization. Some people with Guillain-Barré syndrome need respiratory assistance at some point during the illness. The majority of individuals affected recover completely over a period of months. If you're severely affected, you'll likely need long-term rehabilitation to regain your independence. Some permanent impairment may remain in about 15 to 20 percent of cases.

Treatment

There's no cure for Guillain-Barré syndrome. But two treatments have been shown to speed the recovery from and reduce the severity of the disorder:

- **Plasmapheresis.** This treatment — also known as plasma exchange — is a type of "blood cleansing" in which damaging antibodies are removed from your blood. Plasmapheresis consists of removing the liquid portion of your blood (plasma) and separating it from the actual blood cells. The blood cells are then put back into your body, which manufactures more plasma to make up for what was removed. It's not clear why this treatment works, but scientists believe that plasmapheresis rids plasma of certain antibodies that contribute to the immune system attack on the peripheral nerves.
- **Intravenous immunoglobulin.** Immunoglobulin contains healthy antibodies from blood donors. High doses of immunoglobulin can block the damaging antibodies that may contribute to Guillain-Barré syndrome.

Each of these treatments is equally effective. Mixing the treatments or administering one after the other is no more effective than using either method alone.

Although some people can take months and even years to recover, most cases of Guillain-Barré syndrome follow this general timeline:

- Following the first symptoms, the condition tends to progressively worsen for about two weeks.
- Symptoms reach a plateau and remain steady for two to four weeks.
- Recovery begins.

Treatment with plasmapheresis or intravenous immunoglobulin can shorten the time period before

---

INTEGRATIVE MEDICINE

Several drug-free therapies and techniques may help relieve pain associated with peripheral neuropathy. These therapies are frequently used in conjunction with medications, but some may be effective on their own. Integrative therapies used in the treatment of peripheral neuropathy include:

- Biofeedback
- Acupuncture
- Hypnosis
- Relaxation techniques

For information on these therapies, see Chapter 37, "Pain Management," and Chapter 38, "Integrative Medicine."

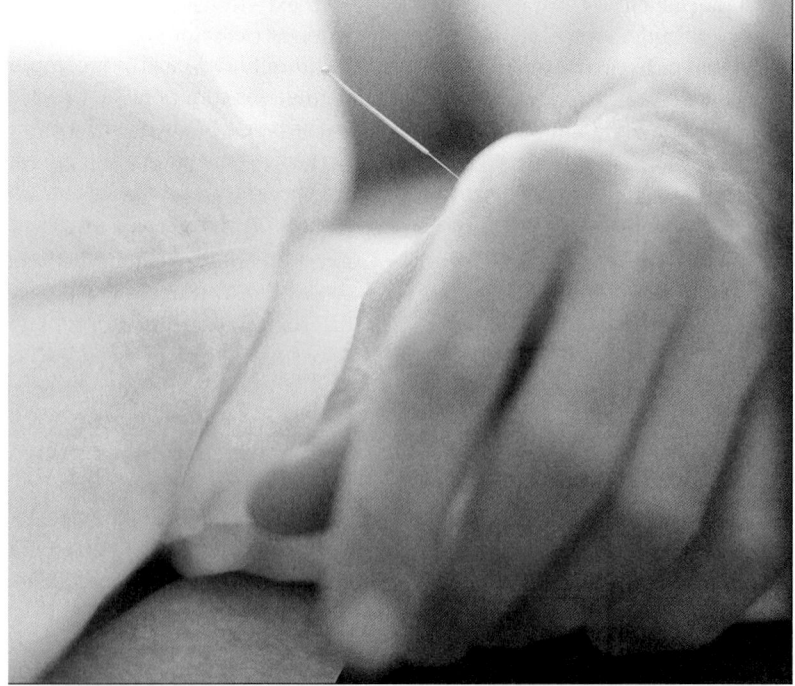

recovery begins by as much as 50 percent.

Before recovery begins, caregivers may need to manually move your arms and legs to help keep your muscles flexible and strong. After recovery has begun, you'll likely need physical therapy to help regain strength and proper movement.

Charcot-Marie-Tooth disease

Signs and symptoms
- Weakness in the legs and, to a lesser degree, the arms
- Absence of muscle-stretch reflex
- Foot deformity

Charcot-Marie-Tooth disease is a broad term for a group of hereditary disorders caused by degeneration of peripheral nerve fibers or the insulating covering (myelin sheath) over the fibers. The disease is named after the three doctors who simultaneously described it over a century ago — Jean Martin Charcot, Pierre Marie and Howard Henry Tooth.

The disorder most often affects the legs, feet and hands. It generally results in muscle weakness and loss of muscle bulk. In some cases, it may cause a mild loss of sensation. Initial signs include foot abnormalities, such as an excessively high arch or flexed toes. It may be difficult to lift your foot.

Signs and symptoms frequently become obvious between mid-childhood and age 30, but they may also appear late in life. They tend to develop slowly and sometimes appear to stabilize spontaneously. The disorder affects approximately 1 in 2,500 people in the United States. Usually, individuals with the disorder don't experience nerve pain.

Diagnosis
A diagnosis of Charcot-Marie-Tooth disease generally includes a physical and neurological examination, electromyography and, rarely, a biopsy of a nerve in the leg. Genetic tests are now available that may help diagnose some of these neuropathies. Electromyography and nerve conduction studies can help guide which genetic test to order.

How serious is Charcot-Marie-Tooth disease?
The disorder isn't life-threatening. The severity of signs and symptoms varies from person to person, but foot abnormalities and difficulty walking are generally the most serious problems. Only rarely is a wheelchair necessary. Most people with this disorder can lead active, vigorous lives.

Treatment
Vocational counseling or leg braces may be needed. Some individuals may require an orthopedic operation or corrective shoes to improve walking. Future treatment could possibly include use of gene replacement therapy.

Syringomyelia

Signs and symptoms
- Gradual loss of sensation in the nape of the neck, shoulders and upper arms
- Weakness of the arms or legs

In syringomyelia, a fluid-filled cavity forms on the spinal cord, usually in the neck area. The cavity may gradually expand along the spinal cord. Pressure from the cavity may damage the cord, producing various signs and symptoms. Initially, the sense of heat or touch may be reduced, followed by the wasting of muscles.

Syringomyelia may result from spinal cord trauma, a tumor or a congenital defect that triggers the disease.

Diagnosis
A neurological examination by a doctor can reveal loss of sensation or movement. Magnetic resonance imaging (MRI) is the best test to determine the severity and location of the cavity.

How serious is syringomyelia?
Often, the progression of signs and symptoms is slow, but if untreated, severe disability can develop.

Treatment
Surgical therapy to drain the cavity and decompress the spinal cord frequently stops progression of the disorder. About half the individuals with syringomyelia improve significantly after the operation.

Myelomeningocele

Signs and symptoms
- A sac protruding from the spinal cord on a newborn's back
- Weakness of the lower limbs

Myelomeningocele (open spina bifida) is a congenital defect that leaves a baby's spinal canal open along several vertebrae in the lower or middle back. It's a severe form of spina bifida, a condition where a baby's neural tube — the embryonic structure that develops into the spinal cord — fails to develop or close properly.

In myelomeningocele, the spinal cord and membranes protrude at birth because of the opening, forming a sac on the baby's back. In some cases, skin covers the sac. In other cases, tissues and nerves are directly exposed, making the baby prone to life-threatening infections. Either partial or complete paralysis is common.

The cause of the disorder is unknown, although factors that may increase risk of myelomeningocele include a neural tube defect in a previous child, lack of folic acid during pregnancy, certain anti-seizure medications and diabetes.

Diagnosis
The condition is apparent at birth. In some cases, prenatal testing to check for spina bifida may be warranted.

How serious is myelomeningocele?
Most babies survive, although they may experience physical and

neurological problems, including lack of normal bowel and bladder control, and partial or complete paralysis of the legs. Most babies born with myelomeningocele also have excess fluid in the brain (hydrocephalus).

Children with both myelomeningocele and hydrocephalus may have learning disabilities. Other congenital malformations are often associated with myelomeningocele, such as syringomyelia, clubfoot or hip dislocation. Meningitis can occur with a leaking sac, so this defect should be promptly treated with surgery.

Treatment

Myelomeningocele usually requires surgery within hours to days after birth. Early surgery can help minimize the risk of infection associated with exposed nerves. It may also help protect the spinal cord from additional trauma.

During the procedure, a neurosurgeon places the spinal cord and exposed tissue inside the body and covers them with muscle and skin. Sometimes, a ventriculoperitoneal shunt, a tube that allows fluid in the brain to drain into the abdomen, is placed during the operation on the spinal cord. At times, the shunt placement isn't needed until weeks to months later.

Paralysis and bladder and bowel problems usually occur with this disorder. Treatment for those conditions usually begins soon after birth.

In case of partial paralysis, special exercises that work the baby's legs and feet may be prescribed. They help prepare the child for walking with braces or crutches when he or she is older.

Many babies with myelomeningocele have spinal cords that are less able to properly expand in length as they grow. This progressive tethering can cause loss of muscle function to the legs, bowel or bladder. Spinal cord surgery may allow the child to regain a normal level of functioning.

Postherpetic neuralgia

Signs and symptoms

- Sharp and jabbing, burning, or deep and aching pain
- Extreme sensitivity to touch and temperature change
- Itching and numbness
- Headaches

Postherpetic neuralgia is a painful condition affecting your nerve fibers and skin. Postherpetic neuralgia is a complication of shingles, a second outbreak of the varicella-zoster virus, which initially causes chickenpox.

During an initial infection of chickenpox, some of the virus remains in your body, lying dormant inside nerve cells. Years later, the virus may reactivate, causing shingles.

Once reactivated, the virus travels along nerve fibers, causing pain. When the virus reaches your skin, it produces a rash and blisters. A case of shingles (herpes zoster) usually heals within a month. But some people continue to feel pain long after the rash and blisters heal — a pain called postherpetic neuralgia.

Postherpetic neuralgia results when nerve fibers are damaged during an outbreak of shingles. Damaged nerves aren't able to send messages from your skin to your brain as they normally do. Instead, the messages become confused and exaggerated, causing chronic, often excruciating pain that may persist for months — or even years — in the area where shingles first occurred.

This complication of shingles occurs much more frequently in older adults. About half of adults older than age 60 experience postherpetic neuralgia after shingles, whereas only 10 percent of all people with shingles do.

Diagnosis

The disorder is usually diagnosed based on your symptoms and having had a recent outbreak of shingles.

How serious is postherpetic neuralgia?

Although the pain may be severe at times and bothersome, the condition isn't life-threatening. Although some people must live with postherpetic neuralgia the rest of their lives, most people can expect the condition to gradually disappear during the first three months. For about 15 percent of people with postherpetic neuralgia, the pain may persist for a year or more.

Treatment

Finding an effective treatment to relieve the pain can sometimes be frustrating. You may have to work with your doctor and sometimes other specialists to try a variety of treatments before you find something that helps. Possible options include:

- **Antidepressants.** Your doctor may prescribe antidepressants for postherpetic neuralgia, even if you're not depressed. These drugs affect key brain chemicals, including serotonin and norepinephrine, which play a role in both depression and how your body interprets pain. Doctors typically prescribe antidepressants for postherpetic neuralgia in smaller doses than they do for depression. Drugs that inhibit the reuptake of norepinephrine and serotonin — including tricyclic antidepressants, such as amitriptyline, desipramine (Norpramin), nortriptyline (Pamelor) and duloxetine (Cymbalta) — may not eliminate the pain, but they can make it more tolerable.
- **Certain anticonvulsants.** Medications for treatment of seizures also can lessen the pain associated with postherpetic neuralgia. These medications stabilize abnormal electrical activity in your nervous system caused by injured nerves. Doctors may prescribe gabapentin (Gralise, Neurontin), pregabalin (Lyrica) or another anticonvulsant to help control burning and pain.

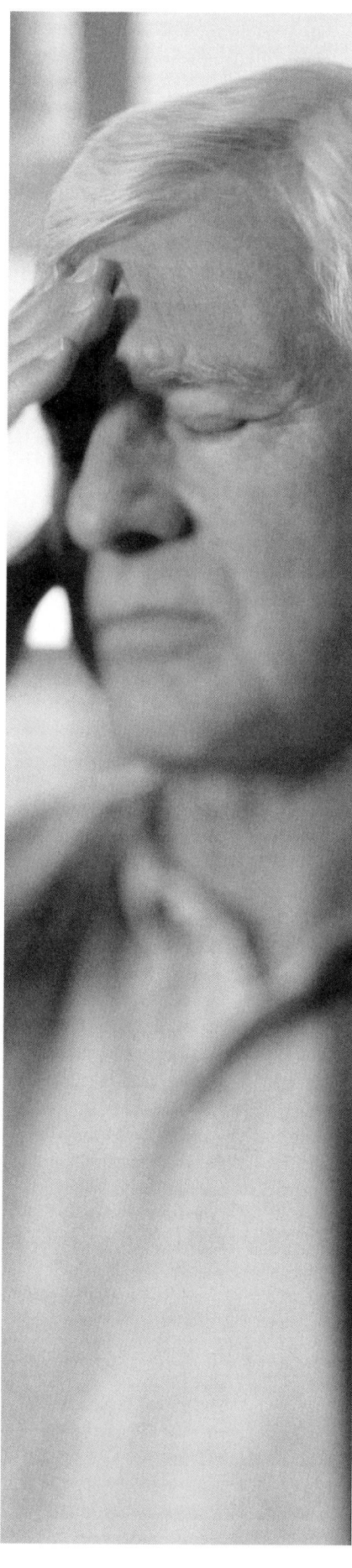

- **Injected steroids.** Corticosteroid medications injected into the area around the spinal cord may help relieve the persistent pain of postherpetic neuralgia. This treatment is usually reserved until after the pustular skin rash associated with shingles has gone away.
- **Painkillers.** Your doctor may prescribe painkillers such as tramadol (Ultram) or drugs containing oxycodone, either in short-acting formulations such as Percocet or in long-acting formulations such as OxyContin. However, these drugs are narcotics and can be addictive. Although this risk is generally low, discuss it with your doctor.
- **Transcutaneous electrical nerve stimulation (TENS).** This treatment involves the placement of electrodes over the painful area. The electrodes deliver tiny, painless electrical impulses to nearby nerve pathways. You turn the TENS unit on and off as needed to control pain. Exactly how the impulses relieve pain is uncertain. One theory is that the impulses stimulate production of endorphins, your body's natural painkillers. This treatment doesn't work for everyone.
- **Spinal cord or peripheral nerve stimulation.** These devices are similar to TENS, but are implanted underneath the skin. Like with TENS units, you can turn these units on and off as needed to control pain. Before the device is surgically implanted, doctors do a trial using a thin wire electrode. The trial is done to ensure that the stimulator will provide effective pain relief. The electrode is inserted through your skin into the epidural space over the spinal cord for a spinal cord stimulator or under your skin above a peripheral nerve in the case of a peripheral nerve stimulator. If a permanent stimulator is implanted, the stimulator's pulse generator is placed under the skin, usually in the upper buttocks, but occasionally in other locations. Some areas, such as your chest, abdomen and some areas of your face, are less amenable to treatment using this method.
- **Lidocaine skin patches.** These are small, bandage-like patches that contain the topical, pain-relieving medication lidocaine. These patches can be cut to fit the affected area. You apply the patches, available by prescription, directly to painful skin to deliver temporary relief. Don't use patches containing lidocaine on your face.

Prevention

Two vaccines are now available that may help prevent shingles and subsequent postherpetic neuralgia — the chickenpox (varicella) vaccine and the shingles (varicella-zoster) vaccine.

Trigeminal neuralgia

Signs and symptoms
- Occasional twinges of mild pain
- Episodes of severe, shooting or jabbing pain that may feel like an electric shock
- Spontaneous attacks of pain or attacks triggered by things such as touching the face, chewing, speaking and brushing teeth
- Bouts of pain lasting from a few seconds to several seconds
- Episodes of several attacks lasting days, weeks, months or longer — some people have periods when they experience no pain
- Pain in areas supplied by the trigeminal nerve (nerve branches), including the cheek, jaw, teeth, gums, lips, or less often the eye and forehead

Imagine having a jab of lightning-like pain shoot through your face when you brush your teeth or put on makeup. Sound excruciating? If you have trigeminal neuralgia, attacks of such pain may occur frequently.

You may initially experience short, mild attacks, but trigeminal neuralgia can progress, causing longer, more frequent bouts of searing pain. These attacks can be spontaneous or provoked by even mild stimulation of your face.

The trigeminal nerve carries sensation from your face to your brain. In trigeminal neuralgia, also called tic douloureux, the nerve's function is disrupted. Usually, the problem is contact between a normal artery or vein and the trigeminal nerve, at the base of your brain. This contact puts pressure on the nerve, causing it to malfunction.

Trigeminal neuralgia can occur as a result of aging, or it can be related to multiple sclerosis or a similar disorder that damages the myelin sheath protecting certain nerves. Less commonly, trigeminal neuralgia can be caused by a tumor compressing the trigeminal nerve. In other cases, a cause cannot be found.

Diagnosis

Your doctor will review your medical history and ask you to describe your pain — how severe it is, what part of your face it affects, how long it lasts and what seems to trigger it. You'll also undergo a neurological examination, during which your doctor examines and touches parts of your face to try to determine exactly where the pain is occurring and — if you appear to have trigeminal neuralgia — which branches of the trigeminal nerve may be affected.

You may need to have a magnetic resonance imaging (MRI) scan of your head, which can show if multiple sclerosis is causing trigeminal neuralgia.

Facial pain can be caused by many different disorders, so an accurate diagnosis is important. Your doctor may order additional tests to rule out other conditions.

How serious is trigeminal neuralgia?

Although your pain may be incapacitating, the condition isn't life-threatening. Your attacks may come and go variably, but the time between them may grow shorter as you get older.

Treatment

Medications are usually the first treatment for trigeminal neuralgia, and many people are successfully treated with medication and require no surgical treatment. However, over time, some people with the disorder eventually stop responding to medications, or they experience unpleasant side effects. For these individuals, injections or surgery may provide other treatment options.

Medications

Medications to lessen or block the pain signals sent to your brain are the most common initial treatment for trigeminal neuralgia.

- **Anticonvulsants.** Carbamazepine (Tegretol, Carbatrol), phenytoin (Dilantin, Phenytek) and oxcarbazepine (Trileptal) are the most common anticonvulsant medications used to treat trigeminal neuralgia. Other anticonvulsants include lamotrigine (Lamictal) or gabapentin (Neurontin, Horizant). If the anticonvulsant you're using begins to lose effectiveness, your doctor may increase the dose or switch to another type.

   Side effects of anticonvulsants may include dizziness, confusion, drowsiness, double vision and nausea. Anticonvulsants have been linked to an increased risk of suicidal thoughts and behavior, so be sure to monitor your mood closely if you're taking an anticonvulsant for the first time. Also, carbamazepine can trigger a serious drug reaction in some people, mainly individuals of Asian descent, so genetic testing may be recommended before you start carbamazepine.

- **Antispasticity agents.** Muscle-relaxing agents such as baclofen may be used alone or in combination with carbamazepine or phenytoin. Side effects may include confusion, nausea and drowsiness.

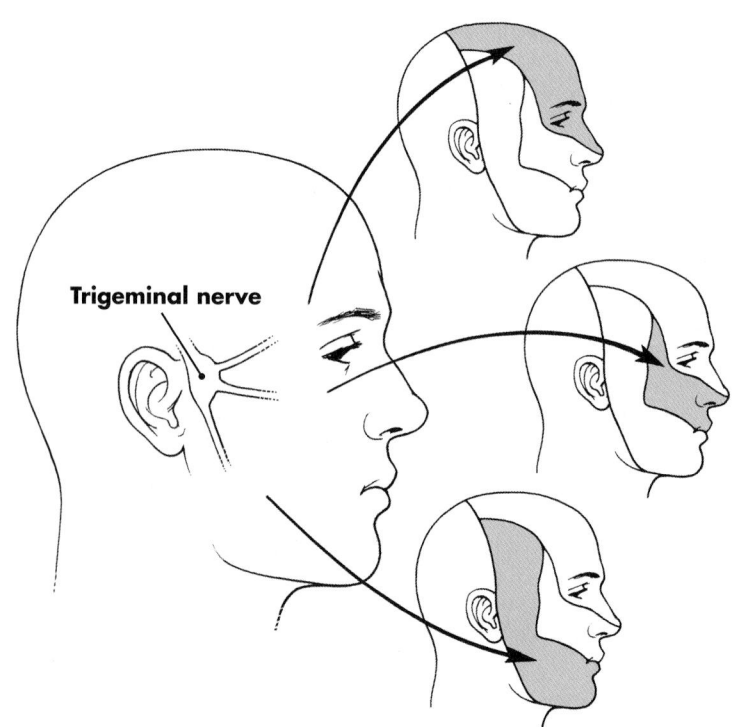

Trigeminal nerve

If you have trigeminal neuralgia, pain may occur in areas supplied by one of the three branches of the fifth cranial (trigeminal) nerve.

Alcohol injection

Alcohol injections provide temporary pain relief by numbing the affected areas of your face. Your doctor will inject alcohol into the part of your face corresponding to the trigeminal nerve branch causing pain. The pain relief isn't permanent, so you may need repeated injections or a different procedure in the future.

Surgery

The goal of surgery for trigeminal neuralgia is either to stop the blood vessel from compressing the trigeminal nerve, or to damage the trigeminal nerve to keep it from malfunctioning. Damaging the nerve often causes temporary or permanent facial numbness, and with any of the surgical procedures, the pain can return months or years later.

Surgical options include:

- **Microvascular decompression (MVD).** Instead of damaging the trigeminal nerve, MVD involves relocating or removing blood vessels that are in contact with the trigeminal root, and separating the nerve root and blood vessels.

  During MVD, your doctor makes an incision behind the ear on the side of your pain. Then, through a small hole in your skull, part of your brain is lifted to expose the trigeminal nerve. Any artery in contact with the nerve root is directed away from the nerve, and the surgeon places a pad between the nerve and the artery. If a vein is compressing the nerve, the surgeon typically will remove it. If no artery or vein appears to be compressing the nerve, your surgeon may sever the nerve instead.

  MVD can successfully eliminate or reduce pain most of the time, but pain can recur in some people. While MVD has a high success rate, it also carries risks. There are small chances of decreased hearing, facial weak-

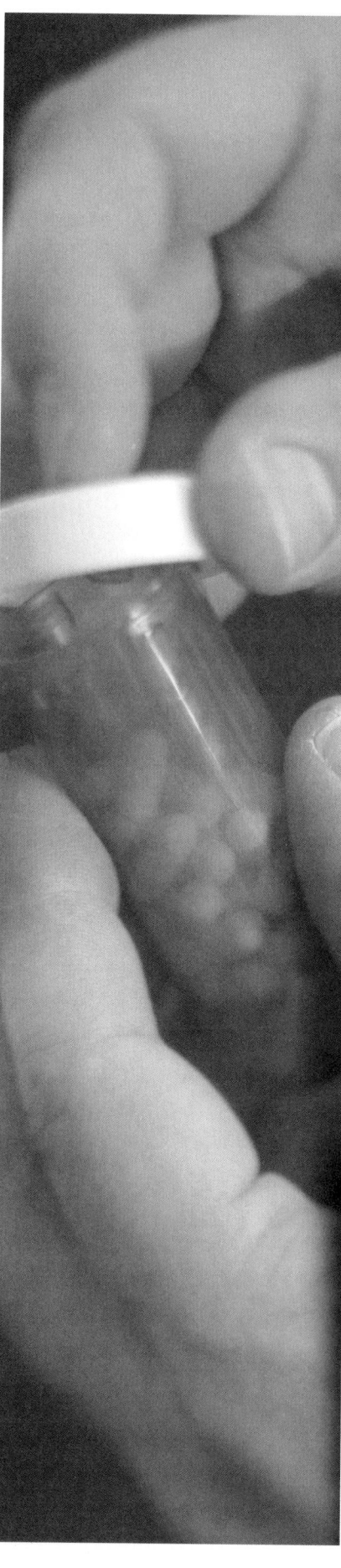

ness, facial numbness, double vision, and even a stroke or death. Since MVD doesn't damage the trigeminal nerve, most people who have this procedure have no facial numbness afterward.

- **Glycerol injection.** During this procedure, called percutaneous glycerol rhizotomy (PGR), your doctor inserts a needle through your face and into an opening in the base of your skull. The needle is guided into the trigeminal cistern, a small sac of spinal fluid that surrounds the trigeminal nerve ganglion — where the trigeminal nerve divides into three branches — and part of its root. Images are made to confirm that the needle is in the proper location, and then a small amount of sterile glycerol is injected. After three or four hours, the glycerol damages the trigeminal nerve and blocks pain signals. Initially, PGR relieves pain in most people. However, some people have a later recurrence of pain, and many experience facial numbness or tingling.

- **Balloon compression.** In percutaneous balloon compression of the trigeminal nerve (PBCTN), your doctor inserts a hollow needle through your face and into an opening in the base of your skull. Then, a thin, flexible tube (catheter) with a balloon on the end is threaded through the needle. The balloon is inflated with enough pressure to damage the nerve and block pain signals. PBCTN successfully controls pain in most people, at least for a while. Most people undergoing PBCTN experience some facial numbness, and more than half experience temporary or permanent weakness of the muscles used to chew.

- **Electric current.** Percutaneous stereotactic radiofrequency thermal rhizotomy (PSRTR) selectively destroys nerve fibers associated with pain. While you're sedated, your doctor places a hollow needle through your face and into an opening in your skull. Once the needle is positioned, an electrode is threaded through it to the nerve root. You're then awakened from sedation so that you can indicate when and where you feel tingling from the mild current pulsed through the tip of the electrode. When the neurosurgeon locates the part of the nerve involved in your pain, you are returned to sedation. Then the electrode is heated until it damages the nerve fibers, creating an area of injury (lesion). If your pain isn't eliminated, your doctor may create additional lesions. Almost everyone who undergoes PSR-TR has some facial numbness after the procedure.

- **Severing the nerve.** A procedure called partial sensory rhizotomy involves cutting part of the trigeminal nerve at the base of your brain. Through an incision behind your ear, your doctor makes a quarter-sized hole in your skull to access the nerve. Because it cuts the nerve at its source, your face will be numb permanently. In some cases, instead of cutting the nerve the surgeon will choose to traumatize the nerve by rubbing it.

- **Radiation.** Gamma Knife radiosurgery involves delivering a focused, high dose of radiation to the root of the trigeminal nerve. The radiation damages the trigeminal nerve and reduces or eliminates the pain. Relief occurs gradually and can take several weeks to begin. Gamma Knife radiosurgery is successful in eliminating pain for the majority of people, but sometimes the pain may recur. The procedure is painless and typically is done without anesthesia. Because this procedure is relatively new, the long-term risks aren't yet known. ■

Eyes and Vision

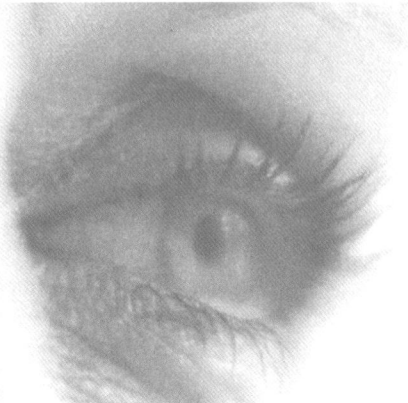

581

Your eyes are a small part of your body, but they play a large role in your life. They're exceptional and unique instruments, able to receive in an instant millions of unrelated pieces of information about the world around you. With your eyes you experience the shape, color and motion of your surroundings.

The eye is often compared to a camera, and there are some similarities. Like a camera, the eye lets light enter through a small opening. An adjustable lens focuses the light onto a layer of light-sensitive cells at the back of the eyeball, comparable to the light-sensitive film in a camera.

This comparison, however, doesn't do justice to your eyes. They're far more complex and sophisticated than any technology developed. Thousands of times a day, your eyes move and focus on images near and far, picking out objects for inspection and interpretation from a vast available field.

Parts of the Eye

The eye is composed of many intricate parts. Each one plays an essential role in the healthy functioning of the eye.

Orbit

Your eyes are cradled in sockets formed by a protective structure of bone known as orbits. The orbits include portions of the bones of the cheek, forehead, temple and nose. Unlike many other bones in your body, these eye protectors usually don't weaken or thin with age. Small deposits of fat cushion the eyeball within the orbit.

The upper and lower eyelids help protect the front of your eyeball by blocking dirt and bright light that can damage your eyes. The eyelids also lubricate your eyeball during each blink. Blinking washes away dust, pollen

and other foreign bodies. The lubricant, familiar to you as tears, comes from lacrimal glands above each eye. Tears drain from each eye into your nose through a tiny opening close to where the eyelids join your nose. From this opening, tears are channeled to your nose by the nasolacrimal ducts.

Sclera

When you look in the mirror and see the white of your eye, you're looking at the sclera. This tough, white, leathery coating forms the circular eyeball shape and protects the eye's delicate internal structures. The sclera has an opening at the front (pupil) that allows light to enter the eyeball.

A thin, moist, clear membrane called the conjunctiva covers the exposed front portion of the sclera. This tissue layer also lines the inside of your eyelids. The conjunctiva helps lubricate your eye.

Cornea

At the front of your eye, covering the opening in the sclera, is a domed layer of clear tissue called the cornea. The cornea juts out from the eyeball as a tiny bulge. Its convex surface bends the light as it enters the eye, helping to focus the images you see. The cornea, in fact, provides about two-thirds of the focusing power of the eye.

The cornea also protects your eye. It's packed with sensitive nerve endings. If even a tiny speck of dust hits the cornea, you feel it instantly. If tears can't wash away the foreign material, continuing pain prods you to locate and remove the material.

Pupil

The pupil lies behind the cornea. The pupil is the dark spot in the center of your eye. It's through the pupil that light passes into your eye.

Sclera
Cornea
Pupil
Iris
Lens
Retina
Choroid
Optic nerve
Macula
Optic nerve head (disk)
Vitreous cavity

Pupil
Iris
Sclera

The eye is a complex and compact structure measuring about 1 inch in diameter. Yet in an instant, the eye can receive millions of pieces of information about the outside world, which are quickly processed by the brain.

Iris

Surrounding the pupil is the iris, the colored part of the eye. Its color comes from a pigment called melanin in the iris tissue. The more pigment, the darker the color. Brown eyes have a lot of pigment. Blue or green eyes have less. Blue eyes are relatively new, due to a gene mutation that occurred 8,000 to 10,000 years ago. Prior to that, all eyes were brown.

In addition to adding color to your eye, the iris contains a ring of muscle fibers that can expand or contract the size of the pupil to control the amount of light that enters the eyeball. In bright light, the iris reduces the size of the pupil. When the light is dim, the iris enlarges the pupil to let in more light.

The space between your cornea and iris is called the anterior chamber. It's filled with a clear fluid called the aqueous humor, which nourishes the cornea and lens, removes waste products, and plays an important role in maintaining normal pressure in the eye. Fluid is continuously produced and circulated through the anterior chamber before draining out of the eye.

Lens

Behind the iris and anterior chamber is the lens, a clear elliptical structure. A circular muscle surrounds the lens. By relaxing or contracting, this muscle changes the lens' curvature to sharpen the focus of whatever you're looking at. When an object is nearby, the muscle contracts and the lens thickens. When an object is farther away, the muscle relaxes and the lens becomes thin. These adjustments allow the lens to change its focusing power. With age, the lens loses its elasticity, making it more difficult for you to focus on close objects.

Vitreous cavity

The vitreous cavity extends from the back of the lens to the retina, which covers the back of the eyeball. The cavity is filled with a colorless, gelatinous substance called vitreous humor. Both the aqueous humor in the anterior chamber and the vitreous humor maintain the pressure and shape of the eyeball.

You may occasionally notice what looks like tiny bits of string or lint moving through your vision. These "floaters" are tiny bits of material suspended in the otherwise clear vitreous humor. Usually, floaters are a result of aging, but they can be a sign of a more serious eye disorder.

Retina

Lining the interior back wall of the eyeball is a thin layer of tissue called the retina. The retina consists of millions of light-sensitive cells and nerve connections that capture the images focused by the cornea and lens.

The light-sensitive cells are shaped like either rods or cones. There are about 20 rod cells for every cone cell. Rod cells allow you to see in dim light, and they assist with your ability to see to the side while looking ahead (peripheral vision), but they can't distinguish colors. Cone cells distinguish color but require more light to function. This is why it can be hard to detect color in dim light. Cone cells are concentrated in the center of the retina and allow you to see sharp detail when looking straight ahead at a well-lit object.

Light striking the rods and cones triggers a chemical reaction. This in turn generates electric impulses that are relayed through the optic nerve and beyond to the visual cortex, the seeing portion of your brain.

The outer portion of the retina is nourished mainly by a layer of arteries and veins called the choroid, which is sandwiched between the retina and sclera. The inner part of the retina receives its nutrition from retinal blood vessels.

Macula and fovea

At the center of the retina is the macula, a small area that's densely packed with cone cells. The macula provides your central vision and allows you to see fine detail. A small depression in the center of the macula, called the fovea, contains only cone cells and provides the sharpest vision.

Optic nerve

Visual information gathered by the retina is transmitted along nerve fibers to the optic nerve, a bundle of more than 1 million nerve fibers that connects the rear of the retina to the brain. The optic nerve serves as a communication pathway between the eyes and brain.

Muscles of the eyeball

Each eye has six muscles attached to the sclera, allowing you to move both eyes and track an object without necessarily turning your head. These eye muscles, working independently or together, allow you to shift your visual field left, right, up, down, around and diagonally. Your brain coordinates these muscles so both eyes move in unison.

How you see

A listing of all of the eye's parts may make the organ seem complicated. Yet the basic mechanism of sight is relatively simple.

Rays of light project through the cornea, the pupil and then the lens. Internal eye muscles help adjust the shape of the lens to focus the light rays on the retina. There, rods and cones turn the light into electrical impulses that are carried by the optic nerve to the brain.

A special part of the brain — the visual cortex — interprets the electrical impulses. The image that the retina receives is upside-down and reversed — just like it is in a camera — because of the optical properties of the cornea and lens. The brain reinterprets the information so that you see the images in their correct orientation. The brain also processes the separate images from each eye and produces a three-dimensional (3-D) image.

Common Vision Problems

You can see an object clearly only when it's properly focused. If the focusing powers of the cornea and lens aren't coordinated with the length or shape of the eyeball, the image is blurry.

The most common eye problems — nearsightedness, farsightedness, astigmatism and presbyopia — are due either to errors of refraction of the lens and cornea or to an abnormal eye shape. Most of these conditions can be corrected with eyeglasses, contact lenses or surgery that changes the curvature of the cornea (refractive surgery).

Nearsightedness

Signs and symptoms
• Distant objects appear blurry
Nearsightedness (myopia) affects about 30 percent of the population. With this condition you can see clearly objects that are near to you, but objects farther away are blurry. If you're nearsighted, your eye is probably too long from front to back, causing the light rays refracted by the cornea and lens to meet in front of — rather than on — the retina.

The degree of your nearsightedness determines your focusing ability. People who are severely nearsighted are able to see clearly only objects that are a few inches from their eyes. Individuals who are mildly nearsighted may see clearly objects that are several yards away.

Occasionally, nearsightedness results not from an elongated eyeball but from too much focusing power in the lens and cornea. The result is the same — the light rays focus in front of the retina.

Nearsightedness often is first detected during childhood, from early school years through the later teens. A child may persistently squint, sit close to the television, movie screen or class chalkboard, hold books very close while reading, and seem to be unaware of distant objects. The condition affects boys and girls equally and tends to run in families. Changes in vision may develop rapidly or slowly and gradually worsen during childhood and adolescence. The condition tends to stabilize during young adulthood.

Treatment
Nearsightedness is easily corrected. An eye specialist will perform a series of tests to determine the extent of the condition and the level of correction needed. Nearsightedness may be treated with eyeglasses or contact lenses. Another option is refractive surgery (see page 593).

Normal Vision

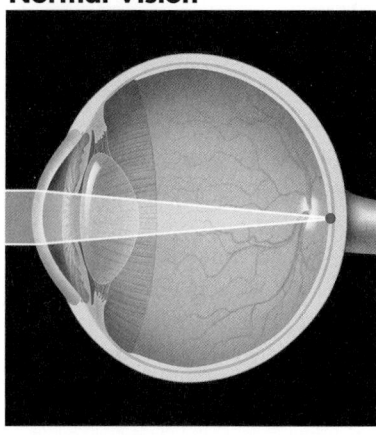

Nearsightedness

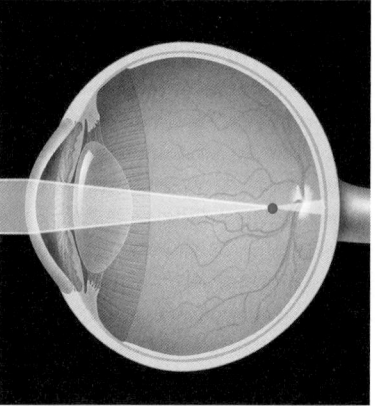

Farsightedness

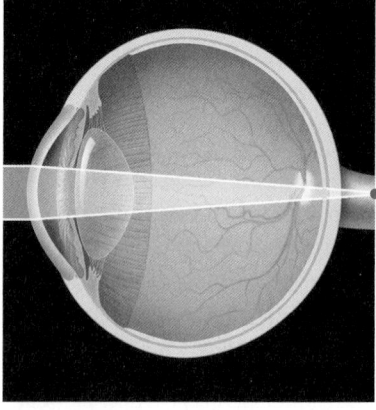

With normal vision, the image is sharply focused onto the retina. In nearsightedness (myopia), the point of focus is in front of the retina, making distant objects appear blurry. In farsightedness (hyperopia), the point of focus falls behind the retina, making close-up objects appear blurry. The dot represents where the image is most clearly focused.

Farsightedness

Signs and symptoms
- Nearby objects appear blurry
- Eyestrain, including aching eyes and headache

Farsightedness (hyperopia) is another common condition. You're able to see objects at a distance clearly but have difficulty focusing on objects that are near.

This condition usually results from the eyeball being too short from front to back. The rays of light coming into your eye aren't focused when they reach the retina, located at the back of the eye. Instead, the point of focus falls behind the retina. Farsightedness may also result from a weakness in the ability of the lens and cornea to focus because one or the other doesn't have a steep enough curvature.

Farsightedness usually is present at birth and tends to run in families. Most young people don't know they have the condition because their lens is flexible enough to compensate for the condition. So most young people with farsightedness don't need corrective lenses. But as they age, the lens becomes less elastic and unable to make the necessary adjustment. By middle age, most farsighted people need corrective lenses to improve their near vision.

Common symptoms of farsightedness include difficulty focusing on objects close at hand and sometimes headaches or eye discomfort after doing close tasks such as reading, writing or drawing.

Treatment
If you're experiencing symptoms of farsightedness, see an eye specialist. He or she will conduct a series of tests to determine the nature and extent of the problem and the level of correction required to improve your vision.

Farsightedness is treated easily with eyeglasses or contact lenses. Surgery to treat farsightedness is available, but it isn't as effective as surgery for nearsightedness.

Astigmatism

Signs and symptoms
- Portions of your visual field are distorted
- Vertical, horizontal or diagonal lines appear blurry

Astigmatism is a refractive error caused by an uneven curvature of the cornea. In a normal eye, the dome of your cornea is curved evenly and smoothly in all directions. In an astigmatic eye, the cornea typically has areas that are steeper or flatter than normal, blurring only some of what you see. In some instances, astigmatism results from abnormalities of the lens inside the eye, and the cornea is normal.

Astigmatism is usually present at birth and may occur in combination with nearsightedness (myopia) or farsightedness (hyperopia). The condition tends to remain constant, neither improving nor deteriorating significantly with age. Sometimes, astigmatism develops after an eye injury, disease or surgery.

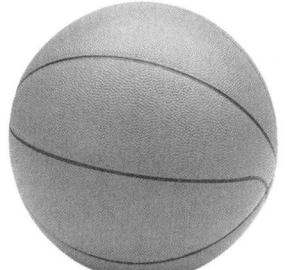 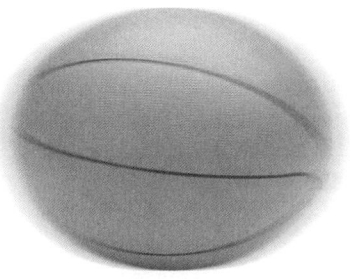

Astigmatism is caused by the uneven curvature of your cornea, which is unable to focus the light entering your eye evenly and creates distorted, blurry vision.

Eye Specialists

There are three main types of eye care professionals. They differ in their level of training and the tasks they perform.

Ophthalmologists
An ophthalmologist is a medical doctor (M.D.) who, in addition to medical school training and a hospital-based general internship, has at least four years of specialized training (residency) in caring for the eyes and diagnosing and treating eye ailments. An ophthalmologist also may receive additional subspecialty training. In addition to providing complete eye examinations, an ophthalmologist treats eye injuries and performs various surgical procedures.

An ophthalmologist is well-trained in the use of specialized instruments to make a correct diagnosis, even if eye problems aren't obvious or are obscure. This can be crucial if the problem is serious and a delay of a few hours may make the difference between good vision and blindness.

Optometrists
An optometrist is trained to diagnose common eye conditions, such as refractive errors, and to prescribe corrective lenses. An optometrist graduates from a school of optometry and earns a doctor of optometry (O.D.) degree.

Optometrists can conduct certain tests, and often they can detect signs of eye disease from examination of the retina. Optometrists may be licensed to prescribe medications to treat eye diseases.

Opticians
An optician is a technician who fills eyeglass and contact lens prescriptions written by ophthalmologists and optometrists. An optician grinds and fits lenses but doesn't examine eyes for refraction problems or disease.

Vision Changes With Age

As you get older, your vision changes. If it doesn't, you're a rare exception. Many of these changes are primarily an annoyance, and most people learn to adjust.

- Often, the retina loses some of its sensitivity to light. To compensate, add brighter lighting to your workstation or your favorite reading chair.
- Lenses in the eye may become less elastic and lose their ability to adjust their focus (presbyopia). You may need reading glasses or a magnifying glass for reading small print.
- Lenses in the eye may become cloudy and cause your visual acuity to decrease, colors to appear dim and glare to form when light shines directly at you (cataract). In this case, you may want to avoid night driving.
- Sometimes, the vitreous humor shrinks, which can produce bothersome floaters in your visual field. With time, most people get used to them. However, if you notice a sudden increase in the number of floaters, you should contact an eye doctor.

Older individuals are also at higher risk of other eye diseases and disorders. Although some vision problems are unavoidable, others can be prevented. And even those that are unavoidable often can be slowed or stopped through early detection and treatment. That's why it's important to have your eyes examined frequently.

Treatment

Minor astigmatism may not cause signs or symptoms. The condition is generally first identified during an eye examination. Astigmatism is treated with a cylindrical corrective lens that corrects for the uneven curvature of the cornea. Hard contact lenses used to correct nearsightedness or farsightedness also correct astigmatism. Another option is surgery to reshape the curvature of the cornea. The procedure is similar to the surgery used to correct nearsightedness and farsightedness.

Presbyopia

Signs and symptoms

- Nearby objects appear blurry
- Eyestrain, including tired eyes and headache

The term *presbyopia* may be unfamiliar to you, but the condition probably isn't. With age, the lens becomes harder and less elastic, making it more difficult for you to see nearby objects clearly. This hardening process is a normal part of life, and it happens to everyone to some degree.

Many people begin to notice a change in their vision around age 40. If you're farsighted, you may encounter this problem even earlier in life. If you're nearsighted, you'll eventually experience presbyopia, although later in life than a normal-sighted person will.

Close-up objects that were once easy to see become blurred. The print in newspapers, books and restaurant menus seems smaller, and you instinctively hold them farther away from your eyes to be able to read them.

Treatment

An eye specialist can easily test your eyes for presbyopia. The condition is usually treated with glasses and only occasionally with contact lenses. As your lenses lose the ability to adjust, you may need a change in prescription every few years until about age 65. At that point, the lenses generally have lost most of their ability to accommodate, so changes in your prescription become less frequent.

If you're nearsighted or have astigmatism, you may need new lenses to counteract the effects of presbyopia. Fortunately, you don't have to constantly shuffle glasses because they can be made with lenses that have two or even three corrections. In a double (bifocal) lens, first introduced by Benjamin Franklin, the upper segment of the lens corrects your distance vision, and the lower segment corrects your near vision (see page 590).

Hereditary Disorders of the Eyes

Some conditions and diseases affecting the eyes can be passed from one generation to the next. These conditions range from simple nearsightedness (myopia) and farsightedness (hyperopia) to more serious eye diseases.

Heredity seems to play a role in the incidence of misaligned and weak eyes (strabismus and amblyopia). Defects of color vision (colorblindness) usually are present from birth. These defects are often passed down through the mother, usually to her sons. Eye diseases with a genetic factor include glaucoma, cataracts, retinitis pigmentosa and retinoblastoma.

Retinoblastoma, a cancerous tumor of the eye that affects young children, has a genetic component in 30 to 40 percent of cases. Other general disorders that can affect vision and have a hereditary component include diabetes and high blood pressure.

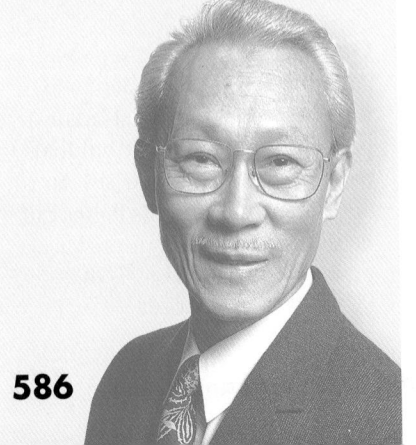

An Eye Examination

It's recommended that everyone have an eye examination from time to time. Individuals who wear glasses or contact lenses should have their eyes checked every year. People who don't wear glasses or contacts don't need an examination as often, unless they have a vision disorder or experience eye symptoms.

Infants usually get an eye exam from their pediatrician between birth and age 3 months and again between ages 6 months and 1 year. It's also recommended that children have their eyes examined at about ages 3 and 5. Children and adolescents should have an eye examination whenever they experience any problems with vision or symptoms of eye trouble.

If you don't wear glasses or contact lenses and don't have an eye disorder, consider having comprehensive eye examinations on the following schedule:
- At least once between ages 20 and 39

- Every three to five years between ages 40 and 50
- Every one to three years beginning at age 51

An eye examination involves a series of tests to evaluate different aspects of your vision, check for signs of disease and assess whether damage has occurred.

Visual acuity test

Acuity refers to the sharpness of your vision — how clearly you see an object. Using a Snellen chart, your eye doctor will check how well you read letters of decreasing size from across the room. Having 20/20 vision means that you can read letters that individuals with normal vision can read from 20 feet away.

Refraction assessment

Refraction refers to how light waves are bent as they pass through your cornea and lens. A refraction assessment helps your eye doctor determine a corrective lens prescription that will give you the sharpest vision.

Your eye doctor may use a computerized refractor to measure your eyes and estimate the prescription you need to correct a refractive error. Or he or she may use a technique called retinoscopy. In this procedure, your doctor shines a light into your eye and measures the refractive error by evaluating the movement of light that's reflected by your retina.

An eye doctor fine-tunes the refraction assessment by asking you to look through a phoroptor, a device that contains wheels of different lenses. You look at the Snellen chart through various lenses and judge which combination of lenses gives you the sharpest vision.

Visual field test

Your visual field is the area in front of you that you can see without moving your eyes. Visual field testing (perimetry) is done in several ways. In one test, you look at a screen on which a computerized machine flashes spots of light in different locations and of varying brightness. You press a button each time you see a flash. The machine records your responses and maps the area you see. Gaps in your field of vision may indicate a serious eye disorder.

Another test uses the Amsler grid, named after the Swiss ophthalmologist who developed it. In the center of a square grid is a black dot. With one eye covered, you focus on the dot and tell your eye doctor whether you can see the entire grid clearly.

Glaucoma test

By measuring the internal pressure of your eye, your eye doctor can determine whether you're developing glaucoma. Two common techniques are used to measure eye pressure — air-puff tonometry and applanation tonometry. Both measure the amount of force needed to momentarily flatten (applanate) your cornea.

Visual Acuity Test

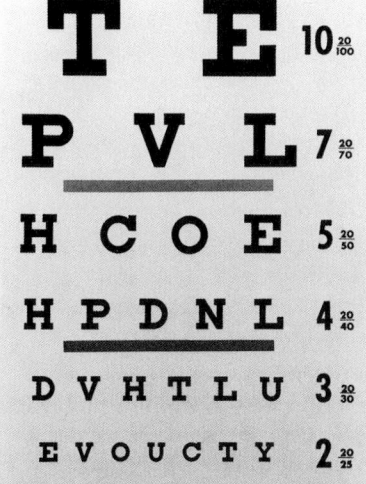

During a visual acuity test, you're asked to read letters of decreasing size on a chart at a fixed distance from you, usually 20 feet.

Refraction Assessment

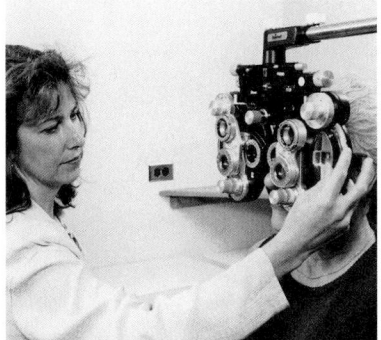

A phoroptor is a device that allows you to view a Snellen chart through different lenses. The lenses are changed until a combination is found that you feel gives you the sharpest vision.

External eye exam

An external eye exam is a quick check of your eyes with no special instruments other than a light. The eye doctor checks your pupils to see if they respond normally, your cornea and iris for clarity and shininess, and your eyes and eyelids for position and movement.

Slit-lamp examination

A slit lamp allows an eye specialist to see the structures at the front of your eye under magnification. The microscope is called a slit lamp because it uses an intense line of light — a slit — to provide a cross-sectional (oblique) view of the cornea, anterior chamber and lens. The illumination allows a doctor to detect and precisely locate any abnormalities.

When examining problems involving the cornea, your doctor may use fluorescein dye. The dye spreads across your eyes and appears bright yellow when hit with blue light. This causes tiny cuts, scrapes, tears, foreign material or infections on your cornea to stand out.

Retinal examination

In a retinal exam, your eye doctor puts dilating drops in your eyes to open your pupils wide and provide a better view of the back of your eye. Using a slit lamp or ophthalmoscope — an instrument that shines a bright light into your eye — an eye doctor can see abnormalities in the structures in the back of the eye, including the retina. This type of exam can help the doctor detect important clues about the presence of disease, such as diabetes and high blood pressure, elsewhere in the body.

Fluorescein angiography

Fluorescein angiography is a diagnostic test used to evaluate diseases of the retina and choroid. Fluorescein

Glaucoma Test

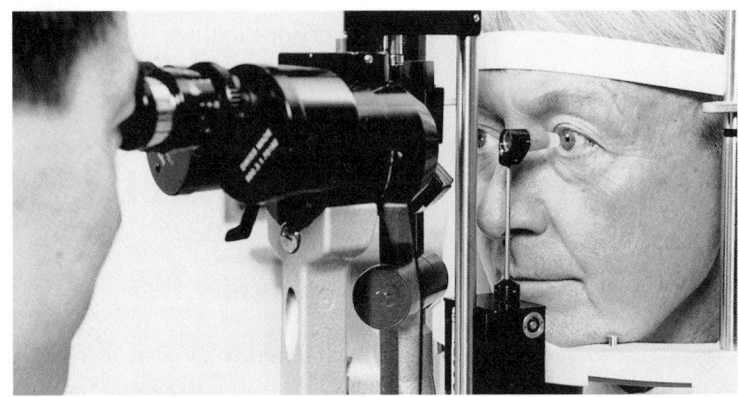

A tiny, flat-tipped cone is mounted on a slit lamp and positioned in front of your eye. By lightly touching the surface of the eye, an eye specialist measures internal eye pressure. High internal pressure may indicate glaucoma.

Slit-Lamp Examination

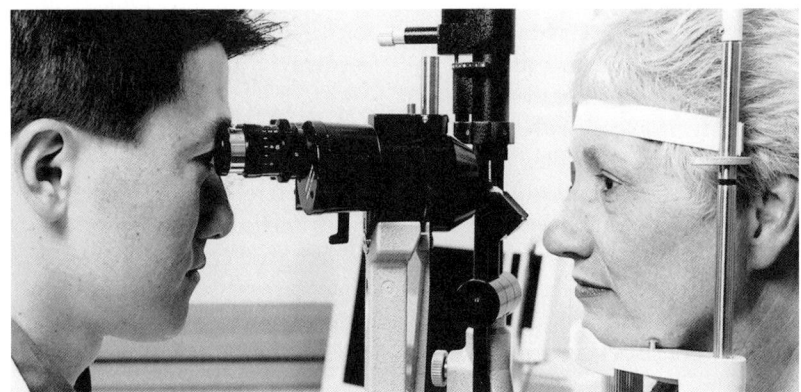

A slit of light is focused to provide an oblique view of the cornea. An eye specialist can also focus this light for a detailed view of the lens.

Retinal Examination

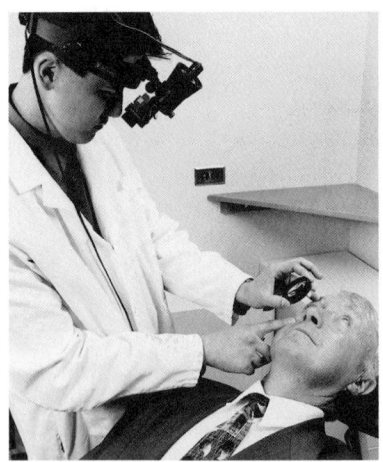

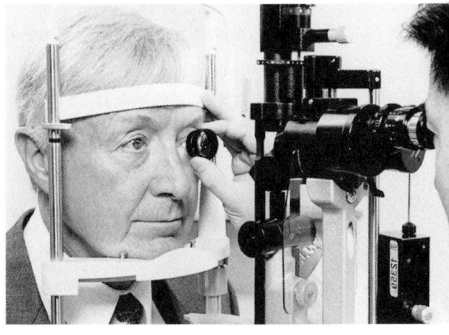

A slit lamp, assisted by a magnifying lens in front of the eye, gives an eye specialist a clear view of the central retina.

With the ophthalmoscope mounted on his head and a powerful lens held in front of the eye, an eye specialist shines a bright light into the eye to examine the entire retina.

dye is injected into an arm vein. As the dye circulates through your eye, the blood vessels in your retina and choroid stand out as bright yellow, and pictures of your retina are taken. The images allow your doctor to assess blood vessel damage and to note the formation of any abnormal blood vessels. This is helpful in diagnosing conditions such as macular degeneration and diabetic retinopathy.

Optical coherence tomography

Optical coherence tomography (OCT) combines the principles of ultrasonography with the high-resolution performance of a microscope. OCT captures infrared light waves reflected off the internal structures of the eye, but with a resolution that's many times greater than what can be achieved with sound waves. The result is a detailed, cross-sectional image that clearly displays the retina and underlying layers.

Sometimes false colors are added to the images to assist in interpretation. The procedure is useful for checking the thickness or thinness of the retina and for diagnosing disorders such as macular holes, macular edema, macular degeneration and inflammation of the retina.

Corneal topography

Also known as videokeratography or corneal mapping, corneal topography is a computer-assisted examination of the clear, front portion of the eye. It's performed by projecting illuminated rings onto the surface of the cornea, which are reflected back and measured. The result is a topographical map of the cornea.

Corneal topography is used to identify the curvature of the cornea and identify distortions or scarring of the cornea. It's helpful in correcting astigmatism, fitting contacts and evaluating individuals undergoing LASIK surgery.

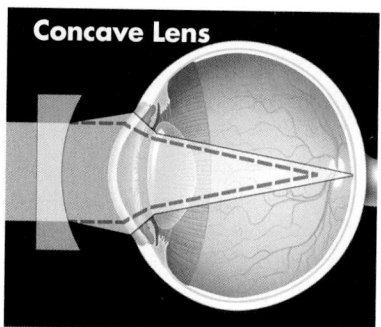 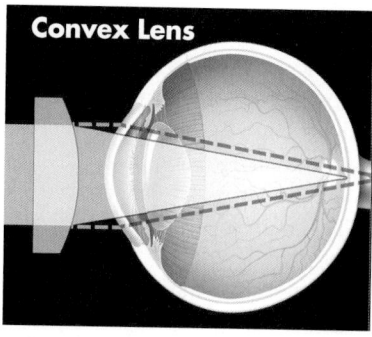

A concave lens (left) corrects for nearsightedness (myopia). The dashed line indicates where the point of focus would be without the corrective lens. A convex lens (right) corrects for farsightedness (hyperopia) and is commonly used in reading glasses. The dashed line indicates where the point of focus would be without the corrective lens.

Correcting Imperfect Vision

If you need to sharpen your vision, whether to see clearly at a distance or to read fine print, you have many options to choose from. These include a variety of eyeglasses and contact lenses and, in some cases, surgery to change your cornea's curvature.

You and your eye doctor can decide which option may work best for you. You'll want to take your individual needs into consideration. If you play sports, are very active or dislike the look and feel of glasses, you may prefer contacts or the more permanent solution of surgery.

How corrective lenses work

Many vision problems are treated with lenses that compensate for abnormalities in the shape of your eye or the curvature of your cornea or lens. There are three basic shapes for corrective lenses:
- **Concave lenses** are thinner in the middle than on the edges. They correct for nearsightedness (myopia).
- **Convex lenses** are thicker in the middle than on the edges, as in a magnifying glass. These

lenses correct for farsightedness (hyperopia) and are commonly used in reading glasses.
- **Cylindrical lenses** are curved more in one direction than the other to compensate for astigmatism.

If after a routine eye exam your doctor determines that you need corrective lenses, he or she will give you a prescription. It indicates the refractive power that each lens needs in order to correct your specific vision problem. The prescription numbers determine the shape and thickness of your lens. The higher the prescription numbers, the stronger the prescription — meaning the more that light must be refracted, the thicker the lens needs to be.

Eyeglasses

About 6 out of 10 Americans wear some kind of corrective lenses. About 8 out of 10 of those needing vision correction choose eyeglasses. Eyeglasses are available in many frame styles and lens designs. You can also purchase them in a variety of locations, including eye doctors' offices, eyeglass shops and discount stores.

Lens materials
Eyeglass lenses can be made of glass or plastic. Most eyeglass wearers choose plastic. Although glass lenses are usually more scratch resistant than plastic lenses,

they can be about twice as heavy. Another drawback of glass lenses is that they're more prone to break or chip, though the lens material must pass a breakage standard set by the Food and Drug Administration.

There are several types of plastic lenses:

- **High-resin plastic.** These plastic lenses are a bit thicker than glass but about half the weight. They're also easy to scratch, and for that reason some manufacturers routinely put a scratch-resistant coating on them.
- **High-index plastic.** This material is lighter and thinner than high-resin plastic lenses. That makes these featherweight lenses ideal for strong corrections. Unfortunately, they cost considerably more than high-resin plastic. They generally include a scratch-resistant coating and ultraviolet (UV) protection.
- **Polycarbonate plastic.** These are the strongest lenses available, which makes them a good choice for active kids and for use in safety glasses and sports glasses. Although they aren't as lightweight as the high-index lenses, they're lighter than high-resin plastic. They generally come with scratch-resistant coating and UV protection.

Lens coatings

Lenses may be coated to offer:

- **Scratch protection.** A clear, hard coating is applied to lenses to make them more resistant to scratching. If you buy high-resin plastic lenses, you may want to pay the extra money for this treatment. Other plastic lenses have already been treated. Have both sides of a lens treated because you can accidentally scratch the inside when cleaning them. Be careful where you store your glasses because scratch-protection coating can crack and peel in extreme temperatures.
- **UV protection.** UV rays may contribute to several age-related eye diseases, such as cataracts

and macular degeneration. When you're outside it's a good idea to wear glasses that filter out 100 percent of both UVA and UVB light. High-index plastic and polycarbonate plastic lenses have UV protection.

- **Anti-reflection coating.** Reflection and glare can make driving difficult, particularly at night. Anti-reflection (AR) coating helps block the light reflected off surfaces such as pavement, water, snow and glass. This is a big help if you have a strong prescription, which increases glare.

AR coating has a few disadvantages. The chemical makeup makes it harder to keep your lenses clean. And frequent, hard cleaning can rub the coating off. Try to wipe them carefully with a lint-free cloth moistened with water or a lens cleaning solution. In addition, the scratch-resistant coating is generally applied before the anti-reflection coating, leaving the AR coating vulnerable to scratches.

Lens treatments

A final consideration in choosing lenses is whether you want any special treatment:

- **Photochromic lenses.** Photochromic lenses are chemically treated so that they automatically become dark in direct sunlight and clear in lower light. However, they won't get dark while you're driving unless the sun is shining directly on your face. So you may need sunglasses or clip-on sunglasses for driving. In addition, this treatment doesn't work as well on plastic lenses as it does on glass.
- **Tints.** Unlike photochromic lenses, which respond to various levels of brightness, tinted lenses remain a constant shade in all lighting conditions. Adding color to your glasses can help if you're especially sensitive to light and wish to use your lenses as sunglasses. Almost any color can be chosen for a tint. Sun-

glasses are often gray or brown. A yellow tint helps keep blue light from entering the lens and can make objects appear sharper.

- **Edge treatment.** If you're very nearsighted, the edges of your lens will be thick and can look unattractive. They also add unnecessary weight to your glasses, especially if you choose large frames. A skilled optician can grind the edges so that they blend into the frame.

Bifocal and trifocal lenses

Many people need only single-vision lenses to correct for nearsightedness (myopia), farsightedness (hyperopia) or astigmatism. Some need multifocal lenses, which are two or more lenses combined into one.

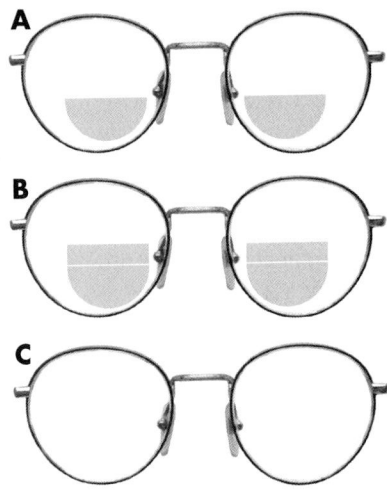

Bifocals (A). With bifocals, the top part of the lens corrects your distance vision, while the lower part (shaded) allows you to read and see objects clearly from a foot or so away.

Trifocals (B). The trifocal lens adds a third power for an intermediate focus between the other two. The added power helps you focus clearly on objects approximately 2 to 4 feet away.

Progressive (C). A progressive lens has no division lines in it. Instead the focal powers change smoothly as your eyes move from top to bottom.

If you're nearsighted or farsighted or have major astigmatism, chances are that by the time you're in your 40s, you'll also need bifocals and eventually trifocals.

In bifocal lenses, the top portion is used for seeing at a distance and the bottom for reading. Trifocals add a third power, to help you see objects at an intermediate distance, such as a computer monitor, items on the grocery store shelf or books on a library shelf.

There are several common designs for multifocal lenses:

- **Flattop semicircle.** The reading, or up-close, section in bifocals

and trifocals appears as a clearly defined semicircle at the bottom of each lens. The line separating the up-close correction from the rest of the lens can be polished out so that people don't know you have multifocal glasses. But your vision will be distorted in the small area where one corrective power merges into the other.

- **Executive style.** Instead of a semicircle, the line dividing the corrective powers runs all the way across the lens. This type of lens gives you the widest possible field of vision for close work and is often used with trifocals.

- **Progressive.** A progressive lens has no division lines. Trifocal correction is built into the lens, and the prescriptions change smoothly as your eyes move from top to bottom. If you require a bifocal correction for the first time, many eye doctors suggest you try progressive lenses to avoid the occasionally bothersome lines separating the segments. One disadvantage of a progressive lens is that there may be some distortion along the bottom edge, near the reading section.

It takes practice getting used to bifocals and trifocals. Be sure your

Eyeglass Frames

When you're looking for new glasses, you may be tempted to start with frames on the display rack. If you want to save time, start by considering your prescription. Your lens may be best suited to a frame that's a certain shape or size. For example, if your prescription calls for a thick lens, a thin wire frame might not be able to support its weight. A skilled optician can tell by your prescription what kinds of frames will work best for you.

When shopping for a pair of frames, keep these tips in mind:

- The size of your frame is important for your vision as well as your appearance. Very large frames can pick up too much glare from overhead lights and distort your vision. If the frame is too small, your field of vision may be limited.

- If you need strong — and, therefore, thick — lenses, choose smaller frames. This will reduce the weight of your glasses and may eliminate distortion created when the size of your lens extends beyond your field of vision.

- Thin metal frames are usually the lightest. But plastic frames tend to be more durable and better able to support thick lenses.

- Both metal and plastic frames come in different grades, or levels of quality. Generally, you'll get what you pay for. Metal frames made of titanium, carbon graphite and Flexon — a titanium-based alloy — are more expensive but are especially durable. Propionate plastic is used in cheaper frames, and Kevlar and Optyl (a resin) are more durable.

- If your glasses fit correctly, they'll feel snug and secure, yet they won't rub behind your ears or irri-

tate the bridge of your nose. If the frames do bother you, they can be adjusted at the hinges, bridge or temples, the side arms that rest on your ears.

- New glasses require a short adjustment period. You may experience some eye ache, but it shouldn't be unbearable or persistent. If your eyes bother you so much that you can't wear the glasses, or the discomfort lasts more than a couple of weeks, check back with the optician. Your frames or prescription may need to be adjusted. It's a good idea to have the fit of your glasses checked every year or so because they become easily misaligned.

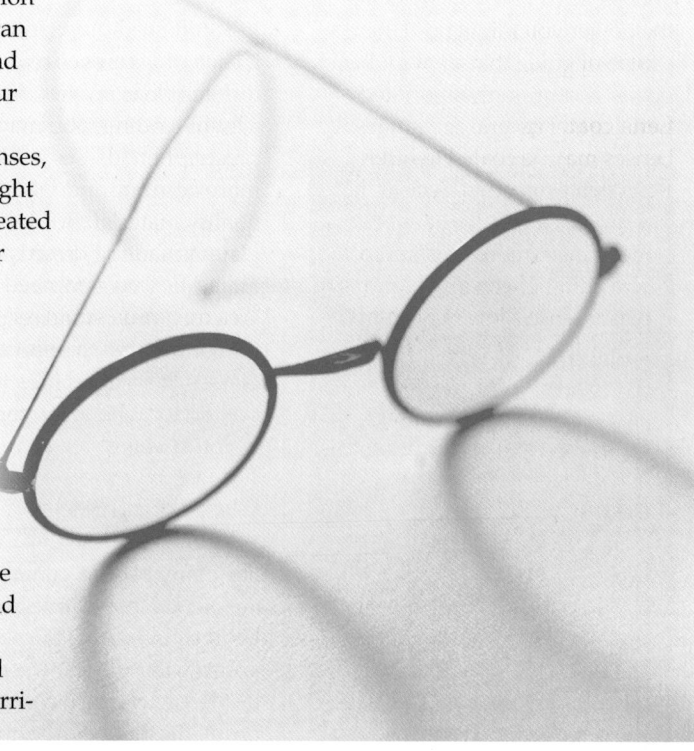

frames are properly adjusted to fit your head. As you tilt your head up and down, your line of vision should move smoothly from one segment of the lens to the other segment in both eyes at precisely the same time.

Nonprescription reading glasses

As you enter your 40s, you may find that you need glasses for reading only. You might be able to save some money by purchasing these glasses at a pharmacy or discount store.

Nonprescription reading glasses with lenses of various strengths are often on display alongside the sunglasses. Reading glasses can also be worn over your contact lenses that correct distance vision.

If your eye doctor has told you the correction that you'll need, look for lenses of that power. Otherwise try the trial-and-error method. The weakest reading lenses are labeled +1.00 diopters, and the strongest are +3.00. Test a few different powers by holding printed material about 14 to 16 inches from your eyes.

When you find a pair that allows you to read comfortably at that distance, that's probably the power you need. To give you an idea of the power you might need, here's a general guide that shows which power is commonly associated with each of several age ranges:

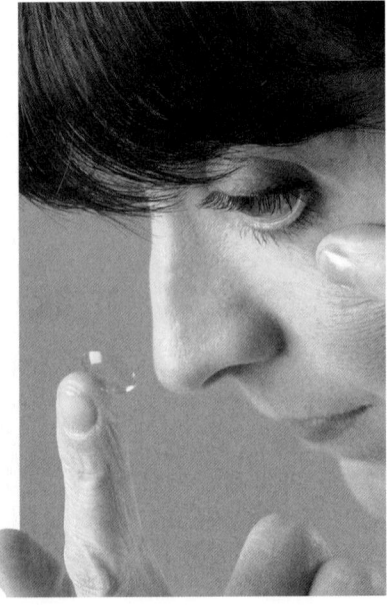

Contact Lens Options

To improve or fine-tune your vision, your eye doctor may recommend one of the following types of contact lenses:

Bifocal
Bifocal soft lenses, like bifocal glasses, have a reading correction and a distance correction on each lens. The lower section of the lens is weighted, so that it stays at the bottom of your cornea and is there when you look down to read. Sometimes, however, when you blink, the lens can momentarily twist around and blur your vision.

Monovision
With monovision lenses, you wear a lens with reading correction in only one eye and a lens with just distance correction in your other eye. Your brain may adjust to this unequal correction, but your vision will be a bit more blurry than normal. Generally, you'll have sharper vision with a bifocal contact lens in each eye.

Toric
Toric lenses are designed to correct astigmatism, as well as nearsightedness or farsightedness. The lenses are weighted to keep them in place. It's important to have toric lenses fitted properly because if the lens moves as you blink or move your eye, your vision won't be sharp.

Ages	Power (in diopters)
40 to 45	+1.25
45 to 50	+1.50
50 to 55	+1.75
55 to 60	+2.00
60 to 65	+2.25
Over 65	+2.50

You'll need prescription glasses if each of your eyes requires a different lens power. If you do a lot of reading, you may prefer prescription glasses, which can be more accurate and made of higher quality material. But inexpensive glasses made of lower quality materials won't damage your eyes. Whether you decide on prescription or nonprescription reading glasses, it's a good idea to see your eye doctor whenever you notice vision changes.

Contact lenses

For many people, contact lenses are a good alternative to glasses. Unlike glasses, contacts don't slide around, fog up or attract dirt. Contact lenses can also correct vision problems that before could only be corrected with eyeglasses. You can even get bifocal contacts.

Contacts are most useful for people with refractive errors such as nearsightedness (myopia), farsightedness (hyperopia) and astigmatism. In addition, some unusual conditions such as keratoconus (cone-shaped cornea) are better treated with contact lenses than with glasses.

As its name implies, a contact lens is worn in contact with the eye. The specially shaped plastic disc sits on the cornea of your eye. The contact lens floats on tears that bathe the eye when you blink. This liquid also allows necessary oxygen to reach the cornea.

Each contact lens is made according to a prescription, just as eyeglasses are. In contrast to eyeglasses, though, contact lenses correct your entire field of vision because all images reaching the eyes pass through the lenses.

Types of contact lenses
Contact lenses have come a long way since the first hard plastic

One of the more common problems with contact lenses is overuse. If you wear them for too long at a time, your corneas may not get enough oxygen. This causes blurry vision, pain, tearing, redness and sensitivity to light.

If you experience such signs and symptoms, remove your lenses immediately. Always keep your lens case readily available so that you can remove and safely store your lenses if your vision becomes blurry or your eyes start to hurt. It also helps to carry a pair of glasses as a backup in case such problems develop.

lenses were developed in the 1940s. That original style of contacts is rarely used anymore. The two basic types of contact lenses used today are rigid, gas permeable lenses and soft lenses.

Rigid, gas permeable lenses

Rigid, gas permeable lenses are slightly flexible hard contacts that are more porous to oxygen. They're comfortable and offer excellent correction for a wide range of vision problems. They're more durable than are soft contacts and may provide sharper vision. But they have several drawbacks. You have to wear them regularly to keep your eyes used to them. They can slip off the cornea and even pop out of your eye more easily than soft contacts. And it's easier for dust to get under gas permeable lenses and irritate your eyes.

Soft lenses

Soft contact lenses hold water, which is what makes them soft and comfortable. Soft contacts allow oxygen to pass through the plastic and nourish your cornea. These contacts are more comfortable and easier to adjust to than are rigid, gas permeable lenses. But they aren't nearly as durable. And the vision they provide is sometimes not as crisp as with rigid, gas permeable lenses. Soft contacts are available in these styles:

- **Daily wear, or conventional.** These plastic lenses conform to the shape of your eye. As the name implies, they're designed to be worn when you're awake and taken out before you go to sleep. You shouldn't wear them overnight. It's important to clean them every day after you wear them and to replace them each year.
- **Disposable, or frequent replacement.** These lenses are thinner and more porous to oxygen than are daily wear lenses, which makes them even more comfortable. As the name suggests, disposables are intended to be replaced at regular intervals. Some are designed to be worn only one day, others two weeks and others one to three months. The length of time you can wear them depends on the design and material and how well you take care of them. Like other soft lenses, disposables can be torn if you handle them roughly. They generally require less care than do conventional soft lenses.
- **Extended wear.** These contacts are usually disposable and are designed for more than 24 hours of wear without being removed. The lenses are approved for up to seven days of continual wear. However, most doctors don't recommend extended-wear contact lenses because, regardless of the material they're made of, your eyes receive less oxygen when you wear contact lenses while sleeping. The lenses also put you at increased risk of an eye infection because bacterial growth on the lenses increases dramatically on them if you wear them overnight.

Buying and fitting contact lenses

Whichever form of lenses you choose, make sure that you have the services of a professional who can determine your exact needs. Good vision, comfort and the health of your eyes require that contact lenses be fitted properly.

Prescribing contact lenses is more complex than it is for eyeglasses. Contacts require measurements for power, curvature, diameter and thickness as well as a selection of design and material. A contact lens prescription is determined after an initial evaluation and a follow-up visit or two.

Caring for contact lenses

Proper care of your contact lenses is vital to eye comfort and the health of your eyes. Each kind of lens has its own requirements, but no matter what type you wear, the first rule is to keep them clean.

1. Before handling your contacts, wash, rinse and dry your hands thoroughly.
2. Use multipurpose contact lens solution with caution. Two brands have been withdrawn from the market in recent years because they were linked to serious eye infections. Don't use any solutions that are discolored or out of date. Gently rubbing the lenses during cleaning enhances the performance of the solution.
3. Replace your contact lenses as recommended.
4. Replace your contact lens case every three to six months. Discard the solution in the case each time you disinfect your lenses.

Refractive surgery

An alternative to wearing glasses or contact lenses is laser surgery to correct the curvature of the cornea. Refractive surgery can correct farsightedness (hyperopia), nearsightedness (myopia) and astigmatism. However, it cannot help with

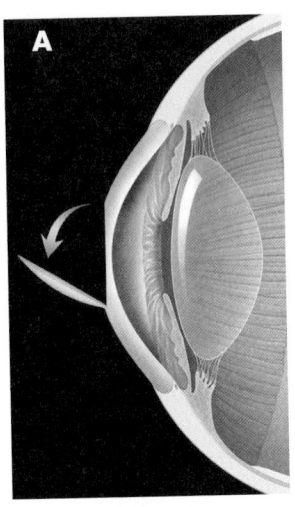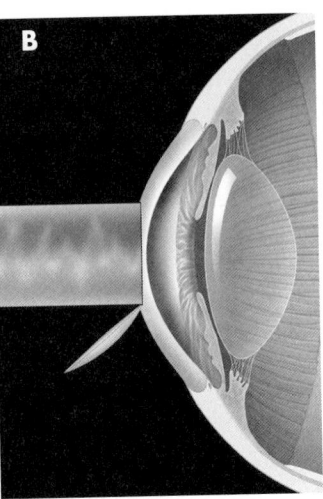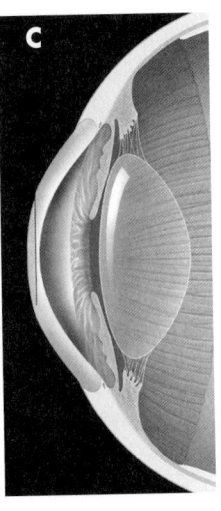

During LASIK surgery: A circular flap of tissue is cut from the cornea and folded back (A). A cool laser (excimer laser) reshapes the underlying layer of the cornea (B). When the reshaping is complete, the corneal flap is returned to its position over the treated area (C).

presbyopia, the waning of your near vision that starts around age 40.

Refractive surgery allows many people to get rid of their glasses or contacts. Yet this type of surgery does have some risks. If you're content with your glasses or contacts, you may not want to take any risks.

Typical candidates for refractive surgery are healthy adults ages 18 to 55 whose vision hasn't changed in the past year and who have mild to moderate nearsightedness, farsightedness or astigmatism. You may not qualify if you have dry eyes, cataracts or other eye problems, or if you're pregnant, because your vision can change during pregnancy.

LASIK surgery

The most common type of refractive surgery is LASIK, short for laser-assisted in-situ keratomileusis. This procedure is currently the gold standard for surgical correction of nearsightedness. The entire procedure takes less than 30 minutes.

LASIK is performed using a laser that's programmed to remove a defined amount of tissue from your cornea. During the procedure you lie on your back in a reclining chair. Numbing drops are placed in your eye and your doctor uses a special instrument to hold your eyelids open. A suction ring is positioned on your eye, which may cause a feeling of pressure and your vision may dim a little.

As the procedure is taking place, you'll be asked to focus on a point of light. Staring at this light helps you keep your eye fixed while the laser reshapes your cornea.

The surgeon uses a laser to cut a circular flap of tissue from the center of your cornea. This flap, still hinged to the cornea, is about the size and shape of a contact lens. The surgeon folds the flap out of the way and uses a laser to reshape the layers of the cornea underneath the flap — removing one microscopic layer at a time. A computer, reading a topographical map of your cornea, tells the surgeon exactly which bits of tissue to remove. After the reshaping is complete, the flap is folded back into place and usually heals without stitches.

Typically, you're able to see after the procedure but your vision may not be better right away. Expect it to gradually improve over two to three months.

Most people who have refractive surgery eventually attain 20/25 vision or better. Your chances for improved vision are based, in part, on how good your vision was before surgery.

Photorefractive keratectomy

Another surgery used with similar success is photorefractive keratectomy (PRK). Instead of sculpting the inner layers of your cornea, the surgeon uses a laser to reshape the outer corneal surface. After removing the thin, protective epithelial layer of the cornea, the surgeon flattens the cornea's curvature. The epithelium grows back and conforms to the new shape of the cornea. There's no flap involved, which must be repositioned after the surgery.

It generally takes up to a week for your eye to regenerate the surface tissue that was removed. It may take three to six months before your vision improves completely.

Benefits and disadvantages of surgery

Refractive surgery allows about 75 percent of nearsighted people to achieve 20/20 vision without corrective lenses. More than 95 percent achieve at least 20/40 vision, the level usually required to pass an eye exam for a driver's license. These percentages continue to rise as a result of improved technology and surgical skill.

Between 5 and 15 percent of recipients undergo a second surgery to further sharpen their vision. This is often referred to as an enhancement.

When the anesthetic drops wear off after LASIK, you may feel a scratchy sensation in your eyes for a day or so. Yet LASIK is the less painful of the two procedures because the exposed nerve endings of your cornea are covered by the corneal flap. With PRK the pain may be more, but the risk of flap problems is avoided.

Possible problems that may arise after refractive surgery include:
- Increased sensitivity to light
- Problems with glare
- Clouded vision, which typically resolves over time
- Decreased night vision and halos around lights
- Intolerance of contact lenses

Selecting the right surgeon

For your surgery, choose an ophthalmologist with special training in the procedure, plenty of experience in the procedure you're having done and a high rate of success. You have only one pair of eyes, so choose carefully whom to trust them with.

Eye Trauma

From time to time, eye injuries happen — from a stray foul ball, a grain of sand or a splash of a household chemical, for example.

Foreign objects

Signs and symptoms
- Sudden pain in the eye
- Sudden decrease in vision
- A red eye

Everyone gets a speck of dust in the eye on occasion, and often just blinking can help wash the particle away. But if you find that this doesn't work or know that something more serious has entered your eye, seek medical attention promptly. A foreign object in the eye can be a serious threat to sight, particularly if the object enters the eye itself or damages the cornea or lens.

Diagnosis
If you go to a doctor for help with a foreign object in your eye, he or she will likely examine your eye with a slit lamp — an instrument with a light source and high magnification. If the object has entered the eye itself, an X-ray or a computerized tomography (CT) scan may be needed.

Treatment
If the object can be seen on the eye surface, the doctor may be able to remove it with surgical tweezers. If the object is no longer present but has scratched the cornea, you may need a topical antibiotic to protect against infection. Your doctor may also suggest that you wear a patch over the eye to protect it until the cornea heals. If an object has entered the eye, surgical removal will likely be necessary.

Chemical burns

Signs and symptoms
- Pain in the eye
- Decreased vision
- Increased sensitivity to light

Chemical burns of the eye can endanger your vision. If your job entails the use of hazardous chemicals, be aware of the dangers, protect your eyes with goggles or protective glasses, and know where the closest source of clean water is in case you need to flush your eyes. Remember that household cleaning products,

Protecting Your Eyes

Myths about eye care are common. For example, the warnings that reading in dim light or sitting too close to the television screen will damage your eyes aren't true. Reading by flashlight is also harmless, as is sitting in the front row of a movie theater. These activities may make your eyes feel tired or strained, but they don't harm them.

However, many other situations can seriously damage your eyes. Some of the most common injuries are the result of accidents while doing everyday tasks such as cooking, cleaning or working in the yard. To help protect your sight:

Wear safety goggles or glasses
Wear safety goggles or glasses while working with industrial chemicals, power tools and hand tools. Make sure that your children also get in the habit of wearing protective eyeglasses when helping with hazardous housework, cooking, gardening or mowing lawn. Teach children early to wear goggles when using tools.

It's also a good idea to wear safety glasses or shields for sports such as racquetball, basketball, squash and tennis. Use appropriate headgear, such as a batter's helmet for baseball and a face mask for hockey. If a hockey puck or racquetball hits your eye, it can cause serious internal damage. Basketball players frequently suffer corneal abrasions from finger pokes.

Be careful when applying makeup
Take care when using anything near your eyes, from brushes to hair spray. You can injure your cornea by hastily applying mascara or accidentally squirting hair spray in the eyes.

Follow instructions
Read the instructions on detergents, ammonia, cleaning fluids and other household chemicals. When using fluids that come in spray containers, point nozzles away from your eyes at all times. Store household chemicals safely and out of children's reach.

Remove dangerous toys
Keep children away from toys that could lead to eye injury. Examples are BB guns, plastic swords or spring-loaded toys that shoot darts. Don't allow children to have fireworks.

Be careful around car batteries
When you're attaching jumper cables, a battery can explode and acid can get into your eyes.

Will wearing sunglasses protect my eyes from disease?

Long-term exposure to ultraviolet (UV) radiation from the sun can contribute to eye disease, particularly some types of cataracts and possibly age-related macular degeneration. The easiest way to protect your eyes from such damage is to wear sunglasses. Generally speaking, you don't need to wear them every time you step outside. But if you spend much time in the sun, wear sunglasses that screen out UV radiation.

Choose sunglasses that provide maximum protection from both ultraviolet A (UVA) and ultraviolet B (UVB) light. The greater the blockage of UV light, the lower your risk of damage. To minimize UV light that can enter from the sides, choose sunglasses that fit close to your face or wraparound glasses. Wear your sunglasses on cloudy days as well as sunny days because clouds don't block all UV radiation.

For activities on water, sand or snow, gray-tinted, polarized lenses can reduce glare. Gray- or green-tinted lenses offer the least color distortion.

particularly those that contain ammonia or bleach, and garden chemicals can be irritating.

Direct contact — a chemical splashed in your eyes — is most hazardous, but concentrated fumes and aerosols also can cause injury. You'll know if a chemical has burned one or both of your eyes. They may hurt or be sensitive to light, and your vision may be blurred.

Treatment
Immediately flush the eye with clean water and continue doing so for 15 to 30 minutes. To flush your eye, hold your head under a water faucet or pour water into your eye from a clean container. Keep your eye open as wide as possible during flushing.

Chemical burns to the eyes are a medical emergency and should be treated promptly. Go to the emergency department at your local hospital or contact your eye doctor. The doctor examining and treating the eye may use a local anesthetic to lessen the pain. Depending on the extent of injury, the eye may be bandaged or treated with an antibiotic and allowed to heal. Serious damage to the conjunctiva, cornea or eyelid may require surgical repair later on.

Black eye

Signs and symptoms
- Bruising around the eye
- Swelling of the lid and tissue around the eye

A bruise around the eye — a so-called black eye — results from bleeding under the skin. The injury may be limited to a small amount of bleeding that provides the characteristic black-and-blue bruising. Sometimes a black eye indicates a more extensive injury, even a skull fracture, particularly if the area around both eyes is bruised or you have a head trauma.

Treatment
Using gentle pressure, apply ice to the soft tissue around the injured

eye for 10 to 15 minutes. Take care not to press on the eye itself.

Seek medical care promptly if you experience vision problems such as double vision or blurring or if you have severe pain or bleeding in the eye or from the nose. A doctor can determine whether more serious damage has occurred.

Blood in an eye

Signs and symptoms
- Bleeding within the front portion of the eye

Bleeding into the front portion of the eye (hyphema) may follow direct trauma to the eye. It can result from a blunt injury or a sharp injury that perforates the eye's coating. At times, hyphema may result from severe inflammation of the iris (iritis), a blood vessel abnormality, cancer within the eye or severe retinal vascular disease. When the bleeding is caused by trauma, the blood is usually absorbed completely within a few days. Recurrent bleeding can reduce vision and damage the cornea. In some cases, glaucoma can result.

Treatment
A doctor may recommend rest and elevating the head of your bed. Eyedrops may be given to lower eye pressure. Other treatments are directed at the underlying cause. For severe bleeding, a doctor may choose to drain the blood through a small opening in the eye. This drain can be reopened later if further bleeding occurs.

Corneal abrasion and injury

Signs and symptoms
- Severe eye pain
- A red eye
- Swollen eyelids

The cornea is the curved, transparent covering at the front of the eye. Along with the cornea, the lens focuses images on the retina.

As the most exposed part of the eye, the cornea is susceptible to injury, ulcers and infections. The most common corneal injury is an abrasion — irritation caused by scratching or rubbing. This can happen when a speck of sand or sawdust scratches the cornea or you wear contact lenses for too long. Your cornea can also be burned from exposure to ultraviolet radiation after you've been sitting in the sun or under a sunlamp for too long or looking into a welding arc without proper eye protection.

Following corneal injury, the tissue around your eye may swell, and the eye itself may redden and hurt intensely. You may blink more than usual. Some people don't feel any symptoms for several hours after the injury, then suddenly find themselves in extreme discomfort for no apparent reason.

Treatment

Eyedrops containing a dye can help a doctor identify damage to the cornea. Simple corneal abrasions and injuries are treated by removing any foreign material, covering the eye with a patch and letting the eye heal itself. The cornea usually heals in as little as a day or two. Your doctor may also apply an antibiotic ointment to prevent infection and prescribe a pain reliever to relieve the discomfort. More serious injury to the cornea may require surgical treatment.

Eyelid Disorders

The eyelids, though thin and delicate, are extremely important in protecting the eyes. Quick and powerful reflexes make the eyelids close when an object nears or when irritating particles are in the air. The eyelids also lubricate the eyes and wash foreign particles from them.

Lacrimal glands located above each eyeball produce tears, which are spread by the eyelids as a thin film. The tears drain from the eyes through nasolacrimal ducts, which have openings at the inner corner of each eyelid. The nasolacrimal ducts carry the tears to the nose — which explains why crying causes your nose to run. The eyelids are lined with the conjunctiva, the transparent mucous membrane that also covers the white surface of the eye.

Sties and lumps

Signs and symptoms
- Painful swelling on the edge of the eyelid
- Slightly blurred vision

A sty (hordeolum) is an infection around the root (follicle) of an eyelash. A sty resembles a pimple or boil. You may get more than one sty at a time or several in succession because bacteria that initially infect one hair follicle can spread and infect others.

A sty usually develops gradually, forming a painful red lump. Eventually, the lump fills with pus and bursts. The release of pus relieves the pain, and after a few more days the sty usually disappears.

Another form of swelling on the lid is called a chalazion. Unlike a sty, a chalazion is relatively painless. It results from a blockage of one of the small glands (meibomian glands) that produce part of the tear layer. Bacteria may grow within the blocked gland. A chalazion develops a little farther up and within the eyelid. Most chalazions are only mildly uncomfortable, but they may be unsightly.

Treatment

Sties and lumps are almost always harmless to the eye and sight. However, if a sty interferes with your vision, doesn't disappear or recurs, see a doctor.

To treat a sty, apply a warm compress to it for about 10 minutes four times a day. To make a compress, soak a clean cloth in warm water and wring it out before applying it to your eye. Warm compresses help relieve the pain. Don't squeeze the sty in an effort to remove the pus. Let the sty burst on its own, then wash your eyelid thoroughly. If the sty is stubborn or you have recurring infections, your doctor may prescribe an oral antibiotic or an antibiotic cream to apply to the eyelid. A persistent sty may need to be lanced and drained.

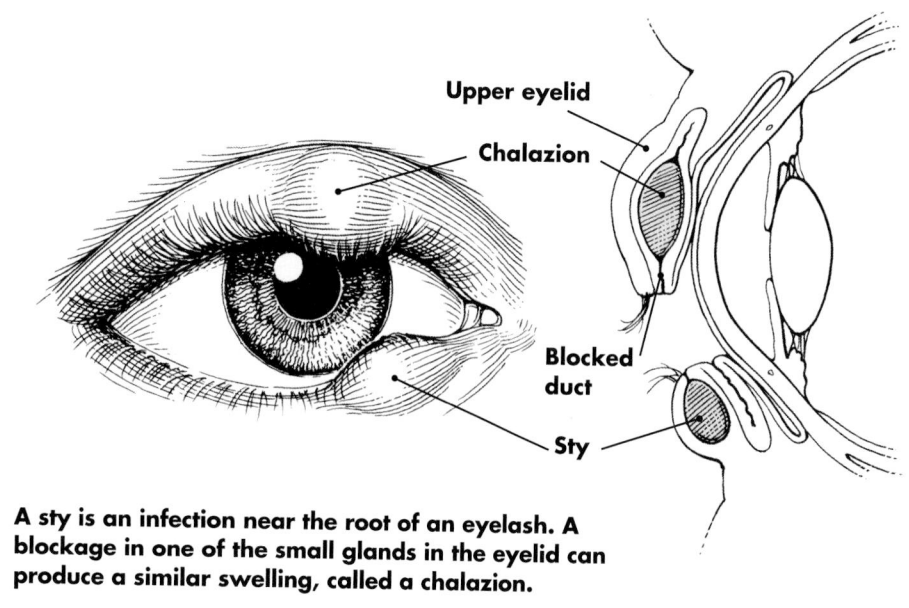

Upper eyelid

Chalazion

Blocked duct

Sty

A sty is an infection near the root of an eyelash. A blockage in one of the small glands in the eyelid can produce a similar swelling, called a chalazion.

Eyedrops

Many brands of eyedrops can be purchased without a prescription. They fall into two general categories: artificial tears and vasoconstrictors.

Artificial tears

Artificial tears contain substances, such as methylcellulose, that hold water and resemble your own tears. One or two drops in each eye usually provide lubrication and comfort for several hours. You can use artificial tears as often as needed.

Vasoconstrictors

Vasoconstrictors (Murine, Visine) contain a medication that causes the tiny blood vessels in the conjunctiva to constrict. If you have bloodshot eyes — redness and visible blood vessels — one or two drops in each eye will usually relieve the redness for several hours and often provide comfort as well. Some vasoconstrictors also contain an antihistamine to provide added relief for allergies.

Vasoconstrictors shouldn't be used more than two or three times a day for more than three days, unless otherwise directed by your doctor. Overuse leads to a rebound effect of increased swelling and redness that persist even after you stop using the drops.

Follow the directions carefully for whatever eyedrops you use. A pharmacist can help you select the type of eyedrops you need and inform you how to use them. After placing eyedrops in your eye, follow these simple steps:

1. Keep the eye closed for 30 seconds. This encourages absorption and minimizes drainage through your tear duct into your nose.
2. Don't blink. Blinking tends to move the liquid from your eye into your tear duct.
3. Use your index finger to apply firm pressure for a minute or two over the junction of your lower eyelid and nose to block the opening of your tear duct.

A chalazion usually disappears without treatment in a month or two. Applying warm compresses may help speed the healing. Your doctor may prescribe an antibiotic ointment. If these methods prove unsuccessful or if the chalazion continues to enlarge, it can be removed surgically. After the procedure the eye usually is covered with a patch for several hours.

Tearing problems

Every time you blink — every few seconds — tears lubricate your eyes. The fluid is essential for your eyes to function properly. Problems may develop with the tear glands that result in continuously watering eyes or dry eyes.

Dry eyes

Dry eyes, caused by an inadequate amount or quality of tears, can lead to an uncomfortable sensation. Your eyes may feel hot and gritty and appear swollen and red. The condition usually affects both eyes.

Dry eyes may result from an allergy to eyedrops used for another condition or from Sjogren's syndrome, a connective tissue disorder often associated with rheumatoid arthritis, or they may occur for no apparent reason. Dry eyes are most common among women after menopause, probably due to hormonal changes.

Problems unrelated to tear production also can cause your eyes to feel dry and scratchy. They include eyelid inflammation (blepharitis); entropion or ectropion (see page 601); eyestrain; environmental irritants, such as smoke, sun, wind and indoor heating; and disruption of the blink reflex.

Common medications, both prescription and over-the-counter, also can cause dry eyes. These include diuretics, antihistamines and decongestants, sleeping pills, tricyclic antidepressants, some drugs for treating acne, and opiate-based pain relievers, such as morphine.

Treatment

Although it generally isn't a threat to your sight, the discomfort of dry eyes may require medical treatment. Your doctor will likely prescribe artificial tears to bathe your eyes whenever needed. Cyclosporine (Restasis) is a prescription medication that helps increase tear production and reduce inflammation. Another treatment option is closing the tear ducts with removable silicone plugs or permanently with surgery.

Watering eyes

Too much tearing can result from either excessive tear production or inadequate drainage by the nasolacrimal ducts, the tubes that drain tears from the eyes to the nose.

Some babies are born with a tear duct that has failed to open. In most of these infants, the ducts open spontaneously within a few weeks. Usually, only one eye is affected by continuous tearing.

PREVENTION TIP

Like any liquid, tears evaporate when exposed to air. These are simple steps you can take to help slow evaporation and minimize problems of dry eyes:

1. Don't direct hair dryers, car heaters, air conditioners or fans toward your eyes.
2. Wear glasses when outside on windy days and goggles while swimming.
3. Keep your home humidity between 30 and 50 percent. In winter a humidifier can add moisture to dry indoor air.
4. Remember to blink. Consciously blinking repeatedly helps spread your own tears more evenly.

Other causes of watering eyes include irritation of the eye due to an abrasion, infection of the eyelid, inward-growing eyelashes, allergies or nasal problems.

Treatment
Your doctor will examine the eye carefully for signs of blockage of a nasolacrimal duct or of excessive tear production. He or she may also ask you questions to identify other possible causes. These might include scarring of the nasolacrimal duct caused by chronic sinusitis, chronic allergies or injury to the nose. Treatment for a blocked duct generally includes probing and irrigating (flushing) the tear drainage system. In some cases, an operation may be needed.

Infection of the tear duct
Occasionally, the nasolacrimal duct can become infected (dacryocystitis). When this happens, the tissues between the inner angle of the eye and the bridge of the nose become swollen, red and tender. Tears can no longer make their way into the nose, causing excessive tearing.

Itchy Eyelid

Itchiness around the eyes often accompanies seasonal allergies, but itchy eyelids may be a manifestation of contact dermatitis, a skin inflammation that results when your fingers come in contact with some irritating or allergy-causing substance and then touch your eyes. Cosmetics also can cause allergic reactions on the sensitive skin of the eyelids.

If your eyelids itch, don't rub or scratch them excessively. Rubbing ultimately can result in eczema, with thickening patches of skin and persistent itching. If your eyelids are sensitive to certain cosmetics or other materials, avoid using them.

Twitchy Eyelid

From time to time, you may experience a twitch in an eyelid. This involuntary quivering usually lasts only a few seconds, but it can be recurrent and irritating and make you wonder if something is wrong with your eyes.

A twitch is almost always harmless. Eye twitches are similar to the common experience of an occasional muscle twitch in a hand, forearm, leg or foot. These muscle flutters (fasciculations) last only a few seconds, although they may happen often.

No one knows exactly what causes most twitches, although they're often associated with fatigue and stress. Very rarely, a twitching eyelid is a symptom of a muscle or nerve disease, but symptoms of these diseases tend to be distinct from an ordinary eye twitch.

You may be able to relieve the twitching by gently massaging the affected eyelid.

Treatment
Your doctor may prescribe an antibiotic for the infection. To relieve discomfort apply a warm compress to your eye several times a day. Soak a clean, lint-free cloth in warm water, wring it out and place it over the affected eye for about 10 minutes.

Once the infection has cleared, a new tear drainage opening may need to be created surgically. In this operation, called dacryocystorhinostomy, the doctor may use thin silicone tubing to keep the new tear duct open while healing occurs. In rare cases, it may be necessary to surgically implant an artificial tear duct in the eyelid. The artificial duct is made of unbreakable glass and is placed in the inner corner of the eyelid.

Blepharitis

Signs and symptoms
- Sticky, crusty and reddened eyelids
- Itchy, burning, swollen eyelids
- Pink eye (conjunctivitis)
- A grainy feeling with blinking
- Loss of lashes

Blepharitis is an inflammation of the eyelid edges that's due to a bacterial infection. When glands near the eyelashes produce excess oil, the oil creates an environment favorable for bacterial growth. The result is a crusty inflammation on the eyelids that's uncomfortable and unsightly but rarely a threat to sight.

You may find that you have to pry your eyes open in the morning, because the sticky secretions seal the eyelids shut overnight. In severe cases, small ulcers may develop on the edges of the lids, and the cornea can become scarred. People with blepharitis often have a history of recurrent sties and chalazions.

Treatment
Cleaning your eyelids carefully is important for treating blepharitis. In the morning, soak a clean, lint-free cloth in warm water, wring it out and place it over the eyes as a compress. This will loosen the crusty scales. Then gently scrub your eyelashes and eyelid edges with a cotton-tipped swab soaked in diluted baby shampoo. This will help remove the crust.

If self-help measures don't clear up the problem, your doctor may prescribe — in addition to eyelid scrubs — an ointment or eyedrops that contain antibiotic and corticosteroid medications. These should help clear up the infection and reduce the swelling. If topical treatment is unsuccessful, it may be necessary to prescribe oral antibiotics.

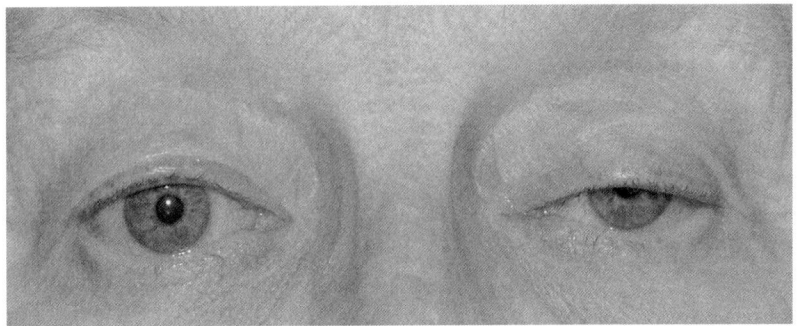

Drooping of the upper eyelid (right side of photo) is known as ptosis.

Drooping eyelid

Signs and symptoms

• Drooping of one or both upper eyelids

Drooping eyelid (ptosis) is caused by a weakness of the muscle that raises the upper eyelid and keeps it open. Some children are born with the condition. When present from birth, it usually affects only one eye. Ptosis often runs in families.

In adults, some drooping of the eyelids can occur as a normal effect of aging, as the eyelid muscles lose tone. Less often, a drooping eyelid may result from an injury or disease, such as diabetes, myasthenia gravis, stroke, a brain tumor or cancer, all which can affect nerve and muscle function. A drooping eyelid that develops suddenly requires immediate attention. It may be a sign of stroke or another acute condition. If the problem develops over several years, it may be due to the effects of aging.

Diagnosis

If your child's eyelids are noticeably uneven, especially to the degree that vision is obscured, have her or him evaluated by a doctor. If you notice that one or both of your own eyelids have gradually become droopy, ask your doctor about it the next time you have an appointment. If the drooping came on suddenly, see your doctor right away. A thorough examination may be needed to determine whether a more general health problem could be the cause.

Treatment

For children born with ptosis, surgical correction may be necessary to prevent poor vision in the affected eye. Among adults, if the drooping is the result of aging or injury, your doctor may recommend that you have an operation to shorten the muscle, lifting (elevating) the lid. If the cause is a more general health problem, such as myasthenia gravis, stroke or diabetes, treatment of the underlying disorder may help relieve the eyelid problem.

Eyelid Surgery

With age, eyelid tissue loses elasticity, strength and tone. Fat accumulates around the eyes. Your eyelids may droop, and you may have bags beneath your eyes. Heredity also can lead to droopy eyelids. Whatever the cause, you may appear to always look tired. Perhaps the sagging skin even interferes with your sight.

Surgery

Blepharoplasty is a surgical procedure to remove excess skin and fat from the upper and lower eyelids. The procedure usually is done using a local anesthetic. The surgeon makes an incision in the fold of the eyelid near the lashes. Excess skin, muscle and fat are removed, and the incision is closed. Mild cases are sometimes treated with laser surgery. In this procedure, the laser shrinks and tightens the skin and muscles without removing them.

Recovery

Blepharoplasty shouldn't interfere with your vision, and you may wear your eyeglasses the day after the procedure. Wearing glasses can also help protect your eyelids from injury. Any swelling, tenderness and pain should subside within two to four weeks.

You may experience some temporary problems. Because many tiny blood vessels are disturbed during the procedure, you may experience areas of blood under the skin (hematomas). These usually subside after a few days and leave no permanent sign. Some people have temporary double vision the first few hours after the operation. Many people report excessive tearing for a few days, but this usually disappears.

An infection after surgery is uncommon but can occur. See your doctor if you experience:

• Excessive swelling that doesn't improve gradually
• Redness that increases over several days
• Tenderness or pain in the eyelid that doesn't resolve gradually
• Problems with vision

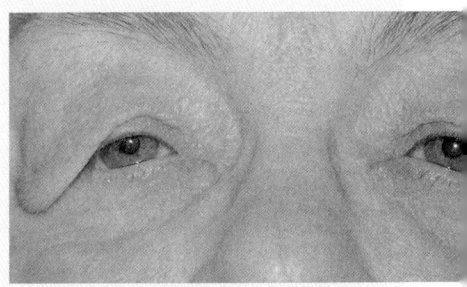

Relaxation of the tissues of the upper eyelid may cause it to droop over the eyelashes and interfere with vision. This is known as blepharochalasis.

Entropion and ectropion

Signs and symptoms
- Eyelashes scratching the eye
- Excessive tearing
- Eye irritation and matter in the eye when you wake up

Entropion and ectropion generally are due to aging. In entropion, the upper or lower lid turns inward, causing the lashes to scratch the eye. In severe cases, this can cause an ulcer or scarring of the cornea. One of the first signs of entropion is irritation and excess matter in the eyes in the morning. This usually improves later in the day. As the disorder advances, the irritation may persist longer or become constant. You may also notice your lashes turning in toward the eyes.

Ectropion — the reverse problem — is often the result of muscle weakness. It also may be related to an underlying condition such as allergic dermatitis or lupus erythematosus.

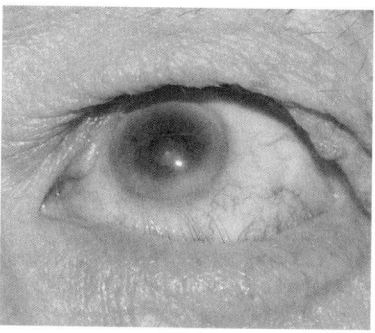

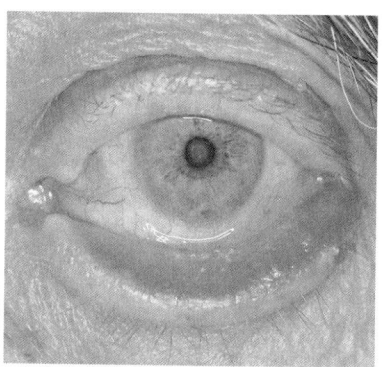

With entropion (top) the eyelid turns inward so that the lashes rub against and irritate the eye. With ectropion (bottom) the eyelid turns outward and sags away from the eyeball.

The lower lid turns outward, sometimes causing tears to flow over the lower lid edge and down your cheek rather than into the tear drainage system.

Treatment
Both entropion and ectropion can be corrected by surgery that repositions the muscles holding the lids in place. The procedures are usually performed on an outpatient basis with a local anesthetic. When an underlying condition is the cause of ectropion, the first step is to treat the underlying cause.

Eye Disorders and Diseases

The eyes are susceptible to various disorders and diseases. Many eye conditions don't seriously affect your ability to see, but they can be annoying or may present more serious risks to your vision over time. Among the most serious disorders are those related to the functioning of the eye. These include glaucoma, cataracts and problems involving the retina, including retinal detachment and macular degeneration.

Colorblindness

Signs and symptoms
- Certain colors are muted and difficult or impossible to see
- An inability to distinguish between certain shades of color
- Seeing everything in shades of gray (extremely rare)

Although most people call it colorblindness, life for a person with poor color vision is usually not black and white. Only rarely is everything seen in shades of gray. Most people with poor color vision are unable to distinguish between certain shades of color.

Your ability to view the world in hundreds of hues begins with just three colors — red, blue and green.

As light rays pass through the lens and the transparent, jellylike substance (vitreous humor) that makes up much of your eye, they interact with light-sensitive chemicals in cone cells in the retina. As long as the cones can accurately distinguish red, blue and green, these colors can be further blended to produce a continuous band (spectrum) of colors. If the cones lack one or more light-sensitive chemicals, you may see only two colors, such as either red and green or blue and yellow. The most common color deficiency is an inability to see red and green.

Defects can be mild, moderate or severe, depending on the amount of light-sensitive substances missing from the cones. In addition, a reduced sensitivity to red is seldom as severe as a reduced sensitivity to green. So more people struggle to see green than red. Interestingly, most people with a red-green deficiency aren't aware of their problem. To them, leaves are green and roses are red, but their "green" may be what normal-sighted people call yellow.

Causes
The causes of color vision deficiencies are as follows:

Genetic
The genetic defect responsible for color vision deficiencies is passed from mother to son. The condition seldom affects women. The gene that carries this defect also determines whether the condition will be mild, moderate or severe. The degree of color deficiency you inherit remains the same throughout your life. Most people who have an inherited color deficiency can see normally in all other respects.

Acquired
Color deficiencies can accompany various forms of eye disease. People may develop problems seeing blue and yellow when the retina is affected by disease.

Disorders of the optic nerve also can affect your color vision. In addition, cataracts can impair color perception.

Age

Aging can bring on color deficiency. During childhood and adolescence, your ability to see colors steadily improves and peaks in your 30s. Color vision then gradually deteriorates as a normal part of aging.

Diagnosis

An ophthalmologist can test for a color deficiency. Many ophthalmologists use a book containing multicolored dot patterns as a simple and accurate screening test for color vision deficiencies. An ophthalmologist can help you find out what type of color deficiency you may have and determine if you have any associated eye disease.

Treatment

No treatment can correct inherited color perception deficiencies. Wearing a colored filter over eyeglasses or a colored contact lens may enhance your perception of contrasts. But such lenses won't improve your ability to discern colors. And because they're usually worn over only one eye, they can distort depth perception.

If you have an acquired color deficiency, it may worsen as the disease that causes it progresses. Treatments that slow or reverse the course of the underlying disease often improve color vision.

Misaligned eyes

Strabismus and amblyopia, conditions that affect eye alignment, are usually first observed during early childhood. Strabismus is the general term for crossed eyes or eyes that are misaligned in some other way. Amblyopia, often called lazy eye, can be a consequence of strabismus.

Babies are born with the ability to see, but, at first, they can't focus. The nerve connections between the eyes and brain haven't yet become fully organized. During the first few weeks of life, your baby's eyes may appear to wander. At times, they may seem to work independently, sometimes crossing and at other times roving outward. This is normal. By the end of the second or third month, however, your baby's eyes should appear to be working in parallel and able to focus on small objects. No one knows why some children's eyes are misaligned, although it tends to run in families.

Strabismus

Normal vision depends on the eyes focusing together, producing binocular vision. When the eyes don't function in tandem, double vision results. In a young child with strabismus, however, the brain will ignore the images from one eye, and the nerve connections between that eye and the brain fail to develop normally.

About 4 percent of children have strabismus. It seems to affect boys and girls equally. If not treated before age 5 or 6, strabismus may cause permanent loss of visual acuity in the nondominant eye.

The most common forms of strabismus in children are cross-eye (esotropia) and walleye (exotropia). Esotropia is characterized by one eye turning inward. Exotropia occurs when an eye turns outward. Sometimes the eye will turn down or up. The deviations may be constant or occasional,

Normal Pattern

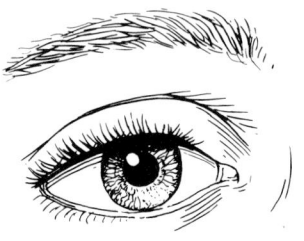 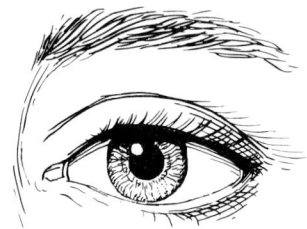

Esotropia

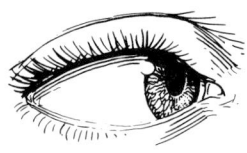 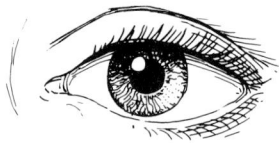

Exotropia

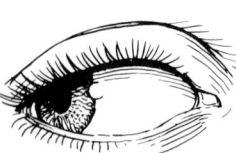 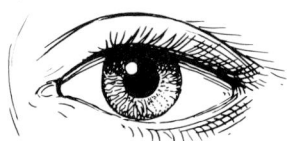

Some children have eyes that are misaligned, a condition called strabismus. Two common forms of strabismus are esotropia, in which an eye turns inward, and exotropia, in which an eye turns outward.

such as when the child is tired and the eye muscles weaken.

The resulting poor vision prevents a child from having normal depth perception, which good binocular vision produces. The affected eye probably won't develop good vision unless it's used. This can be accomplished by surgery to bring the eyes into alignment or perhaps by wearing a patch over the unaffected (dominant) eye, forcing the affected eye to focus and see.

Amblyopia

Amblyopia is a condition in which vision in the nondominant eye is poor, usually as a result of strabismus. Amblyopia can also result from a greater degree of farsightedness (hyperopia), nearsightedness (myopia) or astigmatism in one eye or from the rare occurrence of a childhood cataract. The brain then "turns off" the more affected eye, and the stronger eye becomes dominant and retains good vision.

Diagnosis

The key to treating strabismus and amblyopia is early detection. Strabismus is usually easy to recognize, but amblyopia in a child may not be evident because he or she often doesn't realize that vision is poor in one eye. Testing of visual acuity may be needed to discover amblyopia. Following is a list of things to look for:

1. Do your child's eyes work together? Have your child follow your hand moving back and forth. Notice if the eyes seem to move and follow as one.
2. Cover one of your child's eyes and move your hand or a toy back and forth. Does the uncovered eye follow the object? Cover the other eye and repeat.
3. Can your toddler gauge depth when playing with objects?
4. Does your child seem crosseyed when playing with toys or other close objects but normal when looking into the distance?

5. Does only one eye squint when your child is in the sun?
6. Does your child tend to tilt his or her head to one side?

If you think that your child might have misaligned eyes, check with your doctor. It's never too early to have a child's vision tested for alignment. The key to diagnosing amblyopia in a young child is to identify a difference in vision between the eyes. An ophthalmologist can test your baby's vision by covering one eye and observing your child's responses to the movement of various objects. If one eye is amblyopic, the child might try to remove the patch, or he or she might object to having it over the better eye.

By age 3, vision usually can be measured accurately. Poor vision in one eye doesn't necessarily mean that a child has amblyopia. Poor vision may be due to nearsightedness, farsightedness, astigmatism or another disorder.

Treatment

Ideally, treatment for strabismus and amblyopia begins in early childhood — when the complicated connections between the eye and brain are forming. Depending on the cause and the degree to which your child's eye is affected, treatment may include:

- **Corrective eyewear.** If a condition such as nearsightedness, farsightedness or astigmatism is contributing to strabismus and amblyopia, corrective glasses or contact lenses will likely be prescribed. Sometimes corrective eyewear is all that's needed.
- **Eye patches.** To stimulate the weaker eye, your child may wear an eye patch over the stronger eye — often for two or more hours a day. This helps the part of the brain that manages vision develop more completely.
- **Eyedrops.** A daily or twice weakly drop of a drug called atropine temporarily blurs vision of the stronger eye. This will encourage use of the weaker eye.

Double Vision

Double vision (diplopia) generally results from a nerve or muscle problem. The problem may cause one eye to deviate from the other so that they don't focus in unison. The images the brain receives from the two eyes are positioned differently from each other, causing double vision.

If the eye and brain connections have already become well-established, which usually happens by age 1 or 2, the brain interprets the signals just as it receives them and produces two images. The effect can be confusing and debilitating because objects appear twice in the field of vision.

Sometimes, double vision is a sign of a more serious underlying problem such as diabetes, myasthenia gravis, multiple sclerosis, Graves' disease or a brain injury. In these cases, the underlying disease affects the nerves between the brain and eye muscles or the nerves of the eye muscles themselves. Double vision is usually only one of several symptoms of these disorders.

If you develop double vision, have it checked out as soon as possible. In the meantime, you can alleviate the sensation temporarily by placing a patch over one eye.

Treatment of an underlying disorder may resolve the problem. Sometimes, double vision can be corrected with prescribed eyeglasses that contain prisms — special lenses that align the image seen by one eye with that seen by the other eye. Occasionally, the condition is treated surgically to improve alignment.

- **Surgery.** If your child has crossed or outwardly deviating eyes, the eye muscles may need surgical repair. The surgeon makes a small incision in the tissue that covers the eye. One or more of the eye muscles are then repositioned to achieve proper alignment. Droopy eyelids or cataracts may also need surgical intervention.

For most children, proper treatment improves vision within weeks to several months — the earlier treatment begins, the better. Although research suggests that the treatment window extends through at least age 17, results are better when treatment begins in early childhood. When treatment is completed before age 6, vision often improves to near normal.

Conjunctivitis

Signs and symptoms
- A red eye
- A gritty feeling in an eye
- An itchy eye
- Discharge in an eye that forms a crust during the night
- Blurred vision and sensitivity to light

Conjunctivitis is an inflammation of the transparent membrane (conjunctiva) that lines the eyelids and covers the eyeball up to the edge of the cornea. Commonly known as pink eye, conjunctivitis may result from a bacterial or viral infection, an allergic reaction, or in newborns, an incompletely opened tear duct. Newborns are also susceptible to certain bacteria acquired from the birth canal. This form of conjunctivitis must be treated without delay to prevent loss of vision.

Viral and bacterial conjunctivitis are common among children and are often extremely infectious. Pink eye can spread through a whole classroom of children in a few days. Although conjunctivitis can be irritating, it usually doesn't impair vision. Occasionally, severe conjunctivitis can cause corneal complications in adults.

All forms of conjunctivitis share certain signs and symptoms. The white of the eye becomes red or pink, and the eye feels gritty when you blink. The eye also produces a yellowish discharge that forms a crust during the night. This sticky crust can seal the eyes shut so that you have to pry the lids apart in the morning or soak off the crust.

Viral conjunctivitis usually produces a watery discharge, while the bacterial form often produces thick matter. Allergic conjunctivitis usually causes intense itching, tearing and inflammation of the conjunctiva as well as some itching and watery discharge from the nose.

Treatment
You can soothe the discomfort of conjunctivitis by applying warm compresses to the affected eye or eyes. Soak a clean cloth in warm water, squeeze the water out and apply the cloth to your eyes. You can wipe away discharge with a moistened, disposable tissue or clean cotton ball. Your doctor may prescribe antibiotic eyedrops if the infection is bacterial. Viral conjunctivitis clears up on its own.

Allergic conjunctivitis is often effectively treated with cool compresses. It may also be helped by eyedrops that contain both an antihistamine and an agent that constricts blood vessels.

Prevention
Because bacterial and viral conjunctivitis spread easily and quickly, good hygiene is the best way to prevent pink eye from spreading. If someone in your family has it:
- Keep your hands away from your eyes.
- Wash your hands frequently.
- Change your towel and washcloth daily.
- Change your pillowcase each night. Wash sheets and pillowcases in hot water.
- Discard eye cosmetics, particularly mascara.
- Don't use other people's eye cosmetics.

- Don't share towels, washcloths, pillowcases, handkerchiefs, glasses or utensils with another person.
- Dispose of used tissues immediately.

Scleritis and episcleritis

Signs and symptoms
- Pain in one or both eyes
- Patchy redness on the eye
- Blurred vision
- Swelling of the eye

The sclera is a tough layer of tissue that forms the wall of the eyeball — the part commonly referred to as the white of the eye. The sclera, in turn, is covered by the episclera, a transparent tissue between the sclera and the outer membrane (conjunctiva). Occasionally, the episclera or the sclera becomes inflamed.

Inflammation of the episclera (episcleritis) is a mild, localized inflammation that generally occurs among young adults. Inflammation of the sclera (scleritis) is a less common but more serious disorder, often associated with inflammatory bowel disease or autoimmune diseases such as rheumatoid arthritis. Scleritis primarily affects people between ages 30 and 60.

Both scleritis and episcleritis are characterized by a red or violet patch on the eye or localized swelling on the eye. In both disorders, tiny blood vessels become inflamed. Scleritis may be accompanied by a dull pain. When scleritis occurs at the back of the eye, vision may be impaired.

Treatment
Episcleritis usually disappears on its own after a week or two but tends to recur from time to time. Your doctor may prescribe steroids in drop or ointment form to help reduce the inflammation of episcleritis or scleritis. Pupil-dilating drugs may be used to lessen the chance of damage to the iris and reduce discomfort. If you have scleritis, your doctor may have

What causes a red area on the eye?

The outer covering of the eyeball is filled with tiny blood vessels. Occasionally, one of them may break, appearing as a red spot or area of blood on the white of the eye. The blood from the broken vessel can travel through the space between the conjunctiva and sclera, causing what appears to be a bloody eye. This is called a subconjunctival hemorrhage. It can be alarming when you first see it, but it's nothing to worry about, unless your eye also hurts. If it does, see a doctor right away.

A blood vessel under the conjunctiva may break for no reason or when you cough, sneeze or vomit forcefully. An eye injury also can cause such a hemorrhage. Most subconjunctival hemorrhages disappear after two or three weeks. If hemorrhages recur, see your doctor, who may recommend a more thorough physical examination to detect a possible underlying problem.

you undergo tests to determine if the inflammation is associated with an underlying condition.

Uveitis and iritis

Signs and symptoms
- A red eye
- Blurred vision
- Sensitivity to light

Uveitis is an inflammation of the uvea, the layer of the eye immediately beneath the sclera. The uvea consists of the colored part of the eye (iris), the ciliary body, which produces the fluid inside the eye and helps control lens movement, and the choroid, which lies just within the sclera and lines the eyeball from the iris all around the eye. Thus, inflammation of the uvea may include the area at the back of the eye, the sides and the iris.

When the inflammation involves mainly the iris and ciliary body, it may be called anterior uveitis. When it involves mainly the choroid, it may be called either choroiditis or posterior uveitis. Iritis is inflammation of the iris.

Uveitis may result from an immune reaction provoked by a disease such as Crohn's disease, ulcerative colitis or sarcoidosis, or it may develop after a severe injury. It can also occur with herpes simplex or shingles (herpes zoster).

Treatment
Uveitis can be serious. Early diagnosis and treatment are important to prevent permanent damage. Uveitis and iritis can be treated with several medications. Your doctor may prescribe a cycloplegic drug that paralyzes the iris and keeps the pupil dilated. This relieves pain by preventing the inflamed iris from moving and lessens the chance of scars or adhesions between the lens and back of the iris. Steroid ointment or eyedrops may be prescribed to reduce inflammation. Aspirin or oral steroid medications also may be prescribed to reduce inflammation.

If inflammation from trauma-related uveitis persists for several weeks, complications can occur, including an immune reaction in the uninjured eye. The result may be inflammation of the uvea and, ultimately, a substantial loss of vision in both eyes. For this reason, an ophthalmologist may advise removal of the injured eye if the inflammation doesn't subside as expected.

Orbital cellulitis

Signs and symptoms
- Pain in one eye
- Decreased vision
- Displacement of the eye
- Swelling of the eyelid
- General malaise

Orbital cellulitis is a rare, acute infection of the eye socket. It primarily affects children, and its onset is rapid and severe. Bacteria enter the orbit, often from an infection in the sinuses, a foreign object in the eye, or a boil on the eye or eyelid. The orbit's soft tissue contents become infected. In most cases, only one eye is affected.

The first signs of orbital cellulitis are usually swelling and redness of the eyelid, followed rapidly by pain and decreased vision. The eye may be noticeably displaced due to the swelling, so the eye seems to protrude from its socket. If your child has these signs or symptoms, go immediately to the nearest emergency department.

Diagnosis
Tests, including blood tests, may be conducted to determine the cause of the infection. A computerized tomography (CT) scan may be recommended to determine if the sinuses are involved or if a foreign object is present.

Treatment
Because orbital cellulitis is an acute and dangerous infection, hospitalization may be necessary. Antibiotics will likely be prescribed, based on the specific bacteria involved. Surgical drainage of an abscess may be necessary.

Corneal ulcers and infections

Signs and symptoms
- Impaired vision
- Eye pain
- A red eye
- A visible white patch on the cornea

A corneal ulcer is an open sore on the cornea. An ulcer can result from an infection by a virus, bacterium or fungus or, more commonly, from an abrasion that becomes infected. Viral infections are frequently caused by the herpes

Corneal Transplantation

Transplantation of the cornea can restore good vision after severe corneal injury or scarring. Transplantation, however, isn't an option if you have an infection in your eye.

The cornea to be transplanted is obtained from a deceased person who, before dying, made arrangements to be a donor. Tissue typing can be done to help ensure a good match between the recipient and the donor cornea. Tissue typing is a way to identify proteins on the surface of white blood cells that serve as unique markers distinguishing one person from another.

The operation is performed by removing the central portion of the damaged cornea and replacing it with a clear cornea. Traditionally, the new cornea was placed over the removed portion of the recipient cornea and secured with very fine stitches (sutures). In a newer, more advanced procedure called Descemet's stripping endothelial keratoplasty (DSEK) only the outer damaged cell layer is removed — instead of the entire thickness of the cornea — and replaced with the outer layer from a donor cornea. Due to the small incision there's no need for sutures, which contributes to faster recovery.

The surgery has a high success rate, but some problems can develop, including rejection of the new cornea. Signs and symptoms of rejection include:

- Increased discharge or redness in the eye
- Pain in the eye and sensitivity to light
- Any marked change in vision
- Gray film over the field of vision
- Floaters in the field of vision

simplex virus. Eyelid problems, such as entropion and blepharitis, also can cause an ulcer. Retraction of the lids, as in Graves' disease or ectropion, may expose the cornea so that it's not bathed in tears. This also may result in ulceration.

The signs and symptoms of a bacterial ulcer are generally more severe than are those of a viral one. A bacterial ulcer may be visible as a whitish patch on the cornea. An ulcer caused by the herpes simplex virus is usually invisible unless a staining solution is placed on the cornea. The ulcer that appears resembles the branches of a tree.

Treatment

Corneal ulcers are serious and should be treated as soon as possible. Once your doctor has determined what kind of ulcer you have, appropriate treatment can be prescribed. Bacterial ulcers usually are treated with antibiotic eyedrops. If the ulcer is severe, an antibiotic may be injected near the eye for faster absorption. Additional topical application of corticosteroid drops may lessen the inflammation.

If your infection is viral, antiviral drops or ointment may be prescribed. These will help control the ulcer. However, if it's due to the herpes virus, it may reappear.

Left untreated, an ulcer can permanently damage the cornea. A deep ulcer can even erode through the cornea and cause infection of the entire eyeball. If this happens you'll need surgery. A severely scarred cornea may require surgical replacement (corneal transplantation).

Glaucoma

Glaucoma is sometimes called a silent thief — it can steal your sight before you realize that anything is wrong. The most common form of the disease develops gradually, without warning signs. Many people aren't even aware they have

an eye problem until their vision is already damaged extensively. In the United States, glaucoma is a leading cause of blindness and affects about 3 million people.

Glaucoma actually is a group of diseases. The common feature of these diseases is abnormally high pressure inside the eyeball or optic nerve damage, which may occur with normal eye pressure.

The space between the lens and cornea is filled with a fluid called the aqueous humor. This fluid circulates from behind the colored portion of the eye (iris) through the opening at the center of the eye (pupil) and into the space between the iris and cornea. Aqueous humor is produced constantly, so it must be drained constantly. Drainage is at the place where the iris and cornea meet, known as the drainage angle. From there the fluid is directed into a channel (Schlemm's canal) that leads to small veins outside the eye.

When the drainage angle doesn't function properly, fluid can't drain and pressure builds up within the eye. Pressure is also transmitted to the other fluid in the eye, the vitreous humor behind the lens. The vitreous humor in turn presses on the retina. This increased pressure affects the fibers of the optic nerve.

The optic nerve is a bundle of nerve fibers at the back of the eye. It's like a big electric cable made up of a million individual wires carrying images you see from the retina to the brain. When the optic nerve is damaged, blind spots develop in the visual field, usually starting with side (peripheral) vision. Over time, the result can be a marked loss of vision.

Fortunately, only a small percentage of people with glaucoma ever lose their sight. Medical advances have made it easier to diagnose and treat glaucoma. If treated early, glaucoma need not cause severe vision loss. But you'll need to monitor the disease the rest of your life.

Are You at Risk?

Many people don't notice symptoms of chronic glaucoma until significant, permanent damage has occurred. For this reason, it's particularly important to be aware of the risk factors for the disease.

Age

Chronic glaucoma is rare before age 40. The risk of developing it nearly doubles every 10 years after age 50. Chronic glaucoma is most common in older women.

Race

Black people are three to four times more likely than white people to get glaucoma and six times more likely to have permanent blindness as a result. The reasons for this difference aren't known, but black people may be more susceptible to optic nerve damage or may not respond as well to current treatments. Asians, particularly people of Vietnamese descent, also are at increased risk.

Family history

Glaucoma runs in families. If one parent has glaucoma, you have about a 20 percent chance of developing the disease. If a sibling has it, your chance is 50 percent.

Medical conditions

If you have diabetes, your risk of developing glaucoma is about three times greater than that of people without diabetes. A history of high blood pressure or heart disease also can increase your risk. Other causes include eye inflammations, such as chronic uveitis and iritis, eye tumors, and retinal detachment. Eye surgery also increases your risk.

Nearsightedness

An extensive study found people who were nearsighted (myopic) had a two- or threefold greater risk of developing glaucoma than did people who weren't nearsighted.

Physical injuries

Severe trauma, such as being hit in the eye, can result in increased eye pressure. Injury can also dislocate the lens, closing the drainage angle.

Prolonged corticosteroid use

Corticosteroids used for prolonged periods of time to treat another illness put you at increased risk of glaucoma.

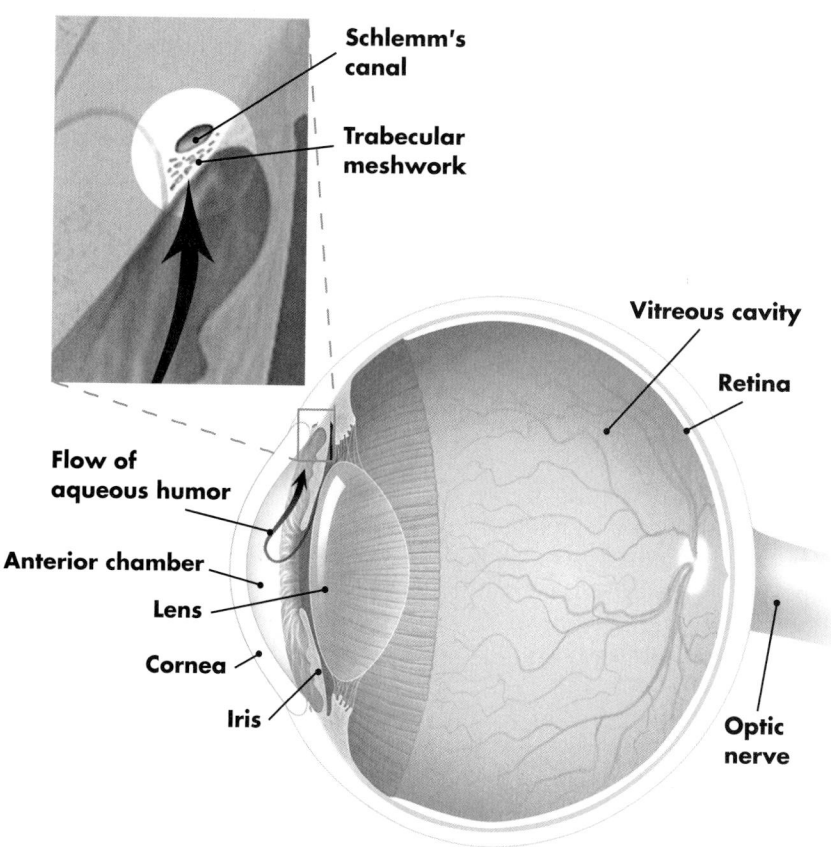

Vision loss caused by glaucoma results from the pressure of built-up fluid within the eye. Aqueous humor normally passes through a narrow space between your iris and lens (see inset), then drains out of your eye through Schlemm's canal. If this outward flow is blocked, pressure can damage your optic nerve and reduce vision.

Glaucoma can be divided into two forms, chronic and acute. The chronic form is by far most common. In addition, there are several rare forms that don't fit into these two main categories.

Chronic glaucoma

Signs and symptoms

- Gradual loss of peripheral vision

Chronic (open-angle) glaucoma often goes undetected for years. With this condition, the drainage angle formed by the cornea and iris remains open, but the aqueous humor drains too slowly. This leads to gradual buildup of pressure within the eye. Damage to the optic nerve is so slow and painless that a large portion of your vision can be lost before you're even aware of it.

The cause of chronic glaucoma remains unknown. It may be that the aqueous humor drains or is absorbed less efficiently with age.

Among some people with glaucoma, intraocular pressure stays within what's considered a normal range but the optic nerve is damaged nevertheless. This is known as normal-tension or low-tension glaucoma. Why the damage occurs is unknown. Some scientists believe people with normal-tension glaucoma may have an abnormally fragile optic nerve or that the blood supply to the nerve is reduced.

Diagnosis

Chronic glaucoma has no early warning signs. The only way to detect glaucoma early is to have regular eye exams once you reach age 40. If you're at increased risk, your doctor may recommend even more frequent monitoring. Tests for glaucoma include:

Tonometry and ophthalmoscopy

Tonometry is an inexpensive and painless test that allows your doctor to determine the pressure within your eye. An ophthalmoscopic examination of the eye's interior can reveal damage to the optic nerve, a sign of glaucoma.

Visual field tests

These tests evaluate your peripheral as well as central vision. With a simple and quick test, a doctor can detect large defects in peripheral vision by asking you to count the number of fingers he or she is holding up while moving his or her hand around the periphery of your vision. Standard, more detailed visual field testing is done with computer-assisted devices.

Imaging tests

Tests may be done to create a three-dimensional (3-D) image of your optic nerve. The image can reveal slight changes to optic nerve fibers, indicating the beginnings of glaucoma. Your doctor may take photographs of the optic nerve to make comparisons at future visits and monitor for changes.

Treatment

It's not always necessary to treat slightly increased eye pressure (intraocular pressure). If no evidence

Measuring the Pressure Within

Glaucoma is one of the leading causes of blindness in the United States. Early detection of the disease won't restore already lost vision, but prompt treatment can stop further deterioration and slow vision loss. A simple testing procedure, called tonometry, can alert your doctor to possible glaucoma.

Tonometry is a method of measuring the pressure within the eyeball. Normal eye pressure (intraocular pressure) is approximately 10 to 22 millimeters of mercury. If tonometry reveals higher pressure, further tests need to be done to determine if you have glaucoma.

Applanation tonometer

The applanation tonometer is a sophisticated device that's usually fitted to a slit lamp, a common instrument for eye examination. For this extremely accurate test, the doctor will numb your eyes with drops. You sit at the slit lamp and a small, plastic plunger pushes lightly against your eyeball. The force required to flatten (applanate) a small area of your cornea translates into a measure of your eye pressure. After the test, your eyes may feel scratchy for a short time.

Air-puff tonometer

An air-puff tonometer uses a puff of air to measure the force needed to indent your cornea. It's not as accurate as the applanation tonometer, but it has the advantage of not requiring the use of anesthetic drops because the instrument doesn't touch the eye.

of optic nerve damage is found, your doctor may suggest monitoring of the condition by having an eye exam several times a year.

If you have elevated eye pressure, your optic nerve shows signs of damage and you've lost peripheral vision, treatment is generally necessary. If you have signs of optic nerve damage and visual field loss, even if your eye pressure is in the normal range, treatment is generally recommended to lower eye pressure further, which may help slow progression of glaucoma.

Glaucoma can be controlled with eyedrops, oral medications or surgical procedures.

Medication

Treatment for chronic glaucoma often starts with medicated eyedrops to help decrease pressure in the eye. For years, the most popular eyedrops to treat glaucoma were those containing adrenaline (epinephrine) or pilocarpine to increase the outflow of fluid.

However, these medications can cause troublesome side effects. As a result, other eyedrops have been developed and are now prescribed. The following list includes eyedrops and medications taken by mouth:

- **Beta blockers.** These eyedrops are remarkably effective. Three drugs commonly used are timolol (Betimol, Timoptic), betaxolol (Betoptic S) and levobunolol (Akbeta, Betagan). Beta blockers can slow heart rhythm and worsen bronchial asthma symptoms. In some circumstances they can leave you feeling fatigued, drowsy, depressed or confused. They can also cause temporary impotence. If you have asthma, bronchitis or emphysema or if you have diabetes and use insulin, beta blockers usually should be avoided.
- **Other eyedrop medications.** These include alpha-adrenergic agents, such as apraclonidine (Iopidine) and brimonidine

(Alphagan P); carbonic anhy-drase inhibitors, such as dorzol-amide (Trusopt); prostaglandin analogues, such as latanoprost (Xalatan); and prostamides, such as bimatoprost (Lumigan). The medications lower eye pressure either by increasing the outflow of fluid from the eye or by reduc-ing the production of fluid. They all have various side effects.

• **Oral medications.** Certain drugs taken by mouth, such as acetazolamide, can lower the pressure within your eye by decreasing the formation of normal eye fluid. This type of medicine can also cause general side effects, and long-term use generally isn't recommended.

Your ophthalmologist under-stands the possible side effects of various medication. If you experience problems, your dosage may be adjusted or you may be switched to another treatment.

Surgery

If medication is unsuccessful in lowering intraocular pressure, your doctor may recommend an operation. Several options are available. In one procedure, a la-ser beam is used to open blocked drainage channels in the front chamber of the eye. For more severe cases, an operation known as a filtration procedure may be recommended. In this procedure, a drainage passage is surgically created between the interior of the eye and the conjunctiva to relieve pressure within the eye.

Acute glaucoma

Signs and symptoms

• Blurred vision, usually in one eye
• Halos appearing around lights
• Eye pain
• A red eye

Acute (closed-angle) glauco-ma is less common than chronic glaucoma. This type occurs when the drainage angle formed by the cornea and iris closes or becomes blocked. The aqueous humor can't exit, resulting in an increase in eye pressure. The increase in pressure can occur suddenly or progress more gradually.

Most people with this type of glaucoma have a very narrow drainage angle, which may be an abnormality from birth. Acute glaucoma is more common among individuals who are farsighted. Normal aging also may cause angle blockage. With age, the lens becomes larger, pushing your iris forward and narrowing the space between the iris and cornea.

A sudden increase in eye pres-sure can result from conditions that cause the pupils to become widely dilated. These may include:
• Darkness or dim light
• Stress or excitement
• Certain medications, such as antihistamines, tricyclic antide-pressants and eyedrops used to dilate the pupil

Attacks of acute glaucoma can develop suddenly or follow warnings weeks or months ahead. The attacks often occur in the evening when the light is dim

and the pupils are dilated. Your vision may become blurred, you may see halos around lights, your eye becomes red, and it may be painful. Although an acute attack often affects only one eye, the other eye is at risk as well.

In a severe attack, the symptoms are more severe and persistent. The pain may be extreme, causing vomiting. The cornea may appear hazy, even gray. The eyeball may be painful and hard to the touch.

An attack of acute glaucoma requires immediate treatment at your local emergency department. Without treatment, it can cause vision loss within hours of onset.

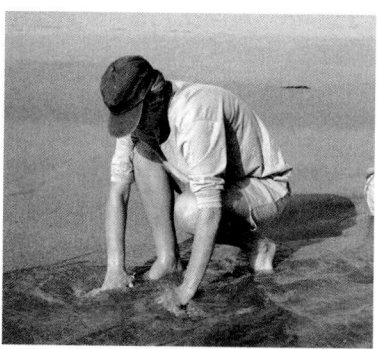 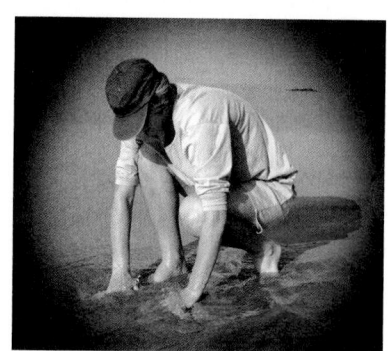 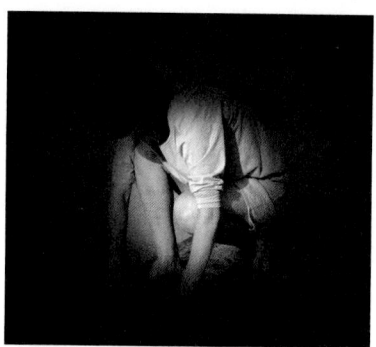

The gradual loss of peripheral vision associated with glaucoma is shown in this sequence from normal vision (left) to early-stage glaucoma (center) to advanced-stage glaucoma (right).

Are You at Risk?

Cataracts are more common among women than men, and more common among black people than white people. However, everyone is at risk of developing cataracts with increasing age. Apart from age, other factors that may increase your risk include:

- Diabetes
- A family history of cataracts
- Previous eye injury or inflammation
- Previous eye surgery
- Prolonged use of cortico-steroid medications
- Excessive consumption of alcohol
- Excessive exposure to sunlight
- Exposure to high levels of radiation, such as cancer therapy
- Smoking

Treatment

Doctors may administer medications to quickly reduce eye pressure. Once your eye pressure is under control, you may need to have an operation called an iridotomy. In this procedure, an ophthalmologist uses a laser beam to create a small hole in the iris that allows aqueous humor to flow more freely within the aqueous cavity. With this technique, a surgeon can create a drainage hole without having to make a surgical incision, avoiding many of the risks generally associated with conventional surgery.

Your doctor may perform an iridotomy on the other eye at a later date because of the high risk that it too will be affected by an acute attack in the future.

Cataracts

Signs and symptoms
- Clouded, blurred or dim vision
- Halos around lights

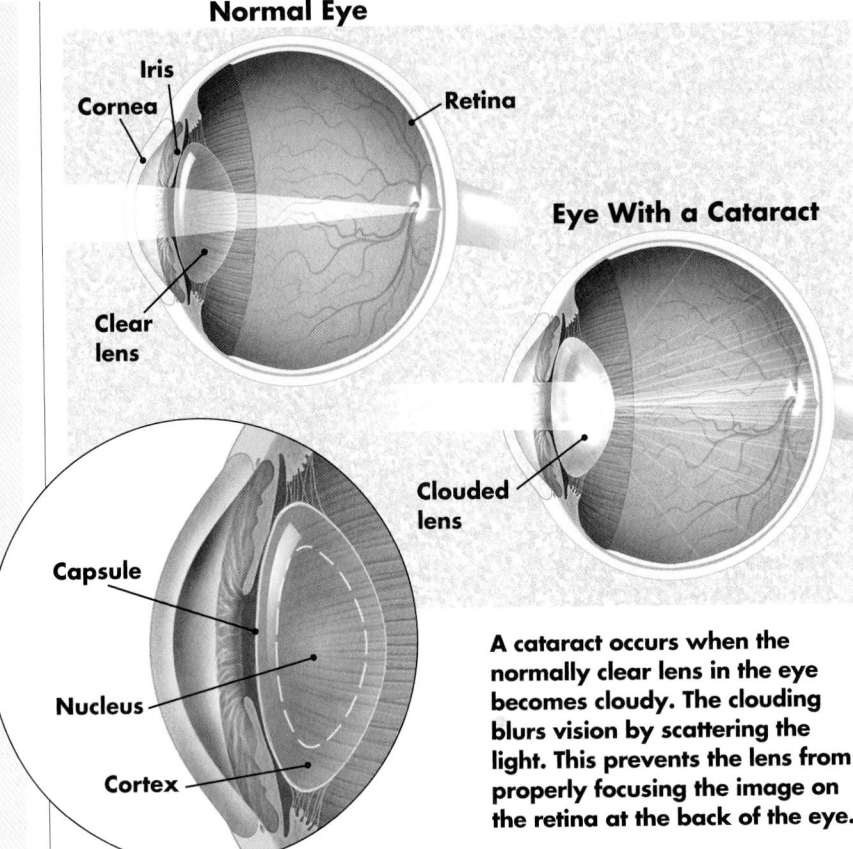

Normal Eye

Iris
Cornea
Retina
Clear lens

Eye With a Cataract

Clouded lens

Capsule
Nucleus
Cortex

A cataract occurs when the normally clear lens in the eye becomes cloudy. The clouding blurs vision by scattering the light. This prevents the lens from properly focusing the image on the retina at the back of the eye.

A cataract can form in any one of the layers of the lens — the nucleus, cortex or capsule.

- Impaired vision at night or in bright light
- Sensitivity to bright light and glare
- A need for brighter light for reading and other activities
- Frequent changes in your eyeglass or contact lens prescription
- Fading or yellowing of colors
- Double vision or multiple vision in one eye

A cataract is a clouding of the normally clear lens of the eye. The lens, one of the two main focusing mechanisms of the eye, lies just behind the pupil. Clouding of the lens blocks the passage of light needed for sight. Although a cataract often starts in only one eye, usually both become involved. Cataracts are accompanied by changes in the chemical composition of the lens, but the cause of these alterations is unknown.

Cataracts are a major cause of vision loss worldwide. In the United States, more than 2 million cataract operations are performed each year. Many people find the idea of cataracts alarming — assuming that if they develop them, they'll become blind. In fact, cataracts are one of the least serious eye disorders because in most instances surgery can restore lost sight.

Everyone develops some clouding of the eye lenses with age. Most people older than age 60 have some degree of cataract formation. But age isn't the only factor in the development of cataracts. Certain diseases, such as diabetes, contribute to the formation of cataracts. People who take corticosteroid medications for a period of years, for diseases such as rheumatoid arthritis, may develop cataracts. People who are exposed to high amounts of ultraviolet radiation from the sun over a period of time also are at increased risk of developing cataracts.

Occasionally, a baby is born with cataracts or develops them shortly after birth. Certain eye disorders, such as iritis or an injury to the eyeball, can lead to the development of cataracts. Cataracts also tend to run in families.

There are three types of cataracts. The most common type, and the one associated with aging, is a nuclear cataract. It occurs in the middle of the lens. A cortical cataract begins as white, wedge-shaped streaks on the outer edge of the lens cortex. A subcapsular cataract starts as a small, opaque area just under the capsule or shell of the lens, usually at the back of the lens.

Most cataracts develop slowly and often don't disturb eyesight in early stages of the disease. Because almost everyone experiences changes in eyesight later in life, the gradual clouding of the lens resulting from cataracts is often ignored. But as the clouding progresses, eventually it can interfere significantly with your vision.

This change in vision is often described as a film-like covering over one or both eyes. You may seem to be looking through fog or a frosty window. Your vision may be worse in both dim and bright light, and you may have problems driving at night. Glare and halos around oncoming lights can make driving after dark especially uncomfortable and dangerous.

Some people experience an improvement in their near vision as the cataract progresses. They may find that they can read without their glasses, a condition known as second sight. In the early stages of development, a nuclear cataract increases the focusing power of the lens. People with a nuclear cataract may need more-frequent changes in their prescription glasses. But as the degree of clouding increases, the temporary improvement in reading ability decreases.

Diagnosis

If you notice changes in your vision, see your eye specialist for a complete examination. Cataracts often aren't visible until they're quite advanced.

Tests to diagnose cataracts include a visual acuity test, a slit-lamp examination and a retinal exam. An ophthalmologist will likely dilate your pupil to examine the lens for signs of a cataract and to determine how dense the clouding is.

Treatment

The only effective treatment for a cataract is surgery to remove the clouded lens and replace it with a lens implant.

Self-care

Medications, dietary supplements or optical devices can't cure cataracts. However, in the early stages when symptoms are mild, you can do a few things to deal with symptoms:

- Make sure your eyeglass or contact lens prescription is the most accurate possible.
- Improve the lighting at home with more or brighter lamps.
- To reduce glare, wear sunglasses during the day when going outside. Some people also wear sunglasses at night to reduce glare from headlights.
- Limit or avoid night driving.
- Use magnifying glasses to read.

These measures may help temporarily, but as the cataract progresses, your vision deteriorates. When vision loss starts to interfere with everyday activities, you may want to consider surgery.

Surgery

Cataract surgery usually is appropriate when failing vision interferes with normal activities. The decision whether and when to have the operation varies with each individual, depending on age, occupation and lifestyle.

In some instances, surgery may be recommended early if there's a risk that the cataract may lead to other eye complications. Years ago, people with cataracts were

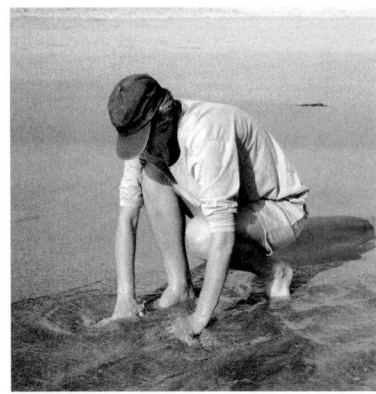

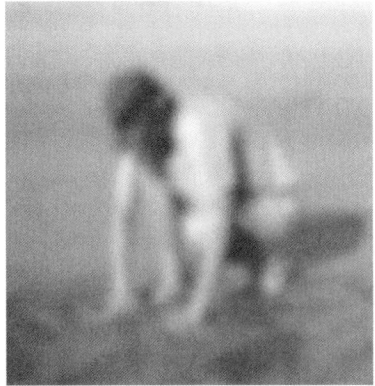

Normal vision (top) becomes blurred as a cataract forms (bottom).

often advised to postpone surgery until the cataract had "ripened," totally clouding the lens. Doctors no longer recommend waiting that long.

Like all surgical techniques, cataract surgery is constantly being improved. Unlike years ago, when cataract surgery was a major operation, the surgery is often done now in an hour or less, without a hospital stay. The lens is removed from the eye and, in most cases, is replaced with an artificial lens. The vast majority of people who have cataract surgery end up with improved vision.

The most common type of cataract surgery is phacoemulsification. In this procedure, the surgeon uses a microscope and ultrasound instruments to remove the cataract, leaving most of the lens capsule in place. The capsule helps support the lens implant. Phacoemulsification requires a very small incision, and the recovery period is short.

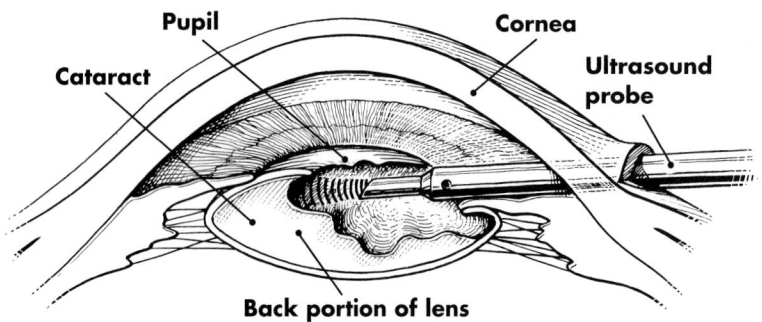

During phacoemulsification the rapidly vibrating tip of the ultrasound hand probe breaks up the cataract, which is then suctioned out.

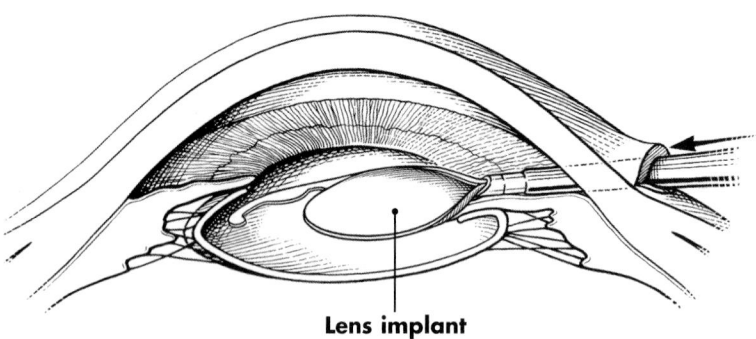

After removing the cataract, the surgeon inserts the lens implant into the empty capsule where the natural lens used to be.

An alternative procedure, called extracapsular cataract extraction, is similar to phacoemulsification but requires a larger incision. It may be needed if your cataract has progressed so far that phacoemulsification can't effectively break up the clouded lens.

After making an opening in the front part of the lens capsule, the surgeon removes the harder center of the lens in one piece and, with suction, removes the more peripheral cloudy lens material. The back portion of the lens capsule is left intact.

Rarely, a surgeon may use a procedure called intracapsular cataract extraction. This procedure involves removal of the entire lens, including the capsule. If a lens implant is performed, the lens will most likely be placed in front of the iris.

Once the cataract has been removed by either phacoemulsification or extracapsular extraction, a clear artificial lens is implanted into the empty lens capsule. This implant, known as an intraocular lens, is made of plastic, acrylic or silicone. You won't be able to see or feel the lens. It requires no care and it becomes a permanent part of your eye.

Most intraocular lenses used today are flexible, allowing a smaller incision that doesn't require stitches. The surgeon folds this type of lens and inserts it into the empty capsule where the natural lens used to be. Once in place, the lens folds to about 1/4 inch in diameter.

Recent advances in intraocular lenses include blue-blocking lenses, which filter out ultraviolet light. Other types of intraocular lenses provide multifocal vision — allowing you to see things both close up and at a distance. The primary goal of multifocal intraocular lenses is to provide you with good visual acuity at more than one distance without the aid of eyeglasses or contact lenses.

Multifocal lenses offer reasonably good near and distance vision. However, vision at the

When Is Surgery the Right Choice?

Cataract surgery restores good vision to thousands of people every day — it's the most common surgery for Americans age 65 and older.

The decision when to have surgery is one that you and your ophthalmologist should make together. In general, consider surgery when your vision starts to hamper your lifestyle.

If you have cataracts and you agree with one or more of the following statements, you may be a candidate for cataract surgery:

- Because of my vision, I don't feel confident when driving.
- Because of my vision, I can't do my best work.
- Because of my vision, I can't read comfortably.
- Because of my vision, I can't do things I enjoy.
- Because of my vision, I'm afraid I'll bump into something or trip and fall.
- Because of my vision, I'm not as independent as I'd like to be.

intermediate range is sometimes less than satisfactory. Some people continue to wear eyeglasses or contact lenses. While vision improves with multifocal lenses, it isn't as sharp as they would like. Glare or halos around lights also can be a problem with multifocal lenses. Improvements are ongoing.

With most cataract surgeries, healing is fast, and vision starts to improve within a few days. If your surgery requires a larger incision with sutures, full healing may take about four weeks.

Other options
There are some alternatives to a lens implant. They include eye-

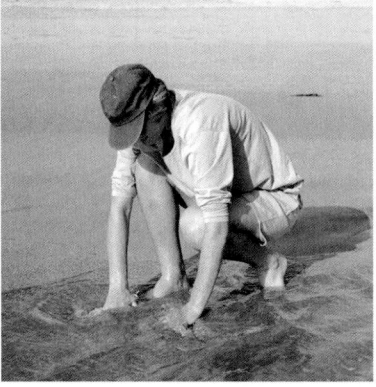 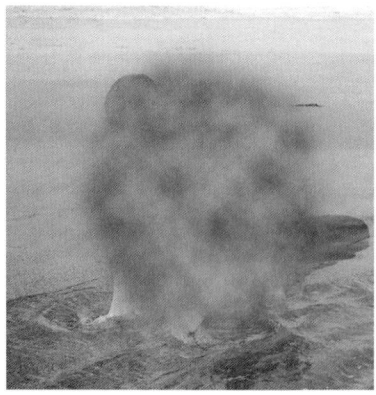

As macular degeneration develops, eyesight becomes impaired by general haziness and a blind spot at the center of the visual field.

glasses and contact lenses. Until the advent of lens implants, thick eyeglass lenses were the only way to correct vision after cataract surgery if contact lenses weren't an option.

Although glasses are helpful, they do have significant drawbacks, including excessive magnification, reduced side vision and limited depth perception.

Contact lenses usually provide better vision than do thick glasses. They're especially helpful if the lens of only one eye is removed. However, some older adults don't care for contact lenses.

Age-related macular degeneration

Signs and symptoms
- A need for bright light when reading or doing close work
- Printed words become increasingly blurry
- Colors appear dull and washed out
- A gradual haziness of overall vision
- Increasingly blurred central vision
- Visual distortions, such as straight lines appearing wavy or crooked

Age-related macular degeneration (AMD) is a chronic disease that occurs if tissue in the macula, the part of your retina that perceives central vision, deteriorates with aging. The result is blurred central vision or even a blind spot in the center of your visual field. Macular degeneration is the leading cause of severe vision loss in people age 50 and older.

The macula (Latin for "spot") is located in the center of the retina and is densely packed with light-sensitive cones and rods. In the early stages of macular degeneration, small deposits called drusen form in this area. As the disease progresses, abnormal blood vessels grow from the choroid, a layer rich in blood vessels under the retina. The retina's supporting tissue (retinal pigment epithelium) also disappears. Both processes damage the light-sensitive cells of the retina, causing loss of reading or central vision.

The first sign of macular degeneration may be a need for more light when you do close-up work. Fine newsprint and street signs may become more difficult to read. Eventually, you may notice that when you look at an object, what should be a smooth, straight line appears distorted or crooked. Gray or blank spots may mask the center of your visual field.

Macular degeneration affects your central vision but not your peripheral vision, so it doesn't cause total blindness. The damage caused by macular degeneration often can't be reversed. But early detection and treatment may help reduce the extent of vision loss.

Types
There are two types of macular degeneration: dry and wet.

Dry
Macular degeneration starts out as the dry form. This occurs when the supporting tissue of the retina begins to thin. The normally reddish-brown color of the macula takes on a mottled appearance, and drusen appear under the retina. Most people have the dry form. It may initially affect only one eye, but usually both eyes eventually become involved.

Wet
Wet macular degeneration develops when new blood vessels grow

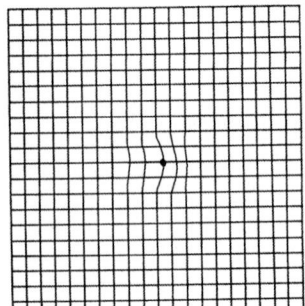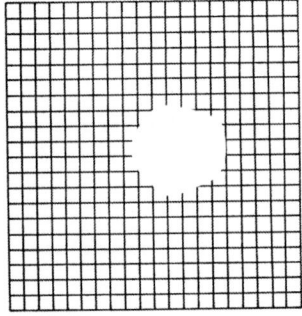

© Amsler M. Earliest symptoms of diseases of the macula. British Journal of Ophthalmology. 1953;37:521.

Someone in the early stages of macular degeneration may see distorted grid lines (left). Someone with a more advanced stage may see a blank spot at the center of the grid (right).

from the choroid underneath the macula. These abnormal vessels leak fluid or blood and cause your central vision to blur. All eyes with wet macular degeneration also show signs of the dry form (drusen and mottled pigmentation). Straight lines appear to be wavy or crooked, and blank spots appear in your field of vision. Vision loss is usually rapid and severe.

Diagnosis
Your eye specialist can test for macular degeneration during a routine eye examination. He or she may begin with a simple test of your central vision using an Amsler grid (see grid above). If you have macular degeneration, some of the straight lines may seem faded, broken or distorted when you look at the grid.

To evaluate the extent of damage to the macula, your doctor may perform a test known as fluorescein angiography to look for abnormal blood vessels. A special dye is injected into a vein of your arm. The dye flows to the blood vessels in the eye. Photographs of the retina are taken and can identify problems with the macula. A similar procedure called indocyanine green angiography may confirm or provide additional information to the fluorescein angiogram.

Optical coherence tomography (OCT) is another diagnostic test that may be used. It creates a cross-sectional image of the eyeball to reveal areas where the retina has thickened or thinned, changes associated with macular degeneration. OCT also can reveal if fluid has accumulated under the retina.

Treatment
A study called the Age-Related Eye Disease Study (AREDS) provides a clear direction for slowing the progression of age-related macular degeneration. It found that a daily supplement containing high doses of vitamin C, vitamin E, beta carotene, zinc and copper reduced by 25 percent the risk of macular degeneration advancing to a more severe stage.

The same research group launched a follow-up study called AREDS2 to see if they could improve the supplement formula. The study found omega-3 fatty acids had no effect on the formulation, and lutein and zeaxanthin together appeared to be a safe alternative to beta carotene, which has been linked to an increased risk of lung cancer in smokers.

For wet macular degeneration, some treatment options are available. The success of treatment often depends on the location and extent of the abnormal blood vessels.

Successful treatment can halt further progress of the disease and may reverse some of the damage.

Anti-angiogenic therapy
When damaged tissue is healing after an injury, new blood

Are You at Risk?

Although researchers don't know the exact causes of macular degeneration, they've identified some contributing factors. These include:

- *Age and race.* The disease is most common in white people older than age 50. It's less common among black people, Asians and American Indians.
- *Family history.* If someone in your family has age-related macular degeneration, you're at greater risk.
- *Cigarette smoking.* Smokers are two to three times more likely than are nonsmokers to develop macular degeneration.
- *Exposure to sunlight.* Long-term exposure to ultraviolet light and blue light — the wavelength just above ultraviolet — may increase your risk. This includes use of sunlamps as well as sunlight.
- *Cardiovascular disease.* This includes circulatory problems, stroke, heart attack and chest pain (angina). Cardiovascular disease that's not well-controlled may contribute to the onset of macular degeneration.
- *Lighter eye color.* People with lighter colored eyes may be at greater risk than people with darker colored eyes.

vessels will form. This process, called angiogenesis, is triggered by the action of proteins — such as vascular endothelial growth factor (VEGF) — that signal blood vessels to grow.

Anti-angiogenic medications work by inhibiting proteins, such as VEGF, that trigger development of new blood vessels. The medications are administered at regular intervals by injecting them directly into the affected eye. This is the most effective way to administer medications to the retina so they reach the target.

A growing body of evidence suggests that the foods you eat may help protect your eyesight. The Age-Related Eye Disease Study (AREDS) and the AREDS2 study highlight the impact of dietary supplements in people at high risk of developing advanced stages of macular degeneration. People in the study groups were able to reduce the risk of progression of macular degeneration, as well as the risk of vision loss, by taking a combination of vitamin C, vitamin E, zinc, copper and either beta carotene or the antioxidants lutein and zeaxanthin. The combination didn't work for early stages of macular degeneration, nor did it affect the development of cataracts.

Vitamins C and E and carotenoids such as beta carotene are antioxidants. Antioxidants are vitamins, minerals and enzymes that help maintain healthy cells and tissues by combating free radicals, unstable oxygen molecules that damage normal cells in a process called oxidation. Oxidation is thought to play a role in the development of cataracts, macular degeneration and glaucoma, as well as many other diseases.

Scientists continue to look at the role that antioxidants may play in the prevention of eye disease. Another study found that people who regularly ate five servings or more a week of dark green leafy vegetables, which are rich in the carotenoids lutein and zeaxanthin, had a markedly lower risk of getting macular degeneration than did study participants who ate smaller amounts or none of these vegetables. A healthy diet may be even more effective in preventing eye disease than taking vitamins.

Reducing your risk generally involves including foods that contain antioxidants in your diet for many years. Your best bet is simply to eat a variety of foods, especially fruits, vegetables and whole grains. Include deep green, dark yellow, red and orange fruits and vegetables. Good choices include collard greens, spinach, green and red peppers, carrots, kale, Swiss chard, cantaloupe, mango, squash, sweet potatoes, broccoli, Brussels sprouts, tomatoes, strawberries, citrus fruits and watermelon.

If you eat a balanced diet, your body will get all of the nutrients it needs. It's fine to take a daily vitamin and mineral supplement, but supplements are no substitute for eating a variety of healthy foods. Excessive doses of vitamins can have dangerous side effects.

The risk of complications from intravitreal injection is low, and the problems are usually temporary and treatable. The most common side effect is redness and scratchiness of the eyeball.

Unlike some other treatments, anti-angiogenic medications also can be used in a broader range of people with wet macular degeneration. Anti-angiogenic therapy is also less likely to cause vision loss than are other therapies.

Laser surgery

A form of laser surgery called photocoagulation can, in some cases, prevent further damage to the macula and halt progression of vision loss for some time. In this procedure, a special lens placed on the eye focuses laser light onto the retina to create small burns, which can seal off and destroy abnormal new blood vessels under your macula.

Whether this surgery is appropriate for you depends on the location and appearance of the blood vessels, the amount of blood that's leaked and the general health of your macula. Very few people with macular degeneration are candidates for laser treatment, and the results are often disappointing — it's successful only about

Spots, Specks and Flashes

Just about everyone occasionally sees what appear to be specks, hairs and fine strings floating freely in the fluid of the eye. These vitreous floaters move in and out of your field of vision. They result from changes in the vitreous humor related to aging and from certain conditions such as nearsightedness (myopia) or inflammation.

As you age, you may notice more and different floaters because the vitreous humor in your eye may shrink and liquefy. The vitreous humor is a jellylike substance that fills the inside of your eye. It's composed almost entirely of water and accounts for three-fourths of the weight of your eye. At the back of the eye, the vitreous cavity attaches to the retina, the light-sensitive tissue of the eye.

When the vitreous cavity shrinks, it gradually leads to the appearance of spots, specks, hairs or strings floating in the fluid. The floaters may be annoying, but they tend to become less conspicuous with time and only rarely affect vision.

If floaters develop or suddenly increase in number, this may signal a serious eye disorder. Consult your ophthalmologist immediately.

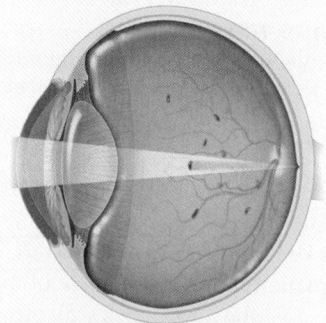

Floaters can interfere with vision by intercepting light entering the eye, casting a shadow on the retina.

50 percent of the time. New blood vessel growth may recur.

If you noticed a dark or gray spot in or near your central vision before laser treatment, the procedure will make vision in that spot completely and permanently blank. With time, you may not notice the blank spot any longer, especially when you use both eyes.

Photodynamic therapy

Photodynamic therapy (PDT) treats damaged areas at the center of the macula while still preserving some central vision. This procedure combines a cold laser and a light-sensitizing dye that's injected into your bloodstream. This dye concentrates in the abnormal blood vessels under the macula. When hit by cold laser light, the dye releases substances that seal the leaking vessels without damaging the macula.

Macular translocation surgery

Macular translocation surgery is an experimental treatment for wet macular degeneration. This surgery may be used if abnormal blood vessels are located directly under the center of the macula (fovea). The procedure shifts the fovea away from the damaged area and moves it over healthy tissue. The surgery is followed by laser treatment to destroy the abnormal blood vessels without damaging the fovea.

Retinal detachment

Signs and symptoms

- A sensation of flashing lights
- Many floaters — spots, specks or lines — in the field of vision
- Blurred vision
- A shadow over a portion of the field of vision

The retina is a thin, transparent membrane that lies smoothly against the inside back wall of your eye. It contains cells that are sensitive to light (cones and rods). It also contains the nerves that carry impulses from the cones and rods to the optic nerve. The optic nerve transports the signals to the brain. A thin layer of tiny blood vessels (choroid) lies under the retina. This layer supplies oxygen and nutrients to the retina, essential for it to function properly.

Retinal detachment results when the retina separates from this layer of blood vessels.

Most cases of retinal detachment are caused by a tear or hole in the retina. The defect may develop from changes in the eye's vitreous fluid caused by aging, or it may develop in weak patches of the retina. The tear allows fluid from the vitreous cavity to leak under the retina and lift it from the choroid. This form of detachment is called rhegmatogenous detachment — caused by a retinal defect.

Occasionally, a tumor or an inflammatory disorder affecting the back portion of the eye also can lead to a separation of the retina from the underlying choroid. Such a detachment is called a serous retinal detachment.

Rhegmatogenous retinal detachment occurs in about 36,000 people in the United States each year. The condition almost always leads to blindness in the affected eye if it's not surgically repaired.

As the vitreous cavity shrinks and sags, it may tug on the retina, producing the sensation of flashing lights. If the tugging is strong enough to cause small holes or tears to develop in the retina, vitreous humor may seep under the retina. This causes hazy vision and the appearance of floaters — spots, specks or lines in the field of vision. As liquid collects, areas of the retina surrounding the holes or tears may pull away from the underlying layer of blood vessels (choroid). The areas where the retina is detached no longer function.

Not all tears and holes lead to retinal detachment. Sometimes, the retina remains attached to the choroid. But detachment that goes undetected and untreated can progress and eventually involve

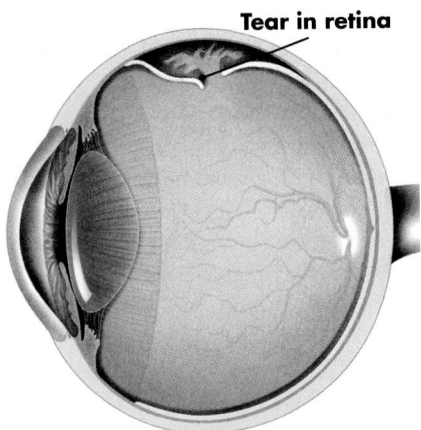

Tear in retina

When vitreous humor leaks through holes in the retina, the retina may start to pull away from the underlying layer of blood vessels. As more liquid accumulates, the detachment may expand, and parts of the visual field may become blurred or lost.

the entire retina, with complete loss of vision in that eye.

Diagnosis

An ophthalmologist can determine if you have a retinal hole, tear or detachment by carefully examining the retina with an ophthalmoscope. If blood in the vitreous humor prevents a clear view of the retina, an ophthalmologist might use sound waves (ultrasound) to get an image of the retina.

Treatment

Surgery is the only effective treatment for retinal detachment. If a tear or hole is treated before detachment occurs or if a retinal detachment is treated before the portion of the retina responsible for central vision (macula) has detached, you hopefully will retain much of your vision.

Surgery for a tear or hole

When a retinal tear or retinal hole hasn't progressed to a detachment, a doctor may use one of two techniques:

- **Photocoagulation.** In this process a laser beam is directed to the area around the retinal defect. The treated area then forms a scar, which usually holds the retina to the underlying tissue.

- **Cryopexy.** This method uses intense cold to freeze the retina around the tear or hole. A freezing probe is applied to the outer surface of the eye directly over the retinal defect. It produces inflammation that leads to the formation of a scar, sealing the defect and holding the retina to the underlying tissue.

Surgery for retinal detachment

Three different surgical procedures are commonly used to repair a retinal detachment. Which of the procedures a surgeon chooses depends on the severity and complexity of the condition:

- **Pneumatic retinopexy.** This technique is used for an uncomplicated detachment in which the retinal defect is located in the upper part of the retina. After freezing the retinal defect (cryopexy), the surgeon injects a bubble of gas into the vitreous cavity. The bubble expands and seals the retinal defect and prevents any more vitreous humor from entering the space below the retina. Fluid that already has collected under the retina is absorbed, and the retina reattaches itself to the back wall of the eye.
- **Scleral buckling.** This is the most common surgery for repairing retinal detachment. First the surgeon treats the tears or holes with cryopexy. Then he or she indents (buckles) the sclera over the affected area by pressing in with a piece of silicone sutured to the outside of the wall of the eye (sclera). The silicone material is either solid or in the form of a soft sponge.

  The buckle closes the tear or hole and helps reduce the circumference of the eyeball, to prevent further pulling and separation. When there are several tears or holes or an extensive detachment, the surgeon may create a scleral buckle encircling the entire circumference of the

eye. The buckle is stitched to the outer surface of the sclera, then covered with the conjunctiva. Once the incision heals, there's little evidence of the operation.

This procedure generally works more than 80 percent of the time with one operation. The success rate exceeds 90 percent with additional operations, if necessary. But it doesn't guarantee normal vision. How well you see afterward depends on the severity of the problem before surgery. There's also a 10 percent chance of some loss of vision due to wrinkling or puckering of the macula.

- **Vitrectomy.** Sometimes, a doctor can't view a detached retina due to clouding of the vitreous by hemorrhage or inflammation. In other instances, scar tissue in the vitreous makes it impossible to repair a retinal detachment with pneumatic retinopexy or scleral buckling alone. In such situations, a procedure called vitrectomy removes the clouded vitreous or scar tissue. The surgeon accomplishes this with a variety of delicate instruments inserted into the eyeball through small openings in the sclera. Following vitrectomy, a scleral buckling procedure may be performed.

  In especially difficult cases, a surgeon may inject air, other gases or silicone oil into the vitreous cavity to help reposition the retina against the wall of the eye. Eventually, your eye absorbs the air or gas and replaces it with fluid that the eye normally produces. Silicone oil, however, isn't absorbed and has to be removed once the retina is reattached and has completely healed.

Retinal vessel occlusion

Signs and symptoms

- Sudden blurring or loss of vision in part or all of one eye

Intricate networks of arteries and veins support the retina. Both networks connect to major blood vessels that enter the eye through the optic nerve. Sometimes, these arteries and veins become blocked, a condition known as retinal vessel occlusion. The condition is common in older adults and can result in reduced vision or loss of vision.

Various factors can obstruct a blood vessel, such as a blood clot, accumulation of fatty deposits (plaques) in a vessel, collapse of a vessel wall and compression of a wall from outside pressure. A blocked vein may rupture and spill blood and fluid into the retina, blurring and clouding vision.

There are four different types of retinal vessel occlusion, determined by the location of the blockage — a vein or artery, a major (central) vessel, or a smaller branch vessel.

The extent of vision damage is generally dependent on the type, as well as how much time elapses before treatment.

Diagnosis

Regular eye examinations are helpful for early detection. A general medical exam that identifies any underlying disorder, such as high blood pressure, diabetes or narrowing of the major artery in your neck that supplies blood to your eyes and brain (carotid artery) also may lead to a diagnosis.

Treatment

Often, little can be done to treat retinal vascular occlusions. However, steps may be taken to prevent further damage and complications that can result from the disorder.

Medications may be administered to reduce pressure within the eye and help prevent further swelling (edema) of the macula. Laser treatment also may be used to relieve pressure and swelling, as well as help prevent the growth of new, abnormal blood vessels that can lead to glaucoma.

For one form of retinal vessel occlusion, called central retinal artery occlusion, experimental treatments aimed at dislodging the obstruction from the blood vessel are being explored. They include ocular massage, removal of aqueous humor from the eye, and inhaling an oxygen and carbon dioxide mixture.

Chances of improved vision are best if treatment occurs within 24 hours of the onset of symptoms.

Optic neuritis

Signs and symptoms
- Acute loss of vision in one eye
- Pain when moving the eye

Optic neuritis is an inflammation of the optic nerve anywhere along its path. The inflammation may stem from a viral illness or certain autoimmune diseases, such as multiple sclerosis. Frequently, the cause of optic neuritis is unknown.

When the condition affects the optic disk, it's known as papillitis. When the inflammation occurs in the portion of the optic nerve behind the eye, it's known as retrobulbar neuritis.

When the optic nerve swells, it blocks visual signals to the brain. The result is a gradual or sudden loss of vision in one or both eyes. With retrobulbar neuritis, eye movement may be painful. In the case of papillitis, loss of vision is usually the only symptom.

Diagnosis
A series of tests will likely be conducted to determine the nature and extent of the problem. Because optic neuritis often is associated with multiple sclerosis in young adults, your doctor may recommend a thorough medical examination.

Treatment
In many cases, optic neuritis gets better on its own without treatment. In some cases, steroid medications are used to treat optic neuritis because they help reduce inflammation of the optic nerve. You may receive steroid medications intravenously, or you may

take an oral pill. In instances in which steroid therapy has failed and severe vision loss persists, a treatment called plasma exchange therapy may help some people recover their vision.

An MRI scan of the brain is often done to determine the risk of multiple sclerosis. If you're at high risk, you may benefit from drugs that help prevent multiple sclerosis. They include interferon beta-1a and interferon beta-1b.

Ischemic optic neuropathy

Ischemic optic neuropathy is a painless swelling of the optic nerve resulting from the loss of blood supply to the nerve. It may be associated with inflammation of arteries in the scalp and head (temporal arteritis) or high blood pressure.

Both eyes may be involved. The inflammation usually resolves. Treatment involves determining and addressing the underlying condition. In the case of arteritis, it may also include the use of corticosteroid medications.

Coloboma

A coloboma is a rare congenital defect in the development of the eye. Parts of the iris, ciliary body, lens, retina, choroid and optic nerve may be absent.

Depending on the extent of the defect, there may be partial or even complete loss of vision in the affected eye. Sometimes, both eyes are affected. It's essential that a child with loss of vision from a coloboma wear protective glasses as soon as possible to protect the unaffected eye from injury.

Choroiditis

Signs and symptoms
- Blurred vision in one eye
- Pain or discomfort in the eye

The choroid is the layer between the retina and sclera of the eye.

It's made up mainly of blood vessels, which nourish the retina. When this layer becomes inflamed (choroiditis), the retina may also become inflamed. This condition is then called chorioretinitis. When the inflammation subsides, the choroid and retina may be scarred. Vision may be impaired if the macula — the center part of the retina responsible for central vision — is involved.

Because the inflammation usually occurs in a spotty fashion, loss of vision is also spotty. Each scarred area will cause a corresponding blind spot, which can be discovered through testing. In many people, the scarring from choroiditis poses no handicap to vision because the blank spots (scotomata) are small and don't involve the macula.

The cause of this condition is often unknown. Occasionally, it may be associated with certain infections, such as histoplasmosis or toxoplasmosis.

Diagnosis
A test may be performed in which dye is injected into a vein in your arm. When it reaches the blood vessels of the eye, a series of photographs of the retina can reveal areas of inflammation. Your doctor may also recommend a general medical examination to rule out the possibility of a serious underlying disorder.

Treatment
Corticosteroid medications may be given to reduce the inflammation. They may be administered in pill form or you may receive an injection in or near the eye. Treatment of any underlying disorder also may improve symptoms.

Retinitis pigmentosa

Signs and symptoms
- Difficulty seeing at night or in reduced light
- Poor central vision
- Loss of side (peripheral) vision

Retinitis pigmentosa is an inherited disorder in which the retina slowly degenerates in both eyes. The structures in the retina called rods are affected the most, causing defective night vision (night blindness). As the disease progresses, peripheral vision also may be lost, producing so-called tunnel vision.

The disease, which is uncommon, may lead to legal blindness. The main criterion for legal blindness is visual acuity of 20/200 or poorer in the better eye while wearing glasses.

Retinitis pigmentosa can be detected in childhood. Reduced night vision may become evident by age 10. If your family has a history of the disorder, have your child tested early.

Diagnosis

During an examination of your eye, an eye doctor may see dark pigmentation of the retina, hence the name pigmentosa. Tests to determine the presence and extent of the disease include a procedure that records the electric response of the retina to light (electroretinography) and another procedure to determine how well the eyes adjust to reduced illumination (dark adaptation).

Treatment

There's no known treatment to cure retinitis pigmentosa, although some research suggests that vitamin A supplements may slow progression of the disease. Use of low vision aids can be helpful.

Some researchers suggest using sunglasses to protect the retina from the harmful effects of visible and ultraviolet light. Experimental devices that widen the field of vision may prove helpful in the future.

Retinoblastoma

Signs and symptoms
- A white color in the center circle (pupil) of the eye
- Cross-eye
- A red, painful eye

- Eye swelling
- White spots on the iris

Tumors can develop anywhere in the body and may be either noncancerous (benign) or cancerous (malignant). Retinoblastoma is a cancer that begins in the retina — the sensitive lining on the inside of your eye. It most commonly affects young children, and only rarely occurs in adults.

Retinoblastoma is often inherited, but the cancer also occurs in children with no family history of the disease. The prognosis for retinoblastoma is good if it's treated early. If someone in your family has had retinoblastoma, be sure to have your children tested early and re-examined periodically.

Children treated for retinoblastoma have a risk of the cancer returning in and around the treated eye. There's also an increased risk of other cancers developing in other parts of the body.

Diagnosis

The key to diagnosis of retinoblastoma is a thorough examination by a specialist experienced in diagnosing and treating retinoblastoma. Examination may be done with the child under general anesthesia to keep him or her still. The pupils are dilated widely so that the doctor can use indirect ophthalmoscopy to check for any growths. Scans and imaging tests help determine if the cancer has spread to other structures around the eye.

Treatment

Treatment of retinoblastoma depends on the number and size of tumors, their location and whether the cancer has spread to areas other than the eye.

Chemotherapy can help shrink a tumor so another treatment, such as external radiation, internal radiation (brachytherapy), cold treatments (cryotherapy), heat treatments (thermotherapy) or laser therapy, can treat the remaining cancer cells. Chemotherapy

is also used to treat cancer that has spread to tissues outside the eyeball.

If a tumor is large and has already destroyed vision, or if it continues to grow despite treatment, the eyeball may be removed and replaced with an implant.

Melanoma of the eye

Signs and symptoms
Conjunctival melanoma
- A brown or black spot on the covering of the eye (conjunctiva)
- A spot on the eye that enlarges or changes color with time

Uveal melanoma
- A dark spot on the iris
- A change in iris color
- Decreased vision
- Visual field defects
- A flickering light sensation
- A red, painful eye

Melanoma is usually seen as a form of skin cancer, but it can also begin in the eye. Melanoma of the eye (ocular melanoma) is a cancer of the pigmented tissues of the eye. It can occur on the surface of the eye (conjunctival melanoma) or inside the eye (uveal melanoma), involving the iris, ciliary body, which produces the fluid inside the eye and helps control lens movement, or choroid, the layer of tissue between the retina and sclera.

Melanoma of the eye is a potentially deadly cancer. As with any type of cancer, early detection and treatment are essential. Melanoma of the eye almost always originates in the eye itself and rarely spreads there from elsewhere in the body.

Diagnosis

The key to diagnosis is a thorough examination by a specialist familiar with the features and variations of eye tumors. In addition to a thorough eye examination, diagnostic tests to determine the extent of the tumor may include an ultrasound examination, a computerized tomography (CT) scan or magnetic resonance imaging (MRI).

How often should I have an eye exam if I have diabetes?

Eye exams are key to detecting problems from diabetic retinopathy. For this reason, regular eye examinations are crucial. The American Academy of Ophthalmology recommends the following:

- *People diagnosed with diabetes before age 30.* This group should have a comprehensive eye exam when diabetes has been present for five years or when the individual is 10 years old, whichever is later.
- *People diagnosed with diabetes at age 30 or older.* This group should have a baseline exam at the time of diagnosis.
- *Women with diabetes who are pregnant or intending to become pregnant.* This group should have an exam before conception or early in the first trimester and thereafter every three months.

Following an initial exam, everyone with diabetes should have his or her eyes checked once a year. If you have other eye diseases, your eye specialist may recommend more frequent monitoring.

Treatment

Treatment may depend on the size and location of the melanoma. Small, nongrowing tumors that cause no visual symptoms may be monitored closely with no immediate treatment.

Melanomas in the conjunctiva are often removed surgically, and the area around the tumor is treated with a freezing procedure (cryotherapy) to destroy any remaining cancer in the area. Small, limited tumors of the iris, ciliary body and choroid also may be treated with surgical removal.

When removing the tumor isn't possible, laser therapy (laser photocoagulation or transpupillary thermotherapy) may be used to destroy small, growing tumors. Radiation therapy and proton beam therapy also may be options.

The eye may have to be removed if the tumor is large, has invaded other parts of the eye or other treatments are unsuccessful. Ocular melanoma, including cancerous cells that have spread to other organs, generally respond poorly to chemotherapy.

Other Diseases and Your Eyes

Some conditions and diseases that affect other parts of the body can also affect your sight. These include stroke, Graves' disease, cranial arteritis, diabetes and high blood pressure.

Diabetic retinopathy

Signs and symptoms
- Blurred or fluctuating vision
- "Spiders," "cobwebs" or tiny specks floating in the eye
- Dark streaks or a red film that blocks vision
- A dark or empty spot in the center of your vision
- Difficulty adjusting from bright to dim light
- Poor night vision
- Eye pain, in advanced cases

The most common and most serious eye complication of diabetes is diabetic retinopathy. Retinopathy is the medical term for damage to the many tiny blood vessels that nourish the retina. Increased blood sugar associated with diabetes can gradually damage the vessels.

The longer you have diabetes, the more likely it is that you'll develop diabetic retinopathy. The disease is most common in individuals with type 1 diabetes who've had diabetes for at least 20 years. Almost everyone who has diabetes shows signs of retinal damage after about 30 years of living with the disease.

Most people with diabetic retinopathy experience only mild vision problems. But the condition can progress and threaten vision. In fact, diabetic retinopathy is a leading cause of blindness among adults in the United States.

Types
There are two types of diabetic retinopathy: nonproliferative and proliferative.

Nonproliferative
Nonproliferative diabetic retinopathy is the most common type. It can be described as mild, moderate or severe. In this condition, the walls of blood vessels in the retina weaken and tiny bulges (microaneurysms) protrude from the vessel walls. The vessels may leak fluid and blood into the retina. Nerve fibers in the retina also may begin to swell. The central portion of the retina (macula) may swell too, reducing blood flow to the macula and causing decreased central vision (macular edema).

Proliferative
Proliferative diabetic retinopathy is the most severe type of diabetic retinopathy. In this condition, abnormal blood vessels grow in the retina. Sometimes the new

blood vessels grow or leak into the clear, jellylike substance (vitreous humor) that fills the center of your eye. Eventually, scar tissue stimulated by the growth of new blood vessels may cause the retina to detach from the back of your eye. If the new blood vessels interfere with the flow of fluid out of the eye, pressure may build in the eyeball. This can damage the optic nerve that carries images from your eye to your brain.

Diagnosis

Diabetic retinopathy can develop with no initial visual problems. That's why annual eye examinations by an ophthalmologist are essential. Your ophthalmologist will examine the retina with an ophthalmoscope, which shines a bright light into the back of the eye

Third Nerve Palsy

Third nerve palsy is a common condition among people with diabetes. This disorder may involve a sudden onset of pain around the eye and double vision. The affected eye turns downward and outward. The pupil usually continues to react normally, enlarging in darkness and contracting in light. The upper eyelid often tends to droop (ptosis).

It's easy to think that these signs and symptoms might indicate a stroke — and in fact the disorder is the result of a temporary interruption of blood flow to the third cranial nerve. This nerve controls the action of some of the muscles that hold the eyeball in its normal position. The pain typically lasts a few days, and double vision and ptosis usually resolve in two to three months. If you have double vision, a droopy eyelid or pain around or in your eye, or if your eye fails to move properly in all directions, see an ophthalmologist promptly.

and allows viewing of the retina. He or she will look for microaneurysms, hemorrhages, fatty deposits and newly formed blood vessels.

In a procedure called fluorescein angiography, dye is injected into a vein of your arm makes its way to the veins in your eyes. As the dye circulates through your eyes, pictures are taken. The images pinpoint blood vessels that are closed, broken down or leaking.

You may also have an optical coherence tomography (OCT) exam. This imaging test provides cross-sectional images of the retina that show its thickness and whether fluid has leaked into retinal tissue.

Treatment

Treatment of diabetic retinopathy begins with managing your diabetes. Tight control of blood sugar slows the onset and progression of retinopathy.

Specific treatment for diabetic retinopathy depends on the severity of the condition and whether your vision is currently impaired or threatened. Mild nonproliferative retinopathy may not require immediate treatment. If you have proliferative diabetic retinopathy, you'll likely need surgical treatment.

Treatment may include one of the following:

Photocoagulation

Photocoagulation, also known as focal laser treatment, can stop the leakage of blood and fluid to the macula in the eye. During the procedure, a high-energy laser beam burns small, pinpoint areas of the retina where leakage is taking place and seals off abnormal blood vessels. Your vision may be blurry for about a day after the procedure. Sometimes small spots caused by the laser burns may appear in your visual field. The spots generally fade and disappear with time.

For proliferative diabetic retinopathy — in which many new blood vessels are forming — a form of laser surgery called pan-

retinal photocoagulation is often used. Another name for this procedure is scatter laser treatment. With this technique, the entire retina, except the macula, is treated with randomly placed laser burns. The burns cause abnormal new blood vessels to shrink and disappear.

Panretinal photocoagulation is usually done in two or more sessions. You may notice some loss of peripheral vision afterward. The treatment is a tradeoff. Some of your side vision may be sacrificed to save your central vision.

Vitrectomy

This procedure may be used to remove blood from the center of the eye (vitreous cavity) and scar tissue that's tugging on the retina.

During the procedure, a surgeon makes tiny incisions in your eye and delicate instruments are used to remove blood-filled tissue and scar tissue. A salt solution is added to maintain your eye's normal shape. Sometimes gas or silicone oil is placed in the eye to help keep the retina attached. The gas dissolves in about three to six weeks. The silicone oil is removed from the eye at a later stage.

Intravitreal injections

There are several medications that may be injected into the eye to treat swelling and new blood vessel growth in the retina. These include steroids and medications called anti-VEGF agents.

Graves' disease

Signs and symptoms
- Bulging or a feeling of pressure around the eyes
- Blurred or double vision
- Tearing
- Red or inflamed eyes
- Sensitivity to light
- Retraction of the eyelids
- Increased nervousness and heat intolerance
- Increased appetite, accompanied by weight loss

Graves' disease is a disorder of the thyroid gland in which too much of the hormone thyroxine is produced. An excess of thyroxine causes a wide range of signs and symptoms, including nervousness, heat intolerance, weight loss despite a healthy appetite, rapid and irregular pulse, and a fine tremor of the hands. For more on Graves' disease, see page 1019.

Immune system abnormalities that stimulate the thyroid also can cause eye problems. Changes in the eyelids and in the muscles that control your eyes may cause double vision and a wide-eyed (bug-eyed) appearance. The eyes may also protrude because of an increase in muscle, fat and other tissues behind the eye. In some cases, enlarged tissues can compress and seriously threaten the optic nerve.

Diagnosis

Eye changes may occur a year or more before or after the onset of the abnormal thyroid function. Protruding eyes and increased distance between the upper and lower eyelids are classic signs of Graves' disease. Sometimes, these eye changes are subtle and not readily apparent.

At times only one eye may seem to be affected, raising concerns about a tumor or sinus infection. Sometimes the most apparent symptom is irritation of the conjunctiva, which may be ascribed to conjunctivitis or an allergic reaction.

The degree of protrusion of the eye can be measured by an ophthalmologist with an exophthalmometer. This is more useful for determining whether the protrusion is worsening or improving than for establishing the diagnosis.

Treatment

Controlling overactivity of the thyroid gland is a key part of treatment to prevent the condition from worsening. If the treatment causes underactivity of the thyroid, you'll likely be given thyroxine tablets to replace the hormone.

Self-care

In many cases, the condition is a mild disorder that requires no treatment. Sleeping with your head elevated may decrease eyelid swelling. Topical ointments and artificial tears can help soothe eye irritation. Glasses with side guards help protect the eyes from dust and wind.

Medication

Temporary treatment with corticosteroid medications can help relieve eye tissue swelling.

Surgery

In more-severe cases, a surgeon may create extra space in a nearby sinus cavity to allow the eye to settle back into a more natural position within the orbit (socket). This procedure often corrects optic nerve changes, which can seriously threaten vision. The surgeon may also correct double vision by repositioning the enlarged muscles that control eye movement.

High blood pressure

Small blood vessels in the retina represent a sample of all of the blood vessels in the body, only they have the advantage of being readily visible. Narrowing of retinal arteries, small hemorrhages and protein deposits (exudates) that leak from affected blood vessels can be evidence of high blood pressure.

It's very unusual for high blood pressure to impair vision, but reduced vision can occur during a hypertensive crisis. Retinal arteries may severely narrow and the retina may swell.

Stroke

The term *stroke* describes several disorders caused by a disturbance in the blood supply to the brain.

The cause may be an insufficient supply of blood due to a blocked brain artery (ischemic stroke) or due to a rupture of an artery that causes bleeding into the brain (cerebral hemorrhage). In many cases, stroke has no warning signs. Only when you're experiencing one do you notice the signs and symptoms of headache, paralysis, sudden weakness and double vision or loss of vision.

If you experience a sudden loss of vision or double vision — or any other signs and symptoms such as sudden weakness on one side of the body, speech difficulty or lack of coordination — seek medical attention immediately.

Treatment

Treatment may include medications or surgery. If atherosclerosis is detected, you may be given anticoagulant medication to keep blood from clotting. If the main arteries in your neck are narrowed by plaques that reduce blood supply to the brain and eyes, surgery may help restore blood flow.

Cranial arteritis

Cranial arteritis, also known as giant cell arteritis or temporal arteritis, is an inflammation of arteries in the head and scalp. The diagnosis is often made by removing a portion of a scalp artery (biopsy) and examining it for inflammation. The inflammation is thought to result from an abnormal immune reaction that thickens the lining of the affected arteries, reducing or blocking blood flow to parts of the body, most commonly the eyes. Vision begins to diminish, and left untreated, the disorder can rapidly cause partial or total blindness.

Cranial arteritis can be treated and blindness prevented with use of oral corticosteroid medications. Symptoms usually improve soon after treatment begins. Treatment must be continued for a year or more and is monitored by blood tests and examinations. ■

Ears, Nose and Throat

Your ears, nose and throat are responsible for a remarkable number of functions. Your ears and their associated nerve mechanisms enable you to hear and to keep your balance. Your nose makes it possible for you to inhale, to warm and filter air, and to smell your surroundings. The structures of your throat enable you to eat, drink, speak and sing.

Your ears, nose and throat are interrelated in their functions and in the disorders that often affect them. An infection of your throat or nose, for example, can easily spread to your ears. An upper respiratory infection may affect your nose, throat and ears.

It's not surprising, then, that each of these is treated by the same specialist, an otorhinolaryngologist. The name derives from the Greek base words for ear (*otos*), nose (*rhinos*) and throat (*larynx*). More commonly, doctors who specialize in this area of medicine are referred to as ENT doctors.

Your Ears

The two main functions of your ears are hearing and balance. Each ear is composed of three parts: the outer ear, middle ear and inner ear.

Outer ear

Your outer ear is made up of the folds of skin and cartilage usually referred to as the ear (pinna), plus your outer ear canal. They carry sound waves to your eardrum and middle ear. The outer ear is the part of the ear you see. Within the outer ear canal are wax-producing glands and hairs that protect the middle ear.

Middle ear

The function of the middle ear is to deliver sound waves to your inner ear, where the vibrations are processed into a signal that your brain recognizes as sound. Your middle ear is a small cavity, with the eardrum (tympanic membrane) on one side and the entrance to your inner ear on the other.

Within your middle ear are three small bones (ossicles) known as the hammer (malleus), anvil (incus) and stirrup (stapes). The names reflect their shapes. These tiny bones act like a system of levers that conduct sound vibrations into your inner ear. The hammer is attached to the lining of your eardrum; the anvil is attached to the hammer; and the stirrup links the anvil to the opening of your inner ear, the oval window.

Your middle ear is connected to your throat by a narrow channel called the eustachian tube. The eustachian tube remains closed until you swallow or yawn; then it opens briefly to equalize the air pressure within your middle ear with the air pressure outside. You may feel a pop when this occurs.

Inner ear

Your inner ear contains the most intricate parts of the hearing mechanism: two chambers called the vestibular labyrinth and cochlea. The vestibular labyrinth consists of elaborately formed canals — three semicircular tubes that connect to one another — that help control your sense of balance. The cochlea, which begins at the oval window, curves into a shape that resembles a snail shell. Tiny hairs attached to auditory nerve endings line the interior of the cochlea. Both the labyrinth and cochlea are filled with fluid.

Sound waves from the world outside cause your eardrum to vibrate. These vibrations continue passing through the bones of your middle ear and into your inner ear through the oval window. They're transmitted into the fluid of the cochlea, where the tiny hairs sense the vibration waves and convert them into electric impulses that are transmitted to your brain by your auditory nerve.

Structures of the Ear

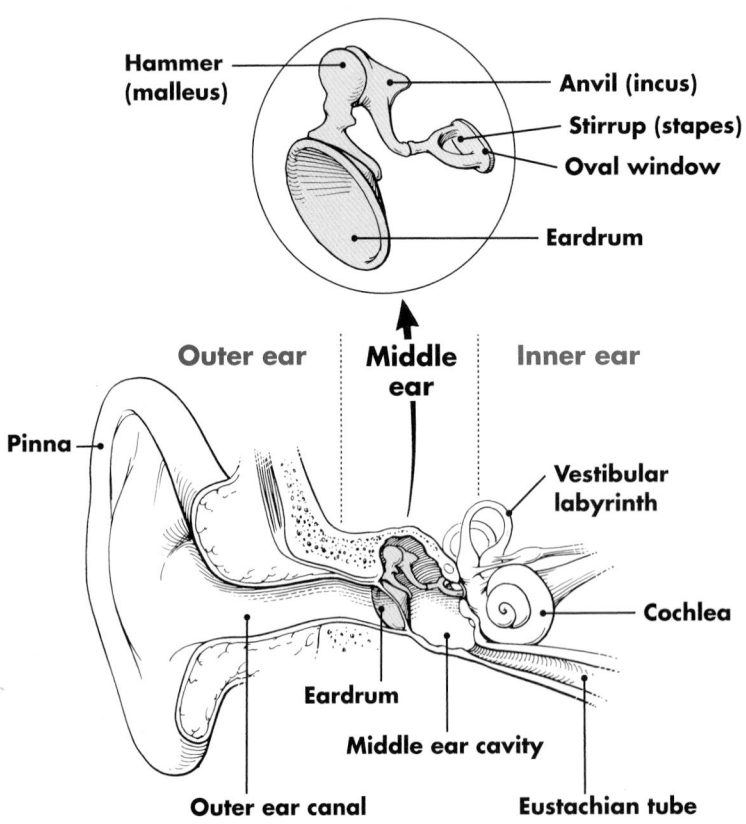

Hammer (malleus)
Anvil (incus)
Stirrup (stapes)
Oval window
Eardrum

Outer ear   Middle ear   Inner ear

Pinna

Vestibular labyrinth

Cochlea

Eardrum

Middle ear cavity

Outer ear canal

Eustachian tube

Your Nose

Your nose is a gateway to your respiratory system. Air that enters your nasal passages moves along the nasal lining and over the top of the structure that separates your nose from your mouth (palate). As you inhale, air passes through to the intersection of your mouth and throat and continues its journey into your lower respiratory system.

Your nose is divided into two nostrils, which are separated by a partition (septum) composed of cartilage and bone and covered by mucous membrane. Thin bony structures covered by mucous membrane (turbinates) protrude into the nasal airway from the sides of your nose toward your septum and increase the surface area in your nasal passages.

Your sinuses, air-filled cavities in your skull, also open into your nasal passages. Your adenoids are a mound of lymphatic tissue located behind your nasal passages.

Protective hairs that help filter the air you breathe are inside the front of your nose. The main cavity of your nose is lined with a mucous membrane that warms, moistens and filters the air.

In addition to these duties, your nose is responsible for your sense of smell and, to a large degree, your sense of taste.

Most of your ability to taste depends on your sense of smell. Smell begins at the very top of your nasal cavity, where small nerve fibers pierce the interface between your brain and your nose. These fibers react with molecules in the air, generating a signal to a larger nerve associated with smell (olfaction). This nerve delivers the signal of smell to your brain.

Your Throat

Your throat (pharynx) is part of the system that delivers air to your lungs, food and drink to your esophagus and stomach, and sounds from your vocal cords to your mouth. Each time you inhale, air passes through your throat on its way to your windpipe (trachea) and lungs. When you swallow food, the muscles at the top of your throat help move the food from your mouth to your esophagus, which is connected to your stomach.

Several organs are located in your throat. Your voice box (larynx), which is above your trachea, contains your vocal cords, which are responsible for generating most of the sounds of speech. When you speak, your throat also helps you shape the sounds you make. Your tonsils are on both sides of the back of your mouth, and your adenoids are above them.

The epiglottis, situated at the very top of the voice box, acts as a lid and diverter for your trachea, closing when you swallow and keeping water and food from "going down the wrong way" and entering your windpipe.

Structures of the Nose

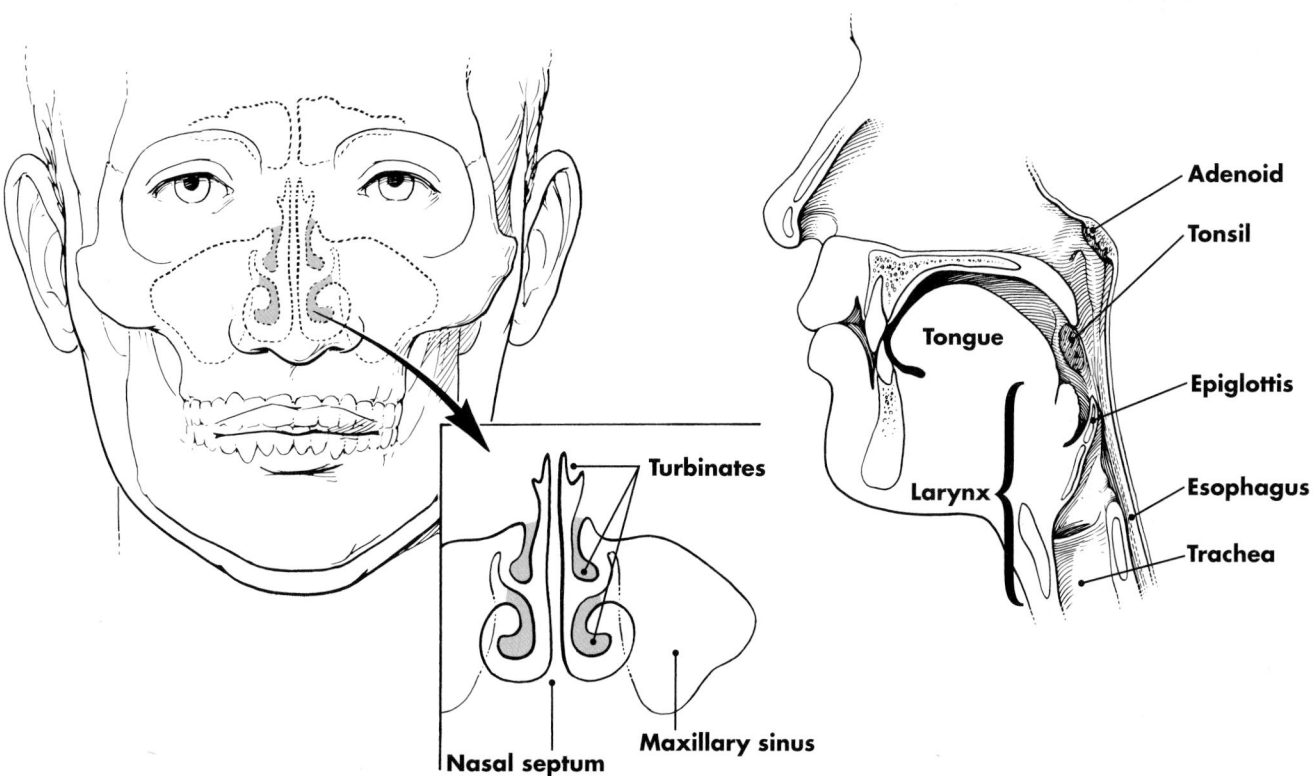

Turbinates

Nasal septum

Maxillary sinus

Structures of the Throat

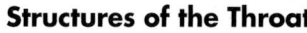

Adenoid

Tonsil

Tongue

Epiglottis

Larynx

Esophagus

Trachea

Disorders of the Ear

The ear is a structural marvel, but its complexity makes it susceptible to infections, congenital disorders, and damage due to accident or noise exposure.

Outer ear infections

Signs and symptoms
- Pain or itching in an ear
- Drainage from an ear canal
- Redness of skin in an ear canal
- Feeling of fullness in the ear

An outer ear infection (external otitis) causes irritation and inflammation of your outer ear canal. It can occur at any age but most commonly affects young adults.

Under normal circumstances, earwax (cerumen) repels water from the surface of your outer ear canal. It also helps maintain a proper acid-alkaline, or pH, balance in your ear to inhibit bacterial growth. If this balance is disrupted, infection may result.

A fungal, viral or bacterial infection can cause external otitis. A bacterium is the most common cause. This type of infection is sometimes referred to as swimmer's ear because it's typically related to moisture problems in the ear canal, which often develop after swimming.

Factors that may spur bacterial growth include:
- **Excessive moisture in the ear canal.** Repeated exposure to water may result in loss of earwax. Unprotected, the ear canal's skin retains moisture and becomes irritated. The normal pH balance also is disrupted, allowing bacteria to grow. Hearing aid use also may promote moisture buildup in the ear canal.
- **Injury or irritation of the skin in the ear canal.** Scratching the ear canal or removing wax with makeshift tools, such as paper clips or hairpins, can damage the skin — providing an entry for bacteria — and even your eardrum. Efforts to clean the canal with cotton-tipped swabs can backfire by forcing excess wax and debris deeper into the ear, possibly causing injury.
- **Chronic skin conditions or allergies.** Skin conditions such as eczema and seborrhea may provide an entry point for bacteria. Allergies to hair dyes or sprays may irritate the skin and lead to infection.

Sometimes, a severe and aggressive infection may develop. This is more commonly seen in people with diabetes, especially older individuals. People with a weakened immune system also are at greater risk of this type of infection.

The infection usually begins as external otitis. But at some point, the bacteria spread from the ear canal skin into nearby tissues, including cartilage and bone. Nerve damage and even facial paralysis may occur.

Diagnosis
If you experience pain in an ear canal or notice fluid or yellowish or yellowish-green pus draining from an ear, see your doctor. Hearing loss can result if the pus or swelling blocks your ear canal.

Your doctor may use a handheld instrument called an otoscope to examine your ear canal. If the outer canal is red and inflamed or pus is present, it's likely you have an outer ear infection.

How serious are outer ear infections?
Most outer ear infections are bothersome, but if treated properly they're not usually dangerous to your general health. Severe external otitis that spreads to nearby tissues can damage underlying bones and cartilage. Left untreated, this condition can be life-threatening.

Treatment
After a diagnosis is made, your doctor will probably clean your ear canal with a suction device or other instrument. This will help relieve irritation and pain. Generally, doctors prescribe eardrops containing some combination of the following:
- An acidic solution to replicate your ear's normal acidic, antibacterial environment
- A corticosteroid to reduce inflammation
- An antibiotic to fight the bacterial infection

If you're in severe pain, your doctor may prescribe a painkiller. Try not to let any water get into your ear while it's healing.

If the infection doesn't show marked improvement after three or four days, your doctor may prescribe an oral antibiotic. He or she can select a drug specifically for the organism causing your infection if a laboratory test (bacterial culture) has identified the organism.

Invasive external otitis is a serious infection of the outer ear and often requires intravenous anti-

---

PREVENTION TIP

An ounce of prevention can help you avoid an outer ear infection:
- Carefully dry your ears with a hair dryer or towel after bathing and swimming because moisture in an ear canal can make it susceptible to infection.
- Put several drops of a 50-50 mixture of water and vinegar or water and rubbing alcohol in the ear canal to aid drying after swimming.
- Avoid excessive ear canal cleaning. Simply wipe out whatever is at the opening of the ear canal.
- Cover your ear canals with cotton balls or something similar when applying hair spray or dye.

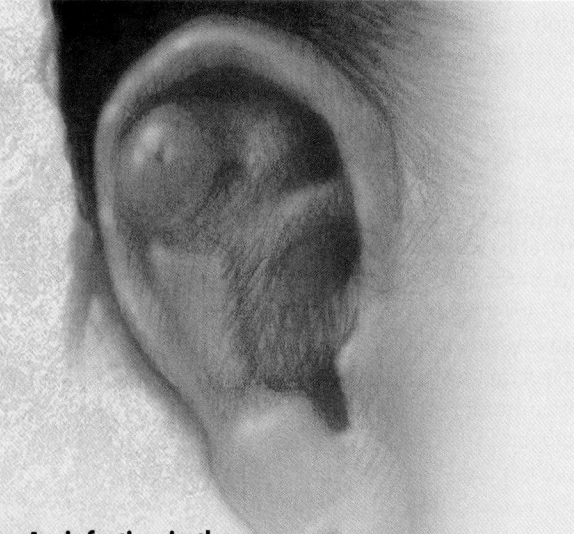

Question and Answer

Is it safe to pierce the upper area of the ear?

Generally, it's best to avoid piercing upper ear cartilage. An infection in the upper ear can lead to cartilage damage that can cause serious, permanent deformity of the ear.

Cartilage determines the shape of your outer ear. It's kept alive by absorbing nutrients from a special tissue that covers it. Inflammation and infection of that tissue lining can peel the nourishing layer off the cartilage, depriving it of nutrients. As a result, the cartilage can be destroyed. Making matters worse, antibiotics are often ineffective because the blood supply isn't adequate to deliver the medication to the cartilage. By contrast, the earlobe has its own blood supply and, if infected, generally responds well to antibiotics.

An infection in the upper ear can cause cartilage damage. Serious deformity of the ear may result.

biotics and hospitalization for several days. Sometimes, surgery is needed to remove dead or infected tissue and bone. After hospitalization, intravenous antibiotics may be continued, or oral antibiotics may be prescribed for several weeks. People who have diabetes or suppressed immune systems require close monitoring.

If you suspect that you have external otitis, you can take steps to relieve the pain while waiting to see your doctor. Placing a warm — not hot — heating pad over your ear may help. Acetaminophen (Tylenol, others), ibuprofen (Advil, Motrin IB, others) or aspirin may help relieve the pain. Aspirin isn't recommended for children.

Benign cysts and tumors

Signs and symptoms
- A lump in your ear canal or in front of or behind your ear
- Accumulation of earwax (cerumen)
- Discomfort in your ear
- Hearing loss

Sebaceous cysts are small sacs filled with cheesy material produced by your skin glands. They commonly develop behind your ear or in your scalp. The cysts are noncancerous (benign)

and often aren't even noticeable. Benign tumors of the ear canal (exostoses or osteomas), caused by an overgrowth of bone, also may occur. The tumors can grow large enough to block your ear canal, trap wax and interfere with hearing. Most benign tumors grow very slowly and often present no problem.

You may feel a semisoft lump on the bony protrusion behind your ear or in front of your ear. These cysts rarely cause discomfort, although they can become infected. Lumps located in front of your ear or under the ear lobe can sometimes be large salivatory gland (parotid) tumors. Most, but not all, are noncancerous.

Diagnosis
If you detect a lump that doesn't go away, visit your doctor. In the case of an osteoma, people are often unaware they have one, and the bony growth usually poses no problem. Occasionally, however, such a growth may partially obstruct an ear canal.

If your ear hurts or you experience hearing loss, consult your doctor. He or she typically will examine your ear canal with an otoscope, which allows full viewing of your outer ear canal.

Treatment
Benign cysts and tumors pose no general threat to health. However, if a benign tumor grows enough to block your outer ear canal, your doctor may recommend that it be surgically removed.

Foreign object in an ear

Signs and symptoms
- Pain in your ear
- Hearing loss
- The sensation of something present in your ear

The assortment of objects that doctors remove from ears is varied — marbles, tiny toys, jewelry, insects, seeds, bits of paper and plastic, and even earplugs. Because of the complicated shape of your ear and ear canal, any small object that you place into your ear can become lodged there.

Diagnosis
Usually, you know when something is stuck in your ear. Your ear hurts or it feels full, and the object may affect your ability to hear. The problem can be a little harder to diagnose when a small child is affected.

Don't attempt to remove the object unless it can be easily grasped with a tweezers. And don't attempt to dislodge an object by probing with a cotton-tipped swab, hairpin, paper clip or another tool. If the object can't easily be grasped, see a doctor.

How serious is a foreign object in an ear?

Most foreign objects don't cause a lasting problem. However, if an object is pushed into your eardrum, the eardrum (tympanic membrane) may tear (rupture) or perforate, and your middle and inner ear may be damaged, creating a potentially serious situation.

Treatment

Before visiting your doctor, you might try these steps at home if the object is clearly visible, pliable and can be grasped with a tweezers:

- If the object isn't an insect, use gravity to dislodge it. Tilt your head to the affected side and gently shake it.
- If the foreign object is an insect, tilt your head so that the ear with the offending insect is upward. Try to float the insect out by pouring mineral, olive or baby oil into the ear canal. The oil should be warm but not hot. Ease the entry of the oil by gently pulling the earlobe backward and upward, straightening the ear canal. The insect should suffocate and float out. Don't use oil to remove an object other than an insect. And don't use this method if you suspect a perforated eardrum, indicated by pain, bleeding or discharge from the ear.

If these methods fail or you continue to experience ear pain, reduced hearing or a sensation of something lodged in the ear, seek medical assistance.

Ruptured eardrum

Signs and symptoms

- Sharp, sudden pain in an ear
- Clear, pus-filled or bloody drainage from an ear
- Hearing loss
- Ringing in the ear

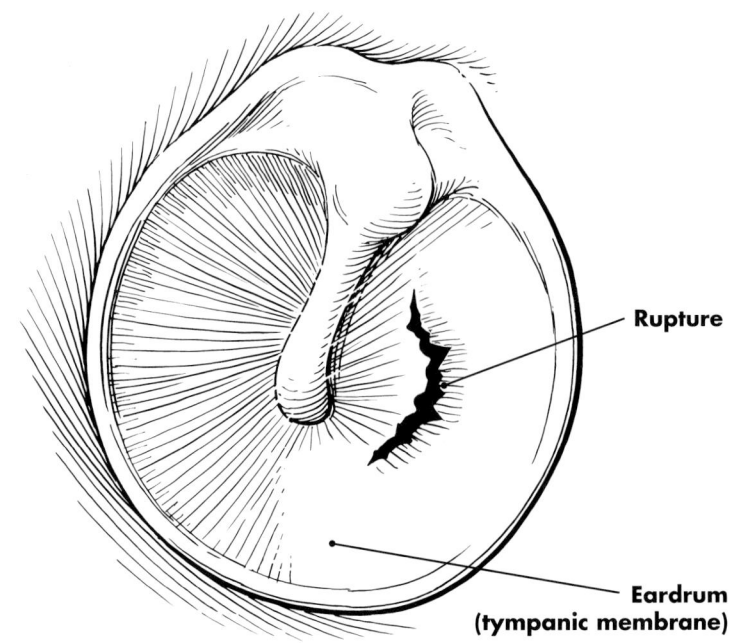

Pain in your ear, hearing loss and discharge from your ear may indicate a tear (rupture) in your eardrum (tympanic membrane).

A ruptured eardrum is a hole, or tear, in your eardrum, the thin drumlike tissue that separates your ear canal from your middle ear. You may puncture your eardrum when you clean or scratch your ear with a cotton-tipped swab or small, sharp object. Other causes of a ruptured eardrum are a hard slap on your ear or an explosion, which can produce a sudden increase in air pressure in your ear.

A middle ear infection (otitis media) can cause inflammation and, sometimes, perforation of part of an eardrum. This is the most common cause of a ruptured eardrum. Small holes may heal, but larger ones can stay open and allow infectious agents to enter your middle ear.

If you experience increased pain and hearing loss in your ear over a period of a day or so, followed by a discharge of blood or fluid — with subsequent relief of the pain — you may have a ruptured eardrum. See a doctor promptly.

Diagnosis

Your doctor will likely examine your inner ear. If your eardrum is ruptured, your doctor should be able to see the injured area.

If there's discharge from your ear, your doctor may order a laboratory culture of the discharge to determine if it stems from a bacterial, viral or fungal infection.

How serious is a ruptured eardrum?

A ruptured eardrum can be painful, particularly at first. Often the rupture heals by itself without complications and with little or no permanent hearing loss. Larger tears may cause recurring inner ear infections and persistent hearing loss.

Treatment

Most ruptured eardrums heal without treatment within a few weeks. If the tear, or hole, in your eardrum doesn't heal by itself, steps need to be taken to close the perforation. These may include an eardrum patch or surgery.

With an eardrum patch, a doctor may apply a chemical to the edges of the tear to stimulate growth and then apply a paper patch over the tear. This procedure may need to be repeated at least once before the tear closes. If the patch doesn't work, a surgeon may graft a tiny patch of your own skin over the eardrum.

Eustachian tube dysfunction

Signs and symptoms
- A plugged ear
- A sensation of fullness or pressure in the ear
- A popping noise in the ear
- Hearing loss

Many ear problems are the result of the eustachian tube not working properly. The eustachian tube has many roles. When you swallow or yawn, it opens briefly to equalize pressure in the ear with the air pressure outside. It also drains the middle ear of fluid.

Most of the time, though, the eustachian tube remains closed. With eustachian tube dysfunction, the tube either doesn't open or close correctly or it's obstructed, preventing it from functioning properly.

Eustachian tube dysfunction can lead to problems with regulating pressure in the ear and problems with clearing the middle ear of secretions. It can cause such conditions as middle ear infection and cholesteatoma, a cyst-like, noncancerous tumor or collection of skin cells. A cholesteatoma is most commonly found in a bone behind your ear (mastoid process) or the middle ear.

This type of dysfunction has many possible causes, including:

- Swelling due to inflammation, infection or allergies
- Failure of the tube to open due to a cleft palate
- Obstruction of the tube due to small growths (polyps)
- Collapse of cartilage around the eustachian tube, which prevents the tube from opening

Diagnosis
Your doctor may use any of several tests to determine whether you have eustachian tube dysfunction and, if so, its cause. For example, he or she may ask you to gently exhale while you hold your nostrils closed and keep your mouth shut. While you do so, your doctor will observe your ear through an otoscope to see if it reacts normally to the change in pressure.

A test called tympanometry evaluates the eardrum's reaction to positive, normal and negative air pressure. A special instrument is used to seal the ear canal and exert sound and pressure. The instrument determines if the eustachian tube is providing proper ventilation to allow the eardrum to vibrate properly.

Your doctor may also view the nasal opening of your eustachian tube using a device called an endoscope. It is a thin, flexible tube with a fiber-optic light that's inserted through your nose.

Treatment
Treatment for eustachian tube dysfunction varies depending on the cause. It may involve decongestant medications or, in rare cases, surgery to treat the underlying cause.

Barotrauma

Signs and symptoms
- Moderate to severe pain in an ear
- A stuffy feeling in an ear
- Slight hearing loss
- Dizziness
- Noise such as a buzzing, ringing or roaring in your ears (tinnitus)

The air pressure in your middle ear usually is the same as that in your outer ear, thanks to a narrow channel (eustachian tube) that connects your middle ear to the top of your throat. When you swallow or yawn, it opens and allows air to flow into or out of your middle ear, equalizing the air pressure of your ear with the outside air pressure.

If a eustachian tube is blocked, differences in pressure occur on the two sides of the eardrum. This can lead to a condition known as barotrauma (barotitis media).

Diagnosis
If you fly in an airplane or scuba dive while you have a congested nose, you may experience the symptoms of barotrauma: ear pain,

---

PREVENTION TIP

If you must fly when your nose and head feel congested, try the following measures to prevent or reduce symptoms:
- Use a nasal decongestant spray and an oral decongestant an hour before takeoff and, if the flight is long, an hour before landing. This may prevent blockage of your eustachian tube.
- During your flight suck candy or chew gum to encourage swallowing. This helps open your eustachian tube to equalize pressure.
- Try using over-the-counter earplugs designed for air travel. They have a small filter to slow the rate of change in air pressure on the eardrum.
- For babies and young children, make sure they're swallowing during ascent and descent. Give the child a bottle or pacifier to encourage swallowing. Have a young child drink or suck on something or chew gum. Decongestants generally aren't recommended for young children.

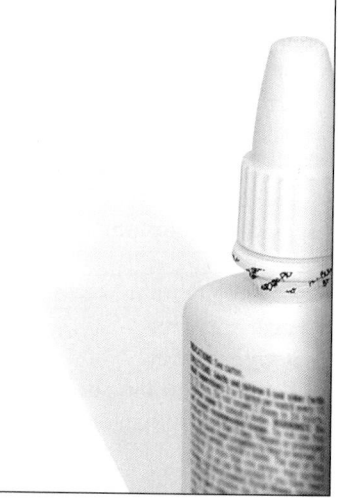

slight hearing loss and a stuffy feeling in your ears. The symptoms are caused by your eardrum bulging outward or retracting inward due to a change in air pressure.

A more severe problem can occur if the air pressure change is great or if a eustachian tube is entirely blocked. The small blood vessels (capillaries) of your middle ear may rupture and bleed, filling your ear with blood and producing hearing loss and a feeling similar to that of being under water.

How serious is barotrauma?

Symptoms of barotrauma usually disappear within a few minutes or hours after they begin. It usually isn't a serious condition and generally doesn't produce permanent hearing loss. In some cases, severe pressure changes can cause bleeding into the middle ear and rupture the eardrum, which can lead to hearing loss. If symptoms don't improve within a few hours after the incident, visit a doctor.

Treatment

If you experience barotrauma, gently blow air out of your nose while your mouth is closed and your nose is slightly pinched.

The symptoms usually clear up on their own. However, if they don't disappear within a few hours, you may be bleeding from the capillaries in your middle ear. See your doctor. Antibiotic treatment may be necessary to prevent infection. On rare occasions, treatment may also involve a surgical incision in your eardrum (myringotomy) and removal of fluid.

Middle ear infections

Signs and symptoms
- Ear pain
- A feeling of fullness in an ear
- Fever and chills

In infant children
- Tugging or pulling on an ear
- Crying more than usual
- Irritability
- Trouble sleeping

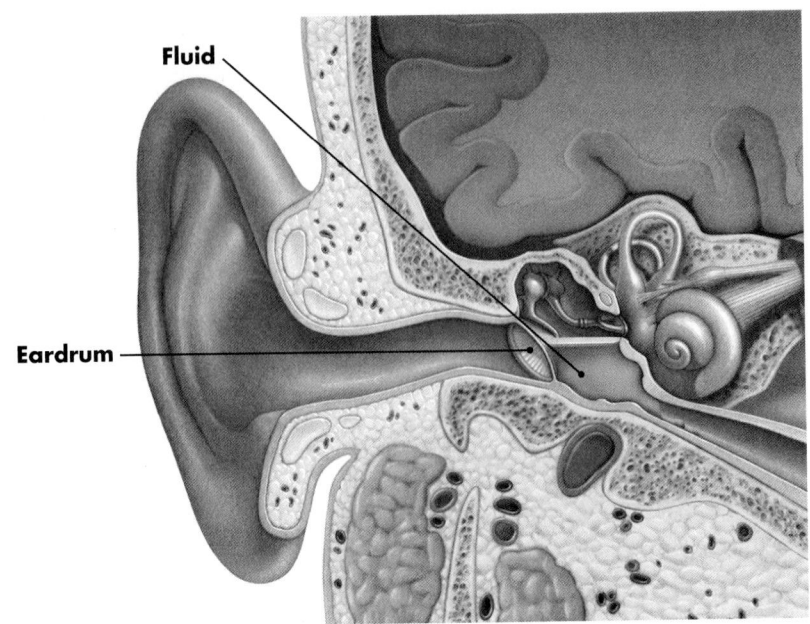

Fluid is trapped behind the eardrum (tympanic membrane).

Middle ear infection (otitis media) is one of the most common illnesses of early childhood. According to the National Institute on Deafness and Other Communication Disorders, 5 out of 6 children have at least one middle ear infection by age 3. While most common in children, middle ear infections can also occur in adults.

A middle ear infection results from inflammation or infection of the middle ear, which is located just behind the eardrum. A middle ear infection often begins with a respiratory infection such as a cold. Colds cause swelling and inflammation in the sinuses and eustachian tubes.

Because children's eustachian tubes are shorter and narrower than those of adults, they're more likely to develop ear infections. The small size increases the chances that inflammation will block the tube completely, trapping fluid in the middle ear. This trapped fluid may cause discomfort, and it creates an ideal environment for bacterial growth. The result can be a severe (acute) infection.

Another factor in ear infections is swelling of the adenoids. These are tissues located in the upper throat near the eustachian tubes. Adenoids contain cells that nor-

mally fight infection, but sometimes the adenoids themselves get infected or enlarged, infecting or blocking the eustachian tubes.

Sometimes, fluid stays trapped in the middle ear after treatment of an infection or because the eustachian tube remains blocked. This can lead to chronic ear infection.

Is Your Child at Risk?

All children are susceptible to ear infections, but statistics show that certain groups of children are at higher risk:
- Boys
- Children whose siblings have a history of recurrent ear infections
- Children with a family history of asthma, allergies or eczema
- American Indian children and children of Native Alaskan or Native Canadian heritage — possibly due to genetic factors that affect the shape of the eustachian tube

When an infection develops, pus generally fills the middle ear. The pressure of the pus may burst the eardrum, causing a discharge of blood and thick pus.

Diagnosis

Your doctor will likely examine the eardrum with an otoscope to determine if there's fluid in the middle ear. The otoscope also allows a doctor to gently blow a small amount of air against the eardrum to see if it moves as freely as it should. If it doesn't, fluid may be in the middle ear. Your doctor will also examine the eardrum for bulging or change of color.

Testing a sample of the fluid can confirm that an infection is present and identify its specific cause, but this isn't practical with young children. To obtain a sample, a small needle is used to penetrate the eardrum and draw off some of the fluid. Young children are unable to hold still long enough for the procedure to be done safely.

Sometimes additional, often pain-free tests for ear infections are recommended, especially if you or your child has had fluid in the middle ear for some time. A test called tympanometry measures eardrum movement. Another test called acoustic reflectometry uses sounds of varying frequencies to help determine how much fluid is inside the ear.

How serious are middle ear infections?

Most middle ear infections don't lead to permanent hearing loss. However, they can sometimes damage the eardrum, ear bones and inner ear structures, causing permanent hearing loss. Infections that aren't treated can spread to other parts of the ear, including the inner ear.

Treatment

Sometimes you can relieve the pain by placing a warm — not hot — heating pad over the ear until you see a doctor. Pain medications such as acetaminophen (Tylenol, others), ibuprofen (Advil, Motrin IB, others) or aspirin also may help, but aspirin generally shouldn't be given to children. Your doctor may recommend one of the following:

Watchful waiting

In some situations, you and your doctor may decide to hold off on using antibiotics and check to see if the ear infection gets better or worse. Most ear infections clear up on their own within a few days.

The American Academy of Pediatrics and the American Academy of Family Physicians recommend watchful waiting for the first 72 hours for children older than 6 months who are otherwise healthy and have mild signs and symptoms or an uncertain diagnosis.

If the fluid in the ear isn't infected or if the infection is viral rather than bacterial, antibiotics provide no benefit. Antibiotics won't help move fluid out of the ear, and they may cause side effects such as nausea, diarrhea or an allergic reaction. In addition, if antibiotics are used only when necessary, they're more likely to be effective when needed to fight future bacterial infections.

Even when there's an obvious ear infection, you may still want to consider watchful waiting as an option before giving antibiotics. If you and your doctor decide to hold off on antibiotics, watch for signs of increased pain or fever or hearing loss. Also be certain to schedule a follow-up visit to be sure the ear infection is improving.

Medication

Treatment with antibiotics is recommended for children younger than 6 months and for children and adults who've had two or more ear infections within the last 30 days.

The antibiotic of choice of many doctors is amoxicillin, although other antibiotics also are effective.

Make sure to take the antibiotic for the full length of the prescription. Stopping the medication too soon could cause the infection to come back.

Chronic ear infections

Signs and symptoms
- Earache
- Periodic drainage of pus from an ear
- Hearing loss

A chronic middle ear infection (chronic otitis media) can be more harmful than an acute infection because its slow, long-lasting effects can cause permanent ear damage. Unlike an acute infection, which develops suddenly, a chronic condition may not be noticed until it's well-established.

Chronic otitis media may result from persistent swelling or inflammation of adenoid tissue behind your nasal passages. This can result in inflammation and blockage of the eustachian tubes.

Adenoid problems most often occur in children. In adults, blockage may stem from nasal allergies or from chronic eustachian tube problems. It can also result from tumors in the back of the nose and throat.

In some cases, an initial acute infection never completely clears after treatment, and a low-level infection continues. It can spread to a bone behind your ear called the mastoid process. Infection in the mastoid process is more difficult to eradicate. A chronic infection can also cause perforation of your eardrum (tympanic membrane) or damage to the small bones in your middle ear.

Diagnosis
An exam typically involves inspection of the ear with an otoscope to identify where the infection is. Your doctor also may arrange a computerized tomography (CT) scan of your head to determine if the infection has spread to the mastoid process.

How serious are chronic ear infections?
Chronic otitis media is uncomfortable and inconvenient, but it rarely causes permanent harm. However, uncorrected, active chronic otitis media can cause permanent hearing damage.

Treatment
The first line of treatment is generally medication. Another option is surgery.

Medication
Medication may be prescribed to treat a chronic ear infection or relieve nasal and sinus congestion if the condition is due to allergies.

If you or your child has had multiple or frequent ear infections — usually three or more ear infections in a six-month period or four infections within 12 months — your doctor may suggest a low-dose antibiotic over a longer time (often a few months) as a preventive measure. Preventive antibiotics won't help clear fluid from the middle ear, but they may prevent bacterial growth. Some studies have found that preventive use of antibiotics reduces the number of ear infections.

Unfortunately, the bacteria commonly responsible for ear infections are becoming increasingly resistant to antibiotics. Even while taking antibiotics, an ear infection can still occur. Because widespread and prolonged use of antibiotics contributes to the growth of drug-resistant bacteria, doctors don't agree on whether antibiotics should be used preventively.

Surgery
Recurrent ear infections that don't respond to antibiotics are sometimes treated by surgically inserting a small plastic tube through a hole made in the eardrum to

Ear Tubes in Children: The Pros and Cons

One way to treat recurrent middle ear infections (otitis media) is to surgically insert a small plastic tube through the eardrum (tympanic membrane), which helps drain fluid, ventilate the middle ear, and equalize the pressure between the outer and middle ear. However, before embarking one this path, discuss the procedure in detail with an ear, nose and throat specialist.

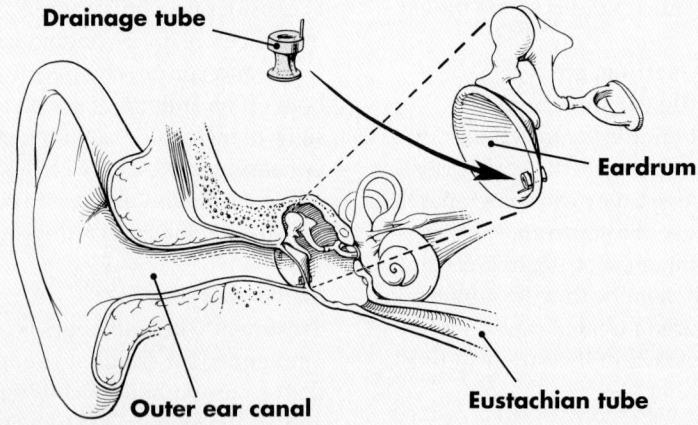

If the infection persists, a doctor may insert a small tube into the eardrum (tympanic membrane) to help drain fluid, ventilate the middle ear, and equalize the pressure between the outer and middle ear.

drain and ventilate the middle ear. Surgery may also be done if fluid persists in the middle ear for more than three months, resulting in hearing loss.

The operation is performed under general anesthesia, and the entire procedure usually takes less than 10 minutes. Working through the ear canal, the surgeon uses a microscope and very delicate instruments to make a small incision in the eardrum, remove any fluid, pus or blood with suction, and then insert a tiny plastic tube into the hole. The procedure is usually performed on both ears. Hearing often improves immediately.

Generally, it's not necessary to come into the doctor's office to have the tube removed. It stays in the eardrum for about 10 months, although this can vary depending on the type of tube used. As a child's eardrum grows, the tube is eventually pushed out into the ear canal where it either falls out or is retrieved by the doctor. About 15 to 25 percent of children with ear tubes need surgery to insert a second set of tubes. A small number of children may even need a third set.

When a tube is in the ear, your doctor may recommend special earplugs for water activities.

If the adenoids are thought to be contributing to the problem, your doctor may recommend surgically removing them (adenoidectomy). If the mastoid bone becomes infected, your doctor may recommend a mastoidectomy — an operation in which the mastoid process is opened surgically to remove infected tissue and prevent recurrence or spread of the infection.

Mastoiditis

Signs and symptoms
- Redness, swelling and tenderness of the mastoid process

- Earache
- Fever
- Discharge of pus from your ear

If a severe (acute) middle ear infection isn't treated, the infection may spread to the bone located behind the outer ear that's connected to the middle ear (mastoid process). When mastoiditis occurs, the infection moves from your middle ear to the mucous membrane lining the mastoid process and the honeycomb-like bone within. If the infection is severe, it can erode this bone and spread further.

Diagnosis
Your doctor may request a culture of any pus apparent in the ear canal and possibly arrange for a computerized tomography (CT) scan or magnetic resonance imaging (MRI) of the head to determine how far any infection has spread.

How serious is mastoiditis?
Before the availability of antibiotics, acute mastoiditis was a leading cause of death in children. Now it's treated successfully with antibiotics, and the health risk is vastly reduced.

Treatment
Antibiotics are used to treat mastoiditis. Curing this infection isn't easy because of the difficulty eradicating infected material from the many, small mastoid cells. It may take several weeks of high-dose antibiotic therapy to eliminate the infection. If antibiotic treatment doesn't work, your doctor may recommend a mastoidectomy, in which part or all of the mastoid bone is surgically opened.

Cholesteatoma

Signs and symptoms
- Hearing loss
- Pus seeping from an ear
- Headache
- Earache
- Dizziness

Cholesteatoma is a cystlike, noncancerous (benign) tumor

The pros
The benefits of tubes include:
- The operation provides ventilation and drainage of the middle ear to prevent fluid from accumulating. It also decreases the risk of permanent changes in the lining of the middle ear that can occur with prolonged infection.
- The procedure usually results in a decrease in the frequency and severity of episodes of middle ear infections.
- Hearing may improve immediately and aid speech development. Studies linking early hearing loss with long-term speech, language and cognitive skill problems have been the basis for a large number of ear tube procedures. However, a more recent study reported that tubes don't appear to have an effect on speech, language and development in children under age 3.

The cons
Reasons against the use of tubes include:
- Although small, a risk of infection and complications is associated with all surgery.
- Complications such as persistent drainage of fluid and perforation or scarring of the eardrum may occur, although this is rare.
- The tube itself can become infected.
- The tubes can fall out.

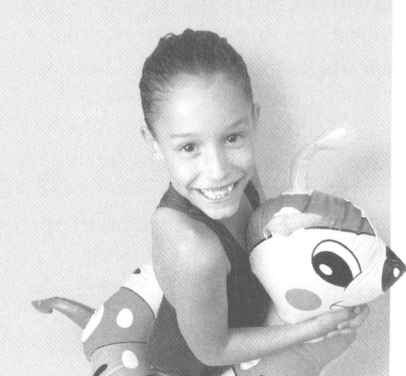

most commonly found in the mastoid bone located behind your middle ear. It occurs as a complication of eustachian tube dysfunction in which the air pressure in your middle ear decreases and your eardrum (tympanic membrane) bends inward.

It can also occur when ear canal skin grows into the middle ear through a hole in your eardrum. In the middle ear, skin cells (epithelial tissue) that would normally be shed are caught, and then they form a cyst. The cyst can damage middle ear bones.

In some people, cholesteatoma results from a congenital problem in which skin cells remain behind the eardrum during fetal development. When a cholesteatoma develops in the ear of a child, it may grow quickly. In adults, the problem usually develops more slowly.

Diagnosis

Your doctor may examine your ear with a small instrument that allows a view of the ear canal (otoscope). You may also receive a hearing test. A computerized tomography (CT) scan of the ear and mastoid may be done to determine the extent of the disease and to aid in planning possible surgery.

How serious is cholesteatoma?

A cholesteatoma isn't cancerous and won't spread to other sites. But it can cause permanent hearing loss and dizziness. If left untreated, it can affect your facial nerve and, rarely, cause meningitis, an infection and inflammation of your central nervous system.

Treatment

Cholesteatoma can only be treated surgically. A large or an advanced cholesteatoma may require an extensive operation or series of operations to correct damage to the bones of the middle ear. A meticulous procedure is necessary to remove every bit of the cyst. Repeat operations may be required because the cyst can recur.

Hereditary Deafness

Hereditary deafness is hearing loss due to a genetic defect that runs in families. In some instances, hereditary deafness occurs alone (non-syndromic deafness). Other times, deafness is only one symptom of a syndrome (syndromic hearing loss). For example, Alport's syndrome is a kidney disorder accompanied by hearing loss. Deafness also can be associated with any number of inherited conditions, including an enlarged thyroid (Pendred's syndrome), malformation of the external ears, skin abnormalities, developmental delay and peripheral neuropathy.

Some causes of deafness are present at birth (congenital) but aren't hereditary. For example, if a mother has German measles (rubella) while pregnant, the newborn child runs a high risk of deafness. Other causes of early hearing loss include prematurity, lack of oxygen during or shortly after birth, blood incompatibilities, and meningitis.

The operation may include rebuilding the bones of the middle ear to restore hearing. Usable portions of natural bone or artificial (prosthetic) devices may be used to reconstruct the middle ear. Sometimes, this leaves a cavity that must be cleaned periodically.

Otosclerosis

Signs and symptoms
- Gradual hearing loss in one or both ears
- Noise such as a buzzing, ringing or roaring in your ears (tinnitus)

In otosclerosis, the bony wall of the inner ear becomes disorganized due to abnormal growth of spongy bone in your inner ear. The stirrup (stapes) — a tiny bone that vibrates to help pass sound waves into the inner ear — may become immobile, resulting in conductive hearing loss.

Conductive hearing loss is failure of the mechanism that passes vibrations through your middle ear via its three connected bones. Unlike nerve deafness (sensorineural deafness), conductive hearing loss often can be treated and reversed with surgery.

Otosclerosis affects more than 3 million Americans. It tends to run in families and is more common in women than in men. Symptoms usually become apparent between the ages of 15 and 35. The hearing loss tends to progress slowly. It can affect one or both ears, and it may be mild or severe. In women with otosclerosis, the degree of hearing loss may increase during pregnancy.

Diagnosis
See your doctor if you notice that your hearing seems to be gradually worsening. Your doctor may examine your ears and refer you to a hearing specialist. Let your doctor know if any close relatives experienced early hearing loss.

How serious is otosclerosis?
Otosclerosis doesn't endanger your general health, and it may be corrected with treatment.

Treatment
Otosclerosis can often be treated successfully with stapedectomy, to replace of the stirrup (stapes) surgically. In this procedure, a surgeon cuts the skin of the ear canal and lifts the eardrum out of the way to replace the stirrup with a tiny wire or prosthesis (see opposite page). The eardrum is returned to its normal position, and the incision usually heals in a week or two.

In some instances, a doctor may use a laser to create a small hole in the bottom of the stirrup. This allows for placement of the prosthesis.

You may experience temporary dizziness for some hours after the operation. Hearing usually improves quickly, and you may be able to resume normal activity within a few weeks. Occasionally, a blood clot blocks sound conduction. The clot usually disappears within a few weeks.

Stapedectomy helps most people with otosclerosis, but a small percentage who undergo the procedure lose all hearing in the ear. This is a matter to consider before proceeding with the operation. If you have otosclerosis in both ears, you might consider having surgery on one ear and then waiting a year to gauge the results before having the other ear done. If your inner ear is impaired, a stapedectomy may not improve hearing.

Noise-induced hearing loss

Signs and symptoms
- Muffled quality of speech and other sounds
- Difficulty understanding words
- Asking others to speak more slowly, clearly and loudly
- Needing to turn up the volume of the television or radio
- Ringing, buzzing or roaring sound

Noise-induced hearing loss is common. It usually occurs as a result of cumulative exposure to loud sounds — 90 decibels or louder — over a period of years. The noise can be occupational, such as at a loud construction site, or recreational, as with firearm use, snowmobiling or listening to loud music, including music from headphones. People at greatest risk have both a noisy job and a noisy hobby — for example, a mechanic who plays in a rock band.

Noise-induced hearing loss is a form of nerve deafness (sensorineural deafness), which is caused by damage to the cochlea. The intense vibration caused by loud sound waves damages the hair cells that line the cochlea of the inner ear. This damage prevents electrical impulses from reaching the auditory nerve, which normally transmits these impulses to the brain to be interpreted as sound.

Sensorineural deafness may also result from a blow to the head or a single exposure to loud impulse noise (acoustic trauma), such as gunfire or an explosion. Other causes include aging, illness, injury, infection, some medications and heredity.

It's crucial to use ear protection whenever possible during exposure to loud sounds. If you work in a noisy environment, your employer should regularly measure noise levels or provide protective devices. Noise-induced hearing loss is usually irreversible, and it often develops insidiously.

Diagnosis
If you notice loss of hearing, see an ear, nose and throat (ENT) specialist and an audiologist. An ENT doctor will examine your ears, and the audiologist will perform tests to determine the nature of your hearing loss. After these examinations, a specialist can recommend a proper course of action.

Treatment
In many cases, the most effective treatment for hearing loss caused by noise is a hearing aid (see page 638).

Age-related hearing loss

Signs and symptoms
- Muffled quality of speech and other sounds
- Difficulty understanding words
- Asking others to speak more slowly, clearly and loudly
- Needing to turn up the volume of the television or radio
- Noise such as a ringing, buzzing or roaring in your ears

Hearing impairment is common among people older than age 65. Almost a third of the people in this age group have noticeable hearing loss. Some lose very little hearing, and others become quite hearing impaired.

Hearing loss due to aging is called presbycusis, from the Latin words *presby*, meaning "old," and *cusis*, meaning "hearing." Typically, the hearing loss begins in middle age and progresses. It affects both ears, particularly for detecting high-frequency sounds. It generally affects men more often and more severely than it does women.

Presbycusis results from changes in the cochlea or the nerves attached to it. The cochlea, the

Hammer (malleus)
Anvil (incus)
Stirrup (stapes)
Oval window
Stirrup removed
Oval window
Wire or prosthesis
Eardrum
Outer ear canal
Eustachian tube

In a stapedectomy, the malfunctioning stirrup (stapes) of the middle ear is replaced with a tiny prosthesis that transmits sound vibrations.

Identifying Dangerous Noise

Sounds are all around you. When sounds become uncomfortable or interfere with daily activities, they're commonly referred to as *noise*, the generic term for any unwanted sound. Exposure to loud noise levels over long periods of time can cause permanent and irreversible hearing loss. A single exposure to loud impulse noise, such as gunfire, also may result in irreversible damage to your hearing. Ringing, buzzing or roaring in your ears (tinnitus) after exposure to loud noise levels is an early indicator of hearing damage. It's crucial to protect your hearing when you're exposed to loud noise.

The loudness of sound (sound intensity) is measured in units called decibels (db). The pitch (frequency) of sound is measured in hertz (Hz). Loudness, pitch and length of exposure are all factors used to predict if noise is damaging to hearing.

Individuals who work in noisy environments fall under the guidelines of the Occupational Safety and Health Administration (OSHA). OSHA requires that employers provide a hearing conservation program, including at least an annual hearing test, to workers exposed to noise that averages 85 db or more during an eight-hour workday. These workers should be offered the use of hearing protectors, such as earmuffs or earplugs. When workers are exposed to noise that averages more than 90 db during an eight-hour day, OSHA requires that they use hearing protectors.

The workplace isn't the only setting for noise exposure. Hazardous noise levels are also associated with commonplace household occurrences and recreational activities. Some examples follow:

Noise source	Approximate decibels
Whisper	30
Normal conversation	60
Ringing telephone	80
Power lawn mower	90
Hair dryer	90
Tractor	96
Chain saw	110
Hammer drill	114
Jet engine at takeoff	140
12-gauge shotgun blast	165

Source: National Institute for Occupational Safety and Health, Centers for Disease Control and Prevention, 2015

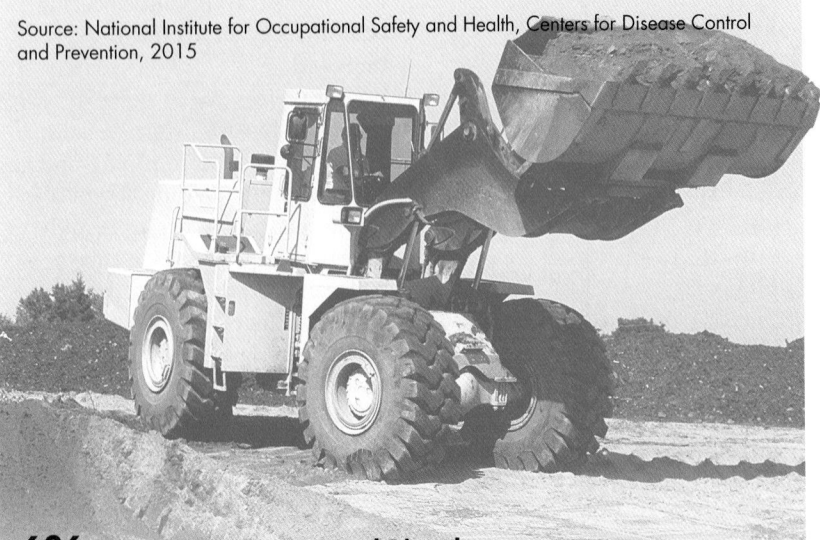

snail-shaped cavity in the inner ear, has thousands of tiny hairs that convert sound vibrations into electric signals. The auditory nerve carries these signals to the brain, where they're interpreted as sound. When some of these hairs or the auditory nerve itself becomes damaged, signals aren't transmitted as efficiently, and hearing loss results. This damage is permanent and can't be reversed medically.

Sometimes, people with presbycusis find that it's more difficult to hear the high-frequency voices of women and children than the lower voices of men. They may also find that it's more difficult to understand conversation in a group than conversation with a single individual.

Diagnosis

If you think that your hearing is diminishing, or a family member suggests that it might be, see your doctor or a specialist for examination and testing. Hearing loss isn't a health threat, but it can interfere with work, cause isolation and be socially debilitating.

Treatment

Age-related hearing loss can't be treated with medication. Often, a hearing aid can be beneficial. In some cases of severe hearing loss, cochlear implantation may be considered. It involves insertion of an electrical device to replicate hearing (see page 640). Other techniques to improve hearing include reading lips, facing the speaker, decreasing background noise — for example, turning off the television or dishwasher and shutting the windows to avoid street noise — and making maximum use of nonauditory clues, such as gestures and facial expressions.

Tinnitus

Signs and symptoms
- Ringing, buzzing, roaring, clicking, whistling or hissing sounds in your ears

Tinnitus — an annoying sensation of noise in your ears — is a common problem, affecting about 15 percent of Americans.

Tinnitus can be a symptom of almost any ear disorder as well as other diseases, including cardiovascular disease, allergies and anemia. It may also result from use of certain drugs, high doses of aspirin, large amounts of caffeine or exposure to loud noise.

Scientists don't fully understand the mechanism that causes these sounds. However, tinnitus is often associated with inner ear damage. When the tiny, delicate hairs in your inner ear become bent or broken, they can "leak" random electrical impulses to your brain. Other common causes of tinnitus include noise-related hearing loss, earwax blockage and stiffening of the bones in the middle ear.

Tinnitus usually occurs in both ears instead of just one. The sounds may be present all of the time or they may come and go. In some cases, the noise can be so loud it interferes with your ability to concentrate or hear.

Diagnosis

If you hear ringing, buzzing, whistling or other sounds when there's no apparent source of such noises, you probably have tinnitus. When evaluating your condition your doctor will likely look for signs of an infectious disease, ear obstruction or hearing disorder. An audiologist may examine your ears, test your hearing, and conduct a series of tests to try and determine the cause of noise. In many instances, an exact cause is never found.

A computerized tomography (CT) scan or magnetic resonance imaging (MRI) may be performed to check for structural abnormalities.

How serious is tinnitus?

Ear noise can be very annoying, but it's usually not a health threat. However, if tinnitus occurs on one side only (unilateral), it could be a

PREVENTION TIP

If you know you'll be exposed to loud noise, it's best to use specially designed ear protection. Hundreds of commercially produced hearing protectors are available, but the best protector is the one that's worn correctly 100 percent of the time when in the presence of loud noise. Earplugs must fit snugly to completely seal off the ear canal. An earmuff cushion must completely encircle the ear.

Commercially made devices that meet federal standards bring most loud sounds down to acceptable levels. You can obtain specially designed earmuffs or custom-molded earplugs made of foam, plastic or rubber. Some earmuffs close out the outside world. Others are fitted with earphones and a microphone that enable you to communicate with other workers. Active electronic hearing protectors, designed for use with firearms, use circuitry that shuts out loud noise almost instantaneously at the sound of gunfire.

Additional steps can be taken to protect your hearing. Identify the source of loud noise and try to reduce the volume. Or distance yourself from the noise. If that isn't possible, take breaks from the noise. Intermittent noise exposure is less damaging than is continuous exposure because it gives the ears time to recover. However, even brief exposure to loud impulse noise, such as gunfire, may cause irreversible damage.

If someone in your home listens to loud music on a headset, use this simple test to determine if the sound is too loud for his or her health: If the individual is wearing the headset and you can identify the music being played, it's too loud. Suggest that he or she listen to the music at a lower volume or for shorter periods of time.

The arm's-length rule provides a good method for gauging potentially damaging noise exposures in everyday life. If you must raise the level of your voice to be heard by someone an arm's-length away, the noise is too loud.

Communication Tips

Here are a few suggestions for communicating effectively with someone who's hearing-impaired:

- Make sure that you have the person's attention before talking. Simply saying the person's name directs his or her attention to you.
- Face the person to whom you're speaking.
- Speak at louder levels if listening conditions are difficult. Politely ask if you're being heard and understood.
- When listening conditions are difficult, talk naturally but a little more slowly and with a few more pauses.
- Stay within a few feet of the person with whom you're speaking.
- If possible, reduce background noise. For example, turn off the radio or television.
- If possible, talk on a one-to-one basis or in a small group.
- Alert your listener to changes in topics of conversation.
- Rephrase your comment if the listener is unsure about what was said.

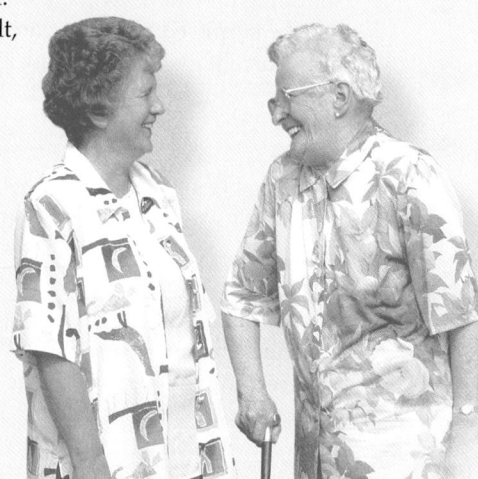

sign of a more serious condition, such as a form of cardiovascular disease or an auditory nerve tumor.

Treatment
Sometimes, tinnitus is easily treated, such as by removing a buildup of earwax. In many instances, though, treating the underlying cause doesn't stop the noise.

One form of treatment for tinnitus is to cover up the unwanted noise with a competing sound, for example, sound from a radio or recorded environmental noise. Another option is a tinnitus masker, a device that's worn like a hearing aid and that produces a different, less annoying noise. In people who also have hearing loss, hearing aids may make tinnitus less noticeable.

Medications can't cure tinnitus, but they may help reduce the severity of symptoms. Possible medications include:
- **Tricyclic antidepressants.** The drugs amitriptyline and nortriptyline (Pamelor) have been used with some success. However, these medications are generally only used for severe tinnitus, as they can cause troublesome side effects, including dry mouth, blurred vision and constipation.
- **Alprazolam (Xanax).** This drug may help reduce tinnitus symptoms, but side effects can include drowsiness and nausea. It also has the potential to become habit-forming.
- **Acamprosate.** This drug used to treat alcoholism is also effective in relieving tinnitus in some

people. However, more research is needed to determine how well it works and its possible side effects.

Meniere's disease

Signs and symptoms
- Recurring episodes of dizziness (vertigo), sometimes accompanied by nausea and vomiting
- Fluctuating hearing loss
- Buzzing, ringing, roaring or hissing in your ears
- Ear fullness or pressure

Meniere's disease is a disorder of the inner ear that causes abnormal sensory perceptions, including dizziness or a sensation of spinning (vertigo). The disease gets its name from the French physician Prosper Meniere who first

Completely in the canal

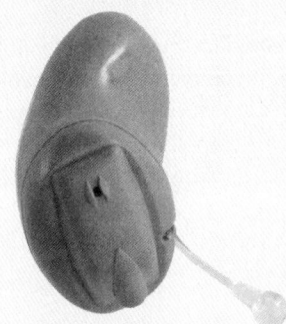

In the canal

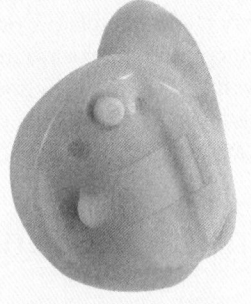

In the ear

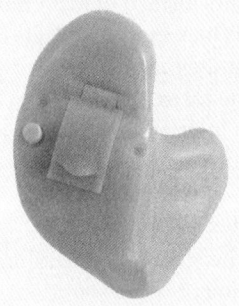

Hearing Aids

If you're thinking about trying a hearing aid for the first time or shopping for a new model, you may be surprised by new technology. Current models are smaller and technologically advanced.

Styles
Hearing aids come in six basic styles, classified by where they're worn:
- Completely in the canal
- In the canal
- In the ear
- Behind the ear
- Receiver in canal or in the ear
- Open fit

The smaller canal styles appeal to individuals concerned with the

appearance of a hearing aid. However, these canal styles may not provide enough amplification if you have severe hearing loss. Generally, the smaller the hearing aid, the less powerful and more likely it is to produce feedback — a high-pitched squeal. In addition, some people find the small controls on canal styles difficult to adjust.

In-the-ear models are suitable for mild to severe hearing loss. They're more powerful than smaller aids and can accommodate more options. A disadvantage is that these types of hearing aids pick up more wind noise because they're not as protected by the ear.

A newer style that's become popular for mild to moderate hearing loss — especially among people

who don't want the hearing aid showing — is the open fit behind-the-ear version. The hearing aid is very small and often is completely obscured behind the outer ear. A clear, thin tube connects the casing to the ear canal, leaving the canal largely open, hence the name. A drawback is that due to the open canal, this style is limited in how much volume it can produce before feedback problems occur.

One vs. two
If you have similar hearing loss in each ear, consider using two hearing aids. Your hearing will be more balanced, and it'll be easier to locate the source of sounds. Plus, you generally hear speech better with two aids.

described its symptoms more than a century ago.

At first, Meniere's disease may affect just one ear, but it eventually affects both ears in up to half the people with the disease. Its cause is unknown, but the condition seems to be associated with an increase of fluid pressure in the inner ear.

The excess pressure is thought to cause tension upon the delicate membranes of the labyrinth — the fluid-filled chamber of the inner ear that controls balance and hearing — distorting and occasionally rupturing them. This trauma produces severe disruption in the senses of balance and hearing.

Periodic attacks characterize Meniere's disease. Between attacks — which may last from several minutes to most of a day — there are far fewer symptoms.

Diagnosis

If you have signs or symptoms associated with Meniere's disease, your doctor likely will ask you questions about your condition and order tests to evaluate your inner ear function and screen for possible causes of the problem. He or she may refer you to an otolaryngologist, or ear, nose and throat (ENT) specialist; a hearing specialist (audiologist); or a nervous system specialist (neurologist).

Hearing assessment

Hearing tests may be performed to assess how well you detect sounds at different pitches and volumes and how well you distinguish between similar-sounding words. The tests not only reveal the quality of your hearing but also may help determine the source of hearing problems.

Balance assessment

Between episodes of vertigo, the sense of balance returns to normal for most people with Meniere's disease. But there may be some degree of ongoing balance problems.

Electronystagmography (ENG) evaluates balance function by assessing eye movement. In an ENG evaluation, electrodes are placed on the skin near the eyes and on the forehead. Then warm and cool water, or warm and cool air, are introduced into the ear canal. Measurements of involuntary eye movements in response to this

Behind the ear

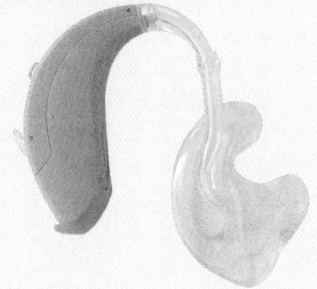

Receiver in the canal or ear

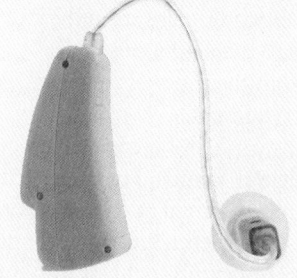

Open fit

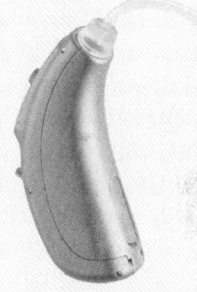

Conventional vs. digital

Conventional (analog) hearing aids aren't recommended. Digital hearing aids offer greater ability to fine-tune sound and reduce feedback and background noise. They're programmed using a computer and can be adjusted to match your preferences. Most digital hearing aids have automatic volume control and noise reduction.

Some devices come with a remote control unit that allows you to reprogram your hearing aids to best fit your current conditions, such as conversation in a quiet room versus a loud restaurant.

Training

Getting used to a hearing aid takes time. The sound you hear is different because it's amplified. In addition, it takes practice to learn how to tune out background noise.

When you get your hearing aid, you may be more comfortable trying it in an ideal situation, such as listening to the television in a quiet room. You may find it discouraging if you first use your hearing aid in a difficult listening situation, such as in a noisy restaurant.

The best way to get accustomed to your hearing aid is to wear it daily, making it part of your routine. This will help you adjust to hearing everyday sounds you don't hear — or don't hear well — without the hearing aid. In addition, ask your audiologist about programs that help teach how to maximize use of all available cues

to improve communication, such as lip reading.

Shopping smart

A hearing aid can be an expensive purchase, so take steps to ensure that you choose a quality product. Begin by selecting a reputable audiologist. If you don't know of one, ask your doctor for a referral.

Make sure that the hearing aid comes with a trial period and a warranty. A typical trial period is 30 to 45 days. The warranty should extend for one to two years and cover both parts and labor. If you're not happy with your hearing aid, return it during the trial period for a refund.

Cochlear Implants

Some children and adults who have severe to profound nerve deafness (sensorineural deafness) and who aren't helped by hearing aids may benefit from a cochlear implant, an electronic device that's implanted under the skin behind the ear.

With nerve deafness the hair cells that line the cochlea of your inner ear have been damaged. Normally, these tiny hairs convert sound vibrations into electric impulses that are carried by the auditory nerve to the brain and then interpreted as sound.

A cochlear implant functions much like the hair cells did before they were damaged. It sends an electric signal via the remaining auditory nerve fibers to the brain. This is altogether different from a hearing aid, which amplifies sound and directs it into the ear canal.

A cochlear implant consists of two sets of components: external and internal. The external component includes:

- A microphone to pick up sound
- A speech processor, which changes sound into a computer code
- A transmitter, which sends electric signals from the speech processor to an internal receiver

The external portion of some cochlear implants looks much like a conventional hearing aid. However, some devices require wearing the speech processor on your body.

The internal component consists of a device that a surgeon implants under the skin behind your ear. It includes:

- A receiver-stimulator, which receives electric impulses from the external transmitter and delivers the impulses to the electrodes
- Electrodes, which receive the impulses from the internal receiver-stimulator and stimulate the auditory nerve fibers

A cochlear implant can't restore normal hearing, but it can help people understand speech and interpret environmental sounds. For many children, a cochlear implant has an impact on the potential to develop normal speech and language. Your brain interprets the electric impulses as speech and environmental sounds. Today, many people with cochlear implants use the telephone and carry on reasonably good communication.

Before you decide to proceed with an implant, have a careful evaluation of your middle and inner ear, including computerized tomography (CT) imaging and a thorough hearing exam by an audiologist. After placement of the implant, you'll be trained in how to best use the device and interpret the sounds it produces.

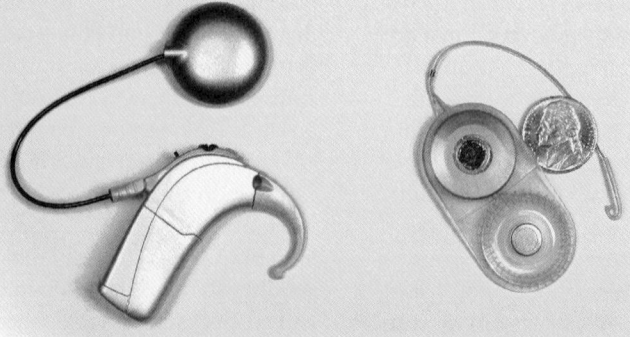

A cochlear implant includes an external component, at left, made up of a microphone, speech processor and transmitter. The internal component, at right, is implanted into your skull and connected directly into the cochlea. The nickel is included only as a size reference.

stimulation are performed. Abnormalities of this test may indicate an inner ear problem.

An ENT specialist may use additional tests that assess function of the inner ear. They include:

- **Rotary chair testing.** Like an ENG, this measures inner ear function based on eye movement. In this case, stimulus to your inner ear is provided by movement of a special rotating chair precisely controlled by a computer.
- **Vestibular evoked myogenic potentials (VEMP) testing.** VEMP testing measures the function of sensors in the vestibule of the inner ear that help you detect acceleration movement. These sensors also have a slight sensitivity to sound. When the sensors react to sound, tiny measurable variations in neck muscle contractions occur. These contractions serve as an indirect measure of inner ear function.
- **Posturography.** This computerized test reveals which part of the balance system — vision; inner ear function; or sensations from the skin, muscles, tendons and joints — you rely on the most and which parts may cause problems. While wearing a safety harness, you stand in bare feet on a special platform and keep your balance under various conditions.

Other tests

Additional tests may be used to rule out disorders that can cause problems similar to those of Meniere's disease, such as a tumor in the brain or multiple sclerosis.

How serious is Meniere's disease?

For most people, the attacks are infrequent, and the disorder is primarily an inconvenience. However, for some individuals, Meniere's disease can lead to complete deafness, and the vertigo and accompanying nausea can be frequent and debilitating.

Treatment

There is no cure for Meniere's disease, but various strategies may help you manage your symptoms.

Medications

Your doctor may prescribe medications to be taken during an episode of vertigo to lessen the severity of the attack:

- Motion sickness medications, such as meclizine or diazepam (Valium), may reduce the spinning sensation of vertigo and ease nausea and vomiting.
- Anti-nausea medications, such as prochlorperazine (Procomp), may control nausea and vomiting during an episode of vertigo.

Your doctor may also prescribe a medication to reduce fluid retention (diuretic). Reducing the amount of fluid your body retains may help regulate the fluid volume and pressure in your inner ear. For some people, diuretics help control the severity and frequency of their symptoms.

Middle ear injections

Medications injected into the middle ear, and then absorbed into the inner ear, may improve vertigo symptoms:

- Gentamicin, an antibiotic that's toxic to your inner ear, reduces the balancing function of your ear, and your other ear assumes responsibility for balance. The procedure often reduces the frequency and severity of vertigo attacks. There is a risk, however, of further hearing loss.
- Corticosteroids, such as dexamethasone, may help control vertigo attacks in some people. Although dexamethasone injections may be slightly less effective than gentamicin, they're less likely than gentamicin to cause further hearing loss.

Surgery

If vertigo attacks associated with Meniere's disease are severe and other treatments don't help, surgery may be an option.

Causes of Dizziness

Dizziness is common in older adults, and for some individuals it can interfere with daily activities. By some estimates, up to 40 percent of Americans will have an episode of dizziness sometime in life that's so severe they'll seek medical attention.

But as common as this complaint is, it often presents a frustrating and complex puzzle to your doctor. Although dizziness may mean one thing to you, to your doctor it's an umbrella term that can signify one of several problems.

Spinning sensation

If you experience a spinning sensation (vertigo), the problem is likely related to the nerves and vestibular system — structures of your inner ear that sense position, movement and changes in your head position. Vertigo can also cause nausea and vomiting. It's almost always accompanied by involuntary, abnormal, rhythmic eye movement called nystagmus. The common causes of vertigo include:

- Benign paroxysmal positional vertigo
- Meniere's disease
- Labyrinthitis
- Acoustic neuroma
- Certain medications, including aspirin, streptomycin and gentamicin, and some medications taken for high blood pressure and heart disease
- Excess caffeine and alcohol

Feeling unsteady

Sometimes, an inner ear disorder can cause loss of balance or a feeling of unsteadiness when walking. A feeling of unsteadiness may also stem from certain medications, such as anti-seizure drugs, sedatives and tranquilizers. Sensory deficits such as failing vision, nerve damage in the arms and legs, osteoarthritis, and muscle weakness also can cause unsteadiness, as can disorders of the central nervous system.

Floating sensation

Many people refer to a sensation of floating as feeling woozy. This sensation is sometimes associated with hyperventilation or an anxiety disorder, such as a panic attack.

Feeling faint

Some people faint at the sight of blood or after hearing bad news or seeing a frightening sight. Feelings of faintness that occur for an unknown reason may be related to a cardiovascular problem. Possible causes include:

- A significant drop in systolic blood pressure on standing (orthostatic hypotension)
- Blocked arteries (ischemia)
- Disease of the heart muscle (cardiomyopathy)
- A rapid or slow heart rate (arrhythmia)

If you experience ongoing dizziness or your dizziness is accompanied by other symptoms, see your doctor. Only about 5 percent of cases stem from a serious condition, but it's important that the cause of your dizziness be identified and serious conditions be ruled out.

- **Endolymphatic sac procedures.** The endolymphatic sac plays a role in regulating inner ear fluid levels. These surgical procedures may alleviate vertigo by decreasing fluid production or increasing fluid absorption. In endolymphatic sac decompression, a small portion of bone is removed from over the endolymphatic sac. Sometimes, this procedure is coupled with the placement of a tube that drains excess fluid from your inner ear (shunt).
- **Labyrinthectomy.** With this procedure, the surgeon removes a portion or all of the inner ear, thereby removing both balance and hearing function from the affected ear. This procedure is only performed if you already have near-total or total hearing loss in your affected ear.
- **Vestibular nerve section.** This procedure involves cutting the nerve that connects balance and movement sensors in your inner ear to the brain (vestibular nerve). The procedure usually corrects problems with vertigo while attempting to preserve hearing in the affected ear.

Hearing aid
A hearing aid in the ear affected by Meniere's disease may improve your hearing. Your doctor can refer you to an audiologist to discuss what hearing aid options would be best for you.

Dietary changes
Modifying your diet can reduce fluid retention and may help decrease fluid in your inner ear. Your doctor may suggest the following:
- **Limit salt.** Consuming foods and beverages high in salt can increase fluid retention. Aim for an intake of 1,000 to 1,500 milligrams (mg) or less of sodium each day.
- **Avoid monosodium glutamate (MSG).** Prepackaged food products and some Asian foods include MSG, a type of sodium.

MSG can contribute to fluid retention.
- **Avoid caffeine.** Foods and beverages that contain caffeine have stimulant properties that can make symptoms worse.

Labyrinthitis

Signs and symptoms
- Extreme dizziness (vertigo)
- Nausea and vomiting
- Involuntary eye movement

Labyrinthitis is an inflammation of the fluid-filled chamber of the inner ear that controls balance and hearing (labyrinth). The condition may result from a bacterial or viral infection.

Diagnosis
A diagnosis is usually made based on the presence of specific signs and symptoms: sensations of nausea and dizziness in which the room seems to be spinning, slow movement of your eyes to one side and then a quick move back to their original position, and the loss of hearing in an ear.

How serious is labyrinthitis?
Signs and symptoms can be frightening, but the condition itself generally isn't dangerous.

Treatment
If you have bacterial labyrinthitis, your doctor will likely prescribe antibiotics. For both bacterial and viral labyrinthitis, your doctor may recommend an anti-nausea drug and a sedative to combat the effects of vertigo. You may need to rest in bed for several days.

Symptoms usually pass within a few days to a week. Feelings of imbalance may persist for several weeks or even months, particularly with quick movements of the head. Recurring episodes of labyrinthitis are rare.

Acoustic neuroma

Signs and symptoms
- Hearing loss in one ear

- Noise such as a buzzing, ringing or roaring in an ear
- Dizziness
- Loss of balance
- Facial numbness and weakness

An acoustic neuroma is a slow-growing, noncancerous (benign) tumor of the auditory nerve. It's usually located near the point where the nerve leaves the cranial cavity and enters the bone structures of your inner ear. The signs and symptoms of acoustic neuroma develop from the tumor pressing on cranial nerves. The tumor may also press on the brainstem.

The only known risk factor for acoustic neuroma is having a rare genetic disorder called neurofibromatosis type 2.

Diagnosis
A diagnosis may involve one or more of the following tests:
- A computerized tomography (CT) scan or magnetic resonance imaging (MRI) of your skull to identify the neuroma
- Hearing tests to check the sharpness and range of your hearing
- Balance tests
- A test called brainstem auditory evoked response, which checks hearing and neurological functions

How serious is an acoustic neuroma?
Although benign in character and slow in growth, this tumor can be a serious threat because it's located next to a number of vital nerves and brain structures. As it grows, it can create pressure that can damage these structures.

Treatment
If you have a small acoustic neuroma that isn't growing or is growing slowly and causes few or no symptoms, you and your doctor may decide to monitor it. Studies indicate more than half of small tumors don't grow after diagnosis and some even shrink. Other options are to remove the

tumor surgically or treat it with a type of stereotactic radiosurgery, such as Gamma Knife radiosurgery. Stereotactic radiosurgery, involves delivering high-dose radiation using a computer's assistance. Your head is immobilized, and focused beams of radiation are aimed precisely at the tumor to avoid harming other parts of the brain.

Surgical removal of an acoustic neuroma involves removing the tumor through an incision in your skull. Care must be taken to preserve the facial nerve to prevent facial paralysis, as well as preserve hearing.

Benign paroxysmal positional vertigo

Signs and symptoms
- Abrupt onset of dizziness when you move your head to certain positions
- Involuntary eye movements

Benign paroxysmal positional vertigo (BPPV) is a common cause of vertigo and more likely to occur in older adults.

BPPV is characterized by sudden, short bursts of vertigo — usually lasting less than a minute — that typically occur after you turn or change the position of your head. You may feel as if you're spinning or floating. Your eyes move back and forth involuntarily (nystagmus) while this happens. You may also experience fatigue and nausea with rare occasions of vomiting. Vertigo associated with BPPV may come and go unpredictably for weeks or even years.

Although the cause is unknown, BPPV is considered a mechanical problem of the balance system — not a neurological problem. Sometimes a blow to the head precedes the condition, but BPPV may also occur spontaneously as a natural result of aging or from damage to the balance organ.

Regardless of the cause, scientists have learned that tiny granules (otoconia) that are nor-

mally located in the utricle of the vestibular labyrinth break loose. Most often, these loose pieces accumulate in one of the semicircular canals.

Certain movements — such as rolling over in bed, sitting up or bending forward — move the particles, disturbing the fluid of the inner ear. This causes the hair cells in the canals to bend, setting off brief episodes of vertigo.

Diagnosis
Your doctor may conduct a series of tests to determine what form of vertigo you have and whether your positional disorientation is a symptom of another disorder. Characteristics of BPPV include vertigo that occurs when you tip your head back or lie on a particular side when sleeping. The vertigo is generally accompanied by involuntary movement of your eyes from side to side. The symptoms usually decrease in less than a minute.

How serious is BPPV?
Benign paroxysmal positional vertigo is an inconvenience but rarely a serious problem, unless you're in an occupation in which even short episodes of vertigo may be disruptive.

Treatment
If BPPV is suspected, a simple office procedure may be all it takes to manage BPPV. The canalith repositioning procedure, which is performed with the assistance of an audiologist, involves specific maneuvers for positioning your head (see page 644). The goal is to progressively move misplaced particles (otoconia) out of the ear canal to an open area near the utricle.

It may be necessary to repeat the procedure several times before feeling the vertigo is eliminated. Afterward, you'll probably need to keep your head upright for the rest of the day to help ensure that the particles stay out of the canal.

The canalith repositioning procedure can be highly effective. However, a recurrence of vertigo frequently happens in the first year after a successful maneuver. If the symptoms do return, repeating the procedure usually is helpful.

Wax blockage

Signs and symptoms
- A sensation that your ear is plugged
- Partial hearing loss

Your outer ear canal is lined with skin that contains hair follicles and glands that produce earwax (cerumen). These hairs and wax trap dust and other foreign particles to prevent them from entering your ear, thereby protecting the delicate mechanisms of your inner ear.

Normally, the small amount of wax that forms makes its way over time to the opening of your ear, where it falls out or is removed as you wash.

Some people, however, produce or accumulate an excessive amount of wax. This extra wax can harden and block the ear canal. Hardened or impacted wax is one of the most common causes of hearing loss among people of all ages.

Diagnosis
If you experience progressive hearing loss over a period of a few weeks or months, your ears feel full, you have an earache, or you hear constant or occasional noises such as ringing in your ears (tinnitus), your doctor will look for signs of earwax blockage.

Treatment
There's an old but wise saying: "Never put anything smaller than an elbow into your ear." Your ear canal and eardrum are delicate, and you can damage them easily by poking around with common items such as cotton-tipped swabs, bobby pins or twisted pieces of

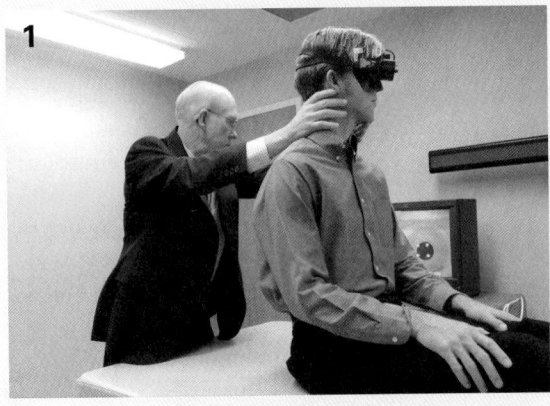

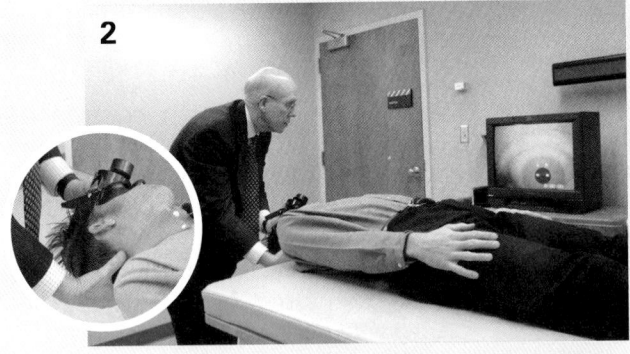

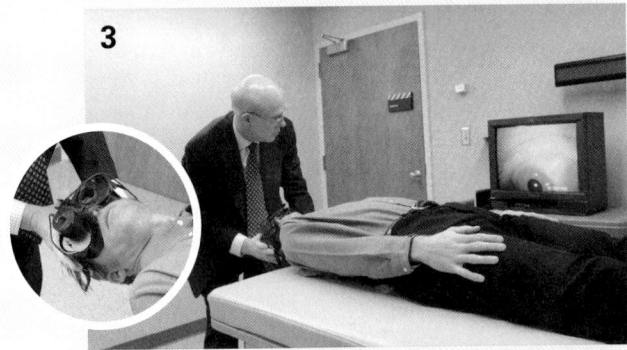

Canalith Repositioning Procedure

To help relieve benign paroxysmal positional vertigo (BPPV), your audiologist may help you perform a series of maneuvers. Each step is held for about 30 seconds. This example is for BPPV on your left side.

1. Start in a seated position with your head turned at a 45-degree angle to the left.
2. Move to a reclining position while your head is kept at the same angle. The audiologist supports your head as it extends over the edge of the table.
3. Still reclined, turn your head to the right.
4. Roll over on your side. Your head is angled slightly as you look down at the floor.
5. Return carefully to a sitting position with your chin tilted down.

Vestibular labyrinth

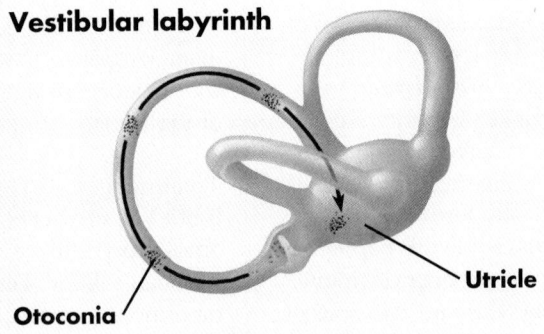

Otoconia

Utricle

As you work through the procedure, the loose otoconia return to the area of the utricle.

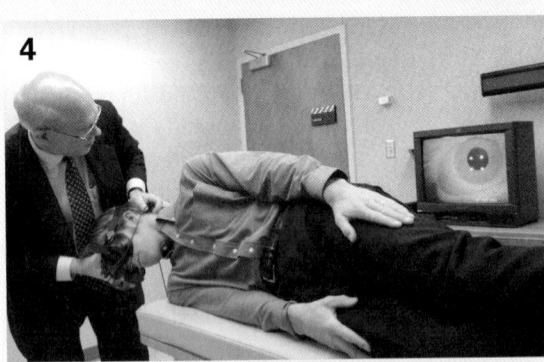

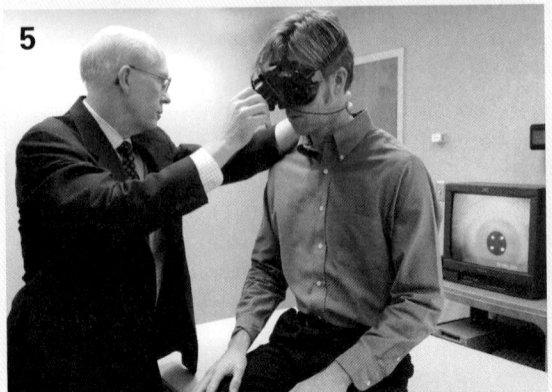

paper. They usually don't remove problem wax and, more importantly, can easily damage your ear canal or eardrum.

If your ear is healthy and excessive earwax recurs, you can use an inexpensive home remedy to remove the wax. Over-the-counter preparations are available, but they're more expensive and often less effective.

To remove problem earwax, follow these steps:

1. Twice a day for several days, place a few drops of baby oil, mineral oil or glycerin in your ear with an eyedropper to loosen the wax. Once you soften the wax well, you can attempt to remove it.
2. Fill a 3-ounce rubber-bulb syringe with water. The water should be at body temperature. If the water is too cool or warm, the following procedure may cause severe, but brief, dizziness.
3. With your head tilted down, pull your outer ear up and back to straighten your ear canal. With the other hand, gently squirt water into the canal, exerting mild pressure but not causing pain.
4. Turn your head to allow the water to drain into a sink or bowl. You may need to flush your ear several times before the wax, usually in the form of a plug, falls out.
5. Dry your outer ear with a towel or a hand-held hair dryer. Place the heat setting and the blower on low.
6. Dry your ear canal by inserting one full eyedropper of rubbing alcohol into the canal. This will absorb the water and destroy bacteria and fungi. Tip your head to the side to drain the alcohol.

Your doctor may use a similar procedure to remove problem earwax. Or he or she may use a special suction device or attempt to scoop the wax out with an instrument called a curet.

Disorders of the Nose and Sinuses

Your nose is the gateway to your respiratory system, with breathing beginning and ending at the nostrils. Normally, your nose filters, humidifies and warms the air as it moves through your nasal passages into your throat and lungs.

Occasionally, your nose is the site of conditions such as a nosebleed, a cold, hay fever (allergic rhinitis) or a sinus infection.

Nosebleeds

Signs and symptoms
Anterior nosebleed
- Sudden bleeding from one nostril

Posterior nosebleed
- Blood streaming down the throat

Most people experience a nosebleed at one time or another. Sometimes, the cause is a blow to the nose, but often a nosebleed is simply the result of a cold, a sinus infection, dry air or a scab being dislodged. If you take a blood-thinning medication, it can exacerbate nosebleeds. Rarely, nosebleeds may be a sign of a serious underlying problem, such as high blood pressure, a bleeding disorder or leukemia.

Nosebleeds are typically thought of as a childhood problem, but they're actually more common in older adults.

Most nosebleeds begin on the anterior septum, the wall of cartilage and bone that separates the two nasal chambers. These are called anterior nosebleeds. This form of nosebleed isn't serious and is usually easy to stop. The front of your septum, just inside your nostril, contains many fragile blood vessels. These vessels are easily damaged, either directly as from a blow or indirectly from crusting in your nose produced by breathing

dry air. A head cold or an allergy also can cause crusting.

Posterior nosebleeds are more serious but less common. They occur when one of the blood vessels in the back (posterior) portion of your nose bleeds. Blood streams down the nasal cavity into the throat rather than out the nostril, so blood loss is more difficult to monitor. Home treatment usually won't stop the bleeding, and a trip to the emergency department often is necessary.

Diagnosis
In most cases, you can stop an anterior nosebleed easily by pinching closed the collapsible portions of your nostrils for about 10 minutes. If the bleeding is hard to stop or occurs frequently, see your doctor.

Your doctor may examine your nose with a flexible tube with a camera at the end (endoscope), to see precisely where the problem lies. If the problem appears to be deep in your nose, your doctor may look for another, more serious problem such as a tumor.

How serious are nosebleeds?
Most nosebleeds are just shirt-staining annoyances. But posterior and recurring anterior nosebleeds can be warning signs of a serious health problem. Frequent nosebleeds in children can be a sign of a noncancerous (benign) tumor (see page 647).

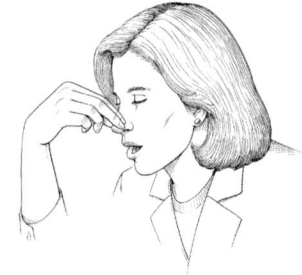

To stop a nosebleed, use your thumb and index finger to squeeze together the soft portion of your nose, located between the end of your nose and the hard, bony ridge.

Treatment

Use these easy steps to stop an anterior nosebleed:

1. Sit up or stand. Don't lie down. An upright position decreases the blood pressure in the veins of your nose, which slows the flow of blood.
2. Pinch the front, soft part of your nose with your thumb and index finger and breathe through your mouth. Do this for about 10 or 15 minutes — the pressure on your bleeding septum should stop the flow of blood.
3. It's not necessary to tip your head backward. Tilting your head slightly forward may prevent blood from streaming into the back of your throat.

To prevent further bleeding, try not to blow your nose for several days after the bleeding episode. If a nosebleed is difficult to stop or occurs frequently, your doctor may use a suction device to remove excess blood and place a medicated cotton ball in your nose. The medication anesthetizes and shrinks your nasal linings.

Cautery

If the bleeding continues, your doctor may recommend that you have the vessel that's causing the problem cauterized. This procedure creates a seal on the vessel by burning it with silver nitrate, electric current or a laser beam. For this procedure, your doctor applies a topical anesthetic to the inside of your nose.

If the bleeding persists after cautery, your doctor may gently pack your nostril with medicated gauze or use a special pack. The packing, which is left in place for several days, exerts pressure on the bleeding site to stop blood flow. When the packing is removed, your vessels may be cauterized again to prevent recurrence of the bleeding.

Surgery

In rare situations when a bent (deviated) septum is thought to contribute to the nosebleeds, doctors may perform a surgical procedure that straightens the wall of cartilage between your nostrils (septoplasty).

For posterior nosebleeds and those caused by an underlying disease that are difficult to stop, one approach is to place a special pack in your nasal cavity. Its placement requires sedation. This procedure is done in a hospital and may involve a short stay for observation. The procedure may be uncomfortable, but it's usually effective in stopping the bleeding. In rare instances, when standard techniques don't work, a doctor may perform surgery to find and treat the bleeding site or block the arteries that supply blood to the nosebleed site.

Prevention

If you have frequent nosebleeds, apply saline gel or petroleum jelly to your nasal septum once or twice each day. Increase the humidity of the air you breathe by using a humidifier or vaporizer.

Nasal obstruction

Signs and symptoms

- An inability to breathe through your nose

Nasal obstruction occurs when the air passageways of your nose become blocked. Everyone experiences a certain amount of temporary blockage when suffering from a cold or an allergy.

Sometimes, nasal obstruction is caused by a deviated septum or excessive use of over-the-counter nasal sprays. Nasal tumors or polyps and enlarged adenoids are other causes. See page 493 for more information on nasal polyps.

Your septum is the cartilage and bony partition that separates your two nasal chambers. Few people have a septum that runs perfectly straight. Most variations are small, but in some people the septum veers significantly to one side or the other, creating the blockage. Such deviations may be the result of an injury, such as a blow to your nose, or they may have been present since birth.

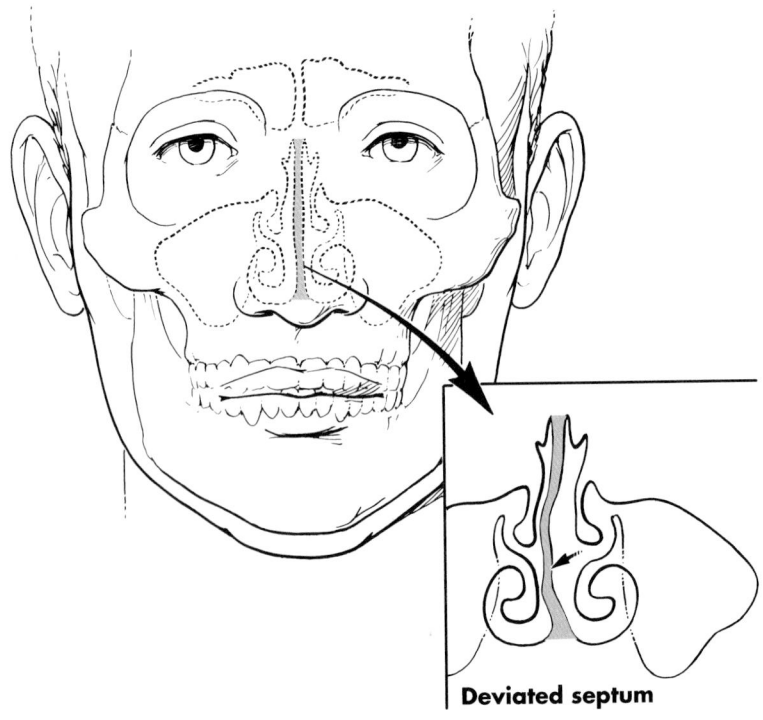

Deviated septum

Your nasal septum separates your nasal chambers. A deviated septum may be a cause of nasal obstruction.

A Simple Remedy for a Stuffy Nose

While in the throes of a cold, who doesn't yearn for a foolproof method to cure a congested nose? Dozens of ads tout products that promise magical cures, but such products rarely live up to their billings. Even when they do relieve the congestion in your nose, they may produce unpleasant side effects such as drowsiness or dry mouth.

One of the best temporary remedies for a stuffy nose doesn't cause complications or cost money. To loosen mucus in your nasal and sinus cavities and relieve congestion, inhale steam. Bring a kettle or pan of water to a boil and inhale the steam for several minutes, taking care not to get so close that you scald yourself. Some people place a towel over their head, making a tent while they inhale the steam. This method is useful for loosening the mucus in your chest too. Similarly, a steaming shower can help clear your head.

Diagnosis

In searching for the cause of the obstruction, your doctor may ask you questions regarding possible injury, allergies and use of nasal sprays. He or she may use a lighted, flexible device that's inserted into your nose to assist in diagnosing the problem. A computerized tomography (CT) scan also can be helpful in some circumstances.

Treatment

For many people, a deviated septum poses little if any inconvenience. However, if the deviation causes a blockage that makes it difficult to breathe normally, a septoplasty may be necessary.

Septoplasty is a surgical procedure that realigns your septum. It generally is done under general anesthesia on an outpatient basis.

If the blockage is a result of overuse of nose drops or a nasal spray, you'll need to stop using the medication and allow time for the rebound swelling to normalize. If allergies are suspected, your doctor may refer you to an allergist for a series of tests to determine what you're allergic to. If the blockage is a result of polyps, enlarged adenoids or a tumor, surgery may be necessary to remove the blockage.

Juvenile angiofibroma

Signs and symptoms
- Frequent nosebleeds
- Nasal obstruction

An angiofibroma is a noncancerous (benign) tumor of the nose that occurs at puberty, particularly in boys. The tumor may shrink on its own after puberty, but it can grow rapidly, obstructing nasal passages and sinuses and causing frequent and often severe nosebleeds. Rarely, the tumor can put pressure on the brain.

Diagnosis

If your child has signs or symptoms suggestive of a juvenile angiofibroma, your doctor may examine the inside of his or her nose for evidence of a tumor. Magnetic resonance imaging (MRI) or a computerized tomography (CT) scan can help determine the size and location of the tumor. If the tumor doesn't shrink on its own, treatment is necessary.

Treatment

The most common treatment for an angiofibroma is surgery to remove the tumor. Before the surgery takes place, doctors frequently use a procedure called embolization.

During embolization, a doctor injects pellets of a glue-like substance into the tumor's blood vessels. The pellets obstruct the tumor's blood vessels, cutting off the blood supply to the tumor. The tumor can then be removed surgically with a significant reduction in bleeding.

It has become common for this type of surgery to be done endoscopically, in which small cameras and surgical tools are guided to the location through natural openings in the nose.

Rhinophyma

Signs and symptoms
- A nose that appears large, bulbous and ruddy

Rhinophyma, which results from a skin condition called rosacea (see page 1075), involves the upper layer of skin (epithelium) on the outer portion of the nose. The skin thickens, causing the nose to be large and bulbous.

The cause of rhinophyma isn't clearly understood. The condition was once thought to result from heavy drinking, but alcohol consumption isn't a factor. People who drink moderate amounts or abstain from alcohol can develop rhinophyma.

Diagnosis

A diagnosis of rhinophyma is made based on the appearance of excessively thick skin on the outer portion of the nose, causing it to take on a large, bulbous shape.

Treatment

The only definitive treatment for rhinophyma is surgery. In this procedure, the surgeon removes excess tissue from the outside of the nose using various surgical instruments or a laser. As it heals, the nose usually resumes its normal shape.

Loss of the sense of smell

Signs and symptoms

- Decreased ability to detect odors
- Decreased nasal breathing

Most people lose their sense of smell when suffering from a head cold, but sometimes the cause isn't so obvious. Loss of the sense of smell (anosmia) results when an obstruction in your nose prevents odors from reaching delicate nerve fibers in your nose that lead to the area of your brain dealing with smell (olfactory area). The most common cause is nasal polyps, pearl-like lumps caused by swelling of nasal membranes, which can block nasal passages (see illustration on page 388).

Loss of the sense of smell may also occur if the olfactory area or its nerve fibers are damaged. A viral infection, allergies or a chronic nose infection can damage these nerves, as can a head injury, nasal surgery or a tumor. Most people who have lost the sense of smell can still distinguish salty, sweet, sour and bitter tastes, which are sensed on the tongue. But they have trouble distinguishing more-subtle flavors and sensations that require both taste and smell.

Diagnosis

If you lose your sense of smell for no apparent reason, consult your doctor. Nasal polyps and chronic nasal allergies are the most common causes of anosmia. Your doctor may check for tumors of the nasal passages.

How serious is loss of the sense of smell?

Most often, anosmia is an inconvenience. Sometimes it can be a symptom of a more serious condition. You may need to have a computerized tomography (CT) scan or magnetic resonance imaging (MRI) to check for polyps, a tumor or signs of a head injury. If you lose your sense of smell after a concussion or other head injury, the blow may be the cause of your anosmia.

Loss of the sense of smell can pose certain dangers. If you have anosmia, be sure to have functioning smoke detectors in your home and workplace because you may not smell the smoke of a fire. In addition, carefully check for food expiration dates and refrigerate food appropriately to avoid ingesting spoiled food, which you may not detect through its smell.

Treatment

If your loss of the sense of smell is due to hay fever (allergic rhinitis) or nasal polyps, treating these conditions will often restore your sense of smell. When the cause isn't readily apparent, as is often the case when a virus is involved, your sense of smell may return when the tissues of your olfactory area regenerate on their own.

Vasomotor rhinitis

Signs and symptoms

- Stuffy or runny nose
- Postnasal drainage
- Coughing

The term *rhinitis* refers to inflammation of the mucous membranes of the nose. Rhinitis can occur for many reasons. The common cold causes nasal membrane inflammation. Allergies are another frequent cause. Nasal inflammation associated with allergies is called allergic rhinitis, commonly known as hay fever. To

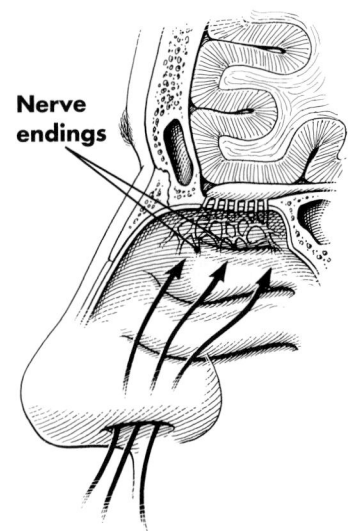

Your sense of smell and, to a large degree, your sense of taste begin with the olfactory nerve endings, found in the upper portion of your nose. These nerves contain sensitive fibers that transmit signals from the olfactory bulb to your brain.

read about hay fever, see Chapter 17, "Allergies and Asthma."

Many people experience nasal stuffiness — sometimes accompanied by sneezing, a runny nose or phlegm in the throat — that isn't related to allergies or an infection, such as a cold. This form of rhinitis is commonly referred to as nonallergic (vasomotor) rhinitis.

Vasomotor rhinitis stems from dilation of blood vessels in the nasal membranes. When the blood vessels expand (dilate), the membranes of the nose swell, taking up more space within an already limited area. This leads to nasal congestion — a stuffy nose.

Many factors may trigger vasomotor rhinitis. They include environmental irritants, such as smoke, dust, smog, dry air or certain odors, such as perfumes. Temperature changes or air conditioning can cause vasomotor rhinitis in some people. Other causes include hormonal changes, anxiety, exercise, spices, beer and wine.

Diagnosis

Rhinitis typically is diagnosed based on your signs and symptoms and when they occur. If you're bothered at a certain time of the year, such as the spring, fall or both, you may have allergic rhinitis. If your nasal congestion doesn't appear to be triggered by allergies, but by other factors, your doctor may determine that you have vasomotor rhinitis.

How serious is vasomotor rhinitis?

Although often annoying, vasomotor rhinitis isn't a worrisome condition. However, to manage your symptoms, you may have to take medication regularly or avoid certain situations, such as smoke-filled rooms or certain foods or beverages.

People with chronic vasomotor rhinitis can also develop nasal polyps and chronic sinusitis.

Treatment

Treatment of the disorder depends on its severity. For mild cases, no treatment may be appropriate. Simply avoiding those factors that seem to trigger the condition is often all that's needed.

Over-the-counter oral decongestants often help. Decongestant nasal sprays can provide temporary relief but they shouldn't be taken regularly because they actually can increase nasal congestion (see page 651).

Prescription corticosteroid nasal sprays are often effective in controlling moderate to severe vasomotor rhinitis. For some people, increased humidity at home and at work also is beneficial. Over-the-counter saline solutions that irrigate your nasal passages often are beneficial. They help by rinsing allergens and irritants off the nasal lining.

Sinusitis

Signs and symptoms
* Pain near the eyes, cheeks or nose
* Tenderness of the sinus areas to pressure or touch
* Headache
* Aching of upper jaw and teeth
* Drainage of yellowish or greenish discharge from nose
* Obstructed nasal breathing
* Bad breath that's unrelated to dental problems
* Reduced sense of taste and smell

Sinusitis results when the cavities around your nasal passages (sinuses) become inflamed and swollen. This interferes with drainage from the sinuses and causes mucus to build up.

There are four pairs of sinuses:
* Frontal sinuses, located in your forehead
* Ethmoid sinuses, located between your eyes
* Sphenoid sinuses, located deeper in your head, behind your nose
* Maxillary sinuses, located in your cheekbones

Each of these cavities has a tiny opening into your nose to allow for exchange of air and mucus. Your sinuses and nose are lined with a continuous mucous membrane. Consequently, anything that causes your nasal passages to swell and clog — such as a cold or an allergic reaction — can affect your sinuses in the same manner. The result is the pain and pressure that people commonly refer to as a sinus infection.

Causes

About two-thirds of sinusitis cases are short-lived (acute). Acute sinusitis is most often caused by the common cold. Sinusitis that lasts more than 12 weeks or keeps coming back is known as chronic sinusitis. Chronic sinusitis may stem from persistent inflammation or infection or from allergies. It's frequently associated with polyps and asthma.

The Sinuses

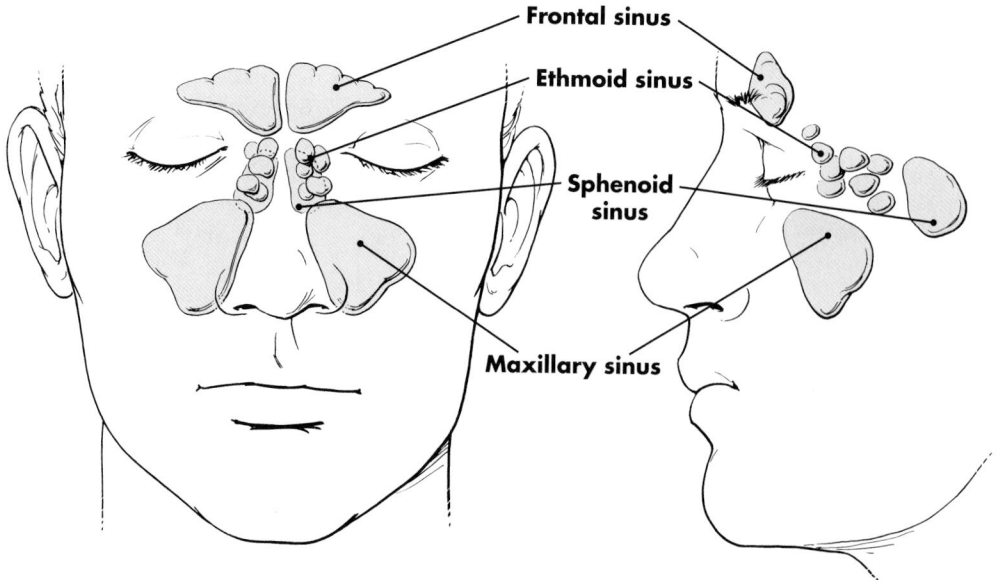

Frontal sinus
Ethmoid sinus
Sphenoid sinus
Maxillary sinus

You may not be able to prevent all sinus problems, but you can take measures to reduce the number and severity of attacks and to help prevent an acute attack from becoming chronic.

- *Wash your hands.* When you've been near someone who has a cold, wash your hands with soap and water to reduce the chance that you'll catch a cold.
- *Keep your distance.* Minimize close contact with people who have colds.
- *Don't smoke.* Tobacco smoke can cause irritation and inflammation of the lining of the sinuses and nose. Inflammation can result in blocked nasal passages.
- *Avoid polluted air.* Contaminants in the air, whether indoors or outdoors, can irritate and inflame your lungs and nasal passageways.
- *Avoid known allergens.* These may include pollen, mold or cat dander. Attach an electrostatic filter to heating and air-conditioning equipment to help remove allergens from the air.
- *Use humidifiers.* This is especially important during the winter when heating systems can make indoor air dry. Be sure to keep humidifiers clean. Contaminated humidifiers can be a source of bacteria and fungi in the air.
- *Use decongestants before airplane travel.* Beware of antihistamine and decongestant drug combinations because antihistamines may cause drowsiness.
- *Talk to your doctor.* Ask your doctor about using a saline nasal spray to keep your nasal passages moist or a prescription medication to reduce inflammation.
- *Avoid alcohol.* It can cause nasal and sinus membranes to swell.

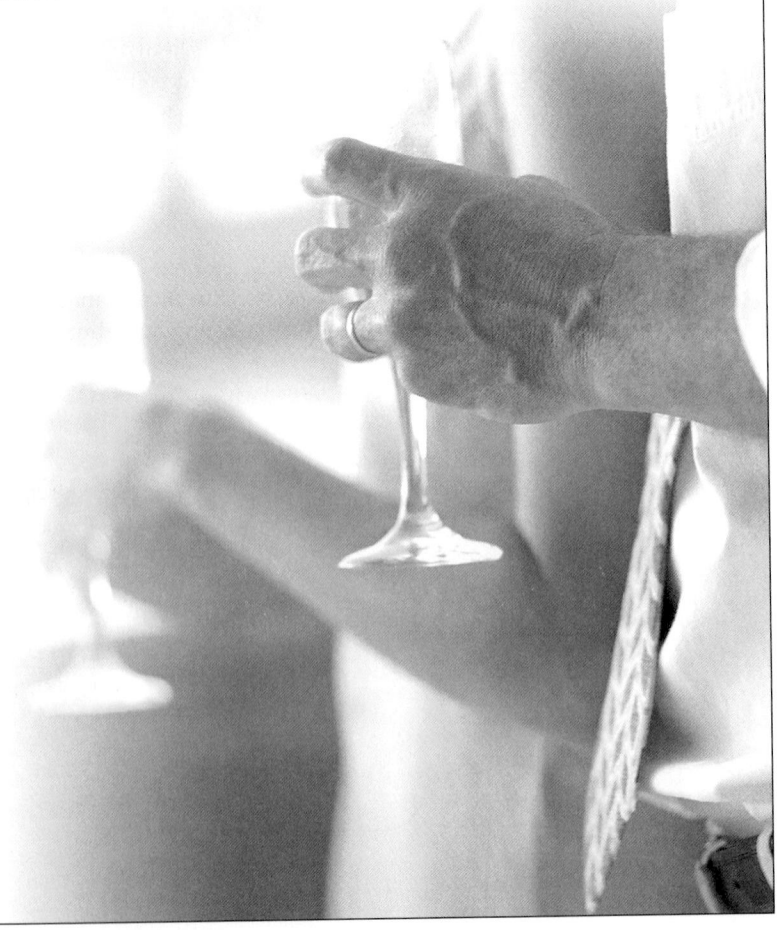

Colds

Most cases of sinusitis start with a cold virus. Sometimes, a cold produces so much mucus that your swollen and congested nasal passages become blocked. Bacteria, which normally reside in your sinuses in small numbers, can begin to multiply and cause bacterial sinusitis.

Allergies

If you're allergic to inhaled allergens such as pollen, pet dander or dust mites, your body mistakes these harmless particles as attackers. Your immune system fights back, causing well-known allergic symptoms, especially a stuffy nose, sneezing and watery eyes. This immune response can lead to sinusitis. Because allergies are frequently persistent, they may cause chronic sinusitis.

Structural abnormalities

Structural abnormalities of the nose include nasal polyps (see page 493) and a deviated septum, in which the cartilage separating the nasal cavities is bent toward one side. These problems can cause the symptoms of nasal obstruction and a decreased sense of smell.

Dental problems

Bacteria associated with dental infections or procedures can invade sinus cavities in the cheekbones. For example, a dental abscess can extend from the root of an upper tooth into a maxillary sinus cavity.

Diagnosis

Sinusitis can be difficult to diagnose because initially it closely resembles the common cold. If your symptoms disappear in five to seven days, you probably had a cold. If symptoms persist and don't respond to decongestants, you may be dealing with a sinus infection. Individuals who have symptoms for an extended period of time or have repeated symptoms may have chronic sinusitis.

If you have repeated (chronic) sinusitis, your doctor may perform a nasal endoscopy. A thin, flexible tube with a fiber-optic light (endoscope) is inserted into your nose, allowing your doctor to visually inspect the openings to your sinuses.

Your doctor may also order a computerized tomography (CT) scan to see which sinuses are involved and if they appear obstructed or inflamed. If mucus or pus is present, a sample of it may be cultured in a laboratory and analyzed.

If allergies are suspected, allergy testing may yield important information about your allergic sensitivities (see page 487).

How serious is sinusitis?

Most cases of sinusitis respond to antibiotics and are easily treated. Only rarely do people develop serious complications. The infection can spread into the membranes that protect your brain (meninges), causing meningitis, which can lead to brain damage. The infection also can spread to the eyes and cause swelling and redness of the eyelids. This more commonly occurs in children.

Treatment

A few home remedies may improve the symptoms of sinusitis:
- Stay indoors in an even temperature.
- Refrain from bending over with your head down. This movement usually increases the pain.
- Try applying warm facial packs, inhaling steam from a kettle or basin of steaming water (be careful not to scald yourself), or taking a warm shower.
- Drink plenty of liquids to help dilute the mucous secretions. Don't drink alcohol, which can worsen nasal and sinus swelling.

Medication

Depending on the cause of your sinusitis and whether it's acute or chronic, your doctor may prescribe one or more of the following medications:

- **Antibiotics.** If your infection is bacterial, your doctor may prescribe a course of oral antibiotic therapy. Chronic sinusitis may require a long period of antibiotic treatment, often using broader spectrum medications than those used for acute sinusitis. A broad-spectrum medication is one that is effective against a wide variety of bacteria.
- **Corticosteroids.** For intense inflammation of the sinuses, your doctor may prescribe a corticosteroid medication. Nasal corticosteroid sprays are commonly used, but severe inflammatory sinusitis may require a corticosteroid injection or pills. After you've had a shot or pills, you might continue using a corticosteroid nasal spray to help prevent the swelling from recurring.
- **Decongestants.** Decongestants reduce stuffiness and help you breathe easier. But over-the-counter decongestant nose drops or sprays shouldn't be used for more than a few days. Otherwise, the medications can cause a rebound effect and lead to even more congestion and swelling. They can also raise your blood pressure and heart rate.
- **Allergy medications.** If allergies are causing your chronic sinusitis, your doctor may prescribe medications to reduce allergy symptoms and hopefully reduce the number and severity of your sinus attacks.
- **Saline nasal spray.** You use it several times a day to rinse your nasal passages of irritants.
- **Pain relievers.** Pain relievers include aspirin, ibuprofen (Advil, Motrin IB, others) and acetaminophen (Tylenol, others).

Surgery

Sometimes, sinusitis persists despite medical treatment. If this happens, a surgeon may perform

Nasal Decongestant Irritation

Your local drugstore sells many products designed to relieve nasal congestion, including decongestant nasal sprays and nose drops (Afrin, Dristan, others). These products provide quick relief by constricting blood vessels and thus shrinking the tissue in your nose. But use these products carefully and only for a limited period, if at all.

When used frequently over several days, decongestant nasal sprays and nose drops can have a rebound effect, causing your nasal tissues to become more swollen and even more congested between applications of the medication. As a result, you'll need greater and more-frequent doses of the spray or drops. Use these products as recommended on the package and for no more than three or four days.

Prolonged use can irritate your mucous membranes, causing a stinging or burning in your nose and a chronic inflammation known as rhinitis medicamentosa.

The way to treat the problem of nasal decongestant overuse is to stop using the sprays or drops. Your condition may become worse for a while, but over a period of weeks your breathing should approach normal as the ill effects of the nasal sprays or drops wear off. Your doctor may recommend a corticosteroid nasal spray or, on occasion, a corticosteroid injection to reduce inflammation and make the transition easier.

651

endoscopic sinus surgery to restore nasal drainage. This type of surgery results in no external incisions or scarring.

During the procedure, your doctor inserts a thin tube equipped with a camera and delicate cutting tools (endoscope) into your nostrils and blocked sinuses. He or she removes polyps and small bone fragments that block your sinuses. The surgeon may also enlarge sinus openings and use a small vacuum to drain trapped fluids or infection.

You may have a mild headache from the operation, and you may need to take antibiotics and pain medication afterward. During the first couple of weeks after surgery, it's normal to have some discomfort and bleeding from your nose. You'll also have to visit your doctor soon after surgery to have dried blood and other secretions removed from your nose.

Occasionally, sinus blockage redevelops, and the surgery must be repeated. Complications of the procedure, although rare, can be serious. They include eye damage, leakage of brain fluid, meningitis (brain abscess), and facial numbness.

Disorders of the Throat

Like other parts of your respiratory system, your throat is susceptible to infection, both bacterial and viral. Your throat is also susceptible to abuse, including overuse while singing or speaking and damage from excessive alcohol consumption or smoking. Gastroesophageal reflux disease (GERD) — a condition in which contents from your stomach reflux into your esophagus — also can affect your throat if the reflux is severe.

Sore throat

Signs and symptoms
- A dry, scratchy or irritated sensation in your throat
- Difficulty swallowing due to pain
- Fever

A sore throat, known medically as pharyngitis, is most often caused by a viral infection, such as a cold or the flu (influenza). Your pharynx is the segment between your adenoids and your voice box (lar-

ynx) — what you commonly think of as your throat.

A sore throat and other accompanying signs and symptoms from a viral infection usually go away on their own in about a week, once your body's antibodies have destroyed the virus.

Bacterial infections are less common but more serious than are most viral infections. Strep throat is the most common bacterial infection. It's caused by the streptococci bacteria and generally is spread by nose or throat secretions.

A sore throat can also stem from allergies and dry air. Constant irritation from smoking, breathing heavily polluted air or consuming too much alcohol can cause a chronic sore throat.

Diagnosis
Most often a doctor will diagnose the cause of a sore throat on the basis of a physical exam and a throat culture. He or she will check your throat for redness and

Postnasal Drip

Mucus produced in your nose and sinuses travels in a thin film to the back of your throat. There, it serves to protect your lungs by humidifying air and by trapping dust and other particles that you inhale. Generally, you're unaware of this process and swallow the mucus and impurities it captures. Swallowing this mucus isn't harmful.

Normally, your nose and sinuses produce a liter or more of mucus daily. However, when smoke or other irritants aggravate your nose, the amount may increase. The extra mucus, secreted to remove more irritants, is often the cause of the discomfort commonly referred to as postnasal drip.

You may become more conscious of mucus in your nose and throat when the air is dry because it may become thicker and more difficult to expel. Drinking plenty of water and humidifying the air you breathe will help keep the mucus thin. Corticosteroid nasal sprays available by prescription also may help relieve postnasal drip.

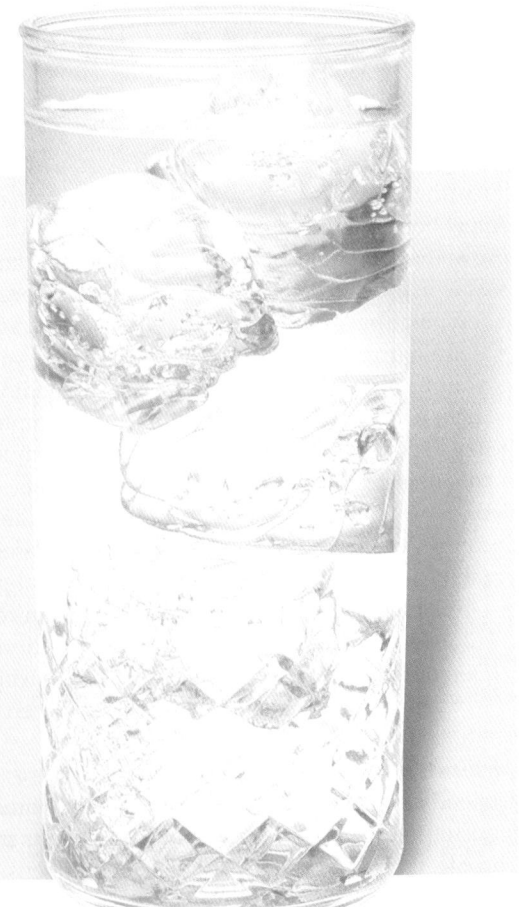

swelling and for white streaks or pus on your tonsils, which are signs of infection. He or she may take a throat culture to check for the presence of bacteria that cause strep throat.

How serious is a sore throat?

Most conditions that cause sore throats aren't serious and go away on their own without causing any complications. However, some bacterial and viral infections can lead to other, more serious problems, such as tonsillitis, strep throat, or a sinus or ear infection.

Treatment

If your sore throat is due to a viral infection, antibiotics won't cure it. Get plenty of rest and double your fluid intake. Fluids may keep your mucus thin and easy to clear.

You can help relieve the pain of a sore throat with acetaminophen (Tylenol, others), ibuprofen (Advil, Motrin IB, others) or aspirin, but don't give aspirin to children because it can trigger a serious condition involving the blood, liver and brain (Reye's syndrome).

Gargling with warm salt water — a half-teaspoon of salt mixed in a glass of warm water — several times a day and using throat lozenges may help relieve the pain to some degree.

If you have a bacterial infection, your doctor will likely prescribe antibiotics to kill the bacteria. Removing the tonsils and the adenoids may prevent recurrent strep infections.

Tonsillitis

Signs and symptoms

- A sore throat
- Red, swollen tonsils
- White patches on the tonsils
- Difficult or painful swallowing
- Fever and chills
- Headache

Tonsillitis occurs when the tonsils — the fleshy pads on each side of the back of the throat — become infected with a virus or bacterium. When organisms such as viruses or bacteria enter your body through your nose or mouth, your tonsils act as a filter, engulfing the organisms in white blood cells. This can cause a low-grade infection in your tonsils. Tonsillitis occurs when the infection gets more serious, and the tonsils become painful and inflamed. When tonsillitis is caused by a specific type of bacteria (group A streptococci), the illness is also known as strep throat.

Diagnosis

Your doctor will likely check your tonsils and the back of your throat for signs of infection, such as redness and pus. He or she may also order a throat culture to check for the bacteria that causes strep throat.

How serious is tonsillitis?

Tonsillitis caused by a viral infection will generally clear up

Adenoid and Tonsil Removal

Your adenoids and tonsils are composed primarily of lymph tissues. Your adenoids are located at the top of your throat just above the soft area at the back of the roof of your mouth (soft palate). Tonsils are located at the back of your mouth. Both act to filter infections from your body and are particularly useful in infants and children up to about 3 years old. In later childhood, the adenoids and tonsils shrink. By puberty, the adenoids have almost disappeared, and the tonsils shrink to the size of almonds.

Many young children and some adults develop bacterial tonsillitis. Occasionally, the adenoids also swell, giving the voice a nasal quality. If you or your child experiences frequent tonsillitis — four to six or more times a year — your doctor may recommend removing the tonsils and adenoids. This combined surgery is known as adenotonsillectomy.

In the past, most children with tonsillitis had their tonsils removed, and often their adenoids as well. Improved antibiotics have made the treatment of tonsillitis much easier and surgery less common. Surgery is still an option when the tonsils become so enlarged that they affect breathing and swallowing, or when an inflamed adenoid causes eustachian tube blockage, leading to a severe middle ear infection (otitis media) and nasal obstruction.

After adenotonsillectomy, the tonsils don't grow back. Sometimes, small remnants of adenoid tissue can enlarge. This rarely causes another problem. After surgery, the throat will be sore. This gradually gets better in 10 to 14 days. Adenotonsillectomy doesn't guarantee freedom from future infections, but the frequency of throat infections usually decreases.

Adenotonsillectomy or adenoidectomy may also be used to treat other conditions. In children, these conditions include:
- Mouth breathing, sleep apnea and snoring (all are caused by chronic upper airway obstruction)
- Recurrent middle ear infection (otitis media)

Conditions that may prompt this type of surgery in an adult include:
- Snoring and sleep apnea
- An abnormal white, stony mass in a tonsil (tonsillar calculus, or tonsillith)
- Recurrent abscess behind a tonsil (peritonsillar abscess)

on its own. Tonsillitis stemming from a bacterial infection that's left untreated can lead to a collection of pus between the tonsil and soft tissues around it (abscess). Rarely, an abscess may spread to the bloodstream or into the neck.

In addition, certain strains of streptococci bacteria that cause tonsillitis may result in later complications, including kidney inflammation (nephritis) or rheumatic fever.

Treatment

If you have tonsillitis, get plenty of rest and drink soothing liquids. Gargling with warm salt water — one-half teaspoon of salt mixed in a glass of warm water — several times a day often helps decrease throat pain. Acetaminophen (Tylenol, others), ibuprofen (Advil, Motrin IB, others) or aspirin also may reduce the pain. Don't give aspirin to children because it could trigger Reye's syndrome, a potentially serious condition.

Medication

If your tonsillitis is caused by a bacterial infection, your doctor will likely prescribe an antibiotic to treat the infection. Signs and symptoms should disappear within a few days, but it's important that you take your full course of medications.

Surgery

At one time, removing the tonsils (tonsillectomy) was a common treatment for recurrent tonsillitis. Today, surgery is recommended only if tonsillitis doesn't get better with other treatment.

Epiglottitis

Signs and symptoms
- A sore throat
- Fever
- A muffled or hoarse voice
- Difficult and painful swallowing
- Difficulty breathing
- Drooling

Epiglottitis is an inflammation of the lidlike structure (epiglottis) that covers your vocal cords and windpipe. When you're not eating or drinking, the epiglottis is slightly lifted so that air can flow into your lungs. When the epiglottis becomes swollen, either from an infection or injury, the airway narrows and may become completely blocked.

Epiglottitis occurs most among children, but adults can get it too.

Vocal Cord Problems

The two vocal cords in your larynx produce the sounds of speech by vibrating. The muscles of your voice box (larynx) control the length, position and tension of the vocal cords, which transmit vibrations to the column of air that passes through your larynx. Your vocal cords can also close, which helps prevent food and water from entering your lungs during swallowing. Like other tissues, vocal cords are susceptible to illness.

Vocal cord polyps

Polyps are small swellings that can develop in the mucous membranes covering your vocal cords. As they grow, they take on a rounded shape. Polyps may extend the full length of your vocal cords or be localized. Vocal polyps may stem from a chronic allergic reaction, or they may form as a result of breathing irritants such as cigarette smoke or industrial fumes.

Polyps can make your voice sound breathy and harsh. Sometimes, a doctor is able to remove them during an examination of your throat with an instrument called a laryngoscope. He or she may biopsy the polyp to be certain that it isn't cancerous (malignant).

Singer's nodules

People who use their voices a great deal, such as professional singers, teachers, auctioneers and members of the clergy, are prone to have nodules on their vocal cords. Such nodules result from excessive voice use.

When you have this condition, your voice may become breathy-sounding and hoarse. A nodule differs from a polyp in that it grows out of the epithelium that covers the mucous membrane, not out of the mucous membrane itself. Thus, it has a structural resemblance to a corn on a toe or a callus on your hand.

Resting your vocal cords by avoiding or minimizing speaking for several weeks may cause the nodules to shrink. Sometimes, surgical removal is necessary. Voice therapy may help eliminate speaking habits that sometimes are responsible for nodule formation.

Contact ulcers

Your vocal cords are subject to developing sores called contact ulcers. This condition results from trauma to your vocal cords. Causes include stomach content backing up into your esophagus and throat (gastroesophageal reflux disease, or GERD), a chronic cough, or insertion of a tube through the mouth or nose into the throat (intubation).

Contact ulcers generally develop at the back of your vocal cords. Signs and symptoms may include pain when swallowing or speaking, hoarseness, and ear pain. Your doctor may take a sample (biopsy) of the ulcerated tissue to be certain no cancer is present. If GERD is the cause, treating the condition should promote healing of the ulcers.

Vocal cord paralysis

Vocal cord paralysis occurs when the nerve impulses to your voice box (larynx) are disrupted. This results

Causes of the condition include burns from hot liquids, direct injury to the throat and various infections. The most common cause is infection with *Haemophilus influenzae* type b (Hib), the same bacterium that causes pneumonia and meningitis.

Fortunately, the number of children with epiglottitis has dropped dramatically since Hib vaccination for infants became routine in the mid-1980s.

Diagnosis

If your doctor suspects that you have epiglottitis, the first priority will be to ensure your airways are open and you're receiving enough oxygen. Once your condition is stable, your doctor will likely examine your throat using a flexible fiber-optic tube. You also may have a throat culture to check for Hib and a blood test to check for a severe blood infection that can accompany epiglottitis (sepsis).

How serious is epiglottitis?

Epiglottitis can begin swiftly and become serious — even life-threatening — within just hours. It can lead to respiratory failure, a life-threatening condition in which the level of oxygen in the blood drops dangerously low or the level of carbon dioxide becomes excessively high. Sometimes the bacteria that cause epiglottitis also cause serious infections elsewhere in the body.

Treatment

Most cases of epiglottitis are treated with antibiotics to kill the bacterial organisms causing the infection. Severe breathing difficulty may require temporary insertion of a tube into the trachea (intubation) by way of your nose or mouth to improve breathing. In extreme cases, a doctor may need to perform a tracheotomy, which allows air into your lungs by bypassing the larynx.

Peritonsillar abscess

Signs and symptoms

- A sore throat and sore soft palate
- Severe pain on swallowing
- Fever
- Tendency to hold your head to one side, away from the pain
- Drooling
- Difficulty opening your mouth

Peritonsillar abscess (quinsy) is a complication of tonsillitis. It's most common in young adults.

in paralysis of the vocal cord muscles. Vocal cord paralysis can affect your ability to speak and even breathe. There are a number of causes of vocal cord paralysis including nerve damage during surgery, viral infections and certain cancers. In some cases, the condition improves on its own. Treatment for vocal cord paralysis usually involves surgery. Voice therapy can sometimes be an option.

Leukoplakia

Leukoplakia is the development of white patches on one or both vocal cords. The patches may be associated with cancer. Once the patches are discovered, your doctor can remove them and have them examined under a microscope to check for cancerous cells. Leukoplakia is often caused by smoking.

Laryngeal papillomatosis

Laryngeal papillomatosis is a disease caused by the human papillomavirus (HPV). These noncancerous (benign), warty tumors (papillomas) grow on the vocal cords, voice box (larynx) or the respiratory tract and cause problems with breathing and swallowing. Most laryngeal papillomas affect young children, usually before age 3.

The papillomas can grow quickly and in large quantities or clusters, making them difficult to remove without damaging the larynx. They may block the airway, causing severe difficulty breathing. In these cases, the tumors need to be treated quickly.

Laser treatment and a shaving procedure with a powered instrument are the primary treatments. Other options include chemotherapy or antiviral therapy.

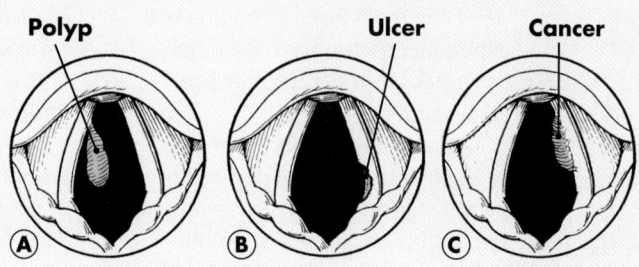

Growths and illnesses that may affect the vocal cords include: a vocal cord polyp (A), a contact ulcer (B) and vocal cord cancer (C).

When a tonsil becomes infected, a collection of pus (abscess) forms between the tonsil and the soft tissues around it. The infection may even extend to the soft area at the back of the roof of your mouth (soft palate), making it possible for the abscess to cover a large area. The infection can also spread to your neck and even farther downward into your chest.

Diagnosis

A diagnosis often is based on the appearance of displaced, inflamed tonsil and swelling at the back of your palate.

How serious is a peritonsillar abscess?

In some cases, the swelling caused by a peritonsillar abscess can become so severe that the roof of your mouth is pushed against your tongue, blocking airflow and making breathing and swallowing very difficult.

Treatment

The infection is treated with antibiotics. If pus is present and the condition doesn't resolve quickly, your doctor may drain the abscess surgically. Because abscesses can recur, your doctor may also recommend a tonsillectomy at the time of the abscess or several weeks after the infection is cured.

Laryngitis

Signs and symptoms

- Hoarseness
- Weak voice or voice loss
- Tickling sensation in throat
- Sore throat
- Dry cough

Laryngitis is an infection or irritation of your voice box (larynx), due to overuse, irritation or infection. Inside the larynx are your vocal cords. In laryngitis the vocal cords become inflamed and irritated. The swelling causes distortion of sounds produced by air passing over them. As a result, your voice sounds hoarse. In some cases, your

voice can become so faint that it's undetectable.

Laryngitis may be short-lived (acute) or long lasting (chronic). Acute laryngitis is usually caused by a virus, and the condition typically disappears without treatment. Acute laryngitis less commonly results from a bacterial infection. However, it often occurs in the course of another illness such as an ordinary cold, flu or pneumonia.

Common causes of chronic laryngitis include constant irritation from excessive alcohol, heavy smoking, or reflux of stomach acid into the esophagus and throat, a condition called gastroesophageal reflux disease (GERD).

Irritations such as excessive talking or singing, allergies, or the breathing in of irritating substances, such as tobacco smoke or chemicals, also can cause hoarseness and loss of your voice.

Diagnosis

A diagnosis is generally made based on the signs and symptoms. The most common sign of laryngitis is hoarseness. If you have chronic hoarseness, your doctor may refer you to an ear, nose and throat (ENT) specialist.

How serious is laryngitis?

For most people, laryngitis is a temporary problem that either resolves on its own or that clears after treatment.

Treatment

Treatment for the condition depends on the type of laryngitis you experience. If you have bacterial laryngitis, your doctor may prescribe antibiotics.

For laryngitis caused by a virus or inhaled irritant, the best treatment is to rest your voice as much as possible, avoid clearing your throat and, if an inhaled irritant is to blame, avoid the irritant. It may also help to inhale steam from a bowl of hot water, teakettle or warm shower.

Drinking warm, noncaffeinated fluids helps keep your throat moist. A humidifier can help moisten the air, but if you use one, make sure to follow the manufacturer's instructions for cleaning the humidifier to prevent bacterial buildup.

To treat chronic laryngitis, you need to remove the underlying cause. If you smoke, stop. If alcohol consumption is responsible, you need to stop drinking.

Throat cancer

Signs and symptoms

- Cough
- Changes in voice, such as hoarseness
- Difficulty swallowing
- Lump or sore that doesn't heal
- Sore throat
- Weight loss

Throat cancer refers to cancerous tumors that develop in your throat (pharynx) or voice box (larynx). Throat cancer can also affect the piece of cartilage (epiglottis) that acts as the lid for your windpipe.

Factors that increase your risk of throat cancer include tobacco use, excessive alcohol use, a sexually transmitted infection called human papillomavirus (HPV) and poor dental hygiene.

Diagnosis

In order to diagnose throat cancer, your doctor may recommend:

- **A throat examination.** Your doctor may use a special lighted scope (endoscope) to get a close look at your throat during a procedure called endoscopy. A tiny camera at the end of the endoscope transmits images to a video screen that your doctor watches for signs of abnormalities in your throat. This scope also can look at the larynx. The procedure is called laryngoscopy.
- **Biopsy.** If abnormalities are found during endoscopy or laryngoscopy, your doctor

Structures of the Larynx

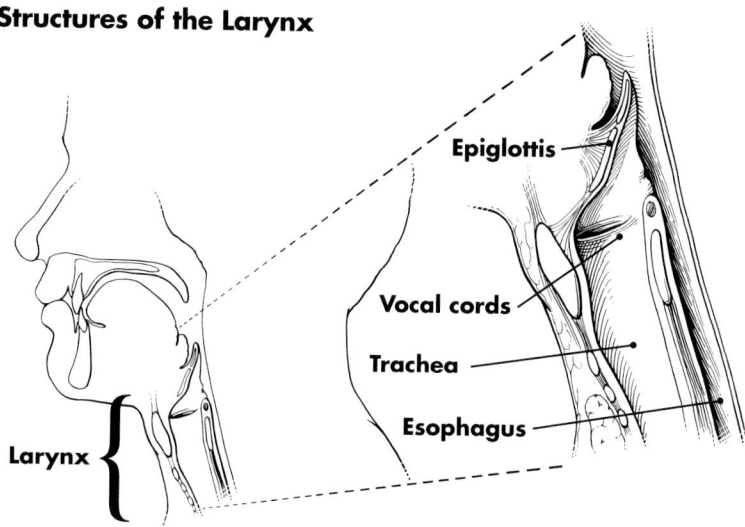

Epiglottis

Vocal cords

Trachea

Esophagus

Larynx

can pass surgical instruments through the scope to collect a tissue sample (biopsy). The sample is sent to a laboratory for testing.

Once throat cancer is diagnosed, the next step is to determine the extent (stage) of the cancer. Knowing the stage helps determine your treatment options.

- **Imaging tests.** Imaging tests, including X-ray, computerized tomography (CT) scans, magnetic resonance imaging (MRI) and positron emission tomography (PET), may help your doctor determine the extent of your cancer beyond the surface of your throat or voice box.

How serious is throat cancer?

Most cancers of the throat can be treated successfully if detected early. If symptoms are ignored, the cancer can spread to other parts of your throat and body.

Treatment

Treatment options are based on many factors and may include:

Radiation therapy

Throat cancers are particularly sensitive to radiation therapy, so treatment for most people with throat cancer includes radiation therapy. For early-stage throat cancers, radiation therapy may be the only treatment necessary. For more-advanced throat

cancers, radiation therapy may be combined with chemotherapy or surgery. In very advanced throat cancers, radiation therapy may be used to reduce signs and symptoms and make you more comfortable.

Surgery

Options may include:

- **Surgery for early-stage throat cancer.** Throat cancer that's confined to the surface of the throat or the vocal cords may be treated using endoscopy. Your doctor inserts a hollow tube into your throat or voice box and passes surgical tools or a laser through the scope. Using these tools, your doctor can scrape off, cut out or, in the case of the laser, vaporize very superficial cancers.
- **Surgery to remove all or part of the voice box (laryngectomy).** For smaller tumors, your doctor may remove only the part of the voice box that's affected by cancer. This may preserve your ability to speak and breathe normally.

  For larger, more extensive tumors, it may be necessary to remove your entire voice box. Your windpipe is then attached to a hole in your throat to allow you to breathe (tracheotomy). If your entire larynx is removed, you have several options for restoring your speech.

- **Surgery to remove all or part of the throat (pharyngectomy).** Smaller throat cancers may require removing only part of your throat during surgery. The use of a transoral robot to carefully dissect the cancer from the back or side of the throat has proved to be a very successful removal method.

  Larger cancers may require an open procedure and reconstruction in order to allow you to swallow food normally.

- **Surgery to remove cancerous lymph nodes (neck dissection).** If throat cancer has spread deep within your neck, your doctor may recommend surgery to remove one or more lymph nodes for laboratory testing.

Chemotherapy

Chemotherapy is sometimes used along with radiation therapy in treating throat cancers. Certain chemotherapy drugs make cancer cells more sensitive to radiation therapy. But combining chemotherapy and radiation therapy increases the side effects of both treatments. Discuss with your doctor the side effects you're likely to experience and whether combined treatments offer benefits that outweigh those effects.

Neck mass

Signs and symptoms

- Lump or mass in the neck that can be felt
- Possible tenderness or pain when touched
- Swelling
- Skin covering the mass may appear red and feel warm

A neck mass refers to a lump or bump under the skin of the neck that can be felt with your fingers. Sometimes, you may have the sensation of a lump in your neck, but you can't actually feel it.

Neck masses can occur for a variety of reasons in people of all ages. Many times, the cause of the mass is noncancerous (benign), but occasionally a neck mass may be associated with cancer.

If you have a lump or bump in your neck that you find worrisome and that persists for more than two weeks, have it evaluated by your doctor.

There are many reasons a mass can occur in your neck, including trauma to the neck, but most neck masses can be divided into three main categories.

Infection

A lump or bump in the neck is often related to an infection. Most often, the mass is associated with an infection elsewhere in the head and neck region that causes one or more lymph nodes in the neck to become inflamed (lymphadenitis). Lymphadenitis can occur anywhere in the neck. In severe cases, it can result in a neck abscess if left untreated.

In addition to a lymph node, infection can occur in other head and neck structures, including a salivary gland or the mastoid bone located behind the ear.

Masses caused by an infection are often tender and the skin above the mass may appear red and feel warm to the touch.

Benign mass

Noncancerous masses such as cysts and lipomas can occur anywhere in the neck. A cyst is a saclike structure usually filled with fluid or pus. A lipoma is a slow-growing, fatty lump.

Thyroid cysts are common and sometimes can be felt. A benign mass also can occur in the parotid or submandibular glands of the neck. Cysts and lipomas tend to be soft and mobile, and a doctor may be able to move the lump under the skin when examining the mass.

Cancer

On occasion, a lump or mass on the neck may be associated with cancer. Often, the cancer originates in other parts of the body, such as the lungs, breasts or gastrointestinal area, and travels to lymph nodes in the neck (metastasizes). Cancer of the lymph glands (lymphoma) also may first develop as a lump in the neck.

Diagnosis

In determining the cause of the lump or mass, your doctor likely will examine your neck and the area surrounding the mass. He or she may feel the mass and try to determine if the lump is soft and pliable or hard and rigid.

You may be asked questions about your health, including if you've recently had a cold or an infection, especially in the head or neck region.

Depending on the situation, your doctor may recommend an imaging test, such as an ultrasound or computerized tomography (CT) scan. If cancer is suspected or the cause is unknown, a biopsy may be performed, in which a thin needle is injected into the mass and a small amount of tissue is removed for examination.

Treatment

Treatment will depend on the cause. In case of an infection, you may be prescribed antibiotics. For a benign mass, your doctor may recommend treatment or observation to see if the mass grows or changes. If the mass is cancerous, treatment will depend on a variety of factors, including the type of cancer. ■

Teeth and Mouth

Your teeth are among your most important assets. Attached to jaws driven by powerful muscles, your teeth enable you to chew your food into a form that aids digestion. Teeth, of course, also have a cosmetic dimension. Frequently, the first thing we notice about other people is their smile. Clean, healthy-looking teeth are a sign the world over of general good health. In the past, a healthy smile belonged only to the young because most people lost their teeth by middle age. Now, however, dental care, improved nutrition and good dental hygiene make it possible for most of us to keep our teeth for our entire lives.

Tooth Development

Most babies are born toothless, or so it appears. Actually, tooth development is well-advanced by the third month of pregnancy, and by the fourth month the hard tissues of baby (primary) teeth, enamel and dentin, have begun to form.

The first teeth erupt in the mouth at about 6 months of age. The time when these first teeth emerge can vary greatly from child to child, but in most infants teeth have broken through the gums by age 1.

In general, the first teeth to emerge are the front teeth (incisors) in the lower jaw, followed by the front teeth in the upper jaw. Next come the first molars, followed by the canines (cuspids). The last to appear are the second molars. Most children have a full set of primary teeth by the age of 3.

Children have 20 primary teeth. Each primary tooth is normally replaced by a permanent tooth, incisor for incisor, canine for canine and premolar for molar. The permanent first molars erupt behind the primary molars.

For many children, the emergence of permanent teeth begins at about age 6. The lower front incisors tend to come in first, followed by the upper front incisors and the first molars. Permanent premolars and canines emerge later.

The process of shedding primary teeth to be replaced by permanent teeth usually continues through the elementary school years. Around 14 years of age, 28 permanent teeth are usually in place. The last four molars, the wisdom teeth, usually emerge in early adulthood, to complete the permanent set of 32 teeth.

Your permanent teeth are divided equally between the top and bottom jaw. From the center of the mouth moving toward the back, they include eight incisors, four canines (cuspids), eight premolars and 12 molars.

Parts of a tooth

The basic structure of each tooth is essentially the same. At the center of the tooth lies the pulp chamber and pulp. The pulp includes the nerves and blood vessels that feed and nourish the tooth. The nerves and blood vessels enter the tooth from the end of the roots.

The pulp is surrounded by hard dentin, the largest portion of the tooth. The dentin, composed of millions of tiny cells arranged in a tubular shape, is sensitive to temperature and touch.

The crown, the part of the tooth that's visible, extends from just beneath the gumline to the end of the tooth. It's covered with enamel, which is the hardest part of the tooth and protects the struc-

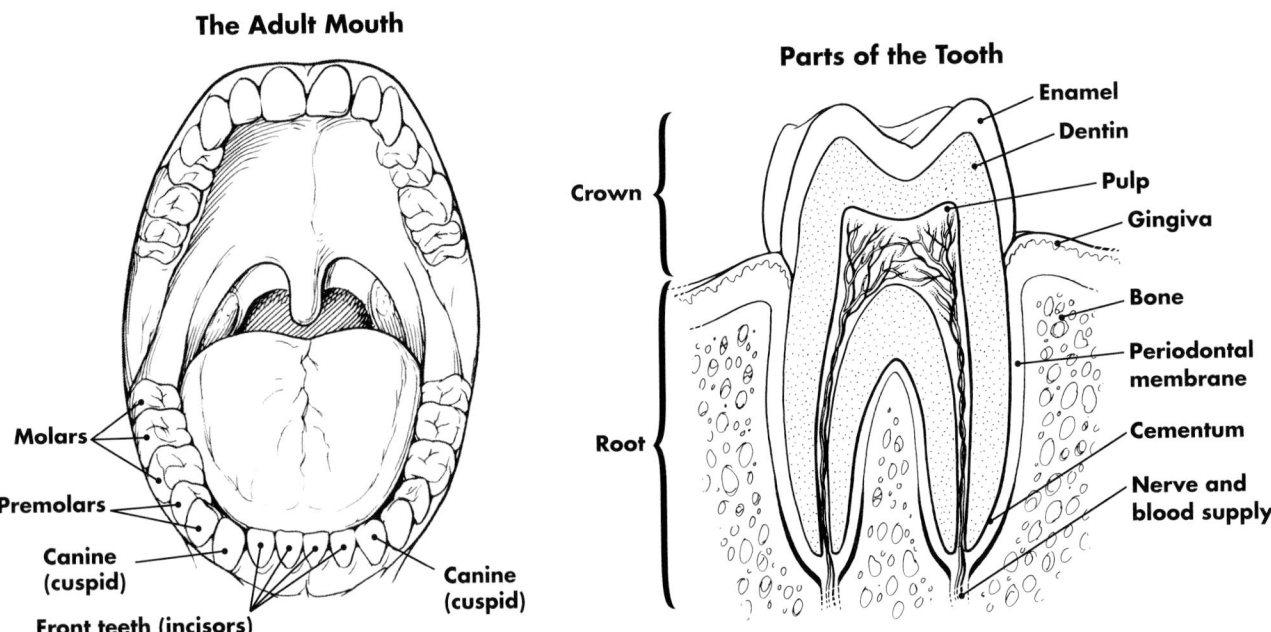

The Adult Mouth

Molars
Premolars
Canine (cuspid)
Front teeth (incisors)
Canine (cuspid)

Parts of the Tooth

Crown
Root

Enamel
Dentin
Pulp
Gingiva
Bone
Periodontal membrane
Cementum
Nerve and blood supply

Sensitive Teeth

When your teeth become painful to certain stimuli — touch, cold, hot, air, sweet or sour foods, or plaque — you may have what's called sensitive teeth (dentin hypersensitivity). This condition is usually caused by enamel erosion or gum recession that exposes the root of the tooth. If you avoid sensitive areas during brushing, flossing, chewing or drinking because of discomfort, you need treatment. Failing to clean your teeth thoroughly because of sensitivity can lead to tooth and gum disease.

After determining the cause of your sensitive teeth, your dentist can treat the troubled area and recommend a maintenance program. This may include using a desensitizing toothpaste, applying a prescribed fluoride solution daily at home or having your dentist cover the exposed areas with bonding agents.

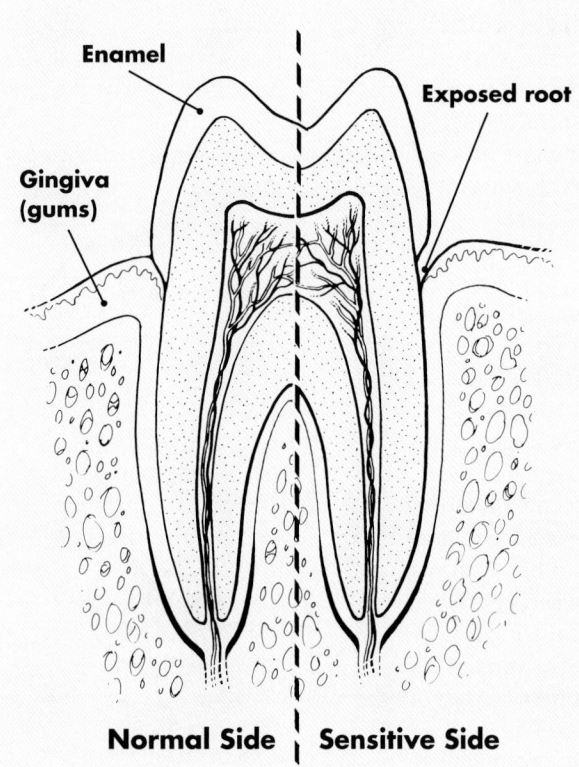

Recession of the gumline that exposes the root of a tooth can cause the tooth to be sensitive to stimuli such as cold and touch.

tures beneath. The crown has no sensation, and it can't heal after an injury.

The root, the part of the tooth below the gums (gingivae), is covered with cementum, which is harder than bone but not as hard as enamel. This rigid connective tissue attaches to the periodontal ligament, which holds the tooth in its socket.

Care of Your Teeth

Essential to maintaining a set of healthy teeth is a lifelong program of good dental hygiene — one that you begin early and practice consistently through the years. This includes brushing your teeth at least twice a day and flossing or using other devices to remove debris and plaque that collects between teeth. It may also include reducing the number of times throughout the day in which you snack on sugary foods or sip sugary beverages.

Good oral care depends more on brushing and cleaning techniques than on use of any particular brand name or product. Rather than paying a premium price for a so-called anti-plaque or anti-tartar toothpaste, your best protection against disease is frequent brushing with a fluoride toothpaste and using floss or other interdental cleaners such as dental picks, pre-threaded flossers, tiny brushes that reach between the teeth, water flossers or wooden plaque removers.

These are the best ways to remove bacteria and food particles before dental problems begin. Floss your teeth once each day and brush them at least twice a day — in the morning and before going to bed. Better yet, brush after each meal or snack. A complete cleaning with a fluoride toothpaste, toothbrush and dental floss should take three to five minutes. It's best to floss first and brush second. This allows you to brush away food particles and bacteria loosened by the flossing.

Floss and other devices

For regular flossing, take at least 18 inches of dental floss — unwaxed or waxed — and wind most of it around the middle finger of one hand. Wind a turn or two around the middle finger of the other hand so that you have 2 to 3 inches of floss between these fingers.

Using a gentle sawing motion, work the floss between your teeth without snapping it into the gums. At the gumline, hold the floss taut, bend it into a C shape, and gently scrape up and down on the side of each tooth. Each stroke should go slightly below your gumline until you feel resistance.

How to Floss and Brush

When flossing and brushing, proper technique is important.

To floss
Wrap the dental floss around the middle fingers of both hands, leaving 2 or 3 inches of floss between these fingers. For upper teeth, position the floss between the thumb of one hand and the index finger of the other, then insert it between your teeth and gently move it back and forth from the top to the bottom of your teeth. For lower teeth, it works best to position the floss between your index fingers.

To brush
Use a soft-bristle brush and minimal pressure. Begin with the outer surfaces of all of your teeth and the inner surfaces of your back teeth. Position your brush horizontally and brush back and forth gently with short — half a tooth wide — strokes at the gumline. Next, brush vertically away from the gumline. To clean the inner surfaces of upper and lower front teeth, brush vertically, moving your toothbrush over both teeth and gums. To clean the junction between your teeth and gums, brush at a 45-degree angle (see insert), keeping the bristles angled against the gumline. Also brush the chewing surfaces with a gentle scrubbing motion and brush your tongue to freshen your breath.

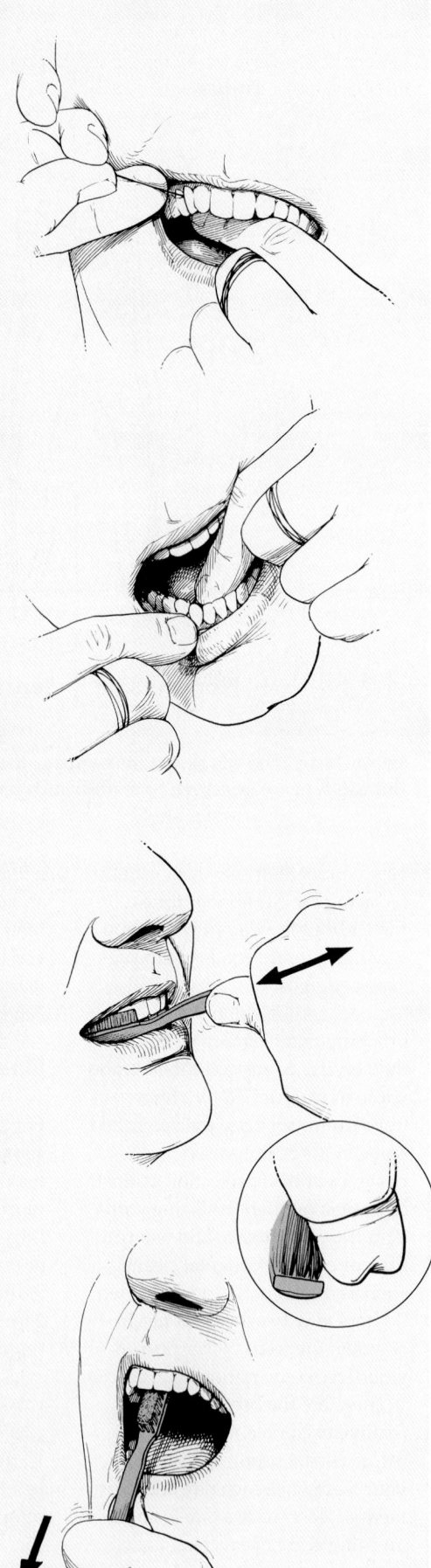

Don't be alarmed if your gums bleed the first few times you floss. If the bleeding continues each time you floss, consult your dentist. The problem may be improper flossing. Your dentist can demonstrate the proper technique.

Other devices you can use to remove debris from between your teeth and help prevent plaque buildup include dental picks, pre-threaded flossers, tiny brushes that reach between the teeth, water flossers or wooden plaque removers.

Brushing

Brush your teeth at least twice daily, once during the day and once in the evening. Using a small amount of fluoride toothpaste, position the toothbrush horizontally on your teeth. To effectively clean the top and bottom surfaces of all teeth, move the brush back and forth horizontally and then vertically away from the gumline in a series of short, gentle strokes.

For surfaces adjacent to your gums, move the brush in short back-and-forth strokes or in a rotary motion over both teeth and gums. Positioning your toothbrush at an angle will help clean the junction between your teeth and gums more effectively. Also brush the chewing surfaces with a gentle scrubbing motion and brush your tongue to freshen your breath.

Toothpaste
With few exceptions, most toothpastes have enough fluoride to protect your teeth against decay. But a growing awareness of dental health has led to a burgeoning array of specialty products. Gone are the days when toothpastes were used only to prevent cavities. Now manufacturers claim their products fight plaque, control tartar, reduce sensitivity and more.

To clean and protect your teeth, what type of toothpaste do you really need? Here's an analysis of some popular claims:

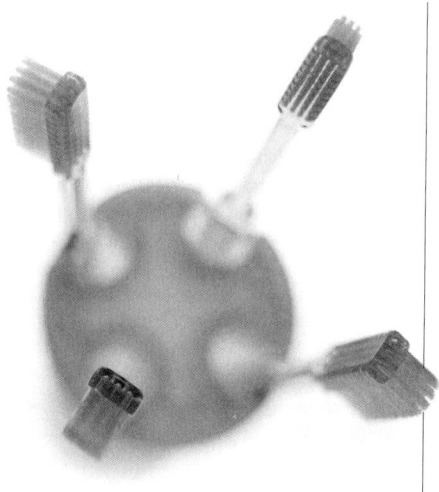

Anti-plaque

Some products claim to remove plaque or kill bacteria that can cause plaque. In reality, all toothpastes remove some plaque if you floss and brush well. Regardless of the product, you can't remove all plaque by brushing. Even if you use a plaque-fighting toothpaste, be sure to have regular checkups.

Tartar control

No toothpaste can remove tartar (calculus) below the gumline. That takes professional cleaning by a dental hygienist. Tartar is the white or yellowish deposit that plaque hardens into when mixed with minerals in saliva.

Anti-tartar toothpastes can help prevent a buildup of tartar on the teeth. Regular flossing and brushing remove plaque, leaving little plaque to harden into tartar. Because anti-tartar toothpastes are more abrasive, they may increase your teeth's sensitivity to cold. If so, change to a product without tartar control.

Baking soda

Baking soda is a mild abrasive and stain remover — but when wet it loses some of its stain-removing power. Some pastes contain hydrogen peroxide to help kill bacteria and loosen plaque. However, effective brushing with a fluoride toothpaste serves the same purpose.

Desensitizing

Desensitizing pastes contain chemicals that block the perception of pain in your teeth. Before using such a product, check with your dentist. Sometimes, sensitive teeth may be a sign of a problem that needs treatment, not cover-up.

Whitening

Before using any kind of whitening gel or polishing cream, ask your dentist for advice. Whitening toothpastes contain ingredients such as peroxide bleach or papaya enzymes, which may be harsh on delicate gum tissue, especially if you have receding gums. Smokers' toothpastes also contain strong abrasives that may be harsh on gum tissue.

Natural

If you use a natural toothpaste product — most don't contain artificial ingredients such as a sweetener — be sure it has fluoride. Without it, natural pastes won't effectively fight decay.

A Dental Checkup

One of the most important steps in keeping teeth healthy is to visit your dentist regularly for a thorough checkup. You and your children — beginning at the eruption of your child's first tooth or no later than age 12 months — should visit the dentist twice a year. You may need more-frequent visits if conditions or problems exist.

People who have several cavities a year and who pay little attention to oral hygiene may need to see their dentists more often, for treatment and cleaning. Even individuals without natural teeth should see their dentists periodically. Your dentist will determine your examination schedule according to your specific needs.

Tooth Whiteners

There's a great deal of interest in obtaining whiter teeth. This is evident in the dental aisle at your local pharmacy or grocery store. All sorts of products promise to make your teeth whiter.

Tooth whitening is a process of changing the color of teeth with the use of peroxide-containing products, which bleach the tooth enamel.

You can whiten your teeth two ways. One is under the supervision of your dentist using various whitening techniques. The other is with over-the-counter products available for general use.

While over-the-counter tooth whiteners are shown to be safe and effective when used properly, it's generally best to partner with your dentist if you use them. You want to assure that your teeth and mouth remain healthy and that your goals are realistic.

Tooth whitening results vary considerably from person to person. Many may be immediately delighted with their outcome, while others may be disappointed. Before you embark on whitening treatment, ask your dentist for a realistic idea of the results you're likely to achieve and how long it should take to achieve them. Expectations play a major role in tooth whitening.

The potentially harmful side effects of tooth whitening include increased sensitivity of the teeth and irritation of the surrounding gums.

Medical history

Before your dentist or hygienist asks you to "Open wide, please," he or she will probably ask a few questions about your general health. The answers can have a direct bearing on your treatment.

For example, certain kinds of heart conditions may make some people susceptible to an infection of the heart valves when their gums are manipulated, such as during a thorough dental cleaning or when a tooth is filled or extracted. These individuals may need an antibiotic before certain dental treatments.

Individuals who are allergic to penicillin can have a reaction when it's prescribed for tooth infections, and people with diabetes whose disease is poorly controlled may require special treatment considerations.

Your dentist or a dental assistant may also ask if you're on any medications so that your dentist doesn't prescribe medications that could cause harmful interactions.

Examination

A dentist typically examines both your mouth and teeth. In your gums and the soft tissues of your mouth, a dentist looks for signs of gingivitis, periodontitis, and less common disorders such as leukoplakia, oral lichen planus and oral cancer.

If you have dentures, your gums will be examined for signs of pressure and uneven wear, indicated by patches of thickened skin, soreness or reddened areas. Your dentist will also check your soft tissues, tongue and lips for lesions or other abnormalities.

A dentist examines each tooth using a dental explorer and a small mirror. He or she looks for signs of decay, including discolored areas and small grooves (fissures) in the tooth enamel.

Existing fillings are checked for deterioration and for signs of new cavities around their edges. To measure signs of bone loss or gum disease, a dentist or hygienist inserts a periodontal probe around the base of each tooth.

X-rays

Almost all individuals who have been to a dentist have had dental X-rays taken. As in other medical fields, these X-rays are used to aid in diagnosing disease or injury. They're useful in identifying the presence and extent of dental cavities. An X-ray can detect decay in a tooth even when the enamel looks intact, particularly if the decay is hidden between teeth or is under the gumline.

X-rays can also help diagnose a tooth abscess, bone damage from periodontal disease, fractures of the jawbone and teeth, and other abnormalities of the teeth and jaw. They also provide a status report on unerupted or impacted teeth.

A dental X-ray may be taken using traditional X-ray film or digital technology. To detect cavities, dentists use bitewing X-rays. A small piece of film is placed in your mouth, next to your teeth. You hold the film in place by biting down on the paper that covers the film. The X-ray machine is then aimed at the tooth, and the exposure is made. A digital image will be available immediately, while a film X-ray takes a few minutes to be developed. Either way, an X-ray image can help your dentist determine an appropriate course of action.

The amount of radiation used during a traditional X-ray is extremely small. The amount of radiation used to make a digital X-ray is even less. Still, no one should have more radiation exposure than is necessary. Discuss with your dentist how often X-rays are necessary. As a precaution against excess radiation, your dentist should fit you with a lead apron that covers you from the chest to lower abdomen.

Cleaning

When your dentist or a dental hygienist cleans your teeth, his or her goal is to remove plaque and hardened plaque (tartar) accumulations. Tartar is a primary cause of gum diseases such as gingivitis and periodontitis. Tartar is most troublesome when it forms below the gumline.

Your dentist or hygienist can remove tartar in one of two ways. The traditional method involves scraping the deposits from your teeth with a sharp instrument known as a scaler. Another method involves use of an ultrasonic device that loosens the tartar through vibration. Whatever method is used, you may experience some gum bleeding. In some people, tartar develops quickly and must be removed every few months.

Once the tartar has been removed, the teeth are polished, which can be helpful in stain removal or in slowing plaque re-accumulation. Polishing is done with a special toothpaste applied by a device with rotating rubber heads. Dentists often finish children's checkups with an application of fluoride to help prevent tooth decay.

Tooth Decay

Tooth decay (caries) is a bacterial disease of teeth. It's one of the most common of all health disorders. Tooth decay affects children and young adults most frequently, although it remains a problem for many individuals throughout their lives.

Decay is the primary cause of tooth loss. Almost half of all children in the United States have some tooth decay by age 4, and many even earlier, despite great improvements in prevention through regular dental checkups, use of fluoride and improved oral hygiene.

Decades ago, few people still had their own teeth beyond middle age. Improved dental care and dentistry advances today make it possible for most people to keep their teeth much longer.

However, this has resulted in a new problem called root caries. Root caries is the decay of a tooth's root and is often associated with receded gums. A lifelong program of appropriate dental care, good nutrition and good oral hygiene can help prevent root caries.

The decay process

Tooth decay is the result of three interacting factors: bacterial growth, dietary sugar and a vulnerable tooth surface.

Your mouth, like many other parts of your body, is host to bacteria. These bacteria convert some of the sugars and carbohydrates you eat into acid. The bacteria and acids they form become part of the sticky deposit — called dental plaque — that clings to the surface of teeth. In addition to bacteria, plaque is composed of saliva and food particles.

Plaque adheres most strongly in pits and grooves (fissures) of the molars and premolars, in the areas just above the gumline, between teeth and at the margins of fillings. The decay-producing acid that forms in plaque attacks the minerals in the tooth's outer enamel surface. The erosion caused by the plaque leads to tiny openings (cavities) in the enamel. The first sign of decay may be a sensation of pain when you eat something sweet, very cold or very hot.

Once the enamel is penetrated, the underlying softer dentin becomes vulnerable. The dentin contains tiny canals leading to the pulp at the core of the tooth.

If bacteria reach the sensitive pulp, the pulp becomes inflamed. Blood vessels within the pulp swell and, because there's no room within the rigid tooth to expand, you experience pain.

In addition, your body sends white blood cells to counteract bacterial invasion from the tooth into the surrounding tissues. This kind of bacterial infection may result in a tooth abscess.

Tooth decay takes time to develop in permanent teeth but less in primary teeth. Fortunately, you're not totally vulnerable to the effects of acid and bacteria. The chemistry and the mechanics of your mouth provide a certain amount of protection: Your saliva and the actions of your tongue wash away some of the destructive material. Today's dentistry also can provide treatment and preventive measures to lessen the effects of dental cavities.

Cavities

Signs and symptoms
- Mild or sharp pain when eating or drinking something sweet, cold or hot
- Toothache

Most cavities are discovered during a dental exam. Detecting and treating tooth decay early can save pain, expense and, most importantly, your teeth. The sooner a cavity is detected, the less pain you'll experience because the enamel and dentin, the outer parts of the tooth, are far less sensitive to pain than is the pulp.

Diagnosis
Your dentist looks for signs of decay by using a dental explorer and a small mirror. Another way to detect a cavity is with X-rays, which provide information about your teeth, gums and bone.

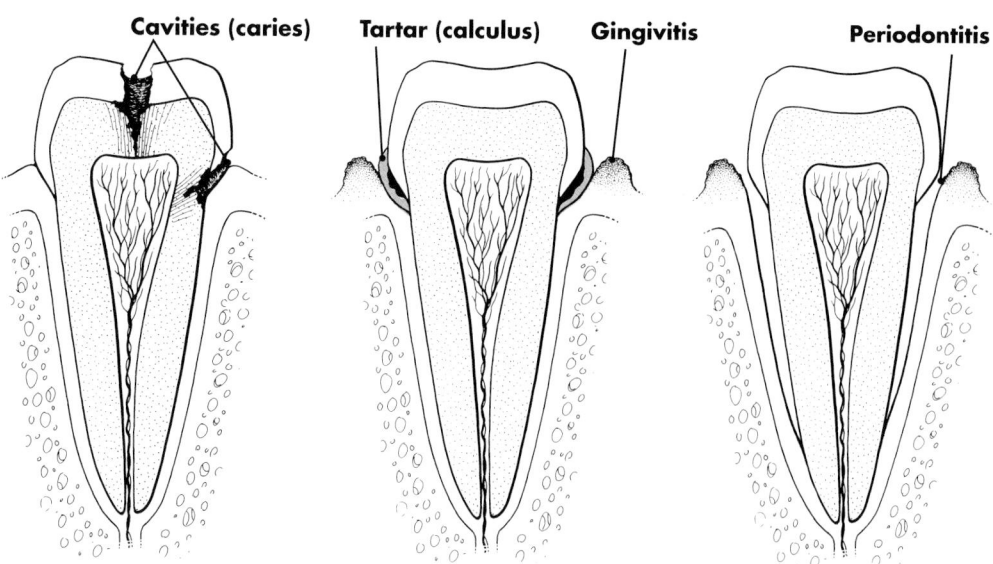

The principal cause of tooth loss is dental cavities (caries). The accumulation of tartar (calculus) can lead to gingivitis and, eventually, detachment of gums from the tooth (periodontitis) — another cause of tooth loss.

Soothing a Toothache

In most children and adults, tooth decay is the primary cause of toothaches. The first sign of decay may be a sensation of pain when you eat something sweet, cold or hot. Until you're able to see a dentist, try these self-care tips:

- Brush and floss to remove any food particles around and between the teeth. You may want to use warm water for brushing your teeth.
- Avoid foods and temperatures that trigger pain.
- Take an over-the-counter pain reliever such as acetaminophen (Tylenol, others), ibuprofen (Advil, Motrin IB, others) or aspirin. Or try an over-the-counter local anesthetic containing benzocaine (Anbesol, Orajel) or oil of cloves. These are available at most pharmacies.

Early stages of tooth decay are often painless. Other times, you may experience mild pain in a tooth when eating something sweet, hot or cold. If you feel a sharp pain, you may have more serious tooth decay.

Treatment

Even if you have a seriously decayed tooth, it often can be saved through procedures such as dental fillings (restorations), crowns and root canals. Before such a procedure, a local anesthetic is typically injected into the nearby gum to deaden the nerve and prevent pain.

Some dentists offer nitrous oxide — sometimes called laughing gas — to decrease discomfort and anxiety. If you're taking any medications, mention this to your dentist before accepting any anesthetic because certain medications and anesthetics taken together can produce adverse reactions.

Fillings

The decay process usually can be halted by removing the decayed portion of the tooth and replacing it with a filling. Sometimes, when decay is extensive, a temporary filling is inserted to provide your dentist an opportunity to observe the tooth's response and sensitivity to treatment. After several weeks, if you've experienced no adverse signs or symptoms, your dentist removes this filling and replaces it with a permanent one.

The kind of filling used depends on the location and function of the tooth. Molars, which do most of the work of chewing, experience the most stress and require more-durable materials than do front (anterior) teeth. Dental amalgam is a filling material used to fill cavities in molars. Dental amalgam is a mixture of metals.

A filling in a front tooth should blend in with the color of the tooth itself. This may be less important

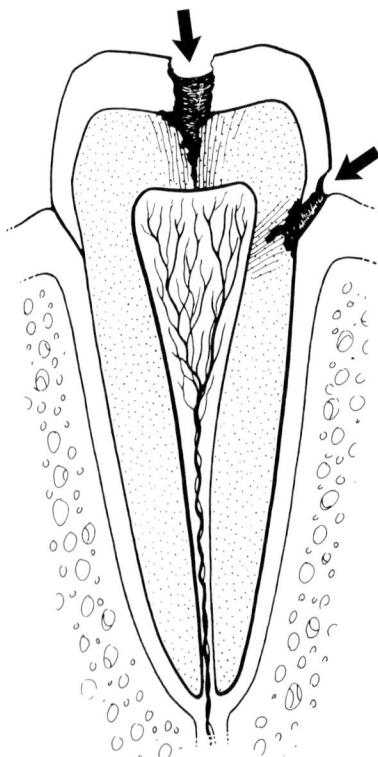

Dental cavities (see arrows) are a common cause of toothache and tooth loss.

with back teeth. Composite resins are typically used in front teeth — and sometimes in back teeth if the decay is small and the area isn't used for heavy chewing. Composite resin fillings are made of a type of plastic (an acrylic resin) reinforced with powdered glass filler. The color of composite resins can be customized to closely match surrounding teeth.

Crowns

If your tooth is so decayed that it can't support several small fillings or a large one without the danger of breaking, your dentist may remove the decay and prepare the tooth to receive a crown, which is placed over the tooth. A crown may be made of porcelain, metal or a combination of the two.

An impression of a digital scan of your tooth provides a model for the crown, which is made in a dental laboratory. When ready, the crown is then fitted, shaped and finally cemented in place on top of what's left of the original tooth.

Root canals

If you have a tooth that's severely infected or that's at risk of severe infection, your dentist or a dental specialist called an endodontist may perform a root canal. It involves removing the nerve and pulp, as well as any associated decayed material, from the root canal and pulp chamber.

In this multistage procedure, the pulp is removed and the opening that's created is disinfected and filled with an inert material (gutta-percha) and sealer. Once that's done, the remaining tooth structure is treated with a filling or crown.

Post and core procedures

Occasionally, when a tooth is fractured or severely damaged, it may need to be rebuilt into shape after a root canal. In this procedure, a filling material is placed around a cemented post, or a custom-shaped gold post is cemented into the tooth, before a crown is fitted.

Tooth abscesses

Signs and symptoms

- Persistent aching or throbbing pain in a tooth
- Sensitivity to sweet, hot or cold foods or liquids
- Pain when chewing
- Swollen lymph nodes in the neck
- A swollen area of the mouth, face or neck
- Fever and general malaise

If tooth decay isn't dealt with promptly and properly, it can lead to a tooth abscess. An abscess

results when bacteria infect the pulp of a tooth, causing the pulp to become swollen and inflamed. Blood vessels in the pulp enlarge and may press on nerves in the area, producing pain.

The infection may spread to the root and into the surrounding bone and cause the tooth to abscess. Despite the body's efforts to fight it off, the infection can overwhelm the pulp, destroying the nerve and blood vessels. The pain may go away, but the infection may remain. The resulting breakdown material (pus) that forms as part of the infection can erode a channel through the jaw and form a swelling or boil on the gum.

Diagnosis

If you have persistent throbbing pain in a tooth, find chewing painful, or are sensitive to sweet, hot or cold foods or liquids, you may have an abscessed tooth. You may have a slight fever and swollen lymph nodes in your neck and feel generally ill.

A swelling that forms on the gum near the sore tooth may at some point burst, releasing into your mouth a thick liquid with a foul taste and smell. Simultaneously, the pain may be relieved. If you experience any of these signs and symptoms, see your dentist.

Treatment

Before you see your dentist, you can help relieve the pain by taking acetaminophen (Tylenol, others), ibuprofen (Advil, Motrin IB, others) or aspirin. Rinsing your mouth with warm salt water — one-half teaspoon of salt dissolved in an 8-ounce glass of warm water — every hour or so also may help soothe the pain.

Your dentist may prescribe an antibiotic to help clear up the infection and keep it from spreading to other parts of your body. He or she can also prescribe pain relief medications to make you more comfortable if the pain is severe.

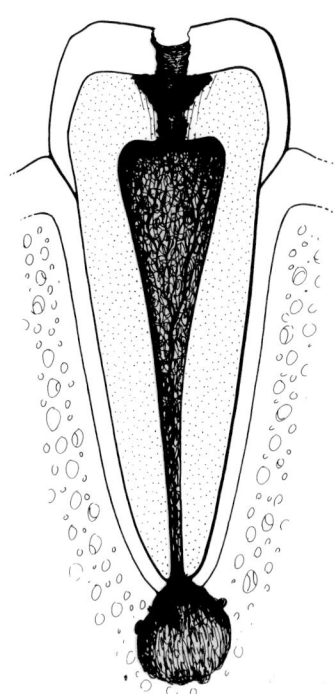

A tooth abscess occurs when bacteria enter through a decayed area and spread inward, infecting the pulp, root and even the bone surrounding the tooth.

At one time, the only treatment for an abscessed tooth was to remove (extract) it. Under certain conditions, extraction still is necessary. However, dentists today can often save an abscessed tooth by performing a root canal. Your dentist may anesthetize the area and then open a hole into the pulp chamber of the tooth. This releases the pressure. The pulp chamber can then be cleared out, disinfected and filled with an inert material.

Next, your dentist may place a temporary filling in your tooth. A permanent filling can be put in place after the infection has cleared. Your dentist most likely will want to see you again in a few months, at which time X-rays may be taken of the tooth to determine if gum and bone tissues are healing after the abscess.

If the tissues appear to be healthy, the treatment is finished. If the infection persists, additional treatment likely is necessary, and your dentist may refer you to a

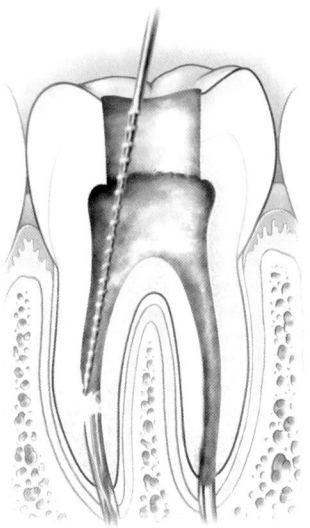
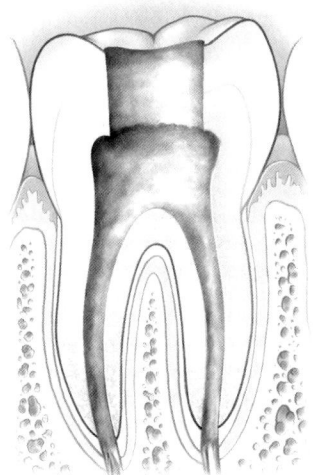
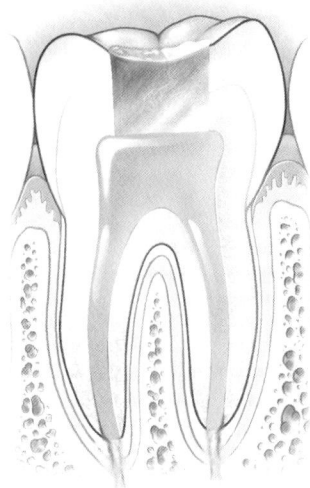

During a root canal, an opening is created into the pulp chamber (left), and the nerves and blood vessels are removed (center). The root canals are cleaned, enlarged, disinfected and filled (right).

specialist who may perform a surgical procedure to remove the diseased tissue, sometimes including a small portion of the root tip.

If swelling persists after an abscessed tooth has been treated, your dentist may want to obtain special cultures or change your medication because of bacterial resistance or the presence of unusual bacteria.

Preventing tooth decay

A successful plan for preventing decay generally involves three steps: taking good care of your teeth, appropriately planning your diet and, in the case of children, applying fluoride and sealant to teeth.

Tooth care
Caring for your teeth includes brushing and flossing thoroughly on a daily basis and seeing your dentist regularly for checkups. In an ideal world, everyone would brush his or her teeth after all meals and snacks. A more realistic goal is to brush at least twice each day — in the morning and before going to bed — and floss at least once a day.

A key to developing good lifelong dental habits is to start early. Teach your children the ritual of brushing even before they have a full set of teeth. Similarly, your child's dentist or hygienist can demonstrate proper methods of flossing.

Diet
The concept that sugar contributes to tooth decay isn't new. But evidence points to all fermentable carbohydrates — not just sugar — as foods that cause tooth decay. Fermentable carbohydrates include all sugars and most cooked starches, including bread, crackers and potato chips.

Because carbohydrates are an important part of a healthy diet, don't cut down on them. And taking care of your teeth doesn't mean that you can't have ice cream, cake, pie or candy. The amount of sugar you eat is less important than how and when you eat it. Sweets eaten between meals do more harm than do those eaten with a meal.

Try to incorporate the following strategies into your eating habits and those of your children:
- **Avoid chewy, sticky, sugary foods, particularly as snacks.** Foods such as candy, candy-coated nuts, dry cereal, doughy bread, raisins and dry fruit cling to your teeth. When you do eat them, try to brush your teeth

within 20 minutes afterward. Acid production by the bacteria that promote tooth decay is most active after this time. If you can't brush your teeth, rinse your mouth with water.
- **Choose snacks carefully.** Snacking on foods that promote tooth decay is worse than eating the same foods during meals. Nibbling on snacks throughout the day allows bacteria to produce a constant supply of acid on your teeth. Don't constantly sip sugar drinks such as soda. Acid-containing soda can cause permanent changes in your teeth due to enamel erosion.

Also, don't chew sugar gum or suck on hard candies, sugar-sweetened breath mints or cough drops. If you do chew gum or suck on hard candies, select those that are sugarless. Sugarless products generally contain xylitol or aspartame, which can help reduce cavity-causing bacteria. Some also have a remineralizing agent that adds calcium and phosphates to teeth.
- **Don't give a baby a bottle of milk or juice at bedtime.** Even babies are at risk of tooth decay, and milk and juice both contain sugar. If your baby needs a bottle to settle down, fill it with

water. Don't allow your baby to feed from a bottle while lying in bed because this can lead to blocked eustachian tubes and may increase the risk of ear infections.

Fluoride

People living in parts of the country where the public water supply naturally contains an optimal amount of fluoride have almost no dental cavities. Too high a fluoride content, however, can cause brown stains on the teeth.

Fluoride was thought to be especially helpful when ingested by children whose teeth were developing. Researchers believed fluoride offered continuing protection by being incorporated into a tooth's enamel structure. They now recognize the benefits of fluoride are mainly the result of chemical reactions on the tooth surface.

Many communities in the United States add small amounts of fluoride to their water supplies because the water is deficient in fluoride. This approach is both cost-effective and safe. Fluoridated toothpastes, gels and rinses are also beneficial.

There's no evidence that fluoride, whether added to water supplies or occurring naturally, is a health risk. If your municipal water supply isn't fluorinated or if you drink primarily bottled or filtered water, ask your dentist about other methods of fluoride application.

Many dentists treat children's teeth with a fluoride solution as a part of regular checkups.

Fluoride is most effective in preventing cavities on the smooth, nonchewing surfaces of your teeth. Consequently, most cavities occur on the chewing surfaces. The reason: These surfaces of your back (posterior) teeth (premolars and molars) have pits and grooves (depressions and fissures) that are almost impossible to clean completely with a toothbrush.

Sealants

Besides good oral hygiene, the single best method to prevent decay on the chewing surfaces of back teeth is a dental sealant. The sealant covers the tooth surface with a thin, plastic-like coating that's usually clear or white.

Application of a sealant is painless and easy. During this procedure, your dentist cleans the chewing surface of your premolars and molars. Then, these surfaces are etched with a mild acid to improve adhesion.

Next, the teeth are thoroughly washed and dried. Your dentist then paints the sealant onto each tooth in much the same way fingernail polish is applied. The sealant hardens into a shield that prevents accumulation of plaque in the pits and fissures.

A dental sealant can last several years, although various conditions may shorten its effectiveness. Regular visits to the dentist permit necessary touch-ups to extend the life of the sealant. If the sealant layer is lost, it can be replaced. If the sealant is damaged, the underlying tooth surface is at no greater risk of cavities than it would be if the sealant had never been applied.

Sealant protection is most appropriate for children and adolescents. It should be applied when the first permanent molars erupt, and again when permanent second molars and premolars erupt. Some older adults also may benefit from a dental sealant.

Developmental Disorders

In many people, teeth develop in a fairly orderly and typical manner. However, problems may occur due to improper prenatal development or environmental or genetic factors.

Fortunately, modern dentistry and oral surgery can often minimize the effects of the developmental disorders.

Impacted teeth

Signs and symptoms
- Pain in the gums, often around the last molar
- Recurrent infection of a partially buried tooth
- Bad breath
- An unpleasant taste in your mouth

Teeth typically emerge through the gums three times during life.

Dental Specialists

Just as the medical field has various specialties, so does dentistry. A dental specialty is an area of dentistry recognized by the American Dental Association as meeting specific requirements. Dental specialists include the following:
- *Pediatric dentists.* They treat children from birth through adolescence.
- *Orthodontists.* They diagnose and treat crowded and misaligned teeth and jaws.
- *Endodontists.* They diagnose and treat diseases and injuries of the tooth pulp and surrounding tissues.
- *Periodontists.* They diagnose and treat diseases of the tissues — gums and bone — that surround and support the teeth.
- *Oral and maxillofacial surgeons.* They extract teeth and diagnose and treat injuries, diseases, and defects of the jaw, face and mouth.
- *Prosthodontists.* They create and fit artificial replacements for defective or missing teeth, including crowns, bridges (fixed partial dentures) and dentures.

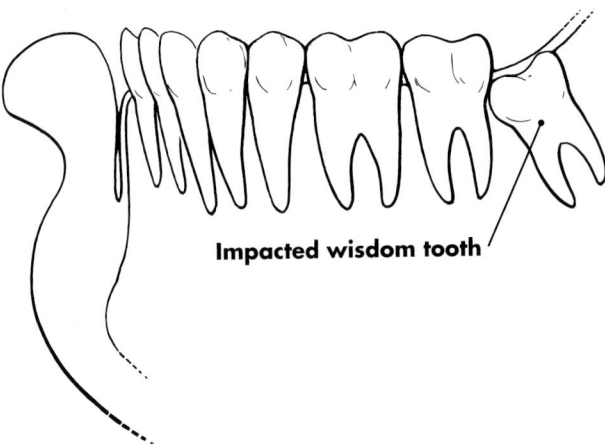

Impacted wisdom tooth

A tooth that doesn't emerge through the gum is called an impacted tooth. This most often occurs with the wisdom teeth at the back of the mouth.

The first time is when the baby (primary) teeth emerge. The second is when permanent teeth emerge during early school years. The third time is when the wisdom teeth (third molars) appear. This is generally during early adulthood.

Frequently, wisdom teeth have trouble emerging because the jaw is often too small. They may become rotated, displaced or tilted as they attempt to emerge. This can cause pain and, occasionally, infection when the tooth traps food debris in the soft gum tissue surrounding it. If the tooth comes in at an angle, it can push on and damage the adjacent tooth, causing pain and contributing to tooth or root decay.

Diagnosis

Impacted teeth don't always cause discomfort. But when they do, the experience is unpleasant. If you feel pain in your gums or have an unpleasant taste when you bite on or near where a wisdom or other unemerged tooth should be, you may have an impacted tooth.

The tooth may be partly visible, and the surrounding gums may be infected. The impacted tooth may press on other teeth, causing pain.

Treatment

Over-the-counter pain relievers such as acetaminophen (Tylenol, others),

ibuprofen (Advil, Motrin IB, others) or aspirin should help relieve the pain from an impacted tooth. Rinsing your mouth with warm salt water — a mixture of one-half teaspoon of salt and 8 ounces of warm water — also may help.

Your dentist can examine your mouth for signs of an impacted tooth. X-rays may be needed to determine the exact location and position of the tooth. If you have an infection around the tooth (pericoronitis), your dentist may prescribe an antibiotic.

The usual treatment for an impacted wisdom tooth is its removal. Wisdom teeth that emerge crooked can affect your bite. Wisdom teeth are also difficult to clean because they're far back in the mouth, and they're prone to decay and disease.

Your dentist may remove the impacted tooth or teeth in his or her office, under local anesthesia. If your case is more complicated, your dentist may refer you to an oral and maxillofacial surgeon. If an impacted tooth lies at a difficult angle or you have several of them, the procedure may be done in a hospital.

Misshapen or discolored teeth

Signs and symptoms
- Misshapen teeth

- Yellowish color on primary or secondary teeth

In rare cases, a child's teeth may not be normal in shape or color. Such abnormalities can result from many factors, including genetics, early illness or trauma, or an environmental factor such as excessive fluoride in the drinking water or the mother's ingestion of tetracycline drugs during pregnancy and nursing. Enamel is completely formed on all but the wisdom teeth by about 8 years of age. Therefore, doctors don't prescribe a prolonged course of the antibiotic tetracycline for children under age 8 or pregnant women.

Other causes of misshapen or discolored teeth include infection, high fever or malnutrition during infancy or early childhood. In rare cases, misshapen teeth are related to serious disorders such as congenital syphilis or Down syndrome.

Most often, abnormalities affect both the primary and secondary teeth. The eight front teeth and the sixth-year molars are the teeth most frequently affected because these develop first. The crowns of the teeth can be pitted or grooved and may be discolored.

Occasionally, the enamel covering the teeth will be imperfect. This can result from several factors, but most often it's due to a genetic trait that recurs in families. The enamel may be discolored, thin or absent. Discoloration can also stem from drinking water with a fluoride content of more than 2 parts per million. In some areas, water naturally contains a high level of fluoride.

Treatment

Misshapen teeth often can be treated by adding a restorative material or by covering them with crowns. Teeth without complete coverings of enamel and some very discolored teeth also may be treated in this manner.

Sometimes this is done on primary teeth if the enamel is so

malformed that serious cavities or wearing occurs. In these instances, the molar teeth often are fitted with stainless steel crowns.

Misaligned or crowded teeth

Signs and symptoms
- Lack of spacing between teeth
- Protruding upper front teeth (overbite)
- Upper and lower front (incisor) teeth that don't touch when biting (open bite)
- Upper teeth, either back or front, that bite inside the lower teeth (crossbite)
- A protruding lower jaw that causes the upper front teeth to bite behind the lower front teeth (underbite)

Few people have perfect bites and symmetrical teeth. Your jaws may be slightly misaligned, perhaps where the upper and lower teeth clamp together to form the bite. Or your teeth may be crowded, sometimes in the front where they're most visible. The technical term for such problems is malocclusion (bad bite).

A minor amount of misalignment or crowding may require little or no attention. But a significant number of children and adults have problems that can benefit from treatment. The branch of dentistry that specializes in the diagnosis, prevention and treatment of dental and facial irregularities is called orthodontics. Orthodontists use appliances, such as braces, to properly align the teeth and jaws and produce an even bite.

In the ideal bite, the teeth of the upper jaw slightly overlap those of the lower jaw. The points of the molars fit into the grooves of the opposing molars. In the ideal jaw, there's room for all teeth to fit neatly, neither crowded nor spaced. There are no rotations of teeth or teeth that twist or lean forward or backward.

Straightening your teeth is important not just for the sake of appearance. When teeth don't fit together properly, they may cause chewing problems and eating and digestion difficulties. Crowded or crooked teeth make it more difficult to control plaque, and may put you at a greater risk of cavities and periodontal disease.

Today, more adults are seeking orthodontic correction of problems that weren't treated when they were younger (see page 672). Treatment time in adults often is longer because tooth movement is slower in mature jaws. Corrective jaw surgery is performed more often on adults than on children.

Diagnosis
Dentists monitor the development of children's secondary teeth and recommend consultation with orthodontists if problems seem imminent. Most alignment problems become apparent once a child's secondary teeth begin to erupt, often as early as age 6. In some instances, problems can be identified and appropriately treated even earlier.

Although teeth can be moved at any time, the American Association of Orthodontists recommends that children be screened at an early age. Some orthodontic problems are more easily corrected when a child is young, before all the permanent teeth come in and before facial growth is complete.

Your orthodontist will examine your or your child's mouth thoroughly to help determine the best treatment. He or she may take a series of X-rays, some of which are used to determine the position of teeth — those that have erupted and those yet to erupt. Special X-rays of the head may help determine the size, position and relationship of the jaw and teeth.

Another diagnostic tool is a plaster model of the teeth. You bite down on a thin, waxlike material to make an impression. This impression is then used to position plaster models accurately to represent the actual bite of the upper and lower teeth. Photographs of the teeth and face and other measurements and recordings also may be needed to make an accurate diagnosis.

If the lower jaw is significantly smaller than the upper jaw, the upper teeth may protrude excessively over the lower teeth (overbite). Similarly, if the lower jaw is larger than the upper, the upper front teeth may bite behind the lower ones (underbite).

When significant discrepancies exist between the upper and lower jaws, an operation called orthognathic surgery may be the best option. Sometimes, the problem can be corrected with various orthodontic appliances.

Treatment
After a thorough examination, an orthodontist generally develops

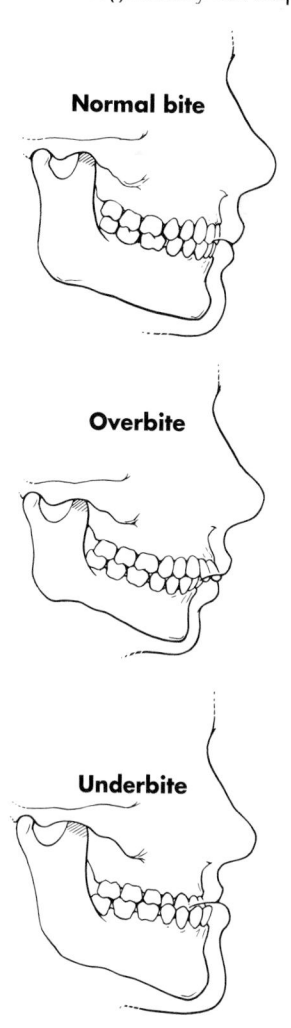

Normal bite

Overbite

Underbite

Adult Orthodontics: It's Never Too Late

As many as 75 percent of adults have some misalignment in their teeth and could benefit from braces. Yet only a small percentage seek orthodontic treatment. Many adults believe they're too old for braces, fear discomfort, think they'll be embarrassed or think they can't afford orthodontics.

Why get braces? Crowded or crooked teeth make it more difficult to control plaque, which leaves you prone to cavities and periodontal disease. If you need restorative work, such as crowns or bridges, having your teeth aligned can make these procedures easier.

Many adults get braces for cosmetic reasons. Aligned teeth look nicer than misaligned teeth. If you think you might benefit from braces, either because your teeth have shifted since you last wore braces or because you never had them, fear not. Braces aren't what they used to be. With advances in orthodontic materials, most adults' fears of wearing braces are unfounded. Here's why:

- Today's wires, made of nickel and titanium, don't need to be tightened as often as those used years ago. Most adults report only mild discomfort for a day or two after each adjustment.
- Ceramic brackets that match your tooth enamel are less obvious than metal brackets. Even metal brackets are smaller and less noticeable than they used to be. Note, however, that ceramic brackets cost more and may result in longer treatment time.
- Clear aligners provide another option. They're made of a clear material that fits over your teeth, exerting pressure on the teeth to move them. You remove the aligners for eating and cleaning.
- There's growing acceptance of adult orthodontics.
- The cost of treatment may be covered by some insurance.

a treatment plan and designs corrective devices. Some devices are removable, and others are cemented or bonded to the teeth.

Braces

If severe overcrowding is the main problem, certain permanent teeth may need to be removed to create room. The remaining teeth can then be realigned by fitting braces to them.

Fixed braces, which can be made of metal, ceramic or plastic, usually are either ringlike bands that encircle the molar teeth or brackets that are attached to the outside surfaces of the premolar and anterior teeth. Clear or tooth-colored braces are sometimes an option.

Wires, springs and other force-producing devices place pressure on the teeth and gradually shift them into new positions. The jaw responds to the pressure by dissolving bone in front of the moving tooth and laying down new bone behind it.

Occasionally, tension will be drawn from the opposite jaw. This often is achieved with elastic bands placed on upper and lower teeth and connected to an opposite tooth.

Other appliances

In growing children and teenagers, several other appliances can be used to direct forces that influence jaw growth and development. For example, headgear that directs pressure to the upper teeth and jaw may be used to influence the speed and direction of upper jaw growth. The appliance is attached to braces in the mouth, and pressure is applied with a strap that wraps around the head. The headgear is usually worn 10 to 12 hours each day, typically during the night.

A Herbst appliance is a device that can't be removed for the duration of the treatment. It's usually attached to the upper and lower molars. It holds the lower jaw forward to help correct severe overbite. A palatal expansion appliance is used when the upper teeth don't fit properly with the lower teeth. The appliance is fixed to the upper back teeth to widen the upper jaw.

Duration of treatment with braces and other appliances ranges from six months to three years. The time varies depending on the growth of the face and mouth, the level of cooperation from the person wearing the braces, and the severity of the problem.

Some individuals — adults and teens — prefer clear aligners instead of braces. These appliances are made of a clear material that fits over your teeth, much like a plastic retainer. The aligner exerts pressure on the teeth to gradually move them. Aligners are removable. You take them out when eating and to clean them.

PREVENTION TIP

Take special care to clean your teeth regularly during the course of orthodontic treatment. Food and plaque can accumulate around orthodontic appliances. If you don't remove these deposits, demineralization occurs and may leave permanent whitish marks (scars) or cavities on your teeth. Brush with a fluoride toothpaste and rinse with a fluoride mouthwash as recommended by your dentist. Although somewhat more difficult to do, flossing also is recommended.

Retainers

After braces are removed, treatment often isn't over. The teeth must be stabilized for months, years or sometimes indefinitely to prevent them from shifting. To accomplish this, the teeth are usually fitted with a retainer. Examples of retainers include:

- **Positioners.** These are rubber-like mouthpieces that you wear at night and bite into for a few hours during the day.
- **Removable retainers.** These are made of plastic material on the inside of the teeth and wires on the outside of the teeth.
- **Removable, clear plastic retainers.** These devices completely cover the sides and biting surfaces of the teeth.
- **Semirigid wires.** These devices most often are fitted to and bonded on the inside of your front teeth.

Corrective surgery

In extreme cases, when conventional orthodontic treatment isn't sufficient to correct a problem, your dentist or orthodontist may recommend corrective surgery. This is more common in adults than in children.

Protrusion of the upper or lower jaw can be corrected by removing a section of bone and setting the remainder in its correct position. Conversely, short jaws can be lengthened, or the height of the lower face can be shortened or lengthened to provide better facial aesthetics and function.

Surgery may also be done to adjust misaligned bites that don't respond fully to orthodontic treatment alone. In addition, surgery may shorten the overall duration of orthodontic treatment.

Corrective surgery usually is performed under general anesthesia and requires hospitalization. It has a relatively short recuperation period. The jaws may be wired together for a few days to a few weeks during the initial healing to curtail movement of the jaws.

Gum Disease

Gum (periodontal) disease is a major cause of tooth loss in adults. Most people experience periodontal disease in some form over the course of their lives, but they don't necessarily lose teeth.

The tissue in which the disease occurs is called the periodontium. This includes the gums (gingivae), the periodontal ligament and the tooth sockets (alveolar bone). These structures support your teeth.

Gum disease results from a combination of factors involving bacterial plaque — the sticky substance found in everyone's mouths — and its long-term effects on the periodontium. It can take several forms, but the result is weakened tooth support. The two most common forms of gum disease are gingivitis, an inflammation of the gums, and periodontitis, a more advanced form with tissue destruction.

Gingivitis

Signs and symptoms
- Swollen, soft, red gums
- Gums that bleed easily, especially when brushing your teeth
- A change in gum color from pink to dusky red

The term *gingivitis* refers to inflammation of the part of your gums around the base of your teeth (gingivae), resulting from a sticky, colorless film of bacteria that coats your teeth (plaque). If allowed to harden (become calcified), plaque turns into white-colored tartar (calculus) that darkens with time. Plaque and tartar buildup can irritate the gingivae. The buildup creates pockets of bacteria between your gums and teeth, which can cause your gums to inflame and bleed easily.

Risk factors
Many people first experience gingivitis during puberty and then at various degrees of severity throughout life. Mild forms of the disease are common among

Complications of Gum Disease

Advanced gum disease (periodontitis) does more than just damage your gums. Mounting evidence suggests it may also put you at greater risk of:

- *Heart disease and stroke.* Research suggests a link between oral bacteria and clogged arteries and blood clots, which can lead to heart attack and stroke. Some evidence shows that people with gum disease are more likely to have a heart attack or stroke than are those with healthy mouths. The more severe the gum disease, the greater the risk.
- *Uncontrolled blood sugar.* Diabetes puts you at greater risk of developing gum disease, as well as other infections. In turn, oral infection makes blood sugar (glucose) levels harder to control.
- *Pneumonia.* If you have serious gum disease and lung problems, inhaling bacteria from your mouth into your lungs may result in pneumonia.
- *Osteoporosis.* Researchers suspect a link between the loss of bone mineral density from osteoporosis and an increased susceptibility to oral bacteria. If osteoporosis also causes the bones of your mouth to lose density, that may increase your risk of gum disease and tooth loss. Sometimes, gum disease or tooth loss may be an indication of osteoporosis.
- *Adverse pregnancy outcomes.* New research suggests that women who have gum disease during pregnancy are at increased risk of giving birth to low-weight, preterm babies.

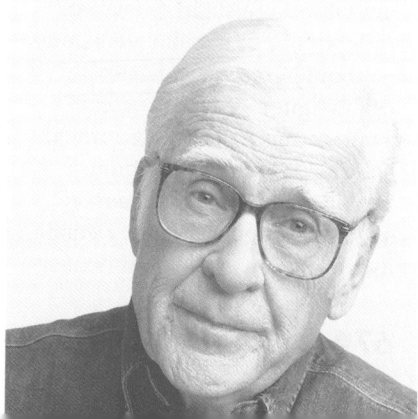

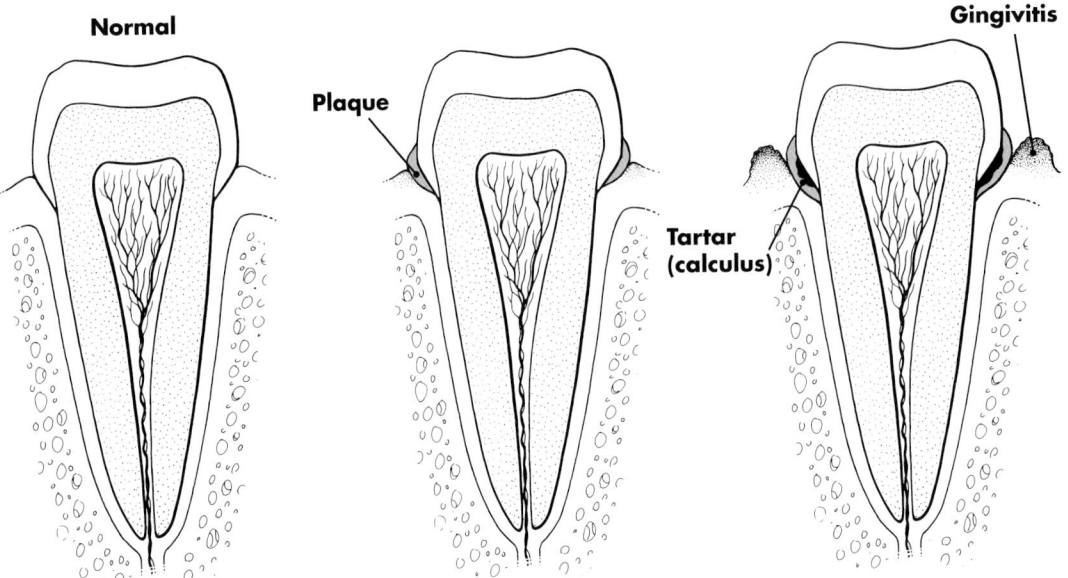

Normal

Plaque

Gingivitis

Tartar (calculus)

If plaque accumulates on a normal tooth and isn't removed promptly, it can harden into a mineral deposit called tartar (calculus). Gradually, the adjacent gums become inflamed and swollen, a disorder known as gingivitis.

adults. The most common contributing factor is a long-term lack of attention to proper oral hygiene, but other factors can increase your risk (see page 676).

Diagnosis

Healthy gums are firm and pale pink. If your gums are swollen, very tender, dusky red and bleed easily, you may have gingivitis.

Often, people first detect a change in their gums when they notice the bristles of their toothbrush are pink after brushing, a sign that their gums are bleeding.

If you have signs and symptoms of persistent gingivitis, consult your dentist. The key to determining the health of your gums is to measure the depth of the groove between your gums and your teeth — the gingival sulcus.

To do this, your dentist inserts a metal probe beneath your gum until it meets a slight resistance. A depth of 2 or 3 millimeters (mm) — about 1/8 inch — indicates a healthy gum. A depth beyond 3 mm means a pocket has formed between your tooth and gum. The deeper the pocket, the more serious your gum disease. Dental X-rays also may help your dentist

gauge the status of your gums by revealing bone loss associated with periodontitis.

How serious is gingivitis?

Gingivitis often is painless and goes unnoticed. If left unchecked, it can lead to periodontitis, a more serious disease that also affects other supporting structures of the teeth and leads to tooth loss.

Treatment

Your dentist may treat your gingivitis by using several techniques. The first step is to thoroughly clean your teeth, including removal of all plaque and tartar. This cleaning can be uncomfortable, particularly if your gums are sensitive or if your teeth are encrusted with heavy tartar. The removal procedure is known as scaling.

Misaligned teeth, overhanging fillings, or poorly contoured restorations such as crowns and bridges can make it difficult to remove plaque, increasing your risk of gingivitis. Teeth can be straightened to minimize plaque accumulation, fillings can be replaced, and restorations can be recontoured.

A long-term program of good oral hygiene is critical to treating

and preventing gingivitis. At first, your gums may bleed after brushing. This should last only a couple of days. Soon your gums should be pink and firm, a sign of their improved health. The program must be followed indefinitely for your gums to remain healthy.

Prevention

If you take good care of your teeth with thorough daily brushing, regular flossing and frequent professional cleaning, your chances of developing serious gingivitis are greatly decreased.

Periodontitis

Signs and symptoms

- Swollen or receding gums
- Bleeding gums
- An unpleasant taste in the mouth
- Bad breath
- Pain in a tooth when eating hot, cold or sweet foods
- Loose teeth
- A change in your bite
- Drainage of pus around one or more teeth

Periodontitis is an advanced stage of gum disease. Plaque-filled pockets form between your teeth and gums, and the gums become inflamed, enlarging the pockets and trapping increasing amounts of plaque. When plaque and tartar extend beneath your gumline, you may develop periodontitis. Gradually, your gums withdraw from around your teeth.

Pockets of infectious material (pus) can form in this dark, airless region and destroy tissue and your tooth sockets (alveolar bone). Left untreated, involved teeth eventually loosen and may fall out.

Periodontitis is usually painless. In some cases, however, an acute infection develops, causing an abscess in one or more of the pockets. This produces pain and erodes bone even more quickly. Generally speaking, the younger a person is when such bone loss begins, the less chance there is of saving the tooth.

Risk factors

Your greatest risk of periodontal disease comes from poor oral hygiene, but other factors increase your risk. People who smoke are more likely to develop periodontitis. They tend to have the problem more severely and respond poorly to treatment. People who grind their teeth also may have more periodontal problems.

Diagnosis

If you experience signs and symptoms of periodontitis, see your dentist. The sooner you do so, the better your chance of healing your gums and preventing loss of teeth.

To determine the health of your gums, your dentist may measure the depth of the groove between your gums and your teeth (gingival sulcus). The deeper the pocket, the more serious your gum disease. Dental X-rays also may help your dentist gauge the health of your gums by revealing bone loss.

Your dentist may also ask a series of questions to determine if a systemic disorder such as diabetes may be contributing to your condition.

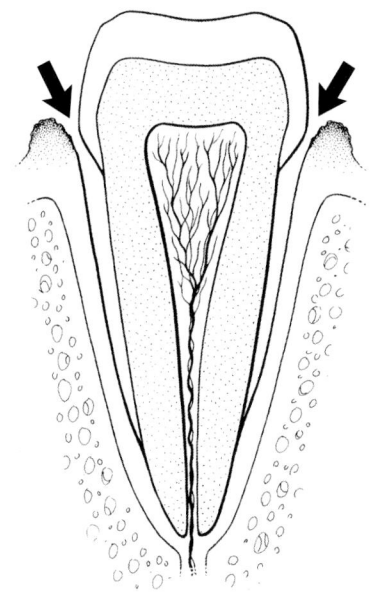

Left untreated, inflammation of the gums (gingivitis) can result in periodontitis, in which an inflamed gum gradually withdraws from the tooth, forming pockets (see arrows). As support for the tooth decreases, it loosens and may eventually fall out.

Treatment

If you have pockets between your gums and your teeth that are 5 millimeters (mm) or less in depth, your dentist may recommend one of the following treatments:

Scaling and root planing

Scaling removes tartar and bacteria from your tooth surfaces and beneath your gums. Sometimes, scaling is done with an ultrasonic device. Root planing smooths the root surfaces, reducing further accumulation of tartar. If followed by good daily oral hygiene, scaling and root planing may be all the treatment you'll need.

Antibiotics

Antibiotics may occasionally be prescribed for periodontal disease, especially for certain aggressive forms of the disease.

Surgery

You may need surgery if you have advanced periodontitis — the depth of the pockets between your gums and teeth exceeds 5 mm. Options include:

- **Flap surgery.** If you have a deep pocket, your dentist can fold up a section of your gum surgically, exposing the roots for more effective scaling and planing. Antibiotics may help control infection.
- **Bone grafting.** If the bone surrounding your tooth root is destroyed, your dentist can obtain sterilized bone segments from a bone bank or synthetic bone grafts to fill the space and keep your tooth in place.
- **Guided tissue regeneration.** This technique allows bone previously destroyed by bacteria to regrow. Your dentist places a special piece of biocompatible fabric between existing bone and your tooth. This material prevents unwanted tissue from entering the healing area. It also stimulates bone to grow back. Sometimes, a bone graft is used in conjunction with the fabric.
- **Gingivectomy.** This procedure involves surgically removing gum (gingival) tissue to decrease the depth of the pockets. After the procedure, the gumline is covered with a protective puttylike packing that serves as a bandage. The dressing allows normal eating and drinking. A surgical procedure to reshape gum tissue also may be used (gingivoplasty). Although gingivectomy procedures were initially developed to treat periodontitis, today they're used more often for cosmetic surgery, such as when medications cause an overgrowth of the gums.

Trench mouth

Signs and symptoms

- Profuse bleeding from and pain in the gums after slight pressure
- A grayish film on the gums

Trench mouth, also known as acute necrotizing ulcerative gingivitis or Vincent's gingivitis,

Are You at Risk?

Everyone is susceptible to gum disease, but the most common contributing factor is long-term lack of attention to good oral hygiene. Other factors also can increase your risk:

- *Smoking.* Smoking reduces your gums' ability to heal by inhibiting the replacement of tissues destroyed by bacteria.
- *Genetics.* Bacteria that lead to gingivitis are more harmful to some people's gums than to others. Those who are susceptible inherit a predisposition to gum disease.
- *Medications.* Some medications decrease the amount of saliva in your mouth, causing a dry mouth. Without the normal cleansing effect of saliva, plaque and tartar can more easily build up. Many antidepressants and cold remedies contain ingredients that decrease the production of saliva. Alcohol has a similar effect.
- *Diabetes.* People with uncontrolled or poorly controlled diabetes are more susceptible to gum disease. Diabetes may cause a thickening of your small blood vessels, making them less able to carry nutrients to your gum tissue and remove wastes. This can leave your gums less healthy and more prone to infection.
- *Pregnancy.* Hormone changes during pregnancy make your gums more susceptible to the damaging effects of plaque.
- *Decreased immunity.* Some illnesses can impair your immune system and make you prone to infection, including gum disease.

is a painful form of gingivitis. It usually affects young adults and can range from mild to severe.

The condition received its name because during World War I it occurred in soldiers who were fighting in trenches under conditions of stress, poor hygiene and poor nutrition.

Trench mouth is characterized by profuse bleeding at the slightest pressure or irritation of the gums. The infection is caused by bacteria that normally inhabit the mouth. It's not passed from one person to another.

Onset of this disease is often sudden. The points of gum tissue between teeth (papillae) are usually damaged, leaving craters that collect plaque and food debris. The area is covered with a grayish layer of decomposing gum tissue. The inflammation and infection may involve other parts of the mouth.

Diagnosis

If you have gum pain and profuse bleeding after slight irritation or pressure on the gums, contact your dentist immediately.

Treatment

Good oral hygiene is crucial to cure the infection. This includes professional cleaning and proper brushing and flossing of your teeth, preferably after each meal and at bedtime.

Your dentist may begin by gently and thoroughly cleaning your teeth and gums. Irrigation of the mouth with a diluted salt or peroxide solution often helps to relieve symptoms. Your dentist may recommend a nonprescription pain reliever to lessen discomfort. You'll also be advised to get plenty of rest, eat a balanced diet, and avoid irritation from smoking or eating spicy foods. Antibiotics may be prescribed if you have a high fever.

Preventing gum disease

As previously noted, gum disease is due in large part to poor dental

hygiene. Inadequate care of your teeth allows plaque and tartar to form and anchor to your teeth. Thorough brushing and flossing are your best defenses.

Brushing and flossing

Follow these tips to keep your gums healthy:

- **Pick the right toothbrush.** Select one with soft, rounded-end or polished bristles that's small enough to allow you to reach your back teeth as well as your front teeth. Replace your brush every three to four months, or sooner if the bristles become bent.
- **Use fluoride toothpaste.** Fluoride toothpaste helps remove plaque and protects against cavities.
- **Brush at least twice daily.** This should include just before bedtime and again each morning. During sleep, saliva flow lessens and allows bacteria to multiply.
- **Brush properly.** To clean the outer surfaces of your teeth and gums, use short, back-and-forth, then up-and-down strokes, covering two teeth at a time. Use vertical strokes to clean the inner surfaces. Be sure to clean the inside of your teeth, the teeth at the back of your mouth, your gums and your tongue. To clean the junction between your teeth and gums, hold your brush at a 45-degree angle to your teeth. This allows the bristles to clean the groove between your gums and your teeth.
- **Floss daily.** Use dental floss or other interdental cleaning aids to clean between your teeth. If you use floss, hold it taut, bend it around each tooth in a C shape, and scrape up and down on the side of each tooth. Each stroke should go slightly below your gumline. Flossing removes plaque between your teeth and helps massage your gums. If you have a bridge, be sure to floss the teeth around it as well as underneath the bridge.

Many toothpaste companies promote tartar-control products. The effectiveness of these products in preventing gum disease is unproved. Tartar-control toothpaste may reduce the formation of tartar on tooth surfaces and make your teeth more cosmetically appealing. However, these products don't help remove tartar below the gumline and between teeth, where gum disease develops.

Other devices

Some people develop plaque in unusual quantities or more rapidly than other people. If you have this problem, your dentist may recommend special toothpicks, stimulators or electric toothbrushes.

Devices that irrigate with water under pressure can be used to flush out toxic products due to buildup of plaque between your teeth. These devices don't remove the plaque but can help prevent some of its effects.

Electric toothbrushes have been found to be superior to regular toothbrushes in removing plaque, but they can be expensive, and manual toothbrushes work well when used properly. Electric toothbrushes can be particularly useful to people with special needs. For example, they may benefit individuals whose manual dexterity is impaired by conditions such as arthritis or people who wear dental appliances, such as braces.

Mouth rinses

Over-the-counter mouth rinses that claim to decrease plaque haven't been proved more beneficial than regular brushing and flossing.

The slick feel that some of these products impart to teeth isn't due to removing tartar and plaque but rather to the glycerin included in the rinse. If you use such a rinse, do so in addition to brushing and flossing.

For people with chronic periodontal problems, a plaque-fighting rinse called chlorhexidine (Peridex, PerioGard) is available by prescription. It's effective, but it isn't a cure for gum inflammation (gingivitis).

Side effects can include an unpleasant taste in your mouth, irritation of the soft tissues of your mouth and staining of your teeth. For these reasons, prolonged use of chlorhexidine products may be undesirable.

Dental cleanings

No matter how careful you are, you're bound to acquire some plaque and calculus. Visit your dentist every six to 12 months for dental cleanings. If you have periodontitis or you develop large amounts of tartar quickly, visit your dentist more often.

Prosthodontics

Among the many stories about George Washington, the first president of the United States, one popular myth holds that he had wooden teeth. It is true that Washington did experience dental disease and tooth loss most of his life. At the time of his inauguration, only one tooth remained.

Dental Care and Diabetes

If you have diabetes, you're at a higher risk of gum disease and infections. Although plaque is the main cause of gum disease, diabetes may make things worse by decreasing your mouth's germ-fighting ability. Poor blood sugar (glucose) control makes gum problems even more likely. The good news is that with proper care, your teeth can last a lifetime.

How often you need to see a dentist depends on many factors — your health, the types of medications you may take, and the condition of your teeth and gums. Some people with diabetes should see a dentist every three months, but others may only need a yearly checkup. Talk to your dentist about what's appropriate for you.

See your dentist if you:
- Experience dry mouth, eating difficulty, or tooth or mouth pain
- Haven't had a dental checkup for over a year
- Notice lesions, sores or lumps in your mouth

When you schedule your visit to a dentist, the American Diabetes Association recommends that you:
- Tell your dentist that you have diabetes, and talk to him or her about any problems you have with infections or controlling your blood sugar.
- Eat before you see your dentist. The best time for dental work is when your blood sugar is within a normal range and the action of your diabetes medication is low.

For example, if you take insulin, a morning visit after a normal breakfast is best.
- Take your usual medications before your dental visit, unless your dentist or doctor tells you to change your dose before dental surgery. Your dentist may consult with your doctor about whether you need to adjust your diabetes medications or if you need an antibiotic before dental surgery to prevent infection.
- Wait to have dental surgery until your blood sugar is under control. If your dental needs are urgent and your blood sugar is poorly controlled, talk to your dentist and doctor about having dental procedures in a hospital or other setting where medical professionals can check on you during and after surgery.

Dentures were an important part of Washington's life, but despite the folklore, they were never made from wood. Hippopotamus, walrus and elephant ivory and other materials such as cows' teeth were used to make his artificial teeth. They were fastened with metal springs that caused excruciating pain.

Before modern dentistry, losing your teeth was an inevitable part of aging. Rare was the person who by old age had any teeth left. The fact that Washington had dentures at all shows that he was one of the lucky few who were able to take advantage of the latest advances in dentistry. Today, the story is different. Fewer people need to have their teeth removed and replaced with dentures.

Partial dentures

If a permanent tooth is lost, there are advantages to replacing it sooner rather than later. Your teeth are positioned such that every tooth has its own place and helps adjacent teeth retain their proper alignment. If you lose a tooth and don't replace it, teeth on either side gradually drift or tilt toward the open space. This can alter your bite, sometimes making it more difficult to chew.

Your dentist will determine what sort of tooth replacement is best suited to meet your needs. If you have a healthy tooth on each side of the missing tooth or teeth, a fixed (nonremovable) partial denture or bridge may be an option. In this procedure, the healthy teeth on each side of the missing tooth or teeth are reshaped to receive a crown. The crowns and an artificial tooth (pontic) or teeth are then joined together, and the bridge is cemented to the supporting teeth.

Another prosthetic device is a removable partial denture. With this device artificial teeth are attached to a metal or plastic base. Clasps or other retainers are incorporated into the partial denture to secure it to the remaining natural teeth. Removable partial dentures are usually less costly than fixed partial dentures, and more teeth can be added in the future if needed.

Partial dentures can trap food, particularly if they don't fit properly. Good oral hygiene is important because retained food particles lead to plaque, tartar, gum disease and decay of the natural teeth. If the partial denture is fixed, be sure to floss and brush it carefully. If it's removable, remove the prosthesis and brush it and the surrounding teeth carefully after every meal. Remove it at bedtime because it's important to allow the gum tissues to rest.

Dentures

If you must have your teeth removed because of serious gum disease or decay, your dentist or a specialist called a prosthodontist can make a set of artificial teeth (dentures).

Dentures can never replace the function and feeling of natural teeth, but they're certainly a better alternative to no teeth at all. You'll lose some of the sensations of eating because the roof of your mouth (hard palate) is covered by the upper denture. In addition, dentures may limit what foods you can eat. Foods such as corn on the cob and whole apples may be difficult to eat because pressure exerted by biting or chewing these foods can cause dentures to loosen.

The chewing pressure you can exert with dentures is much less than you can exert with your natural teeth, which are anchored in your jaw. Well-fitted dentures usually don't require use of denture adhesives.

Fitting dentures

Two standard methods are used for fitting dentures. The teeth can be extracted and the gums and jaw allowed to heal before dentures are fitted. Or the dentures can be prepared in advance and inserted immediately after the extraction.

Not everyone is eligible for immediate dentures. Your dentist will assess the conditions in your mouth and recommend the best approach for you. Immediate dentures save you the inconvenience of being without teeth for a period of time. However, they often must be refitted once the jaw heals, and occasionally new ones must be made if the jaw changes shape significantly after extraction.

A full set of dentures usually consists of complete upper and lower bases that fit over the gums. Another option is an overdenture. When a few acceptable teeth remain in the jaw, the denture can be constructed to cover them. An overdenture may be somewhat more stable than a regular denture and, thus, reduce potential soreness in your mouth. It may be necessary to remove the nerves from the remaining teeth — a procedure called root canal — and then cover them with fillings before constructing the overdenture.

The remaining teeth under the denture must be carefully and regularly maintained to keep them healthy. Your dentist or prosthodontist can advise you on the possibility of using an overdenture.

Whatever kind of removable denture you have, it will need periodic adjustments to keep it comfortable and to help prevent bone loss and mouth sores.

Denture problems

Signs and symptoms
- A persistently loose denture
- Pain in the mouth while wearing dentures
- Inflamed gums
- Sores in the mouth at denture pressure points

First President George Washington once returned an ill-fitting set of dentures to his dentist, writing:

Proper Care of Your Dentures

A dental prosthesis — a removable denture or partial denture — can last from six months to five years or more, depending on the material, how well the denture fits, the condition of your jaw and how well you maintain the denture.

For a prosthesis to be comfortable and durable, you must care for it properly. Good maintenance isn't difficult, particularly if you:

1. Make sure your prosthesis fits properly. If it seems uncomfortable after the initial adjustment period, revisit your dentist or prosthodontist.
2. Remove your prosthesis each night at bedtime. Your gums need a period of rest to remain healthy.
3. Store your prosthesis in water and, when needed, add a denture-cleaning agent. Dentures not stored in water can warp, making them uncomfortable to wear. To avoid damage to the metal clasps of your dentures, don't soak removable dentures with metal bases in a cleansing solution for more than 10 minutes. Soaking them for more than 10 minutes may be fine if it's indicated on the label of the cleansing product.
4. Clean your prosthesis each day, according to your dentist's instructions. Food particles and plaque need to be removed regularly.
5. Each day, brush and floss any remaining natural teeth you have. It's imperative to keep remaining teeth and gums as healthy as possible, particularly if a partial denture is secured to these teeth.
6. Clean and massage your mouth and gums each day using a toothbrush, cloth or your finger. It's as important to keep the gums and soft tissues of your mouth clean and stimulated as it is to keep your teeth clean.

"I must once again resort to you for assistance. The teeth herewith enclosed have by degrees worked loose and, at length, two or three of them have given away altogether. I send them to you to be repaired. ... They are both uneasy on the mouth and bulge my lips out."

Even today, many Americans experience ill-fitting dentures. Natural teeth are supported by a specialized type of bone in the upper and lower jaws. When teeth are lost, the supporting bone begins to shrink. This shrinkage may be accelerated by aging and also by wearing ill-fitting dentures. The result may be loose dentures, which can cause soreness during chewing. In addition, the dentures may become dislodged when you're talking or laughing.

Other problems include mouth sores and inflamed gums. If you're a new denture wearer, you may think that you should expect irritation or sores until you get used to your dentures. But you shouldn't. If you're having problems, your dentist should be able to adjust the denture to eliminate the source of irritation.

If you've worn dentures for a while and begin developing sores, the irritation may be due to a change in the denture or a change in the alignment of your mouth. Less commonly, denture sores can develop if food becomes trapped beneath the denture.

Problems are more common with a lower denture than an upper denture. The lower denture usually doesn't remain in place by itself. Successful use may depend on your ability to control the denture with the muscles of the tongue and cheeks.

Diagnosis

If your dentures are uncomfortable for more than the initial few minutes after you put them in, you experience pain when chewing, or you notice that your gums are red and swollen or have sore, white patches, see your dentist.

How serious are denture problems?

Rarely, persistent or recurring mouth sores can signal a more serious health problem. Therefore, it's important to continue having yearly dental checkups, even if you have no natural teeth.

Treatment

Your dentist may be able to adjust your dentures to relieve the pressure on your gums. Or, if the teeth aren't worn, they can be realigned. If the teeth are worn and the fit is poor, a new set may be needed.

If your gums have shrunk and your dentist has trouble making dentures that fit well, a metallic support (dental implant) can be placed in the bone and used to stabilize the dentures.

If your gums are red and swollen because of a fungal infection, your dentist may prescribe an antifungal medication. Avoid using an over-the-counter ointment to numb denture-induced pain, unless directed to do so by your dentist. Using an ointment won't fix the cause of the sore, and it may mask a more serious problem.

Dental implants

Dental implants are an alternative to dentures, bridgework and missing teeth. They enable you to have permanent replacement teeth — a full mouth or just a few — that stay put when you eat, talk and laugh. Many people are rediscovering the joys of eating and interacting with others without the clicks and wobbles of dentures.

What are dental implants?

Dental implants, available in the United States since the 1980s, serve as artificial "roots." They are metal — usually titanium — posts that are surgically secured in the jawbone beneath the gum tissue. These posts provide stable anchors for artificial replacement teeth, which look like natural teeth and are attached to the implants.

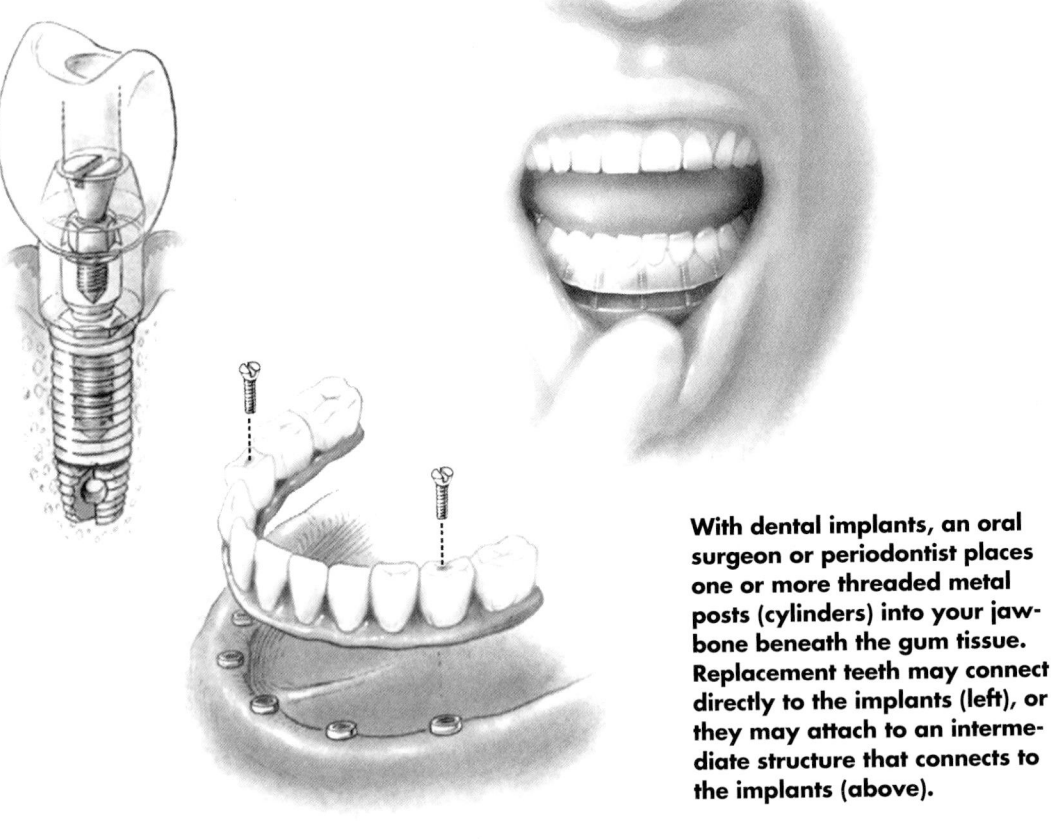

With dental implants, an oral surgeon or periodontist places one or more threaded metal posts (cylinders) into your jawbone beneath the gum tissue. Replacement teeth may connect directly to the implants (left), or they may attach to an intermediate structure that connects to the implants (above).

Dental implants are successful because of a natural process in which the bone grows around and attaches to the metal implant (osseointegration). This provides a solid foundation for artificial teeth. Dental implants feel and function very much like natural teeth.

Are dental implants right for you?

Anyone in good health who's missing teeth — be it one or all — can benefit from dental implants. Those who can't use conventional dentures or bridges because they're missing sections of their jaw might find implants the best option. Bone grafts can be used with implants to reconstruct the jaw and replace missing teeth.

However, implants might not be the best option if you smoke or have a disease such as diabetes. Tobacco use and some diseases, when not properly managed, can interfere with healing and your body's ability to resist or control infection, and they can cause a higher risk of implant failure. On average, about 1 in 20 dental implants fail. Other risks of implanted teeth include nerve damage from the surgery, infection or fracture of bone by implanted posts.

Dental implants are more expensive than conventional dentures. Weigh the pros and cons of implants before you decide which option is right for you.

Type

The endosteal implant is the most commonly used type of implant. The term *endosteal* means "within bone." This type of implant is similar in shape to the root of a natural tooth. It's placed directly into the jawbone, where it becomes solidly anchored through the process of osseointegration.

The procedure

Examinations and consultations by a dentist and implant surgeon can determine if the procedure is appropriate for you. If you are a candidate, your surgeon will use standard or specialized X-rays with computer imaging to plan surgery specific to your situation.

Dental implant surgery is usually performed in an outpatient facility with use of local anesthesia. The procedure involves several steps over a number of months:

Placing the implants

Gum tissue is cut and lifted to expose the bone. Then precisely measured holes are drilled into the bone where each implant will be inserted. The implants are inserted in the holes, and stitches (sutures) are made to close the gum tissue over the bone and implants. Sometimes a surgeon will place a metal healing post in the implant and close the gums around it. The sutures will either dissolve or need to be removed later.

Swelling can be expected for up to 72 hours after the procedure, as well as some discoloration of the skin and gums for a few days. Use of an ice pack in the area during the first 24 hours after surgery may help reduce swelling. Your doctor may prescribe pain medication and antibiotics to control pain and prevent infection.

Minor bleeding is normal on the day of surgery. Report excessive bleeding to your doctor immediately. You'll likely be able to resume normal activity a day or two after surgery.

You'll be given special instructions that explain how you're to clean your mouth during the healing process after surgery. A soft diet is generally recommended to avoid undue pain and stress on the new implants. Most often you're provided with temporary removable teeth during the healing period. In some cases teeth may be attached directly to the newly placed implants. This option is generally only done under special circumstances and can alter the healing process of the implants if not carefully applied.

While the implants are healing it's important not to cause any trauma to the gums in the area of the implants. Therefore, soft foods are encouraged.

Osseointegration occurs gradually as healing progresses. The implants are usually anchored firmly by bone within three to six months after placement.

Attaching metal posts

After healing is complete, if the surgeon did not place healing posts that are visible through the gums, the gums are reopened and metal posts are attached to the implants. Each post has threads like a bolt that support the new artificial tooth. This stage of the implant procedure involves less pain and a healing time of a week or less.

Making new teeth

When the gum tissue has recovered, impressions are made of your mouth, which are used to make models of the jaw and any remaining teeth. New artificial teeth (restorations, or prostheses) are based on these models.

Artificial teeth can be removable, fixed (nonremovable) or a combination of both. A removable prosthesis is similar to a conventional denture, but it has the advantage of being fastened to the implant by clips or magnets. Fixed teeth are screwed into the implants and held firmly in place. They're designed to be removed only by a dentist.

Maintaining dental implants

Self-care is an important part of maintaining dental implants. Follow these guideline:

- **Practice good oral hygiene.** Implants, artificial teeth and gum tissue must be kept clean. Home care aids such as special toothbrushes and floss holders can help.
- **Avoid damaging habits.** Smoking and excessive alcohol consumption as well as chewing hard items such as ice and hard candy may damage an implant.
- **Continue professional care.** Periodic checkup visits are necessary to ensure jawbone health and proper functioning of the implant.

Although the overall success rate of dental implants is 90 to 95 percent, a small percentage fail due to poor maintenance. The implants can also become infected or, rarely, fracture.

Dental implantation is an extensive process that requires serious commitment from those who choose the procedure. For appropriate candidates, dental implants may make eating easier, improve speech and allow a more comfortable life.

Jaw Trauma and Disorders

When an accident happens, the most likely dental and oral injury is a dislocated or fractured jaw or loss of a tooth (tooth avulsion).

Such injuries to the jaw are usually medical emergencies that should be treated without delay.

Broken or dislocated jaw

Signs and symptoms

- Misalignment of the teeth
- An inability to close your mouth
- Intense pain upon moving the jaw

Emergency signs and symptoms

- An obstructed airway
- Profuse bleeding

Most jaw trauma involves the lower jaw (mandible). If you sustain an injury to your mouth or face, seek immediate help from your doctor or the nearest emergency department. If breathing is difficult or considerable blood is present, call for emergency help.

Diagnosis

X-rays and an examination of the jaw are generally the first steps in determining if the bone is fractured. Computerized tomography (CT) scans may be obtained to see if other facial bones have been fractured. Blows that are strong enough to break other bones of your face may also damage your neck and back.

Your doctor may suspect a fracture if you're unable to close your mouth, your teeth are misaligned when your mouth is closed, or you experience tenderness or numbness around your jaw. If you're unable to close your mouth, your jaw may be dislocated. Swelling and bruising are likely to accompany all jaw injuries.

Treatment

Treatment depends on whether you have a dislocation or a fracture:

Jaw dislocation

If your jaw is dislocated, your doctor may move it back into place by manually manipulating it. You may be given an anesthetic before this treatment.

Once the jaw is back in place, it may be stabilized with a bandage to keep your mouth from opening too wide and causing another dislocation. Avoid opening your mouth very wide for up to six weeks after the injury. When you feel a yawn coming on, place your fist under your chin to keep your mouth from opening wide.

If you've dislocated your jaw more than once, you may want to consult a surgeon who specializes in problems of the jaw and the bones of the face (oral and maxillofacial surgeon) to discuss treatment options.

Jaw fracture

If your jaw is fractured, your doctor will immobilize the jaw to reduce discomfort and allow healing. In many cases, surgery is necessary to realign the bones and allow them to heal. After surgery the jaw often needs to be immobilized for six to eight weeks. During this time, you'll be able to eat only soft or liquid foods, and talking may be difficult.

Loss of a tooth

When a permanent tooth is accidentally knocked out, appropriate emergency medical care is required, whether the tooth loss (tooth avulsion) happens to a child or an adult. Permanent teeth that are knocked out sometimes can be reimplanted if you act quickly. A broken tooth, however, can't be reattached. For more information, see page 44.

Temporomandibular joint disorders

Signs and symptoms
- Tenderness of your jaw muscles
- A dull aching pain in front of your ear
- A clicking sound or grating sensation when opening your mouth or chewing
- Locking of the joint, making it difficult to open or close your mouth
- Headache

The temporomandibular joints (TMJs) are the hinge-like joints that connect both sides of your lower jaw (mandible) to your skull. As with many other joints, the bony surfaces are covered with cartilage and are separated by a small disk that prevents the bones from rubbing against one another. Muscles that enable you to open and close your mouth also serve to stabilize these joints, which are located about a half inch in front of each ear canal.

When you open your mouth, the mandible moves downward and forward. For normal jaw function, both TMJs must work in synchrony. If the movement of both joints isn't coordinated, the disk that separates the lower jaw from the skull can slip out of position, resulting in jaw malfunction. Should your mouth be forced open rapidly or too far, the jaw can become dislocated.

As with other joints, the TMJ is susceptible to various disorders such as osteoarthritis, rheumatoid arthritis and other forms of inflammation. Other causes of TMJ pain include wear and tear on the joint, injury, stress, an improperly aligned bite, and poorly fitting braces or other dental appliances. In rare instances, tumors may arise in this area.

Chronic tension and anxiety may cause you to habitually maintain a clenched jaw or grind your teeth — a condition called bruxism. Many people are unaware that they grind their teeth because it often happens while sleeping.

This overuse of your TMJ and supporting muscles may cause jaw pain and a headache when you awake in the morning. The pain associated with temporomandibular disorders can vary from minor to severe, and the condition can be temporary or chronic.

Diagnosis
Your doctor or dentist may listen for any sounds your jaw makes and observe its range of motion.

Examining your bite can reveal abnormalities in the alignment of your teeth and in the movement of your jaw. Conditions such as a high filling, a tipped tooth, teeth displaced due to earlier loss of other teeth or certain inherited characteristics may produce misalignments and subsequent pain.

In addition, by examining wear patterns, your dentist can determine if you chronically grind your teeth. Feeling the joint while you move it also may help your dentist determine the cause of the condition. An X-ray or magnetic resonance imaging (MRI) can help your doctor or dentist check for abnormalities.

Treatment
Often jaw problems are temporary and they resolve with time and simple steps such as rest and medication. Aside from asking you to avoid overusing your jaw, your doctor or dentist may suggest one or more of the following:

Anti-inflammatory medications
To reduce inflammation, your doctor or dentist may advise taking aspirin or a nonsteroidal anti-inflammatory drug (NSAID), such as ibuprofen (Motrin IB, Advil, others). For severe pain and inflammation, your doctor or dentist may inject a corticosteroid drug into the joint.

Bite plate
If the temporomandibular joint is misaligned, your dentist may recommend use of a plastic bite plate (splint) that's worn over your teeth to help align your upper and lower jaws.

Night guard
If you grind your teeth in your sleep, a night guard — a soft or firm device that you insert over your teeth — can help protect your teeth during grinding.

Corrective dental treatment
Your dentist may be able to im-

prove your bite by balancing the biting surfaces of your teeth or by replacing missing teeth, fillings or crowns.

Surgery

If other approaches don't work, surgery to repair or remove the disk between your mandible and temporal bone may be necessary, but this is rare.

Self-care

In addition to medical treatments, these self-care approaches can help prevent overuse and inflammation of your temporomandibular joint:

- Don't chew gum.
- Avoid sticky foods and foods that require a lot of chewing, such as caramels, tough meat and celery.
- Try not to sleep on your side with your hand under your jaw.
- When yawning, avoid opening your mouth too wide.
- If stress is causing you to habitually grind your teeth or clench your jaw, relaxation therapy or a night guard worn while you sleep may provide relief.

Teeth grinding

Signs and symptoms

- Severe or loud teeth grinding or clenching that occurs during sleep or during times of anxiety or stress
- Tips of teeth that are worn down, flattened or chipped
- Worn tooth enamel that exposes the inside of a tooth
- Increased tooth sensitivity
- Jaw clenching or muscle contractions
- Jaw pain or tightness in the jaw muscles
- Popping, clicking or locking of the jaw joint
- Earache due to jaw muscle contractions
- Dull morning headache
- Chronic facial pain
- Chewed tissue on the inside of the cheek

Bruxism is the medical term for grinding, gnashing or clenching of your teeth during sleep or during situations that make you feel anxious or tense. This condition may be mild and occur only occasionally, or it may happen frequently and be violent.

Bruxism most often occurs in the early part of the night and can disturb sleep partners. Some people grind their teeth so loudly that they can't duplicate the sound while awake. Others make no sound and deny having the condition, even when there's tooth or jaw damage.

Your bite (occlusion) affects the health of your teeth and jaw. It's estimated that about 10 percent of Americans are affected by bruxism and that the condition occurs in as many as 15 percent of children.

Some individuals grind or clench their teeth with enough force to fracture dental fillings or crowns or cause other types of tooth damage. Severe bruxism may also cause tension-type headaches, facial pain and temporomandibular disorders, which occur in the temporomandibular joint (TMJ) located just in front of your ear.

Some people with bruxism clench their teeth only now and then. They might go days or weeks without doing so. People with bruxism may also habitually bite their fingernails, pencils or the insides of their cheeks.

Bruxism is a common sleep disorder. Research indicates that people who grind or gnash their teeth are more likely to snore, have pauses in breathing during sleep and develop sleep apnea. Bruxism is more prevalent in women than in men. In addition, women are more prone to tissue damage in the jaw joint resulting from teeth grinding and clenching.

Causes

The causes of bruxism are not well-understood. The condition is thought to mainly stem from a variety of psychological and physical causes. These include:

- Suppressed anger or frustration
- An aggressive, competitive or hyperactive personality type
- Anxiety, stress or tension
- A movement driven by the central nervous system

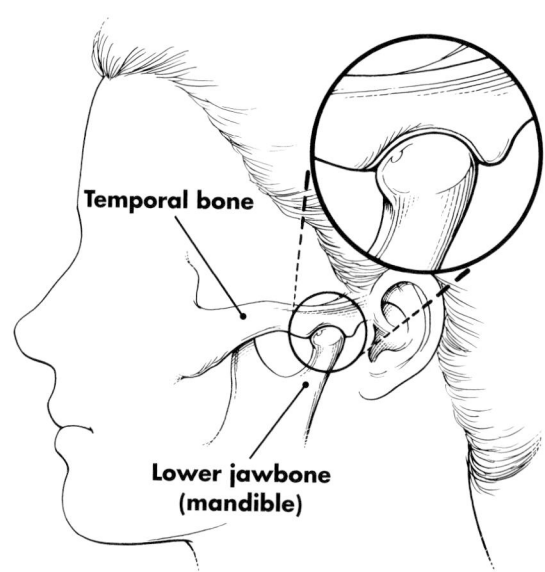

Your temporomandibular joints (TMJs) are hinge-like joints. One is situated on each side of your head where the lower jawbone (mandible) connects with the temporal bone of your skull. Inflammation, injury or dislocation of this joint can cause pain.

Temporal bone

Lower jawbone (mandible)

- Abnormal alignment of upper and lower teeth (malocclusion)

Bruxism can sometimes occur as a complication of severe brain injury or as a symptom of rare neuromuscular diseases involving the face. It can also be caused by an uncommon side effect of some psychiatric medications, including antidepressants such as sertraline (Zoloft), paroxetine (Paxil) and fluoxetine (Prozac, Sarafem).

Stimulants such as tobacco and caffeine may cause your body to produce more adrenaline (epinephrine), which can worsen the condition. There's little evidence to support that bruxism is related to hereditary or genetic factors.

In children, bruxism may be related to growth and development. Some children grind or clench their teeth because their top and bottom teeth are misaligned. Others do so as a response to pain such as from an earache or teething.

Although most children outgrow bruxism, even short-term teeth grinding or clenching can damage permanent teeth. Of children who begin grinding their teeth between the ages of 3 and 10, more than half stop spontaneously by age 13.

Diagnosis

During regular dental exams, a dentist usually checks for evidence of bruxism. If your dentist notices signs, the condition may be observed over several visits to be sure of the problem before therapy is started.

Your dentist might ask about stresses in your life, your general dental health and any medications you take. He or she may also want to know whether you routinely drink beverages containing alcohol or caffeine, especially in the evening. Your dentist may want to ask your roommate or bed partner about your sleep habits, especially about any unusual grinding sounds heard during the night.

To evaluate the extent of the problem, your dentist or a specialist may perform a physical examination of your mouth and jaw. During this exam, he or she will check for tenderness in your jaw muscles and any obvious dental abnormalities, such as broken or missing teeth and poor teeth alignment.

In addition to checking your bite and examining your teeth, your dentist will likely check underlying bone and the inside of your cheeks for damage caused by bruxism. Mouth and jaw X-rays may be taken.

Treatment

The goal of treatment is to prevent permanent damage to your teeth and reduce pain caused by bruxism. Learning to rest your teeth, tongue and lips properly may help you to change your behavior and relieve bruxism. Resting your tongue upward with your teeth apart and lips closed can relieve discomfort by keeping your teeth from grinding or your jaw from clenching.

Other forms of treatment vary depending on the cause:

Stress

If your condition is related to stress, various strategies to help you relax may help reduce your bruxism. Sometimes a muscle relaxant medication is prescribed to temporarily reduce the spasm within a clenched jaw.

Dental problems

If your bruxism is related to a dental problem, your dentist may treat it with a mouth guard. Or he or she may recommend a protective dental appliance if the problem is severe enough to cause extensive tooth damage.

Brain injury or neuromuscular illness

Bruxism stemming from a brain injury or neuromuscular illness can be difficult to control. You may receive a mouth guard to help control bruxism.

Medication

If you develop bruxism as a side effect of medication, your doctor may change your medication or prescribe an additional medication to counteract your bruxism. Studies indicate that gabapentin (Neurontin) may successfully treat bruxism caused by antidepressant therapy.

Oral Infections and Diseases

Almost everyone experiences some sort of infection or disease of the mouth on occasion. Many times the problem is a passing irritation, such as an occasional canker sore. Other conditions are more debilitating or serious.

Canker sores

Signs and symptoms

- Small, painful, white ulcers in the mouth

Canker sores are common but annoying ulcers in the mouth. They occur singly or in clusters on the inside surface of the cheeks and lips, on the tongue, at the base of the gums, and on the movable flesh at the back of the roof of the mouth (soft palate).

Despite a great deal of research, the cause of canker sores remains elusive. Current thinking suggests that either stress or tissue injury may cause common canker sores to erupt. Some researchers think certain foods — for example, citrus fruits, tomatoes and some nuts — may complicate the problem. A minor injury, such as biting the inside of your mouth, may trigger a canker sore.

Canker sores can be simple or complex. A simple type of canker sore may appear three or four times a year and last four to seven days. The first occurrence is usually between the ages of 10 and 20, but it can occur in younger children.

As a person reaches adulthood, the sores occur less frequently and may stop developing altogether. Women seem to get them more often than men, and the condition seems to run in families.

Complex canker sores are less common but much more of a problem. People with this condition may have these sores 50 percent of the time. As old sores heal, new ones appear.

Treatment

There's no cure for either simple or complex canker sores, and effective treatments are limited. However, the following practices may provide temporary relief:

- Avoid abrasive, acidic or spicy foods, which may increase the pain.
- Apply ice to the canker sore.
- Brush your teeth carefully to avoid irritating the sore.
- Use an over-the-counter topical anesthetic.
- Rinse your mouth with over-the-counter preparations, such as diluted hydrogen peroxide.
- Use an over-the-counter pain reliever.

For severe attacks of canker sores, your dentist or doctor may prescribe an antibacterial paste called amlexanox, an antibacterial mouthwash, a corticosteroid salve or an anesthetic solution containing lidocaine hydrochloride. See your dentist if you have sharp tooth surfaces or dental appliances that may be causing the sores.

Gingivostomatitis

Signs and symptoms

- Mouth and gum sores
- Bad breath
- Fever and a feeling of malaise

Gingivostomatitis is a viral infection of the gingivae and oral mucus that occurs mostly in children. It often accompanies an up-per respiratory infection such as a cold. Gingivostomatitis infections range from mild to severe and generally last about two weeks.

Diagnosis

Signs indicating gingivostomatitis include sores on the gums or on the insides of the cheeks, bad breath, and a fever. A doctor or dentist may examine your child's mouth and check for any underlying infection, particularly of the chest or throat. A sample may be taken for culture.

Treatment

Treatment of an underlying infection or disorder may help clear the mouth infection. A medicated oral rinse may help relieve the pain and promote healing.

Good oral hygiene and a nutritious diet of soft foods and plenty of fluids are important. Using a mouthwash made of one-half teaspoon of salt dissolved in 8 ounces of water or an over-the-counter mouthwash may be soothing.

Oral thrush

Signs and symptoms

- Creamy-white sore patches in the mouth or throat

Your mouth houses many different kinds of germs. One of them, the fungus *Candida albicans*, can reproduce uncontrollably, causing an infection known as oral thrush (candidiasis). The infection may extend downward into the esophagus.

This fungus is also responsible for vaginal yeast infections that many women experience. Oral thrush tends to occur most often when your natural resistance to disease has been weakened by illness or when your mouth's natural balance of microbes has been upset by medications such as antibiotics, immunosuppressants or corticosteroids.

The infection is most common among babies, young children and older adults, although it can occur at any time of life. Thrush likes to develop in moist spots that may be chafed or sore, such as under poorly fitting dentures. You're also at increased risk if you smoke.

Diagnosis

If slightly raised, creamy-white painful patches develop in your mouth or on your tongue, you may have oral thrush. The patches may be brushed off when you clean your teeth or eat. Brushing may cause increased soreness and slight bleeding. The infection can spread to the roof of your mouth and your gums, tonsils, and throat.

Your doctor or dentist will likely examine your mouth and throat to look for an underlying cause.

How serious is oral thrush?

Oral thrush can be painful, but ordinarily it's not a serious disorder. However, it can interfere with eating.

Treatment

Your doctor or dentist will likely prescribe a seven- to 10-day course of oral antifungal medication. Any underlying disorder, if present, must be treated as well.

Leukoplakia

Signs and symptoms

- A thickened, firm, white patch on a cheek or your gums or tongue

The term *leukoplakia* comes from a Greek word meaning "white plate," an apt description of the white patches that characterize this disorder. Leukoplakia is the mouth's reaction to chronic irritation, such as from tobacco between the cheek and gum, ill-fitting dentures, or a rough tooth rubbing against a cheek or gum.

Over the course of several weeks, you may notice a white or grayish patch developing on the inside of one cheek or on your tongue or gums (see the illustration on page 400). At first it may not cause problems. After a while, it may become rough and sensitive to hot or spicy foods.

When a white patch develops in the mouth of a smoker, the condition is called smoker's keratosis. These patches are the body's natural protection against the heat of tobacco smoke. They also occur where a cud of chewing tobacco or snuff is held within the mouth for extended periods.

Leukoplakia is most common among older adults.

Diagnosis

Your doctor or dentist will likely examine the patch and try to determine the cause of the irritation. He or she may also take a specimen of the area for examination under a microscope (biopsy). A small percentage of leukoplakias are either cancerous (malignant) upon diagnosis or will develop into cancer within 10 years if not treated properly.

Treatment

Treating leukoplakia involves removing the source of irritation, if possible. If a rough tooth or denture is the cause, the offending tooth can probably be filed down or replaced. If the patch is linked to smoking or chewing tobacco, your best option for successful treatment is to quit the habit.

Once the source of irritation is removed, the patch usually clears up within weeks or months. If the area doesn't clear, a biopsy may be taken to make sure it's not oral cancer.

Oral lichen planus

Signs and symptoms

- Small, pale pimples that form a lacy network on the tongue or inside the cheeks
- Shiny, red, slightly raised patches on the tongue or cheeks
- A sore or burning mouth
- Dry mouth
- A metallic taste in your mouth
  Oral lichen planus may be limited to a network of pale pimples or shiny, red, raised patches on the

Bad Breath

Everyone would like to have breath that's always "kissing sweet." Because fresh breath is important to most people, mints and mouthwashes constitute a multimillion-dollar industry.

Sadly, these products don't always succeed in curing bad breath (halitosis) and actually may be less effective than rinsing your mouth with water and brushing and flossing your teeth.

What causes bad breath?

There are many causes of bad breath. First, your mouth itself may be the source. Bacterial decomposition of food particles and other debris in and around your teeth can produce a foul odor composed of volatile sulfur compounds. Pockets of infection, as in periodontitis, are obvious causes of odor. A dry mouth, such as occurs during sleep or as the result of some drugs or smoking, enables dead cells to accumulate on your tongue, gums and cheeks. These decompose and cause odor.

Bad breath is sometimes associated with small stones that form on the tonsils that are covered with bacteria and produce an odor. Infections of inflammation of the nose, sinuses or throat, which can contribute to postnasal drip, also can cause bad breath.

Another cause of bad breath is eating foods containing volatile oils with a strong, distinctive odor. Onions and garlic are the best-known examples, but other vegetables and spices also can cause bad breath. After such foods are digested, the volatile substances are absorbed into your bloodstream and carried to your lungs. Here they're exhaled in your breath. Alcohol behaves in the same fashion, thus allowing measurement of blood alcohol levels by breath tests.

Lung disease can cause bad breath, as can chronic infections in the lungs. Gastroesophageal reflux disease also can cause bad breath. Several general health problems can cause a distinctive breath odor. Kidney failure can cause a urine-like odor, and liver failure may cause an odor sometimes described as fishy. Acetone in the breath causes a fruity odor and may occur in people with diabetes who are developing excessive blood acids (ketoacidosis).

Preventing bad breath

For most people, bad breath can be improved by:

- Brushing your teeth after every meal.
- Brushing your tongue to remove dead cells.
- Flossing once a day to remove food particles from between your teeth.
- Drinking plenty of water — not coffee, soda pop or alcohol — to keep your mouth moist.
- Avoiding strong foods that cause bad breath. Brushing your teeth or using a mouthwash only partially disguises odors of garlic or onion, which come from your lungs.
- Changing your toothbrush every three to four months.
- Rinsing your mouth after using inhaler medications.
  In other situations, bad breath can be eliminated by treating the underlying condition, such as reflux, lung disease, liver failure or kidney failure.

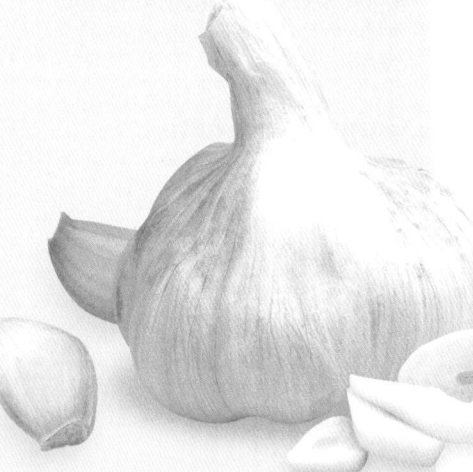

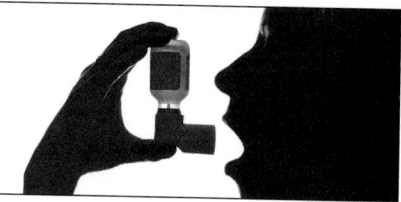

sides of the tongue or inside the cheeks, or it may advance into a painful erosive lesion. Your mouth may be sore and dry and have a metallic taste. Some people experience no signs or symptoms other than the raised pimples or bumps.

The cause of oral lichen planus is uncertain. Emotional stress seems to trigger the response in some people. In others, it may be associated with any of a number of medications, such as antibiotics, diuretics, iodides, phenothiazines, chloroquine, quinacrine or quinidine.

Some cases have been linked to infections, such as hepatitis. Any adult can develop this rare disorder, but it affects middle-aged women more frequently than other groups.

There seems to be a relationship between the oral form and the skin form of lichen planus because almost half of those with the oral condition also have it on the skin.

How serious is oral lichen planus?
Oral lichen planus usually isn't a serious condition. However, people with persistent oral lesions are at increased risk of squamous cell carcinoma — a form of skin cancer. In these cases, a doctor may advise regular examinations to monitor any changes in the lesions. It's also important to stop any tobacco use, which raises your risk of squamous cell carcinoma.

Treatment
Treatment may not be necessary. If the cause is a certain medication, your doctor or dentist may advise you to stop using it and perhaps prescribe another medication.

Other treatments focus on relieving symptoms. They include: :

- A corticosteroid ointment or cream
- Phototherapy with ultraviolet light, in some cases
- Oral corticosteroid medications, in severe cases
- Immune-modulating therapy, in severe cases

Tongue disorders

Signs and symptoms
- The tongue becomes smooth, dark red and sometimes sore
- The tongue becomes discolored, black or dark brown
- The tongue appears hairy or furry

A number of conditions can affect your tongue. Most are minor, but if the symptoms persist for

> **? Question and Answer**
>
> ### Can oral piercing cause a serious infection?
>
> Piercing isn't always a healthy choice. Some people don't realize that oral piercing — piercing a tongue or lip — can land them in the doctor's office or the emergency department.
>
> An oral piercing provides an opportunity for the millions of bacteria in your mouth to cause infection. Other complications include swelling, increased saliva flow, injuries to the gum tissue, uncontrollable bleeding and nerve damage.
>
> Blood poisoning (septicemia) and blood clots can also occur. Tongue swelling is common and, if severe, can block the airway and obstruct breathing.

more than 10 days, visit your doctor or dentist for an examination.

Inflammation of the tongue
Normally, the surface of your tongue is covered with small, hairlike projections of tissue called papillae. Inflammation of the tongue (glossitis) harms the papillae and may cause a range of other tongue changes to occur, including discoloration. Specifically, the tongue loses its usual pink and velvety character, and it may become sore.

Various factors can cause glossitis, including a bacterial or fungal infection, iron deficiency anemia, and pernicious anemia, which is due to a vitamin B-12 deficiency.

Acute glossitis
Acute glossitis can occur as the result of a local infection, a burn or trauma. It may develop quickly with swelling and tenderness. It can interfere with chewing, swallowing and speaking.

If your tongue swells a great deal, it can obstruct your air passages. If this happens, immediately go to the nearest emergency department or call for emergency medical help. Immediate corticosteroid treatment usually relieves the swelling.

Geographic tongue
Geographic tongue is characterized by absence of papillae in patches, which makes the tongue appear smooth and bright red within those patches (see the illustration on page 400). Soreness or burning may occur. Its cause isn't completely understood.

Geographic tongue may vary from day to day or be persistent.

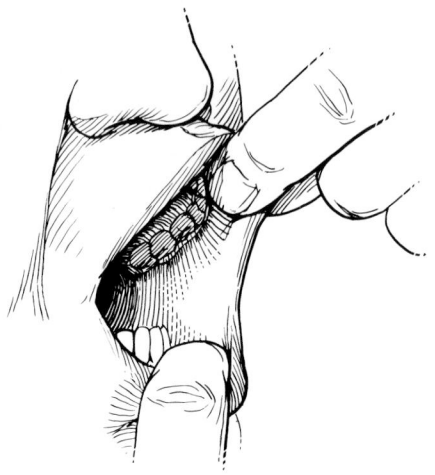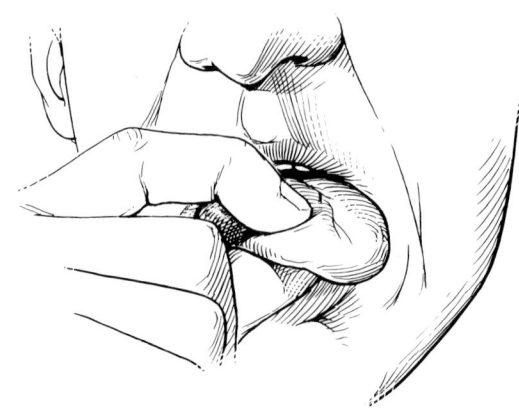

Routine self-examination of your mouth and tongue may enable you to see or feel an oral cancer when it's small and when treatment is most effective.

There's no specific treatment. Avoid hot or spicy foods, tobacco, and alcohol.

Black, hairy tongue
Long, hairlike projections caused by altered shedding of surface cells can allow bacteria and debris to collect on the surface of the tongue. These bacteria may accumulate on the papillae of the tongue, commonly turning the tongue black (see the illustration on page 400). The cause of this condition isn't clear, but it may be related to:
- Fungal growth after antibiotic use, which changes the normal bacterial content of the mouth
- Use of medications containing bismuth, such as Bismatrol and Pepto-Bismol
- Smoking or using chewing tobacco

Other possible causes for hairy tongue include excessive use of prescription mouthwashes that contain chlorhexidine, decreased saliva flow or poor oral hygiene.

The condition isn't serious, and it usually clears after discontinuing use of the offending medication or mouthwash. You can remove the discoloration and hairlike growths by gently brushing your tongue with your toothbrush twice a day.

Diluted hydrogen peroxide — 1 ounce hydrogen peroxide to 5 ounces water — may help bleach the color. You can gargle with it or apply it with a toothbrush. Avoid swallowing the solution. Rinse your mouth afterward. If this doesn't resolve the problem, consult your doctor or dentist.

Oral cancer

Signs and symptoms
- A mouth sore that doesn't heal or increases in size
- Persistent pain in your mouth
- Lumps or white, red or dark patches inside your mouth
- Thickening of your cheek
- Difficulty chewing or swallowing or moving your tongue
- Difficulty moving your jaw
- Swelling or pain in your jaw
- Soreness in your throat or a feeling that something is caught in your throat
- Numbness of your tongue or elsewhere in your mouth
- A lump in your neck
- A change in your voice

Each year, almost 50,000 new cases of oral cancer — cancer of the lips, mouth, tongue, gums and salivary glands — and cancer of the upper throat (oropharyngeal cancer) occur in the United States.

About 9,700 Americans die of these cancers annually.

Most oral cancers arise on the tongue or on the floor of the mouth. They also may occur inside your cheeks, on your gums or on the roof of your mouth.

Periodic self-examination of your mouth is the best way to detect early signs of oral cancer. An early indication of oral cancer is a change in the way the soft tissues of your mouth look or feel. When detected early and treated adequately, oral cancer is almost always curable. Unfortunately, more than half of all oral and upper throat cancers are advanced by the time a diagnosis is made.

Causes
Oral cancer appears to occur as a result of situations that damage the cells in your mouth so that they reproduce rapidly as cancer cells. A variety of factors that you can control increase your risk of oral cancer.

Use of tobacco
Tobacco can damage cells in the lining of the oral cavity and upper throat. Smokers are six times more likely than nonsmokers to develop oral or upper throat cancers. The majority of people who develop

these cancers use some form of tobacco. People who use smokeless tobacco are at high risk of cancers of the cheek and inner surface of the lips. Oral cancer is twice as common in men as in women.

Excessive alcohol consumption

Alcohol can damage cells inside your mouth and upper throat. Many people with oral and upper throat cancers consume alcohol frequently. The combination of alcohol and tobacco use increases risk.

Prolonged exposure to ultraviolet light

Too much ultraviolet light can damage the cells on your lips and increase your risk of lip cancer.

Leukoplakia

Most of the time white patches on the inside of the cheek or tongue (leukoplakias) aren't dangerous. But on occasion they may be early indicators of cancer. A large percentage of oral cancers occur in areas adjacent to leukoplakia. Leukoplakia may result from a variety of causes, including smoking or chewing tobacco products, ill-fitting dentures, a rough spot on an adjacent tooth, or habitual cheek biting.

Diagnosis

To determine if a suspect area in your mouth is cancerous, your doctor will need to take a small tissue sample for examination under a microscope (biopsy).

Almost all oral cancers are of the squamous cell type. Squamous cells are firm and flat, and they form the lining of the oral cavity and upper throat as well as the surface of the skin. Squamous cell cancer begins with abnormal cells located only on the surface.

As the cancer progresses, the malignant cells invade deeper layers of the oral cavity and upper throat and may spread to the lymph nodes as well as to other parts of the body.

For your doctor to determine whether or how far the cancer has spread, you may need dental X-rays, X-rays of your head and chest, a computerized tomography (CT) scan, magnetic resonance imaging (MRI) or an ultrasound scan.

Treatment

Surgery at an early stage provides the best chance for cure with the fewest side effects. If a tumor can't be completely removed, your doctor may recommend radiation. Sometimes, doctors recommend chemotherapy before surgery or in combination with radiation therapy.

Surgery

The type of surgery performed depends on the size and location of the tumor. Tumors that haven't invaded nearby tissues can be

Smokeless Doesn't Mean Harmless

If you think that smokeless tobacco won't hurt you, chew on this — one pinch held between your cheek and gum for 30 minutes puts the same amount of nicotine in your body as does smoking three cigarettes. Your body also absorbs several toxic chemicals, including arsenic and formaldehyde.

Spit tobacco — also known as chew, snuff or dip — causes cancer. Each year, millions of Americans put their health at risk by using spit tobacco. The risk of developing oral cancer among long-term spit tobacco users is up to 50 times higher than for nonusers.

Tobacco companies have coined the term *smokeless tobacco*, which implies to some that it's less harmful and less addictive than are cigarettes. This makes an already dangerous product sound safer and more acceptable than other tobacco products.

Who uses it?

The majority of spit tobacco users are under age 18, despite the product being illegal for this age group in most states. High school-aged boys are some of the biggest users. Contrary to popular belief, major league baseball players aren't the only ones who use spit tobacco regularly. Other occupational groups have started using spit tobacco more frequently due to new "No smoking" regulations that prevent them from smoking on the job or at work sites.

What it does to you

Spit tobacco can get you hooked on nicotine. Research indicates that spit tobacco can be as addictive as morphine or cocaine.

Spit tobacco isn't made of only tobacco or natural products. Each time you use it, you absorb a number of toxic chemicals, many of which can cause cancer (carcinogens). These include:

- Nitrosamines — the most powerful cancer-causing chemicals known
- Polonium — radioactive particles
- Formaldehyde — a chemical used in embalming fluid
- Arsenic and cadmium — poisonous metals

As early as one week after you start using spit tobacco, you may develop small white patches called leukoplakia inside your mouth (see page 400). Within a few months of regular use, many spit tobacco users have these white patches, which can be an early sign of cancer. Red patches called erythroplakia are even more likely to become cancerous.

surgically removed with relatively few side effects. However, if the tumor has invaded nearby tissues, the surgery may be more extensive. Sometimes, surgeons need to remove bone from the jaw or tissue from the roof of the mouth.

To treat a cancer located on the tongue or upper part of your throat, a surgeon may need to remove tissues used for swallowing and, in some cases, the voice box (larynx). If the cancer has spread beyond the mouth, lymph nodes in the neck also may be removed.

Radiation

Radiation therapy uses high-energy waves to kill cancer cells. A doctor may advise treatment with radiation therapy if the tumor is small. Radiation may be used along with surgery to destroy small amounts of cancer cells that couldn't be removed during surgery.

Chemotherapy

Chemotherapy uses drugs to destroy cancer cells. You typically receive the medication either through your veins (intravenously) or orally. The type of drugs and the length of treatment generally depend on the size, type and location of the tumor. Chemotherapy may be used before surgery to shrink a tumor. In the case of a large and invasive tumor, it may be used in combination with radiation therapy instead of surgery.

Reconstructive surgery

After the removal of an extensive tumor, reconstructive surgery may enhance your recovery and rehabilitation. The goal of reconstructive surgery is to improve your appearance and to help you adjust to difficulties you may have chewing, swallowing, speaking or breathing.

When portions of the jaw need to be removed to control the disease, the jaw can be reconstructed with healthy bone from other regions of the body.

If you've had extensive neck surgery, you may need surgery to create a hole in your neck (tracheotomy) to help you breathe more easily. If muscles you need for swallowing have been removed, you'll need surgery to create access to your stomach (gastrostomy) in order to receive food directly through a feeding tube.

Salivary Gland Disorders

Saliva, produced by your salivary glands, serves several purposes. It helps clean your mouth and teeth, it aids in swallowing, and it contains enzymes that aid digestion and help control infection.

There are three major sets of salivary glands located throughout your mouth, as well as numerous smaller glands. The parotid glands are located in each cheek. The submandibular glands are located under your jaw, and the sublingual glands are in the floor of your mouth (see page 692). Each set has its own tube (duct) carrying saliva from the gland to your mouth.

Malfunctions of the salivary glands may cause either excessive secretion or decreased salivation.

Dry mouth

Signs and symptoms

- A sensation of dryness in your mouth
- Saliva that seems thick and stringy
- Sores or cracked skin at the corners of your mouth
- Bad breath
- Difficulty speaking or swallowing
- A burning or tingling sensation on the tongue
- An altered sense of taste
- Increased plaque on your teeth
- Increased tooth decay or gum disease

Lack of saliva is a common problem that may seem little more than a nuisance. But don't ignore it. Persistent dry mouth can affect how food tastes and even the health of your teeth. Although many things can cause dry mouth, it's often a side effect of medication.

The saliva in your mouth serves many purposes. Most noticeably, it makes it easier to talk. It also enhances your ability to taste food, makes it easier to swallow and aids in digestion.

The minerals found in saliva help repair early tooth decay, and saliva helps prevent decay by washing away food and plaque from your teeth, limiting bacterial growth that can dissolve tooth enamel and neutralizing damaging acids in your mouth

On any given day, a healthy adult produces about 3 pints of saliva. Saliva production generally goes unnoticed unless too little is produced. The result is dry mouth (xerostomia).

Causes

At one time, dry mouth was thought to be part of aging. It's now recognized that most cases of dry mouth are related to the medications taken by older adults rather than their age. Many common medications, including some over-the-counter drugs, produce dry mouth as a side effect.

Among the more likely drugs to cause problems are some depression and anxiety medications, antihistamines, high blood pressure medications, anti-diarrheals, muscle relaxants, drugs for urinary incontinence, and medications for Parkinson's disease.

Another cause of dry mouth is cancer therapy. Chemotherapy drugs can change the nature of saliva and the amount produced. Radiation treatments to the head and neck can damage salivary glands.

Nerve damage to the head and neck area can also result in dry mouth. Other conditions that can lead to dry mouth include salivary gland problems, endocrine disorders, Alzheimer's disease, stroke and Sjogren's syndrome, an autoimmune disorder.

In addition, smoking or chewing tobacco can affect saliva production, aggravating dry mouth. Snoring and breathing with your mouth open also can contribute to the problem.

Diagnosis

Your doctor or dentist likely will examine your mouth and go over your medical history. Sometimes, blood tests and imaging scans of the salivary glands are needed to identify the cause.

Treatment

If medication is believed to be the cause, your doctor may adjust your dosage or switch you to another medication that doesn't cause dry mouth. If a medical disorder is causing dry mouth, treating the underlying condition may help.

Other Health Risks

In addition to oral cancer, smokeless products such as spit tobacco and e-cigarettes increase your risk of:

Tooth and gum disorders

To speed the delivery of nicotine into your blood, spit tobacco contains abrasives such as sand. These substances make tiny cuts in your gums, causing you to lose gum tissue and even teeth. Gum recession isn't reversible and exposes the roots of your teeth, which makes them four times more prone to cavities.

Cardiovascular disease

Using spit tobacco increases your risk of high blood pressure, heart attack and stroke.

Other cancers

Using spit tobacco increases your risk of cancers of the esophagus, throat (pharynx), voice box (larynx), stomach, pancreas and prostate.

Quitting

Quitting is possible — either gradually or abruptly — and your doctor can help. Quitting spit tobacco use can be just as difficult as stopping smoking, and most people attempt it many times before quitting for good.

You'll probably experience withdrawal symptoms: cravings, irritability and difficulty concentrating. These steps may help you kick your spit tobacco habit:

- *Pick a stop date.* Mark the date on your calendar and stick to it.
- *Use less.* Even before you quit, cut back on the number of times you dip each day, increase the time between each dip, and leave the dip in your mouth for less time.
- *Avoid peer pressure.* Surround yourself with people who support your decision.
- *Use spit tobacco substitutes.* Other products may help keep you from returning to spit tobacco use. Try sugarless gum or hard candy, sunflower seeds, or beef jerky. Nontobacco chews and pouches, herbal chews, or certain dietary supplements also may help curb your cravings.
- *Don't give in to cravings.* Each craving usually lasts only three to five minutes. During a craving, divert your attention with deep breathing, exercise or munching on substitutes.
- *Talk to your doctor or dentist or call a tobacco quit line.* Your doctor or dentist can help you plan a strategy.
- *Medication.* Studies have shown that bupropion (Zyban) may help people quit spit tobacco. Nicotine gum, patch, inhaler or nasal spray also may be helpful. Consult your doctor about these products.

You can improve saliva flow by sucking on sugar-free hard candy or chewing sugar-free gum. Avoid lemon-flavored hard candy because it makes saliva acidic, increasing the risk of tooth decay. Your doctor may also consider prescribing the drug pilocarpine (Salagen) to stimulate saliva production.

In addition, you might try:
- Sipping water regularly throughout the day
- Using over-the-counter liquid or gel saliva substitutes that are sprayed or rubbed in the mouth to add moisture
- Breathing through your nose, not your mouth
- Adding moisture to the air at night with a bedroom humidifier

Salivary gland infections

Signs and symptoms
- Swelling in the floor of the mouth, under the jaw or in front of the ears
- Decreased saliva flow
- Peculiar tastes in the mouth
- Pain in the mouth

Viral infections, such as mumps, commonly affect the salivary glands. Bacterial infections may occur after obstruction of a salivary gland or may be associated with poor oral hygiene.

The enlarged gland may be quite painful and may limit your ability to open your mouth widely. A doctor or dentist may also notice pus at the opening of the duct.

Treatment generally involves antibiotics to clear the infection. Warm saltwater rinses — one-half teaspoon of salt mixed in 8 ounces of warm water — can often aid in removing the pus.

Salivary gland stones

Signs and symptoms
- Swelling under the chin or in front of the ear
- Lack of saliva, particularly when eating
- Pain in the mouth

Sialolithiasis is the medical term for a stone or stones in a salivary gland or its duct. Caused by chemicals from the saliva that harden (calcify) into a solid material, these stones can block the submandibular, sublingual or the parotid glands.

When the stone partially blocks a duct, you may experience pain, particularly during mealtimes when large quantities of saliva are needed. The engorged gland may become swollen, which may lead to gland infection.

Diagnosis
Your doctor may check for swelling under your chin or in front of your ear, which could indicate a blocked salivary duct. Other indications are lack of saliva and pain in the bottom of your mouth. An X-ray of your mouth can often help identify a blocked duct.

Treatment
A stone in a salivary duct can be removed by one of two methods: manipulation or excision. Your doctor may be able to push the stone out of the salivary duct. If not, the stone can be removed by a surgical procedure. Occasionally, a gland that has had repeated infections and recurrent salivary duct stones may need to be surgically removed.

Salivary duct tumors

Signs and symptoms
- Swelling under the jaw or in front of your ear

Rarely, cells in one of the salivary glands — usually one of the

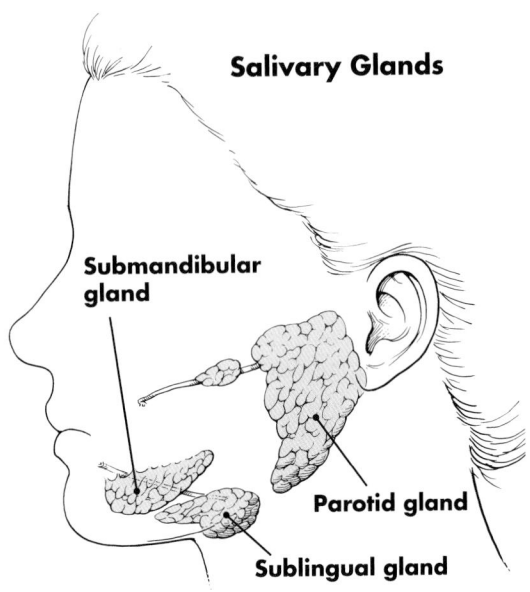

Salivary Glands

Submandibular gland

Parotid gland

Sublingual gland

parotid glands in the cheeks or submandibular glands under the jaw — multiply to form a tumor. In most cases, the growth is non-cancerous (benign) and self-contained. These tumors develop over a period of years and cause the gland to gradually swell.

People who've had radiation exposure to the jaw or neck are at increased risk of cancerous tumors in the salivary glands. Tobacco use also may increase the risk.

Diagnosis
A special X-ray called a sialogram is most often used to detect a salivary gland tumor. This test detects dye that's injected into the gland, revealing the flow of saliva into the mouth. Removal of some tumor tissue for examination (biopsy) is the only way to establish a cancer diagnosis.

Treatment
Treatment usually involves surgical removal of the involved gland. If the tumor is cancerous (malignant), radiation therapy or additional surgery may be recommended, as well, to help prevent spread of the cancer. ■

Heart and Blood Vessels

About the size of your fist, your heart is a hollow, muscular organ located under your rib cage beneath and to the left of your breastbone. Hard-working and powerful, the heart pumps blood to all parts of the body — each cell, muscle, bone and organ.

Every minute of your life, your heart beats approximately once a second and considerably faster when you're engaging in physical activity. It weighs about a pound yet pumps 5 or more quarts of blood a minute. Each day, your heart pumps the equivalent of about 2,000 gallons of blood through your circulatory system.

The blood your heart pumps provides individual cells with oxygen and nutrients they need. The circulatory system through which your blood passes consists of two main types of vessels. Arteries and their branches carry freshly oxygenated blood away from the heart to tissues throughout the body. Veins and their branches carry blood containing waste products, such as carbon dioxide, back to the heart and then to the lungs. The lungs remove the carbon dioxide and provide a fresh supply of oxygen.

If the pumping of your heart and the circulation of blood stops for more than a few minutes, life ends. In fact, all too often the first sign of heart and blood vessel (cardiovascular) disease is sudden death. This is a major reason so much emphasis is given to prevention of cardiovascular disease.

Your Heart

Your heart lies inside a thin sac of fibrous tissue called the pericardium. The heart has three layers of tissue: the epicardium, myocardium and endocardium.

The epicardium is a thin, shiny membrane covering the surface of the heart. Under the epicardium is a thick layer of muscle called the myocardium. The inside of the heart is lined with a smooth, shiny membrane called the endocardium. It covers the inside of the chambers of the heart, the heart valves and muscles in the heart chambers that attach to the valves.

The heart is made up of four chambers. The top two chambers are called the right and left atria (plural for atrium). The two lower chambers, the ventricles, are larger, thick-walled chambers that do the work of pumping blood to the lungs and the rest of the body.

The septum is a muscular wall that divides the right atrium from the left atrium and the right ventricle from the left ventricle. The septum prevents blood from passing directly from one side of the heart to the other. The right atrium and right ventricle are referred to as the right heart. The left atrium and left ventricle together are called the left heart.

Four flexible structures called valves keep blood flowing in the proper direction through the heart, to the lungs and then to the body.

Double pump

You might think of your heart as a double pump operating in a parallel fashion. One pump, the right heart, receives blood from all parts of the body through two large veins called the superior vena cava and inferior vena cava. Blood headed for the right heart has just delivered oxygen and nutrients to the body. Because it has less oxygen, this blood is called deoxygenated blood. The right heart pumps

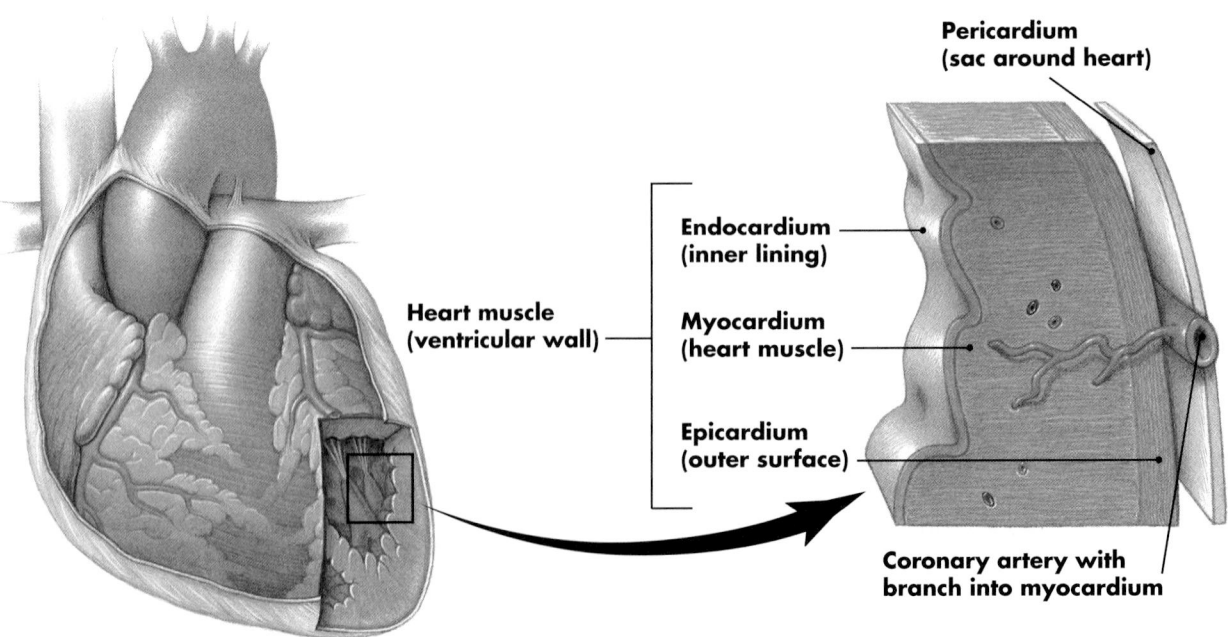

Heart muscle (ventricular wall)

Pericardium (sac around heart)

Endocardium (inner lining)

Myocardium (heart muscle)

Epicardium (outer surface)

Coronary artery with branch into myocardium

this blood to the lungs, where it picks up additional oxygen from air sacs (alveoli). Blood then leaves the lungs and returns to the heart, arriving in the left atrium. From there it's pumped to the left ventricle and then to the body by way of the aorta, the largest blood vessel in the body. The aorta divides into several branches to supply blood to various parts of the body.

These parts of the heart work together to create the double-pump action of the heart. It receives blood from veins, pumps it to the lungs, receives it back from the lungs and pumps it into the body by way of arteries. This cycle is repeated thousands of times each day.

Cardiac cycle

On the right side of the heart, the tricuspid valve allows blood to flow from the right atrium into the right ventricle and prevents blood from flowing in the opposite direction.

From the right ventricle, the blood is pumped through the pul- monary valve to the lungs, where it picks up oxygen from the air sacs and disposes of carbon dioxide and other waste products into them.

From the left atrium, the blood flows through the mitral valve into the left ventricle. From the left ventricle, the blood is pumped through the aortic valve and then to the rest of your body, includ- ing your brain, other organs and extremities.

In this cycle, the atria serve as the priming pumps and the ventricles as the main pumps responsible for circulating blood. While many people can live without effective atrial function, death ensues within minutes if the ventricles cease to function.

Systole and diastole

Contraction of the ventricles, which forces blood out to the lungs and other parts of the body, is called systole. Relaxation of the ventricles to allow blood to enter them is referred to as diastole. The right and left chambers contract and relax simultaneously.

The rate at which the heart con- tracts and relaxes varies, depend- ing on your body's activities at the moment. When you're at rest, your heart pumps more slowly. When you run or climb stairs, the pace of your heart increases to provide your muscles and other tissues with additional oxygen.

Natural pacemaker

Unlike other muscles in your body, which rely on brain or spinal cord nerve connections to receive the electrical stimulation they need to function, your heart has its own electrical stimulator — a natural pacemaker that transmits electric impulses signaling the heart to beat.

These electric impulses course through a network of specialized fibers within the heart, stimulat- ing the atria to contract and move blood into the ventricles, and the ventricles to contract and force blood out to the lungs and the rest of the body.

With each heartbeat, blood circu- lates throughout body. The typical heart rate is about 72 beats a minute, and with each beat 2 to 3 ounces of blood are pumped into the arterial system. At this rate, the heart beats about 104,000 times daily.

Your Blood Vessels

Your vascular system consists of the blood vessels in your body. Its name comes from the Latin word *vasculum* for "a small vessel."

The further a blood vessel extends from the heart, the smaller it becomes. The aorta, the principal blood vessel in your body, delivers blood from your heart to the larger arteries. These arteries, in turn, branch into smaller arteries, which become tiny arterioles. They even- tually become so small that only a

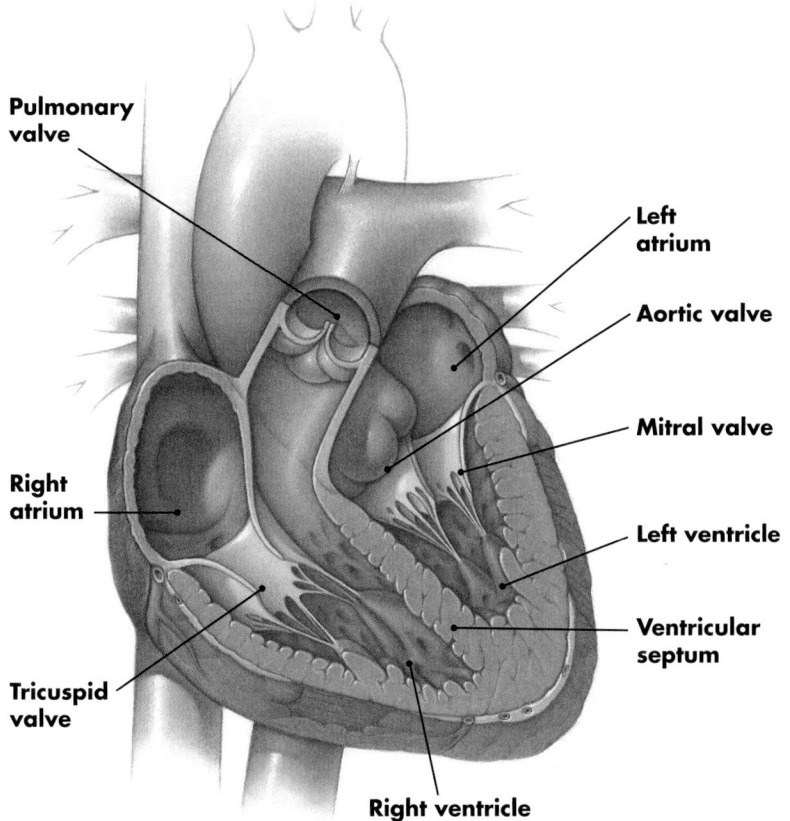

Pulmonary valve

Right atrium

Tricuspid valve

Right ventricle

Left atrium

Aortic valve

Mitral valve

Left ventricle

Ventricular septum

Diastole   **Systole**

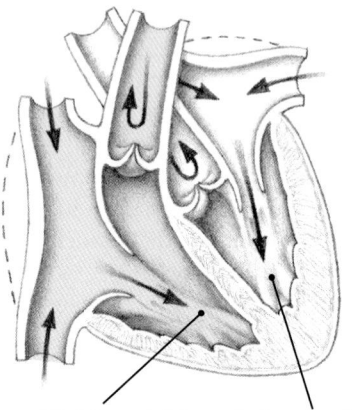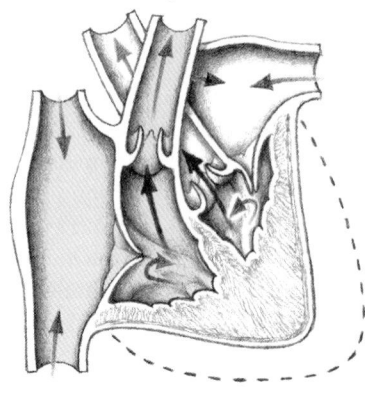

Right ventricle   Left ventricle

The heart pumps in two stages. The ventricles relax during diastole so that blood can enter the heart. They contract during systole to pump blood out.

single blood cell can pass through at a time. These smallest vessels are called capillaries. Capillaries deliver oxygen and nutrients to your tissues and pick up waste, such as carbon dioxide, from your cells.

Blood begins its return trip to your heart through tiny veins called venules. Blood flows from venules to larger and larger veins until it reaches the right atrium. Your veins, which are under less pressure, aren't as muscular and elastic as your arteries.

Like all muscles in your body, your heart needs oxygen and nutrients from blood to survive. Thus, it has its own pair of arteries, called coronary arteries. These special heart vessels are the first branches off the aorta just as it leaves the heart. The right coronary artery supplies blood to the bottom and back of the heart. The left coronary artery supplies the top, front and left sides, as well as an area of the back of the heart (see the illustration on page 716).

Blood pressure

To keep blood moving, there must be pressure in your blood vessels

Interpreting Your Heartbeat

For most of us, the feel of a stethoscope on our chest is familiar. Less familiar is the bass drum heart thumping your doctor hears through the other end of the hearing device. Heart sounds can provide your doctor with considerable information about your heart and your health.

When listening to your heart, your doctor may ask you to breathe in and out naturally or perhaps in a deliberately rhythmic fashion. He or she may move the stethoscope in small steps from one location to another over your chest.

A normal heartbeat has a consistent pattern represented by the syllables *lubb* and *dupp*. These sounds correspond to closure of the heart valves. *Lubb* is followed by a short pause, and *dupp* is followed by a longer pause.

Differences in the intensity of these heart sounds may provide clues to possible disease involving your heart or lungs. Obesity, emphysema or fluid around the heart can muffle the heart's pumping sounds.

Other sounds also may be detected. Murmurs are the result of turbulence in the blood during the heartbeat. Depending on the location and character of the murmur and its relationship to the lubb-dupp sounds, your doctor can often identify a structural change in the heart that's responsible for the turbulence.

The presence of abnormal sounds during the relaxation (diastole) phase of your heart rhythm suggests an alteration in the function of the heart muscle. Sounds heard during the contraction (systole) phase, often called clicks, combined with a murmur identify specific types of valve abnormalities.

A heart murmur may be a sign of anemia, a leaky valve or other problems. Some murmurs are benign and aren't associated with a heart condition. In children, murmurs that aren't the result of a structural abnormality can sometimes be heard. Called innocent murmurs, they're typically faint, often heard only intermittently and detected in only a small area of the chest. Innocent murmurs are harmless and may disappear by adulthood.

When your doctor listens to your heartbeat, he or she is gathering clues regarding the health of your heart.

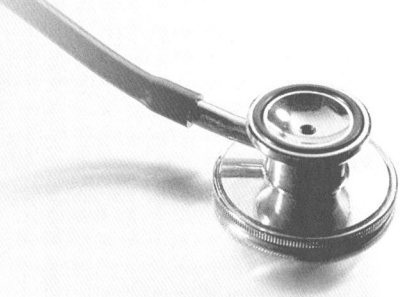

at all times. During the contraction (systole) phase — when the left ventricle pumps blood into the arteries — the pressure rises (systolic pressure). This is the moment of highest pressure. During the relaxation (diastole) phase — between heartbeats while the left ventricle is refilling — the pressure falls (diastolic pressure). This is the moment of lowest pressure.

A blood pressure cuff (sphygmomanometer) is the instrument used to measure blood pressure in units of millimeters of mercury (mm Hg). Your blood pressure is written like a fraction — the systolic number is on the top, and the diastolic number is on the bottom. When stated verbally, the word *over* is generally used to separate the two numbers. For example, a blood pressure reading of 120/80 mm Hg would be described as "120 over 80."

Risk Factors

Heart and blood vessel (cardiovascular) disease has been the No. 1 killer in the United States every year since 1900, except for 1918 when an influenza epidemic briefly claimed the spot.

About 1 in 5 Americans has some form of cardiovascular disease, whether it's high blood pressure, coronary artery disease, a stroke or congestive heart failure.

Because of its serious nature and wide prevalence, a tremendous amount of research is being directed at improving doctors' understanding of cardiovascular disease, which should continue to result in better treatments and, perhaps more important, prevention.

Researchers continue to investigate the cause-and-effect relationships between our behavior, genes and aging processes and the ways our hearts function and malfunction. Many ongoing, long-term medical studies, such as the Multiple Risk Factor Intervention Trial

---

? Question and Answer

How is cardiovascular disease different from heart disease?

The phrase *cardiovascular disease* is often used interchangeably with *heart disease*. However, *cardiovascular* is a more inclusive term than *heart* because it takes into account not only the heart but also all of the arteries, capillaries and veins that are directly or indirectly connected to the heart. In this sense, the term *cardiovascular disease* includes not only diseases of the heart but also of the blood vessels, such as a stroke.

---

and the Framingham Heart Study, have brought about a new level of understanding as to why cardiovascular disease is so common.

The findings are persuasive. A remarkably high percentage of people with cardiovascular disease have a history of certain risk factors. Risk factors are lifestyle habits or family characteristics that increase your likelihood of developing a certain disease.

Risk factors for cardiovascular disease include some things in life over which you have no control — sex, age and heredity — and aspects of your life that you often can control — tobacco use, body weight, physical activity, blood cholesterol levels, high blood pressure and elevated blood sugar (glucose).

As you read through the following pages, remember that ways of controlling cardiovascular disease are constantly evolving. As investigators search for the best forms of prevention and treatment, conflicting findings sometimes result.

Some studies suggest that causal relationships exist between certain dietary habits and cardiovascular disease, and others conclude

---

there's no clear-cut evidence of this. Still, studies are consistently finding that your lifestyle habits are likely to have an important effect on the health of your heart and blood vessels.

Also keep in mind that risk refers to odds or chances, not to inevitability. Risk factors can affect your chances of having cardiovascular disease, but they don't automatically guarantee that you'll develop it.

Smoking

Since the Surgeon General announced that smoking tobacco is a health hazard, cigarette manufacturers have been required to place a printed warning of the hazards of smoking on every package of cigarettes sold in the United States. In the years since, that warning has been made more emphatic — and an immense amount of clinical, statistical and other research has reinforced the original point.

Smoking is harmful — not only because of the association between smoking and lung cancer but also because smoking is high on the list of risk factors for cardiovascular disease.

If you smoke cigarettes, your risk of a heart attack or stroke is at least double that of nonsmokers. The risk increases with the number of cigarettes you smoke each day. Cigarette smokers who have a heart attack are more likely to die and die suddenly — within an hour — than are nonsmokers. Cigars, pipes and chewing tobacco seem to increase your risk as well, but to a lesser degree.

When smoking is combined with other risk factors, such as high blood pressure, high blood cholesterol or a family history of heart problems, the risk of cardiovascular disease appears to increase greatly.

Complications
Smoking a cigarette causes your adrenal glands to secrete a hormone that temporarily increases your blood pressure and makes

your heart work harder. In addition, smoking decreases the amount of oxygen available to your heart. As a result, every cigarette places a small but unnecessary load on your heart and blood vessels.

Smokers also have more fatty deposits (plaques) in their arteries (atherosclerosis) than nonsmokers do. This is likely because smoke increases the clumping of certain blood cells (platelets), which stimulates the deposit of cholesterol in arteries. Because the process of atherosclerosis is accelerated by both high blood pressure and smoking — likely due to the harmful effects of nicotine and carbon monoxide on blood vessels — a smoker with high blood pressure is at much greater risk of atherosclerosis.

Damage to arteries that supply blood to your limbs can also lead to claudication, a condition that produces leg pain and muscle cramping while walking. Claudication can also affect your arms. In severe cases, claudication can severely interrupt blood flow in your legs and feet, increasing the risk of amputation.

Tobacco smoke contains carbon monoxide gas. When inhaled, carbon monoxide binds to hemoglobin, the oxygen-carrying pigment in blood, and takes the place of oxygen. The result is that blood traveling to all parts of your body carries less oxygen to your cells. Often, as much as 8 percent of a smoker's hemoglobin may be occupied by carbon monoxide, making it unable to carry out its normal function of transporting oxygen.

Research suggests that carbon monoxide may have a direct, degenerative effect on the heart muscle itself, on the blood vessels and perhaps even on the clotting of your blood. Low-tar, low-nicotine cigarettes also can produce carbon monoxide and thus can't be considered safe.

Benefits of quitting smoking

The cumulative harmful effects of smoking on your body's organs argue convincingly for quitting. Furthermore, quitting smoking may actually reverse some of the damage smoking caused initially.

After a year of not using tobacco, your risk of coronary artery disease, including heart attacks and chest pain (angina), is reduced by half. After 15 years of abstinence, your risk is similar to that of someone who has never smoked. And the earlier you quit, the more years you can expect to add to your life.

It's not easy to quit tobacco. It generally takes most people three to four attempts before they're successful. However, each try increases your chances of future success. See page 313 for more information.

Obesity

If your weight exceeds a "desirable" level for your height and sex by 20 percent or more, you're considered to be seriously overweight, or obese.

Defining *overweight* and *obese*

Doctors define desirable weight by means of body mass index (BMI). Your BMI is a sex-based estimate of body fat that's calculated from your weight and height. It's a better measure of your health risks than is your weight alone or than weight tables based only on your height. See the BMI chart on page 267.

A BMI between 25 to 29 is considered overweight. Obesity is defined as a BMI of 30 or more. If you're very muscular, you may be an exception because BMI doesn't account for heavily muscled people with relatively little body fat.

By BMI definitions, 70 percent of the adult population is overweight, and about 38 percent is obese. Childhood obesity also is at an all-time high. Obesity figures have reached epidemic proportions.

Complications

As you put on weight, you gain mostly fatty tissue. Like other parts of your body, this tissue requires oxygen and nutrients from your blood. As demands for oxygen and nutrients increase, the amount of blood circulating through your body also must increase. Being overweight or obese increases your risk of high blood pressure.

Excess body fat is also associated with elevated blood levels of low-density lipoprotein (LDL, or "bad") cholesterol and triglycerides and a reduced level of high-density lipoprotein (HDL, or "good") cholesterol. Over time, these changes in blood fats can contribute to the buildup of fatty deposits (plaques) in your arteries, a condition called atherosclerosis. Atherosclerosis puts you at risk of coronary artery disease and strokes.

Obesity has other harmful effects. It's a major cause of type 2 diabetes and gallstones, and it can worsen sleep apnea and degenerative joint disease. Several types of cancer are associated with being overweight as well. In women, these include cancer of the breast, uterus, colon and gallbladder. Overweight men have a higher risk of colon and prostate cancer.

Benefits of losing weight

Even small amounts of weight loss are beneficial. The amount of weight you need to lose to improve your health may be much less than what you feel you need to lose. Losing just 10 percent of your current weight if you're obese can have a positive effect on your health. Slow and steady weight loss of 1 or 2 pounds a week is considered the safest way to lose weight and keep it off. For more information on healthy weight loss, see Chapter 8, "Nutrition and Weight."

Physical inactivity

Physical inactivity is a major risk factor for cardiovascular disease. It also contributes to other risk factors, including obesity, diabetes, high blood pressure and a low level of high-density lipoprotein (HDL, or "good") cholesterol.

Complications

Being inactive approximately doubles your risk of coronary artery disease and is comparable to the risk observed with high blood cholesterol, high blood pressure or cigarette smoking. In addition, sedentary people have a greater risk of developing high blood pressure.

Benefits of physical activity

Regular, moderate-to-vigorous exercise plays an important role in preventing cardiovascular disease. Even modest levels of physical activity are beneficial if done regularly and over the long term.

Daily physical activity can decrease your risk of cardiovascular disease. It increases the amount of "good" cholesterol in your blood, decreases the levels of "bad" cholesterol and triglycerides, reduces high blood pressure, improves the efficiency of your heart muscle, and helps you control your weight. Regular exercise can also reduce the risk of a second heart attack and death.

In addition to benefiting your heart and blood vessels, physical activity benefits other parts of your body. It builds healthy bones, muscles and joints and reduces the risk of colon cancer. Physical activity also brings psychological benefits. It reduces feelings of depression and anxiety, improves mood, and promotes a feeling of well-being.

Aerobic and anaerobic exercise

Not all types of exercise have the same effect on your body. Aerobic exercise, which includes activities such as moderate-paced walking, jogging, bicycling and swimming, improves cardiovascular fitness by causing your body to continuously use extra oxygen and calories while exercising.

Your heart rate and depth of breathing increase, and your body becomes warmer. If the exercise is sufficiently long and vigorous, you'll perspire.

Anaerobic exercise, such as weight training, strengthens and tones your muscles through short periods of intense exercise. Anaerobic activities generally aren't as beneficial to your heart because they often don't challenge your heart and lungs to deliver oxygen in a sustained fashion to your body's tissues.

To benefit from regular physical activity, you don't need to develop a formal fitness plan or sign up for an organized activity — unless, of course, that's the only way you'll commit to regular conditioning. What's important is regular exercise, which should include three parts: warm-up, aerobic conditioning and cool-down.

Choose an exercise routine that's frequent enough, intense enough, of sufficient duration and of the appropriate type to gradually improve your health. Many people do a lot of walking at work or frequently move about during the day. However, for exercise to be of benefit, it needs to be uninterrupted and of adequate duration.

In general, try to burn about 1,000 to 2,000 calories a week with exercise. Walking 10 to 20 miles a week accomplishes that goal for the average person. Unless you're trying to lose weight, there's no evidence that you'll reduce your cardiovascular risks further by burning off more than 2,000 calories a week. For more information on how to develop a fitness program, see Chapter 9, "Fitness."

Are You an Apple or a Pear?

If you're overweight, observing where your fat is concentrated can help you assess your risk of obesity-related diseases. If your weight is concentrated around your abdomen, giving you an apple shape, your risk may be higher than if your weight is concentrated around your hips and thighs, resembling a pear shape.

To find out if you're an apple or a pear, measure your waist circumference just above your hipbones and your hip circumference at the widest part of your buttocks. Then divide your waist measurement by your hip measurement. A waist-to-hip ratio greater than 0.95 for men or 0.80 for women indicates an apple shape.

Undesirable blood fats

Cholesterol is a substance found in the bloodstream and in all of your body's cells. It's an important part of a healthy body because it's used to form cell membranes, some hormones and other needed tissues. But an undesirable blood cholesterol level is a major risk factor for coronary artery disease, which can lead to a heart attack.

Cholesterol comes from two sources. It's produced in your body, primarily by the liver, and it's found in foods that come from animals, such as meats, poultry, fish, seafood and dairy products. Fish is generally lower in cholesterol than are other meats. Foods from plants, such as fruits, vegetables, grains, nuts and seeds, don't contain cholesterol.

Triglycerides are a form of fat that circulate in your blood and are a source of energy. A high level of triglycerides is linked to coronary artery disease and possibly inflammation of the pancreas (pancreatitis).

Types

Important substances and fat found in blood include:

Low-density lipoprotein

Low-density lipoprotein (LDL) cholesterol is the major cholesterol carrier in the blood. LDL transports cholesterol to sites throughout your body, where it's either deposited or used to repair cell

Before You Start

For most people, the health advantages of regular physical activity far outweigh possible risks. However, if you have a chronic health condition or several risk factors for cardiovascular disease, some special precautions might apply. Check with your doctor before you begin an exercise program if you:

• Have heart, lung or kidney disease, diabetes or arthritis
• Are age 40 or older
• Are obese
• Have parents or siblings who've experienced coronary artery disease before age 55
• Are unsure of your health status

Your doctor may advise you to have an exercise stress test to help determine if physical activity is likely to cause an insufficient supply of blood and oxygen to reach your heart or to provoke heart rhythm abnormalities (see page 731). Discuss with your doctor any exercise limitations that he or she would suggest because of a health condition that you have.

If you've previously been sedentary, start with five- to 10-minute sessions of physical activity and gradually build up to your desired level of activity. Your doctor can help you determine a desirable (target) heart rate to strive for while exercising. Achieving this target heart rate brings you the maximum benefit from the activity. As your fitness improves, your target heart rate may change.

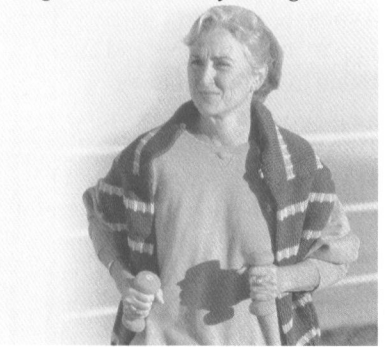

membranes. But like hard water that causes lime to build up inside plumbing, LDL cholesterol promotes accumulation of cholesterol in the arteries feeding your heart and brain.

Combined with other substances, LDL cholesterol can form thick, hard deposits (plaques) that clog the arteries and cause them to narrow (atherosclerosis), increasing your risk of a heart attack and stroke. This is why LDL cholesterol is often called the "bad" cholesterol.

High-density lipoprotein

Think of high-density lipoprotein (HDL) as a scavenger or clean-up form of cholesterol. It helps decrease the amount of LDL cholesterol in your blood. For this reason, HDL cholesterol is thought of as the "good" cholesterol.

Higher values of HDL cholesterol mean a lower risk of atherosclerosis. Your HDL cholesterol level tends to increase with exercise and weight loss, but considerable amounts of exercise may be needed before significant results are seen.

Triglycerides

Triglycerides are a type of blood fat. An excess amount of triglycerides in your blood is called hypertriglyceridemia. This condition is thought to favor development of atherosclerosis, but this relationship isn't nearly as clear as that for LDL cholesterol and total cholesterol values.

Causes

Some people appear to have a genetic predisposition to an abnormal cholesterol or triglyceride level. One rare hereditary disorder, called familial hypercholesterolemia, causes such high levels of cholesterol that the affected person may experience a heart attack in childhood. Those who inherit a lesser form of this disorder have very high cholesterol levels and often have heart attacks by midlife

or earlier. The trend to a high triglyceride level also may be in one's genetic makeup.

Diseases such as hypothyroidism, diabetes and kidney failure may influence blood fat levels. Some medications may have an adverse effect. For many people, though, abnormal blood-fat levels are a result of an unhealthy diet and too little exercise.

Measuring blood fats

Early detection of high blood cholesterol or triglycerides allows you to take steps to improve your health and prevent cardiovascular disease. The only way to find out your cholesterol and triglyceride levels is by having them measured with a blood test. To get the best results, it's important to fast prior to having a cholesterol test.

A typical lipids test measures total cholesterol, HDL cholesterol and triglycerides. Tests that measure only total cholesterol can be misleading because some people have a low level of HDL cholesterol and a high level of triglycerides but a normal or even high level of LDL cholesterol. In these cases, a total cholesterol measurement might appear normal, and you and your doctor would be unaware of cardiovascular disease risks posed by the abnormal levels that weren't measured. Even with a desirable total cholesterol level, if you have a low HDL level, you may be at increased risk of heart disease.

Desirable ranges for cholesterol levels depend on your age, sex, family history and overall health status. There's no magic number that separates risky levels from safe levels. Rather, researchers and doctors have identified lipid levels above which your risk of developing heart and blood vessel complications is high enough to warrant lifestyle changes.

Benefits of managing blood fats

If you have a family history of high cholesterol and triglyceride levels or a heart attack or stroke at an early age, you're at greater risk of developing atherosclerosis. You can't do anything to change your heredity, but you can take precautions by having your blood cholesterol measured regularly as recommended by your doctor, and by following a healthy diet, controlling your weight and avoiding tobacco.

The primary goal of cholesterol management is to reduce an abnormally high level of LDL cholesterol. After assessing your cholesterol levels, major cardiovascular risk factors and your 10-year risk, your doctor can help you establish an LDL goal.

Lifestyle changes are usually the first line of treatment. You want to try this approach first. If lifestyle changes don't work or if your LDL cholesterol is very high, medication is generally recommended.

Reduce fat and cholesterol intake
Keep all types of fat — saturated, polyunsaturated, monounsaturated and trans fats — within a range of 25 to 30 percent of your daily calories. Eat monounsaturated and polyunsaturated fats, which can help lower your LDL cholesterol, limit saturated fat and avoid trans fats.

In addition, limit your daily cholesterol intake to less than 200 milligrams. You can accomplish this goal by limiting or avoiding concentrated sources of cholesterol, such as fatty or heavily processed meats, egg yolks and whole milk products.

Eat foods with soluble fiber
Soluble fiber can help lower your total blood cholesterol level. Foods high in soluble fiber include oat bran, oatmeal, beans, peas, rice bran, barley, citrus fruits, strawberries and apple pulp.

Eat whole grains
A variety of nutrients found in whole grains promote heart health. Choose whole-grain

What Do the Numbers Mean?

Results are listed as a set of numbers in milligrams per deciliter (mg/dL) indicating total cholesterol, low-density lipoprotein (LDL, or "bad") cholesterol and high-density (HDL, or "good") cholesterol and triglyceride levels. The chart below can help you determine which numbers are acceptable and which ones may carry increased risk. As you compare your numbers with these values, remember that numbers alone don't tell the whole story. Ask your doctor to interpret your test results.

Cholesterol and triglyceride classifications

Total cholesterol

Mg/dL*	What your level means
<200	Desirable
200-239	Borderline high
≥240	High

LDL ('bad') cholesterol

Mg/dL	What your level means
<70	Best if you have heart disease or diabetes
<100	Optimal
100-129	Near optimal
130-159	Borderline high
160-189	High
≥190	Very high

HDL ('good') cholesterol

Mg/dL	What your level means
<40 (men) <50 (women)	Poor
50-59	Better
≥60	Best

HDL cholesterol protects against cardiovascular disease, so for HDL, higher numbers are better.

Triglycerides

Mg/dL	What your level means
<150	Desirable
150-199	Borderline high
200-499	High
≥500	Very high

*Milligrams per deciliter

Adapted from *Journal of Clinical Lipidology*, 2015;9:129 and *Circulation*, 2014;129 (suppl 2).

Know Your Fats

Foods contain several different kinds of fats.

Saturated fats

Most saturated fats come from foods of animal origin — meats, milk and milk products. Plant sources of fat include the tropical oils: coconut oil, palm kernel oil, palm oil and cocoa butter. Unlike other plant oils, tropical oils are composed predominantly of saturated fatty acids. They're common ingredients in commercial cakes, cookies and other snack foods. Saturated fats contribute to low-density lipoprotein (LDL) cholesterol (the "bad" cholesterol).

Monounsaturated fats

Olive, peanut and canola oils are sources of monounsaturated fats. Unlike saturated fats, monounsaturated fats, in recommended amounts, help lower total blood cholesterol and resist oxidation, the process that enables cells in your arteries to absorb fats and cholesterol.

Polyunsaturated fats

Like monounsaturated fats, polyunsaturated fats are found in many vegetable oils and help to lower your total and LDL blood cholesterol levels. Unlike monounsaturated fats, however, polyunsaturated fats are vulnerable to oxidation.

Trans fats

Trans fats (trans-fatty acids) are often produced when polyunsaturated fats undergo the chemical process of hydrogenation. One example is margarine. When it's hydrogenated, some of its polyunsaturated fatty acids are converted to saturated fats or trans fats. This process makes the fat more solid. The greater the degree of hydrogenation, the more saturated the fat becomes.

Research indicates that trans fats raise your total cholesterol and LDL cholesterol level, and lower your high-density lipoprotein (HDL) cholesterol (the "good" cholesterol) level. Some of the main sources of trans fats include margarine and vegetable shortening, as well as products made from them, such as cookies, desserts, crackers and other prepared foods.

breads, whole-wheat pasta, whole-wheat flour and brown rice. Oatmeal and oat bran are other good choices.

Eat fruits and vegetables

Fruits and vegetables are rich in dietary fiber, which can help lower cholesterol. Snack on seasonal fruits.

Eat heart-healthy fish

Some types of fish — such as cod, tuna and halibut — have less total fat, saturated fat and cholesterol than do meat and poultry. Salmon, mackerel and herring are rich in omega-3 fatty acids, which help promote heart health.

Drink alcohol only in moderation

Moderate use of alcohol may increase your levels of HDL cholesterol — but the benefits aren't strong enough to recommend alcohol for anyone who doesn't drink already. If you choose to drink, do so in moderation. This means no more than one drink a day for women and one to two drinks a day for men.

Exercise regularly

Regular physical activity, such as brisk walking, jogging, bicycling or cross-country skiing, helps increase your level of HDL cholesterol. An exercise program can also help you lose weight, which in turn decreases your risk of cardiovascular disease.

Don't smoke

Cigarette smoking damages the walls of your blood vessels, making it easier for cholesterol to accumulate. It may also lower your level of HDL cholesterol.

Atherosclerosis

When fatty deposits (plaques) and other substances accumulate in your arteries and cause them to narrow, blood flow becomes restricted. This condition is called atherosclerosis. It's a leading cause of blockage of the blood vessels to your heart (coronary arteries), which can result in a heart attack or chest pain (angina).

When the inner wall of an artery is injured, blood cells called platelets often clump at microscopic sites of injury. At these sites, fatty deposits also collect. Initially, the deposits are only streaks of fat-containing cells, but as they progress, they invade some deeper layers of the arterial walls, causing scarring and calcium deposits. Larger accumulations of plaques are the principal characteristic of atherosclerosis.

Complications

The greatest danger from these deposits is the narrowing of the channel through which the blood flows. When this occurs, body tissues supplied by an affected artery don't receive their full quota of blood, particularly during exercise, when demand is greatest. Pieces of the fatty deposits may dislodge, travel with the blood flow and obstruct an artery at some distant point — a condition called arterial embolism.

Atherosclerosis is one form of arteriosclerosis, but the two terms are often used interchangeably. The term *arteriosclerosis* refers to hardening of the arteries. As calcium is deposited in an artery, its walls may become more rigid or hardened. Sometimes, arteries in the forearms can be felt and may resemble small, hard pipes.

To some extent, your body can protect itself from narrowing of an artery by gradually developing additional arterial connections that detour blood around the narrowed point. This is referred to as collateral circulation.

If you have a significant amount of atherosclerosis in one part of your body, you're more likely to have some degree of the disease in another part. For instance, a person who has poor arterial circulation in his or her legs is more vulnerable to angina or a heart attack because of similar narrowing of the coronary arteries.

Treatment may involve procedures to open narrowed segments of your arteries or surgery to bypass the plaques, as well as steps to control further accumulations of plaques through dietary measures and, possibly, use of medication. For more information on the treatment of atherosclerosis, see page 719.

High blood pressure

Your blood pressure is the force that's exerted on your artery walls as blood passes through. You might compare it to the pressure inside a garden hose. Your heart, arteries and kidneys all work together to control the amount of pressure put on your artery walls. When this complex system malfunctions, too much pressure can develop within your arteries. If this condition continues on a

Cholesterol Medications

The specific choice of medication or combination of medications depends on various factors, including your individual risk factors, your age, your current health and possible side effects. Common choices include:

Statins
Statins are among the most commonly prescribed drugs for lowering cholesterol. They block a substance your liver needs to make cholesterol. This causes your liver to remove cholesterol from your blood. Statins may also help your body reabsorb cholesterol from built-up deposits on your artery walls, potentially reversing coronary artery disease.

Examples include atorvastatin (Lipitor), fluvastatin (Lescol XL), lovastatin (Altoprev), pitavastatin (Livalo), pravastatin (Pravachol), rosuvastatin (Crestor) and simvastatin (Zocor).

Bile-acid-binding resins
Your liver uses cholesterol to make bile acids, a substance needed for digestion. The medications cholestyramine (Prevalite), colesevelam (Welchol) and colestipol (Colestid) lower cholesterol indirectly by binding to bile acids. This prompts your liver to use excess cholesterol to make more bile

acids, which reduces the level of cholesterol in your blood.

Cholesterol absorption inhibitors
Your small intestine absorbs the cholesterol from the food you eat and releases it into your bloodstream. The drug ezetimibe (Zetia) helps reduce blood cholesterol by limiting the absorption of dietary cholesterol. Ezetimibe can be used in combination with a statin drug.

Injectable medications
A new class of drugs can help the liver absorb more LDL cholesterol — which lowers the amount of cholesterol circulating in your blood. The medications alirocumab (Praluent) and evolocumab (Repatha) may be used in people who have a genetic condition that causes very high levels of LDL. They also may be prescribed for individuals with a history of coronary disease who have an intolerance to statins or other cholesterol medications.

Most of these medications are well-tolerated, but effectiveness varies from person to person. The common side effects are muscle pains, stomach pain, constipation, nausea and diarrhea. Your doctor may recommend liver function tests to monitor the medication's effect on your liver.

persistent basis, it's called high blood pressure (hypertension). Often, high blood pressure causes no symptoms.

Complications
High blood pressure is an important risk factor for cardiovascular disease. Left uncontrolled over a period of years, high blood

pressure can damage arteries throughout your body so that their walls become thickened and stiff (arteriosclerosis) and obstructed (atherosclerosis), thus decreasing blood flow to vital organs.

Your body responds to this threat by increasing blood pressure to maintain an adequate flow of blood. The increase in blood

Cardiovascular Disease: Men vs. Women

Women sometimes think that concerns about cardiovascular disease don't really apply to them. True, men tend to develop heart disease earlier than women do. However, over time, women and men are equally likely to die of a heart attack.

Until puberty, males and females have roughly the same level of "good" — high-density lipoprotein (HDL) — cholesterol. However, during puberty, the level of HDL cholesterol in males decreases, making them more susceptible to cardiovascular disease.

In females, the hormone estrogen tends to increase the level of "good" cholesterol and lower the level of "bad" — low-density lipoprotein (LDL) — cholesterol, thus providing a potentially protective effect against cardiovascular disease. Following menopause, when estrogen levels are decreased, women become increasingly likely to have heart attacks and related problems.

Before the age of 60, men are the most likely candidates for heart attacks. After age 60, the difference in risk between men and women narrows. However, these patterns could change. Due to an increase in the number of women who smoke, women are beginning to experience heart attacks at earlier ages.

pressure in turn results in further blood vessel damage, setting a vicious cycle in motion. This cycle exacts a toll on your heart, too, because your heart is forced to work harder. The heart muscle may thicken — called cardiac hypertrophy — to accommodate its added load. Aside from affecting your heart, high blood pressure can affect blood vessels in your kidneys, eyes and brain.

For information on diagnosis and treatment of high blood pressure, see page 708. Many of its complications can be avoided with proper management, which may include lifestyle changes and medication.

Diabetes

Diabetes is characterized by a lack of insulin or your body's resistance to this hormone, resulting in the body's inability to process sugars found in your diet. The use of insulin and other medications has made the disease manageable, but diabetes remains an important risk factor for cardiovascular disease.

Complications

Increased blood sugar (glucose) levels are often accompanied by increased cholesterol and triglyceride levels and blood vessel problems. Men with diabetes have about twice the normal risk of coronary artery disease, and women with diabetes have five times the risk. An individual with diabetes who smokes is at particularly high risk of cardiovascular disease.

If you have diabetes, careful management of your blood sugar levels can reduce your risk of heart and blood vessel problems. For more information on diabetes, see Chapter 28, "Endocrine System."

Family history

Your genes help determine your risk of developing cardiovascular disease, but heredity factors are complex. In simple terms, if one of your parents or another close relative had a heart attack at a young age — for a man, younger than age 55, and for a woman, younger than age 65 — then your risk of coronary artery disease is significantly greater than that of someone with no family history of cardiac problems. This doesn't mean that you're destined to suffer the same fate. It argues strongly, though, for taking every preventive advantage offered to minimize the risk factors that you can control.

If you don't have a family history of cardiovascular disease, you can still develop the condition. Therefore, individuals without a strong genetic link also need to pay attention to cardiovascular risk factors.

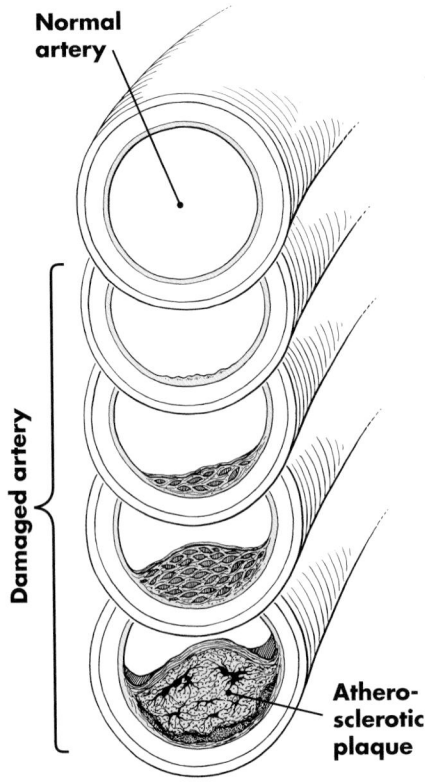

Atherosclerotic fatty deposits (plaques) gradually develop in the lining of the arteries. As plaques form, blood circulation decreases. This increases the risk of a heart attack, stroke and other serious vascular problems.

Emerging risk factors

As researchers gain a better understanding of cardiovascular disease and its causes and treatment, other potential risk factors are emerging. If you have a strong family history of cardiovascular disease, your doctor may recommend monitoring one or more of the following blood substances:

Homocysteine
Homocysteine is a natural byproduct of your body's use of protein. Research indicates a relationship between high homocysteine levels in your blood and an increased risk of coronary artery disease. Folic acid and vitamins B-6 and B-12 can help lower homocysteine levels, although it hasn't yet been proved that such treatment decreases the risk of coronary artery disease.

Lipoprotein lipase
Lipoprotein lipase is an enzyme that regulates the metabolism of lipids and lipoproteins. The way it operates isn't well-understood. Some evidence links elevated levels of lipoprotein lipase in the blood to premature heart attacks.

C-reactive protein
The level of C-reactive protein (CRP) in your blood increases when inflammation is present. Some studies show that the process of inflammation — your body's reaction to injury — plays a role in the buildup of fatty deposits (plaques) in your arteries (atherosclerosis). If this is true, then an elevated CRP level may be an indicator of atherosclerosis and a potential predictor for first heart attacks.

Fibrinogen
Fibrinogen is a protein made by the liver that's important in blood clotting. In some studies, an elevated level of fibrinogen in the blood has been associated with a greater risk of cardiovascular disease. Other cardiovascular risk factors, including smoking, advancing age, obesity, physical inactivity and high cholesterol levels, seem to increase the fibrinogen level. This indicates that controlling other risk factors may also help to control the level of fibrinogen.

Although these factors seem to provide new information about cardiovascular disease, more research is needed to establish their relationship with the workings of the heart and blood vessels. In addition, the methods used to measure these substances in the blood require further investigation and fine-tuning.

High Blood Pressure

Throughout this book, medical disorders are generally accompanied by a list of their signs and symptoms. With high blood pressure, that approach doesn't work. Initially, most people have no symptoms. Even a doctor can't readily tell that you have high blood pressure until he or she actually measures the pressure of the blood flow in your arteries. Some people think that headaches, dizziness and nosebleeds are signs and symptoms of high blood pressure, but this isn't necessarily true. These signs and symptoms generally don't occur until blood pressure has reached an advanced — even life-threatening — stage.

High blood pressure and *hypertension* are interchangeable terms that refer to a condition in which your blood is traveling through your arteries at a pressure that's too high for good health. The incidence of high blood pressure increases with age. High blood pressure is more common in blacks than in whites or Hispanics. More men than women have high blood pressure in young adulthood and early middle age. Thereafter the situation reverses.

? Question and Answer

Should I take a daily aspirin to reduce my risk of heart problems?

It's well-known that aspirin inhibits platelets, blood cells that contribute to clotting. By doing this, aspirin reduces the tendency of blood to clot. Thus, it may help reduce or prevent narrowing of your blood vessels due to atherosclerosis. Your doctor may recommend that you take an aspirin daily:

- If you have a cardiovascular condition such as atherosclerosis, angina, high blood pressure or atrial fibrillation, each of which puts you at increased risk of a heart attack or stroke
- To avoid a second heart attack
- If you've had a coronary artery bypass operation, to reduce the likelihood that the bypass grafts will become blocked by a blood clot and accumulation of plaques

Taken in low doses, aspirin is inexpensive, generally safe and easy to take. But if you don't have cardiovascular disease, it's not clear that aspirin offers any benefits for your heart and blood vessels. Aspirin can cause stomach irritation and bleeding, although that's uncommon when it's taken in low doses. This risk can be decreased by taking coated aspirin, which dissolves in your small intestine rather than your stomach. Discuss daily aspirin use with your doctor.

ASPIRIN

250 TABLETS
325 MG EACH

Although high blood pressure generally doesn't produce any symptoms, this doesn't mean that it's not dangerous. The risk lies in the long-term damage the disease can produce. High blood pressure is a leading cause of strokes, heart attacks, heart failure, kidney failure, dementia and premature death.

The past 30 years have brought important advances in detecting and treating high blood pressure. Greater attention to this illness is one of the main reasons that deaths from strokes have gone down significantly and deaths from heart and blood vessel (cardiovascular) disease are down more than 50 percent. Still, half or less of all Americans with high blood pressure are receiving treatment, and even fewer have their blood pressure under control.

There's no cure for high blood pressure, but the condition is both preventable and treatable. Lifestyle adjustments and medication can help you control your blood pressure and keep it at a safe level.

Blood pressure basics

Blood pressure is determined by the amount of blood your heart pumps out and the resistance to this blood flow within your arteries. Organs and substances that help to regulate blood pressure include:

Your heart
The pumping action of your heart needs to create a certain amount of force in order to eject blood into your main artery (aorta). The harder your heart muscle has to work to eject the blood, the greater the force exerted on your arteries.

Your arteries
To accommodate the surge of blood with each heartbeat, your arteries are lined with smooth muscles that allow them to expand and contract as blood courses through. The more elastic your arteries are, the less resistant they are to the flow of blood and the less force

that's exerted on their walls. When arteries lose their elasticity or they become narrowed, resistance to blood flow increases, and additional force is needed to push blood through the vessels, thus raising the pressure.

Your kidneys
Your kidneys regulate the amount of sodium your body retains and hence the volume of water circulating in your body. Sodium retains water. Therefore, the more sodium that's in your body, the more water that's contained in your blood. This extra fluid in blood can increase blood pressure.

Others
Other organs and substances that influence blood pressure include your central nervous system and many hormones and enzymes. Within the walls of your heart and various blood vessels, tiny structures called baroreceptors continuously monitor your blood flow and send signals to your brain regarding the status of your blood pressure. The brain responds by signaling the release of hormones and enzymes that affect the

---

? Question and Answer

What causes an adrenaline rush?

One of the most significant hormones to affect blood pressure is adrenaline (epinephrine). Adrenaline is released into your body during periods of high stress or tension, such as when you're frightened or in a hurry. When this happens, your arteries narrow, and your heart contractions become stronger and faster, increasing pressure in your arteries. The feeling created by the release of this hormone is often referred to as an adrenaline rush.

---

functioning of your heart, blood vessels and kidneys.

Measuring your blood pressure

Your blood pressure is measured with a sphygmomanometer, which includes an inflatable cuff that's wrapped around your upper arm, an air pump, and a standardized pressure gauge or electronic meter.

Blood pressure is expressed as two numbers in units of millimeters of mercury (mm Hg). The top or first number is the systolic pressure — the amount of pressure in your arteries when your heart contracts and forces blood into the aorta. The bottom or second number is the diastolic pressure, the pressure that remains in your arteries between beats when your heart muscle is relaxing and filling with blood. During this time, your blood pressure decreases. A blood pressure reading below 120/80 mm Hg (120 over 80) is considered normal (optimal).

Your blood pressure normally fluctuates throughout the day. It increases during periods of activity and decreases when your body is at rest. Before you receive a diagnosis of high blood pressure, your doctor usually determines your average blood pressure by taking two or more readings at each of two or more visits after an initial screening.

Normal vs. high blood pressure
A newborn's blood pressure is usually about 90/60 mm Hg. During childhood, it slowly increases. As an adult, you want to keep your blood pressure lower than 120/80 mm Hg. If you have a systolic blood pressure between 120 and 129 mm Hg with a diastolic pressure less than 80 mm Hg, your blood pressure is classified as elevated. Elevated blood pressure increases your risk of cardiovascular disease.

Your blood pressure is considered high if your systolic pressure

Blood Pressure Classifications

	Systolic pressure (mm Hg*)		Diastolic pressure (mm Hg)
Normal **	lower than 120	and	lower than 80
Elevated	120 to 129	and	lower than 80
Stage 1 hypertension	130 to 139	or	80 to 89
Stage 2 hypertension	140 or higher	or	90 or higher
Hypertensive crisis	higher than 180	and/or	higher than 120

*Millimeters of mercury
**Based on the average of two or more readings taken at each of two or more visits after an initial screening

Source: Whelten PK, et al. 2017 Guideline for the Prevention, Detection, Evaluation, and Management of High Blood Pressure in Adults.

is consistently 130 mm Hg or higher or your diastolic pressure is consistently 80 mm Hg or higher, or both. In the past, diastolic pressure was assumed to be a better indicator of potential heath risks than systolic pressure. But long-term studies have shown that a high systolic reading is an equally important — if not more serious — risk factor, especially in older adults.

High blood pressure is separated into three stages, with hypertensive crisis being the most serious. See a doctor immediately if your blood pressure meets the criteria for hypertensive crisis (see chart above). The terms *mild* and *moderate* are no longer used to describe high blood pressure so people won't mistakenly dismiss mild or moderate high blood pressure as not being a serious health threat.

High blood pressure usually develops gradually. In most instances, people start out with normal blood pressure that slowly progresses to elevated and, eventually, to stage 1 high blood pressure.

Left untreated, excessive pressure can eventually damage many of your organs and tissues. Even stage 1 high blood pressure can be harmful if it continues over months to years.

Causes

In most people with high blood pressure, no cause for the increase in blood pressure can be found. This is known as primary (essential) hypertension.

In the few cases where the cause can be established, the condition is known as secondary hypertension. This term is used because the increased pressure is the result of, or secondary to, another condition or factor. These might include:
- Over-the-counter cold remedies, nasal decongestants, appetite suppressants, pain relievers, and some prescription medications such as oral contraceptives and steroids.
- Kidney disorders such as kidney failure, kidney artery narrowing (stenosis) and inflammation of the glomeruli (glomerulonephritis)

- Adrenal gland overactivity
- Thyroid problems
- Blood vessel abnormalities
- Preeclampsia, a complication of pregnancy
- Illicit drug use

Sometimes, if the primary problem is taken care of, the secondary hypertension goes away.

Complications

The symptoms of high blood pressure may be silent, but the dangers are very real. Left untreated over a period of years, high blood pressure can damage various body organs. Heart attacks, heart failure, kidney failure, strokes, dementia and loss of vision are some of the complications that can result.

Coronary artery disease
The major cause of death in people with high blood pressure is coronary artery disease. High blood pressure accelerates the buildup of fatty deposits (plaques) in your arteries and leads to narrowing of these blood vessels (atherosclerosis). This can result

in a heart attack, stroke or other complications.

When blood pressure is elevated, the heart is forced to work harder to maintain blood flow to the tissues. Over time, the heart muscle may thicken (hypertrophy) in order to keep pushing blood out of the heart against increased resistance.

The left ventricle is the chamber of the heart that pumps oxygenated blood to other parts of the body. Thus, this muscle thickening is called left ventricular hypertrophy. Left ventricular hypertrophy is associated with a higher risk of sudden death and heart attacks.

Heart failure

Over time, high blood pressure can cause the heart muscle (myocardium) to wear out, and congestive heart failure may result. With this condition, your heart can't push forward all of the fluid returning to it from your veins. Fluid accumulates in your lungs, legs and other tissues.

Controlling your blood pressure can greatly reduce your risk of cardiovascular diseases, such as congestive heart failure. If blood pressure is controlled for at least five years, your risk of heart failure decreases by more than 50 percent.

Stroke

Elevated blood pressure in the arteries leading to your brain can either slow blood flow to your brain or cause a blood vessel in your brain to burst; either can cause a stroke.

High blood pressure is the most important risk factor for a stroke. When blood pressure is decreased with appropriate treatment, the risk of a stroke is decreased as well — about 40 percent over two to five years.

Dementia

Research indicates that high blood pressure can lead to significant memory impairment (dementia).

The onset of dementia varies from a few years to several decades following diagnosis of high blood pressure and may result from experiencing several "ministrokes."

There's increasing evidence that drug treatment to lower elevated blood pressure may lower this risk. Further research is still necessary to confirm an association between high blood pressure and dementia.

Kidney disease

About one-fifth of the blood dispersed to your body with each pump of your heart goes to your kidneys. The kidneys filter waste products from the blood and help to maintain a proper balance of salts, acids and water in your blood.

High blood pressure can injure your kidneys and impair their ability to perform normal functions, one of which is to help control blood pressure. So damage to these organs can worsen high blood pressure. This leads to a destructive cycle that, ultimately, results in increasing blood pressure and less ability of the kidneys to remove impurities from the blood.

Lifestyle changes

Although the precise cause of high blood pressure often remains unknown, the condition can usually be treated effectively. With proper medical attention and advice, most or all of the potentially dire consequences of high blood pressure can be avoided.

Depending on your blood pressure, your doctor may begin your treatment by recommending lifestyle changes alone or lifestyle changes with medication.

Even with drug treatment, making changes in your daily habits are important to managing your disease. Lifestyle adjustments may include losing weight, adjusting your diet, restricting use of alcohol and caffeine, quitting smoking, and increasing your level of physical activity.

Physical activity

Physical activity is very important in controlling your blood pressure because it makes your heart stronger. As a result, your heart is able to pump more blood with less effort. The less your heart has to work to pump blood, the less force that's exerted on your arteries.

Isolated Systolic Hypertension

If the top number in your blood pressure reading (systolic blood pressure) is consistently high (130 mm Hg or above) but your bottom number (diastolic blood pressure) is in the normal range (lower than 80 mm Hg), you may have isolated systolic hypertension (ISH). This condition affects a number of people older than age 60 with high blood pressure.

Doctors once thought that ISH was a harmless result of aging and were reluctant to treat it because of a lack of evidence of benefits and the risk of possible side effects, along with the cost of treatment. However, several studies have shown that treating this form of high blood pressure can prevent thousands of strokes and other severe cardiovascular problems each year.

If you've received a diagnosis of ISH, get accurate, regular readings of your blood pressure. Ask your doctor about medications to control the problem and follow the prescription carefully. Address the lifestyle factors that can add to your risk of ISH: smoking, obesity, a high-sodium diet, lack of regular exercise and the use of alcohol.

Aerobic activity that increases your heart rate and your need for oxygen has the greatest beneficial effect on blood pressure. As your body becomes accustomed to this level of activity, your heart becomes stronger, and your blood pressure drops. Regular aerobic activity can reduce your blood pressure by 5 to 10 mm Hg. It can also help with weight loss. For more information on physical activity, see Chapter 9, "Fitness."

Diet

Eating a nutritionally balanced diet also benefits your blood pressure. And eating well doesn't mean focusing on calories and giving up all of your favorite foods. Rather, it means enjoying a variety of foods that help to ensure the right mix of nutrients your body needs to be healthy. Emphasizing plenty of grains, fruits, vegetables

Risk Factors

Certain genetic traits and lifestyle habits can increase your chances of developing high blood pressure. Generally, the more of these risk factors that you have, the greater your odds of having high blood pressure during your lifetime. By managing risk factors that are controllable, you can reduce your risk.

Uncontrollable risk factors

Risk factors you can't change include:

Race
High blood pressure occurs more frequently in blacks than in whites and Hispanics. In blacks, high blood pressure generally develops at an earlier age, is more severe and tends to progress more rapidly.

Age
Your risk of high blood pressure increases with age, particularly among Americans age 65 and older.

Family history
If high blood pressure is common in your family, your chances of developing it are increased.

Sex
Among young and middle-aged adults, men are more likely to have high blood pressure than women are. After about age 50, when most women are beyond menopause, high blood pressure becomes more common in women than in men.

Controllable risk factors

Risk factors that you can change include:

Obesity
Excess body mass requires more blood to supply tissues with oxygen and nutrients. More blood flowing through your blood vessels creates extra force on artery walls.

Inactivity
Lack of physical activity increases your risk of being overweight, which increases your risk of high blood pressure. People who are inactive also tend to have higher heart rates, and their hearts work harder to pump blood.

Tobacco use
Nicotine makes your heart work harder by temporarily constricting your blood vessels and increasing your heart rate and blood pressure. In addition, carbon monoxide in cigarette smoke replaces oxygen in your blood, causing your heart to work harder to supply adequate oxygen to your body's organs and tissues.

Sensitivity to sodium
People who are sodium sensitive retain sodium more easily, leading to fluid retention and increased blood pressure. Salt is a major source of sodium.

Low potassium intake
Potassium helps balance the amount of sodium in your body. If your diet doesn't include enough potassium or your body isn't able to retain a proper amount, too much sodium can accumulate, increasing your risk of high blood pressure.

Excessive alcohol consumption
Having two or more drinks in a sitting can temporarily raise your blood pressure. Over time, heavy drinking can also damage your heart.

Stress
Stress doesn't cause persistent high blood pressure, but a high level of stress can lead to temporary, dramatic increases in blood pressure. If these temporary episodes occur often enough, they can eventually damage your blood vessels, heart and kidneys in the same manner as persistent high blood pressure.

Chronic illness
Certain illnesses can contribute to increased blood pressure or make high blood pressure more difficult to control. These include atherosclerosis, diabetes, sleep apnea and heart failure.

and low-fat dairy foods can help you control your blood pressure and possibly avoid the need for medication.

The DASH diet

Dietary Approaches to Stop Hypertension (DASH) is a diet recommended for people with high blood pressure and those with prehypertension, who are at risk of developing high blood pressure.

DASH stresses fruits and vegetables plus ample grains and low-fat dairy products. A study of DASH found that individuals who followed the diet experienced an average decrease of 11.4 mm Hg in systolic pressure and 5.5 mm Hg in diastolic pressure, which is about the same effect as achieved with some medications.

Although researchers aren't certain why the combination diet fared better, they believe it may be because the diet promotes weight loss and because it's rich in potassium, calcium and magnesium, minerals linked with lower blood pressure.

A follow-up study called the DASH-Sodium study found that reductions in sodium consumption reduced blood pressure even more.

Reducing sodium

Sodium plays a critical role in maintaining the right balance of fluids in the body. It also helps to transmit nerve impulses that influence contraction and relaxation of your muscles.

If too much sodium accumulates in your blood, blood volume increases because sodium attracts and holds water. Your heart has to work harder to move the increased volume of blood through blood vessels, increasing pressure on your arteries. Some people are simply more sensitive to high levels of sodium in their blood. You're more likely to be sodium sensitive if you're black, age 65 or older, or have diabetes.

There's been some controversy over whether salt restriction can help to reduce blood pressure. Some studies have found little to support this theory. Other studies, including the DASH-Sodium study, indicate that reducing sodium does reduce blood pressure.

Many health professionals and organizations support a reduced-sodium diet. The National High Blood Pressure Education Program, sponsored by the National Institutes of Health, recommends that all Americans limit sodium to no more than 2,400 milligrams a day. However, reducing sodium intake to 1,500 milligrams a day can have an even more dramatic effect on your blood pressure.

If you have high blood pressure and you're sodium sensitive, consuming less sodium can help lower your blood pressure. Limiting sodium in combination with other lifestyle changes may be enough to keep you off medication. Even if you take blood pressure medication, limiting sodium can help

Stocking Your Kitchen

You'll be able to find everything you need for the DASH diet at a well-stocked supermarket. Having the right ingredients at your fingertips makes it easier to whip up healthy dishes. Here are some examples of foods to stock up on:

Dairy products
- Low-fat or fat-free milk
- Low-fat or reduced-fat cottage cheese or ricotta
- Reduced-fat cheeses
- Reduced-fat or fat-free sour cream
- Tub or squeeze margarine

Grains
- Bread, bagels and pita bread
- Low-fat flour tortillas
- Plain cereal
- Brown or white rice
- Pasta

Fruit
- Standard fresh varieties
- Seasonal fresh fruits
- Canned fruit in juice or water
- Frozen fruit without added sugar
- Dried fruit

Vegetables
- Standard fresh varieties
- Seasonal fresh vegetables
- Frozen vegetables without added butter or sauces
- Canned tomato products low in sodium
- Canned vegetables or vegetable soups low in sodium

Legumes
- Lentils
- Black beans
- Red (kidney) beans
- Navy beans
- Chickpeas (garbanzos)

Meat
- White meat, skinless chicken and turkey
- Unbreaded fish
- Pork tenderloin
- Extra-lean ground beef
- Round or sirloin beef cuts

Baking items
- Imitation butter, flakes or buds
- Cooking spray
- Canned evaporated milk, fat-free or reduced-fat
- Cocoa powder, unsweetened
- Angel food cake mix

Condiments, seasonings and spreads
- Low-fat or fat-free salad dressings
- Herbs
- Spices
- Flavored vinegars
- Salsa or picante sauce

The DASH Diet

Food	Benefits	Serving examples
Grains 7-8 daily servings*	Grains include breads, cereals, rice and pasta. In addition to being low in fat, grains are rich in complex carbohydrates and nutrients. Whole grains provide even more fiber and nutrients than refined varieties do. Avoid adding high-fat toppings to your breads and pasta, such as butter and sauces made with cream and cheese. Instead, choose fruit spreads or honey for your breads and use fresh vegetable or tomato-based toppings for your pasta.	• ½ cup, or 3 ounces (oz.), cooked cereal, rice or pasta • ½ cup (1 oz.) ready-to-eat cereal • 1 slice whole-grain sandwich bread • ½ bagel or English muffin
Fruits and vegetables 8-10 daily servings	Fruits and vegetables are virtually fat-free and low in calories, so load up on these. They also provide fiber and a variety of nutrients, including potassium and magnesium, as well as phytochemicals, substances that can reduce your risk of cardiovascular disease and some cancers. Replacing high-fat, high-calorie foods with fruits and vegetables is an easy way to improve your diet without cutting back on your portions. Just don't smother them with dips or sauces that contain a lot of fat.	• ¼ cup (1½ oz.) raisins • ¾ cup (6 fluid oz.) 100% fruit juice • 1 medium apple, banana or other fruit • 12 grapes • 1 cup (2 oz.) raw leafy green vegetables • ½ cup (3 oz.) cooked vegetables • 1 medium potato
Dairy products 2-3 daily servings	Dairy products are key sources of calcium, vitamin D and protein, but they can be high in fat. Choose low-fat or fat-free varieties. This way you'll get the health benefits minus the fat.	• 1 cup (8 fl. oz.) low-fat or fat-free milk or 1 cup (8 oz.) yogurt • 1½ oz. reduced-fat or fat-free cheese
Meat, poultry and fish 2 or fewer daily servings	Meat, poultry and fish are rich in protein, B vitamins, iron and zinc. Choose lean cuts, such as tenderloin, round or sirloin. Remove all visible fat from meats and skin from poultry. Fish is one of the leanest animal proteins you can choose. The fat it does contain is mainly omega-3 fatty acids, which may help lower your blood pressure, thin your blood and reduce your risk of blood clots.	• 2-3 oz. cooked skinless poultry, seafood or lean meat
Legumes, nuts and seeds 4-5 servings a week	Legumes include beans, dried peas and lentils, which are low in fat, contain no cholesterol and are an excellent source of protein. They also provide a variety of nutrients, including magnesium, potassium, phytochemicals and fiber. Although nuts and seeds contain fat, most of it is monounsaturated, the type that may help protect against coronary artery disease.	• ½ cup (3½ oz.) cooked legumes • ¼ cup (1 oz.) seeds • ⅓ cup (1 oz.) nuts

*Serving amounts are based on a diet of 2,000 calories a day. Most Americans need between 1,600 and 2,400 calories daily, depending on age and activity. To include fewer or more servings, talk to a registered dietitian.

Adapted from National Institutes of Health

Shaking Out the Sodium

Here are some ways to reduce sodium in your diet:

- *Eat more fresh and fewer processed foods.* Fresh foods usually have less sodium than do processed foods.
- *Look for lower sodium products.* Some processed foods that are typically high in sodium, such as soups, broths, canned vegetables and condiments, are also prepared in lower sodium versions.
- *Read labels.* Read the nutrition facts labels on food products that you're considering purchasing or consuming. Each label tells you how much sodium is in a serving of that particular product.
- *Don't add salt to food.* If you think your food needs more flavor, try another seasoning, such as lemon, pepper, cilantro, or other herbs and spices.
- *Limit your use of condiments.* Salad dressings, sauces, dips, ketchup, mustard and relish all contain sodium. So do pickles and olives.
- *Rinse canned foods.* Rinsing canned vegetables and meats helps to remove about one-third of the sodium.

Before you try a salt substitute, check with your doctor. Some salt substitutes or "lite" salts contain a mixture of sodium chloride (salt) and other compounds. To achieve that familiar salty taste, you may end up using more of the salt substitute than you do regular salt and not reducing your sodium intake.

In addition, potassium chloride is a common ingredient in salt substitutes. Too much potassium can be harmful if you have kidney problems or if you're taking certain high blood pressure or heart failure medications.

the medication be more effective.

Weight control

If you have high blood pressure — or if you're at increased risk of it — it's not critical that you become "thin." But you should try to achieve and maintain a weight that improves control of your blood pressure and lessens your risk of other health problems. In general, blood pressure increases with weight gain and decreases with weight loss.

If your body mass index (BMI) is 25 or more, try to lose some weight (see BMI chart on page 267). Losing as few as 10 pounds can reduce your blood pressure. For some people, weight loss alone is enough to avoid blood pressure medication. To learn more about achieving a healthy weight, see Chapter 8, "Nutrition and Weight."

Tobacco, alcohol and caffeine

High blood pressure combined with tobacco use increases the risk of fatty deposits in your arteries (atherosclerosis), a major risk factor for a heart attack.

Reducing use of alcohol may reduce your blood pressure. If you drink alcohol, limit your consumption to a moderate level. For younger and middle-aged men, that generally means no more than two drinks a day. Moderate consumption for women and all individuals over age 65 is no more than one drink a day.

Caffeine may increase your blood pressure. If you have high blood pressure, limit daily caffeine to no more than two cups of coffee, four cups of tea or four cans of caffeinated soda. Also avoid caffeine right before activities that naturally increase your blood pressure, such as exercise or hard physical labor.

Stress

The effects of stress are usually only temporary. But if you experience stress regularly, it can produce increases in blood pressure that may gradually damage your arteries, heart, brain, kidneys and eyes. Changes in your daily routine and use of relaxation techniques may help you avoid or better cope with stress (see Chapter 10, "Stress").

Medications

Changing your lifestyle can go a long way toward controlling high blood pressure. But sometimes lifestyle changes aren't enough. In addition to diet and exercise, your doctor may recommend medication to lower your blood pressure. Which category of medication your doctor prescribes depends on your stage of high blood pressure and whether you also have other medical problems.

The major types of medication used to control high blood pressure include:

- **Thiazide diuretics.** Diuretics, sometimes called "water pills," are medications that act on your kidneys to help your body eliminate sodium and water, reducing blood volume. Thiazide diuretics are often the first — but not the only — choice in high blood pressure medications. But diuretics often are not prescribed. If you're not taking a diuretic and your blood pressure remains high, talk to your doctor about adding one or replacing a drug you currently take with a diuretic.

  If you're age 80 or older, a special type of thiazide diuretic, indapamide, may be particularly effective in lowering your blood pressure. In this age group, indapamide has been shown to reduce deaths from strokes, heart failure and other cardiovascular disease causes.

- **Beta blockers.** These medications reduce the workload on your heart and open your blood vessels, causing your heart to beat slower and with less force.

Among blacks, beta blockers don't work as well when they're prescribed alone, but they're effective when combined with a thiazide diuretic.

- **Angiotensin-converting enzyme (ACE) inhibitors.** These medications help relax blood vessels by blocking the formation of a natural chemical that narrows blood vessels. ACE inhibitors may be especially important in treating high blood pressure in people with coronary artery disease, heart failure or kidney failure.

  Like beta blockers, ACE inhibitors don't work as well in blacks when prescribed alone, but they're effective when combined with a thiazide diuretic.

- **Angiotensin II receptor blockers.** These medications help relax blood vessels by blocking the action — not the formation — of a natural chemical that narrows blood vessels. Like ACE inhibitors, angiotensin II receptor blockers often are useful for people with coronary artery disease, heart failure and kidney failure.

- **Calcium channel blockers.** These medications help relax the muscles of your blood vessels. Some slow your heart rate. Calcium channel blockers may work better for blacks than do ACE inhibitors or beta blockers.

  A word of caution for grapefruit lovers. Grapefruit juice interacts with some calcium channel blockers, increasing blood levels of the medication and putting you at higher risk of side effects. Talk to your doctor or pharmacist if you're concerned about interactions.

- **Renin inhibitors.** The medication aliskiren (Tekturna) slows down the production of renin, an enzyme produced by your kidneys that starts a cascade of chemical steps that increases blood pressure. Tekturna works by reducing the ability of renin to begin this process. Aliskiren

is still being studied to determine its ideal use and dosage for people with high blood pressure.

If you're having trouble reaching your blood pressure goal with combinations of the above medications, your doctor may prescribe one of the following drugs:

- **Alpha blockers.** Alpha blockers reduce nerve impulses to blood vessels, reducing the effects of natural chemicals that narrow blood vessels.

- **Alpha-beta blockers.** In addition to reducing nerve impulses to blood vessels, alpha-beta blockers slow the heartbeat to reduce the amount of blood that must be pumped through the vessels.

- **Central-acting agents.** These medications work by preventing your brain from signaling your nervous system to increase your heart rate and narrow your blood vessels.

- **Vasodilators.** Vasodilators work directly on the muscles in the walls of your arteries. They prevent the muscles from tightening and your arteries from narrowing.

Once your blood pressure is under control, your doctor also may have you take a daily aspirin to reduce your risk of cardiovascular disorders.

To reduce the number of daily medication doses that you need, your doctor may prescribe a combination of low-dose medications rather than larger doses of one single blood pressure drug. In fact, two or more blood pressure drugs often work better than one drug alone.

Sometimes, finding the most effective medication — or combination of medications — is a matter of trial and error. Try to be patient as you and your doctor work together to find the best treatment for you.

Resistant Hypertension

If your blood pressure remains stubbornly high despite taking at least three different types of high blood pressure drugs, you may have resistant hypertension — blood pressure that's resistant to treatment.

Having resistant hypertension doesn't mean your blood pressure will never get lower. If you and your doctor can identify what's behind your persistently high blood pressure, there's a good chance you can meet your blood pressure goals with the help of more-effective treatment. You may need to see a hypertension specialist if your primary care doctor isn't able to pinpoint the cause. It may also be that another condition you have that you may not be aware of — such as sleep apnea or kidney problems — is causing your high blood pressure.

Your doctor or a hypertension specialist can evaluate whether the medications and doses you're taking for your high blood pressure are appropriate. You may have to fine-tune your medications to come up with the most effective combination and doses. Your doctor may also prescribe other medications, including a more potent or longer acting diuretic if you're not already taking one. Your doctor may also suggest a nonthiazide diuretic, such as spironolactone (Aldactone) or eplerenone (Inspra), which changes the way your body absorbs sodium and excretes potassium by blocking the hormone aldosterone.

In addition, your doctor may review the medications you're taking for other conditions. Some medications, foods or supplements can worsen high blood pressure or prevent high blood pressure medications from working effectively. Be open and honest with your doctor about all of the medications you take.

Hypotension

Hypotension is low blood pressure. If blood pressure falls to dangerously low levels and blood can't be effectively circulated to vital tissues, shock occurs, a condition that can be life-threatening. Shock may result from significant loss of fluid or blood and, rarely, from serious infections. A major goal of emergency treatment for hypotension is to increase your blood pressure to more normal levels.

Chronic low blood pressure — when your blood pressure is below average but not symptomatically or dangerously so — isn't uncommon and may reduce your risk of cardiovascular disease. It can be a normal finding or may result from medications given for high blood pressure. Conditions such as pregnancy, diabetes or arteriosclerosis also can produce low blood pressure.

One potentially dangerous type of low blood pressure is called postural hypotension. Dizziness or faintness that occurs on standing up quickly from a seated position is the key symptom. Typically, this type of low blood pressure isn't serious, but it may increase the risk of falls and injury. Taking precautions can help you to avoid danger: Stand up slowly from a seated position and wait a few seconds before walking. If episodes seem to occur after you've been in the sun for prolonged periods or after fasting, avoid such circumstances.

Home monitoring

If you have high blood pressure, monitoring your blood pressure at home may be a necessary part of your treatment. A variety of devices to measure blood pressure (sphygmomanometers) are available. The recommended type is an automatic, cuff-style, upper-arm (bicep) monitor.

When you're taking your blood pressure, it's important that you use proper technique. To get an accurate reading with an upper arm device, make sure that the cuff fits properly.

Before you purchase a sphygmomanometer, have your doctor or other health care professional measure your arm to determine the correct cuff size for you. Then after you buy one, bring it to your next appointment and ask your doctor or one of his or her staff to show you how to use it and make sure that it's working properly. Some health care facilities offer classes in home blood pressure monitoring.

If you use a home blood pressure monitor, make sure to verify its accuracy yearly. To do this, bring it to your doctor's office. If the reading is off more than 3 millimeters of mercury (mm Hg), replace the unit.

If your blood pressure is under control and you're willing to monitor it at home, it's possible you may be able to make fewer visits to your doctor.

Benefits
Monitoring your blood pressure yourself can help:
- **Track your treatment.** Because high blood pressure often has no symptoms, the only way to make sure lifestyle changes or medications are working is to check your blood pressure regularly.
- **Promote better control.** When you take the initiative to measure your own blood pressure, this responsible act tends to rub off on other areas. It can give you added incentive to eat more healthfully, increase your activity level and take your medication properly.
- **Identify white-coat hypertension.** Simply going to a doctor's office can create stress in people

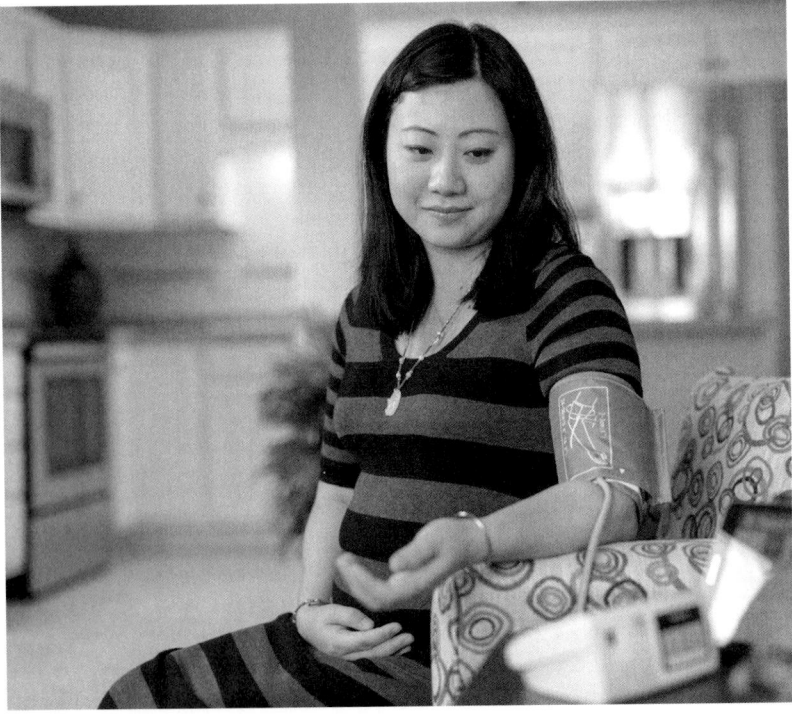

An electronic blood pressure monitor enables you to take your own blood pressure without the use of a stethoscope. Your blood pressure reading appears on a digital screen.

Taking Your Own Blood Pressure

Learning to take your blood pressure correctly isn't hard, but it takes training and a little practice. Here are some tips to improve the accuracy of your measurements:

- Don't measure your blood pressure right after you get up in the morning. Wait until after you've been active for an hour or more. If you exercise after you awaken, check your blood pressure before you exercise.
- Wait to measure your blood pressure for at least a half-hour after you've eaten, smoked, or used caffeine or alcohol. All of these factors can increase your blood pressure.
- Empty your bladder first. A full bladder increases your blood pressure slightly.
- Sit quietly for five minutes before taking a reading. Repeat once after several minutes.
- Remember that your blood pressure varies throughout the day. Readings are often a little higher in the morning. Your mood also can affect your blood pressure. If you've had a difficult day, don't be alarmed if your blood pressure rises.
- Measure your blood pressure at work as well as at home, to ensure that it remains in your target range. Keep in mind, though, that measurements taken at places other than at home tend to be slightly higher.

and increase their blood pressure (white-coat hypertension). Home monitoring can help determine if you have high blood pressure or white-coat hypertension.

- **Save money.** Monitoring your blood pressure at home may save you the cost of going to your doctor's office to have your blood pressure taken. This is especially true when you first start to take medication and you need to have your blood pressure checked frequently to adjust the dose.

Types of monitors

Not all blood pressure monitors are the same. Some are easier to use. Others are more reliable. In addition, some monitors are inaccurate and a waste of your money.

Spring-gauge monitors

Spring-gauge monitors (aneroid manometers) are fitted over your upper arm and feature a round dial activated by a spring-pressure gauge. Each scale for the needle is set to match millimeters of mercury. They're the type most often used by your doctor or nurse.

Spring-gauge models are generally inexpensive and easy to transport. Some gauges are extra large, for easier reading, and some models have a built-in stethoscope for easier use.

Standard spring-gauge monitors aren't recommended if you have trouble hearing or if you have poor dexterity in your hands, because they require that you listen to a stethoscope and operate a bulb pump simultaneously.

Electronic monitors

Electronic (digital) monitors are the most popular and the easiest to use. They're also the most expensive, although the price is declining.

Electronic blood pressure monitors generally require that you do two things: Put the cuff on your arm and push a button. The cuff automatically inflates with air and

slowly deflates. Unlike spring-gauge models, electronic monitors detect artery motion, not sound. Your blood pressure measurements are shown as numbers on a screen.

If you have an irregular heart rhythm, check with your doctor before purchasing an electronic monitor.

Finger or wrist monitors

Some models are available that measure blood pressure in your wrist or finger instead of in your upper arm. This makes them more compact and easier to use but they're generally not recommended because they're not as precise.

The bottom line: Avoid finger monitors because they're inaccurate. Wrist monitors can be fairly accurate as long as you make sure that your wrist is supported at the level of your heart when you take your blood pressure measurement. Also, it's more difficult to validate the accuracy of wrist monitors than upper arm monitors.

Coronary Artery Disease

Coronary artery disease causes more deaths, disability and economic loss than any other form of heart and blood vessel (cardiovascular) disease. It often develops gradually and silently, typically over many years. In fact, this condition can go virtually unnoticed until it suddenly produces a heart attack. Approximately 735,000 Americans have heart attacks each year, of which about 116,000 are fatal.

The coronary arteries are part of your heart's circulatory system. They provide the muscles of your heart with a steady supply of blood carrying oxygen and nutrients. The coronary arteries encircle the heart like a crown and send branches downward to the tip of the heart. When disease develops or damage occurs in these arteries, the condition is known as coronary artery disease.

The diagnosis and treatment of coronary artery disease have seen a great deal of innovation. Newer and better tests to identify coronary artery disease — particularly in its early stages — are continuously being developed.

Treatments also are improving. Specialized procedures can open narrowed coronary arteries. Bypass operations to direct blood around narrowed or blocked arteries also continue to be refined. In addition, the introduction of new medications to improve the flow of blood to the heart muscle have proved helpful in minimizing symptoms and have contributed to longer life in those who have coronary artery disease.

Despite these advances, you still play a critical role. Greater awareness of the disease and better control of its risk factors are likely behind the decreased death rate from coronary artery disease.

Most common cause

Coronary artery disease usually results from an accumulation of fatty deposits (plaques) in the lining of arteries. Plaques contain substances such as cholesterol, platelets, scar tissue and calcium. They narrow the arteries and create a condition called atherosclerosis. As plaques increase within the arteries, the flow of blood is blocked. This often occurs in an irregular fashion, with more blockage at some points than at others.

Plaques also increase the chances that a blood clot will develop in an artery. When a clot blocks the flow of blood through a coronary artery, your heart muscle doesn't receive its proper supply of blood, oxygen and nutrients. This is called myocardial ischemia. If the death of heart muscle tissue occurs, this is a heart attack (myocardial infarction).

Symptoms of atherosclerosis such as chest pain (angina) and fatigue are more likely to occur during exercise than at rest, at least initially. When you stop and rest, the discomfort usually resolves in a few minutes. However, blockages can be so severe that even resting your muscles doesn't allow adequate blood flow, and you may experience symptoms such as chest pain with only minimal exertion. On the other hand, many people with atherosclerosis experience no symptoms until serious complications arise.

Factors that contribute to the development of atherosclerosis include high blood cholesterol levels, high blood pressure, diabetes and tobacco use.

Diagnosis and detection

One of the challenges faced by doctors is detecting coronary artery disease before serious signs and symptoms or complications occur. Your doctor can't detect blocked coronary arteries simply by listening to your heart with a stethoscope. To diagnose coronary artery disease, more-specialized tests are generally needed.

Electrocardiogram

The electrical activity of your heart is characterized by a pattern of changing impulses. These can be recorded through electrodes attached to the surface of your body. The electrical activity of the heart — represented by characteristic waves — can be evaluated instantaneously on a monitor or studied later on graph paper printouts.

The electrocardiogram (ECG) procedure is safe and painless. While you're relaxing on a bed or examining table, 12 to 15 electrodes are attached to the skin of your legs, arms, neck and trunk.

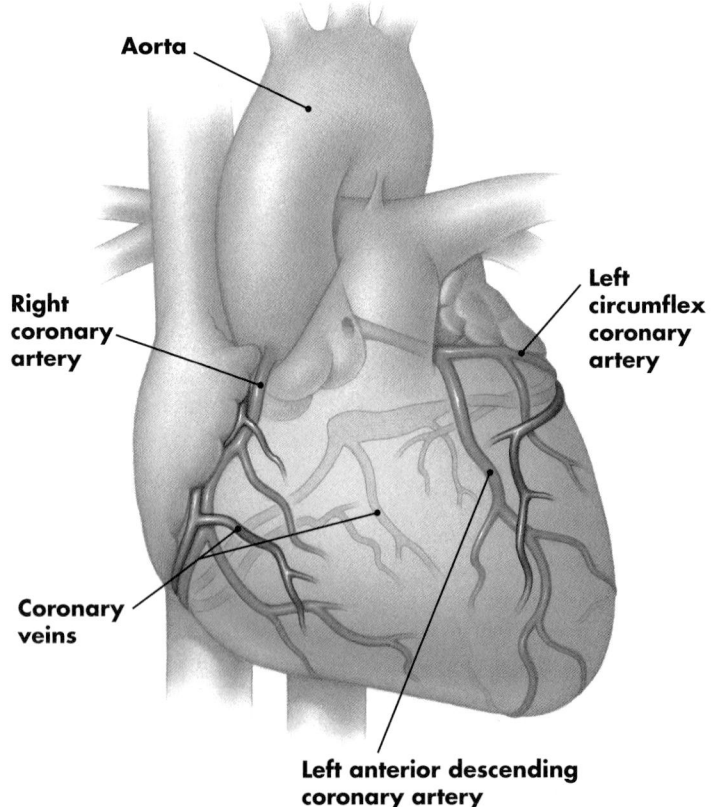

The coronary arteries emerge from the aorta and extend along the surface of your heart. Branches extend into your heart's wall to supply cells with oxygen and nourishment. The blood returns to your heart through your coronary veins.

The recording process then takes only a few minutes.

Analysis of an ECG involves looking for indications of heart rhythm abnormalities, a past heart attack or a heart attack in progress. If you have narrowed arteries but haven't had a heart attack, an exercise ECG (cardiac stress test) may be helpful. Your doctor may want an ECG of your heart when you're 30 to 40 years old and in good health to provide a basis for comparison if heart problems develop.

ECG recordings taken continuously over a 24-hour period or longer may help detect conditions such as rhythm disturbances or inadequate blood flow to the heart muscle (myocardial ischemia). This technique, called Holter monitoring (ambulatory electrocardiography monitoring), involves use of a portable monitor that's slightly larger in size than a deck of cards.

Electrodes attached to your chest are connected to the monitor, which is hooked to your belt or carried on a shoulder strap. You wear the monitor for 24 hours as you go about your normal activities. Information on your heart's activity is stored in the monitor and retrieved later by medical personnel.

Blood tests

A sample of your blood may be taken for analysis. Your doctor may want an analysis of your blood cholesterol levels.

Too much low-density lipoprotein (LDL or "bad") cholesterol or too little high-density lipoprotein (HDL or "good") cholesterol puts you at greater risk of atherosclerosis, an accumulation of fatty deposits in your blood vessels.

Other tests may include measurement of your blood sugar (glucose) for indications of diabetes, and of thyroid hormone — abnormal levels of these substances can increase your risk of cardiovascular disease. Elevated levels of certain enzymes in the bloodstream that are released from injured or dying heart muscle tissues, such as creatine kinase and troponin, also may indicate heart damage during a heart attack.

Cardiac stress test

A cardiac stress test helps measure how well your heart muscle is functioning and whether it's receiving an adequate blood supply. A stress test may be used to evaluate symptoms such as chest pain or shortness of breath during

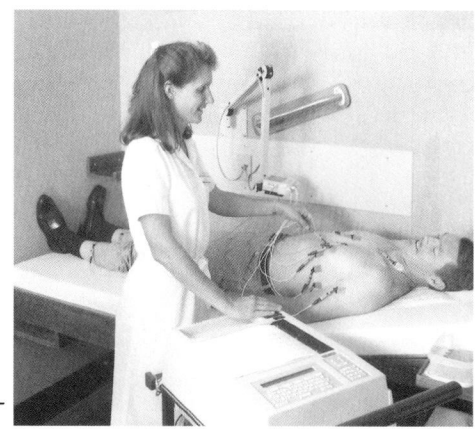

An electrocardiogram (ECG) records electrical activity of your heart. Electrodes convey impulses to a device that produces a graphic representation of your heart's activity. This can be studied for patterns and abnormalities.

exertion. In some people with several risk factors for coronary artery disease, the test may be used as a screening tool.

A stress test accurately identifies the presence of significant coronary artery disease, and it also helps identify people who don't have significant coronary artery disease.

If you've had a heart attack, your doctor may order a stress test to determine the extent of your coronary artery disease. Stress tests are also recommended before you begin a program of vigorous exercise, particularly if you have any cardiovascular risk factors. Before you enter a cardiac rehabilitation program, you'll likely undergo a stress test.

The two main types of stress tests are exercise and nonexercise (pharmacologic). A pharmacologic test may be combined with imaging tests to help visualize your heart under a workload.

Exercise stress test

With an exercise stress test, electrodes are placed on various parts of your chest, and a blood pressure cuff is placed on your arm. You then walk on a treadmill while an ECG records your heart's response to an increasing workload. As the

Heart Glossary

angina. Chest pain or pressure that results from lack of blood supply.

cardiovascular disease. Any disease that affects the heart or blood vessels.

coronary artery disease. Disease in the coronary arteries, which supply blood to the heart.

heart attack (myocardial infarction). Myocardial ischemia that lasts long enough to cause death in the area of the heart muscle supplied by a blocked coronary artery.

myocardial ischemia. Insufficient blood and oxygen reaching the heart muscle due to blockage of the coronary arteries.

silent ischemia. Myocardial ischemia that causes no symptoms.

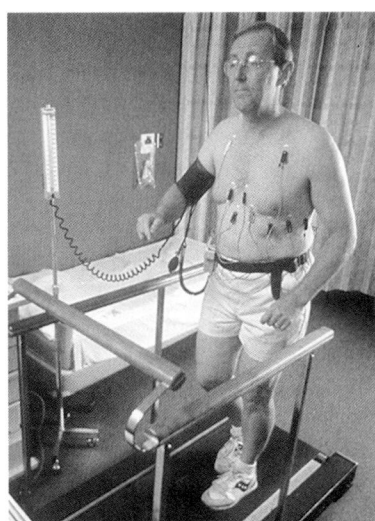

A treadmill test measures the activity of your heart while you exercise.

speed and grade of the treadmill are gradually increased and the workout becomes more demanding, your heart rate increases.

Problems rarely occur during the test because doctors recommend these tests only for people for whom they believe the testing will be safe. In addition, the health care professional overseeing the test will be monitoring your heart rate, blood pressure and electrocardiographic tracings.

If a problem should occur, a medical facility is probably the safest place to have it happen, because the condition can be diagnosed and treated appropriately and quickly. For individuals who can't walk on a treadmill, other forms of exercise, such as pedaling a stationary bicycle or doing arm exercises, are sometimes used instead.

Nonexercise stress test
A nonexercise (pharmacological) stress test is used in individuals who can't exercise due to conditions such as arthritis in the hip or knee. A medication is injected into your bloodstream that increases your heart rate, mimicking the effects of exercise. The effects of the medication are observed with imaging tests.

If the test indicates that your heart's activity was unaffected by

the stress, the chances are excellent that your heart will function properly when you work out on your own. If the test indicates problems, the results can be useful in establishing exercise limits and developing a specialized medication and fitness program. If the test produces any abnormal patterns on the electrocardiographic tracings or other special images ordered, your doctor may advise additional evaluations.

Chest X-ray
A chest X-ray produces an image that includes your heart and blood vessels. It can be useful in identifying the presence of an enlarged heart, which may develop after a heart attack or during heart failure. It can also show calcium deposits in some of the large arteries. A chest X-ray may also detect changes in your lungs that are related to abnormal functioning of your heart.

Coronary angiography
Coronary angiography has long been considered the definitive test for coronary artery disease. This test reveals specific sites of narrowing in the coronary arteries.

A hollow, flexible tube (catheter) is inserted into an artery in your groin or wrist and is threaded back through your main artery (aorta) into your heart. The tip of the catheter is then guided into a coronary artery. A dye (contrast agent) is injected through the catheter. As the dye flows through coronary arteries, your doctor can see narrowed segments and blockages with the help of X-ray movies (angiogram).

Angiography can be performed on many other blood vessels in the body. When it's done on the coronary arteries, the test is called coronary angiography.

Nuclear scan
A nuclear scan is a noninvasive test that helps identify blood flow problems to your heart. The pro-

cedure involves injecting a trace amount of radioactive material, such as thallium, into your bloodstream, often during a treadmill test. A special scanning device then records a series of pictures registering the locations of the radioactive material in the heart muscle. Dark areas on the scans indicate portions of your heart to which blood flow is impaired. However, this test doesn't provide an image of the actual blocked artery.

Echocardiography
Echocardiography, another noninvasive test, uses ultrasound sound waves that reflect (echo) off the surfaces of your heart's structure (see the photo on page 743). A computer then constructs an image of your heart or analyzes its blood flow. By assessing how well blood moves with each heartbeat, it can help identify if an area of your heart muscle has been damaged.

When combined with a stress test, echocardiography can help identify areas of diminished blood flow to the heart. For example, when a portion of the heart muscle receives insufficient

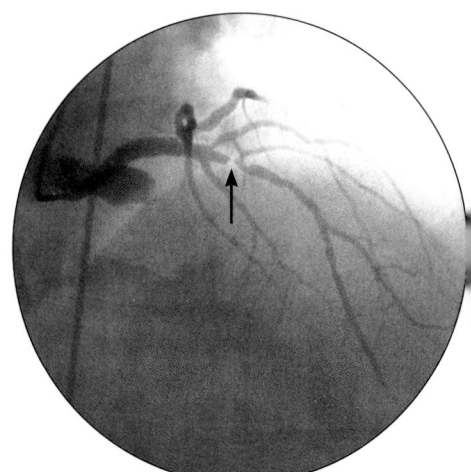

A coronary angiogram outlines the major arteries of the heart. It can show a blockage in an artery (see arrow) due to accumulation of atherosclerotic fatty deposits (plaques).

blood flow during exercise, it develops an abnormal weakened contraction pattern that can be recognized by comparing the images of the contractions at rest before exercise and immediately following exercise.

Coronary calcium scan

A coronary calcium scan can detect calcium deposits within coronary arteries. Calcium deposits (calcifications) are indicators of atherosclerosis, the leading cause of coronary artery disease.

If a substantial amount of calcium is discovered, coronary artery disease is likely. Calcium deposits appear as light spots on the scans and can be measured. However, the presence of coronary calcium doesn't necessarily mean you'll have a heart attack, nor does the absence of calcium deposits exclude coronary artery disease.

A coronary calcium scan is most useful in people who have risk factors for coronary artery disease but are reluctant to change behaviors or use preventive medications, such as statins. If positive, the scan can be used to guide them.

Heart scan. Computerized tomography (CT) technologies can help your doctor see calcium deposits in your arteries that can narrow the arteries. If a substantial amount of calcium is discovered, coronary artery disease may be likely. A CT coronary angiogram, in which you receive a contrast dye injected intravenously during a CT scan, also can generate images of your heart arteries.

Treatment

Treatment of coronary artery disease involves identifying and treating the underlying cause — in most cases, the cause is atherosclerosis. Changing your daily habits may be the single most effective way to treat atherosclerosis and prevent coronary artery disease from progressing.

The most beneficial changes that you can make include:
- **Diet.** Eating a diet low in fat — especially saturated fat — and cholesterol helps reduce high blood cholesterol, a primary cause of atherosclerosis. In fact, maintaining healthy cholesterol levels following a heart attack helps lower your risk of having another one. Eating less fat can also help you lose weight. If you're overweight, losing weight can help you further lower blood cholesterol.
- **Exercise.** A program of regular walking can stimulate the formation of collateral vessels around a narrowed artery, thus bypassing the blockage and increasing circulation. Although collateral vessels won't return circulation to normal, they may reduce symptoms enough to eliminate or delay the need for more-aggressive treatment.
- **Quitting smoking.** Smoking increases the tendency for blood to clot and obstruct the flow of blood. It also reduces your high-density lipoprotein (HDL or "good") cholesterol and deprives your heart muscle of the oxygen it needs to function properly. Quitting smoking dramatically lowers your risk of complications from atherosclerosis.

Medication

Various drugs can be used to treat coronary artery disease, including:

Cholesterol medications. By decreasing the amount of cholesterol in the blood, especially low-density lipoprotein (LDL, or the "bad") cholesterol, these drugs decrease the primary material that deposits on the coronary arteries. Your doctor can choose from a range of medications, including statins, niacin, fibrates and bile acid sequestrants.

Aspirin. Your doctor may recommend taking a daily aspirin or other blood thinner. This can reduce the tendency of your blood to clot, which may help prevent obstruction of your coronary arteries. If you've had a heart attack, aspirin can help prevent future attacks. There are some cases where aspirin isn't appropriate, such as if you have a bleeding disorder or you're already taking another blood thinner.

Beta blockers. These medications slow your heart rate and decrease your blood pressure, which decreases your heart's demand for oxygen. If you've had a heart attack, beta blockers can reduce the risk of future attacks.

Nitroglycerin. Nitroglycerin tablets, sprays and patches can control chest pain by temporarily dilating your coronary arteries and reducing your heart's demand for blood.

Angiotensin-converting enzyme (ACE) inhibitors and angiotensin II receptor blockers (ARBs). These similar medications decrease your blood pressure and may help to prevent progression of coronary artery disease.

Revascularization procedures

In some cases, medications don't provide adequate relief, and the blocked artery must be widened (dilated) to allow adequate blood flow. This is done with a procedure called coronary angioplasty.

During the procedure, your doctor inserts a long, thin tube (catheter) into the narrowed part of your artery. A wire with a deflated balloon is passed through the catheter to the narrowed area. The balloon is then inflated, compressing the deposits against your artery walls.

A tiny wire-mesh tube (stent) is often left in the artery to help keep the artery open. Some stents slowly release medication to help keep the artery open.

Coronary Angioplasty

Coronary angioplasty, also called percutaneous coronary intervention (PCI), is a common medical procedure used to open clogged heart arteries.

Coronary angioplasty can improve symptoms associated with blocked arteries, such as chest pain and shortness of breath, or it can be used during a heart attack to quickly open a blocked artery and minimize heart damage.

Angioplasty involves temporarily inserting and expanding a tiny balloon at the site of your blockage to help widen a narrowed artery. Angioplasty is usually combined with implantation of a small metal coil called a stent in the clogged artery to help prop it open and decrease the chance of it narrowing again (restenosis).

Who is angioplasty for?

When medications or lifestyle changes aren't enough to reduce the effects of artery blockages, or if you have a heart attack, worsening chest pain or other symptoms, your doctor might suggest angioplasty. First you'll have an imaging test called a coronary angiogram to determine if your blockages can be treated with angioplasty.

You may be a good candidate for angioplasty if:

- Your blockage is small
- Your blockage can be reached by angioplasty
- The artery affected isn't the main vessel supplying blood to the left side of your heart
- You don't have heart failure
  If the main artery supplying the left side of your heart is narrowed, if your heart muscle is weak or if you have small, diffusely diseased blood vessels, then coronary artery bypass graft (CABG) may be a better option. In addition, if you have diabetes and multiple blockages,

your doctor may suggest coronary artery bypass surgery.

The decision of angioplasty versus bypass surgery will depend on the details of your heart disease and overall medical condition.

What happens during angioplasty?

Angioplasty is performed by a heart specialist (cardiologist) and a team of specialized cardiovascular nurses and technicians, usually in a cardiac catheterization laboratory. The procedure isn't considered surgery because it's less invasive — your body isn't cut open except for a very small puncture in a blood vessel in the leg, arm or wrist through which a small, thin tube (called a catheter) is threaded and the procedure performed. The entire procedure can take 30 minutes to several hours.

Angioplasty is commonly performed through an artery in your groin (femoral artery). Less commonly, it may be done using an artery in your arm or wrist area.

- Before the procedure, the area is prepared with antiseptic solution.
- A local anesthetic is injected into your groin to numb the area.

- Small electrode pads are placed on your chest to monitor your heart rate and rhythm.

General anesthesia isn't needed, so you're awake during the procedure. You'll receive fluids and medications for relaxation and mild sedation through an intravenous catheter. Blood-thinning medications (anticoagulants) are used to reduce blood clotting, and then the procedure begins:

- After numbing the incision area, a small cut is made, usually in your leg, to access an artery. Your doctor will then insert a thin guide wire into the artery and thread it through the artery from the incision area up to your blockage.
- Once the guide wire reaches the blockage, a small, thin tube (catheter) is passed over the wire until it reaches the blockage. You might feel pressure in your groin while this is being done, but you shouldn't feel sharp pain. You also won't feel the catheter in your body.
- A small amount of contrast agent, or dye, is injected through the catheter. This helps your doctor look at the blockage on X-ray images called angiograms.

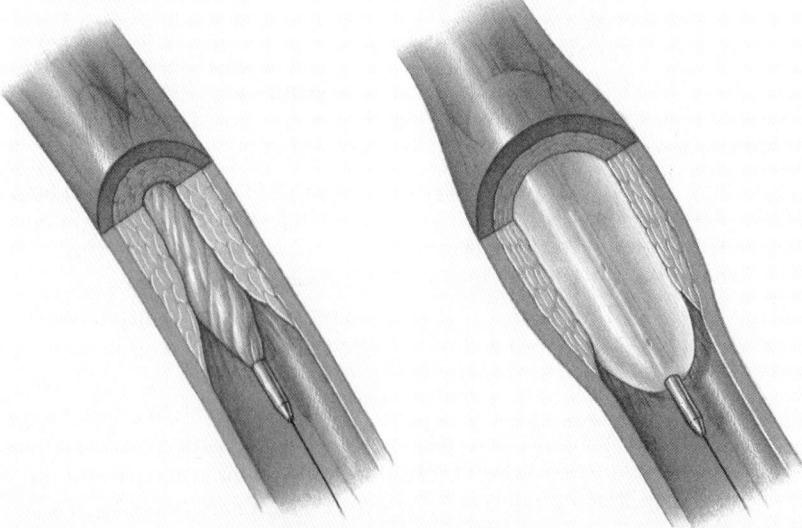

During coronary angioplasty, a balloon-tipped tube is inserted through a catheter and directed to the narrowed portion of the artery (left). The balloon is inflated, compressing deposits and widening the artery (right).

- A small balloon at the end of the catheter is inflated, widening the blocked artery. The balloon stays inflated for up to several minutes at the site of the blockage, stretching out the artery before it's deflated and removed. Your doctor might inflate and deflate the balloon several times before it's removed, stretching the artery a bit more each time to widen it.

Because the balloon temporarily blocks blood flow to part of your heart, it's common to experience chest pain while it's inflated. If you have several blockages, the procedure may be repeated at each site.

Stents provide added support

Once the artery is widened, a device called a stent is usually placed in the artery to act as scaffolding to help prevent it from re-narrowing. The stent looks like a very tiny coil of wire mesh. Stents can be coated with medication that's slowly released to help prevent arteries from re-clogging. These coated stents are called drug-eluting stents, in contrast to noncoated versions, which are

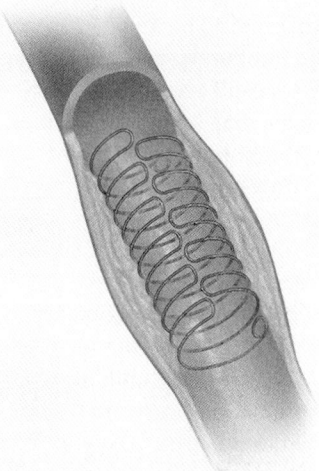

After angioplasty, a fine, metallic mesh tube (stent) is often placed in the artery to prevent renarrowing (restenosis).

called bare-metal stents. The stent remains in the artery permanently to hold it open and improve blood flow to your heart.

Anticoagulant medications are prescribed to prevent blood clots, relax your arteries and protect against coronary spasms.

Results

For most people, coronary angioplasty greatly increases blood flow through the previously blocked artery and reduces or eliminates chest pain. Lifestyle modifications can help you maintain your good results. They include:
- Stopping smoking
- Maintaining a healthy weight
- Getting regular exercise
- Lowering your cholesterol levels
- Controlling other conditions, such as diabetes and high blood pressure

Successful angioplasty also means you might not have to undergo a more invasive surgical procedure called coronary artery bypass surgery. During a bypass, an artery or a vein is removed from a different part of your body and sewn to the surface of your heart to allow blood to flow around (bypass) the blocked coronary artery. It requires a large incision in the chest, and recovery is usually longer and more uncomfortable.

If you have many blockages or narrowing of the main artery leading to the heart, reduced heart function, or diabetes, your doctor may recommend bypass surgery instead of angioplasty and stent placement. In addition, for technical reasons some blockages may be better treated with bypass surgery.

Benefits of angioplasty

As with most medical procedures, angioplasty has benefits and risks. Among the benefits are:
- It doesn't require a major incision.
- General anesthesia isn't needed.
- Major complications are uncommon.

- It can relieve your symptoms, such as chest pain.

Risks of angioplasty

The most common risks include:
- *Re-narrowing of your artery (restenosis).* With angioplasty alone — without stent placement — restenosis happens in about 30 percent of cases. Stents were developed to reduce restenosis. Bare-metal stents reduce the chance of restenosis to about 15 percent, and the use of drug-eluting stents reduces the risk to less than 10 percent.
- *Blood clots.* Blood clots can form within stents even after the procedure. These clots can close the artery, causing a heart attack. It's important to take aspirin, clopidogrel (Plavix), prasugrel (Effient), ticagrelor (Brilinta) or another medication that helps reduce the risk of blood clots exactly as prescribed to decrease the chance of clots forming in your stent. Talk to your doctor about how long you'll need to take these medications, and never discontinue them without discussing it with your doctor.
- *Bleeding.* You may have bleeding in your leg or arm where a catheter was inserted. Usually this simply results in a bruise, but sometimes serious bleeding occurs and may require a blood transfusion or surgical procedures.

Other risks:
- Though rare, you may experience a heart attack.
- Your coronary artery may be torn or ruptured (dissected).
- The dye used during angioplasty and stent placement can cause kidney damage, especially in people with kidney problems.
- A stroke can occur if plaques break loose when the catheters are being threaded through the aorta. Blood clots also can form in catheters and travel to the brain if they break loose. A stroke is an extremely rare complication of coronary angioplasty.

Surgery

Severe blockages or those in places that are too difficult to reach using a catheter may require surgery. In these cases, a doctor may recommend an operation to bypass the blocked arteries, thereby providing an alternate route for blood flow (see page 725).

Angina

Signs and symptoms
- Pain — a tight, band-like, crushing, suffocating sensation — that's usually centered beneath the breastbone (sternum) and may spread to the throat, jaw or arm
- A sensation of heaviness or tightness in the chest that is less than pain
- Chest pain brought on by exercise or emotional stress

Angina is a type of chest pain or discomfort caused by reduced blood flow to the heart. Angina is a symptom of coronary artery disease. When your heart muscle doesn't get enough oxygen-rich blood, you may have chest pain.

Angina pectoris, the medical term for angina, gets its name from the nature of the pain. The Latin word *angere*, for "choke," describes the characteristic suffocating sensation, and the term *pectoralis*, for "chest," indicates where it's located.

Angina is often one of the warning signs of coronary artery disease. When the attacks come frequently and without physical activity, they may be warning signs of an impending heart attack and require urgent treatment.

The discomfort usually lasts from two to 15 minutes. The pain may be severe and may be accompanied by a constricting feeling behind the breastbone and extending into the throat, jaw or arm. People sometimes describe it as mild heaviness, tightness or burning discomfort. Angina may be referred, which means that your brain confuses the pain impulses, causing you to feel the discomfort in your throat, jaw or arm rather than in your chest.

Angina is usually brought on by exertion such as heavy lifting, sexual activity or strenuous exercise. When you exert yourself, your heart requires more oxygen to do the extra work. When narrowed coronary arteries that serve your heart are unable to provide increased blood flow demanded by the exercise, nerves in your heart transmit pain messages to your brain.

Extreme cold or emotions such as intense fear, anger, grief and frustration can bring on the pain, as can ingestion of a heavy meal.

Types
The severity, duration and type of angina can vary. It's important to recognize if you have new or changing chest pain because it may signal a more dangerous form of angina or a heart attack. With each type the pain may vary:

Stable angina
- Develops predictably when your heart works harder, such as when exercising or climbing stairs
- Is usually similar to previous types of chest pain you've had
- Lasts a short time, perhaps five minutes or less
- Disappears when you rest or take your angina medication
- May feel like indigestion
- May be triggered by mental or emotional stress

Unstable angina
- Occurs even at rest
- Is a change from your usual pattern of angina
- Is unexpected
- Is more severe and lasts longer, maybe as long as 30 minutes
- May not disappear with rest or the use of angina medication

Variant angina
- Usually happens unpredictably during rest
- Is often severe
- May be relieved by angina medication

Stable angina is the most common form of angina. If this is a new symptom for you, it's important to see a doctor or health care professional to establish a diagnosis and proper treatment. If your stable angina gets worse or changes, becoming unstable, seek medical attention immediately. Variant angina is caused by a spasm of the muscles in the wall of the coronary arteries.

Diagnosis
A diagnosis of angina is usually suspected based on a person's history of chest discomfort and the setting in which it occurs. There's no specific laboratory test for the diagnosis of angina. Your doctor may want to obtain an electrocardiogram to see if a heart attack has occurred or is occurring. He or she may also order certain blood tests to rule out other disorders that may force your heart to beat faster, use more oxygen and, therefore, precipitate angina. A stress test can measure how your heart and blood vessels respond to exertion, which may indicate if your pain is related to your heart (see page 717).

How serious is angina?
The decrease in blood flow to your heart caused by angina is partial and temporary, so muscle damage doesn't occur. In some cases, angina may serve as a warning of a future or impending heart attack. If you have angina, see your doctor.

Treatment
If you experience angina, try to stop the activity that precipitated the attack. This should lessen the load on your heart and reduce its need for increased oxygen. Your pain and other symptoms will probably improve within a few minutes. If the discomfort doesn't stop within several minutes or if the frequency or severity of the attacks increases, seek prompt medical attention.

One of the first steps in treating angina is to modify factors that may trigger or worsen the condition. If you smoke, stop. If you're overweight, lose the extra pounds. Eliminating obesity or stopping smoking may decrease or even end your symptoms.

Exercise

Having angina doesn't need to make you sedentary. In fact, exercise is a key part of managing your condition. The exercise must be compatible with the limitations imposed by your pain and is often suggested after your angina is under control with medications. Your symptoms and your doctor will help you determine how much exercise is appropriate.

Medication

The type of medication your doctor recommends will depend on your particular symptoms. You may need more than one medication to get the best effect.

- **Nitrates.** Nitrates are often used to treat angina. Nitrates relax and widen your blood vessels, allowing more blood to flow to your heart muscle. You might take a nitrate when you have angina-related chest discomfort, before doing something that normally triggers angina (such as physical exertion), or on a long-term preventive basis. The most common form of nitrate used to treat angina is with nitroglycerin tablets put under your tongue.
- **Aspirin.** Aspirin reduces the ability of your blood to clot, making it easier for blood to flow through narrowed heart arteries. Preventing blood clots can also reduce your risk of a heart attack. But don't start taking a daily aspirin without talking to your doctor first.
- **Clot-preventing drugs.** Certain medications, such as clopidogrel (Plavix), prasugrel (Effient) and ticagrelor (Brilinta), can help prevent blood clots from form-

ing by making your blood platelets less likely to stick together.
- **Beta blockers.** Beta blockers work by blocking the effects of the hormone epinephrine, also known as adrenaline. As a result, the heart beats more slowly and with less force, thereby reducing blood pressure. Beta blockers also help blood vessels relax and open up to improve blood flow, thus reducing or preventing angina.
- **Statins.** Statins are drugs used to lower blood cholesterol. They work by blocking a substance your body needs to make cholesterol. They may also help your body reabsorb cholesterol that has accumulated in plaques in your artery walls, helping prevent further blockage in your blood vessels. Statins also have many other beneficial effects on your heart arteries.
- **Calcium channel blockers.** Calcium channel blockers, also called calcium antagonists, relax and widen blood vessels by affecting the muscle cells in the arterial walls. This increases blood flow in your heart, reducing or preventing angina.
- **Ranolazine (Ranexa).** Ranexa can be used alone or with other angina medications, such as calcium channel blockers, beta blockers or nitroglycerin. Unlike some other angina medications, Ranexa can be used if you're taking oral erectile dysfunction medications.

Surgery and other procedures

If angina continues despite lifestyle changes or the use of medications or it occurs more often or with greater intensity (unstable angina), your doctor may consider a procedure called coronary angiography to look at the anatomy of your coronary vessels. This test can help your doctor evaluate whether you're a candidate for coronary angioplasty (see page 720) or coronary artery bypass surgery (see page 725).

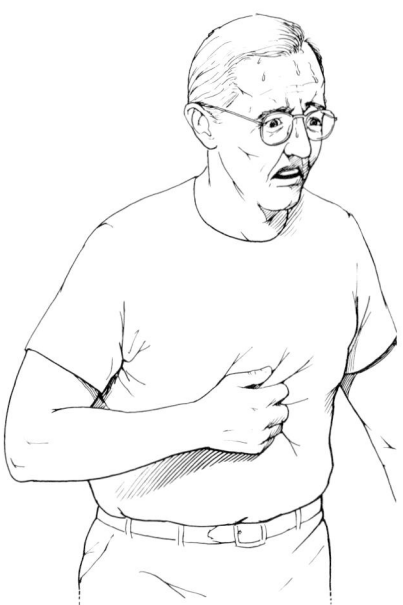

The pain of a heart attack varies from person to person, but typically you'll experience a profound squeezing sensation in the chest, accompanied by profuse perspiration. Pain may radiate to the left shoulder and arm, to the back and even to the jaw and teeth.

Heart attack

Emergency signs and symptoms

- Pressure, fullness or squeezing pain in the center of the chest lasting more than a few minutes
- Pain that extends beyond the chest to the left shoulder and arm, the back, and even the teeth and jaw
- Pain in the upper abdomen
- Shortness of breath
- Sweating
- Nausea and vomiting
- Impending sense of doom
- Fainting

A heart attack causes injury to your heart muscle from loss of blood supply. It usually occurs when a blood clot blocks blood flow through a coronary artery. Years ago, a heart attack was often fatal. Thanks to better awareness of signs and symptoms and improved treatments, most people who have a heart attack now survive.

The medical term for a heart attack is *myocardial infarction. Myo* means

What to Do in Case of a Heart Attack

If you think you or someone you're with is having a heart attack, promptly take the following steps:

1. *Seek urgent medical attention.* Call for emergency medical help or take the sick person to the nearest emergency department. Each year thousands of people die because they didn't seek medical help in time. Don't worry about confusing a heart attack with indigestion or something else. If in doubt, don't wait before calling for help.

2. *Have the sick person chew an aspirin.* Aspirin prevents blood from clotting and may help restore blood flow through clogged arteries, significantly improving the odds of surviving. Chewing the aspirin instead of swallowing it whole speeds absorption into the system.

3. *Use cardiopulmonary resuscitation (CPR).* If you're with someone who stops breathing, begin CPR immediately. After a person stops breathing, he or she can live only a few minutes without CPR.

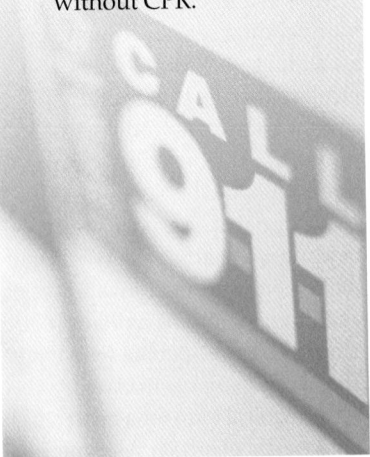

"muscle," *kardia* means "heart" and *infarct* refers to an area of dead tissue that's caused by lack of oxygen.

Most often the clot that causes a heart attack forms in a coronary artery narrowed by an accumulation of cholesterol and other fatty deposits in atherosclerotic plaques.

A plaque consists of a firm shell that may contain calcium with areas of fatty material. The center consists of soft cholesterol. The shell may crack or fissure, exposing the inner portion. When this happens, a blood clot tends to develop at that site. If the clot blocks blood flow in a coronary artery for longer than 20 minutes to two hours, it causes a heart attack.

Rarely, a heart attack can occur when a blood clot from inside a diseased heart breaks loose and lodges in a coronary artery. Another uncommon cause of a heart attack is a spasm of a coronary artery that shuts down blood flow to the heart. Drugs such as cocaine can cause such a life-threatening spasm. A condition called spontaneous coronary artery dissection (SCAD) also can result in a heart attack. It's an uncommon emergency condition that results when a tear forms in a heart blood vessel.

A heart attack isn't a static, one-time event. It's a dynamic process that typically evolves over four to six hours. With each passing minute, more heart tissue is deprived of oxygen and deteriorates or dies, forming scar tissue and causing pain and pressure. If blood flow can be restored quickly, damage to the heart can be prevented or limited.

If you think that you or someone you're with is having a heart attack, call for emergency medical assistance or take the sick person to the nearest hospital emergency department. Don't delay in seeking medical help — it's a mistake that takes thousands of lives every year. Some people think the pain will disappear on its own or they're having a bout of indigestion.

A heart attack may be preceded by a series of angina attacks, or it may occur suddenly with no advance warning. Unlike angina, however, the pain doesn't cease when the exercise or stress that caused it is discontinued.

The pain may be constant, or it may come and go. Occasionally, the pain doesn't fit any particular pattern. This is especially true in older adults and people with diabetes. In these individuals, it's not unusual for a heart attack to occur with no symptoms. These silent heart attacks may be detected only when a routine electrocardiogram reveals a change in the pattern of transmission of electrical impulses through the heart.

In some people, a primary symptom of a heart attack is a sudden onset of shortness of breath. Among a few people, the only symptom is a sudden fainting spell.

Factors that put you at increased risk of a heart attack include smoking, obesity, lack of physical activity, high blood pressure, high cholesterol, diabetes, family history, excessive use of alcohol and stress. Men are usually at higher risk of heart attacks than are women. However, the risk for women increases after menopause.

Diagnosis

If you're having a heart attack or suspect you're having one, you'll likely be asked to describe your symptoms and have your blood pressure, pulse and temperature checked. You'll be hooked up to a heart monitor and will almost immediately have tests done to determine if you're having a heart attack. These tests may include:

- **Electrocardiogram (ECG).** An electrocardiogram records the electrical activity of your heart via electrodes attached to your skin. Because injured heart muscle doesn't conduct electrical impulses normally, the ECG may show that a heart attack occurred or is in progress.
- **Blood tests.** Certain heart enzymes slowly leak out into your blood if your heart has been

Bypass Surgery

Heart attacks, angina and other heart-related problems can occur as the result of narrowed or blocked coronary arteries that supply blood to the heart muscle. In certain situations, coronary artery bypass surgery may provide an alternate route for blood flow to your heart muscle. Bypass surgery is most often performed when your symptoms don't respond to other medical treatment or when you have multiple blockages of the coronary arteries.

Procedure

To create a bypass, a surgeon transplants (grafts) a blood vessel from another part of your body to a coronary artery. He or she may use one of three blood vessels: the internal mammary artery from the chest, the saphenous vein from the inner side of the leg or the radial artery from the forearm. These are blood vessels that your body doesn't need. Some doctors may use a combination of these grafts.

In most cases, the internal mammary artery is used as the bypass. This artery lies inside the front wall of the chest. There's one on each side of the breastbone. The lower end of this artery is freed from the inside surface of the chest wall and sewn to the coronary artery beyond the blockage. The other end is left attached and blood is rerouted into the coronary arteries. The major advantage of this type of graft is its tendency to resist later formation of fatty deposits (plaques).

To create a bypass graft with the saphenous vein or the radial artery, a segment of the vein or artery is removed. One end of the vein or artery is attached to the aorta above the blocked coronary artery. The other end of the vein or artery is connected to the coronary artery beyond the blocked area. Thus, the diseased part of the artery is bypassed.

For a portion of the operation, the functions of your heart and lungs are assumed by a heart-lung machine.

Results

The goal of bypass surgery is adequate blood flow to the heart muscle, which generally is reestablished. Improved blood flow often relieves angina or other coronary artery problems.

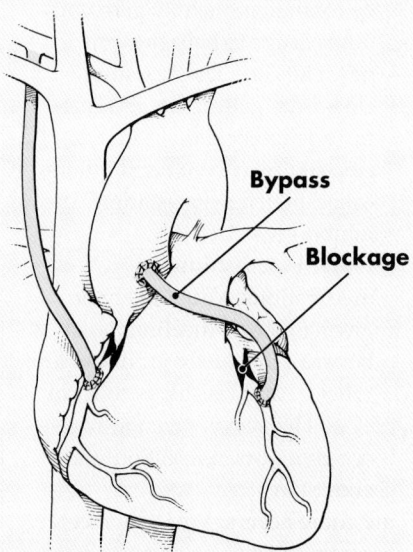

Bypasses around blockage sites can be surgically constructed out of blood vessels taken from the leg (saphenous veins) or forearm (radial arteries) or from arteries arising near the collarbone (internal mammary arteries).

Bypass operations are done frequently by experienced surgical teams. However, as with any operation, there are risks. In general, if you're under age 65, you have a normal left ventricle — the heart's major pumping chamber — and you're in relatively good health, your chance of surviving the operation and recovery is 99 percent.

Recovery and rehabilitation

A five- to seven-day stay in the hospital is usual following bypass surgery. Immediately after the operation, you may spend 24 to 36 hours in a special coronary (cardiac) care unit (CCU) or intensive care unit (ICU). There the rate and rhythm of your heart and other vital signs are closely monitored.

Your doctor or surgeon will advise you about the degree of exertion your activities can involve for the next several weeks of recovery and the gradual resumption of normal activities.

Who's a candidate?

If you have mild angina on exertion or have recovered from a heart attack with no continuing symptoms, you may be best treated with medication or by other means.

Bypass surgery is generally considered appropriate for the following people:

- Individuals with a blocked left main coronary artery
- Individuals with disease in multiple arteries and poor function of the left ventricle
- Individuals with incapacitating angina

For such people, a bypass procedure is of clear value and life is prolonged in most cases.

---

damaged. Medical personnel will likely take samples of your blood to test for the presence of these enzymes.

You may undergo additional tests, including and an echocardiogram and coronary catheterization (angiogram). An echocardiogram can help determine if a part of your heart has been damaged. An angiogram can show if your coronary arteries are narrowed or blocked.

How serious is a heart attack?

A heart attack may lead to sudden death, either because so much of the heart tissue dies that the heart no longer can function or because a fatal heart rhythm disorder develops. Most people who die of a heart attack have severe blockages of more than one coronary artery.

If the area of damaged tissue is small and the electrical system that controls your heart isn't damaged, your chances of surviving a heart attack are good. The sooner you get to a hospital, the more that can be done to limit the amount of heart muscle damage.

Damage to only a small portion of the ventricle muscle may lead to a decrease in the amount of blood that your heart can eject during each contraction. The reduction in heart function is mild, so you can usually expect a return to a reasonably normal lifestyle.

If a moderate amount of heart muscle is damaged, congestive heart failure may develop. If a significant amount of the heart muscle is damaged — half the muscle, or more — shock or death may occur.

Treatment

As early as the initial minutes of a heart attack, ventricular fibrillation can occur. This unstable heart rhythm produces an ineffective heartbeat, and the heart muscle quivers uselessly.

Without immediate treatment, ventricular fibrillation usually leads to sudden death. Use of automatic external defibrillators (AEDs) that can shock the heart back into a normal rhythm can provide emergency treatment before reaching the hospital.

These lifesaving, portable devices are increasingly available in ambulances, police cars, commercial airplanes and some public facilities. They come with plainly worded instructions and require little training to use.

If you encounter someone who is unconscious from a presumed heart attack, call for emergency medical help and, if you've received training in emergency procedures, begin cardiopulmonary resuscitation (CPR). If you're not trained in emergency procedures, skip mouth-to-mouth rescue breathing and proceed directly to chest compressions. See Chapter 1"First Aid and Emergency Care," for more information.

Medication

Initial treatment of a heart attack generally involves medications such as:

- **Aspirin.** The 911 operator may instruct you to take aspirin, or emergency medical personnel may give you aspirin immediately. Aspirin reduces blood clotting, thus helping maintain blood flow through a narrowed artery.
- **Thrombolytics.** These drugs, also called clotbusters, help dissolve a blood clot that's blocking blood flow to your heart. The earlier you receive a thrombolytic drug after a heart attack, the greater the chance that you'll survive and with less heart damage.
- **Antiplatelet agents.** Emergency room doctors may give you other drugs to help prevent new clots and keep existing clots from getting larger. These include medications, such as clopidogrel (Plavix) and others, called platelet aggregation inhibitors.
- **Other blood-thinning medications.** You'll likely be given other medications, such as heparin, to make your blood less "sticky" and less likely to form clots. Heparin is given intravenously or by an injection under your skin.
- **Pain relievers.** You may receive a pain reliever, such as morphine, to ease your discomfort.
- **Nitroglycerin.** This medication, used to treat chest pain (angina), can help improve blood flow to the heart by widening (dilating) the blood vessels.
- **Beta blockers.** These medications help relax your heart muscle, slow your heartbeat and decrease blood pressure, making your heart's job easier. Beta blockers can limit the amount of heart muscle damage and prevent future heart attacks.
- **ACE inhibitors.** These drugs lower blood pressure and reduce stress on the heart.

Surgical and other procedures

In addition to medications, one of the following procedures may be necessary to treat a heart attack:

- **Coronary angioplasty and stenting.** Doctors insert a long, thin tube (catheter) that's passed through an artery, usually in your leg or groin, to a blocked artery in your heart. This procedure is often done immediately after a cardiac catheterization, a procedure used to locate blockages.

  The catheter is equipped with a special balloon that, once in position, is briefly inflated to open a blocked coronary artery. A metal mesh stent may be inserted into the artery to keep it open long term, restoring blood flow to the heart. Depending on your condition, your doctor may opt to place a stent coated with a slow-releasing medication to help keep your artery open.
- **Coronary artery bypass surgery.** In some cases, doctors may perform emergency bypass surgery at the time of a heart attack. If possible, your doctor may suggest that you have bypass surgery after your heart has had time to recover from your heart attack — about three to seven days. Bypass surgery involves sewing veins or arteries in place beyond a blocked or narrowed coronary artery, allowing blood flow to the heart to bypass the narrowed section.

  Once blood flow to your heart is restored and your condition is stable following your heart attack, you may be hospitalized for observation. Because physical exertion and emotional upset place stress on your heart, be sure to rest. Visitors are usually limited to family members and close friends.

Rehabilitation

The goal of emergency treatment of a heart attack is to restore blood flow and save heart tissue. The purpose of subsequent treatment is to promote healing of your heart and prevent another heart attack.

Sex Following a Heart Attack

Having a heart attack doesn't mean that you'll never be able to have sex again. Usually, all that's required is a sensible lapse, perhaps of a few weeks after your heart attack.

The demands placed on your heart when you have sexual relations are roughly the same as taking a brisk walk or climbing a flight or two of stairs. Your heart rate, breathing rate and blood pressure increase. Therefore, sexual activities need to be approached as any other physical activities: sensibly, with caution but without fear.

Take it easy

In order to minimize the stress on your heart, it may help to resume sexual activity with your partner under circumstances you're already accustomed to. You'll probably feel more relaxed making love in a familiar setting. If you find certain positions less strenuous than others, choose the less taxing route.

Communicate

Talk to your partner, both before and after sexual activity, to reassure yourself and your partner. Shared fears and concerns may be alleviated if lines of communication are open. Talk to your doctor if you have any questions. It's quite normal for your needs to change temporarily. You may experience either increased or reduced desire for sexual activity.

Be aware

If you experience chest pain, extreme shortness of breath or an irregular heart rhythm during sexual activity, stop. Men should avoid the use of sildenafil (Viagra), a medication taken for erectile dysfunction, until their doctor has approved its use. Using Viagra while also taking nitrates, such as nitroglycerin or isosorbide, may increase the chance of serious cardiovascular events and a severe drop in blood pressure.

Some hospitals offer cardiac rehabilitation programs that may start while you're in the hospital and, depending on the severity of your attack, continue for weeks to months after you return home. You may undergo a wide variety of rehabilitative strategies involving a varied group of professionals.

Cardiac rehabilitation usually involves the use of medication to keep your heart functioning as near normal as possible and help prevent a second heart attack. Rehabilitation also involves lifestyle readjustments. In addition to mentally and emotionally adjusting to your situation, you may need to make other important changes in your life. The rehabilitation team can assist you, particularly as you begin to implement new habits.

- **Don't smoke.** If you smoke, the single most important thing you can do to improve your heart's health is to stop. It's very hard to stop smoking by yourself, so ask your doctor to prescribe a treatment plan to help you kick the habit.
- **Check your cholesterol.** Have your blood cholesterol levels checked regularly, through a blood test at your doctor's office. If "bad" cholesterol levels are undesirably high, your doctor can prescribe changes to your diet and medications to help lower the numbers and protect your cardiovascular health.
- **Get regular medical checkups.** Some of the major risk factors for a heart attack — high blood cholesterol, high blood pressure and diabetes — cause no symptoms in their early stages. If you have one of these conditions, you and your doctor can manage it early to prevent complications that can lead to a heart attack.
- **Control your blood pressure.** Have your blood pressure checked every two years. Your doctor may recommend more frequent measurement if you have high blood pressure or a history of coronary artery disease.
- **Exercise regularly.** Regular exercise helps improve heart muscle function following a heart attack. Exercise is a major component of a cardiac rehabilitation program. It helps prevent a heart attack by helping you achieve and maintain a healthy weight and control diabetes, elevated cholesterol and high blood pressure. Exercise doesn't have to be vigorous. Walking 30 minutes a day, five days a week can improve your health.
- **Maintain a healthy weight.** Excess weight strains your heart and can contribute to high cholesterol, high blood pressure and diabetes. Losing weight can lower your risk of heart disease.
- **Eat a heart-healthy diet.** Too much saturated fat and cholesterol in your diet can narrow arteries to your heart. If you've had a heart attack, limit fat and cholesterol — and sodium. A diet high in sodium can raise your blood pressure. Follow your doctor's and dietitian's advice on eating a heart-healthy diet. Fish is part of a heart-healthy diet. It contains omega-3 fatty acids, which help improve blood cholesterol levels and prevent blood clots. Eat plenty of fruits and vegetables. Fruits and vegetables contain antioxidants — nutrients that help prevent everyday wear and tear on your coronary arteries.
- **Manage stress.** To reduce your risk of a heart attack, reduce stress in your day-to-day activities. Rethink workaholic

habits and find healthy ways to minimize or deal with stressful events in your life.

- **Consume alcohol in moderation, if at all.** Drinking more than one to two alcoholic drinks a day raises blood pressure, so cut back on alcohol consumption if necessary. For men, moderate alcohol consumption is one to two drinks daily. For women, it's one alcoholic beverage a day. One drink is equivalent to 12 ounces of beer, 4 ounces of wine or 1.5 ounces of an 80-proof liquor.

Surviving a heart attack doesn't mean that life as you knew it is over. On the contrary, most people lead full, active lives after a heart attack. But it may mean making some changes in your daily habits, being patient as you recover and adopting a can-do attitude.

Heart Failure

Heart failure is a serious problem, but it doesn't mean that the heart isn't working at all. Heart failure has various degrees of severity, depending on what the problem is and how long it has existed.

Congestive heart failure

Signs and symptoms
- Weakness and fatigue
- Shortness of breath
- Rapid or irregular heartbeat
- Persistent cough or wheezing
- Swelling in legs, ankles and feet
- Swelling in abdomen

Congestive heart failure typically develops slowly and is a chronic, long-term condition. In heart failure, your heart can't pump enough blood to meet your body's needs.

Over time, conditions such as coronary artery disease or high blood pressure can leave your heart too weak or stiff to fill and pump efficiently. The term *congestive* refers to blood backing up into — or congesting — the liver,

abdomen, lower extremities and lungs. In acute heart failure, which is less common, symptoms develop suddenly.

Congestive heart failure mainly affects older adults. If failure occurs in the left pumping chambers of your heart, blood collects in your lungs, which causes them to become congested with fluid. This congestion is responsible for the sensation of breathlessness common in congestive heart failure.

If the right side of your heart fails, blood backs up into your legs and into your liver, which become congested. This produces swelling (edema) that's usually most obvious in the lower legs and ankles. Often, both the left and right sides of the heart fail simultaneously.

Inadequate blood flow to the muscles reduces endurance. Therefore, people with congestive heart failure often experience fatigue when they exert themselves physically.

The heart's loss of pumping efficiency in congestive heart failure may be the result of:
- Narrowed coronary arteries (coronary artery disease)
- Weakened heart muscle tissue from a heart attack
- Diseases directly affecting the heart muscle, such as cardiomyopathy
- Mechanical problems in the valves of the heart
- Prolonged high blood pressure
- Stiffening and constriction of the sac that surrounds the heart (pericardium), which may occur after inflammation of the pericardium (pericarditis)
- Abnormal heart rhythms
- Heart defects present at birth

Diagnosis
If your doctor suspects heart failure, he or she will likely listen to your heart and lungs with a stethoscope to detect sounds associated with heart failure. Your doctor may also look for swollen or distended neck veins, an enlarged liver and swelling of the

feet, all of which may be signs of heart failure.

After a physical exam your doctor may order one or more of the following tests:
- **Blood tests.** Your doctor may take a sample of your blood to check your kidney and thyroid function and to look for indicators of other diseases that affect the heart. In addition, your doctor may check your blood for specific chemical markers of heart failure, such as a hormone called brain natriuretic peptide (BNP). Although first identified in the brain, BNP is secreted by the heart at high levels when it's injured or overworked.
- **Chest X-ray.** X-ray images help your doctor see the condition of your lungs and heart. In heart failure, your heart may appear enlarged and fluid buildup may be visible in your lungs. Your doctor can also use an X-ray to diagnose conditions other than heart failure that may explain your signs and symptoms.
- **Electrocardiogram (ECG).** This test records the electrical activity of your heart through electrodes attached to your skin. Impulses are recorded as waves and displayed on a monitor or printed on paper. This test helps your doctor diagnose heart rhythm problems and damage to your heart from a heart attack that may be underlying heart failure.
- **Echocardiogram.** An important test for diagnosing and monitoring heart failure is the echocardiogram. It uses sound waves to produce a video image of your heart. This image can help doctors determine how well your heart is pumping by measuring the percentage of blood pumped out of your heart's main pumping chamber (the left ventricle) with each heartbeat. This measurement is called the ejection fraction.

In a healthy heart, the ejection fraction is about 60 percent — meaning 60 percent of the blood

Kawasaki Disease

Kawasaki disease is named for the Japanese doctor, Tomisaku Kawasaki, who first described this childhood illness. This condition is capable of producing coronary artery disease in children, and rarely it can cause heart attacks and death. The number of children affected by the illness has increased, and it's now one of the leading causes of acquired heart disease in children — a position once occupied by rheumatic fever.

Four of every five people who acquire Kawasaki disease are less than 4 years old. People of Asian descent, even if they've lived in the United States for generations, are more susceptible than are people of other ethnicities.

Signs and symptoms include:
- A high, spiking fever for more than five days
- Swollen, watery eyes
- Reddened, cracked and swollen surfaces on the lips, tongue, mouth and throat
- Swollen, reddened hands and feet, followed by peeling of the skin in these areas
- A measles-like rash
- Swollen lymph glands of the neck

No one is certain what causes the condition. No infectious agent has been identified with it, although it tends to occur in outbreaks, especially in winter and spring. Some experts suspect that an unusual virus or other germ may be the cause or that toxic agents may be involved. Most of the hallmarks of Kawasaki disease are related to inflammation, and the damage that sometimes occurs in the coronary arteries or heart muscle may be an immune response.

In about one out of five children with Kawasaki disease who aren't treated, heart-related problems develop. The most common is expansion of sections of coronary arteries (aneurysms). In some children, an aneurysm can become obstructed by a blood clot and cause a heart attack. However, this is rare, especially when the condition has been treated.

Although the illness can be harrowing, and despite its effect on the coronary arteries, Kawasaki disease is usually a self-limited illness. The death rate in treated children is well below 1 percent. Even among those in whom coronary problems develop, most have substantial improvement with time.

The goal of treatment is to reduce inflammation and prevent damage to the heart and coronary arteries. This may be accomplished with anti-inflammatory medications and injections of purified human antibodies (immunoglobulin).

---

that fills the ventricle is pumped out with each beat. Other imaging tests may be used to measure ejection fraction, including cardiac catheterization, a multiple gated acquisition (MUGA) scan, magnetic resonance imaging (MRI) and computerized tomography (CT).

In addition to the physical examination, blood tests, chest X-ray and echocardiogram, your doctor may recommend one or more tests to help diagnose heart failure, determine its underlying cause and guide treatment. They include:

- **Stress test.** You may have one of a variety of stress tests either using an exercise bike or treadmill or medications that stress the heart. In some stress tests, pictures are taken of your heart with either nuclear medicine or echocardiographic techniques to determine if you have blockages in your heart arteries causing your heart failure. You may also have an oxygen uptake stress test, which helps your doctor know how well your body is compensating for your condition.

- **Cardiac CT or MRI scan.** These tests are now being used with increased frequency for people with heart failure, not only to measure ejection fraction but to check the heart arteries and valves, determine if you have had a heart attack, and look for unusual causes of heart failure.

- **Coronary catheterization (angiogram).** In this test, a thin, flexible tube (catheter) is inserted into a blood vessel at your groin or arm and guided through the aorta into your coronary arteries. A dye injected through the catheter makes the arteries supplying your heart visible on an X-ray. This test helps doctors identify narrowed arteries to your heart (coronary artery disease) that can be a cause of heart failure. The test may include a ventriculogram — a procedure to determine the strength of the left ventricle (the heart's main pumping chamber) and the health of the heart valves.

How serious is congestive heart failure?

Untreated congestive heart failure can be fatal. However, lifestyle adjustments and proper medication can improve heart function, relieve symptoms and prolong life.

Treatment

The goal of treatment often is to prevent further damage to your heart and help it pump as efficiently as possible.

Self-care

Your doctor may recommend that you get plenty of rest to help you conserve energy. However, this doesn't mean that you should retire to your bed. On the contrary, maintaining your mobility and an exercise regimen can be a key component of the treatment program. Motion improves circulation.

Your doctor may also give you specific nutritional guidelines to follow. In general, you restrict the amount of sodium you consume to help reduce accumulation of fluid. A dietitian may advise you to eat salt-free or reduced-sodium foods. You may also need to avoid alcoholic beverages and, if you're overweight, to lose weight.

Medication

Several types of drugs are useful in the treatment of heart failure. Depending on your symptoms, you might take one or more of the following:

- **Angiotensin-converting enzyme (ACE) inhibitors.** They help people with systolic heart failure live longer and feel better. ACE inhibitors are a type of vasodilator, a drug that widens blood vessels to lower blood pressure, improve blood flow and decrease the workload on the heart. Examples include enalapril (Vasotec), lisinopril (Zestril) and captopril (Capoten).
- **Angiotensin II receptor blockers.** These drugs, which include losartan (Cozaar) and valsartan (Diovan), have many of the same benefits as ACE inhibitors. They may be an alternative for people who can't tolerate ACE inhibitors.
- **Beta blockers.** This class of drugs not only slows your heart rate and reduces blood pressure but also limits or reverses some of the damage to your heart if you have systolic heart failure. Examples include carvedilol (Coreg), metoprolol (Lopressor) and bisoprolol (Zebeta). These medicines reduce the risk of some abnormal heart rhythms and lessen your chance of dying unexpectedly. Beta blockers may reduce signs and symptoms of

heart failure, improve heart function and help you live longer.
- **Diuretics.** Often called water pills, diuretics make you urinate more frequently and keep fluid from collecting in your body. Diuretics, such as furosemide (Lasix), also decrease fluid in your lungs so you can breathe more easily. Because diuretics make your body lose potassium and magnesium, your doctor also may prescribe supplements of these minerals. Your doctor will likely monitor potassium and magnesium levels in your blood with regular blood tests.
- **Aldosterone antagonists.** These drugs include spironolactone (Aldactone) and eplerenone (Inspra). These are potassium-sparing diuretics that have additional properties that may help people with severe systolic heart failure live longer. Unlike some other diuretics, spironolactone and eplerenone can raise the level of potassium in your blood to dangerous levels, so talk to your doctor if increased potassium is a concern, and learn if you need to modify your intake of food that's high in potassium.
- **Inotropes.** These are intravenous medications used in people with severe heart failure in the hospital to improve heart pumping function and maintain blood pressure.
- **Digoxin (Lanoxin).** This drug, also known as digitalis, increases the strength of your heart muscle contractions. It also tends to slow the heartbeat. Digoxin reduces heart failure symptoms in systolic heart failure. It may be more likely to be given to someone with a heart rhythm problem, such as atrial fibrillation.
- **Valsartan and sacubitril (Entresto).** This combination drug is approved for use in certain people with chronic heart failure. The medication helps reduce the risk of needing to be hospitalized when symptoms worsen and helps lower the risk of death from heart failure.

- **Ivabradine (Corlanor).** Ivabradine helps to regulate your heart rate. It's also taken to lower the chance of having to be hospitalized for worsening heart failure.

Your doctor may prescribe other heart medications as well — such as nitrates for chest pain, a statin to lower cholesterol or blood-thinning medications to help prevent blood clots.

Surgery and medical devices

In some cases, surgery is needed to treat the underlying problem that led to heart failure. For example, a damaged heart valve may be repaired or coronary bypass surgery may be performed to treat severely narrowed arteries contributing to heart failure. Other treatments being studied and used include:

- **Implantable cardioverter-defibrillators (ICDs).** An ICD is a device implanted under the skin and attached to the heart with small wires. The ICD monitors the heart rhythm. If the heart starts beating at a dangerous rhythm, the ICD shocks it back into normal rhythm. Sometimes a biventricular pacemaker is combined with an ICD for people with severe heart failure.
- **Cardiac resynchronization therapy (CRT) or biventricular pacing.** A biventricular pacemaker sends timed electrical impulses to both of the heart's lower chambers (the left and right ventricles), so that they pump in synchrony and in a more efficient, coordinated manner. As many as half the people with heart failure have abnormalities in their heart's electrical system that cause their already-weak heart muscle to beat in an uncoordinated fashion. Sometimes a biventricular pacemaker is combined with an ICD for people at greatest risk of rhythm problems.
- **Heart pumps.** These mechanical devices, called left ventricular assist devices (LVADs), are implanted into the abdomen and

attached to a weakened heart to help it pump. Doctors first used heart pumps to help keep heart transplant candidates alive while they waited for a donor heart. LVADs are now sometimes used as an alternative to transplantation.

- **Heart transplant.** Heart transplants can dramatically improve the survival and quality of life, but candidates for transplantation often have to wait a long time before a suitable donor heart is found.

Pulmonary edema

Emergency signs and symptoms
- Severe shortness of breath
- Restlessness, anxiety and a feeling of suffocating
- Cough that produces frothy sputum
- Perspiration
- Pale skin

Pulmonary edema occurs when increased pressure in the veins and capillaries of your lungs forces fluid out of the capillaries and into the lungs' air sacs (alveoli). The result is that your lungs are filled with fluid, making it difficult for them to supply your body with oxygen and eliminate carbon dioxide. This is an emergency situation and requires urgent care.

Pulmonary edema is usually caused by heart problems such as an extensive heart attack, disease of the heart valves or uncontrolled high blood pressure. Rarely, it may result from noncardiac causes such as high-altitude exposure or a lung infection.

Diagnosis
Severe shortness of breath is the primary symptom of pulmonary edema. You may feel as if you're starving for air or drowning. This is often accompanied by anxiety and restlessness.

Chest X-rays can detect engorgement in your lungs' blood vessels. X-rays don't pass through fluid as easily as they

pass through air, so fluid that has leaked into lung tissue is often visible on an X-ray. Other diagnostic tests check for valve or heart muscle problems or determine the amount of pressure in your lungs.

Treatment
Pulmonary edema is a life-threatening condition. Immediate hospitalization and treatment are required. Treatment typically consists of receiving supplemental oxygen. If you're having extreme difficulty breathing, it may be necessary to insert a breathing tube into your trachea and provide temporary mechanical ventilation.

You may also receive one or more of the following medications:

- **Preload reducers.** Doctors commonly use nitroglycerin and diuretics, such as furosemide (Lasix), to treat pulmonary edema. These medications dilate the veins in your lungs and elsewhere in your body, which decreases fluid pressure going into your heart and lungs.
- **Morphine.** This narcotic may relieve shortness of breath and associated anxiety, but the risks of morphine use need to be weighed against the drug's benefits.
- **Afterload reducers.** These drugs dilate the peripheral vessels and take a pressure load off the left ventricle. Some examples of afterload reducer medications include nitroprusside (Nitropress), enalapril (Vasotec) and captopril (Capoten).
- **Aspirin.** Your doctor may recommend aspirin therapy if you're not already taking it. Aspirin helps thin your blood so that it moves through your small blood vessels more easily.
- **Blood pressure medications.** If you have high blood pressure when you develop pulmonary edema, you'll be given medications to lower your blood pressure. If your blood pressure is too low, you're likely to be given drugs to raise it.

Heart Rate and Rhythm Disorders

The pumping of your heart must be continuous. If the process becomes disordered or interrupted, your heart may fail to deliver the blood that your tissues require for life.

Your heart consists of four chambers — two upper chambers (atria) and two lower chambers (ventricles). Within the upper right chamber (right atrium) is a group of cells called the sinus node. The sinus node acts as your heart's natural pacemaker, producing electrical impulses that cause the heart muscle to contract and pump blood. This contraction is heard as a heartbeat.

The rate at which your heart muscle pumps (beats) varies depending on your activity at any given moment.

When you're at rest, your heart pumps more slowly and at a regular rate, about 60 to 100 beats a minute. When you run, climb stairs or otherwise exert yourself, the sinus node issues electrical stimuli that increase the pace of your heart in order to provide your muscles and other tissues with additional blood and oxygen. Depending on your age and level of fitness, your heart rate may increase to 200 beats a minute if you exert yourself strenuously.

If something goes wrong with the functioning of the sinus node, disturbing the normal pacing of your heart, one of a number of disorders of the heart rhythm may occur. Too rapid a heartbeat is called tachycardia. Too slow a heart rate is bradycardia.

Arrhythmias

Signs and symptoms
- Fluttering in your chest
- A racing heartbeat
- A slow heartbeat

Supraventricular Tachycardia

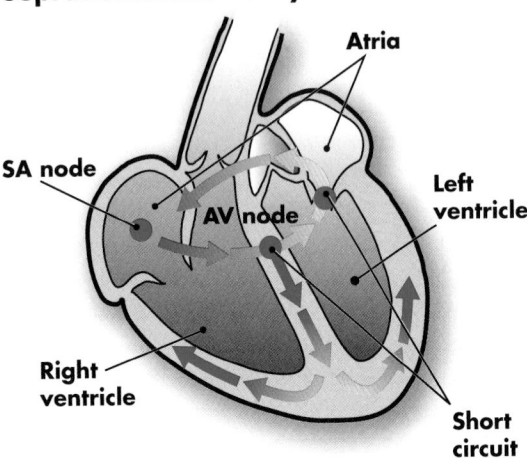
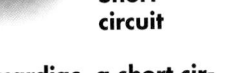

In some supraventricular tachycardias, a short circuit stops some of the electrical signals before they reach the ventricles.

Atrial Fibrillation

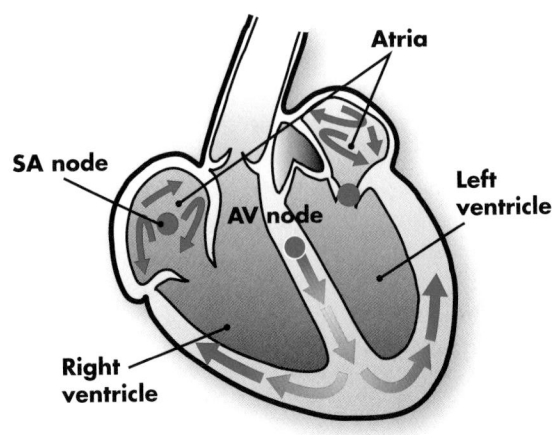

In atrial fibrillation, the upper chambers of the heart (atria) quiver due to chaotic, uncoordinated electrical activity.

- Chest pain
- Shortness of breath
- Lightheadedness
- Dizziness
- Fainting or near fainting

Heart rhythm problems (arrhythmias) occur when the electrical impulses in your heart that coordinate your heartbeats don't function properly, causing your heart to beat too fast, too slow or irregularly.

Arrhythmias are common and usually harmless. Most people have occasional, irregular heartbeats that may feel like a skipped heartbeat or a fluttering or racing heart. However, some heart arrhythmias can cause bothersome — sometimes even life-threatening — signs and symptoms.

Millions of Americans, especially older adults, experience recurrent or symptom-producing heart arrhythmias. Recurrent heart arrhythmias may cause frequent heart palpitations, chest pain and lightheadedness. Some arrhythmias produce no symptoms but are detected during a physical exam or a heart checkup. Not all arrhythmias require treatment.

Causes

In a healthy person with a healthy heart, it's unlikely for a sustained arrhythmia to develop without some outside trigger, such as an electrical shock or the use of illicit drugs. That's primarily because a healthy person's heart is free from any abnormal conditions, such as an area of scarred tissue.

However, in a heart with some evidence of disease or deformity, the initiation or conduction of the heart's electrical impulses may be destabilized, making arrhythmias more likely to develop. Any pre-existing structural heart condition can lead to arrhythmia.

These pre-existing heart conditions may include:

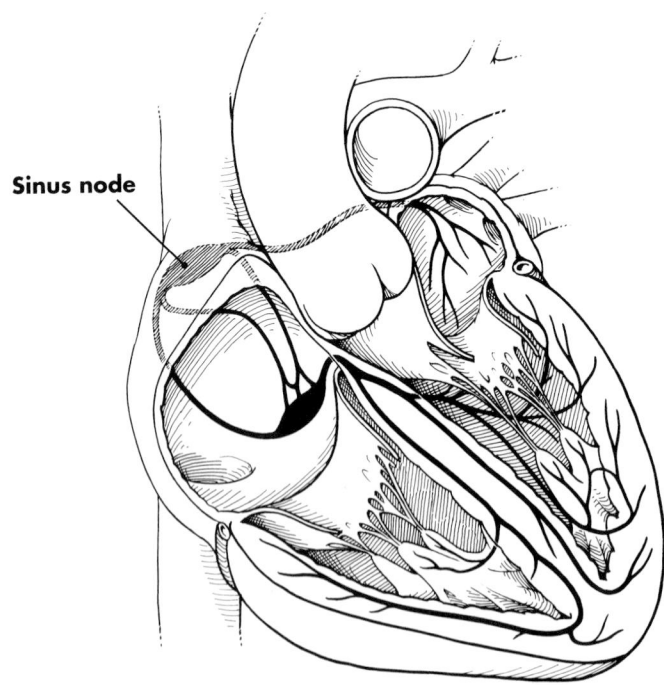

The sinus node, located in the right atrium, acts as your heart's pacemaker, controlling its contractions by issuing nerve impulses along electrical pathways throughout the heart.

Ventricular Fibrillation

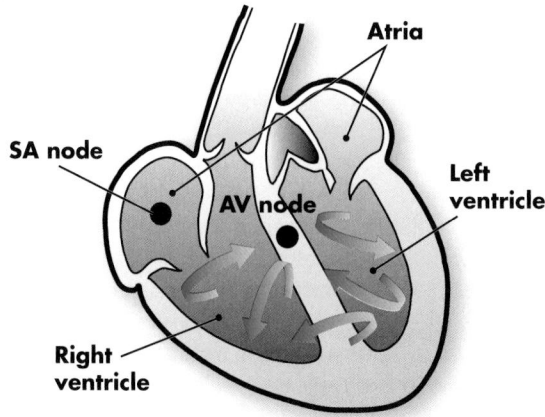

Ventricular fibrillation is associated with chaotic activity of the ventricles, which requires immediate treatment.

Heart Block

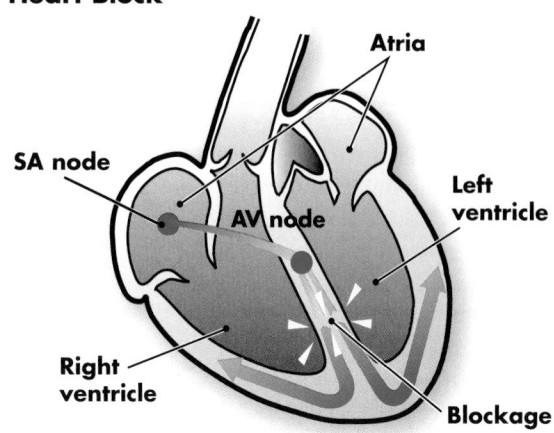

Slow heart rates can result from defects in the heart's conduction system that prevent electrical impulses from reaching the ventricles. This is called heart block.

- **Coronary artery disease (CAD).** Although it has been linked to many arrhythmias, CAD is most closely associated with ventricular arrhythmias and sudden cardiac death. Narrowing of the arteries that occurs with CAD can progress until a portion of the heart dies as a result of lack of blood flow (heart attack). A previous heart attack leaves behind a scar. Electrical short circuits around the scar can prevent normal heart function by causing the heart to beat dangerously fast or to quiver.
- **Cardiomyopathy.** Cardiomyopathy refers to disease of the heart muscle. It occurs primarily when the heart's ventricular walls stretch and enlarge or when the left ventricle wall thickens and constricts. In either case, cardiomyopathy decreases your heart's blood-pumping efficiency and often leads to heart tissue damage.
- **Valvular heart diseases.** Leaking or narrowing of your heart valves can lead to stretching and thickening of your heart muscle (myocardium). When the chambers become enlarged or weakened due to the added stress caused by the tight or leaking valve, arrhythmia can develop.

Types of arrhythmias

Doctors classify arrhythmias not only by where they originate (atria or ventricles) but also by the speed of heart rate they cause:
- **Tachycardia.** This refers to a fast heartbeat — a heart rate greater than 100 beats a minute.
- **Bradycardia.** This refers to a slow heartbeat — a resting heart rate less than 60 beats a minute.

Not all tachycardias or bradycardias indicate disease. For example, during exercise it's normal to develop sinus tachycardia as the heart speeds up to provide your tissues with more oxygen-rich blood.

Tachycardias in the atria

Tachycardias originating in the atria include:
- **Atrial fibrillation.** This fast and chaotic beating of the atrial chambers is a common arrhythmia. It mainly affects older people. Your risk of developing atrial fibrillation increases past age 60, mostly due to the wear and tear that may affect your heart's function as you age, especially if you've had high blood pressure or other heart problems. During atrial fibrillation, the electrical activity of the atria becomes uncoordinated. The atria beat so rapidly — as

fast as 350 to 600 beats a minute — that instead of producing a single, forceful contraction, they quiver (fibrillate). Atrial fibrillation can be intermittent (paroxysmal), lasting a few minutes to an hour or more before returning to a regular heart rhythm. It can also be chronic, causing an ongoing problem. Atrial fibrillation is seldom a life-threatening arrhythmia, but over time it can lead to more-serious conditions, such as stroke.
- **Atrial flutter.** Atrial flutter is similar to atrial fibrillation. Both can coexist in your heart, coming and going in an alternating fashion. The key distinction is that more-organized and more-rhythmic electrical impulses are called atrial flutter. These occur because atrial flutter, unlike atrial fibrillation, arises from a short circuit. In typical atrial flutter, this short circuit exists in the right atrium. This is an important distinction because typical right atrial flutter is more responsive to treatment.
- **Supraventricular tachycardia (SVT).** SVT includes many forms of arrhythmia originating above the ventricles (supraventricular). SVTs usually cause a burst of rapid heartbeats that

Sick Sinus Syndrome

The function of the sinus node is to regulate your heartbeat. Sometimes the sinus node fails to adequately perform its role as your heart's pacemaker. When this occurs, the condition is called sick sinus syndrome.

In this condition, the sinus node initiates heartbeats too slowly, pauses too long between beats or stops producing beats. If it stops producing beats, a different part of the heart must take over the pacemaker function, which it usually does at a rate that's substantially slower than normal.

To further complicate the situation, sinus nodes that are sick may also have a tendency to beat too fast at times, and occasionally they beat in an irregular fashion, such as in atrial fibrillation. Thus, the signs and symptoms of sick sinus syndrome can be those associated with slow heartbeats, such as fatigue, lightheadedness and blackouts, alternating with symptoms of fast heartbeats, such as palpitations. Either the slow or fast rhythms can cause shortness of breath, lightheadedness, blackouts and fatigue.

Therapy for sick sinus syndrome can be complex because the condition often involves slow and fast components. Medications may be given to slow the rapid heartbeat. In addition, a pacemaker may be required to prevent symptoms of too low a heart rate.

begin and end suddenly and can last from seconds to hours. These often start when the electrical impulse from a premature heartbeat begins to circle repeatedly through an extra pathway. Although generally not life-threatening in an otherwise normal heart, symptoms from the racing heart may feel uncomfortable. These arrhythmias are common in young people.

- **Wolff-Parkinson-White syndrome.** One cause of SVT is Wolff-Parkinson-White syndrome. This arrhythmia results from an extra electrical pathway between the atria and the ventricles. This pathway may allow electrical current to pass between the atria and the ventricles without passing through the AV node, leading to short circuits and rapid heartbeats.

Artificial Cardiac Pacemakers

If your heart is unable to maintain a fast enough heartbeat or if it occasionally pauses, the solution may be an artificial cardiac pacemaker. This may be either a short-term treatment or a permanent solution.

Symptoms that may suggest a problem requiring a pacemaker include blackout spells, near faints, shortness of breath (especially during physical activity) and undue fatigue. A slow heartbeat or pauses can occur with various types of heart disease and even in an otherwise apparently normal heart.

An artificial pacemaker is an electrical device that causes the heart to beat with a series of electric discharges. It replaces the function of your heart's own rate control system, the sinus node and conduction system. An implanted pacemaker mimics the electrical impulses of a healthy heart and re-

stores a sufficiently fast heartbeat. At times, your heartbeat may be fast enough on its own. When this occurs, the pacemaker automatically goes on standby.

Equipment

The pacemaker itself is small, weighing about $1\frac{1}{2}$ ounces, and is powered by a lithium battery that lasts up to 10 years. Other models that are generally used only for short periods aren't implanted but instead are carried outside the body (external pacemakers).

Procedure

The pacemaker usually is implanted beneath the skin just below your collarbone. The device is connected to one or two insulated, flexible wire leads. These are usually passed into the right side of the heart by way of a large vein beneath the collarbone. There, an electrical contact (electrode) discharges impulses to the inner surface of the right side of the heart to stimulate its contractions when the heart rate slows.

Applications

An artificial cardiac pacemaker isn't a solution to all heart problems, but it can be used to treat a number of heart disorders. Its primary application is to control or prevent slow arrhythmias of the ventricles. Many pacemakers are designed to increase the heart rate automatically during activity or stress, just as in the normal heart.

Two-wire pacemakers — with one wire located in the top chamber (atrium) of the heart and one wire in the bottom chamber (ventricle) — are called dual chamber pacemakers. They ensure that the heart beats in a normal sequence. When medications aren't effective, some specialized devices can treat specific types of fast arrhythmias. Some pacemakers have three wires. They're generally used to treat heart failure.

Living with a pacemaker

Modern pacemakers may be affected by outside electrical interference in some circumstances. If you have a pacemaker, talk

Tachycardias in the ventricles

Tachycardias occurring in the ventricles include:

- **Ventricular tachycardia (VT).** This fast, regular beating of the heart is caused by abnormal electrical impulses originating in the ventricles. Often, these are due to a short circuit around a scar from a previous heart attack and can cause the ventricles to contract more than 200 beats a minute. VT generally occurs in people with some form of heart-related problem. Sometimes, ventricular tachycardia lasts for 30 seconds or less (unsustained) and is often harmless. Still, an unsustained VT may be a predictor for more-serious ventricular arrhythmias, such as longer lasting (sustained) VT. An episode of sustained VT is a medical emergency. It may

be associated with palpitations, dizziness, fainting or even death.

- **Ventricular fibrillation.** About 300,000 Americans die every year of sudden cardiac death believed to be caused by ventricular fibrillation. With ventricular fibrillation, rapid, chaotic electrical impulses cause your ventricles to quiver uselessly instead of pumping blood. Without an effective heartbeat, your blood pressure plummets, instantly cutting off blood supply to your vital organs — including your brain. Most people lose consciousness within seconds and require immediate medical assistance. Without cardiopulmonary resuscitation (CPR) or defibrillation, death can result in minutes. Ventricular fibrillation is often triggered by a heart attack.

- **Long QT syndrome.** This syndrome may be either an acquired or an inherited condition. On an electrocardiogram, the letter *Q* marks the point where an electrical impulse signals the ventricles to contract. The letter *T* marks the point where the cells of your ventricles have electrically recharged for the next heartbeat. When the QT interval is prolonged, people with the condition are prone to palpitations and fainting spells, and may have an increased risk of sudden death.

Bradycardias

Although a heart rate below 60 beats a minute while at rest is considered bradycardia, a low resting heart rate doesn't always signal a problem. If you're physically fit, you may have an efficient heart

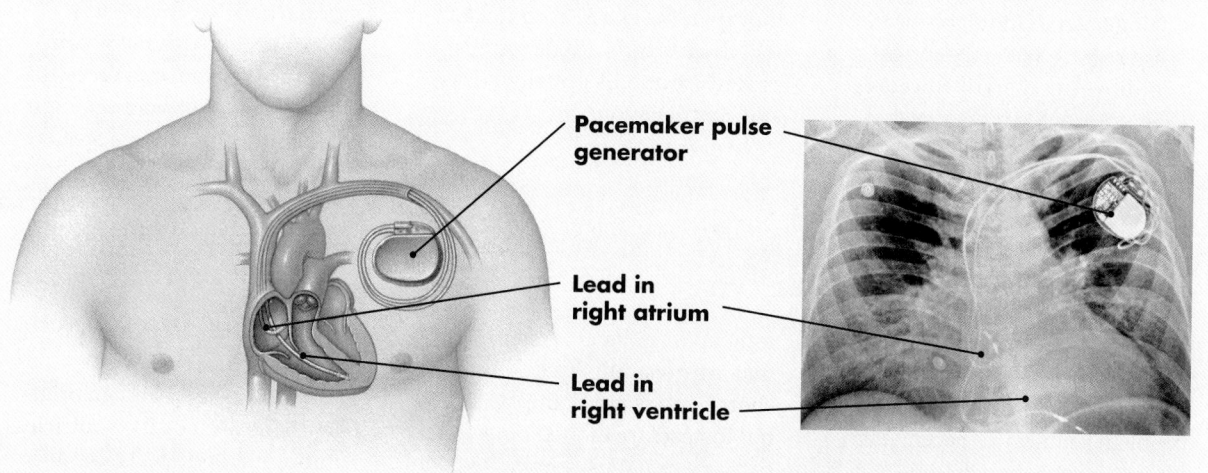

Pacemaker pulse generator

Lead in right atrium

Lead in right ventricle

If your heart's internal pacing system fails to control your heartbeat, an artificial pacemaker may be surgically implanted. The battery-powered device is inserted beneath the skin of your chest. Flexible wire leads are threaded into the right side of the heart to deliver electrical impulses.

to your doctor before doing arc welding or mechanical work on a running car engine, because electromagnetic fields may interfere with your pacemaker's function. Although cellphones rarely cause problems, it's best to hold it to the ear farthest from your pacemaker and to not carry the phone in a pocket over your pacemaker.

Avoid electromagnetic fields such as those found near high-voltage transmission lines or substations. Don't linger in doorways armed with electromagnetic anti-theft or surveillance devices.

Pacemakers can also pose problems during a magnetic resonance imaging (MRI) scan or an operation in which electrocautery is

used to control bleeding. If you need one of these procedures, be sure to tell your doctor you have a pacemaker. Avoid hard contact to the pacemaker, such as might occur while playing football or firing a rifle from the shoulder near the pacemaker. Modern pacemakers aren't affected by microwave ovens.

Internal Cardioverter Defibrillator

Ventricular fibrillation is a life-threatening rhythm disturbance. Unfortunately, people who experience ventricular fibrillation are at risk of recurrence. In addition, individuals with ventricular tachycardia may have serious symptoms, such as loss of consciousness. And the tachycardia may proceed to the more dangerous ventricular fibrillation.

Because no medication is 100 percent effective for preventing or treating any recurrence, special measures are often warranted. Internal cardioverter defibrillators are increasingly being used to fulfill this need.

Like pacemakers, internal cardioverter defibrillators are battery-powered devices that are implanted in the body. They're implanted beneath the skin of the upper chest.

Wire electrodes that are inserted through veins attach the pulse generator to the heart. Internal cardioverter defibrillators continuously sense the heart's rhythm and respond in a fashion that's designed to convert the heart to a normal rhythm.

The devices function like a regular pacemaker, should the need arise. They can also detect when ventricular tachycardia occurs and then attempt to correct the rhythm with a small electric pacing current. If several of these attempts are unsuccessful or if ventricular fibrillation develops, the internal cardioverter defibrillator shocks the heart directly.

The shock may feel different for each person in each event. It may feel like a kick or a thump in the chest. Your doctor will discuss indications for this procedure and its potential risks and complications.

capable of pumping an adequate supply of blood with fewer than 60 beats a minute at rest. However, if you have a slow heart rate and your heart isn't pumping enough blood, you may have one of several bradycardias including:

- **Sick sinus.** If your pacemaking sinus node isn't sending impulses properly, your heart rate may be too slow, or it may speed up and slow down intermittently. Sick sinus can be caused by an impulse block near the sinus node that's slowing, disrupting or completely blocking conduction.
- **Conduction block.** A block of your heart's electrical pathways can occur in or near the AV node or along pathways that conduct impulses to each ventricle. Depending on the location and type of block, the impulses between your atria and ventricles may be slowed or partially or completely blocked. If the signal is completely blocked, certain cells in the AV node or ventricles are capable of initiating a steady, although usually slower, heartbeat. Some blocks may cause no signs or symptoms, and others may cause skipped beats or bradycardia.

Premature heartbeats

Premature heartbeats can originate in the atria or the ventricles. Although it often feels like a skipped heartbeat, a premature heartbeat is actually an extra beat between two normal heartbeats. Premature heartbeats occurring in the ventricles come before the ventricles have had time to fill with blood following a regular heartbeat.

Although you may feel an occasional premature beat, it seldom indicates a more serious problem. Still, a premature beat can trigger a longer lasting arrhythmia — especially in people with heart disease. These types of arrhythmias are commonly caused by

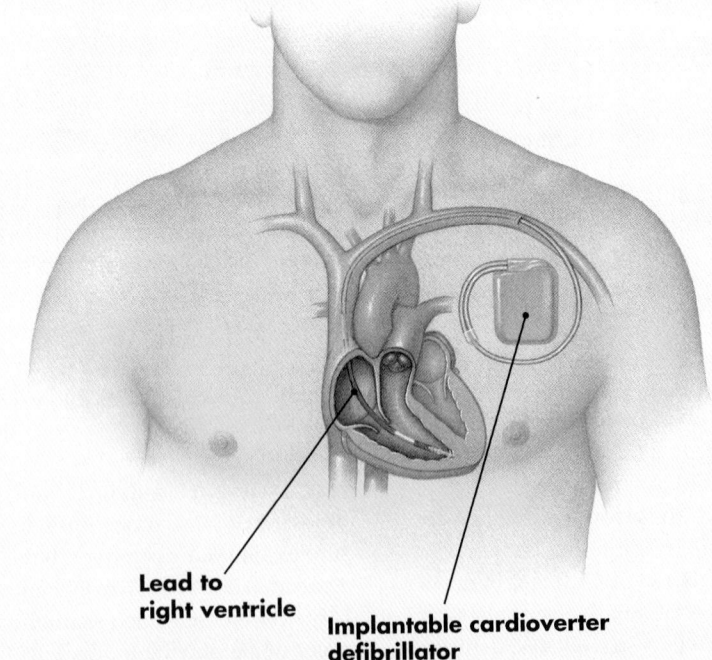

Lead to right ventricle

Implantable cardioverter defibrillator

Internal cardioverter defibrillators can both pace and deliver shocks that can treat ventricular fibrillation or ventricular tachycardia.

stimulants, such as caffeine from coffee, tea and soft drinks, over-the-counter cold remedies containing pseudoephedrine, and some asthma medications.

Diagnosis

Methods used to diagnose arrhythmias include:

- **Electrocardiogram (ECG).** Sensors that can detect the electrical activity of your heart are attached to your chest and sometimes to your limbs. An ECG measures the timing and duration of each electrical phase in your heartbeat.
- **Holter monitor.** This portable ECG device is worn for a day or more to record your heart's activity as you go about your routine.
- **Event monitor.** For sporadic arrhythmias, you keep this portable ECG device at home, attaching it to your body and activating it only when you experience symptoms of an arrhythmia. This permits your doctor to determine your heart rhythm at the time of your symptoms, to see if there's an association.
- **Echocardiogram.** A hand-held device (transducer) placed on your chest uses sound waves to produce images of your heart's size, structure and motion.

Heart monitoring tests that your doctor may use to induce an arrhythmia include:

- **Stress test.** Some arrhythmias are triggered or worsened by exercise. During a stress test, you exercise on a treadmill or stationary bicycle while your heart activity is monitored by an ECG. Your doctor may also use a drug to stimulate your heart in a way that's similar to exercise. This may be particularly helpful if you have difficulty exercising, and it can also be used to detect coronary artery disease.
- **Tilt table test.** Your doctor may recommend this test if you've had recurrent fainting spells. Your heart rate and blood pres-

sure are monitored as you lie flat on a table. The table is then tilted as if you were standing up. Your doctor observes how your heart and the nervous system that controls your heart responds to the change in angle.
- **Electrophysiological testing and mapping.** In this test, thin, flexible tubes (catheters) tipped with electrodes are threaded through your blood vessels to a variety of spots within your heart. Once in place, the electrodes can precisely map the spread of electrical impulses through your heart. In addition, your cardiologist can use the electrodes to stimulate your heart to beat at rates that may trigger — or halt — an arrhythmia. This allows your doctor to observe the location of the arrhythmia and the mechanisms that may be causing it.

How serious are arrhythmias?

Many arrhythmias rarely cause complications, but some can be serious, especially if untreated. A heart that's not beating normally may not be able to pump blood efficiently. If blood flow to the brain is inadequate, you can faint. A heart that beats very fast for a prolonged period may become weakened, leading to congestive heart failure.

Certain arrhythmias, such as atrial fibrillation, may allow small blood clots to form in a chamber of your heart. If one or more clots break loose and are carried by way of your bloodstream to your brain, they could cause a stroke.

In general, arrhythmias are more serious if you have other heart-related conditions.

Treatment

Treatment may or may not be necessary, depending on your situation. Usually, it's required only if the arrhythmia is causing significant symptoms or if it's putting you at risk of a more serious arrhythmia or complications.

Treating bradycardias

If bradycardias that produce symptoms don't have a cause that can be corrected, doctors often treat them with a pacemaker (see page 734). If your heart rate is too slow or if it stops, the pacemaker sends out electrical impulses that stimulate your heart to beat at a steady, proper rate. The newest pacemakers can monitor and pace your atria or ventricles — or both — in proper sequence to maximize the output of blood from your heart.

Treating tachycardias

For tachycardias originating in the atria or ventricles, treatments may include one or more of the following:

- **Vagal maneuvers.** You may be able to stop a supraventricular tachycardia (SVT) by using particular maneuvers, which include holding your breath and straining, dunking your face in ice water, or coughing. Your doctor may be able to recommend other maneuvers to halt a fast heartbeat. These maneuvers affect the nervous system that controls your heartbeat, often causing your heart rate to slow.
- **Medications.** Many types of tachycardias respond well to anti-arrhythmic medications. Though they don't cure the problem, they can reduce episodes of tachycardia or slow down the heart when an episode occurs. Some medications can slow down your heart so much that you may need a pacemaker. It's very important to take any anti-arrhythmic medication exactly as directed by your doctor in order to avoid complications.
- **Cardioversion.** If you have an atrial tachycardia, including atrial fibrillation, your doctor may use cardioversion, which is an electric shock used to reset your heart to its regular rhythm. Usually this is done externally in a monitored setting, and you're given medication to sedate you during the procedure.

Fainting Spells

A fainting spell can be frightening. Often, however, there's no reason to panic.

A fainting spell (syncope) is a sign, not a disorder. When you faint, it means that your brain isn't getting sufficient oxygen to function properly. The signs and symptoms of impending syncope may include nausea, perspiration or a graying-out of your vision. The key sign, however, is a loss of consciousness.

What are the causes?

Fainting is often classified into three broad categories:

- *Vasodepressive.* Fainting due to a temporary internal nervous system (autonomic) imbalance.
- *Cardiac.* Fainting that results from an electrical or mechanical problem in the heart.
- *Neurological.* Fainting related to a seizure or, less commonly, a stroke.

In healthy individuals, most fainting spells are harmless and often due to a temporary autonomic imbalance, such as standing too quickly. Syncope can also be triggered by the sight of blood and nausea. In people with heart and blood vessel (cardiovascular) disease, the cause may be more serious and should be evaluated by a doctor.

What are the risks?

Once you're lying flat, blood flow is quickly restored and you usually regain consciousness. Recovering consciousness quickly after a fainting spell means that little or no damage is sustained by your brain due to the shortage of oxygen. In fact, the most serious risk of syncope is usually from the fall itself. Fractures or head injuries may result.

What should you do?

If you experience a fainting spell that doesn't have an apparent cause — such as extreme heat or suddenly moving from a lying position to a standing position — consult your doctor. He or she may perform tests to try to determine a cause and treat the condition appropriately.

- **Cardiac ablation.** In this procedure, one or more catheters are threaded through your blood vessels to your inner heart. They're positioned on areas of your heart identified as causing your arrhythmia. Electrodes at the catheter tips are heated with radiofrequency energy. Another method involves cooling the tips of the catheters, which freezes the problem tissue. Either method destroys (ablates) a small spot of heart tissue and creates an electrical block along the pathway that's causing your arrhythmia.

Implantable devices

Implantable devices used to treat arrhythmias include:

- **Pacemaker.** A pacemaker helps regulate slow heartbeats (see page 734).
- **Internal cardioverter defibrillator (ICD).** Your doctor may recommend this device if you're at high risk of developing a dangerous ventricular tachycardia (VT) or ventricle fibrillation (VF). Implantable defibrillator units designed to treat atrial fibrillation also are available. An ICD is a battery-powered unit that's implanted near the left collarbone (see page 736). An ICD may lessen your chance of having a fatal arrhythmia.

Surgical treatments

In some cases, surgery is performed:

- **Maze procedure.** It involves making a series of surgical incisions in the atria, which heal into carefully placed scars. The scars form boundaries that force electrical activation to proceed in an orderly manner from top to bottom. The procedure has a high success rate, but because it requires open-heart surgery, it's usually reserved for people who don't respond to other treatments. The surgeon may use a cryoprobe — an instrument for applying extreme cold to tissue — or a hand-held radiofrequency probe to create the scars.
- **Ventricular aneurysm surgery.** In some cases, a bulge in a heart blood vessel (aneurysm) is the cause of an arrhythmia. Surgery may be needed to remove the aneurysm.

- **Coronary bypass surgery.** If you have severe coronary artery disease in addition to frequent ventricular tachycardia, your doctor may recommend coronary bypass surgery. It may improve the blood supply to your heart and reduce the frequency of ventricular tachycardia.

Conduction system disease

Signs and symptoms

- Breathlessness and a feeling of exhaustion

Emergency signs and symptoms

- Extreme breathlessness and weakness
- Loss of consciousness, convulsions

Your heart rate is controlled by electrical impulses issued by the sinus node in the right atrium. These pacemaker cells produce electrical impulses that travel throughout both atria, causing their muscular walls to contract. The electrical impulses travel from the atria through a small bed of specialized tissue called the atrioventricular (AV) node to a band of specialized fibers (the bundle of His) that conducts the impulses to the muscle fibers of the ventricles. These muscles then contract.

In conduction system disease (heart block), the electrical impulse passes through the atrioventricular node and the bundle of His slowly, intermittently or not at all. This can result for various reasons:
- Scarring in the path of the specialized conduction fibers
- Coronary artery disease, including a heart attack
- Congenital heart disease
- Effects of certain medications, including some heart medications
- Some rheumatologic disorders, such as dermatomyositis
- Infections such as Lyme disease and diphtheria

Diagnosis
Many people with heart block have no obvious symptoms. In severe cases, you may experience a sudden loss of consciousness due to dramatic slowing of your heart rate.

Heart block is classified by degrees. First degree heart block causes no symptoms and is evident only on an electrocardiogram as a delay in the transmission of the impulse from the atria to the ventricles. It requires no treatment.

In second degree heart block, some of the impulses fail to reach the ventricles. The result is an irregular pulse. In many cases, second degree heart block is a result of excessive medications, and the heartbeat often returns to normal with the withdrawal of the medication. Sometimes, use of a pacemaker is necessary.

In third degree heart block, no impulses reach the ventricles, and the ventricles are forced to beat with their own intrinsic rhythm. The beating is often so slow that flow of blood to the brain and other parts of the body is insufficient. Loss of consciousness may result.

Treatment
For first degree heart block and many forms of second degree

heart block, observation or withdrawing or reducing the medication responsible may be all the treatment that's necessary. When the heart is no longer able to pace itself, an artificial cardiac pacemaker may be required (see page 734).

Sudden cardiac arrest

Signs and symptoms
- Sudden collapse
- Loss of consciousness
- No pulse or breathing

Sudden cardiac arrest is the sudden, unexpected loss of heart function, breathing and consciousness. It usually results from an electrical disturbance in your heart that disrupts its pumping action and causes blood to stop flowing to the rest of your body. This is different from a heart attack in which just a portion of the heart muscle is deprived of blood.

The vast majority of people who experience sudden cardiac death have heart problems, even if they don't experience any symptoms. Heart conditions that can lead to sudden cardiac arrest include coronary artery disease, a heart at-

tack, an enlarged heart, heart valve disease, congenital heart disease and electrical system disorders.

Treatment
Sudden cardiac arrest requires immediate emergency action. If the heart ceases to function, cardiopulmonary resuscitation (CPR) is required to maintain some oxygenation of the blood and some flow of blood to the brain. CPR temporarily restores circulation. However, to get the heart beating again and restore a spontaneous heartbeat, an electric shock may need to be delivered to the heart. A defibrillator is used to shock the heart, which stops the ventricular fibrillation and allows a normal heart rhythm to return.

After resuscitation, medications called anti-arrhythmics may be prescribed to prevent recurrent episodes. Most individuals who survive sudden cardiac arrest also receive an internal cardioverter defibrillator (see page 736), which monitors the heart rhythm. If it detects ventricular tachycardia or ventricular fibrillation, the device delivers a shock to stop the arrhythmia.

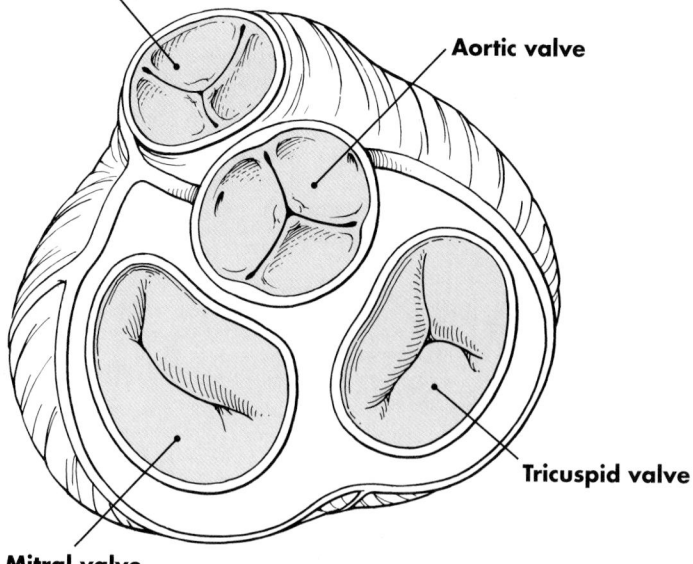

Pulmonary valve

Aortic valve

Tricuspid valve

Mitral valve

Each heart valve consists of two or three flaps (leaflets) of tissue. When closed, a valve prevents blood from flowing to the next chamber or from returning to the previous one. When open, blood flows freely.

Heart Valve Disorders

The human heart consists of four chambers and four valves. Two of the valves — the mitral and tricuspid valves — regulate the flow of blood from the upper chambers (atria) to the lower chambers (ventricles). The other two valves — aortic and pulmonary valves — regulate the flow of blood out of the ventricles for circulation to other parts of the body.

The mitral valve links the atrium to the ventricle on the heart's left side. The aortic valve, which is also on the left, opens to allow blood to flow from the left ventricle into the body's main artery (aorta).

On the right side, the tricuspid valve regulates flow from the atrium to the ventricle, and the pulmonary valve allows blood to exit from the heart's right ventricle into the lungs by way of the pulmonary artery (see the illustration on page 361).

The valves allow blood to flow in only one direction. Each valve consists of two or three strong, thin flaps (leaflets) of tissue. When closed, a valve prevents blood from flowing to the next chamber or from returning to the previous one.

When the valve opening becomes narrowed and flow through it is limited, the condition is called stenosis. Each of the heart's valves may be subject to stenosis or obstruction. In addition, a valve may lose its shape and begin to bulge (prolapse) or fail to close completely (leak), causing a backflow of blood (regurgitation).

Valve problems may occur as a result of infection, a congenital abnormality, a heart attack, a disease of the heart muscle or deterioration due to aging.

Mitral valve problems

Signs and symptoms
- Often, none
- Breathlessness, especially after exercise
- Fatigue
- Frequent bouts of bronchitis
- Chest discomfort or palpitations

On the left side of your heart, the mitral valve links the upper chamber (atrium) to the lower chamber (ventricle). When the opening of the mitral valve becomes narrowed and the passage of blood through it is restricted, the condition is termed mitral valve stenosis. When the mitral valve fails to close properly and blood leaks back into the atrium from the ventricle, the disorder is called mitral valve regurgitation or incompetence.

Mitral valve stenosis
Mitral valve stenosis occurs when the heart's mitral valve is narrowed, preventing the valve from opening properly and obstructing blood flow. Too much blood accumulates in the left atrium. Pressure builds up in the left atrium, and the chamber may enlarge. Blood may back up into the lungs, leading to lung congestion (pulmonary edema). Mitral valve stenosis commonly leads to a heart rhythm irregularity called atrial fibrillation.

Mitral valve stenosis is almost always due to rheumatic fever, a complication of streptococcal throat infection (strep throat). But some babies are born with an already narrowed mitral valve and develop

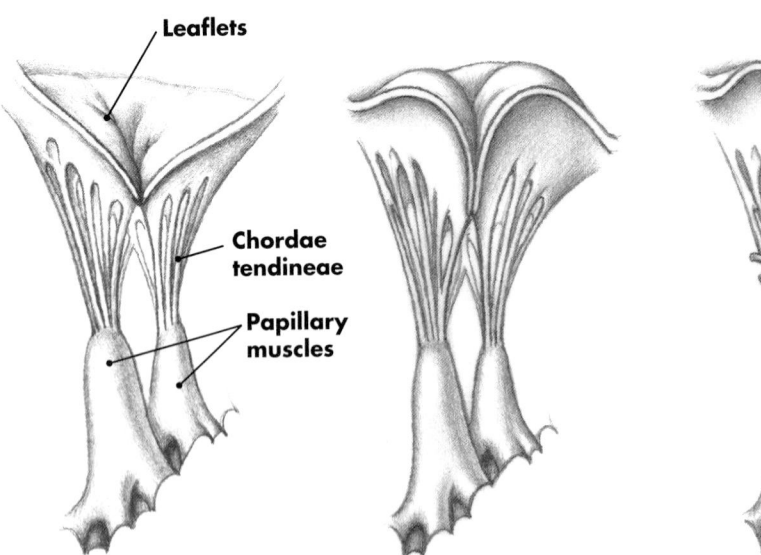
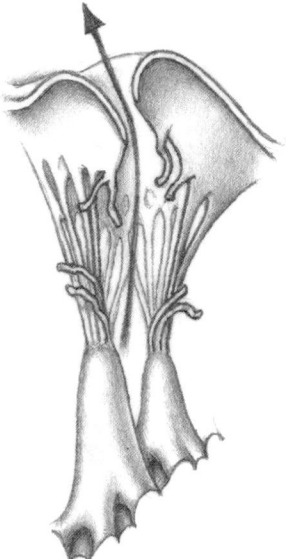

Leaflets

Chordae tendineae

Papillary muscles

A normal mitral valve (left) closes tightly to prevent leakage of blood. A prolapsed mitral valve (center) causes the thin flaps (leaflets) of tissue that control the flow of blood to bulge (prolapse) upward during closure. This may occur because the leaflets are too large or the valve's tendons are too long. Mitral valve regurgitation (right) may result if some of the valve's tendons break, causing leaflets to flail and allowing blood to leak back into the atrium.

Balloon Valvuloplasty

A narrowed heart valve (stenosis) can limit blood flow and lead to complications such as heart failure. The problem may be treated by open-heart surgery or a procedure called balloon valvuloplasty.

The decision to proceed with valvuloplasty is based on the risk of the procedure versus the risk of surgery. Less calcified and less severely deformed valves carry a very low risk from balloon valvuloplasty. Balloon valvuloplasty is more commonly used for mitral valve stenosis than aortic valve stenosis. In the case of aortic valve stenosis, balloon valvuloplasty is generally used only if aortic valve surgery is thought to be too risky for you or if you have some other serious medical problem that requires treatment before aortic valve replacement.

Procedure

During balloon valvuloplasty of the mitral valve, a catheter is inserted through a vein, most often in the groin area. The catheter is guided through your blood vessels to the right side of the heart and to the mitral valve. A balloon at the tip of the catheter is gently inflated to widen the valve opening, thus improving blood flow. Sometimes, two balloons are inflated.

The procedure for aortic valvuloplasty is similar except that a catheter is inserted into an artery and advanced backward across the aortic valve. When the tip is in the opening of the diseased valve, the balloon is inflated.

Recovery

As with any heart procedure, there are risks. But the result may be immediate relief of symptoms such as breathlessness. The hospital stay and recovery time for balloon valvuloplasty are substantially less than for open-heart surgery.

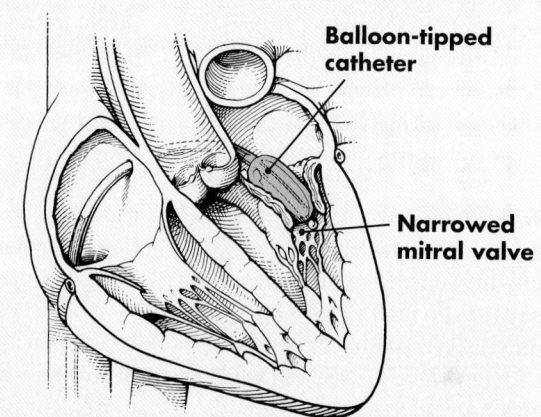

Mitral valve stenosis may be effectively treated by threading a catheter with an inflatable balloon through a vein and across the atrial septum. The balloon is positioned through the tight mitral opening and then inflated, forcing the valve leaflets apart to produce a wider opening.

---

mitral stenosis early in life. These babies usually require surgery to correct the valve. Others are born with a malformed mitral valve that puts them at risk of developing mitral valve stenosis later in life.

Mitral valve prolapse

Mitral valve prolapse occurs when the valve between your heart's left upper chamber (left atrium) and left lower chamber (left ventricle) doesn't close properly. When the left ventricle contracts, the valve's leaflets bulge (prolapse) upward or back into the atrium. The condition sometimes leads to blood leaking backward into the left atrium (mitral valve regurgitation). The flow of blood backward produces a sound called a murmur.

In most people, the condition is harmless and doesn't require any treatment. In some people, though, the prolapse can gradually reach a point where treatment of the leakage is necessary to prevent other heart-related disorders, such as heart failure.

Mitral valve regurgitation

In this condition, the heart's mitral valve doesn't close properly, allowing blood to flow backward into the heart. Because of this, blood can't move through your heart or the rest of your body as efficiently. The left ventricle — the heart's main pumping chamber — pumps harder to try to compensate for the decreased blood flow. Consequently, the left ventricle may become enlarged and eventually may fail.

Mitral valve regurgitation has several possible causes. It can be the result of damage sustained during a bout of rheumatic fever. It can be present from birth. Or it can result from a ballooning out (prolapsing) of the mitral valve or from damage to the cords that anchor the flaps (leaflets) of the mitral valve to the heart wall. Other causes include an infection of the heart's inner lining (endocarditis), age-related wear and tear, or a prior heart attack.

Diagnosis

Breathlessness, especially with mild exertion or at night when lying in bed, is a common symptom of mitral valve problems. In advanced cases, backing up of blood may lead to accumulation of fluid in the ankles, causing them to swell.

Many of the signs and symptoms of mitral valve regurgitation are similar to those of mitral valve stenosis. To make the diagnosis, your doctor will likely listen to your heart to try to detect the sound of a characteristic heart murmur. A chest X-ray also can help your doctor determine if the left ventricle is enlarged. Lung congestion also is visible on an X-ray.

Often, mitral valve prolapse is discovered during a routine stethoscope examination of your heart. Your doctor may confirm the diagnosis with a test called an echocardiogram, used to help detect heart rhythm irregularities. Tests such as a transesophageal echocardiogram or cardiac catheterization can provide even more detailed information about the state of your heart valves.

How serious are mitral valve problems?

If your valve disease is mild, you may remain well or have only minimal symptoms for decades.

Severe valve disease can weaken your heart to the point where it's unable to pump enough blood to meet your body's needs, a condition called congestive heart failure. There's also a risk of atrial fibrillation, in which the heart beats in a rapid and uncoordinated fashion. This can lead to the dangerous formation of a blood clot that can travel to other parts of the body and cause serious damage.

Treatment

Treatment depends on the severity and progression of your condition. In general, the focus is on maximizing your heart's function, minimizing your signs and symptoms, and avoiding future complications.

Medications

No medications can correct a defect in the mitral valve. However, certain drugs can minimize symptoms by easing your heart's workload and regulating your heart's rhythm.

Your doctor may prescribe diuretics to reduce fluid accumulation in your lungs or elsewhere. Anticoagulants can help to prevent blood clots from forming in a heart with a damaged valve. Your doctor may also prescribe drugs to treat atrial fibrillation or other rhythm disturbances associated with mitral valve disorders.

Previous guidelines suggested that if you had mitral valve stenosis, you might need to take antibiotics before certain dental or medical procedures to prevent a heart infection known as endocarditis. Current guidelines indicate that's not necessary in most cases.

Discuss preventive antibiotic use with your doctor.

Surgery

If you have more-severe disease, you may need to repair or replace the valve. Procedures include:

- **Balloon valvuloplasty.** This procedure — which doesn't involve open-heart surgery — uses a soft, thin tube (catheter) tipped with a balloon to open up the mitral valve passageway. A doctor guides the catheter through a blood vessel in your arm or groin to your heart and into your narrowed mitral valve. Once in position, a balloon at the tip of the catheter is inflated. The balloon pushes open the mitral valve and stretches the valve opening, improving blood flow. The balloon is then deflated, and the catheter with the balloon is guided back out of your body.

Balloon valvuloplasty can relieve mitral valve stenosis and its symptoms. But it may not be appropriate if the valve is both tight (stenotic) and leaky (regurgitant). Balloon valvuloplasty may improve the blood flow for a while. However, over time the narrowing may recur.

Echocardiogram

Before the development of echocardiography, a doctor generally had to rely on a medical history, a physical examination, an electrocardiogram and an X-ray to evaluate how well an individual's heart was functioning. Now it's possible to "look" directly at a person's heart without ever penetrating the skin.

Echocardiography is a special application of ultrasonography, or ultrasound. The concept behind ultrasound is the same as that used in depth finders on boats.

A wand-like device called a transducer sends sound waves into your body and receives echoes from the surfaces of internal structures, such as your heart muscle and heart valves. A machine called an echocardiograph analyzes the waves to determine how far away the structures are from the transducer. Using this information, a computer calculates the time it takes the sound waves to travel to and from your heart and then reconstructs an image of the heart. The image (echocardiogram) of your heart is displayed on a monitor and is stored digitally.

Echocardiography allows the heart to be seen in action and can be used to diagnose various heart disorders. On the screen, your

doctor can observe the heart's main pumping chamber, its movement (contractility), the shape and thickness of the chamber walls, the valves, the heart's external covering (pericardium), and the large veins and arteries that lead into and out of the heart. The velocity and direction of blood flow through the heart valves and chambers also can be recorded by a technique called a Doppler ultrasound to determine narrowing and leakage of the valves.

Procedure

When you undergo echocardiography, you lie on your back and perhaps turn slightly to your left. A special jelly is applied to your

- **Mitral valve repair.** To repair a leaky valve, a surgeon may separate valve flaps (leaflets or cusps) that have fused, replace the cords that support the valve, remove excess valve tissue so that the leaflets or cusps can close tightly, or patch holes in a valve. The surgeon may tighten or reinforce the ring around a valve (annulus) by implanting an artificial ring.
- **Mitral valve replacement.** The narrowed mitral valve is removed and replaced with a mechanical valve or a tissue valve from a pig, cow or human cadaver donor. Pigs and cows have heart tissue similar to that of humans. Mechanical valves, made from metal, are durable, but they carry the risk of blood clots forming on or near the valve. If you receive a mechanical valve, you must take an anticoagulant medication, such as warfarin (Coumadin), for life to prevent blood clots. Tissue valves rarely raise your risk of blood clots, but they tend to wear out faster than mechanical valves and may need to be replaced. Your doctor can discuss the risks and benefits of each with you.

Aortic valve problems

Signs and symptoms
- Fatigue and weakness, especially during exertion
- Shortness of breath
- Chest pain or tightness
- Dizziness and fainting
- Heart palpitations
- Swollen ankles and feet

The aortic valve controls the flow of blood out of the heart's main pumping chamber (left ventricle) into the main artery of the body (aorta), which transports oxygen-laden blood to the rest of the body.

The aortic valve consists of three cup-shaped folds of tissue (cusps) that come together to prevent blood from flowing backward into the ventricle between contractions.

Aortic stenosis
In this condition the aortic valve is narrowed, preventing it from opening fully and obstructing blood flow. The left ventricle is forced to pump harder to maintain normal blood output. This results in thickening of the muscle of the left ventricle, a condition called left ventricular hypertrophy. Over time, the left ventricle muscle becomes less efficient, enlarged and flabby.

Because your heart can only pump a limited amount of blood, your body's tissues, including your muscles, don't receive the increase in blood flow needed for activities such as exercise.

Aortic regurgitation
A different sort of problem occurs when the aortic valve fails to shut tightly between contractions. In aortic valve regurgitation, blood leaks back into the ventricle. Consequently, the flow of blood to the rest of the body decreases, and the heart must pump harder in an attempt to compensate for the decreased blood flow. The left ventricle becomes enlarged over time, and the muscle of the ventricle may wear out and become flabby.

Both aortic stenosis and aortic regurgitation can result from a congenital abnormality or damage to the aortic valve from rheumatic fever. In the United States, aortic stenosis most commonly occurs in older adults and results from degeneration and calcification of the aortic valve.

chest to increase the conductivity of the ultrasound waves. The transducer is maneuvered to different locations and in different positions on your chest to view your heart from various angles.

Although the test is noninvasive and usually painless, you may feel some pressure as the transducer occasionally must be held firmly against your chest. A thorough examination may take from 15 minutes to more than an hour, depending on the complexity of the problem.

Advantages
The procedure requires no X-ray exposure. The equipment is portable, so the test can be done in your hospital room, in your doctor's office or even in the operating room.

Variation
If your doctor needs a clearer picture, he or she may request a variation of the test called transesophageal echocardiography. In this test, a transducer is threaded down your throat into your esophagus. The proximity of the esophagus to the heart and major blood vessels in your chest (aorta) can overcome some limitations — such as body shape and weight — that accompany traditional echocardiography, and provide an even better view of the heart.

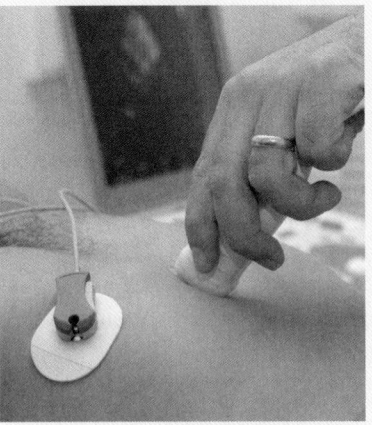

During an echocardiogram, a technician or doctor holds a wand-like device (transducer) over your chest wall. The transducer produces images of your heart that can be seen on a monitor.

Diagnosis

Your doctor may suspect either of these disorders while listening to your heart with a stethoscope. He or she may order one or several tests, including a chest X-ray, electrocardiogram, echocardiogram and cardiac catheterization. These tests can help your doctor determine how damaged your aortic valve may be and how well your heart is pumping.

How serious are aortic valve problems?

Aortic valve stenosis puts a strain on the heart. Left unchecked, aortic valve problems can lead to heart failure, a serious condition in which your heart is unable to pump sufficient blood to meet your body's needs. Severe aortic valve stenosis can ultimately be life-threatening.

Aortic valve stenosis also puts you at risk of endocarditis, an infection of your heart's inner lining (endocardium). This membrane lines the four chambers and four valves of your heart. If the aortic valve is narrowed, it's more prone to infection than a healthy valve is.

Doctors used to recommend some people with aortic valve stenosis take antibiotics before certain dental or medical procedures to prevent endocarditis, but not anymore. In 2007, the American Heart Association issued new guidelines saying, in part, antibiotics were no longer necessary in most cases for someone with this condition. Your doctor can tell you if antibiotics are necessary for you before such procedures.

Treatment

In most cases, neither aortic stenosis nor regurgitation means that you need to change your lifestyle. While you many need to avoid strenuous activity, reasonable physical activity is usually encouraged.

Medication

There is encouraging information suggesting that cholesterol-lowering medications, such as statins, may prevent aortic valve stenosis or slow its progress in certain individuals. Ask your doctor if you need cholesterol-lowering medications. In addition, your doctor may prescribe certain medications to control heart rhythm disturbances associated with aortic valve disorders.

Surgery

Surgery is the primary treatment for aortic valve problems. Surgical procedures include:

- **Aortic valve replacement.** This is the most common surgical treatment for aortic valve stenosis and regurgitation. Surgeons remove the narrowed aortic

Heart Valve Surgery

In some cases, open-heart surgery may be the best option for individuals with heart valve problems. The term *open-heart surgery* implies opening the chest and using a heart-lung machine to support the person's breathing and blood flow while the abnormality of the heart is being repaired. Open-heart procedures include coronary artery bypass surgery, correction of congenital abnormalities of the heart, heart valve surgery and removal of some heart tumors.

Valve repair

Your doctor will, if possible, repair the natural valve rather than insert an artificial (prosthetic) valve because the results with natural valve repair are usually better and longer lasting. And with this type of surgery, you may not need to take anticoagulant medications, as is necessary with artificial valves. A surgeon may repair the leaky valve by reconnecting the valve leaflets to the tendons that anchor the valve to the heart muscle or by cutting out excess tissue so that the leaflets can close snugly. Sometimes, repair includes cinching the surrounding ring of heart tissue tighter to ensure that the leaflets close adequately.

Valve replacement

Replacement of the mitral valve with an artificial valve is necessary if either repair or balloon valvuloplasty is unlikely to provide a satisfactory result. Valve replacement is also the preferred treatment for aortic valve disease that needs treatment beyond medication. To replace a damaged heart valve, the surgeon removes it and sutures an artificial valve in its place.

Your doctor will discuss with you what type of prosthetic valve would be best for you. Each type has some advantages and disadvantages. Mechanical prosthetic valves are constructed from metal and synthetic materials. These are extremely durable, but if you have one implanted, you'll need to take an anticoagulant such as warfarin (Coumadin) for the rest of your life because blood has a tendency to clot on the valve.

Biological tissue valves (bioprostheses) are made from animal or human tissue. An animal tissue bioprosthesis is usually made from a pig's heart valve, or it is fashioned from the pericardium or outer lining of the heart of a cow. A human tissue bioprosthesis (homograft) consists of a heart valve obtained from someone who has died. The advantage of bioprostheses is that they rarely require anticoagulation medication. However, they're not as durable as mechanical valves.

Procedure

When you undergo heart valve surgery, you'll be given a general

valve and replace it with a mechanical valve or a tissue valve from a pig, cow or a deceased human donor.

Mechanical valves are made from metal and are durable, but they carry the risk of blood clots forming on or near the valve. If you receive a mechanical aortic valve, you must take an anticoagulant medication for life.

Tissue valves, such as those from a pig, cow or human cadaver, rarely increase your risk of blood clots, but they tend to wear out faster than mechanical valves do. Another type of tissue valve replacement is autograft, in which your own pulmonary valve — another heart valve — is used to replace the aortic valve.

Replacement of the aortic valve involves open-heart surgery, performed with general anesthesia.

• **Transcatheter aortic valve replacement (TAVR).** This is a minimally invasive nonsurgical procedure. It's also sometimes called transcatheter aortic valve implantation (TAVI).

During TAVR, your doctors may access your heart through a blood vessel in your leg or a small incision in the chest. A hollow tube (catheter) is guided through your veins to the aortic valve. Once it is positioned correctly, a balloon-expandable or self-expandable replacement aortic valve is inserted.

TAVR may be an option for people considered to be at intermediate or high risk of complications from surgical aortic valve replacement. It may also be an option if you have an existing biological tissue valve that was previously inserted to replace the aortic valve, but it isn't functioning well anymore.

Tricuspid and pulmonary valve problems

Signs and symptoms
• Fatigue
• Breathlessness
• Lightheadedness
• Fainting
• Fluid retention
• Swelling in arms, legs and liver
• Discomfort in the upper right abdomen
• Nausea and vomiting

The valves on the right side of the heart (tricuspid and pulmonary) are much less affected by disease than are those on the left side, and when they are, the problem is often better tolerated.

Blood returning from the body flows into the right atrium, through the tricuspid valve to the right ventricle below. Then it exits from the right ventricle through the pulmonary valve to the pulmonary artery, which

anesthetic. Through an incision the length of your breastbone (sternum), your heart is exposed and connected to a heart-lung machine that takes over the functions of breathing and maintains blood circulation during the procedure. The damaged heart valve is repaired or replaced.

Recovery
After the operation, you'll likely spend one or more days in an intensive care unit (ICU). During recuperation, therapists, dietitians, patient educators and your doctor will assist your recovery and return to a productive life.

All prosthetic valves are prone to infection, which is difficult to treat with antibiotics once it develops. If you have a prosthetic valve, it's extremely important to take appropriate precautions, which generally involve taking antibiotics before any dental or surgical procedure.

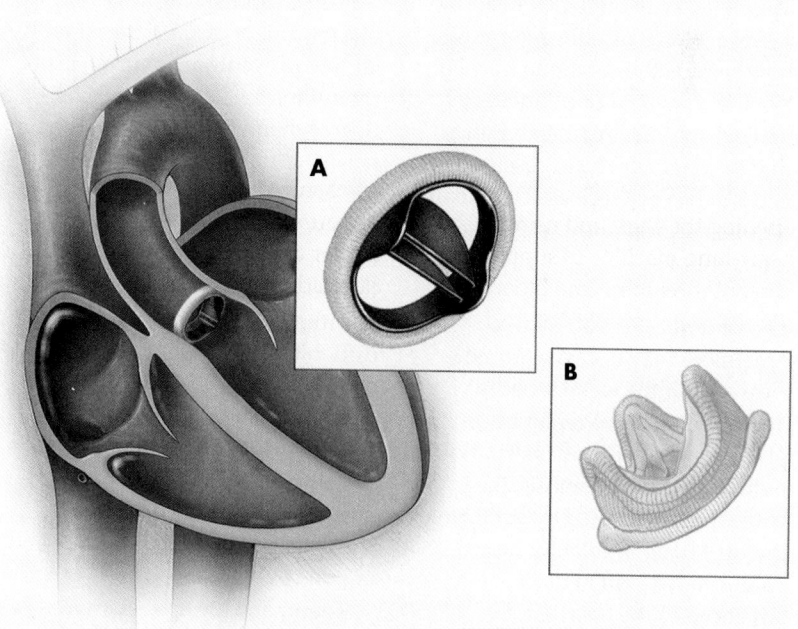

During heart valve replacement surgery, a surgeon removes the damaged valve and replaces it with a mechanical valve (A) or a biological tissue valve made from animal or human tissue (B).

carries the blood to the lungs for oxygenation.

The tricuspid and pulmonary valves, like the aortic and mitral valves, can have problems in which the valve opening narrows, restricting the flow of blood (tricuspid stenosis and pulmonary stenosis). In some cases, the valve fails to close properly, allowing blood to flow back through the valve (regurgitation).

Tricuspid and pulmonary valve problems are usually caused by rheumatic fever or congenital abnormalities.

Diagnosis

Often, these conditions are discovered by doctors during routine examinations. Your doctor may recommend tests — such as a chest X-ray, electrocardiogram and echocardiogram — to determine the status of blood flow and your heart's pumping ability.

How serious are tricuspid and pulmonary valve problems?

Tricuspid valve problems are often associated with left-sided heart disease, which usually determines how serious the condition may be. Isolated tricuspid or pulmonary valve disorders are rare and often due to congenital heart disease and can be very serious. They may require surgical or catheter-based interventions.

Treatment

Treatment may not be required. However, if the valve is badly deteriorated, valve repair or replacement may be necessary. With pulmonary valve stenosis, the valve may be opened by stretching it with a balloon catheter inserted through a vein in the leg and advanced to the heart.

Rheumatic fever

Signs and symptoms

A diagnosis of rheumatic fever requires two major criteria or one major criteria with two minor criteria, with evidence of a streptococcal infection.

Major criteria
- Inflammation of the heart, sometimes manifested by weakness and shortness of breath
- Arthritis that tends to migrate from one joint to another
- Uncontrolled movement of limbs and face
- Raised, red patches on the skin
- Lumps under the skin

Minor criteria
- Joint aches without inflammation
- Fever
- Previous rheumatic fever or evidence of rheumatic heart disease
- Abnormal heartbeat on electrocardiogram (ECG)
- A blood test indicating the presence of inflammation

Rheumatic fever is a serious inflammatory condition that appears to be the result of an immune reaction of the body to specific strains of streptococcal bacteria. A week or two after a streptococcal throat infection (strep throat), symptoms of rheumatic fever may appear.

Prompt and appropriate antibiotic treatment of strep throat will largely prevent the occurrence of rheumatic fever. In fact, prevention of rheumatic fever is the main reason antibiotics are prescribed for strep throat.

One of the problems in preventing rheumatic fever, however, is that sore throats that result from harmless viral infections are often difficult to distinguish from those caused by streptococci. To be sure that strep throat infections are treated properly, throat cultures are obtained to identify the organisms. If the culture is positive, the doctor will likely prescribe an antibiotic.

Rheumatic fever is relatively rare. It isn't as common in the United States today as it was before the widespread use of penicillin. But several outbreaks were reported in U.S. cities during the late 1980s. Rheumatic fever is still common in developing countries.

Most strep throat infections don't lead to rheumatic fever. When rheumatic fever does occur, it usually occurs in children.

Diagnosis

No laboratory test can confirm that your child has rheumatic fever. A diagnosis is generally based on his or her symptoms, classified by the several major and minor criteria listed earlier.

In some cases, your child's doctor may take a blood sample to test for the presence of antibodies to streptococcal bacteria. He or she may also recommend an ECG to check for any abnormal heart rhythms.

How serious is rheumatic fever?

Rheumatic fever can result in inflammation in one or several organs. Most often, several joints are affected with arthritic swelling, redness and the sensation of heat.

About half of people having a first attack of rheumatic fever have heart inflammation, which may resolve with no permanent damage. In some cases, however, permanent scarring of one or more heart valves may occur, which can cause obstruction to blood flow (stenosis) or backflow of blood (regurgitation).

Over a period of months or years, valve function may be seriously compromised, and surgery may be necessary to repair or replace the damaged heart valve or valves.

Rheumatic fever can also produce disk-like raised and red areas on the skin (erythema marginatum). Lumps or nodules may form beneath normal-appearing skin.

Treatment

Antibiotics are given to eliminate any remaining streptococcal organisms. Administration of low-dose penicillin, orally or by monthly injection, effectively prevents recurrences of rheumatic fever.

Nonsteroidal anti-inflammatory drugs (NSAIDs) can help reduce inflammation of the heart or joints. For severe heart inflammation, a corticosteroid medication can help reduce the inflammation.

Endocarditis

Signs and symptoms

- Fever
- Chills
- New or changed heart murmur
- Fatigue, aching joints and muscles
- Night sweats
- Shortness of breath
- Pale skin color
- Persistent cough

The inside of your heart contains four chambers and four valves lined by a thin membrane called the endocardium. Endocarditis is an infection of this inner lining.

Endocarditis typically occurs when bacteria or other germs from another part of your body, such as your mouth, spread through your bloodstream and attach to damaged areas of your heart. Left untreated, endocarditis can damage or destroy your heart valves, and it can be life-threatening.

Endocarditis is uncommon in people with normal, healthy hearts. People at greatest risk of such an infection are those with a damaged heart valve, an artificial heart valve or other heart defects. There may be a roughened and abnormal surface within the heart where the infecting organisms can congregate, multiply and, potentially, spread to other parts of the body.

Certain bacteria that commonly inhabit the mouth and upper respiratory tract may cause endocarditis. They may enter the bloodstream during everyday activities such as brushing your teeth or chewing food, especially if your teeth or gums are in poor condition. Dental or surgical procedures such as a tooth extraction, tonsillectomy or another operation that involves bleeding in the mouth or throat also can provide an entry point.

Intestinal bacteria, called enterococci, may enter your bloodstream during an instrumental examination or surgery in areas such as the prostate, bladder, rectum or female pelvic organs. A catheter — a thin tube inserted into your body as part of medical treatment — can serve as an entry point for bacteria.

Individuals who inject drugs into a vein with unsterilized needles are also vulnerable to endocarditis.

Diagnosis

Endocarditis may develop rapidly, usually with a fever and chills, but this isn't always the case, especially in older adults. Less serious conditions can cause similar signs and symptoms but you won't know for sure until you see a doctor. Your doctor may suspect endocarditis based on your signs and symptoms and your medical history. He or she may listen for a new heart murmur or a change in an already existing murmur.

Your doctor may order a series of blood cultures to identify bacteria in the bloodstream. Blood tests

can also help identify anemia — a shortage of healthy, red blood cells that can be a sign of endocarditis. Your doctor may also request an echocardiogram, an ultrasound procedure that allows him or her to see the heart's valves.

How serious is endocarditis?

Without treatment and elimination of the infecting organism, endocarditis is usually fatal. Left untreated, endocarditis can damage your heart valves and permanently destroy the heart's inner lining.

Even if you're cured of the bacterial infection, you may have continued heart symptoms due to additional valve damage from the infection. Complications such as cardiac or renal failure may develop as well.

A more common danger with endocarditis is that clumps of bacteria and cellular debris (vegetations) may form in your heart at the site of the infection and break loose and block blood vessels elsewhere in your body. This can cause a variety of problems including a stroke or other organ damage.

Treatment

Even with the availability of powerful modern antibiotics, treatment of endocarditis can be difficult and the results uncertain. Furthermore, many types of bacteria have become resistant to antibiotics.

Medication

Antibiotic therapy depends on the type of microorganism causing the disease. Blood cultures are used to determine which antibiotic is most appropriate. Often, a combination is used, with penicillin commonly being one of them. The medication is often given through a vein continually over a period of several weeks to eradicate the infection.

Surgery

If the infection causes major damage to the heart valves, valve replacement may be necessary.

Diseases of the Heart Muscle and Lining

The heart's wall is composed of three layers:

- The epicardium, a thin, smooth covering on the outside of the heart
- The myocardium, the heart muscle itself
- The endocardium, the smooth inner lining of the heart that's in contact with the blood

Surrounding the heart on the outside is the pericardium, a fibrous sac.

Like the rest of your body, the heart muscle and its associated linings are subject to disease. Although relatively rare, diseases that can damage the heart muscle and the heart's linings do occur. They may develop as isolated problems or be consequences of disorders that affect other organs.

Cardiomyopathy

Signs and symptoms
- Shortness of breath, even at rest
- Swelling of legs, ankles and feet
- Abdominal bloating
- Fatigue
- Rapid or fluttering irregular heartbeats
- Dizziness and fainting

Preventing Endocarditis

People with the following heart conditions are at risk of more-serious outcomes from endocarditis:

- Artificial (prosthetic) heart valve
- Previous endocarditis infection
- Certain types of congenital heart defects
- Heart transplant complicated by heart valve problems

People with these conditions may need to take preventive antibiotics before certain medical or dental procedures to prevent endocarditis.

Preventive antibiotics

Certain dental and medical procedures may allow bacteria to enter your bloodstream. Antibiotics taken before these procedures can help destroy or control the harmful bacteria that may lead to endocarditis.

However, antibiotics are no longer recommended before *all* dental procedures, as they once were, or for procedures of the urinary tract or gastrointestinal system.

Current guidelines reserve preventive antibiotic treatment only for those people who would have the worst outcomes if they get infective endocarditis. As a result, the list of procedures for which antibiotics are recommended has grown shorter. Antibiotics are now recommended only before the following:

- Dental procedures that manipulate gum tissue or part of the teeth
- Procedures involving the respiratory tract, infected skin or musculoskeletal tissue

If you've had to take preventive antibiotics in the past before your dental exams, you were likely told to get antibiotics because of a concern that common dental procedures increased your risk of endocarditis. But as doctors have learned more about endocarditis prevention, they've realized that endocarditis is more likely to occur from exposure to random germs than from a typical dental exam or surgery.

As a result of this new knowledge, considerably fewer people take preventive antibiotics before a dental exam. Part of the reason for the change is that although the risk of receiving antibiotic treatment is small, adverse reactions and even life-threatening reactions can occur.

This doesn't mean it's not important to take good care of your teeth through brushing and flossing. There is some concern that infections in your mouth from poor oral hygiene might increase the risk of germs entering your bloodstream. In addition to brushing and flossing, regular dental exams — at least get a yearly exam — are an important part of maintaining good oral health.

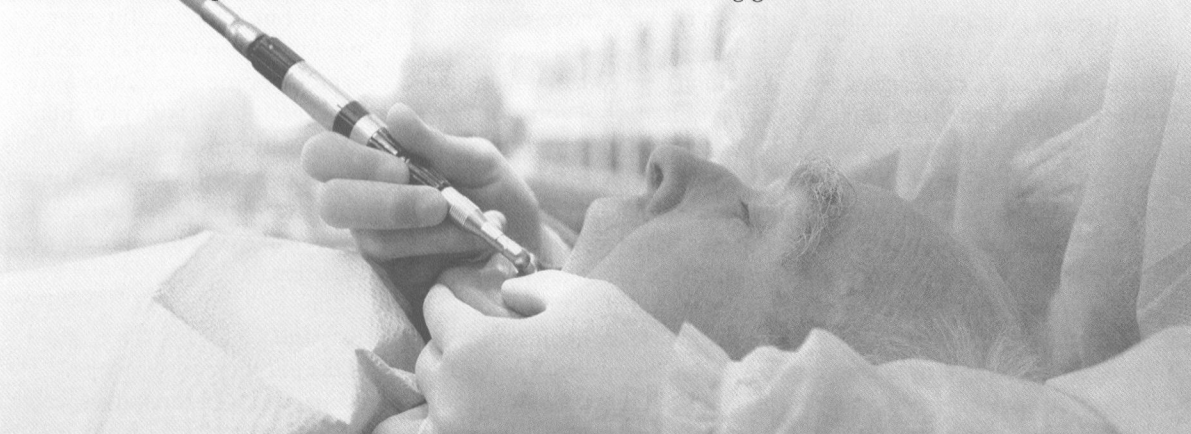

When the muscle of the heart is damaged or defective, the disorder is called cardiomyopathy. The term comes from Greek roots for "heart" (*kardia*), "muscle" (*myo*) and "disease" (*pathos*).

There are many causes of cardiomyopathy including coronary artery disease and heart valve disorders. Sometimes, the cause is unknown.

Types

There are three main forms of cardiomyopathy:

- **Dilated cardiomyopathy.** This is the most common type of cardiomyopathy. In this disorder, your heart's main pumping chamber — the left ventricle — becomes enlarged (dilated), its pumping ability becomes less forceful, and blood doesn't flow as easily through the heart. Although this type can affect people of all ages, it occurs most often in middle-aged people, and is more likely to affect men. Some people with dilated cardiomyopathy may have a family history of the condition.
- **Hypertrophic cardiomyopathy.** This type involves abnormal growth or thickening of your heart muscle, particularly affecting the muscle of your heart's main pumping chamber. As thickening occurs, the heart tends to stiffen and the size of the pumping chamber may shrink, interfering with your heart's ability to deliver blood to your body. Hypertrophic cardiomyopathy can develop at any age, but the condition tends to be more severe if it becomes apparent during childhood. Most affected people have a family history of the disease, and some genetic mutations have been linked to hypertrophic cardiomyopathy.
- **Restrictive cardiomyopathy.** The heart muscle in people with restrictive cardiomyopathy becomes rigid and less elastic, meaning the heart can't properly expand and fill with blood between heartbeats. While restrictive cardiomyopathy can occur at any age, it most often tends to affect older people. It's the least common type of cardiomyopathy and can occur for no known reason (idiopathic). The condition may also be caused by diseases elsewhere in the body that affect the heart, such as amyloidosis, a rare condition in which abnormal proteins present in the blood are deposited into the heart.

Diagnosis

In diagnosing cardiomyopathy, your doctor will consider your symptoms and will likely perform other tests.

A chest X-ray will show whether your heart is enlarged. Your doctor may recommend an ultrasound procedure (echocardiography) to examine the size of your heart and its motions and beats (see page 742). An echocardiogram often can determine what form of cardiomyopathy is present. In some cases, a procedure called cardiac catheterization may be needed. This test can measure pressure within the chambers of your heart to see how forcefully blood pumps through it. During this procedure, your doctor may also obtain a tissue sample (biopsy) from the heart for microscopic examination.

How serious is cardiomyopathy?

In most cases, cardiomyopathy poses no symptoms until the disease is quite advanced. The condition can lead to heart failure but rarely does it cause sudden death.

Treatment

The goals of treatment for cardiomyopathy are to manage your signs and symptoms, prevent your condition from worsening, and reduce your risk of complications.

Treatment varies by which type of cardiomyopathy you have.

Dilated cardiomyopathy

Your doctor may recommend medications, surgically implanted devices or a combination of both.

The medications you may be prescribed include:

- Angiotensin-converting enzyme (ACE) inhibitors to improve your heart's pumping capability, such as enalapril (Vasotec, Epaned), lisinopril (Zestril, Prinivil), ramipril (Altace) or captopril (Capoten)
- Angiotensin receptor blockers (ARBs) for those who can't take ACE inhibitors, such as losartan (Cozaar) and valsartan (Diovan)
- Beta blockers to improve heart function, such as carvedilol (Coreg) and metoprolol (Lopressor, Toprol-XL)

Another option for some people is a special pacemaker that coordinates the contractions between the left and right ventricle (biventricular pacing).

In people who may be at risk of serious arrhythmias, drug therapy or an internal cardioverter defibrillator (ICD) may be options. ICDs are small devices — about the size of a box of matches — implanted in your chest to continuously monitor your heart rhythm and deliver electric shocks when needed to control abnormal, rapid heartbeats. The devices can also work as pacemakers (see page 736).

Hypertrophic cardiomyopathy

Your doctor may recommend beta blockers to relax your heart, slow its pumping action and stabilize its rhythm. These medications include beta blockers or calcium channel blockers, such as verapamil (Calan, Isoptin, others).

In some cases, your doctor may recommend a pacemaker or an ICD. In advanced cases of hypertrophic cardiomyopathy, a surgeon may remove a portion of the thickened muscle wall that blocks normal blood flow. This procedure, called septal myectomy, can reduce symptoms in most cases.

Another type of therapy is called alcohol ablation. This nonsurgical procedure, which uses injected alcohol to destroy extra heart muscle, may reduce muscle thickening and improve blood flow. It's usually reserved for individuals who have other conditions that make them too high a risk for surgical septal myectomy.

Restrictive cardiomyopathy

Treatment for restrictive cardiomyopathy focuses on improving symptoms. Your doctor will likely recommend that you pay careful attention to your salt and water intake and monitor your weight. He or she may also prescribe a diuretic if sodium and water retention becomes a problem. You may be prescribed medications to lower your blood pressure and control fast or irregular heart rhythms.

Heart transplantation

If you have severe cardiomyopathy and medications can't control your symptoms, a heart transplant may be an option. Because of the shortage of donor hearts, even people who are critically ill may have a long wait before having a heart transplant.

In some cases, a mechanical heart-assist device can help critically ill people as they wait for an appropriately matched donor heart. These devices, known as ventricular assist devices (VADs), can support circulation for a prolonged period of time and may allow you

Heart Transplantation

In some situations, the heart becomes so damaged or weak that conventional medical treatment can do little to improve its functioning. In such cases, a heart transplant may be considered.

During the past 30 years, heart transplantation has become a relatively common procedure in many medical centers. More than 5,000 heart transplants are performed worldwide each year. Results have improved so that current one-year survival rates at experienced medical centers are from 85 to 95 percent. Survival without a transplant in this group is dismal. Most people who undergo a transplant enjoy a full and active life, and many return to full-time employment.

Who qualifies?

Almost anyone from a newborn infant with a serious congenital heart defect to an older adult with end-stage heart disease can be considered for heart transplantation. Potential heart transplant candidates should be motivated for transplantation and have good function of all other vital organs, including the liver, kidneys and lungs. Candidates need to be free of other noncardiac diseases, such as blood disorders, severe diabetes or cancers that reduce life expectancy.

People most likely to benefit are usually those younger than age 65 with irreversible heart disease in which the life expectancy without transplantation would be less than two or three years.

Available organs

Unfortunately, nearly one-third of the people waiting for a heart transplant die before a donor heart becomes available because of the shortage of hearts for transplant. Educational efforts to inform the public of the need for more donor hearts is a high priority. Although no one should want another person to die so that a heart will be available for transplantation, when deaths occur, families often find comfort in helping others through organ donation.

Procedure

Before a heart transplant operation, a donor heart must be available. Most often, this heart comes from a healthy person who died of an accident that didn't damage the heart. A nationally maintained waiting list uses a computer to match a patient in the region of the donor with a compatible blood type and acceptable size range for the donor heart. Once doctors remove the heart from the donor, ideally it should be transplanted into the recipient within four hours.

The donated heart is transported in a special cold solution to the recipient hospital. The recipient's chest cavity is opened, and the diseased heart is removed. During this portion of the procedure, the supply of oxygenated blood to the recipient is maintained by a heart-lung machine, as is done in many other types of heart surgery. The donated heart is then placed into the recipient's chest cavity and delicately connected to the major blood vessels.

Rejection

All transplanted organs are susceptible to rejection. The body's immune system recognizes the transplanted tissue as foreign and produces antibodies to attack it, just as the immune system might attack a virus or bacterium.

To minimize the risk of rejection of a transplanted heart, medications that suppress the body's normal immune response are needed. Some of these immunosuppressant medications are used for only a short time after the operation. Others must be taken for the rest of a person's life.

Immunosuppressant medications also decrease your body's ability to recognize and resist infections. Dosages must be monitored carefully to minimize side effects. Periodic biopsies of your heart tissue can aid your doctor in assessing rejection. The biopsy speci-

to live outside the hospital while you wait for a donor organ. In individuals who aren't candidates for a heart transplant, VAD therapy may provide long-term support.

Myocarditis

Signs and symptoms
- Chest pain
- Rapid or abnormal heartbeat
- Shortness of breath
- Swelling of legs, ankles and feet
- Fatigue

Myocarditis is an inflammation of the myocardium, the middle layer of the heart wall. The condition is uncommon and is most often caused by a viral infection. In severe cases, myocarditis can weaken the heart's ability to pump, so it can't deliver adequate blood to the body.

Diagnosis
Your doctor may check you for myocarditis if you've recently had a viral or other type of infection and you develop signs and symptoms that suggest a swollen heart muscle. Diagnostic tests may include a chest X-ray, echocardiogram, electrocardiogram (ECG) and blood tests.

How serious is myocarditis?
Myocarditis can be very serious, but the outcome depends on the cause. Severe cases can lead to cardiac failure and death, but most often the inflammation clears and good health follows.

men is obtained by way of a catheter that's placed in a vein and advanced to the heart.

Recovery
Most people who have had a successful heart transplant can live a relatively normal life. Many live for more than a decade and some for more than 20 years following their heart transplant.

Long-term complications
Now that transplant recipients are living longer, doctors have found that some problems appear years after transplantation. The transplanted heart's coronary arteries may develop widespread narrowing (atherosclerosis). Because the nerves have been cut in the transplanted heart, recipients don't usually feel chest pain (angina) when their coronary arteries don't supply enough oxygen to the heart muscle. Therefore, doctors may perform annual coronary angiography and intracoronary ultrasound to look for possible narrowing of the coronary arteries.

Doctors also continue to examine recipients for any evidence of tumor formation, especially of the skin and lymph glands, because immunosuppressant medications can increase the chances of these types of cancers (malignancies).

Recent developments
The greatest challenge in heart transplantation is solving the serious donor shortage. It doesn't appear that there will ever be enough human donors to satisfy the need, therefore, alternative strategies are being explored:

Ventricular assist devices
One such effort involves the use of a left ventricular assist device to perform the work of the main pumping chamber of the heart (left ventricle). Weakness of the left ventricle is the cause of heart failure symptoms in most people. Assist devices are used in many major centers to keep heart transplant candidates alive while they wait for a donor heart. Several ventricular assist devices and full artificial hearts have been studied as an alternative to transplantation among individuals who aren't candidates for transplantation. The devices are proving effective and ultimately may offer hope for long-term treatment of people with heart failure.

Xenotransplantation
Another approach is developing animals, particularly pigs, whose organs have been genetically engineered to be used for human transplantation (xenotransplantation). This work is still in its early phases. If this research is successful, this type of transplantation could prove to be a long-term solution to the donor shortage.

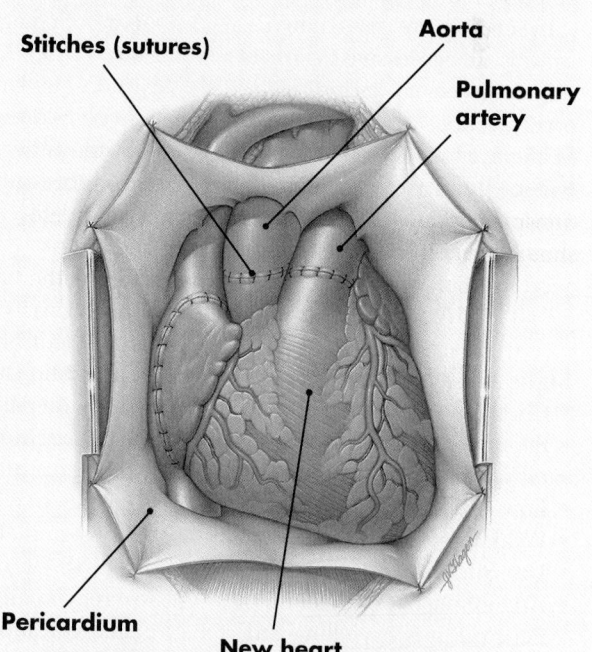

During a heart transplant operation, the ventricles and part of the atria, together with the heart valves and coronary arteries, are transplanted.

Treatment

In mild cases, your doctor may tell you to rest and prescribe medications to help your body fight off the infection causing myocarditis while your heart recovers. If bacteria are causing the infection, your doctor will prescribe antibiotics. Certain rare types of viral myocarditis respond to corticosteroids or other medications to suppress the immune system.

Once your heart inflammation has improved, you can gradually resume a more active lifestyle. In the meantime, your doctor may recommend that you limit the amount of salt in your diet, and avoid alcohol, tobacco use and vigorous exercise. Taking these steps can reduce the workload on your heart.

If you have rapid or irregular heartbeats, your doctor may hospitalize you. You'll likely receive drugs to regulate your heartbeat. If your heart is weak, your doctor may prescribe medications to strengthen its pumping ability, reduce your heart's workload or help you eliminate excess fluid.

In some severe cases of myocarditis, an aggressive treatment may be necessary, including use of intravenous drugs, placement of a pump in the aorta (intra-aortic balloon pump), use of a temporary artificial heart (assist device) or, possibly, heart transplantation.

Pericarditis

Signs and symptoms

- Chest pain
- Shortness of breath when reclining
- Low-grade fever
- Weakness, fatigue or feeling sick
- Dry cough
- Abdominal or leg swelling

Pericarditis is a swelling and irritation of the pericardium, the thin sac-like membrane that surrounds your heart. It occurs primarily in men between the ages of 20 and 50, often after a respiratory infection. Pain is felt when the pericardium and the heart's outermost layer rub against each other. There also may be an accumulation of excess fluid between the pericardium and the heart (pericardial effusion). Too much fluid can put pressure on the heart so that it doesn't fill properly.

The cause of pericarditis is often hard to determine. In some cases a viral infection may lead to the condition. Pericarditis can also develop after a major heart attack or trauma to your heart or chest.

One of the aftereffects of some cases of pericarditis is a permanent thickening, scarring and contracture of the pericardium.

Diagnosis

Your doctor may have you undergo a variety of tests — including a chest X-ray, electrocardiogram (ECG) and echocardiogram — in order to differentiate pericarditis from a heart attack. Blood tests also may be obtained. Although recurrences are common, most episodes of pericarditis last two to six weeks and resolve without further problems.

For both diagnosis and treatment, a procedure called pericardiocentesis may be of benefit. It involves draining excess fluid from the pericardial cavity using a small tube (catheter).

Treatment

Your doctor may recommend limited activity until you're feeling better. Medications to reduce the inflammation and swelling associated with pericarditis are often prescribed. Most pain associated with the condition responds well to treatment with aspirin or another nonsteroidal anti-inflammatory drug (NSAID). If your pain is severe, you might need stronger pain medications, such as a narcotic, for a short time.

The anti-inflammatory medication colchicine (Colcrys) may be prescribed for acute pericarditis or as a treatment for recurrent signs and symptoms. It can reduce the length of signs and symptoms or decrease the risk the condition will recur. The drug is not recommended for people with certain pre-existing conditions, including liver and kidney disease.

About 1 in 5 people with pericarditis will have a recurrence of symptoms within months of the original episode. If the symptoms don't respond to NSAIDS or colchicine, sometimes steroid medications are used.

When a bacterial infection is the underlying cause of pericarditis, you'll be treated with antibiotics and drainage if necessary.

When an excess amount of fluid has accumulated in the pericardial cavity, you may undergo a technique called pericardiocentesis to drain the fluid. In this procedure, a doctor uses a sterile needle or a small tube (catheter) to remove and drain the fluid. A local anesthetic is generally given before undergoing the procedure. The drainage may continue for several days during the course of your hospitalization.

In more-severe cases, you may need to undergo a surgical procedure (pericardiectomy) to remove the entire pericardium that has become rigid and is compromising the functioning of your heart.

Circulatory Problems

Your circulatory (vascular) system, the circuit through which your blood travels, consists of all the blood vessels in your body. It has two loops. The shorter loop handles lung (pulmonary) circulation. It begins at the right side of your heart, delivers blood to your lungs and then returns the oxygenated blood to your heart.

The longer loop is for whole-body (systemic) circulation. It begins at the left side of the heart, which receives blood oxygenated

Gangrene

When the supply of blood to any tissue is severely impaired, the supply of oxygen and nutrients is also restricted. If blood flow isn't restored, the tissue may die. This condition is called gangrene.

Blood flow to the legs can cease abruptly or slowly. In either situation, the foot becomes pale and cold. The pain is variable.

Forms of gangrene

The two main types of gangrene are dry and wet. With dry gangrene, the tissue has died but has not become infected. With wet gangrene, the tissue has died and become infected with bacteria.

Dry gangrene

Tissue affected with dry gangrene is cold to the touch and gradually becomes black. At first, it's painful, but as the affected tissue dies, the pain decreases. Over time, the tissues dry and drop off, but the gangrene doesn't usually spread. However, there's some risk of wet gangrene developing.

Dry gangrene is more prone to occur in people who've had diabetes for a long time, hardening of the arteries (arteriosclerosis) or a recent case of severe frostbite.

Wet gangrene

Wet gangrene, which is also called moist gangrene, involves a bacterial infection. At first, the involved tissues may be red and hot as a result of inflammation. With time, the tissues become cold and blue and pus may ooze from the area. Eventually, the tissues begin to slough off.

Wet gangrene tends to spread rapidly as the bacteria contribute to tissue breakdown. If the bacteria produce a gas that has a strong, disagreeable odor as it destroys the tissue, the condition is called gas gangrene. If not promptly treated, a person with gas gangrene may die in a matter of days.

Prevention

If you have diabetes or advanced arteriosclerosis, proper care of your extremities, especially your feet, is essential. Even minor injuries must be treated with special attention. Careful control of your blood sugar (glucose) level is important if you have diabetes. If you smoke, choose to stop. Every cigarette causes additional damage to blood vessels.

If you sustain a wound or injury, be sure it's properly treated. If virulent bacteria are present, wet gangrene may result from even a minor limb injury in which the blood supply is decreased.

Treatment

If you think you may have gangrene, consult your doctor right away. Treatment should be initiated immediately. Surgery to open or bypass blocked arteries may be possible. Tissues affected by dry gangrene may shrivel up and not be a problem, but surgical removal of the dead tissue often is needed.

Antibiotic medications are usually prescribed to prevent or treat wet gangrene. Tissue affected by wet gangrene may need to be removed surgically.

---

in the lungs. From the left side, this blood is pumped to body tissues through a series of arteries that become smaller and smaller: Arteries branch into smaller arterioles, and the arterioles branch into tiny capillaries that deliver blood to the tissues. After the blood in the capillaries collects carbon dioxide and other waste products from the tissues, it begins its trip back to your heart by way of small venules and, eventually, veins.

The total amount of blood within your body is relatively constant — about 7 percent of your body weight. The distribution of blood within blood vessels varies considerably with exercise and exposure to heat and cold. During exercise blood flow to active muscles is increased. After you eat, your stomach and intestines require more blood to assist in digestion.

Changes in the surrounding temperature also affect the flow of blood. Warmer temperatures produce increased flow to the outer layers of your skin, which helps you to get rid of heat. Alternatively, your body responds to cold by redistributing blood flow into the inner vessels, to conserve heat.

This complex system is subject to a wide range of malfunctions — some the result of heart disorders, others because of disorders that directly affect the blood vessels.

Arteriosclerosis

Signs and symptoms

- Pain in the feet, legs, buttocks or hips that develops during activity and resolves after the activity is stopped
- Numbness or pain in the feet or toes when at rest
- Ulcers or gangrene on the feet or toes

Arteriosclerosis is a disease of the arteries, the blood vessels that carry oxygen and nutrients from your heart to the rest of your body. In arteriosclerosis, the walls of your arteries lose their elasticity and become thick and stiff. As a result, blood flow may be reduced, and your organs and tissues don't receive adequate amounts.

The effects of arteriosclerosis generally appear first in your legs or feet. Major arteries that deliver blood to your legs and feet become narrowed, and blood flow decreases. Smaller blood vessels assume

What's the difference between arteriosclerosis and atherosclerosis?

The distinction between the two terms isn't always clear. *Arteriosclerosis* refers to the abnormal thickening and hardening of the walls of your arteries.

Atherosclerosis is one form of arteriosclerosis, but it's often used to describe many forms of arteriosclerosis. *Atherosclerosis* refers to the accumulation of fatty deposits (plaques) in your arteries. Atherosclerosis that occurs in your coronary arteries is called coronary artery disease.

some of the load, but the physical activity of walking even a block or two can create an unmet need for increased blood flow and produce pain in your legs or feet. The discomfort often disappears when you rest. This sequence of walk-pain-rest is called intermittent claudication.

Sometimes, blockages can develop in your arteries. If the blockage occurs suddenly, as when a fragment of a fatty deposit (plaque) or clot lodges at a fork of your leg artery (arterial embolism), you may experience sudden and severe pain and your leg may become pale and cold below the level of the blockage. The accumulation of fatty deposits (plaques) in your arteries is known as atherosclerosis.

The limited blood supply can cause inflammation and damage to the nerves. In severe cases, gangrene may occur. Gangrene is a condition in which tissue dies.

Circulation problems are common in people with diabetes. In addition, people with diabetes may have nerve damage (diabetic neuropathy). The decreased sensitivity to touch that often accompanies diabetic neuropathy makes the person more likely to injure the affected foot.

Diagnosis

A key aspect to diagnosis of arteriosclerosis is observing the nature and timing of your discomfort. Does the pain occur only with exercise? Is it relieved by rest? Does it recur when activity is resumed? If so, your doctor may suspect arteriosclerosis. He or she may take your blood pressure in an ankle and compare it with the blood pressure in your arm. If pressure in your ankle is much less than in your arm, it may indicate that the arteries in your legs are narrowed.

Other tests, including an ultrasound scan, angiogram and blood tests may be ordered. An angiogram can help your doctor determine where the blockage is located. For this procedure, an X-ray is taken during and after a dye is injected into the artery that supplies the affected area.

How serious is arteriosclerosis?

For many people, arteriosclerosis in one or both legs can be serious because it may be an indication of problems elsewhere in the body. Appropriate care can prevent severe disability or loss of a limb. Among people with diabetes, circulatory problems are more common.

Treatment

Lifestyle changes, such as eating a healthy diet, exercising and stopping smoking, are often the first line of defense in treating arteriosclerosis.

Foot care is essential for people with arteriosclerosis of the legs or feet. Wear shoes that fit properly. Even minor cuts or scrapes may require immediate attention because decreased circulation means that the tissues heal more slowly. If left untreated, even a minor injury to the skin of your lower leg or foot can lead to infection, gangrene and possibly amputation.

Are You at Risk?

Your risk of arteriosclerosis of the legs and feet increases if you:
- Smoke
- Are a man
- Are a woman past menopause
- Are at least 60 years old
- Have high blood pressure
- Have high blood cholesterol
- Are overweight
- Are sedentary
- Have diabetes

Not smoking is the best way to prevent or reduce this condition. Regular exercise can improve blood flow in the smaller arteries of your legs and condition your muscles so that they require less oxygen.

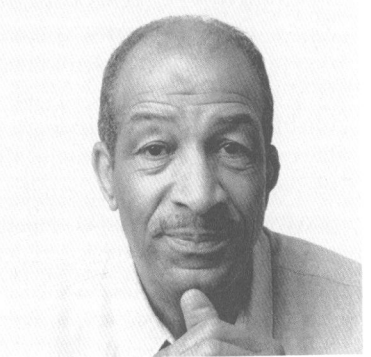

Sometimes, medication or surgical procedures may be recommended as well.

Medications

Various drugs can slow — sometimes even reverse — the effects of ateriosclerosis due to accumulation of plaques (atherosclerosis). Here are some common choices:
- **Cholesterol medications.** Lowering your low-density lipoprotein (LDL, or "bad") cholesterol can slow, stop or even reverse the buildup of fatty deposits in your arteries. Boosting your high-density lipoprotein (HDL, or "good") cholesterol may help, too. Your doctor can choose from a range of cholesterol medications.

- **Anti-platelet medications.** Your doctor may prescribe anti-platelet medications, such as aspirin, to reduce the likelihood that platelets will clump in narrowed arteries, form a blood clot and cause further blockage.
- **Anticoagulants.** An anticoagulant, such as heparin or warfarin (Coumadin), can help thin your blood to prevent clots from forming.
- **Blood pressure medications.** Medications to control blood pressure — such as beta blockers, angiotensin-converting enzyme (ACE) inhibitors and calcium channel blockers — can help slow the progression of atherosclerosis.
- **Other medications.** Your doctor may suggest certain medications to control specific risk factors for atherosclerosis, such as diabetes. Sometimes medications to treat symptoms of atherosclerosis, such as leg pain during exercise, are prescribed.

Surgery
Sometimes more-aggressive treatment is needed. If you have severe symptoms or a blockage that threatens muscle or skin tissue survival, you may be a candidate for one of the following procedures:
- **Angioplasty.** Your doctor inserts a long, thin tube (catheter) into the blocked or narrowed part of your artery. A wire with a deflated balloon is passed through the catheter to the narrowed area. Once in place, the balloon is inflated, compressing the deposits against your artery walls and opening up the vessel. Angioplasty may also be done with laser technology.
- **Endarterectomy.** In some cases, fatty deposits must be surgically removed from the walls of a narrowed artery. When the procedure is done on arteries in the neck (carotid arteries), it's known as carotid endarterectomy.
- **Thrombolytic therapy.** If you have an artery that's blocked by

a blood clot, your doctor may insert a clot-dissolving drug into your artery at the point of the clot to break it up.
- **Bypass surgery.** A surgeon may create a graft bypass using a vessel from another part of your body or a synthetic tube. This allows blood to flow around the blocked or narrowed artery.

Arterial embolism

Signs and symptoms
- Sudden pain
- Pale, cool skin
- Numbness

An embolus is a clot that has moved from its point of origin to a new location and is blocking the flow of blood. An embolus isn't the same as a thrombus. A thrombus is a clot that forms in the vessel and remains stationary.

Emboli may be multiple and small, or they may be single and massive. Emboli can be life-threatening, such as when they lodge in the brain and cause a stroke, or they can lead to tissue death in an arm or leg if not treated within a few hours. Arterial emboli may originate in the left atrium of the heart among people experiencing an abnormal heart rhythm (atrial fibrillation) or in the left ventricle following a heart attack.

When embolization occurs, flow of blood to the affected areas may abruptly stop or gradually slow. If a clot or debris from fatty deposits

(plaques) in the aorta is carried with the flow of blood to an artery in the thigh, it may plug the artery at the level of the knee, where the larger artery splits into several small ones. This can cause sudden pain and pale skin in the lower leg and foot.

Diagnosis
Your doctor will measure the blood pressure in the affected limb and also may try to locate the embolus with an ultrasound examination or arteriography, a test in which dye is injected into the affected blood vessels and X-rays are taken.

How serious is an arterial embolism?
If the clot or debris isn't surgically removed within a matter of hours, the tissue below that level may die and amputation may be necessary.

When embolism occurs, it's important to protect the limb from any injury by wrapping it loosely with a soft blanket and gauze. It's tempting to apply heat, but this may worsen already damaged tissue. However, protecting the limb from loss of heat by using a blanket, gauze or other wrap is safe and important.

Treatment
Once a diagnosis of an arterial embolism is reached, clot-dissolving medication may be given to try to break up the embolus, perhaps

---

PREVENTION TIP

Sitting during a long airplane flight or automobile ride commonly causes swollen ankles. The inactivity also increases your risk of thrombosis in the veins of your legs. To help prevent a blood clot from forming:
- Take a walk around the airplane cabin once an hour or so. If you're driving, stop every hour and walk around to stretch your legs.
- While seated, flex your ankles.
- Wear support hose (compression stockings). They help compress your leg veins to promote blood flow. Wear them if you're prone to swollen legs and ankles.
- If you're not allergic to aspirin, consider taking one just before a long trip. It may help prevent clot formation. Before using aspirin on a regular basis, consult your doctor.

delivering it directly to the affected artery through the use of a catheter. This is called thrombolysis. Long-term use of aspirin or another anticoagulant medication may be appropriate in order to prevent the development of more clots.

If the health of a limb is in danger, immediate surgical removal of the clot may be attempted. This is usually done with a balloon-tipped catheter inserted into the artery. As it's being withdrawn, the inflated balloon pulls the clot out. Occasionally, replacement or bypass of the blocked vessel is necessary.

Aortic aneurysm

Signs and symptoms
- Pulsating feeling near the navel, if the aneurysm is in the abdomen
- Tenderness or pain in abdomen or chest
- Back pain

An aortic aneurysm is a weakened and bulging area in the aorta, the major blood vessel that feeds blood to the body. The aorta runs from your heart through the center of your chest and abdomen.

Most small and slow-growing aortic aneurysms don't rupture, but large, fast-growing aortic aneurysms may. A ruptured aortic aneurysm can cause life-threatening bleeding.

Abdominal aortic aneurysms
About 75 percent of all aortic aneurysms occur in the part of your aorta that's in your abdomen. Although the exact cause of abdominal aortic aneurysms is unknown, a number of factors may play a role, including:
- **Tobacco use.** In addition to the damaging effects that smoking causes directly to the arteries, smoking contributes to atherosclerosis and high blood pressure, and causes aneurysms to grow faster.
- **High blood pressure.** High blood pressure, especially if poorly controlled, increases the risk of developing an aortic aneurysm.
- **Vasculitis.** In rare cases, an aortic aneurysm may be caused by an infection or inflammation that weakens a section of the aortic wall.

Thoracic aortic aneurysms
About 25 percent of aortic aneurysms occur higher up in your chest (thoracic area). The same risk factors associated with abdominal aortic aneurysms can contribute to thoracic aortic aneurysms. Additional factors that can lead to a thoracic aortic aneurysm include:
- **Marfan syndrome.** People who are born with this genetic condition are particularly at risk of a thoracic aortic aneurysm. Those with Marfan syndrome may have a weakness in the aortic wall that makes them more susceptible to aneurysms. Related disorders that are less common include Loeys-Dietz syndrome and Ehlers-Danlos syndrome.

- **Previous injury to the aorta.** You're more likely to have a thoracic aortic aneurysm if you've had previous problems with your aorta, such as a tear in the wall of the aorta (aortic dissection).
- **Traumatic injury.** Some people who are injured in falls or motor vehicle crashes develop thoracic aortic aneurysms.

Diagnosis
Often, aortic aneurysms have no symptoms. In advanced cases, pain may be present in the abdomen and lower back.

Your doctor may detect the pulsating vessel during a routine examination of your abdomen. In some cases, an X-ray taken for another reason will reveal an aneurysm. Its presence is usually confirmed with an ultrasound exam or a computerized tomography (CT) scan or magnetic resonance imaging (MRI).

Because aortic aneurysms often don't cause symptoms, anyone

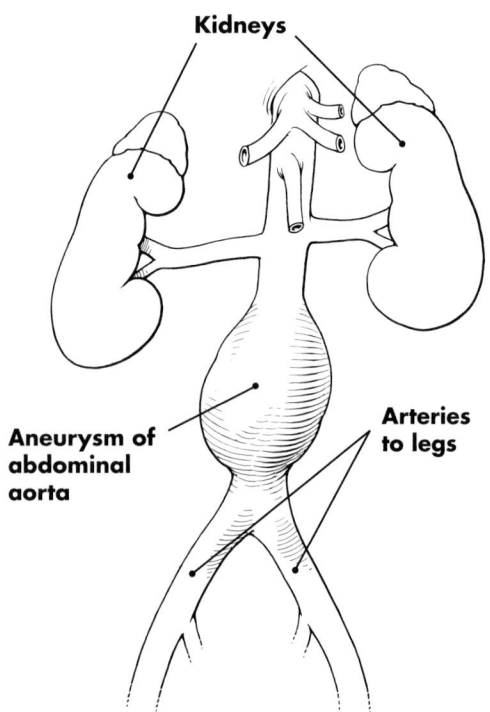

Kidneys

Aneurysm of abdominal aorta

Arteries to legs

An aneurysm, an abnormal widening of an artery, can occur in any location, but commonly occurs in the abdominal aorta just below the kidneys. The weakened wall of the aorta balloons out over time, usually growing at a rate of ⅛ to ¼ inch a year.

age 60 and older with risk factors for developing an aortic aneurysm should consider screening for the condition. Men ages 65 to 70 who have ever smoked should have a one-time screening for abdominal aortic aneurysm. Men age 60 and older with a family history of the condition also should be screened.

Treatment

The goal of treatment is to prevent your aneurysm from rupturing. Generally, your treatment options are to watch and wait or to have surgery. That decision generally depends on the size of the aneurysm and how fast it's growing. Surgery is generally recommended for large or faster growing aneurysms.

A traditional operation on an aortic aneurysm involves opening the abdomen or chest and stopping blood flow in the aorta so that the damaged section can be replaced with a synthetic tube graft.

A minimally invasive procedure called endovascular surgery uses a synthetic graft attached to the end of a catheter. The catheter usually is inserted into your bloodstream through an artery in your leg. It's threaded upstream to your aorta and used to position the graft at the site of the aneurysm. Once in place, the graft is expanded and fastened with small hooks or pins. The graft reduces pressure on the walls of the aorta. This type of surgery reduces recovery to days instead of weeks.

Thrombophlebitis

Signs and symptoms
- Tenderness and pain
- Redness and swelling

Thrombophlebitis is the medical term for inflammation in a vein caused by a blood clot. Often, the name is shortened to *phlebitis*. Typically, the condition occurs in the legs. On rare occasions it can affect veins in your arms or neck. It may affect either the deep or the superficial veins.

Potential causes include prolonged inactivity, such as from bed rest after surgery or sitting for a long period on an airplane or in a car. Inactivity decreases blood flow and may cause a clot to form. Paralysis, certain types of cancer and use of the hormone estrogen also may lead to thrombophlebitis.

Diagnosis

When the clot and inflammation occur in a vein near the surface of the skin (superficial phlebitis), your doctor can make the preliminary diagnosis on the basis of discomfort in the area and a hard, usually tender, cord-like clot that can be felt and seen. Superficial phlebitis is most often seen in varicose veins.

When thrombophlebitis occurs in a deep vein in the leg or, more rarely, in the arm, the condition is called deep vein thrombosis. To confirm this diagnosis, your doctor may perform one or more special tests including an ultrasound examination, computerized tomography (CT) scan, or venography, in which dye is injected into the affected veins and X-rays are taken.

How serious is thrombophlebitis?

Superficial thrombophlebitis rarely leads to serious complications. With deep vein thrombosis, the principal danger is the clot breaking loose, moving upstream and lodging in a blood vessel in your lungs — a condition called pulmonary embolism.

Treatment

If thrombophlebitis occurs in a superficial vein, your doctor may recommend self-care steps that include applying heat to the painful area, elevating the affected leg and using a nonsteroidal anti-inflammatory drug. The condition usually subsides within a week or two.

Your doctor may also recommend these treatments:

- **Medications.** If you have deep vein thrombosis, injection of a blood-thinning (anticoagulant) medication, such as low molecular weight heparin or fondaparinux (Arixtra), will prevent clots from enlarging. After the initial treatment, taking the oral anticoagulant warfarin (Coumadin, Jantoven, others) or the drug rivaroxaban (Xarelto) for several months continues to prevent clots from enlarging.
- **Support stockings.** They help prevent recurrent swelling and reduce the chances of complications of deep vein thrombosis.
- **Filter.** In some instances, especially if you can't take blood thinners due to a bleeding condition, a filter may be inserted into the main vein in your abdomen (vena cava) to prevent clots that break loose in leg veins from lodging in your lungs.
- **Varicose vein stripping.** Your doctor can surgically remove varicose veins that cause pain or recurrent thrombophlebitis in a procedure called varicose vein stripping. Removing the vein won't affect circulation in your leg because veins deeper in the leg take care of the increased volumes of blood. This procedure is also commonly done for cosmetic reasons.
- **Clot removal or bypass.** Sometimes, surgery is necessary to remove an acute clot blocking a pelvic vein or an abdominal vein. Your doctor may recommend surgery to bypass the vein, or a nonsurgical procedure called angioplasty to open up the vein. Once angioplasty has opened up the vein, your doctor inserts a small wire mesh tube (stent) to keep the vein open.

Varicose veins

Signs and symptoms
- Achy, heavy feeling in legs
- Burning, throbbing, cramping and swelling in lower legs

- Itching around one or more veins
- Skin ulcers near the ankles

Varicose veins are twisted and enlarged veins close to the surface of the skin. Any vein may become varicose, but the veins most commonly affected are those in your legs and feet. Varicose veins are common, affecting both men and women.

For many people, varicose veins are a cosmetic concern, but for some people they can cause pain and discomfort. Sometimes, the condition can lead to serious problems.

Varicose veins occur as a result of a malfunction of the valves in the veins. Normally, the valves help prevent blood from flowing backward, but they can become stretched as a result of pregnancy, thrombophlebitis, congenital weakness, obesity or standing for long periods of time. When the valves are weakened and are no longer able to close normally, blood pools in the veins. As a result, the veins enlarge and become varicose.

Spider veins are a mild version of varicose veins. They're smaller, closer to the surface and may look like a spider web.

Diagnosis

In making a diagnosis, your doctor will examine your legs while you're standing and look for swelling. He or she may also perform an ultrasound test to see if the valves in the veins are functioning normally.

How serious are varicose veins?

Varicose veins can be associated with complications of venous insufficiency. These can include a brownish discoloration, thickening of the skin and ulcerations near the ankle. If skin ulcers develop, contact your doctor. Ulcers require medical attention.

Treatment

Self-help measures — such as exercising, losing weight, not wearing tight clothes, elevating your legs, and avoiding long periods of standing or sitting — can ease pain and prevent varicose veins from getting worse. Varicose veins that develop during pregnancy generally improve without medical treatment within three months after delivery.

If you don't respond to self-help or if your condition is more severe, your doctor may advise one of these varicose vein treatments:

- **Sclerotherapy.** In this procedure, your doctor injects varicose veins with a solution that scars and closes those veins. In a few weeks, treated varicose veins should fade. Although the same vein may need to be injected more than once, sclerotherapy is effective if done correctly.
- **Laser surgeries.** Doctors are using new technology in laser treatments to close off smaller varicose veins and spider veins. Laser surgery works by sending strong bursts of light onto the vein, which makes the vein slowly fade and disappear. No incisions or needles are used.
- **Catheter-assisted procedures.** Your doctor inserts a thin tube (catheter) into an enlarged vein and heats the tip of the catheter. As the catheter is pulled out, the heat destroys the vein by causing it to collapse and seal shut. This is usually done for larger varicose veins.
- **Vein stripping.** This procedure involves removing a long vein through small incisions. Removing the vein won't affect circulation in your leg because veins deeper in the leg take care of the larger volumes of blood.
- **Ambulatory phlebectomy.** Your doctor removes smaller varicose veins through a series of tiny skin punctures. Scarring is generally minimal.
- **Endoscopic vein surgery.** This is generally done only in advanced cases involving leg ulcers. A surgeon inserts a thin device with an attached video camera in your leg to visualize and close varicose veins, and then removes the veins through small incisions.

Vascular skin ulcers

Signs and symptoms
- Swelling in legs or feet
- A wound or sore that doesn't heal on a leg or foot

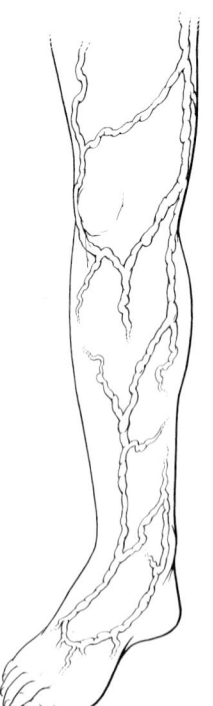
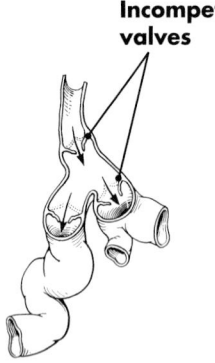

Incompetent valves

Varicose veins are enlarged veins that are easily seen beneath the surface of the skin of the legs and feet. These twisted veins may be caused by incompetent valves, which allow blood to flow backward.

Lymphedema

Lymphedema is an abnormal accumulation of lymph fluid in the extremities. It causes painless swelling, which usually starts in the toes and feet and progresses toward the trunk. This form of swelling (edema) may initially improve with bed rest and elevation of the leg, but as it progresses, the improvement may be minimal.

In some situations, the cause is obvious. For example, it occurs after some types of traumatic injury, operations and radiation therapy. It might also result from an infection, particularly in tropical climates. A more serious cause of lymphedema is a cancer that obstructs the flow of lymph fluid back into the abdominal cavity. Thus, if you develop lymphedema for unexplained reasons in an extremity, your doctor may perform tests to rule out cancer.

- An aching or burning sensation at the sore site
- Paleness of a leg or foot or discoloration of a foot
- Numbness or tingling in a leg, foot or toes

Vascular skin ulcers usually start out as a small sore on the foot or an itchy patch of skin near the ankle from which fluid eventually seeps. These ulcers result from impaired circulation in the arteries or veins in your feet and legs, which may be caused by conditions such as atherosclerosis, diabetes, excess weight or pregnancy.

The two main types of vascular skin ulcers are:

- **Venous ulcers.** These are the most common type of vascular skin ulcers. They're associated with circulatory problems in veins, and they typically develop on the inside area of your leg's lower calf or near your ankle. One-way valves that keep blood from flowing backward in the veins may become stretched or damaged, allowing blood to pool. Swelling (edema) may result and weaken surrounding tissues. Skin may become bluish or brownish in color and leathery before it gives way to an open wound.
- **Ischemic ulcers.** Ischemic skin ulcers can occur when the flow of oxygenated blood is reduced in arteries serving the legs and feet. The main cause of ischemic ulcers is atherosclerosis. As

arteries become progressively more narrow, blood flow to the legs and feet may be significantly reduced. This can lead to temporary cramping or pain in your muscles after walking (intermittent claudication).

Diagnosis

Tests may be needed to determine the cause of the ulcer and its severity. These may include the use of blood pressure cuffs on your legs and ultrasound imaging.

If surgery is being considered, your doctor may use X-ray imaging with a contrast dye to view your veins (venogram) or your arteries (arteriogram).

How serious are vascular skin ulcers?

Once recognized, most vascular ulcers can be treated, and they eventually heal. Left untreated, a skin ulcer has the potential to become very deep — affecting fat tissue, muscle and even bone.

Treatment

Regular cleaning and dressing changes are an important part of treatment. For venous ulcers, elastic compressive wraps also may be used to improve blood flow and decrease swelling while the ulcer heals.

If an ulcer isn't responding to such standard treatment, is recurrent or particularly deep, more-

intensive measures may be needed. These include:

- **Mechanical pumps.** A sleeve attached to a small pump fits over your leg. The sleeve compresses intermittently, forcing blood and fluid out of swollen tissues to promote venous blood flow.
- **Hyperbaric oxygen.** This treatment involves periodically spending about 90 minutes in a chamber where you breathe pure oxygen at high pressure to promote wound healing.
- **Human growth factors.** A topical paste that contains growth factors found in human blood platelets is applied to a wound. The growth factors help stimulate new tissue formation.
- **Skin grafting.** Skin grafting involves removing healthy skin from another area of your body and grafting it to the area affected by the ulcer. Or your doctor may use artificial skin (human skin equivalent), a cellular skin substitute that includes cells derived from human tissues. It provides wound protection and fosters growth of new skin.
- **Surgery.** Only a small percentage of people with venous ulcers are candidates for surgery. If a blocked artery is the cause of the ulcer, balloon angioplasty may be used to open a narrowed artery. A stent — a small metallic mesh tube that's positioned in an artery following dilation of the blocked area — also may be placed in the artery to keep it open.

Surgery may also be performed to remove fatty deposits (plaques) and blood clots in blocked arteries, or to bypass a blocked artery.

Raynaud's disease

Signs and symptoms

- White fingers or toes on exposure to cold, with numbness or stinging pain
- Blue or red skin

Named after the French doctor who described it, this disease results from changes in circulation in your hands or feet. It's normal for the blood vessels in your extremities to constrict when exposed to cold temperatures, but in people with Raynaud's disease, this response to cold is exaggerated. Stress can also trigger the symptoms.

Arteries to the fingers and toes go into what's called vasospasm. This constricts the vessels temporarily, but dramatically limits blood supply. Over time, these same small arteries may thicken slightly, further limiting blood flow. The affected skin turns pale and dusky-colored due to the lack of blood flow. Once the spasms subside and blood returns to the area, the tissue may turn red or blue before returning to a normal color.

Women are more likely to develop the problem than are men. The first episode often occurs between ages 15 and 25.

You can have Raynaud's without any underlying disease associated with it, called primary Raynaud's. This is the most common form. Or you can have it as part of another disease, in which case doctors may refer to it as secondary Raynaud's. Secondary Raynaud's is associated with conditions such as:

- Connective tissue diseases, including scleroderma and lupus
- Rheumatoid arthritis
- Sjogren's syndrome
- Diseases of the arteries, including atherosclerosis
- Carpal tunnel syndrome
- Use of certain medications, including beta blockers, ergotamine preparations and over-the-counter cold remedies
- Exposure to certain chemicals

Diagnosis

Your doctor may be able to diagnose Raynaud's disease directly from a description of your symptoms and from examining affected parts, such as your fingers and toes for characteristic changes.

Blood tests may be performed to check for certain antibodies found in people with autoimmune disorders, such as scleroderma or lupus, and for inflammation.

How serious is Raynaud's disease?

For most people, Raynaud's disease is more of a nuisance than a disability. But people with secondary Raynaud's may experience complications including skin ulcers and even tissue death (gangrene).

Treatment

Prevention is key to reducing the number and severity of attacks of Raynaud's disease. In more-severe cases, medication may be prescribed to help widen narrowed blood vessels and promote circulation. Rarely is surgery performed.

Prevention

To avoid attacks of Raynaud's disease, adequate protection from the cold is essential. Other steps also can help.

- Dress warmly when exposed to the cold, making sure to keep your feet and hands warm.
- Don't smoke. Nicotine in tobacco decreases skin blood flow.
- Avoid caffeine because it causes your blood vessels to narrow and it may increase the signs and symptoms of Raynaud's.
- Use insulated glasses for cold drinks.
- Warm up your car before driving in cold weather.
- Try to avoid stressful situations.
- Exercise. It increases your energy level and improves blood flow.
- Avoid over-the-counter cold remedies, which can worsen symptoms.
- If you use birth control pills, switch to another method of contraception because they affect your circulation and may make you more prone to attacks.

Buerger's disease

Signs and symptoms

- Pain or weakness in the hands or feet

- Swelling in feet or hands
- Pale, red or bluish skin of affected areas
- Open sores on your fingers or toes

Buerger's disease is named after American doctor Leo Buerger, who first described it in 1908.

It's a rare disease of the blood vessels in the arms and legs. Your blood vessels swell and can become blocked with blood clots. The skin of the hands and feet becomes tender and, over time, pain and ulcers develop.

The disease characteristically strikes men between ages 20 and 40. For unexplained reasons, there appears to be a direct link between tobacco use and Buerger's disease. One theory is that the chemicals in tobacco may irritate the lining of the blood vessels, causing them to swell.

Diagnosis

Your doctor may be able to diagnose Buerger's disease by looking at the affected hands or feet. Usually, two or more limbs are affected. Tests may be needed to check blood flow through your arteries and veins and to look for blockage of blood vessels.

How serious is Buerger's disease?

In some cases, gangrene may develop and amputation of the affected limb may be necessary.

Treatment

Eliminating the use of tobacco usually results in a cure. Avoid cold temperatures and other conditions that may impair circulation.

Warmth and gentle exercise may increase circulation. Medications to relax the muscles in the walls of blood vessels, improve blood flow and dissolve blood clots may be prescribed. A surgical procedure may be performed to cut the sympathetic nerves in the affected area to control pain and improve circulation. However, the operation isn't always successful. ■

Lungs and Respiratory System

Your lungs are part of your respiratory system. This system includes a network of organs and nerves that enable you to breathe. Your lungs are enclosed by your chest wall and your diaphragm. The chest wall is made up of ribs, cartilage and the muscles between them. The diaphragm consists of sheets of muscle that separate your chest cavity (thoracic cavity) from your abdominal cavity.

The lungs are soft and spongy. If you're healthy, they're usually a mottled pinkish-gray color. However, even healthy lungs can become blackened from carbon particles in polluted air. Your right lung is divided into three sections (lobes), and your left into two lobes. Your heart is between your lungs.

The pleura is a membrane with lubricating fluid between its two layers. The pleura covers the surface of each lung and the inside of the chest wall. The slippery pleural surfaces allow your lungs to move easily within the chest cavity as you breathe.

Your windpipe (trachea) branches into two main airways, called bronchial tubes. Each bronchial tube then branches into smaller passageways that divide several times more, finally forming much smaller tubes called bronchioles. The branching gives the airways of your respiratory system the appearance of an upside-down tree.

The smallest bronchioles end in tiny closed elastic air sacs (alveoli). Your lungs contain approximately 300 million alveoli. If they all could be stretched out on a flat surface, they would cover an area approximately the size of a tennis court.

Tiny blood vessels, called capillaries, carry blood to the alveoli. Capillaries release carbon dioxide into the alveoli and absorb inhaled oxygen into your bloodstream.

How Your Lungs Work

The primary function of your lungs is to supply oxygen to and remove carbon dioxide from your blood. To reach your lungs, air enters through your mouth and nose, travels through the back of your throat (pharynx), through your voice box (larynx) and down your windpipe (trachea), and into air passages called bronchi.

When you inhale, the muscles between your ribs contract, causing your ribs to move upward and outward. At the same time, your diaphragm contracts, pushing down toward your abdomen. These two actions increase the size of your chest cavity, causing your lungs to expand so that air is drawn into them. Individual alveoli also fill with air. During normal breathing, a healthy adult draws about a pint of air into the lungs with each breath. However, during deep breathing, you can draw as much as 3 to 6 quarts of air into your lungs.

When you exhale, your diaphragm and rib muscles relax and return to their original positions. This decreases the size of your chest cavity, compressing your lungs slightly and forcing stale air — now carrying carbon dioxide — out of your body. The whole process of breathing in and out occurs automatically without your having to think about it.

Your lungs are connected to your heart by the pulmonary arteries and veins. The term *pulmonary* comes from the Latin word *pulmo*, for "lung." After traveling through your body, blood returns to the right side of your heart, where the bottom-right chamber (right ventricle) pumps it through the pulmonary artery to your lungs. Blood then passes through the arteries of the lungs into smaller and smaller vessels, similar to the branching of the bronchi. Finally, it flows into the capillaries, which are situated in the walls of the alveoli.

After gases are exchanged in the alveoli, blood — now carrying oxygen — passes into the smallest veins. These veins merge to form larger vessels until the pulmonary veins reach the heart. The pulmonary veins carry oxygen-rich blood from the lungs back to the lower-left side of your heart (left ventricle). The left ventricle then pumps the blood back to the cells and organs of your body.

The Chest Cavity

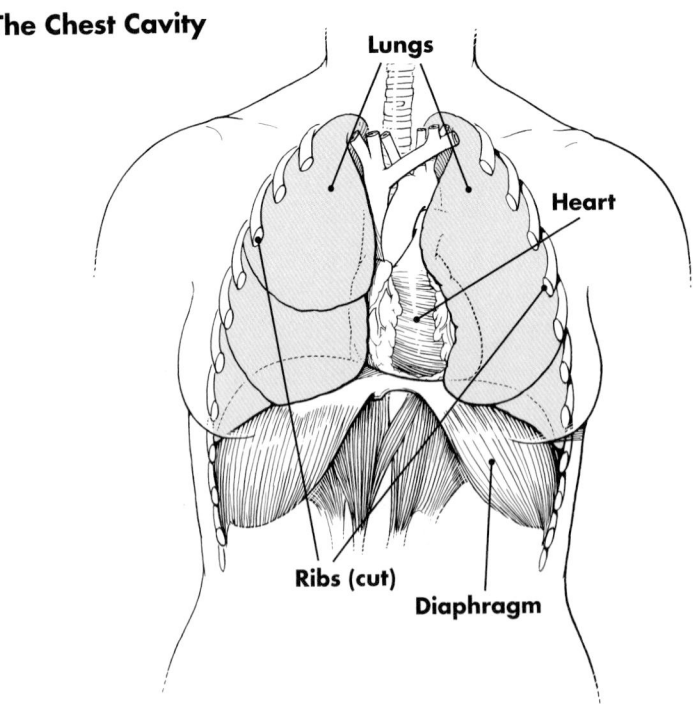

Lungs

Heart

Ribs (cut)

Diaphragm

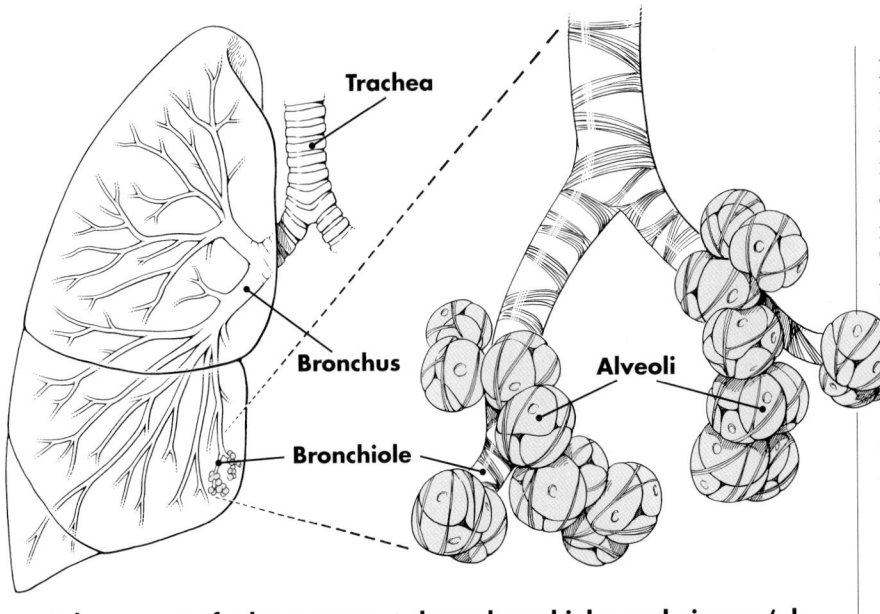

Enlargement of a lung segment shows bronchioles and air sacs (alveoli). Within these air sacs, your blood releases carbon dioxide as it absorbs oxygen.

Natural defenses

Your respiratory system has several defense mechanisms that prevent foreign material from entering your lungs. The hairs and mucus in your nose trap larger particles. Special cells in your trachea and bronchial tubes secrete mucus that helps keep the airways moist and lubricated. The mucus also traps bacteria, dust and other foreign material.

Cilia are microscopic hair-like projections that line your airways. The cilia continuously beat so that mucus moves upward, away from your lungs and toward your throat, to help keep air passageways clean. Some substances, such as cigarette smoke, interfere with their function. Inhaling cigarette smoke causes cilia to stop beating and increases mucus production.

Respiratory Infections

If bacteria, viruses or fungi enter the lungs and become established there, they can cause several diseases, ranging from common and usually benign illnesses such as a chest cold to more-serious illnesses such as bronchiolitis, pneumonia and tuberculosis.

Bronchiolitis

Signs and symptoms
- Runny or stuffy nose
- Wheezing
- Rapid or difficult breathing
- Rapid heartbeat
- Fever
- Bluish skin

Bronchiolitis is a common infection of the lungs' airways, often caused by a virus. It most frequently occurs in infants and young children. Bronchiolitis starts out with symptoms similar to those of a common cold but then progresses to coughing and wheezing. For severe symptoms, hospitalization may be necessary. The condition is contagious.

Diagnosis
Usually, bronchiolitis is preceded by mild nasal congestion. Gradually, breathing becomes more difficult and may become rapid with more vigorous exhalation. Wheezing, a rapid heartbeat and a cough also may develop. A fever may develop. In some cases, an infant's lips and fingernail beds become blue — a condition called cyanosis — due to a decrease in blood oxygen.

How serious is bronchiolitis?
Bronchiolitis usually isn't serious in older children and adults, but it can be serious in infants because their air passages are much narrower than are those of adults. The air passages of an infant may become partly or completely blocked, making it difficult for him or her to breathe. In rare cases the condition can be fatal.

Treatment
Treatment generally consists of using a humidifier to moisten the air and sitting in an upright position to make breathing easier. Have your child drink plenty of fluids to prevent dehydration.

Hospitalization may be necessary, especially for an infant younger than 2 months who has cyanosis, has had repeated attacks of bronchiolitis, or is breathing rapidly and shallowly. Treatment consists of providing warm, moist air, perhaps with extra oxygen.

Use of medications depends on the nature and severity of the illness.

About half the children who contract bronchiolitis have later episodes of wheezing and may become more susceptible to respiratory infections.

Bronchitis

Signs and symptoms
- Soreness and a feeling of constriction or burning in the chest
- Difficulty breathing
- Wheezing
- Coughing
- Production of mucus
- Chills
- Malaise and a slight fever

When mucous membranes that line the main air passageways of the lungs (trachea and large bronchi) become inflamed, the condition is called bronchitis. Virtually everyone experiences bronchitis at some time, just as everyone catches the common cold. So it's reasonable to expect that you may have bronchitis occasionally.

A Cough

Coughing is both normal and common. Often more annoying than serious, a cough is a normal protective reflex, designed to defend your respiratory system against irritants.

However, a forceful or nagging cough can be painful and bothersome. Some of these coughs need your doctor's attention. Others respond to simple self-care techniques and nonprescription medicine.

What causes a cough?

The mucus that lines your nose and airways increases in response to irritants so that it can trap them. The irritants stimulate the cough receptors in your nose, throat or chest, and the receptors send messages to your brain that lead to coughing to help clear out the irritants by expelling the mucus.

Cold and flu viruses are the most common causes of a cough. Generally, the cough goes away when the infection clears. Other coughs may be triggered by:

- *Postnasal drip.* Overproduction of mucus that slowly trickles from the back of your nose down into your throat may be due to allergies, inflamed mucous membranes within sinuses (sinusitis) or other causes.
- *Environmental irritants.* These may include cigarette smoke, smog, dust, home aerosol sprays and other scents, and cold or dry air.
- *Asthma.* Because asthma inflames and constricts air passages, it could cause you to cough, especially if attacks occur during the night, after exercise, or when you're exposed to cold air or irritants. Although wheezing is a common symptom of asthma, many people with this condition don't wheeze, they cough.
- *Gastroesophageal reflux disease.* GERD is the result of acid from your stomach working its way up the esophagus when you lie down. Although heartburn is the most common symptom of GERD, some only experience a cough. You also can have both heartburn and a cough.
- *Some medications.* These include angiotensin-converting enzyme (ACE) inhibitors and some beta blockers prescribed for high blood pressure or heart disease.
- *A foreign body in a bronchial tube.* Rarely, a foreign body, such as a piece of food, can lodge in a bronchial tube, producing a cough.
- *Coughing itself.* Some people cough out of habit. There's no medical explanation for their coughing, and sometimes they're not even aware they're doing it. For some, it may be a way of releasing nervous tension or expressing anger. Whatever the reason, one cough can irritate your throat and lead to another, setting up a vicious cycle.

Treatment

Treatment depends on the type of cough you're experiencing.

Dry, hacking coughs

Dry, hacking coughs generally go away within a week or two. Drinking fluids, especially water, keeps your throat lubricated. If a persistent cough irritates your throat, suck on sugar-free hard candy or throat lozenges or drink hot tea sweetened with honey to soothe your throat.

If a cough caused by GERD disrupts your sleep, try antacids and raise the head of your bed 6 to 8 inches by putting blocks under

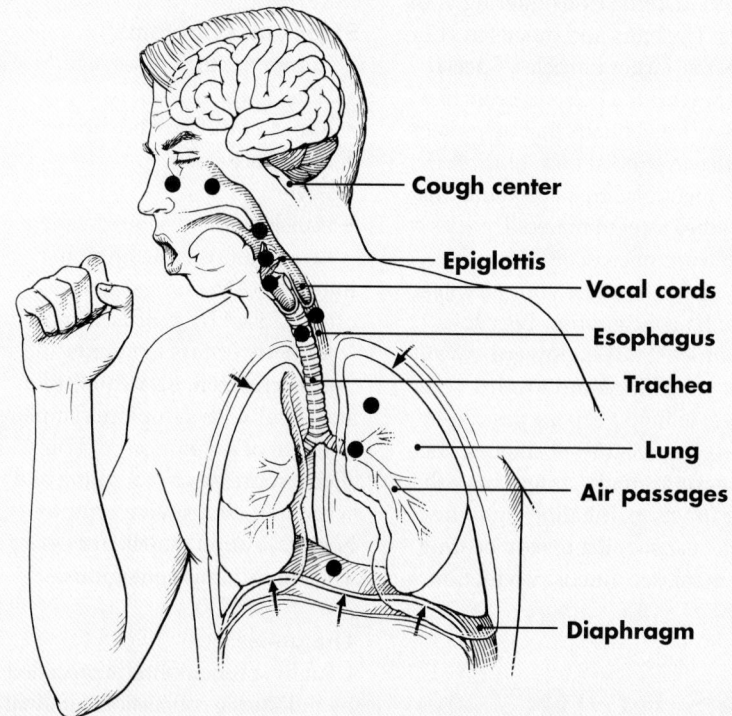

Cough center
Epiglottis
Vocal cords
Esophagus
Trachea
Lung
Air passages
Diaphragm

A cough begins when irritants reach one of the cough receptors in your nose, throat or chest (see large dots). The receptor sends a message to the cough center in your brain, signaling your body to cough. After you inhale, your epiglottis and vocal cords close tightly, trapping air within your lungs. Your abdominal and chest muscles contract forcefully, pushing against your diaphragm (see arrows). Finally, your vocal cords and epiglottis open suddenly, allowing trapped air to rush outward.

the front legs of the bed. If symptoms persist, see your doctor, who may prescribe medication to prevent reflux.

To temporarily reduce the frequency of your cough, take an over-the-counter cough suppressant. Although codeine is one of the most effective cough suppressants, it's a narcotic, so in most states cough formulas containing codeine are available only by prescription. Cough medicines aren't recommended for children.

Productive coughs

Productive coughs are those that raise mucus to help remove irritants from your lungs and air passages. It's best not to suppress a productive cough. Drinking fluids, especially water, helps thin and loosen mucus to make your cough more productive. However, if your cough continually disrupts your sleep, then you can take just enough suppressant to decrease the frequency and severity of your cough but not enough to get rid of it altogether.

Antihistamines may help dry up secretions associated with allergies, sinusitis and postnasal drip, but they can make you sleepy. Don't take antihistamines in combination with alcohol or tranquilizers or when you need to stay alert.

Chronic coughs

If your cough lasts longer than two or three weeks, you may have a chronic cough. Managing a chronic cough requires careful evaluation and treatment of the underlying cause, when possible.

When to see a doctor

If your cough is accompanied by shortness of breath, wheezing, a fever, sweating at night, weight loss or bloody phlegm, see your doctor. Also see a doctor if your cough persists more than two to three weeks.

In most cases, this common ailment is acute — it's caused by a viral infection similar to those that cause the common cold. The infection spreads to the bronchi, producing a deep cough.

Sometimes, bronchial tube inflammation and thickening can become permanent. This is known as chronic bronchitis. The most common culprits of chronic bronchitis are smoking, air pollution, dust and toxic fumes.

Diagnosis

To diagnose bronchitis your doctor will likely listen to your chest using a stethoscope. He or she may request a chest X-ray, sputum culture or other tests to rule out other causes. If you have chronic lung or heart problems, such as asthma, emphysema, chronic bronchitis or congestive heart failure, and think you have bronchitis, it's especially important that you see your doctor.

How serious is bronchitis?

In virtually all cases, acute bronchitis improves in a matter of days with no lasting effects. In some people, the condition can lead to pneumonia. Repeated bouts of bronchitis may signal chronic bronchitis, asthma or other lung disorders.

Treatment

Because bronchitis is most often the result of a viral infection, antibiotics usually aren't effective. Getting plenty of rest, drinking adequate fluids, taking acetaminophen (Tylenol, others) for a fever and taking a nonprescription cough medicine are generally the cornerstones of treatment.

In addition, avoid irritants to the airways, such as tobacco smoke. You don't have to confine yourself to bed while you have acute bronchitis, but it's wise to remain in a warm environment in which the air is somewhat humid, perhaps from the use of a vaporizer.

Your doctor may prescribe a bronchodilator drug to help open narrowed passages in your lungs.

Prevention

If you have repeated attacks of bronchitis, you may be able to trace their occurrence to your environment. For example, cold, damp conditions combined with tobacco smoke or air pollution can make you more susceptible to bronchitis.

Respiratory syncytial virus

Signs and symptoms
- Congested or runny nose
- Dry cough
- Low-grade fever
- Sore throat
- Mild headache
- Discomfort (malaise)

Respiratory syncytial virus (RSV) is a common respiratory infection in children. Most children have been infected with the virus at a young age. Adults also may become infected. RSV may affect the upper or lower respiratory tract.

RSV enters the body through the eyes, nose or mouth and spreads easily. If you inhale infectious respiratory secretions, such as those spewed by coughs or sneezes, or touch objects contaminated with oral or nasal secretions and then touch your mouth, nose or eyes, you're likely to acquire the virus.

The peak season for catching the virus typically begins in the fall and ends in the spring.

Diagnosis

Your child's doctor may suspect respiratory syncytial virus based on a physical exam, during which he or she may listen to your child's lungs with a stethoscope to check for wheezing or other abnormal sounds. A nasal swab test can confirm the presence of the virus.

How serious is respiratory syncytial virus?

In adults and older, otherwise healthy children, the infection typically mimics the common cold. Symptoms usually improve in seven to 10 days.

In some infants, children with underlying heart or lung conditions, or children who were born prematurely, the infection may be more severe, even life-threatening, and the child may require hospitalization.

Some infants and young children infected with RSV for the first time may develop symptoms of pneumonia and bronchiolitis. Middle ear infection (otitis media) is another complication.

Treatment

Because respiratory syncytial virus causes a viral infection, antibiotics are of no use, unless a bacterial infection also is present, such as an inner ear infection or bacterial pneumonia.

In cases of severe infection, infants and children may need hospitalization so that they can be treated with humidified oxygen to get sufficient oxygen to the blood, intravenous fluids to prevent dehydration and, sometimes, a ventilator to support breathing.

Medication

Over-the-counter medications such as acetaminophen (Tylenol, others) may reduce symptoms. In severe cases, a doctor might prescribe a bronchodilator or ribavirin (Virazole), an antiviral medicine.

Self-care

To help ease breathing, use a cool-mist humidifier or vaporizer to humidify air. Sitting upright makes breathing easier. Offer the sick person plenty of fluids to drink, including warm ones such as soup. Over-the-counter saline nasal drops may ease congestion.

Prevention

There's no vaccine against this disease, but the medication palivizumab (Synagis) may decrease the risk of hospitalization and limit the severity of the illness. It's given monthly to children at high risk during the peak season for the infection.

Pneumonia

Signs and symptoms
- Coughing that may produce colored or bloody sputum
- High fever and chills with shaking
- Difficulty breathing
- Chest pain that increases with deep breathing and coughing
- Headache
- Loss of appetite
- Nausea and vomiting
- Bluish skin
- Fatigue

Pneumonia is a common, potentially serious inflammation of the lungs that causes difficulty breathing. Each year in the United States about 1 million people are hospitalized due to pneumonia.

There are many types of pneumonia, which range in severity from mild to life-threatening. Pneumonia can affect one or both lungs. Inflammation of both lungs is sometimes called double pneumonia.

Causes

Pneumonia has more than 50 causes. Infectious pneumonia can be caused by viruses, bacteria such as pneumococci, staphylococci and streptococci, or other organisms. Viruses, including those that cause the flu (influenza), are responsible for half the cases of pneumonia.

Chemical irritants, parasites and certain types of fungi also can cause pneumonia. The *Mycoplasma pneumoniae* organism causes symptoms similar to both viral and bacterial pneumonia, although the symptoms appear more gradually and often are milder.

Pneumonia is sometimes classified according to where or how you're exposed to the disease. These classifications include:

Community-acquired pneumonia

Community-acquired pneumonia gets its name from the way it's acquired — from the community at large rather than in the hospital. Common causes of community-acquired pneumonia are pneumococci bacteria, mycoplasmas and the influenza virus.

Hospital-acquired pneumonia

Your risk of developing pneumonia increases if you're hospitalized, especially if you're on a mechanical ventilator, in an intensive care unit (ICU) or have a compromised immune system. In a hospital, many types of potentially infectious organisms are present, and they may be more severe than those you encounter in everyday life. Hospital-acquired pneumonia can be extremely serious, especially for older adults and young children.

Aspiration pneumonia

Aspiration pneumonia is the result of inhaling (aspirating) foreign matter into the lungs. This can occur accidentally during swallowing or vomiting.

Opportunistic pneumonia

This type of pneumonia is caused by opportunistic organisms that strike people with compromised immune systems. Opportunistic organisms don't ordinarily cause illness in healthy people, but they can be extremely dangerous to people with human immunodeficiency virus (HIV) or AIDS, or in individuals on medications that suppress their immune systems.

Diagnosis

Because pneumonia often mimics a cold or the flu, many people don't realize they have it. Symptoms can vary depending on the organism causing the pneumonia.

Your doctor listens to your lungs with a stethoscope to check for abnormal bubbling or crackling sounds (rales) and coarse rattling sounds (rhonchi). These sounds may indicate inflammation caused by infection. Your doctor may order a chest X-ray to determine the location and extent of the infection.

A sample of your sputum may be tested to help identify the infecting agent. Usually, you can produce a sample that's sufficient for the test by coughing. In some cases, it may be necessary to use other means to obtain a sample, including inserting a bronchoscope into your airway. Your doctor may also request blood tests to check your white cell count or a blood culture to look for the presence of viruses, bacteria or other organisms.

How serious is pneumonia?

In the United States, about 50,000 people die of pneumonia every year. The seriousness of this disorder depends largely on your overall health and the type of pneumonia you contract. Healthy people generally have sufficient defense mechanisms to neutralize most infectious agents. In young people, pneumonia might be a mild, undiagnosed illness that's regarded as simply a cold.

If alcoholism, aging, injury, use of immunosuppressant drugs or other medical conditions have impaired your natural defense mechanisms, you may be more susceptible to pneumonia. In older adults and people weakened by disease — especially people with heart failure, asthma or emphysema — pneumonia can be fatal.

Pneumonia becomes deadly when inflammation from the disease fills so many of the air sacs within your lungs (alveoli) that it interferes with your ability to breathe or causes a blood infection (sepsis).

Sometimes, fluid accumulates between the layers of the pleural membrane, which covers the surface of the lung and lines the inside of the chest wall. This condition is known as a pleural effusion. When your lungs are infected, this accumulating fluid also can become infected.

Treatment

Pneumonia treatments vary, depending on the severity of your symptoms and the type of pneumonia you have.

- **Bacterial.** Doctors usually treat bacterial pneumonia with antibiotics. Although you may start to feel better shortly after beginning your medication, be sure to complete your entire course of antibiotics. Stopping medication too soon may cause your pneumonia to return. Doing so also helps create strains of bacteria that are resistant to antibiotics — an increasingly serious problem in the United States.
- **Viral.** Antibiotics aren't effective against most viral forms of pneumonia. And although a few viral pneumonias may be treated with antiviral medications, the recommended treatment is generally the same as for the flu — rest and plenty of fluids.

> **? Question and Answer**
>
> ### What's walking pneumonia?
>
> *Walking pneumonia* isn't a specific medical term. The term is typically used to describe pneumonia that isn't severe enough to confine you to bed. In fact, many people with walking pneumonia don't feel sick enough to seek medical care.
>
> If you've been told that you have walking pneumonia, the illness may be due to a tiny organism called mycoplasma. This community-acquired pneumonia spreads easily among people who spend a lot of time together, such as school-aged children. Walking pneumonia usually affects people younger than age 40.
>
> Mycoplasma causes symptoms similar to those of both bacterial and viral pneumonia. However, the symptoms often appear more slowly and they're often milder.

- **Mycoplasma.** Mycoplasma pneumonias are treated with antibiotics. Even so, recovery may not be immediate. In some cases fatigue may continue long after the infection itself has cleared. Many cases of mycoplasma pneumonia go undiagnosed and untreated. The signs and symptoms mimic those of a bad chest cold, so some people never seek medical attention.
- **Fungal.** If your pneumonia is caused by a fungus, you'll likely be treated with an antifungal medication.

In addition to these treatments, your doctor may recommend over-the-counter medications to reduce fever, treat your aches and pains, and soothe the cough associated with pneumonia. You don't want to suppress your cough completely, though, since coughing helps clear your lungs. If you must use a cough suppressant, use the lowest dose that helps you get some rest.

If you have severe pneumonia, you'll likely be hospitalized and treated with intravenous antibiotics and put on oxygen. If you don't need oxygen, you may recover as quickly at home with oral antibiotics as in the hospital, especially if you have access to qualified home health care. Another option is to spend three or four days in the hospital receiving intravenous antibiotics and then continue to recover at home with oral medication.

Your doctor will most likely schedule a follow-up X-ray and an office visit after your initial diagnosis and treatment. By that time your infection should have cleared, but it's important for your doctor to see you, even if you're feeling better. Follow-up appointments and X-rays are especially important for smokers. If you're not feeling better, the follow-up visit is an opportunity for your doctor to schedule tests to determine more specifically what's causing your symptoms.

Prevention

You usually don't "catch" pneumonia from someone else. Instead, you develop the disease because your immune system is temporarily weakened, often for no known reason. The following suggestions can help keep you healthy:

- **Get vaccinated.** Because pneumonia can be a complication of the flu, getting a yearly flu shot is a good way to prevent viral influenza pneumonia, which can lead to bacterial pneumonia. In addition, there are two available vaccines to prevent pneumonia: PCV13 and PPSV23. Ask your doctor if you should have these vaccines. Recommendations are based on age and the existence of other health issues. Generally, vaccination is recommended for infants and adults age 65 and older.
- **Wash your hands.** Your hands are in almost constant contact with germs that can cause pneumonia. Washing your hands thoroughly and often can help reduce your risk.
- **Take care of yourself.** Proper rest and a diet rich in fruits, vegetables and whole grains along with moderate exercise can help keep your immune system strong.

Syndromes That Can Mimic Pneumonia

Some rare lung disorders that aren't caused by infectious agents may mimic pneumonia. These include:

Pulmonary alveolar proteinosis

Pulmonary alveolar proteinosis occurs when fluid builds up within the air sacs of the lungs (alveoli). It occurs primarily in men between the ages of 20 and 50 who aren't known to have lung disease. The cause is unknown.

In pulmonary alveolar proteinosis, fluid-filled alveoli inhibit the lungs' ability to transfer oxygen to the blood, causing shortness of breath with exertion and sometimes at rest. Most nonsmokers with this disorder also develop an unproductive cough, and smokers develop a cough that produces sputum. A chest X-ray may reveal shadowy areas on both lungs.

People with few or no symptoms don't require treatment. For others, a procedure called whole-lung lavage, performed under general anesthesia, may be used to rinse material within the alveoli from the lungs.

People with this disease usually recover, although occasionally the disorder may recur.

Goodpasture's syndrome

The precise cause of Goodpasture's syndrome is unknown, although it's more likely to occur in young, male smokers. It causes bleeding (hemorrhage) of the lungs and a type of kidney inflammation called glomerulonephritis (see page 906).

Although a lung hemorrhage can be life-threatening, the effect on the lung can range from mild to severe. The diagnosis is made by a biopsy of either the lung or kidney. The course of the disease varies considerably.

Your doctor may prescribe corticosteroids or cyclophosphamide to control the disorder. In addition, your doctor might recommend removing antibodies from your blood that may play a role in causing this disease.

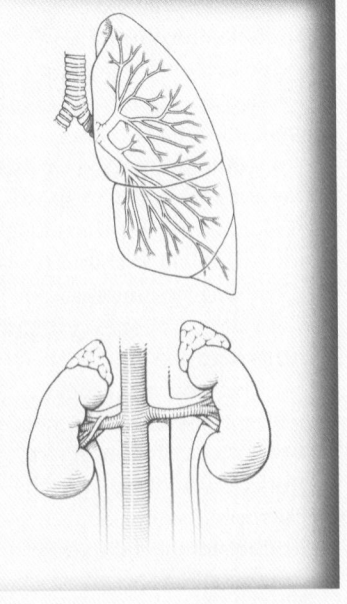

Tuberculosis

Signs and symptoms

- Persistent coughing that may produce discolored or bloody sputum
- Slight fever
- Fatigue
- Loss of appetite and weight
- Night sweats
- Pain with breathing or coughing

Tuberculosis (TB) is a life-threatening infection that primarily affects your lungs. Every year, TB kills about 2 million people worldwide. Although the incidence of TB declined greatly during most of the last century, there's been an increase since the 1980s. It's been found among people living in poor and cramped living conditions in inner cities, people infected with the human immunodeficiency virus (HIV), and people immigrating to the United States.

TB is a long-lasting (chronic) infection. It results from the bacterium *Mycobacterium tuberculosis.* These bacteria can attack any part of your body, but most commonly they invade your lungs.

TB spreads through airborne droplets when a person with the infection coughs, talks or sneezes. In general, you need prolonged exposure to an infected person before becoming infected yourself. Even then, you may not develop symptoms of the disease or they may not show up until years later.

Although your body may harbor the TB bacteria, your immune system can prevent you from becoming sick. For that reason, doctors make a distinction between:

- **TB infection.** This condition, sometimes called latent TB, causes no symptoms and isn't contagious.
- **Active TB.** This condition makes you sick and can spread to others. However, the infection may not display symptoms for years, even though it's active and causing damage.

Diagnosis

The most commonly used diagnostic tool for TB is a simple skin test. A tuberculin skin test can determine whether you've ever been infected with the TB organism. This test involves injecting a small amount of a substance called PPD into your skin. If you've been infected by the TB organism, the injection causes a reaction in your skin within 48 to 72 hours. Your doctor or a nurse will interpret the results of the test two to three days after the injection.

In some cases the test can produce a false-positive result, suggesting you have TB when you don't. This is most likely to occur if you're infected with a mycobacterium other than the one that causes TB or you've been vaccinated with a TB vaccine rarely used in the United States called bacillus Calmette-Guérin.

Another test to check for TB has been approved by the Food and Drug Administration. It uses a blood sample to detect the presence of white blood cells (lymphocytes) that have been sensitized to TB bacteria. The sensitized lymphocytes indicate the person has been infected with TB bacteria.

Other tests that may be used when making a diagnosis include a chest X-ray and culture tests. The diagnosis is confirmed by growing (culturing) the organism in the laboratory. Your sputum is usually the easiest sample to obtain for culture. Other common sources are urine and stomach secretions. Stomach secretions are collected by passing a small tube through the nose, down the back of the throat, through the esophagus and into the stomach. Culture results may not be available for up to six to eight weeks because the TB bacterium grows slowly.

Culture results can also provide important information as to how well or poorly the bacterium may respond to treatment. Some strains of the TB organism require different or more-intensive treatments than do other strains.

How serious is tuberculosis?

TB can be deadly, but in the United States more than 95 percent of individuals recover completely. You'll show no subsequent evidence of disease except for changes seen on a chest X-ray and a positive tuberculin skin test or a blood assay test. Once you have TB, your skin test and blood test remain positive even after the disease is cured.

Treatment

Drugs offer the most effective therapy for TB. In recent years, though, an increasing number of TB organisms have become resistant to drugs commonly used in treatment. It's important to determine the sensitivity to anti-tuberculosis drugs in every newly diagnosed case so that each case is treated with the most effective medications.

If you have active TB, treatment commonly starts with the drugs isoniazid (Laniazid), rifampin (Rifadin) and pyrazinamide — which can be combined in one tablet (Rifater) — and the drug ethambutol (Myambutol). The medications are usually given under close observation by a public health nurse to reduce the chance of the tuberculosis organism developing resistance to the medications and making the disease more difficult to treat. Normally, you take the medications for six to 12 months to completely destroy the bacteria.

All medications used for TB have some potential toxicity. Both rifampin and isoniazid may cause a noninfectious form of hepatitis and jaundice, which are generally reversible after you stop taking the medication. Rifampin may cause your urine, sweat and tears to take on an orange or brownish color.

Some forms of TB are multi-resistant, meaning they can't be treated with the most common and powerful TB drugs. Multi-resistant TB can be treated, but it requires at least two years of therapy with second line medications that can be highly toxic. Even with this treatment, some people don't survive.

Prevention

If you have a positive tuberculin skin test, especially if you've recently been in close contact with a person with TB, your doctor may consider giving you the medication isoniazid to decrease your risk of developing active TB. The drug must be taken for six to nine months. Your doctor may also give the medication or a similar one to others in your household.

Legionnaires' disease

Signs and symptoms

- Headache
- Muscle pain
- Fever and chills
- Shortness of breath
- Coughing that may produce mucus or blood
- Chest pain
- Fatigue
- Nausea, vomiting and diarrhea

Legionnaires' disease was first identified when a sudden, virulent outbreak of pneumonia occurred primarily among delegates attending an American Legion convention at a hotel in Philadelphia in July 1976 — hence its name. More than 200 people became ill with severe pneumonia of unknown cause, and 34 died.

The cause eventually was identified as a previously unknown bacterium that was later named *Legionella pneumophila.* Children have developed the disease, but most cases occur in middle-aged or older adults, particularly those who smoke or have weakened immune systems.

The legionella bacterium also causes Pontiac fever, a milder illness resembling the flu. Separately or together, the two illnesses are sometimes called legionellosis.

Legionella bacteria thrive in warm, damp environments. The bacteria can develop in water systems, whirlpool spas and air conditioning systems. Most outbreaks have occurred in large buildings, perhaps because complex air conditioning and ventilation systems allow the bacteria to grow and spread more easily.

Diagnosis

Special tests are needed to distinguish Legionnaires' disease from other types of pneumonia. To identify the presence of legionella bacteria, your doctor may use a test that checks your urine for legionella antigens. You may also have blood tests, a chest X-ray, and tests on a sample of your sputum or lung tissue.

How serious is Legionnaires' disease?

Typically, Legionnaires' disease causes pneumonia severe enough to require hospitalization. Although most people recover fully, a small percentage of those who get the disease die of respiratory failure.

Treatment

Legionnaires' disease is treated with antibiotics. The sooner antibiotic therapy is started, the less likely the chance of serious complications. In some cases, you may need intravenous (IV) fluids because the high fever can cause dehydration. Supplemental oxygen may be necessary to help you breathe.

Pontiac fever generally goes away on its own without treatment and causes no lingering problems.

Bronchiectasis

Signs and symptoms
- Persistent mild or severe coughing that may produce thick, foul-smelling sputum, usually gray-green, that may contain blood
- Loss of appetite and weight
- Anemia and general weakness
- Recurring attacks of pneumonia

Bronchiectasis is long-lasting, abnormal expansion (dilation) of the walls of bronchial tubes. This dilation can also result from chronic bronchitis, but the dilation is more pronounced in bronchiectasis.

Some people are born with the condition, but most people with bronchiectasis develop it as a complication of cystic fibrosis or from diseases such as whooping cough, pneumonia and tuberculosis. Rare causes of bronchiectasis include defects of the microscopic hair-like projections (cilia) lining the breathing (bronchial) tubes and low levels of blood antibodies (gamma globulin). Bronchiectasis occurs primarily in children and young adults under 21. It has become much less common since the introduction of antibiotic treatment of pneumonia.

Diagnosis

A doctor may have you undergo X-rays or a high-resolution computerized tomography (CT) scan to confirm the diagnosis.

How serious is bronchiectasis?

The bronchial tube damage is irreversible, and areas of the bronchial walls may be destroyed. Severe cases can cause scarring and loss of lung blood vessels, affecting the heart.

Inhalation Anthrax

Anthrax is a disease caused by the bacterium *Bacillus anthracis*, which is housed in a hardy spore. The disease usually affects livestock, but it can affect humans as well.

Anthrax occurs in three forms: skin (cutaneous), intestinal, and inhalation (pulmonary), which infects your lungs. Inhalation anthrax is the deadliest form. It's caused by inhaling sufficient quantities of anthrax spores to cause infection. Once the infection spreads, inhalation anthrax is fatal in the majority of cases.

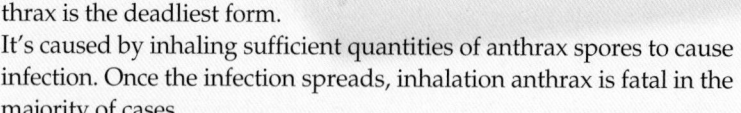

After lodging in the respiratory tract, the spores can take from a day to two months to become active, at which time signs and symptoms develop. Initially, the infection may feel like a cold or the flu, with a sore throat, muscle aches and mild chest discomfort. These first symptoms may last for a few hours to a few days before they may seem to briefly subside. However, within a few days of the onset of symptoms, the disease leads to a high fever and breathing problems. The disease destroys lung tissue and may spread to the brain, causing meningitis.

Fortunately, all three forms can be prevented or treated with antibiotics. With inhalation anthrax, antibiotics can reduce the risk of death, especially if started within the first few days of symptoms.

For more information on anthrax, see page 461.

Treatment

Your doctor may suggest chest physiotherapy to help treat the condition. This includes positioning the body to help lung drainage (postural drainage) and vibrating the chest wall (chest percussion), as shown below. Breathing exercises also can help improve the functioning of your lungs. Avoid dust, smoke and other respiratory irritants. Get plenty of exercise because deep breathing helps raise secretions. Eat a nutritious diet. Drinking fluids helps to dilute the sputum in your lungs.

Unless your doctor advises against it, get pneumococcal

Postural Drainage and Chest Percussion

Respiratory conditions such as bronchiectasis, cystic fibrosis and lung abscesses may cause a large volume of secretions to accumulate in your lungs. Postural drainage and chest percussion help empty your lungs of the unwanted secretions. These therapies are especially important for individuals with cystic fibrosis. Your doctor may recommend a sequence that combines both methods for maximum effect.

Postural drainage

Postural drainage uses gravity to help clear your lungs of secretions. You position yourself to allow the secretions to move to your windpipe (trachea) so that you can cough them out. Because the branches of your lungs point in various directions, it may be necessary for you to assume various positions to drain different areas of the lungs.

Some doctors recommend a time-consuming series of positional changes for individuals with cystic fibrosis. Others have found that compliance with these instructions tends to decrease as the child who has cystic fibrosis gets older. Therefore, the recommended positions may be limited to those that drain areas of the lungs where secretions are most likely to lodge, usually the lower portions of the lungs.

Cystic fibrosis

If you have cystic fibrosis, your doctor or a trained therapist can provide you with specific instructions on postural drainage. Remember to cough during each position change to aid in raising the sputum.

Bronchiectasis

Bronchiectasis is uncommon in the upper lobes of the lungs because they drain well when you're in an upright position. Therefore, postural drainage for bronchiectasis may be simpler than it is for some other conditions. You can drain lower portions of your lungs quite well by kneeling or lying facedown on a bed or couch and putting your hands on the floor. Stay in this position for about 10 minutes, coughing periodically.

Collect the expectorated sputum and note its color and approximate amount. You may stop postural drainage when you produce no more sputum, and resume it later when you notice that you're producing sputum again. This is a valuable technique because antibiotics work better and remain effective longer if you keep your airways as free of secretions as possible.

Chest percussion

Chest percussion helps loosen secretions in your lungs. Lie on your back on a firm surface. Cup your hands and rapidly strike your chest wall with one hand and then with the other. You may want to protect your skin with a bath towel. Be careful not to strike the heart area, breasts, lower ribs, shoulders or kidneys.

This technique may be more effective applied to the back. Parents and others concerned with a child's care should learn this technique. Adults also may need someone to help them use this technique on their backs.

Some people loosen secretions with the aid of an electric chest clapper, known as a mechanical percussor. Some use an inflatable vest with a machine attached that vibrates at high frequency to help the user cough up secretions.

The postural drainage technique uses gravity to help clear your lungs of unwanted secretions. The position shown here is designed to clear the lower lungs.

vaccines and a yearly flu shot. You may need a repeat pneumonia vaccine after five years.

Medication

Because bacterial infections are associated with production of pus in bronchiectasis, your doctor will likely prescribe an antibiotic. It's generally not recommended that you use an antibiotic continuously. At times, it may be advisable to take two or three kinds of antibiotics on a rotating basis. Alternating medications can help prevent the development of an antibiotic-resistant bacterial strain.

Your doctor may also prescribe a bronchodilator to relieve spasms in your bronchial tubes.

Surgery

If you have inadequate response to other treatments or if you're coughing up blood, surgical removal of the affected portions of the lungs may be necessary. However, this is an option only if the disease is localized in one or two areas of the lungs and there's adequate lung function to allow removal of part of your lungs.

Lung abscess

Signs and symptoms
- A high and irregular fever
- Sweats and chills
- Shortness of breath
- Coughing that produces sputum containing pus and sometimes blood
- Malaise
- Loss of appetite and weight
- Chest pain

A lung abscess is a cavity that develops in your lungs and fills with pus. Usually, inhaling infectious material from your mouth or throat (aspiration) causes the infection to localize in your lungs. Dental disease is often the source of the infection.

In middle-aged or older people who smoke, lung cancer may cause a lung abscess by obstructing a bronchial tube. Sometimes,

a lung abscess occurs as a complication of pneumonia. More rare causes of lung abscesses are infections caused by tuberculosis or by fungal or parasitic organisms.

In most cases, a single abscess develops in one lung, but occasionally multiple abscesses appear.

Diagnosis

Signs and symptoms of a lung abscess develop slowly over several days or weeks. Initially, they're similar to those of pneumonia. A cough develops after the abscess ruptures into a bronchial tube. Depending on the type of organism causing the infection, the sputum may be foul smelling.

In addition to giving you a physical examination, your doctor may request a chest X-ray and a computerized tomography (CT) scan of the lung and may take a sample of your sputum to check for bacteria or other organisms if he or she suspects a lung abscess. Such information can lead to more-effective treatment with specific antibiotics or other therapy.

How serious is a lung abscess?

A lung abscess is generally a temporary (acute) disease, although if not treated adequately it can become long term (chronic). With treatment, most people with an acute abscess recover completely without surgery.

Treatment

Treatment usually involves a combination of medication and drainage techniques.

Medication

Antibiotics are generally needed. The antibiotic prescribed will depend on the bacterium causing the infection. If the abscess is the result of another organism, such as a fungus, your doctor may prescribe a different type of medication.

Other therapies

Postural drainage and chest percussion may be used to help

drain a lung abscess. If your lung abscess doesn't respond to antibiotics or drainage and percussion, a bronchoscopy may be recommended (see page 785). If the abscess has been present for several weeks, has a thick wall or has spread into the space between the membranous layers surrounding your lungs (pleural space), surgery may be necessary.

Empyema

Signs and symptoms
- A dry or productive cough
- Fever and night sweats
- Weight loss
- Shortness of breath
- Chest pain on deep breathing

Normally, only a tiny amount of clear, lubricating fluid is present between the membranous layers surrounding your lungs (pleural space). In empyema, pus collects in the pleural space as the result of an infection. It's typically a complication of bacterial pneumonia, a lung abscess, an open wound in the chest or chest surgery.

You may experience chest pain due to inflammation in the pleural space (pleurisy) early in the course of the disease. As fluid accumulates in the pleural space, the pain may gradually disappear. A collection of infected fluid — up to a pint or more — can compress your lungs.

Diagnosis

To confirm a diagnosis, your doctor may perform thoracentesis. In this procedure, a needle is inserted between your ribs to remove fluid from your pleural cavity. Often, the procedure is done with guidance from an ultrasound image.

Treatment

Treatment consists of antibiotic medications and drainage of the infected fluid from the chest.

If the fluid in the pleural space flows through a needle, repeated thoracentesis may remove it. To achieve adequate fluid removal, a tube thoracostomy is often necessary. For this procedure, you're given local anesthesia, and a doctor makes a small incision in your chest wall and inserts a chest tube for drainage. Medications may be placed down the tube to improve drainage.

If a thoracostomy is unsuccessful, you may need a thoracotomy. While you're under general anesthesia, an opening is made in the chest wall to remove all of the infected fluid. If thickening of the pleura restricts expansion of your lung, surgical removal of the thickened tissue may be necessary.

Pleurisy and pleural effusion

Signs and symptoms
- Shortness of breath
- Chest pain during breathing
- A dry cough
- Fever and chills

Pleurisy occurs when the double membrane (pleura) that lines the chest cavity and surrounds each of your lungs becomes inflamed. As the inflamed layers rub against each other during breathing, sharp pain occurs. Between breaths, you feel almost no pain. Coughing, sneezing or deep breathing may make the pain worse.

If an accumulation of fluids (pleural effusion) is associated

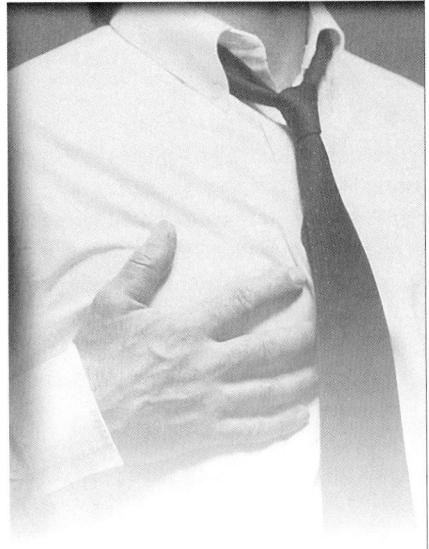

with pleurisy, the pain usually disappears because the fluid serves as a lubricant. However, if enough fluid accumulates, it puts pressure on your lungs and interferes with their function, causing shortness of breath. Sometimes you develop a dry cough, fever and chills, particularly if the fluid in the pleural space is infected.

Pleurisy and pleural effusions occur as complications of an underlying disease such as tuberculosis, pneumonia, pulmonary embolism, cancer or congestive heart failure, as well as from trauma to the chest.

Diagnosis
Your doctor may use the following diagnostic procedures to determine the underlying cause of pleurisy:
- **Imaging.** A chest X-ray or computerized tomography (CT) scan produces images of your lungs to help identify fluid or inflammation. Sometimes doctors want a special type of chest X-ray in which you lie on your side where the pleurisy is to see if there's any fluid that doesn't appear on a standard chest X-ray. This is called a decubitus chest X-ray. Your doctor may also use ultrasound to determine whether you have a pleural effusion.
- **Blood test.** A blood test may tell your doctor if you have an infection and, if so, what type of infection you have.
- **Thoracentesis.** In this procedure, your doctor first injects a local anesthetic, then inserts a needle through your chest wall between your ribs to remove fluid. In addition, a sample of tissue (pleural biopsy) for microscopic analysis may be obtained to help determine the cause of the condition. If only a small amount of fluid is present, your doctor may insert the needle with the help of ultrasound over the site of the fluid.
- **Video-assisted thoracic surgery.** Another way of obtaining a sample of pleural tissue is by a surgical procedure called

video-assisted thoracic surgery. A tube is inserted to collapse a lung to about a quarter of its normal size. This creates space for your doctor to insert a pen-sized instrument through your chest wall to take a tissue sample under video guidance. You'll need general anesthesia for this procedure.

How serious are pleurisy and pleural effusion?
The outcome of these conditions primarily depends on the seriousness of the underlying disease. If the underlying disease can be treated effectively, pleurisy and pleural effusion generally resolve.

Treatment
First, it's important to treat the underlying condition or illness causing the pleurisy or pleural effusion. For example, if the cause is a bacterial infection, an antibiotic may control the infection. In some cases, a pleural effusion needs to be drained through a chest tube for several days.

Pain relievers (analgesics) and anti-inflammatory medications may help relieve some of the signs and symptoms. Codeine may be prescribed to help control a cough.

Fungal Diseases of the Lungs

If yeast and the spores of certain fungi are inhaled, they can infect the lungs, causing disease. Most of these ailments cause a fever, cough and malaise.

Histoplasmosis

Signs and symptoms
- Fever
- Cough
- Headache
- Fatigue
- Chest pain

- Sweats
- Weight loss

Histoplasmosis results from inhaling airborne spores that you breathe in when you work around soil that contains a fungus called *Histoplasma capsulatum.* Farmers, landscapers, construction workers, and people who have contact with bird or bat droppings are especially at risk.

There are several types of histoplasmosis infections, which can range from mild to severe. If the fungus spreads from the lungs through the blood, it may cause enlargement of the liver, lymph nodes or spleen and, less frequently, oral or gastrointestinal ulcers.

Histoplasmosis can become long lasting (chronic), producing an illness similar to chronic tuberculosis. At its most severe, histoplasmosis spreads (disseminates) throughout the body. People with a weakened immune system are at highest risk of disseminated histoplasmosis.

Diagnosis
To confirm the diagnosis of histoplasmosis, your doctor likely will obtain specimens of sputum, lymph nodes, bone marrow, liver, blood, urine or oral ulcerations to check for the fungus. The specimen is placed on a medium that enhances growth of the fungus (fungal culture). Other similar tests also may be used.

Your doctor may also order a chest X-ray or computerized tomography (CT) scan or perform an examination of your windpipe (trachea) and the air passages in your lungs, a procedure called a bronchoscopy.

How serious is histoplasmosis?
Mild histoplasmosis usually requires no treatment. More-severe forms of the disease can be fatal if not treated promptly.

Treatment
If you don't have symptoms, treatment may be unnecessary. If you do have symptoms, your doctor may prescribe an oral antifungal agent such as itraconazole (Sporanox).

Treatment generally eliminates the fungus, but the lesions it produces on your lungs remain. Normally, they calcify and don't cause any long-term problems.

Cryptococcosis

Signs and symptoms
- Low-grade fever
- Chest pain
- Coughing that may produce sputum
- Malaise
- Lesions in the lungs
- Increasingly severe headaches
- Nausea
- Vertigo
- Loss of appetite
- Vision disorders
- Mental deterioration

Cryptococcosis is caused by the yeast *Cryptococcus neoformans,* which lives in soil and on pigeon droppings. Disease results when a person inhales the organism. The yeast may remain in the lungs, or it may spread, particularly to the central nervous system. Some pulmonary cases produce only mild symptoms. More-serious cases resemble bronchitis, and lesions develop in the lungs.

Diagnosis
Your doctor may request a chest X-ray and samples of sputum, pus or spinal fluid to check for presence of the yeast.

How serious is cryptococcosis?
People who have a weakened immune system or individuals taking immunosuppressant drugs are most susceptible to the disease. Some mild cases resolve without treatment, but for people with a weakened immune system, cryptococcosis can lead to death, especially if it spreads beyond the lungs.

Treatment
Treatment includes medication and, rarely, surgery. Milder cases may respond to oral antifungal medications. For individuals with a suppressed immune system, treatment may require the intravenous antifungal drug amphotericin B or the oral medication flucytosine (Ancobon).

Coccidioidomycosis

Signs and symptoms
- Fever and chills
- Malaise
- Backache
- Headache
- Chest pain
- A red, spotty rash
- Swelling of the knees and ankles
- Coughing
- Nasal congestion

Coccidioidomycosis is caused by inhaling spores of the fungus

Aspergillosis

Aspergillus is a genus of fungi that's found virtually everywhere. It may be present in nasal discharges and respiratory secretions of people regularly exposed to it from the soil or farm dust, but it rarely causes problems.

In people with asthma, however, aspergillus can produce an allergic response. In other susceptible individuals, such as those with a weakened immune system, it can cause an unusual form of pneumonia. Both of these conditions, called aspergillosis, can be treated effectively with corticosteroids or antifungal medication, such as itraconazole (Sporanox).

In people whose lungs are damaged, aspergillus may collect within the lungs and cause coughing and bloody sputum, weight loss and a mild fever. Often, surgery is needed to control bleeding. If aspergillosis occurs in an individual with leukemia, the prognosis is poor.

Coccidioides immitis, which lives in the soil in certain arid parts of the southwestern United States, Mexico, and Central and South America.

Nine of every 10 people who move to the desert areas of the southwestern part of the United States test positive for this fungus within four to five years.

Most often, coccidioidomycosis causes no symptoms, but a small percentage of infected people develop symptoms, often referred to as "valley fever." Symptoms usually begin 10 to 30 days after exposure to the fungus. Chest discomfort, a fever, chills and other flu-like symptoms may occur. Nasal congestion and a mild cough may be followed by bronchitis. One to two days after the fever begins, a red, spotty rash may appear, and your knees and ankles may swell.

Coccidioidomycosis can affect anyone, but people with a weakened immune system are especially vulnerable.

Diagnosis
Your doctor may order a chest X-ray and tests of blood, sputum and spinal fluid to determine the presence of the fungus.

How serious is coccidioidomycosis?
Usually, the disease clears without complications, although in some cases lesions formed in the lungs can be difficult to cure. In rare cases, the disease may recur after weeks or months. Occasionally, the infection spreads throughout the body, causing lesions in the bones and other organs as well.

Treatment
If you have no symptoms, treatment usually is unnecessary. For flu-like symptoms, your doctor may recommend bed rest and over-the-counter medications to relieve the signs and symptoms.

For more-severe illness, your doctor may prescribe the intravenous medication amphotericin

B, which is often effective. Ketoconazole (Nizoral) or a similar medication taken orally may be used in localized pulmonary disease. Surgical drainage of lung abscesses or pleural fluids is sometimes necessary.

Chronic Lung Conditions

Three common chronic lung disorders restrict the flow of air out of the bronchial passages: chronic bronchitis, emphysema and asthma.

Chronic bronchitis causes a persistent inflammation of the lining of the bronchial tubes, which are the two main branches of the windpipe (trachea). Emphysema is characterized by enlargement of the air sacs (alveoli) and the destruction of the walls between them. Some degree of bronchitis is usually associated with emphysema.

Doctors often refer to emphysema and chronic bronchitis as chronic obstructive pulmonary disease (COPD).

Asthma involves inflammation of the airways and excess mucus production that contribute to airway obstruction. With asthma, the bronchial passages narrow too much and too easily in response to a wide variety of provoking stimuli. Obstruction of the outflow of air tends to be variable and episodic, often occurring in attacks of wheezing and shortness of breath.

Chronic obstructive pulmonary disease

Signs and symptoms
- Persistent cough that usually produces mucus
- Shortness of breath
- Wheezing
- Chest tightness
- Frequent respiratory infections

Chronic obstructive pulmonary disease (COPD) is the overall term for a group of chronic lung conditions that obstruct the airways in your lungs. COPD is very common. In the majority of cases, it's caused by long-term smoking.

COPD develops gradually and produces few symptoms in its early stages. In addition, because people typically become less active as they get older, it becomes easier

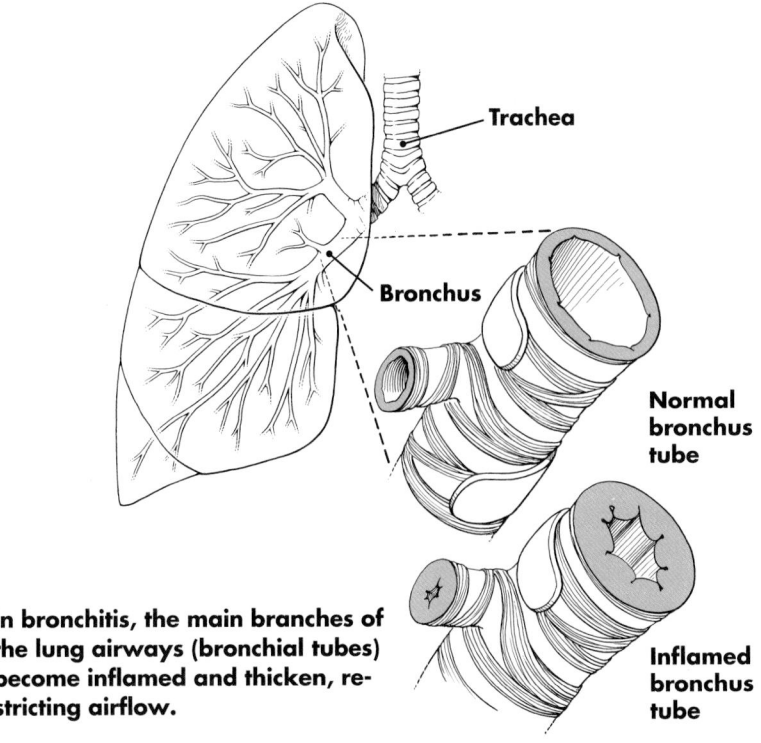

Trachea

Bronchus

Normal bronchus tube

Inflamed bronchus tube

In bronchitis, the main branches of the lung airways (bronchial tubes) become inflamed and thicken, restricting airflow.

to blame COPD symptoms on age or being out of shape.

Most people with COPD have both chronic bronchitis and emphysema.

Chronic bronchitis

Chronic bronchitis is a chronic inflammation and thickening of the lining of the bronchial tubes.

This disorder can narrow air passages enough to interfere with breathing and induce spells of coughing. The inflammation also causes the glands of the bronchial tubes to produce excessive amounts of mucus, increasing lung congestion that further hampers breathing.

As the disease worsens, relapses of the cough become more frequent and more severe. Shortness of breath develops late in the course of the disease, especially if smoking has caused significant lung damage.

Emphysema

Your lungs normally contain about 300 million elastic air sacs (alveoli). In the alveoli is where oxygen is added to the blood and carbon dioxide is removed.

The inflammation from emphysema damages the walls of the alveoli, causing them to lose elasticity, become overstretched and rupture. Several adjacent alveoli may rupture, forming one large space instead of many small ones. Larger spaces can combine into an even bigger cavity, called a bulla.

Damage to alveoli means fewer and less elastic sacs are helping force air out of your lungs. Air that you aren't able to exhale before you need to inhale again gets trapped in your lungs, and you become short of breath. In addition, damage to alveoli walls can disrupt the oxygen and carbon dioxide transfer.

Emphysema usually produces no symptoms until the disease is far advanced. At that point, shortness of breath may occur, along with less capacity for exertion.

What It Feels Like to Have COPD

To get an idea of what it feels like to have chronic obstructive pulmonary disease (COPD), try this exercise with a thin straw, but only if your lungs are healthy: First, inhale normally without the straw, then exhale fully through the straw. Likely you'll feel the need to inhale again before you're done exhaling. If you continue the exercise, you won't be able to empty your lungs, your breathing will become shallow and you'll become short of breath.

Causes

COPD most often occurs in people age 40 and older who are current or former smokers. Inhaled tobacco smoke paralyzes the microscopic hairs (cilia) that line the bronchial tubes. As a result, irritants and germs caught in mucus remain in the bronchial tubes because the cilia can't sweep them out. This results in the inflammation of bronchial membranes, eventually resulting in chronic obstruction.

Although smoking is the most common cause of COPD, occupational exposure to chemical fumes or dusts from grain, cotton, wood, coal or other sources also can put you at risk. In addition, air pollution and toxic gases in the environment, such as smog, can contribute to the development of COPD in smokers.

Diagnosis

To determine if you have COPD, your doctor may recommend these tests:

- **Pulmonary function tests.** Spirometry is the most common lung function test. During this test, you'll be asked to blow into a large tube connected to a spirometer. This machine measures how much air your lungs can hold and how fast you can blow the air out of your lungs. Spirometry can detect COPD even before you have symptoms of the disease. It can also be used to track the progression of disease and to monitor how well treatment is working.
- **Chest X-ray.** A chest X-ray can suggest the presence of emphysema. It can also rule out other lung problems or heart failure.
- **Arterial blood gas analysis.** This blood test measures how well your lungs are bringing oxygen into your blood and removing carbon dioxide.
- **Sputum examination.** Analysis of the cells in your sputum can help identify the cause of your lung problems and help rule out some lung cancers.

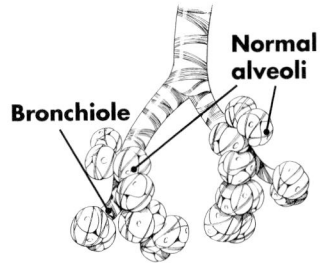

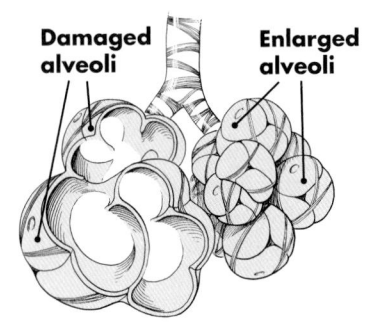

In emphysema, the air sacs of the lungs (alveoli) lose elasticity, enlarge and may rupture. This decreases the exchange of oxygen and carbon dioxide in your blood.

- **Computerized tomography (CT) scan.** A CT scan is an X-ray technique that produces more-detailed images of your internal organs than those produced by conventional X-rays. A CT scan of your lungs can help detect emphysema and help determine if you might benefit from surgery for COPD.

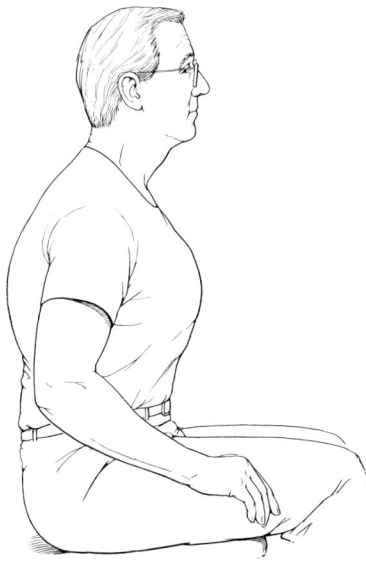

An enlarged chest is one characteristic sign of emphysema.

How serious is COPD?

COPD is extremely serious. A severe case is likely to shorten your life span. If the disease is detected early and you stop smoking if you're a smoker, your outlook improves greatly. If you stop smoking before you experience symptoms, you may prevent further progression of the disease.

As COPD progressively decreases lung function, some people don't get enough oxygen in their blood, a condition called hypoxemia. Signs and symptoms of hypoxemia include a decreased ability to exercise, fatigue, memory loss, depression, confusion and poor nighttime sleep with frequent awakenings.

Treatment

There's no cure for COPD. And it's impossible to undo damage to your lungs. But COPD treatments can control symptoms, reduce the risk of complications and slow the progression of emphysema.

Smoking cessation

The most essential step in any treatment plan for smokers with COPD is to stop smoking. It's the only way to keep COPD from getting worse. Talk to your doctor about nicotine replacement products and medications that might help, as well as how to handle relapses.

Medications

Doctors use three basic groups of medications to treat the symptoms and complications of COPD. You may take some medications on a regular basis and others as needed:
- **Bronchodilators.** These medications — which usually come in

Smoking and Genetics

Smoking is clearly the primary risk factor for emphysema. A rare inherited condition known as alpha-1-antitrypsin deficiency also can cause emphysema.

Alpha-1-antitrypsin is a protein in the blood that circulates to the lungs, where it limits damage to the air sacs (alveoli) during episodes of infection or inflammation. If you're deficient in this protein, this protection is lacking, so you're more likely to develop emphysema

at a young age — usually in your 30s and 40s — if you smoke. If you don't smoke and you have this genetic deficiency, you may not develop emphysema until much later in life, if at all.

About 1 in 2,500 people have alpha-1-antitrypsin deficiency, which can be detected with a blood test. The test isn't performed routinely, but if you have family members who weren't smokers but developed COPD or who smoked and developed the disease at a young age, you might want to discuss this testing with your doctor.

How Smoking Damages Your Lungs

Tobacco smoke contains thousands of substances, including chemicals, gases and tiny droplets of tar, many of which can cause cancer. Irritants in tobacco smoke cause your air passages to constrict and your bronchial tubes to produce excess mucus. These irritants may also impair the function of the immune system cells in your lungs and upset the normal balance of pulmonary enzymes, making you more susceptible to respiratory disease. Finally, inhaled tobacco smoke stops the movement of the tiny hair-like projections (cilia) in

your windpipe (trachea) and bronchial tubes that help expel foreign material from your lungs.

Tobacco smoke also contains carbon monoxide, a toxic gas that combines with hemoglobin to form carboxyhemoglobin, which blocks the transport of needed oxygen to your tissues. Many smokers have carboxyhemoglobin levels of 8 to 10 percent in their blood, whereas a nonsmoker commonly has only up to 1.5 percent.

Because some cigar and pipe smokers don't inhale smoke directly, many believe they have a lower risk of developing lung disease than cigarette smokers do. This is only partly true. Smoking-related diseases are also more common in cigar and pipe smokers than in nonsmokers.

an inhaler — relax the muscles around your airways. This can help relieve coughing and shortness of breath and make breathing easier. Depending on the severity of your disease, you may need a short-acting bronchodilator before activities, a long-acting bronchodilator that you use every day or both.

- **Inhaled steroids.** Inhaled corticosteroid medications can reduce airway inflammation and help you breathe better. But prolonged use of these medications can weaken your bones and increase your risk of high blood pressure, cataracts and diabetes. They're usually reserved for people with moderate or severe COPD.
- **Antibiotics.** Respiratory infections, such as acute bronchitis, pneumonia and influenza, can aggravate COPD symptoms. Antibiotics can help fight bacterial infections. Azithromycin is an antibiotic with anti-inflammatory properties. It may help prevent sudden worsening of the disease in some people.
- **Emerging medications.** A number of promising COPD medications are in the testing stages of development. Researchers hope these new medications will provide longer or more effective relief of COPD symptoms.

Surgery
Surgery is an option for some people with some forms of severe emphysema who aren't helped sufficiently by medications alone:

- **Lung volume reduction surgery.** In this surgery, your surgeon removes small wedges of damaged lung tissue. This creates extra space in your chest cavity so that the remaining lung tissue and the diaphragm work more efficiently.
- **Lung transplant.** Lung transplantation may be an option for certain people with severe emphysema who meet specific criteria. Transplantation can

improve your ability to breathe and be active. Among some people with severe disease, lung transplantation may prolong life expectancy.

Other therapies
Doctors often use these additional therapies for people with moderate or severe COPD:

- **Oxygen therapy.** If there isn't enough oxygen in your blood, you may need supplemental oxygen. Several devices can deliver oxygen to your lungs, including lightweight, portable units that you can take with you to run errands and get around town. Some people with COPD use oxygen only during activities or while sleeping. Others use oxygen all the time. Talk to

your doctor about your needs and options.

- **Pulmonary rehabilitation program.** Comprehensive pulmonary rehabilitation may be able to decrease the length of hospitalizations, increase your ability to participate in everyday activities and improve your quality of life. These programs typically combine education, exercise training, nutrition advice and counseling. If you are referred to a program, you'll probably work with a range of health care professionals, including physical therapists, respiratory therapists, exercise specialists and dietitians.

Managing exacerbations
Even with ongoing treatment, you may experience times when symp-

Protecting Your Lungs From Everyday Hazards

If you have COPD, you need to protect yourself from hazards in the air and exposure to infectious agents. Here are some suggestions:

Eliminate smoke from your environment
- Don't let anyone smoke in your home.
- When in public, look for nonsmoking establishments or sit in nonsmoking areas.
- Avoid wood smoke and cooking smoke.

Prevent respiratory infections
- As much as possible, avoid exposure to anyone who has a cold or the flu (influenza). Avoid crowds when colds and the flu are common.
- Wash your hands frequently, especially before you eat or take medicine, because viruses are often passed from hand to mouth.
- Unless your doctor advises against it, get a yearly flu shot and pneumococcal pneumonia vaccinations. You may need a repeat pneumonia vaccination five years after your first one.

Limit pollutants in your home
- Change your furnace and air conditioner filters according to manufacturers' instructions.
- Keep windows closed when it's dusty or smoky outside.
- Keep the humidity level in your home at 40 to 50 percent. If you use a humidifier, clean it frequently to prevent molds and bacteria from growing and potentially aggravating your lung condition.
- Limit your use of cleaning chemicals and avoid aerosol sprays and irritants such as paint fumes.
- Wear a dust mask when cleaning.

toms suddenly worsen. This is called an acute exacerbation, and it may cause lung failure if you don't receive prompt treatment. Exacerbations may result from a respiratory infection or a change in temperature or air pollution. Seek prompt medical help if you notice more coughing, a change in your mucus or if you have a harder time breathing.

When exacerbations occur, you may need additional medications, supplemental oxygen or treatment in the hospital.

Asthma

Signs and symptoms
- Shortness of breath
- Coughing
- Tightness in the chest
- Wheezing

Emergency signs and symptoms
- Extreme difficulty breathing
- Bluish lips and nails
- Severe shortness of breath
- Increased pulse rate
- Sweating
- Severe coughing

Asthma is a form of chronic lung disease characterized by inflammation of the lung airways (bronchial

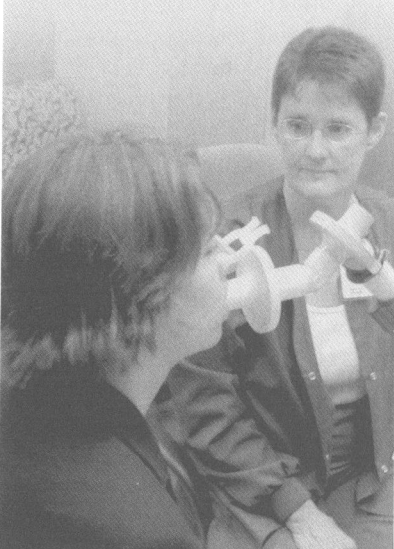

? Question and Answer

What are pulmonary function tests?

Pulmonary function tests detect lung disease and indicate its severity. The tests typically involve use of a device called a spirometer that you blow into to determine how much air you can take into your lungs and how fast you can blow it out.

You may be asked to blow into a spirometer before and after you use inhaled medications to test your response to them. This may include inhalants such as albuterol (Proventil HFA, Ventolin HFA), which can open bronchial tubes, or methacholine (Provocholine), which can constrict your bronchial tubes briefly and indicate if your airways have an asthma-type reaction.

Diaphragmatic Breathing

If you have chronic obstructive pulmonary disease (COPD) or another chronic lung disorder, a regular program of aerobic exercise, such as walking or bicycling, is the most effective way to improve your lung function — after you quit smoking, that is. In addition to exercise, practicing diaphragmatic breathing also may be helpful. The following exercise can help you learn to breathe more efficiently. You might want to practice this breathing exercise at least once a day.

1. Lie on your back with your head and knees supported by pillows. Begin the exercise by breathing in and out slowly and smoothly in a rhythmic pattern. Relax.
2. Place the fingertips of one or both hands on your abdomen, just below the base of your rib cage. As you inhale slowly, you should feel your diaphragm lifting your hand.
3. Practice pushing your abdomen against your hand as your chest becomes filled with air. Make sure your chest remains motionless as you inhale through your mouth for a slow count of three. Then purse your lips, which helps to increase the amount of air that can be exhaled, and exhale through your mouth while counting slowly to six.
4. After you can take 10 to 15 consecutive breaths in one session without tiring, practice the exercise while lying on your side, and then on your other side. Progress to doing the exercise while sitting in a chair, while standing up, while walking and, finally, while climbing stairs.

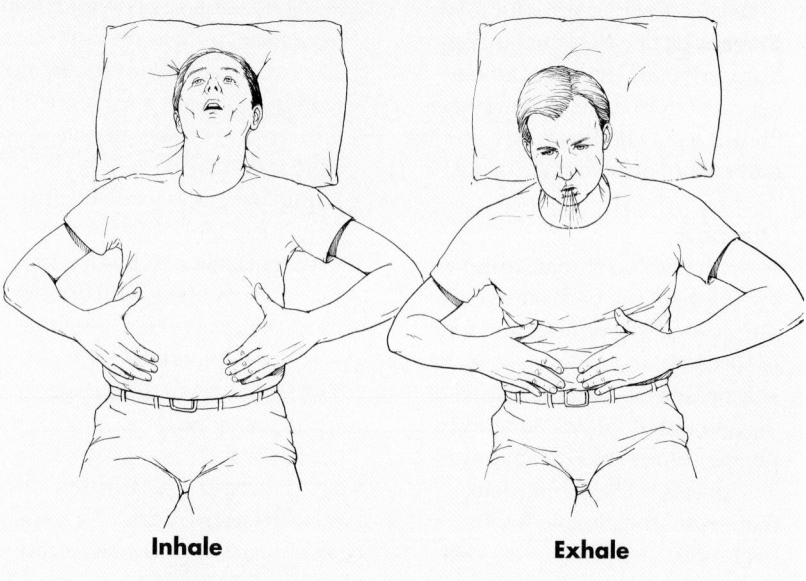

Inhale   **Exhale**

tubes) that causes them to narrow. Signs and symptoms of asthma may be persistent or occur periodically. For more information on asthma, see Chapter 17, "Allergies and Asthma."

Cystic fibrosis

Signs and symptoms

- Salty taste to the skin
- Blockage in bowels
- Foul-smelling, greasy stools
- Cough or wheezing
- Thick sputum
- Frequent chest and sinus infections with recurring pneumonia or bronchitis
- Delayed growth

Cystic fibrosis is an inherited condition that affects the respiratory and digestive systems. It's the most common potentially fatal hereditary disease among white children in the United States, occurring equally in boys and girls.

Cystic fibrosis affects the cells that produce mucus, sweat, saliva and digestive juices. Normally, these secretions are thin and slippery, but in cystic fibrosis a defective gene causes them to become thick and sticky. Instead of acting as a lubricant, the secretions plug up tubes, ducts and passageways, including the lungs. Respiratory failure is the most dangerous consequence of cystic fibrosis.

The greatest risk factor for cystic fibrosis is a family history of the disease. If both you and your partner come from families with cystic fibrosis, your children have a one in four chance of having the disease.

Diagnosis

If your child has chronic respiratory or digestive problems, your physician may perform lung function or stool tests. He or she may also order a sweat test to measure the amount of salt in your child's perspiration. A blood test is available to detect the genetic defect that causes the disease. Because babies may not produce enough sweat for a reliable diagnosis,

Supplemental Oxygen

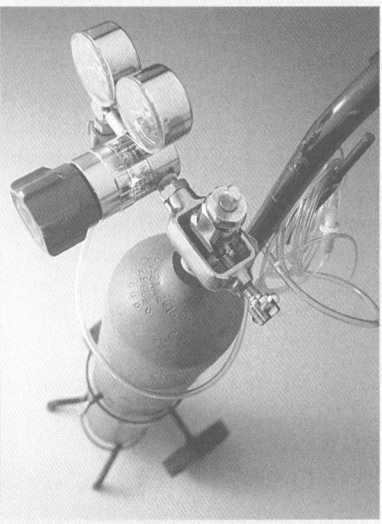

If you have a chronic lung disease and appropriate testing reveals a significant lack of oxygen in your blood, your doctor may prescribe supplemental oxygen.

Supplemental oxygen may decrease shortness of breath and improve your sense of well-being, but it's prescribed primarily to support the heart because inadequate blood oxygen can seriously disturb heart function.

You might need oxygen only at certain times, such as when you exercise or sleep, or you may need to use it all of the time. Three sources of supplemental oxygen are available. Your doctor will help you determine which type is best for you.

- Compressed oxygen comes in a tank with a flow meter and a regulator attached so that you can adjust the flow. The oxygen is stored under pressure, so you must handle the tank carefully. This may be your best choice if you don't need supplemental oxygen all of the time.
- An oxygen concentrator, which operates on electricity, takes oxygen from the air and concentrates it for your use. This may be your best bet if you need oxygen all of the time. Portable units are available for use in recreational vehicles and campers. Backup is necessary in case of an electrical outage.
- Liquid oxygen is available in a tank. Most tanks come with a light, portable unit that you can fill easily and take with you. The most portable option, this may work best for you if you want to stay active but need oxygen during activity.

Taking proper precautions

Fire burns faster in an oxygen-rich environment, so take special care

when using oxygen in your home. Keep objects that produce sparks, flames or intense heat well away from the area where you keep oxygen equipment. Keep flammable materials away from the area too. Never expose the oxygen tank and its attachments to temperatures above 125 F.

Be sure that the oxygen cylinders are well-secured to prevent them from tipping over. When not in use, seal the tank's connections properly with protective caps.

When installing the regulator, follow instructions precisely. Before the regulator is attached, open the valve slightly and then close it immediately. This clears out dust or combustible material.

If you require oxygen 24 hours a day, your doctor may recommend use of a portable oxygen device that allows you to travel beyond the reach of the large tank and its hose. The rules and regulations cited above apply equally to portable tanks.

Portable containers carry only a limited amount of oxygen. Longer trips require preparation to ensure a continuous oxygen supply. Plan where you'll need to stop to refill your tanks and check to make sure you can get a refill when you need it. Your oxygen supplier can help you determine your oxygen needs for travel.

doctors usually don't perform a sweat test until an infant is several months old.

How serious is cystic fibrosis?

Cystic fibrosis is serious and may be fatal. About half the individuals with this disease live beyond age 30. As techniques for treating cystic fibrosis improve, many people are living much longer. Mild forms of the disease may not produce symptoms until adulthood.

Treatment

Many treatments exist. The main goal is to prevent infections, reduce the amount and thickness of secretions in the lungs, improve airflow, and maintain adequate calories and nutrition.

Medication

Medications include:

- **Antibiotics.** Newer antibiotics may more effectively fight the bacteria that cause lung infections in people with cystic fibrosis. Among these are aerosolized antibiotics that send medication directly into airways. One of the major drawbacks of long-term use of antibiotics is the development of bacteria that are resistant to drug therapy. In addition, using antibiotics over a long period of time can lead to fungal infections of the mouth, throat and respiratory tract.
- **Mucus-thinning drugs.** The aerosolized drug dornase alfa (Pulmozyme) is an enzyme that fragments DNA, making mucus thinner and easier to cough up. Side effects of the drug may include airway irritation and a sore throat.
- **Bronchodilators.** Use of medications such as albuterol, which can be delivered by an inhaler or a nebulizer, may help keep open the bronchial tubes by clearing thick secretions.
- **CFTR modulators.** These are newer medications designed to correct the function of defective protein made by the cystic fibro-

sis transmembrane conductance regulator (CFTR) gene.

Bronchial airway drainage

People with cystic fibrosis need a way to physically remove thick mucus from their lungs. This is often done by manually clapping with cupped hands on the front and back of the chest — a procedure that's best performed with the person's head over the edge of the bed so that gravity helps clear the secretions.

In some cases an electric chest clapper, or mechanical percussor, is used. An inflatable vest that vibrates at high frequency also can help people with cystic fibrosis cough up secretions.

Many adults and children with pulmonary cystic fibrosis need to have bronchial airway drainage at least twice a day for 20 to 30 minutes. Older children and adults can learn to do this themselves, especially if they use mechanical aids. Young children need the help of another individual.

Oral enzymes and good nutrition

Cystic fibrosis can cause you to become malnourished because the pancreatic enzymes needed for digestion don't reach your small intestine, preventing food from being absorbed. As a result, you may need many more calories than you otherwise would. Supplemental high-calorie nutrition, special fat-soluble vitamins and enteric-coated oral pancreatic enzymes can help you maintain or even gain weight.

Lung transplantation

Your doctor may suggest lung transplantation if you have declining lung function or increasing resistance to antibiotics. Whether you're a good candidate for the procedure depends on a number of factors, including your overall health and certain lifestyle factors. Because both lungs are affected by cystic fibrosis, both need to be replaced.

Sarcoidosis

Signs and symptoms

- Persistent cough
- Shortness of breath
- Discomfort and fatigue
- Fever
- Weight loss
- Small red bumps on face, arms or buttocks
- Red, watery eyes

Sarcoidosis is a chronic disease characterized by abnormal collections of inflammatory cells (granulomas) that can form in different areas of your body. Sarcoidosis can affect virtually any organ, but it most commonly affects the lungs, lymph nodes, eyes and skin.

Doctors believe that sarcoidosis results from an abnormal immune response. The course of the disease varies from person to person. It often goes away on its own, but in some people symptoms may last a lifetime.

Diagnosis

A chest X-ray may reveal inflamed patches in the lungs or lymph node enlargement. To confirm the diagnosis, your doctor may perform a lung biopsy using a fiber-optic bronchoscope to obtain tissue for examination (see page 785). Lung function tests indicate how much air your lungs can hold.

If the skin, lymph nodes or sclera of the eye are involved, tissue may be taken from these organs for diagnosis instead because the retrieval process is less invasive.

Sarcoidosis may cause an abnormally high level of calcium in your blood. Blood tests may be performed to check calcium levels and other substances that may be present in blood.

How serious is sarcoidosis?

Most people recover completely or have only minor lingering effects, even without treatment. Some, though, have chronic disease that stays active or comes and goes intermittently for many years. Rarely, sarcoidosis leads to the need for a lung transplant or death, usually after having had the disease for many years.

Treatment

If you don't have signs or symptoms or they aren't bothering you, you may not need treatment. If you have pronounced symptoms or if the disease doesn't resolve spontaneously after a few months, your doctor may prescribe medication.

The most commonly used drugs are corticosteroids to relieve inflammation. If prolonged treatment is required, other medications may be prescribed to lessen the chance of steroid-related side effects.

If you aren't able to tolerate corticosteroids, your doctor may prescribe other medications that reduce inflammation. The drug hydroxychloroquine (Plaquenil) may be helpful for skin disease.

As the disease improves — as demonstrated by chest X-rays or other tests — your doctor likely will taper you off the medications.

Interstitial lung disease

Signs and symptoms
- Shortness of breath, particularly with exertion
- A dry cough
- Fatigue and malaise

Interstitial lung disease refers to a large group of diseases that are long lasting (chronic) but aren't cancerous or infectious. These diseases are characterized by infiltration of inflammatory cells into the air sacs of your lungs (alveoli). The result is formation of scar tissue in the connective tissues that support the alveoli, impairing the transfer of oxygen to the blood. If the disease progresses, the scarring can advance to the point of destroying the lungs.

Interstitial lung disorders most often occur in people older than age 50. Their causes aren't known.

Sarcoidosis is a common form of interstitial lung disease. Another

more common form is idiopathic pulmonary fibrosis.

Idiopathic pulmonary fibrosis

This chronic disorder causes progressive shortness of breath. Males and females get the disorder in equal numbers. It commonly develops in the middle years of life, but it can occur at any age. The air sacs become inflamed and eventually damaged and scarred. The sacs behave like stiff balloons — they thicken and won't inflate well. It takes more effort to breathe as scar tissue interferes with oxygen transfer.

A variant of interstitial lung disease is desquamative interstitial pneumonia. It has the same symptoms, but the lung tissue, when seen under a microscope, looks different.

Lymphoid interstitial pneumonia, another variant, generally affects the lower lobes of the lung. It tends to develop in people with Sjogren's syndrome and sometimes in children and adults with human immunodeficiency virus (HIV) infection.

Certain typical sounds heard through a stethoscope, characteristic patterns seen on a chest X-ray and results of lung function tests can be of help in the diagnosis. However, a lung biopsy by a bronchoscope or surgery also may be necessary. If the affected person has a history of occupational exposure to asbestos, there is an increased risk of lung cancer.

How serious is interstitial lung disease?

The course of the disease depends on the type. Some are progressive and ultimately fatal. Others resolve spontaneously or stabilize. Some have a fluctuating course.

Treatment

Idiopathic pulmonary fibrosis is treated with anti-fibrotic agents that may slow the progression of the disease. Anti-GERD therapy also appears to be beneficial in

treating this form of the disease. Treatment of other interstitial lung diseases may involve corticosteroid medications, cytotoxic drugs or immunosuppressant medications.

Additional therapies include oxygen therapy, pulmonary rehabilitation and, in some cases, lung transplantation.

Lung collapse

Signs and symptoms
- Shortness of breath
- Fever
- Decreased blood pressure and a rapid heartbeat
- Shock
- Pain on the side of the affected lung
- A severe, hacking cough

Atelectasis is the medical term for collapse of portions of a lung or, rarely, an entire lung. The collapse can occur slowly when it's due to a growing tumor in the lung, or it may happen suddenly.

The collapse may result from an infection, from an obstruction of bronchial passages in the lungs — commonly by a plug of thick mucus — by accidental inhalation of a foreign object, by outside pressure from a tumor, aneurysm or enlarged lymph node, or from pneumothorax. Sometimes, lung collapse occurs as a complication of surgery, when breathing is shallow and portions of the lung don't expand.

Diagnosis

A chest X-ray will show an airless portion of the lung.

Treatment

If the collapse is due to an obstruction, the first goal is to remove the cause of the obstruction, if possible. If coughing, suctioning or other therapeutic measures don't work, a doctor may perform a bronchoscopy (see page 785). If your doctor suspects that you have an infection, he or she may prescribe antibiotics.

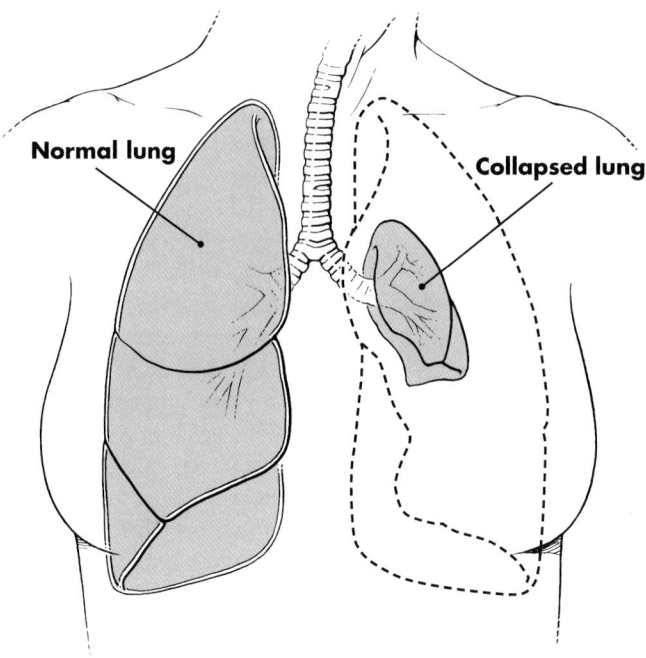

Normal lung

Collapsed lung

A portion of a lung or, rarely, an entire lung may collapse for a variety of reasons, including an obstruction of lung airways, pneumothorax, an infection or a complication of surgery.

Prevention
Lung collapse is much less likely to occur after surgery if during recovery you get up and walk around as soon as possible and take frequent deep breaths. You may be given a device to help you draw more air into your lungs rapidly and forcefully.

Pneumothorax

Signs and symptoms
• Sudden, sharp chest pain
• Shortness of breath
• Chest tightness
• Rapid heart rate
 Pneumothorax is a type of lung collapse that occurs when air leaks into the area between your lungs and chest wall (pleural space). A pneumothorax can stem from a chest injury, certain medical treatments, lung disease or a break in an air blister on the lung's surface. An entire lung can collapse, but a partial collapse is more common.

Diagnosis
A chest X-ray will show an airless portion of the lung.

How serious is pneumothorax?
A small, uncomplicated pneumothorax may heal on its own in a week or two. When the condition is more severe, the excess air is usually removed by inserting a tube or needle between the ribs into the pleural space. If air continues to build up, the increasing pressure can push on your heart and blood vessels, compressing both your lung and heart. This is life-threatening and requires immediate care.

Treatment
The goal in treating pneumothorax is to relieve the pressure on the lung, allowing it to re-expand, and to prevent recurrences.
 If your lung is less than 20 to 25 percent collapsed, your doctor may simply monitor your condition with chest X-rays until the air is completely reabsorbed and your lung has re-expanded.
 When your lung has collapsed more than 25 percent, your doctor may remove the air by inserting a needle or small tube through the chest wall into the pleural space.

Chest tubes are often attached to a suction device that continuously removes air from the chest cavity. Recurrent pneumothorax may require more-aggressive surgical treatment to repair the air leak in the lung.

Lung Cancer

Lung cancer is the leading cause of cancer deaths in the United States in both men and women. According to the American Cancer Society, about 85,000 men and 71,000 women die of lung cancer each year.

Signs and symptoms

Lung cancer usually doesn't cause any symptoms until the disease is advanced. When symptoms do occur, they may include:
• A new cough that doesn't go away
• Changes in a chronic cough or "smoker's cough"
• Coughing up blood
• Shortness of breath
• Chest pain
• Wheezing and hoarseness
• Weight loss
 Lung cancer is among the most preventable of all cancers. Cigarette smoking accounts for nearly 90 percent of lung cancers. Other risk factors include secondhand smoke, exposure to asbestos and other occupational carcinogens, and high concentrations of radon.
 Cancer that develops in the lungs is uncommon in nonsmokers. Secondary lung cancer — cancer that spreads (metastasizes) to the lungs from other organs, such as the breast, colon, prostate, testicle, kidney, thyroid or bone — can occur in smokers and nonsmokers.

Types of tumors

A cancerous (malignant) tumor is an abnormal growth of cells that can invade and destroy nearby

Normal Lung

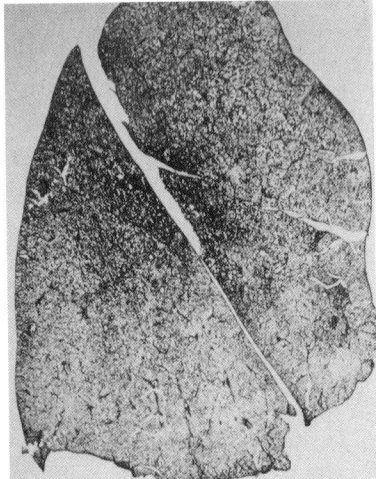

Cancerous Lung

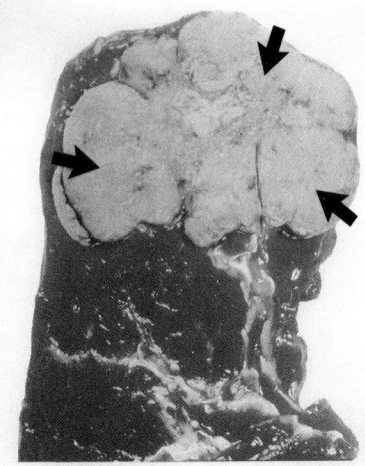

tissue and organs and can spread to other parts of the body. The two main types of lung cancer are small cell and non-small cell.

Small cell lung cancer

Small cell lung cancer, also called oat cell carcinoma, develops in the central areas of the lung. Named for the small, round or oval shape of the cancer cells that resemble oats when viewed under the microscope, it's one of the more aggressive cancers and is found almost exclusively in smokers. It can cause narrowing of air passageways (bronchi) by compressing them. Small cell lung cancer is less common than non-small cell.

Non-small cell lung cancer

Non-small cell lung cancer is an umbrella term for several types of lung cancer that behave in a similar way. Non-small cell cancers include the following:

- **Adenocarcinoma.** This type is the most common form of lung cancer in women and people who've never smoked. It usually develops in the mucus-producing cells of the lung. It may spread to the lymph nodes in that area of the lung or through the bloodstream to other organs.
- **Squamous cell cancer.** Squamous cell lung cancer is most commonly found in men. The majority of squamous cell can-

cers arise from cells lining the largest air passages of the lungs.

- **Large cell carcinoma.** Large cell carcinoma appears in the periphery of the lung and spreads through the bloodstream. It's the least common of the three.

Diagnosis

Some lung cancers are discovered on a routine chest X-ray or a chest X-ray taken for another condition. However, chest X-rays aren't an effective screening tool for identifying early-stage lung cancer.

A computerized tomography (CT) scan can reveal small lesions in your lungs. A low-dose CT scan of the chest may be useful in older individuals with a significant smoking history. Ask your doctor if you should be screened.

Magnetic resonance imaging (MRI) and positron emission tomography (PET) may be used to detect the spread of the cancer.

If you have a cough and are producing sputum, looking at the sputum under a microscope can sometimes reveal the presence of cancer cells.

In a biopsy procedure, a sample of tissue cells are removed from the lungs for examination. A lung biopsy may be performed using a number of techniques.

Smoking and Lung Cancer

The vast majority of lung cancer cases can be traced to smoking. People who smoke more than one pack of cigarettes a day have a 20 times greater risk of developing lung cancer than do people who never smoked. A person who smokes two packs of cigarettes or more daily for 20 years has a 60- to 70-fold increase in risk of developing lung cancer compared with a nonsmoker.

Because some cigar and pipe smokers don't inhale smoke directly, many believe that they have a lower risk of developing lung cancer than cigarette smokers do. This is only partly true. Smoking-related diseases are also more common in cigar and pipe smokers than in nonsmokers.

Currently, lung cancer is more common in men than in women. Unfortunately, more women are smoking, so their incidence of lung cancer is increasing rapidly. Lung cancer now surpasses breast cancer as the most common cause of cancer deaths in American women.

The tar in cigarette smoke contains numerous substances that cause cancer (carcinogens) as well as substances that accelerate the production of cancer cells (cocarcinogens). Small cell lung cancer and squamous cell cancer are most strongly associated with cigarette smoking.

Cancer risk decreases when you quit smoking. Ten years after quitting, individuals who smoked more than 20 cigarettes a day can expect their early death rate to decrease by two-thirds. Unfortunately, many people don't quit until they've already developed symptoms of respiratory disease or have lung cancer.

Staging

Once your lung cancer has been diagnosed, your doctor will work to determine the extent, or stage, of your cancer. Your cancer's stage is important in determining what treatment would be the most appropriate.

Staging tests may include imaging procedures that allow your doctor to look for signs that cancer has spread beyond your lungs, such as magnetic resonance imaging (MRI), positron emission tomography (PET) and bone scans. Not every test is appropriate for every person, so talk with your doctor about which procedures are appropriate for you.

Non-small cell lung cancer stages are as follows. Stages I through IV contain subgroups.

- **Stage 0.** The cancer is limited to the thin layer lining the airways and hasn't invaded deeper into lung tissue or other areas.
- **Stage I.** Cancer at this stage has invaded the underlying lung tissue but it hasn't spread to the lymph nodes.
- **Stage II.** Stage II means the cancer has spread to neighboring lymph nodes or it has invaded the chest wall.
- **Stage III.** The cancer has spread from the lung to lymph nodes in the center of the chest. Or the cancer has spread locally to areas such as the heart, blood vessels, trachea and esophagus — all within the chest — or to lymph nodes in the area of the collarbone or to the tissue that surrounds the lungs within the rib cage (pleura).
- **Stage IV.** The cancer has spread to other parts of the body, such as the liver, bones or brain.

Small cell lung cancer is sometimes described as being limited or extensive. Limited indicates the cancer is limited to one lung. Extensive indicates the cancer has spread beyond one lung.

Prognosis

Lung cancer is a serious disease that often has a poor prognosis. Overall, approximately 18 percent of people with the disease survive for five years. However, the outcome depends on a number of factors, including the extent of the disease when discovered, your general health and age, the type of cancer, how rapidly it grows, and the therapy used.

Only a small percentage of lung cancers are detected before the cancer has spread. Once signs or symptoms of lung cancer appear, the disease may be advanced and not treatable by surgery. In fact, most lung cancers can't be removed surgically at the time of initial diagnosis.

Small cell lung cancer is extremely serious because of its tendency to spread before signs or symptoms are apparent.

Treatment

The treatment options for lung cancer are surgical removal of the tumor and surrounding tissue, chemotherapy, radiation therapy or some combination of these. Targeted therapies are sometimes used. Targeted therapies are medications that are designed to destroy the cancer by targeting specific molecular pathways involved in its development and spread.

Bronchoscopy

A bronchoscopy is a procedure in which a specially designed tube is passed down your airway to allow your doctor to see the inside of your air passages. A bronchoscopy enables your doctor to look for tumors, foreign objects, areas of internal bleeding and abnormalities of your lungs and air passageways. A bronchoscope also has an open channel through which a doctor can remove secretions and obtain biopsy specimens.

There are two types of bronchoscopes: the fiber-optic bronchoscope, which is flexible and 3 to 7 millimeters in diameter, and the rigid bronchoscope, which is larger and more difficult to use. The flexible fiber-optic bronchoscope is used more often. It contains glass fibers that transmit light and return a magnified picture of the passageways of your lungs. Your doctor watches the progress of the bronchoscope through an eyepiece or on a small television-like monitor.

You shouldn't eat for at least 6 to 12 hours before you undergo a bronchoscopy. Just before the procedure, you may be given a local anesthesia, or general anesthesia may be used. The anesthetic agent, which suppresses your cough and swallowing reflexes, is usually administered through your nostrils or mouth. Your doctor may also give you a sedative to help you relax.

During the procedure, you'll either be sitting or lying down. The bronchoscope is inserted through your mouth or nose. Lidocaine jelly serves as an oral anesthetic and a lubricant to protect your air passages.

A flexible bronchoscopy usually is painless and seldom causes complications. After the procedure, you shouldn't eat or drink anything for about an hour, until your swallowing and coughing reflexes return to normal.

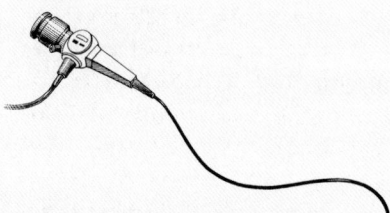

During a procedure called a bronchoscopy, your doctor can see the inside of your airways by passing a flexible tube (bronchoscope) into them.

Surgery

During surgery a surgeon works to remove the cancer and a margin of healthy tissue. Procedures to remove lung cancer include:

- Wedge resection to remove a small section of lung that contains the tumor along with a margin of healthy tissue
- Lobectomy to remove an entire lobe of one lung
- Pneumonectomy to remove an entire lung

If you undergo surgery, your surgeon may also remove lymph nodes from your chest in order to check them for signs of cancer. If your lymph nodes contain cancer cells, this usually indicates that cancer has spread, even if cancer hasn't been detected outside of your chest.

Lung cancer surgery carries risks, including bleeding and infection. Expect to feel short of breath after lung surgery. Your lung tissue will expand over time and make it easier to breathe. You may also feel pain in the muscles of your chest and in your arm on the side where you had the operation. Your doctor may recommend physical therapy or a rehabilitation program to help you restore your strength and range of motion.

Chemotherapy

Chemotherapy uses drugs to kill cancer cells. One or more chemotherapy drugs may be administered through a vein in your arm (intravenously) or taken orally. A combination of drugs usually is given in a series of treatments over a period of weeks or months, with breaks in between so that your body can recover.

Chemotherapy can be used as a first line treatment for lung cancer or as additional treatment after surgery. In some cases, chemotherapy can be used to lessen side effects of your cancer.

Radiation therapy

Radiation therapy uses high-powered energy beams, such

Lung Cancer Surgery

Surgical removal (resection) of a cancerous tumor may be performed in people with lung cancer that hasn't spread to other parts of the body. Depending on the extent of the cancer, people with squamous cell cancer, large cell carcinoma or adenocarcinoma are candidates for surgical treatment. Surgery is seldom performed for small cell lung cancer because it spreads too rapidly and too extensively to be removed completely with surgery.

The procedure

The surgeon removes the tumor and the tissue that's immediately surrounding it. The most common surgery is a lobectomy, in which the involved lobe is removed. Other types of lung surgery include a wedge resection, in which a small portion of a lobe is removed, a segment resection, which involves removal of a larger portion of a lobe, and pneumonectomy, removal of the entire lung. Usually, the surgeon also removes those lymph nodes that drain the involved lung.

The hospital stay after the surgery usually lasts five to seven days, although it'll take longer for you to recover completely. Many people are able to resume their normal activities in four to six weeks. However, the rate and degree of recovery depend on the general condition of your lungs, the amount of lung tissue removed and your overall health.

The outlook

Of individuals whose cancer is detected early, approximately 75 percent are alive at five years after the operation. After surgery, it's important to have regular medical checkups to detect possible recurrence of the cancer, either within the lung or in other parts of your body. If the cancer recurs, chemotherapy or radiation therapy may decrease the size of the tumor, prolong life, and relieve pain and other symptoms.

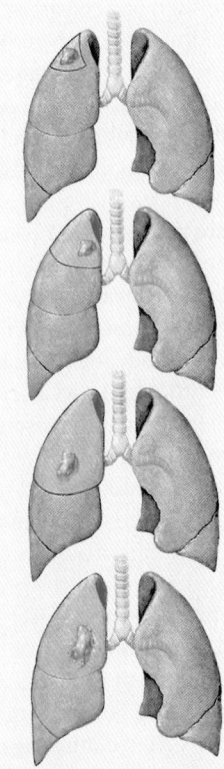

Wedge resection is removal of a small portion of a lobe.

Segment resection is removal of a larger portion of a lobe.

Lobectomy is removal of an entire lobe.

Pneumonectomy is removal of an entire lung.

as X-rays, to kill cancer cells. Radiation therapy can be directed at your lung cancer from outside your body (external beam radiation) or it can be put inside needles, seeds or catheters and placed inside your body near the cancer (brachytherapy).

Radiation therapy can be used alone or along with other lung cancer treatments. Sometimes it's administered at the same time as chemotherapy. Radiation therapy can also be used to lessen side effects of lung cancer.

Targeted drug therapy

Targeted therapies are cancer treatments that work by targeting specific abnormalities in cancer cells. Targeted therapy options for treating lung cancer include:

- **Bevacizumab (Avastin).** Bevacizumab stops a tumor from creating a new blood supply. Blood vessels that connect to tumors can supply oxygen and nutrients to the tumor, allowing it to grow. Bevacizumab is usually used in combination with chemotherapy and is approved for advanced and recurrent non-small cell lung cancer. Bevacizumab carries a risk of severe bleeding.
- **Erlotinib (Tarceva).** Erlotinib blocks chemicals that signal the cancer cells to grow and divide. Erlotinib is approved for people with advanced and recurrent non-small cell lung cancer who haven't been helped by chemotherapy. Side effects include a skin rash and diarrhea.

Occupation-Related Lung Disease

Hazardous materials in the workplace that are inhaled on a regular or significant basis can cause lung disease. Perhaps the best known of these diseases are asbestosis, black lung and silicosis. In addition, various industrial and agricultural dusts and some fungi cause lung diseases, which are usually named after the occupation in which they're most likely to occur or the type of dust inhaled.

Asbestosis

Signs and symptoms
- Shortness of breath
- Decreased exercise tolerance
- Coughing
- Chest pain

Asbestos was used extensively as insulation in building construction for many years in the mid-1970s, when it was replaced by other materials, such as fiberglass and slag wool. There are four types of asbestos fibers that can cause respiratory disease if large amounts of fine asbestos fibers accumulate in your lungs.

Millions of workers may be at risk of asbestosis. People who were exposed to asbestos include workers in the mining, milling and manufacturing of asbestos and its products, as well as those who installed asbestos products. People who installed asbestos products include pipe fitters, boilermakers, shipbuilders and construction workers.

The problem with asbestos is that its particles flake off. When disturbed, the tiny fibers release from the surface. These loose fibers may stay airborne for some time. The vast majority of the people who work in or go into buildings containing easily crumbled asbestos have a very small risk of contracting respiratory illness from the fibers, but the safe level of asbestos exposure is uncertain.

Various federal, state and local government regulations now require asbestos control or removal, particularly in schools. Many insurance companies won't cover buildings that contain asbestos.

The lung disorder asbestosis generally results when asbestos fibers accumulate around small air passageways in the lungs (bronchioles). Your lungs react to the fibers by forming small masses of scar tissue (fibrosis). Symptoms

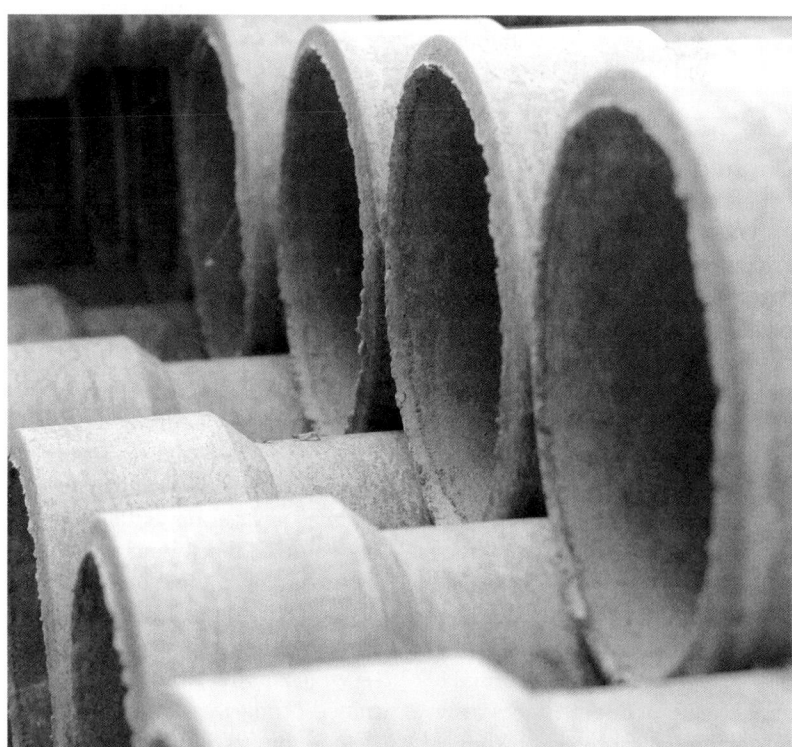

Asbestos used in pipe covering can be hazardous to your health. Removal requires care and expertise.

Mesothelioma

In addition to impairing lung function, asbestosis can increase your risk of a rare cancer of the lining of the lung called mesothelioma.

Mesothelioma may develop 20 to 40 years after exposure to asbestos fibers and can occur even if you were exposed only for one or two years or less. Some people with mesothelioma have no history of exposure to asbestos.

Signs and symptoms include significant chest pain, shortness of breath and weight loss. In about half of those with mesothelioma, the disease spreads, producing tumors in other parts of the body. In other cases, the tumors are limited to the chest. An accumulation of fluid between the two layers of the pleural membrane (pleural effusion) often contributes to shortness of breath and chest pain.

The chance of recovery depends on the size and location of the cancer, whether and how far it has spread, and how it responds to treatment. Mesothelioma is usually treated with surgery to remove the cancer, radiation therapy, chemotherapy or some combination of these therapies.

appear when the scar tissue causes your lungs to lose their elasticity. The first symptom of asbestosis may be the gradual onset of shortness of breath on exertion.

On a chest X-ray, the scar tissue may appear as small, scattered, opaque areas. These areas are generally first evident in the lower parts of the lung, but gradually spread upward as the disease progresses. Eventually, your entire lung may develop a honeycomb appearance on an X-ray.

Another result of prolonged exposure to asbestos may be the development of pleural plaques around your lungs. These areas of thickening of the membrane that surrounds your lungs (pleura) usually occur along the lower part of the chest wall or near the diaphragm. The presence of pleural plaques is strong evidence that you've been exposed to asbestos, but it doesn't mean that your lungs are impaired, unless you have other signs and symptoms.

Diagnosis

An abnormal chest X-ray may suggest that you have been exposed to asbestos, but it doesn't necessarily mean you have asbestosis. Your doctor may also have you undergo a computerized tomography (CT) scan to view your lungs in more detail and pulmonary function tests to determine how well your lungs are functioning. Symptoms of debilitating pulmonary fibrosis, including the abnormal development of scar tissue, are also necessary in making a diagnosis.

Treatment

There's no treatment to reverse the effects of the disorder. Treatment is usually for slowing progression of the disease and easing symptoms. Oxygen therapy or draining fluid from around the lungs may improve your breathing.

Black lung and silicosis

Signs and symptoms

- Shortness of breath
- Coughing that produces sputum

Black lung (coal miner's pneumoconiosis) and silicosis result from inhaling industrial particles that become permanently lodged in the lungs. Black lung is caused by inhaling coal dust for several years. The disease is more common in miners of anthracite coal — which, in the United States, is mined primarily in the East — than in miners of bituminous coal, which is mined primarily in the West.

Silicosis is caused by the inhalation of free silica (crystalline quartz). Free silica exposure occurs in occupations such as mining, stonecutting, quarrying (especially of granite), sandblasting, rock blasting, road building and industries that manufacture abrasives.

It usually takes 15 to 20 years of exposure before symptoms develop. Unprotected workers in occupations with intense exposure to silica may develop silicosis in less than a year.

Diagnosis

In most cases, both black lung and silicosis cause no respiratory symptoms, unless you smoke cigarettes. The diseases are generally diagnosed when small, irregular, opaque areas are seen on a chest X-ray, and they can be attributed to a history of exposure to coal dust or silica. With long-term exposure, the irregular areas become larger and combine into rounded nodules.

Both black lung and silicosis may develop into significant scarring of lung tissue, called progressive massive fibrosis.

How serious are black lung and silicosis?

In their early stages, black lung and silicosis don't cause respiratory impairment, which usually occurs with development of massive fibrosis. Despite avoidance of further exposure, massive fibrosis can cause death. Survival time may be less than two years. In addition, people with silicosis have a greater than average risk of tuberculosis.

Treatment

There's no specific treatment for either of these diseases, although lung transplantation may be an option in some cases.

If you have either condition, avoid additional exposure to the causative dust. If you smoke, stop. In addition, limit exposure to respiratory irritants such as irritating fumes or cold, dry or extremely humid air. If you have silicosis and your tuberculin skin test is positive, you'll need treatment for tuberculosis, even if you have no symptoms.

Occupational asthma

Signs and symptoms
- Shortness of breath
- Coughing
- Tightness in the chest
- Wheezing

Emergency signs and symptoms
- Extreme difficulty breathing
- Bluish lips and nails
- Severe shortness of breath
- Increased pulse rate
- Sweating
- Severe coughing

In a small percentage of people with asthma, the cause is related to their occupation or environment.

Some agents known to cause asthma are paints, wood dust, grain dust, pollens, synthetic dyes, gum arabic and rosin (soldering flux). Inhalation of one of these agents doesn't mean you'll develop asthma, but in some individuals they can trigger the disease.

Diagnosis
The signs and symptoms of occupational asthma are the same as those of nonoccupational asthma. Testing may include a bronchial provocation test, in which you're exposed to the suspected allergen or irritating substance in a laboratory so that your airway reaction to it can be measured.

Treatment
Treatment generally consists of medications to help keep your airways open. Avoiding the substance that causes your asthma is also important. For more information on asthma, see Chapter 17, "Allergies and Asthma."

Hypersensitivity pneumonitis

Signs and symptoms
- Persistent coughing that produces large amounts of sputum
- Wheezing
- Shortness of breath
- Decreased pulmonary function

Causes
This disease is caused by exposure to organic dusts. It goes by many names, usually relating to the occupation in which it's acquired:
- Farmer's lung, caused by exposure to dust from moldy hay
- Byssinosis, caused by dust from cotton or, to a lesser extent, flax, jute, or hemp yarn or rope
- Humidifier lung, caused by dust or moisture from humidifiers, heating systems and air conditioners contaminated by a fungus
- Bagassosis, caused by fungi in moldy sugar cane fiber (bagasse)
- Suberosis, caused by inhaling cork dust
- Sequoiosis, caused by redwood sawdust
- Maple bark stripper's disease, caused by dust from rotting maple tree logs and bark
- Mushroom worker's lung, caused by dust from moldy compost
- Detergent worker's lung, caused by dust from enzyme additives

Diagnosis
All of these organic dusts cause the same symptoms in those individuals who are sensitive to them. Making a diagnosis is the first step in treatment. To help in this process, doctors often use pulmonary function tests.

Industrial Bronchitis

Bronchitis that occurs in coal miners and workers exposed to cotton, flax or hemp dust is called industrial bronchitis. Fumes from ammonia, strong acids, certain organic solvents, chlorine, hydrogen sulfide, sulfur dioxide and bromine also may cause bronchitis.

Common signs and symptoms include shortness of breath and a chronic cough that produces sputum.

It's not clear whether exposure to the dusts causes bronchitis in these workers or whether the exposure aggravates bronchitis from other causes, such as smoking. The disease generally clears up with rest, drinking plenty of liquids and eliminating exposure to the irritant that caused it. Sometimes, the use of a humidifier or vaporizer is helpful.

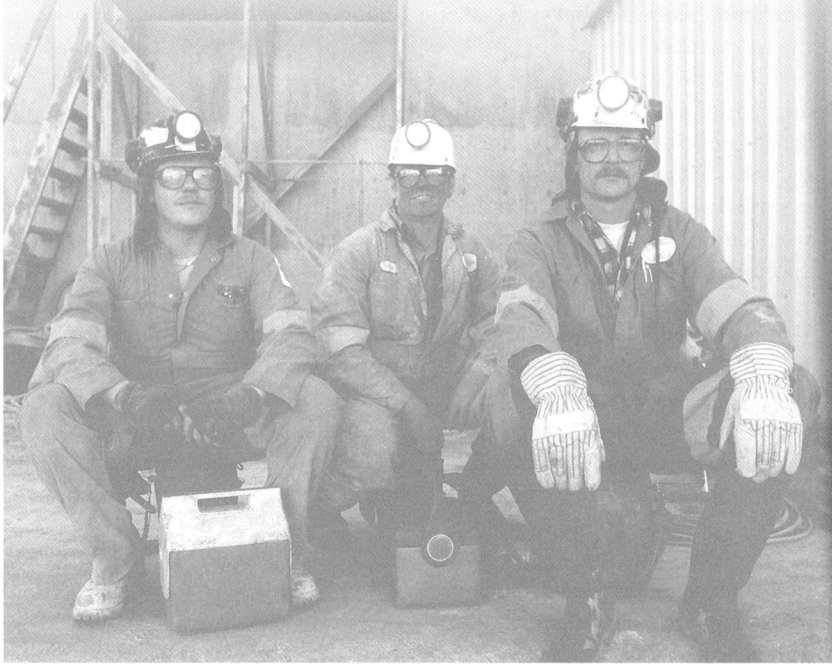

Treatment

The first line of treatment is to avoid inhaling the offending substance. For some individuals, corticosteroid medications may be prescribed. Chronic and progressive forms of the disease may require lung transplantation.

Byssinosis

Signs and symptoms

- Tightness in the chest

Byssinosis is an asthma-like disease that's sometimes found in workers who produce cotton or, to a lesser extent, flax, jute, or hemp yarn or rope.

Also known as brown lung and Monday fever — a misnomer because it doesn't cause a fever — byssinosis results from inhaling dust from the raw plant bales. Those who work with cotton and other fibers during the cleaning processes — blowing, mixing and carding (straightening) — that precede spinning are at greatest risk.

Diagnosis

The disease may develop right after the first exposure or after years of working in the industry. You may feel tightness in your chest toward the end of the day on Monday, the first day after the weekend, assuming that you had the weekend off.

At first, the symptoms don't appear during the rest of the week, but in some individuals the chest tightness eventually persists for several days, then throughout the week and into the weekend and vacation periods.

How serious is byssinosis?

Byssinosis generally isn't serious. But if the disease persists or gets worse, it can lead to chronic illness such as emphysema or chronic bronchitis.

The best way to avoid damage to your lungs is to stop working in that industry. When you stop being exposed to the fibers, the illness resolves.

Treatment

Bronchodilators and antihistamines help control the symptoms.

Farmer's lung

Signs and symptoms

- Fever
- Chills
- Coughing that produces sputum
- Worsening shortness of breath on exertion
- Fatigue
- Nausea and vomiting
- Loss of appetite and weight

Farmer's lung is a type of lung disease caused by repeated inhalation of dust from moldy hay that contains spores of a fungus. Only a small percentage of people exposed to the spores develop the disease, and then only after considerable exposure.

Diagnosis

A medical history and physical examination, along with a chest X-ray and pulmonary function tests, may be used to confirm the diagnosis. The results of blood tests for antibodies associated with the disease can strongly suggest farmer's lung, but the results aren't diagnostic.

How serious is farmer's lung?

In temporary (acute) cases, avoiding exposure to moldy hay usually reduces the severity of symptoms within hours, although it may take weeks for a complete recovery. The disease can also become persistent (chronic), particularly if you're continually exposed to low levels of the fungus over long periods.

Treatment

Avoiding exposure to the dust from moldy hay is the only sure way to prevent progression to chronic disease. If you can't avoid contact with moldy hay, you might purchase a special type of protective dust mask that you wear when working with the hay. If you have a severe case of the disease, your doctor may prescribe a corticosteroid medication.

Silo filler's lung

Signs and symptoms

- An irritated, runny nose
- Coughing
- Shortness of breath

Silo filler's lung is an acute illness that results from inhalation of nitrous oxide fumes given off by moist silage. When inhaled, the gas irritates the bronchi and lungs.

How serious is silo filler's lung?

The severity of the illness depends on the length of exposure. A farmer can die after spending an extended period of time in a silo filled with the yellowish gas and acrid odor of oxides and nitrogen. Less exposure may cause only irritation of the respiratory tract.

If you've been exposed, see your doctor promptly. Irritation to the lungs from nitrous oxide fumes can lead to a collection of fluid in the lungs (pulmonary edema), which can result in permanent lung damage or be fatal. Exposure may also produce inflammation of the tiny airways near the alveoli (bronchiolitis), which can cause permanent damage to your lungs if you don't seek prompt treatment.

Treatment

Your doctor may prescribe a corticosteroid medication to prevent permanent damage to the lungs.

Fumes, Gases, Smoke and Air Pollution

Exposure to high concentrations of toxic fumes and gases, indoor and outdoor air pollutants, and smoke can cause various respiratory symptoms.

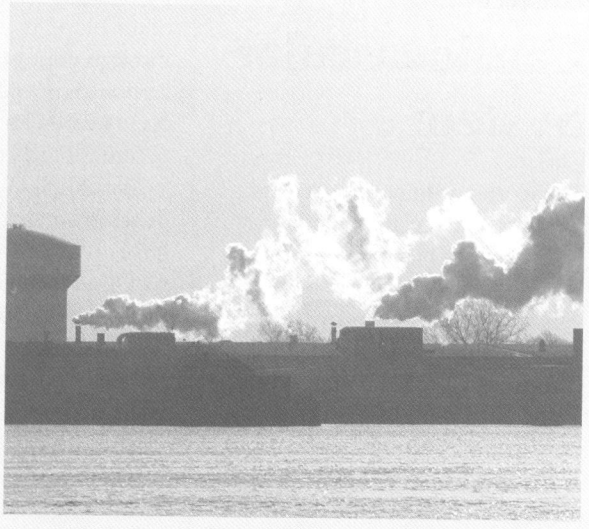

Industrial fumes and gases

Long-term, low-level exposure or accidental exposure to high levels of industrial toxic chemicals can cause various temporary (acute) and, sometimes, long-lasting (chronic) respiratory problems. Usually, the lower respiratory tract is affected, causing symptoms such as shortness of breath and coughing and possibly leading to chronic bronchitis. A sampling of toxic chemicals includes ammonia, cyanides, formaldehyde, hydrogen sulfide, diazomethane, halides, nitrogen dioxide, phosgene, phthalic anhydride and sulfur dioxide.

The industrial process of heating certain metals, such as cadmium, chromium, nickel and beryllium, to high temperatures and quickly cooling them releases fumes that can cause various respiratory diseases if inhaled. Signs and symptoms usually appear several hours after exposure and clear up within 24 hours, only to return with repeat exposure.

If you work in an industrial trade that uses high heat, such as welding, brazing, smelting, pottery making and furnace work, you may be at risk. Using nonhazardous compounds, ensuring adequate ventilation, and using safe machinery and work practices can help prevent exposure to toxic fumes.

Workers exposed to these fumes and gases and who also smoke have a greatly increased risk of developing lung cancer.

Outdoor air pollutants

Air pollution, such as that caused by automobiles, power plants and factories, can increase levels of ozone and sulfur dioxide in the air. Exposure to this pollution can cause wheezing in people who have asthma and may cause shortness of breath in older adults, young children and people with chronic cardiopulmonary disease. On days when the ozone level is high, usually after a long stretch of hot, humid weather, it may be best for individuals at risk to stay indoors.

Indoor air pollutants

Energy efficiency concerns have led to the construction of houses that are more tightly sealed than older houses were, and many codes now require outside air intake into heating and air conditioning systems. Therefore, fumes that once were of little concern may build up in the house instead of escaping to the outside. One example is cigarette smoke, which, besides having major health effects on the smoker, also affects nonsmokers who are exposed to it. Secondhand (passive) cigarette smoke has been shown to increase respiratory infections and decrease lung function in children whose parents smoke.

For people with asthma, poorly ventilated areas, wood smoke from wood-burning furnaces and fumes from kerosene floor heaters can aggravate symptoms.

Another potentially hazardous agent is formaldehyde. It's present in urethane foam insulation and in some types of flooring used in construction of new houses, mobile homes and furniture. New products made with formaldehyde may have a pungent odor due to formaldehyde fumes, which may irritate the eyes, nose, throat and airways. The formaldehyde gradually evaporates within a few months, after which it should cause no problem. But before it evaporates, it may worsen symptoms for people with respiratory disease.

Smoke

Whenever anything containing carbon burns, it produces carbon monoxide that, when inhaled, interferes with transportation of oxygen by the blood. All smoke contains some of this odorless gas. Be careful, therefore, when you have any fire indoors, such as from a wood-burning stove or fireplace. The effects of inhaling carbon monoxide are so subtle as to be unnoticeable, and you can become unconscious without realizing anything is wrong. Smoke that contains a heavy concentration of floating particles also irritates the lungs.

Many plastics, polyurethanes and other synthetic materials used in home furnishings give off toxic gases when they burn. They're particularly harmful to the lungs and may cause severe, temporary illness. Firefighters and others who have long-term exposure to smoke may have an increased risk of chronic illness, although this is difficult to measure.

Your Lungs and Cardiovascular System

The workings of your heart and lungs are interrelated. Blood travels from your heart through your lungs to be oxygenated.

If a blood clot forms in your veins and travels through your bloodstream, the clot may eventually become lodged in an artery in your lungs (pulmonary embolism). Chronic lung disease also can lead to heart failure of the right ventricle (cor pulmonale).

Pulmonary embolism

Signs and symptoms
- Sudden shortness of breath
- Chest pain that may mimic a heart attack
- Coughing that produces bloody or blood-streaked sputum
- Rapid heartbeat
- Wheezing
- Clammy or bluish-colored skin
- Leg swelling

The term *embolism* refers to blockage in an artery caused by an embolus. Usually, an embolus is a clot of blood, but sometimes it may be a globule of fat, an air bubble, tissue from a tumor or a clump of bacteria. This clot is carried into a blood vessel in the lungs, where it becomes lodged and interrupts blood flow.

Most emboli originate from blood clots (thrombi) in the veins of the lower extremities or pelvis. If they break free, the veins carry them up through the right side of the heart to a lung. Emboli may also arise from the walls of the heart. If a clot arises in the left side of the heart, then the embolus will go to the brain or some other part of the body, rather than to the lung. Tissue death (infarction) occurs when the clot blocks blood supply to tissues.

An embolism can occur in any small artery, but the lungs are particularly vulnerable because all of the blood in your body passes through your lungs. Pulmonary embolism is a condition that occurs when an artery in a lung becomes blocked.

About half the people who develop abnormal blood clots have an inherited tendency to do so. Other factors that may cause an unwanted clot to form include surgery and long periods of inactivity, such as occurs with prolonged bed rest or long airplane or car trips. In addition, any increase in the tendency of your blood to clot, including certain types of cancer, makes you more susceptible.

Signs and symptoms resulting from the blockage depend on the size of the embolus and the health of your cardiopulmonary system.

Diagnosis
A pulmonary embolism can be difficult to diagnose, especially in people with underlying lung or heart disease. A chest X-ray, a specialized computerized tomography (CT) scan of the chest, a lung scan or pulmonary angiogram may be used to detect the clot.

A lung scan called a ventilation-perfusion scan uses small amounts of radioactive tracers (radioisotopes) to study airflow and blood flow in your lungs. The radioisotopes are attached to substances known as radiopharmaceuticals so that a special device (gamma camera) can show images of air movement in your lungs and the movement of blood in the lungs' blood vessels. It can be useful in diagnosing pulmonary embolism. However, the findings of about half of all such lung scans are indeterminate. For this reason, CT angiography (CTA) is often used instead.

Pulmonary angiography is the most accurate test for detecting emboli in the lung. During a pulmonary angiogram, a dye is injected into a vein of an arm or leg. As it circulates into the arteries of the lung, the arteries are highlighted so that they show up better on an X-ray and clots, if present, can be seen. Your doctor may recommend other tests as well.

How serious is a pulmonary embolism?
In most cases, a pulmonary embolism isn't fatal. With appropriate diagnosis and treatment, the outlook is good. You should return to normal health within a few weeks unless you have another serious health condition.

Each year, the condition affects as many as 900,000 people in the United States and causes as many as 100,000 deaths. Once you've had a pulmonary embolism, you're at increased risk of another.

Treatment
Prompt treatment is essential in order to prevent serious complications or death.

Anticoagulants
Initially you may receive the fast-acting anticoagulant heparin, administered intravenously or under your skin (subcutaneously), which immediately helps prevent existing clots from enlarging and stops the formation of new ones. Your doctor may also prescribe the anticoagulant warfarin, a pill that's given by mouth. Warfarin also helps stop clot formation, but because it works less quickly than heparin does, both drugs must be overlapped for at least five days, until the warfarin effect alone is enough to prevent clot formation.

A newer class of anticoagulants, referred to as novel oral anticoagulants (NOACs), has been tested and approved for treatment of venous thromboembolism, including pulmonary embolism. These medications work quickly and have fewer interactions with food or other medications. Some NOACs have the advantage of being given by mouth, without the need for overlap with heparin. However, all anticoagulants have side effects, with bleeding being the most common.

After the original clot has dissolved, you'll likely continue to take an anticoagulant medication. How long depends on your particular case. If you have a chronic disorder that puts you at high risk of pulmonary embolism, you may need to stay on these drugs indefinitely. In general, though, you take them for at least three to six months.

As with all medications, the benefits of anticoagulants need to be weighed against the risks. Heparin, warfarin and NOACs reduce your chance of developing blood clots, but because they may also prevent normal blood coagulation, they increase your risk of bleeding complications. Many of these complications are minor, such as bleeding from your gums, but some may be severe and life-threatening.

If you're taking warfarin, you'll likely need periodic blood tests to check how well the drug is working.

During anticoagulant therapy, avoid using aspirin unless you have heart disease and your doctor instructs you to continue taking a low dose. Also avoid other nonsteroidal anti-inflammatory drugs such as ibuprofen (Advil, Motrin IB, others), which also affects your blood's ability to clot. Because more than 100 other drugs, including over-the-counter medications and some herbs, can interact with warfarin, be sure your doctor knows all the medications you're taking.

When pulmonary embolism is life-threatening

If you experience a massive pulmonary embolism, if you have worsening cardiopulmonary disease or if other treatments aren't effective, one of the following therapies may be an option:

- **Clot-dissolving (thrombolytic) therapy.** Rather than simply preventing clot formation, medications are prescribed to dissolve clots. They work by activating an enzyme that breaks down blood clots and are sometimes popularly referred to as "clotbusters."

  You're not a candidate for these drugs if you're pregnant, have had a recent stroke, have severe high blood pressure or have undergone surgery within the past 10 days. Thrombolytic medications increase your risk of bleeding. Some bleeding may be fatal, especially if bleeding occurs in the brain.
- **Vein filter.** In an attempt to block clots from being carried into the pulmonary artery, you may have a filter placed in the main vein (inferior vena cava) in your abdomen leading from your legs and pelvis to the right side of your heart. This is done by inserting the filter on the tip of a catheter through a vein in your groin or neck.

  Surgery is rarely is necessary to remove a large, obstructing blood clot.

Prevention

Anytime you have surgery, it's important to move around as soon as possible or to perform active and passive leg exercises to help prevent formation of a blood clot.

When sitting for long periods of time, such as on an airplane or in a car, make sure to walk periodically or at least wiggle your toes and move your feet. If you're immobilized, elevate your legs and perhaps wear support stockings. All of these can help prevent pooling and clotting of blood in your leg veins, a frequent cause of emboli.

If you're at risk of a recurrent pulmonary embolism, heparin, warfarin, an NOAC or an antiplatelet drug such as aspirin may be prescribed.

Lung Transplantation

A lung transplant is a surgical procedure to replace a diseased or failing lung with a healthy lung, usually from a deceased donor. A lung transplant is reserved for people who have tried other medications or treatments, but their conditions haven't sufficiently improved.

Depending on your medical condition, a lung transplant may involve replacing one of your lungs or both of them. In some situations, the lungs may be transplanted along with a donor heart.

Lung transplantation may be an option for individuals with end-stage lung disease who have a poor quality of life or a poor future prognosis or both.

Individuals considered for transplant are carefully screened to ensure they can tolerate the surgery and recovery, including immunosuppressant medications required afterwards.

A lung transplant may not be appropriate if you:
- Have an active infection
- Have a recent personal medical history of cancer
- Have serious diseases such as kidney, liver or heart diseases
- Are unwilling or unable to make lifestyle changes necessary to keep your donor lung healthy, such as not drinking alcohol or not smoking

People who are candidates for a transplant are listed according to blood type, size, and whether they require a heart-lung, bilateral-lung or single-lung transplant. The median wait time for a transplant is about four months.

Among individuals who undergo a lung transplant, the average survival is about 5.5 years, although long-term survival is possible.

Pulmonary hypertension

Signs and symptoms

- Shortness of breath while exercising and eventually at rest
- Fatigue
- Dizziness or fainting spells
- Chest pressure or pain
- Swelling in ankles and legs
- Bluish color to your lips and skin
- Racing pulse or heart palpitations

Pulmonary hypertension is a type of high blood pressure that affects the arteries in your lungs and the right side of your heart.

In one form of the disease, tiny arteries in your lungs, called pulmonary arterioles, and capillaries become narrowed, blocked or destroyed. This makes it harder for blood to flow through your lungs, and raises pressure within lung arteries. As the pressure builds, your heart's lower right chamber (right ventricle) must work harder to pump blood through your lungs, eventually causing your heart muscle to weaken and fail.

Diagnosis

Pulmonary hypertension is hard to diagnose early. Even when more advanced, its signs and symptoms are similar to those of other heart and lung conditions.

Tests used to help diagnose pulmonary hypertension include an echocardiogram, electrocardiogram, chest X-ray and a procedure called right heart catheterization, in which a thin tube (catheter) is threaded to your right ventricle and pulmonary artery and pressure in the artery is measured.

How serious is pulmonary hypertension?

Some forms of the disease are serious conditions that become progressively worse and can even be fatal.

Treatment

Pulmonary hypertension can't be cured, but treatments are available to control symptoms and help you manage the condition.

Medications

A variety of medications are used to treat the condition. They include blood vessel dilators (vasodilators) to open narrowed blood vessels.

Medications called endothelin receptor antagonists are designed to reverse the effect of endothelin, a substance in the walls of blood vessels that causes them to narrow. These drugs may improve your energy level and symptoms.

The medications sildenafil (Revatio, Viagra) and tadalafil (Cialis, Adcirca) are sometimes used to treat pulmonary hypertension. These drugs work by opening blood vessels in the lungs to allow blood to flow through more easily.

Other medications include anticoagulants to help prevent the formation of blood clots within the pulmonary arteries, diuretics to eliminate excess fluid in your body, and the drug digoxin (Lanoxin) to help your heart beat stronger and pump more blood. It can also help control arrhythmias.

Oxygen

You may need to breathe pure oxygen, a treatment known as oxygen therapy, especially if you live at a high altitude or have sleep apnea. Some people with pulmonary hypertension eventually require continuous oxygen.

Surgery

If medications don't control your pulmonary hypertension, open-heart surgery might be an option. In a procedure called atrial septostomy, a surgeon creates an opening between the upper left and right chambers of your heart (atria) to relieve the pressure on the right side of your heart. In some cases, a lung or heart-lung transplant might be an option.

Cor pulmonale

Signs and symptoms

- Swelling of the lower extremities
- Shortness of breath during exertion
- Bulging of the veins in the neck
- An enlarged and tender liver
- Weakness and fatigue

Cor pulmonale is enlargement and eventual failure of the lower right chamber of the heart (right ventricle) due to pulmonary disease. Because the heart and lungs are closely associated in function, diseases of the lungs often affect the heart as well.

Blood goes from the right side of the heart into the lungs, where carbon dioxide is removed and oxygen added to it. Normally, it doesn't take a great deal of pressure to move blood into the lungs, so the muscular walls of the right ventricle aren't as strong as those on the left side, which pumps blood under high pressure to the rest of the body. However, when emphysema, fibrosis or other severe chronic lung disease impairs your lungs, it requires more pressure to pump blood into them. Although the heart may compensate for a while, eventually it fails.

Diagnosis

Tests used to help diagnose cor pulmonale may include a pulmonary function test, chest X-ray, electrocardiogram and echocardiogram.

How serious is cor pulmonale?

Once symptoms of cor pulmonale appear, survival on average is two to five years. If the underlying cause is uncomplicated emphysema, survival may be considerably longer.

Treatment

An important step is to treat the underlying disease causing cor pulmonale, when possible. In addition, your doctor may advise the use of oxygen and restriction of salt and fluids. He or she might prescribe diuretic medications to control fluid accumulation in tissues or medications to dilate the pulmonary vessels. ■

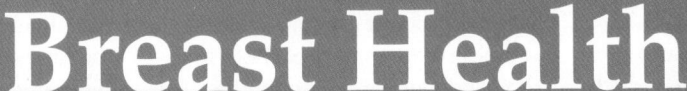

Breast Health

The structure of the human female breast is remarkable and complex. For the most part, female breasts consist of fat and connective tissue. This tissue houses a network of blood vessels, ducts and milk-producing glands called lobules.

During lactation, the glands secrete milk into a system of ducts — milk passages that connect the lobules to the nipples. The breasts are attached to the muscles of the chest wall by ligaments and connective tissue.

Nipples may be flat, but the tissue they're composed of contains nerves that cause the tissue to become erect (protrude) with certain types of stimulation, such as when they're cold or during sexual arousal. Some women's nipples are always erect, and other women's are turned inward (inverted). Having any of these types of nipples is perfectly normal.

Encircling the nipple is the areola, a ring of tissue the same color as the nipple. Oil glands in the areola lubricate the nipple during breast-feeding. In some women, these glands are visible as small bumps. Many women have hairs growing at the edges of the areola.

Blood vessels and lymph vessels also run throughout the breasts. Blood in the blood vessels nourishes breast tissues and cells. Lymph vessels carry a fluid called lymph, which contains immune system cells and drains waste products from tissues. Lymph vessels lead to pea-sized collections of tissue called lymph nodes.

Some women are self-conscious about their breasts. They think that their breasts are either too small or too large or are concerned because one breast is larger than the other.

Actually, breast size makes no difference either in sexual responsiveness or the ability to nurse a baby. It's also normal for a pair of breasts to differ somewhat from each other in size and shape.

Normal Breast Changes

To understand the diseases and conditions that can affect breasts, it's helpful for you to know how a normal breast functions. Hormones play a major role both in breast development and in the changes breasts undergo at different stages of life.

From puberty until after menopause, breasts change as hormones fluctuate. At puberty, when a girl's body first produces estrogen in quantity, her breasts rapidly develop both a framework of connective tissue (stroma) and a system of glands, ducts, blood vessels, lymph channels and nerves. At the same time, breasts develop fat cells, which make up the bulk of breast tissue.

The lymph system is made up of lymph, lymphatic vessels and lymph nodes. Lymph is a clear fluid containing tissue waste products and immune system cells. Lymphatic vessels are similar to very small veins, but they carry lymph instead of blood. Most of the lymphatic vessels of the breast drain into underarm (axillary) lymph nodes, which are largely collections of immune system cells.

After puberty, breasts change each month. During the first half of the menstrual cycle, the female ovaries release estrogen, which causes new cells to grow in glands, ducts and other breast tissue. Blood flow to the breasts also increases.

During the second half of the cycle, after ovulation, glands in the breasts are stimulated by progesterone as well as estrogen, and

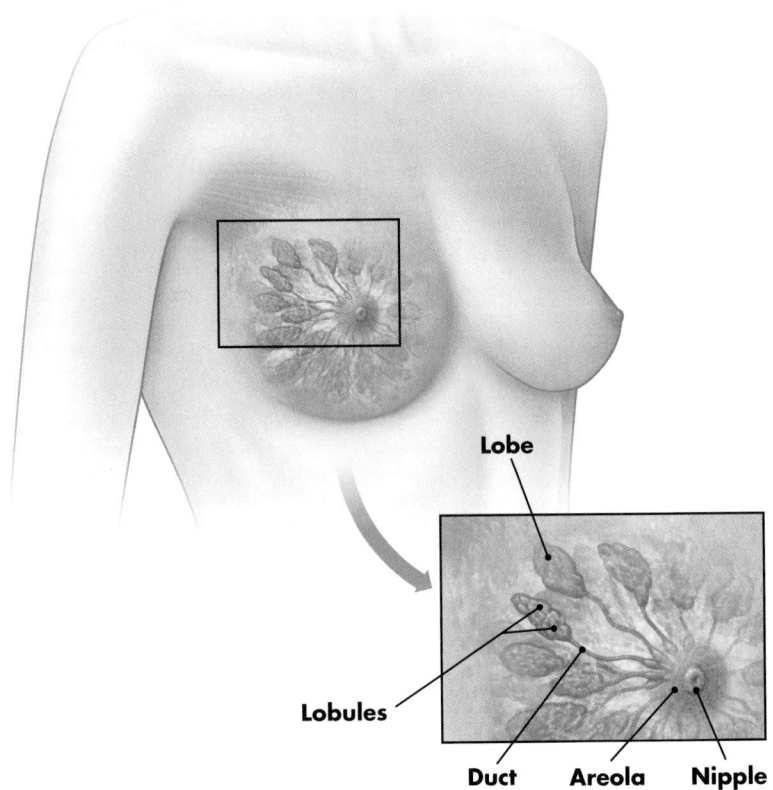

Lobe

Lobules

Duct   Areola   Nipple

The female breast includes milk-forming units called lobes. Each lobe is made up of smaller structures (lobules) that end in tiny bulbs. The lobes, lobules and bulbs are linked by a network of tubes called ducts. The ducts drain toward the nipple and areola.

Breast Reduction

Breast size can be much more than a cosmetic issue. Very large breasts can cause a host of problems, including:
- Chronic upper back, neck and shoulder pain
- Poor posture
- Persistent skin rash under the breasts
- Grooves worn in shoulders from bra straps
- Difficulty exercising

Such problems may be one reason why breast reduction surgery (reduction mammoplasty) has increased.

A large analysis of women who had breast reduction surgery indicated that the procedure significantly improved their physical symptoms and, for most of the women, their quality of life.

Benefits included decreased headache, back, neck, shoulder and breast pain, and reduced hand pain and numbness caused by pressure on the shoulders from bra straps.

The most commonly used technique for breast reduction surgery involves making an incision around the dark part of the breast (areola) and down to the crease under the breast so that the surgeon can remove tissue. Typically, the surgeon removes 1 to 3 pounds of breast tissue from each breast. The surgery leaves permanent scars, which can be covered by a bra or swimsuit.

As with any surgery, breast reduction surgery has a small risk of infection and adverse reaction to anesthesia. You may end up with breasts of slightly different sizes or unevenly positioned nipples. You may experience a permanent loss of sensation in the nipples and breasts.

Some breast reduction techniques can preserve enough of the milk duct system to allow future breast-feeding.

Recovery usually takes about six weeks. The surgery may be medically indicated and covered by medical insurance, but it usually requires prior authorization from the insurance company.

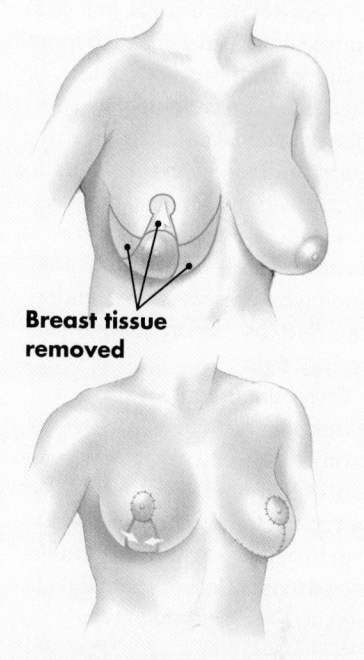

Breast tissue removed

The most commonly used breast reduction technique involves making an incision around the dark part of the breast (areola) and down to the crease under the breast. Typically, the surgeon removes 1 to 3 pounds of tissue from each breast.

---

they begin to secrete substances that are the precursors of breast milk. Unless pregnancy occurs, levels of these hormones decrease, the female body absorbs both the secretions and the new cells, and the blood supply to the breasts diminishes.

Some women's breasts become engorged and can be painful just before their menstrual period. Other women have water-filled cysts in their breasts that may enlarge at that time. Birth control pills also can cause breast tenderness and swelling, although most women who take birth control pills don't experience such side effects.

During pregnancy, the breasts gradually enlarge. Together they may gain as much as a pound. Their duct systems and lobules — stimulated by hormones produced

by the placenta and the pituitary gland — grow and branch. The body creates more cells in the stroma and adds fat cells. The nipple and areola often grow larger and become darker.

Once the baby is born, additional hormones affect the breasts. Prolactin, produced by the pituitary gland, regulates milk production. Even before the baby is weaned and breast stimulation ends, prolactin production tapers off.

After weaning, the flow of breast milk ceases, and the breasts return to nearly their pre-pregnancy state.

At menopause, breast changes that occur during the reproductive cycle generally cease. Problems such as cystic breast lumps often diminish or disappear. However, the risk of breast cancer increases at this time.

Become familiar with monthly breast changes and learn to identify new changes that may require medical evaluation. This is even more important after menopause.

Breast Disorders

Breast conditions range from uncomfortable but harmless menstrual swelling to breast cancer.

Premenstrual tenderness and swelling

Signs and symptoms
- Swelling in the breast
- Lumpiness in the breast
- Breast discomfort

During each menstrual cycle, you may experience temporary changes in your breasts. Just as the uterine lining thickens each month in preparation for a possible pregnancy, breasts develop new cells in their glands and ducts over the course of the month to prepare for breast-feeding. Thus, in the week or so before menstruation, your breasts become engorged. For some women, this causes tenderness and discomfort, known as cyclical pain.

Breast engorgement also is a symptom of premenstrual syndrome (PMS). No one knows what causes this syndrome, but it may be related to hormonal changes that take place near the end of your menstrual cycle. For more information on PMS, see page 1195.

Diagnosis

Your doctor may ask you to keep a record of premenstrual symptoms for a few months, noting the day your breasts become uncomfortable, the day your discomfort ends and the day your period starts. Although it can be painful, premenstrual breast engorgement isn't considered serious.

Treatment

Medications and self-care techniques may ease the discomfort of premenstrual symptoms.

Medication

If you have severe breast pain, taking a nonsteroidal anti-inflammatory drug (NSAID), such as ibuprofen (Advil, Motrin IB, others), before your period begins may provide some relief.

Self-care

You may feel more comfortable if you cut down on salt before the end of your cycle because excessive salt can contribute to and worsen breast engorgement. Caffeine may contribute to breast tenderness, so you might want to cut your intake or switch to decaffeinated products.

A comfortable bra worn 24 hours a day may help as well. An underwire bra can exacerbate tender breasts. If you wear this type of bra, try switching to one without an underwire during this time of the month.

Breast infections

Signs and symptoms

- Tenderness and redness of the skin on the breast
- Painful swelling or a lump in your breast
- Swelling of nearby lymph glands in your underarm area
- Flu-like symptoms
- Fever (uncommon)

Breast infection, also known as mastitis, is common in women who are nursing a baby or who've recently stopped breast-feeding. The condition is caused by bacteria that enter one or both breasts.

If the infection is severe, it can form an abscess. Surrounding tissues protect themselves by secreting a substance that creates a wall around the infection. Pus collects inside, and the overlying skin is often red and tender.

Diagnosis

If you're breast-feeding, the signs and symptoms listed above strongly suggest mastitis. Breast infections can also develop in women who aren't breast-feeding. If you develop such an infection your doctor will likely want to see you soon after your treatment is complete to make sure that the infection has cleared up.

Persistent or frequent recurrences of a breast infection require prompt evaluation to rule out cancer. The evaluation may include a mammogram, an ultrasound and a biopsy procedure.

How serious are breast infections?

Breast infections usually respond quickly to treatment. If they don't, an abscess may form, which could require surgical care.

Treatment

Antibiotic medication will usually clear up a breast infection. However, sometimes medication may not be completely effective and a surgical procedure known as incision and drainage is necessary.

Medication

Your doctor will likely prescribe an antibiotic and perhaps an analgesic for pain and fever. If you're breast-feeding, continue to do so. These drugs shouldn't have any harmful effects on your milk supply or on your baby.

Self-care

Get adequate rest and increase your intake of fluids. Applying warm compresses to the affected area also may help reduce pain.

? Question and Answer

What is a yeast infection of the breast?

Yeast (candida) is a fungal organism that may infect your nipples and breasts during breast-feeding. You may experience pain in your nipple or breast, even when your baby is correctly positioned and sucking properly. The pain can be in one nipple or breast or in both.

Signs and symptoms include red, itchy, flaky skin on the nipple or the dark area surrounding it (areola). Cracked nipples that don't heal may be due to a yeast infection. Other symptoms may include a burning, throbbing pain in your breast during or after feeding. Your baby may have no signs or symptoms or may have thrush or a diaper rash caused by a yeast infection.

Yeast infections also can occur after antibiotic treatment. See your doctor.

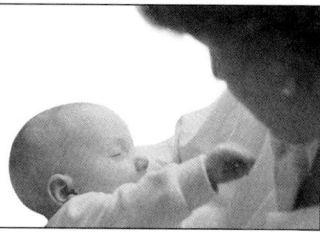

Surgery

Usually, an antibiotic is sufficient treatment, but if an abscess forms, it needs to be drained. Your doctor may aspirate the abscess with a needle or drain it by making a small incision.

Nipple disorders

Signs and symptoms

- Discharge from your nipple
- A nipple that's newly inverted
- Lumps in the area surrounding your nipple (areola)
- Scaling of your nipple

It's wise to pay attention to changes in your nipples. Although most often the cause is noncancerous (benign), some changes are cancer related.

Yellow, green, brown or gray fluid that leaks from multiple ducts in both your nipples is likely due to either fibrocystic changes of the breasts (see page 801) or dilated ducts (mammary duct ectasia). Whitish fluid from multiple ducts is probably breast milk, especially if it comes from both nipples.

A discharge that's dark red or black likely contains blood. It may indicate a tiny, benign tumor growing in a milk duct, although breast cancer is a remote possibility. A discharge that's clear (watery) also can indicate an underlying cancer.

Inverted nipples are normal if you've had them since puberty. A nipple that inverts later in life can be a sign of cancer.

Small lumps in your areola generally are cysts caused by blocked oil glands. If an infection develops, a cyst may turn into a boil.

Scaling of a nipple is usually due to benign changes. If scaling persists, you may need a biopsy to rule out an underlying cancer. Paget's disease of the breast is a type of breast cancer that usually appears first as a red, scaly or itchy nipple. It may also appear on the areola. It may be misdiagnosed as eczema, a type of skin disease.

Diagnosis

If you notice any unusual changes in your nipples or breasts, see your doctor for a breast examination. For a newly inverted nipple or a bloody discharge, diagnostic tests may include a mammogram, ultrasound and biopsy procedure.

How serious are nipple disorders?

Nipple discharge and inverted nipples are rarely serious. However, they can be an indication of cancer, so it's important to have an evaluation by your doctor to evaluate new changes and determine the cause.

Treatment

If the changes aren't cancer related, you may not need treatment. In the case of an infected cyst or persistent inflammation, your doctor will likely prescribe an antibiotic. Whether surgery is necessary depends on the underlying problem.

Galactorrhea

Signs and symptoms

- Whitish discharge from your nipples, usually from both breasts
- Missed menstrual periods (amenorrhea)

Normally, you produce breast milk only after giving birth, for as long as you continue breast-feeding. Some women, though, will have milky discharge persist for several months to a year after completion of breast-feeding. If your nipples leak milk at other times, you may have an uncommon condition called galactorrhea. The name comes from the Greek words *gala*, for "milk," and *rhoia*, for "flow."

Approximately 25 percent of women with galactorrhea have a type of pituitary tumor called a prolactinoma. The tumor is usually noncancerous (benign) but secretes prolactin, the hormone that regulates production of breast milk. Galactorrhea also may be caused by medication or a chest wall injury.

Medications that can cause galactorrhea include certain antipsychotics, antidepressants, sedatives and stimulants, as well as anti-nausea drugs and some opioid medications.

Diagnosis

If you're experiencing signs and symptoms, see your doctor for a breast examination. To help determine the cause of the problem, your doctor may run some tests, including those to check your prolactin and thyroid hormone levels. Other tests may include magnetic resonance imaging (MRI) of your hypothalamus and pituitary gland.

How serious is galactorrhea?

Galactorrhea isn't threatening to your health unless it's caused by a pituitary tumor. Such tumors grow slowly, and some eventually stabilize. They often can be treated successfully with medication. If that fails, your doctor may recommend surgery or radiation.

Treatment

The type of treatment you receive for galactorrhea will depend on the cause of the disease. The two main types of treatment are medication and surgery.

Breast-Feeding

Women choose to breast-feed because of the health benefit to their babies and for the mother-baby bonding opportunity it offers. Breast milk is biologically complex. It provides your baby with unique protection against infections and stimulates the development of the baby's immune system.

The sticky, yellowish fluid secreted by your breasts for the first several days after you give birth (colostrum) contains hormones and antibodies that benefit your baby. After three to five days, your pituitary gland directs your breasts to produce mature milk, which contains essential nutrients. The removal of milk from your breasts sustains your milk production.

The let-down reflex controls the flow of breast milk. When a baby suckles, the nipples respond by sending sensory impulses to the brain. The pituitary gland releases hormones, principally oxytocin, into the bloodstream. When the hormones reach the breasts, they cause the cells surrounding the cavities where milk is produced (alveoli) to contract, expressing milk into the ducts.

Initially, this process may take several minutes. Once you establish breast-feeding, the let-down reflex triggers easily, often merely in response to your baby's cry.

Expect some temporary nipple tenderness initially. You shouldn't experience pain, which is generally a sign that something is wrong. Make sure your baby's mouth is centered on the nipple area. You can help avoid nipple injury by positioning your baby properly while nursing.

Breast-feeding should be enjoyable for both you and your baby. Using a breast pump intermittently can enable you to have a more flexible lifestyle.

You may experience a plugged milk duct when you breast-feed, or you may develop a breast lump that's hot and painful. For relief, try heat, rest, massage and prolonged, frequent nursing. If the lump does not get better with these measures, you may have mastitis.

Mastitis is a breast infection usually caused by bacteria. Signs and symptoms include fever, flu-like symptoms, and breast pain and redness. For relief, increase fluids, get more rest and apply heat to the affected area. In addition, notify your doctor, who will likely prescribe an antibiotic.

Weaning your child from breast milk should be a gradual process. Abrupt weaning can be difficult for you and your baby and can result in engorged breasts. Starting your baby on solid food at about six months can begin the weaning process.

Prolactin, the hormone that helps prepare your breasts for breast-feeding, offers some protection from pregnancy. But don't rely solely on it for birth control. You may ovulate while breast-feeding, even if you don't menstruate.

Medication

For hypothyroidism, your doctor is likely to prescribe the medication levothyroxine (Levoxyl, Synthroid, others). If you have a pituitary tumor that's causing the problem, treatment will depend on the size of the tumor and the management of symptoms, such as vision changes or low sex hormone levels. Medications such as cabergoline or bromocriptine (Parlodel) are recommended as the first line of treatment to shrink the tumor and reduce prolactin levels.

Surgery

For a large pituitary tumor, surgery may be necessary. Because such tumors tend to recur, you may need long-term treatment with bromocriptine or a course of radiation.

Intraductal papilloma

Signs and symptoms
- Watery or bloody discharge from your nipple
- A very small lump under your nipple

An intraductal papilloma is a tiny, noncancerous (benign) tumor that grows within a milk duct of your breast — usually under the areola or the nipple.

These uncommon tumors are often too small to feel. An intraductal papilloma may be detected on ultrasound.

Diagnosis

Your doctor will likely go through diagnostic procedures to make sure you don't have breast cancer. These may include a mammogram or an ultrasound. He or she may apply gentle pressure in the area around your nipple to try to reproduce the discharge to help determine which duct may contain a papilloma. Although intraductal papillomas are benign, they should be biopsied or surgically removed to be sure the lump is a papilloma and not cancer.

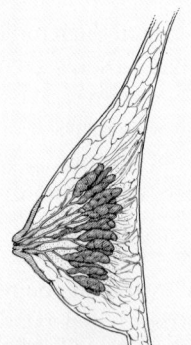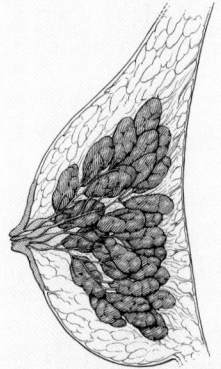

When breast-feeding, the system of ducts and glands within the breast expands as milk is produced, a process called lactation.

Treatment

Treatment may be necessary if your doctor can feel a lump. When no lump is present, but a bloody discharge persists from a single duct, your doctor may recommend a procedure called a duct exploration, in which milk ducts beneath the nipple are removed.

If the discharge occurred only once, careful follow-up may be recommended. This may include a clinical breast exam, a mammogram, an ultrasound exam of the breast, or a combination of these procedures.

Breast lumps

Signs and symptoms

- A change or thickening of breast tissue that makes it feel different from surrounding tissue
- One or more lumps in a breast that may or may not be painful
- Dimpling of the skin
- A greenish or straw-colored discharge from your nipple

Most breast lumps aren't cancerous, but some are. That's why it's important to have them evaluated promptly.

Cysts

A breast lump that occurs around the time of menstruation often is a harmless cyst. A breast cyst is a fluid-filled sac that tends to enlarge near the end of your menstrual cycle, when your body is retaining more fluid. After menstruation, this type of lump often disappears.

Some cysts are tiny, but others can be as large as an egg. Cysts are often round with smooth edges, and they typically can be moved under the skin. The cyst may feel like a soft grape or a water-filled balloon. Sometimes a cyst may feel firm.

Breast cysts develop when an overgrowth of glands and connective tissue block milk ducts, causing them to dilate and fill with fluid. You're most likely to develop cysts when in your 30s

and 40s, years before menopause. Because cysts generally disappear after menopause, changes in ovarian hormones probably cause the fluctuations in size.

A lump that persists and doesn't decrease in size after two to three menstrual cycles should be evaluated by a doctor.

Fibrocystic breasts

Fibrocystic breasts are more common in women in their 20s and 30s. This condition is also known as fibrocystic breast changes or chronic cystic mastitis.

In this condition, growth or proliferation of fibrous connective tissue and ducts — in combination with cyst development — causes glandular tissue in the breast to thicken. The result is dense, lumpy breast tissue.

The thickened tissue usually is more prominent in the upper, outer region of your breast. This condition is also associated with variations in hormonal levels during your menstrual cycle, and it can be painful.

If an area of thickening increases, persists or doesn't lessen after a menstrual cycle, have the breast evaluated.

Fibroadenomas

Breast lumps that are neither cysts nor cancer are most likely to be fibroadenomas. These noncancerous (benign) tumors most often develop in women in the first half of their childbearing years.

A fibroadenoma has a firm, smooth, rubbery feeling and a well-defined shape. It can be moved about under the skin. It develops when connective tissue grows within the glands or lobules of the breast.

Others

Other types of breast lumps include those caused by infection (abscess) or by bleeding from an injury (hematoma). A lump caused by a tumor of the fatty tissues is called a lipoma. A lump may also

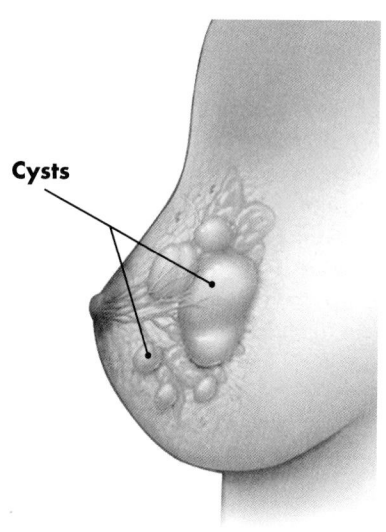

Cysts

Many women have lumpy (fibrocystic) breasts. The condition is most often associated with hormonal changes that occur with menstruation.

stem from an intraductal papilloma, especially if the papilloma is blocking a duct, causing a cyst. None of these conditions increases your risk of breast cancer.

Diagnosis

Your doctor's main focus will be on making sure the lumps in your breast aren't cancerous.

Cyst aspiration

If you have a single lump that feels like a cyst, your doctor may try to draw (aspirate) fluid from it by using a thin needle. If fluid can be aspirated, the lump may disappear, an indication that it was a cyst.

If the fluid found in a cyst is straw-colored or yellow, it may not need to be analyzed. If the fluid appears bloody or abnormal, or if the lump doesn't disappear after the fluid is aspirated, then your doctor may send the liquid that's removed to a laboratory to be analyzed for evidence of cancer. Your doctor may also recommend further evaluation of the lump with ultrasound and mammography.

Know Your Breasts

Becoming familiar with your breasts can be lifesaving because it can alert you to cancerous (malignant) breast lumps. Studies suggest that breast self-examination can cause needless worry and anxiety and lots of breast biopsies that come back negative — that don't detect cancer. It's true that most breast lumps are noncancerous (benign). However, if you find a lump and it is cancerous, the earlier treatment begins the better your chance for a successful outcome.

All women should try to examine their breasts periodically and become familiar with what is normal for them. If you haven't reached menopause, the best time is a few days after your period ends because your breasts are less likely to be tender or swollen then. If you're no longer menstruating, then pick a day of the month and try to do the examination on that date.

Here are things to look for:

1. Stand nude in front of a mirror. With your arms at your sides, look at your breasts for puckering or dimpling or for changes in their size, shape or skin color (redness or pitting). Unless your nipples are normally inverted, make sure they haven't turned inward. Rest your hands on your hips, then place them behind your head. Check for the same signs in each position.

2. When you're in shower and your breasts are wet, place your left hand behind your head and examine your left breast with your right hand. Think of your breast as the face of a clock and place your right hand at 12 o'clock, at the top of the breast, approximately $1/2$ inch below your collarbone. Hold your hand flat, fingertips pressed together, and, using the pads of your three middle fingers (not the fingertips), move your fingers toward the nipple. Move your hand to 1 o'clock and do the same, to 2 o'clock, and so on — like the spokes on a wheel. Use this pattern until you have checked every part of your breast, including the nipple. This procedure also can be done lying on your back instead of in the shower.

3. To check for nipple discharge, make a V shape with your thumb and first finger and place to the left and right of your nipple. Push down on the areola and gently pull up once. Then change the position of the V shape so that the thumb and finger lie on the areola above and below the nipple. Push down and gently pull up.

4. Examine the area adjacent to your breast, under your armpit, because it also contains breast tissue and lymph nodes that drain the lymph channels in the breast tissue.

5. Do the same examinations using your left hand on your right breast.

6. If your breasts are normally lumpy because of fibrocystic changes, make a note of how many lumps you have, where they're situated and approximately what size they are. Each month, check for changes. Once you know what's normal for your breasts, if you find a new lump or lumps that persist for two or three menstrual cycles or increase in size, see your doctor.

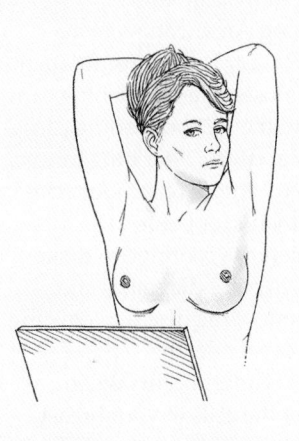

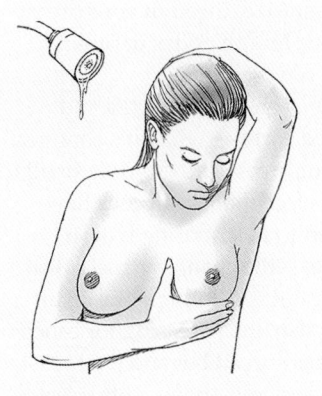

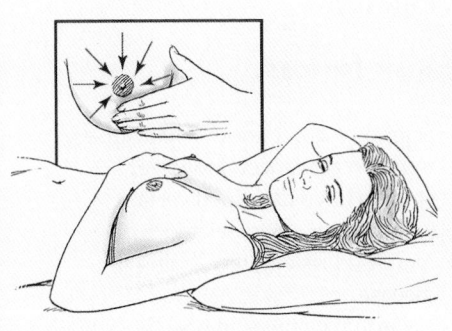

Use your eyes and hands to examine your breasts for skin changes, lumps, thickened areas or swelling. Feel for lumps in your breasts while you're standing or lying down.

Ultrasound

Ultrasound also may be used in an initial evaluation of a lump. When performed by an experienced operator, an ultrasound exam can reliably detect a cyst. If confirmed by ultrasound, a cyst doesn't need to be aspirated as long as you have no symptoms. However, if your cyst is painful, then aspiration may relieve your discomfort.

Mammography

If aspiration fails to find fluid in a lump, your doctor may recommend a mammogram. If a mammogram indicates a lump, or if an ultrasound procedure shows a solid area rather than a fluid-filled cyst, the next step may be a biopsy to remove some or all of the lump and examine it under a microscope.

Biopsy

Several types of needle biopsies can be used to help evaluate a breast lump.

- **Fine-needle aspiration.** Fine needle aspiration tends to be the least accurate because it may not be performed with imaging guidance, creating the risk of not sampling the lump in question. In addition, the technique only samples cells and it may not adequately sample the tissue.
- **Core biopsy.** A core biopsy, performed by a radiologist or surgeon using ultrasound guidance is considered very accurate. The procedure is done while using local anesthesia. A stereotactic biopsy, also performed by a radiologist and with local anesthesia, involves use of special mammogram imaging for guidance.
- **Surgical biopsy.** A surgical biopsy (excisional biopsy, or lumpectomy), which involves removing the whole lump, is another way to determine the cause of a lump. A surgical biopsy is done in a hospital or an outpatient surgical facility, using either local or general anesthesia.

How serious are breast lumps?

The majority of lumps aren't cancerous. Benign lumps usually aren't harmful beyond causing occasional discomfort. All lumps, though, need to be taken seriously until cancer has been excluded.

Some breast lumps, such as complex fibroadenomas, are associated with an increased risk of breast cancer. Most fibrocystic changes don't increase breast cancer risk. However, women with lumpy breasts may have more trouble detecting a cancerous tumor, if one were to develop.

Check for changes or thickening when you examine your breasts. If you find anything new that persists, increases in size or changes consistency, notify your doctor promptly.

Treatment

Depending on the type of lumps you have, they may be treated with medications or a medical procedure. Self-care measures also may be useful.

Medication

Some women take mild pain relievers, such as aspirin or ibuprofen (Advil, Motrin IB, others), for pain associated with cysts or fibrocystic breast changes. The medications danazol and bromocriptine (Parlodel) may relieve breast pain, but both can have unpleasant side effects and are expensive.

Vitamin E is sometimes taken to relieve symptoms, but there's no definitive evidence it works. Evening primrose oil may relieve cyclical breast pain in some women.

Self-care

Good breast support with a well-fitted bra, worn even at night, can be effective at relieving some breast discomfort.

If you drink caffeinated beverages, you may want to cut back on how much you consume or switch to decaffeinated products. Although the evidence is inconclusive, some women report that their

Lifestyle and Breast Cancer

Can the decisions you make about exercise, alcohol use and managing your weight affect your risk of breast cancer? Growing evidence suggests they may.

Exercise

Several studies indicate that low levels of physical activity — being sedentary — may increase breast cancer risk. Evidence also suggests that moderate to vigorous physical activity is associated with lower risk.

Exercise may influence hormone levels and is thought to boost the body's natural immune function.

Alcohol

Studies have consistently shown that women who consume two or more alcoholic beverages every day are at increased risk of breast cancer compared with nondrinkers. To reduce your risk, drink alcohol in moderation.

Weight

Being overweight or obese increases the risk of breast cancer in postmenopausal women. The more overweight you are, the greater the risk. Fat increases your estrogen levels, which may increase your breast cancer risk.

Additional studies are needed to confirm these relationships, but making healthy dietary and exercise decisions certainly can't hurt because they result in many other known health benefits.

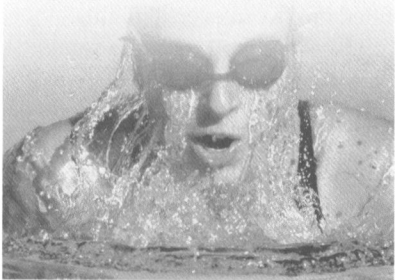

lumps subsided after they gave up caffeine or reduced its intake.

Medical procedure
If the cysts are painful or they're filled with blood, your doctor may aspirate them. If they aren't painful or bothersome — and diagnostic imaging results are consistent with your cysts and aren't worrisome — it's not necessary to remove the fluid. It's possible the cysts may recur or enlarge following aspiration.

Any solid-appearing lump, even if it has a benign appearance on an ultrasound image or a mammogram, is typically biopsied to exclude cancer. A lump that's been confirmed by biopsy to be a fibroadenoma may be left in place unless it's uncomfortable or increases in size. You and your doctor will want to check it regularly to see if it continues to grow.

A fibroadenoma that continues to grow is usually removed surgically because of a small risk of cancer and, in case of a phyllodes tumor, to prevent further growth. A phyllodes tumor is a rare, rapidly growing breast tumor. It's usually noncancerous (benign), but some contain cancer (malignant) cells.

Breast Cancer

Signs and symptoms
- A new lump or thickening in your breast, which may not be painful
- Clear or bloody discharge from a nipple
- Retraction or indentation of a nipple
- A change in the size or contours of your breasts
- Any dimpling or puckering of the skin of your breast
- Redness or pitting of breast skin

An estimated 255,000 new cases of female breast cancer are diagnosed yearly in the United States. Approximately 1 in 8 women

(about 12 percent) will develop invasive breast cancer over the course of their lifetimes.

Among American women, breast cancer is the most frequently diagnosed life-threatening cancer, and the second-leading cause of cancer death, after lung cancer. Yet there's more reason for optimism than ever before. Doctors and scientists continue to make strides in early diagnosis and treatment of the disease, reducing breast cancer deaths.

Breast cancer occurs when some of the cells in your breast begin growing abnormally. These cells divide more rapidly than do healthy cells and they can spread (metastasize) through your breast to your lymph nodes or other parts of your body.

If the cancer is detected and treated early — while it's confined to your breast, the tumor is small, and before malignant cells have spread to neighboring lymph nodes — the chance of successful treatment is very high. Survival odds also are increasing for cancer that has spread beyond the breast.

Fortunately, today, with greater use of mammography and other cancer-screening methods, doctors often can detect breast cancer at an early stage.

Risk factors

Scientists don't know what causes most breast cancer. However, studies have identified certain factors that are associated with increased risk of developing the disease.

Certain changes in breast tissue are thought to precede the development of breast cancer. If these changes are identified in your breast tissue, your risk of breast cancer is higher than it is for women who don't have these "markers." Precancerous breast changes are often discovered after a breast biopsy done for another reason.

Types of precancerous changes include:

- **Atypical hyperplasia.** Abnormal cells associated with this condition may develop in either a duct or lobule. Women with atypical hyperplasia have about a fourfold increased risk of developing breast cancer compared with women who don't have the condition.
- **Lobular carcinoma *in situ* (LCIS).** This condition occurs within the lobules located at the end of the breast ducts. Most experts don't consider LCIS to be a cancer in and of itself. Rather, it's seen as an area of abnormal tissue growth that signals increased risk of developing invasive cancer later on. This increased risk applies to both breasts.

Other risk factors include:

- **Age.** Your chances of developing breast cancer increase with age.
- **Personal history.** If you've had breast cancer in one breast, you have an increased risk of developing it in the other breast.

- **Family history.** You have a significantly higher risk than do most women if you have a mother, sister or daughter with breast cancer, especially if it was diagnosed before age 50.
- **Genetic predisposition.** Between 5 and 10 percent of breast cancers are inherited. Defects in one of several genes — especially the BRCA1 or BRCA2 genes — put you at greater risk of developing breast, ovarian and colon cancers.
- **Radiation exposure.** If you received radiation treatments to your chest as a child or young adult, you're more likely to develop breast cancer later in life.
- **Excess weight.** The relationship between excess weight and breast cancer is complex. In general, weighing more than is healthy increases your risk.
- **Early onset of menstruation or late menopause.** If you got your period at a young age, especially before age 12, or if you still are experiencing menstruation

after age 55, you have a greater likelihood of developing breast cancer. Experts attribute the increased risk to prolonged exposure of breast tissue to the hormone estrogen.
- **Late pregnancy or no pregnancy.** Your risk is somewhat increased if you've never had children or if you were older than age 35 when you had your first child.
- **Breast density.** Women with denser breasts have a higher cancer risk than do those with less dense breasts.
- **Environment.** Interaction between your genetic makeup and the environment may play a role.

Interestingly, most breast cancers develop in women with no identifiable risk factors.

Screening

To increase your chances of detecting breast cancer at an early stage — when chances of successful treatment are highest — it's important to be screened. Early detection of breast cancer, while the tumor is small and before it spreads, is key to survival. Screening includes:

Breast awareness
Beginning around age 20, become familiar with your breasts — their usual appearance and how they feel (see page 802). Awareness of how your breasts normally look and feel may help in detecting early signs of breast cancer. If you notice a change, promptly bring it to your doctor's attention.

Clinical breast exam
In women with no family history of breast cancer, many professional organizations no longer recommend that doctors perform a yearly clinical breast exam. If you have a strong family history of breast cancer or other factors that place you at high risk, talk to your doctor about having a yearly

Inherited Breast Cancer: Are You at Risk?

An estimated 5 to 10 percent of breast cancer is thought to be inherited. Several breast cancer susceptibility genes have been identified, including breast cancer genes 1 and 2 (BRCA1 and BRCA2). A blood test may be helpful in determining if you carry a breast cancer gene mutation. Clues that may point to inherited breast cancer include a strong family history of breast cancer on either your mother's side or father's side, multiple women on one side diagnosed with the disease, and development of the disease before age of 50.

Being diagnosed with a breast cancer susceptibility gene doesn't mean you'll get cancer, but your risk is greater. Different therapies to prevent breast cancer caused by gene abnormalities are being explored. In the meantime, if you have a genetic alteration, be vigilant about monitoring for signs of breast cancer. Be sure to do breast self-exams and discuss with your doctor how often you should have clinical breast exams, mammograms and, possibly, breast magnetic resonance imaging (MRI). Women with a gene alteration should begin annual breast mammograms and MRI at age 30.

Some women at high risk choose to have their breasts removed. This preventive procedure is called prophylactic surgery. It significantly reduces the risk of breast cancer, but doesn't eliminate it entirely because some breast tissue remains.

clinical breast exam. During a clinical exam, your doctor examines your breasts for lumps and discrete areas of firm or thickening tissue.

Mammography

A mammogram is an X-ray of the breast that uses low doses of radiation to view breast tissue. It can detect tumors even before you or your doctor can feel them.

Mammography saves lives by identifying breast cancer at an early stage when it's the most curable. However, the test isn't infallible.

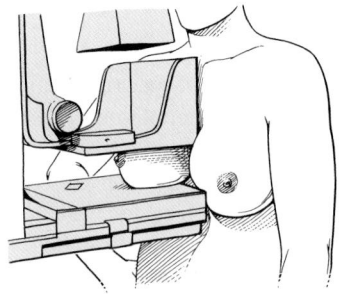

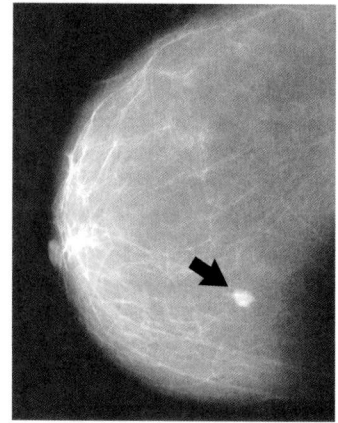

Mammograms are produced by a special X-ray device (top) that can detect tumors before you or your doctor can feel them. The mammogram image at right shows breast cancer (see arrow).

Advances in Detection

Mammography is the most commonly used method to screen for breast cancer so that the disease can be detected early.

However, standard mammography can miss about 15 percent of cancers, especially in women with dense breast tissue. Conversely, approximately 3 out of 4 areas that look like a cause for concern on a mammogram will end up being noncancerous (benign).

Advances in screening hope to detect more cancers earlier and prevent false-positives.

Computer-aided detection

After a radiologist reviews a mammogram, a sophisticated form of computer technology — mammography enhanced by computer-aided detection (CAD) — scans the film for suspicious areas and highlights them for a closer look.

Research indicates that CAD identifies more suspicious areas than does standard mammography, but many of the suspicious areas often prove to be noncancerous. CAD is now commonly performed in most mammography centers.

Digital mammography

An electronic process is used to collect and display X-ray images on a computer screen — as opposed to on film. This allows a radiologist to alter contrast and darkness, making it easier to identify subtle differences in tissue.

In addition, digital images can be transmitted electronically so women living in remote areas can have their mammograms more easily and quickly transmitted to and read by an expert located elsewhere. Studies have found digital images to be most helpful in evaluating dense breast tissue in women in their 40s.

Magnetic resonance imaging

Magnetic resonance imaging (MRI) can reveal tumors that are too small to be detected through a physical examination and difficult to see on conventional mammograms. In addition, it can help distinguish between noncancerous and cancerous (malignant) tumors. MRI is used in addition to, not in place of, traditional mammography.

Using magnetic fields and radio waves linked to a computer, MRI takes pictures of the inside of the breast. Unlike mammography, it doesn't pick up microcalcifications, tiny calcium deposits that can serve as an early sign of breast cancer.

Although MRI isn't used for routine screening, studies have found it's a valuable tool for women at very high risk of developing breast cancer. This includes women who:
- Carry a BRCA1 or BRCA2 gene mutation or other known hereditary breast cancer gene mutations
- Have a strong family history of breast or ovarian cancer with a family member known to have a genetic mutation
- Have a greater than 20 to 25 percent lifetime risk of developing breast cancer based on risk calculation models that take family history into account
- Received radiation to the chest wall before age 30

Ultrasound examination

Your doctor may use this technique to evaluate an abnormality seen on a mammogram or found during a clinical exam. Ultrasound uses sound waves to produce images of structures deep within the body. It's a safe diagnostic tool that can help determine whether an area of concern is a cyst or a solid tissue.

Breast ultrasound isn't used for routine screening because it has a high rate of false-positive results — it indicates problems where none exist.

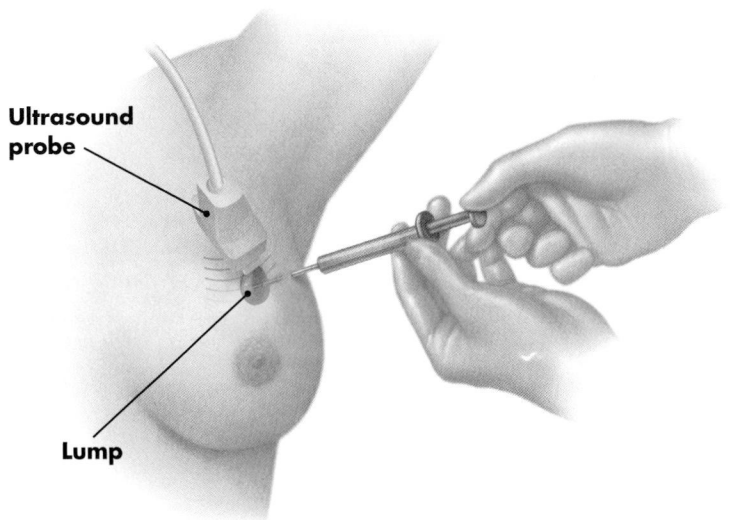

During fine-needle aspiration and core needle biopsy, a needle is inserted into a suspicious mass (lump) and tissue is removed for examination. A larger needle is used in core needle biopsy than in fine-needle aspiration. Ultrasound may be used to guide the needle to the location.

Occasionally, it fails to show a tumor, especially in dense breasts, and at other times it can indicate a problem when none exists. There are two types of mammograms:

- **Screening mammograms.** Screening mammograms are performed on a regular basis — approximately every one to two years — to check your breast tissue for any changes since your last mammogram.
- **Diagnostic mammograms.** Your doctor may recommend a diagnostic mammogram to evaluate a breast change detected by you or your doctor. During a diagnostic mammogram, the radiologist performing the exam will likely take additional views to evaluate the area of concern more closely.

During mammography, it's necessary to compress the breast between two plates on the X-ray device. This can cause some brief discomfort, but it smooths the breast tissue, making it easier for the radiologist to detect abnormalities.

In addition, a compressed breast receives less radiation, and compression reduces movement, which can create a blurry image. If the breast is inadequately com-

pressed, then overlapping normal breast tissue can create the appearance of an abnormality where none exists.

There's disagreement within the medical profession about the age at which women should begin having regular mammograms. In young women breast cancer isn't as common, and their breasts often are so dense that they don't X-ray well. Most medical experts agree that women younger than 35 who aren't in a high-risk category don't need mammograms and that women older than 50 should have them regularly.

Controversy has centered on whether screening is necessary for women in their 40s. Studies indicate that regular mammograms do save lives among women in their 40s. Presently, the best advice is:

- If you're younger than age 40, you probably don't need a mammogram unless you develop a breast problem or you're at high risk.

Women with a family history of breast cancer should begin having regular mammograms beginning five to 10 years before the age the youngest first-degree relative with breast cancer received her diagnosis.

- If you're between the ages of 40 and 49, talk with your doctor about how often you should have a mammogram, based on your risk factors, personal preferences and your understanding about the benefits and limitations of mammography.
- If you're age 50 or older, have a mammogram every one to two years.
- If you're age 75 or older, talk with your doctor about how long to continue having mammograms. In general, mammograms are recommended for women with a life expectancy greater than five to 10 years.

Diagnosis

Unlike screening tests, diagnostic procedures help to further characterize breast abnormalities found by some other means, such as feeling a lump or seeing a spot on a mammogram or magnetic resonance imaging (MRI).

Your doctor also may squeeze your areola area gently to see if any discharge comes from the ducts leading to the nipple, and feel your armpits for signs your lymph nodes might be involved. Breast cancer commonly spreads through the lymph channels.

A diagnostic mammogram or an ultrasound exam may be performed. During an ultrasound exam, if the area in question doesn't appear to be a simple benign cyst, the doctor performing the exam may use a thin needle to try to draw (aspirate) fluid from it. This fluid is analyzed for cancerous (malignant) cells. If the lump can't be aspirated, it should be evaluated with a needle biopsy.

Biopsy

In a biopsy, a small sample of tissue is removed for analysis in a laboratory. It's the only test that can tell for certain if cancer is present. Biopsies also provide

Breast Cancer Staging

Staging takes into account how far the cancer has spread and the biology of the tumor, which includes tumor type, hormone receptor status and proliferation factors. This information is gathered primarily from surgical findings and diagnostic tests, which may include bone scans, computerized tomography (CT) scans, X-rays and blood tests. Staging is one of the most important factors in determining optimum treatment, and the most significant factor in predicting prognosis or outcome.

In general, breast cancer is grouped into five stages:

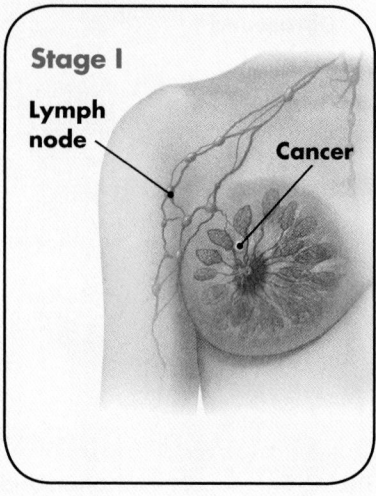

Stage I

Lymph node

Cancer

- **Stage 0** (noninvasive, or *in situ*). This is very early breast cancer that hasn't spread within the breast. It includes ductal carcinoma *in situ* (DCIS), in which abnormal cells remain within the duct. Lobular carcinoma *in situ* (LCIS) is not included in this staging system because it's considered a marker, not a cancer.

- **Stage I.** The diameter of the tumor is less than 2 centimeters (cm) — 2.5 cm equal 1 inch — and the cancer hasn't spread beyond the breast.

- **Stage II.** This stage is divided into two substages. In stage IIA, the tumor is smaller than 2 cm, but the cancer has spread to the lymph nodes under the arm, or the tumor is between 2 and 5 cm, but the cancer hasn't spread to the lymph nodes under the arm.

  In stage IIB, the tumor is between 2 and 5 cm, and the cancer has spread to the lymph nodes under the arm, or the tumor is larger than 5 cm, but the cancer hasn't spread to the lymph nodes under the arm.

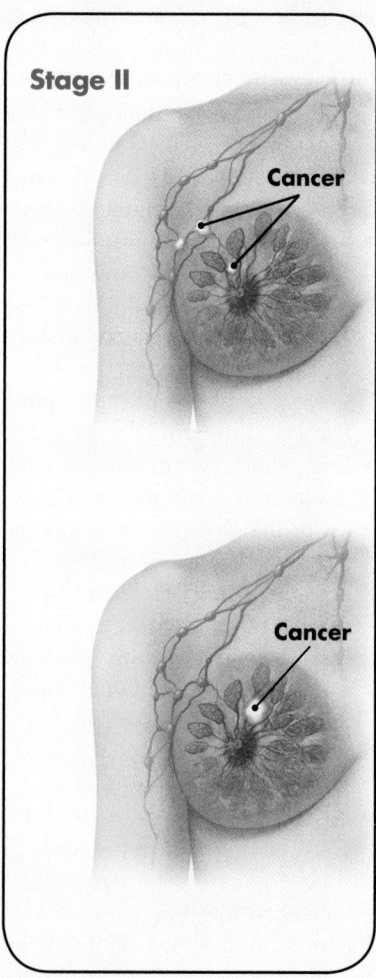

Stage II

Cancer

Cancer

- **Stage III.** This stage is also divided into substages. In stage IIIA, the tumor is smaller than 5 cm (2 inches), and the cancer has spread to lymph nodes under the arm in a way that the lymph nodes are matted together, or the tumor is larger than 5 cm, and the cancer has spread just to lymph nodes under the arm.

  Stage IIIB signifies a tumor of any size in which the cancer has spread to tissues near the breast — skin, chest wall, muscles or ribs — or has spread to lymph nodes inside the chest wall along the breastbone.

- **Stage IV.** The cancer, regardless of its size, has spread (metastasized) to distant sites, such as bones, the lungs, the liver or lymph nodes not near the breast.

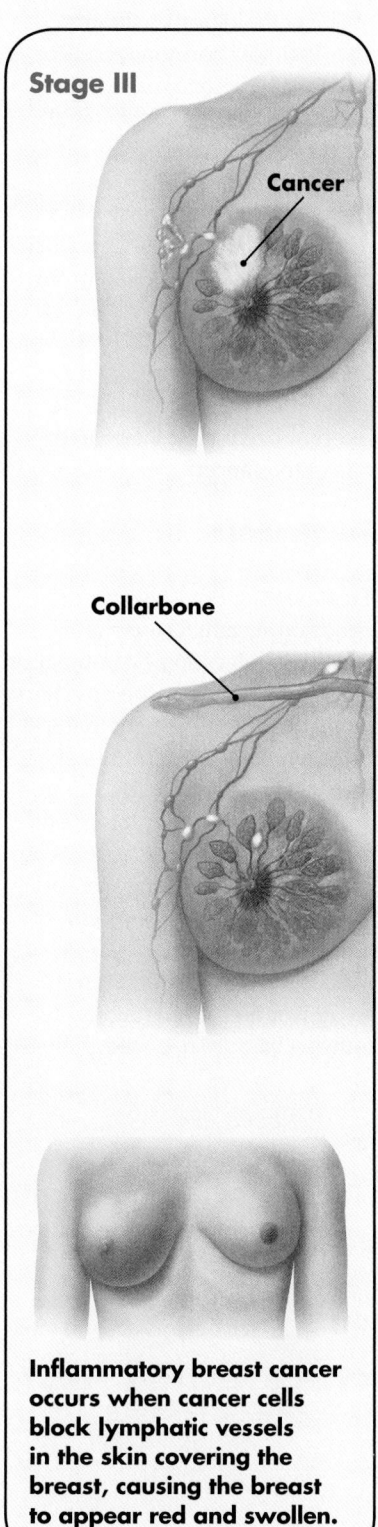

Stage III

Cancer

Collarbone

Inflammatory breast cancer occurs when cancer cells block lymphatic vessels in the skin covering the breast, causing the breast to appear red and swollen.

Stage IV

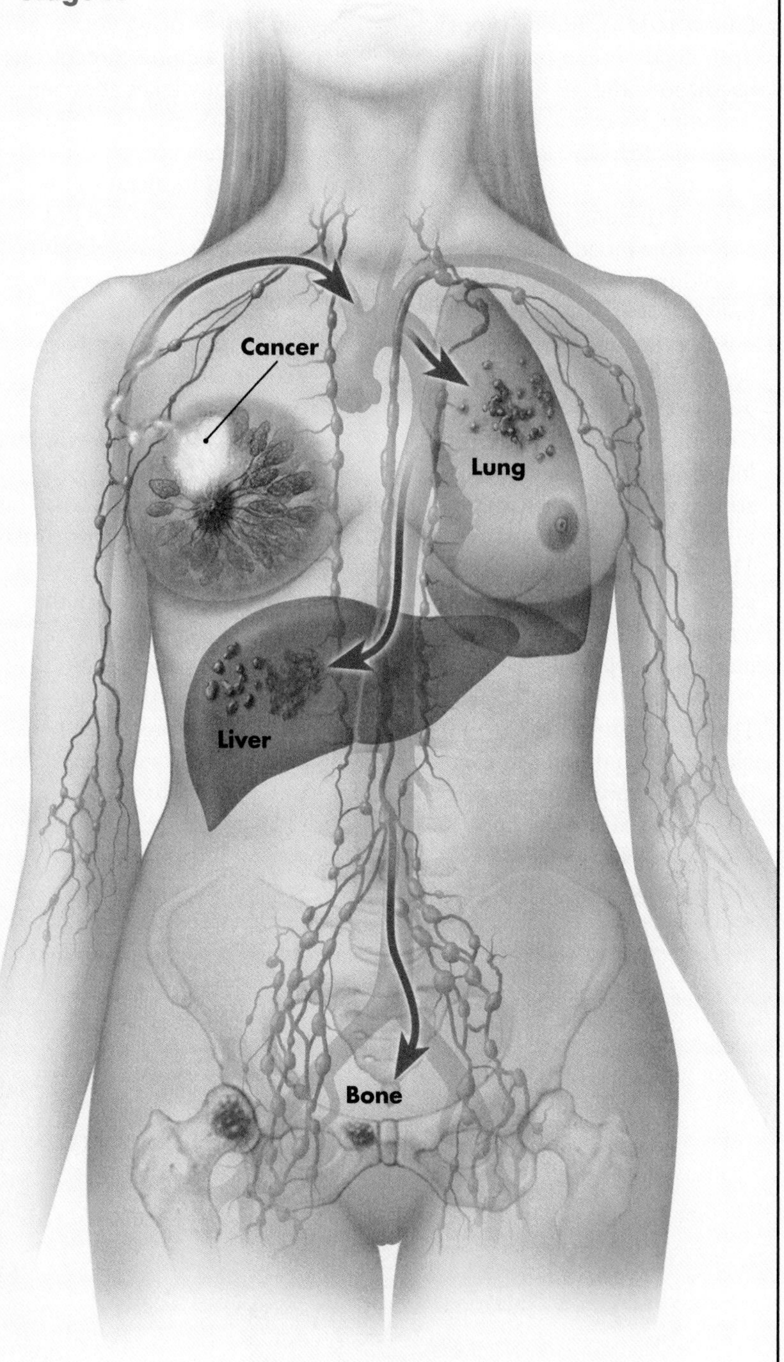

Cancer

Lung

Liver

Bone

important information about unusual breast changes, and they help determine whether surgery may be needed.

Types of biopsies include:

- **Fine-needle aspiration biopsy.** Your doctor uses a thin, hollow needle to withdraw tissue from the lump. He or she then sends the tissue to a lab for microscopic analysis. The procedure takes about 30 minutes and is similar to drawing blood. A similar procedure — fine-needle aspiration — is typically performed to remove the fluid from a painful cyst, but it can also help distinguish a cyst from a solid mass.
- **Core needle biopsy.** Following local anesthesia, a radiologist or surgeon uses a hollow needle to remove tissue samples from a breast lump. As many as 15 samples, each about the size of a grain of rice, may be taken and sent to a pathologist to be analyzed for cancerous cells. The advantage of a core needle biopsy is that it removes more tissue for analysis. Often, ultrasound is used to help guide the placement of the needle.
- **Stereotactic biopsy.** This technique is used to sample and evaluate an area of concern, such as microcalcification, that can be seen on a mammogram but can't be felt or seen on an ultrasound. During the procedure, a radiologist takes a core needle biopsy, using your mammogram as a guide. Stereotactic biopsy usually takes about an hour and is performed with local anesthesia.
- **Wire or seed localization.** A doctor may recommend this technique when a worrisome lump is seen on a mammogram but can't be felt or evaluated with other surgical guidance procedures. A thin wire is placed in your breast and, using your mammogram as a guide, its tip is directed to the lump or area of concern to be tested. This procedure is usually performed before a surgical biopsy.
- **Surgical biopsy.** It's generally recommended only in cases where a needle biopsy can't be performed. During the procedure, a surgeon removes all or part of a breast lump. In general, a small lump will be completely removed (excisional biopsy). If the lump is large, only a sample will be taken (incisional biopsy). The procedure is generally performed on an outpatient basis in a clinic or hospital.

The pathological evaluation also includes hormone receptor tests and tests for a marker known as the HER2 receptor protein. If cancer cells have receptors for the hormones estrogen or progesterone or both, your doctor may recommend treatment with a drug that prevents the hormone from binding to these sites. If you test positive for excess HER2 protein, your doctor may recommend medication that binds to HER2 receptors, reducing the growth rate of the cancer.

Treatment

Treatment for breast cancer depends on several factors, but it usually involves some combination of surgery, radiation therapy, hormone therapy and chemotherapy.

Depending on the results of breast surgery and follow-up tests, you may need further treatment, which may include radiation, chemotherapy or hormone therapy.

Mammography isn't necessary after some surgeries — simple mastectomy, skin-sparing mastecomy or nipple-sparing mastectomy — because not enough breast

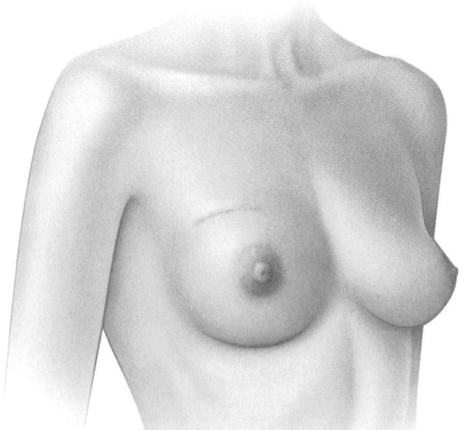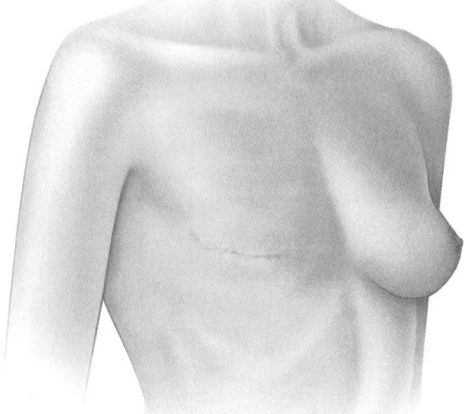

In a lumpectomy (upper left), the tumor is removed along with some healthy tissue around the tumor. In a simple mastectomy (upper right), the breast is removed, as well as the nipple and areola tissue. There may be a second incision under the arm where the sentinel node(s) are removed or axillary dissection performed.

tissue remains to screen. Breast self-exams and skin and chest wall examinations are important.

Breast surgery

Routine mammography and heightened awareness among women and their doctors about breast cancer have contributed to an increase in the number of people who are diagnosed with breast cancer at an earlier stage.

When discovered at its earliest stage, breast cancer is highly curable with surgery. Surgical procedures for breast cancer include:

Lumpectomy (breast conservation)

This operation saves as much of your breast as possible by removing only the lump and a small amount of surrounding tissue. For a small tumor that's detected early, a lumpectomy to remove the tumor may be all the breast surgery that's necessary. If the tumor is larger, a lumpectomy may not be ideal.

In general, lumpectomy — also known as breast conservation surgery — is usually followed by radiation therapy to destroy any remaining cancer cells. Studies show survival rates for breast conservation surgery plus radiation are similar to those for mastectomy.

Simple mastectomy

During a simple mastectomy the surgeon removes all of your breast tissue — the lobules, ducts, fatty tissue and skin, including the nipple and areola. Mastectomy is needed when the cancer is in multiple sites within the breast or the tumor is large, relative to the size of the breast. Some women choose to have a simple mastectomy instead of lumpectomy.

Skin-sparing mastectomy

During this operation, the surgeon removes all of your breast tissue, including the nipple and areola, but preserves the skin of the breast. This procedure is used in women having mastectomy and immediate breast reconstruction.

Axillary Surgery

Because breast cancer first spreads to the lymph nodes under the arm, all women with invasive cancer need to have these nodes examined during breast surgery.

A procedure called sentinel node biopsy is used to determine if the cancer has spread to one or more lymph nodes. The sentinel lymph node(s) is the first lymph node(s) to which a tumor drains, and therefore the first place where cancer is likely to spread. During surgery, one or more sentinal nodes are located and removed for evaluation of cancer.

Research indicates that if the sentinel node(s) is cancer-free, it's unlikely the cancer has spread, and removal of additional lymph nodes typically isn't necessary. If any sentinel nodes contain cancer, further node removal and examination may be necessary to determine the extent of lymph node involvement.

To identify the sentinel node(s), blue dye, a radioactive solution or both are injected near the tumor. The dye travels to and accumulates in one or more sentinel nodes. Once these nodes are identified, they're removed and sent to a laboratory for examination.

If one or more sentinel nodes test positive for cancer, axillary dissection may be recommended. Axillary dissection involves the removal of a majority of lymph nodes under your armpit. This may result in arm swelling (lymphedema) and diminished arm mobility.

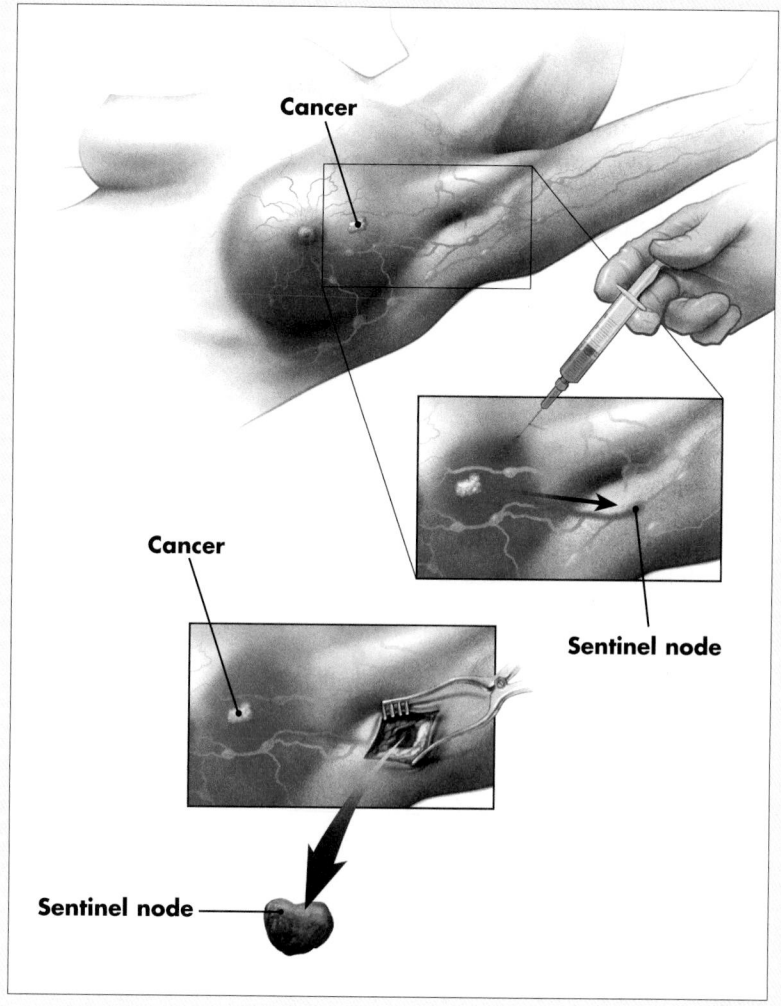

Nipple-sparing mastectomy

A nipple-sparing mastectomy removes the breast tissue while preserving the skin and the nipple and areola. Nipple-sparing mastectomy may be an option depending on the size and location of the tumor and the size of the breast. The operation is used in select individuals undergoing mastectomy with immediate breast reconstruction.

Breast reconstruction

Not all women who have a mastectomy choose to have breast reconstruction. Some may choose to have a breast prosthesis worn in their bra. Women who choose to undergo breast reconstruction basically have two options: reconstruction with a synthetic breast implant or reconstruction using their own body tissue.

You can have breast reconstruction at the time of your mastectomy (immediate) or as a separate procedure at a later date (delayed), depending on your preference and that of your surgeon.

- **Reconstruction with implants.** This technique uses artificial material — silicone gel or saline, in an implantable, leak-proof silicone shell — to replace surgically removed breast tissue. Often a surgeon will use a tissue expander, which is an empty implant shell that inflates as fluid is injected. It's placed under your skin and muscle, and your doctor gradually fills it with fluid — usually over a period of several months. When your muscle and skin have stretched enough, the expander is removed and replaced with a permanent (either silicone or saline) implant.
- **Reconstruction with a tissue flap.** One option is a transverse rectus abdominal muscle (TRAM) flap. This surgery reconstructs your breast using tissue — including skin, fat and muscle — from your abdomen. Sometimes, surgeons may

use tissue from your back or buttocks instead. Because the procedure is fairly complicated, recovery may take six to eight weeks. Complications include the risk of hernia and tissue death.
- **Deep inferior epigastric perforator (DIEP) flap reconstruction.** In this procedure, skin and fat tissue from your abdomen is used to create a natural-looking breast. Because your abdominal muscles are left intact, you're less likely to experience abdominal complications than with the TRAM procedure. You may also experience less pain and a speedier recovery. If you have a low amount of body fat, your surgeon may decide this type of surgery isn't an option.
- **Reconstruction of your nipple and areola.** After your initial surgery with either tissue transfer or an implant, you may have further surgery to make a nipple and areola. Using tissue from elsewhere in your body or from the mastectomy site, your surgeon creates a small mound that resembles a nipple. He or she may then tattoo the skin around the nipple to create an areola.

Understanding DCIS

Ductal carcinoma *in situ* (DCIS) signals the presence of abnormal cells inside a milk duct within a breast. The cancer is noninvasive, meaning it hasn't spread outside the duct to other parts of the body.

On a mammogram, DCIS often appears as small clusters of calcifications that have irregular shapes and sizes. DCIS is considered the earliest form of breast cancer and it's common. It accounts for about 1 in 5 breast cancers diagnosed each year. Increased and more advanced screening for breast cancer in recent years has led to a rise in this very early-stage cancer.

A diagnosis of DCIS can be confusing to some women who may be told they have stage 0 cancer but that they need surgery to remove the cancer and, possibly, additional treatment.

While DCIS isn't life-threatening, left untreated it eventually could become invasive. Most women with DCIS are effectively treated with breast-conserving surgery (lumpectomy) and radiation. In certain cases — such as a very large area or more than one area of DCIS within a breast — mastectomy may be recommended.

Palliative surgery

If you have widespread cancer that has gone beyond the confines of your breast and underarm area — such as to your bones, brain or liver — palliative surgery, which includes mastectomy, may be recommended. It's done to provide tissue for laboratory analysis and some degree of tumor control. The intent of this surgery isn't to cure the cancer but to control its growth and reduce complications.

Radiation therapy

Radiation therapy uses high-energy X-rays to kill cancer cells and shrink tumors. It's administered by a radiation oncologist at a radiation center. In general, radiation is the standard of care after a lumpectomy for both invasive and noninvasive breast cancers. Oncologists are also likely to recommend radiation after a mastectomy for a large tumor, inflammatory breast cancer, cancer that has invaded the chest wall or cancer that has spread to several lymph nodes in your armpit.

If your doctors also recommend chemotherapy, it's usually administered before radiation therapy. Radiation treatments often are done five days a week for five to six consecutive weeks. Newer, more-intense treatments may be completed more quickly. Radiation treatments are painless and are similar to getting an X-ray. The effects are cumulative, however, and you may become tired toward the end of the series. Your breast may be pink, puffy and somewhat tender, as if it's been sunburned.

In a small number of women, more-serious problems may occur, including arm swelling, damage to the lungs, heart or nerves, or a change in the appearance and consistency of breast tissue. Radiation therapy also may increase your risk of developing another tumor. For these reasons, it's important to learn about the risks and benefits of radiation therapy when deciding between lumpectomy and mastectomy. You may also want to talk to a radiation oncologist about clinical trials investigating shorter courses of radiation or focal application of radiation.

Chemotherapy

Chemotherapy uses drugs to destroy cancer cells. The size of the tumor, characteristics of the cancer cells, your age and premenopausal status, and the extent of spread of the cancer determine if you need chemotherapy.

If your cancer has a high chance of returning or spreading to another part of your body, your doctor may recommend chemotherapy after surgery to decrease the chance that the cancer will recur. This is known as adjuvant systemic chemotherapy. If your cancer has already spread to other parts of your body, chemotherapy may be recommended to try to control the cancer and decrease any symptoms the cancer is causing.

Treatment often involves receiving two or more drugs in different combinations every two to three weeks. These may be administered intravenously, in pill form or both. You may have between four and eight treatments spread over three to six months.

Because chemotherapy affects healthy cells as well as cancerous ones, side effects are common. Your digestive tract, hair and bone marrow — all composed of fast-growing cells — tend to take the brunt of this toxicity, leading to hair loss, nausea, vomiting and fatigue. Not everyone has all of these side effects, however, and methods to control chemotherapy side effects have improved greatly in recent decades. Notably, more-effective drugs can help prevent or reduce nausea and vomiting.

Depending on the chemotherapy drugs your doctor recommends, other side effects may occur, including damage to the heart, nerves, kidneys and other organs. Chemotherapy may temporarily affect your white blood cells — cells that fight off infection.

Another possible side effect is chemobrain, the common term for memory and concentration problems that happen to some people during and after chemotherapy. Chemobrain is associated with difficulties involving specific thought processes, including word finding, memory and multitasking.

Premature menopause and infertility also are potential side effects of chemotherapy. The older you are when you begin treatment, the greater the likelihood that your reproductive cycle will be affected. In rare cases, certain chemotherapy medications may lead to cancer of the white blood cells (acute myeloid leukemia) — often years after treatment ends.

Hormone therapy

Hormone therapy — perhaps more properly termed hormone blocking therapy — is often used to treat women whose cancers are sensitive to hormones. These are known as estrogen and progesterone receptor positive cancers.

Cancer Prevention Drugs

Advances in breast cancer research have led to the use of synthetic drugs to reduce cancer development in women at high risk but with no prior history of breast cancer. For example, the drug tamoxifen (Soltamox) can reduce the risk of breast cancer in high-risk women by about 50 percent. Tamoxifen belongs to a class of drugs known as selective estrogen receptor modulators (SERMs), which block the effects of estrogen on the breast. Unfortunately, tamoxifen has an estrogen-like effect on the uterus, increasing the risk of uterine cancer and blood clots. Tamoxifen is approved for use in both premenopausal and postmenopausal women at high risk of breast cancer. It's generally taken for five years.

The drug raloxifene (Evista) also has been shown to decrease the risk of invasive breast cancer in high-risk postmenopausal women, as well as help prevent and treat osteoporosis. It also is taken for five years.

Aromatase inhibitors are another class of medications available to postmenopausal women. They've been shown to reduce the development of breast cancer in high-risk women by about 60 percent.

Your doctor can help you decide which medication may be more suitable for you based on your breast cancer risk, your personal health, and side effects and risk of the medications.

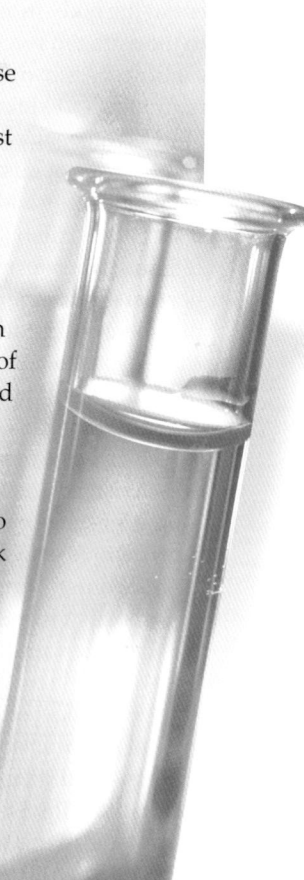

Breast Cancer in Men

Although male breast cancer is rare, it happens. Having a father or brother with the disease puts you at higher risk, whether you're male or female. To learn more about breast disorders in men, see Chapter 28, "Endocrine System."

Similar to chemotherapy, this treatment is used to decrease the chance of your cancer returning. If the cancer has already spread, hormone therapy may shrink and control it.

Two classes of medications are used in hormone therapy: selective estrogen receptor modulators (SERMs) and aromatase inhibitors.

• **Selective estrogen receptor modulators (SERMs).** SERMs act by blocking any estrogen present in the body from attaching to the estrogen receptor on the cancer cells, slowing the growth of tumors and killing tumor cells. SERMs can be used in both pre- and postmenopausal women.

The most common SERM used is tamoxifen (Soltamox). It's prescribed for women with hormone-sensitive (estrogen or progesterone positive) breast cancer. You take tamoxifen daily, in pill form, for up to 10 years to reduce the risk of recurrence.

It also may be used for hormone-sensitive metastatic breast cancer. And it's been approved for use as a preventive drug for women at increased risk of breast cancer.

Tamoxifen is less toxic than most anti-cancer drugs, but it isn't trouble-free. Women taking tamoxifen may experience menopausal symptoms such as night sweats, hot flashes and vaginal discharge. More-serious side effects, including blood clots and endometrial cancer, occur infrequently.

• **Aromatase inhibitors.** This class of drugs, which includes anastrozole (Arimidex), letrozole (Femara) and exemestane (Aromasin), blocks the conversion of a hormonal substance (androstenedione) into estrogen. This effectively stops estrogen production in cells other than the ovaries. Fat cells, the adrenal gland and other normal cells all make small amounts of estrogen.

Aromatase inhibitors may be taken for up to 10 years to reduce the risk of cancer recurrence. The drugs are only effective in postmenopausal women or in women receiving medication to stop production of estrogen by the ovaries.

In several randomized, controlled trials, women receiving aromatase inhibitors fared slightly better than have those receiving tamoxifen. Women treated with aromatase inhibitors also had a lower incidence of blood clots and endometrial cancer. The primary drawbacks of aromatase inhibitors are an increased risk of osteoporosis, vaginal dryness and joint pain.

Talk to your doctor about the best medication or sequence of medications for you.

Biological therapy

As scientists learn more about the differences between normal cells and cancer cells, treatments aimed at these differences — called biological therapy — are being developed. Immunotherapy is a type of biological therapy targeted at repairing or stimulating your natural immune response to cancer.

Biological therapies for breast cancer include the following:

• **Monoclonal antibodies (MoAbs).** MoAbs enhance the immune system of a person with cancer, interfering with the growth of cancer cells. They also work with anti-cancer drugs to deliver toxin directly to a tumor in an effort to destroy it.

Trastuzumab (Herceptin) is a biological therapy approved by the Food and Drug Administration that uses monoclonal antibody technology to attack a protein (HER2) that's overproduced in about 1 out of every 4 breast cancers. The drug is effective on tumors that produce excess amounts of HER2, located on the surface of cancer cells. By attacking this protein, Herceptin kills cancer cells on its own and in conjunction with chemotherapy or hormone therapy.

• **Pertuzumab (Perjeta).** It's a monoclonal antibody sometimes taken in with Herceptin to treat overproduction of HER2.

• **Lapatinib (Tykerb).** Like Herceptin, Tykerb zeros in on and blocks the effects of the HER2 protein. But while Herceptin blocks HER2's action from the outside of the cell, Tykerb is a smaller molecule that works on the inside of the cell. Tykerb works for some women for whom Herceptin is no longer effective. The drug is only approved for use in conjunction with chemotherapy and in women with advanced, metastatic breast cancers.

• **Palbociclib (Ibrance).** This medication slows the growth of hormonally sensitive cancer that's already spread outside the breast and adjacent lymph nodes. It's used in conjunction with hormone-blocking therapy.

• **Everolimus (Afinitor).** It inhibits a tumor pathway called mTOR and helps control hormonally sensitive metastatic cancer when given in combination with the aromatase inhibitor exemestane.

• **Trastuzumab-emtansine, or T-DM1 (Kadcyla).** Called an antibody conjugate medication, it links Herceptin to a strong chemotherapy drug for treatment of metastatic cancer with overproduction of HER2.

For more on cancer treatment advances, see Chapter 15. ■

Digestive System

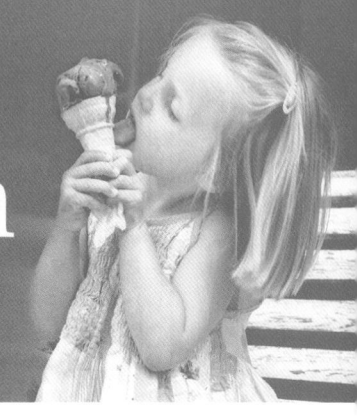

Heartburn, cramps, nausea, diarrhea, constipation — these are just a few of the ways the organs that make up your digestive system let you know when they aren't well. Most people experience these signs and symptoms on occasion. Often, they last just a day or two and then disappear. For many people, though, digestive signs and symptoms linger and become a daily annoyance.

It's estimated that around 20 percent of Americans — perhaps even more — regularly battle some kind of digestive problem. You can see the evidence in your local drug, grocery or discount store. Shelves are lined with an increasing array of medicines for digestive conditions: antacids, acid blockers, laxatives, fiber supplements and anti-diarrheal agents.

A general overview of how digestion works might help you understand why digestive problems are so common.

Your digestive system is much more than your stomach and intestines. It's a complex system of organs that convert the food you eat into the energy you need. Because of this, digestion is one of the critical functions your body performs.

Your Digestive System at Work

Digestion begins even before you take your first bite. The aroma of the food you're about to eat — or even the mere thought of eating — is enough to start saliva flowing in your mouth.

Once you take a bite, your salivary glands kick into high gear pumping out juices that begin to chemically break down the food. Not all of the work is chemical, though. Your teeth crunch and grind the food, while your tongue mixes it with saliva.

Your saliva contains the enzyme ptyalin that begins to change starches (carbohydrates) into sugars. Chewing reduces the food to a mushy consistency. When you swallow, the food is propelled into the back part of your throat, past the opening of the voice box (larynx), and into the upper part of your esophagus.

Food is prevented from entering your larynx and air passages by a flap of soft tissue (epiglottis) that closes as food passes into the esophagus. If the epiglottis fails to close completely, a brief coughing fit may result, commonly referred to as food having "gone down the wrong way." This coughing has a protective function in that it brings food and saliva back into your mouth, preventing this material from going down your windpipe (trachea) and into your lungs.

Esophagus

The esophagus is a tube approximately 10 inches long that leads directly into the stomach. The food is moved into your esophagus by muscles in the back of your throat (pharynx). When it enters the main part of the esophagus, muscles there undergo a series of wavelike contractions, called peristalsis, to move the food into your stomach. Peristalsis is also the mechanism by which the food moves throughout the remainder of its trip through your digestive tract until the waste products reach the muscles of the anus.

A muscle that encircles the bottom portion of the esophagus (lower esophageal sphincter) is critical in the passage of food into your stomach. When this valve-like sphincter relaxes, it opens and permits food to enter your stomach. It then closes, preventing the food from re-entering your esophagus (regurgitating). When the sphincter fails to work properly, acidic stomach contents can regurgitate into the esophagus, damaging its sensitive lining. If

this occurs, you may experience the symptoms of heartburn. Frequent heartburn is a symptom of a common condition called gastro-esophageal reflux disease (GERD).

Stomach

The walls of your stomach consist primarily of various layers of powerful muscles. These muscles cause the stomach to churn, breaking food into smaller and smaller pieces. At the same time, gastric juices manufactured by glands that line your stomach mix with the food particles. These juices contain pepsin, a digestive enzyme that breaks down proteins in the mixture, and hydrochloric acid, which provides pepsin with the proper chemical environment.

There's a delicate balance in your stomach between the acid produced by its glands and the resistance of your stomach lining to that acid. If this balance is upset, the result may be damage to the stomach lining, causing a peptic ulcer or a diffuse inflammation known as gastritis.

Food leaves your stomach in two phases. The upper portion of your stomach contracts first, pushing liquid material into your small intestine. The more-solid contents leave later, primarily by the action of the muscles in the lower part of your stomach. This partially processed food (chyme) then travels through the adjoining pyloric canal into the first portion of your small intestine, called the duodenum. Very little food is actually absorbed by your stomach — only small amounts of alcohol, simple sugars and some medications.

Small intestine

The small intestine (small bowel) is a tube whose length in adults is approximately 20 feet, depending on the tone of its muscular wall and the way it's measured.

The small intestine is divided into three parts. The duodenum is

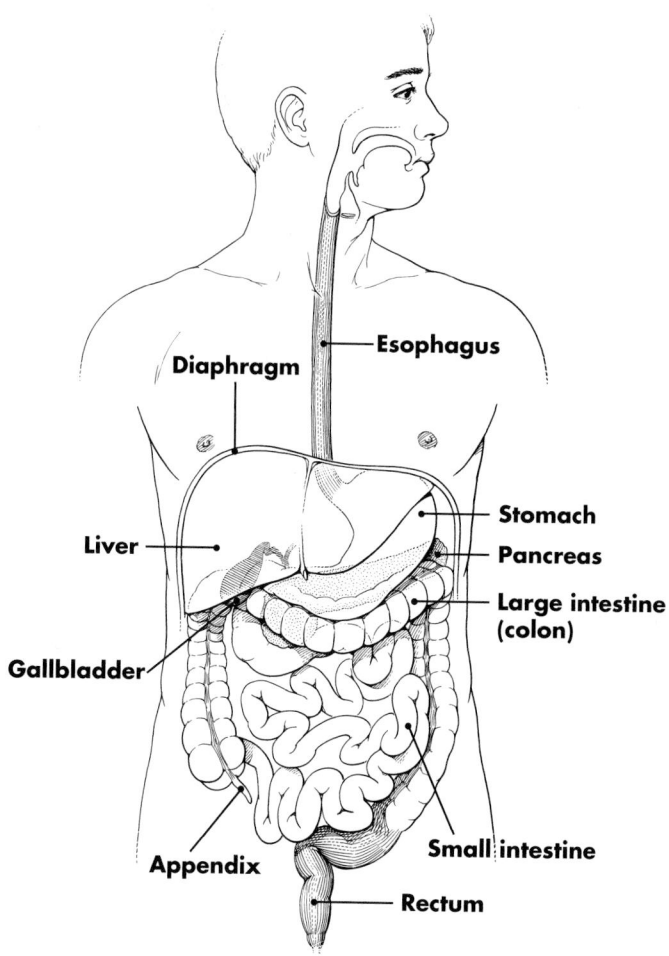

Diaphragm

Esophagus

Liver

Stomach

Pancreas

Large intestine (colon)

Gallbladder

Appendix

Small intestine

Rectum

Large intestine

Once food residue reaches the large intestine (large bowel, or colon), the role of your digestive system changes. Now its job is to process waste, consisting mainly of undigested and nonabsorbed food, fiber and water.

Liquid from the small intestine is carried into the colon where most of it is absorbed into the bloodstream. Your colon, which is about 5 feet long, is very efficient at this process. Of the approximately 1 quart of fluid that enters it every day, nearly 80 percent is absorbed before reaching the anus.

The rest of the waste material moves through the three major segments of your colon — right (ascending), transverse and left (descending) colon — then into the S-shaped sigmoid colon located in your lower left abdomen. Finally, the waste material moves into the last 4 to 6 inches of the colon (rectum). Here the material collects until defecation.

Liver

Your liver produces bile, a fluid containing cholesterol and bile acids. Bile flows from the liver and through the cystic duct into your gallbladder, where it's concentrated and stored. Bile is eventually emptied into the duodenum after meals, where it performs its major function of assisting in the absorption of fats through the lining of the small intestine into the bloodstream. Bile acids are then reabsorbed by the small intestine — mostly in the ileum — and recycled into the liver to be used again.

The liver has other functions as well. One of these is the storage of glycogen, a complex carbohydrate that's converted to sugar for release into your bloodstream when your blood sugar level falls. Glycogen is deposited in the liver when the level of sugar in the blood increases. Many proteins are synthesized in the liver.

the first and shortest part. It's here that the absorption process truly begins. The jejunum, the middle and largest portion of the small intestine, is where the majority of absorption takes place. The final section of the small intestine, the ileum, also has important absorptive functions (vitamin B-12, for example). It's also responsible for the passage of food into the large intestine.

The duodenum contributes to the mixing of food material and also neutralizes acid coming from your stomach. Bile tubes (ducts) from the liver and gallbladder and the pancreatic duct from the pancreas empty their digestive juices into the duodenum to prepare the chyme for maximum absorption.

As the semisolid food continues its movement through your small intestine, it undergoes further

digestion by various enzymes. In this process, the food is broken into smaller components that can be absorbed through the lining of the small intestine and enter your bloodstream.

Starches are converted to simple sugars, and proteins are broken down into amino acids. Fats are broken down by enzymes from the pancreas. Because of their detergent-like properties, bile acids from the liver make the fat molecules soluble in water so that they can then be absorbed into your bloodstream. In addition, minerals, vitamins, water and electrolytes, such as sodium and calcium, are absorbed through the wall of the small intestine and into your bloodstream.

By the time the food is ready to pass into your large intestine, most of its nutrients have already been absorbed.

The liver also helps determine the amount of nutrients that are sent to the rest of your body. It converts nutrients from food into substances your body can use. In addition, your liver breaks down some medications to enable them to be eliminated in the stool. Alcohol is metabolized in the liver to supply energy or to be deposited as fat.

Gallbladder

The gallbladder is a pear-shaped organ that sits beneath the liver. It's a storage site for much of the bile produced in the liver. Bile enters the gallbladder through the cystic duct and is stored there until needed for the digestion of fats.

Although the gallbladder serves a useful function, it's not vital to maintaining normal body functions because bile can be delivered directly from the bile ducts into the duodenum.

Pancreas

Shaped somewhat like a banana only wider, the pancreas stretches from your duodenum to your spleen. This organ produces two kinds of secretions — those that are released into the duodenum and those that pass directly into your bloodstream. The first type is called pancreatic juice. It aids in the digestion of fats, proteins and some carbohydrates. The other type includes the hormones insulin and glucagon, which regulate the metabolism of blood sugar (glucose).

Esophageal Disorders

Your esophagus is the muscular tube that leads directly into your stomach, transporting food from your throat to your stomach. Many conditions can affect the esophagus and interfere with swallowing or the transport of food from your mouth to your stomach.

Gastroesophageal reflux disease

Signs and symptoms
- A burning sensation in the chest, often radiating from the upper abdomen into the neck
- Regurgitation of sour or bitter-tasting material into the throat and mouth, especially when lying down
- Chest pain
- Persistent coughing
- Difficulty swallowing

Nearly everyone experiences heartburn, that burning sensation in the chest — and sometimes the throat — from stomach acid that washes back into the esophagus. An occasional episode of heartburn is generally nothing to worry about. Many people, though, battle heartburn regularly, even daily. Frequent heartburn can be a serious problem that deserves medical attention. Most often, frequent heartburn is a symptom of gastroesophageal reflux disease (GERD).

When you eat, food travels down your esophagus to a muscular valve that separates your lower esophagus and stomach. Called the lower esophageal sphincter, this valve opens to allow food to pass into your stomach and then closes again.

Sometimes, though, the sphincter muscle relaxes (opens) at the wrong time, allowing acidic stomach contents to re-enter the esophagus, producing the symptoms commonly referred to as heartburn. When the acid regurgitates into your upper esophagus, it leaves a sour taste in your mouth and may cause you to cough.

The constant backwash of acid can irritate the lining of the

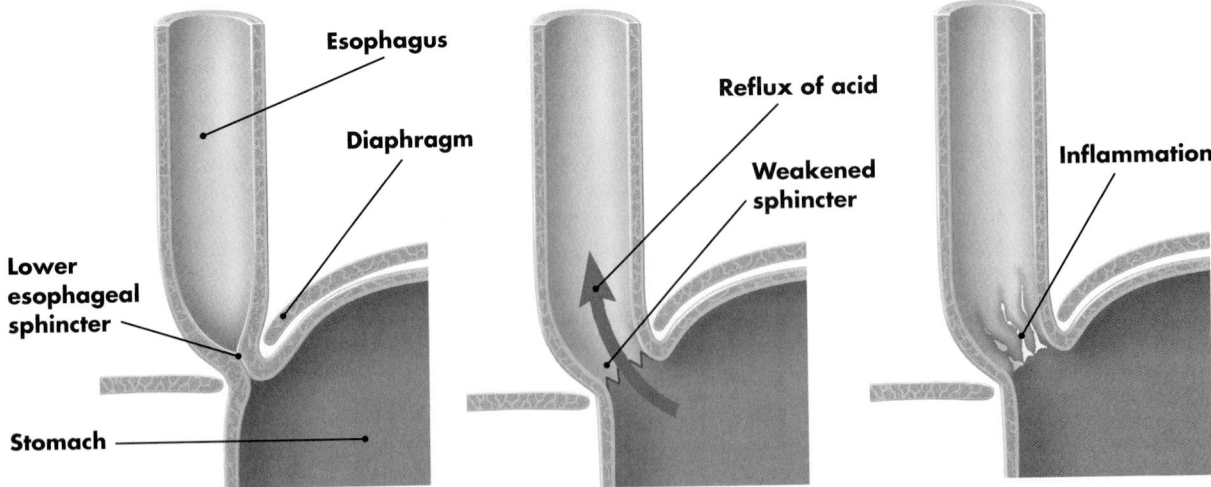

Normally, the lower esophageal sphincter remains closed, preventing acidic stomach contents from washing into the esophagus. If the sphincter weakens or relaxes, stomach contents can flow back (reflux) into the esophagus, causing heartburn and tissue inflammation.

Hiatal Hernia

Your chest is separated from your abdomen by a dome-shaped sheet of muscle called the diaphragm. To reach your stomach, your esophagus has to pass through an opening (hiatus) in the diaphragm.

When tissues around the hiatus weaken, part of the stomach may protrude through the opening into the chest cavity. This is termed hiatal hernia. Hiatal hernia is thought to result from a weakening of the anchoring tissues at the junction to the diaphragm, possibly due to increased pressure within the abdomen, such as with obesity.

Hiatal hernias are common. About 25 percent of people older than age 50 have a hiatal hernia. Because the majority of these hernias produce no signs or symptoms, they usually go undetected. In fact, they're often found incidentally on a chest X-ray where part of the stomach can be seen in the chest cavity. Hiatal hernias are frequently found in people with heartburn who undergo barium X-ray studies. It's unlikely that a small hiatal hernia will cause serious problems, and by itself it isn't a dangerous ailment.

Large hernias, in which a substantial portion of the stomach is above the diaphragm, can cause slow bleeding and iron deficiency anemia. One potential

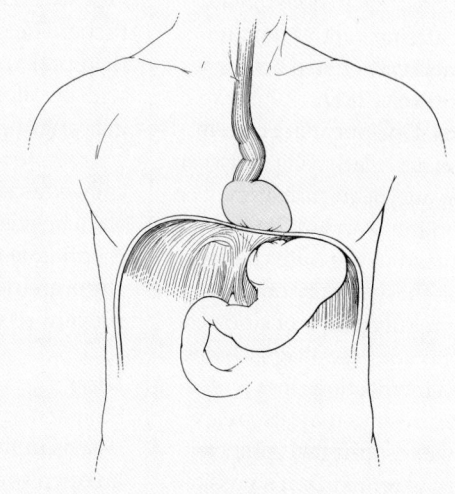

In hiatal hernia, a portion of the stomach protrudes through the diaphragm into the chest cavity.

but extremely rare danger of a very large hernia is strangulation of the stomach, in which the herniated stomach becomes so tightly constricted that its blood supply is severely reduced. Symptoms typically include persistent chest pain and difficulty swallowing. This is a medical emergency and may require prompt surgery.

esophagus causing it to inflame, a condition called esophagitis.

Over time, the inflammation can narrow or erode the esophagus, causing difficulty swallowing or chest pain. Gastroesophageal reflux disease is the name for chronic acid reflux that causes esophagitis.

Anyone can have GERD, even children and infants. However, the condition is more common in people older than age 40. It's also common in pregnant women because of hormonal changes and increased pressure within the abdomen.

Factors that can significantly increase GERD include:

- **Being overweight.** Many, but not all, people with GERD are overweight. Excess weight puts extra pressure on your stomach and diaphragm, the large muscle that separates your chest and abdomen, forcing open the lower esophageal sphincter. Eating very large or high-fat meals may produce similar effects.

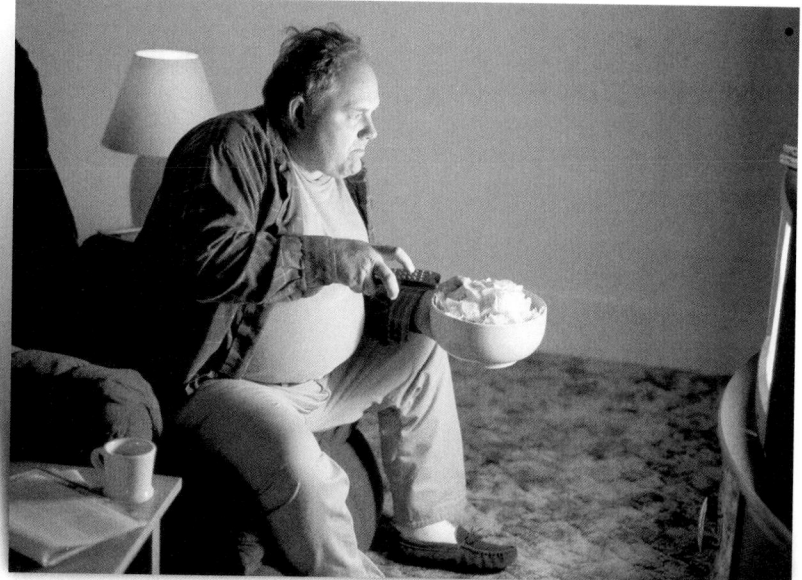

- **Hiatal hernia.** Hiatal hernia is a condition in which part of your stomach protrudes into your lower chest, and your diaphragm is no longer able to support the lower esophageal sphincter. A large hiatal hernia can worsen acid reflux.

Smoking. Smoking may increase acid production and aggravate reflux.
- **Excessive alcohol.** Alcohol reduces pressure on the lower esophageal sphincter, allowing it to relax and open. Alcohol may also irritate the esophageal lining.

- **Certain foods.** Foods such as fatty foods, spicy foods, chocolate, caffeine, onions, tomato sauce and carbonated beverages can worsen GERD.
- **Asthma.** Doctors aren't certain of the exact relationship between asthma and heartburn. It may be that coughing and difficulty exhaling lead to pressure changes in your chest and abdomen, triggering regurgitation of stomach acid into your esophagus. Some asthma medications that widen (dilate) airways may also relax the lower esophageal sphincter and allow reflux. Or it's possible that the acid reflux that causes heartburn may worsen asthma symptoms.
- **Diabetes.** One complication of diabetes is gastroparesis, a disorder in which your stomach takes too long to empty. If left in your stomach too long, stomach contents can regurgitate into your esophagus and cause heartburn.

Diagnosis

Often, a description of symptoms is all a doctor needs to establish the diagnosis of GERD. However, if symptoms are particularly severe or don't respond to treatment, tests such as a barium X-ray of the esophagus and stomach or an endoscopic examination of your upper gastrointestinal tract may be necessary. An ambulatory acid (pH) probe also may be done to measure the acid levels in your upper and lower esophagus.

How serious is gastroesophageal reflux disease?

Occasional heartburn, though uncomfortable, generally isn't a serious problem. GERD, however, is a serious condition that requires treatment. Left untreated it can lead to one or more of the following:

Esophageal narrowing
Some individuals with GERD experience esophageal narrowing (stricture). Damage to the lining of the lower esophagus from acid exposure leads to formation of scar tissue. The scar tissue narrows the food pathway and can interfere with swallowing, causing food to get caught in the narrowing.

Treatment for stricture typically consists of a procedure that stretches tissues and widens the esophagus followed by acid-suppressing medication to help prevent re-narrowing.

Ulcer
Stomach acid can severely erode tissues in the esophagus, causing an open sore to form. The ulcer may cause pain and make swallowing difficult. Rarely, it may bleed. Medication and lifestyle changes to control stomach acid reflux can cure an ulcer by giving damaged tissues time to heal. For more information on ulcers, see page 828.

Barrett's esophagus
Persistent acid reflux can damage the normal lining of the esophagus, replacing it with a lining that resembles that of the stomach or small intestine. This abnormal development of tissue is called metaplasia.

Metaplasia is brought on by repeated and long-term exposure to stomach acid and is associated with an increased risk of esophageal cancer. About 5 to 10 percent of people with GERD have Barrett's esophagus. Once you have it, your chances of developing esophageal cancer are significantly greater than that of the general population.

Management of Barrett's esophagus generally includes lifestyle changes and medication to control acid reflux. Your doctor may also want to periodically examine the lining of your esophagus to increase the chance of detecting and treating abnormal (precancerous) cells at an early stage.

If tests indicate that you have a precancerous condition known as high-grade dysplasia, your doctor may recommend treatment to prevent the development of cancer. Treatment may involve burning away the abnormal tissue or surgery to remove a portion of the esophagus.

Other
Other complications of GERD include laryngitis, bronchitis and aspiration pneumonia.

Treatment

Regardless of the severity of the disease, the first step in managing GERD is to change certain lifestyle habits. For mild symptoms, a

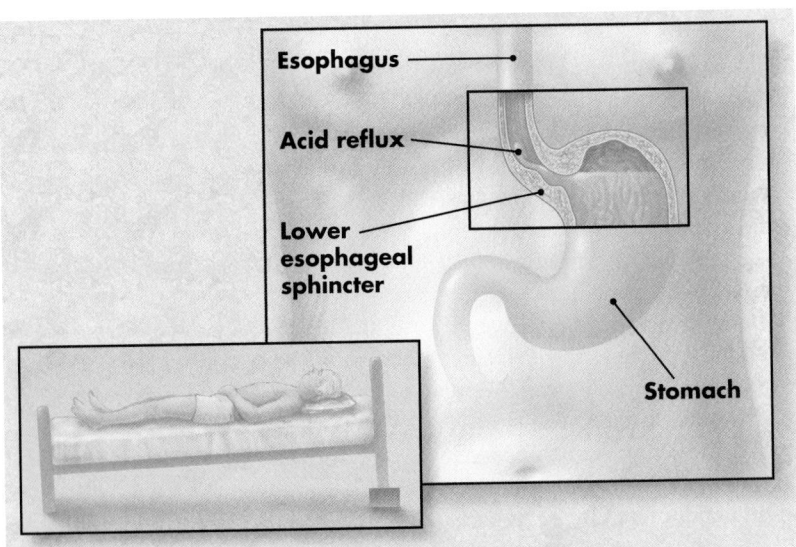

Esophagus
Acid reflux
Lower esophageal sphincter
Stomach

Raising the head of your bed helps keep acid in your stomach while you sleep. Place a 6-inch block under the feet at the head of the bed.

change in habits may be all that's needed to manage the disease. For more-severe symptoms, lifestyle changes can make your condition easier to control with medication.

Self-care

You can take several steps to help relieve GERD symptoms:

- **Don't smoke.** Smoking increases acid reflux and dries your saliva. Saliva helps protect your esophagus from stomach acid.
- **Eat smaller meals.** This reduces pressure on the lower esophageal sphincter, helping to prevent the valve from opening and acid from washing back into your esophagus.
- **Sit up after you eat.** After eating wait at least three hours before going to bed or taking a nap. By then most of the food in your stomach will have emptied into the small intestine, so it can't flow back into your esophagus.
- **Don't exercise immediately after a meal.** After a meal wait two to three hours before engaging in strenuous activity.
- **Limit fatty foods.** Studies show a link between fat consumption and GERD. Fatty foods relax the lower esophageal sphincter, allowing stomach acid into the esophagus. Fat also slows stomach emptying, increasing how long acid can regurgitate.
- **Avoid problem foods and beverages.** These may include caffeinated drinks, chocolate, onions, spicy foods and mint. They tend to increase production of stomach acid and relax the lower esophageal sphincter. Also limit citrus fruits and tomatoes and tomato-based foods. They're acidic and can irritate an inflamed esophagus, making GERD symptoms worse.

- **Limit or avoid alcohol.** Alcohol relaxes the lower esophageal sphincter and may irritate the esophagus, worsening symptoms.
- **Lose excess weight.** Heartburn and acid regurgitation are more likely to occur when there's added pressure on your stomach from excess weight.
- **Elevate the head of your bed.** Raise the head of your bed 6 to 9 inches. This provides a gradual incline from your feet to your head and helps prevent acid from flowing back into your esophagus as you sleep. Place a foam wedge under the mattress to raise it. Or put blocks of wood under the legs at the head of your bed.
- **Avoid tightfitting clothes.** They put pressure on your stomach.

Medication

For people with more-severe symptoms, medication is generally the main line of treatment. Drugs used to treat GERD include:

- **Antacids.** Available over-the-counter, antacids (Maalox, Rolaids, others) neutralize gastric acid and provide quick, temporary relief. Antacids can relieve your symptoms, but they don't eliminate all reflux. These products are generally safe, but if taken regularly they can cause side effects such as diarrhea and constipation. Some of them can also interfere with other medications taken for kidney or heart disease.
- **Acid blockers.** Also known as histamine (H-2) blockers, these medications are available both over-the-counter and by prescription. Instead of neutralizing acid, they reduce acid secretion. Acid blockers include cimetidine (Tagamet HB), ranitidine (Zantac), famotidine (Pepcid AC)

and nizatidine (Axid AR). The advantage of acid blockers is that they help prevent acid secretion, rather than just neutralizing acid. Acid blockers are generally safe, but some may interact with other medications. Check with your doctor or pharmacist for possible drug interactions.

- **Proton pump inhibitors.** These medications are most often prescribed for severe symptoms. They're the most effective in preventing acid secretion and in treatment of GERD. Examples of proton pump inhibitors include lansoprazole (Prevacid), omeprazole (Prilosec), rabeprazole (Aciphex), pantoprazole (Protonix), esomeprazole (Nexium) and dexlansoprazole (Dexilant). They inhibit acid production and allow time for damaged esophageal tissue to heal. In clinical trials, proton pump inhibitors have been found safe to use for at least 10 years. Using the lowest effective dosage can help prevent side effects of the medication, such as abdominal pain, diarrhea and headache.

Surgery

Between 10 and 40 percent of people with GERD don't respond to medication. Surgery may be an option for individuals helped by proton pump inhibitors but who don't want to take high doses of medication the rest of their lives. Surgery generally isn't recommended for people not helped by drug therapy.

The most common surgery for GERD is a procedure called Nissen fundoplication. It involves tightening the lower esophageal sphincter by wrapping the very top portion of the stomach around the outside of the lower esophagus. Often, this surgery can be performed laparoscopically — a less invasive form of surgery in which a few small incisions are made in the abdomen instead of one large one.

Recently, doctors began performing an incisionless variation

Hiccups

Holding your breath, swallowing water from the wrong side of the glass, breathing in and out of a paper bag, eating a spoonful of sugar, or having someone startle you. These all are common — and not necessarily successful — methods of getting rid of the hiccups, a generally minor complaint that afflicts almost everyone from time to time.

For the most part, hiccups are harmless and resolve in a short time. On rare occasions, hiccups may persist for days or even weeks. When this occurs, they can interfere with eating and sleeping. After major surgery, a prolonged case of the hiccups can impede the healing of an abdominal wound. In a few instances, persistent hiccups can be a sign of a serious disorder.

Although almost everyone has had hiccups, few people know exactly what they are. Very simply, hiccups are repeated, involuntary contractions of your diaphragm, the muscle that separates the chest from the abdomen. The phrenic nerves control the smooth, coordinated, normal contraction of the two flaps of the diaphragm for breathing. The phrenic nerves extend from the neck to the chest. Hiccups may result from irritation anywhere along the path of a phrenic nerve. Reflex contraction of the diaphragm similarly can be the result of irritation to nerves.

Hiccups are more likely to occur when your stomach is distended, typically after eating a big meal or drinking an over-abundance of alcohol.

As for a cure, try this: Massage the back portion of the roof of your mouth with a cotton-tipped swab, moving the swab gently back and forth for a minute or so. There's no guarantee this method will work, but it often does.

of the procedure, called MUSE. An endoscope equipped with a tiny camera, surgical endostapler and ultrasound sensor is used to wrap the top of the stomach around the lower end of the esophagus.

An alternative procedure involves a ring of tiny magnetic titanium beads that is wrapped around the junction of the stomach and esophagus. The magnetic attraction between the beads is strong enough to keep the opening between the two closed to refluxing acid, but weak enough so that food can pass through it. Known as the LINX device, it can be implanted using minimally invasive surgery methods.

Other causes of esophagitis

In addition to GERD, other disorders can cause inflammation of the esophagus.

Scleroderma of the esophagus

Scleroderma is a disease characterized by an overgrowth of scar-like tissue, causing stiffening and hardening of tissues. This condition can weaken the lower esophageal sphincter, allowing acid to reflux into the esophagus and causing symptoms and complications similar to those of GERD. The contraction (peristalsis) of the esophagus also is diminished, further contributing to reflux symptoms.

Your doctor may prescribe an acid-blocking medication to reduce acid reflux. He or she may also instruct you in self-care measures to prevent reflux (see page 821). If constriction of the esophagus prevents or retards the passage of food, a procedure to widen (dilate) the esophagus may be necessary.

Herpes simplex esophagitis

Infection from the herpes simplex virus can cause inflammation and ulcers in the esophagus. People who develop this condition are often debilitated from another dis-

ease or have a weakened immune system. The antiviral drug acyclovir (Zovirax) may be helpful in treating herpes simplex esophagitis.

Candida esophagitis

The fungus candida growing in the esophagus can cause inflammation and painful swallowing. This is called candida esophagitis. Such an infection often occurs in people whose immune systems are weakened, for example, as a result of medications used to fight cancer. Several antifungal medications can treat candida esophagitis.

Radiation esophagitis

Esophagitis can result from radiation treatment for cancer, most commonly lung or esophageal cancer, that causes the esophagus to narrow. Symptoms include heartburn and pain when swallowing. The likelihood of this disorder increases in direct relation to the amount of radiation received. With the help of medication, the inflammation usually resolves once the radiation treatment ends.

Pill esophagitis

Acute pain in the front of the chest made worse by swallowing can result from pills or capsules that stick in the esophagus and dissolve or break open before entering the stomach. Common culprits include tetracycline antibiotics, potassium, vitamin C, iron medications, and some arthritis and osteoporosis drugs. The condition is preventable by taking medications with plenty of water and not lying down right after taking a medication. Pill esophagitis usually gets better on its own within a few days.

Swallowing difficulties

Signs and symptoms
- Liquids and solid foods stick in the throat or chest
- Regurgitation of food
- A gurgling sound in the throat
- Chest discomfort on swallowing

Emergency signs and symptoms
- An inability to swallow liquids or solids
- Drooling saliva

The causes of persistent swallowing problems vary. Damage or malfunction of the muscles in the wall of the throat or esophagus can cause swallowing difficulties. Ulcers or scar tissue in the esophagus as the result of acid reflux can be another cause.

Pouches (diverticula) may form in the esophageal lining and interfere with the movement of food down the esophagus. Sometimes, swallowing difficulties are associated with diseases such as myasthenia gravis and cancer. In addition, the muscles that line your esophagus and propel food to your stomach can weaken with age, making it more difficult for you to swallow.

Swallowing difficulty may be transient and unimportant, but it's always possible that the problem is an indication of a serious medical condition. Therefore, see your doctor if you continue to have painful or difficult swallowing.

Achalasia

Achalasia is a rare disorder of the esophagus caused by lack of coordinated movement of the muscles of the esophagus and the sphincter muscle at the lower end of the esophagus. The disorder makes it very difficult for food and liquids to pass into the stomach.

People with achalasia often regurgitate food. Sometimes, particularly in the early stages, drinking a large amount of liquid helps to push the food into the stomach. Eventually, however, this fails to help. Some chest discomfort or pain also may occur, although heartburn is unusual.

If you have signs or symptoms of achalasia, your doctor may order a series of tests, possibly including a barium X-ray or an esophageal muscle test, to determine if the esophageal muscles are functioning properly. A procedure

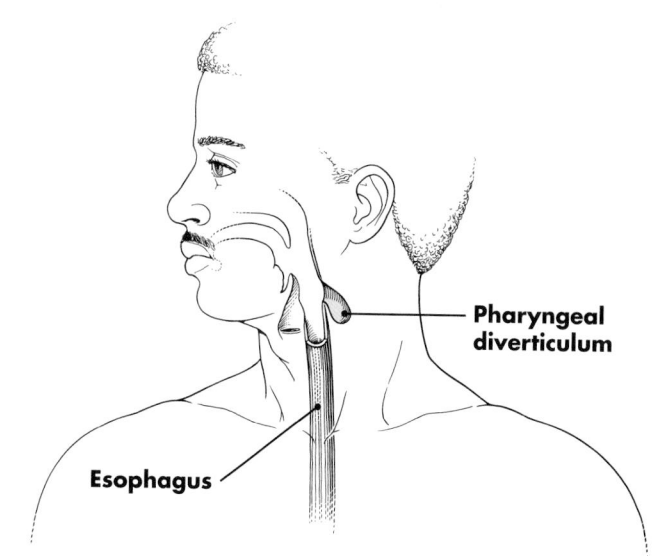

When the muscular wall of your throat (pharynx) weakens, a small pouch, called a pharyngeal diverticulum, may form and trap food or liquids.

called upper endoscopy also may be done to rule out cancer.

Individuals with achalasia are at increased risk of esophageal cancer. Malnutrition, weight loss and aspiration of food into the lungs, leading to pneumonia, are other problems associated with achalasia. Sometimes, a muscle relaxant derived from botulinum toxin (Botox) can be injected by endoscopy into the lower end of the esophagus, allowing food to pass more easily.

A form of treatment for achalasia involves mechanical stretching of the esophageal muscles. A slender tube with a balloon attached is passed down the esophagus to the narrowed area. The balloon is filled with water or air to expand the balloon and stretch open (dilate) the passageway. Balloon dilation weakens the lower esophageal sphincter so that food can pass down the esophagus by gravity. After this treatment, most people can swallow better.

A surgical procedure called esophagomyotomy is another option. In this procedure, a surgeon opens the chest and partially cuts the muscles at the lower end of the esophagus to allow easier passage of food. Risks of this operation

are low, and long-term results generally are good. Some newer techniques involve less invasive (laparoscopic) surgery, allowing speedier recovery.

Diffuse spasm

Diffuse spasm is the term for multiple high-pressure, poorly coordinated contractions of the esophagus that usually occur after swallowing. This is another rare disorder of unknown cause that affects the smooth (involuntary) muscles in the walls of the lower esophagus.

Signs and symptoms can be mild and may even disappear without treatment. You may mistake the symptoms for simple heartburn or heart-related conditions. Sometimes, acid reflux can trigger spasm. With this condition, signs and symptoms often occur intermittently over a period of years. Treatment may include acid-reducing medications. A procedure called balloon dilation can widen (dilate) the esophagus and may produce relief initially. Surgery is rarely, if ever, necessary.

Pharyngeal diverticula

When muscles in the wall of the throat (pharynx) weaken, especially with aging, pouches called diverticula can form, sometimes becoming large enough to trap food. This is especially true when the upper esophageal sphincter doesn't function properly.

With pharyngeal diverticula, also known as Zenker's diverticulum, your throat may become irritated, you may notice a gurgling sound, and you may regurgitate food particles shortly after eating. As the pouches grow larger, food that's retained for days may give you bad breath. There's also a risk that fluid and regurgitated food will be inhaled into the lungs (aspirated), increasing the risk of a lung infection, such as pneumonia.

For large diverticula that produce troublesome symptoms, the most common treatment is removal of the diverticula, often combined with cutting the upper esophageal sphincter, either surgically or endoscopically. Diverticula can also occur in the esophagus, but they rarely cause problems.

Pharyngeal paralysis

The principal characteristics of pharyngeal paralysis are weakness and lack of coordination of the muscles of the throat (pharynx), which cause swallowing difficulty. A person with this problem has trouble getting food from his or her mouth into the throat and esophagus. In addition to swallowing difficulty and throat discomfort, this disorder may result in inhalation of food or fluids (aspiration) into the windpipe (trachea) or regurgitation of food or fluids into the nose.

The symptoms are thought to be the result of faulty transmission of nerve impulses to the muscles in the pharynx and are often due to one of several neurological or muscular disorders.

Tests to establish a diagnosis of pharyngeal paralysis may include a barium X-ray or an esophageal motility study. A procedure called upper gastrointestinal endoscopy may be performed to rule out other possible causes.

Gastrostomy

When the swallowing mechanism of your throat (pharynx) or upper esophagus is disabled, you may be unable to eat properly, preventing you from getting adequate nutrition. Another method is needed to deliver food to your stomach.

This can be done by placement of a tube into the stomach, a procedure called gastrostomy. The tube bypasses the pharynx and esophagus, allowing nutrients to go directly into the stomach, where they pass into the small intestine for digestion and absorption. Sometimes, an extension of this tube is placed directly into the small intestine.

With this type of feeding mechanism, often referred to as a feeding tube, you can receive adequate calories to maintain

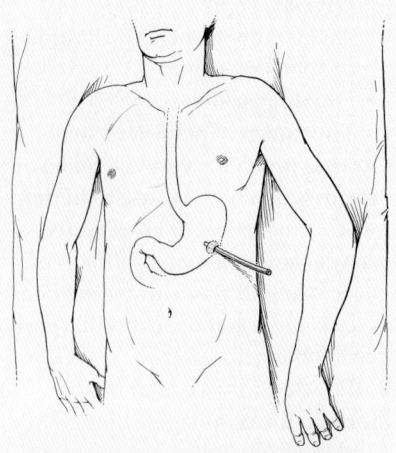

A gastrostomy (feeding) tube allows an individual to receive food directly into the stomach.

nutrition. Your doctor or dietitian will instruct you in proper feeding techniques, including the amount of calories to be infused to ensure adequate nutrition.

If the ability to swallow returns, the feeding tube can be removed.

If the paralysis is due to a neurological disease, it may respond to treatment for the disease. People recovering from a stroke often experience improvement over time. Surgery is rarely effective.

Many people with pharyngeal paralysis require a temporary feeding tube (nasogastric tube), which runs through the nose to the stomach.

Sometimes, a feeding tube is placed directly through the abdominal wall into the stomach, a procedure called gastrostomy. This bypasses the affected area in the pharynx or esophagus and allows use of the remaining gastrointestinal tract for proper digestion.

Globus

Some people experience the sensation of a lump in their throat without having any problem swallowing their food. This disorder is called globus. At times, it may be the result of stress or related to the reflux of acid.

If your doctor suspects globus, he or she may ask you to identify any possible source of stress in your life. Often times, relief of stress eliminates the problem.

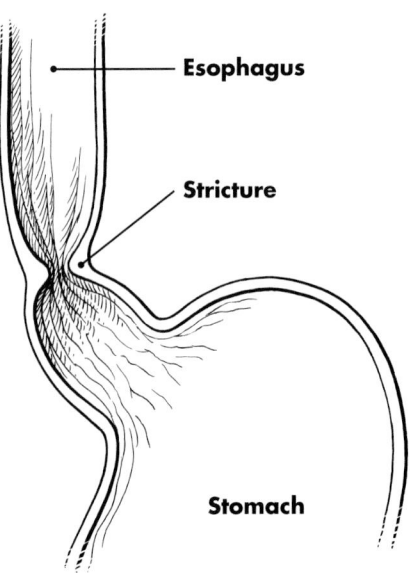

Esophagus

Stricture

Stomach

Narrowing of the passageway of the esophagus is called an esophageal stricture. This can cause difficulty in swallowing.

Esophageal stricture

Signs and symptoms
- Difficulty swallowing

Esophageal stricture is a narrowing of the passageway of the esophagus, so food and, eventually, liquids can't pass through without difficulty. The main cause of a stricture in adults is scar tissue caused by reflux of stomach acid (see page 818). Scar tissue can also result from other causes, including radiation, previous esophageal surgery or ingestion of caustic chemicals.

An esophageal web, a network of thin membranes across the esophagus, also can narrow the upper end of the esophagus. For unknown reasons, this condition is more likely to appear in middle-aged women and may be associated with iron deficiency. It may lead to difficulty swallowing solid foods.

Another condition that can cause esophageal stricture is a mucosal ring. This may occur near the lower esophageal sphincter. This disorder also causes difficulty in swallowing solids.

Diagnosis
To determine the cause of your swallowing difficulty and to identify a stricture, your doctor may perform a variety of tests, including an upper endoscopic examination and a barium X-ray.

Treatment
One form of treatment for an esophageal stricture is a procedure in which the narrowed passageway is opened with a dilator. The dilator stretches the scar tissue, web or ring.

Before this procedure, you need to fast for at least six to eight hours. A topical anesthetic may be applied to the lining of your throat. You may also receive a sedative. A thin, flexible instrument called an upper endoscope is inserted into your esophagus to perform the procedure.

In one method, a guide wire is inserted through the endoscope and then the endoscope is withdrawn. Progressively larger dilators are threaded along the length of the wire and through the stricture, to force open the passageway. At times, balloons are passed through the scope and moved to the point of the narrowing. There they are inflated, helping to open the passageway.

Dilation is generally quite safe, but for a few hours after the procedure you may feel tightness or discomfort in your chest or some pain when you swallow. Rarely, a tear may occur in the wall of the esophagus. The benefit of dilation is that it permits blocked food and fluids to move freely through the esophagus and into the stomach. Repeat dilations may be necessary from time to time. Acid-reducing medications are prescribed after dilation to prevent recurrence of the stricture. Surgery is rarely necessary to treat a stricture.

Foreign bodies

Signs and symptoms
- Difficulty swallowing

Emergency signs and symptoms
- A complete inability to swallow liquids or solids
- Drooling saliva
- Inability to breathe or to utter a sound
- Pale and clammy skin

Sometimes, food, such as a large piece of meat, or another object can become lodged in your throat or esophagus. Older adults with dentures and people who have difficulty chewing their food properly are prone to obstruction of the throat or esophagus. Children are prone to swallowing pins, coins, pieces of their toys or other small objects that can become stuck.

Blockage of the throat may cut off the airway, prompting a medical emergency. The Heimlich maneuver (see page 14) should be performed to dislodge the offending piece of food or object. A more common situation occurs when food is stuck farther down the esophagus, blocking the passage into your stomach. If the obstruction is partial, you may be able to drink liquids. If the obstruction is total, you may spit up saliva.

Many foreign objects actually may pass into the stomach and through the gastrointestinal tract without complications. However, if the object is sharp-edged, it may scratch or perforate the esophagus, stomach or intestine on its way through.

If an obstruction causes an inability to swallow or interferes with your ability to breathe, call for emergency help or have someone take you to the nearest emergency department immediately. If you're able to breathe satisfactorily but have difficulty swallowing water or food, go to the emergency department right away.

Diagnosis
Your doctor may use a variety of tests, including endoscopy, in which a fiber-optic tube is inserted down your throat, to identify the location and severity of the obstruction. Before the instrument is inserted, you will likely receive a sedative.

Treatment
Often, a doctor can retrieve a foreign object lodged in the throat or esophagus with an endoscope. He or she might push the object into the stomach if it's something that will likely pass all the way through the digestive tract. Once the object has been removed from the esophagus, your doctor may want to inspect your esophagus to determine if some type of abnormality contributed to the obstruction.

Esophageal tumors

Signs and symptoms
- Progressive difficulty in swallowing
- Weight loss
- Regurgitation

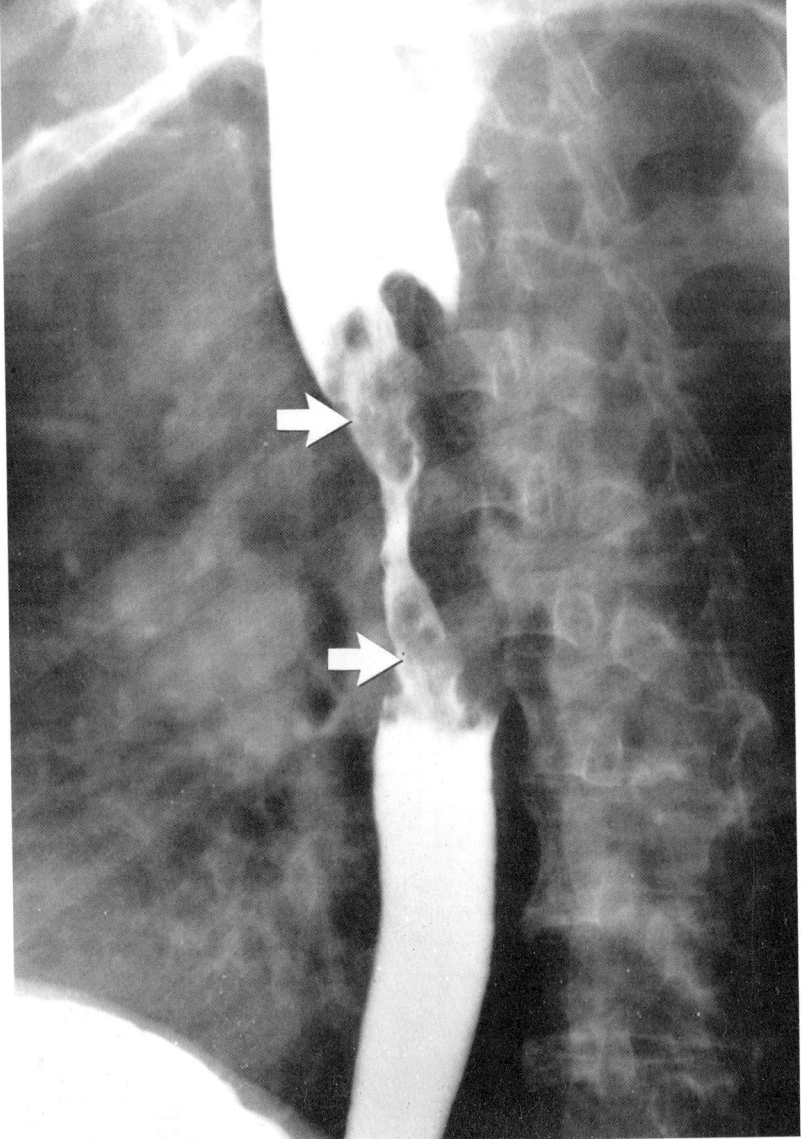

A barium X-ray reveals narrowing of the esophagus (see arrows) caused by a cancerous tumor.

analyzed in a laboratory. Your doctor may also order a computerized tomography (CT) scan or an endoscopic ultrasound exam to determine the extent of the tumor.

How serious are esophageal tumors?

Most tumors in the esophagus are malignant. Because the disease is often far along in its development before the cancer is identified, the cure rate is poor. Early detection is key to successful treatment.

Treatment

The most common surgical treatment for esophageal cancer is to remove the cancerous section of the esophagus and reconnect the remaining healthy sections.

If a large portion of your esophagus is removed, your surgeon may form a new passageway from your throat to your stomach using a segment of your intestine.

If your cancer is very small, confined to the superficial layers of your esophagus and hasn't spread, your surgeon may recommend removing the cancer using an endoscope that's passed down your throat and into your esophagus.

Chemotherapy and radiation are sometimes used, alone or in combination, to ease signs and symptoms, shrink the tumor or kill cancerous cells that have spread beyond the esophagus.

To improve swallowing, sometimes a hollow tube (stent) is inserted into the esophagus. The tube helps increase the opening through the obstructing cancer, making eating easier.

Esophageal varices

Signs and symptoms
- Vomiting of blood
- Faintness, sweating and pallor

With esophageal varices, veins that line the esophagus become abnormally enlarged (varicose). Pressure within the expanded varicose veins (varices) of the esophagus can cause them to

Most esophageal tumors form in the middle or lower portion of the esophagus, and nearly 90 percent of them are cancerous (malignant). The principal symptom of an esophageal tumor, whether noncancerous (benign) or malignant, is progressive difficulty in swallowing. The difficulty often begins with solid foods but eventually includes liquids. As the condition worsens, weight loss, regurgitation of food and foul-smelling breath often occur.

Because swallowing becomes progressively worse over a relatively long period of time, many people delay seeing a doctor. Con-

sequently, in many cases by the time the person receives a diagnosis of esophageal tumor, the tumor is large enough to fill about half the diameter of the esophagus.

Malignant tumors are twice as likely to occur in men as in women. Individuals at the highest risk are those between the ages of 50 and 60 who are heavy smokers and drink excessive amounts of alcohol.

Diagnosis

The diagnostic test used to identify an esophageal tumor is an upper endoscopic examination. If a tumor is found, a sample of tissue (biopsy) may be removed and

rupture. Heavy bleeding can result in shock. Esophageal varices occur infrequently and usually result as a complication of liver disease.

How serious are esophageal varices?

Although uncommon, esophageal varices are serious. The bleeding can be life-threatening.

Treatment

Treatment depends in large part on the location of the bleeding and its severity. Often, drugs are used initially to slow the rate of bleeding. To control bleeding, small rubber bands are placed over the enlarged veins. Less commonly, a physician may inject a solution into the vein that initially obliterates and then inflames and scars the varicose vein, a process called variceal sclerotherapy. These methods often stop the bleeding but may need to be repeated.

Yet another procedure, called transjugular intrahepatic portosystemic shunt (TIPS), involves placing a mesh tube (stent) between your liver (hepatic) vein and your portal vein to shunt blood away from the portal vein and reduce pressure on the connecting esophageal veins. Decreased portal vein outflow due to liver disease is often the cause of increased pressure in your esophageal veins.

If these methods fail, surgery may be necessary to shunt blood away from the ruptured veins.

Esophageal trauma

Signs and symptoms
- Chest pain
- Rapid, shallow breathing
- Sweating
- Vomiting blood

A tear or puncture can sometimes occur in the esophagus. The injury may result from swallowing a foreign object or from a diagnostic procedure in which an instrument is inserted into the esophagus. It may also be a complication of another disorder or, rarely, a result of an episode of forceful vomiting.

Esophageal trauma may produce some blood in vomit. In more severe cases, such as a large perforation, breathing can become shallow and rapid, accompanied by severe chest pain.

Treatment

The first step typically involves diagnostic tests to determine the presence and location of the tear. This is typically done with X-rays. If the perforation is large, surgery may be necessary to repair the esophagus. For less serious injuries, such as a superficial tear, the condition may be treated with a hollow tube (stent) inserted into the esophagus, intravenous (IV) fluids and antibiotics until the injury heals.

Stomach Disorders

A hollow, J-shaped sac, the stomach rests in the left-central section of your upper abdomen, just below your rib cage. It receives food from the esophagus, reducing it to a semiliquid mixture. Most of the stomach's contents trickle into the small intestine for further digestion and absorption.

The stomach is a remarkable organ, but it doesn't always function smoothly. Problems primarily affecting the lining of the stomach can lead to illness. The lining of the stomach generally is resistant to injury, but at times its resistance can break down.

Indigestion

Signs and symptoms
- Discomfort or a feeling of fullness in the upper abdomen
- Nausea
- A sensation of bloating, often relieved by belching

Indigestion (dyspepsia) is not a disease but rather a collection of symptoms you may experience, such as heartburn, bloating, belching and nausea.

If you eat too much of any food, you can have an upset stomach, particularly if you overindulge in fatty or spicy foods. Eating too quickly has the same effect. Alcohol and stress can also take a toll.

Persistent indigestion may point to other digestive conditions such as heartburn, peptic ulcers, gastritis, gallstones or stomach cancer.

Additional causes of indigestion may include a reaction to certain drugs or supplements. Aspirin or nonsteroidal anti-inflammatory drugs (NSAIDs) such as ibuprofen (Advil, Motrin IB, others) and naproxen sodium (Aleve) can cause ulcers and gastritis. These medications may irritate your digestive system without producing visible stomach or intestinal damage. The same may be true for other medications and supplements, including antibiotics, steroids, minerals and herbs.

Acid-secreting cells in the stomach may produce higher than normal amounts of digestive juices that irritate gastric tissues. Or tissues in the stomach and duodenum may be overly sensitive to normal acid levels and become easily irritated. It's also possible that nerve signals between your stomach and brain may be altered, causing an exaggerated response to normal changes that take place during digestion.

Diagnosis

Because indigestion can be a vague term, it's important that you be specific about your symptoms when describing them to your doctor. Where is the discomfort located? Does it occur before, during, shortly after or several hours after a meal? How long do the symptoms last? Because indigestion can be caused by problems anywhere in the digestive system, answers to these questions can help your doctor pinpoint the affected area.

Diagnostic tests may include an upper endoscopic examination, a barium X-ray, or an ultrasound or computerized tomography (CT) scan of your pancreas, liver and gallbladder. Your doctor may test you for a certain bacterium called *Helicobacter pylori*, which can cause indigestion, gastritis or ulcers.

How serious is indigestion?
In itself, indigestion is more of a discomfort than a serious problem. However, because it can be a symptom of a major underlying disease, treat your indigestion seriously, particularly if it's of recent onset. It's important to see a doctor so that more-serious problems can be ruled out.

Treatment
If a specific cause such as a peptic ulcer or gastritis is responsible for your indigestion, treating that condition will likely relieve your symptoms. When a cause can't be found, lifestyle adjustments and medication are often the most common treatments for indigestion.

Self-care
Your doctor may advise you to eliminate or limit certain foods or beverages that may be causing your indigestion. He or she might also discourage the use of cigarettes, alcohol or NSAIDs, which can contribute to indigestion.

In addition, your doctor may suggest techniques to help reduce stress, if stress appears to be a possible cause of your symptoms. Efforts should be directed at changing those factors that may relieve your symptoms.

Medication
Your doctor may elect to have you try a few weeks of treatment with an acid blocker or a proton pump inhibitor, such as omeprazole (Prilosec), lansoprazole (Prevacid), rabeprazole (Aciphex) or esomeprazole (Nexium), to see if symptoms improve.

He or she may also recommend a medication such as sucralfate (Carafate), which works by protecting the lining of the stomach. It has varying success and may be associated with side effects.

Peptic ulcers

Signs and symptoms
- A burning, aching, gnawing, or pain or discomfort in the upper abdomen or lower chest
- A bloated feeling after meals
- Nausea and vomiting

Emergency signs and symptoms
- Cold, clammy skin and fainting, suggesting excessive blood loss
- Vomiting of bright red blood
- Black, tarry, foul-smelling stools

Peptic ulcers are open sores in the inner lining of the stomach, duodenum or lower esophagus. Peptic ulcers are not uncommon in our society.

Causes
Peptic ulcers form as a result of an imbalance between destructive forces and protective mechanisms in the stomach and duodenum. The lining of the stomach and duodenum is normally resistant to injury and kept intact by a balance of stomach acid and neutralizing substances. When the balance breaks down, the result may be a peptic ulcer.

In the United States, the bacterium *Helicobacter pylori* is a common cause of peptic ulcers, especially in areas characterized by crowded conditions and a low socioeconomic standard of living.

Regular use of nonsteroidal anti-inflammatory drugs (NSAIDs), such as naproxen sodium (Aleve) or ibuprofen (Advil, Motrin IB, others), also can irritate or inflame the lining of your stomach and small intestine and lead to an ulcer. About 20 percent of people who take NSAIDs regularly develop an ulcer.

Smoking decreases healing of ulcers and can increase complications related to them.

Types
The most common peptic ulcer is a duodenal ulcer. It appears in the first part of the small intestine (duodenum). A gastric ulcer (stomach ulcer) is usually found on the lower portion of the stomach.

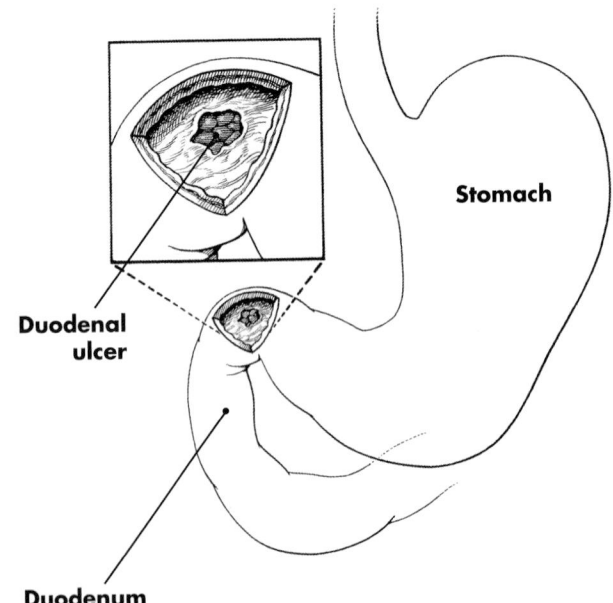

Stomach

Duodenal ulcer

Duodenum

A peptic ulcer that occurs in the upper portion of the small intestine (duodenum) is called a duodenal ulcer.

Duodenal ulcer

There's no one symptom that will tell you that you have a duodenal ulcer. A possible indication, however, is a burning, aching, gnawing or hungry sensation in the upper middle section of your upper abdomen or a pain under the lower part of your breastbone that comes and goes. If the ulcer is located on the back wall of your duodenum, you may feel pain in your midback. If scarring results from a long-standing ulcer, it can obstruct the outlet of the stomach (pylorus). Your stomach may feel distended after meals, and you may vomit or regurgitate stomach acid.

Some people don't experience any pain with an ulcer. Bleeding may be the only sign. The stools may be black, tarry and foul smelling, or maroon colored.

Gastric ulcer

Excessive gastric acid may contribute to the formation of a gastric ulcer. However, in most cases it's believed that a gastric ulcer develops because the mucus and protective lining of the stomach are defective and unable to resist the usual amount of stomach acid.

It's not easy to distinguish between a duodenal ulcer and gastric ulcer on the basis of symptoms. The pain from a gastric ulcer may be less likely to be relieved by eating. In some cases, eating actually increases the pain of a gastric ulcer.

Esophageal ulcer

An esophageal ulcer is usually located in the lower section of the esophagus. It's often associated with chronic gastroesophageal reflux disease (GERD).

Diagnosis

If your doctor suspects that you have an ulcer, he or she may conduct an upper endoscopic examination. Using an endoscope, a sample of tissue (biopsy) is removed and sent for laboratory analysis to check for bacteria that can cause ulcers and to exclude cancer. An upper gastrointestinal X-ray may also be used. In this test you swallow a white, metallic liquid, which outlines your esophagus, stomach and duodenum.

In addition to a biopsy, other tests also may determine if the cause of your ulcer is *H. pylori* infection. These include a breath test and stool antigen test.

How serious are peptic ulcers?

With early detection and proper treatment, most people recover from an ulcer within a few weeks. However, early treatment doesn't guarantee a cure because some people treated for ulcers have a recurrence.

Several potentially serious complications are associated with peptic ulcers. Sometimes, an ulcer will bleed (hemorrhage), necessitating hospitalization. If the bleeding is only slight but continues over a period of time, iron deficiency anemia may develop.

Perforation, another serious complication, occurs when the ulcer erodes through the wall of the stomach or duodenum into the abdominal cavity. This produces sudden onset of intense, persistent abdominal pain. A long-standing ulcer may cause an obstruction at the outlet of the stomach.

Treatment

Because many ulcers stem from *H. pylori* bacteria, doctors use a two-pronged approach to peptic ulcer treatment: Kill the bacteria and reduce the level of acid in your digestive system to relieve pain and encourage healing. Accomplishing these goals requires the use of three or four of the following medications:

- **Antibiotics.** Doctors use combinations of antibiotics to treat *H. pylori* because one antibiotic alone isn't always sufficient to kill the organism. Antibiotics prescribed for treatment of *H. pylori* include amoxicillin (Amoxil), clarithromycin (Biaxin) and metronidazole (Flagyl).

Combination drugs that include antibiotics together with an acid suppressor or cytoprotective agent (Prevpac, Pylera) have been designed specifically for the treatment of *H. pylori* infection.

- **Acid blockers.** Also called histamine (H-2) blockers, these medicines reduce the amount of hydrochloric acid released into your digestive tract, which relieves ulcer pain and encourages healing. Acid blockers work by keeping histamine from reaching histamine receptors. Histamine is a substance normally present in your body. When it reacts with histamine receptors, the receptors signal acid-secreting cells in your stomach to release hydrochloric acid. Available by prescription or over-the-counter (OTC), acid blockers include the medications ranitidine (Zantac), famotidine (Pepcid), cimetidine (Tagamet HB) and nizatidine (Axid AR).

- **Antacids.** Your doctor may include an antacid in your drug regimen. An antacid may be taken in addition to an acid blocker or in place of one. Instead of reducing acid secretion, antacids neutralize existing stomach acid and can provide rapid pain relief.

- **Proton pump inhibitors.** Another way to reduce stomach acid is to shut down the "pumps" within acid-secreting cells. Proton pump inhibitors block the action of these tiny pumps. These drugs include the prescription and over-the-counter medications omeprazole (Prilosec), lansoprazole (Prevacid), rabeprazole (Aciphex) and esomeprazole (Nexium). The drug pantoprazole (Protonix) can be taken orally or administered intravenously in the hospital. Doctors frequently prescribe proton pump inhibitors to promote the healing of peptic ulcers. Proton pump inhibitors also appear to inhibit *H. pylori*. However, long-term use of proton pump inhib-

What About Diet and Stress?

Before the bacterium *Helicobacter pylori* was discovered and the association was made with NSAIDs, ulcers were thought to be a result of certain lifestyle factors, such as diet and stress.

There's no clear evidence that people who are under a lot of stress or eat hurried, irregular meals or spicy foods are more likely to have ulcers. And now that these factors have been eliminated as causes, they no longer figure in treatment. For example, eating a bland diet with plenty of milk is no longer advised. In fact, drinking large quantities of milk is discouraged because foods rich in protein and calcium tend to stimulate acid production.

It's still a good idea, though, to avoid spicy foods and reduce stress while an ulcer is healing. Even though stress and food don't cause an ulcer, they can exacerbate ulcer pain. Stress also slows digestion, allowing food and digestive acids to remain in your stomach and intestines for a longer period.

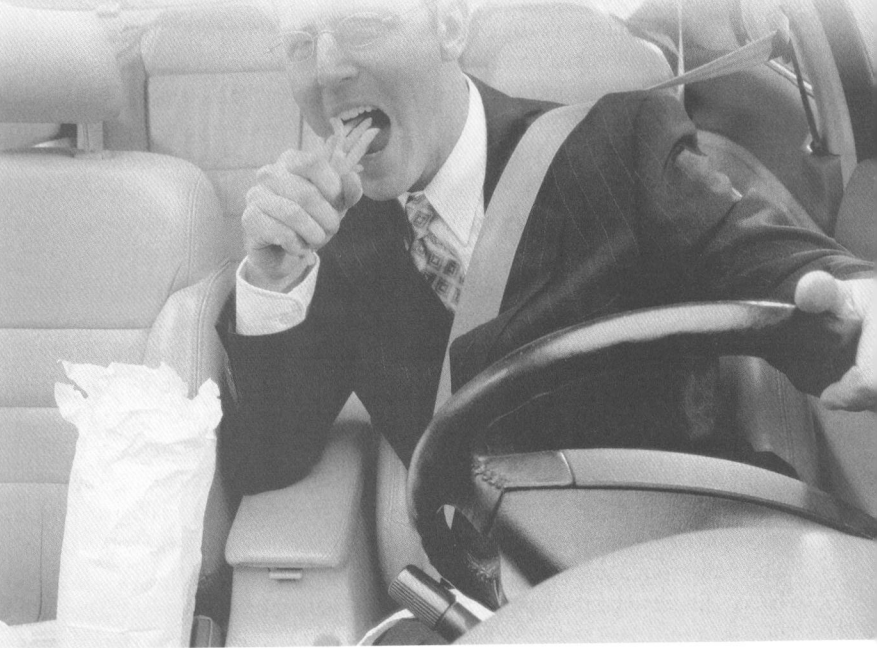

itors, particularly at high doses, may increase your risk of hip fracture. Research suggests they may also put people at higher risk of chronic kidney disease.

- **Cytoprotective agents.** These medications help protect the tissues that line your stomach and small intestine. They include the prescription medications sucralfate (Carafate) and misoprostol (Cytotec). A nonprescription cytoprotective agent is bismuth subsalicylate (Pepto-Bismol).

Peptic ulcers that don't heal with treatment are called refractory ulcers. Treatment for refractory ulcers generally involves eliminating factors that may interfere with healing, along with stronger doses of ulcer medications. Surgery is necessary only when the ulcer doesn't respond to aggressive drug treatment.

Prevention
The delicate balance of acid in your stomach and gastrointestinal tract can be disrupted by aspirin and other pain relievers. If you need to take pain relievers regularly, ask your doctor about acetaminophen (Tylenol, others). It doesn't cause ulcers and stomach

upset as do other pain relievers. Anti-inflammatory prescription medications called COX-2 inhibitors (Celebrex) may be less damaging to your digestive system.

If you have a history of ulcers, mention this whenever a doctor prescribes a medication for you. If an ulcer-provoking drug is absolutely necessary to treat another condition, your doctor can prescribe a second medication to reduce the risk of a recurrent ulcer.

Zollinger-Ellison syndrome

Signs and symptoms
- Ulcer-like symptoms in the upper abdomen
- Severe, persistent ulcer-like symptoms that aren't relieved by antacids
- Diarrhea
- Heartburn and acid reflux

Zollinger-Ellison syndrome is a rare condition in which tumors, called gastrinomas, form most commonly in the pancreas or duodenum. The tumors secrete a substance called gastrin, which stimulates excessive acid secretion by the stomach.

As a result, most people with Zollinger-Ellison syndrome have a peptic ulcer at some point during their disease. Ulcers associated with Zollinger-Ellison syndrome are typically more persistent and less responsive to treatment than usual peptic ulcers are. The syndrome may occur at any age, but signs and symptoms are more likely to appear between ages 30 and 60.

Diagnosis
If you have symptoms that suggest Zollinger-Ellison syndrome, your doctor may perform blood tests to see if the gastrin level in your blood is increased. Generally, a person with Zollinger-Ellison syndrome has an abnormally high serum gastrin level, which causes production of excessive amounts of stomach acid. Your doctor may also order an upper endoscopic examination of your stomach to search for evidence of ulcers.

Gastrinomas are often small and difficult to locate, but recent advances in diagnostic techniques have improved identification and localization of these tumors. Techniques include ultrasound that can be used in the operating room and nuclear medicine scans, which use a tiny dose of radioactive material that binds to the tumor and shows as a hot spot on the scan.

How serious is Zollinger-Ellison syndrome?
Zollinger-Ellison syndrome can be serious. The tumors may slowly spread, most commonly to the lymph nodes and liver. In addition, ulcers associated with the syndrome are usually severe and not easily treated with conventional medication or surgery. As with most serious illness, the earlier you receive a diagnosis, the better the chances of a favorable outcome.

Treatment
Ulcers associated with Zollinger-Ellison syndrome typically are resistant to standard doses of medication. Especially if you're young and in good health, your doctor may elect to perform an operation to identify and remove the one or more tumors responsible for the excess production of acid. Sometimes, these tumors are so small or multiple in nature that they can't be identified and removed.

If your surgeon is unable to remove the gastrinomas, you'll need to take an acid-reducing medication. The most effective drug is a proton pump inhibitor, such as omeprazole (Prilosec), lansoprazole (Prevacid), rabeprazole (Aciphex), pantoprazole (Protonix) or esomeprazole (Nexium), which has the advantage of virtually eliminating acid production for a period of time. With this type of ulcer, you may need to take larger and more frequent doses than you would for an ordinary peptic ulcer. Usually, these medications are taken indefinitely to prevent recurrence of signs and symptoms.

You'll also need follow-up examinations to watch carefully for growth or spread of the tumors.

Gastritis

Signs and symptoms
- Upper abdominal discomfort
- Nausea and, occasionally, vomiting
- Loss of appetite
- Belching or bloating

The term *gastritis* is used to describe a group of conditions characterized by inflammation of the lining of the stomach. Gastritis can result from a number of causes, each of which may produce somewhat different signs and symptoms.

Acute gastritis occurs suddenly and is more likely to cause nausea and burning pain or discomfort in your upper abdomen. Chronic gastritis develops gradually and is more likely to cause a dull pain and a feeling of fullness or loss of appetite after a few bites of food.

Gastritis can occur as a result of acid-induced damage to the lining of the stomach when no ulcer is present. Excessive smoking or alcohol consumption is known to produce gastritis or to aggravate existing signs and symptoms.

Gastritis can also be a side effect of many prescription drugs. One form, erosive gastritis, is often associated with the ingestion of aspirin or pain medications such as ibuprofen (Advil, Motrin IB, others) or naproxen sodium (Aleve). Gastritis may also result from infection with the organism *Helicobacter pylori*. Severe stress due to burns, trauma, surgery or shock may produce stress gastritis.

Interestingly, gastritis is sometimes seen in people whose stomachs don't produce acid. In such cases, the lining of the stomach is atrophied. This condition, called atrophic gastritis, may be associated with vitamin B-12 deficiency and occurs in many older adults.

Diagnosis

Your doctor may be able to make a diagnosis based on a description of your symptoms. Your doctor may inquire about your eating habits and use of medications. He or she may also want to know if you're a heavy drinker or you smoke regularly.

In addition, your doctor may request a barium X-ray of your stomach. However, the results of this study are often normal. A diagnosis of gastritis can best be confirmed with an upper endoscopy examination, which reveals typical findings. A biopsy of stomach tissues also can be helpful in confirming the diagnosis and can indicate the cause.

Other tests can determine if the cause of your gastritis may be *H. pylori* infection. These include a breath test and stool antigen test. A positive test indicates you've come in contact with the bacteria at some point, but it doesn't necessarily indicate current infection.

How serious is gastritis?

In most cases, symptoms of gastritis are relatively mild and short-lived, pose no real danger, and have no lasting effect, especially if you receive an early diagnosis and the condition is treated. Occasionally, gastritis may cause bleeding.

Treatment

Treatment of gastritis depends on the specific cause. Acute gastritis caused by NSAIDs or alcohol may be relieved by stopping use of those substances. Chronic gastritis caused by *H. pylori* infection is treated by eradicating the bacteria. Most gastritis treatment plans also incorporate medications that treat stomach acid to reduce your signs and symptoms and promote healing in your stomach.

Medications to treat stomach acid
Stomach acid irritates inflamed tissue in your stomach, causing pain and further inflammation. That's why, for most types of gas-

tritis, treatment involves taking drugs to reduce or neutralize stomach acid, such as:

- **Antacids.** Over-the-counter antacids (Maalox, Mylanta, others) in liquid or tablet form are a common treatment for mild gastritis. Antacids neutralize stomach acid and can provide fast pain relief.
- **Acid blockers.** When antacids don't provide enough relief, your doctor may recommend a medication, such as cimetidine (Tagamet HB), ranitidine (Zantac), nizatidine (Axid AR) or famotidine (Pepcid), that helps reduce the amount of acid your stomach produces.
- **Proton pump inhibitors.** They reduce acid by blocking the action of tiny pumps within the acid-secreting cells of your stomach. This class of medications includes omeprazole (Prilosec), lansoprazole (Prevacid), rabeprazole (Aciphex) and esomeprazole (Nexium).

Medications to treat H. pylori
Several regimens may be used to treat *H. pylori* infection. Most include a combination of two antibiotics and a proton pump inhibitor. Sometimes bismuth subsalicylate (Pepto-Bismol) is added to the mix. The antibiotics help destroy the bacteria. The proton pump inhibitor relieves pain and nausea, heals inflammation and may increase the antibiotics' effectiveness.

Gastrointestinal tract bleeding

Signs and symptoms

- Red blood in the stool, creating maroon-colored stool
- Black, tarry stool
- Vomiting of blood
- Fatigue from iron deficiency

Gastrointestinal tract bleeding may result from a variety of conditions, including a peptic ulcer, gastritis, esophageal varices, esophageal trauma, inflammatory bowel disease, cancerous (malignant) tumors, diverticular disease, hemorrhoids and vascular lesions.

Red or maroon stool can indicate several problems, such as colon cancer, Crohn's disease or ulcerative colitis. One of the more common explanations for heavy bleeding in stool in people older than age 60 is bleeding from pouches (diverticula) or blood vessels in the colon.

Red blood in the stool may also indicate blood loss from the stomach or duodenum, particularly if the bleeding is heavy and rapid. Slow bleeding that occurs in the stomach or duodenum and passes through the gastrointestinal tract causes black and sticky stools that resemble tar. Ingestion of iron or bismuth subsalicylate (such as Pepto-Bismol) also may turn your stool black.

If you notice blood in your stool or in the toilet bowl, consult your doctor. The source of the blood may be as simple as hemorrhoids, but you want to rule out other conditions such as colon cancer.

Vomited blood, on the other hand, suggests that the bleeding is from the esophagus, stomach or upper small intestine (duodenum). Blood that enters the intestines below the duodenum usually doesn't reflux back into the stomach but passes in stool.

Vomiting of bright red blood generally indicates that the bleeding began shortly before you vomited. Blood that has been in your stomach for a longer time is generally dark red or brown in color or has the texture and color of old coffee grounds.

Diagnosis

For bleeding that occurs in the upper portion of the gastrointestinal tract, your doctor may perform a procedure called upper gastrointestinal endoscopy, in which a small fiber-optic tube is inserted down your esophagus and into your stomach to look for the source of the bleeding. For bleeding in the lower gastrointestinal tract, your doctor may perform a colonoscopy, which is similar to upper endoscopy, only the tube is inserted through the rectum and threaded up through the colon.

Often, blood in the stool can be detected only by diagnostic tests because the amount is too small to see. This is called occult blood.

Treatment

Treatment depends on the cause and severity of the bleeding. For variceal bleeding in the esophagus, various techniques stop the bleeding. If the bleeding is from a diverticulum, injecting medication adjacent to the diverticulum may stop the bleeding.

For bleeding related to an ulcer, gastritis or hemorrhoids, treating the condition will often stop the bleeding. At times, the use of an electric current or laser light delivered through an endoscope may stop bleeding in the stomach, duodenum or colon. In some cases, such as if the bleeding resists these treatments, specialized radiologic tests or surgery may be required.

Stomach cancer

Signs and symptoms
- Discomfort in the upper or middle regions of the abdomen
- Black, tarry stools
- Vomiting of blood
- Vomiting after meals
- A bloated feeling after meals
- Weight loss
- Anemia

Most tumors that develop in the stomach are noncancerous (benign) growths (polyps) that have little if any potential to turn cancerous. Much less common are adenomas, which infrequently become cancerous as they grow in size. Stomach cancer affects twice as many men as women, usually between the ages of 50 and 70. It's rare to find this type of cancer in people younger than age 40.

The cause of all cancerous stomach tumors isn't certain. However, infection with *Helicobacter pylori* and the presence of atrophic gastritis are considered risk factors. Genetic factors also may have some influence. Stomach tumors are two to four times more common in members of the immediate family of people with the disease. In addition, stomach cancer is much more common in some countries, such as Japan. It's interesting to note, though, that the children of Japanese parents who migrate to the United States have a much lower incidence of stomach cancer, suggesting that environmental influences, such as diet, also may be potential causes.

Diagnosis

No one symptom is suggestive of stomach cancer. Some people with cancerous stomach tumors have symptoms similar to individuals with peptic ulcers.

If persistent indigestion develops for the first time in your life, along with unexplained weight loss and nausea, your doctor may want to perform an upper endoscopic examination to determine if your symptoms are due to cancer or to some other abnormality. During an endoscopic examination, your doctor may remove a small piece of tissue from your stomach for analysis (biopsy). If cancer is found, he or she may also want to obtain a computerized tomography (CT) scan or endoscopic ultrasound examination to determine if the cancer has spread (metastasized).

How serious is stomach cancer?

Stomach cancer can be difficult to treat. If the cancer is confined to the stomach, chances of successful treatment are good. If the disease has spread, the chance of cure is significantly decreased.

Treatment

Surgery offers the best chance for treating stomach cancer. The likelihood of success depends almost exclusively on whether the cancer has spread to other organs or areas of the body. If the cancer is detected early and surgery can remove all of the affected areas, full recovery is possible. Even when surgery may not offer a cure, treatment with chemotherapy and radiation therapy can prolong survival. Chemotherapy and radiation may also prevent recurrence of the cancer after surgery.

Even when a cure isn't possible, surgery still may help alleviate pain, bleeding or obstruction.

Ménétrier's disease

Signs and symptoms
- Stomach pain
- Nausea and vomiting
- Weight loss
- Intestinal bleeding
- Swelling of the hands, feet or legs

Ménétrier's disease usually develops after age 50 and is of unknown origin. In this condition, the lining of the stomach overdevelops (hypertrophies) and creates large folds, which may have tiny breaks (erosions). Some erosions can develop into ulcers and cause bleeding from the stomach. Protein may be lost from the folds, causing low blood proteins and swelling in the extremities (edema).

X-rays can reveal the enlarged stomach folds. To rule out any possibility of cancer, your doctor may perform other tests such as an upper gastrointestinal endoscopic examination or an endoscopic ultrasound exam. Under certain conditions, a doctor may opt to make a small surgical opening

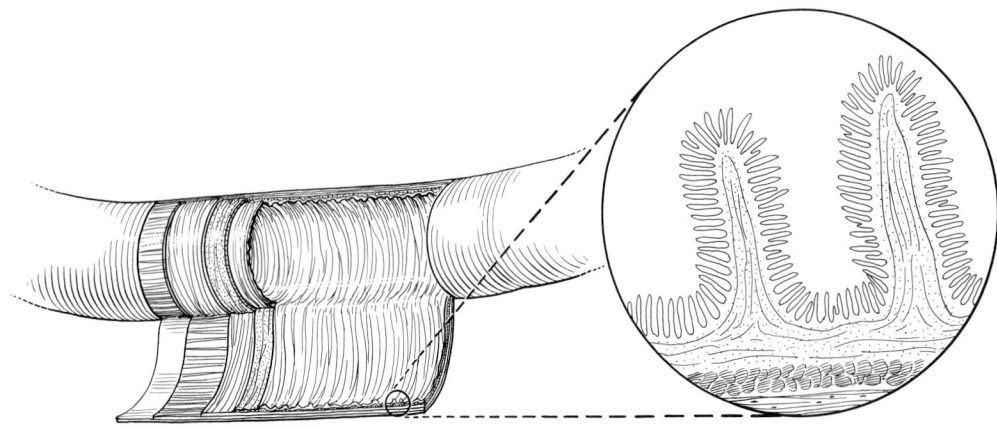

The wall of the small intestine is lined with many small projections called villi (see inset). Villi increase the surface area through which nutrients can be absorbed.

in the abdomen (laparotomy) to confirm the diagnosis.

There's no single treatment for all people with this disease. Your doctor may urge you to eat a high-protein diet to compensate for any protein loss. If you develop associated problems such as ulcers or protein deficiency, they also need to be treated. The use of acid-suppressing medications may be helpful, particularly if erosions or ulcers are present. A variety of other medications can sometimes be helpful. In severe cases, surgery may be necessary to remove at least a portion of the stomach.

Eosinophilic gastroenteritis

Signs and symptoms
- Abdominal pain
- Nausea and vomiting
- Intermittent diarrhea, possibly bloody
- Weight loss and a failure to thrive and grow

This is a rare disease in which the lining of the stomach and the intestinal tract become infiltrated with a type of white blood cell (eosinophils). A diagnosis can be made by a biopsy of tissue in the stomach and intestinal tract.

Treatment
Corticosteroid medications are usually effective in treating the disease. Individuals should also be assessed for food allergies.

Intestinal Disorders

The small intestine consists of three parts: the duodenum, the jejunum and the ileum. This organ continues the processes of digestion and absorption that began in your stomach. Bile from the liver and juices from the pancreas enter the small intestine to aid in the process of digestion.

Most of the nutrients in the food you eat are absorbed into your bloodstream by way of the small intestine. The wall of the small intestine is lined with numerous small projections called villi. These projections significantly increase the surface area through which food can be absorbed.

The small intestine is connected to the large intestine at the ileocecal valve. Through this valve, semi-liquid material from the small intestine passes into the first part of the large intestine (cecum). The shape of the large intestine resembles an upside-down U in that it runs up, across and down in the abdomen.

The ascending colon starts on the right side of the abdomen at the cecum and moves up near the liver. The portion of the colon that crosses the abdomen from right to left is the transverse colon. The descending colon is the section on the left that extends to the sigmoid colon. Shaped like the letter S, the sigmoid colon curves into the pelvis, where it joins the rectum. The rectum is a relatively straight 4- to 6-inch tube that leads to the anus.

In the large intestine, food waste is solidified and prepared for excretion. What passes from the small intestine into the large intestine is generally a mixture of unabsorbed fiber, water and electrolytes, such as sodium. As this mixture proceeds through the large intestine, much of the water and salt are absorbed through the lining of the large intestine. Once the water is removed, the residue becomes a semisolid mass that's passed out the anus as stool (feces). By the time waste products reach the anus, about 80 percent of the liquid that originally entered the colon has been absorbed.

Gastrointestinal infections

Signs and symptoms
- Watery, sometimes bloody, diarrhea
- Cramping abdominal pain
- Fever
- Nausea and vomiting
- Muscle aches and headache

Emergency signs and symptoms
- Profuse diarrhea to the point of dehydration

Gastrointestinal tract infections are extremely common throughout the world. In developing countries, diarrhea caused by infection is among the leading causes of death in children. Improvements in sanitation and hygiene have had a significant impact on preventing many of these infections, particularly those transmitted by contaminated food and water. Even so, the Centers for Disease Control and Prevention estimates that foodborne diseases cause approximately 48 million illnesses and 3,000 deaths in the United States each year.

Viruses account for well over half the infections of the gastrointestinal tract. Other gastrointestinal infections are the result of bacteria and parasites.

Viral infections

Acute viral gastroenteritis — the stomach flu — is the second most common disease in the United States, with upper respiratory tract infections being the most common. Signs and symptoms usually include diarrhea, nausea, vomiting, a low-grade fever, abdominal cramps and muscle pains.

Viral gastroenteritis is often the cause of considerable discomfort and of time lost from school or work. In some people — especially in infants, older individuals, and individuals whose immune systems are suppressed by disease or certain medications — signs and symptoms can be severe.

Many of the viruses responsible for acute viral gastroenteritis are passed by fecal-oral transmission. Hand-washing is key to preventing transmission of the virus to others. Generally, the infection resolves over time.

Many types of viruses can cause acute viral gastroenteritis. However, the most common are those caused by the rotavirus and the Norwalk virus.

Rotavirus

Rotavirus is frequently identified as the cause of diarrhea in children younger than 2 years. It's also the most common source of diarrhea in children attending child care centers. Rotavirus occasionally causes epidemics of infection among older adults in nursing homes. The peak frequency of rotavirus infections in the United States is during the winter. The virus is transmitted from one person to another.

The incubation period is one to three days. Typical signs and symptoms include watery, nonbloody diarrhea, vomiting and a low-grade fever lasting five to eight days. There's no specific treatment for rotavirus gastroenteritis, but getting plenty of fluids is critical.

Norwalk virus

The Norwalk virus is an important cause of outbreaks of gastroenteritis in families and communities, particularly in older children and adults. This ailment is also called winter vomiting disease. In addition to diarrhea, nausea and vomiting, many people with this disorder experience muscle aches.

This virus usually is acquired by ingesting contaminated food or water. The incubation period from the time of ingestion of the contaminated food or water to the onset of signs and symptoms ranges from four to 72 hours.

Other causes

Cytomegalovirus is a cause of diarrhea in people with a weak immune system. A medication called ganciclovir may be effective in treating cytomegalovirus-induced diarrhea.

Gastrointestinal infections with herpes simplex can occur in individuals who engage in anal intercourse, especially the receptive participant, and in immuno-suppressed individuals. Generally, people infected with the herpes simplex virus experience anal pain, constipation and sometimes mild, bloody diarrhea. These people may also develop neurological symptoms, including numbness or tingling of the buttocks, upper thighs or anal area.

Treatment often consists of soaking in a warm bath and taking pain relievers and stool softeners. The antiviral drug acyclovir (Zovirax) can decrease the severity of the attack and the chance of relapses.

The Large Intestine

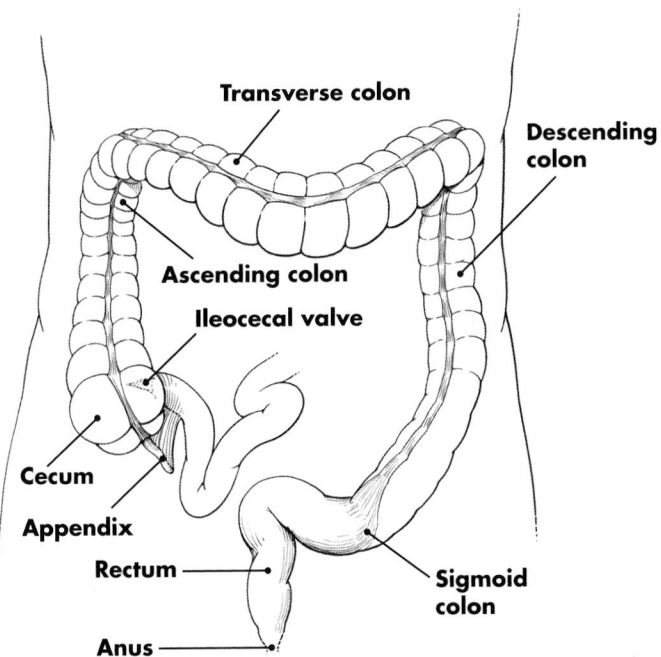

Transverse colon

Descending colon

Ascending colon

Ileocecal valve

Cecum

Appendix

Rectum

Anus

Sigmoid colon

Dehydration is the main complication of diarrhea-causing diseases such as gastrointestinal infections. In infants and children, dehydration can be fatal in a matter of days. If you have diarrhea, be sure to drink plenty of fluids, and if your child has it, keep him or her hydrated. Water usually doesn't supply all of the needed minerals lost in diarrhea, so a sports drink or electrolyte solution may be a better alternative.

In case of severe diarrhea or persistent vomiting, fluids may need to be administered intravenously in a hospital.

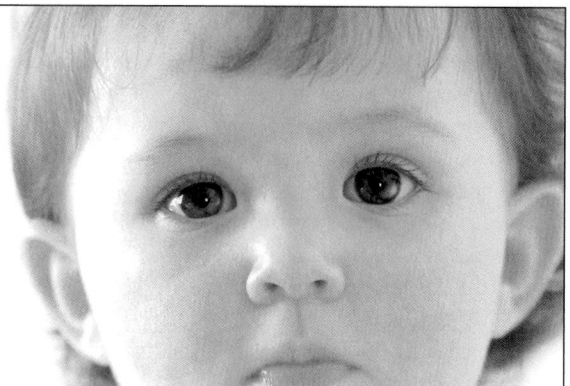

Bacterial infections

Gastrointestinal infections resulting from bacteria often are easier to identify than are viral causes. Bacterial infections are commonly referred to as food poisoning because they generally result from contaminated food. The illness generally improves on its own without need for specific treatment.

Campylobacter

Campylobacter infections occur in all age groups, but most occur in children younger than a year and in young adults. Infections with this organism generally occur in the summer and fall.

The most common source of campylobacter appears to be contaminated food, particularly poultry and unpasteurized milk. The incubation period from exposure to onset of signs and symptoms is two to four days. The illness may have an abrupt onset and include abdominal pain, nausea, a low-grade fever, headache and muscle pains. You may experience many loose bowel movements each day. In severe cases, the stools may be bloody.

This illness rarely lasts longer than a week. Occasionally, you may experience a relapse or a prolongation of your illness. Antidiarrheal agents aren't recommended because they may delay clearing of the organism from your system and prolong the illness. An antibiotic such as erythromycin may be given if the signs and symptoms are severe.

Salmonella

Salmonella has been implicated as responsible for about one-third of cases of diarrhea from contaminated food. Salmonella generally originates from contamination of the food itself, as opposed to the hands of infected food handlers.

Some evidence suggests that salmonella may occur in animals treated with antibiotics, possibly increasing the risk of salmonella infection in individuals who consume meats from these animals.

Salmonella bacteria are commonly found in raw or undercooked meats, poultry, eggs, unpasteurized cheese and milk, chocolate made from contaminated cocoa beans, and contaminated marijuana. Some reptile pets also can be a source of infection. The disease can be passed by the fecal-oral route. For example, if you change your infected baby's diaper, fail to wash your hands properly and then sit down to dinner, you could become infected.

When salmonella-infected food isn't cooked adequately or thawed properly, you may acquire the infection directly from the food. Signs and symptoms of salmonella infection include abdominal cramps, diarrhea, nausea, vomiting and fever.

In most cases, the infection clears on its own and only supportive treatment, such as drinking plenty of fluids, is needed. In some people, salmonella can cause a severe, prolonged illness, and antibiotic treatment may be necessary.

Shigella

Shigella is an important cause of bacterial gastroenteritis in the developing world and in travelers to these areas. It also occasionally occurs in outbreaks in the United States. The ailment is most common in children ages 1 through 5.

Shigella is transmitted primarily from person to person by the fecal-oral route. Outbreaks can occur in child care centers. Occasionally, outbreaks can be caused by contamination of food by infected food handlers. The usual signs and symptoms are watery diarrhea associated with cramping abdominal pain, fever, and sometimes, blood and mucus in the stool.

Generally, the disease improves on its own. Antibiotics may be effective in shortening the duration of the diarrhea and in eliminating shigella from the gastrointestinal tract. The usual drug of choice is sulfamethoxazole-trimethoprim (Bactrim, Septra) or azithromycin (Zithromax, Zmax). They can be given orally after appropriate stool cultures have been obtained. Other possible medications include trimethoprim, ciprofloxacin (Cipro) and ampicillin.

Escherichia coli

The organism called *Escherichia coli* has various subgroups. The source of this infection usually is contaminated food and water. A particular strain of this bacterium named *E. coli* O157:H7 is sometimes found in undercooked beef, particularly ground beef, and in infected produce. In a small percentage of cases, particularly in the very young and very old, *E. coli* O157:H7 can lead to a serious complication called hemolytic uremic syndrome. A potentially fatal condition, this syndrome destroys red blood cells and causes kidney failure.

If the diarrhea is mild, generally no treatment is necessary other than rehydration. For more-severe or prolonged signs and symptoms, an antibiotic such as sulfamethoxazole-trimethoprim (Bactrim, Septra) or ciprofloxacin (Cipro) is often prescribed. Anti-diarrheal medications generally are not used because they delay elimination of the organism.

Cooking meats properly, especially ground meat, can help prevent an *E. coli* O157:H7 infection. It's also important to wash hands and cooking utensils after working with raw meat and to avoid having the meat come into contact with other foods. For more on *E. coli* O157:H7, see page 453.

Clostridium perfringens

Another common cause of food poisoning is the bacterium *Clostridium perfringens* and its toxin. The infection is usually acquired by ingesting contaminated food — particularly inadequately cooked and refrigerated meat that has been insufficiently reheated.

Signs and symptoms include severe abdominal cramps and diarrhea, which begin about eight to 24 hours after consuming foods containing large amounts of the bacteria. Diagnosis is obtained by identifying the bacteria in an infected person's stool. The illness usually resolves on its own and usually lasts no more than a day. During the illness it's important to drink plenty of fluids to prevent dehydration, a potential complication of diarrhea.

Outbreaks most often occur in places such as school cafeterias, nursing homes and hospitals, where large quantities of food are prepared ahead of time and stored for future meals. A potentially fatal type of this bacterial infection is known as pig-bel disease (enteritis necroticans), but it's very rare in the United States.

Staphylococcus

Staphylococcal food poisoning often results from eating foods such as egg, dairy and poultry products, sandwich fillings, and egg, chicken, tuna, potato and macaroni salads, which are commonly found to harbor the bacteria. The bacteria are usually transmitted through the food handler and thrive when the food hasn't been kept hot or cold enough.

Onset of signs and symptoms, including nausea, vomiting, diarrhea, loss of appetite and fever, is usually swift after the ingestion of contaminated food. The illness may last from 24 to 48 hours, but typically resolves on its own. Anti-diarrheal medication generally isn't necessary and may prolong the infection by preventing elimination of the bacteria. To avoid dehydration, make sure to consume plenty of fluids.

Washing of your hands and food utensils carefully before and after food preparation can help prevent infection. Also, don't let food sit out. Refrigerate it promptly.

Parasitic infestations

Parasitic infestations are the least common of the three major causes of diarrheal diseases:

Giardia lamblia

This parasitic organism causes giardiasis, which is probably the most common parasitic cause of diarrhea in the United States. Outbreaks of giardiasis can occur in communities where the water supply is contaminated by raw sewage.

Giardiasis may also be contracted by swimming in pools, lakes and water parks

Food Poisoning

Food poisoning is caused by the ingestion of contaminated food. Its signs and symptoms usually include diarrhea and nausea. Vomiting and abdominal pain also may occur.

The most common cause of food poisoning is the toxin produced by the bacterium *Staphylococcus aureus*. When this organism contaminates certain foods — especially cream pastries, mayonnaise-containing foods, or potato, chicken, egg or tuna salad — it multiplies rapidly. This explains why staphylococcal food poisoning often occurs in outbreaks. Contamination most often occurs from the hands of a food handler.

What to do?
Usually, the discomforts of food poisoning pass in a few hours. After the vomiting or diarrhea ends, consume clear liquids for the first 12 hours. Then limit food intake to bland foods for the next 24 hours. For very young children, older adults and individuals who have other ailments, consult a doctor.

Prevention
The best strategy is to avoid contaminated food. Keep all meats and leftovers refrigerated. Don't allow food to come into contact with uncooked meat juices. Wash fruits and vegetables thoroughly.

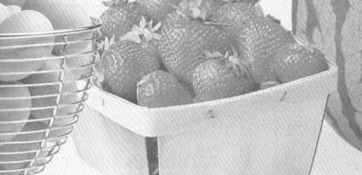

or by drinking water from lakes or mountain streams.

As many as two-thirds of people with giardiasis have no signs or symptoms. However, they may pass the infestation to others. Those who do develop signs and symptoms typically have watery diarrhea, abdominal cramps and, sometimes, weight loss. Generally, these signs and symptoms occur one to three weeks after exposure. The stools may be foul smelling, greasy looking and floating. Bloating and distention also may occur. A low-grade fever may be present. These signs and symptoms usually last for five to seven days, although some people have problems for months.

Diagnostic tests may identify the parasite. Giardiasis is usually treated with metronidazole (Flagyl). Individuals with certain immune deficiencies may be at increased risk of recurrent giardia infections.

Entamoeba histolytica

Entamoeba histolytica is a common cause of diarrheal disease throughout the world, although it's relatively uncommon in the United States. Infection generally occurs from person to person through the fecal-oral route. Your doctor may treat the infection with metronidazole (Flagyl). Other drugs are sometimes used.

Cryptosporidium

Cryptosporidium is a common cause of diarrhea in people with AIDS. It can also cause illness in otherwise healthy people. Epidemics have occurred as a result of contaminated public water supplies. Signs include prolonged watery diarrhea with up to 25 bowel movements a day. In otherwise healthy individuals, the infection resolves without treatment in one to two weeks.

In people with AIDS, the infection can be severe. For severe diarrhea, the medication nitazoxanide (Alinia) may be combined with azithromycin (Zithromax, Zmax).

Treatment

The initial danger of gastrointestinal infections is dehydration after the loss of fluids and electrolytes in stool. Therefore, the primary goal of treatment is replacement of fluids and essential electrolytes.

For some infections, the use of anti-diarrheal agents isn't recommended because they may delay the elimination of the causative organism and prolong the disease. Most parasitic infections require specific treatments to eradicate the organism.

Antibiotic-associated diarrhea

Signs and symptoms

- Diarrhea occurring during or shortly after antibiotic therapy
- Abdominal cramps
- Fever

Antibiotics, especially clindamycin (Cleocin), ampicillin, cephalosporins and the aminoglycosides, can cause diarrhea. Usually, the diarrhea is a result of the antibiotic having altered the environment of the bowel, which permits certain bacteria to flourish. This can cause inflammation of the colon.

Antibiotic-associated diarrhea is fairly common, affecting up to 25 percent of clindamycin users and up to 10 percent of those who take ampicillin. The most serious form of antibiotic-related diarrhea is pseudomembranous colitis, caused by a toxin secreted from an organism called Clostridium difficile.

Typically, diarrhea begins four to 10 days after the antibiotic treatment is started. However, in as many as 25 percent of people, signs and symptoms don't develop until the antibiotic has been discontinued.

Diagnosis

If your doctor suspects that your diarrhea is related to the use of antibiotics, he or she may perform tests on a sample of stool.

How serious is antibiotic-associated diarrhea?

Many people improve after discontinuing the antibiotic. Others become extremely ill and have persistent diarrhea and dehydration. On occasion, pseudomembranous colitis can develop into a life-threatening situation.

Treatment

Your doctor will likely stop treatment with the antibiotic that may be causing your diarrhea. The medications metronidazole (Flagyl) or vancomycin (Vancocin HCL) can be used for treatment, if necessary.

For recurrent C. difficile infection, a procedure called fecal microbiota transplant (FMT) is being studied. FMT restores healthy intestinal bacteria by placing another person's (donor's) stool in your colon, using a colonoscope or nasogastric tube. Donors and their stools are carefully screened for viruses, parasites and other infectious bacteria before being used in FMT. The procedure isn't yet approved by the Food and Drug Administration, but its success rate for treating C. difficile infections is greater than 90 percent.

For people with severe illness, surgery may be necessary to remove the diseased portion of the colon.

Malabsorption disorders

Signs and symptoms

- Weight loss
- Diarrhea
- Abdominal cramps, gas and bloating
- Weakness
- Foul-smelling and yellowish stools that may be fatty or oily

During digestion the nutrients contained in the food you eat must be broken down (digested) into molecules that can be absorbed into your bloodstream. For various reasons, these nutrients may not be completely digested and their absorption is impaired. When this occurs, vital nutrients needed by your body are instead eliminated in stool. The result of this malabsorption can be malnutrition.

Malabsorption can stem from many different problems. In the case of pancreatic disease, enzymes necessary to digest certain foods may be absent. This is often called maldigestion. Maldigestion can also occur with chronic liver disease.

A principal sign of malabsorption is fatty (steatorrheal) stools. This results from fat not being properly digested and absorbed during digestion and being eliminated in stool. Stool may be yellow or pale and somewhat larger than normal. The excessive fat content may cause stool to be more malodorous than normal. Protein also may be lost in stool, resulting in swelling (edema) of the legs or arms. Malabsorption can also lead to deficiencies in vitamins A, B-12, D, E, K and folate.

Celiac disease

Celiac disease, also known as celiac sprue, is a common cause of malabsorption. This disease is caused by sensitivity to gluten, a protein found in wheat, and similar-acting proteins found in rye and barley. Oats don't contain gluten, but depending on where they're manufactured cross-contamination can occur. The intolerance to gluten causes the lining of the intestine to lose its tiny folds (villi) through which nutrients are absorbed.

Signs and symptoms include foul-smelling diarrheal stools, bloating, weight loss and anemia. In mild cases, signs and symptoms may be limited to anemia or early-onset osteoporosis and not include any digestive signs or symptoms. Sometimes, celiac disease may mimic irritable bowel syndrome.

In children, the most dramatic signs often are weight loss and failure to grow. Bony changes similar to those in rickets may be seen in some children. In adults, demineralization of bone (osteomalacia) may occur with bone pain and tenderness.

If celiac disease is suspected, your doctor will likely order a blood test. If the results are suggestive of celiac disease, the next step is to have an upper endoscopy procedure in which tissue samples (biopsies) are taken from the small bowel. A positive biopsy is needed to confirm the diagnosis.

Celiac disease is treated by eliminating foods from your diet that contain gluten. Your doctor or a dietitian will instruct you in how to follow a gluten-free diet. If a gluten-free diet is carefully followed, the villi of the small intestine hopefully will resume their normal shape and regain their absorption ability over a period of several months. Your stools should return to normal, and you should stop losing weight. To correct certain nutrient deficiencies, initially you may be given vitamin and mineral supplements.

Tropical sprue

Tropical sprue affects visitors to tropical regions of the world, particularly in the Caribbean and Southeast Asia. People with tropical sprue may experience diarrhea, weight loss, anemia and an inability to gain weight.

Signs and symptoms can appear months or even years after you return from the area. The cause of the disease is uncertain, but it may be an infectious microorganism.

In many ways the illness appears identical to celiac disease, but with tropical sprue antibody testing of blood will be negative. Treatment for tropical sprue generally consists of vitamin supplementation and an antibiotic such as tetracycline. Usually, no special diet is required. Depending on the severity of the disease, you may take antibiotics for up to six months.

Bacterial overgrowth

Normally, overgrowth of bacteria in the small intestine isn't a problem because the constant muscular movement of the intestine (peristalsis) removes the bacteria.

However, under certain conditions, intestinal bacteria may grow to a point where they cause malabsorption.

This condition can occur in people with diabetes. Other illnesses that may predispose a person to bacterial overgrowth include the development of pouches (diverticula) in the small intestine, narrowed areas (strictures) of the small intestine and radiation damage to the intestine (radiation enteropathy). Bacterial overgrowth may also occur in individuals with abnormal bowel contractions or motility and those who don't produce stomach acid. Age also may be a factor. In addition, bacterial overgrowth can occur after bowel surgery in which segments of the small bowel are bypassed.

The diagnosis is made from cultures taken from the small bowel or sometimes through indirect tests that involve collecting your breath. The condition is generally treated with antibiotics.

Scleroderma

When scleroderma affects the intestine, it causes stiffening of its muscular walls, which can impair absorption of nutrients and affect peristalsis. Because the disease is progressive and can spread to other organs, medically it's known as progressive systemic sclerosis (PSS). The cause of this chronic disease is unknown. PSS may cause pouches (diverticula) to form in the intestine, and it may restrain peristalsis in the small bowel, leading to an overgrowth of bacteria. This overgrowth may, in turn, lead to severe diarrhea. Antibiotics taken in cyclical fashion, often one week each month, may be helpful.

AIDS

Acquired immunodeficiency syndrome (AIDS) can cause malabsorption. The primary signs, diarrhea and weight loss, are thought to be the result of infections in the small intestine and colon.

Whipple's disease

Whipple's disease is an extremely rare malabsorption disorder that primarily affects men older than age 45. The disease is likely caused by a recently identified infectious organism, the *Tropheryma whipplei* bacterium. Signs and symptoms such as diarrhea, abdominal pain, progressive weight loss and a darkening of the skin may occur. The infection also may cause a low-grade fever.

A diagnosis is often made by performing a biopsy of the small bowel, in which a sample of tissue is taken for laboratory examination. Long-term — 12- to 18-month — use of antibiotics typically is effective in correcting malabsorption due to Whipple's disease.

Amyloidosis

Amyloidosis results from a protein — called amyloid — that's present in excessive amounts in various tissues and locations. Depending on where the protein deposits occur in the body, the consequences can range from insignificant to severe. For example, amyloid in the small intestine will make the lining rubbery, firm and waxy and result in serious malabsorption.

Diagnosis of this condition is made by a small bowel biopsy. There's no method of preventing the formation of amyloid deposits. Treatment is geared toward relieving signs and symptoms or treating an underlying disorder that sometimes is responsible for the condition. Such disorders include tuberculosis, Hodgkin lymphoma and rheumatoid arthritis.

Lactose intolerance

Lactose, the principal sugar in cow's milk, requires the enzyme lactase for its digestion. Lactose intolerance occurs when the lining of your small intestine produces reduced amounts of this enzyme.

The condition causes abdominal cramps, bloating, diarrhea and excessive gas when more than a certain amount of milk or a milk product is ingested. Small amounts of milk usually don't produce signs and symptoms.

Lactose intolerance is very common worldwide. Low lactase levels may occur in association with other malabsorptive diseases, such as celiac or tropical sprue, viral or bacterial infections of the small intestine, and cystic fibrosis.

If you have lactose intolerance, you don't need to eliminate all dairy products from your diet unless your signs and symptoms are severe. Rather, decrease your consumption of milk products. Drink milk only during meals and try to get your calcium from cheese and yogurt, dairy products lower in lactose than milk. Another alternative is to buy a commercial lactase preparation, such as Lactaid or Dairy Ease, which can be mixed into your milk. These preparations convert lactose into simple sugars that are easily absorbed.

Short-bowel syndrome

A number of situations can reduce the surface area of your small intestine. Surgical removal of a portion of the intestine is one of the most common. Damage from radiation therapy or a disease that affects the intestine also can reduce the length of your bowel.

Because of reduced surface area, absorption of nutrients may be impaired. In some people, this can lead to malabsorption problems, called short-bowel syndrome.

Because different nutrients are absorbed in different areas of the small intestine, the type of malabsorption depends on how much and what part of the intestine was removed. For example, removal of the last portion of the small intestine — the main location for bile acid and vitamin B-12 absorption — may lead to excess bile acids spilling over into the colon and vitamin B-12 deficiency. If bile acids enter the colon, they may irritate or inflame the lining of the colon, causing watery diarrhea.

Appendicitis

Signs and symptoms
- Abdominal pain, usually starting around the navel and settling in the lower right side of the abdomen
- Loss of appetite
- Nausea and, sometimes, vomiting
- Mild fever

The appendix, a hollow worm-shaped structure that's attached to the first section of the large intestine (cecum), is about $3\frac{1}{2}$ inches long. It's function isn't certain, but it may play a role in bowel immunity. It's not always clear why the appendix can become inflamed, swollen and filled with pus, but many times appendicitis is associated with an obstruction.

Diabetic Intestinal Disorders

Long-standing diabetes can cause decreased function of the autonomic nerves that control the muscular activity of the stomach. A condition called diabetic gastroparesis diminishes the mixing and propelling activity by the stomach. Gradually, the stomach begins to resemble a limp bag and enlarges. Signs include vomiting rather large amounts of fluid and partially digested food that was eaten as long as a day or two before. Medications such as metoclopramide (Reglan) or erythromycin sometimes are effective in treating this disorder.

Similar deterioration of nerves in the intestines can impair the propulsive action of the intestines. Diarrhea tends to occur at night, and because of impaired sensation and function of the anal sphincter, there may be fecal incontinence especially during sleep. Some degree of malabsorption also may be seen.

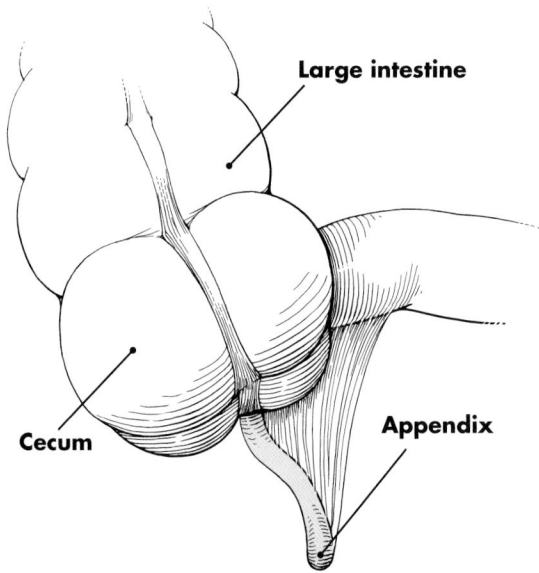

The worm-shaped appendix is attached to the cecum. The appendix can become inflamed and, without prompt treatment, burst.

Individuals most likely to have acute appendicitis are between the ages of 10 and 30, although the condition can occur at almost any age. Appendicitis can be especially difficult to diagnose in infants and people who are very old.

Diagnosis
Your doctor may ask you questions about your symptoms, including your appetite, location of the pain and fever. On examination of your abdomen, tenderness is an important sign. Depending on your symptoms, a blood test and an ultrasound or computerized tomography (CT) scan of the abdomen may be done.

How serious is appendicitis?
Most cases of appendicitis aren't life-threatening, but the condition warrants prompt treatment. Peritonitis, a serious infection of the abdominal cavity, may develop if the appendix becomes extremely inflamed and bursts.

Treatment
The standard procedure is to remove the infected appendix surgically. This can sometimes be done with a less invasive form of surgery called laparoscopy.

Meckel's diverticulum

A diverticulum is a pouch that develops in tubular organs such as the bowel. Meckel's diverticulum is a specific type of diverticulum present at birth. The pouch generally forms in the lower part of the small intestine (ileum) and is typically about 2 inches long.

Although this fairly common disorder frequently causes no signs and symptoms, the pouch can become inflamed and bleed. In some cases, especially among young children, bleeding may occur as the result of an ulcer that has formed at the same site.

If inflammation of a Meckel's diverticulum becomes severe, it can perforate the intestinal wall. A Meckel's diverticulum may also twist or herniate, causing a bowel obstruction. Treatment may include surgical removal of the diverticulum if problems arise.

Intussusception

Signs and symptoms
- Sudden, severe abdominal pain
- Vomiting, often with bile
- Bloody stools that may resemble currant jelly
- Faintness, sweating and pallor

Intussusception is a rare disorder in which a portion of the intestine, usually the small intestine, telescopes into another segment of the intestine. It's the most common cause of intestinal obstruction in children between the ages of 3 months and 6 years. The cause is unknown, but in some cases there may be a correlation between intussusception and certain viral infections.

Typically, intussusception strikes abruptly in a previously well child. The child suddenly has a severe, colicky abdominal pain that occurs at frequent intervals. At first, the child may play normally between the pains but soon becomes weaker and lethargic.

Intussusception in adults is uncommon and, unlike in children, usually associated with an intestinal disease.

Diagnosis
The signs and symptoms and physical findings may be sufficient to establish a diagnosis, but often further tests, such as an abdominal X-ray or computerized tomography (CT) exam may be needed.

How serious is intussusception?
Left untreated, the condition can become very serious. Most children recover if treatment starts within 24 hours after the initial signs and symptoms.

Treatment
In many cases, surgery is necessary. Generally, there's no recurrence after surgery.

Protein-losing enteropathy

Signs and symptoms
- Diarrhea
- Generalized swelling of tissues

Some gastrointestinal disorders cause protein in your blood to leak into your gastrointestinal tract and be excreted in your stool. The protein may pass into the gastrointestinal tract through an inflamed or ulcerated intestinal lining, as with the diseases Crohn's disease and ulcerative colitis. The result is low blood protein, which in turn can cause swelling (edema) of tissues.

Primary intestinal lymphangiectasia is a type of protein-losing intestinal disease in which swelling of the lymph channels of the small intestine leads to loss of protein and fat from these lymph channels into the intestines. Children and young adults are most commonly affected by this disorder. The principal treatment is a low-fat, high-protein, medium-chain triglyceride diet.

Inflammatory bowel disease

Inflammatory bowel disease is a term generally used to describe two disorders that involve the gastrointestinal tract and for which no cause has been found. These disorders are Crohn's disease and ulcerative colitis.

Signs and symptoms of Crohn's disease
- Long-term (chronic) diarrhea
- Abdominal cramps and pain
- Blood in the stool
- Fever
- Fatigue
- Reduced appetite and weight loss
- Joint pain
- Skin lesions

Crohn's disease is a chronic inflammation of the intestine. It often involves the lower part of the small intestine (ileum). However, it can also affect the colon or any other part of the digestive tract. The inflammation often affects the entire thickness of the bowel wall.

Anyone may be affected, but people with this disease typically first receive a diagnosis between the ages of 15 and 35, although the disease may also initially present itself in individuals more than 60 years old. No one is quite sure what triggers Crohn's disease.

Diagnosis
Signs and symptoms of Crohn's disease may include persistent diarrhea, abdominal pain, fever and general fatigue. Occasionally, there may be blood in the stool. Weight loss also may occur.

To establish the diagnosis your doctor will likely perform a procedure called colonoscopy to examine the lining of the colon and the last several inches of the ileum. A specially designed computerized tomography (CT) scan may show irregular segments of bowel, fibrotic masses or an abscess. Blood tests may also aid in the diagnosis.

How serious is Crohn's disease?
The course of Crohn's disease varies greatly from one person to another. Some people with Crohn's disease remain without signs and symptoms (asymptomatic) after the initial one or two episodes. Others have recurrent episodes of abdominal pain, diarrhea and fever. Crohn's disease is usually long-term (chronic), but you may have long periods of remission.

The complications of Crohn's disease are many and varied. Progressive obstruction, particularly of the small bowel, is the most common reason for surgical treatment of Crohn's disease. Obstructive symptoms generally develop gradually over a long period.

Fistulas and fissures in and around anal and rectal areas are common. A fistula is an abnormal passage between two segments of the intestine or from the intestine to the skin. Fistulas can also develop from the intestine to the vagina or bladder. An anal fissure is a crack or cleft in the anus or skin around the anus. Intestinal bleeding also may occur with Crohn's disease.

Other complications may include arthritis, particularly of large joints, or inflammation involving an eye or your skin. Occasionally, you may experience inflammation of the bile ducts (primary sclerosing cholangitis). In addition, the development of kidney stones and gallstones is common with Crohn's disease.

Treatment
The goal of treatment is to reduce the inflammation that triggers your signs and symptoms. In some cases, this may lead not only to symptom relief but also to long-term remission. Treatment for Crohn's disease often involves drug therapy or, in certain cases, surgery.

Doctors use several categories of drugs that control inflammation in different ways. But medications that work well for some people may not work for others, so it may take time to find one that helps you. In addition, because some drugs have serious side effects, you'll need to weigh the benefits and risks of drug treatment.

Anti-inflammatory drugs
Anti-inflammatory drugs are often the first step in the treatment of Crohn's disease. They include:
- **Corticosteroids.** Corticosteroids can help reduce inflammation anywhere in your body, but they have numerous side effects, including a puffy face, excessive facial hair, night sweats, insomnia and hyperactivity. More-serious side effects include high blood pressure, type 2 diabetes, osteoporosis, bone fractures, cataracts and an increased susceptibility to infections. Long-term use of corticosteroids in children can lead to stunted growth.

Also, these medications don't work for everyone with Crohn's disease. Doctors generally use corticosteroids only if you have moderate to severe inflammatory bowel disease that doesn't respond to other treatments. A newer type of corticosteroid, budesonide (Entocort EC), works faster than do traditional steroids and appears to produce fewer side effects. However, it is only effective for Crohn's disease that's in certain parts of the bowel.

Corticosteroids aren't for long-term use. They can be used for short-term symptom improvement for about three to four months. They're also used in conjunction with other medications as a means to induce remission. For example, corticosteroids may be used with an immune system suppressor — the corticosteroids can induce remission, while the immune system suppressors can help maintain remission.

Occasionally your doctor may prescribe steroid enemas if you have disease in your lower colon or rectum. These also are only for short-term use.

- **Oral 5-aminosalicylates.** These drugs were widely used in the past but now are considered of limited benefit. They may be helpful if Crohn's disease affects your colon, but they aren't helpful treating disease in the small intestine. They include sulfasalazine (Azulfidine), which contains sulfa, and mesalamine (Asacol HD, Delzicol, others). These drugs, especially sulfasalazine, have a number of side effects, including nausea, diarrhea, vomiting, heartburn and headache.

Immune system suppressors
These drugs also reduce inflammation, but they target your immune system, which produces the substances that cause inflammation. For some people, a combination of these drugs works better than one drug alone:

- **Azathioprine (Imuran, Azasan) and mercaptopurine (Purixan, Purinethol).** These are the most widely used immunosuppressants for treatment of inflammatory bowel disease. Taking them requires that you follow up closely with your doctor and have your blood checked regularly to look for side effects, such as a lowered resistance to infection.

Short term, they also can be associated with inflammation of the liver or pancreas and bone marrow suppression. Long term, although rarely, they are associated with certain infections and cancers including lymphoma and skin cancer. They may also cause nausea and vomiting. Your doctor will use a blood test to determine whether you can take these medications.

- **TNF inhibitors.** This includes the medications infliximab (Remicade), adalimumab (Humira) and certolizumab pegol (Cimzia). Also called "biologics," they work by neutralizing an immune system protein known as tumor necrosis factor (TNF). They're used in adults and children with moderate to severe Crohn's disease to reduce signs and symptoms. They also may induce remission.

TNF inhibitors may be used soon after diagnosis, particularly if your doctor suspects that you're likely to have more severe Crohn's disease or if you have a fistula. Sometimes they're used after other drugs have failed. They also may be combined with an immunosuppressant in some cases, but this practice is somewhat controversial.

People with certain conditions can't take TNF inhibitors. Tuberculosis and other serious infections have been associated with the use of immune-suppressing drugs. Talk to your doctor about your potential risks and have a skin test for tuberculosis, a chest X-ray and a test for hepatitis B before starting these medications. They are also associated with certain cancers, including lymphoma and skin cancers.

- **Methotrexate (Trexall).** This drug, which is used to treat cancer, psoriasis and rheumatoid arthritis, is sometimes used for people with Crohn's disease who don't respond well to other medications.

Short-term side effects include nausea, fatigue and diarrhea, and rarely, it can cause potentially

Nutrition and Crohn's Disease

The ability to absorb adequate nutrients is often limited in people with Crohn's disease, particularly if the disease affects significant portions of the small bowel or if portions of the small bowel have been surgically removed.

Your doctor may advise specific replacement of certain vitamins or minerals if there's evidence of a deficiency. It's not uncommon for people with Crohn's disease to have a deficiency of vitamin B-12, which is absorbed in the lowest segment of the small bowel (ileum). Vitamin B-12 can be easily replaced with monthly injections.

Bile acids also are absorbed in this portion of the small bowel. If bile acids aren't absorbed from the small bowel, they may cause diarrhea by irritating the colon lining and interfering with the absorption of water. A bile acid binder, such as cholestyramine, may decrease the amount of free bile acid in stool.

Avoiding foods and beverages that aggravate signs and symptoms is helpful, especially during a flare-up of the disease. Other dietary suggestions include limiting dairy products, trying low-fat foods, eating small meals, and drinking plenty of liquids that aren't caffeinated, alcoholic or carbonated.

Some doctors advocate the use of supplements consisting of liquid preparations containing simple sugars, amino acids and minerals, particularly for people with active Crohn's disease who are malnourished. Some people need to receive all of their nutrition intravenously for weeks, or even months, during severe bouts of Crohn's disease.

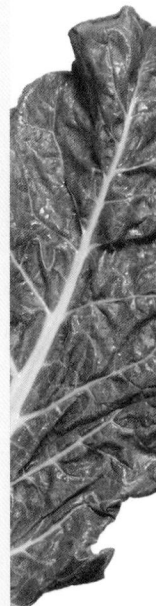

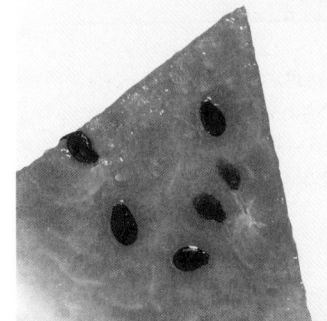

life-threatening pneumonia. Long-term use can lead to bone marrow suppression, scarring of the liver and sometimes to cancer. You'll need to be followed closely for side effects.

- **Cyclosporine (Gengraf, Neoral, Sandimmune) and tacrolimus (Astagraf XL).** These potent medications, often used to help heal Crohn's-related fistulas, are normally reserved for people who haven't responded well to other medications. Cyclosporine has the potential for serious side effects, such as kidney and liver damage, seizures, and fatal infections. These medications aren't for long-term use.
- **Natalizumab (Tysabri) and vedolizumab (Entyvio).** Natalizumab works by stopping certain immune cell molecules — integrins — from binding to other cells in your intestinal lining. Natalizumab is approved for people with moderate to severe Crohn's disease with evidence of inflammation who aren't responding well to other drugs.

Natalizumab is associated with a rare but serious risk of progressive multifocal leukoencephalopathy (PML) — a brain disease that usually leads to death or severe disability. Therefore, you must be enrolled in a special distribution program to use it.

Vedolizumab works through a mechanism similar to natalizumab, but it's gut specific and it hasn't been shown to enter the brain. In large clinical trials, vedolizumab wasn't associat-

Colostomy, Ileostomy and Ileoanal Anastomosis

Colostomy, ileostomy and ileoanal anastomosis are surgical treatments for diseases such as Crohn's disease, ulcerative colitis and colon cancer. All three procedures alter the normal route for the elimination of waste.

Colostomy

During a colostomy, the surgeon makes an incision to examine the colon and possibly remove diseased areas. Sometimes, the anus and rectum are removed and the anal area permanently closed. A separate incision is made in the abdomen, and a section of colon is pulled through this opening (stoma). A small bag is securely fastened over the opening. The feces then flow into the bag, which is emptied periodically.

Colostomies are identified by the portion of the colon that's brought out through the stoma. For example, a sigmoid colostomy involves the sigmoid colon. The consistency of the stool also depends on where the intestine has been interrupted. If the initial portion of the colon empties into the pouch, the stool will be loose. If the lower end of the colon is brought through the stoma, the stool will be more formed because more liquid has been absorbed in the colon.

Although many colostomies are permanent, sometimes a temporary colostomy is done to allow a portion of the bowel to heal after injury or disease. After the area is healed, the stoma is closed and the bowel is reconnected so that the normal waste elimination can continue.

Ileostomy

This procedure usually follows the entire removal of the colon and rectum. During a conventional ileostomy, a portion of the small intestine is brought out through the stoma created in the abdominal wall. As with a colostomy, an ileostomy requires that a bag be worn over the stoma to collect the waste, which in this case has a liquid consistency because the colon has been removed, where much of the liquid normally is absorbed. Sometimes, an ileostomy may be a temporary procedure to allow the bowel time to heal.

A variation of the standard ileostomy is called a continent ileostomy (Kock pouch), which uses a portion of the small intestine to construct an internal pouch and valve for waste. This pouch can store your waste internally for several hours at a time, eliminating the need for an outside bag. You can then drain the pouch at your convenience using a thin tube (catheter) inserted into the stoma.

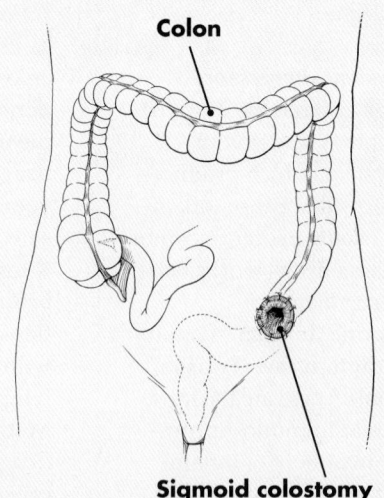

Colon

Sigmoid colostomy

In performing a sigmoid colostomy, the surgeon alters the normal route for waste excretion. The remaining intestine is brought through an opening (stoma) in the abdominal wall. Stool is eliminated into a small bag worn securely over the opening.

ed with PML. Vedolizumab is given intravenously — more frequently at first, then every eight weeks thereafter.

- **Ustekinumab (Stelara).** This drug is used to treat psoriasis. Studies have shown it's useful in treating Crohn's disease as well and may be used when other medical treatments fail.

Antibiotics

Antibiotics can heal fistulas and abscesses in people with Crohn's disease. Researchers also believe antibiotics help reduce harmful intestinal bacteria and suppress the intestine's immune system, which can trigger symptoms. Frequently prescribed antibiotics include:

- **Metronidazole (Flagyl).** Once the most commonly used antibiotic for Crohn's disease, metronidazole can sometimes cause serious side effects, including numbness and tingling in your hands and feet and, occasionally, muscle pain or weakness. If these side effects occur, stop the medication and call your doctor. Other side effects include nausea, a metallic taste in your mouth, headache, dizziness and loss of appetite. Avoid alcoholic beverages while taking this medication because a severe reaction may result.

- **Ciprofloxacin (Cipro).** This drug, which improves symptoms in some people with Crohn's disease, is now generally preferred to metronidazole. Ciprofloxacin may cause fainting, an irregular heartbeat, abdominal pain, diarrhea, fatigue and tendinitis.

The ileostomy and Kock pouch procedures are being done less frequently, having been replaced in large part by ileoanal anastomosis.

Recovery

With either colostomy or ileostomy, there's a period of adjustment. A stomal therapist can be helpful in this period.

- During the six to eight weeks immediately after the operation, avoid lifting, pushing or pulling more than 5 to 10 pounds. In general, simple exercises such as walking and swimming are good activities to firm your muscles and keep your digestive tract working properly.

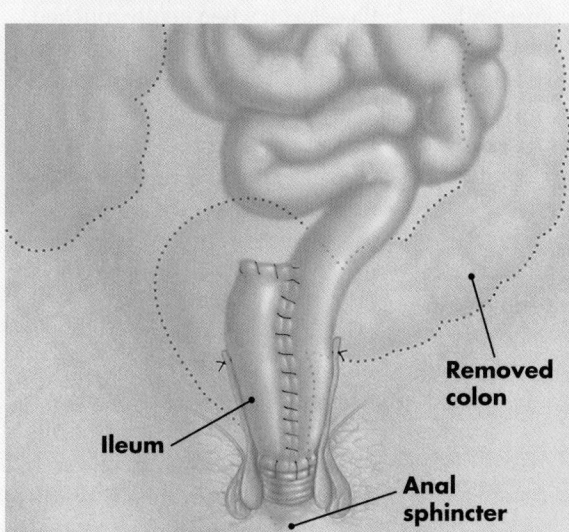

In ileoanal anastomosis, a surgeon removes the colon and innermost lining of the rectum, creates a J-shaped pouch out of the last section of the small intestine (ileum), then reattaches the pouch near the anal sphincter. Leaving the anal sphincter and rectal muscles intact preserves near-normal passage of stool.

Ileum

Removed colon

Anal sphincter

- Most doctors advise abstaining from sexual activity for a while after this operation. Sexual dysfunction may occur immediately after the operation. If pain in the vagina or an inability to achieve erection occurs, it may be temporary. If the problem persists, discuss it with your doctor.

Ileoanal anastomosis

An ileoanal anastomosis is the most common surgical procedure for ulcerative colitis. It involves the removal of the colon and rectum through an incision in the abdomen. The surgeon removes the inner lining from the anus but carefully preserves the sphincter muscles. A small J-shaped pouch is made from the end of the ileum to collect fecal material to decrease the number of bowel movements you have. A temporary ileostomy is necessary to divert feces away from the ileal pouch until this new area of intestine has time to heal — about two to three months.

Recovery

After some initial pain, you'll likely start feeling better soon. Many people debilitated by their disease are surprised to notice weight gain and increased strength so quickly after their operation. By the time they return to the hospital to have the ileostomy closed, they often feel better than they have in years.

Once the ileostomy is closed, expect to have frequent bowel movements for several months. Usually, the first bowel movement occurs about three days after the stoma is closed. The pouch made at the end of the ileum slowly increases in size. As this pouch becomes larger, it can store more stool and the number of bowel movements a day decreases.

If incontinence is a problem, your doctor may prescribe a medication to slow down your bowel and thicken the consistency of the stool.

Other medications

In addition to controlling inflammation, some medications may help relieve your signs and symptoms. Depending on the severity of your Crohn's disease, your doctor may recommend:

- **Anti-diarrheals.** A fiber supplement, such as psyllium powder (Metamucil) or methylcellulose (Citrucel), can help relieve signs and symptoms of mild to moderate diarrhea by adding bulk to your stool. For more severe diarrhea, loperamide (Imodium) may be effective. Use anti-diarrheals with great caution and only after consulting your doctor, because they increase the risk of toxic megacolon, a life-threatening inflammation of your colon.
- **Pain relievers.** For mild pain, your doctor may recommend acetaminophen (Tylenol, others). Don't use aspirin or nonsteroidal anti-inflammatory drugs (NSAIDs), such as, ibuprofen (Advil, Motrin IB, others) or naproxen sodium (Aleve). They are likely to make your symptoms worse. Also avoid narcotics (opioids). There's strong data to suggest individuals who take narcotics don't do as well in the long term.
- **Iron supplements.** If you have chronic intestinal bleeding, you may develop iron deficiency anemia. Taking iron supplements may help restore your iron levels to normal and reduce this type of anemia once your bleeding has stopped or diminished.
- **Vitamin B-12 shots.** Vitamin B-12 helps prevent anemia, promotes normal growth and development, and is essential for proper nerve function. It's absorbed in the terminal ileum, a part of the small intestine often affected by Crohn's disease. If inflammation of your terminal ileum is interfering with your ability to absorb this vitamin, you may need monthly B-12 shots for life.
- **Calcium and vitamin D supplements.** Most people with Crohn's disease need to take a calcium supplement with added vitamin D. This is because Crohn's disease itself and steroids can increase your risk of osteoporosis.

Surgery

If diet and lifestyle changes, drug therapy, or other treatments don't relieve your signs and symptoms, your doctor may recommend surgery to remove a damaged portion of your digestive tract or to close fistulas or remove scar tissue.

In Crohn's disease, surgery may provide a temporary improvement in your signs and symptoms. During surgery, your surgeon removes a damaged portion of your digestive tract and then reconnects the healthy sections. He or she may also close fistulas or drain abscesses. One of the most common surgeries for Crohn's is strictureplasty, a procedure that widens a segment of the intestine that has become too narrow. Laparoscopic surgery using small incisions can lead to improved outcomes and shorter hospital stays for some people with Crohn's disease.

Even so, the benefits of surgery for Crohn's are only temporary. The disease often recurs, frequently near the reconnected tissue or elsewhere in the digestive tract. Nearly 3 of 4 people with Crohn's disease eventually need some type of surgery. Of those, as many as half will need a second procedure, and still others may require a third operation.

Signs and symptoms of ulcerative colitis

- Bloody diarrhea that may contain mucus
- Abdominal pain
- Painful, urgent bowel movements
- Fever
- Weight loss
- Joint pain
- Skin lesions

Unlike Crohn's disease, which can involve any portion of the intestinal tract, ulcerative colitis is confined to the colon. Similar to Crohn's disease, the cause of ulcerative colitis is largely unknown.

Ulcerative colitis is a long-term (chronic) condition in which an inflammatory reaction characterized by tiny ulcers and small abscesses occurs in the inner lining of the colon. The reactions almost always involve the rectum and may extend into the entire colon. The amount of colon affected varies from person to person. If the inflammation is limited to the rectum, the term *ulcerative proctitis* may be used.

Although ulcerative colitis can strike at any time of life, it's most common between the ages of 15 and 35.

Diagnosis

Ulcerative colitis is often identified during a procedure called colonoscopy, in which a thin, flexible tube with an attached camera is inserted into the colon. If tissues are inflamed, bowel walls will bleed even when gently touched by the probe. A tissue specimen may be taken from the area for analysis (biopsy). A similar procedure called a flexible sigmoidoscopy may be performed in place of a colonoscopy. It examines just the lowest part of the colon. Blood tests or X-rays also may be done.

How serious is ulcerative colitis?

In approximately 20 percent of people with ulcerative colitis, the disease involves the entire colon and may cause severe bloody diarrhea, fever and abdominal pain. The disease more often presents itself as proctitis, which is limited to the rectum, or as left-sided colitis. Signs and symptoms that progressively worsen may even constitute a medical emergency because of risk of dilation of the colon (toxic megacolon) and perforation of the markedly inflamed colon.

Ulcerative colitis may cause various signs and symptoms in other areas of the body. These may include pain or inflammation of large joints, most often the knees, ankles and wrists. Skin abnormalities that can occur with ulcerative colitis include chronic skin ulcers and tender, red bumps that turn into dark areas that look like bruises. Acute eye inflammation also may develop. Although uncommon, the disease can also affect the flow of bile from the liver, a condition called primary sclerosing cholangitis.

Among people who've had the disease for at least eight to 10 years and in whom more than half of their colon is affected, there's also increased risk of colon cancer.

You'll need more frequent screening for colon cancer because of this increased risk. The recommended schedule will depend on the location of your disease and how long you've had it.

If your disease involves more than your rectum, you may need a colonoscopy examination every one to two years. It's generally recommended that you have a colonoscopy as soon as eight years after your diagnosis if the majority of your colon is involved, or 10 years if only the left side of your colon is involved.

Treatment

The goal of medical treatment is to reduce the inflammation that triggers your signs and symptoms. In the best cases, this may lead not only to symptom relief but also to long-term remission. Ulcerative colitis treatment usually involves either drug therapy or surgery.

Doctors use several categories of medications that control inflammation in different ways. But medications that work well for some people may not work for others, so it may take time to find a drug that helps you. In addition, because some drugs have serious side effects, you'll need to weigh the benefits and risks of any treatment.

Anti-inflammatory drugs

Anti-inflammatory drugs are often the first step in treatment. They include the following medications:

- **Mesalamine (Asacol HD, Rowasa, others).** These medications tend to have fewer side effects than sulfasalazine has. You take them in tablet form or use them rectally in the form of enemas or suppositories, depending on the area of your colon affected by ulcerative colitis. Mesalamine enemas can relieve signs and symptoms in more than 80 percent of people with ulcerative colitis in the lower left side of their colon and rectum.
- **Balsalazide (Colazal).** This is another formulation of mesalamine. Colazal delivers anti-inflammatory medication directly to the colon. The drug is similar to sulfasalazine, but uses a less toxic carrier and may produce fewer side effects.
- **Corticosteroids.** Corticosteroids can help reduce inflammation, but they have numerous side effects, including a puffy face, excessive facial hair, night sweats, insomnia and hyperactivity. More-serious side effects include high blood pressure, type 2 diabetes, osteoporosis, bone fractures, cataracts and an increased susceptibility to infections. Long-term use of these drugs in children can lead to stunted growth.

  Doctors generally use corticosteroids only if you have moderate to severe inflammatory bowel disease that doesn't respond to other treatments. Corticosteroids aren't for long-term use and are generally prescribed for a period of three to four months.

  Occasionally, a doctor may also prescribe steroid enemas to treat disease in your lower colon or rectum. These, too, are only for short-term use.

Immune system suppressors

These drugs also reduce inflammation, but they target your immune system rather than treating inflammation itself. Because immune suppressors can be effective in treating ulcerative colitis, scientists theorize that damage to digestive tissues is caused by your body's immune response to an invading virus or bacterium or even to your own tissue. Immunosuppressant drugs include:

- **Azathioprine (Azasan, Imuran) and mercaptopurine (Purinethol, Purixam).** These are the most widely used immunosuppressants for treatment of inflammatory bowel disease. Taking them requires that you follow up closely with your doctor and have your blood checked regularly to look for side effects, including effects on the liver and pancreas. Additional side effects include lowered resistance to infection and a small chance of developing cancers such as lymphoma and skin cancers.
- **Cyclosporine (Gengraf, Neoral, Sandimmune).** This drug is normally reserved for people who haven't responded well to other medications. Cyclosporine has the potential for serious side effects, such as kidney and liver damage, seizures, and fatal infections, and isn't for long-term use. There's also a small risk of cancer, so let your doctor know if you've previously had cancer.
- **TNF inhibitors.** This includes the medications infliximab (Remicade), adalimumab (Humira) and golimumab (Simponi). Also called "biologics," they work by neutralizing an immune system protein known as tumor necrosis factor (TNF). The medications are for people with moderate to severe ulcerative colitis who don't respond to or can't tolerate other treatments. People with certain conditions can't take TNF inhibitors. Tuberculosis and other serious infections have been associated with the use of immunosuppressant drugs.

These drugs also are associated with a small risk of developing certain cancers such as lymphoma and skin cancers. Also, because infliximab (Remicade) contains mouse protein, it can cause allergic reactions in some people, which may be delayed for days to weeks after starting treatment.

- **Vedolizumab (Entyvio).** This medication was recently approved for treatment of ulcerative colitis in people who don't respond to or can't tolerate biologics and other treatments. It works by blocking inflammatory cells from getting to the site of infection. It's also associated with a small risk of infection and cancer.

Nicotine patches
These skin patches — the same kind smokers use — seem to provide short-term relief from flare-ups of ulcerative colitis in some people, especially people who formerly smoked. How nicotine patches work isn't exactly clear, and the evidence that they provide relief is contested among researchers. Talk to your doctor before trying this treatment. And don't take up smoking as a treatment for ulcerative colitis.

Other medications
In addition to controlling inflammation, some medications may help relieve your signs and symptoms. Depending on the severity of your ulcerative colitis, your doctor may recommend one or more of the following:

- **Anti-diarrheals.** A fiber supplement such as psyllium powder (Metamucil) or methylcellulose (Citrucel) can help relieve signs and symptoms of mild to moderate diarrhea by adding bulk to your stool. For more severe diarrhea, loperamide (Imodium A-D) may be effective. Use anti-diarrheal medications with great caution, however, because they increase the risk of toxic megacolon.

- **Pain relievers.** For mild pain, your doctor may recommend acetaminophen (Tylenol, others). Don't use aspirin or nonsteroidal anti-inflammatory drugs (NSAIDs) such ibuprofen (Advil, Motrin IB, others) or naproxen sodium (Aleve). They may make your symptoms worse.
- **Iron supplements.** If you have chronic intestinal bleeding, you may develop iron deficiency anemia. Iron supplements may help restore your iron levels to normal and reduce the anemia once the bleeding has stopped.

Surgery
If diet and lifestyle changes, drug therapy or other treatments don't relieve your signs and symptoms, you may need surgery.

Surgery can often eliminate ulcerative colitis. But that usually means removing your entire colon and rectum (proctocolectomy). In the past, after this surgery you would wear a small bag over an opening in your abdomen (ileostomy) to collect stool. But a procedure called ileoanal anastomosis eliminates the need to wear a bag. Instead, your surgeon constructs a pouch from the end of your small intestine. The pouch is then attached directly to your anus. This allows you to expel waste more normally, although you may have as many as five to seven soft or watery bowel movements a day

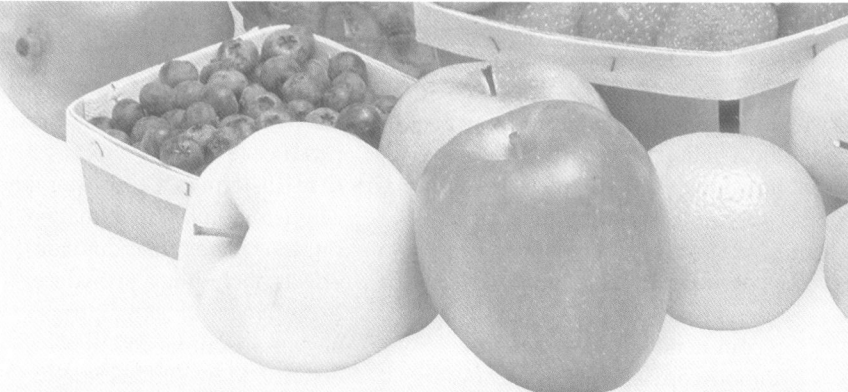

Fiber in Your Diet

In recent years, Americans have become increasingly aware of the need for more fiber in their diets. A high-fiber diet helps prevent constipation, and it may lower your risk of specific disorders, such as hemorrhoids, diverticular disease and irritable bowel syndrome. Other benefits of fiber include a possible lowering of cholesterol and, in people with diabetes, a slowing of sugar absorption, which may decrease the need for insulin.

The role of fiber in the prevention of colon cancer remains unclear. Some studies suggest a high-fiber diet reduces the risk of colon cancer, but other studies don't show evidence of benefit.

Fiber and digestion
High-fiber foods — often referred to as bulk or roughage — include whole-grain products, fruits, vegetables and legumes, such as beans and lentils. These may be better sources of fiber than fiber supplements.

Unlike most components of food, fiber isn't affected by digestive enzymes. It passes virtually unchanged through the stomach and small intestine and into the colon. In the colon, some forms of fiber are fermented by bacteria. Others resist fermentation and are eliminated in stool unchanged, which increases the weight and size of the stool, in

because you no longer have your colon to absorb water.

If you have surgery, your doctor may discuss whether an ileostomy or an ileoanal pouch is right for you. Between 25 and 40 percent of people with ulcerative colitis eventually need surgery.

Diverticulosis and diverticulitis

Signs and symptoms
- Pain
- Abdominal tenderness
- Fever
- Nausea
- Constipation or diarrhea

Diverticulosis is the name for the development of small pouches (diverticula) in the colon wall. Most people with diverticulosis experience no signs or symptoms, and typically the condition goes undiscovered or is identified when diagnostic tests are performed for other reasons. Occasionally, a pouch will bleed, alerting a doctor to the condition.

When inflammation or infection occurs in or around one or more pouches, the condition is called diverticulitis. Diverticulitis is more likely to occur in the lower (sigmoid) portion of your colon and may result from undigested food and bacteria lodging in a pouch. The inflammation can compromise the blood supply to the pouch, making it susceptible to an invasion by bacteria. The result can range from a small abscess to a massive infection or perforation. The process resembles that of appendicitis except that it occurs in the lower left side of the colon.

Symptoms of diverticulitis include cramping pains, which are usually most severe on the left side. Fever and nausea also may be present. Sometimes, an inflamed diverticulum can rupture, spilling intestinal material into the abdominal cavity. This is a medical emergency.

Causes

Diverticula usually develop when naturally weak places in your colon give way under pressure. This causes pouches to protrude through the colon wall.

Risk of diverticular disease increases with age, perhaps because the outer muscular wall of the colon thickens over time, narrowing the internal passageway and increasing pressure in the colon. Pressure on the colon wall can also be increased by straining to pass hard stools, which may result from too little fiber in your diet. Lack of exercise has also been associated with a greater risk of diverticula.

Treatment

For diverticulosis without signs and symptoms, treatment is generally unnecessary. A high-fiber diet with plenty of fluid may reduce the risk of complications and the development of more diverticula.

Oral antibiotics are often prescribed to treat diverticulitis if the inflammation is mild and the diverticulum hasn't ruptured. Follow a liquid diet for a few days while your bowel heals. Once your symptoms improve, you can gradually add solid food to your diet.

For a severe attack, or if you have other health problems, you may need to be hospitalized. Treatment generally involves intravenous antibiotics. A tube may be inserted to drain an abscess, if one has formed.

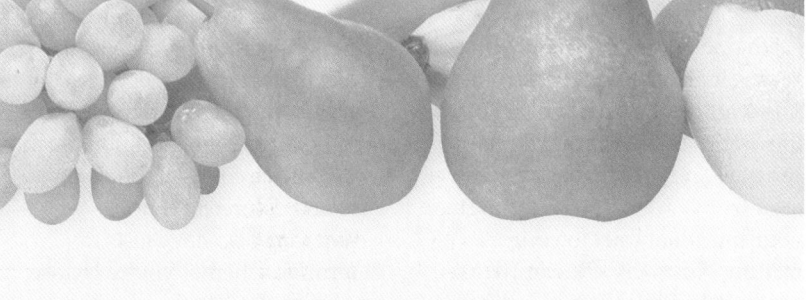

addition to softening it. A bulky stool is easier to pass, decreasing the chance of constipation. If you have loose, watery stools, fiber may help to solidify the stool because it absorbs water and adds bulk to stool.

Fueling up on fiber

Americans typically consume 10 to 15 grams of fiber daily. Dietary guidelines recommend twice that amount. To help ensure adequate dietary fiber, follow these suggestions:

- *Get your fiber from food.* Sometimes, people assume that if they take a fiber supplement, they need not pay attention to their diets. A supplement may be helpful, but natural fiber found in food may be better.
- *Eat a varied diet.* Include high-fiber foods such as grains, vegetables, fresh fruits and legumes. High-fiber snack foods include nuts, seeds, popcorn, fresh and dried fruits, and whole-grain crackers.
- *Limit your consumption of processed foods.* These often contain little fiber. The refining process often removes the outer coat (bran) from grain. This is why whole-grain products are higher in fiber content than are those made of refined flour. In a similar fashion, removing the skin from fruits and vegetables decreases their fiber content.
- *Increase your fiber intake gradually.* This will help your digestive system adjust to the increased levels of this bulking agent. A gradual increase will also help prevent problems with bloating and gas.

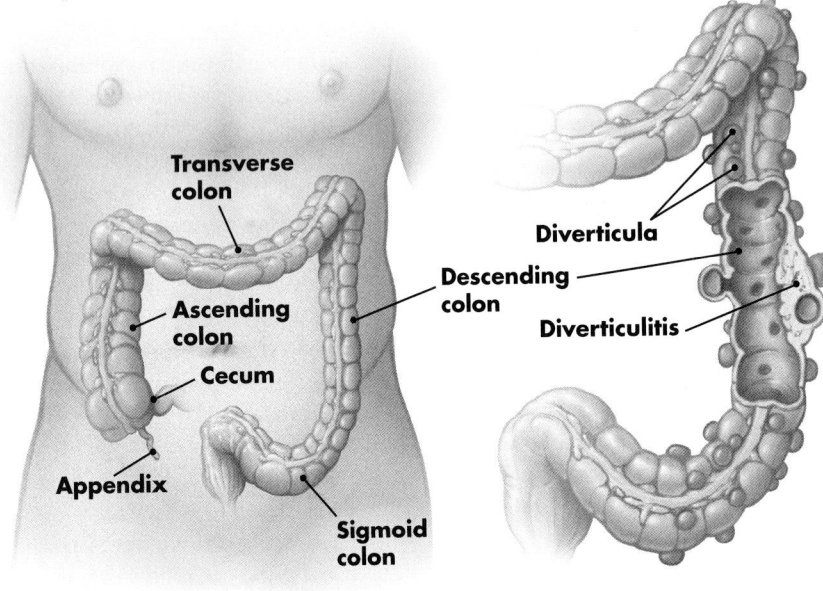

The most common location for development of small pouches (diverticula) is the large intestine (colon). When a pouch becomes inflamed or infected, the condition is called diverticulitis.

In case of a rupture or widespread infection, surgery may be necessary to remove the diseased segment of colon. For severe signs and symptoms, a temporary colostomy (see page 844) may be necessary while the colon heals. Later, after healing has occurred, a second operation to reconnect the colon is performed.

Irritable bowel syndrome

Signs and symptoms
- Abdominal pain or discomfort
- Bloating and gas
- Diarrhea
- Constipation
- Mucus in the stool

Irritable bowel syndrome (IBS) is one of the most common disorders that doctors see. Yet it's also one that many people aren't comfortable talking about because the signs and symptoms may be embarrassing.

It's estimated that between 25 million and 45 million Americans are affected by IBS, but only a small percentage of people with the condition experience severe signs and symptoms.

No one knows exactly what causes irritable bowel syndrome. The walls of the intestines are lined with layers of muscle that contract and relax as they move food from your stomach through your intestinal tract to your rectum. Normally, these muscles contract and relax in a coordinated rhythm. But if you have irritable bowel syndrome, the contractions may be stronger and last longer than normal. As a result, food is forced through your intestines more quickly, causing gas, bloating and diarrhea. In some cases, the opposite occurs. Passage of food slows, and stools become hard and dry.

For reasons that aren't clear, if you have IBS you probably react strongly to stimuli that don't bother other people. Triggers for IBS can range from gas or pressure on your intestines to certain foods, medications or emotions.

- **Foods.** Many people find that their signs and symptoms worsen when they consume certain foods or beverages. This may include chocolate, dairy products, alcohol, carbonated beverages, foods or beverages with caffeine or artificial sweeteners, some fruits and vegetables, and fatty foods.
- **Stress.** If you're like most people with IBS, you probably find that your signs and symptoms are worse or more frequent during stressful events, such as a change in your daily routine or family arguments. But while stress may aggravate symptoms, it doesn't cause them.
- **Other illnesses.** Sometimes another illness can trigger IBS.

Diagnosis
A diagnosis of irritable bowel syndrome depends largely on a complete medical history and physical examination to exclude more-serious problems. Your doctor may also recommend conducting several tests, including stool studies to check for infection or malabsorption problems. He or she may perform a flexible sigmoidoscopy or colonoscopy. These tests help rule out conditions such as ulcerative colitis, Crohn's disease and colorectal cancer.

You may also have tests to determine whether you're lactose intolerant. Lactase is an enzyme needed to digest the sugar found in dairy products. If you lack this enzyme, you may have signs and symptoms similar to those caused by irritable bowel syndrome, including abdominal pain, gas and diarrhea. Lactose intolerance may coexist with irritable bowel syndrome.

Because there are usually no physical signs of disease in irritable bowel syndrome, diagnosis is often a process of elimination. To help in this process, researchers have developed diagnostic criteria, known as Rome criteria, for irritable bowel syndrome and other functional gastrointestinal disorders — conditions in which the bowel appears normal but doesn't function normally.

According to these criteria, you must have certain signs and symptoms before receiving a diagnosis of irritable bowel syndrome. The most important signs and symptoms are abdominal pain and diarrhea or constipation lasting at least three months. You also need to have at least two of the following signs and symptoms a quarter or more of the time:

- A change in the frequency or consistency of your stool. For example, you may change from having one normal, formed stool every day to several loose stools. Or you may have only one hard stool every three to four days.
- Straining, urgency or a feeling that you can't empty your bowels completely.
- Mucus in your stool.
- Bloating or abdominal swelling.

Treatment

Often times, you can successfully control mild signs and symptoms of irritable bowel syndrome by learning to manage stress and making changes to your diet and lifestyle. But if your problems are moderate or severe, you may need more than what lifestyle changes can offer. Your doctor may suggest:

- **Fiber supplements.** Taking fiber supplements such as psyllium powder (Metamucil) or methylcellulose (Citrucel) with fluids may help control constipation.
- **Anti-diarrheal medications.** Over-the-counter medications such as loperamide (Imodium A-D) can help control diarrhea. However, in the long run, these medications can cause problems if you don't use them correctly. The same is true of laxatives. If you have any questions about them, check with your doctor or pharmacist.
- **Eliminating high-gas foods.** If you have bothersome bloating or are passing significant amounts of gas, your doctor may also ask you to cut out such items as carbonated beverages, salads, raw fruits and vegetables, cabbage, broccoli, and cauliflower.

- **Anticholinergic medications.** Some people need medications that affect certain activities of the nervous system (anticholinergics) to relieve painful bowel spasms.
- **Antidepressant medications.** If your symptoms include pain or depression, your doctor may recommend a tricyclic antidepressant, such as nortriptyline (Pamelor) or amitriptyline. It may help relieve depression as well as inhibit the activity of neurons that control the intestines. If you have diarrhea and abdominal pain without depression, your doctor may suggest a lower than normal dose. Side effects of these drugs include drowsiness and constipation.
- **Counseling.** You may benefit from counseling if you have depression or if stress tends to worsen your symptoms.

Medication specifically for IBS
Medications that have been approved to treat IBS include:

- **Alosetron (Lotronex).** Alosetron was removed from the market just nine months after its approval when it was linked to at least two deaths and severe side effects in 113 people. In 2002, the Food and Drug Administration (FDA) allowed alosetron to be sold again — with restrictions. The drug can be prescribed only by doctors enrolled in a special program and is intended for severe cases of diarrhea-predominant IBS in women who haven't responded to other treatments. Alosetron is not approved for use by men.
- **Lubiprostone (Amitiza) and linaclotide (Linzess).** They work by increasing fluid secretion in your small intestine to help with the passage of stool. The medications are approved for adults who have IBS with constipation. Side effects may include nausea, diarrhea and abdominal pain. The drugs are generally prescribed in cases of severe con-

stipation when other treatments haven't been successful.

- **Rifaximin (Xifaxan).** Rifaximin is an antibiotic that fights bacterial infection only in the intestines. It works differently from other antibiotics because it passes through your stomach and into your intestines without being absorbed into your bloodstream. Rifaximin may be used to treat IBS in some adults whose main symptom is diarrhea. Side effects may include swelling (edema), headache, dizziness and fatigue.
- **Eluxadoline (Viberzi).** Eluxadoline may be used to treat IBS when the main sign is diarrhea. It works directly in your intestines to slow the movement of food during digestion. It also makes the nerves in your intestines less sensitive to stimulation. Side effects may include constipation, nausea and stomach pain.

Chronic constipation

Signs and symptoms
- Passage of hard stools less than three times a week
- Occasionally, abdominal bloating and discomfort

Many people believe that constipation is the inability to have a daily bowel movement. In fact, it's not necessary to have a bowel movement every day. For some, regularity means having a bowel movement three times a week. For others, it may be three times a day. Chronic constipation refers to bowel movements that occur infrequently — generally less than three times a week — and in which the stool is hard and difficult to pass.

Alterations in the speed at which waste passes through the colon or in the amount of water removed from the waste can affect normal bowel function and cause chronic constipation. The condition can also occur from use of medications, including some used to treat Parkinson's disease,

Laxative Abuse

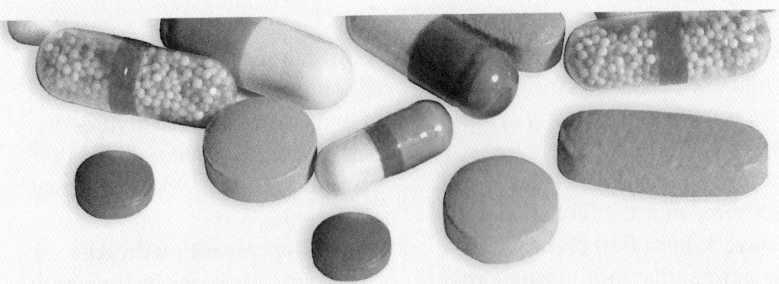

It's rare for anyone to need a laxative on a daily basis, yet many people use them regularly. Some people take laxatives to fight constipation. Others take them regularly as a preventive measure even though they aren't really constipated. Still others take laxatives in an attempt to lose weight.

Kinds of laxatives

One of the oldest laxatives is castor oil. It undergoes chemical transformation within the small intestine to become an acid that stimulates intestinal activity and prevents the intestinal wall from absorbing water. However, prolonged use of castor oil can damage the cells that line your intestinal tract.

Some laxatives act by inhibiting water absorption. Other laxatives work by increasing water content within your colon and are less irritating to your bowel. These include milk of magnesia and stool softeners.

Bulk-forming agents or so-called natural laxatives (psyllium and methylcellulose) don't stimulate your digestive system. Instead, they expand when they come into contact with water in the colon. These agents generally are safe for long-term use and can help prevent hard stools.

What are the risks of overuse?

When taken in excess, laxatives can flush out necessary medications, vitamins and other nutrients before they're fully absorbed. Some laxatives also can lead to an electrolyte imbalance, especially after prolonged use. Electrolytes — which include calcium, chloride, potassium, magnesium and sodium — regulate a number of body functions.

If you're dependent on laxatives to have a bowel movement, ask your doctor for advice on how best to treat your constipation.

depression, hypertension and some heart disorders. In addition, constipation often becomes more common with advancing age.

Diagnosis

If your constipation is a recent development or your stool habits differ from what you consider normal, see your doctor. He or she will first want to rule out other causes, such as an obstruction to the passage of stool. Diagnostic tests may include a colonoscopy or sigmoidoscopy examination.

Treatment

Treatment of constipation generally involves changes in eating and lifestyle habits:

- Drink at least six to eight glasses of water or other noncaffeinated liquids every day.
- Gradually increase fiber in your diet by eating more fresh fruits and vegetables. If you're intolerant of high-fiber foods, ask your doctor about using a bulk former.
- Incorporate physical exercise into your day. Exercise helps stimulate bowel contractions.

- Set aside a specific time every day for a bowel movement. Even if you don't feel like you have to have a bowel movement, try.
- Don't resist the urge to have a bowel movement.
- Avoid enemas. Thorough "cleansing" of the colon, by either repeated enemas or laxatives, can disrupt your body's normal balance of minerals. Many people with constipation rely on laxatives to relieve their problem. However, regular laxative use can lead to even more constipation. It could also damage your bowel.
- If your constipation doesn't improve, see your doctor.

Fecal impaction

Signs and symptoms

- An intense urge to have a bowel movement
- An inability to have a bowel movement
- Rectal pain and abdominal cramping
- Nausea and vomiting

A fecal impaction is a mass of stool that can't be eliminated by a normal bowel movement. It can occur after an extended period of constipation and most often poses a problem for older adults, especially those who are bedridden, and young children.

Symptoms may include an intense desire to have a bowel movement and pain in the anal region, rectum and center of the abdomen. Nausea, vomiting and loss of appetite also may occur.

Causes

Inadequate consumption of liquids and dietary fiber can lead to a fecal impaction. Other causes include:

- Medications such as codeine-containing pain relievers, antidepressants and aluminum-containing antacids
- Chronic health problems such as hemorrhoids, kidney disease, cancer, cardiovascular disease and neurological disorders
- Immobility, especially bed rest
- Failing to heed the call when your body tells you it's time for a trip to the bathroom, a habit

that's most common among young children

Treatment

A fecal impaction can generally be removed manually by a doctor or other medical professional. To prevent recurrence:

- Drink two or more glasses of water with each meal and one between meals.
- Eat a high-fiber diet.
- Heed the first urge to go to the bathroom.
- If possible, avoid prolonged bed rest and medications that increase your risk of fecal impaction.

Megacolon

Signs and symptoms

- Severe constipation
- Abdominal enlargement (distension)

From either congenital or acquired causes, the colon can become so enlarged that it becomes unable to move stool, a condition referred to as megacolon or giant colon. Nerve damage or deficiencies in the colon or rectum frequently are the cause of megacolon.

Hirschsprung's disease is a congenital disorder in which babies are born without normal nerve cells in a segment of their rectum. These infants are unable to have a bowel movement because the segment of the colon nearest the anus is unable to relax to permit the passage of feces. Hirschsprung's disease occurs more often in males than in females and often runs in families.

A type of acquired megacolon is psychogenic megacolon, which usually develops at the time of toilet training, causing severe and chronic constipation. In Central and South America, an infection called Chagas' disease causes megacolon. The infection destroys the ganglion nerve cells of the colon to create a condition similar to Hirschsprung's disease.

Other conditions that can cause megacolon are severe neurological disorders such as a spinal cord injury or Parkinson's disease and some medications, including opioids (narcotics). Toxic megacolon may also result as a complication of severe colon inflammation.

Diagnosis

Diagnosis of Hirschsprung's generally involves an examination of the rectum, a full-thickness rectal biopsy, and possibly a test called anorectal manometry. For this test a balloon is dilated in the rectum to check for the rectoanal inhibitory reflex, which is absent in someone with Hirschsprung's disease.

Treatment

The most effective treatment for Hirschsprung's disease is surgery to remove the affected portion of the colon. This usually restores normal bowel movements. For acquired causes, the key is education on proper bowel habits, such as drinking plenty of fluids, increasing the fiber content of your diet and not resisting the urge to have a bowel movement.

Your doctor may suggest treatments to help retrain your bowel. Decreasing the use of opioid-containing medication also may be recommended. Toxic megacolon requires surgical intervention to prevent bowel perforation.

Peritonitis

Signs and symptoms

- Increasing abdominal pain
- A distended and tender abdomen
- Nausea and vomiting
- An inability to pass feces or gas
- Fever
- Low blood pressure

Peritonitis is an inflammation, either confined or widespread, of the peritoneum, the membrane that covers the abdominal organs and lines the abdominal cavity.

Peritonitis most often is due to bacterial infection of the peritoneal cavity. Typically, bacteria enter from a perforation in the gastrointestinal tract, such as that from a ruptured appendix or trauma to the abdomen, as with a penetrating wound. Peritonitis can also result from a severe reaction related to the release of pancreatic enzymes, digestive enzymes or bile. People with systemic lupus erythematosus sometimes have bouts of peritonitis.

The most frequent causes of peritonitis are perforations related to appendicitis, diverticulitis or a peptic ulcer. Obstruction of the bowel with subsequent gangrene and bowel perforation also can cause peritonitis.

How serious is peritonitis?

Peritonitis is a medical emergency that must be treated immediately. Blood tests and X-rays may be done to help establish the diagnosis.

Treatment

Surgery is usually necessary, either to remove the cause of the problem, such as a ruptured appendix, or to repair an injury, such as a perforation in the stomach or intestine. Antibiotics are given to fight the infection. Because the intestines don't function during peritonitis, a tube may be inserted through your nose into the stomach to drain secretions and air that accumulate.

Intestinal obstruction

Signs and symptoms

- Abdominal distention
- Spasmodic pain or cramping, usually in the midabdomen
- Vomiting
- An inability to pass feces or intestinal gas

An intestinal obstruction is a partial or complete blockage in either the small intestine or colon. It prevents contents from completing their journey through the intestines.

If you have a blockage in your small intestine, you may feel cramplike pain in the middle of your abdomen and have bouts of vomiting. Failure to pass feces can occur no matter how high up the obstruction is located. If your intestine is totally blocked, you may not be able to pass gas. A partial intestinal obstruction may stimulate your intestines to contract and secrete more fluid than can be absorbed, resulting in diarrhea.

A dramatic feature of intestinal obstruction is abdominal distention. The abdomen will protrude more and more as the condition worsens. The swelling is produced by intestinal gas and fluid trapped within the obstructed segment of the intestine.

Several things can cause an obstruction. The most common cause in the small intestine is scar tissue from a prior operation. Hernias and a knotted or twisted intestine (volvulus) also are common causes of small bowel obstruction. In the colon, a tumor may create a blockage. These are called mechanical obstructions because they physically block movement of contents through the bowel.

Sometimes, abdominal swelling (distention) and an inability to have a bowel movement result not from a physical blockage but from failure of the intestines to move waste along the digestive tract as they normally should. This is called adynamic (paralytic) ileus and sometimes occurs after an abdominal injury or operation.

Other causes include pancreatitis, peritonitis, injury to the abdominal blood supply and metabolic disturbances, such as low blood potassium levels. Narcotics such as morphine also may result in adynamic ileus.

Diagnosis

If your doctor believes that your signs and symptoms suggest an intestinal obstruction, he or she may order various tests, possibly including abdominal X-rays, sigmoidoscopy, colonoscopy or a barium X-ray.

How serious is an intestinal obstruction?

If the obstruction blocks the blood supply to the intestine, the tissue may begin to die. This increases the possibility of gangrene or perforation of the intestine. Both are life-threatening.

Treatment

Your doctor may begin treatment by placing a small tube through your nose and into your stomach or small intestine. Suction is applied to remove intestinal secretions and air through the tube (nasogastric suction). This often relieves distention of the abdomen. Lost fluids are replaced with intravenous (IV) feedings.

Sometimes, the cause of an obstruction resolves spontaneously after the swelling has been relieved. If the obstruction doesn't resolve, surgery may be necessary to correct the blockage, such as removal of scar tissue or untwisting an intestinal knot. An underlying cause may then be identified.

Primary intestinal pseudo-obstruction

Signs and symptoms
- Sudden attacks of abdominal pain
- Abdominal swelling
- Nausea and vomiting
- Weight loss

Primary (idiopathic) intestinal pseudo-obstruction isn't a true intestinal obstruction. Rather, it's a motility disturbance that causes intestinal malfunction similar to an actual obstruction. The intestines become distended, and you may experience sudden, severe (acute) attacks of abdominal pain, nausea and vomiting. Malabsorption may accompany this disorder, with subsequent weight loss.

Because the cause of the condition is unknown, doctors sometimes call this condition idiopathic intestinal pseudo-obstruction — the term *idiopathic* refers to a disease with no recognizable

cause, and *pseudo* means "false." When an underlying disease such as scleroderma or diabetes is the cause, the term *secondary intestinal pseudo-obstruction* is used.

Treatment of intestinal pseudo-obstruction is difficult. In a procedure called nasogastric suction, a tube is placed through the nose into the stomach to remove air from (decompress) the bowel. People with intestinal pseudo-obstruction often need nutritional support to prevent malnutrition and weight loss. If intestinal pseudo-obstruction is related to an illness or medication, treatment involves addressing the underlying illness or stopping the medication.

Treatment may also include medications, such as antibiotics to treat bacterial infections, pain medication, and medication to treat intestinal muscle problems. In severe cases, surgery might be necessary.

Vascular problems of the bowel

A vast network of blood vessels nourishes the organs located in your abdomen. Sometimes, a blood vessel or abdominal disorder can reduce the blood supply to the intestines. When this happens, the affected area becomes deficient in nutrients and oxygen, and the tissue can die. Three vascular problems of the bowel include:

Mesenteric ischemia

This disorder is characterized by a partial or complete lack of blood flow to the intestines. This vascular obstruction may occur gradually from accumulation of cholesterol-containing deposits (plaques) in the linings of arteries supplying oxygen to the intestines. The main symptom is severe, midabdominal pain. The pain is usually aggravated by eating and relieved by fasting.

Another type of vascular obstruction is a blood clot (embolus) that passes from the heart into the arteries supplying blood to the intestines. The result is sudden, complete blockage of blood flow to a portion of the intestines. The condition often causes severe and sudden abdominal pain and is a medical emergency.

Examination of blood vessels in the abdomen (angiography) can determine the site of a vascular obstruction. This is generally followed by an operation to remove the segment of intestine that has lost its blood supply. If there hasn't been permanent damage, the clot can be removed or the affected artery reconstructed or bypassed.

Ischemic colitis

In ischemic colitis, blood supply to the colon is decreased, often stemming from congestive heart failure or low blood pressure (hypotension). The condition most often affects older adults. Signs and symptoms include cramping lower abdominal pain and rectal bleeding.

Surgery may be required in severe cases, but most often the problem resolves spontaneously as heart failure or low blood pressure is corrected. A narrowing of the colon (stricture) can occur later at the site of the prior ischemia.

Angioectasia of the colon

This condition is characterized by dilation, distortion or thinning of blood vessels in the inner wall of the colon or small intestine. It's most common in older adults.

Rectal bleeding is a common sign, which is often managed with cautery, injection or clipping procedures. Severe bleeding (hemorrhage) is infrequent. It often can be stopped by blocking an affected vessel during a diagnostic procedure called arteriography. For massive bleeding or bleeding from multiple sites, surgical removal of the affected portion of the colon or small intestine may be necessary.

Carcinoid syndrome

Signs and symptoms
- Flushing of the skin
- Diarrhea

Carcinoid tumors are slow-growing, potentially cancer-causing growths that usually occur in the appendix or ileum, the lowest section of the small intestine. These tumors may spread (metastasize) to the liver, lungs and other organs. Occasionally, they can cause flushing of the skin, asthma and diarrhea, called carcinoid syndrome. Excessive levels of a normal body chemical or metabolite in urine is an important biochemical indicator of carcinoid tumors.

The objective of treatment is to decrease the mass of one or more tumors by either chemotherapy or surgery. Treatment generally relieves the signs and symptoms of carcinoid syndrome. Some people recover fully after surgery, depending on how soon the cancer is detected and where it's located. In the case of advanced cancer, medication such as octreotide (Sandostatin) may be used to control the episodes of flushing and diarrhea and to try to retard tumor growth.

Tumors of the small intestine

Signs and symptoms
- Abdominal cramps and pain
- Nausea and vomiting
- Weight loss
- Bloody stools

It's uncommon for tumors to occur in the small intestine. When they do occur, most are noncancerous (benign) and they're usually discovered between the ages of 40 and 60. The most frequent signs and symptoms are pain, bloody stools, and nausea and vomiting.

There are several types of benign tumors, including lipomas, leiomyomas, angiomas and adenomas. These tumors don't spread. Often, they're found when an

X-ray is taken related to another condition.

A small percentage of tumors of the small intestine are cancerous (malignant). The most prevalent primary small intestinal tumors are adenocarcinomas, neuroendocrine neoplasms, lymphomas and gastrointestinal stromal tumors.

Signs and symptoms of a malignant tumor may include weight loss, abdominal pain, bloody stools, and nausea and vomiting. Your doctor may feel an abdominal mass during a physical examination.

Diagnosis
A specialized computerized tomography scan (CT enterography) is most often used to detect small intestinal tumors. Sometimes, the image can't distinguish a benign from a malignant tumor, and surgical exploration of the abdomen may be necessary to establish the diagnosis. Occasionally, the tumors are identified by accident during testing for another condition.

How serious are tumors of the small intestine?
Benign tumors aren't life-threatening, but they can cause dangerous signs and symptoms, such as bleeding and obstruction. Malignant tumors are dangerous, can be life-threatening and require prompt treatment.

Treatment
Surgery is usually recommended for all benign tumors that cause signs and symptoms, as well as for cancerous (malignant) tumors that haven't become too widespread. When a tumor has spread (metastasized) to such an extent that surgery isn't effective, some medications, as well as chemotherapy and radiation — either individually or in combination — may be used.

Colon polyps

Signs and symptoms
- A recent change in bowel movements

- Blood in stool, often in microscopic amounts

As many as 30 percent of middle-aged and older adults have one or more colon polyps — a small clump of cells that forms on the colon lining.

Colon polyps usually don't cause any signs and symptoms and are discovered incidentally, often during a screening test for colorectal cancer or during a test to diagnose another disorder. The great majority of colon polyps are harmless, but some may become cancerous over time.

Types

The three main types of colon polyps are:

Adenomatous polyps
Adenomatous polyps (adenomas) are quite common. They're classified into five varieties based on their microscopic features: tubular, tubulovillous, villous, traditional serrated and sessile serrated. The most common are tubular adenomas, which generally are less than ½ inch in diameter. Once an adenomatous polyp grows beyond the size of a pencil eraser it has the potential to become cancerous (malignant). That's why these polyps are generally removed.

Hyperplastic polyps
These polyps, which also are common, occur most often in your left (descending) colon and rectum. Hyperplastic polyps are generally less than ¼ inch in diameter and they're rarely cancerous.

Inflammatory polyps
Inflammatory polyps are thought to result from injury to or inflammation of the lining of the colon, such as in ulcerative colitis or Crohn's disease. These are uncommon and typically not a significant health risk.

Diagnosis

Colon polyps are most frequently found during a colon screening examination or during an evaluation of the colon to identify the cause of rectal bleeding, a change in bowel habits or abdominal pain. Depending on the type of polyps detected, your doctor may recommend periodic checkups or removal of the polyps.

How serious are colon polyps?

An adenomatous polyp has the potential to become cancerous. Most, if not all, colorectal cancers seem to develop from adenomas. In addition, sometimes colon polyps may cause problems such as bleeding and obstruction.

Treatment

Although some types of colon polyps are far more likely to become malignant than are others, a pathologist usually must examine a polyp under a microscope to determine whether it's potentially cancerous. For that reason, your doctor is likely to remove all polyps discovered during a bowel examination.

The great majority of polyps can be removed during colonoscopy or sigmoidoscopy by snaring them with a wire loop that simultaneously cuts the stalk of the polyp and cauterizes it to prevent bleeding. Some small polyps may be cauterized or burned with an electrical current. Risks of polyp removal (polypectomy) include bleeding and perforation of the colon.

Polyps that are too large to snare or that can't be reached safely are usually surgically removed — often using laparoscopic techniques. This means your surgeon performs the operation through several small incisions in your abdominal wall, using instruments with attached cameras that display your colon on a video monitor. Laparoscopic surgery may result in a faster and less painful recovery than traditional surgery using a single large incision. Once the section of your colon that contains the polyp is removed, that

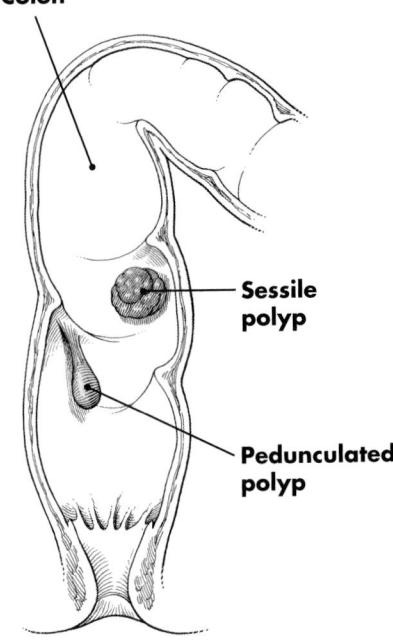

Colon

Sessile polyp

Pedunculated polyp

Polyps are small growths that may appear in the colon and rectum. In most cases, they're noncancerous (benign). They may assume various shapes. Polyps that grow on fleshy stalks are pedunculated polyps. Those that have a broad base are sessile polyps.

polyp can't recur, but you have a moderate chance of developing new polyps in other areas of your colon. For that reason, follow-up care is extremely important.

In cases of rare, inherited syndromes, such as familial adenomatous polyposis (FAP), your surgeon may perform an operation to remove your entire colon and rectum (total proctocolectomy). Then, in a procedure known as ileoanal anastomosis (J pouch) surgery, a pouch is constructed from the end of your small intestine (ileum) that attaches directly to your anus. This allows you to expel waste normally, although you may have several watery bowel movements a day.

Colorectal cancer

Signs and symptoms
- A change in bowel habits
- Rectal bleeding or blood in stool
- Abdominal pain or cramping

- Weakness or fatigue
- Unexplained weight loss

Cancer of the colon and rectum (colorectal cancer) is one of the most common forms of cancer in both men and women. Each year, more than 135,000 Americans receive a diagnosis of this disease, and approximately 50,000 die of it.

A complex mix of factors, including lifestyle, environment and genetics, may be responsible. Researchers theorize that most people have dormant genes that can produce cancerous cells. These genes stay dormant until they're activated by an outside agent, such as an infection, tobacco or pollutants.

Most cases of colorectal cancer begin as small, noncancerous (benign) clumps of cells called adenomatous polyps. Over time, some of these polyps become colon cancers.

Most gastrointestinal cancers occur in the colon and rectum, where food residue moves more slowly and toxins linger. Colorectal cancer risk appears to be more common in people who eat a high-fat, low-fiber diet. Risk of colorectal cancer is also higher in individuals who smoke, consume large amounts of alcohol and are physically inactive.

A small percentage of colorectal cancer — between 5 and 10 percent — is considered hereditary. One type of inherited cancer is called hereditary nonpolyposis colorectal cancer (HNPCC). People with this disorder have a 50 percent chance of passing on the gene to their children. They also have a significantly higher risk of developing colon cancer, and at a younger age than normal.

Another inherited condition called familial adenomatous polyposis (FAP) produces hundreds, even thousands, of tiny precancerous growths (polyps) in the colon and rectum. Cancer almost always develops in one or more of these polyps, typically between the ages of 30 and 50.

Diagnosis

Colorectal cancer increasingly is being detected with periodic screening examinations. Rectal bleeding, a change in bowel habits, unexplained weight loss and abdominal pain also can be warnings of the disease. If you experience these signs and symptoms, your doctor may advise diagnostic testing.

If cancer is identified, other tests, including blood tests and a computerized tomography (CT) scan, may be done to determine if it has spread to adjacent tissues or other organs.

How serious is colorectal cancer?

Colorectal cancer is the third most common cancer in men and women in the United States and accounts for about 10 percent of cancer deaths. When detected and treated at an early stage, chances for cure are high. Mortality rates for colorectal cancer have declined in the past 20 years, probably due to increased screening and polyp removal. Unfortunately, many people still don't seek medical attention even when such warning signs as rectal bleeding and a change in bowel habits occur.

Inherited Gene Mutations

A small percentage of colon cancers result from gene mutations. These cancers are autosomal dominant, meaning you need to inherit only one defective gene from either of your parents. If one parent has the mutated gene, you have a 50 percent chance of inheriting the mutation. Although inheriting a defective gene greatly increases your risk, not everyone with a mutated gene develops cancer.

One genetic defect that plays a key role in colon cancer occurs in the adenomatous polyposis coli (APC) gene. When the APC gene is normal, it helps control cell growth. But if it's defective, cell growth accelerates, leading to the formation of multiple adenomatous polyps in your intestinal lining. Conditions related to APC gene defects include:

- **Familial adenomatous polyposis (FAP).** This is a rare, hereditary disorder that results from an APC gene defect. FAP causes you to develop hundreds, even thousands, of polyps in the lining of your colon beginning in your teenage years. If these go untreated, your risk of developing colon cancer is nearly 100 percent. The encouraging news about FAP is that in some cases, genetic testing can help determine whether you're at risk of the disease.
- **Gardner's syndrome.** This syndrome is a variant of FAP. This condition causes polyps to develop throughout your colon and small intestine. You may also develop noncancerous tumors in other parts of your body, including your skin (sebaceous cysts and lipomas), bone (osteomas) and abdomen (desmoids).
- **Hereditary nonpolyposis colorectal cancer (HNPCC).** This is the most common form of inherited colon cancer. It, too, results from a defect in the APC gene, but unlike people with FAP or Gardner's syndrome, people with hereditary nonpolyposis colorectal cancer tend to develop relatively few colon polyps. They do, however, often have tumors in other organs. Hereditary nonpolyposis colorectal cancer includes Lynch I and Lynch II syndromes. People with Lynch I syndrome usually develop a small number of polyps that quickly become malignant. Those with Lynch II syndrome tend to develop tumors in the breast, stomach, small intestine, urinary tract and ovaries as well as in the colon.

For more on genetic testing, see Chapter 14, "Genetics and Disease."

Treatment

The type of treatment your doctor recommends will depend largely on the stage of your cancer — stage 0 is the earliest stage and stage IV is the most advanced. The three primary treatment options are surgery, chemotherapy and radiation.

Surgery (colectomy) is the main treatment for colorectal cancer. How much of your colon is removed and whether other therapies, such as radiation or chemotherapy, are an option for you depend on the location of your cancer, how far cancer has penetrated into the wall of your bowel, and whether it has spread to your lymph nodes or other parts of your body.

Surgical procedures

Your surgeon removes the part of your colon that contains the cancer, along with a margin of normal tissue on either side of the cancer to help ensure that no cancer is left behind. Nearby lymph nodes are usually also removed and tested for cancer. Your surgeon is often able to reconnect the healthy portions of your colon or rectum.

But when that's not possible, for instance, if the cancer is at the outlet of your rectum, you may need to have a permanent or temporary colostomy. This involves creating an opening in the wall of your abdomen from a portion of the remaining bowel for the elimination of body waste into a special bag. Sometimes the colostomy is only temporary, allowing your colon or rectum time to heal after surgery. In some cases, however, the colostomy may be permanent.

Side effects of colon cancer surgery may include short-term pain

Screening for Colorectal Cancer

A number of tests can identify early colorectal cancer or potential cancer-causing polyps (adenomas) before they produce signs and symptoms. The American Cancer Society recommends that all adults have one or a combination of the following screening tests beginning at age 50. Screening may be done earlier for individuals at higher than average risk.

Digital rectal exam

In this simple office exam, your doctor inserts a gloved finger into your rectum to feel for polyps or masses. Although simple and safe, this test is limited to examination of your rectum. Thus, it's usually done in conjunction with other screening tests.

Fecal occult blood test

A fecal occult blood test checks for microscopic amounts of hidden (occult) blood in stool. It can be performed in a doctor's office or at home. The problem is that some cancers and most polyps don't bleed and aren't detected with this test. In addition, positive test results don't necessarily mean that you have cancer or polyps. The bleeding may be from other sources, such as hemorrhoids or gastritis. In addition, the test may be affected by your diet and certain medications. For these reasons, many doctors recommend alternative or additional screening methods.

Stool DNA test

This test involves analyzing several DNA markers, which come from cells that are shed by colon cancers or precancerous polyps into stool. For the test, you receive a collection kit from your doctor, collect a bowel movement at home and send the kit to a laboratory for analysis. Cologuard currently is the only stool DNA test approved for use in the United States.

Sigmoidoscopy

A sigmoidoscopy allows your doctor to see and inspect the lower portion of your colon (sigmoid and rectum). The test requires one or two enemas for preparation. It doesn't require sedation, and it takes about five to 10 minutes to perform. A flexible, lighted tube with a fiber-optic camera (sigmoidoscope) is inserted into your rectum and threaded through your rectum and sigmoid colon. About one-third to one-half of all colorectal cancers or polyps can be seen during such an examination. If a polyp or suspicious area is identified, samples of tissue are taken with the instrument for microscopic examination.

Colonoscopy

A colonoscopy is considered the gold standard of colorectal cancer screening. In general, it's the preferred test for all individuals, but particularly those at higher than average risk of colorectal cancer. A flexible, lighted tube with a tiny camera attached is used to examine your entire colon and rectum. The tube is inserted into your rectum and threaded through the rectum and entire length of your colon (see image at right). If polyps or suspicious areas are detected, your doctor can painlessly remove them and take tissue samples for laboratory analysis (biopsy). Preparation for the test generally involves a clear liquid diet, a special laxative preparation and, sometimes, enemas to cleanse the colon for better viewing. Most people also receive sedation just before the examination.

Barium enema

A barium enema allows your doctor to view your large intestine on an X-ray. Barium, a chalk-like contrast medium, is inserted into your colon. The

and tenderness, and temporary constipation or diarrhea. If you have a colostomy, you may develop an irritation on the skin around the opening (stoma).

Surgery for early-stage cancer
If your cancer is small, localized in a polyp and in a very early stage, your surgeon may be able to remove it completely during a colonoscopy. If the pathologist determines that the cancer in the polyp doesn't involve the base — where the polyp is attached to the bowel wall — then there's a good chance that the cancer has been completely eliminated.

Some larger polyps may be removed using laparoscopic surgery. In this procedure, your surgeon performs the operation through several small incisions in your abdominal wall, inserting instruments with attached cameras that display your colon on a video monitor. He or she may also take samples from the lymph nodes that drain the area where the cancer is located. Studies have found that people who have this procedure don't have higher rates of recurrence than those who choose the open surgery.

Surgery for advanced cancer
If your cancer is very advanced or your overall health very poor, an operation to relieve a blockage of your colon or other conditions in order to improve your symptoms may be the best option. This type of surgery is referred to as palliative surgery. The goal of palliative surgery isn't to cure your cancer, but to relieve signs and symptoms, such as bleeding and pain.

barium coats the lining of the colon, creating a clear silhouette of your colon, and then an X-ray is taken. The test takes about 20 minutes. A barium enema is often combined with sigmoidoscopy.

CT colonography (virtual colonography)
A CT colonography is an X-ray test performed with techniques similar to a computerized tomography (CT) scan. It allows detailed inspection of the colon to look for polyps or masses. The same type of bowel preparation is required as with a colonoscopy, but there's no device that's inserted into the colon. If polyps are seen, traditional colonoscopy is necessary to remove the growths.

What test is best?
The best screening method for you depends on your age, your overall health and if you have other risk factors that put you at higher than average risk of colorectal cancer. Discuss these with your doctor, and together the two of you can determine the best course of action. Proper screening and early detection can go a long way in preventing and treating this disease.

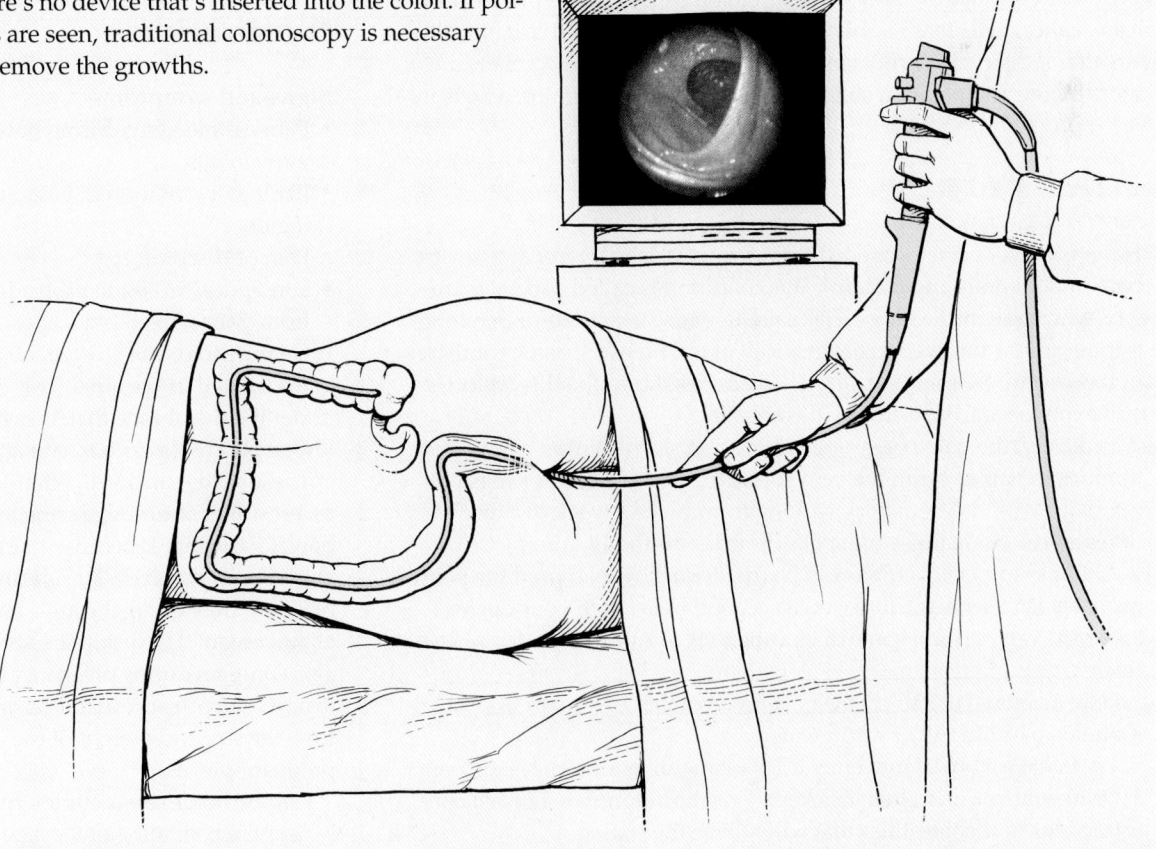

In specific cases where the cancer has spread only to the liver and if your overall health is otherwise good, your doctor may recommend surgery to remove the cancerous lesion from your liver. Chemotherapy may be used before or after this type of surgery.

Chemotherapy

Chemotherapy medications may be used to destroy cancer cells after surgery, to control tumor growth or to relieve symptoms of colon cancer. Your doctor may recommend chemotherapy if your cancer has spread beyond the wall of the colon. In some cases, chemotherapy is used along with radiation therapy.

Possible side effects of chemotherapy include nausea and vomiting, mouth sores, fatigue, hair loss, and diarrhea. Discuss the side effects and risks as well as the potential benefits with your doctor.

Radiation therapy

Radiation therapy uses powerful energy sources, such as X-rays, to kill any cancer cells that might remain after surgery, to shrink large tumors before an operation so that they can be removed more easily, or to relieve symptoms of colon cancer and rectal cancer.

Radiation therapy is rarely used in early-stage colon cancer, but it is a routine part of treating early-stage rectal cancer, especially if the cancer has penetrated through the wall of the rectum or traveled to nearby lymph nodes. Radiation therapy, usually combined with chemotherapy, may be used after surgery to reduce the risk that the cancer may recur in the area of the rectum where it began.

Side effects of radiation therapy may include diarrhea, rectal bleeding, fatigue, loss of appetite and nausea.

Targeted drug therapy

Drugs that target specific defects that allow cancer cells to grow are available to people with advanced colon cancer. These medications can be given along with chemotherapy or administered alone.

Targeted therapies are typically reserved for people with advanced colon cancer. Some people are helped by targeted drugs, while others are not. Researchers are working to determine who is most likely to benefit from targeted medications. Until then, doctors carefully weigh the limited benefit of targeted drugs against the risk of side effects and the expensive cost when deciding whether to use these treatments.

Prevention

Healthy lifestyle changes such as eating a low-fat, high-fiber diet, limiting alcohol, stopping smoking and getting regular exercise can reduce your risk of colon cancer.

Anorectal Disorders

The anus is the muscular canal that's the outlet for the rectum. It's a relatively simple structure, in contrast to the other parts of the digestive system. However, it, too, can be a site for significant problems, collectively referred to as anorectal disorders.

Hemorrhoids

Signs and symptoms

- Painless bleeding during bowel movements
- Itching or irritation in your anal region
- Pain or discomfort
- Soft "piles" of tissue protruding from your anus

Hemorrhoids are clusters of veins located in the anus, just under the membrane that lines the lowest part of the rectum and anus.

These veins can swell, often as a result of straining during a bowel movement. Because these veins are thin and easily ruptured, bleeding may occur during a bowel movement. Hemorrhoids are also common during pregnancy due to increased pressure in the veins from the size and weight of the pregnant uterus.

Hemorrhoids can occur internally near the beginning of the anal canal or externally, where they pro-

Anal Pain

Have you ever been awakened from a sound sleep by a sharp, severe pain in your anus and rectum? This condition is called proctalgia fugax, which means fleeting rectal pain. Its cause isn't well-understood, but the pain is believed to be the result of an intense spasm of muscles in the lower pelvis and rectum. The pain resembles the discomfort you experience from a cramp in your calf.

Typically, the pain begins at night during sleep. Within a few minutes to half an hour, the pain subsides. It may recur at irregular intervals, with the frequency varying from twice a week to a few times a year. Sometimes the spells disappear entirely.

Although proctalgia fugax can be frightening, rest assured the pain probably isn't serious. However, it's a good idea to see your doctor. He or she can perform some diagnostic tests to rule out a more serious cause.

Here are some tips to try the next time you have this sort of pain:
- Sit in a bathtub full of warm water.
- Try to have a bowel movement. This sometimes eliminates the pain.
- Drink warm water or eat crackers. This may stimulate normal contractions in the intestines that will relieve the spasm.

Rectal Bleeding

Rectal bleeding can be a sign of cancer, but more often it indicates a bowel problem that isn't life-threatening and responds well to treatment. Other causes of bleeding in the lower gastrointestinal tract include:

- Proctitis or colitis, an inflammation of the inner lining of the rectum or colon
- Colon or rectal polyps, small noncancerous (benign) growths in the lining of the lower intestine
- Hemorrhoids, enlarged veins in the lining of the anus
- Anal fissure, a tear in the lining of the anus
- Anal fistula, an abnormal channel between the anal canal and the skin around the opening to the anus
- Rectal prolapse, a condition in which a portion of the rectum protrudes through the anus
- Diverticular disease, small pouches (diverticula) that form in the large intestine
- Angioectasia, weakened blood vessels in the colon lining

Rectal bleeding requires prompt evaluation by your doctor to establish its cause and, more importantly, to exclude cancer.

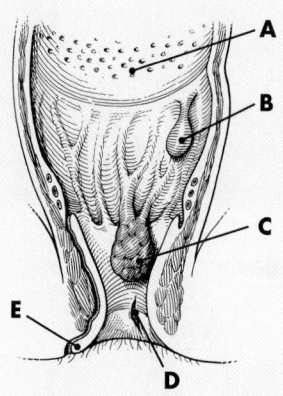

This cross-sectional view of the anus and rectum shows some common causes of rectal bleeding: proctitis (A), polyp (B), hemorrhoids (C), anal fissure (D) and anal fistula (E).

trude outside the anus. Both types are common and both may bleed.

Hemorrhoids can become especially painful if a blood clot forms in a swollen vein, a condition referred to as a thrombosed hemorrhoid. These clots generally occur in external hemorrhoids and cause a painful lump at the anal opening.

Itching and anal pain can occur with a complication of hemorrhoids such as thrombosis or irritation or inflammation of the skin surrounding the anus.

Diagnosis

Visual examination of the anus by a doctor usually reveals external hemorrhoids. The interior of the anus can be examined with a rubber-gloved finger, but because hemorrhoids are very soft, a definite diagnosis may not be made. Sometimes, a doctor will use a short scope to view inside the anus and rectum.

All episodes of rectal bleeding should be investigated. Don't assume that rectal bleeding is from hemorrhoids until other potential sources of bleeding, such as a colon polyp or colorectal cancer, have been excluded.

Treatment

Often, treatment for hemorrhoids involves steps that you can take on your own, such as lifestyle modifications. Sometimes, medications or surgical procedures are necessary.

Medications

If your hemorrhoids produce only mild discomfort, your doctor may suggest over-the-counter creams, ointments, suppositories or pads. These products contain ingredients, such as witch hazel or hydrocortisone, that can relieve pain and itching, at least temporarily.

Don't use an over-the-counter cream or other product for more than a week unless directed by your doctor. They can cause side effects, such as skin rash, inflammation and skin thinning.

Minimally invasive procedures

If a blood clot has formed within an external hemorrhoid, your doctor can easily remove the clot with a simple incision, which may provide prompt relief.

For persistent bleeding or painful hemorrhoids, your doctor may recommend another minimally invasive procedure. These treatments can be done in your doctor's office or other outpatient setting.

- **Rubber band ligation.** Your doctor places one or two tiny rubber bands around the base of an internal hemorrhoid to cut off its circulation. The hemorrhoid withers and falls off within a few days. This procedure is effective for many people. It can be uncomfortable and may cause bleeding, which might begin two to four days after the procedure but is rarely severe.
- **Injection (sclerotherapy).** In this procedure, your doctor injects a chemical solution into the hemorrhoid tissue to shrink it. While the injection causes little or no pain, it may be less effective than rubber band ligation.
- **Coagulation (infrared, laser or bipolar).** These techniques use laser or infrared light or heat. They cause small, bleeding, internal hemorrhoids to harden and shrivel. While coagulation has few side effects, it's associated with a higher rate of hemorrhoids coming back (recurrence).

Surgical procedures

If other procedures haven't been successful or you have large

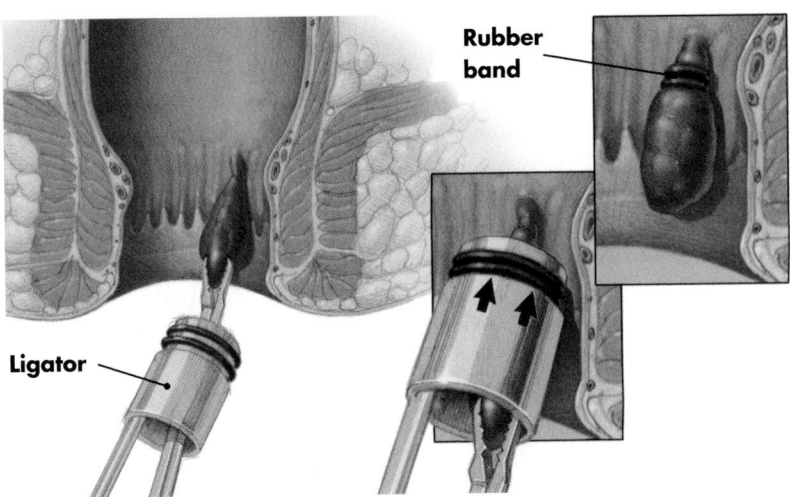

To remove an internal hemorrhoid with a rubber band, a doctor first attaches a special instrument (ligator) to the hemorrhoid and stretches it downward (left). A rubber band is then placed around the hemorrhoid to cut off its blood supply (right).

hemorrhoids, your doctor may recommend a surgical procedure. Surgery can be performed on an outpatient basis, or you may need to stay in the hospital overnight.

- **Hemorrhoidectomy.** Your surgeon removes excessive tissue that causes bleeding. Various techniques may be used. Hemorrhoidectomy is the most effective and complete way to remove hemorrhoids, but it also has the highest rate of complications. These may include temporary difficulty emptying your bladder and urinary tract infections related to this difficulty. Most people experience some pain after the procedure.
- **Stapling.** This procedure, called stapled hemorrhoidectomy or stapled hemorrhoidopexy, blocks blood flow to hemorrhoidal tissue. Stapling generally involves less pain than does hemorrhoidectomy and it allows an earlier return to work. Compared with hemorrhoidectomy, however, stapling has been associated with a greater risk of recurrence and rectal prolapse, in which part of the rectum protrudes from the anus. Talk with your doctor about what might be the best option for you.

Anal itch

Anal itch (pruritus ani) is a common, distracting and potentially embarrassing problem. Almost everyone is afflicted at one time or another. A persistent anal itch is a more common problem for children and older adults. In children, it's frequently caused by pinworms. Among older adults, the cause usually is dry, aging skin.

For most of the rest of the population, the cause isn't always easily identified. Your doctor will look for signs of a skin condition such as psoriasis or a yeast infection and may also check for hemorrhoids or an anal fissure or fistula, which may cause itching and irritation. The precise cause often remains a mystery, but it usually isn't associated with any serious disorder.

Additional factors also can cause anal itching:
- Some people scrub their anus with a harsh soap and rough washcloth. This can lead to irritation and itching. On the other hand, inadequate cleansing following a bowel movement also can cause irritation and itching.
- Some people use over-the-counter products to relieve anal itching. These products may actually increase itching

by irritating and sensitizing the skin.
- Some doctors believe that stress may be a factor.
- Sometimes, the muscles and sphincter that normally keep the anus closed can become lax, allowing stool to seep out and irritate the surrounding skin.

Treatment

If anal itching is a problem for you, try the following measures. If they don't help, see your doctor for an evaluation.

- **Stop scratching.** As hard as this may be, summon your willpower and try it. Continued scratching leads to persistent inflammation and damage to the delicate tissue. The more you scratch, the more you itch.
- **Keep the area clean.** Cleanse the area gently in the morning, in the evening and after a bowel movement. Use moistened, unscented, white toilet paper or cotton balls. Pat the area dry rather than rubbing it.
- **Pad the area.** To prevent skin irritation caused by leakage of stool, place a cotton pad between your buttocks, up against the anus. Replace the pad as necessary.
- **Drink extra fluid.** Try to drink six 8-ounce glasses of water each day. This will help make your stool soft and bulky. A hard stool can irritate your anus further.
- **Take a stool-bulking supplement.** Once or twice a day, take a stool-bulking supplement (Citrucel, Metamucil, others) mixed with water to prevent your stool from being uncomfortably hard.
- **Avoid certain foods and beverages.** Try eliminating alcohol, coffee, tea, soda, nuts, popcorn, chocolate, tomatoes, citrus juices and milk from your diet for about a month. Then reintroduce these items one at a time into your diet. If resumption of the itching corresponds to

consumption of an item, avoid the item.
- **Use hydrocortisone.** Try a cold pack and a 0.5 percent hydrocortisone cream or ointment (available without a prescription) to relieve the discomfort.

Anal fissures and fistulas

Signs and symptoms
- Pain during and after bowel movements
- Bright red blood in the stool or on the toilet paper
- Seepage of stool or mucus through the skin around the anus

Anal fissure
An anal fissure is a relatively minor cut or crack in the lining of the anal canal in an area adjacent to the tailbone, scrotum or vagina. It starts at the anal opening and extends up into the canal.

Adding more fiber to your diet and using stool softeners or bulking agents can often help heal a temporary (acute) anal fissure and relieve the pain. If the cut is deep, the pain may be more intense, both during and after passage of stool because the affected tissue may cause the anal sphincter muscle to spasm. A warm bath can relax the sphincter muscle and reduce painful muscle spasm. For severe pain, your doctor may recommend a nitroglycerin ointment or paste. An operation to repair the cut generally is only performed if other measures fail.

Anal fistula
An anal fistula is an abnormal tubelike passageway from the anal canal to a hole in the skin around the opening to the anus. A fistula usually results from an anorectal abscess that has drained, although it may result from inflammation of the lower colon or a previous surgery involving the lower colon. An anal fistula or anorectal abscess may also result from Crohn's disease.

Pus and debris can collect in the fistula tract, causing pain and swelling. This often drains spontaneously, and signs and symptoms resolve until the opening again becomes clogged.

Treatment of fistulas usually consists of making an incision through the skin, fat and muscle overlying the fistula tract. This is usually done with a local anesthetic. The wound is left open and usually heals in four to six weeks. An abscess may be drained by lancing the skin overlying the collection of pus.

Anorectal abscess

Signs and symptoms
- Discomfort in or around the anal opening
- Swelling and redness near the anus
- Discharge of pus
- Fever

Anorectal abscesses affect the area immediately around the anus. Most are the result of infected tissue around the anus and rectum.

An abscess that's easily accessible near the anus can be pierced and drained. Deep abscesses are less accessible, their diagnosis is more difficult, and potential complications are more serious. Deep rectal abscesses warrant careful attention because they may stem from a fistula due to Crohn's disease or from diverticulitis. In addition to draining the abscess, your doctor may give you antibiotic and pain medication if needed.

Proctitis

Signs and symptoms
- Blood, mucus or pus in the stool
- Constipation
- Diarrhea
- Severe rectal pain
- Fever

Proctitis is an inflammation of the rectum. It may result from a bacterial or viral infection or be a feature of inflammatory bowel disease.

In some instances, proctitis can stem from a sexually transmitted infection (STI) acquired by anal intercourse. An individual with proctitis from an STI can spread the disease to other sexual partners. Radiation treatment, such as for prostate cancer, also can cause proctitis, as can reduced blood flow to the rectum (ischemia).

A repeated urge to defecate or an inability to move your bowels may occur. If the inflammation is higher in your bowel (proctocolitis), signs and symptoms may be more severe.

Diagnosis
Sometimes, signs and symptoms associated with proctitis are a clue to the possible cause of the infection. If herpes simplex virus has caused the infection, you may experience extreme anal pain and ulcers or blister-like elevations around the anus. Skin around your anus may burn and itch.

Your doctor may examine the skin around your anus, analyze the stool for infection and conduct an examination of the rectum using a flexible, fiber-optic tube (endoscope) inserted into the rectum.

How serious is proctitis?
Depending on the cause, the inflammation may or may not be easily treated. Bacterial infections usually respond to antibiotics, but viral infections don't.

Treatment
Treatment for a bacterial infection generally includes an antibiotic. Other forms of proctitis may be treated with enemas that contain anti-inflammatory medications.

There's no medication available to cure proctitis caused by the herpes virus, although your doctor may prescribe agents that can control the spread of the infection and ease the signs and symptoms. For proctitis caused by other STIs, such as gonorrhea, treatment of the infection helps cure the proctitis.

Proctitis associated with inflammatory bowel disease can be treated with 5-aminosalicylic acid (5-ASA) or corticosteroid suppositories. For radiation-induced proctitis, if persistent bleeding occurs, laser treatment may be used to seal the affected blood vessels.

Fecal incontinence

Fecal incontinence refers to the inability to retain stool between bowel movements. The problem can be due to an underlying condition such as an abscess, inflammation or past trauma in the rectum, anus or perianal area.

Fecal incontinence is also frequently seen after a previous operation in the area or, in women, from trauma to the anal sphincter during childbirth. In some cases, fecal incontinence is related to a spinal cord injury or nervous system disorder.

In older adults, fecal incontinence may result from the aging of the sphincter and pelvic floor muscles and ligaments. Fecal impaction, which is more common in older adults, is another possible cause of fecal incontinence.

To determine a cause, your doctor may ask a number of questions, including if the incontinence occurs with sneezing or coughing or if it occurs only at night. He or she may examine your anal sphincter to see if the sphincter muscles are intact and order tests to determine various pressures in the rectal and anal regions.

Treatment

In some adults, a bowel retraining program can improve fecal continence, particularly if the anal sphincter is intact.

Your doctor may advise you to take time each day to have a bowel movement. This often results in continence during the remainder of the day. He or she may also advise you to eat more fresh fruits and vegetables. This sometimes helps produce a more normal stool

Hernia Surgery

Surgery is the preferred treatment for most abdominal hernias, with the exception of an umbilical hernia in an infant, which usually corrects itself in one or two years.

The procedure

Hernia surgery consists of replacing any protruding intestine into the abdomen and surgically repairing the weakened or torn tissues to prevent the intestine from breaking through again.

Surgery may be postponed if you have a cold and cough because the spasmodic pressure in the abdomen may weaken the incision before it can heal properly.

Before the operation you'll be given some type of anesthetic — local, spinal or general, depending on the type and severity of the hernia. A small incision is then made in the area of the

and decreases the number of times you have to pass stool.

If the sphincter muscle has been damaged by trauma, childbirth or prior surgery, an operation may be necessary to repair the damage.

Hernias

A hernia occurs when one part of your body — usually the small intestine — protrudes through a gap or weak spot into another part of your body. Several types of hernias can affect the abdomen: inguinal, femoral, umbilical, hiatal and incisional. A hiatal hernia (see page 819) is a protrusion of part of the stomach through the esophageal opening (hiatus) of the diaphragm.

People tend to associate hernias with heavy lifting, but in fact, hernias often have no apparent cause. Even a baby can be born with one.

hernia, and the herniated tissue is returned to the abdominal cavity. This type of surgery is called a herniorrhaphy. If the herniated intestine is strangulated and gangrenous, that section of the intestine will be removed (resected), and the healthy ends will be sutured together. The operation is concluded by repairing the tissues of the abdominal wall. Your surgeon may elect to strengthen a weakened abdominal wall by placing a synthetic mesh patch over the tissue to keep it from protruding again. This procedure is called a hernioplasty.

Sometimes, hernia repair is performed laparoscopically. Instead of making a large incision in your abdomen, the surgeon makes several small incisions of $\frac{1}{2}$ to 1 inch in length. Flexible, tubelike instruments (laparoscopes), one of which has an attached miniature camera, are inserted through the incisions,

Inguinal hernia

In men, a hernia commonly develops in the groin — the region where the spermatic cord and blood vessels to the testicles pass out of the abdominal cavity and into the scrotum (see page 866). The area where these structures pass through the abdominal muscles is called the inguinal canal.

When a loop of bowel passes out of the abdomen along with the spermatic cord, this is called an indirect inguinal hernia. A bulge directly through the abdominal wall in this area is called a direct inguinal hernia. The vast majority of groin hernias are inguinal.

Men are more likely to have an inherent weakness along the inguinal canal because of the way males develop in the womb. In the male fetus, the testicles form within the abdomen and then move down the inguinal canal into the

allowing the surgeon to see inside your abdomen, guide the protruding intestine back into place, and repair weakened tissue and muscle. Because only small incisions are made, the procedure often results in a quicker recovery than with conventional surgery.

Recovery

Hernia surgery is usually done on an outpatient basis. After the operation you'll be urged to move about as soon as you're able, usually within the first day. Some soreness is typical, but many people go back to work within a few days. Recovery may last anywhere from one to six weeks, depending on the type of surgery you had and your occupation.

Your doctor may have specific activity restrictions, but in general it's best to avoid contact sports and heavy lifting or straining for at least three weeks to allow the incision to heal.

If you notice any redness or discomfort around the site of the incision, report it to your doctor. It may be a sign of infection.

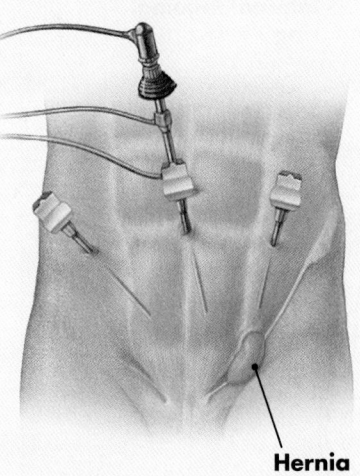

Hernia

Laparoscopic surgery involves inserting instruments through several small incisions. Traditional surgery uses one larger incision.

scrotum. Shortly after birth, the inguinal canal closes almost completely, leaving just enough room for the spermatic cord to pass through, but not large enough to allow the testicles to move back into the abdomen.

Sometimes, however, the canal doesn't close properly, leaving a weakened area. There's less chance that the inguinal canal won't close after birth in female babies. In women, an inguinal hernia more often develops at the point where the connective tissue supporting the uterus exits from the abdomen to join with the tissue near the vaginal opening. Women are also more likely to develop hernias in the femoral canal, an opening near the inguinal canal where the femoral artery, vein and nerve pass through.

Whether or not you have a pre-existing weakness, extra pressure in your abdomen can cause a hernia. This pressure may result from:

- Straining during bowel movements or urination
- Heavy lifting
- Fluid in the abdomen (ascites)
- Pregnancy
- Excess weight

Signs and symptoms of an inguinal hernia include discomfort while bending or lifting and a tender lump in the groin area. In men, the protruding intestine sometimes enters the scrotum, causing pain and swelling of the scrotum.

Diagnosis

See your doctor if you have a painful or noticeable bulge in the area on either side of your pubic bone. Usually, a doctor can diagnose an inguinal hernia by examination. Minor hernias are often detected during routine physical exams.

How serious is an inguinal hernia?

A hernia that can't be replaced into the abdomen by application

of gentle pressure may be trapped (incarcerated). Without treatment, the hernia can strangulate and cut off the blood supply to the intestine. This can cause gangrene in a section of the bowel, a life-threatening condition requiring immediate surgical attention.

Treatment

The best treatment for an inguinal hernia that's causing signs and symptoms is an operation in which the intestine is pushed back into the abdomen and weakened muscles in the abdominal wall are reinforced. Today's hernia surgery isn't the same as your father may have had — with a large abdominal incision, a long hospital stay and weeks of immobility. Instead, many inguinal hernias can be successfully repaired with a technique that uses several small incisions, leading to a faster, less painful recovery (see "Hernia Surgery").

Wearing a truss or support device doesn't provide a good long-term solution for a hernia. However, your doctor may suggest that you wear one before surgery to prevent the condition from worsening.

Femoral hernia

A femoral hernia forms along the canal that carries the principal blood vessels (femoral artery and vein) into the thigh. This hernia usually produces a bulge that's slightly lower than where an inguinal hernia tends to appear.

Femoral hernias are more common in women than in men, and these types of hernias are more likely to become strangulated.

Umbilical hernia

Does your baby's bellybutton protrude when he or she cries? This is a classic sign of an umbilical hernia — a common and typically harmless condition. Umbilical hernias are most common in infants, but they can affect adults as well.

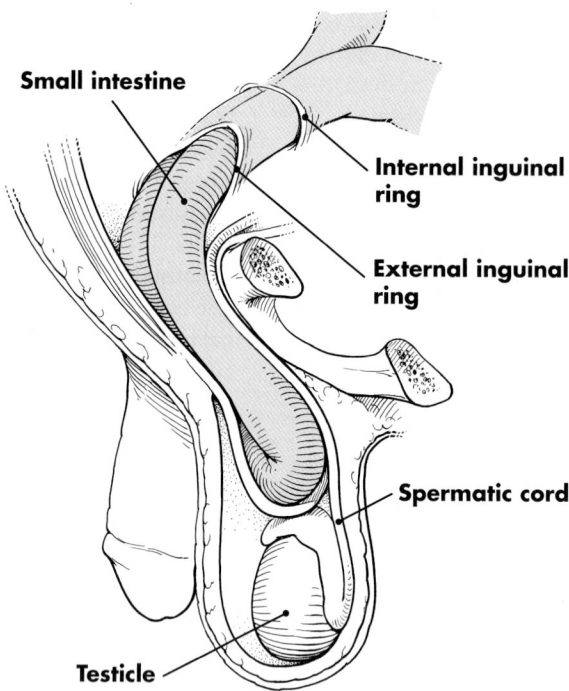

Small intestine

Internal inguinal ring

External inguinal ring

Spermatic cord

Testicle

In an inguinal hernia, the small intestine protrudes into the scrotum. It commonly occurs in men at the point where the spermatic cord that suspends the testicles passes out of the abdomen into the scrotum.

With this type of hernia, a bulge appears at the navel (umbilicus) because of a weakness in the abdominal wall surrounding the umbilicus allowing part of the bowel to remain outside of the abdominal cavity. These hernias often don't cause any signs and symptoms and may resolve on their own. In adults, umbilical hernias may become sore or painful.

Most umbilical hernias close on their own by age 1, though up to 10 percent may take longer to heal. Umbilical hernias that don't disappear by age 4 or those that appear during adulthood may need surgical repair.

Incisional hernia

A surgical incision in the abdominal wall can lead to an incisional hernia. Incisional hernias usually pose only a minor risk of complications, although at times portions of your intestine may protrude (prolapse) through the hernia and cause discomfort.

Gallbladder and Bile Duct Disorders

The gallbladder is a pear-shaped sac that's attached to the underside of the liver on your right side. The gallbladder stores bile that's produced in your liver and discharges it into the upper part of your small intestine (duodenum) after a meal. Bile facilitates the digestion of fats. Several conditions can affect the gallbladder and bile ducts.

Gallstones

Signs and symptoms
- Intense and sudden pain in the upper abdomen
- Pain that moves around to the right shoulder blade area
- Chronic indigestion
- Nausea and vomiting
- Fever

Gallstones are solid deposits of cholesterol or calcium salts that form in the gallbladder or nearby bile ducts. They can be as small as a grain of sand or larger than a golf ball, smooth and round, or irregular with many edges. Some people have only one gallstone, and others have hundreds.

Gallstones develop in many people and they usually don't cause signs and symptoms. But some people with gallstones have a gallbladder attack that can cause symptoms, such as nausea and an intense, steady ache in the upper middle or upper right abdomen.

As the pain subsides, you may have a mild aching sensation or soreness in the upper abdomen, which may last for up to a day. Gallbladder attacks can be infrequent, occurring no more than a few times a year.

Yellowing of your skin and eyes (jaundice), especially if it's accompanied by pain, suggests that a stone may have migrated into the common bile duct. The presence of a high fever or shaking chills usually indicates a complication such as inflammation of the gallbladder (cholecystitis), acute pancreatitis or infection in the bile duct (cholangitis) due to an obstruction.

Sometimes, signs and symptoms of gallbladder disease occur after eating, but they can occur anytime.

The likelihood of gallstones increases with age and obesity. Extreme, rapid weight loss also is associated with gallstone formation.

Types
Not all gallstones are made of the same material. Most contain a mixture of substances. Among Americans, about 80 percent of gallstones are composed primarily of undissolved cholesterol. The remaining 20 percent contain mostly calcium salts of bile pigment. Pigment stones form when your bile contains too much bilirubin, a residue from the breakdown of red blood cells.

Diagnosis

If a severe, persistent pain develops in your upper abdomen, your doctor may want to check for gallstones. Your doctor may palpate your abdomen to see if your gallbladder is tender or has become swollen (distended) because of obstruction of the duct.

Tests used to diagnose gallstones generally include blood tests and tests that create pictures of your gallbladder or that check your bile ducts for gallstones.

These tests may include a hepatobiliary iminodiacetic acid (HIDA) scan, magnetic resonance imaging (MRI) or endoscopic retrograde cholangiopancreatography (ERCP). Gallstones discovered using ERCP can be removed during the procedure.

Treatment

Because the majority of gallstones produce no symptoms, they require no treatment. If your gallstones cause symptoms, however, several possible treatments are available.

Surgery

Gallbladder surgery (cholecystectomy) is one of the most common surgeries performed in the United States. The surgery can be performed in two ways:

- **Laparoscopic surgery.** Most often gallbladder surgery is performed using a laparoscope, a pencil-thin tube with its own lighting system and miniature video camera. The video camera produces a magnified view of the inside of your abdomen on a television monitor. This allows the surgeon to see the surgery in detail. To remove your gallbladder, he or she uses tiny instruments that are inserted through several other small abdominal incisions.

    Because laparoscopic cholecystectomy uses smaller incisions, you'll likely have less postoperative pain, less scarring and an earlier return to your normal activities. Laparoscopic removal of the gallbladder is effective in the majority of cases.

- **Open surgery.** In open surgery, the gallbladder is removed through a large abdominal incision. This may be the best option in severe cases. It may also be used when the gallbladder walls are thick and hard, the gallbladder is obviously infected, or scar tissue is present from earlier abdominal operations.

    If you have stones in the bile duct as well as your gallbladder, your doctor may recommend surgical removal of both the duct stones and your gallbladder. In some cases, your doctor may suggest removing the stones in the bile duct with the ERCP procedure. The same procedure may be used to remove a stone from a blocked pancreatic duct.

Nonsurgical options

Stones usually recur when nonsurgical treatments are used. But if surgery isn't an option, your doctor may recommend one of the following:

- **Bile salt tablets.** This medication, ursodiol (Actigall), dissolves cholesterol stones over a period of time. The treatment works best on small cholesterol stones, but is effective only about 50 percent of the time.

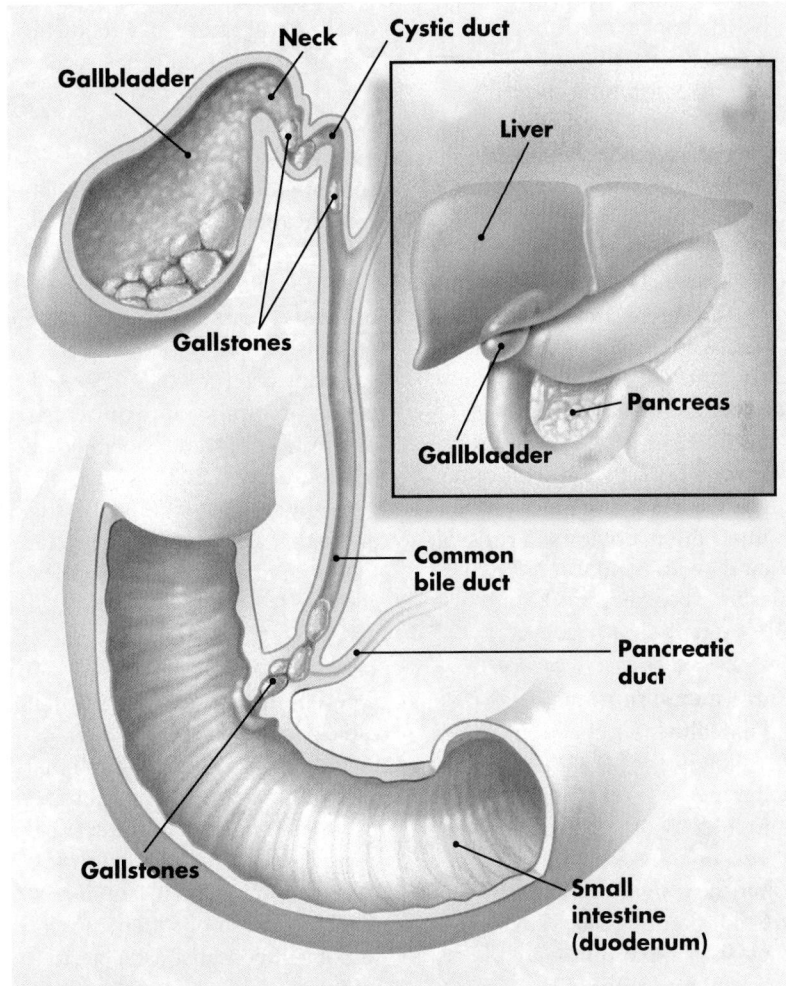

The gallbladder is located behind the liver on the right side of the upper abdomen. A gallbladder attack occurs when stones that form in the gallbladder lodge in the neck of the gallbladder or the cystic duct leading to the main (common) bile duct. Gallstones that obstruct the common bile duct or pancreatic duct can cause inflammation of the bile ducts (cholangitis) or pancreatitis.

- **Sound wave therapy (extracorporeal shock wave lithotripsy).** This treatment uses high-frequency sound waves to break up gallstones. You then take ursodiol tablets (Urso) to dissolve the fragments. Sound wave therapy is appropriate for only a small percentage of people with gallstones.
- **Percutaneous electrohydraulic lithotripsy.** This procedure relies on a catheter that's inserted into the gallbladder several weeks prior to the treatment. A small probe is inserted into the catheter to deliver short bursts of energy to break up the stones. This is the only nonsurgical treatment option that can be used on any type of gallstone. Because this procedure is time-consuming and isn't widely available, it's usually considered only for people with a high risk of surgical complications.
- **Topical gallstone dissolution.** In this procedure, a small catheter is inserted into the gallbladder. A solution that dissolves cholesterol gallstones is then delivered through the catheter into the gallbladder over a several-hour period. This option has lower recurrence rates than medication, but it's still considered experimental.

Bile duct obstruction

Signs and symptoms
- Pain in the upper abdomen
- Yellowing of the skin and eyes
- Itching
- Light gray or tan stools
- Tea- or coffee-colored urine

Emergency signs and symptoms
- Cold, clammy, pale skin and a weak or rapid pulse
- High fever with chills
- Mental confusion

The common bile duct is the main passageway for transporting bile into the duodenum. An obstruction is the common bile duct can occur for these reasons:

Gallstones
The most common cause of a bile duct obstruction is a gallstone that has lodged in the duct. One or more stones may obstruct the narrow duct and cause episodic pain in the upper abdomen. Spiking fevers with shaking chills and yellowing of your skin and eyes (jaundice) may signal a severe (acute) bile duct obstruction.

An obstruction in the common bile duct at the location where it's joined by the pancreatic duct can cause inflammation of the pancreas (pancreatitis). Pancreatic enzymes aren't able to flow out of the pancreas and become trapped inside, damaging the organ. Obstruction of the common bile duct can lead to a medical emergency requiring immediate relief of the obstruction.

Narrowing of a duct
Narrowing (stricture) of the common bile duct is a potential complication of gallbladder or bile duct surgery. The stricture may develop immediately after surgery or several years later. Strictures may also develop following a gallstone obstruction. A special endoscopic procedure called endoscopic retrograde cholangiopancreatography (ERCP) is often performed to help widen the area and a tiny tube (stent) is placed in the location until the narrowing is corrected.

Hemobilia
Blood in the bile duct (hemobilia) can clot and obstruct the duct. Hemobilia is a rare condition that may occur as a result of trauma to the liver or bile duct during surgery. People with hemobilia often have abdominal pain, jaundice and blood in stool. Often, the clot dissolves spontaneously, but it might need to be removed with an endoscopic procedure.

Primary sclerosing cholangitis
The term *sclerosis* refers to hardening and thickening of tissue. A chronic disorder called primary sclerosing cholangitis causes tissues in the bile duct wall to harden and thicken. This can partially block the duct and lead to formation of bile duct stones. Either the obstruction or resulting stones can cause the same signs and symptoms as gallstones in the bile duct, including jaundice, itching, pain in the right side of the abdomen, and episodes of fever and chills.

Primary sclerosing cholangitis can also lead to cirrhosis, liver failure, bile duct cancer or bleeding from veins in the esophagus. Frequently, sclerosing cholangitis is associated with an underlying disease such as ulcerative colitis.

Bile duct cancer
A cancerous (malignant) tumor in the bile duct can cause obstruction. Signs and symptoms of bile duct cancer may include jaundice, weight loss, light-colored stools and, less commonly, abdominal pain.

Other disorders
Sometimes, the common bile duct can become partially or completely obstructed by external pressure. This can occur as a complication of pancreatitis, pancreatic cancer, lymphoma or cancer that has spread (metastasized) from another part of the body. The principal sign is jaundice. Treatment is directed at the underlying disorder.

Diagnosis
Because the early signs and symptoms of a bile duct obstruction are similar, regardless of the cause, your doctor may use many of the same diagnostic tests used to identify gallstones. Two other diagnostic procedures, called percutaneous transhepatic cholangiography and endoscopic retrograde cholangiopancreatography (ERCP), involve injection of a contrast material into the common bile duct.

How serious is a bile duct obstruction?
Bile duct blockage is a serious

Detecting Duct Obstructions

Bile and pancreatic ducts are small and located deep in the abdomen, so standard diagnostic tests often aren't beneficial in examining them. To identify a possible obstruction in a duct, a doctor may use one of the following procedures:

Endoscopic ultrasound

Endoscopic ultrasound (EUS) involves the use of a small ultrasound probe that's attached to a thin, flexible instrument called an endoscope. While you're sedated the endoscope is inserted through your mouth and threaded down your throat to your stomach and upper small intestine (duodenum).

The ultrasound probe is used to view internal organs and structures that are adjacent to the stomach and intestines, including the gallbladder, pancreas and liver. EUS can help diagnose disorders affecting these organs, including obstructions in the pancreatic and bile ducts. This procedure provides clear pictures without having to inject contrast materials into the ducts, reducing the risk of complications. If a growth is detected, tissue samples can be taken (biopsies) for laboratory analysis.

Endoscopic retrograde cholangiopancreatography

Endoscopic retrograde cholangiopancreatography (ERCP) is another procedure used to identify the cause of a bile duct obstruction, such as a gallstone, damaged bile duct tissue or tumor.

While you're sedated, an endoscope is threaded into your mouth, down your throat, through your stomach and into the first part of your small intestine (duodenum). Air is injected to inflate the duodenum to help identify the tiny opening through which the bile and pancreatic ducts drain. Once this opening is found, a hollow tube (catheter) is passed through the endoscope and into the bile and pancreatic ducts. A dye or contrast solution is injected through this catheter into the ducts. X-rays are then taken of the ducts.

Other types of catheters may be placed through the endoscope to take tissue samples or treat specific

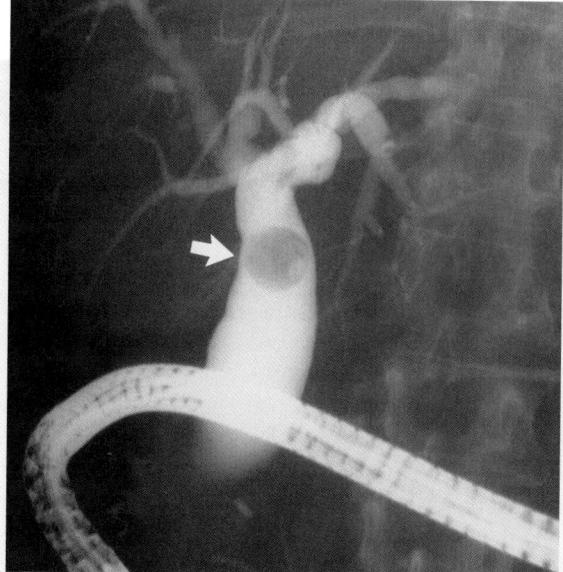

This **X-ray image taken during an endoscopic retrograde cholangiopancreatography procedure shows a dilated common bile duct containing a gallstone (see arrow).**

abnormalities identified on the X-rays, such as removing any obstructing stones.

Percutaneous transhepatic cholangiography

Percutaneous transhepatic cholangiography is an X-ray procedure that uses a contrast material to provide pictures of the bile duct. Before the test you lie down on an X-ray table that can be rotated into vertical and horizontal positions. A tube is inserted into a vein in your arm for administration of a sedative and antibiotic. The skin over your liver is cleansed with an antiseptic, and a local anesthetic is injected below the skin.

Once the area where the anesthetic was injected becomes numb, a long, thin needle is inserted into your liver. Most people don't feel the needle pass into the liver. When X-ray images indicate that the needle has reached the bile duct, a contrast medium is injected through the needle. A series of X-rays is taken as you're rotated into different positions to provide varying views of your liver. You may need to stay in the hospital overnight for monitoring in case bleeding or infection develops. This test is usually performed if the bile duct has a known obstruction that can't be managed with ERCP.

and even life-threatening problem that requires prompt treatment. Blood cultures during episodes of fever may reveal the presence of bacteria that have entered into the bloodstream from the obstructed and infected bile duct. Blood infection (sepsis) can lead to shock.

Treatment
The principal goal of treatment is to relieve the blockage.

Surgery
If the cause of the obstruction is one or more gallstones within the bile duct and you have gallstones in

your gallbladder, your doctor may recommend surgical removal of the gallbladder once the stones lodged in the duct have been removed.

If the obstruction is due to narrowing (stricture) of the bile duct, the duct may be widened and a tiny tube (stent) inserted into the area to help keep the duct open and allow passage of bile.

Because late-stage primary sclerosing cholangitis typically causes multiple narrowings that can't be treated, presently there's no specific surgical therapy for that disorder. If the disorder results in severe liver failure, a liver transplant may be an option.

Endoscopic retrograde cholangiopancreatography

Bile duct obstructions are generally treated with endoscopic retrograde cholangiopancreatography (ERCP), a procedure in which a flexible tube (endoscope) is threaded into your digestive tract to where the common bile duct enters into the upper portion of the small intestine (duodenum). A cutting device attached to the tube can be inserted through the entrance of the bile duct, enlarging the entrance to permit passage of the obstructing stone. A tiny tube (stent) may be temporarily placed in the duct to keep it open.

Medication

Itching is often a predominant symptom with chronic obstruction of the bile ducts. It can be successfully managed with medication. Your doctor may also prescribe vitamins A, D, E and K, which are poorly absorbed in people with bile duct obstruction. If fever and chills are present, you may be given an antibiotic.

Choledochal cysts

Cysts can sometimes form in the bile duct. Cysts that result from a birth defect that causes expansion of the duct are called choledochal cysts. A choledochal cyst can lead to obstruction or infection of the bile duct, which causes a narrowing (stricture) of the duct. Because the process is very gradual, many people experience occasional symptoms of abdominal pain and irritation for years before an obstruction develops.

Once such a cyst is identified, it's generally removed surgically. People who have had a choledochal cyst have an increased risk of developing bile duct cancer.

Pancreatic Disorders

The pancreas lies horizontally behind the lower part of the stomach. Its head rests against the wall of the first portion of the small intestine (duodenum), and its tail extends toward the spleen.

The pancreas produces and secretes digestive enzymes and alkaline material (sodium bicarbonate) into the pancreatic duct, which then flow into the duodenum. The alkaline secretion makes it possible for digestive enzymes to break down nutrients into smaller units, enabling them to be absorbed into the bloodstream by the small bowel.

The pancreas also produces and secretes the hormones insulin and glucagon into the bloodstream, which are important to help regulate your metabolism, including your level of blood sugar (glucose).

Infections, injury and tumors can damage the pancreas and affect its functions. If, for example, secretion of the hormone insulin is diminished, diabetes may result.

Pancreatitis

Signs and symptoms
- Nausea and vomiting
- Fever
- Weight loss
- Oily, malodorous stools
- Rapid pulse
- Swollen, tender abdomen

Pancreatitis is a term used to describe inflammation in the pancreas. The pancreas is a long, flat gland that sits tucked behind the stomach in the upper abdomen. The pancreas produces enzymes that help digestion and hormones that help regulate the way your body processes sugar (glucose).

Pancreatitis can occur as acute pancreatitis — meaning it appears suddenly and lasts for days. Or pancreatitis can occur as chronic pancreatitis, which describes pancreatitis that persists over many years. Mild cases of pancreatitis may go away without treatment, but severe cases can cause life-threatening complications.

During normal digestion, inactivated pancreatic enzymes move through ducts in your pancreas and travel to the small intestine where they become activated and help with digestion. In pancreatitis, the enzymes become activated while still in the pancreas. This causes the enzymes to irritate the cells of your pancreas, causing inflammation and the signs and symptoms associated with pancreatitis.

A number of causes have been identified for acute pancreatitis and chronic pancreatitis, including:
- Alcoholism
- Gallstones
- Abdominal surgery
- Certain medications
- Endoscopic retrograde cholangiopancreatography (ERCP), when used to treat gallstones
- Family history of pancreatitis
- Cystic fibrosis
- High calcium levels in blood (hypercalcemia)
- High parathyroid hormone levels in blood (hyperparathyroidism)
- High triglyceride levels in the blood (hypertriglyceridemia)
- Infection
- Injury to the abdomen
- Pancreatic cancer
- Ulcer

How serious is pancreatitis?
In most cases, signs and symptoms of mild acute pancreatitis subside within a week. Severe pancreatitis, however, can be life-threatening. Major complications include breathing problems, malnutrition, diabetes, infection, kidney problems and development of pancreatic cancer.

The Pancreas

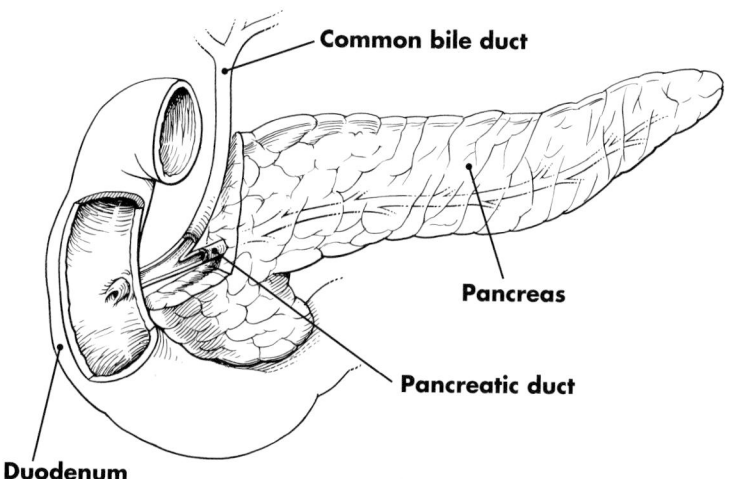

Common bile duct

Pancreas

Pancreatic duct

Duodenum

Diagnosis

During a physical examination, your doctor may elicit pain by pressing the abdominal area. A sample of your blood may be taken to check for specific abnormalities, such as excessive levels of certain pancreatic enzymes, a high white blood cell count, high blood sugar (hyperglycemia) and low calcium levels (hypocalcemia). Other tests may include stool tests, a computerized tomography (CT) scan, abdominal ultrasound, endoscopic ultrasound and pancreatic function tests. If your doctor suspects a malabsorption problem, you may have a pancreatic function test to measure the ability of your pancreas to secrete substances necessary for digestion.

Your doctor may recommend other tests depending on your particular situation.

Treatment

Pancreatitis usually requires hospitalization. Once your condition is stabilized in the hospital and inflammation in the pancreas is controlled, doctors can treat the underlying cause of your pancreatitis.

Hospitalization

If you're experiencing pancreatitis, your doctor may admit you to the hospital for care. Initial treatments to help control the inflammation in

your pancreas and make you more comfortable may include:

- **Resting your pancreas.** You'll stop eating for a couple of days in the hospital in order to give your pancreas a chance to recover. Once the inflammation in your pancreas is controlled, you may begin drinking clear liquids and eating bland foods. With time, you can go back to your normal diet.
- **Pain medications.** Pancreatitis can cause severe pain. Pain medications help control the pain.
- **Intravenous (IV) fluids.** As your body devotes energy and fluids to repairing your pancreas, you may become dehydrated. For this reason, you'll receive extra fluids through a vein in your arm during your hospital stay.

How long you stay in the hospital will depend on your situation. Some people recover quickly and others develop complications that require a longer hospitalization.

Procedures and surgery

Once your pancreatitis is brought under control, your health care team can treat the underlying cause of your condition. Treatment will depend on the cause of your pancreatitis and may include:

- **Procedures to remove bile duct obstructions.** Pancreati-

tis caused by a narrowed or blocked bile duct may require procedures to open or widen the bile duct. A procedure called endoscopic retrograde cholangiopancreatography (ERCP) uses a long tube with a camera on the end to examine your pancreas and bile ducts. The tube is passed down your throat, and the camera sends pictures of your digestive system to a monitor. ERCP can aid in diagnosing problems in the bile duct and also in making repairs.

- **Gallbladder surgery.** If gallstones caused your pancreatitis, your doctor may recommend surgery to remove your gallbladder (cholecystectomy).
- **Endoscopic necrosectomy.** This procedure is often used to drain fluid from your pancreas or to remove diseased tissue.
- **Treatment for alcohol dependence.** Drinking several drinks daily over many years can cause pancreatitis. If this is the cause of your pancreatitis, your doctor may recommend you enter a treatment program for alcohol addiction. Continuing to drink can worsen your pancreatitis and lead to serious complications.

Additional treatments

Chronic pancreatitis may require additional treatments, depending on your situation. They may include:

- **Pain management.** Chronic pancreatitis can cause persistent abdominal pain. Your doctor may recommend medications to control your pain and may refer you to a pain specialist. Severe pain may be relieved with surgery to block nerves that send pain signals from the pancreas to the brain.
- **Enzymes to improve digestion.** Pancreatic enzyme supplements can help your body breakdown and process the nutrients in the foods you eat. Pancreatic enzymes are taken in tablet form with each meal.

- **Changes to your diet.** Your doctor may refer you to a dietitian who can help you plan low-fat meals that are high in nutrients.

Pancreatic cancer

Signs and symptoms
- Abdominal pain that may radiate to your back
- Loss of appetite and weight
- Yellowing of the skin and eyes
- Itching
- Nausea and vomiting
- Depression

Although pancreatic cancer accounts for only a small percentage of all cancers in the United States, it's one of the leading causes of cancer deaths. The reason it's so deadly is that it's usually diagnosed too late. The cancer typically produces no signs and symptoms until it's advanced and incurable.

Pancreatic cancer occurs when cells of the pancreas grow uncontrollably and form a tumor. Much about why or how this cancer develops is unclear. Several factors may increase your risk:
- **Smoking.** Cigarette smokers are two to three times more likely to get pancreatic cancer than are nonsmokers.
- **Being overweight.** People who are overweight or obese are more likely to get pancreatic cancer than those who aren't.
- **Family history.** Cancer of the pancreas seems to run in families.
- **Age.** Most people are between ages 60 and 80 when they receive a diagnosis of this disease.
- **Race.** Black people are more likely to get the disease than are people of other racial groups.
- **Chronic pancreatitis.** People with long-term inflammation of the pancreas (chronic pancreatitis) may have an increased risk of developing pancreatic cancer.

Diagnosis
Because the pancreas is located deep in the abdomen and behind other organs, it's almost impossible for a doctor to feel a lump on examination. Possible evidence of pancreatic cancer on a physical exam includes abdominal tenderness, jaundice or liver enlargement.

If your doctor suspects pancreatic cancer, you may have one or more of the following tests to diagnose the cancer:
- **Ultrasound.** Ultrasound uses high-frequency sound waves to create moving images of your internal organs, including your pancreas. The ultrasound sensor (transducer) is placed on your upper abdomen to obtain images.
- **Computerized tomography (CT) scan.** CT scan uses X-ray images to help your doctor visualize your internal organs. In some cases you may receive an injection of dye into a vein in your arm to help highlight the areas your doctor wants to see.
- **Magnetic resonance imaging (MRI).** MRI uses a powerful magnetic field and radio waves to create images of the pancreas.
- **Endoscopic retrograde cholangiopancreatography (ERCP).** This procedure uses a dye to highlight the bile ducts in your pancreas (see page 869).
- **Endoscopic ultrasound (EUS).** EUS uses an ultrasound device to make images of your pancreas from inside your abdomen. The ultrasound device is passed through an endoscope into your stomach in order to obtain the images. Your doctor may also collect a sample of cells (biopsy) during EUS.
- **Percutaneous transhepatic cholangiography (PTC).** This procedure involves injecting a dye into your liver to highlight your bile ducts. Your doctor carefully inserts a thin needle into your liver and injects the dye into the bile ducts in your liver. A special X-ray machine (fluoroscope) tracks the dye as it moves through the ducts.
- **Biopsy.** During a biopsy, your doctor obtains a small sample of tissue from the pancreas for examination under a microscope. A biopsy sample can be obtained by inserting a needle through your skin and into your pancreas (fine-needle aspiration). Or it can be done using endoscopic ultrasound to guide special tools into your pancreas where a sample of cells can be obtained for testing.

How serious is pancreatic cancer?
The survival rate with pancreatic cancer is generally poor. By the time the cancer is identified, it often has spread (metastasized) beyond the pancreas. The median survival of advanced pancreatic cancer is about three to six months from the time of the diagnosis.

Treatment
Treatment for pancreatic cancer depends on the stage and location of the cancer as well as on your age, overall health and personal preferences. The first goal of pancreatic cancer treatment is to eliminate the cancer, when possible. If that isn't an option, the focus may be on preventing the cancer from growing or causing more harm. When pancreatic cancer is advanced and treatments aren't likely to offer a benefit, your doctor may suggest ways to relieve symptoms and make you as comfortable as possible.

Surgery
Only a small portion of pancreatic cancers are resectable — that is, they have a good chance of being removed completely with surgery. Once the cancer has spread beyond the pancreas to other organs, lymph nodes or blood vessels, surgery is usually no longer an option.

If your pancreatic cancer is located in the head of the pancreas, you may consider an operation called a Whipple procedure (pancreatoduodenectomy). The Whipple procedure involves removing the head of your pancreas, as well as a portion of your small intestine (duodenum), your gallbladder

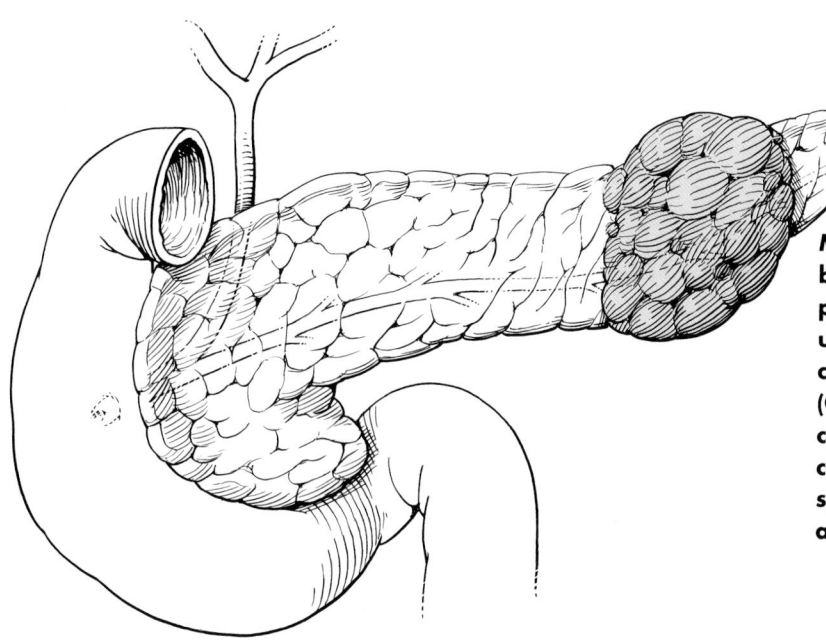

Most pancreatic cancer begins in the lining of the pancreatic ducts and grows undetected for years. The computerized tomography (CT) scan below shows a cancerous tumor in the pancreas (black arrow) that has spread to the liver (white arrow).

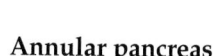

and part of your bile duct. Part of your stomach may be removed as well. Your surgeon reconnects the remaining parts of your pancreas, stomach and intestines to allow you to digest food.

Whipple surgery carries a risk of infection and bleeding. It can cause temporary diabetes until your pancreas recovers from surgery. And some people experience nausea and vomiting that can occur if the stomach has difficulty emptying after surgery (delayed gastric emptying). Expect a long recovery after the Whipple procedure.

Surgery to remove the tail of the pancreas or the tail and a small portion of the body is called distal pancreatectomy. Your surgeon may also remove your spleen.

Expect a long recovery after any of these procedures. Research shows pancreatic cancer surgery tends to cause fewer complications when done by experienced surgeons. Don't hesitate to ask about your surgeon's experience.

Radiation therapy

Radiation therapy uses high-energy beams to destroy cancer cells. You may receive radiation treatments before or after cancer surgery, often in combination with chemotherapy. Or, your doctor may recommend a combination of radiation and chemotherapy treatments when your cancer can't be treated surgically.

Chemotherapy

Chemotherapy uses powerful drugs to kill cancer cells. The drugs can be injected into a vein or taken orally. You may receive only one chemotherapy drug or a combination of drugs. Chemotherapy can also be combined with radiation therapy. This is called chemoradiation. Chemoradiation is typically used to treat cancer that has spread beyond the pancreas, but only to nearby organs and not to distant regions of the body. It may also be used after surgery to reduce the risk that cancer may recur.

Targeted drug therapy

Targeted drug therapy is an emerging area of cancer treatment. Targeted drugs attack specific abnormalities within cancer cells in an attempt to stop the cancer from growing and proliferating. Many targeted drug treatments are under investigation in clinical trials (see page 427).

Congenital pancreatic abnormalities

Occasionally, problems with the pancreas occur at birth.

Annular pancreas

An annular pancreas is a rare, ring-shaped formation of pancreatic tissue that surrounds the first portion of the small intestine (duodenum) and may cause an intestinal obstruction. The condition most often affects children.

You may feel exceptionally full after meals and later have pain in the pit of your stomach that may cause nausea and vomiting. Because the symptoms may be mild and tolerable, many people go for years before they receive a diagnosis of this condition.

Once you receive a diagnosis of this condition and are experiencing symptoms, the problem will likely be corrected surgically.

Pancreas divisum

Pancreas divisum is a congenital defect in which two parts of the pancreas fail to grow together. As a result, the pancreas must drain its secretions through a smaller secondary duct. Most people with this condition have no signs and symptoms,

You can take a number of precautions to avoid viral forms of hepatitis.

Immunization

Effective vaccines for preventing hepatitis A and B are available. Depending on the type of vaccine used, a series of two or three injections offers about 20 years of protection from hepatitis A. A series of three or four injections protects you for at least 10 years against hepatitis B.

Americans considered to be at high risk of hepatitis B virus infection include:

- Individuals who inject illicit drugs with needles
- Individuals with multiple sex partners
- Sexually active individuals who are gay or lesbian
- Sexual partners of individuals with hepatitis B
- People with hemophilia
- People who undergo hemodialysis for kidney failure
- Dental and medical health professionals
- Male prison inmates

Most infants now receive hepatitis B vaccination as part of their routine childhood immunization series. Preadolescents, adolescents, college students and young adults also should receive the vaccine if they haven't been previously immunized.

The Occupational Safety and Health Administration (OSHA) requires some employers to offer hepatitis B vaccine at no cost to employees such as health care workers, public safety personnel and others who might be exposed to blood in the course of their work.

Prior to certain foreign travel, vaccination against hepatitis A may be recommended. In individuals with pre-existing liver disease of any kind leading to cirrhosis, vaccination against hepatitis A and B should be offered to prevent future liver injury.

Food preparation

Follow these safe food handling tips:

- Always wash fruits and vegetables.
- Cook foods thoroughly.
- When in developing countries, use only bottled water or boil tap water for at least 10 minutes, even for brushing your teeth. Avoid ice cubes.

Workplace precautions

In health care settings, follow all infection control procedures, including washing your hands and wearing gloves. In child care settings, wash your hands thoroughly after changing or handling diapers.

Other precautions

Practice good health habits:

- If you have sexual relations with multiple partners, use a latex condom with each sexual contact.

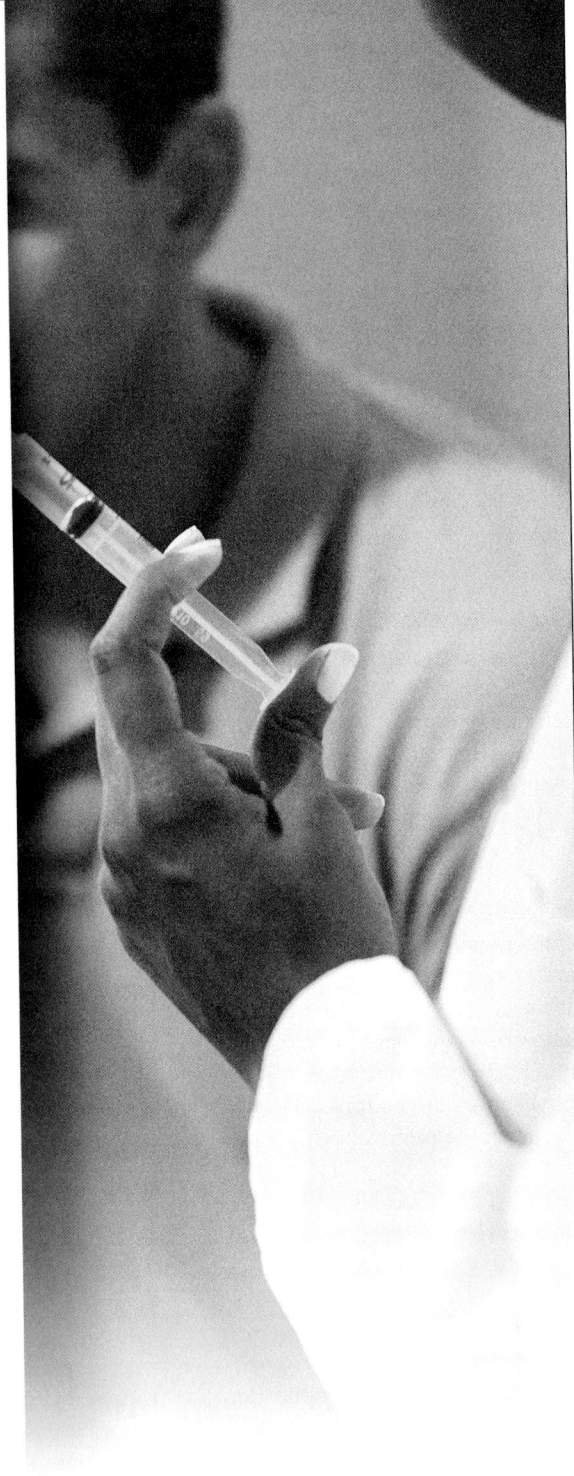

- Don't share drug syringes.
- If you undergo acupuncture, body piercing or tattooing, make sure the needles are sterilized.
- Don't share toothbrushes, razors or other items that may come into contact with blood.

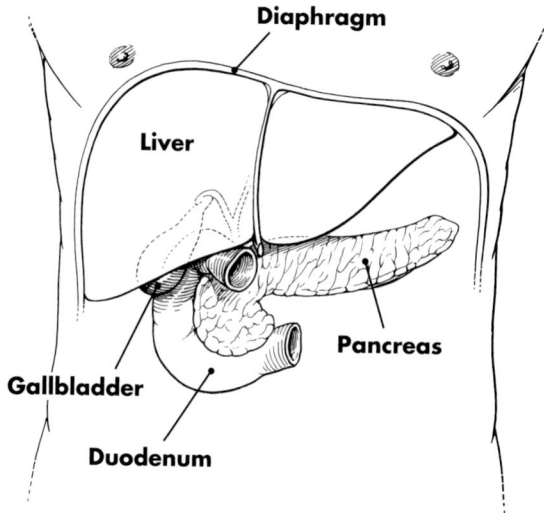

Diaphragm

Liver

Pancreas

Gallbladder

Duodenum

but some develop inflammation of the pancreas (pancreatitis).

Liver Disorders

The liver is the largest single internal organ, and the most complex. Weighing as much as 4 pounds, the liver performs many complicated tasks essential to proper functioning of the entire body. These functions may be grouped into three categories: regulation, metabolism and detoxification.

- **Regulation.** The liver regulates the composition of your blood, in particular the amounts of sugar (glucose), protein and fat that enter the bloodstream. The liver also removes a substance called bilirubin from the blood. Bilirubin comes from the breakdown of red blood cells. Once bilirubin enters the liver, it's chemically changed so that it becomes soluble in water, added to bile and eliminated in the stool.
- **Metabolism.** The liver processes most of the nutrients absorbed from the intestines. In addition to converting many nutrients into forms that can be used by the body, the liver serves as a storage center for other nutrients, such as vitamin A and iron.

It also manufactures cholesterol, blood-clotting substances, specific proteins and bile, a fluid that facilitates the digestion of fat.
- **Detoxification.** The liver detoxifies blood. It removes some drugs and potentially harmful substances from the bloodstream and converts them so that they can be excreted in bile, and subsequently in stool. Because of its complexity and exposure to many potentially harmful substances, the liver is especially vulnerable to injury. However, nature protects the organ in two key ways. First, the liver is capable of regeneration — it can heal itself by repairing or replacing injured tissue. Second, it has many units that are responsible for the same task. Thus, if tissue in one section of the organ is injured, other cells can perform the functions of the injured section.

Hepatitis

Signs and symptoms
- Fatigue
- Loss of appetite
- Nausea and vomiting
- Yellowing of the skin and eyes
- Low-grade fever
- Mild abdominal discomfort

The most common disease to affect the liver is hepatitis, an inflammation of the liver. It can take several forms:

Acute vs. Chronic Hepatitis

Hepatitis signs and symptoms may last for a short period of time and then disappear (acute hepatitis), or they may persist indefinitely (chronic hepatitis).

Acute hepatitis
Acute hepatitis generally causes little or no permanent liver damage. It may develop suddenly or gradually, but it usually subsides in six months or less. As your body's defenses overcome the virus, liver inflammation and associated signs and symptoms gradually subside and disappear. Hepatitis A and E are acute forms. Hepatitis B also is acute, but in a few cases the inflammation can become chronic. Infants born with hepatitis B usually have chronic disease.

Chronic hepatitis
In chronic hepatitis, the liver remains inflamed even though you may have no signs and symptoms. Some people have hepatitis for more than 20 years without realizing it. In others, the inflammation may gradually cause formation of scar tissue in the liver (cirrhosis) and lead to liver failure. People with chronic hepatitis are at increased risk of liver cancer.

Nonalcoholic steatohepatitis is a common cause of chronic hepatitis. Hepatitis C may begin as an acute infection but often becomes chronic.

Chronic hepatitis can take different routes. It may progress very slowly with limited damage, or it may progress rapidly, causing extensive liver damage.

Alcohol- or drug-induced hepatitis

Alcohol- or drug-induced hepatitis is the most common form of this disease, occurring in people who drink excessive alcohol or take certain medications. The inflammation stems from toxic chemicals that your body produces as it breaks down alcohol and drugs. Over time, these chemicals can damage liver cells and interfere with your liver's ability to do its job.

Up to 35 percent of heavy drinkers develop alcoholic hepatitis. Someone with a severe case of alcoholic hepatitis may run a high fever and develop an enlarged, painful liver. Recovery often is slow, even after complete abstinence from alcohol.

Medications that most commonly lead to drug-induced hepatitis include both nonprescription and prescription drugs and herbs and supplements:

- **Over-the-counter pain relievers.** Nonprescription pain relievers such as acetaminophen (Tylenol, others), aspirin, ibuprofen (Advil, Motrin IB, others) and naproxen sodium (Aleve) can damage your liver, especially if taken frequently or combined with alcohol.
- **Prescription medications.** Some medications linked to serious liver injury include the statin drugs used to treat high cholesterol, the combination drug amoxicillin-clavulanate (Augmentin), isoniazid, sulfur antibiotics, nitrofurantoin (Macrobid, Furadantin), phenytoin (Dilantin, Phenytek), azathioprine (Azasan, Imuran), niacin (Niaspan, Niacor), ketoconazole, certain antivirals and anabolic steroids. There are many others.
- **Herbs and supplements.** Some herbs considered dangerous to the liver include aloe vera, black cohosh, cascara, chaparral, comfrey, kava and ephedra.

Hepatitis A

Hepatitis A is caused by a virus most commonly encountered during international travel. This highly infectious disease is transmitted mainly by contaminated food or water. The virus may be present in your stools, blood and bile for two to three weeks before any signs and symptoms develop. The virus disappears once yellowing of the skin and eyes (jaundice) develops or within two to three weeks afterward.

The vast majority of people with hepatitis A recover completely. The liver is often entirely healed within one to two months. In a few cases, especially in older adults, hepatitis A may cause severe signs and symptoms requiring medical therapy and perhaps hospitalization. In rare cases, it can be fatal.

Hepatitis B

Hepatitis B is a more serious form of viral liver infection. Up to 2 million people in the United States have hepatitis B infection. Worldwide, about 240 million people have this form of hepatitis.

Its signs and symptoms are much the same as those of hepatitis A, but this disease can be more severe and last longer. As a result, there's a greater possibility of liver damage. Most individuals with uncomplicated hepatitis B recover within four to five months. In some individuals, the disease progresses from acute to chronic hepatitis. Individuals with chronic hepatitis or cirrhosis from hepatitis B are at increased risk of liver cancer.

Hepatitis B is highly contagious. It's found in blood, semen, vaginal fluid and saliva and can survive for seven days or more outside the body. It's most often transmitted through sexual contact, contaminated syringes and needles, and blood products. People at greatest risk of the disease are users of illicit drugs, those who practice unprotected sexual intercourse, and hospital workers who are exposed to blood and blood products.

Some people (carriers) infected with the hepatitis B virus never experience signs and symptoms but are still capable of passing the virus to others.

Hepatitis C

Hepatitis C is the most common cause of viral hepatitis in the United States, affecting more than 3 million people. The majority of people with acute hepatitis C are without signs and symptoms or have only mild fatigue. Often, an abnormal result on a routine liver test alerts a doctor to the possibility of chronic hepatitis C.

Hepatitis C is spread through blood and blood products and contaminated needles. Users of illicit intravenous (IV) or intranasal drugs who share drug paraphernalia account for a high percentage of new infections. People who received blood transfusions before

---

A Liver Biopsy

In the course of evaluating liver disease, your doctor may perform a liver biopsy. This is a diagnostic procedure that's used in various liver disorders, including cirrhosis, hepatitis and tumors.

For the procedures, you'll be positioned flat on your back and given a local anesthetic to numb the area where the procedure will take place. A thin needle is then inserted between or below your ribs into your liver. Small samples of tissue are taken from the liver for laboratory analysis. A liver biopsy is often done with the help of ultrasound guidance. Infrequently, there's some discomfort following the procedure.

Laboratory tests on the liver tissue may reveal the presence or absence of certain disorders. Liver biopsy can be helpful in evaluating the progress of disease.

1992 also are at increased risk. In 1992 blood banks began screening for the hepatitis C virus. The virus can now be identified with a blood test.

Commonly, hepatitis C may lead to chronic liver diseases such as cirrhosis, liver cancer and liver failure. It ranks close to alcoholism as the main cause of liver disease and is the leading reason for liver transplants in the United States.

Hepatitis D
To get this bloodborne virus, you must already have had hepatitis B. The hepatitis D virus survives and replicates by attaching itself to the hepatitis B virus. Hepatitis D isn't common in the United States, except among users of illicit drugs.

Hepatitis E
A foodborne virus similar to that of hepatitis A, the hepatitis E virus is prevalent in Asia and South America. Most cases of hepatitis E reported in the United States are in travelers to parts of the world where the virus is common. Pregnant women with hepatitis E are at increased risk of serious complications.

Autoimmune hepatitis
Autoimmune hepatitis is believed to result from an agent that triggers the immune system to attack liver cells. The disease is more common among women than among men and typically occurs between ages 15 and 40.

Nonalcoholic steatohepatitis
With nonalcoholic steatohepatitis (NASH), your liver contains excessive fatty deposits, similar to alcohol-induced hepatitis. But the condition isn't associated with alcohol abuse.

NASH most often occurs in people who are obese, or who have diabetes or high cholesterol levels. It can also occur in people who take steroids or are malnourished. NASH is a common cause of abnormal liver test results and is a common cause of chronic hepatitis.

Diagnosis
To determine the type of hepatitis you may have, your doctor will likely ask you a number of questions about medications you're taking, about your sex life, whether you've traveled outside the United States, whether you had any blood transfusions before 1992, whether you used illicit drugs.

A physical examination may reveal an enlarged, shrunken or hardened liver. Blood tests and imaging tests can help identify liver disease, including hepatitis.

To confirm the diagnosis, your doctor may remove and examine a sample of liver tissue (biopsy). A biopsy specimen also helps your doctor to identify the specific type of hepatitis you have and determine the severity of the inflammation and the extent of any permanent liver damage.

How serious is hepatitis?
Nearly all people who are healthy before contracting hepatitis A recover from the illness, and it doesn't become chronic. Approximately 95 percent of individuals with acute hepatitis B recover completely. Hepatitis C and nonalcoholic steatohepatitis often give rise to chronic hepatitis.

In alcohol- or drug-induced hepatitis, if the individual stops drinking early enough or avoids the medications causing the condition, the liver can heal itself. But, recovery is often long and requires complete abstinence from alcohol.

Treatment
Treatment depends on the type of hepatitis you have. If you have hepatitis A, you probably won't need medications. However, you may need to abstain from alcohol use, at least during your recovery. Alcohol and some drugs can cause more injury to the already damaged liver.

Hospitalization may be required if you're pregnant, an older adult, dehydrated or experiencing other health problems. In the rare

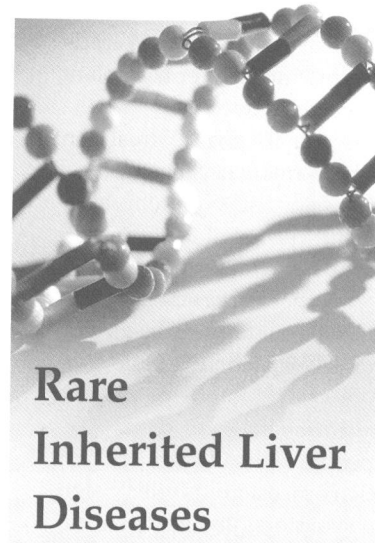

Rare Inherited Liver Diseases

Two uncommon inherited liver disorders are:

Wilson's disease
Wilson's disease is an inherited disorder in which copper accumulates in various organs of the body, especially the brain, eyes, kidney and liver. It may be characterized by tremors, a copper ring near the cornea of the eye, and signs and symptoms of acute or chronic hepatitis. If untreated, cirrhosis and neurological problems may result.

Treatment involves removing the deposits of copper with use of medication. This treatment usually is continued for life. If you have Wilson's disease, your blood relatives should be screened for evidence of the disease. Liver transplantation may be necessary in severe acute disease.

Alpha-1-antitrypsin deficiency
Alpha-1-antitrypsin deficiency results from a genetic defect that causes your body to produce abnormal forms of alpha-1-antitrypsin, an enzyme inhibitor. The deficiency may lead to liver and lung disease. A liver transplant is the only treatment that can halt the liver damage.

situation when hepatitis A leads to liver failure, a liver transplant may be necessary.

The primary goals of treatment of other forms of hepatitis are to relieve signs and symptoms and prevent scarring of the liver (cirrhosis). For viral forms of hepatitis, another important goal is to reduce the amount of the virus (viral levels) in body fluids.

Medication

In people with autoimmune hepatitis, corticosteroids relieve signs and symptoms about 80 percent of the time. Steroids reduce liver inflammation by suppressing the immune system. The most commonly prescribed medication is prednisone. Because of the side effects associated with corticosteroids, your doctor may gradually reduce the dosage to the lowest possible amount needed. Corticosteroids aren't prescribed for viral forms of hepatitis because suppressing your immune system may allow the virus to multiply more rapidly.

Hepatitis B and C may be treated with the following:

- **Antiviral medications.** Several antiviral medications — including lamivudine (Epivir), adefovir (Hepsera), telbivudine (Tyzeka) and entecavir (Baraclude) — can help fight the virus and slow its ability to damage your liver. Talk to your doctor about which medication might be right for you.
- **Interferon alfa-2b (Intron A).** This synthetic version of a substance produced by the body to fight infection is used mainly for young people with hepatitis B who don't want to undergo long-term treatment or who might want to get pregnant within a few years. It's given by injection.

Researchers are making significant advances in treatment for hepatitis C using new "direct-acting" antiviral medications, sometimes in combination with existing ones. As a result, people experience better outcomes, fewer side effects and shorter treatment times — some as short as eight weeks. The choice of medications and length of treatment depend on the hepatitis C genotype, presence of existing liver damage, other medical conditions and prior treatments.

Liver transplantation

When liver damage is extensive and medications are no longer helpful, your doctor may discuss the possibility of a liver transplant (see page 883). Hepatitis C is the most common indication for liver transplantation in the United States. If you have hepatitis C or B, the hepatitis virus might recur in the transplanted liver. Immunoglobulin injections and medication may reduce this risk.

Hemochromatosis

Signs and symptoms

- Fatigue
- Joint pain
- Impotence or loss of sex drive
- Increased skin pigmentation (bronzing)
- Diabetes
- Hypothyroidism

Hemochromatosis is due to a genetic abnormality that causes your intestines to absorb too much iron from the food you eat, leading to iron overload. The extra iron enters the bloodstream and builds up in certain organs, primarily the liver, heart and pancreas. In rare cases, iron overload results from repeated blood transfusions or overconsumption of dietary iron.

The most common cause of the disease is a flawed gene discovered in 1996, called the HFE gene that leads your intestines to absorb excessive amounts of iron. It's estimated that approximately 1 in 10 Americans, most commonly those of Northern European descent, carries a flawed HFE gene. People with just one copy of the abnormal gene generally don't experience problems. Hemochromatosis tends to develop among people with two abnormal copies, usually inheriting an abnormal gene from each parent.

Diagnosis

Doctors can detect iron overload with two blood tests:

- **Serum transferrin saturation.** This test measures the amount of iron bound to a protein (transferrin) that carries iron in your blood. Transferrin saturation values greater than 45 percent are considered too high.
- **Serum ferritin.** This test measures the amount of iron stored in your body. If the results of your serum transferrin saturation test are higher than normal, your doctor will check your serum ferritin. Because a number of infectious and inflammatory conditions other than hereditary hemochromatosis can cause elevated ferritin, both tests are needed to diagnose the disorder. You may need the tests repeated for the most accurate results.

To confirm a diagnosis of hereditary hemochromatosis, your doctor may recommend genetic testing or a liver biopsy.

How serious is hemochromatosis?

Left untreated, hemochromatosis can lead to organ damage, including cirrhosis and congestive heart failure. It can also increase your risk of liver cancer and diabetes. The good news is that hemochromatosis is easily treated. If discovered early, permanent damage can usually be prevented.

Treatment

Doctors can treat hemochromatosis safely and effectively by removing blood from your body (phlebotomy) on a regular basis, just as if you were donating blood. But in this case, the goal is to reduce your iron levels to normal. The amount of blood drawn depends on your age, your overall health and the severity of iron overload. Some people need many phlebotomies to achieve normal iron levels.

- **Initial treatment schedule.** Initially, you may have a pint of blood taken once or twice a week. This process shouldn't be too uncomfortable. While you recline in a chair, a needle is inserted into a vein in your arm. The blood flows from the needle into a tube that's attached to a blood bag. Depending on the condition of your veins and the consistency of your blood, the time needed to remove a pint of blood can range from 10 to 30 minutes.
- **Maintenance treatment schedule.** Once your iron levels have returned to normal, you may need to have blood drawn only four to six times a year.

Cirrhosis

Signs and symptoms
- Fatigue
- Bleeding easily
- Easy bruising
- Accumulation of fluid in the abdomen and legs and feet
- Loss of appetite and nausea
- Weight loss

Cirrhosis is the term used to describe scarring of the liver. It occurs in response to chronic liver damage. With mild cirrhosis, your liver can make repairs and continue its functions. With more advanced cirrhosis, more and more scar tissue forms in the liver, making it impossible for the organ to function.

Causes
A wide variety of diseases and conditions can damage the liver and lead to cirrhosis, including:
- Chronic alcohol abuse
- Hepatitis B
- Hepatitis C
- Cystic fibrosis
- Destruction of the bile ducts (primary biliary cholangitis)
- Fat that accumulates in the liver (nonalcoholic fatty liver disease)
- Hardening and scarring of the bile ducts (primary sclerosing cholangitis)
- Inability to process sugars in milk (galactosemia)
- Iron buildup in the body (hemochromatosis)
- Liver disease caused by your body's immune system (autoimmune hepatitis)
- Poorly formed bile ducts in babies (biliary atresia)
- Too much copper accumulated in the liver (Wilson's disease)

Diagnosis
By examining your abdomen, your doctor may be able to determine if your liver is enlarged and firm, a sign that you may have liver disease. As cirrhosis progresses, however, your liver may shrink. When that happens, blood flow may be impaired, resulting in an enlarged spleen. Abnormal blood test results may be the first sign of liver injury.

To determine the extent of your disease, your doctor may want to evaluate your liver with ultrasound, computerized tomography (CT) or magnetic resonance imaging (MRI). A sample of liver tissue (biopsy) for microscopic examination can reveal the extent and possibly the cause of the liver damage. Most cases can be diagnosed without the need for a liver biopsy. Your doctor may also recommend blood tests, such as a complete blood count, bilirubin test and specific tests to help determine the cause of cirrhosis.

How serious is cirrhosis?
There's no cure for cirrhosis, as it causes irreversible liver damage. The good news is that it often progresses slowly. In the United States, cirrhosis results in about 38,000 deaths annually. People with cirrhosis have an increased risk of a certain type of liver cancer (hepatocellular cancer).

Cirrhosis may lead to several serious complications:
- **More-frequent infections.** If you have cirrhosis, your body

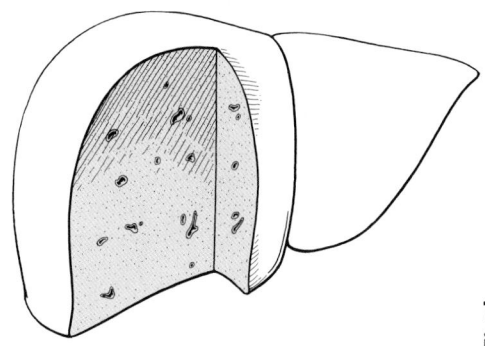

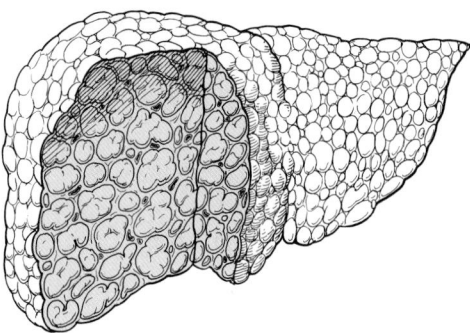

These cross-sectional illustrations show a normal liver (top) with no sign of scarring, and a cirrhotic liver (bottom) with extensive scarring.

may have difficulty fighting infections.

- **Malnutrition.** Cirrhosis may make it more difficult for your body to process nutrients. This can lead to weakness and weight loss.
- **High levels of toxins in the blood (hepatic encephalopathy).** A liver damaged by cirrhosis isn't able to clear toxins from the blood as well as a healthy liver can. Toxins in the blood can cause confusion and difficulty concentrating. With time, hepatic encephalopathy can progress to unresponsiveness or coma.
- **Increasing pressure in the main vein bringing blood to the liver (portal hypertension).** Scar tissue can make it difficult for blood to flow freely through the liver. This causes increased pressure in the portal vein, which causes blood to be redirected to smaller veins near the liver. Those smaller veins may become overwhelmed by the pressure and can burst, causing serious bleeding. Building pressure in the veins of your esophagus is called esophageal varices. In the stomach this is called gastric varices.
- **Increased risk of liver cancer.** Cirrhosis can increase your risk of liver cancer. For this reason, your doctor may recommend regular ultrasound examinations to look for abnormalities.

Treatment

The main focus of medical care often is treating and preventing complications. Self-care measures and medication can help decrease further damage to the liver. If liver failure occurs, liver transplantation may be an option.

Self-care

The damage caused by cirrhosis is irreversible, but you can take steps to reduce further liver damage:

- **Stop using alcohol.** Some of the chemicals contained in alcohol are toxic to your liver.
- **Limit medications.** Your damaged liver is unable to detoxify and eliminate medications normally from your system. Discuss all medications that you take, including nonprescription ones, with your doctor. Don't combine pain relievers with alcohol, as this can be especially damaging to your liver.
- **Take measures to prevent yourself from getting sick.** When your liver is damaged, you're unable to fight off infections as well as healthy people can. Avoid sick people and get vaccinated for hepatitis A and B, flu (influenza) and pneumococcal pneumonia.
- **Eat plenty of fresh fruits, vegetables and whole grains.** They're high in nutrients, including vitamins A, C and E. Cirrhosis tends to deplete these important vitamins. Your doctor may prescribe supplemental vitamins K, A and D, which may be depleted in your body as well.
- **Monitor dietary protein.** Many individuals with cirrhosis are malnourished. Daily protein is important, but you don't want

Liver Cysts and Noncancerous Tumors

Liver cysts are common and usually are detected in the course of examining the liver by computerized tomography (CT) or ultrasonography for another condition. Liver cysts don't become cancerous (malignant) and rarely cause signs and symptoms. Treatment is unnecessary except in the rare instances when they cause significant abdominal discomfort.

Some liver tumors are noncancerous (benign). The most common is hemangioma. Often, hemangiomas are discovered incidentally during study of the liver for another reason. Benign liver tumors often don't cause signs and symptoms or require treatment. Hepatic adenoma, another benign tumor, can occur in women who have taken oral contraceptives for a long time. When the birth control pill is discontinued, the tumors may become smaller. Hepatic adenomas may cause pain or rupture and require surgical removal.

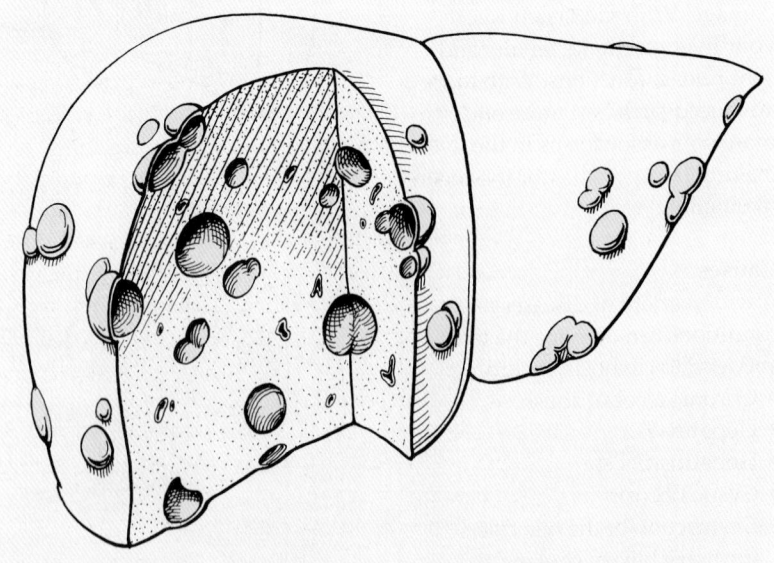

Cysts commonly occur in the liver. Most often they're harmless.

too much. A dietitian can help you consume the right amount.
- **Restrict salt.** Reducing salt can help reduce fluid buildup.

Medication

To help prevent esophageal and gastric varices from rupturing and bleeding, your doctor may recommend a medication to lower the pressure within the varices. Other options include a procedure to prevent blood from flowing into them or a procedure to destroy them.

Diuretics help reduce accumulation of excess abdominal fluid. To reduce fluid retention, you also may need to avoid salt. Sometimes, abdominal fluid may become infected, causing pain and fever. If this occurs, your doctor may insert a long, thin tube (catheter) into your abdomen to remove a fluid sample so that the infecting organism can be identified (cultured) and the proper antibiotic prescribed.

Cholestyramine and rifampin (Rifadin, Rimactane) are often prescribed to reduce itching caused by metabolites in the blood.

The medication lactulose can help lower blood ammonia levels. Your doctor may also recommend an antibiotic to reduce the level of bacteria in your intestines that produce ammonia.

Liver transplantation

A liver transplant is generally considered when the disease has advanced to the point where the liver can no longer adequately function. The success rate of liver transplantation continues to improve, approximately 90 percent of people who receive transplants are still alive a year later. The problem is, when cirrhosis is related to viral hepatitis, there's a chance the disease will recur in the new liver. For more information on transplantation, see page 883.

Liver cancer

Signs and symptoms
- Loss of appetite and weight

- Abdominal pain, especially in the upper right part of the abdomen
- General fatigue and weakness
- Nausea and vomiting
- Abdominal swelling
- An enlarged liver
- A yellow discoloration of the skin and eyes (jaundice)

Primary liver cancer begins in the cells of the liver itself, as opposed to secondary liver cancer in which the cancer starts elsewhere in the body and spreads (metastasizes) to the liver. The liver is especially vulnerable to invasion by cancerous cells and, with the exception of the lymph nodes, is the most common site of cancer metastasis. Cancers that commonly spread to the liver include colon, lung and breast.

In the United States, approximately 41,000 new cases of primary liver cancer occur each year. While many cancers are declining in the United States, new cases of primary liver cancer are increasing. Primary liver cancer is about twice as common in men as it is in women.

Primary liver cancer is divided into several types based on the type of cells that become cancerous. Types include hepatocellular carcinoma (HCC), cholangiocarcinoma, hepatoblastoma, and angiosarcoma or hemangiosarcoma. Factors that increase risk of primary liver cancer include chronic liver disease, such as cirrhosis; hepatitis B or C infection; hemochromatosis; long-term use of anabolic steroids; exposure to certain toxins, such as aflatoxin and vinyl chloride; and excessive alcohol consumption.

Diagnosis

A thorough physical examination and blood tests are generally the first steps in diagnosing liver cancer. Additional tests may include images of the liver by a computerized tomography (CT) scan, ultrasound examination or magnetic resonance imaging (MRI). All of these imaging tests can detect masses within the liver.

A liver biopsy, in which a sample of liver tissue is removed for laboratory analysis, can provide even more information. If a liver biopsy doesn't provide a definitive diagnosis, an abdominal operation may be necessary.

How serious is liver cancer?

Both primary and secondary liver cancer often are fatal, especially secondary liver cancer, which is a sign that the primary cancer has already spread (metastasized). Early detection poses the best chances for successful treatment.

Treatment

Treatments for primary liver cancer may include one or more of the following therapies:
- **Surgery.** The best treatment for localized resectable cancer is usually an operation known as surgical resection. In some cases, the area of the liver where the cancer is found can be completely removed. You aren't a candidate for surgical removal of liver tumors if you have cirrhosis or only a small amount of healthy liver tissue. Even when resections are successful, there is a chance the cancer can recur elsewhere in the liver or in other areas within a few years.
- **Alcohol injection.** In this procedure, pure alcohol is injected directly into tumors, either through the skin or during an operation. Alcohol dries out the cells of the tumor and eventually the cells die. Each treatment consists of one injection, although you may need a series of injections for the best results. Alcohol injection has been shown to improve survival in people with small hepatocellular tumors. It may also be used to help reduce symptoms in cases of metastatic liver cancer. The most common side effect is leaking of alcohol onto the liver or into the abdominal cavity.
- **Radiofrequency ablation.** In this procedure, electric current

in the radiofrequency range is used to destroy malignant cells. Using an ultrasound or CT scan as a guide, several thin needles are inserted into small incisions in your abdomen. When the needles reach the tumor, they're heated with an electric current, destroying the malignant cells. Radiofrequency ablation may be an option for people with small, unresectable hepatocellular tumors and for some types of metastatic liver cancers.

- **Chemoembolization.** Chemoembolization is a type of chemotherapy treatment that supplies strong anti-cancer drugs directly to the liver. Chemoembolization isn't curative, but it can shrink tumors in a certain percentage of people, which may provide symptom relief and improve survival. During the procedure, the hepatic artery — the artery from which liver cancers derive their blood supply — is blocked, and chemotherapy drugs are injected between the blockage and the liver. The idea is that by targeting the tumor directly, doctors can use potent doses of drugs without creating as many side effects as occur with systemic chemotherapy. But the fact is that chemoembolization causes many of the same side effects as other forms of chemotherapy, including abdominal pain, nausea and vomiting.

- **Cryoablation (cryosurgery or cryotherapy).** This treatment uses extreme cold to destroy cancer cells. Cryoablation may be an option for people with inoperable primary and metastatic liver cancers. It may also be used in addition to surgery, chemotherapy or other standard treatments. During the procedure, your doctor places an instrument (cryoprobe) containing liquid nitrogen directly onto liver tumors. Ultrasound images are used to guide the cryoprobe and monitor the freezing of the cells. Side effects include

damage to the bile ducts and major blood vessels, leading to bleeding or infection.

- **Radiation therapy.** This treatment uses high-powered energy beams to destroy cancer cells and shrink tumors. Radiation may come from a machine outside your body or from radiation-containing materials inserted into your liver. Radiation may be used on its own to treat localized unresectable cancer. Or you may have radiation therapy after surgical removal of a tumor to help destroy any remaining malignant cells. Radiation side effects may include fatigue, nausea and vomiting.

- **Chemotherapy.** This treatment uses powerful drugs to kill cancer cells. The medications may be given intravenously or injected. Chemotherapy is generally not effective in treating liver cancer, but may be a treatment option in certain cases.

- **Liver transplantation.** In this procedure, a diseased liver is removed and replaced with a healthy, donated organ. Liver transplantation may be an option for some people with small, early-stage liver tumors and for certain people with bile duct tumors. In other cases, especially when tumors are larger or blood vessels are involved, a transplant may not improve long-term outlook because the cancer may recur outside the new liver.

- **Sorafenib (Nexavar).** Sorafenib was approved by the Food and Drug Administration for use in advanced inoperable liver cancer. Sorafenib is a targeted therapy designed to interfere with a tumor's ability to generate new blood vessels. Sorafenib has been shown to slow or stop advanced liver cancer from progressing for a few months longer than with no treatment. More studies are needed to better understand how targeted therapies may be used to control advanced liver cancer.

Liver abscesses

Signs and symptoms
- Persistent fever
- Chills
- Nausea and vomiting
- Weakness
- Weight loss
- A tender liver

Abscesses — fluid- or pus-filled cavities — sometimes form within the liver as a result of infection by a bacterium or parasite. Those of bacterial origin generally have a more rapid course with fever and chills. An abscess from a parasite tends to develop more slowly.

Diagnosis
Liver abscesses can generally be identified with a computerized tomography (CT) scan or ultrasound examination of your liver. From the image produced, a doctor often can determine the size, location and number of abscesses. Blood tests also may be helpful, particularly if your doctor suspects the abscess may be caused by a parasite.

Fluid from the abscess can often be obtained for examination by insertion of a needle into the abscess, using ultrasound or a CT scan for guidance. However, if your doctor suspects that the abscess is caused by a parasite such as amoeba, other testing is preferred to avoid spreading the infection.

How serious are liver abscesses?
A liver abscess, particularly one caused by bacteria, is potentially fatal and requires immediate treatment.

Treatment
If the abscess is the result of a bacterial infection, your doctor may advise drainage of the abscess with a tube (catheter) and intravenous (IV) antibiotics to kill the infection. Antibiotics may be required for several weeks. Sometimes, surgical drainage of the abscess or even removal of the

portion of the liver containing the abscess is required.

If the cause is a parasite, your doctor may advise treatment with medications aimed at eliminating the parasite.

Genetic liver disorders

Some inherited liver abnormalities cause increased concentrations of bilirubin in the blood (hyperbilirubinemia) and produce yellowing of the eyes and skin (jaundice).

Gilbert's syndrome

Gilbert's syndrome is an inherited disorder in which bilirubin isn't processed normally in the liver for excretion in stool. Bilirubin has to chemically combine (conjugate) with another substance in the liver in order to make it water-soluble and capable of being excreted through the bile.

In Gilbert's syndrome, bilirubin is usually left unconjugated because of an enzyme deficiency or liver function defect. Gilbert's syndrome may be the most common cause of hyperbilirubinemia.

Signs and symptoms generally are mild. In some cases, the disorder is detected only during a routine blood test. Gilbert's syndrome doesn't lead to liver damage, and no treatment is necessary.

Crigler-Najjar syndrome

This rare disorder causes two types of hyperbilirubinemia: type 1 and type 2. Type 1, the more severe form, is due to an absence of an enzyme needed to conjugate bilirubin. Type 2 involves only a partial enzyme deficiency and is less severe.

Crigler-Najjar syndrome is caused by a different genetic mutation than is Gilbert's syndrome and is generally much more severe.

The mainstay of treatment for Crigler-Najjar syndrome type 1 is phototherapy. Your bare skin is exposed to intense light, while your eyes are shielded. This helps to change the bilirubin molecules

in the skin, so that they can be excreted in bile without conjugation. Plasmapheresis may be used on occasion. It involves removing blood plasma from your body by withdrawing blood, separating it into plasma and cells, and transfusing new or treated plasma back into your bloodstream. Liver transplantation is the only definitive treatment for individuals with Crigler-Najjar syndrome type 1. Type 2 hyperbilirubinemia can be treated successfully with medication.

Dubin-Johnson syndrome

Some genetic disorders cause elevated concentrations of predominately conjugated (chemically combined, water-soluble) bilirubin. One such inherited disorder is Dubin-Johnson syndrome, also known as chronic idiopathic jaundice. People with this disorder often will have either no signs and symptoms or vague gastrointestinal symptoms. In some cases, the liver is enlarged and pigmented. This disorder generally requires no treatment.

Benign recurrent cholestasis

This rare disorder usually becomes apparent in childhood. Sometimes called Summerskill syndrome, it's characterized by recurrent episodes of jaundice and itching that last for days or months. There's no treatment, but episodes usually resolve spontaneously and don't cause lasting liver damage.

Liver transplantation

In the past two decades, liver transplantation has emerged as the best option for many people with life-threatening complications or debilitating signs and symptoms of severe liver disease. The survival rate for people who receive a liver transplant is steadily improving. Based on today's national averages, about 90 percent of people who receive a liver transplant are alive a year later, and about 75

percent are alive five years after the procedure.

Advances in the preservation of donor organs have improved survival rates, as have refinements in surgical techniques, anti-rejection medications and postoperative care. This success has led to a wider application of this procedure. For example, in the past, liver transplantation wasn't an option for people with cancer. Now, transplantation is sometimes considered for individuals with a certain type of liver cancer (hepatocellular carcinoma) and for individuals with some neuroendocrine cancers — tumors that originate in the complex body system where nervous and endocrine systems interact — that have spread to the liver.

Methods of transplantation

The main factor that limits use of liver transplantation is a shortage of donor organs. The waiting time has increased from about a month to more than a year. In the meantime, many people become increasingly ill, and some die while waiting for a donor liver.

Thus, alternatives to traditional liver transplantation are being pursued. In one procedure, about 60 percent of a healthy liver is removed from a living donor, generally a relative. In the person with liver disease, the failing liver is removed and replaced with portions of healthy liver. Because liver tissue normally regenerates, within a few weeks to a few months the liver usually returns to normal size in both the donor and the recipient.

Living-donor liver transplantation achieved initial success in children in the early 1990s. Today, many pediatric transplantations are done using living donors. Studies of adult-to-adult living-donor liver transplantations have been positive, and this method is now becoming acceptable therapy. Adults require more liver mass than children do, but even so, the graft regenerates rapidly in the recipient, as does the remaining portion left in the donor.

The risks to recipients of living-donor liver transplantation are similar to those of traditional transplantation, such as bleeding, poor function of the transplanted liver, infection and rejection of the new organ.

Risk to the donors is generally minimal. Immediately after removal of a portion of their liver, donors may experience temporary jaundice, and it may take longer for blood to clot. Bile leakage also is a risk. But the liver usually returns to full size in two to four weeks.

As with all major surgeries, there is a very small risk of fatality for both the recipient and donor.

Medication

You'll take a number of medications after your liver transplant, many for the rest of your life. Drugs called immunosuppressants help keep your immune system from attacking your new liver. They include medications such as prednisone, cyclosporine (Neoral, Sandimmune, Gengraf), tacrolimus (Astagraf XL, Prograf), azathioprine (Azasan, Imuran) and 6-mercaptopurine.

Other drugs help reduce the risk of other complications after your transplant.

Who's a candidate?

Adults under age 65 and children are the best candidates. Individuals selected for transplantation generally have liver disease that's progressive and incurable by other medical or surgical means and they don't have other life-threatening illnesses.

The procedure

Liver transplantation is a complex procedure. It can take three to five hours and is performed mainly in large medical centers where experienced personnel and extensive facilities can yield the best results.

Recovery

Rehabilitation may take up to four months. Lifelong therapy with immunosuppressant drugs to prevent organ rejection is necessary. Use of these drugs also requires lifelong monitoring for complications. ■

Kidneys and Urinary Tract

The kidneys are part of the urinary tract, a complex system whose primary function is to remove excess fluid and waste material from blood. In addition, the kidneys function as endocrine glands — releasing hormones important to the production of red blood cells, regulation of blood pressure and formation of bone.

In addition to the kidneys, the urinary system includes two ureters, two major renal arteries and renal veins, a bladder, and a urethra. The kidneys, a pair of bean-shaped organs, are located against the back of the abdominal wall, one on each side of the spine at the level of the lowest ribs.

The ureters are muscular tubes that propel urine from each kidney to the bladder. The bladder is a muscular bag that stores urine. The urethra is the narrow tube through which urine leaves the bladder during urination.

The kidneys vary their activities from day to day in response to changes in the kinds and amounts of food and fluids you consume. For example, suppose that one day you drink large amounts of water and juice and the next day you drink almost nothing. Your kidneys adapt accordingly, allowing your tissues to be neither flooded nor depleted. They do this by carefully controlling the amount of fluid and salts excreted in your urine. Although other organs, such as the skin, lungs and intestines, also remove fluid, the kidneys are by far the most important organ for fluid excretion.

Blood enters each kidney from its renal artery, a major branch of the aorta, which is the body's main artery. Although the kidneys account for less than 1 percent of the body's weight, 20 percent of the blood pumped from the heart passes through them.

Within the kidneys, blood passes through filtering systems called nephrons. These are the main functioning units of the kidneys. Each kidney contains more than 1 million nephrons, each consisting of a cluster of small blood vessels (glomerulus) and attached small tubes (renal tubules).

As blood passes through the glomeruli, blood cells, proteins, large particles and some water remain in the bloodstream. Everything else, including a large percentage of the water, filters out and passes into the tubules.

Waste products, such as urea, creatinine and uric acid, along with excess salts and water, remain within the tubules. Cells that make up the walls of the tubules absorb and return salt, water, and other substances to the bloodstream in precisely the right amounts needed by the body. Thus, the composition of urine is determined by both the need to get rid of unwanted substances and the need to retain others.

Urine that emerges from the lower end of each tubule enters the renal pelvis, then the ureter and then the bladder, where it's stored. When the nerves of the bladder signal a feeling of fullness, urine is voided through the urethra, usually voluntarily. On average, about $1\frac{1}{2}$ quarts of urine are excreted every day. This is only a small fraction of the fluid initially filtered through the glomeruli into the tubules.

Blood that leaves the kidneys contains salts, protein, sugar, calcium and other substances vital to maintaining normal body function. This blood travels through the renal veins and back to the heart to recirculate throughout the body.

The Kidneys and Urinary Tract

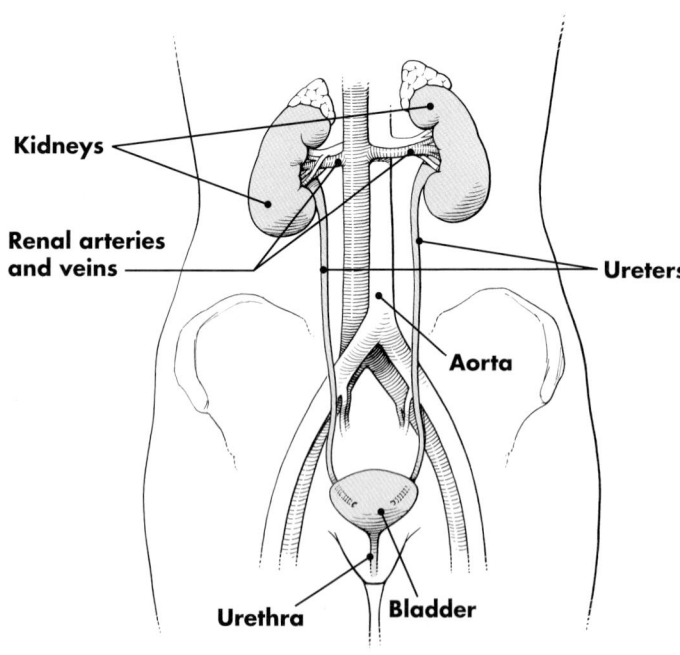

Kidneys

Renal arteries and veins

Ureters

Aorta

Urethra

Bladder

Cross Section of a Kidney

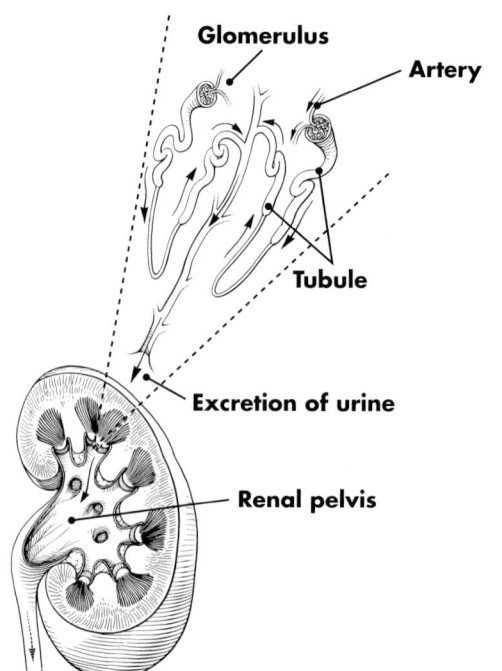

Glomerulus

Artery

Tubule

Excretion of urine

Renal pelvis

Most of the time this complex process is performed flawlessly. Sometimes, however, problems impair the kidneys' ability to filter or reclaim fluid and chemicals. For example, if the tubules are defective, valuable substances that should be returned to the bloodstream may be excreted in urine. Or glomeruli may leak enough protein into the urine to cause a disorder called nephrotic syndrome.

Diabetes, trauma, high blood pressure, toxins, kidney stones, tumors, some drugs and even infections in other parts of the body can cause kidney damage. Unfortunately, many kidney diseases cause no notable symptoms until substantial and even irreparable damage has occurred.

Congenital Kidney Disorders

Some infants are born with an abnormal kidney that doesn't function properly, or even with only one kidney. Fortunately, human beings can lead normal lives with just one functioning kidney. Many of the following anatomical abnormalities cause no symptoms and may go undetected, at least initially. They're typically diagnosed when tests are done for other purposes.

Medullary sponge kidney

Signs and symptoms
- Pain in the side
- Burning pain during urination
- Blood in the urine
- Kidney infection or stones

Medullary sponge kidney results from an abnormal widening of the ducts (papillary ducts) that drain into the urine-collecting portion of the kidney (renal pelvis). Often this condition produces no signs or symptoms in the people who have it. If it does, the signs or symptoms typically occur in adolescence or early adulthood. Often, the condition can be diagnosed with a kidney X-ray.

Treatment
Treatment involves relieving symptoms, if some are present. If you aren't experiencing symptoms, your doctor will likely recommend that you drink adequate quantities of water. This reduces the chance of kidney infection and the chance of kidney stone formation. If kidney stones are present, treatment also may involve correcting urine abnormalities contributing to stone formation.

Vesicoureteral reflux

Signs and symptoms
- Recurrent urinary tract infections
- A scarred or small kidney on a kidney X-ray
- Excess protein in the urine
- High blood pressure

Vesicoureteral reflux is the abnormal flow of urine from the bladder back into the ureters. It's the single most common urinary tract problem in children. It often results from anatomical abnormalities of the valve that normally prevents the backflow of urine from the bladder.

Diagnosis
A doctor may suspect vesicoureteral reflux if a child has recurrent urinary tract infections. The definitive test for this problem is voiding cystourethrography. It shows if fluid stays in the bladder or flows back up (refluxes) to the kidney.

If your child has reflux, additional tests may be performed to determine if the kidneys have been scarred or sustained other damage.

How serious is vesicoureteral reflux?
The reflux can be mild, moderate or severe. If your child has mild reflux, there's a good chance the problem will disappear as he or she grows. Moderate or severe reflux is less likely to disappear with time.

Kidney damage is a real danger with this condition, particularly in infants and children younger than age 5. Reflux can be harmful to the kidneys because it creates abnormal pressure and, most important, it may cause bacteria from the bladder to back up into the kidneys. The kidneys can become infected and, ultimately, damaged.

Reflux is one of the most common causes of severe high blood pressure and end-stage kidney (renal) failure in children and young adults.

Treatment
Treatment for the condition depends on its severity.

Medication
Initially — particularly if the reflux is mild to moderate — low doses of antibiotics may be prescribed long term to keep the urine free of bacteria, thus preventing the refluxed urine from infecting the kidneys. Urine samples may be taken at regular intervals to ensure no bacteria are present.

Surgery
An operation to correct vesicoureteral reflux may be considered if:
- A child has severe reflux
- A child has moderate reflux that over time shows no sign of resolving
- Urinary infections occur despite continuous antibiotic treatment
- Other urinary abnormalities make continued reflux likely

Urinary tract infections continue to occur in a small number of cases despite an apparently successful operation. Children who undergo this operation often receive antibiotics for several months after the operation.

Other anatomical abnormalities

Additional kidney abnormalities that may be present at birth include:

Solitary kidney

Solitary kidney is a condition in which one kidney is missing at birth. The lone kidney performs the work of two. Usually this disorder doesn't pose any problems.

Horseshoe kidney

Horseshoe kidney is a condition in which the lower ends of the two kidneys are connected, forming a horseshoe appearance. Horseshoe kidney often goes undetected until diagnostic tests are performed for another condition or because of signs and symptoms.

Blood in urine, kidney stones, urinary obstruction and increased susceptibility to infection are complications of horseshoe kidney. These signs and symptoms can be treated if they occur. The condition itself rarely leads to kidney (renal) failure.

Kidney duplication

Kidney duplication is a condition in which the urine-collecting portion of the kidney (renal pelvis) is divided into separate compartments, each with its own ureter. This may occur in one or both kidneys, and may be partial or complete.

People with this condition may not have any signs or symptoms, but the disorder carries with it an increased risk of infection and urinary obstruction.

Congenital ureteropelvic junction obstruction

Congenital ureteropelvic junction obstruction is a disorder that involves an obstruction in the area where the ureter leaves the kidney. Typically, this occurs on one side.

Abdominal pain or infection may lead to the diagnosis. The obstruction is sometimes detected after the passage of bloody urine, often after a blow to the kidney area. Sometimes, this disorder is detected in a fetus during a prenatal ultrasound.

Pressure from obstructed drainage can lead to scarring of the kidney and cause loss of function

Kidney and Bladder Tests

The following tests may be used to detect a kidney or bladder condition:

Renal ultrasound

Renal ultrasound uses sound waves to make images of the kidneys, ureters and bladder. During the examination, an ultrasound machine sends sound waves into the kidney area and images are recorded on a computer. The black-and-white images show the internal structure of the kidneys and related organs.

Computerized tomography (CT) urogram

This imaging exam is used to evaluate your urinary tract, including the kidneys, the bladder and the tubes (ureters) that carry urine from your kidneys to your bladder. A CT urogram uses X-rays to generate multiple images of a slice of the area in your body that's being studied, including bones, soft tissues and blood vessels. The images are sent to a computer and reconstructed into detailed 2-D images.

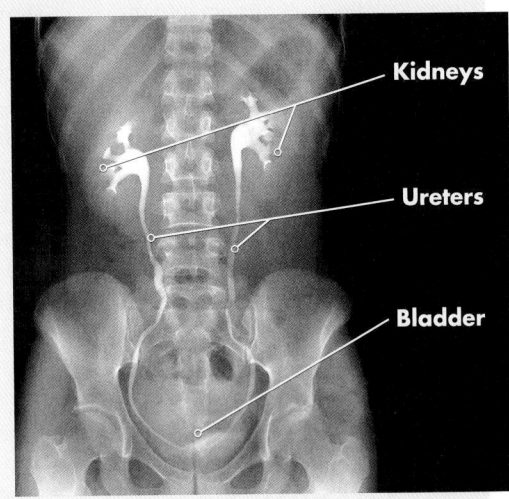

During a CT urogram, an X-ray dye (iodine contrast solution) is injected into a vein in your hand or arm. The dye flows into your kidneys, ureters and bladder, outlining each of these structures. X-ray pictures are taken at specific times during the exam, so your doctor can see your urinary tract and assess how well it's working or look for any abnormalities.

Intravenous pyelography

Intravenous pyelography (IVP, or excretory urography) is an X-ray examination that provides detailed pictures of the kidneys and lower urinary tract. The examination begins with the injection of a contrast agent into a vein in your arm. This substance makes the kidneys and urinary tract visible on X-rays. IVP is useful for identifying congenital abnormalities, tumors, scarring of the kidneys and stones in the urinary tract. An ultrasound exam, computerized tomography (CT) scan or magnetic resonance imaging (MRI) may be used to further define any abnormal IVP findings.

The success of IVP depends on the ability of each kidney to concentrate the contrast agent and move it throughout the urinary system. Thus, it's difficult to obtain a good IVP study when the kidneys don't filter properly.

Voiding cystourethrography

With this procedure X-rays are taken while the bladder is filled with X-ray contrast fluid and subsequently emptied during urination. A small, flexible tube (catheter) is inserted through the urethra into the bladder to introduce the contrast fluid. This test reveals whether any of the fluid flows back (refluxes) into the ureters or kidneys. Voiding cystourethrography is most often used to check the structure and function of the bladder and urethra. It can detect faulty bladder emptying or an anatomical abnormality.

on the affected side. Minimally invasive surgery, such as laparoscopy, may be required to eliminate the obstruction and prevent further kidney damage.

Multicystic dysplasia

Multicystic dysplasia is caused by abnormal growth of tissue in the kidney. It's characterized by multiple fluid-filled sacs (cysts).

Sometimes, this disorder is detected in a fetus during a prenatal ultrasound. On an X-ray, the affected kidney often resembles a bunch of grapes. It commonly functions poorly, if at all.

Multicystic dysplasia may spontaneously regress with time. The other kidney typically functions satisfactorily, so this condition doesn't interfere with normal growth and development.

Inherited Kidney Disorders

Some kidney disorders run in families. If a doctor diagnoses an inherited kidney disease in a family member, other family members may be tested — even if they have no symptoms — to see if they also have the disease.

Polycystic kidney disease

Signs and symptoms
- High blood pressure
- Pain in the side or back
- Abdominal pain
- Increase in size of abdomen
- Blood in urine
- Frequent urination

In polycystic kidney disease, the kidneys contain clusters of round, hollow, fluid-filled sacs (cysts) that interfere with kidney function and enlarge the kidneys. The disease can occur in children and adults but is much more common in adults. It usually doesn't cause problems until the second or third decade of life or later.

Types

Abnormal genes cause polycystic kidney disease, and the genetic defects mean the disease runs in families. The disease has two types, caused by different genetic flaws.

Autosomal dominant

Signs and symptoms of this form often develop between the ages of 30 and 40. This type was once called adult polycystic kidney disease, but in a small number of instances children do develop the disorder. Only one parent needs to have the disease in order for it to pass along to the children. If one parent has autosomal dominant polycystic kidney disease (ADPKD), each child has a 50 percent chance of getting the disease.

This form accounts for 85 to 90 percent of cases of polycystic kidney disease. In 25 to 40 percent of cases, a person with ADPKD has no known family history of the disease. Most often, someone in the affected person's family did have the disease, but didn't show signs or symptoms before dying of other causes. In a smaller percentage of cases where no family history is present, ADPKD results from a spontaneous gene mutation.

Autosomal recessive

This form is far less common than ADPKD. The signs and symptoms often appear shortly after birth. Sometimes, symptoms don't appear until later in childhood or during adolescence. Both parents must have abnormal genes to pass on this form of the disease. If both parents carry the genes for this disorder, each child has a 25 percent chance of getting the disease.

Diagnosis

An ultrasound examination, computerized tomography (CT) or magnetic resonance imaging (MRI) is used to diagnose the

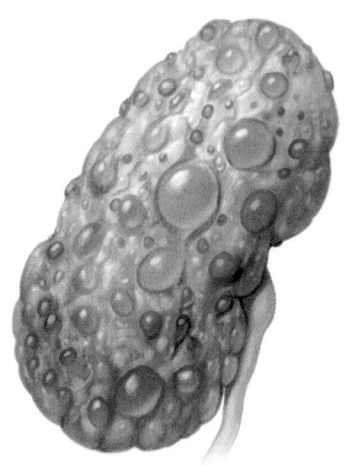

Development of many fluid-filled sacs (cysts) in kidney tissues causes polycystic kidneys, which may progress to kidney failure.

disease. Your doctor may recommend genetic testing to determine if you carry a gene associated with polycystic kidney disease.

How serious is polycystic kidney disease?

With autosomal dominant polycystic kidney disease, high blood pressure and progressive loss of kidney function often develop during adulthood. Most people with the severe form of this disease reach end-stage kidney (renal) disease by the time they're in their 40s or 50s, but some experience it earlier. Others may have only a mild to moderate loss of renal function throughout their lives.

Once end-stage kidney disease is reached, either kidney dialysis or kidney transplantation is necessary to sustain life. Many adults with this disease also have liver problems, including cysts that can become infected and cause fever and other symptoms.

Autosomal recessive polycystic kidney disease is very serious and may result in death in infancy or childhood.

Treatment

No treatment is currently available in the United States to prevent the cysts from forming and enlarging. Outside the U.S., the drug tolvaptan (Samsca) is prescribed for some people with rapidly progressing disease. Other measures can alleviate the symptoms and complications of polycystic kidney disease. If you have high blood pressure, managing your blood pressure can help preserve remaining kidney function. If you get a urinary tract infection, seek prompt treatment to prevent additional kidney damage.

A doctor may puncture and drain the cysts because of pain, bleeding, infection or obstruction or because massive enlargement of the kidneys is affecting other abdominal organs. Occasionally, this procedure is done in an attempt to improve or stabilize kidney function.

When end-stage kidney disease ensues, kidney dialysis or transplantation is your best option for successful treatment.

The childhood form of the disease requires careful and consistent medical attention to monitor any complications. Most children with polycystic kidney disease reach end-stage kidney disease during childhood. Thus, dialysis or transplantation is used much earlier than in the adult form. Associated liver disease is often severe, as well.

Cystinuria

Signs and symptoms

- Blood in the urine
- Pain
- Kidney stones

With cystinuria, the kidneys' tubules don't adequately reabsorb certain protein elements (amino acids). Excessive amounts of the amino acids lysine, arginine, ornithine and cystine are excreted in the urine. This inheritable disorder occurs in 1 in 7,000 people and is characterized by stones in the kidneys, ureters and bladder.

Diagnosis

A urine analysis can reveal the presence of excessive amounts of amino acids. If you pass a kidney stone, your doctor may have it tested to determine its composition. If the stone contains cystine, it's likely you have cystinuria.

Blood in Urine

Blood in urine (hematuria) may be visible to the eye (gross hematuria) or apparent only when the urine is examined under a microscope (microscopic hematuria). Hematuria is often detected when a urinalysis is performed for some other reason, such as a screening test at the time of a routine physical examination.

Hematuria may result from a wide variety of kidney or urinary tract problems, such as infection, stones, cysts or tumors. However, many people with hematuria have no evidence of any of these problems, despite thorough evaluation. They have what's called benign hematuria, which isn't associated with kidney damage.

Benign hematuria has two forms: recurrent (sporadic) and familial (inherited). Benign recurrent hematuria typically is detected in childhood but may not become apparent until later in life.

Aside from the presence of blood in the urine, all other findings related to the urine, blood and kidneys are normal. Treatment is unnecessary, and often the blood eventually disappears.

Benign recurrent hematuria is fairly common among athletes, particularly long-distance runners. The exact cause of blood in the urine isn't clear, but the incidence of exercise-induced hematuria is directly related to the duration and intensity of physical activity. The hematuria usually goes away within 24 hours after exercise stops.

How serious is cystinuria?

Cystinuria is a long-lasting (chronic) disease. People with it are likely to form cystine stones, which may damage the kidneys by causing ureteral obstruction or infection. Some people produce many such stones and need surgical operations

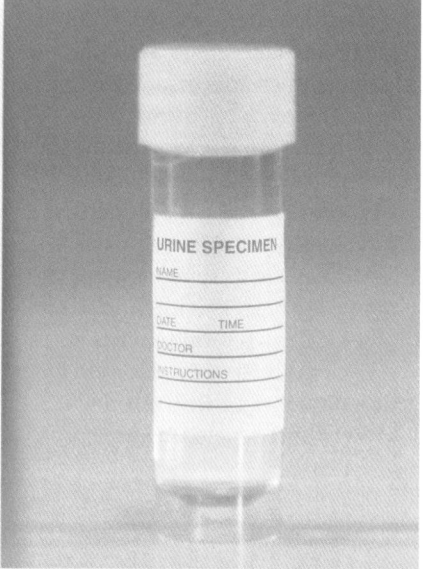

The familial form is acquired from a parent — a single gene inherited from either parent is capable of causing the disorder. If one parent has the condition, his or her child has a 50 percent chance of inheriting it. In such situations, several members of a family are usually affected.

In many cases, a kidney biopsy is necessary to confirm the diagnosis of benign familial hematuria and distinguish it from other conditions. Benign familial hematuria commonly is recognized in childhood. Typically, it persists throughout life but causes no kidney damage or other problems.

No treatment is necessary. In some children with isolated hematuria, a high concentration of calcium is found in the urine (hypercalciuria) and is believed to be the cause of the hematuria. These children may have an increased risk of kidney stones.

to remove them. Occasionally, cystinuria can cause kidney failure and lead to other organ damage.

Treatment
If you have cystinuria, drink plenty of water — up to a gallon every 24 hours — and drink one-third of it at night. This isn't always easy to do, but it'll help dilute the concentration of cystine in your urine.

Because cystine is more soluble in an alkaline solution, your doctor may also advise you to ingest a sodium bicarbonate or sodium citrate solution to keep the urine alkaline. If you don't respond to treatment with water and alkaline salts, your doctor may prescribe other medications that decrease cystine excretion. However, because of possible adverse effects, these are used only if other methods fail.

Renal tubular defects

In some cases of inherited kidney disease, the small tubes (tubules) contained in the kidneys' microscopic filtering units (nephrons) are the main parts affected. Renal tubules play a key role in your kidneys' absorption of nutrients and removal of waste.

Renal tubular acidosis
Renal tubular acidosis refers to several disorders that can be inherited or can result from an autoimmune disease, diabetes or certain medications that cause the kidneys to not remove enough acid from the bloodstream or to reclaim a base, such as bicarbonate, in excessive amounts. This disrupts the normal acid-base balance (pH) of the body.

Under these circumstances, the kidneys often lose an abnormal amount of potassium, calcium and sodium in the urine. The blood becomes acidic, and chloride levels increase in the blood.

In children, such tubular defects are often manifested by impaired growth. In adults, kidney stones may result. People with diabetes often have a type that leads to higher blood potassium levels. Treatment generally consists of giving enough sodium bicarbonate or potassium citrate to keep the blood within its normal range of alkalinity.

Vitamin D-resistant hypophosphatemic rickets
Vitamin D-resistant hypophosphatemic rickets is an inherited disorder in which the kidneys are unable to retain phosphate normally. The result is impaired growth, rickets and shortened adult stature. Treatment with phosphate and vitamin D preparations is often necessary.

Bartter's and Gitelman syndromes
Bartter's and Gitelman syndromes are rare, inherited conditions known as urinary wasting disorders.

Bartter's syndrome is generally diagnosed in childhood. It's characterized by an excessive amount of potassium in the urine. The condition is thought to result from a defect in the kidneys' ability to reabsorb sodium chloride. Signs and symptoms include muscle cramping and weakness, constipation, increased urination, and growth failure.

Gitelman syndrome is similar in many respects to Bartter's syndrome. However, it also causes loss of magnesium in urine. In addition, it's usually diagnosed in adulthood and is often milder than Bartter's syndrome.

Alport's syndrome

Alport's syndrome is a rare, inherited disorder that damages the tiny blood vessels in the kidneys. It also causes hearing loss and eye problems. It's caused by a defect (mutation) in a gene for a protein in the connective tissue, called collagen. Based on inheritance patterns, the syndrome affects men more severely than women.

In males, the usual course of the syndrome is progressive loss of kidney function. Females may have minimal symptoms, if any, but they can pass on the genetic defect to their children.

Congenital nephrotic syndrome
Congenital nephrotic syndrome is evident shortly after birth and is most commonly found in children of Finnish origin. Its manifestations are low birth weight, large amounts of protein in the urine (proteinuria) and massive fluid retention.

Infection, malnutrition or kidney failure can result in death during the first year of life. Early treatment, including kidney transplantation, has been successful therapy for some children.

Sickle cell disease

People with sickle cell disease (sickle cell anemia) have a blood abnormality and can experience a delay in growth, and in infants, failure to thrive. It occurs most frequently in black people. Associated kidney problems include susceptibility to urinary tract infection, blood in the urine and loss of the kidneys' ability to concentrate urine, which causes dehydration.

People who inherit only one gene for the disease carry the sickle cell trait but don't develop the disease, although they may notice blood in their urine and they may be at higher risk of kidney failure. See page 1042 for more on sickle cell anemia.

Blood Vessel Problems

The aorta is the largest blood vessel in the body, originating directly from the heart. Its branches carry blood to different parts of the body. Each kidney receives blood from one or more branches of the renal arteries. Twenty percent of the volume of blood pumped from the heart at any given time passes through the kidneys.

After the kidneys perform their filtering function, the blood returns by way of the renal veins to the major vessel that carries blood from the lower body back to the heart (inferior vena cava).

Disorders of either the renal arteries or the renal veins not only can affect the way the kidneys function but also can be a major cause of high blood pressure.

Acute arterial occlusion

Signs and symptoms
- Abrupt onset of side or abdominal pain
- Blood in the urine

Acute arterial occlusion of the kidney occurs when a renal artery is obstructed by a blood clot (thrombus). It usually occurs in people with known cardiovascular disease, primarily mitral or aortic valve disease or atrial fibrillation.

Diagnosis
A test called arteriography can help pinpoint the location of the obstruction in the renal artery. A small, flexible tube (catheter) is inserted through your groin into the aorta and manipulated into the renal artery. A contrast agent is injected and X-rays are taken.

Occasionally, a diagnosis is made using a renal scan, which uses tiny amounts of radioactive materials called tracers (radiopharmaceuticals). The tracers emit radiation that's detected by a special camera that produces detailed images of the kidneys and measures blood flow to the kidneys.

How serious is acute arterial occlusion?
The danger of acute arterial occlusion is that the affected kidney may cease to function. The other kidney can take over the process of eliminating wastes, but if arterial occlusion occurs in a person with only one kidney, or if it affects both kidneys, kidney failure may occur.

Treatment
Sometimes the blood clot dissolves spontaneously. If the artery has been blocked for only a few hours, your doctor may give you clot-dissolving medications or anticoagulant medications that prevent your blood from clotting.

In some cases, the blockage may be removed using a catheter that can be threaded through the arterial system into the affected artery. Occasionally, surgery is necessary to repair the artery.

Renal artery stenosis

Signs and symptoms
- High blood pressure
- A history of hard-to-control blood pressure

Renal artery stenosis is a narrowing or blockage of the renal artery before it enters the kidney, which impedes blood flow to the kidney and can cause chronic kidney failure or high blood pressure.

In older adults, renal artery stenosis most often develops as a result of a buildup of fatty deposits (atherosclerotic plaques) in the renal artery. Renal artery blockage can also occur as a result of beadlike thickening of the artery wall (fibromuscular dysplasia), a condition most commonly seen in women 20 to 40 years of age.

Diagnosis
Your doctor may suspect renal artery stenosis if he or she hears a sound called a bruit when listening with a stethoscope over your kidneys. Tests may include a kidney X-ray called intravenous pyelography or a computerized tomography (CT) angiogram.

A kidney ultrasound examination, which measures blood flow, may be helpful in identifying narrowing of the arteries. Magnetic resonance imaging (MRI) or an X-ray test called arteriography may be used to determine the exact location and extent of the blockage. A small, flexible tube (catheter) is inserted through the groin into the aorta and manipulated into the renal artery. A contrast agent is injected and X-rays are taken, at which time treatment such as stenting or angioplasty may be performed.

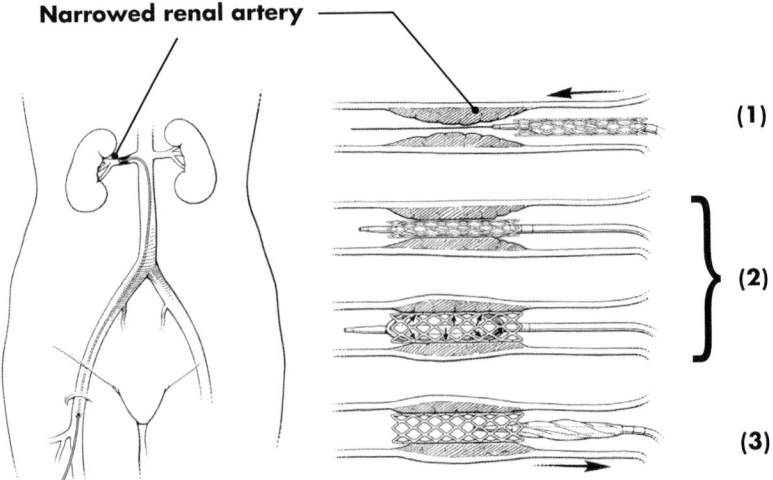

Narrowed renal artery

(1)

(2)

(3)

Percutaneous transluminal angioplasty (balloon angioplasty) may be used to open a narrowed renal artery. (1) During the procedure, a catheter containing a balloon that's enclosed within a mesh framework (stent) is threaded up an artery in the thigh and into the narrowed renal artery. (2) The artery is widened by inflating the balloon situated at the tip of the catheter. (3) The balloon and catheter are removed, but the stent stays in place to help keep the artery open.

Treatment

Sometimes, surgery is needed to remove or bypass the obstruction or narrowing of the renal artery. Surgery is done to prevent progressive renal failure and improve control of high blood pressure. Another treatment consists of passing a special catheter into the renal artery and inflating the balloon at the tip of the catheter to open the artery (percutaneous transluminal angioplasty, or balloon angioplasty), with or without placement of a stent. This has been particularly successful in women with fibromuscular dysplasia. Some people still need medication to control high blood pressure.

Renal vein thrombosis

Signs and symptoms
- Severe pain in the lower back and side
- Large quantities of protein in the urine

In this condition, a blood clot (thrombus) develops in the vein leaving the kidney. The clot may develop shortly after significant trauma to the abdomen or back.

Renal vein thrombosis may also be the result of a tumor blocking blood flow in the renal vein, or it may be associated with nephrotic syndrome. In some cases, particularly in infants, severe dehydration may be responsible for the condition.

Diagnosis

Your doctor may use a test in which a contrast agent is injected through the groin into the major vein that returns blood from the lower part of your body to your heart (inferior vena cava), and then into the renal vein. The intent is that the agent will outline the blood clot in the renal vein, allowing it to show up on an X-ray.

Sometimes, a doctor can make a diagnosis with the use of an ultrasound technique called Doppler imaging, which can detect evidence of a blood clot in the vein.

Treatment

Most often, the treatment for renal vein thrombosis consists of anticoagulant medications that prevent blood from clotting. Generally, over time the renal vein reopens unless the obstruction is due to tumor growth into the vein from extension of a kidney cancer.

Kidney Failure

Kidney (renal) failure occurs when the kidneys are unable to adequately perform their task of filtering waste out of the blood. This may happen suddenly (acute renal failure), such as with a blood vessel obstruction, or as a result of the slow and silent destruction (chronic renal failure) of the kidneys' filtering units (nephrons).

Because the kidneys have so many nephrons — approximately a million per kidney — symptoms of chronic kidney failure may go unnoticed until substantial damage has occurred. Kidney function generally drops at least 80 percent before serious complications result.

Diabetes and high blood pressure, when untreated or uncontrolled, cause almost two-thirds of adult cases of kidney failure in the United States. Other causes of kidney failure include infection, injury, exposure to toxins and drugs, and various kidney diseases.

In addition, systemic lupus erythematosus, sickle cell anemia, glomerulonephritis, polycystic kidney disease, cancer and obstruction of urine flow can cause kidney failure.

Acute kidney failure

Signs and symptoms
- Decreased urine output
- Swelling of legs, ankles or feet
- Drowsiness
- Shortness of breath
- Confusion

Acute kidney (renal) failure is a condition in which the kidneys rapidly lose their ability to remove waste products and excess fluid from your blood. Acute kidney failure is most common in people who are hospitalized. It tends to occur after a complicated surgery, a severe injury, antibiotic use for an infection, contrast dye exposure or when blood flow to the kidneys is disrupted.

Causes
Three types of conditions can cause acute kidney failure:
- **Prerenal conditions.** These include extremely low blood pressure or poor heart function that can decrease blood flow to the kidneys.
- **Renal conditions.** These include conditions such as inflammation of the kidneys, toxic injury or atherosclerosis, which directly damages the structures of the kidneys.
- **Postrenal conditions.** These include conditions such as a ureter or bladder obstruction that interferes with the excretion of waste from the kidneys' filtering process.

Diagnosis
If your doctor suspects kidney failure, he or she will likely request blood and urine tests to check for abnormal levels of waste products normally removed from your blood.

You may also have an X-ray to check for fluid in your lungs (pulmonary edema), as well as tests to rule out other potential causes of your signs and symptoms.

An abdominal ultrasound examination may be necessary to rule out an obstruction. In some cases, computerized tomography (CT) or magnetic resonance imaging (MRI) may be used. Sometimes a biopsy of the kidney is needed for correct diagnosis and treatment.

How serious is acute kidney failure?
Although acute kidney failure is a potentially serious condition that

may require hospitalization and intensive care, the kidneys generally are able to recover and resume normal function over a period of a couple of weeks to a few months. But it can take as long as a year to regain normal kidney function.

In some people, acute kidney failure may progress to chronic kidney failure. If left untreated, acute kidney failure can be lethal. Factors that can adversely affect the outcome of acute kidney failure are old age, infection and gastrointestinal bleeding.

Treatment

The goal is to treat the illness or injury that originally damaged your kidneys. Once that's under control, the focus will be on preventing the accumulation of excess fluids and wastes in your blood while your kidneys heal. This is best accomplished by limiting your fluid intake and following a high-carbohydrate, low-protein, low-potassium diet.

Your doctor may prescribe calcium, glucose or sodium polystyrene sulfonate (Kalexate, Kionex) or other potassium-lowering drugs to prevent the accumulation of high levels of potassium in your blood. Too much potassium in the blood can cause dangerous irregular heartbeats (arrhythmias).

Dialysis

In case of severe acute kidney injury, you may need to undergo temporary hemodialysis — often referred to simply as dialysis — to help remove toxins and excess fluids from your body while your kidneys heal (see page 896). Dialysis, which is a mechanical way of filtering waste from your blood, is an imperfect but lifesaving substitute for kidney function.

In acute kidney failure, dialysis is usually done at a hospital or dialysis center, not at home. The treatment relies on an artificial kidney (dialyzer) to take over kidney function. Blood is pumped out of your body into the artificial

kidney through one of two routes — a catheter placed surgically in one of your main blood veins, or a surgically created junction between a vein and artery in your arm. Inside the artificial kidney, your blood moves across membranes that filter out waste before the blood is returned to your body.

Your overall health will be monitored for evidence of complications such as infection, cardiac or neurological problems, high blood pressure, or gastrointestinal bleeding. Laboratory tests can indicate the development of uremic poisoning or other chemical imbalances.

In some cases of acute kidney failure requiring hospitalization, a type of dialysis called continuous renal replacement therapy may be used until the individual can be switched back to standard dialysis.

Chronic kidney disease

Signs and symptoms

- High blood pressure
- Decreased urine output
- Dark-colored urine
- Anemia
- Headache
- Nausea or vomiting
- Loss of appetite and weight change
- Discomfort (malaise)
- Fatigue and weakness
- Itching (pruritis)
- Headaches
- Sleep problems
- Decreased mental sharpness
- Pain alongside kidney or mid- to lower back

Chronic kidney disease is a gradual loss of your kidneys' filtering ability, usually due to high blood pressure or diabetes.

Unlike acute kidney failure, chronic kidney disease generally develops over a number of years as the kidneys' filtering units (nephrons) are progressively destroyed.

The National Kidney Foundation (NKF) has divided chronic kidney disease into five stages — with stages 1 and 2 being the mildest and stage 5 the most severe.

When a doctor knows what stage of kidney disease a person has, he or she can provide the best care, as each stage calls for different tests and treatments.

Often the disease causes no signs or symptoms in its early stages. In many cases, no symptoms are apparent until kidney function has decreased to less than 25 percent of what's considered normal.

Causes

In addition to diabetes and high blood pressure, chronic kidney disease may result from obstruction of urine flow, ongoing exposure to toxins such as fuels or solvents, or other kidney diseases, such as polycystic kidney disease or kidney infection.

Diagnosis

If you have diabetes, your doctor may schedule an annual test to measure small amounts of protein in your urine (microalbuminuria). This can screen for early signs of kidney damage related to diabetes (diabetic kidney disease). If you have another chronic condition that increases the risk of kidney disease, such as high blood pressure, your doctor may want to monitor your kidney function on a regular basis.

Blood tests and urine analyses are the most common tests used to measure kidney function. Blood tests can detect elevated amounts of waste products such as creatinine in blood. Urine studies measure protein leakage into the urine over the course of a day. A comparison of urine creatinine and blood creatinine levels allows your doctor to measure how much blood the kidneys are filtering per minute.

To confirm a diagnosis of chronic kidney disease, your doctor may request an ultrasound examination of your kidneys to determine the shape and structure of the kidneys and reveal any obstructions. He or she may also order other imaging tests, such as computerized tomography (CT) or magnetic resonance imaging (MRI). In some cases, a small sample of kidney tissue may be taken for analysis in a laboratory (biopsied).

How serious is chronic kidney disease?

Chronic kidney disease affects almost all of the body systems. Fluid retention from the disease can cause congestive heart failure, high blood pressure and swelling of body tissues (edema).

Healthy kidneys produce a hormone called erythropoietin that stimulates your bone marrow to produce new red blood cells. Red blood cells carry oxygen to all of the tissues and organs in your body. When the kidneys are damaged, they may not be able to make enough erythropoietin, causing a decreased production of red blood cells. This results in anemia.

Other problems that may occur include stomach ulcers, miscarriage, changes in skin color and weakening of the bones, which makes them susceptible to fracture. Even the central nervous system can be affected so that individuals with chronic kidney disease have difficulty with concentration or memory and have problems with the nerves and muscles in their arms and legs.

The condition eventually can progress to end-stage kidney disease. When this occurs, the kidneys aren't capable of sustaining life and either dialysis or kidney transplantation is the only option to preserve life.

Complications in children

In children, one of the most serious consequences of chronic kidney disease is failure to grow properly. In addition to regulating fluids and ridding the body of waste, the kidneys regulate the interaction of calcium and vitamin D, which are essential for bone growth.

Complications during pregnancy

Women with chronic kidney disease who become pregnant face a number of potential complications because the kidneys must work especially hard to deal with the demands of pregnancy. This can lead to worsening high blood pressure and an increase in waste products circulating in the blood.

Chronic high blood pressure can decrease the amount of blood the baby receives through the placenta, which can seriously affect fetal development. And waste products in the mother's bloodstream also may harm the baby's health.

Pregnant women with chronic kidney disease are also at high risk of preeclampsia, a serious complication occurring in late pregnancy. Preeclampsia causes a dangerous rise in blood pressure.

Treatment

Chronic kidney disease has no cure, but treatment can help control signs and symptoms, reduce complications, and slow the progress of the disease. If you have chronic kidney disease, your primary doctor will likely refer you to a kidney specialist (nephrologist), if you aren't seeing one already.

Treating the underlying condition

The first priority is controlling the disorder responsible for your condition. If you have diabetes or high blood pressure, for instance, that means carefully following your doctor's recommendations for diet and exercise and taking any medications as directed.

Most people with chronic kidney disease are treated with medications to lower their blood pressure — commonly angiotensin-converting enzyme (ACE) inhibitors or angiotensin II receptor blockers — and to preserve kidney function. Because these medications can initially increase serum potassium and decrease overall kidney function, you may have frequent blood tests to check your potassium levels.

Over the long term, these medications tend to both lower blood pressure and preserve kidney function. To protect kidney function, your blood pressure may need to be lower than if your kidneys were functioning normally.

In addition, you'll likely need to limit the amount of salt in your diet to help control high blood pressure. And, over time, you may need to restrict the amount of potassium and phosphorus you consume. Finally, you'll need to avoid medications that can further damage your kidneys, such as nonsteroidal anti-inflammatory drugs (NSAIDs).

Treating complications

Complications of chronic kidney disease need to be addressed. For example, anemia may require supplements of the hormone erythropoietin to induce production of more red blood cells. In addition, your doctor may prescribe a form of vitamin D (calcitriol) to prevent weak bones, as well as a phosphate-binding medication to lower the amount of phosphate in your blood. Lowering phosphate will increase the amount of calcium available for your bones to help prevent weakening and fracture.

Kidney dialysis

Dialysis is an artificial means of removing waste products and extra fluid from your blood when your kidneys aren't able to perform these functions (see page 896). It's not a miracle treatment, and it presents significant risks, including infection. Still, it can help prolong life for people with end-stage kidney disease.

Kidney transplant

If you have no other life-threatening medical conditions, a kidney transplant is usually a better option than dialysis, although you may need to undergo dialysis temporarily until a suitable donor kidney becomes available.

A successful kidney transplant depends on finding the best immunological match possible. Ideally, you and the kidney's donor will have the same blood type, cell-surface proteins and antibodies. The more closely these features are matched, the lower the risk that your body will reject the new kidney. A sibling is often the best donor. If that's not possible, a blood relative, or even a nonblood-related adult may be considered.

When a living donor isn't available, tissue-typing centers throughout the country may search for a kidney from an accident victim or another person who has offered to donate organs after his or her death.

End-stage kidney disease

Signs and symptoms
- Kidney function permanently deteriorates to a level unable to sustain life
- Uremia and many resulting complications, which may include high blood pressure, congestive heart failure, anemia, bone disease, gastrointestinal problems, urinary tract infection and dementia

End-stage renal disease occurs when the kidneys have lost about 90 percent of their ability to function normally. This means that the kidneys are incapable of sustaining life and that their function must be replaced by kidney dialysis or a kidney transplant.

More than 450,000 people in the United States receive kidney dialysis, and approximately 200,000 people are alive because they had kidney transplant surgery.

Diabetes is the most common cause of end-stage kidney disease in the United States. Other causes include high blood pressure, various kidney diseases and a urinary tract problem called vesicoureteral reflux (see page 887).

Kidney Dialysis

Dialysis is an artificial means of removing waste products and extra fluid from blood. For many people with irreversible kidney failure, kidney dialysis provides the opportunity to live long after their kidneys have ceased to function. Currently in the United States, more than 450,000 people are receiving dialysis.

The different forms of dialysis are as follows:

Hemodialysis
Hemodialysis is the most common form of dialysis. It uses a machine (kidney dialyzer) to remove extra fluid, chemicals and waste from your blood.

Before you can undergo hemodialysis, a surgeon must create an access point in your blood vessels for blood to leave and re-enter your body during dialysis. Usually, the access is in the forearm. The procedure increases blood flow by enlarging a blood vessel (arteriovenous fistula) or creating an artificial one (arteriovenous graft). If your blood vessels are not suitable for a fistula or a graft, you may instead use a large, intravenous catheter that tunnels under your skin and exits out your chest wall.

When you're connected to the dialysis machine, your blood is pumped from the access point into the machine, where it flows across membranes that let waste compounds filter through. A solution in the machine helps remove excess fluid and regulates substances left in the blood. The blood then flows back into you. Less than 1 cup of blood is outside your body at a time.

As a rule, most people on dialysis require nine to 12 hours of dialysis a week. These are usually divided into three sessions.

Peritoneal dialysis
When you undergo peritoneal dialysis, instead of using a dialyzer, you use the vast network of tiny blood vessels located in your abdomen (peritoneal cavity), known as capillaries, to filter your blood.

First, a surgeon creates an access by placing a small, flexible tube (catheter) into your abdominal cavity. Dialysis solution is introduced into the abdominal cavity through the catheter. Small blood vessels in the inside lining of your abdomen filter waste products and water from your blood into the dialysis solution. After a set period of time, the solution is drained out of your abdomen, taking with it excess waste and fluid.

Each of these cycles is called an exchange. You need several exchanges each day. Exchanges can be done as you go through your daily routine, or at night if you have a home peritoneal dialysis machine. The machine fills and empties fluid automatically while you sleep.

Continuous ambulatory peritoneal dialysis
You can perform continuous ambulatory peritoneal dialysis (CAPD) at home by using a permanently implanted catheter in your abdomen to exchange the dialysis solution four times a day, seven days a week. In this way, the solution is in your abdomen continuously. In between exchange sessions, you're not attached to anything. You can move about freely while the dialysis solution is in the peritoneal cavity.

Continuous cycling peritoneal dialysis
Continuous cycling peritoneal dialysis (CCPD), also called nocturnal cyclical peritoneal dialysis (NCPD), uses a machine that automatically infuses dialysis solution into your peritoneal cavity — through an implanted catheter — and drains several times over the course of the night while you sleep. This allows

How serious is end-stage kidney disease?

End-stage kidney disease is fatal unless dialysis is initiated or kidney transplantation is performed. Both have serious risks.

Treatment

Once a person reaches end-stage kidney disease, conservative measures used to manage chronic kidney disease — treating the underlying cause, dietary restrictions and medications — no longer suffice. If kidney transplantation isn't possible because of poor general health, remaining treatment options include hemodialysis, peritoneal dialysis or conservative therapy, which treats underlying symptoms associated with kidney failure but doesn't clean the bloodstream.

Stones, Cysts and Tumors

Kidney stones can develop in overly concentrated urine. Bladder stones are usually the result of lower urinary tract blockage. Kidney cysts — hollow, fluid-filled, benign lesions — are common and typically produce no symptoms. More than half of older adults have at least one kidney cyst. Malignant tumors also can develop in or invade the kidneys, ureters or bladder, but they're much less common.

Kidney stones

Signs and symptoms

- Pain in the side and lower back
- Fluctuating pain intensity, with periods of pain lasting 20 to 60 minutes
- Waves of pain radiating down to the abdomen and groin

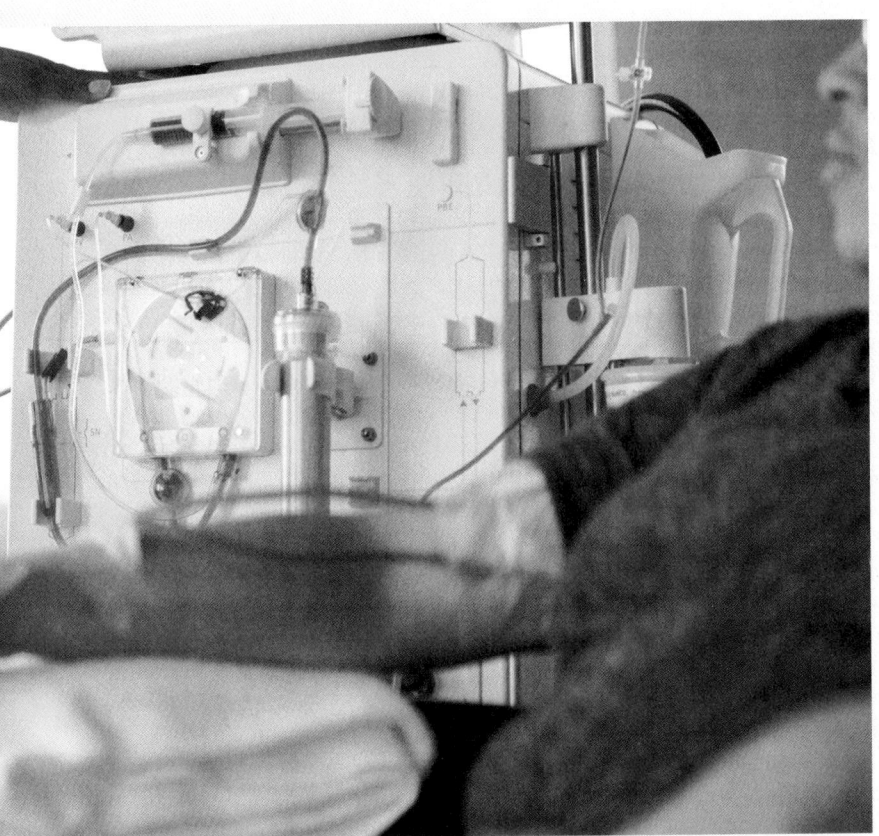

A dialysis machine (kidney dialyzer) artificially cleanses waste products from the blood of people whose kidneys are no longer able to do so.

your days to be free, but you need to be attached to the machine at night.

Your doctor can help you decide which type of dialysis is best for you. Mostly it depends on your particular needs and what's available in your community.

Dialysis can be used as a temporary measure during acute kidney injury, preventing the buildup of waste in blood while the kidneys heal. In acute situations, dialysis may be performed in a hospital dialysis unit or in an intensive care unit. Blood dialysis in a hospital may be done over a three- to five-hour time frame (typical hemodialysis) or it may be performed continuously for 24 hours (continuous renal replacement therapy) in an intensive care unit. Dialysis may also be a temporary measure for young and otherwise healthy individuals awaiting a kidney transplant.

For individuals with chronic kidney disease for whom transplantation isn't an option because of age or other medical problems, dialysis may be a permanent form of treatment. When does a person with chronic kidney disease need dialysis? Every one is different. As a rule, most doctors try to manage the condition for as long as possible with conservative measures, such as dietary modifications and medication. Most people begin dialysis when kidney function falls below 10 percent of normal or if they have poor kidney function and symptoms such as nausea, vomiting, fatigue, itchy skin and swollen legs.

Inevitably, though, there comes a time when the benefits of dialysis outweigh the risks. Complications associated with dialysis include malfunction of the dialysis machine, infection of the access point and nutritional deficiencies.

Kidney Transplantation

More than 200,000 people who received kidney transplants are living in the United States. Kidney transplantation provides the best alternative for most individuals with end-stage kidney (renal) failure. With the increased use of living-donor organs for this procedure, many people today can receive a transplant before they need kidney dialysis.

Who's eligible?

Most people with end-stage renal disease are candidates for kidney transplantation. But those with a recent history of cancer or another severe medical condition may not be considered suitable for a transplant. Today, kidney transplantation — especially with a kidney from a living donor — is a relatively safe procedure that can be performed even among people with significant medical problems, such as cardiovascular disease or diabetes.

Living vs. deceased donor

The surgical technique used to perform a kidney transplant has been well-established for years. With the development of new immunosuppressant medications designed to prevent organ rejection, only a relatively small number of people undergoing a kidney transplant have significant problems with rejection.

During an evaluation, the person receiving the transplant is generally presented with two options — receiving a kidney transplant from a living donor or being placed on a list and waiting until a kidney from a deceased donor becomes available. The best option, when available, is a living donor because a living donor presents the possibility for an immediate transplant, reducing or, in many cases, completely eliminating the need for dialysis.

Compatibility and matching between the donor's and the recipient's tissue types has become less important in recent years. This is due to significant improvements in anti-rejection medications. Currently, it's common to perform kidney transplants between husband and wife, where one spouse is the donor and the other is the recipient. Because no genetic relationship exists between the two, the tissue types are usually completely different (mismatched). This hasn't been associated with worse outcomes. Success rates are comparable to those of people who receive a kidney transplant from a sibling.

Finding a donor

The primary qualification to be a kidney donor is to be healthy, with no relevant medical problems that may put you at risk of complications during or after the surgery. Generally, the blood type of the donor and of the recipient has to be compatible to prevent hyperacute rejection at the time of the transplant. However, some medical centers, including Mayo Clinic, are performing kidney transplants between friends and relatives of incompatible blood types. This requires special techniques, which include removal of blood antibodies by a process called plasmapheresis. This is a good option for individuals whose only potential donor happens to have an incompatible blood type.

Paired donation is another type of living kidney donation if you have a willing kidney donor whose organ isn't compatible with you or doesn't match well for other reasons. Rather than donating a kidney directly to you, your donor may give a kidney to someone who may be a better match. Then you receive a compatible kidney from that recipient's donor.

When a living donor isn't available, the person in need of a transplant gets placed on a transplant waiting list and is called when an organ from a deceased donor becomes available. The average waiting time is three to five years. Once a kidney is located, it's usually transplanted within 48 hours of removal from the donor.

After transplantation

Individuals undergoing kidney transplantation usually stay in the hospital for four to six days after surgery. Kidney rejection used to be a significant hurdle during the days after the surgery, but with new immunosuppressant drugs this has become less of a problem. Kidney transplant success rates at one year are in the neighborhood of 97 percent for living-donor transplants and 96 percent for deceased-donor transplants.

The medications administered after the transplant can have some side effects. Your doctor will look for and address the side effects if they appear. A combination of immunosuppressant medications must be taken for life. In addition, anti-lymphocytic preparations are sometimes used during the first few days after the transplant. During the first few weeks or months after transplantation, most people receive antibiotics and antiviral and antifungal drugs. These medications help prevent some of the most common infections that tend to occur in transplant recipients.

Recent advances

The development of the laparoscopic donor nephrectomy technique has resulted in a significant increase in the number of kidney transplantations performed in recent years. This technique allows for removal of the living-donor kidney through a very small incision and a quick recovery time for the person donating the kidney.

The kidney paired donation program also is making it possible for more people to receive donated kidneys.

- Bloody, cloudy or foul-smelling urine
- Pain when urinating
- Persistent urge to urinate
- Nausea and vomiting

Few who have passed a kidney stone ever forget the experience. Most people who have gone through it agree that it was one of the most painful episodes in their lives. Occasionally, though, a kidney stone passes with minimal or no symptoms.

Kidney stones are small, hard deposits of mineral and acid salts on the inner surfaces of your kidneys. Normally, the substances that make up kidney stones are dissolved in the urine. When urine is concentrated, though, minerals may crystallize, stick together and solidify. Most kidney stones contain calcium.

The pain usually occurs when the stone dislodges and blocks drainage of urine from the kidney. The pain starts in your back or your side just below your lower ribs. As the stone moves down the ureter toward your bladder, the pain may radiate down to your groin.

Kidney stones are common. About 11 percent of men and 6 percent of women in the United States have kidney stones at least once during their lifetimes.

Certain types of stones tend to run in families. In addition, some kidney stones are associated with other medical conditions, such as overactive parathyroid glands, renal tubule defects, cystic kidney disease, chronic urinary tract infections and rare metabolic disorders.

Gout, inflammatory bowel disease, blockage of the urinary tract and too much vitamin D also can increase your risk of kidney stones, as can certain AIDS medications, diuretics and excessive use of calcium-based antacids. However, the exact cause of kidney stone formation often is unknown.

Types

Several different types of stones may develop in the kidneys:

- **Calcium stones.** Roughly 4 out of 5 kidney stones are calcium stones, usually in the form of calcium oxalate. Oxalate is found in some fruits and vegetables, but the liver produces most of the body's oxalate supply. Dietary factors, high doses of vitamin D, intestinal bypass surgery and several different metabolic disorders can increase the concentration of calcium or oxalate in urine.
- **Struvite stones.** Found more often in women, struvite stones are almost always the result of urinary tract infections. Struvite stones may be large enough to fill most of a kidney's urine-collecting space, forming a characteristic stag horn shape.
- **Uric acid stones.** These stones are formed of uric acid, a by-product of protein metabolism. You're more likely to develop uric acid stones if you eat a high-protein diet. Gout also may lead to uric acid stones. Certain genetic factors and disorders of the blood-producing tissues also may predispose you to the condition.

- **Cystine stones.** These stones represent only a small percentage of kidney stones. They form in people with a hereditary disorder that causes the kidneys to excrete excessive amounts of certain amino acids (cystinuria).

Diagnosis

Tests that may be used to diagnose a kidney stone include an ultrasound exam, a computerized tomography (CT) scan or a special kidney X-ray called intravenous pyelography (see page 888).

Once the stone has been passed or removed, your doctor may send your stone to the laboratory for analysis to determine its composition. This information may suggest the cause of the stone and help with developing a plan to prevent new stones from forming.

If you have recurrent or multiple stones, your doctor may request a chemical analysis of your blood and a 24-hour collection of urine to measure the clearance of waste products from the kidneys.

How serious are kidney stones?

Although passing a stone is

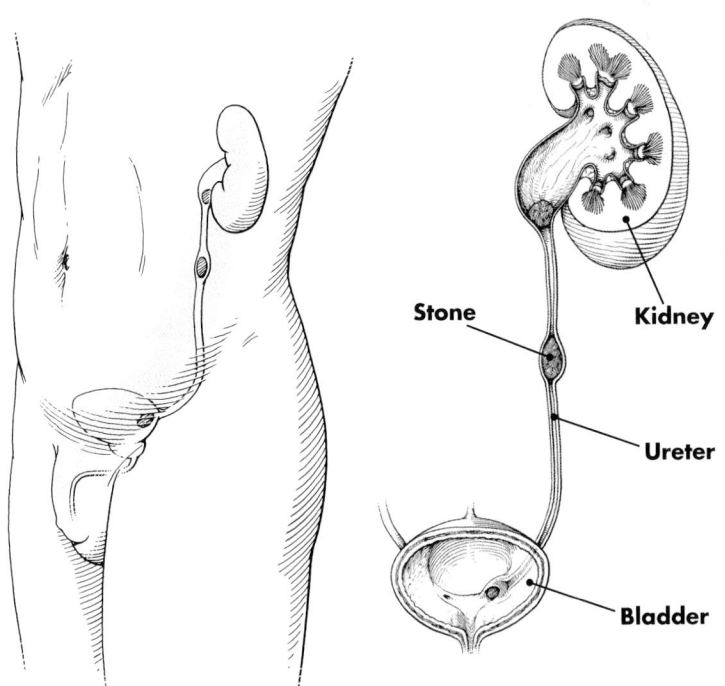

Stone

Kidney

Ureter

Bladder

The blue-tinted zone on the torso is where the pain of kidney stones most often occurs. Stones originate in the kidneys and can travel down into the ureters and bladder.

painful, most kidney stones pass through the ureter and into the bladder without causing permanent damage. If complications develop, such as ureteral obstruction or urinary tract infection, kidney damage may result.

Treatment

Treatment for kidney stones varies, depending on the type of stone and the cause. You may be able to move a stone through your urinary tract simply by drinking plenty of water — as much as 2 to 3 quarts a day — and by staying physically active. Passing a small stone can cause some discomfort. Pain relievers may help to relieve mild pain.

Stones that can't be treated with more-conservative measures — either because they're too large to pass on their own or because they cause bleeding, kidney damage or ongoing urinary tract infections — may need professional treatment. Options to remove problem kidney stones include:

- **Medical therapy.** Your doctor may give you a medication to help pass your kidney stone. This type of medication, known as an alpha blocker, relaxes the muscles in your ureter, helping you pass the kidney stone more quickly and with less pain.
- **Surgery.** A procedure called percutaneous nephrolithotomy involves surgically removing a kidney stone using small telescopes and instruments inserted through a small incision in your back. You'll receive general anesthesia during the surgery and be in the hospital for one to two days while you recover. Your doctor may recommend this surgery if other treatments were unsuccessful.
- **Scope procedure.** To remove a smaller stone in your ureter or kidney, your doctor may pass a thin, lighted tube (ureteroscope) equipped with a camera through your urethra and bladder to your ureter. Once the

stone is located, special tools can snare the stone or break it into pieces that will pass in your urine. Your doctor may then place a small tube (stent) in the ureter to relieve swelling and promote healing. You may need general or local anesthesia during this procedure.

- **Sound wave therapy.** For certain kidney stones — depending on size and location — a procedure called extracorporeal shock wave lithotripsy (ESWL) may be used. ESWL uses sound waves to create strong vibrations (shock waves) that break the stones into tiny pieces that can be passed in your urine. The procedure lasts about 45 to 60 minutes and can cause moderate pain, so you may be under sedation or light anesthesia to make you comfortable.

ESWL is less commonly performed today than it once was. It can cause blood in the urine, bruising on the back or abdomen, and bleeding around the kidney and other adjacent organs.

Bladder stones

Signs and symptoms

- Lower abdominal pain
- Pain or discomfort in the penis
- Painful urination
- Frequent urination
- Difficulty urinating or interruption of urine flow
- Urine leakage
- Blood in urine
- Abnormally dark-colored urine

Bladder stones are small masses of minerals that form in your bladder. They often develop when concentrated urine sits in your bladder. As urine stagnates, minerals in urine form various crystals that may combine to form stones.

Bladder stones usually develop as a result of another condition, such as an enlarged prostate gland or a urinary tract infection. Occasionally, bladder stones are caused by long-term use of catheters that are left in place, causing

an associated infection and stone formation on the catheter.

Diagnosis

If you have a bladder stone, a test of your urine (urinalysis) will usually reveal blood in the urine. Generally, a stone can be seen on an X-ray or with computerized tomography (CT) or magnetic resonance imaging (MRI).

How serious are bladder stones?

Bladder stones may pass without intervention if they're small. If they don't pass, they should be removed. Your doctor will want to identify and treat the underlying cause of the bladder stones in order to prevent a recurrence.

Treatment

Bladder stones are usually removed during a procedure called a cystolitholapaxy. During this procedure, your doctor inserts a small tube with a camera at the end (cystoscope) through your urethra and into your bladder to view the stone. Your doctor may use a laser, ultrasound or mechanical device to break the stone into small pieces. The pieces are then flushed from your bladder.

You'll likely have regional or general anesthesia prior to the procedure to make you comfortable. Complications from a cystolitholapaxy aren't common, but urinary tract infections, fever, a tear in your bladder and bleeding can occur. After a cystolitholapaxy, sometimes a doctor may check to make sure that no stone fragments remain in the bladder.

Occasionally, bladder stones that are large or too hard to break up are removed through open surgery. In such circumstances, a surgeon makes an incision in your bladder and removes the stones. Any underlying condition causing the stones, such as an enlarged prostate gland, may be corrected at the same time that the stones are removed.

Kidney cysts

Signs and symptoms
- Pain in the side
- Blood in the urine

Kidney cysts are noncancerous (benign) lesions of the kidney. They're usually round and contain water-like fluid. Cysts can vary in size from small to large and may contain quarts of fluid. Unlike cancer, a cyst generally enlarges slowly and stops growing when it attains a certain size.

Cysts in the kidney are common. Up to half the people older than age 50 have at least one kidney cyst. The fact that infants and children rarely have cysts suggests kidney cysts usually aren't inherited.

Diagnosis
Your doctor can usually distinguish between benign cysts and kidney cancer by using ultrasound, computerized tomography (CT) or magnetic resonance imaging (MRI).

How serious are kidney cysts?
Most kidney cysts are noncancerous (benign) and don't cause symptoms. Only when a cyst is extremely large may it require treatment due to compression of organs around the kidney. Bleeding may occur within the cyst. An infection or, rarely, cancer can develop in a cyst. Kidney cysts rupture very infrequently.

Treatment
Usually, no treatment is required. In rare instances, fluid must be removed from a cyst by way of laparoscopic surgery or an aspiration to relieve pressure or pain and to prevent damage to the kidney.

Kidney or ureter cancer

Signs and symptoms
- Blood in the urine
- Back pain just below the ribs
- Weight loss
- Fatigue
- Intermittent fever
- An abdominal mass

Kidney cancer is diagnosed in approximately 64,000 Americans each year, and about 14,000 die of the disease annually. Yet if kidney cancer is detected and treated early, the chances for a full recovery are good. Cancers that originate in the collecting system of the kidney are relatively rare, accounting for less than 5 percent of renal tumors.

For reasons that aren't totally clear, the rate of kidney cancers has been increasing. Part of the increased diagnosis may be related to greater use of computerized tomography (CT) and magnetic resonance imaging (MRI) for other conditions.

Your kidneys are part of the urinary system, which removes waste and excess fluid and electrolytes from your blood, controls the production of red blood cells, and regulates your blood pressure. Inside each kidney are more than a million small filtering units called nephrons.

As blood circulates through your kidneys, the nephrons filter out waste products as well as unneeded minerals and water. This liquid waste (urine) flows through two narrow tubes (ureters) into your bladder, where it's stored until it's eliminated from your body through another tube, called the urethra.

Unfortunately, kidney cancer often gives no warning signs in its early stages. As the tumor grows, your doctor may feel a mass in the kidney during a physical examination of the abdomen, and blood may be detected in your urine.

Types
Just what causes kidney cells to become cancerous isn't clear. But researchers have identified certain factors that appear to increase the risk of kidney cancer.

The most common types of kidney cancer include:
- **Renal cell carcinoma.** This type of kidney cancer usually begins in the cells that line the small tubes of each nephron. In most cases, renal cell tumors grow as a single mass, but you may have more than one tumor in a kidney or develop tumors in both kidneys.
- **Urothelial carcinoma.** This type of kidney cancer develops in the lining that forms the drainage system, which includes the kidney, ureter, bladder and urethra. Urothelial carcinomas can also begin in the ureters or in the bladder.
- **Wilms' tumor.** Wilms' tumor is a type of kidney cancer that occurs in young children.

Diagnosis
Tests that might be used to diagnose kidney or ureter cancer include a special kidney X-ray procedure called intravenous pyelography (see page 888), or an ultrasound exam, computerized tomography (CT) scan, or magnetic resonance imaging (MRI).

Sometimes, a doctor may recommend a procedure to remove a small sample of cells (biopsy) from a suspicious area on a kidney. Additional tests may include a chest X-ray, a bone scan or liver tests to determine if the cancer has spread to other organs or tissues. A special examination of urine (cytology) may reveal cancer cells shed in the urine.

How serious is cancer of the kidney or ureter?
The outcome in individuals with renal cell carcinoma depends on the extent to which the tumor has spread. If the tumor is in its earliest stage, 85 to 95 percent of those affected are cured. If the lymph nodes around the kidney or other organs are involved, the five-year survival rate drops to 30 to 50 percent.

If a urothelial carcinoma hasn't spread, five-year survival rates are very high. If the cancer has spread, the chance of surviving the next five years is significantly diminished.

Children with Wilms' tumor generally have a good chance

of survival if the disease hasn't spread. Overall, more than 90 percent are cured.

Treatment

Together, you and your medical team will discuss all of your treatment options. The best approach for you may depend on a number of factors, including your general health, the kind of kidney cancer you have, whether the cancer has spread and your own preferences for treatment.

Many kidney tumors are detected incidentally and don't need immediate treatment. If your tumor is small, your doctor may recommend surveillance of the tumor to gauge how aggressive it is and whether you'll need treatment. Surveillance typically requires periodic CT scans, MRIs or ultrasounds to see if the tumor is growing.

Surgery

Surgery is the initial treatment for the majority of kidney cancers. Surgical procedures used to treat kidney cancer include:

- **Removing the affected kidney (radical nephrectomy).** Radical nephrectomy involves the removal of the kidney, a border of healthy tissue and the adjacent lymph nodes. The adrenal gland also may be removed.

  Most often this surgery is done laparoscopically using several small incisions in your abdomen to insert a video camera and tiny surgical tools. In some cases, it may be done using robot-assisted surgery, which means the surgeon uses hand controls that tell a robot how to maneuver surgical tools to perform the operation. Occasionally, if the tumor is particularly large or involves nearby structures, the surgery is performed as an open operation with a larger incision in your abdomen.

- **Removing the tumor from the kidney (nephron-sparing surgery).** Small tumors that don't take over the majority of the kidney may be removed without removing the entire kidney. During this procedure, also called partial nephrectomy, a surgeon removes the tumor and a small margin of healthy tissue that surrounds it, rather than removing the entire kidney. Nephron-sparing surgery can be an open procedure, or it may be performed laparoscopically or with robotic assistance. When possible, this type of surgery is often preferred because it retains as much kidney tissue as possible, reducing your risk of potential complications later on.

Other therapies

For some people, surgery isn't an option. Treatment may involve:

- **Treatment to freeze cancer cells (cryoablation).** A special needle is inserted through your skin and into your kidney tumor using X-ray guidance. Gas in the needle is used to cool down or freeze the cancer cells. The procedure is typically reserved for people who can't undergo other surgical procedures and those who have small kidney tumors.

- **Radiofrequency ablation.** This procedure uses heat rather than cold to kill cancer cells. A small probe is guided into the center of the cancerous tumor. The probe is connected to a radiofrequency generator that delivers heat energy to the tumor. The heat causes cancer cells to shrink and die.

Mayo Clinic studies have demonstrated that both radiofrequency ablation and cryoablation may be effective for small kidney tumors.

Advanced or recurrent cancer

Kidney cancer that recurs and kidney cancer that spreads to other parts of the body may be curable. In these situations, treatments may include:

- **Surgery.** If it is possible to remove all of the cancer with surgery, sometimes an operation may be performed. This can be a big operation with several teams of surgeons. It's important to discuss with your surgeon whether the cancer can be removed entirely or in part.

- **Immunotherapy.** Immunotherapy uses your body's immune system to fight the cancer. Kidney cancers can produce proteins that make the cancer invisible to your immune system. Drugs that block formation of these proteins allow your immune system to identify and attack the cancer. Drugs in this category include interferon, aldesleukin (Proleukin) and nivolumab (Opdivo).

- **Targeted therapy.** Targeted treatments block specific abnormal signals present in kidney cancer cells that allow them to proliferate. These drugs have shown promise in treating kidney cancer that has spread to other areas of the body. The targeted drugs axitinib (Inlyta), bevacizumab (Avastin), pazopanib (Votrient), sorafenib (Nexavar) and sunitinib (Sutent) block signals that play a role in the growth of blood vessels that provide nutrients to cancer cells and allow cancer cells to spread. Temsirolimus (Torisel) and everolimus (Afinitor, Zortress) block a signal that allows cancer cells to grow and survive. Targeted therapy drugs can cause side effects, such as a rash that can be severe, diarrhea and fatigue.

  Targeted drugs, as well as immunotherapy, can be very expensive.

- **Radiation therapy.** Radiation therapy uses high-powered energy beams, such as X-rays, to kill cancer cells. Radiation therapy is sometimes used to control or reduce symptoms of kidney cancer that has spread to other areas of the body, such as the bones.

Upper tract urothelial cancer

Treatment for upper tract urothelial cancer typically involves chemotherapy followed by surgery or surgery alone.

Chemotherapy may be useful in treating some cancers that have spread or that recur. Chemotherapy uses chemicals to kill rapidly growing cells, such as cancer cells. Other rapidly growing cells, such as those in your gastrointestinal tract and your hair follicles, also may be destroyed by the drugs. That's why people who undergo chemotherapy can experience certain side effects, including nausea, vomiting and hair loss.

Bladder cancer

Signs and symptoms
- Blood in the urine
- Frequent urination
- Painful urination
- Abdominal pain
- Back pain

Nearly 77,000 new cases of bladder cancer are diagnosed annually in the United States. This disease is responsible for approximately 16,000 deaths each year. Bladder cancer rarely occurs in people younger than age 40. It's three times more common in men than in women.

Factors that increase your risk of bladder cancer include smoking; exposure to certain chemicals, such as those used in some manufacturing; prior radiation therapy to the pelvis; and treatment with certain chemotherapy drugs, such as cyclophosphamide and ifosfamide. Long-term catheter use may also increase your cancer risk.

Types
Different types of cells in your bladder can become cancerous. The type of cell involved in your cancer determines the type of treatments that may work best for you. Types of bladder cancer include:
- **Urothelial carcinoma.** Urothelial carcinoma occurs in the cells that line the inside of your bladder. Urothelial cells expand when your bladder is full and contract when your bladder is

empty. These same cells line the inside of your ureters and your urethra, and tumors can form in those places as well. Urothelial carcinoma is the most common type of bladder cancer in the United States.
- **Squamous cell carcinoma.** Squamous cells appear in your bladder in response to infection and irritation. Over time they can become cancerous. Squamous cell bladder cancer is rare in the United States. It's a more common type of bladder cancer in areas of the world where a certain parasitic infection (schistosomiasis) is a more prevalent cause of bladder infections.
- **Adenocarcinoma.** Adenocarcinoma begins in cells that make up mucus-secreting glands in the bladder. Adenocarcinoma of the bladder is rare in the United States.

Some bladder cancers include more than one type of cell.

Diagnosis
Your doctor may have you provide a urine sample to be examined for malignant cells (cytology). Other procedures may include a computerized tomography (CT) scan, a kidney X-ray procedure called intravenous pyelography (see page 888) and a cystoscopic examination in which a thin, flexible fiber-optic tube is inserted through the urethra and into the bladder so that your doctor can see inside (see page 904).

If a tumor is seen within the bladder, it may be removed with a procedure called transurethral resection of bladder tumor (TURBT). You receive anesthesia during the procedure. Once the tumor is removed, it's sent to a laboratory to determine the type.

If cancer is found, your doctor may order a computerized tomography (CT) scan or magnetic resonance imaging (MRI) of the abdomen or pelvis to help determine the extent of the cancer and whether it has spread.

How serious is bladder cancer?
If the tumor is noninvasive — it's small and hasn't deeply invaded tissues within the bladder wall — the chances of recovery are excellent. Approximately three-quarters of bladder cancers are detected at this early stage. These tumors usually aren't deadly, but they do have a tendency to return, so it's important to have periodic cystoscopic examinations to look for tumor recurrence.

Tumors that invade into or through the bladder wall can be aggressive and spread throughout the body. These cancers are treated much more aggressively.

Treatment
Treatment options for bladder cancer depend on a number of factors, including the type and stage of the cancer, your overall health, and your personal preferences. Discuss your options with your doctor to determine what treatment is best for you.

Most people with bladder cancer undergo surgery to remove the cancerous cells. The types of surgical procedures available to you may be based on factors such as the stage of your bladder cancer, your overall health and your personal preferences.

Early-stage bladder cancer surgery
If your cancer is small and hasn't invaded the wall of your bladder, your doctor may recommend:
- **Surgery to remove the tumor.** Transurethral resection of bladder tumor (TURBT) is often used to remove bladder cancers that are confined to the inner layers of the bladder. During TURBT, your doctor passes a resectoscope with a small wire loop through your urethra and into your bladder. The loop is used to burn away cancer cells with an electric current. Sometimes, a high-energy laser may be used instead of electric current. A catheter may be left in the bladder for several days afterward.

TURBT may cause painful or bloody urination for a few days after the procedure.

- **Surgery to remove the tumor and a small portion of the bladder.** During partial cystectomy, the surgeon removes only the portion of the bladder that contains cancer cells. Partial cystectomy may be an option if your cancer is limited to one area of the bladder that can be removed without harming bladder function. This surgery may be performed with open surgery, involving one large incision, or with robotic assistance, in which a couple of smaller incisions are made in the lower abdomen. The surgery typically involves a short hospital stay.

You may experience more frequent urination after partial cystectomy because the operation reduces the size of your bladder. Over time this may improve, but in some people it's permanent.

Invasive bladder cancer surgery
If your cancer has invaded the deeper layers of the bladder wall, your options may include:

- **Surgery to remove the entire bladder.** A radical cystectomy is an operation to remove the entire bladder, as well as surrounding lymph nodes. In men, radical cystectomy typically includes removal of the prostate gland and seminal vesicles. In women, radical cystectomy involves removal of the uterus, ovaries and part of the vagina.

Cystectomy carries a risk of infection, bleeding, blood clots and bowel obstruction. In men, removal of the prostate gland and seminal vesicles will cause infertility. In most cases, the surgeon will take care to spare the nerves necessary for an erection. Removal of the ovaries causes infertility and premature menopause in women who haven't experienced menopause prior to this surgery.

Radical cystectomy is a complex operation. It may be performed with open surgery, involving a large incision, or robotically, with several smaller incisions.

- **Surgery to create a new way for urine to leave the body.** Immediately after a radical cystectomy, the surgeon works to create a new way for your body to expel urine. Several options exist. Which is the best for you depends on your cancer, your health and your preferences. Your surgeon may create a tube (urinary conduit) using a piece of your intestine. The tube is connected to both ureters and transports urine outside of your body, where it drains into a pouch (urostomy pouch) that you wear on your abdomen.

In another procedure, the surgeon uses a section of intestine to create a small reservoir to hold urine inside your body (cutaneous continent urinary diversion). A few times each day, you can drain urine from the reservoir using a catheter through a hole in your abdomen.

Cystoscopy

Diagnostic cystoscopy is an important technique for direct examination of the urethra, the inside of the bladder and, in men, the prostate gland. In adults, the procedure is done using local anesthesia. Just before the procedure, the area around your urethral opening is anesthetized, and you remain awake during the examination. Children are usually given a general anesthetic. A flexible, narrow tube made of metal or rubber (cystoscope) is inserted through the urethra into your bladder. This tube carries a lens and a fiber-optic light so that your doctor can examine the structures through which the scope passes.

A sample of bladder tissue may be removed and examined for cancer or other diseases or a small stone. All of this can be done through the cystoscope with use of general or spinal anesthesia. Cystoscopy is useful for evaluating a range of bladder problems, including recurring infection, painful urination and cancer. In men, the procedure is used to evaluate the degree of obstruction resulting from an enlarged prostate gland.

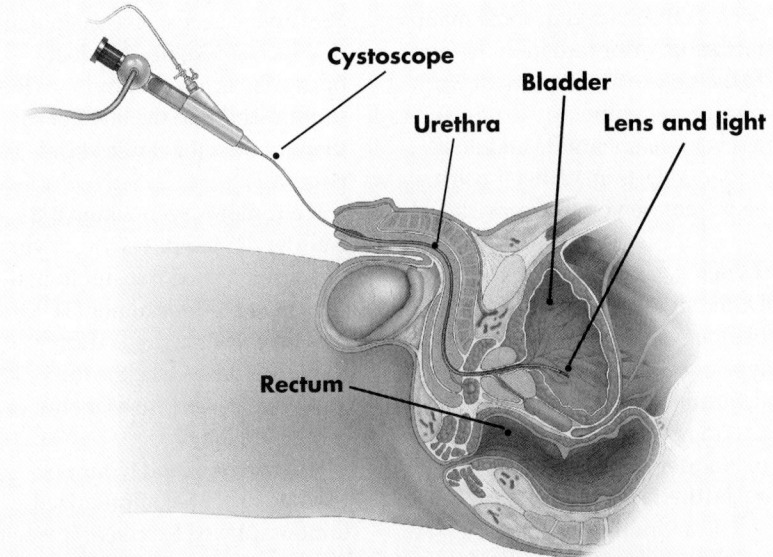

Cystoscopic examination can reveal a stone in the bladder and help identify other diseases, such as cancer. This simple procedure is most often done using local anesthesia.

In select cases, a surgeon may create a bladderlike reservoir out of a piece of your intestine (neobladder). This reservoir sits inside your body and is attached to your urethra, which allows you to urinate normally. You may need to use a catheter to drain all the urine from your new bladder. Nighttime incontinence is common with this procedure.

Intravesical therapy

Individuals with noninvasive urothelial carcinoma at high risk of tumor recurrence may undergo specific treatment in an attempt to reduce recurrence. This may include one of the following:

- **An immune-stimulating bacterium.** Bacille Calmette-Guérin (BCG) is a bacterium used in tuberculosis vaccines. BCG can cause bladder irritation and blood in your urine. Some people feel as if they have the flu after treatment with BCG.
- **A synthetic version of an immune system cell.** An interferon is a type of cell your body uses to fight infections. A synthetic version of interferon, called interferon-alfa, may be used to treat bladder cancer. Interferon-alfa is sometimes used in combination with BCG. Interferon-alfa can cause flu-like symptoms.

Intravesical chemotherapy

Several different types of chemotherapy medications are available that may be placed inside the bladder to reduce the risk of noninvasive bladder cancer recurrence. These drugs can cause irritation of the bladder, which usually gets better once the treatment is complete. The drugs are administered in a doctor's office using a urethral catheter.

Radiation therapy

In some cases, radiation therapy may be used after surgery to kill any remaining cancer cells.

Injury and Inflammation

The kidneys and other parts of the urinary tract are subject to many types of injuries and inflammation. Because of the kidneys' protected location within the body, direct traumatic injury to them is uncommon, but they are quite susceptible to injury by toxic substances. Inflammation of the urinary tract, including the kidneys, can be associated with drugs, an infection or disorders of other organs.

Injury of the kidney

Signs and symptoms

- A history or evidence of physical injury
- Blood in the urine
- Severe pain in the side
- Nausea and vomiting
- Swelling of the abdomen
- Fever
- Internal bleeding
- Shock

Traumatic injury to the kidney occurs mainly from athletic activities or industrial or motor vehicle accidents. Such injuries are relatively rare because the kidneys are protected by the rib cage and large back muscles.

Diagnosis

If you have signs or symptoms of kidney injury, your doctor will likely order blood and urine laboratory tests. He or she may also have you undergo a kidney X-ray, computerized tomography (CT), magnetic resonance imaging (MRI) or an X-ray of the arteries leading to your kidneys. This last test is useful in determining whether blood flow to your kidneys is blocked or reduced.

How serious is kidney trauma?

When a kidney is injured, most often it's merely bruised, and the bleeding stops spontaneously. Sometimes, however, complica-tions such as severe hemorrhage, infection and shock develop. After an injury to its blood vessels, a kidney's ability to function may be lost within just a few hours. In most cases, kidney injuries require hospitalization.

Treatment

Often, treatment for kidney trauma includes bed rest, pain relievers and intravenous (IV) administration of fluids to control blood pressure and stimulate urine production. Within six to 12 weeks after the injury, a CT scan may be done to make sure that the kidney is properly healed.

Rarely, if the kidney is more severely injured, it may need to be repaired or removed. Drainage of the space surrounding the kidney and repair of lacerations or a torn ureter also may be necessary. A small percentage of people with traumatic injuries to the kidneys require emergency surgery to control massive bleeding.

Injury of the bladder or urethra

Signs and symptoms

- A history of trauma
- An inability to urinate
- Blood in the urine
- Pain in the lower abdomen
- Shock

Direct traumatic injury to the bladder is uncommon because of the organ's location deep within the pelvis. The bladder may be ruptured by bone fragments after pelvic fracture, an injury that might occur, for example, in a motor vehicle accident. The bladder may also be injured during an operation such as hernia repair.

Rupture of the urethra, the narrow tube that carries urine from the bladder, is rare but requires immediate realignment or placement of a special tube. In men, most injuries to the urethra occur when a catheter is passed into an obstructed urethra for bladder drainage. In women, urethral damage is rare.

Diagnosis

If your signs and symptoms suggest a bladder or urethral injury, your doctor likely will perform a thorough examination of your abdomen and rectum. He or she may also order an X-ray to help determine if your bladder or urethra is torn.

Your doctor may also do a cystoscopic examination, which involves passing a thin, flexible fiber-optic tube up the urethra and into the bladder. Cystoscopy allows your doctor to visually inspect this part of the lower urinary tract.

How serious is injury of the bladder or urethra?

The most serious situation is a ruptured bladder that leaks urine into the abdominal cavity. This is a life-threatening situation, and it requires emergency surgery to repair the bladder wall and to remove the urine from the abdominal cavity.

A long-term complication of urethral injury is formation of a stricture. This is a severe narrowing of the urethra produced by stiffening of scar tissue. The scar tissue develops during healing and remains after the injury has healed.

Treatment

The first step is to treat shock or bleeding that may accompany the injury. They are treated with blood transfusions and fluid replacement given through a vein (intravenously). Antibiotics may be given to prevent infection.

If the bladder is ruptured, you'll need surgery. If your urethra is injured, your doctor or a urologic surgeon may need to pass a small, flexible tube (catheter) through the urethra into the bladder to provide an exit route for urine while you heal. The catheter can usually be removed after several weeks.

Urethral injuries sometimes require immediate repair, but often treatment of the injury is delayed.

Acute interstitial nephritis

Signs and symptoms
- Blood in the urine
- Excess protein in the urine
- High blood pressure
- Fever
- A rash
- Weight gain
- Fluid retention

Acute interstitial nephritis is an inflammation of the kidney that affects the tubules and small blood vessels (glomeruli) of the nephrons and the spaces between these structures (see the illustration on page 886). Most often, the inflammation is confined to the spaces.

Acute interstitial nephritis is generally associated with an allergic reaction to a drug or to a kidney condition called analgesic nephropathy. Some drugs that may cause acute interstitial nephritis include penicillin, ampicillin, medications for stomach acid reflux called proton pump inhibitors, and nonsteroidal anti-inflammatory drugs such as indomethacin (Indocin), ibuprofen (Advil, Motrin IB, others) and naproxen sodium (Aleve).

Diagnosis

In this condition, damage to the kidneys allows red blood cells and proteins to leak into the urine. Thus, a urine analysis is the first step toward making the diagnosis. Your doctor likely will also order blood tests to help assess your kidney function. He or she may also perform a kidney biopsy to confirm the diagnosis and to evaluate the extent of the damage.

How serious is acute interstitial nephritis?

Kidney damage that results from acute interstitial nephritis is often reversible. If the condition stems from use of a drug, discontinuing

use of that drug usually allows the kidney to heal. Sometimes, short-term dialysis is needed (see page 896). Near-complete recovery is the rule, although progression to chronic kidney failure may occur in rare cases.

Treatment

The first step in your treatment is to avoid drugs known to cause acute interstitial nephritis. You can reduce fluid retention and swelling by restricting your intake of salt, water and other beverages. Your doctor may prescribe medication for high blood pressure. You may need dialysis for a short time if you experience acute kidney failure. In some cases, corticosteroid drugs such as prednisone are beneficial.

Glomerulonephritis

Signs and symptoms
- Cola- or tea-colored urine
- Foamy urine
- High blood pressure
- Swelling of face, hands, feet and abdomen
- Fatigue
- Less frequent urination

Glomerulonephritis is a medical term for inflammation of the small blood vessels (glomeruli) of the kidneys' filtering structures (nephrons). The inflammation damages the membrane of the glomeruli, allowing some of the proteins and red blood cells that flow through them to be lost in the urine. It can also interfere with the glomeruli's filtering of waste products, increasing waste products in the blood.

Acute vs. chronic

The two main categories of glomerulonephritis are acute and chronic. Acute glomerulonephritis is a sudden attack of inflammation of the glomeruli. Chronic glomerulonephritis is characterized by persistent inflammation of the glomeruli and is associated with gradual kidney failure.

Causes

There are many causes of glomer-ulonephritis. It may result from conditions related to infections, immune diseases and inflammation of the blood vessels (vasculitis), as well as those that scar the glomeruli, such as high blood pressure or diabetic kidney disease.

Chronic glomerulonephritis sometimes develops after a bout of acute glomerulonephritis. Infrequently, it runs in families.

Diagnosis

Specific signs and symptoms may suggest glomerulonephritis, but the condition often comes to light when a routine urinalysis is abnormal. The urinalysis may show red blood cells, an indicator of possible damage to the glomeruli; white blood cells, a common indicator of infection; or increased protein, which may indicate nephron damage.

Other indicators such as increased blood levels of creatinine or urea also are red flags. Or, your hard-to-control high blood pressure may cause your doctor to suspect glomerulonephritis.

If your doctor suspects glomerulonephritis, you may undergo one or more of the following procedures, in addition to urine testing:

- **Blood tests.** These can provide information about kidney damage and impairment of the filtering mechanisms by measuring levels of waste products, such as creatinine and blood urea nitrogen.
- **Imaging tests.** If your doctor detects evidence of damage, he or she may recommend diagnostic studies that allow visualization of your kidneys, such as a kidney X-ray, an ultrasound examination or a computerized tomography (CT) scan.
- **Kidney biopsy.** This procedure involves using a special needle to extract small pieces of kidney tissue for microscopic examination to help determine the cause of the inflammation. A kidney biopsy is almost always necessary to confirm a diagnosis of glomerulonephritis.

How serious is acute glomerulonephritis?

In instances of acute glomerulonephritis, most children make a complete recovery and show no evidence of chronic renal disease later in life, although a very small percentage of them develop the chronic form of glomerulonephritis that may end in renal failure.

Adults generally don't do as well as children after acute glomerulonephritis. The reasons for this are unclear. Adults who've had a particularly severe initial acute form that leads to high blood

The Kidneys and Toxic Injury

The kidneys are particularly vulnerable to toxic injury because of the vast quantity of blood circulating through them at any given time. If you've been exposed to a toxin, the effect may be greater on your kidneys than on any other organs. The four most common types of toxic injury to the kidney are:

Analgesic nephropathy

Analgesic nephropathy results from long-term, excessive use of nonsteroidal anti-inflammatory drugs (NSAIDs) — such as indomethacin (Indocin) and ibuprofen (Advil, Motrin IB, others) — and long-term, excessive use of phenacetin-containing medications, which are no longer produced in the United States. Some doctors believe that excessive amounts of acetaminophen (Tylenol, others) also may damage the kidneys, but this hasn't been definitively proved.

Analgesic nephropathy occurs more often in women than in men. Incidence has decreased significantly since phenacetin was removed from most over-the-counter drugs. Signs and symptoms of analgesic nephropathy include white blood cells in the urine, anemia and high blood pressure.

Lead nephropathy

In children, lead nephropathy usually results from ingestion of lead-based paint. Adults generally

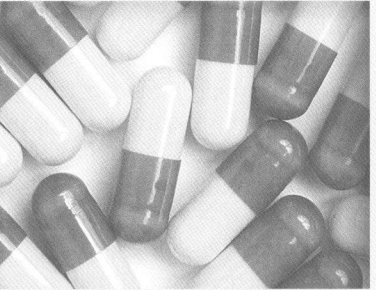

are poisoned from inhaling vapors produced when metal covered with lead-based paint is welded. Alcohol illegally distilled in an apparatus made from car radiators is another source of lead poisoning.

In children, signs and symptoms of lead poisoning may include irritability, weight loss, sluggishness and abdominal pain. Signs and symptoms of lead poisoning in adults may include gouty arthritis, high blood pressure, abdominal pain and anemia.

Acute uric acid nephropathy

Acute uric acid nephropathy results from overproduction of uric acid. It most often occurs in individuals with bone marrow and lymph node malignancies who've been treated with certain cancer medications. Signs and symptoms include diminished urine output and the presence of blood and uric acid crystals in the urine.

Solvent and fuels nephropathy

Carbon tetrachloride and other solvents and fuels have the potential for causing kidney damage. This is the reason for the warning on many commercial cleaners and sprays stating that they be used only in well-ventilated environments.

pressure or large amounts of protein in the urine are more prone to chronic kidney failure. Those who've had one attack of the disease generally recover once the kidneys heal.

Although recurrent attacks are unusual, one-third to one-half of those who do experience repeated attacks progress to renal failure.

As for chronic glomerulonephritis, the outlook depends on the cause of the disease and the severity of the complications, particularly high blood pressure and protein loss in the urine.

Most forms of chronic glomerulonephritis develop slowly and gradually lead to the loss of kidney function (chronic kidney failure). Chronic kidney failure often can be delayed through management of symptoms.

Treatment

Treatment and outcome of glomerulonephritis depend on whether you have an acute or chronic form of the disease, on the underlying cause, and on the type and severity of your signs and symptoms. Some cases of acute glomerulonephritis, especially those that follow a strep infection, often improve on their own and require no specific treatment.

To control your high blood pressure and slow the decline in kidney function, your doctor may prescribe one of several medications, including:

- Diuretics
- Angiotensin-converting enzyme (ACE) inhibitors
- Angiotensin II receptor agonists
- Calcium channel blockers
- Beta blockers

You also may receive medications such as corticosteroids or other therapies to treat the underlying cause of glomerulonephritis.

Therapies for associated kidney failure

For acute glomerulonephritis and acute kidney failure, temporary dialysis can help remove excess fluid and control high blood pressure. The only long-term therapies for end-stage kidney disease are kidney dialysis and kidney transplantation. When a transplant isn't possible, often because of poor general health, dialysis and conservative measures to help provide comfort are the remaining options.

Nephrotic syndrome

Signs and symptoms

- Large amounts of protein in the urine
- Swelling of the eyelids, feet and abdomen
- Fluid retention
- Poor appetite
- High cholesterol
- Low blood protein

Nephrotic syndrome is a group of signs and symptoms that often accompany many diseases that affect the filtering function of the kidneys' glomeruli. The syndrome is characterized by high levels of protein in urine and low levels of protein in blood, high cholesterol, and swelling of the eyelids, feet and abdomen.

The most common causes of nephrotic syndrome are diabetes, glomerulonephritis, focal segmental glomerulosclerosis, membranous nephropathy, amyloidosis, systemic lupus erythematosus and nonsteroidal anti-inflammatory drugs (NSAIDs).

In children, the average age at onset is 3 to 4 years. The majority of these children have a form of nephrotic syndrome called minimal change disease (also known as lipoid nephrosis, nil disease and foot process disease).

Minimal change disease is characterized by the signs and symptoms of nephrotic syndrome but little or no changes in the structure of the glomeruli when examined by a standard microscope. About 15 to 20 percent of the adults who have nephrotic syndrome have this form.

Diagnosis

Diagnostic tests for nephrotic syndrome include blood and urine studies. If these show large amounts of protein in the urine, your doctor may recommend removal of a sample of kidney tissue (biopsy) for evidence of a specific cause and for formulating the best treatment plan. Children less often require a renal biopsy.

How serious is nephrotic syndrome?

The seriousness of this syndrome depends on its cause and complications. As a rule, if you have minimal change disease, you can expect both remissions and relapses of excessive protein in urine. The vast majority of children and adults with minimal change disease don't progress to kidney failure.

When the syndrome is caused by infection or drugs, it often resolves after the infection is cured or the drug is discontinued. Some of the other causes of nephrotic syndrome don't have such a favorable outcome. The more persistent the nephrotic syndrome, the worse the long-term outcome.

Treatment

Treatment is aimed at alleviating symptoms and preventing complications. Predictors of a good outcome depend on how well your treatment:

- Reduces or eliminates high protein levels in your urine
- Controls your high blood pressure
- Controls or improves your decreased renal function

Several medications may be useful in reaching these goals. A corticosteroid such as prednisone is often prescribed to decrease the protein content of urine. In minimal change disease, corticosteroid therapy enhances the body's tendency toward natural remission.

Treatment usually consists of daily oral doses of prednisone for two months. When you're ready to discontinue the medication, your doctor may reduce the dosage gradually to prevent relapse.

Prednisone is a potent drug with significant side effects. The most common effects are increased appetite, weight gain and facial puffiness. Some children may require so much of the drug that their growth is temporarily delayed.

Immunosuppressive drugs such as cyclophosphamide or rituximab (Rituxan) may be given if there's no improvement with prednisone. However, these medications may cause serious side effects.

Angiotensin-converting enzyme (ACE) inhibitors also may be prescribed. Other treatment measures include restricting sodium in your diet and diuretic drugs to control fluid retention and high blood pressure.

Urinary Tract Infections

Urinary tract infections (UTIs) are common — especially among women — and lead to about 8 million doctor visits annually in the United States. A female's lifetime risk of having at least one UTI ranges from 40 to more than 50 percent.

The majority of urinary tract infections affect the lower urinary tract (bladder and urethra). Most bacteria enter the urinary tract by way of the urethra.

Under normal circumstances, these bacteria are flushed out during urination or controlled by the antibacterial properties of urine. However, certain factors increase the chance that these bacteria will take hold and multiply into a full-blown infection.

Sexual intercourse, pregnancy, urinary obstruction and the virulent nature of some bacteria all contribute to the likelihood of an infection.

The general term *urinary tract infection* is often used to describe infections that begin in the bladder (cystitis), kidney (pyelonephritis) or urethra (urethritis).

Bladder infection

Signs and symptoms
- Frequent and urgent urination
- Burning during urination
- Pressure in the lower abdomen
- Blood in the urine
- Malodorous urine

Bladder infection (cystitis) refers to inflammation of the bladder, usually from an infection. Cystitis commonly occurs in women and is often caused by sexual intercourse.

During sexual activity, bacteria that are frequently present in the lower urethral and vaginal areas are pushed up into the bladder. Once inside the bladder, the bacteria begin to multiply. Usually, the body can remove such bacteria by urination, but when it can't, cystitis may occur.

Although sexually active women between 20 and 50 years of age are the most likely to acquire cystitis, even young girls are susceptible to lower urinary tract infections because the anus, a constant source of bacteria, is so close to the female urethral opening. The vast majority of cystitis episodes are due to *Escherichia coli* (*E. coli*), a species of bacteria commonly found in the colon and rectum.

Bladder infections are uncommon in men because of the male anatomy — the urethra is much longer in men than in women, making it more difficult for bacteria to reach the bladder. When men do develop cystitis, it's often related to a problem with emptying of the bladder, such as with an enlarged prostate.

Diagnosis
A urine sample is generally used to diagnose cystitis. To collect a urine sample for laboratory analysis, you wash the vaginal area or the tip of the penis with a disinfectant, pass a small amount of urine into the toilet to flush out the urethra and then collect the next portion of voided urine midstream in a sterile cup for examination. This is called a midstream collection.

A urine culture can reveal an abnormal bacterial count and determine the type of bacteria present so that appropriate treatment can be initiated.

How serious is a bladder infection?
Although a bladder infection is uncomfortable and annoying, it isn't a serious disease.

Treatment
Some minor cases of bladder infection resolve without treatment. Most people are treated with a three- to five-day course of oral antibiotics. The symptoms usually improve within 24 to 48 hours after the first dose. More-severe cases may require treatment for up to 10 days before there's improvement.

Individuals who have more than three infections within six months may benefit from long-term, low-dose antibiotic therapy as a way to decrease the number of infections. Some women who are prone to bladder infection may further reduce their risk by taking a low dose of an antibiotic after sexual intercourse.

Other steps to reduce infections include drinking plenty of water, urinating frequently, emptying your bladder as soon as possible after sexual intercourse and wiping from front to back after a bowel movement.

Urethral infection

Signs and symptoms
- Frequent urination
- Burning pain during urination
- Pus in the urine
- In men, penile discharge

The urethra is the tube that drains urine from the bladder during urination. Urethral infection (urethritis) can be caused by the same organisms that infect the bladder, including *Escherichia coli* (*E. coli*) bacteria.

In addition, some sexually transmitted infections cause urethral infection. In women, because of the urethra's proximity to the vagina, infections caused by the herpes simplex virus or chlamydia bacteria are possible.

In men, gonococci and chlamydia bacteria cause most urethral infections. Reiter's syndrome is a combination of urethritis, arthritis and conjunctivitis (an eye inflammation) that's usually acquired through sexual contact.

Diagnosis

In women, it's difficult to differentiate a urethral infection from a bladder infection (cystitis) because the signs and symptoms of these conditions are similar. A urine sample can help in the diagnosis.

Approximately one-third of women with painful and frequent urination don't have a significant number of bacteria in their urine. This indicates that the inflammation may be in the urethra or that it may not be the result of a bacterial infection.

Your doctor will question you about your signs and symptoms. Bloody urine, a sudden onset of illness of short duration and a history of previous similar infections suggest that a bacterial infection is causing the inflammation. If the illness began gradually more than seven days before the examination and no blood is in your urine, the symptoms may be from chlamydia infection, particularly if you've recently changed sex partners.

How serious is a urethral infection?

In most cases of urethritis, the infection goes away after treatment. When urethritis caused by gonorrheal or chlamydial infection is left untreated, it can lead to much more serious problems, such as pelvic inflammatory disease, stricture of the urethra, prostatitis,

epididymitis, sterility, arthritis, meningitis and inflammation of the heart.

Chlamydia and gonorrhea are sexually transmitted infections. If you have them, notify your sexual partner or partners. During treatment, abstinence or the use of condoms can help prevent spread of the infection.

Treatment

Treatment for urethritis depends on the cause of the infection. For chlamydia infection, an antibiotic such as tetracycline may be taken for a week or so. For gonorrhea, the drugs ceftriaxone and azithromycin are often prescribed. Some strains of gonorrhea are resistant

to penicillin. If laboratory tests indicate that this is the case, a different medication is prescribed. Antibiotics may also be prescribed for other bacterial infections. In some situations, your doctor may advise that your sexual partner also be treated.

Acute kidney infection

Signs and symptoms

- Pain in the side
- High fever
- Shaking chills
- Vomiting
- Burning pain during urination
- Needing to urinate frequently

Sometimes bacteria travel up the ureters to the upper urinary

Urinary Tract Infections and Sexual Intercourse

Some women experience frequent, painful urination after sexual intercourse. The symptoms generally last for a day or two and then disappear, only to recur the next time they have sex.

This problem is a bladder infection that's sometimes called honeymoon cystitis, although it's actually a form of chronic urethral infection (urethritis). It's generally the urethra, not the bladder, that's inflamed. Sometimes laboratory tests don't reveal any microorganisms that could be responsible, and some women, even after treatment with an antibiotic, continue to experience symptoms whenever they have intercourse.

To make these infections less likely, there are a few things that you can do. Follow safe sex practices. Empty your bladder immediately after intercourse and drink plenty of water to help flush bacteria out of your urethra. You might also try using a water-soluble lubricant during intercourse to make penetration easier and urethral inflammation less likely.

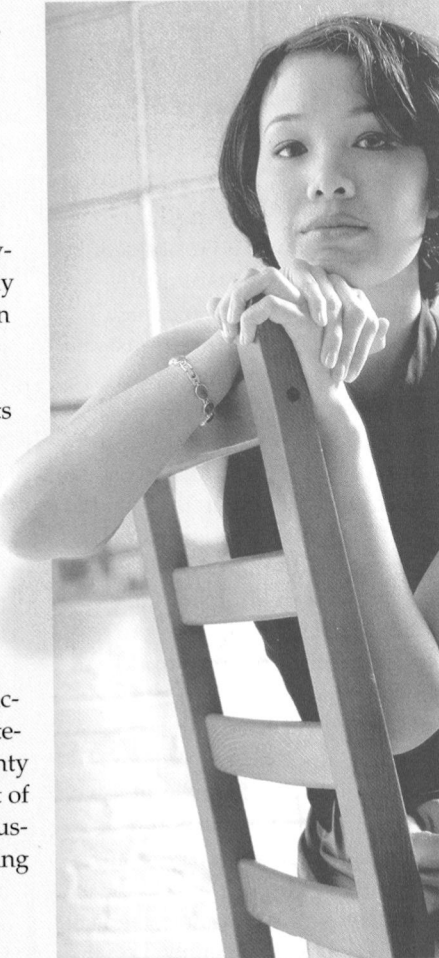

tract, which includes the kidneys, causing an acute kidney infection (acute pyelonephritis).

Diagnosis
Providing a urine sample and taking a culture of the sample should reveal if you have a bacterial infection. There's no simple test to differentiate a kidney infection from a lower urinary tract infection, but the presence of fever and side pain suggests that the infection extends into the kidney.

How serious is an acute kidney infection?
When properly treated, an acute kidney infection rarely progresses to chronic kidney (renal) disease, but it can lead to a bloodstream infection (sepsis) and be life-threatening in an older adult in poor health or an individual with a weakened immune system. A kidney infection can also recur if the bacteria aren't totally eradicated.

Treatment
Antibiotics are the first line of treatment. When recurrences are frequent or the kidney infection becomes chronic, your doctor may look for an underlying problem, such as an obstruction or urine flowing backward from the bladder into the ureter (vesicoureteral reflux). He or she may use a computerized tomography (CT) scan, an ultrasound examination or other diagnostic tests to search for a hidden cause.

Urinary Tract Infections in Men

Although urinary tract infections (UTIs) are more common in women, they also affect men.

The classic symptoms are a painful sensation when you urinate and difficulty urinating. Even when you feel the urge, you may not be able to pass urine freely, or you release only a small amount. The urge quickly returns. Most UTIs aren't dangerous if you get proper care. If you have pain in your abdomen or back, chills, fever, or vomiting, your kidneys may be infected. A kidney infection is a more serious medical condition requiring prompt treatment.

The most common cause of UTIs is the *Escherichia coli* (*E. coli*) bacterium. It resides in your intestinal tract and may migrate through your lymph system to your bladder. Inflammation of the bladder (cystitis) is frequently due to infection with *E. coli*. Some other factors also can promote urinary tract infections in men:

Prostate problems
Your prostate gland is the size of a walnut and situated below your bladder, surrounding your urethra. A urinary tract infection can occur if your prostate gland enlarges and constricts your urethra, preventing your bladder from emptying completely. Leftover (residual) urine creates a breeding ground for bacteria. Enlargement of the

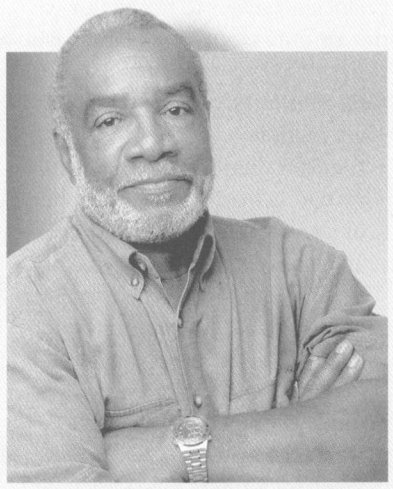

prostate gland is a normal part of aging, but infection isn't.

Invasive medical procedures
A catheter inserted into the urethra can introduce bacteria, especially if the catheter stays in place for several days.

Narrowed urethra
Frequent inflammation of your urethra (urethritis) can lead to scarring of your urethra (urethral stricture). In years past, strictures were usually associated with recurrent bouts of a sexually transmitted infection, such as gonorrhea. Today, they're more commonly associated with trauma from catheters or instruments used to evaluate or treat urologic problems.

Dehydration
An inadequate intake of fluids can lead to concentrated (stagnated) urine and possibly a UTI.

Other Urinary Disorders

Although urinary tract infections are the most common urinary disorders, other conditions also can cause urinary problems.

Urinary incontinence

Signs and symptoms
- Involuntary urination
- Small amounts of urine escaping under pressure, such as during a cough or sneeze

Urinary incontinence refers to the inability to keep urine in your bladder until you decide to void, resulting in an accident. The problem has varying degrees of severity. Some people experience occasional, minor leaks of urine. Others wet their clothes frequently.

Urinary incontinence can have several causes. The muscular and neurological systems that control the retention and release of urine are complex. These systems can be affected by illness, medications, urinary tract infections, prostate gland problems or complications of an operation. Neurological disorders such as Alzheimer's disease, Parkinson's disease, multiple sclerosis and stroke are some conditions that can cause incontinence.

In children, bed-wetting is common. After puberty, however, urinary incontinence is rare until the later decades of life. Many people age 65 and older experience incontinence. In general, urinary incontinence is more frequent in women than in men.

Types

Often, incontinence occurs either because your bladder muscle contracts involuntarily or because your pelvic muscles and tissues are too weak to withstand the pressures in the bladder. The two main types of urinary incontinence are stress incontinence and urge incontinence. A combination of the two is called mixed incontinence.

Stress incontinence

With stress incontinence, leakage occurs in response to some kind of physical activity that increases pressure on your abdominal area, such as sneezing, coughing or lifting something heavy.

Women past menopause and those who have given birth are especially susceptible to stress incontinence. It's often associated with a loss of strength in pelvic support tissues. This weakening can result in a downward displacement (prolapse) of the uterus and vaginal tissues or a shift of the bladder and urethra. Being overweight and having some chronic medical conditions also can cause stress incontinence.

Urge incontinence

With urge incontinence, leakage occurs when your bladder contracts on its own and overpowers your urinary sphincter, which is the circular band of muscle fibers in your urethra that holds back urine flow. Prevalence of this condition increases with age. This type of incontinence may also stem from a low-grade urinary infection or an abnormality of the bladder muscle.

Diagnosis

A complete physical examination, focusing on your abdomen and genitals, may give clues to your incontinence. Your doctor will look for reasons for your incontinence, such as a urinary tract infection, a mass or compacted stool. If the cause of your incontinence is harder to find, your doctor may want to do some tests.

Common tests

They include:
- **Bladder diary.** Your doctor may go over a bladder diary that he or she has asked you to complete at home over several days. You record how much you drink, when you urinate, the amount of urine you produce, whether you had an urge to urinate and the number of incontinence episodes. To measure your urine, your doctor may give you a pan that fits over your toilet rim. The pan has markings like those on a measuring cup. Keeping a bladder diary can be tedious, but it gives your doctor important information.
- **Urinalysis.** A sample of your urine is sent to a laboratory, where it's checked for signs of infection, traces of blood or other abnormalities. For the sample to be collected, you're asked to urinate into a container. A urine culture is a lab test that specifically checks for signs of infection in your urine. A urine cytology involves a check of your urine for cancer cells.
- **Blood test.** Your doctor may have a sample of your blood drawn and sent to a laboratory for analysis. Your blood is checked for various chemicals and substances related to causes of incontinence.

Specialized tests

If further testing is needed, you'll likely be referred to a doctor who specializes in urinary disorders (urologist). Women might be referred to a doctor who focuses on urological problems in women (urogynecologist). You may undergo additional testing such as:
- **Postvoid residual (PVR) measurement.** This test helps your doctor determine whether you have difficulty emptying your bladder. For the procedure, you're asked to urinate (void) into a funnel-like container that allows your doctor to measure your urine output. Then your doctor measures the amount of residual urine in your bladder using a catheter — a small, flexible tube that's inserted into your urethra and bladder to drain any remaining urine — or an ultrasound device. For the ultrasound test, a computer transforms sound waves into an image of your bladder so that your doctor can see how full or empty it is. A large amount of leftover (residual) urine in your bladder may mean that you have an obstruction in your urinary tract or a problem with your bladder nerves or muscles.
- **Pelvic ultrasound.** Ultrasound may be used to view other parts of your urinary tract or genitals to check for abnormalities.
- **Stress test.** For this test, you're asked to cough vigorously or bear down as your doctor watches for loss of urine.
- **Urodynamic testing.** These tests measure pressure in your bladder both at rest and when filling. A doctor or nurse inserts a catheter into your urethra and bladder. The catheter is used to fill your bladder with water while a pressure monitor measures and records the pressure within your bladder. This test helps your doctor measure the strength of your bladder muscle and the health of your urinary sphincter.
- **Voiding cystourethrogram.** For this X-ray of your bladder,

a catheter is inserted into your urethra and bladder. Through the catheter, your doctor injects a fluid containing a special dye. As you urinate and expel this fluid, images show up on a series of X-rays. These images help reveal problems with your urinary tract.

- **Cystoscopy.** In this procedure, a thin tube with a tiny lens (cystoscope) is inserted into your urethra. With the aid of this device, your doctor can check for — and potentially remove — abnormalities in your urinary tract.

How serious is urinary incontinence?

Although bothersome, urinary incontinence generally isn't medically serious. However, in trying to determine the cause of the leakage, your doctor may find underlying disorders that may require treatment.

Treatment

Treatment for urinary incontinence depends on the type of incontinence, the severity of your problem and the underlying cause. Your doctor will recommend the approaches best suited to your condition. Often a combination of treatments is used. Most people treated for urinary incontinence see a dramatic improvement in their symptoms. The success of your treatment depends most of all on the right diagnosis.

Behavioral techniques

Behavioral techniques and lifestyle changes work well for certain types of urinary incontinence. Your treatment may include:

- **Pelvic floor muscle exercises.** These exercises strengthen your urinary sphincter and pelvic floor muscles — the muscles that help control urination. Your doctor may recommend that you do these exercises frequently to treat your incontinence. They are especially effective for stress incontinence, but may also help urge incontinence. To do pelvic floor muscle exercises (Kegels), see "Strengthening Your Pelvic Muscles," below.
- **Bladder training.** Bladder training involves learning to delay urination after you get the urge to go. You may start by trying to hold off for 10 minutes every time you feel an urge to urinate. Then try increasing the waiting period to 20 minutes. The goal is to lengthen the time between trips to the toilet until

Strengthening Your Pelvic Muscles

If you urinate involuntarily at times, it may be a result of weakened muscles. Exercise can improve pelvic muscle condition and tone, allowing you greater control over your bladder.

Although these exercises are best taught by a doctor, nurse or therapist, here are some tips on how to do them.

Women

Bladder training exercises for women are sometimes called Kegel exercises, after the physician who developed them in the 1950s.

- Starting with an empty bladder, contract the muscles that you use when you try to stop urine flow. When you contract them, you should feel a pulling. An effective Kegel exercise will cause the vagina to tighten.
- Pull in the muscles and hold for a count of three. Then relax for a count of three. Work up to 10 to 15 repetitions each session.
- For best results, do the exercises at least three times a day and in different positions — standing, lying down and sitting.

It may take three to six weeks to notice an improvement in bladder control. As the tone in your pelvic floor muscles increases, you should have better bladder control. As a bonus, many women find that they also become more sexually responsive.

Men

Weakened pelvic muscles in men sometimes occur after prostate surgery.

To improve your bladder control, you need to exercise two groups of muscles: those that you tighten when you want to stop a bowel movement or hold back gas in the rectum and those at the base of the penis that you use to expel final drops of urine or ejaculate semen.

- Tighten the muscles you use to stop a bowel movement.
- While tightening these muscles, tighten muscles at the base of the penis. You may feel your penis pull in slightly toward your body.
- Hold both sets of muscles.
- Relax the muscles.

Perform this exercise once a day before going to bed, preferably in a sitting position. Don't overexercise, as your muscles may become tired and you may experience more leakage. Once you achieve urinary control, continue to perform this exercise to keep these muscles in good condition.

you're urinating only every two to four hours.

Bladder training may also involve double voiding — urinating, then waiting a few minutes and trying again. This exercise can help you learn to empty your bladder more completely to avoid overflow incontinence.

- **Scheduled toilet trips.** This means timed urination — going to the toilet according to the clock rather than waiting for the need to go. After this technique, you go to the toilet on a routine, planned basis.
- **Fluid and diet management.** Sometimes, you can regain control of your bladder by modifying your daily habits. This may involve cutting back or avoiding alcohol or caffeine, if either causes you incontinence. If acidic foods irritate your bladder, you may want to cut back on such foods to see if that rids you of your problem. For some people, reducing the amount of liquid they drink before bedtime is all that's needed.

Medications
Sometimes, urinary incontinence can be corrected with the help of medications. Often, medications are used in conjunction with behavioral techniques. Medications used to treat incontinence include:

- **Anticholinergic (antispasmodic) drugs.** These prescription medications calm an overactive bladder, so they may be helpful for urge incontinence. Examples include oxybutynin (Ditropan XL), tolterodine (Detrol), darifenacin (Enablex), fesoterodine (Toviaz), solifenacin (Vesicare) and trospium. The drugs can be effective at controlling incontinence, but dry mouth is a side effect with some. To combat dry mouth, you may be tempted to drink more water, but that may not help your incontinence. Some of the medications come in extended-release forms or as a skin patch. These forms may have fewer side effects.
- **Mirabegron (Myrbetriq).** Used to treat urge incontinence, this medication relaxes the bladder muscle and can increase the amount of urine your bladder can hold. It may also increase the amount you are able to urinate at one time, helping to empty your bladder more completely.
- **Alpha blockers.** In men with urge or overflow incontinence, these medications relax bladder neck muscles and muscle fibers in the prostate and make it easier to empty the bladder. Examples include tamsulosin (Flomax), alfuzosin (Uroxatral), silodosin (Rapaflo), terazosin and doxazosin (Cardura).
- **Topical estrogen.** Applying low-dose, topical estrogen in the form of a vaginal cream, ring or patch may help tone and rejuvenate tissues in the urethra and vaginal areas. This may reduce some of the symptoms of incontinence.

Electrical stimulation
In this procedure, electrodes are temporarily inserted into your rectum or vagina to stimulate and strengthen pelvic floor muscles. Gentle electrical stimulation can be effective for stress incontinence and urge incontinence, but it takes several months and multiple treatments to work. And it can cause side effects, such as abdominal cramps, diarrhea and bleeding. Electrical stimulation is usually reserved for people with severe urge incontinence who don't respond to other therapies.

Medical devices
Several medical devices are available to help treat incontinence. They're designed specifically for women and include:

- **Urethral inserts.** These are small, tampon-like disposable devices or plugs that are inserted into the female urethra — the narrow tube where urine exits the body — to prevent urine from leaking out. Urethral inserts aren't for everyday use. They work best for women who have predictable incontinence during certain activities, such as playing tennis. The device is inserted before the activity. If you need to urinate, you simply removes the device. Urethral inserts are available by prescription.
- **Pessary.** Your doctor may prescribe a pessary — a stiff ring that you insert into your vagina and wear all day. The device helps hold up your bladder, which lies near the vagina, to prevent urine leakage. You need to regularly remove the device to clean it. You may benefit from a pessary if you have incontinence due to a dropped (prolapsed) bladder or uterus.

Interventional therapies
These treatments include the following:

- **Bulking material injections.** Some women and men with stress incontinence benefit from urethral injections of bulking agents. This procedure involves injecting bulking materials — such as collagen, carbon particle beads or synthetic sugars — into the tissue surrounding the urethra or the skin next to the urinary sphincter. The injection tightens the seal of the sphincter by bulking up the surrounding tissue. The procedure is done with minimal anesthesia and typically takes about two to three minutes. It usually needs to be repeated after several months, because the effect can be lost over time. There is a risk of rejection or infection.
- **Botulinum toxin type A (Botox).** Injections of Botox into the bladder muscle may benefit people who have an overactive bladder. Botox is generally prescribed to people only if other first line medications haven't been successful.

- **Nerve stimulators.** A device resembling a pacemaker is implanted under your skin to deliver painless electrical pulses to the nerves involved in bladder control (sacral nerves). Stimulating the sacral nerves can control urge incontinence if other therapies haven't worked. The device may be implanted under the skin in your buttock and connected directly to the sacral nerves or may deliver pulses to the sacral nerves via a nerve in the ankle.

Surgery

If other treatments aren't working, surgery may be necessary. Surgical procedures include:

- **Sling procedure.** The most popular and common surgery for women with stress incontinence is the sling procedure. During this procedure, a surgeon removes a strip of abdominal tissue and places it under the urethra. Or the surgeon may use a strip of synthetic mesh material or a strip of tissue from a donor (xenograft). The strip acts like a hammock, compressing the urethra to prevent leaks that occur with the activities of daily living. Sling procedures improve or cure incontinence in most cases. There are varying techniques for the sling procedure, so talk with your doctor about what procedure is planned and why.
- **Bladder neck suspension.** In this procedure, your surgeon makes a small incision in your lower abdomen. Through this incision, he or she places stitches (sutures) in the tissue near the bladder neck and secures the stitches to a ligament near your pubic bone (Burch procedure) or in the cartilage of the pubic bone itself (Marshall-Marchetti-Krantz operation). This has the effect of bolstering your urethra and bladder neck so that they don't sag. The downside of this procedure is

that it involves major abdominal surgery performed under general anesthesia. Recovery takes about six weeks, and you'll likely need to use a catheter until you can urinate normally.
- **Prolapse surgery.** In women with mixed incontinence and pelvic organ prolapse, surgery may include a combination of a sling procedure and prolapse surgery.
- **Artificial urinary sphincter.** This small device is particularly helpful for men who have weakened urinary sphincters from treatment of prostate cancer or an enlarged prostate gland. It's rarely used in women with stress incontinence. Shaped like a doughnut, the device is implanted around the urethra. The fluid-filled ring keeps your urinary sphincter shut tight until you're ready to urinate. To urinate, you press a valve implanted under your skin that causes the ring to deflate and allows urine from your bladder to be released. This surgery is the most effective procedure for male stress incontinence associated with treatment of prostate cancer or an enlarged prostate gland.

Chronic urethral infection

Signs and symptoms
- Discomfort during urination that persists or recurs
- Frequent urination
  Sometimes the urethra may remain irritated and inflamed for weeks or months, with or without evidence of a bacterial infection. This is known as chronic urethral infection (chronic urethritis). You may feel the need to urinate frequently, and doing so is uncomfortable. As your inflamed urethra undergoes periods of healing, it may gradually narrow.
  Inflammation that extends into the bottom of your bladder is called trigonitis.

Diagnosis
In order to determine whether you have chronic urethritis and trigonitis, your doctor will probably insert a thin, flexible fiber-optic tube (cystoscope) into your urethra and bladder. A urinalysis can indicate the presence of bacteria. Your doctor also may ask you if you use any douches, washes or laundry detergents that may contain irritating chemicals.

How serious is chronic urethral infection?
Left untreated, chronic urethral infection may eventually lead to narrowing of the urethra and kidney infection. Most of the time, a cause can be identified and the condition properly treated.

Treatment
If an infection is present, your doctor may prescribe antibiotics or sulfa drugs. If no infection is evident, your doctor may prescribe phenazopyridine (Pyridium) to relieve your discomfort. Your doctor may also advise you to discontinue using any possible irritants to see if your condition improves.

Interstitial cystitis

Signs and symptoms
- Persistent, urgent need to urinate
- Frequent urination
- Pelvic pain
- Pelvic pain during sexual intercourse
  Interstitial cystitis is an inflammation of the bladder wall, but with no apparent cause. This uncommon condition usually affects women in their childbearing years. The symptoms are similar to those of a bladder infection (cystitis), including a frequent urge to urinate and burning or cramping while voiding. Intercourse may be painful as well. Men may experience painful ejaculation. The condition isn't the result of an infection, but it's also

not a more serious problem such as cancer.

It's likely that many people with interstitial cystitis have a defect in the protective lining (epithelium) of the bladder. A leak in the epithelium, for example, may allow toxic substances in urine to irritate the bladder wall.

Diagnosis

A diagnosis of interstitial cystitis is generally arrived at by ruling out all other possible causes for the symptoms, such as infection, cancer or bladder overactivity. Your doctor may examine your bladder lining and determine your bladder's capacity with a thin, flexible fiber-optic instrument called a cystoscope. In some cases, he or she may take a sample of tissue for microscopic analysis (biopsy).

Another test sometimes done is a potassium sensitivity test. Your doctor places two solutions — water and potassium chloride — one at a time into your bladder. If you feel more pain or urgency with the potassium solution than with the water, you may have interstitial cystitis. People with normal bladders can't tell the difference between the two solutions.

How serious is interstitial cystitis?

Interstitial cystitis isn't life-threatening, but the difficulty in identifying the disorder and the lack of a specific treatment can make it a disabling condition.

Treatment

No simple treatment exists to eliminate the signs and symptoms of interstitial cystitis, and no one treatment works for everyone. You may need to try various treatments.

Oral medications

Medications that may improve the signs and symptoms of interstitial cystitis include ibuprofen (Advil, Motrin IB, others) and other non-steroidal pain medications

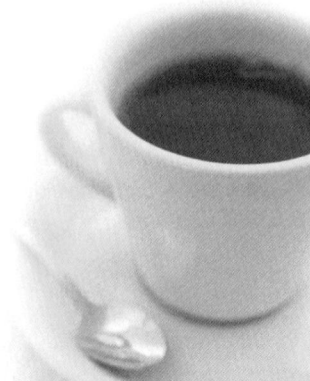

to relieve discomfort. Tricyclic antidepressants, such as amitriptyline or imipramine (Tofranil), may help relax your bladder and block pain. Antihistamines may provide symptom relief for some people.

Your doctor may also prescribe pentosan (Elmiron), an oral medication approved by the Food and Drug Administration specifically for interstitial cystitis. How it works is unknown, but it may restore the inner surface of the bladder, which protects the bladder wall from substances in urine that could irritate it. It may take two to four months before you begin to feel pain relief and up to six months to experience a decrease in urinary frequency.

Nerve stimulation

Nerve stimulation techniques include:

- **Transcutaneous electrical nerve stimulation (TENS).** With TENS, mild electrical pulses relieve pelvic pain and, in some cases, reduce urinary frequency. TENS may increase blood flow to the bladder. This may strengthen the muscles that help control the bladder or trigger the release of substances that block pain. Electrical wires placed on your lower back or just above your pubic area deliver electrical pulses — the length of time and frequency of therapy depends on what works best for you.

- **Sacral nerve stimulation.** Your sacral nerves are a primary link between the spinal cord and nerves in your bladder. Stimulating these nerves may reduce urinary urgency associated with interstitial cystitis. With sacral nerve stimulation, a thin wire placed near the sacral nerves sends electrical impulses to your bladder, similar to what a pacemaker does for your heart. If the procedure decreases your symptoms, you may have a permanent device surgically implanted. This procedure doesn't manage pain from interstitial cystitis, but may help to relieve some symptoms of urinary frequency and urgency.

Bladder distention

Some people notice a temporary improvement in symptoms after undergoing cystoscopy with bladder distention. Bladder distention is the stretching of the bladder with water or gas. If you have long-term improvement, the procedure may be repeated.

Medications instilled into the bladder

In bladder installation, your doctor

places the prescription medication dimethyl sulfoxide (Rimso-50) into your bladder through a small, flexible tube (catheter) inserted through the urethra. The solution sometimes is mixed with other medications, such as a local anesthetic, and remains in your bladder for about 15 minutes. You urinate to expel the solution.

You might receive dimethyl sulfoxide (DMSO) treatment weekly for six to eight weeks, and then have maintenance treatments as needed — such as every couple of weeks, for up to one year.

A newer approach to bladder instillation uses a solution containing the medications lidocaine, sodium bicarbonate, and either pentosan or heparin.

Surgery

Doctors rarely use surgery to treat interstitial cystitis because removing the bladder doesn't relieve pain and can lead to other complications.

People with severe pain or those whose bladders can hold only very small volumes of urine are possible candidates for surgery, but usually only after other treatments fail and symptoms affect quality of life.

Surgical options include:

- **Fulguration.** This minimally invasive procedure involves inserting an instrument through the urethra to burn off ulcers present with interstitial cystitis.
- **Resection.** This is another minimally invasive method that involves insertion of instruments through the urethra to cut around any ulcers.
- **Bladder augmentation.** In this procedure, a surgeon increases the capacity of your bladder by putting a patch of intestine on the bladder. However, this is performed only in very specific and rare instances. The procedure doesn't eliminate pain, and some people need to empty their bladders with a catheter many times a day.

Overactive bladder

Signs and symptoms

- A strong, sudden urge to urinate
- Involuntary loss of urine
- Frequent urination

An unstable (overactive) bladder is one that contracts uncontrollably at times. It's one of the causes of urge incontinence. You may need to urinate so suddenly and urgently that you can't make it to the bathroom. This problem is fairly common. Sometimes, an infection is to blame, but often the cause remains unclear, although aging is frequently suggested as a primary cause.

Diagnosis

The first step in diagnosing overactive bladder is to rule out other causes of urinary leakage, such as infection. To do this, your doctor will likely want a urine specimen for laboratory analysis. You may also have a special kind of X-ray (intravenous pyelogram or computerized tomography) to visualize your bladder, kidneys and urinary drainage structures.

Other tests may include viewing the inside of the bladder and urethra, measuring the pressure and function of the bladder (urodynamic testing), and determining if your bladder empties completely when going to the bathroom.

How serious is an overactive bladder?

An overactive bladder can be distressing, but it isn't dangerous.

Treatment

Your doctor is likely to recommend a combination of treatments.

Behavioral interventions

Behavioral interventions can help you manage overactive bladder. If you experience urge incontinence, these interventions alone aren't likely to result in complete dryness, but they will likely reduce the number of incontinence episodes. The interventions include watching your fluid consumption, training your bladder to delay voiding when you feel an urge to urinate, scheduling toilet trips so that you urinate at the same time every day, and doing pelvic floor muscle exercises, called Kegel exercises (see page 913). If you're overweight, losing weight may help ease symptoms.

Medications

Medications that relax the bladder can be helpful for relieving symptoms of overactive bladder and reducing episodes of urge incontinence. These drugs include tolterodine (Detrol), oxybutynin (Ditropan XL), trospium, solifenacin (Vesicare), darifenacin (Enablex), mirabegron (Myrbetriq) and fesoterodine (Toviaz).

Side effects of many of these drugs include dry eyes and dry mouth, but drinking water to quench thirst can aggravate symptoms of overactive bladder. Constipation — another potential side effect — can aggravate your bladder symptoms. Some of the drugs are available in extended release forms or as a skin patch or gel and may cause fewer side effects.

Sucking on a piece of sugar-free candy or chewing sugar-free gum may help relieve dry mouth. Use eyedrops to keep your eyes moist.

Bladder injections

OnabotulinumtoxinA (Botox) is a toxin from the bacteria that cause botulism illness. Used in small doses directly injected into bladder tissues, this protein partially paralyzes muscles.

Clinical research shows that it may be useful for severe urge incontinence. The temporary effects generally last five months or more, but repeat injections are necessary.

About half of people who receive Botox injections experience side effects, including urinary retention. If you're considering Botox treatments, you should be willing and able to catheterize yourself if urinary retention occurs.

Nerve stimulation

Regulating the nerve impulses to your bladder can improve overactive bladder symptoms.

One procedure uses a thin wire placed close to the sacral nerves — which carry signals to your bladder — where they pass near your tailbone. This surgical procedure is often done with a trial of a temporary wire or as an advanced procedure in which the permanent electrode is implanted and a longer trial is performed prior to a surgical placement of the battery-powered pulse generator. Your doctor then uses a device connected to the wire to deliver electrical impulses to your bladder, similar to what a pacemaker does for the heart.

If the treatment successfully reduces your symptoms, the wire is eventually connected to a small battery device that's placed under your skin.

Surgery

Surgery to treat overactive bladder is reserved for people with severe symptoms who don't respond to other treatments. The goal is to improve the bladder's ability to store urine and reduce pressure in the bladder. However, these procedures won't help relieve bladder pain. Interventions include:

- **Surgery to increase bladder capacity.** This procedure uses pieces of your bowel to replace a portion of your bladder. This surgery is used only in cases of severe urge incontinence that doesn't respond to other, more-conservative treatments. If you have this surgery, you may need to use a catheter intermittently for the rest of your life to empty your bladder.
- **Bladder removal.** This procedure is used as a last resort and involves removing the bladder and surgically constructing a replacement bladder (neobladder) or an opening in the body (stoma) to attach a bag on the skin to collect urine.

Urethral stricture

Signs and symptoms

- A slow, weak urine stream
- Dribbling
- Split stream

A urethral stricture is a narrowing of the tube that transports urine from the bladder to the outside. In extreme instances, the urethra can become totally obstructed. The condition is most common in men.

Causes of urethral stricture include an infection or a disease that produces scar tissue in the urethra and, in men, injury to the penis. Urethral stricture may develop years after an acute episode of gonorrhea.

Diagnosis

Your doctor will likely perform various tests to rule out other causes, including examination of the urethra with a thin, flexible instrument called a cystoscope.

How serious is urethral stricture?

The stricture may narrow to the point that it blocks urine flow, causing acute urinary retention. This requires quick relief. Treatment usually works well, but recurrence of the stricture is common.

Treatment

Often, the first approach is to stretch the urethra by dilating it with progressively wider instruments that are inserted into the urethra. This treatment often must be repeated a number of times. If the passageway doesn't remain open after repeated dilations, surgery may be necessary.

In one procedure, the surgeon uses a knife to cut away the fibrous tissue that's blocking the urethra. A special type of laser also may be used.

Another other option is to remove the affected section of the urethra. The healthy ends are then reattached or a graft is used to replace the damaged urethra. ■

Bones, Joints and Muscles

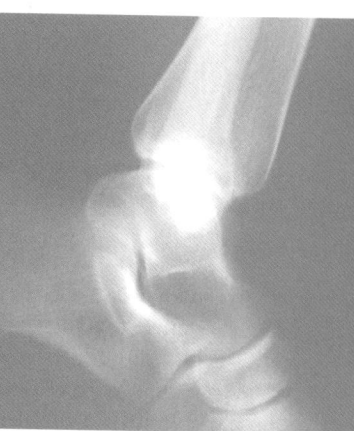

How Your Bones, Joints and Muscles Work

The musculoskeletal system is a marvel of mechanics. Made up of muscles, bones, ligaments and tendons, it allows you to move in myriad ways — walking, running, bending, stretching, sitting and much more.

Most bones in this remarkable system are interconnected by joints, essentially hinges that allow the bones to move. Some joints move differently. The hips and shoulders are ball-and-socket joints, and the backbone (vertebral column) has limited movement.

Besides providing mobility, your musculoskeletal system also protects your internal organs. Your ribs surround your lungs and heart, your skull protects your brain, and your spine protects your spinal cord.

Until this amazing system breaks down — whether due to accident, disease, or general wear and tear over time — it's easy to take the workings of your bones, joints and muscles for granted. Breakdowns can occur at any time and for various reasons.

Components of your musculo-skeletal system work together to keep the human body functioning. Here's a look at the various roles they play.

Bones

Your body houses 206 bones. They're composed of osseous tissue, which is made of various substances, including proteins, minerals and bone cells. The proteins form a framework into which minerals — especially calcium and phosphate — become incorporated.

Bone is made up of two types of tissue. The spongy inner layer is called cancellous bone. The hard outer layer is known as cortical bone.

Despite its stable appearance, bone is always changing in a process called remodeling. It's constantly being torn down by cells called osteoclasts, reabsorbed and then rebuilt by cells called osteoblasts.

Your bones provide support for your body and function as your body's storehouse for important minerals. Inside certain bones is the marrow, a soft core that manufactures blood cells.

Joints

The ends of bones that meet in a joint are cushioned with a layer of cartilage, which absorbs some of the shock or weight involved in movement.

Your joints also contain a liquid called synovial fluid, a membrane, a protective casing called the capsule and bands of fibrous tissue called ligaments. Ligaments join bones together and help make the joint stable.

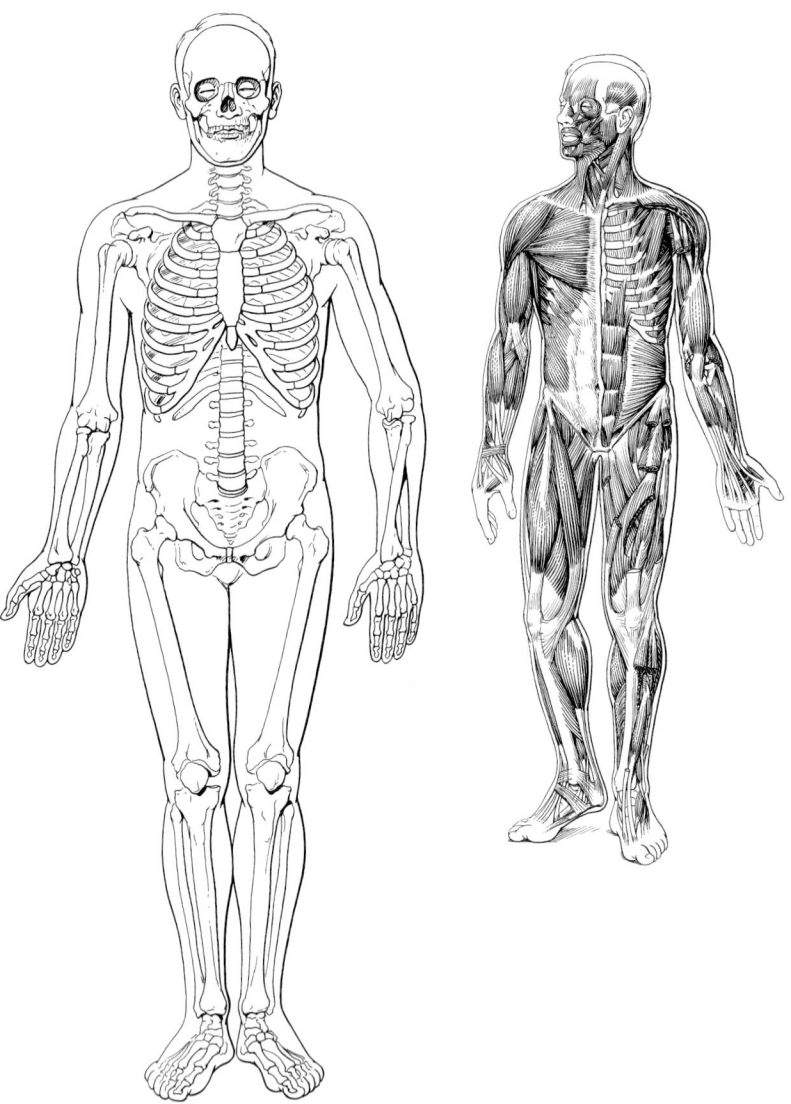

Your bones are living tissue and are always changing. They provide support for your body and function as your body's depository for important minerals.

Many of your skeletal muscles are paired, enabling your body to move. Tendons connect skeletal muscles to your bones.

Musculoskeletal Specialists

Several types of medical specialists deal with problems of the musculoskeletal system.

Rheumatologists

A rheumatologist is a doctor who has special training in diagnosing and treating diseases of the muscles and joints, especially inflammatory or autoimmune illnesses, such as rheumatoid arthritis or lupus erythematosus.

Orthopedists

An orthopedist is a surgeon who has special training in managing disorders of the body's moving parts, including the skeleton, joints, muscles, ligaments and cartilage. An orthopedist may recommend nonsurgical or surgical treatment.

Physiatrists

A physiatrist is a specialist in physical medicine and rehabilitation — a doctor who is specially trained to help restore and maximize the function of injured or damaged joints, muscles, and limbs. Physiatrists also teach methods to condition the musculoskeletal system and protect joints from further injury. Physiatrists provide nonsurgical management of musculoskeletal injuries and often work closely with physical and occupational therapists.

Endocrinologists

An endocrinologist is a doctor who has special training in diagnosing and treating diseases of the hormone system, including metabolic bone diseases due to hormone excess or deficiency. This includes diseases such as osteoporosis, osteomalacia and Paget's disease.

Physical therapists

A physical therapist is a licensed professional who designs programs — including therapeutic exercise and pain management strategies — to help in rehabilitation and recovery after an injury or illness. Physical therapists aren't medical doctors, and they can't prescribe medications.

Occupational therapists

An occupational therapist is a licensed professional who focuses on the function of the upper limbs. Often, occupational therapists work in collaboration with physical therapists. Occupational therapists offer training in how to perform daily tasks following an injury or illness that has impaired upper body movement.

Muscles

Some 650 muscles primarily help move your body. Your muscles are made of fibers that can contract, which enables them to shorten and lengthen, producing movement. Tendons connect your muscles to your bones.

Most muscles are paired with another muscle that works in opposition to it, such as the biceps and triceps muscles in your arm. When you bend your arm at the elbow, your biceps contract, and when you extend your arm, the opposing triceps contract.

Not all muscles move your skeleton. In addition to the skeletal (striated) muscles, you have smooth (nonstriated) muscles. You can find smooth muscles in internal organs, such as the stomach, uterus and bladder, and in the walls of blood vessels. They're usually arranged in sheets. Doctors call them involuntary muscles because they're under autonomic rather than conscious control. The heart (myocardium) is a special type of involuntary muscle. Smooth muscles and the heart muscle aren't part of the musculoskeletal system.

Common Injuries

Although the body's musculoskeletal system is extremely durable, muscle and bone injuries are common. A fall or an accident can stress and break a bone, overstretch muscles, and extend a joint beyond its usual range of motion.

Whether from falling out of the backyard apple tree as a child or from tripping while playing tennis as an adult, most people experience a variety of musculoskeletal injuries during their lifetimes — though often minor, some can be severe.

Bone fracture

Signs and symptoms

- A swelling or bruising over a bone
- Deformity of a limb
- Localized pain that intensifies when the affected area is moved or pressed
- Loss of function in the area of the injury
- A bone that perforates the skin

When a bone can't withstand the physical force exerted on it, it breaks (fractures). Fractures are common. Most people sustain one or more during their lifetimes.

Fractures can be classified into several categories. A simple fracture is one in which the bone breaks into two pieces. A comminuted fracture is one in which the bone fragments into several pieces. When the bone protrudes through the skin, it's called an open (compound) fracture (see page 36).

Fractures are also categorized according to the way the bone breaks. If the bone snaps completely into two or more parts, it's called a complete fracture. If the bone cracks but doesn't separate, it's an incomplete fracture. If one fragment of bone is embedded into another fragment of bone, it's called an impacted fracture.

Another type of fracture occurs in people with bones weakened by disease. When diseased, bones may fracture spontaneously or with only minor stress exerted on them. Such breaks are termed pathologic fractures because the principal cause is an underlying disease or a cancer that has spread to the bone.

Severity of fractures often increases with age. Children's skeletons are flexible, so their bones are more likely to bend than to break. As a result, when a child fractures a bone, it's often an incomplete fracture. Conversely, falls or other accidents that generally don't affect younger bones can cause complete fractures in older adults, whose bones are more likely to be brittle.

A stress fracture, another type of break, is really a hairline crack that often is invisible on an X-ray for up to six weeks after the onset of pain.

When a bone breaks, damaged blood vessels between the ends of the broken bone will clot, preventing further bleeding. Cells called osteoclasts reabsorb the damaged bone. A soft callus made of fibrous protein (collagen) develops as the bone begins to regenerate with the help of cells called osteoblasts. These cells build a mesh of spongy bone on the collagen, creating an internal splint that links the fractured bone ends. Eventually, this mesh is replaced by denser bone, resulting in a healed fracture.

Diagnosis

A bone protruding from the flesh makes the diagnosis obvious. In some instances, though, identifying a fracture isn't easy. Soft tissue injuries and fractures often produce similar signs and symptoms.

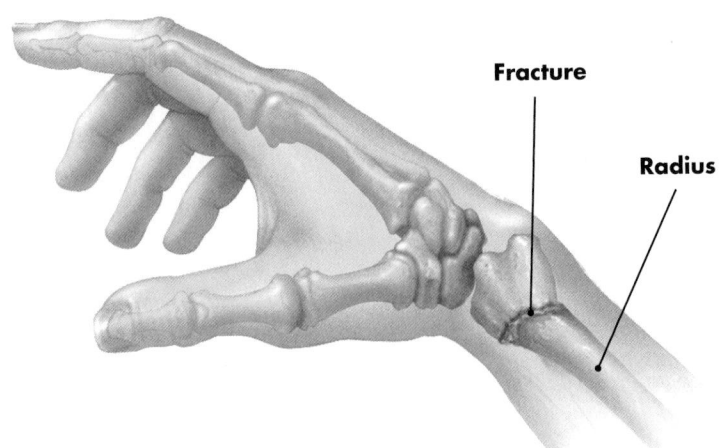

Fracture

Radius

A Colles' fracture is a common type of fracture. It occurs at the end of the radius, just below the wrist. You may feel a sharp pain in your wrist, especially when moving your hand in a circular motion.

An X-ray taken from two or more angles helps confirm the diagnosis (see image on page 1266). In the case of a suspected skull fracture or the fracture of a vertebra, a doctor may order a computerized tomography (CT) scan or magnetic resonance imaging (MRI). An MRI or a bone scan is sometimes used to detect a stress fracture.

How serious is a bone fracture?

The seriousness of a bone fracture depends on the location of the break and the damage to the bone and adjacent tissues. Some fractures require only temporary protection, such as using crutches to bear weight or a splint to immobilize the broken bone. For more-serious fractures, dangerous complications can occur if you don't receive medical treatment.

With any fracture, your doctor should examine the adjacent area carefully to establish if there's additional damage to nerves or blood vessels. Injuries to the skull or spine might put you at risk of brain injury or spinal cord damage.

The time it takes a broken bone to heal varies with the age and health of the person with the fracture and the nature and location of the fracture. In children, a minor break may heal within a few weeks. In older adults, a serious fracture often requires months to heal.

Sometimes a fracture that's healing particularly slowly may require a procedure in which tissue taken from another bone is grafted onto the fracture to fill in bone and stimulate healing. The source of bone for a graft is often the pelvis (iliac bone). With prompt and proper treatment and a good rehabilitation program, you can usually expect a complete recovery.

Treatment

All suspected fractures should be treated with proper first aid and evaluated by a doctor. To heal properly, a bone that has been displaced must be put back (set) in its proper position. Setting (realignment) of the bone is called reduction. When this can be done without surgery, it's called a closed reduction. You're given an anesthetic to numb the area so that your doctor can reposition the bone using X-rays as a guide.

Surgery

When surgery is necessary to set or repair a fracture, the procedure is called an open reduction. You're given an anesthetic, and the doctor makes an incision to gain access to the broken bone so that it can be restored to its proper position.

A fracture that's unstable or one that's immediately adjacent to or extending into a joint may require a device such as a rod, pin, plate or screw to hold it in place. During a surgical procedure, an orthopedic surgeon fastens the device to the bone to position and stabilize the broken parts. Advantages of this approach include early mobility of the joint and some use of the injured limb within weeks rather than months.

In rare instances, it's better to insert an artificial joint, especially in an older adult with osteoporosis or another disorder that has led to deterioration of the bone or joint.

Casts and splints

If you have a broken arm or leg, your doctor may put a cast on it to immobilize it. Preventing motion between the two ends of the bone reduces pain and facilitates healing.

First, a layer of soft material is applied to cover your arm or leg, protecting the skin from irritation. Next, the arm or leg is covered with a layer of bandages saturated with plaster, fiberglass or plastic. As the cast dries, it becomes rigid. Be careful to avoid changing the cast's shape while it dries. Because flattening the cast can put pressure on your skin beneath the plaster, don't rest the cast on a flat surface. Use pillows instead.

For some fractures, a doctor may apply a splint. This device immobilizes and supports an injured, displaced, or deformed limb or joint. Often, splints are used instead of a cast to prevent motion of a dislocated joint or of the ends of a fractured joint.

In some cases, no device is needed. The mass of chest muscles that surround a broken rib, for example, hold it in place. With a broken finger, your doctor may simply tape it to an adjacent finger.

Ultrasound

If a fracture isn't healing properly, your doctor may use low-intensity ultrasound, applied to the skin over a fracture through a transducer for about 20 minutes a day. The sound wave pulses jiggle the bone, a motion that is believed to promote healing.

Electromagnetic stimulation

Although controversial, electromagnetic stimulation may be another way to aid healing. An electromagnetic current is directed to the area over the fracture site for several hours a day. At the same time, a cast is usually worn for several months to stabilize the fracture. A person with a fracture that fails to heal may opt for electromagnetic stimulation in the hopes of avoiding surgery.

Rehabilitation

After the bone has been set in its proper position and immobilized, the next step in treatment is rehabilitation. This process begins as soon as possible, even with the broken bone still in a cast.

A rehabilitation program generally follows the principle of relative rest, meaning the injured tissue rests while the rest of your body engages in exercise or activity. Movement of adjacent tissues increases blood flow, enhances healing and prevents the formation of potentially dangerous blood clots, which can form in the vessels of immobilized limbs. Movement also helps maintain muscle tone. And it can limit wasting (atrophy) of muscles and withering of bones from prolonged immobilization. Rehabilitation also helps prevent stiffness that can occur in unused joints.

Medication

In most cases, a doctor will prescribe medication to relieve pain and, on occasion, antibiotics to reduce the risk of infection.

Hip fracture

Signs and symptoms
- Severe pain in your hip or groin
- Inability to bear weight on your injured leg
- Bruising and swelling in and around your hip area
- Shorter leg on the side of your injured hip
- Turning inward or outward of your leg on the side of your injured hip

You can break your hip at any age, but 90 percent of hospitalizations for hip fractures are for people older than age 65. As you age, your bones slowly lose minerals and become less dense. Gradual loss of density weakens bones and makes them more likely to fracture.

Hundreds of thousands of Americans are hospitalized each year because of hip fractures. Doctors expect that number to grow as the U.S. population ages. Women are two to three times more likely than men to fracture a hip. That's because women lose bone density at a greater rate than men do. The drop in estrogen levels in women during and after menopause accelerates bone loss and increases the risk of hip fractures.

The direct cause of a hip fracture often is an accident or a fall, even a relatively minor fall. The underlying cause, especially as you get older, is likely to be osteoporosis.

In osteoporosis, your bones don't contain adequate calcium and other minerals and your bone structure weakens. Loss of bone strength tends to be greatest in your spine, lower forearms and upper thighbones (femurs), the site of hip fractures.

Diagnosis

Often, your doctor can determine that you have a hip fracture based on a history of injury and your symptoms and by observing the abnormal position of your hip and leg. An X-ray can confirm that you have a fracture and show exactly what part of your hip is fractured.

Most hip fractures occur in one of two locations along your femur, the long bone that extends from your pelvis to your knee:
- **The femoral neck.** The femoral neck is located in the upper

portion of your femur, the ball part of the ball-and-socket joint.

- **The intertrochanteric region.** This region is the portion of your upper femur that juts outward.

How serious is a hip fracture?

A hip fracture is a serious injury, particularly if you're older. Although the fracture itself is treatable, complications can be life-threatening, especially in older adults.

Doctors rarely treat unstable (displaced) hip fractures without surgery because bed rest and traction are associated with serious complications. The risk of traction is that it keeps you immobile for a long period, during which you can develop blood clots in one or both legs. You can also develop a blood clot in a leg after hip surgery, especially if you don't get up and move around. This blood clot can break off and travel to and become lodged in a lung artery, blocking blood flow to lung tissue. This condition, called pulmonary embolism, can be fatal unless treated promptly.

Fortunately, surgery to repair a hip fracture is usually very effective, although recovery often requires time and patience. Most people, even those older than age 80, make a good recovery from a hip fracture. Generally, the better your health and mobility, the better your chances for a full recovery.

Treatment

Surgery is almost always the best way to repair a broken hip. Doctors typically use nonsurgical alternatives only if the fracture is stable or you have other medical problems that make surgery too risky. The type of surgery you have generally depends on the nature and severity of the hip fracture and your age.

Femoral neck fractures
Surgeons generally repair this type of fracture by one of three methods:

- **Internal fixation.** If, following the break, bones can be properly aligned, your doctor may insert metal screws or a plate and screws into the bone to hold it together while the fracture heals. This is called internal fixation.
- **Partial hip replacement.** If the ends of the broken bone are severely damaged and the blood supply to the femoral head is compromised, your doctor may remove the head of the femur and replace it with a metal prosthesis. This is known as hemiarthroplasty.
- **Total hip replacement.** This procedure involves replacing your upper femur and the socket in your pelvic bone with artificial prostheses. Total hip replacement is a common operation to treat severe arthritis of the hip joint, but it's rarely used to treat a hip fracture.

In general, the more complex the fracture and the older you are,

Hip Fractures
Most hip fractures occur in one of two locations — the femoral neck or the intertrochanteric region.

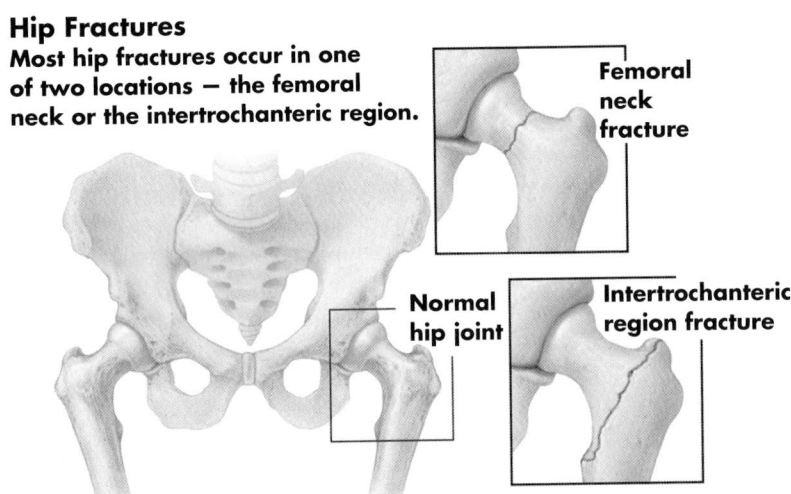

Femoral neck fracture

Normal hip joint

Intertrochanteric region fracture

Hip Fracture Repair Techniques
For a fracture in the femoral neck, total hip replacement, partial hip replacement or internal fixation may be used.

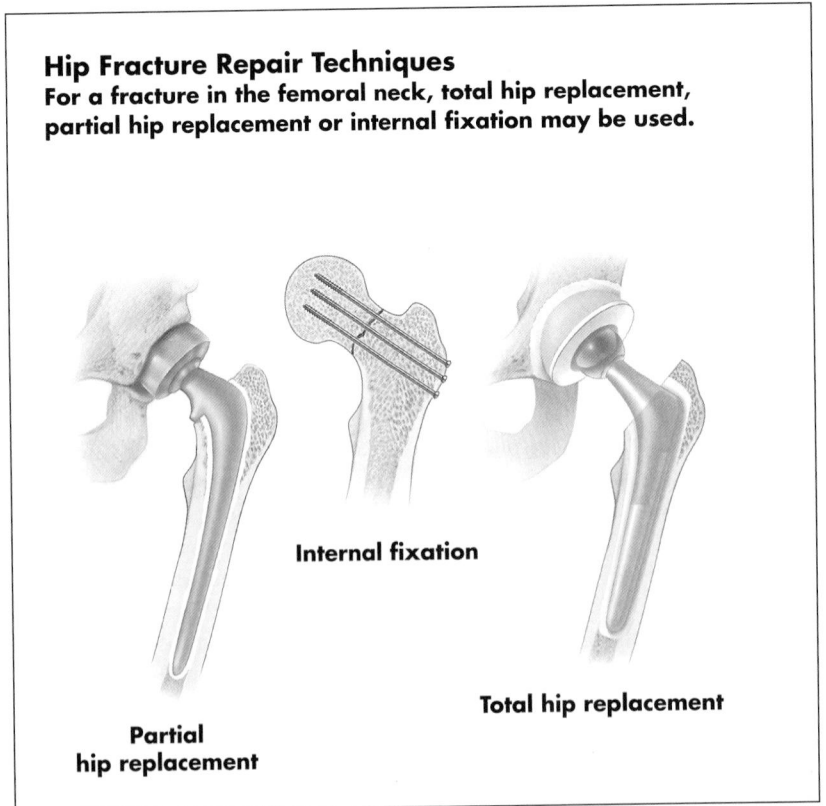

Internal fixation

Partial hip replacement

Total hip replacement

Hip Protectors

A step that won't prevent you from falling but may protect you if you do is to wear a hip protector. These padded, externally worn protectors are similar to what hockey players wear to avoid injury. One study involving active older adults found that wearing hip protectors reduced the risk of a hip fracture from a fall by more than 60 percent.

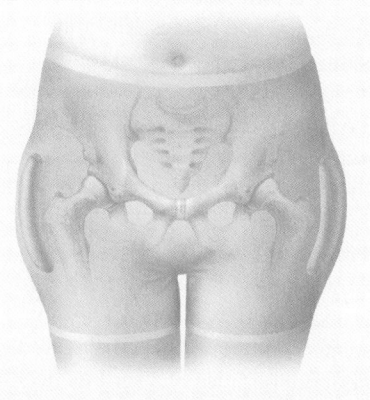

The protectors are small enough that they can be worn under a skirt or pants, and they don't limit activity such as walking or sitting.

the more likely you are to receive a hip prosthesis. Internal fixation is used more in younger people and for fractures that are less complex and well-aligned.

Intertrochanteric region fractures
To repair this type of fracture, a doctor usually inserts a metal plate and screw device to fix the fracture. The screw is attached to a plate that runs down alongside the femur and is attached with other screws to help keep the bone stable. As the bone heals, the screw allows the bone pieces to compress, so the edges grow together. Another method of fixing this type of fracture is to insert a long rod inside the bone. Cross screws help stabilize the rod within the bone to promote healing.

Recovery
Recovering from a hip fracture involves a lengthy period of rehabilitation. The goal of rehabilitation is to help you regain full mobility. You'll learn how to gradually place more weight on your hip until it can bear your full weight. You'll also learn how to sit, stand and walk so that you don't re-injure your hip or damage your prosthesis, if you have one.

After a hip fracture, you'll likely need the help of a walking aid, such as a cane, walker or crutches, for several months. You may

also need help getting around your home and doing daily tasks. About half the people older than age 65 who break a hip enter an extended-care facility for at least part of their recuperation because they need assistance that's unavailable at home.

Prevention
These steps can help you guard against hip fracture by reducing your risk of falls:

- **Fall-proof your home.** Keep your home well-lit and free of situations that might cause you to trip and fall. Avoid area rugs and exposed electrical cords. Place furniture where you're unlikely to bump into it. Consider installing grab bars in your bathroom, stair treads on steps and handrails along stairways.
- **Wear sensible shoes.** If you're older, wear thinner, hard-soled, flat shoes. Resilient-soled athletic shoes may impair your

balance and contribute to falls. Avoid wearing high heels or sandals with light straps. Avoid wearing shoes that are either too slippery or too sticky.

- **Avoid dangerous activities.** Be careful doing tasks that require you to climb a ladder or step-ladder. Avoid lifting heavy objects, climbing and engaging in unusually vigorous activities.
- **See your eye doctor.** Poor eyesight is a common cause of falls. If you're having trouble seeing, have your eyes checked.
- **Be mindful of medication side effects.** Feeling weak or dizzy is a side effect of many medications. This can increase your risk of falling. Talk to your doctor about possible side effects caused by your medications.

Joint dislocation

Signs and symptoms
- A joint that slips out of place after being subjected to a blow, fall or other trauma
- Swelling, intense pain and, frequently, immobility of the affected joint

A joint dislocates when the ends of bones are forced from their normal positions. As a result, the joint no longer functions properly. In addition, the displaced bones may damage the structure in or around the joint, including muscles, ligaments, nerves and blood vessels.

In some cases, the cause of a dislocation is an underlying disease or disorder, such as rheumatoid arthritis or a defective ligament. Some people who sustain repeated

Nursemaid's Elbow

Nursemaid's elbow is a common and often misdiagnosed dislocation of part the elbow. It typically occurs in children younger than age 5, usually when an adult or another child pulls or jerks a child's arm. The immature elbow dislocates easily because it can't withstand the stress.

The child typically experiences pain and limited mobility in the elbow. An X-ray may be taken to rule out any other problems. As the bones are easily returned to their proper position, the pain resolves.

dislocations have such a congenital weakness, which may allow some joints to dislocate spontaneously.

Diagnosis

After you sustain a dislocation, it becomes difficult, if not impossible, to move your joint. Trying to move it is likely to intensify the pain. Usually, you can see a change in the alignment of the joint and there's swelling.

If your doctor suspects a dislocation, an X-ray usually helps him or her confirm the diagnosis and determine if you also have an accompanying fracture.

How serious is a joint dislocation?

It depends on which joint is affected. A serious neck or back injury may result in a dislocated vertebra, which poses a risk of spinal cord damage and paralysis. A serious shoulder or hip dislocation could result in nerve damage.

In many cases, a doctor can correct a simple dislocation nonsurgically without damage to surrounding nerves and tissues. The joint is immobilized for a short time — typically about two weeks — while the injury heals. Some dislocations require surgery to repair or reconstruct damaged ligaments.

Treatment

Any suspected dislocation should be examined by a doctor. If you suspect someone has a dislocated vertebra because of a serious neck or back injury, don't move the injured person. Wait for emergency medical personnel to arrive.

A dislocation usually needs treatment as quickly as possible. The displaced bones in the joint must be returned to their proper positions by a procedure called reduction. If the injury remains untreated for more than half an hour, increased swelling and pain often makes it more difficult to reduce the dislocation.

Immobilize the affected area and transport the injured person to a doctor or hospital emergency department. It's important that only a person with proper training provide treatment because improper attempts at repositioning the joint can cause additional damage to the joint and adjacent structures.

Immobilization

After a joint has been returned to its normal position, it may be necessary to immobilize it. Most often a splint is used.

Rehabilitation

Rehabilitation begins after the joint is back in its proper position and immobilized, even if the joint is in a cast. Movement stimulates blood flow in adjacent tissues and enhances the healing process. Movement also helps maintain muscle tone and limits the wasting of muscles and weakening of bone from prolonged immobilization. It also helps prevent the joint stiffness that extended disuse may cause.

Follow your doctor's advice about limiting physical activity of the affected joint. Returning to full

Absence or Loss of a Limb

Some people are born without one or more of their limbs, generally because of a developmental defect. Other individuals lose a limb because of an injury or disease. Doctors perform surgical amputations for a variety of reasons. Some people with advanced diabetes develop poor circulation in their extremities that can result in ulcers and gangrene and necessitate amputation of a foot or leg.

The best treatment for certain bone cancers may require amputation of an arm or a leg. Removing a limb through amputation is a major operation. In addition to drawing on the body's healing capacity, an amputation also requires significant psychological adjustment — learning to live with altered physical capacities and an altered body image.

Risks

Amputation that results from an accident has additional risks, including blood loss and shock. As with any invasive procedure, there's also the risk of infection, which is greater if a limb is severed in an accident than if it's removed surgically.

In most cases, though, an amputation isn't life-threatening. The biggest challenge often is dealing with the consequences of the amputation, which range from coping with the pain of the surgery to making major adjustments to your lifestyle.

Surgical removal of a body part can also be emotionally demanding. There may be pain in the residual limb or the sensation that the limb or part of the limb is still present (phantom limb sensation). In addition, amputation can affect an individual's self-image, self-confidence and sense of self-worth.

Reattaching a severed body part

Surgeons have made remarkable advances in recent years in reattaching severed fingers, hands and even limbs. With the help of a microscope, surgical repairs and reattachments of tiny structures, such as blood vessels and nerves, are possible. The results depend on many factors, but tend to be more successful for hand or finger reattachments than for arms, and more successful for arms than for legs.

If the severed body part has had proper care and a trained surgeon is readily available, chances of a successful reattachment are good. The function of the reattached finger, hand or limb varies from person

activity too soon increases your risk of re-injuring the joint.

Medication

To manage the pain, your doctor may recommend that you take a pain reliever (analgesic).

Severed tendon

Signs and symptoms

* A deep cut in an arm or leg
* An inability to move a finger, toe or whatever joint is near the cut

A deep cut in a hand, foot, arm or leg can damage the fibrous tissues that connect muscle to bone called tendons. Severing a tendon may result in an inability to move the affected joint.

A severed tendon requires two kinds of attention. First, the wound must be cleansed and closed to aid healing and prevent infection. Second, the tendon must be repaired surgically. Sometimes, both can be done in one procedure, when the wound is treated. However, in some cases, the cut should heal before an operation to repair a tendon is performed. Generally, reattachment is done within a week of the injury.

Diagnosis

The key sign suggesting a severed tendon is an inability to move a finger, toe or other joint in the area of an injury. Your doctor may want an X-ray of the affected area in case you also have a fracture.

How serious is a severed tendon?

In most cases, timely repair of a severed tendon allows the affected area to return to nearly normal. However, you may experience stiffness and a decrease in the range of movement of a related joint.

Treatment

A severed tendon usually requires surgery and rehabilitation.

Surgery

When a tendon is severed, one part may retract and be difficult for a surgeon to retrieve. As a result, a long surgical incision may be required. In some instances, doctors use tissue from another tendon to repair the damaged one.

Rehabilitation

After an operation, the area you've injured probably will be immobilized. Your doctor may recommend an exercise program when it's time for you to resume physical activity.

Doctors often recommend passive exercise during the recovery period to help prevent long-term stiffness. These exercises involve movements that place minimal stress on the injured tendon.

Muscle strain

Signs and symptoms

* Localized pain when a muscle injury occurs, followed by tenderness and possibly swelling
* Stiffness or tenderness a day after you overwork the muscles in an area of your body

to person. In some instances, the reattached part regains most or all of its usefulness. In others, sensitivity, flexibility and strength remain impaired.

Use of a prosthesis

If a severed limb can't be reattached or if your limb is amputated due to disease, a replacement part (prosthesis) is generally the next best option. A prosthesis can never replicate the movement, flexibility, strength and sensitivity of your original body part. Yet once you adjust to it, a prosthesis can help you live more fully.

As the surgical wounds heal, exercises are important for keeping your remaining muscles in condition and your joints mobile. Then the process of fitting you for a prosthesis begins, starting with a temporary one. A training process helps you master the different movements involved in using the prosthesis.

Gradually, you'll be able to wear the prosthesis all day. After you've adjusted to the temporary prosthesis, a specially designed prosthesis can be fabricated. A permanent prosthesis is tailored to meet your

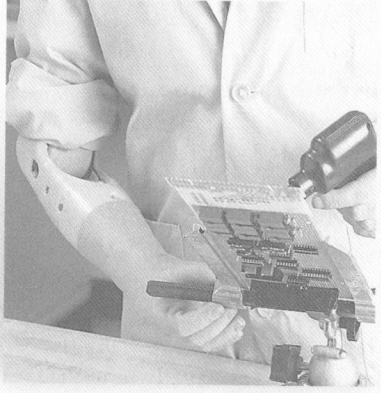

specific needs. It can strike a balance between physical demands for mobility and strength and concern with appearance.

In general, leg prostheses work better than arm prostheses. A person with a prosthetic leg is more likely to use his or her prosthesis than is someone with a prosthetic arm.

Rehabilitation

After an amputation, a doctor or physical therapist can outline a program of rehabilitation. Frequently, it's a team approach that involves physical and occupational therapists under the guidance of a physician who specializes in physical medicine and rehabilitation (physiatrist).

The goal of rehabilitation is to help you achieve as normal a life as possible. The program may include exercises to help you maintain or increase the strength of your remaining muscles. If you need a prosthesis or other equipment, the program may include additional exercises. Other components generally include counseling, detailed instruction on proper use of a prosthesis and learning new ways to perform daily tasks.

Sports Injuries

Most injuries that occur during athletic activity result from unusual demands placed on bones, muscles or other tissues. A novice runner who completes five miles the first day will likely have undreamed-of aches and pains the next morning. The over-40 former athlete who comes out of retirement for the company softball game is an excellent candidate for sprains and strains.

You can't expect to go through life without injury. However, a few sensible rules will help you avoid inconvenient, painful, expensive and, at times, disabling injuries.

Warm up first
Give your muscles a chance to warm up before you exercise. Before you start running, for instance, walk or march in place for five minutes and then stretch your muscles for another five minutes. Don't stretch cold muscles before warming them up. The increased blood flow reduces tension in your muscles, improves their range of motion and flexibility, and may even increase your level of performance. This reduces your risk of muscle strains and other injuries.

Cool down afterward
It's just as important to cool down your muscles after a workout as it is to warm them up before you exercise. The muscles you use contract during a workout, and repetitive activities can cause them to shorten. Stretching after the workout is critical for maintaining flexibility.

Muscles that aren't kept flexible through stretching are more likely to sustain strains.

Pace yourself
Sudden and unfamiliar exertion increases the risk of injuries. If you want to improve your performance, do so at a sensible pace.

Don't increase your distance or the duration of your exercise by more than 10 percent a week. Develop a program that allows your body to adjust gradually to the challenges you're giving it.

Select an appropriate activity
If you have a painful back or perpetually sore knees, the pounding of running isn't for you. You might try swimming or riding a stationary bicycle instead. Whatever activity you choose, make sure your technique is as good as possible. Take lessons and have an expert watch you perform. Imperfect technique and overuse often lead to injury.

Make it a habit
Working out only once a week, no matter how vigorous the activity, fails to provide you with maximal aerobic and conditioning benefits and puts you at risk of injury. Try to establish a schedule of at least 30 minutes of activity most days of the week. And keep this advice in mind: Don't play your sport to get in shape. Get in shape to play your sport.

Give injuries their due
If you do sprain an ankle or twist a knee, get medical advice. Then follow it. A key to recovery is what doctors commonly refer to as the tincture of time. Allow the injury to heal before you use that body part too vigorously. Make sure the injury is properly rehabilitated and ready to withstand the stresses of your sport or activity.

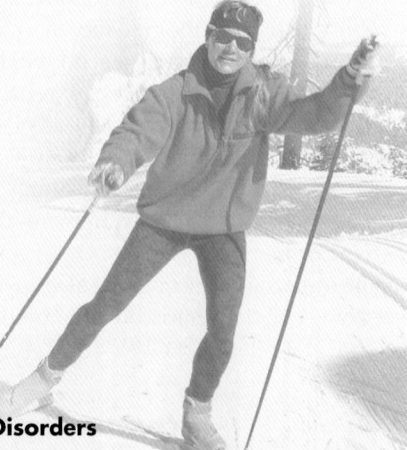

- An inability to use the muscle

Excessive demand on a muscle may strain it. This is also known as a pulled muscle. Overstretching or overworking a certain area of your body may cause minor muscle strains. The muscle doesn't lose strength, but it's sore.

A more serious muscle strain occurs when some of the fibers of a muscle actually tear, causing your muscle to contract and bleed internally. Occasionally, the muscle may rupture, either partially or, in rare instances, entirely.

One of the most common muscle strains occurs in the group of muscles at the back of the thigh (the hamstrings), especially in people who run or water ski.

The hamstrings enable you to flex your knee and extend your thigh, motions used in running. Pain or muscle weakness at the back of your thigh may indicate an injury to your hamstrings.

A second common muscle injury is a groin pull. When you sustain a groin pull, the tendons and muscles in your groin — including the lower abdominal, leg and pelvic muscles — may be stretched or torn. This may result from repetitive overuse or a single injury and cause pain or muscle spasms in the groin area.

Diagnosis
Discomfort in the involved area, which may include tenderness, muscle spasms and swelling, is the key to diagnosis. An X-ray can rule out bone injury as a cause of the problem at the site of the tendon attachment.

How serious is a muscle strain?
Muscle strains often respond to rest and simple self-care measures. But if you suspect that a muscle has ruptured or a bone is fractured, or if the pain persists for more than a few days, see a doctor.

Treatment
Apply ice or cold packs to the injured area for about 20 minutes

at a time several times a day for the first few days after injury. You may be able to prevent or reduce swelling by elevating the injured limb and using a compression wrap such as an elastic bandage. Don't bind it tightly. Try not to use the injured muscle until the pain subsides.

Medication

For minor muscle pulls, acetaminophen (Tylenol, others), aspirin or an over-the-counter nonsteroidal anti-inflammatory drug (NSAID) such as ibuprofen (Advil, Motrin IB, others), may help reduce the pain. Use aspirin only if there's no sign of bleeding. For moderate or more-severe muscle strains, your doctor may prescribe an anti-inflammatory drug, a muscle relaxant or a prescription pain reliever, depending on the injury.

Surgery

If the injury is severe enough to rupture the muscle, surgical repair is usually needed.

Prevention

You can avoid many muscle strains with appropriate conditioning that includes warming up before exercising and stretching afterward. If you experience recurrent muscle pulls, then you may benefit from a program of muscle development to strengthen weak muscles.

Sprain

Signs and symptoms

- Rapid swelling, sometimes accompanied by discoloration of the skin
- Impaired joint function or a feeling of instability
- Pain and tenderness in the affected area
- An audible popping sound
- Difficulty using the joint

A wide range of injuries are referred to as sprains, but a true sprain involves damage to the ligaments, the tough bands of connective tissue that attach bone to bone

Heat vs. Cold

After you sprain a ligament or strain a muscle, it's best to use cold treatment for one to three days after the injury to reduce swelling and inflammation. Swelling damages cells by decreasing the oxygen supply to surrounding tissues. Cold applications slow metabolism of cells within the area and allow the tissue to survive a temporary lack of oxygen. This promotes the renewal or repair of cells and speeds healing. Cold also constricts blood vessels to minimize bleeding and relieves pain by acting as a local anesthetic. Most bleeding associated with acute inflammation resolves within one to three days.

To relieve muscle spasms, minor sprains and strains, apply cold treatment intermittently for 24 to 72 hours. After this time period, some people find that heat lessens pain from the injury and improves stiffness. If you try heat, apply it only after swelling and bleeding have stopped. Heat may complicate early recovery by causing more swelling and bleeding. For chronic symptoms, use either heat or ice, whichever feels better.

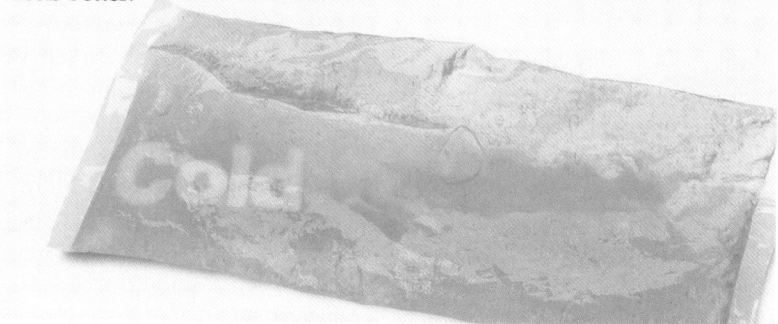

in a joint. Sprains most commonly occur in the ankles and knees.

A sprain occurs when a traumatic event, such as a fall or collision, causes your joint to move beyond its normal range of movement and a ligament stretches or tears.

Diagnosis

You can sprain any joint. With a sprain, the joint may be able to function or may feel unstable. Movement and pressure over the ligament are painful.

If the joint can't function, the injury may include a fracture or dislocation. If you suspect a fracture or serious ligament damage — or if the pain and your difficulty in moving the joint don't go away within two or three days — seek medical care. Your doctor may order an X-ray to check for a fracture.

How serious is a sprain?

In general, the greater the pain, the more serious the injury. Sprains

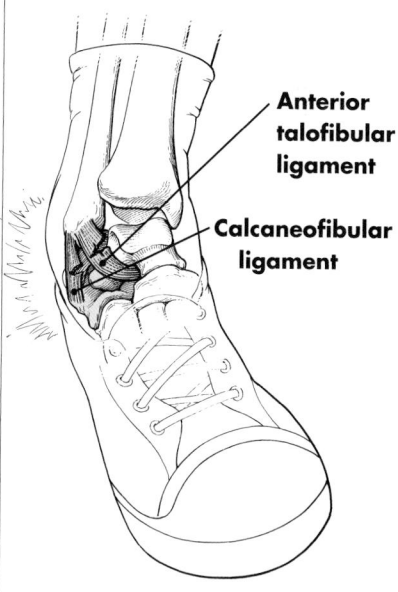

Anterior talofibular ligament

Calcaneofibular ligament

An ankle sprain occurs when ligaments that support your ankle stretch or tear. The anterior talofibular and calcaneofibular ligaments are the ones most likely to be injured.

R.I.C.E.

If you sustain a minor soft tissue injury, remember these words — *rest, ice, compression, elevation* — and the acronym, *R.I.C.E.* R.I.C.E. is a self-help treatment that can help speed your recovery. Follow these steps:

Rest
Avoid activities that cause pain or swelling. Rest is essential to promote tissue healing, but try to keep uninjured body parts moving and active to prevent significant deconditioning.

Ice
To decrease pain, swelling or muscle spasm, immediately apply ice to the injured area for approximately 15 to 20 minutes. Ice packs, slush baths and ice massage to smaller areas of injury are all useful. Re-apply ice periodically for as long as the swelling lasts.

Compression
Swelling can result in loss of motion in an injured joint. To control swelling, compress the injured area with wraps or elastic bandages until the swelling has stopped.

Elevation
Raise the swollen arm or leg above the level of your heart to reduce swelling. This is especially important at night.

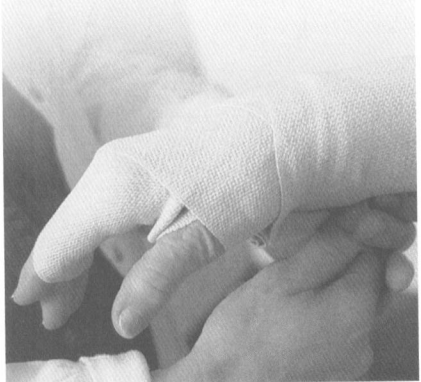

range in severity from minor to severe.

- **Mild sprain.** A mild sprain occurs when fibers within ligaments overstretch or tear slightly. You may feel pain and tenderness when touching or moving the joint. There's little or no swelling. You can usually put weight on the joint, and X-rays of the joint are normal.

  Repeated minor sprains can lead to a weakened joint. In most cases, a mildly sprained joint will be able to bear weight within approximately 24 hours and be fully healed within about two weeks.

- **Moderate sprain.** When ligament fibers tear without rupturing completely, you have a moderate sprain. Pain and tenderness are moderate, but you may hesitate to use the injured part because of a feeling of instability. You may experience some swelling and black-and-blue discoloration.

- **Severe sprain.** If one or more ligaments tear completely, you have a severe sprain. The area is painful, swollen and black-and-blue. You can't move your joint normally or stress it. If you try to use it, the joint may seem unstable.

Treatment
For a simple sprain, apply ice during the first 24 hours after the injury to reduce swelling. Support the joint with a supportive wrap such as an elastic bandage, and rest the joint in an elevated position.

Slowly resume normal activity, testing the injured joint gradually after a day or more has passed.

Medication
You may want to take acetaminophen (Tylenol, others) or aspirin for pain or a nonsteroidal anti-inflammatory drug (NSAID), such as ibuprofen (Advil, Motrin IB, others), to relieve pain accompanied by swelling. Be aware, however, that use of aspirin and NSAIDs may increase bleeding.

Surgery
If your sprain is serious enough that the joint is unstable, you may need an operation to repair ligaments that are torn or detached from the bone. Your doctor may also elect to stabilize the sprained joint in a brace, cast or splint. Rehabilitation may involve a supervised physical therapy program and an exercise program to strengthen the muscles surrounding the sprained joint.

Prevention
Taping, bracing or wrapping knees, ankles, wrists or elbows hasn't been shown to effectively prevent a sprain, but these tools may be used in rehabilitating injuries. Exercises, especially stability training, are critical for strengthening muscles weakened by injury and for stabilizing a joint to help prevent reinjury.

Shin splints

Signs and symptoms
- Pain over the front part of the leg above the ankle and below the knee and the inner side of the shinbone (tibia)
- Occasionally, swelling

  Pain on the front, inside portion of the tibia, the large bone of your lower leg, may be the result of shin splints (also called medial tibia stress syndrome). Shin splints occur when fibers of the membrane that ties muscles to the front and side of your tibia become irritated and inflamed, producing pain and occasional swelling. Often, shin splints occur when you stress and overload the inner portion of the tibia, but the stress isn't enough to cause a stress fracture.

  Shin splints usually result from repeated pounding on hard surfaces during activities such as running, marching or playing basketball, soccer or tennis.

Diagnosis
In addition to examining your leg, your doctor may order an X-ray

Neck Pain

Your neck supports a weight equivalent to that of a bowling ball year after year. No wonder it occasionally becomes stiff and sore.

When your neck muscles stiffen and movement becomes painful, your muscles automatically tense to prevent further movement. But tense neck muscles can cause painful spasms, strain your ligaments and cause radiating pain.

Sometimes, tight neck muscles can irritate or impinge on scalp (occipital) nerves that are close to the muscles. This can cause pain to radiate up the back of the neck, behind an ear and to the side of the scalp, a condition called occipital neuralgia. To combat a flare of neck pain, try the following approaches.

Medication
Acetaminophen (Tylenol, others), aspirin or a nonsteroidal anti-inflammatory drug (NSAID), such as ibuprofen (Advil, Motrin IB, others) or naproxen sodium (Aleve, others), may provide temporary relief.

Rest
Lie down during the day to ease neck strain. But avoid prolonged inactivity. It can increase stiffness.

Cold and heat
A cold pack often dulls the pain for the first day or two. Apply a cold pack to the back of your neck several times a day for 20 minutes or less each time. After that, use either heat or cold to relieve discomfort. Don't use cold or hot packs if you have severe heart or circulation problems.

Exercises
Certain exercises can help you maintain proper posture and reduce neck pain and stiffness. Exercises can also improve your overall fitness, helping to prevent recurrence of neck pain. Try the following:
- *Shoulder squeeze.* Squeeze your shoulder blades together and hold for about three seconds. Repeat as often as is comfortable.
- *Shoulder shrug.* Gently raise your shoulders tightly to your neck, hold for five to 10 seconds, then slowly relax to a normal position.
- *Seated rowing.* Sit on the floor or on a stool or weight bench and pull your arms back and forth in a rowing motion.
- *Fly.* Grasp light dumbbells (1 to 2 pounds), bend forward at your hips keeping your back straight, and let your arms hang straight down. Gently raise and lower the weights as if you were flying. If you can't keep your back straight, lie on your stomach on a table or weight bench.

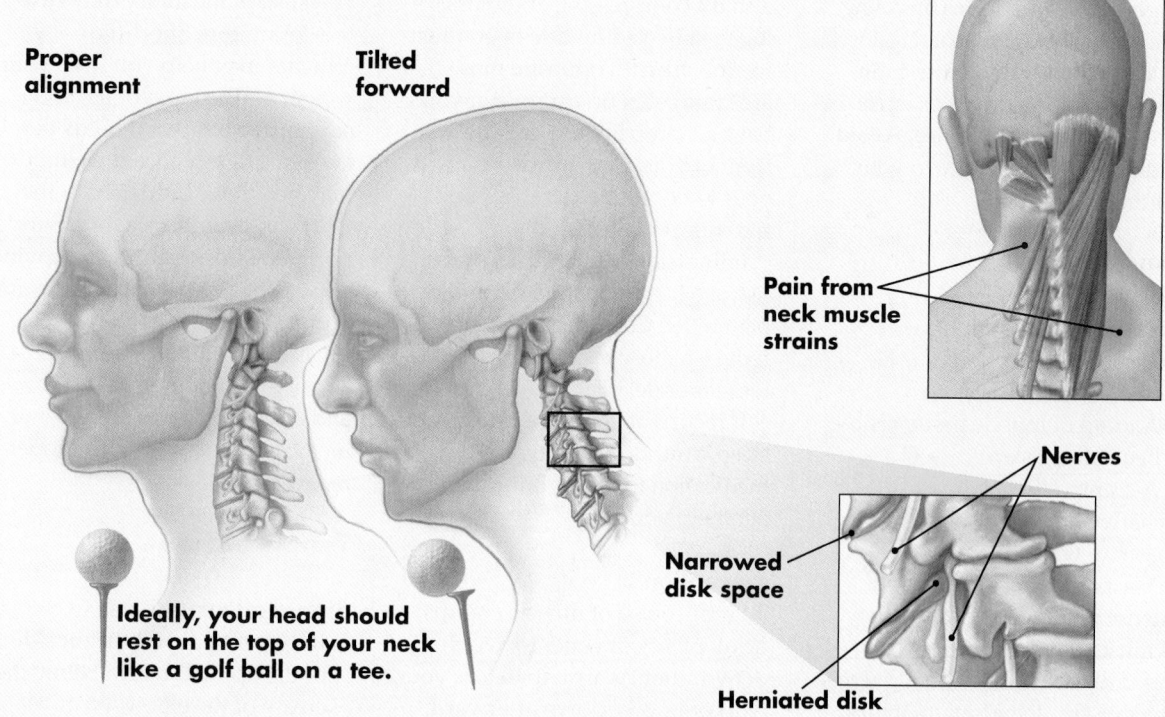

Proper alignment

Tilted forward

Ideally, your head should rest on the top of your neck like a golf ball on a tee.

Pain from neck muscle strains

Nerves

Narrowed disk space

Herniated disk

A variety of factors can cause neck pain, including improper alignment, muscle strains, narrowed disk spaces, herniated disks and pinched nerves.

to check for a hairline crack of the tibia or a magnetic resonance imaging (MRI) scan or bone scan to rule out a stress fracture from prolonged overuse activity.

Treatment

Similar to other minor musculoskeletal injuries, shin splints are treated with rest and ice. Acetaminophen (Tylenol, others) or an over-the-counter anti-inflammatory medication may help reduce pain.

Other therapies

In some cases, putting a soft insert in your shoe can reduce some of the shock during vigorous physical activity. Your doctor may prescribe a specially fabricated device (orthotic) if your foot has a structural factor that's predisposed to injury, such as an excessively high arch or a flatfoot.

You may be able to eliminate the problem by avoiding exercise that involves a persistent pounding of the legs, such as running or basketball, for two weeks to two months and substituting a lower impact activity, such as bicycling or swimming. Also, when training, build up slowly and cross-train, mixing the low-impact exercise with your impact exercise. Avoid adding time or distance to your routine too quickly.

Muscle cramp

Signs and symptoms

- A sudden and sharp muscle pain, often in a leg
- A lump of muscle tissue visible beneath the skin

A cramp — sometimes called a charley horse — is actually a spasm in which a muscle contracts, producing sudden and intense pain. A common variety of muscle cramp occurs in your calf muscles during sleep. Overuse of a muscle, dehydration, injury, muscle strain or simply holding a position for prolonged periods may result in a muscle cramp. Athletes who become fatigued and dehydrated while participating in warm-weather sports frequently develop muscle cramps.

How serious is a muscle cramp?

Almost everyone experiences a muscle cramp at some time. For most people, it's an occasional inconvenience. For some individuals, muscle cramps, especially at night, can be recurrent and severe. If you experience frequent and severe cramps that interfere with sleep, consult a doctor.

Intermittent claudication is a distinct form of cramplike discomfort in the legs associated with exercise and relieved with rest. It's caused by inadequate blood supply to muscles in the calves. Nerve compression in the spine also can cause another form of exercise-related pain. See your doctor if you repeatedly have cramping or pain in your legs when you exercise.

Treatment

When a cramp occurs, gently stretching the contracted muscle usually provides relief. You might also try compressing and massaging the affected muscle or contracting the muscles opposite those that are cramped. For example, if you have a cramp in your calf, flex the front of your foot upward toward your knee and hold it there until the cramp improves.

Immersion in a hot bath or the use of a heating pad may provide pain relief. Cold packs also may reduce a muscle spasm or relax a tense muscle.

If recurrent cramps disturb your sleep, your doctor may prescribe a medication to relax your muscles and help you sleep.

Prevention

To reduce risk of muscle cramps, drink plenty of water to avoid dehydration, warm up before your workouts, cool down afterward, and don't overfatigue your muscles. If you get cramps at night, stretch your legs before going to bed.

Thigh bruise

Signs and symptoms

- Sudden pain and tenderness in the muscles at the front of the thigh from a blow to the thigh
- Discomfort aggravated by movement

Physical contact can cause a bruise in the muscles on the front of your thigh that allow you to extend your leg at the knee (quadriceps).

Diagnosis

Pain and swelling of the front part of the thigh and reduced ability to bend the knee of the affected leg usually indicate a thigh bruise (contusion). You may notice discoloration under the skin, beginning with redness and progressing to the characteristic black-and-blue of a bruise after several days.

This injury may take a week or months to heal. X-rays can rule out a bone fracture.

Treatment

Applying ice to the bruise with the leg bent immediately after you sustain the injury may ease the discomfort. Short-term use of crutches may help you keep your weight off the injured leg, and a supportive wrap that holds the knee in a tightly flexed position may help limit the extent of the injury and speed recovery. Supportive wraps or tape can provide some protection when you resume normal activities.

Deep thigh bruises from sports activity require medical care, and often a physical therapist or medical trainer to ensure proper recovery.

Tennis elbow

Signs and symptoms

- Recurrent pain on the outside of the upper forearm below the crease of the elbow
- Sometimes, pain extending down the forearm toward the wrist

You don't have to play tennis to experience tennis elbow.

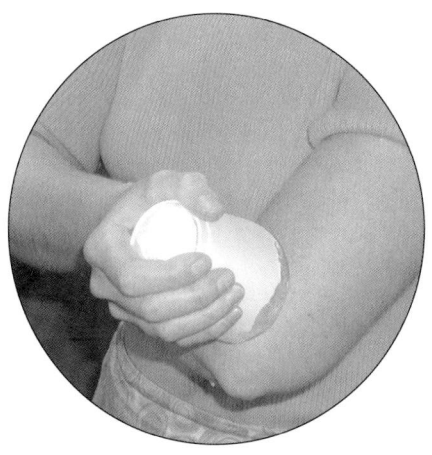

To help relieve pain, freeze water in a plastic foam cup, peel away the top of the cup and rub the ice over the affected area.

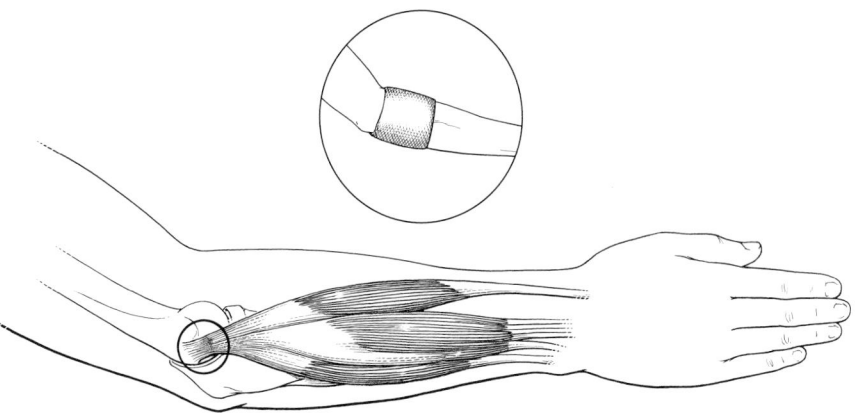

Tennis elbow produces pain on the outside of your forearm near your elbow when you exercise the joint. Tiny tears in tendon tissue cause the discomfort (see small circle). In some cases, you can get relief from a forearm support band (see inset) worn just below your elbow.

Both tennis elbow and a related ailment called Little League elbow are pains that likely result from repeated, tiny tears in the tendons that attach the muscles of your lower arm at the elbow.

The tears can result from a variety of activities involving repeated rotary motion of the forearm and repeated wrist movement. Hitting a backhand in tennis, painting a house or twisting a screwdriver all can precipitate tennis elbow. Little League elbow usually affects the inside of the elbow in youngsters and is often brought on by the strain of throwing a baseball.

In adults, tendinitis over the inside of the elbow is called golfer's elbow because a golf swing, especially with improper technique, may strain these tendons.

Diagnosis
To rule out other possible causes of your symptoms, your doctor may order an X-ray of the area.

How serious is tennis elbow?
In most cases, the discomfort improves in six to 12 weeks. A youngsters with Little League elbow shouldn't use the arm in ways that may injure the growth plate.

Treatment
Discontinue the activity associated with the pain. Apply ice to the injured elbow for 15 to 20 minutes at a time and repeat every two to three hours, except while you're sleeping.

Massaging the area and stretching the forearm muscles also are appropriate. Depending on the severity of your injury, your doctor may refer you to a physical therapist.

Exercise
Exercise can strengthen the wrist muscles to speed healing and may prevent a recurrence. Once the pain has subsided, you can do strengthening exercises with a light hand weight. Holding the weight in your hand, with your elbow bent and your palm down, lift and slowly lower your wrist.

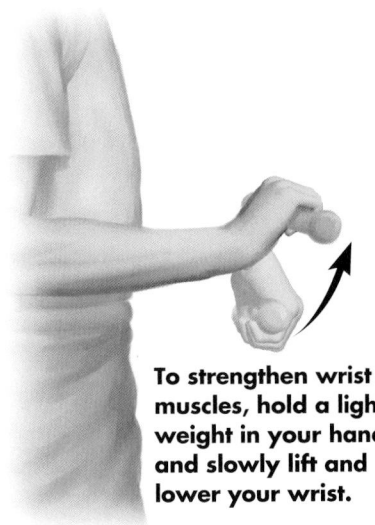

To strengthen wrist muscles, hold a light weight in your hand and slowly lift and lower your wrist.

Medication
Acetaminophen (Tylenol, others) or an over-the-counter nonsteroidal anti-inflammatory drug (NSAID) can reduce the pain of tennis elbow. In certain cases, your doctor may inject a corticosteroid drug into the painful area to help reduce the swelling.

Prevention
To avoid recurring episodes of tennis elbow, pay special attention to your technique when engaging in the particular activity that provoked the injury. A stable and comfortable wrist position in sports and other activities is critical. Also make sure your equipment fits you properly.

Baseball finger

Signs and symptoms
- Swelling and pain in the last joint of a finger
- An inability to straighten a finger
Baseball finger (mallet finger) occurs when the tendon that connects the muscles to the end of your finger is forcibly separated from the bone. This often results when a thrown or batted baseball strikes the tip of a finger.

Diagnosis
This injury often is the result of trauma, so an X-ray may be ordered to rule out a fracture.

Rehabilitation From an Athletic Injury

The goal of a sports rehabilitation program is to return the injured athlete to normal physical activity, good health and full function. Various factors, including your age, level of physical activity, body structure and conditioning program at the time of injury, influence the approach of rehabilitation and determine how quickly you'll recover from the injury.

The rehabilitative process generally has four stages. Skipping any of them may put you at risk of re-injury or prolong your recovery.

Stage 1
Stage 1 involves controlling the inflammation and pain of the acute injury, usually through R.I.C.E. — rest, ice, compression and elevation.

Stage 2
Stage 2 involves restoring the full range of motion to the injured joint. A physical therapist may recommend exercises that you can do alone or with an assistant moving the extremity at the injured joint. Muscle-strengthening exercises follow — usually beginning with isometrics, in which you tighten and release the muscles without moving the extremity. This may be followed by light resistance training.

When you've regained substantial strength and normal range of joint motion, additional exercises, including ones that promote agility and stability, may be added. You'll also begin a general cardiovascular endurance program, perhaps involving long-distance biking, swimming or running, to prevent deconditioning.

Stage 3
In stage 3 you return to movement patterns related to your specific sport. For example, a baseball pitcher recovering from an operation on the arm would resume throwing a baseball.

Stage 4
When you regain your pre-injury level of conditioning and can resume normal activity, your doctor or physical therapist may prescribe a program to enable you to maintain and improve flexibility, strength and endurance.

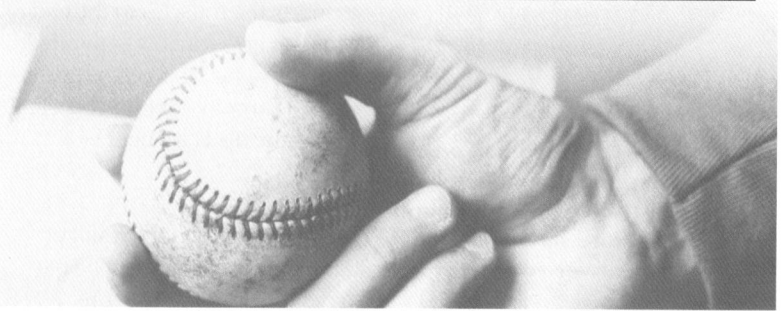

How serious is baseball finger?
With proper treatment, you should be able to use the injured finger normally within about eight weeks. However, your finger may be permanently deformed.

Treatment
Treatment generally involves immobilizing the finger and taking medication to control the pain. Surgery usually is necessary only when a bone is fractured.

To immobilize the affected finger, your doctor will probably splint the last joint in an extended position for about six weeks to allow the tendon to repair itself. After the splint is removed, gradually try to return the finger to its normal position. Your doctor may recommend gentle range-of-motion exercises.

Jumper's knee

Signs and symptoms
- Pain at the front of the knee
- Pain with pressure to the tendon just below the kneecap (patella)
- Swelling

Many athletes develop pain at the front of the knee known as patellar tendinitis — commonly called jumper's knee.

Inflammation of tendons (tendinitis) or microtrauma to tendon fibers in the knee causes the pain, which may occur in one or both knees. Knee inflammation is usually the result of overuse or misuse rather than a single traumatic event. The pain usually isn't constant, but occurs when you jump, run, squat or climb stairs.

Diagnosis
A doctor often makes a diagnosis on the basis of a physical examination and the degree of discomfort.

How serious is jumper's knee?
Given proper rest and treatment, pain from patellar tendinitis usually disappears in a matter of weeks. If you don't address the cause of the problem, it may recur.

Treatment

Apply ice to the sore knee and avoid the activity that caused the discomfort. Avoid jumping, repetitive stair climbing and running until symptoms subside. Acetaminophen (Tylenol, others) and nonsteroidal anti-inflammatory drugs (Advil, Motrin IB, others) can help reduce the pain.

Prevention

Some common causes of knee pain are overuse, improper training and muscle inflexibility or weakness. You may prevent recurrences by reviewing and altering your training program with someone knowledgeable about sports medicine.

Some people switch from running to swimming or bicycling, activities that put less stress on their knees. Orthotic devices may help correct flatfeet or other alignment problems in your legs. If alignment problems seem to be causing your symptoms, your doctor may refer you to a physiatrist, podiatrist or physical therapist.

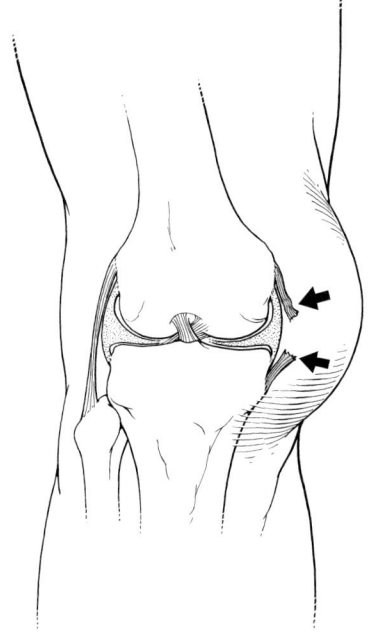

A torn ligament (see arrows) is a common form of knee injury. The knee swells, and the joint becomes unstable.

Support for your kneecap in the form of a light brace also may help. A strap across your patellar tendon may help reduce the pressure. Another key strategy is to stretch and strengthen the muscles at the front of your thigh (quadriceps).

Knee injury

Signs and symptoms
- Pain and swelling in your knee
- Instability of the knee
- A popping sound, a snapping sensation or locking of the joint

Three key factors make the knee joint susceptible to injury. First, its location leaves it exposed to trauma. Second, you use it constantly. Third, the structure of your knee is complex. More than a hinge, a knee's range of motion is unique among body joints. It must slide, glide and swivel, as well as bend.

Knee injuries result from a variety of causes. Acute knee injuries often occur during sports. Wear and tear over time can produce chronic knee problems, such as osteoarthritis in a knee joint. Knee injuries also can result from an accident or simply a mistaken step that causes the joint to extend beyond its normal range of motion.

Knee Braces

If your knee is swollen or unstable, your doctor may recommend that you wear a knee brace, especially when you're participating in activities that may stress the joint.

One type of brace available in medical supply stores is a rubbery neoprene or elastic sleeve that slips over your knee. Be aware, though, that the brace may seem to offer more support than it actually does. The warmth and compression the brace provides can make your knee feel better, but it doesn't necessarily protect you from injury. Some braces — especially those designed for medial and lateral support — may even increase your risk of injury. It's best to avoid them even if they ease discomfort.

Your doctor might also recommend another type of brace if you have osteoarthritis of the knee. It shifts the load on your knee, protecting the joint and helping to ease discomfort.

If you tear your anterior cruciate ligament (ACL) — the most common knee ligament injury — and you don't choose surgical reconstruction, your doctor may prescribe a functional brace to help stabilize your knee during certain activities. A knee brace can't take the place of a fully functioning ACL, but it can keep your knee properly aligned during activities such as skiing, playing tennis or hiking. These braces usually are custom fitted or custom tailored, so they can be costly. Depending on your situation, your insurance provider may or may not cover the cost. Check with your insurance provider.

Factors a doctor considers in deciding if you need a brace include your age, lifestyle and injury. With the aid of a brace, most people can continue to participate in many of their favorite activities that don't involve jumping, turning sharply and pivoting. People who wear knee braces report fewer episodes of instability or giving way. But your knee may continue to be unstable during certain types of activities, even with a brace. Repeated episodes of instability can damage the knee further.

The best way to protect your knees against further injury is to strengthen the muscles in the thighs — hamstring and quadriceps — because these strong muscles support your knees.

Diagnosis

If you sustain a knee injury, your doctor will likely examine your knee in a variety of positions to assess the joint's internal structure and the damage it has sustained.

Traditional X-rays are a common method of evaluating a knee injury. If necessary, magnetic resonance imaging (MRI) provides much more detailed images of the structures of the knee, including its soft tissues.

How serious is a knee injury?

The severity of a knee injury depends on the type of damage the joint has sustained.

Most knee injuries fall into one of three classifications: a meniscal tear, a torn ligament or a bone or cartilage injury. Each of these can produce pain and swelling of the knee joint.

Meniscal tear

The meniscus is the crescent-shaped cartilage in your knee situated between the ends of the bones of your thigh and lower leg. Certain types of impact and twisting injuries can produce tears in the meniscus, causing pain in the joint.

Often, a meniscal tear causes you to collapse due to acute, severe knee pain. In some cases, you'll be able to get up and even resume activity, but more likely the tear will cause swelling and persistent pain. The pain may subside over a period of weeks, but symptoms may recur if you participate in activities that involve rotating or pivoting the knee joint.

Torn ligament

Ligaments are dense bands of tissue that surround a joint and provide stability to the joint. Occasionally, a ligament in a knee may stretch and tear, causing immediate pain, tenderness over the injury site and swelling of the knee. You may also experience a feeling of instability and loss of trust in the knee.

Other Causes of Knee Pain

The most common sources of knee pain are injuries, the constant stress of excess weight on your knees, and general wear and tear.

When the smooth tissue that covers the ends of bones in the knee (articular cartilage) gradually deteriorates, it's called osteoarthritis. Another source of knee pain is the softening and the loss of smooth cartilage covering the backside of the kneecap (chondromalacia patella). This condition can be aggravated by a condition in which the kneecap isn't centered in the femoral groove and slides over leg bones when bending or straightening the knee. Moving the knee causes pain, especially when you kneel or go down stairs.

When the inner soft tissue lining (synovium) of the knee becomes inflamed due to arthritis, the knee swells with fluid. Some of this fluid may be pushed into a area at the back of the knee and called a Baker's cyst (popliteal cyst). The cyst itself is not dangerous, but indicates that there's something wrong inside the knee joint.

Arthroscopy

Before the development of the arthroscope in 1972, injuries of the knee and other joints often required traditional surgery through a long incision. This type of surgery often involved an extended hospital stay and a long, painful period of recuperation. Although some joint conditions still require incisions to open and reconstruct the joint, doctors can now correct many injuries by using an arthroscope.

Arthroscope comes from the terms *arthro* for "joint" and *scope*, meaning "to view." The device consists of a slender tube, an optical system of magnifying lenses and a fiber-optic light source.

Before the procedure, you're given a local, regional or general anesthetic. The surgeon then makes a small incision into the

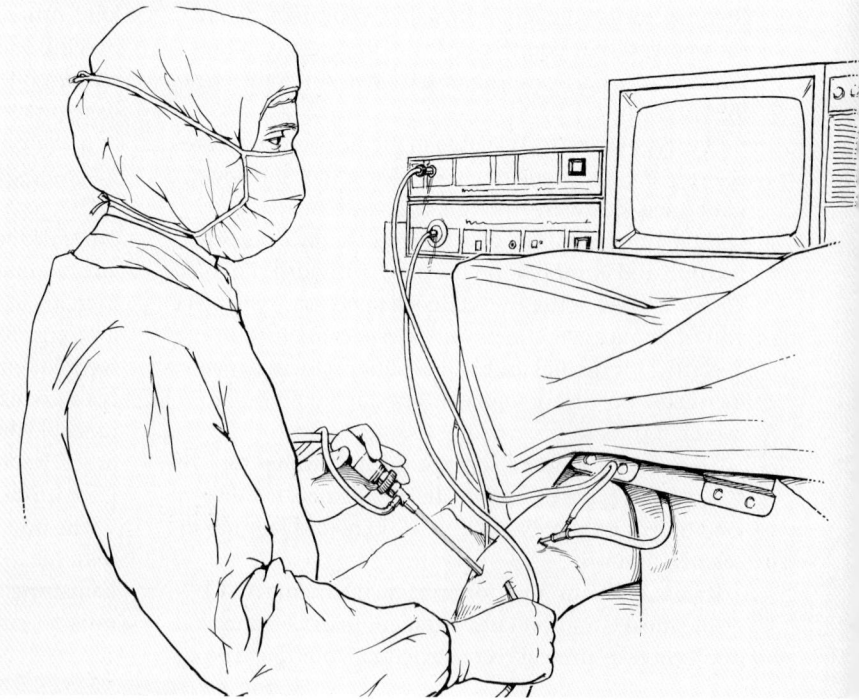

Knee Swelling

Occasionally, a knee may swell for no clear reason. The swelling is sometimes associated with pain when you move your knee, and your knee may be tender and appear red or inflamed. Knee swelling may also occur without pain, tenderness or inflammation. Significant swelling causing discomfort or making it difficult to move the knee should prompt you to see your doctor to determine the cause.

If your knee is inflamed or reddened, you have a fever, and it hurts to move your knee, see your doctor right away. These signs and symptoms may indicate infection in the joint. Occasionally, knee swelling, tenderness and pain may be initial manifestations of gout, which can be effectively treated once a diagnosis is made.

Sometimes, isolated knee swelling may be an initial symptom of a physical illness, such as inflammatory bowel disease, or it may be related to a systemic disease, such as rheumatoid arthritis or Lyme or other tick-borne diseases.

affected joint to insert the arthroscope. Other small incisions are made, as needed, to insert surgical instruments. Often, the incisions are so small that stitches aren't required.

Sterile fluid distends the joint space during the procedure to enhance visibility. Once the arthroscope is in place, the surgeon can view the inside of your joint on a monitor. Small instruments can be inserted into the joint to remove floating bits of cartilage or bone, repair the meniscus, or reconstruct ligaments.

Recovery from an arthroscopic procedure generally requires less time than does recovery from traditional surgery. Many people go home the same day. Be careful not to subject the joint to vigorous physical activity for several weeks after surgery. Many people can, however, resume most normal activities within a few days.

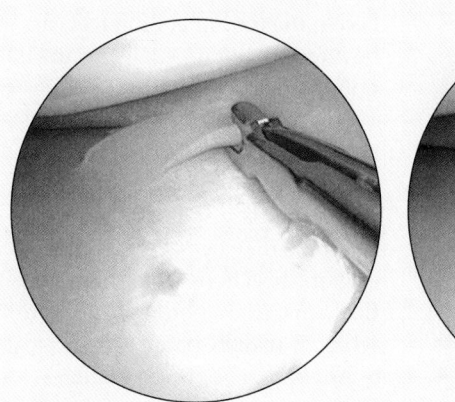 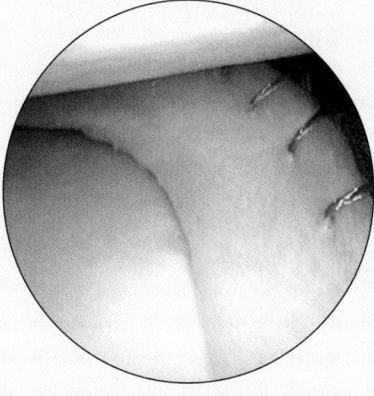

Using an arthroscope, a surgeon can see inside your knee or another joint to examine the joint or repair it without major surgery. Above are arthroscopic views of a meniscus trimming (left) and a suture repair of the meniscus (right).

Bone or cartilage injury

Some knee injuries involve pieces of cartilage or bone that have broken away from their proper positions and are floating about in the joint space, producing pain and swelling.

Sometimes, the loose pieces can get pinched between the moving parts of the knee. This can cause the knee to get stuck, or "lock," so that it can't be straightened. This is a very painful condition.

Treatment

The treatment for a knee injury depends on the injury. For relatively minor knee injuries, the proper treatment approach is R.I.C.E.: rest, ice, compression and elevation (see page 930). Stop using your knee after you injure it. Use ice and compression to limit swelling, and keep your leg elevated to help reduce the pain and swelling.

If your knee joint has sustained major damage, you may need reconstructive surgery. A dislocated or fractured bone may need to be reset and repaired.

A ruptured ligament may need to be reattached or reconstructed. Often, the damage can be repaired surgically with a procedure called arthroscopy, which requires a few small incisions in the knee rather than one large incision. Arthroscopy causes less tissue disruption than traditional surgery, and it generally results in more rapid rehabilitation.

Rehabilitation

After surgery, your doctor may apply a splint or brace to the knee for a brief period of time. Once you're allowed to move your knee, you'll likely receive a series of exercises to restore range of motion to your joint and to help strengthen it.

You may be referred to a physical medicine and rehabilitation specialist or to a physical therapist who will oversee your rehabilitation program.

Problems of the Feet

Your feet are highly specialized structures. Each foot has 26 bones held together with ligaments, muscles and tendons. As you walk, your muscles work the bones like levers, making movement possible.

As long as your feet take you where you want to go without pain, you probably don't think much about them. You may even mistreat them unwittingly by squeezing them into too-tight shoes, often with high heels and pointy toes. However, if you're lucky and you wear properly fitted, comfortable footwear, your feet will cause you little worry.

If you develop foot problems that cause pain or discomfort, you may want to seek guidance from your doctor, an orthopedist or a podiatrist. A podiatrist is a licensed professional whose area of expertise is the diagnosis, prevention and treatment of foot disorders.

Achilles tendinitis

Signs and symptoms
- A dull ache or pain in the Achilles tendon, especially when running or jumping
- Mild swelling or tenderness over the tendon
- Difficulty walking or running due to pain over the tendon
Achilles tendinitis refers to inflammation or microtearing of a tendon known as the heel cord (Achilles tendon). This tendon links your leg muscles to the back of your heel bone. Tiny tears in the tendon during strenuous exercise can cause pain and inflammation. More-severe injury results when the tendon is torn more extensively or fully torn (ruptured).

Diagnosis
Your doctor will examine your foot and may X-ray the area to rule out other possible causes.

How serious is Achilles tendinitis?
Conservative treatments such as rest, ice, stretching and special exercises should allow the tendon to repair itself over a period of weeks. You may have to alter your exercise program. Left untreated, the tendon could continue to sustain small tears through exercise and repeated movement and eventually rupture. A ruptured tendon is a serious injury that affects your ability to walk and often requires surgical repair.

Treatment
Resting your ankle is the best treatment for Achilles tendinitis. Applying ice to the tendon can provide relief. A temporary orthotic device that elevates the heel within the shoe may relieve strain on the stretched tendon. Acetaminophen (Tylenol, others) and nonsteroidal anti-inflammatory drugs (NSAIDs) can reduce pain and discomfort.

Once the pain is gone, gently stretch the heel cord and the hamstring muscles at the back of your thigh. Strengthening the calf muscles is key to healing and preventing recurrence. Until the tendon is fully healed, it may be best to take part in nonimpact or low-impact exercises.

Surgery
A complete rupture of an Achilles tendon usually requires surgery. The procedure generally involves making an incision in the back of the leg and stitching the torn tendon together. Recovery involves spending about six to 12 weeks with your leg in a walking boot, cast, brace or splint.

If the tendon is only partially torn, treatment may involve wearing a cast or walking boot and allowing the ends of the torn tendon to reattach without surgery. Studies indicate that this method can be effective and doesn't have the same risk of complications, such as infection, that can occur with surgery. However, the incidence of re-rupture is higher with the nonsurgical approach, and recovery can take longer.

Heel pain

Signs and symptoms
- Pain in the bottom of the heel of the foot when you bear weight on the foot
- Pain that's worse with the first few steps after awakening or when climbing stairs or standing on tiptoe
The heel pad consists of fibrous tissue that cushions the underlying structure of the foot when you bear weight on it.

Pain in the heel may result from a pinched nerve or a chronic condition, such as arthritis. But a common cause of heel pain is a condition called plantar fasciitis, an inflammation of the fibrous plantar fascia along the bottom of your foot that runs from your heel bone (calcaneus) to your toes. The pain may stem from stretching of the plantar fascia, causing inflammation or tears in the tissue.

Heel pain usually develops gradually, but it can come on suddenly and be severe. It tends to be worse when you get out of bed in the morning. Both feet can be affected, but it usually occurs in only one foot.

The pain generally subsides once your foot limbers up, but it can recur if you stand or sit too long. Climbing stairs or standing on tiptoe may be painful. Tension on your heel bone from this condition can cause a bone spur to form, which is usually painless.

Anyone can develop plantar fasciitis, but it tends to be more common with age as the arch of your foot begins to sag. Carrying excess weight, wearing poorly fitted shoes and having a foot abnormality can increase your risk.

Diagnosis
Your doctor will likely ask if the pain is constant or occurs only

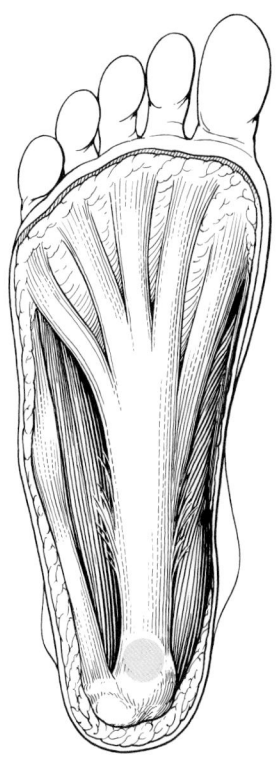

Heel pain may result from small tears or inflammation of your heel pad where the tissue attaches to your heel bone (see highlighting). Bone spurs may form but rarely cause pain.

when you put weight on your heel. An X-ray or magnetic resonance imaging (MRI) may be done to rule out a stress fracture.

Sometimes, an X-ray shows a spur of bone projecting forward from the heel bone. In the past, bone spurs often were blamed for heel pain and removed surgically, but doctors have found that they're typically not the cause of pain. Surgery to remove such a spur is rare.

How serious is heel pain?
In most cases, the pain gradually improves or disappears. It can recur, though, especially if you walk barefoot or wear poorly fitted shoes or shoes that lack cushioning at the heel when performing weight-bearing exercise.

Some people find that the only way to avoid a recurring problem is to modify their activity, such as

Exercises to Help Strengthen the Heel

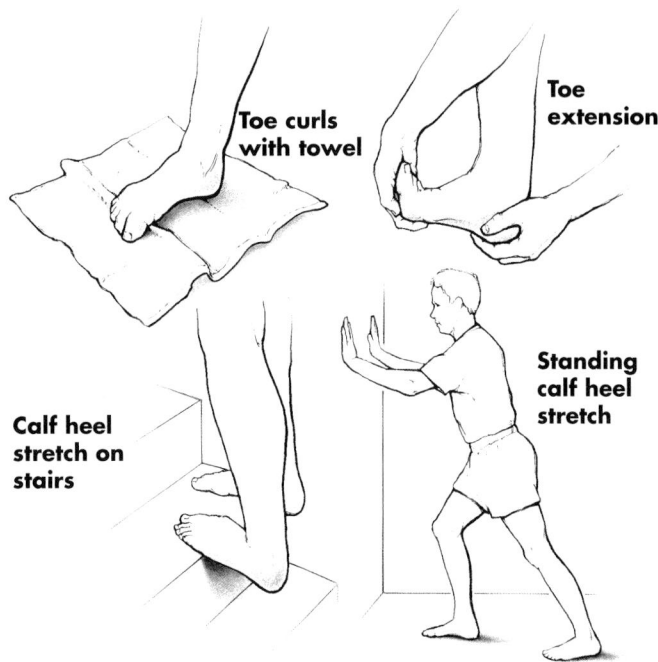

Toe curls with towel

Toe extension

Calf heel stretch on stairs

Standing calf heel stretch

These exercises stretch or strengthen your plantar fascia, Achilles tendon and calf muscles. Hold each for 20 to 30 seconds and do one or two repetitions two to three times a day.

switching from running or playing tennis to swimming or bicycling. For most people, a complete recovery is often possible with appropriate treatment.

Treatment
Self-care measures may help to relieve the pain and inflammation, but recovery may take six months or longer. If self-care measures are ineffective, your doctor may refer you to a physical therapist.

Medication
To relieve the pain, try acetaminophen (Tylenol, others) or an over-the-counter nonsteroidal anti-inflammatory drug (NSAID).

Your doctor may inject a type of steroid medication into the tender area to provide temporary pain relief. Multiple injections aren't recommended because they can weaken your plantar fascia and possibly cause it to rupture. More recently, platelet-rich plasma has been used, under ultrasound guidance, to provide pain relief with less risk of tissue rupture.

If other conservative measures fail, a minimally invasive procedure may be performed that removes the scar tissue of plantar fasciitis without the need for surgery.

Self-care
Self-care steps to treat plantar fasciitis include:
- Apply ice to the area for up to 20 minutes after an activity that causes pain.
- Massage and gently stretch the arch and calf muscles. Stretching increases flexibility in the plantar fascia, Achilles tendon and calf muscles. Stretching your foot as soon as you wake up also helps reverse tightening of the plantar fascia that sets in overnight.
- Do daily exercises to strengthen your arch and the muscles in your foot (see above illustrations).
- Wear soft-soled shoes when running. Your doctor may prescribe an arch support to wear in your shoes or a night splint to stretch the arch and calf overnight.

Shopping for Shoes

Improperly fitted shoes are the source of many foot problems. Choosing shoes carefully can help you avoid many problems with your feet. When buying shoes, look for the following:

- *Wide toe box.* Buy shoes with a wide toe box that provides adequate toe room. Pointy, narrow-toed shoes can cramp your feet and lead to ingrown toenails, calluses, corns and bunions.
- *Low heels.* Select shoes with heels of no more than 2 inches. High heels place extra stress on your knees and back. They force you to lean back to compensate for the forward tilt of your heel. High heels can contribute to tightness of the Achilles tendon and toe pain.
- *Laces.* Lace-up shoes generally offer more room and adjustable support.
- *Breathable materials.* Soft leather or suede allows perspiration to evaporate from your feet, whereas vinyl and plastic inhibit evaporation of perspiration.

Shop for shoes in the afternoon to get a fit that accommodates your feet as they swell throughout the day. However, you don't want a shoe to be so roomy that your foot slips around inside. Measure the size of both of your feet. As you age or gain weight, your shoe size may increase.

Don't buy shoes that need breaking in. If they're not comfortable in the store, they're not likely to be comfortable later on. Ask to have the shoes stretched at any pressure point.

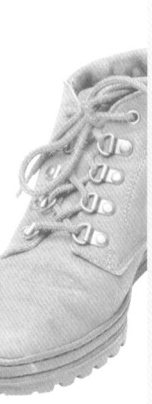

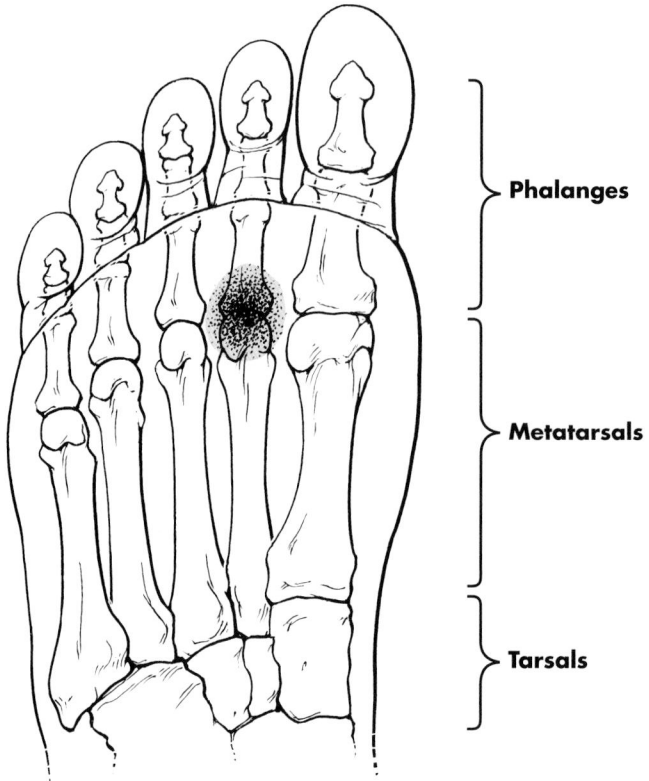

The pain of metatarsalgia can occur at any of the joints that separate the phalangeal and metatarsal bones in your foot. The highlighted area shows the joint most commonly affected.

- For everyday wear, buy shoes with a low heel (no higher than 2 inches), good arch support and shock absorbency.
- Put soft heel pads in your shoes.

Surgery

When pain is severe and all else fails, surgery is sometimes performed to detach the plantar fascia from the heel bone. Side effects include a weakening of the arch in the foot.

Metatarsalgia

Signs and symptoms

- Pain in the ball of the foot
- The sensation of walking on pebbles

The term *metatarsalgia* means pain in the ball (metatarsal area) of your foot.

You have five metatarsal bones in each foot. Each has a narrow shaft and a rounded tip. The bones link your ankle and heel bones (tarsals) with the bones in your toes (phalanges). Hinge joints between the metatarsals and phalanges let your toes move up and down and, to a lesser extent, sideways.

Although metatarsalgia may affect males and females from adolescence to older adulthood, the condition is most common among middle-aged women.

This condition has multiple causes. Having narrow, high-arched feet can put excessive stress on the balls of your feet, as can certain types of flatfeet. If your legs are unequal in length, the metatarsal-phalangeal joints of the shorter leg receive additional stress.

Other contributing factors include rheumatoid arthritis, stress fractures, fluid accumulation, muscle fatigue, excess weight from pregnancy or obesity, and prolonged standing or walking.

Diagnosis

Your doctor or podiatrist will likely examine your feet and legs

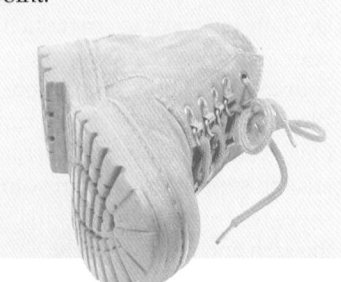

and ask about your pain. He or she may want to know if the pain tends to occur in certain situations.

Treatment

Simple self-care measures usually reduce the pain. Avoid wearing tight, thin-soled or high-heeled shoes. Your doctor might suggest that you wear a foot pad or an arch support, a type of orthotic device that relieves pressure under the painful area.

An over-the-counter pain medication can often help relieve the pain. Your doctor may inject a corticosteroid medication into the tender area. Surgery is seldom necessary.

Burning feet

Signs and symptoms

- Nearly constant burning and stinging in the feet

This condition tends to be most common among people older than age 65. The discomfort ranges from mild irritation to severe pain. Possible culprits include irritating fabrics, poorly fitted shoes or a fungal infection, such as athlete's foot.

Diagnosis

The cause of burning feet is often difficult to pinpoint. If a nerve or blood disorder is responsible, you may also have a prickling feeling in your feet, weakness or change of sensation in your legs, nausea, diarrhea, or loss of urine or bowel control.

Damaged peripheral nerves (neuropathy) can cause persistent burning or tingling. Peripheral neuropathy has many possible causes, including inherited disorders, diabetes, pernicious anemia, malnutrition, side effects of medications, exposure to toxins, chronic kidney failure and liver disease.

How serious are burning feet?

Although generally not serious, this condition can signal a serious underlying problem.

Treatment

Self-help measures may help improve your symptoms. Wear socks made from synthetic fibers such as acrylic or polypropylene. Select well-fitting shoes made of natural materials that breathe. Reduce or eliminate activities that aggravate your condition, such as standing in one place for a long period. Cool your feet in cool tap water for 15 minutes twice a day. Or soak your feet in cool water and then in hot water, a method called contrast foot soaks.

If nerve damage is the cause, your symptoms may take months to subside because nerves heal slowly. Prescription and over-the-counter pain relievers may provide pain relief.

Morton's neuroma

Signs and symptoms

- Burning pain in the ball of the foot that may radiate into the toes
- Numbness in the toes

Morton's neuroma is a noncancerous (benign) tumor of a nerve. Also called plantar neuroma, it's actually a thickening of the tissue that surrounds the digital nerve

leading to the toes. This condition may occur in response to irritation, pressure or injury. Morton's neuroma is more common in women than in men.

Diagnosis

Typically, there's no outward sign of this condition, such as a lump. A doctor may feel a palpable mass or notice a clicking between the bones upon examination of the affected foot.

How serious is Morton's neuroma?

The condition causes discomfort but otherwise isn't serious.

Treatment

Usually, treatment involves self-care. Make sure to wear sandals or well-fitting shoes with adequate room in the toe box. Avoid high heels. Custom shoe inserts or pads may help reduce pressure on the nerve.

A doctor may recommend injections with steroid medications to reduce swelling and inflammation of the nerve. In rare cases, surgery to remove the benign growth may be indicated.

To avoid an ingrown toenail, don't clip your toenails too short (A). Clip them straight across. When a toe takes on a claw-like, clenched appearance, the condition is called hammertoe (B). Hammertoe most often affects the second toe, which frequently develops a corn due to pressure from shoes. To help avoid hammertoe, ingrown toenails and other foot problems, wear shoes that fit properly.

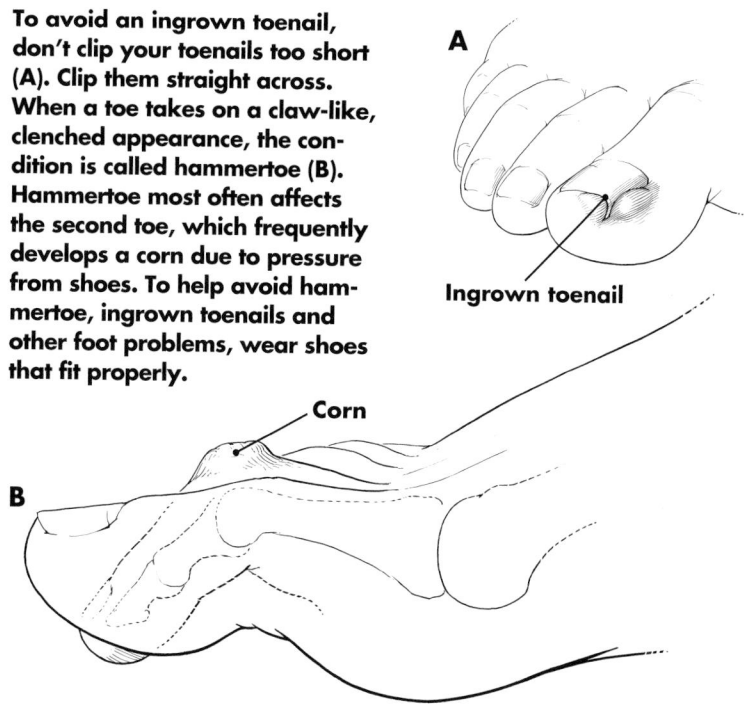

A

Ingrown toenail

Corn

B

Ingrown toenail

Signs and symptoms
- Pain
- Swelling and redness around a toenail

An ingrown toenail is a condition in which the toenail grows into the flesh of a toe, often the big toe. This can result from unusually curved toenails, poorly fitted shoes or toenails that are cut improperly. The tissue around the nail may become infected.

Treatment
If the tissue around the nail is infected, your doctor may prescribe an antibiotic and trim the portion of the nail that has grown into the toe. This minor procedure can be done in a doctor's office. Your doctor may recommend soaking your foot in warm water and resting the foot.

Prevention
To avoid chronic recurrence of ingrown toenails, don't clip your nails too short. Cut them straight across rather than curving them to match the shape of your toes.

It's also important to wear socks and shoes that fit properly without putting excessive pressure on your feet and toes.

Corns and calluses

Signs and symptoms
- A thickened layer of skin
- With corns, pain

Corns and calluses are the result of pressure or friction, causing the skin to protect itself by thickening and hardening. Corns typically are smaller — less than 1/4 inch in diameter — than calluses and have a hard center. They usually develop on the tops and sides of your toes and can be painful. Calluses, which may be rough but are rarely painful, usually develop on your soles and palms.

Shoes that fit poorly are often the cause of corns or calluses on your feet. Calluses on your hands usually result from the pressure or friction of hand tools. For instance, over time, daily use of a shovel will line your hands with calluses.

How serious are corns and calluses?
Although corns and calluses can be unsightly, they need treatment only if they cause discomfort. If you have diabetes, you're at an increased risk of complications from a corn or callus. See your doctor if a corn or callus becomes painful or ulcerated.

Treatment
In most cases, you can prevent corns and calluses by wearing shoes that fit properly. Protect your hands by wearing gloves when using tools. Often, you can treat corns or calluses on your own. If a large corn persists or is painful, your doctor may pare it down.

The problem can be more serious if you have an underlying foot deformity. Your doctor may be able to correct the situation with surgery or with custom-made padded shoe inserts (orthotics), which prevent recurring corns.

Hammertoe and mallet toe

Signs and symptoms
- A clawlike or mallet-like clenched appearance of a toe

- Pain and difficulty moving the toe

Unlike a bunion, which affects only the big toe, hammertoe can affect any toe. Most commonly, it occurs in the second toe. Generally, both toe joints are affected, causing the toe to bend upward in the middle, giving it a clawlike appearance. Wearing shoes that are too short can cause hammertoe. The condition tends to run in some families. The deformity may occur in people with muscle and nerve damage from diabetes. A mallet toe is characterized by a deformity at the end of the toe that gives it a mallet-like appearance.

How serious are hammertoe and mallet toe?
Both conditions can cause pain with walking and other movements.

Treatment
Your doctor or a podiatrist may prescribe an orthotic device to reposition the toe and relieve the pressure and pain. It's also important to wear shoes that fit properly and that have a wide toe box. In severe cases, the condition may require surgery.

Bunions

Signs and symptoms
- A bony protrusion at the base of your big toe

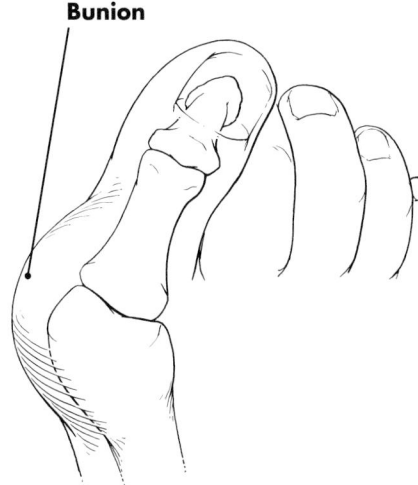

Bunion

When the base of your big toe extends beyond the normal profile of your foot, the bump that results is called a bunion. To prevent a bunion, avoid shoes with narrow toes or high heels.

- Pain and limitation of motion

A bunion develops when the big toe bends toward the next toe or overlaps it, causing deformity of the foot. The base of the big toe juts out beyond the normal profile of the foot, producing a bump known as a bunion. A bunion is often subjected to constant rubbing that, in turn, results in thickening of the skin.

Women are much more likely to develop this common problem than are men. Some people are genetically predisposed to getting bunions, but the problem can also develop as a result of wearing tight, high-heeled shoes with pointed toes.

Diagnosis

Your doctor may be able to diagnose a bunion simply by looking at your foot. However, he or she may request X-rays to evaluate the problem and treatment options.

How serious is a bunion?

Typically, a bunion causes only minor discomfort, but sometimes the pain can be severe. Accompanying bursitis or osteoarthritis can develop in the toe joint, causing pain and stiffness. Because a bunion distorts the shape of your foot, finding suitable shoes can be difficult.

Treatment

The best way to relieve a painful bunion — or to prevent the condition — is to wear shoes that fit properly and that have a wide toe box that provides ample room for your toes. To provide more room in a leather shoe for a bunion deformity, take your shoes to a shoe repair shop and have them stretched.

Treating corns and calluses in the area of the bunion may reduce discomfort. If you develop bursitis, wearing an old shoe with a hole cut in the area over the bunion may provide relief. Felt pads also may be helpful.

Surgery generally isn't necessary unless the deformity is severe or causes severe pain. During surgery, a surgeon realigns the bones by removing excess bone.

Flatfeet

Signs and symptoms

- No visible arches in your feet when placing your weight on them

The intricate alignment of bones, muscles, ligaments and tendons in your feet form side-to-side (metatarsal) and lengthwise (longitudinal) arches. As you walk, these springy, elastic arches help distribute your body weight evenly across each of your feet. Your arches play an integral role in how you walk.

Everyone has flatfeet at birth. Your arches usually develop fully by age 12 or 13, but some people's arches never form properly. Many people with flatfeet have no problems because alignment elsewhere in their lower extremities compensates for their flatfeet.

Some people with flatfeet, however, experience inflammation and pain in the ligaments in the bottoms of their feet, Achilles tendinitis, stress fractures, shin splints, bunions and calluses. Flatfeet can lead to muscular imbalances and joint problems in their ankles, knees, hips and lower back.

Most flatfooted people develop arch problems as a result of continual stress on the feet. Excessive weight, postural abnormalities, weakened supportive tissue or overuse may weaken the ligaments and muscles supporting the arch that runs lengthwise in your foot, causing it to fall. Prolonged stress on the balls of your feet or walking, standing or exercising on hard surfaces may weaken or flatten the metatarsal arch at the front of your foot. This places additional pressure on nerves and blood vessels in the area, causing pain and irritation.

Diagnosis

A medical doctor or podiatrist can diagnose flatfeet by examining your feet.

Treatment

If you experience chronic pain as a result of flatfeet, wearing a custom-designed arch support might provide relief. You slip this orthotic device into your shoe, and it helps support and re-form the arch of your foot.

Corrective orthotic devices help align your foot in a better weight-bearing position. They also absorb shock and help control excessive inward or outward rotation (pronation or supination) of your longitudinal arch when you walk. To get custom-made orthotic devices, you need to see your doctor or podiatrist. Flexible models are available for people who can't tolerate the more rigid corrective orthotic devices.

Foot ulcer

Signs and symptoms

- An open sore on the skin surrounded by inflamed tissue
- Pus from the ulcer, if the tissue is infected

A foot ulcer can result from a foot wound or from skin irritation caused by wearing improperly fitting shoes. Foot ulcers are most common in individuals with diminished circulation or nerve deterioration due to diabetes.

See your doctor if you develop a foot ulcer. Several treatments are available to treat the condition, and only rarely is surgery necessary. For more information on foot ulcers, see pages 758 and 1001.

Back Pain

The spine is one of the strongest parts of the body. It's made up of more than 26 bones, 24 of which are called vertebrae. You have seven cervical vertebrae in your neck, 12 thoracic vertebrae in the middle of your back behind your chest and five lumbar vertebrae in your lower back. The other two bones are the sacrum, made up of five fused vertebrae between your pelvic bones, and your tailbone (coccyx), which is made up of three to five fused bones at the end of your spinal column.

Your vertebrae stack on top of one another to form your backbone, the flexible column that runs from the base of your skull to your tailbone. Between your vertebrae are spongy cushions called disks. They have a strong, fibrous outer covering that protects a gel on the inside. The joints of your vertebrae are reinforced by strong ligaments and surrounded by many sturdy muscles.

The intricate structure of your back bends and twists and bears the weight of your body and the loads you carry. Your backbone also protects your spinal cord.

The complex structure of your spine contributes to its potential for problems. Seemingly minor changes in the alignment or balance of any part — whether a disk, vertebra, joint or muscle — can make movements painful. When the nerves or spinal cord that travels through your backbone (spinal canal) is affected, there's a risk of pain or numbness in parts of your body. A serious back injury can cause permanent damage to your spinal cord and paralysis (see page 568).

Fortunately, it's difficult to damage the spine. Usually, when your back hurts, there's an irritation of one of the spine's components. For example, your disks may have a poor blood supply. As a result, adults are susceptible to disk cracking and dehydration (degeneration) over time. All adults' disks degenerate to some degree with age.

Risk factors that may make some people more prone to back problems and slow recovery are lack of physical activity, poor posture, being overweight, being under physical or mental stress, and having weak trunk muscles that support your spine. Work-related risk factors include heavy physical labor, frequent bending or twisting, or static work postures, such as standing still, sitting in one place or bending over for long periods of time.

Back strain and spasm

Signs and symptoms
- Back pain and stiffness
- Difficulty moving

Back problems are among the most common human ailments. Most people experience back discomfort in their lifetimes. It most often occurs from strained muscles and ligaments, from improper or heavy lifting, or after a sudden awkward movement. Sometimes a muscle spasm can cause back pain.

Structural problems
In some cases, back pain may be caused by structural problems, such as:
- **Bulging or ruptured disks.** Disks act as cushions between the vertebrae in your spine. Sometimes, the soft material inside a disk may bulge out of place or rupture and press on a nerve. But many people who have bulging (herniated) disks experience no pain.
- **Sciatica.** If a bulging (herniated) disk presses on the main nerve that travels down your leg, it can cause sharp, shooting pain through the buttock, back of the leg and even into the foot.
- **Arthritis.** The joints most commonly affected by osteoarthritis are the hips, hands, knees and lower back. In some cases arthritis in the spine can lead to a narrowing of the space around the spinal cord and nerves, a condition called spinal stenosis.
- **Skeletal irregularities.** Back pain can occur if your spine curves in an abnormal way. If the natural curves in your spine become exaggerated, your upper back may look abnormally rounded or your lower back may arch excessively. Scoliosis, a condition in which your spine curves to the side, also may lead to back pain.
- **Osteoporosis.** Compression fractures of your spine's vertebrae can occur if your bones become porous and brittle.

In rare cases, back pain may be related to serious neurological problems, cancer in the spine or an infection of the spine.

Sometimes, you may feel pain at the moment you strain the muscle or sprain the ligament. At other times, soreness may develop gradually. You may awaken with the discomfort. Regardless of how the pain develops, it's often difficult for your doctor to determine the exact cause.

Diagnosis
Diagnostic tests aren't usually necessary to confirm the cause of your back pain. However, if you do see your doctor for back pain, he or she will examine your back and assess your ability to sit, stand, walk and lift your legs. He or she may also test your reflexes with a rubber reflex hammer.

These assessments help determine exactly where the pain comes

Structures of Your Spine

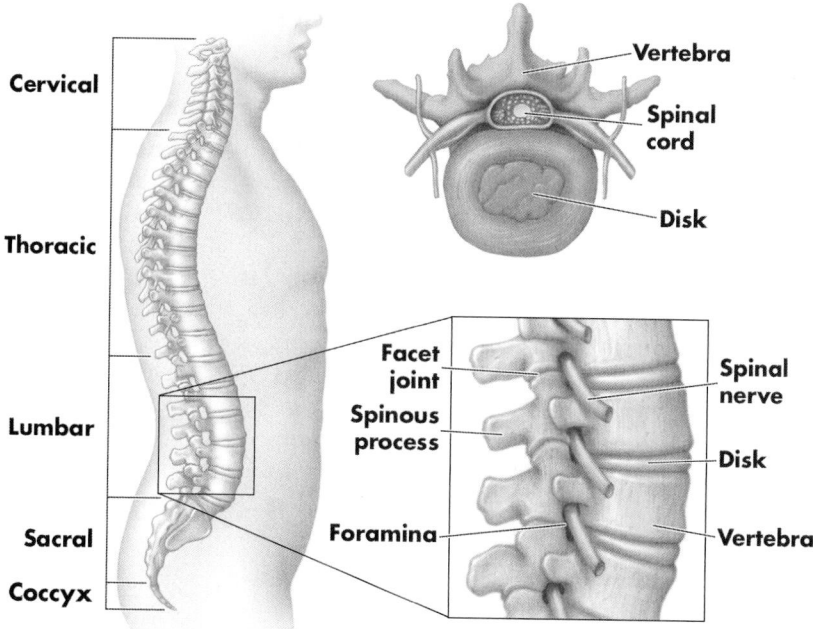

Cervical

Thoracic

Lumbar

Sacral

Coccyx

Vertebra

Spinal cord

Disk

Facet joint

Spinous process

Foramina

Spinal nerve

Disk

Vertebra

from and what types of activities are best for you. They can also help rule out more-serious causes of back pain.

If there's reason to suspect that you have a tumor, a fracture, an infection or other specific condition that may be causing your back pain, your doctor may order tests such as an X-ray, computerized tomography (CT) scan, magnetic resonance image (MRI) or bone scan.

How serious are back strain and spasm?

There's no ignoring the discomfort that accompanies a sore back. Most often the problem subsides given time and rest. Unfortunately, recurring episodes of back pain are the rule rather than the exception.

See a doctor if you experience:
• Severe pain
• Fever, chills, night sweats or unexplained weight loss — these signs and symptoms may indicate a spinal infection or tumor
• Pain that awakens you at night or severely limits your day-to-day activities

• Signs or symptoms that don't improve within a week or two
  See a doctor immediately if you experience pain that radiates down one of your legs along with associated weakness in the leg or bowel or bladder changes.

Diagnosing the cause of back pain often isn't easy, but it's important to rule out certain underlying causes. Once that's done, knowing precisely what's causing the pain probably won't change the approach to treatment.

Treatment

Most back pain gets better with a few weeks of home treatment and careful attention. Over-the-counter pain relievers may be all that you need to improve your pain. A short period of bed rest is OK, but more than a couple of days actually does more harm than good.

If this doesn't help, see your doctor. He or she may suggest stronger medications or other therapies.

Medications

Your doctor may prescribe non-steroidal anti-inflammatory drugs

or in some cases, a muscle relaxant, to relieve mild to moderate back pain that doesn't get better with over-the-counter pain relievers. Narcotics, such as codeine or hydrocodone, may be used for a short period of time with close supervision by your doctor.

Low doses of certain types of antidepressants — particularly tricyclic antidepressants, such as amitriptyline — have been shown to relieve chronic back pain, independent of their effect on depression.

Physical therapy and exercise

A physical therapist can apply a variety of treatments, such as heat, ice, ultrasound, electrical stimulation and muscle-release techniques, to your back muscles and soft tissues to reduce pain. As pain improves, the therapist can teach you specific exercises to increase your flexibility, strengthen your back and abdominal muscles, and improve your posture. Regular use of these techniques can help prevent the pain from coming back.

Injections

If other measures don't relieve your pain and if your pain radiates down your leg, your doctor may inject cortisone — an anti-inflammatory medication — into the space around your spinal cord (epidural space). A cortisone injection helps decrease inflammation around the nerve roots, but the pain relief usually lasts less than six weeks. In some cases, your doctor may inject medication near or into the small joints (facet joints) at the back of the spine, which are often affected by arthritis.

Surgery

Few people ever need surgery for back pain. There are no effective surgical techniques for muscle- and soft tissue-related back pain. Surgery is usually reserved for pain caused by a herniated disk placing pressure on a nerve.

If you have unrelenting pain or progressive muscle weakness caused by nerve compression, you may benefit from surgery. Types of back surgery include:

- **Fusion.** This surgery involves joining two vertebrae to eliminate painful movement. A bone graft is inserted between the two vertebrae, which may then be splinted together with metal plates, screws or cages. A drawback to the procedure is that it increases the chances of arthritis developing in adjoining vertebrae.
- **Disk replacement.** An alternative to fusion, this surgery inserts an artificial disk as a replacement cushion between two vertebrae.
- **Partial removal of disk.** If disk material is pressing or squeezing a nerve, your doctor may be able to remove just the portion of the disk that's causing the problem.
- **Partial removal of a vertebra.** If your spine has developed bony growths that are pinching your spinal cord or nerves, surgeons can remove a small section of the offending vertebra, to open up the passage.

Self-care

Self-care that you can perform at home is the most common approach to resolving back pain.

- **Heat and cold.** Hot baths and hot and cold compresses can soothe sore and inflamed muscles. Use cold treatments first, several times a day, for no longer than 20 minutes each time to avoid injury to the skin. Use ice wrapped in a plastic bag and then in a cloth or towel to protect your skin. Check your skin every five minutes or so during treatment. It will redden with the use of ice. If it begins to lose its redness, stop icing the area because the loss of color may indicate frostbite.

  After the pain subsides a bit — usually in a day or two — apply heat with a heating pad or heat lamp. Avoid falling asleep while using a heating pad because the pad may get hotter the longer it's on. You don't want to burn yourself. Limit heat applications to 20 minutes. Avoid using heat or ice on areas of skin with decreased sensation or poor circulation.
- **Exercise.** Exercise is one of the primary keys to recovery. Do whatever you can do, such as walking, riding an exercise bike or swimming. Start with a small amount of exercise and increase by small increments.
- **Rest.** In the past, doctors recommended staying on your back in bed for a number of weeks. Now the recommendation is for, at most, one or two days, and only in severe cases. Prolonged bed rest is generally not good for your back because it decreases strength and endurance.

Prevention

The best way to deal with back pain is to prevent it. If you've already had episodes of back pain, you may be able to prevent a recurrence. If your pain does recur, you may be able to lessen its duration and severity.

Exercise daily

Regular exercise is your most potent weapon against back problems. Activity can increase your aerobic capacity, improve your overall fitness, strengthen back and abdominal muscles, and help you shed excess pounds, which can stress your back. Stretching and strengthening your muscles also can help reduce wear and tear on your back.

Stretching after warming up and after you exercise reduces your risk of injury by increasing flexibility in

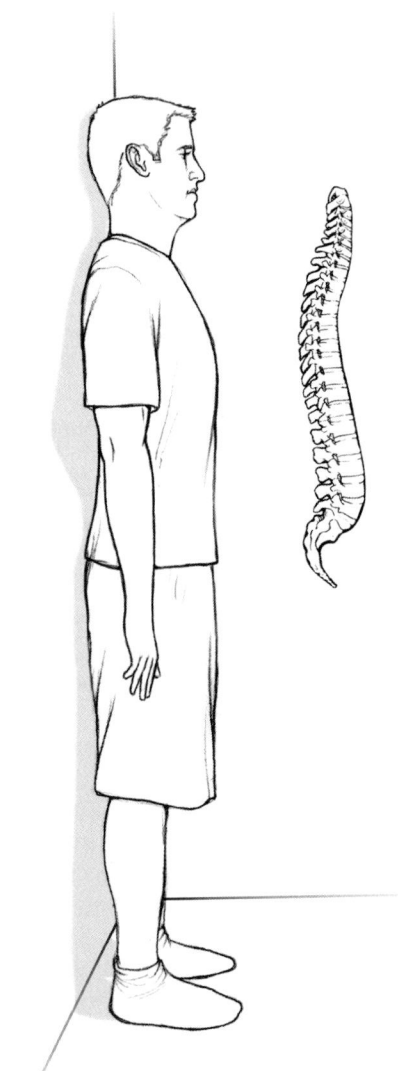

For proper posture, stand straight and imagine that a string extends from your earlobe to your instep.

Back-Strengthening Exercises

The following exercises can help stretch and strengthen the muscles in your back and prevent spinal fractures.

Hamstring Stretch

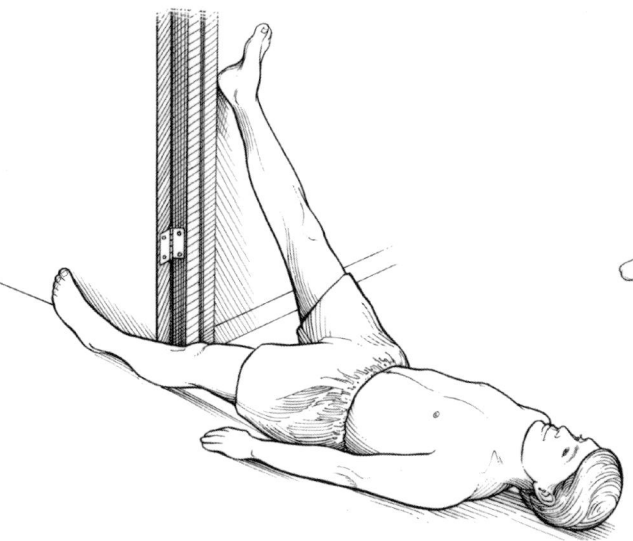

Lie on the floor in front of a doorway and extend your left leg across the threshold. Place the leg to be stretched up against the wall and straighten the leg. Hold for 30 seconds. Repeat, reversing leg positions. Don't lock your knee.

Knee-to-Chest Stretch

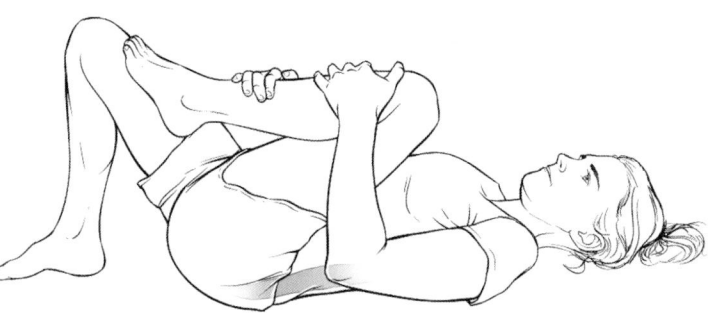

Lie with your knees bent and feet flat on the floor. Pull your left knee toward your chest with both hands. Hold for 30 seconds. Switch legs. Repeat with each leg.

Bridge

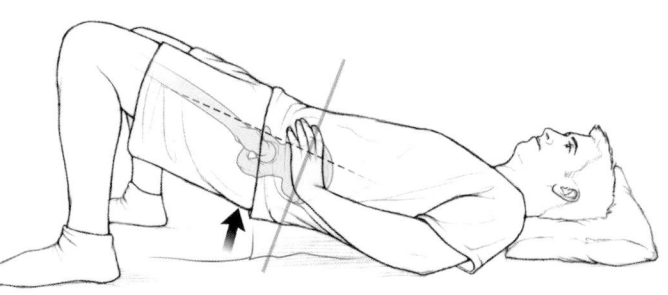

Lie on a mat with your feet flat, about shoulder-width apart. Raise your buttocks off the mat, keeping a level line from your knees to your hips. Keep your shoulders, head and neck relaxed on the mat. Hold the position until you become fatigued and can no longer comfortably keep your knees and hips in a straight line.

Standing Extension

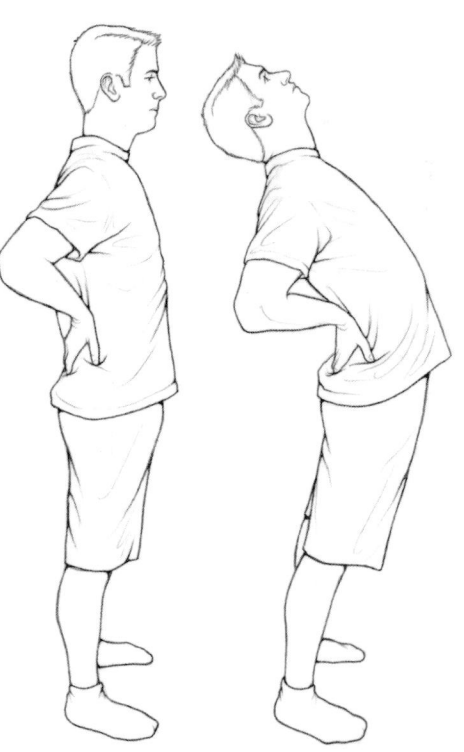

Stand tall. Place your hands on your lower back. Slowly lift your chest up and over your hands to gently arch your back. Follow the same path to return to the starting position. Repeat.

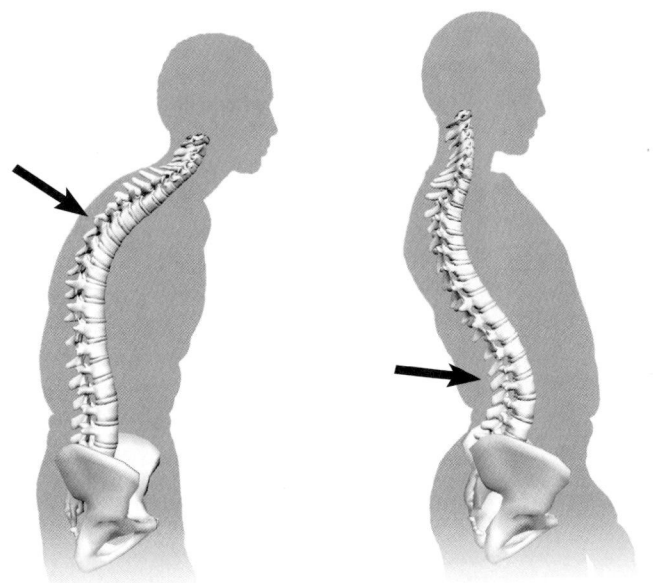

Two common forms of improper posture are slouching your shoulders (kyphosis), left, in which shoulders roll forward, and swayback (lordosis), right, in which your abdomen sticks out too far in front and your buttocks too far in back.

your muscles. Strengthening your arms, legs, abdomen and lower body can help prevent or relieve back pain and decrease your risk of falls and other injuries.

Ask your doctor or a physical therapist for advice before beginning an exercise program, especially if you've hurt your back before or if you have other health problems, such as osteoporosis.

If you're out of condition from lack of activity, your back muscles may be weak and susceptible to injury. Start slowly and pace yourself. As you become stronger, work up to 30 minutes of exercise daily.

Swimming and other water exercises place minimal strain on your lower back. Using a stationary bike, treadmill, elliptical trainer or cross-country ski machine will jar your back less than running will.

Practice good posture
Poor posture can lead to back pain, inhibit your breathing and fatigue your muscles. Good posture supports and protects all parts of your body. By keeping your muscles, ligaments, tendons and bones in

their natural positions, you reduce stress on your back.

You normally have three spinal curves: an inward (forward) curve at the neck, an outward curve at the upper back and an inward curve at the lower back. Slouching or rolling your shoulders forward (kyphosis) shortens your chest muscles and reduces their flexi-

bility. Swayback (lordosis) causes your abdomen to stick out in front and your buttocks to stick out in back, creating an exaggerated curve between your pelvis and ribs and stressing your lower back.

Practice good posture by becoming aware of how you sit and stand and correcting your position when necessary. When standing, keep your shoulders back and your head high. Pull in your abdomen and buttocks, and tuck in your chin. When sitting, make sure your thighs are parallel to the ground and that your head isn't slumped forward.

Lift correctly
When lifting, bend your knees, not your back. Whether the object you want to pick up weighs a fraction of an ounce or 50 pounds, squat with your back straight and let your legs do the lifting. Hold the load close to your body and increase the tension on your muscles gradually. Don't jerk or lunge to lift the load.

Maintain a healthy weight
A major cause of backache is being overweight. Extra pounds at the midriff stress your back. If you're overweight, try to achieve and maintain a healthy weight and establish an exercise program.

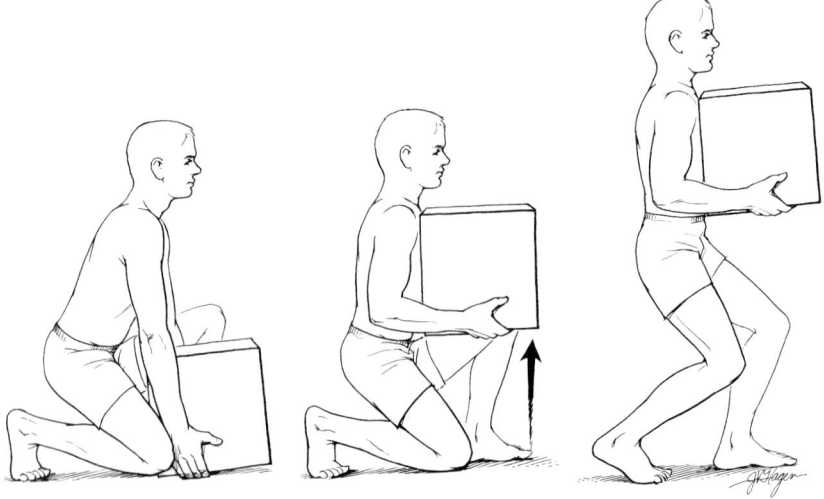

When lifting any object, let your legs do the work. Bend your knees rather than your back. Hold the object close to your body and lift gently. Avoid jerking or lunging upward.

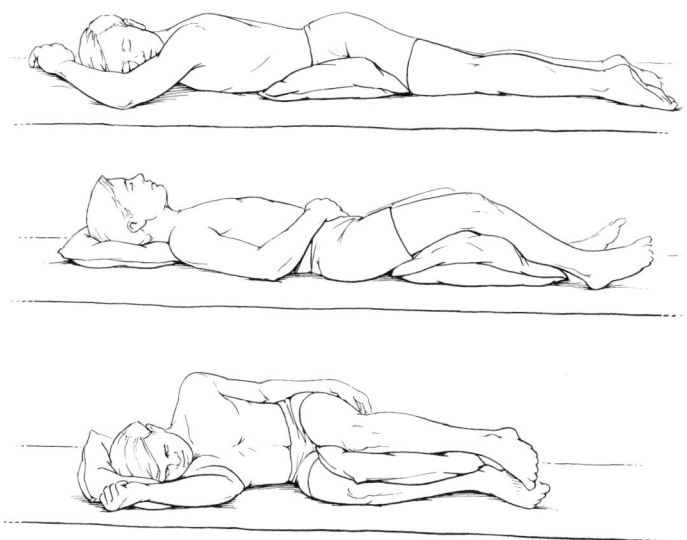

To avoid aggravating a back problem: When you sleep or lie down, don't sleep on your stomach unless you cushion your abdomen with a pillow (top). If you sleep on your back, use pillows to support your knees and neck (middle). The best option is to sleep on your side with your legs drawn up slightly toward your chest (bottom) and with a pillow between your knees.

Herniated disk

Signs and symptoms

- Mild to severe pain in your neck or back
- Numbness or weakness of an arm or hand and serious neck, shoulder and upper extremity pain, which might indicate a herniated disk in the neck
- Numbness or weakness in the buttocks, legs or feet, which might indicate a herniated disk in the middle or lower part of the back
- Shooting pain during coughing, sneezing or straining
- Usually, one arm or one leg affected significantly more than the other
- Sudden change in bowel or bladder function, such as incontinence

Your spinal column is made up of bones (vertebrae) that are cushioned by small disks consisting of a tough outer layer (annulus) and a soft, jellylike inner layer (nucleus). These disks act as shock absorbers, protecting the spine and nerves from the stress of everyday tasks as well as strenuous work such as heavy lifting.

When a disk herniates, a tear or weakness in the annulus allows the jellylike nucleus to push out into the spinal canal. If it puts pressure on a spinal nerve, the herniated disk can cause pain, numbness or weakness in the back, legs or arms, depending on where the disk is located.

Herniated disks are most common in the lower (lumbar) spine, but about 10 percent occur in the neck (cervical spine). Anyone can get herniated disks, but herniations in the lumbar spine are most common between 35 and 45 years of age. Cervical disk herniation is more common between 50 and 60 years of age.

You can have a herniated disk without knowing it. Bulging (herniated) disks sometimes show up on spinal images of people who have no symptoms of a disk problem. But some herniated disks can be painful.

Disk herniation is most often the result of gradual, age-related wearing of the disks. As you age, your spinal disks lose some of their water content. That makes them less flexible and more prone to tearing or rupturing.

Diagnosis

Your doctor will likely take your medical history and perform a physical exam. In most herniated disk cases, a physical exam is all that's needed to make a diagnosis. If your doctor suspects another condition or needs to see which nerves are affected or if there is no symptom improvement after four weeks of conservative treatment, one or more of these diagnostic tests may be performed:

- **Magnetic resonance imaging (MRI) scan.** MRI uses a magnetic field and radio waves to create images of your body. This test can be used to confirm the location of the herniated disk and to see which nerves are affected.

Back Braces

Custom-fitted back braces (corsets) are available by prescription. Some are sold over-the-counter at most full-service pharmacies and medical supply stores. Worn properly, they relieve muscle strain by restricting motion in your lower back when you sit or stand. They can provide warmth, comfort and support to your back.

Unfortunately, many back braces have stiff stays and uncomfortable shoulder straps. They can also be unattractive and expensive. More important, because the support comes from the brace rather than from your own muscles, a back brace may actually weaken your back muscles, especially if you wear it for long periods. Most doctors recommend using a back brace only for short periods during back-straining activities or after some types of back surgeries.

- **Computerized tomography (CT) scan.** An X-ray unit creates cross-sectional images of your spinal column and the structures around it.
- **Myelogram.** A dye is injected into the spinal fluid, and then X-rays are taken. This test can show pressure on the spinal cord or nerves due to multiple herniated disks or other conditions.
- **X-rays.** Plain X-rays don't detect herniated disks, but they may be performed to rule out other causes of back pain, such as an infection or a broken bone.

How serious is a herniated disk?

In many people, a herniated disk will repair itself given time — usually two to six weeks — and proper rest. In some instances, an operation is necessary.

Treatment

Conservative treatment — mainly avoiding painful positions and following a planned exercise and pain-medication regimen — relieves symptoms in 9 out of 10 people with a herniated disk. Within a couple of months of starting this treatment, you should be back to normal. Imaging studies show that the protruding or displaced portion of the disk shrinks over time, corresponding to the improvement in symptoms. Depending on your symptoms, your doctor may recommend:

- **Modified activity.** Take it easy when you have back pain. Try to avoid activities that aggravate your symptoms, such as improper reaching, bending and lifting, and prolonged sitting.

  However, intermittent activity to maintain fitness and minimize stiffness is very important, so physical therapy and exercises to increase flexibility and strength may be prescribed. Physical activity shouldn't be avoided. In fact, staying at work is best, even if you need to reduce your workload or assume lighter duties.

  Over several weeks, your activity level can gradually increase until you're comfortable with everyday tasks.
- **Physical therapy.** A physical therapist can apply heat, ice, traction, ultrasound and electrical stimulation for pain relief. A physical therapist can also show you positions and exercises designed to minimize the pain of a herniated disk. As the pain improves, your physical therapist can advance you to a rehabilitation program of core strength and stability to maximize your back health and help protect against future injury.

- **Heat or cold.** Initially, cold packs can be used to relieve pain and inflammation. After a few days, you may switch to gentle heat to give relief and comfort.
- **Pain medication.** If your pain is mild to moderate, your doctor may recommend analgesic medication, such as aspirin, ibuprofen (Advil, Motrin IB, others), acetaminophen (Tylenol, others) or naproxen sodium (Aleve, others). Muscle relaxants such as diazepam (Valium) or cyclobenzaprine (Amrix) may be prescribed for a few days if you have back or limb spasms.

  If your pain doesn't improve with these medications, your doctor may prescribe a stronger medication to help relieve your pain. In addition, inflammation-suppressing corticosteroids may be prescribed orally or given by injection directly into the area around the spinal nerves.
- **Bed rest.** Constant, severe back pain from a herniated disk

Sciatica

Inflammation of a nerve or compression of a nerve root in your lower back can cause sciatica. The condition is named after the sciatic nerve that extends down each leg from your hip to your heel. Only 1 or 2 percent of people with back pain have sciatica.

The disorder is characterized by pain radiating from your lower back down through your buttock to your lower leg. The nerve compression also can cause tingling, numbness or muscle weakness. Coughing, sneezing and other activities that exert pressure on your spine can aggravate sciatica.

Usually, the pain resolves on its own. However, severe nerve compression can cause progressive weakness of affected muscles and require surgical intervention.

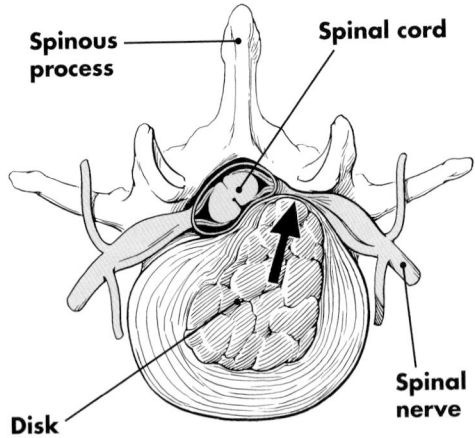

Spinous process

Spinal cord

Disk

Spinal nerve

If a disk in your back ruptures, a portion of its jelly-like interior may protrude, putting pressure on a spinal nerve (see arrow) or on the spinal cord.

sometimes requires one or two days in bed on a firm surface or mattress. Strict bed rest for longer than a day or two, however, can inhibit recovery by causing loss of muscle tone.

- **Time.** Herniated disk symptoms generally take four to six weeks to significantly improve. If your symptoms have not resolved after six weeks, more-aggressive therapies may be effective and prevent you from needing surgery.

Surgery

A small percentage of people with herniated disks eventually need surgery. You may be a good candidate for surgery if conservative treatment fails to improve your symptoms after four to six weeks. Surgery also may be considered if a disk fragment lodges in the spinal canal, pressing on a nerve, or if you're having trouble standing or walking.

The most common surgery for a herniated disk is a microdiskectomy. This procedure has the best success rate among healthy people with single disk herniations.

Microdiskectomy is related to standard (open) diskectomy, a spinal surgery that involves cutting away some of the spinal bones (vertebrae) to access the herniated disks and compressed nerve roots. In microdiskectomy, surgeons use a surgical microscope or magnifying lens to allow smaller incisions in the skin, muscles and bone overlying a herniated disk. Smaller incisions and less disruption to surrounding tissue lessen pain and shorten recovery time.

Spondylosis

Signs and symptoms

- Back pain and tenderness
- Difficulty moving your back
- Pain in the back of your thighs when standing
- In mild cases, none

Spondylosis is a disorder in which, over time, the spine becomes stiff and loses its flexibility. Spondylosis may result from excessive wear and tear, an injury, or simply aging.

Whatever the cause, the disks between the vertebrae become worn, and the spaces between them narrow. The facet joints of the spine are usually affected as well, and bone spurs may develop. The result is pain and stiffness.

Spondylosis is sometimes referred to as degenerative joint disease or osteoarthritis of the spine. Spondylosis that occurs in the neck is known as cervical spondylosis. It's not the same condition as ankylosing spondylitis (see page 980).

Diagnosis

An X-ray of your spine can often reveal the condition of your vertebrae. If you've had a herniated disk, you may be more susceptible to spondylosis.

How serious is spondylosis?

For many people, the condition isn't serious, but learning to deal with the discomfort can take time.

In rare cases, spondylosis in the lower back can lead to difficulty with bladder and bowel control and with walking.

Treatment

Depending on the severity of the condition and your symptoms, your doctor may recommend a combination of physical therapy, self-care measures such as heat, cold and gentle massage, and pain relievers.

Treatment of more-severe cases may involve taking muscle relaxants or injecting corticosteroid medications into the joints between the vertebrae to reduce pain and inflammation.

If neurological signs and symptoms develop or worsen, such as weakness in the arms or legs, surgery may be necessary to remove bone spurs or other irregularities that are placing pressure on the spinal cord.

Spinal stenosis

Signs and symptoms

- Pain or cramping in legs when walking or standing for long periods
- Radiating pain that starts in a hip or buttock and extends down the back of the leg
- Progressive numbness or weakness in a leg
- Pain in neck or shoulders
- Trouble with bladder and bowel control

Spinal stenosis is a narrowing of an area in your spinal canal that can cause compression of your spinal cord and nerve roots. You may first notice an ache in a buttock, thigh and calf when you walk or stand.

Symptoms are often subtle and similar to those associated with other causes of back and leg pain. However, if you bend forward at your waist or sit for a few moments, the pain goes away.

Spinal stenosis typically affects adults beyond age 50. It can develop because of a congenital defect, but it usually results from osteoarthritis.

Wear and tear, a previous injury, or aging can slowly deteriorate the protective tissue (cartilage) covering joint surfaces in your spine. Disks between vertebrae in your spine may become worn, and spaces between vertebrae may narrow. Bony outgrowths (spurs) also may develop. These changes can cause vertebrae and soft tissue to move inward into the spinal canal, compressing nerves.

Ligaments in your back may become stiff and thick over time. This loss of elasticity may shorten your spine, narrowing the spinal canal and compressing nerve roots.

Pressure may develop on roots of your sciatic nerve. This may cause pain to radiate from your lower back down your buttock to your calf. Numbness or weakness in your legs may eventually develop. Occasionally, nerves to the bladder and bowel become compressed, which leads to incontinence.

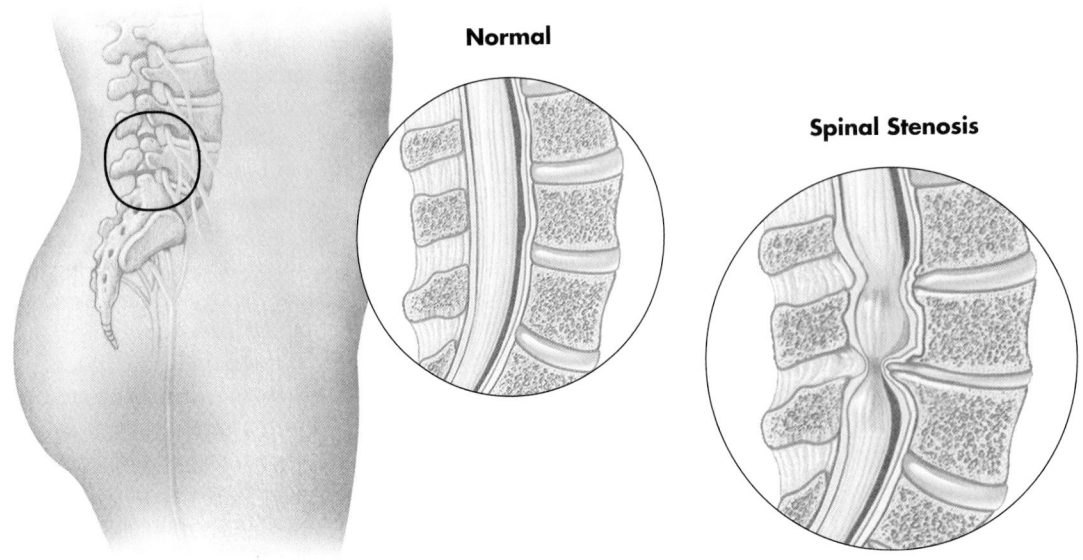

Normal

Spinal Stenosis

In spinal stenosis, an area of the spinal canal is narrowed, often from a herniated disk. The narrowing may place pressure on the spinal cord and compress nerve roots.

Bending forward at your waist or sitting relieves the pain because these positions increase the diameter of your spinal canal, reducing pressure on spinal nerves. In severe cases of narrowing, the pain may persist regardless of activity or position.

Diagnosis

Spinal stenosis can be difficult to diagnose because its signs and symptoms are often intermittent and because they resemble those of many age-related conditions. To help diagnose spinal stenosis and rule out other disorders, your doctor will ask about your medical history and perform a physical exam that may include checking your peripheral pulses, range of motion and leg reflexes.

You're also likely to undergo one or more tests, including a spinal X-ray, magnetic resonance image (MRI) scan or computerized tomography (CT) scan, to look for an abnormality such as a herniated disk or bone spur that's putting pressure on your spinal cord.

Sometimes a doctor may inject an individual with a spinal nerve block or epidural steroids. If your symptoms improve after the injection, spinal stenosis is likely the cause of your discomfort. The problem with this approach is that a negative finding doesn't mean you don't have spinal stenosis.

How serious is spinal stenosis?

Symptoms differ depending on what part of your spine is involved and how large an area it affects. If the pressure on your nerve roots can be effectively relieved with treatment, symptoms may not progress any further and may even improve.

In some cases, spinal stenosis can lead to disabling pain or other symptoms that require surgery.

Treatment

Many people are effectively treated with conservative measures. But if you have disabling pain or your ability to walk is severely impaired, your doctor may recommend spinal surgery. Acute loss of bowel or bladder function is usually considered a medical emergency and requires immediate surgical intervention.

Nonsurgical treatments

Before considering surgery, your doctor is likely to recommend trying one or more of the following for at least three months:

- **Physical therapy.** Working with a physical therapist can build up your strength and endurance and help maintain the flexibility and stability of your spine.
- **Nonsteroidal anti-inflammatory drugs (NSAIDs).** They include over-the-counter and prescription medications, such as ibuprofen (Advil, Motrin IB, others) or indomethacin (Indocin), to reduce inflammation and pain. Although they can provide relief, NSAIDs have a "ceiling effect" — there's a limit to how much pain they can control.

What's more, NSAIDs can cause serious side effects, including stomach ulcers that may bleed. If you take these medications, talk to your doctor so that you can be monitored for potential problems.
- **Analgesics.** This group of pain relievers includes acetaminophen (Tylenol, others). Analgesics don't reduce inflammation, but they can effectively treat pain. Yet chronic overuse of acetaminophen can cause kidney and liver damage. Drinking alcohol increases your risk of serious side effects.
- **Rest or restricted activity.** Moderate rest followed by a gradual

return to activity may improve symptoms. Swimming is a good exercise, especially for people with neurogenic claudication, but biking also is recommended because it keeps your back in a flexed position rather than in an extended one.

- **A back brace (corset).** This helps provide support and may especially benefit people who have weak abdominal muscles or degeneration in more than one area of the spine.
- **Epidural steroid injections.** In some cases, your doctor may inject a corticosteroid medication into the spinal fluid around your spinal cord and nerve roots.

Corticosteroids suppress inflammation and can be especially helpful in treating pain that radiates down the back of your leg. But because corticosteroids can cause a number of serious side effects, the number of injections you can receive is limited.

Surgery
The goal of surgery is to relieve pressure on the spinal cord or nerves and to maintain the integrity and strength of your spine. This can be accomplished in several ways. The most common surgical procedures include:

- **Decompressive laminectomy.** In this procedure, your surgeon removes all of the lamina — the back part of the bone over the spinal canal — to create more space for the nerves and to allow access to bone spurs or ruptured disks that may also be removed.
- **Laminotomy.** In this procedure, just a portion of the lamina is removed to relieve pressure or to allow access to a disk or bone spur that's pressing on a nerve. The risks are the same as for laminectomy.
- **Fusion.** This procedure may be performed on its own or at the same time as laminectomy. It's used to permanently connect (fuse) two or more vertebral bones in your spine and may be

especially indicated when one vertebra slips over another. To fuse the spine, small pieces of extra bone are needed to fill the space between two vertebrae. This may come from a bone bank or from your own body, usually your pelvic bone. Wires, rods, screws, metal cages or plates also may be used, especially if your spine is unstable or the operation takes place to correct a deformity.

Back surgery can relieve pressure in your spine, but it's not a cure-all spinal stenosis treatment. You might continue to have pain for a period of time. For some people, recovery can take weeks or months and may require physical therapy. What's more, surgery won't stop the degenerative process, and symptoms may return — sometimes within just a few years.

Scoliosis

Signs and symptoms
- A sideways curvature of the spine
- An asymmetric rib cage with one shoulder blade protruding

Scoliosis is a painless, abnormal curvature of the spine. Usually, a curve to one side develops, followed by a compensating bend in the opposite direction, forming an S-like configuration — as seen from the back.

A small percentage of cases result from a congenital spinal defect. The cause of most cases is unknown, although heredity may play a role. The deformity may begin during infancy or in the preschool or early grade school years, but often the condition is detected in adolescence. Because the onset is gradual and the condition doesn't cause pain, significant curvature can develop without a child or parent noticing it. Many schools have screening programs to detect scoliosis.

Diagnosis
A visual examination of the spine is usually sufficient to identify

scoliosis, although your doctor may want an X-ray of your spine to help determine the extent of the curvature.

How serious is scoliosis?
Mild cases generally cause few problems and don't require treatment, but they need close monitoring because the condition can worsen.

In more-severe scoliosis, vertebrae may rotate, resulting in widely separated ribs on one side of the body and narrowed spaces on the other. Lung problems may develop as a result of the disease.

Treatment
Small curves don't require treatment. More-pronounced curves may require treatment with a brace, especially in growing adolescents. The brace helps correct the deformity and straighten the spine. More-severe curvature may require surgery. In general, exercises have no effect on scoliosis.

Bone Diseases

Your bones are living, changing tissues. The marrow within the bones produces blood cells, and the bones act as a storehouse for the minerals calcium and phosphate. Some of the diseases that affect bone, such as osteoporosis, are common, and others are rare.

Osteoporosis

Signs and symptoms
- Back pain
- Loss of height with stooped posture
- A bone fracture, including a vertebral compression fracture

Osteoporosis, which means "porous bones," causes bones to become weak and brittle — so brittle that even mild stresses such as bending over, lifting a vacuum cleaner or coughing can cause a fracture. In most cases, bones weaken when you have low levels of calcium, phosphorus and other minerals in your bones.

A common result of osteoporosis is fractures — most of them in the spine, hip or wrist. Although it's often thought of as a female disease, osteoporosis also affects many men. In addition to people who have osteoporosis, many more have low bone density.

When you're young, your body makes new bone faster than it breaks down old bone, and your bone mass increases. You reach your peak bone mass in your mid-30s. After that, bone remodeling continues, but you lose slightly more than you gain.

At menopause, when estrogen levels drop, bone loss in women increases dramatically. Although many factors contribute to bone loss, the leading cause in women is decreased estrogen production during menopause.

The higher your peak bone mass, the more bone you have "in the bank" and the less likely you are to develop osteoporosis as you age. Not getting enough vitamin D and calcium in your diet may lead to a lower peak bone mass and accelerated bone loss later.

Diagnosis

Osteopenia refers to mild bone loss that isn't severe enough to be called osteoporosis, but that increases your risk of osteoporosis. Doctors can detect osteopenia or early signs of osteoporosis using a variety of devices to measure bone density.

The best screening test is dual energy X-ray absorptiometry (DXA). This procedure is quick, simple and gives accurate results. It measures the density of bones in your spine, hip and wrist — the areas most likely to be affected by osteoporosis — and it's used to accurately follow changes in these bones over time.

Other tests that can accurately measure bone density include ultrasound and quantitative computerized tomography (CT).

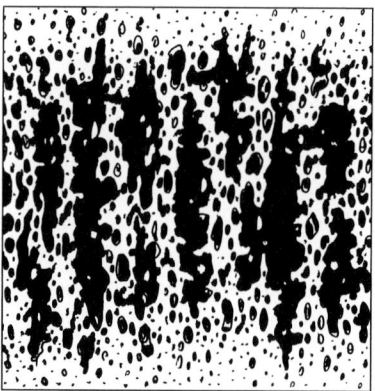 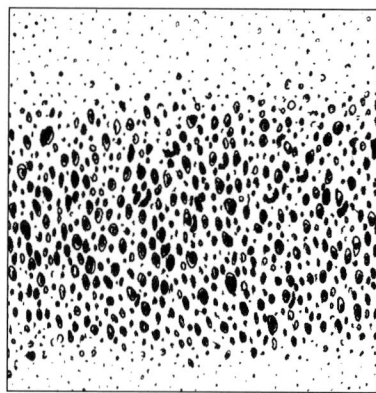

Osteoporotic bone (left) is weaker, more porous and more prone to fracture than is normal bone (right).

Should you be tested?

The National Osteoporosis Foundation recommends that women who aren't taking estrogen have a bone density test if any of the following apply:

- You're older than age 65.
- You're postmenopausal and have at least one risk factor for osteoporosis, including having fractured a bone.
- You have a vertebral abnormality.
- You use medications, such as prednisone, that can cause osteoporosis.
- You have type 1 diabetes, liver disease, kidney disease, thyroid disease or a family history of osteoporosis.
- You experienced early menopause.

Doctors don't generally recommend osteoporosis screening for men, unless they're at high risk, because the disease is less common in men than it is in women.

Results are reported in T-scores, which reflect the difference between your bone density and that of a healthy, young adult. The lower your bone density, the higher your risk of fractures.

If your T-score is greater than -1, you have normal bone density. A reading between -1 and -2.4 means that you have low bone density (osteopenia) that puts you at greater risk of developing osteoporosis or fracturing a bone. A T-score at or below -2.5 indicates osteoporosis.

How serious is osteoporosis?

If your bones are severely weakened, osteoporosis can be dis-abling. Fractures are the most common consequence of osteoporosis. Osteoporotic bones can break with little or no unusual stress. Each year, osteoporosis leads to approximately 1.5 million fractures in the United States.

Vertebral compression fractures due to osteoporosis rarely require surgery. Severe pain often begins abruptly, centers on your back, possibly radiates around the trunk, is aggravated by movement and relieved by heat, and gradually subsides within a month or two. Over a period of years, however, a sequence of spinal compression fractures can lead to dowager's hump (widow's hump) and increasingly stooped posture.

Treatment

A number of treatments may be used to treat or prevent reduced bone density. Lifestyle factors also play a significant role.

Medication

Hormone therapy was once the mainstay of treatment for osteoporosis. But because of concerns about its safety and the availability of other treatments, the role of hormone therapy in managing osteoporosis is changing. It's typically used for bone health in younger women or in women whose menopausal symptoms also require treatment.

- **Hormone-related therapy.** Raloxifene (Evista) mimics estrogen's beneficial effects on bone density in postmenopausal women, without some of the risks associated with estrogen. Taking this drug may also reduce the risk of some types of breast cancer. Hot flashes are a common side effect. Raloxifene also may increase your risk of blood clots.

In men, osteoporosis may be linked with a gradual age-related decline in testosterone levels. Testosterone replacement therapy can help improve symptoms of low testosterone, but osteoporosis medications have been better studied in men to treat osteoporosis and thus are recommended alone or in addition to testosterone.

- **Bisphosphonates.** Much like estrogen, they inhibit bone breakdown, preserve bone mass, and even increase bone density in your spine and hip. They include the medications alendronate (Fosamax), risedronate (Actonel, Atelvia), ibandronate (Boniva) and zoledronic acid (Reclast, Zometa).

Bisphosphonates may be especially beneficial for postmenopausal women, men and young adults. They're also used to help prevent osteoporosis in people who require long-term steroid treatment for a disease such as asthma or arthritis.

Side effects include nausea, abdominal pain and heartburn-like symptoms. These are less likely to occur if the medicine is taken properly. Intravenous forms of bisphosphonates don't cause stomach upset but can cause fever, headache and muscle aches for up to three days. It may be easier to schedule a quarterly or yearly injection than to remember to take a weekly or monthly pill, but it can be more costly.

Using bisphosphonate therapy for more than five years has been linked to a very rare problem in which the middle of the thighbone cracks and in

Bone Density Testing

Bone density can be measured in several painless and noninvasive ways. Various types of bone density tests include:
- *Central dual energy X-ray absorptiometry.* Called DXA, this test (shown below) uses low-level X-rays to assess your spine, hip or total body. This is the preferred method, but it may be available only in a hospital or clinic.
- *Peripheral dual energy X-ray absorptiometry.* Called pDXA, this test uses low-level X-rays to measure bone mass in your wrist, finger or heel. Your doctor's office may be more likely to offer this than a central DXA, making it more accessible.
- *Quantitative ultrasound.* A QUS test transmits sound waves through your heel, shinbone and kneecap. This equipment is portable and inexpensive, which makes it potentially accessible to more people. Its accuracy compared with DXA is being studied.
- *Quantitative computerized tomography.* A QCT test is most commonly used to measure your spine.

How often you need repeat testing depends on the results. If you're taking medication for osteoporosis or osteopenia, you may have measurements every two to three years to determine the effectiveness of your treatment.

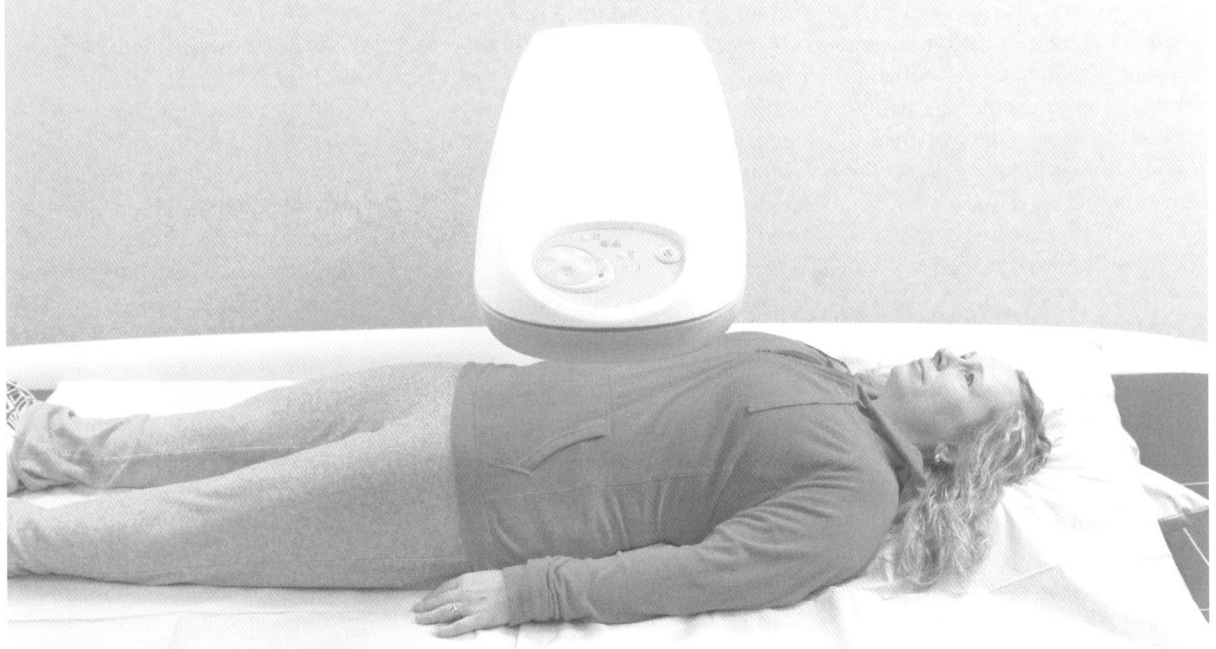

some cases might even break completely.

Bisphosphonates also have the potential to affect the jawbone. Osteonecrosis of the jaw is a rare condition that can occur typically after a tooth extraction in which a section of jawbone fails to heal where the tooth was pulled. You should have a recent dental examination before starting bisphosphonates.

If you can't tolerate the more common medications used to treat osteoporosis — or if they don't work well enough to treat your condition — your doctor might suggest that you try one of the following:

- **Denosumab (Prolia).** Compared with bisphosphonates, denosumab produces similar or better bone density results and reduces the chance of all types of fractures. Denosumab is delivered via a shot under the skin every six months.

- **Teriparatide (Forteo).** This powerful drug is similar to parathyroid hormone and stimulates new bone growth. It's given by daily injection under the skin. After two years of treatment with teriparatide, another osteoporosis drug is taken to maintain the new bone growth.

Exercise

A regular exercise program is important in the management and prevention of osteoporosis. Weight-bearing exercise and strength training can help maintain bone density. Back-strengthening exercises help you maintain good posture. Exercise also strengthens your muscles, which may improve your balance and help you avoid falls and fractures.

Select your exercise carefully. A good weight-bearing exercise is walking. Start out slowly, and gradually increase the pace and duration. Paradoxically, the serious female competitive athlete is often vulnerable to osteoporosis because leanness and excessive exercise may decrease estrogen production.

Stabilizing fractures

Fractures of vertebrae may require a procedure known as vertebroplasty to stabilize the bone. Physical therapy is often a key part of the recovery from any fracture.

Prevention

Indications are that the more calcium a woman has stored in her skeleton before menopause, the less risk she has of developing significant osteoporosis. So starting at a young age, women should eat a calcium-rich diet with plenty of vitamin D to aid absorption of calcium.

Foods high in calcium include dairy products, leafy green vegetables, beans, nuts and whole-grain cereals. Many doctors advise tak-

Vertebroplasty

Vertebroplasty is a procedure used to relieve pain that can accompany compression fractures of the vertebrae. It entails injecting plastic cement into the involved vertebrae. The cement hardens within hours, stabilizing the fractures and relieving pain.

Spinal compression fractures are most often the result of acute stress on bones weakened by osteoporosis. Less frequently, the fractures are the result of cancerous (malignant) tumors that involve the spine.

Vertebroplasty often provides pain relief when standard care for compression fractures — which includes rest, pain medications and a brace — doesn't. It may be most effective in fractures that are less than six weeks old.

A similar procedure is kyphoplasty, in which a balloon-like device is inserted into a compressed vertebra to expand the vertebra before the cement is injected. Most people who undergo vertebroplasty experience significant pain relief within 48 hours.

Who's a candidate?

Many people with compression fractures get significant pain relief after several weeks of standard care. But for some, pain persists, limiting mobility and interfering with daily activities. For them, vertebroplasty may be a good alternative.

If you're a candidate for the procedure, you'll likely need to have spinal X-rays as well as more- specialized radiographic imaging such as magnetic resonance imaging (MRI) or a bone scan to help determine which vertebrae are involved and the age of the fractures.

People who may not be good candidates for vertebroplasty are those who have medical conditions that prevent them from lying on their stomachs for up to two hours and those who have bleeding disorders or who can't be taken off anticoagulant medication.

What does the procedure involve?

You'll be asked to lie on your stomach, and you'll receive a sedative. An injection of a local anesthetic will numb the skin over the affected vertebrae. Some individuals may receive general anesthesia.

A radiologist — a doctor who specializes in the use of X-rays and other radiographic procedures — inserts a specially designed needle into the involved vertebra, using an X-ray to provide guidance. When the needle is in the correct position in the vertebra, the radiologist injects the bone cement.

ing a calcium supplement to ensure that you get adequate calcium in your diet. A calcium intake of at least 1,000 milligrams (mg) a day from your diet or a supplement may help you maintain maximal calcium status. If you're older than 50, aim for 1,200 mg a day.

It's also important that you get adequate vitamin D. All individuals should get a minimum of 400 international units (IU) every day.

Regular weight-bearing and strength training exercises are important for prevention of osteoporosis. Weight-bearing exercises include running, walking, tennis, dancing, weightlifting and almost any activity that combines movement with stress on your limbs.

Additional precautions also may be beneficial. Don't smoke, limit caffeine consumption to no more than 3 cups of caffeine-containing beverages a day and avoid consuming excessive amounts of alcohol.

Osteomalacia

Signs and symptoms
- Pain in the bones of your arms, legs, spine and pelvis
- Progressive weakness
- Bowlegs, projection of the chest (pigeon breast) and, in children, protrusion of the stomach

Osteomalacia means softening of the bones. The softening stems from an inability of the skeleton to incorporate adequate minerals into the bones. The bones become flexible so that body weight and other forces gradually mold them, often resulting in deformities. In children, osteomalacia is known as rickets.

Osteomalacia may be due to malabsorption of fat, a condition called steatorrhea. Instead of being absorbed in the small intestine, fat passes out of the body in your stool. As a result, vitamin D, a fat-soluble vitamin, is poorly absorbed. This hinders the intestinal absorption of the minerals calcium and phosphorus, which rely on vitamin D for their absorption.

Another cause of osteomalacia is a dietary deficiency of vitamin D. In the United States, people get vitamin D by drinking milk, which is supplemented with it. In addition, your body naturally produces vitamin D when your skin is exposed to sunlight. Inadequate vitamin D is most common in countries where the vitamin isn't added to foods or where people get little sun exposure.

A rare cause of osteomalacia is an increased amount of acid in the body fluids due to abnormal kidney function. This problem, called renal tubular acidosis, occurs in people with congenital or acquired kidney disorders. The increased acid gradually dissolves the skeleton, just as vinegar softens an eggshell.

Several rare hereditary forms of osteomalacia can lead to shortened

Following the procedure, you'll be asked to lie flat on your back for about three hours while the cement hardens. You may return home either later that day or the next morning.

What are the risks?
The primary risk associated with vertebroplasty is that bone cement may leak into surrounding tissues and vessels and put pressure on the spinal cord or nerve roots, causing pain and weakness. Another risk is that if bone cement enters blood vessels, it could travel to the lung and lodge in a lung artery (pulmonary embolism), causing chest pain and breathing difficulties. These risks are rare, however.

A person with soft bones may fracture a rib lying stomach-down during the procedure. Other risks include infection, bleeding and further injury to the vertebra from needle placement.

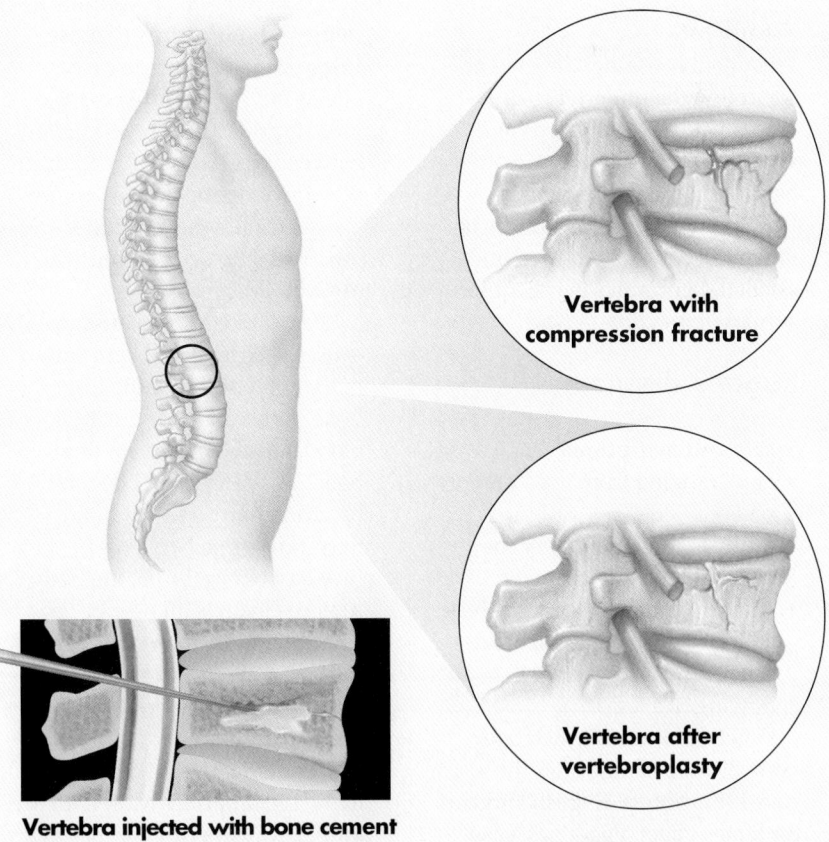

Vertebra with compression fracture

Vertebra after vertebroplasty

Vertebra injected with bone cement

adult stature. Vitamin D-resistant disease is due to an inability of body tissues to respond to vitamin D.

Diagnosis

Blood tests to measure levels of calcium, phosphorus and vitamin D and X-rays of the affected bones are often the first steps in a diagnosis of osteomalacia (rickets). Infrequently, a tiny piece of hipbone is removed (biopsied) for examination in a laboratory.

Once osteomalacia is diagnosed, typically the next step is to determine the cause, such as an intestinal problem (malabsorption) or a kidney abnormality.

How serious is osteomalacia?

In many cases, correcting the mineral deficiency eliminates the signs and symptoms. In children and adults, appropriate treatment can correct most of the mineral depletion in the bones, and the skeletal deformities may improve over time.

Treatment

Treatment is usually directed at correcting the underlying problem. Calcium, phosphorus and vitamin D supplements are often part of treatment. In vitamin D-resistant rickets, high doses of vitamin D may be required and skeletal deformities may require surgical correction.

Paget's disease

Signs and symptoms

- Pain, ranging from mild to more severe
- Warmth in the skin over the affected area
- Neurological problems, such as hearing loss, blindness, headache and weakness
- Bowing of a leg

Paget's disease is a metabolic bone disease named after the mid-19th-century English surgeon Sir James Paget. Paget's disease of the bone isn't related to Paget's disease of the breast, a type of breast cancer.

Many people think the human skeleton stops changing once it reaches full growth. That's not true. Bone is living tissue engaged in a continuous process of renewal.

Paget's disease disrupts the normal process of bone loss and formation, resulting in the breakdown of excess bone tissue and increased new bone formation. This leads to an abnormal structure in the affected bone because new bone is laid down in a disordered pattern and may be softer and weaker than normal bone.

Skeletal Disorders of Childhood

Numerous skeletal problems are unique to children. Fortunately, most of them are rare. These disorders include:

Legg-Calvé-Perthes disease

Legg-Calvé-Perthes disease affects boys more often than girls. It usually becomes evident between ages 3 and 10. Children who develop the disease before age six usually have a better outcome than do children who develop it later.

Legg-Calvé-Perthes disease causes progressive deterioration of the top portion of the thighbone (femoral head) due to poor blood supply to the growing bone. The cause isn't clear, but heredity, hormones and injury may play a role.

After bone cells die, the body replaces them with new bone cells. But while these new bone cells are forming, the bone is unstable and may break and become deformed.

A child may complain of pain in the hip and may walk with a limp. Because a number of other childhood conditions may cause hip pain and a limp, it's important to identify the cause.

The cause of Paget's disease isn't clear. Some experts believe that it may be due to a viral infection of certain bone cells called osteoclasts. In addition, some people may be genetically predisposed to the disease.

People older than age 40 are the most likely to develop Paget's disease, although in rare instances it occurs in younger adults. Occasionally, it runs in families.

The disease frequently affects the skull, arms, legs and spine. It may affect only one or two areas within the skeleton, or it may be widespread.

The focus of treatment is to protect the bone and joint from further stress and injury during the natural healing process, which may last up to three years. Treatment depends on the severity of the disease, but may include bed rest, range-of-motion exercises, crutches and nonsteroidal anti-inflammatory drugs (NSAIDs). Traction on the bone to immobilize it may help it heal. Bracing and surgery may be necessary.

Most children with this disorder resume normal function but may continue to limp for several years. Children with severe cases are more likely to develop osteoarthritis of the hip joint.

Slipped capital femoral epiphysis

During the growth spurt just before puberty, the growth plate of the ball of the hip may slip. The thighbone rotates outward and slides upward relative to the ball of the hip. This unusual condition is called a slipped capital femoral epiphysis.

Common symptoms are pain in the knee, thigh or hip and a limp that involves lurching to the side and turning the foot outward.

Diagnosis

Often, the first indication of the condition is an elevated alkaline phosphatase level found through routine blood testing. Alkaline phosphatase is an enzyme involved in new bone formation. If you haven't had a blood test and your doctor suspects Paget's disease, he or she will probably order one. Your doctor may also order X-rays and bone scans. A sample of affected bone tissue (biopsy) may be obtained for laboratory analysis.

How serious is Paget's disease?

Most people with the disease have no symptoms. Among people with symptoms, usually only one area of the body is affected, most commonly the spine, skull, pelvis, thighs or lower legs. However, multiple sites can be involved. The affected bones can become deformed and subject to fracture. In most cases, the disease progresses very slowly.

In rare cases, serious, long-term complications occur. These range from deafness to congestive heart failure or spinal cord injury. Rarely, a bone cancer known as osteosarcoma may develop in bones affected by Paget's disease.

Treatment

If you don't have symptoms, you probably won't need treatment. If you have symptoms, your doctor may recommend medication.

In its early stages, Paget's disease may produce pain and inflammation. Pain relievers such as acetaminophen (Tylenol, others) and nonsteroidal anti-inflammatory drugs (NSAIDs), such as ibuprofen (Advil, Motrin IB, others), often suffice.

If the disease progresses, your doctor may prescribe a bisphosphonate drug, such as zoledronic acid (Reclast, Zometa), pamidronate (Aredia), alendronate (Fosamax), risedronate (Actonel, Atelvia), tiludronate (Skelid) or etidronate, to help reduce bone loss and increase bone density. They're usually taken for several months. Calcitonin (Miacalcin), a naturally occurring hormone involved in calcium regulation and bone metabolism, is another effective medication. Rarely, surgery is necessary to repair deformities.

Fibrous dysplasia

Signs and symptoms
- Bone pain, especially in the lower leg
- Difficulty walking
- Rarely, fractures and multiple bone deformities
- Often, none

Fibrous dysplasia resembles Paget's disease in that it's characterized by abnormal growth of bone tissue. In the case of fibrous dysplasia, however, the bone tissue is fibrous rather than bony. The condition typically first appears in childhood and affects one or more bones. The abnormal growth usually stops at puberty.

The cause of fibrous dysplasia is unknown. Severe cases in which bones deform or fracture can seriously affect quality of life.

Diagnosis
The presence of fibrous dysplasia generally is confirmed with X-rays

---

Symptoms usually evolve gradually over weeks or months, but they can also appear suddenly in association with an injury.

The condition is most common in boys between ages 11 and 14, particularly those who are overweight. In one-fourth of cases, it affects both hips.

A slipped capital femoral epiphysis requires surgery to correct the problem or prevent further displacement. If the slip progresses until it's severe, it can deform the hip and interfere with normal walking.

Osgood-Schlatter disease

Osgood-Schlatter disease affects children between 11 and 15 years of age, especially boys, and is characterized by pain and swelling at the bony protuberance on the shinbone (tibia), just below the kneecap. This is where the tendon from the kneecap attaches to the tibia. This disease is associated with overuse and is much more common than other conditions discussed in this section.

Icing, stretching and rest from impact activities such as running and jumping are usually the best treatment for Osgood-Schlatter disease. A strap across the kneecap tendon can help take the force away from the bony protuber-

ance. Anti-inflammatory medications, such as ibuprofen (Advil, Motrin IB, others), also may be helpful. The condition usually resolves as the skeleton matures.

Congenital dislocation of the hip

Congenital dislocation of the hip, also called developmental dysplasia of the hip, is caused by a hip socket that's too shallow at birth, making the joint susceptible to dislocation. The problem can lead to an altered shape of the bones of the joint, which may require surgery later in life.

Even if a baby appears to be entirely healthy, a doctor should be on the alert for this condition during the first year of a child's life. Early diagnosis allows for simple treatment with splinting, which is usually successful. Congenital dislocation of the hip tends to recur in families, so alert your doctor if you or your spouse had the condition.

Clubfoot

Clubfoot, technically known as talipes equinovarus, is a deformity of the foot present at birth. It may be hereditary. It can be treated with casts or splints in the first few weeks of life, often with good results (see page 172).

of your bones or by removing samples of bone for laboratory analysis.

Treatment

Although fibrous dysplasia isn't curable, surgery to remove fibrous growths from affected bones may help. Bisphosphonate drugs may be used to treat bone pain if surgery isn't needed.

Osteogenesis imperfecta

Signs and symptoms

- Fragile bones resulting in fractures
- Bluish coloration in the white part of the eye (sclera)
- Limb deformities, particularly bowing
- Early tooth loss
- Flatfeet
- Short stature

Osteogenesis imperfecta is a rare, inherited disease in which bones are abnormally brittle and fragile due to collagen abnormalities. Collagen is a fibrous protein found in bone, connective tissue and cartilage. Fractures may be present at birth or occur later when the child begins to walk. Hearing impairment also is common.

Diagnosis

X-ray studies of the bones often can confirm the diagnosis. A skin biopsy may also be taken for collagen analysis.

How serious is osteogenesis imperfecta?

This disease takes several forms. The more-severe forms often are fatal. In less severe forms, the number of fractures decreases markedly once a child reaches adolescence.

Treatment

The treatment for less severe forms of this disease involves reducing the risk of fractures. It's important to set all fractures promptly and to correct skeletal deformities. Parents of a child with the condition

Endocrine Disorders and the Bones

Your endocrine system is made up of hormone-secreting glands that affect virtually all body functions and parts, including bones. The following endocrine disorders affect your bones. For more information on these conditions, see Chapter 30, "Endocrine System."

Acromegaly

This condition is the result of the pituitary gland secreting too much growth hormone in adults. People with acromegaly have characteristically large hands and feet, as well as a large jawbone and skull.

Gigantism

Gigantism is a rare condition caused by too much growth hormone before a child reaches full growth. The condition causes accelerated growth resulting in excessive height.

Hypopituitarism

Hypopituitarism occurs when the pituitary gland produces too few or no hormones. When a child with the disorder receives too little growth hormone, dwarfism results.

Hyperparathyroidism

In this condition, your body produces too much parathyroid hormone. Your bones then release too much calcium, causing a weakening of the skeleton.

might consider genetic counseling before another pregnancy.

Osteomyelitis

Signs and symptoms

- Intense pain and increased heat over the affected bone
- Tenderness and swelling
- Fever
- Fatigue

Osteomyelitis is a bone infection caused by bacteria or, rarely, fungi. The infectious organism may be acquired through a wound, fracture or other injury and carried to the bone by the blood. The condition can lead to destruction of bone and surrounding tissue.

Osteomyelitis is rare in the United States and is more common in children than in adults. It's usually treated successfully with antibiotics, but it can recur.

Diagnosis

If your doctor suspects osteomyelitis, blood tests or imaging tests may help with the diagnosis. Your doctor may also perform a biopsy, in which a sample of bone, pus or other tissue is removed for analysis and culture.

Treatment

A course of antibiotics is the usual treatment, along with adequate bed rest. In some instances, surgery may be necessary to remove the infected tissue.

Bone tumors

Signs and symptoms

- A hard lump on the surface of a bone
- Pain
- Fracture of the involved bone

Tumors that begin in bones are rare. The majority of bone tumors are noncancerous (benign), but some are cancerous (malignant). Both types may grow and impinge on healthy bone tissue, but benign tumors don't spread and rarely are life-threatening.

If the tumor is cancerous, most often the cancer has spread to the bone from elsewhere in the body (metastasized). Exceptions are a type of blood cancer called multiple myeloma that begins in bone marrow and osteosarcoma, the most common primary bone cancer. Osteosarcoma develops in new tissue in growing bones, most commonly in the knees, upper legs and upper arms. It occurs mostly in children, adolescents and young adults ages 10 to 25.

The exact cause of bone cancer is unknown. Children and young adults who've had radiation or chemotherapy treatments for other conditions are at increased risk of developing osteosarcoma. Adults with Paget's disease of the bone also may be at increased risk.

Diagnosis

Many times, X-rays are helpful in diagnosing a bone tumor, but they may not provide a conclusive diagnosis. Your doctor may perform a biopsy, in which a small sample of the tissue is removed for laboratory examination.

How serious is a bone tumor?

A benign growth rarely presents a serious health risk. If the tumor is a cancer that originated in bone (primary tumor) and hasn't spread, it may be curable with a combination of treatments. Bone cancer that has spread to another site or cancer that has metastasized to bone from another site is rarely curable.

Treatment

Benign tumors may require no treatment, but some are removed surgically if they cause pain or other symptoms. A cancerous tumor may require a combination of treatments, including surgery, radiation and chemotherapy. Amputation of the affected limb sometimes is necessary, but preoperative and postoperative chemotherapy is making it possible for a surgeon to preserve the limb by removing only the diseased portion of the bone and reconstructing the extremity. A program of rehabilitation often follows.

For cancer that has spread, generally the focus is on relieving pain and maintaining quality of life.

Muscle, Tendon and Soft Tissue Disorders

Your muscle fibers are elongated and contractible. When you move an arm, leg, hand or foot, one muscle contracts to produce the movement. To return the limb to its original position, the opposite muscle must contract.

Equally important to movement are tendons, which connect muscles to bones. In most parts of your body, tendons either intertwine with the muscles or take the form of short connectors between the ends of the muscles and bones. Tendons in your hands and feet are long and cordlike. Throughout your body fibrous tendons convey the movement of the muscles to the bones. Contract a muscle and it causes the attached tendons and bones to move.

Your muscles, tendons and soft tissues can be affected by a number of common disorders, from the discomfort of tendinitis to the crippling effects of muscular dystrophy.

Tenosynovitis

Signs and symptoms

- Tenderness and pain
- Movements accompanied by a crackling sound or feeling
- Pain when you move the affected area
- A joint that's hot and inflamed

Long, cable-like tendons run through your hand and into each finger. Each tendon is enclosed within a sheath lined with a membrane called the synovium. The synovium secretes fluid to lubricate the joints and the tendon sheaths and to nourish cartilage.

The function of the tendon sheath is to keep the tendon from adhering to tissues along its path. In tenosynovitis, the synovium becomes inflamed or infected.

Tenosynovitis may be related to underlying arthritis, but most often the cause is unknown or is related to overuse or overload of the tendon and its corresponding muscle. The condition may be aggravated by repetitive activity, but it occurs no more frequently in people who perform repetitive tasks, such as factory workers and computer keyboard operators, than in those who don't.

Tenosynovitis can occur in the wrist, hand, ankle and, more commonly, the bicipital tendon in the shoulder. It's most common in women at or beyond middle age.

Diagnosis

Your doctor will likely examine the affected area to determine if the synovium is infected. He or she may order an X-ray to rule out other bone problems, such as a bone growth or deformity, that may be causing your symptoms.

How serious is tenosynovitis?

Rarely, tenosynovitis may result from an infection. If the pain is accompanied by fever, an infection is a possibility. See a doctor to have your symptoms evaluated.

Treatment

Medication and, in some cases, surgery may relieve your discomfort and restore function to the affected area.

When tenosynovitis is aggravated by overuse, treatment may include resting and modifying your activities. Proper technique in sports and work activities is important to preventing overload of the tissue.

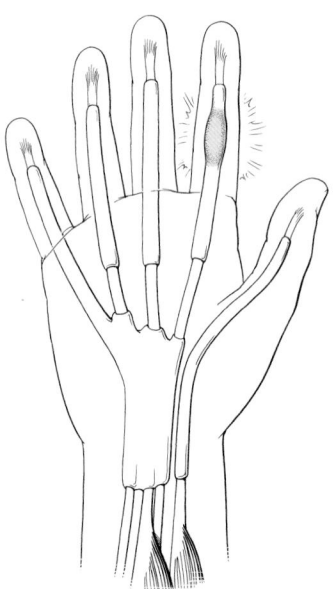

Each of the cable-like tendons in your hand is surrounded by a protective sheath called the synovium. When the synovial membrane is inflamed or infected (see highlighting), tenosynovitis results. Treatment varies but may include rest, medication or even surgery.

Medication
For noninfectious tenosynovitis, a pain reliever, such as acetaminophen (Tylenol, others) or a nonsteroidal anti-inflammatory drug (NSAID), such as ibuprofen (Advil, Motrin IB, others), may reduce the pain. If an infection is causing the discomfort, your doctor will likely prescribe an antibiotic.

Injection of a steroid drug, such as cortisone, may relieve symptoms. An injection is most often used when more-conservative measures aren't helpful.

Splint
A protective splint that limits movement can provide needed rest and support for a hand or wrist affected by tenosynovitis.

Surgery
In some cases of infectious tenosynovitis, surgery may be performed to drain pus at the infection site and to limit the spread of the infection.

Carpal tunnel syndrome

Signs and symptoms
- A numbness or tingling sensation in your fingers or hand, especially your thumb and index and middle fingers
- Wrist pain that may extend into your forearm, the palm of your hand or your fingers
- Hand weakness
- A loss of feeling in some fingers

The eight wrist (carpal) bones and the tendons that overlie them form a tunnel-like structure in your wrist. Bounded by bones and ligaments, the carpal tunnel protects the nerves and tendons that extend into your hand.

Swelling or inflammation of tissues within the tunnel can compress the median nerve — the nerve that provides sensation to your thumb, index and middle fingers, and part of your ring finger. Pressure on the nerve produces a specific pattern of numbness and pain that characterizes carpal tunnel syndrome. Many times it affects both wrists.

Although carpal tunnel syndrome often develops without a specific cause, a number of factors can predispose you to developing it. They include arthritis, obesity, smoking, pregnancy and certain occupations that require forceful, repetitive, and awkward or stressed motions of your hands and wrists. This may include carpenters, meat cutters, pianists, mechanics and, occasionally, hobbyists such as golfers, canoeists and bicyclists.

Carpal tunnel syndrome may also accompany some endocrine disorders, such as diabetes, acromegaly and, rarely, hypothyroidism, as well as rheumatoid arthritis.

In addition, inherited physical characteristics, such as the shape of your wrist, may make you more susceptible. In general, women approaching middle age are most likely to develop carpal tunnel syndrome.

Diagnosis
A key symptom that helps in making a diagnosis is that the numbness in your fingers doesn't include the little finger. Your doctor may perform certain tests to determine if electric impulses traveling along the median nerve slow in the carpal tunnel, indicating that the nerve is being compressed.

Tingling or shooting pain into your hand or forearm when tapping on the palm side of your wrist may also be an indication of carpal tunnel syndrome. In addition, you may have loss of bulk in the muscles of your thumb.

How serious is carpal tunnel syndrome?
Proper treatment can relieve the pain and numbness and usually prevent permanent damage to your hand and wrist. Untreated, the syndrome can lead to permanent nerve and muscle damage.

Treatment
Conservative treatment generally involves avoiding or modifying certain activities. A splint often helps, especially in relieving nighttime pain, by preventing the wrist from flexing, which pinches the median nerve in the carpal tunnel. Applying ice and stretching your wrist muscles may relieve symptoms.

Medication
Acetaminophen (Tylenol, others) or nonsteroidal anti-inflammatory drugs (NSAIDs), such as ibuprofen (Advil, Motrin IB, others) or naproxen sodium (Aleve, others), can help relieve the discomfort.

Sometimes a doctor may inject the carpel tunnel with a corticosteroid medication, such as cortisone, to relieve the pain. Corticosteroids decrease inflammation, relieving pressure on the median nerve.

Surgery
When the symptoms of carpal tunnel syndrome persist despite other treatments, an operation to open

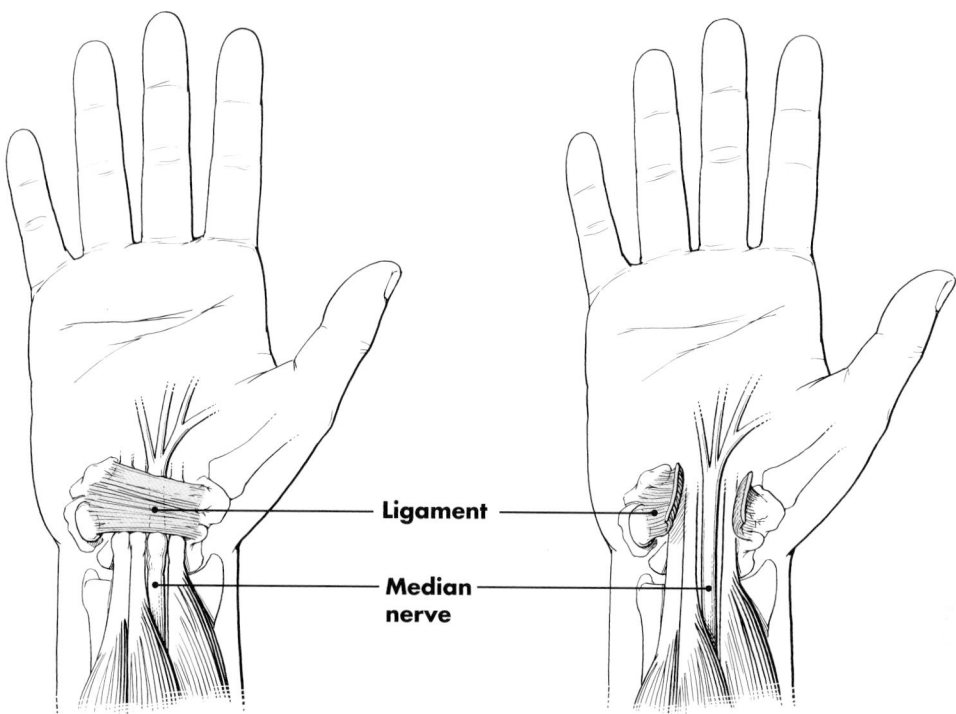

Ligament

Median nerve

A narrow tunnel through your wrist — the carpal tunnel — protects the median nerve, which provides sensation to your thumb, index and middle fingers, and a portion of your ring finger. Swelling or inflammation of tendon sheaths within the carpal tunnel or swelling of tissues around the carpal tunnel can compress the median nerve, producing pain and numbness. If conservative treatment isn't effective, the carpal tunnel may be surgically cut (right) to relieve the compression.

the tunnel and create more room for the median nerve may be the best option. Frequently, this surgery can be done through a small instrument called an endoscope. Full use of the wrist and hand usually returns within several weeks to a few months.

In some cases, some numbness may persist, and it's not uncommon to continue to experience discomfort with certain activities.

Prevention

When engaging in activities that require repetitive, forceful motion with your wrists flexed, take some precautions. Stop every 15 to 20 minutes and gently stretch and bend your hands and fingers. If possible, change activities and do something else for a while. Avoid gripping too hard when driving, writing or using small hand tools.

Using oversized, soft grip adapters on pens, pencils and tools may help.

Ganglion cyst

Signs and symptoms
- A generally painless lump, usually on your wrist or hand
- Possible pain, especially when your wrist is extended or flexed

A ganglion cyst is a noncancerous fluid-filled lump that appears beneath your skin, usually on the back of your wrist. In some cases, it may occur on the front of your wrist or on your fingers or a foot. Ganglion cysts contain an accumulation of a jellylike substance from a joint or tendon sheath and are generally rubbery to the touch.

Diagnosis

Your doctor will feel the lump and may order an X-ray or other tests

to rule out other problems. An ultrasound examination may help confirm the diagnosis.

How serious is a ganglion cyst?

A ganglion cyst is essentially harmless. However, if you find a lump on your wrist or foot, consult your doctor so that he or she can check for more-serious causes.

Treatment

In most cases, the lump doesn't interfere with your lifestyle and requires no treatment. If the cyst is painful, your doctor may take steps to relieve the discomfort. Sometimes, a doctor may inject a ganglion cyst with a corticosteroid drug or drain it with a needle. Often, though, it recurs after the drainage. Immobilizing the wrist or hand with a splint or brace may help the cyst decrease in size.

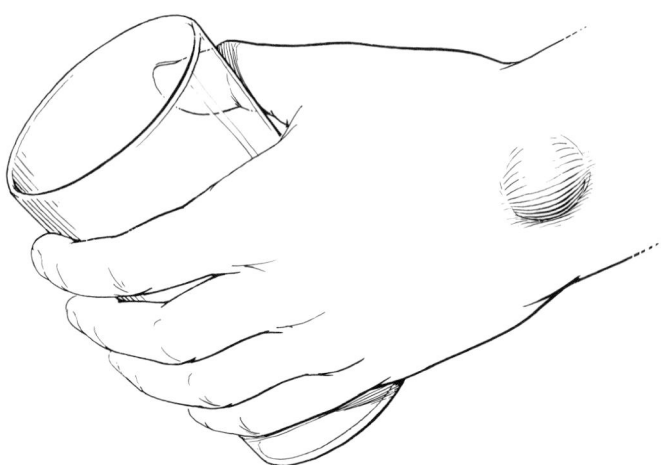

A ganglion cyst is a harmless swelling beneath the skin, usually on the back of the wrist.

Surgery
If a ganglion cyst is painful and doesn't respond to other measures, it can be removed surgically.

Dupuytren's contracture

Signs and symptoms
- A small lump, cord or area of tightness in the palm of your hand
- Dimpling of the skin over the affected area
- An inability to straighten one or several fingers

Named after the early 19th-century French surgeon Guillaume Dupuytren, this disorder is characterized by a hardening of tissue beneath the skin of the palm of the hand (palmar fascia), which can lead to an involuntary, fixed contraction of one or more fingers.

Dupuytren's contracture usually isn't painful, but it may progressively deform your hand. A similar hardening and shrinkage of tissue may affect the soles of your feet. Dupuytren's contracture most commonly involves the ring and little fingers, but it can affect any finger, the thumb or the feet.

The cause of Dupuytren's contracture isn't known, but there appears to be a strong genetic component. Many people with the condition are middle-aged men of Scottish, Irish or Scandinavian descent.

There also appears to be some predisposition associated with alcoholism and epilepsy, although the reason for the linkage is unknown. The condition isn't related to a traumatic event.

Diagnosis
A physical examination usually is adequate to diagnose Dupuytren's contracture. Dimpling of the skin over the affected area is characteristic of the disorder. A cord of immobile tissue may lie beneath the skin.

Your doctor may ask you to place your hand palm down on a tabletop or other flat surface. If you're unable to hold your fingers and hand flat, you may need treatment. Even if you can perform this task, you should repeat it periodically to monitor the progression of the condition. If the result indicates that your condition has worsened, surgery may be advisable.

How serious is Dupuytren's contracture?
Although the disorder is rarely painful, decreasing flexibility of your fingers can be debilitating. Many times, surgery can restore most, if not all, normal movement, although the problem may recur.

Treatment
In many cases, treatment isn't required. When treatment is necessary, surgery is usually recommended.

Medication
A corticosteroid injection may shrink the nodules. Some doctors are experimenting with an injection of enzymes or other medications to treat Dupuytren's contracture.

Surgery
Surgical treatment involves removing the thickened tissue. Extreme cases may require skin grafting or other surgical intervention.

Your hand will be bandaged with your fingers straight for a few days or weeks, after which you may begin physical therapy that includes finger and hand exercises. Usually, the hand is splinted at night for several months after surgery, as well.

Tendinitis

Signs and symptoms
- Pain, tenderness and stiffness near a joint
- Pain aggravated by movement
- A fever
- Redness, swelling or warmth over the affected area

Tendinitis is inflammation or irritation of a tendon. This condition — which causes pain and tenderness just outside a joint — is most common around the shoulders, elbows and knees, but it can also affect the hips, back of the ankles and wrists.

Tendons are thick, fibrous cords that attach muscles to bone. Usually, a tendon is surrounded by a sheath of tissue (synovium) similar to the lining of the joints. The most common cause of tendinitis is injury to a tendon or overuse from work or recreational activities. Rarely, an infection within the tendon sheath causes the inflammation. Tendinitis also may be associated with diseases such as rheumatoid arthritis.

Diagnosis

If pain interferes with your normal activities or doesn't improve, see your doctor. An X-ray of the area of soreness and other tests may reveal the cause of the problem.

How serious is tendinitis?

Tendinitis may become a chronic problem and can cause permanent damage to or rupture of a tendon. If the overuse that causes the soreness continues, what was a vague discomfort at age 30 can lead to loss of flexibility and decreased strength due to tissue scarring later in life. The natural tendency to favor the painful area can lead to joint stiffness.

Sometimes the discomfort of tendinitis disappears within a few weeks, especially if you rest the affected joint.

In individuals who continue to overuse the affected area and in older adults, the condition tends to heal more slowly or progress to a chronic problem. The ligaments and tendons around your shoulder may gradually stiffen, which leads to a loss of movement. Severe loss of range of motion in a shoulder is called frozen shoulder (see page 984).

Treatment

The goals of treatment are to relieve pain and reduce inflammation.

Ulnar Nerve Dysfunction

If you've ever hit your "funny bone" on your elbow and felt a tingling sensation down your arm into your hand, you've bumped your ulnar nerve. The ulnar nerve travels down the arm and aids in sensation and movement of the wrist and hand. At the elbow, the nerve passes close to the skin surface. Because of this vulnerable location, this nerve is easily damaged by repeated leaning on or trauma to the elbow. It also is stretched every time you bend your elbow. Over time, this repeated stretching can cause problems with the ulnar nerve. Sometimes, abnormal bone growth in the elbow or swollen tendons or ligaments can compress the ulnar nerve, damaging its protective covering (myelin sheath) or the nerve itself.

Ulnar nerve dysfunction is the result of ulnar nerve damage, whether from direct pressure or stretching. The most characteristic problem is numbness and tingling in the ring and little fingers, aggravated by leaning on your elbow or holding your elbow bent for a long period of time, such as when talking on the telephone or sleeping. You may also have difficulty moving your ring and little fingers, and you may experience tenderness along the inside of the elbow. Persistent ulnar nerve dysfunction (ulnar neuropathy) can lead to muscle degeneration (atrophy) in the affected hand and some difficulty fully straightening the ring and little fingers.

Treatment depends on the cause. Often, no treatment is required except to avoid pressure on the elbow. Recovery is spontaneous. In case of trauma, a splint or elbow pad may be used to prevent further injury and to allow the nerve to heal. In some cases, surgery may be necessary to relieve the pressure on the ulnar nerve. To eliminate the effect of stretching, the surgeon may shift the path of the nerve from behind to in front of the elbow.

Ulnar nerve dysfunction can result in complete loss of sensation in the hand or fingers and complete loss of hand or wrist movement. However, if the cause of the dysfunction can be identified and successfully treated, full recovery is possible. Early diagnosis and treatment increase the chances of a successful outcome.

Trigger Finger

A condition sometimes confused with tenosynovitis is a more common condition called trigger finger. The characteristic symptom is a clicking sensation in the finger as you bend or straighten it. In addition, when you try to point your finger, rather than responding smoothly, it seems to hesitate, then suddenly straightens with a snap. Left untreated, the condition can lead to an inability to straighten the finger.

The usual cause of trigger finger is a thickening and narrowing of the sheath that protects the tendon and helps guide it as it moves. What causes the sheath to thicken is unknown, but the condition is more common in older adults and people with diabetes.

Corticosteroid injections usually are effective in treating trigger finger. A protective splint that limits movement of the affected finger may be used in mild cases. Sometimes, surgery is necessary. An incision is made in the tendon sheath of the affected finger. This often relieves the constriction and restores full movement.

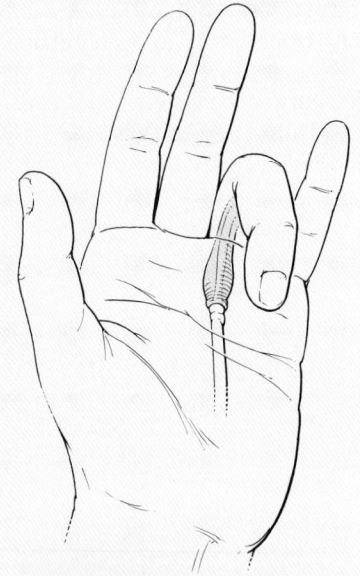

A condition sometimes confused with tenosynovitis is called trigger finger. The sheath that protects the tendon thickens, making it difficult to straighten the affected finger.

Medication

Short-term use of an over-the-counter nonsteroidal anti-inflammatory drug (NSAID), such as ibuprofen (Advil, Motrin IB, others), may help reduce your discomfort. If symptoms persist, your doctor may inject the area with a steroid drug, such as cortisone, to reduce the inflammation.

Self-care

Don't use the affected area for several days, but move other parts of your body. Elevating and applying ice to the area may help reduce discomfort and swelling.

Although rest is a key part of treating tendinitis, prolonged inactivity can cause stiffness in your joint. After you've rested the injured area for a few days, do gentle range-of-motion exercises four times a day to help you maintain flexibility in the joint. Movement is especially important for the shoulder, which tends to lose mobility quickly when it isn't used.

Surgery

Surgeons can repair tendon tears to reduce pain, restore function and, in some cases, prevent complete tendon rupture. Surgery may also be necessary to clean inflamed tissue out of the tendon sheath or relieve pressure on the tendon by removing a portion of bone.

Prevention

To reduce your chance of developing acute or recurrent tendinitis, warm up before you exercise or engage in physical labor and cool down afterward. Avoid activities that place excessive stress on your tendons. Strengthening exercises may also help.

Consider taking lessons or getting professional instruction when starting a new sport or using exercise equipment. Improper technique in either a sport or a work activity is one of the most common causes of tendinitis. A well laid out workstation may prevent stressing or overloading your joints and tendons. An "ergonomic assessment" can help identify a proper workspace.

Fibromyalgia

Signs and symptoms

- Widespread pain on both sides of your body above and below the waist
- Fatigue
- Troubles with focus, attention and concentration

Tendons

The shoulder joint is a complex structure. Strong tendons attach muscle to bone. Inflammation or irritation of a tendon causes tendinitis.

Fibromyalgia is a disorder characterized by widespread musculoskeletal pain accompanied by fatigue, sleep, memory and mood issues. Researchers believe that fibromyalgia amplifies painful sensations by affecting the way your brain processes pain signals.

Doctors don't know what causes fibromyalgia, but it most likely involves a variety of factors working together. These may include:

- **Genetics.** Because fibromyalgia tends to run in families, there may be certain genetic mutations that may make you more susceptible to developing the disorder.
- **Infections.** Some illnesses appear to trigger or aggravate fibromyalgia.
- **Physical or emotional trauma.** Fibromyalgia can sometimes be triggered by a physical trauma, such as a car accident. Psychological stress may also trigger the condition.

Symptoms sometimes begin after physical trauma, surgery, an infection or significant psychological stress. In other cases, symptoms gradually accumulate over time with no single triggering event.

Women are more likely to develop fibromyalgia than are men. Many people who have fibromyalgia also have tension headaches, temporomandibular joint (TMJ) disorders, irritable bowel syndrome, anxiety and depression.

While there is no cure for fibromyalgia, a variety of medications can help control symptoms. Exercise, relaxation and stress-reduction measures also may help.

Diagnosis

In the past, doctors would check 18 specific points on a person's body to see how many of them were painful when pressed firmly. Newer guidelines don't require a tender point exam. Instead, a fibromyalgia diagnosis can be made if a person has had widespread pain for more than three months — with no underlying medical condition that could cause the pain.

While there is no lab test to confirm a diagnosis of fibromyalgia, your doctor may want to rule out other conditions that may have similar symptoms. Blood tests may include a complete blood count, erythrocyte sedimentation rate test, cyclic citrullinated peptide test, rheumatoid factor test and thyroid function tests.

How serious is fibromyalgia?

The disorder is chronic but not progressive, crippling or life-threatening. It shouldn't lead to disability, and it generally doesn't lead to other, more serious disorders. However, it can cause depression and interfere with sleep and your overall quality of life.

Treatment

In general, treatments for fibromyalgia include both self-care and medication. The emphasis of treatment is on minimizing symptoms and improving general health. No one treatment works for all symptoms.

Self-care

Regular physical activity is important to ease sore muscles and maintain range of motion. If you don't already exercise regularly, start slowly and build up. Swimming, walking, stretching, participating in water aerobics and stationary bicycling are all good choices.

Establishing a regular sleep routine and getting adequate sleep each night are also important. You may need occasional rest breaks throughout the day. If you're overweight, achieving a healthy weight may reduce the pain.

Many people find stress management techniques and complementary forms of medicine, such as acupuncture, meditation or biofeedback, to be helpful. For more information, see Chapter 10, "Stress," and Chapter 38, "Integrative Medicine."

Medication

Medications can help reduce the pain of fibromyalgia and improve sleep. Common choices include:

- **Pain relievers.** Over-the-counter pain relievers such as acetaminophen (Tylenol, others), ibuprofen (Advil, Motrin IB, others) or naproxen sodium (Aleve, others) may be helpful. Your doctor might suggest a prescription pain reliever such as tramadol (Ultram). Narcotics are not advised, because they can lead to dependence and may even worsen the pain over time.
- **Antidepressants.** Duloxetine (Cymbalta) and milnacipran (Savella) may help ease the pain and fatigue associated with fibromyalgia. Your doctor may prescribe amitriptyline or the muscle relaxant cyclobenzaprine to help promote sleep.
- **Anti-seizure drugs.** Medications designed to treat epilepsy are often useful in reducing certain types of pain. Pregabalin (Lyrica) was the first drug approved by the Food and Drug Administration (FDA) to treat fibromyalgia. Gabapentin (Neurontin, Gralise) is sometimes helpful in reducing fibromyalgia symptoms.

Therapy

A variety of different therapies can help reduce the effect that fibromyalgia has on your body and your life. Examples include:

- **Physical therapy.** A physical therapist can teach you exercises that will improve your strength, flexibility and stamina. Water-based exercises might be particularly helpful.
- **Occupational therapy.** An occupational therapist can help you make adjustments to your work area or the way you perform certain tasks that will cause less stress on your body.
- **Counseling.** Talking with a counselor can help strengthen your belief in your abilities and teach you strategies for dealing with stressful situations.

Complex regional pain syndrome

Signs and symptoms

- Continuous burning or throbbing pain, usually an arm or leg
- Skin sensitivity
- Changes in skin temperature, color and texture
- Changes in hair and nail growth
- Joint stiffness, swelling and damage
- Decreased ability to move the affected body part

Formerly called reflex sympathetic dystrophy syndrome, complex regional pain syndrome is an uncommon, chronic condition that usually affects an arm or a leg. You may experience intense burning or aching pain along with swelling, skin discoloration, altered temperature, abnormal sweating and hypersensitivity in the affected area.

The cause of complex regional pain syndrome isn't clearly understood. Women are more likely to be affected than are men. The condition typically develops after an injury, surgery, a stroke or a heart attack, but the pain is out of proportion to the severity of the initial injury.

Complex regional pain syndrome occurs in two types, with similar signs and symptoms, but different causes:

- **Type 1.** Also known as reflex sympathetic dystrophy syndrome, this type occurs after an illness or injury that didn't directly damage the nerves in your affected limb. About 90 percent of people with complex regional pain syndrome have type 1.
- **Type 2.** Once referred to as causalgia, this type follows a distinct nerve injury.

It's not well-understood why these injuries can trigger complex regional pain syndrome. Researchers believe it may be due to a dysfunctional interaction between your central and peripheral nervous systems and inappropriate inflammatory responses.

Diagnosis

Tests that measure perspiration, temperature or circulation can help confirm the diagnosis by showing abnormal patterns in response to cold or other stimuli. A bone scan may show increased circulation to the joints in the affected area. In later stages, X-rays may reveal a loss of minerals (osteopenia) in affected bones.

Treatment

The focus in treatment is to provide pain relief and to get the affected joints moving. Maintaining range of motion is essential. A physical therapy program that includes heat and cold and exercise may help relieve pain and tenderness.

Your doctor may recommend a medication depending on the severity and location of your pain. Various medications are used to treat the symptoms.

- **Pain relievers.** Over-the-counter pain relievers — such as aspirin, ibuprofen (Advil, Motrin IB, others) and naproxen sodium (Aleve, others) — may ease pain and inflammation. Your doctor may prescribe stronger pain relievers if these aren't helpful.
- **Antidepressants and anticonvulsants.** Sometimes antidepressants, such as amitriptyline, and anticonvulsants, such as gabapentin (Gralise, Neurontin), are used to treat pain that originates from a damaged nerve (neuropathic pain).
- **Corticosteroids.** This includes prednisone, which may be prescribed to reduce inflammation.
- **Osteoporosis medications.** Medications such as alendronate (Fosamax) and calcitonin (Miacalcin) may be given to reduce bone loss.
- **Sympathetic nerve-blocking medication.** An injection of an anesthetic to block pain fibers in your affected nerves may relieve pain in some people.

If medications aren't effective or you prefer not to take medication, other forms of treatment include:

- **Heat and cold.** Applying cold may relieve swelling and sweating. If the affected area is cool, applying heat may offer relief.
- **Topical analgesics.** Various topical treatments are available that may reduce hypersensitivity, such as nonprescription capsaicin cream or prescription lidocaine patches (Lidoderm, others).
- **Physical therapy.** Gentle, guided exercising of the affected limbs may help decrease pain and improve range of motion and strength. The earlier the disease is diagnosed, the more effective exercises may be.
- **Transcutaneous electrical nerve stimulation (TENS).** Chronic pain is sometimes eased by applying electrical impulses to nerve endings.
- **Biofeedback.** In some cases, biofeedback techniques may help. In biofeedback, you learn to become more aware of your body so that you can relax your body and relieve pain.
- **Spinal cord stimulation.** Tiny electrodes are inserted along your spinal cord. A small electrical current delivered to the spinal cord results in pain relief.

Chest wall pain

Signs and symptoms

- Pain in the front of the chest where your ribs join your breastbone (sternum)
- Pain that intensifies when you push on your sternum
- Swelling at the pain site

Chest wall pain (costochondritis) is an inflammation of the cartilage of the rib cage that causes pain and soreness. It's most likely to affect the cartilage that joins your rib cage to your sternum. A blow or other trauma to the rib cage, physical exertion or upper body strain may cause the inflammation, but often the cause is unknown. Movement of the ribs and pressure exerted directly on the affected area often intensify the pain.

The pain associated with this condition is often mistaken for a heart attack because it can be intense and come on suddenly. The difference between chest wall pain and a heart attack is that with chest wall pain, it hurts when you push on your sternum or on your ribs near your sternum. Chest wall pain isn't a medical emergency, but the sudden onset of severe chest pain should be evaluated by a doctor to rule out a heart attack.

Diagnosis

Tenderness at the junction of the ribs and breastbone suggests chest wall pain, but without actual swelling that you or your doctor can feel, it's difficult to be sure. Your doctor may have you undergo chest X-rays, electrocardiograms, blood tests and other tests to exclude other unrelated disorders that could produce similar pain.

Treatment

Given time and rest, the symptoms may disappear. In the meantime, applying ice or heat may help ease your discomfort. Exercise may aggravate the symptoms, so avoid activities that worsen the pain. Your doctor may refer you to a physical therapist for guidance on use of ice and heat and proper exercises.

Acetaminophen (Tylenol, others) and nonsteroidal anti-inflammatory drugs (NSAIDs), such as ibuprofen (Advil, Motrin IB, others), may reduce your discomfort. Sometimes, a doctor will inject a steroid drug, such as cortisone, into the affected area.

Abdominal wall pain

Signs and symptoms

- Sharp pain in the abdomen
- Increased pain when you push directly over a tender spot
- Increased pain and tenderness when abdominal muscles are tensed and improvement when the muscles are relaxed

Abdominal wall pain is a chronic pain that originates in the abdominal wall. Often the source of the pain is a strained muscle or an irritated nerve ending. The pain may also result from structural conditions, such as lesions associated with endometriosis, an abdominal wall hernia or a muscle tear.

The abdomen typically is tender to the touch in a specific location. Pushing on that spot (trigger point) produces moderate to severe pain. Movements that tense the abdominal muscles — such as when moving from a lying to a sitting position or when doing leg lifts or situps — increase pain and tenderness. Symptoms generally improve when the muscles are relaxed.

Diagnosis

A diagnosis is often based on your medical history and an examination of your abdomen. Increased pain in the abdomen when you lift your head and shoulders off the examining table and pain when a doctor pushes on the trigger point while your muscles are tensed are often positive indications of the condition.

Treatment

Given time and rest, the symptoms may disappear. In the meantime, applying ice or heat may help ease your discomfort. Acetaminophen (Tylenol, others) and nonsteroidal anti-inflammatory drugs (NSAIDs), such as ibuprofen (Advil, Motrin IB, others), may reduce pain. Sometimes, a doctor may inject a local anesthetic with or without cortisone into the affected area. Reassurance that there's nothing seriously wrong is often treatment in and of itself.

Muscle tumors

Signs and symptoms
- A lump in a muscle, perceptible on the surface of the skin
- Pain in the affected area
- Rapid growth of a lump in a muscle

Most lumps located under the skin are lipomas, which consist of fat and are situated between the skin and the muscle layer. Often they're easy to identify because they move readily with slight finger pressure. They're rubbery to the touch and usually not tender. It's not unusual to have several lipomas.

Muscle tumors are rare. Most muscle tumors are noncancerous (benign), but some can be cancerous (malignant). A malignant muscle tumor (rhabdomyosarcoma) can be life-threatening and requires prompt treatment.

Diagnosis
Your doctor will examine the lump and may order an X-ray, magnetic resonance imaging (MRI) scan or a computerized tomography (CT) scan of the area. A biopsy of the lump, in which a sample of tissue is removed for laboratory analysis, may be necessary.

How serious are muscle tumors?
A benign tumor isn't serious. A malignant tumor requires prompt treatment.

Treatment
A benign tumor may be left alone or surgically removed. A cancerous tumor requires removal, which may be followed by radiation or chemotherapy.

Muscular dystrophy

Signs and symptoms
- Muscle weakness
- Lack of coordination of motor movements
- A clumsy gait
- An inability to lift the arms overhead
- Progressive muscle weakening, causing loss of mobility and an inability to do everyday tasks

Muscular dystrophy is a rare, progressive disease involving mostly the voluntary muscles. The most common and severe form of the disease is Duchenne's muscular dystrophy (pseudohypertrophic muscular dystrophy). In this disease, muscles appear to be deficient in the protein dystrophin, which is essential to muscle function. Without this protein, the muscles grow progressively weaker, but may appear larger than normal because fat and connective tissue replace lost muscle fibers.

An inherited disorder that strikes only males, Duchenne's muscular dystrophy may be passed from mother to son through one of the mother's genes. It usually begins at an early age, often before age 5.

Becker's muscular dystrophy, a milder form of the disease, usually strikes older boys and young men. Also passed from mother to son, it progresses more slowly, usually over several decades.

There are many other less common types of muscular dystrophy, characterized by different patterns of muscle weakness. Some are passed along in the same inheritance pattern that marks Duchenne's and Becker's muscular dystrophies. Other types may be handed from one generation to the next, affecting males and females alike. Still others require a defective gene from both parents.

Diagnosis
In a toddler, loss of mobility — such as difficulty walking, climbing stairs or rising to a standing position — or difficulty in lifting his or her arms overhead may signal muscular dystrophy. Your child's doctor may review your family's health history, perform an examination and order blood tests.

In electromyography, a needle electrode is inserted through the skin into the muscle to measure electrical activity to confirm a muscle disease. Your doctor may also order a biopsy of the muscle, in which a small sample of tissue is removed for analysis. Some forms of muscular dystrophy can be diagnosed by analyzing a blood sample for an abnormal gene.

Although much still remains to be learned about muscular dystrophies, it's clear that they're usually inherited disorders. Because females carry the affected genes for Duchenne's and Becker's muscular dystrophies — the two most common forms of the disease — women with a family history of muscular dystrophy should seek genetic counseling before deciding on pregnancy. The odds are that half of all the male children of a carrier will have the devastating disorder.

How serious is muscular dystrophy?

Duchenne's muscular dystrophy is a crippling disease. In most cases, the arms, legs and spine become progressively deformed. By their teenage years, most boys with Duchenne's muscular dystrophy need a wheelchair. Duchenne's also can cause cardiovascular and respiratory problems. Increased susceptibility to respiratory infections often causes early death.

Other forms of muscular dystrophy are less severe, and they generally don't have such a devastating effect on physical functioning and survival.

Treatment

There's no cure for muscular dystrophy. Treatment may include a combination of medication and physical therapy. If respiratory muscles become weakened, a ventilator may become necessary.

Medications

Medications that may help manage the muscle spasms, stiffness and weakness associated with this condition include mexiletine, phenytoin (Dilantin, Phenytek), baclofen (Lioresal, Gablofen), dantrolene (Dantrium, Revonto) and carbamazepine (Tegretol, Carbatrol). Corticosteroid medications may be used in an attempt to slow the progression of Duchenne's muscular dystrophy.

Physical therapy

Physical therapy can help maximize muscle function. Exercises can prevent contractures of muscles and joints and may reduce or delay curvature of the spine. Occupational therapy can help people with the disease maintain independence.

Surgery

To release the contractures that may develop and that can position joints in painful ways, doctors can perform a tendon release surgery. This may be done to relieve tendons of your hip and knee and on the Achilles tendon at the back of your foot. Surgery also may be needed to correct curvature of the spine.

Arthritis and Other Joint Disorders

In every joint, a layer of cartilage cushions the ends of your bones. Cartilage has a smooth surface, allowing for uninhibited movement of bones within a joint.

Surrounding the joint space is a membrane called the synovial membrane. It produces synovial fluid that lubricates the joint. Encasing the synovial membrane is a fibrous, protective layer called the joint capsule.

Bands of fibrous tissue called ligaments bind the parts of a joint together and help keep the joint stable.

A problem in a joint may be the result of mechanical failure, or it may stem from inflammation produced by an infection, disease or some unknown cause.

Osteoarthritis

Signs and symptoms

- Pain in a joint during or after use or following periods of inactivity
- Stiffness in one or more joints, especially in the morning after waking
- Tenderness in a joint when you apply light pressure
- Loss of flexibility in a joint

Osteoarthritis, also known as degenerative joint disease, is the most common form of arthritis. It affects more than 46 million Americans.

Osteoarthritis may initially strike only one joint, such as a knee or hip, or it may involve multiple joints, such as the joints of the fingers. Wear and tear on cartilage in a joint, affecting the joint's mobility, is a principal feature of the disease.

With age, slippery, lubricated cartilage that normally cushions the ends of the bones in a joint gradually changes. Cartilage may lose its elasticity, making the joint more vulnerable to damage from injury or overuse. The smooth surface also roughens and loses its cushioning effect. The breakdown of cartilage causes the lining in a joint (synovium) to become inflamed. The inflamed tissue releases enzymes that further damage cartilage. As the ends of the bones become exposed from cartilage loss, they thicken and form bony growths (spurs, or osteophytes), and bone rubs against bone. Each of the steps in this process produces pain.

Normal joint deterioration, however, doesn't necessarily result in osteoarthritis, and osteoarthritis isn't an inevitable part of aging.

In addition to age, injury to a joint is another factor in the development of osteoarthritis. People with joint injuries due to sports, work-related activity or accidents may be at increased risk of developing osteoarthritis. A major factor that leads to osteoarthritis of the knees is obesity. Genetics also plays a role in development of osteoarthritis, particularly in the hands. Some people are born with defective cartilage or with slight defects in the way their joints fit together. As they age, these defects can cause early cartilage breakdown in joints.

Diagnosis

Pain in one or more joints is a prominent symptom of osteoarthritis. Your doctor will likely ask you about your symptoms and examine your joints. An X-ray may be taken to confirm the diagnosis.

Bone spurs (osteophytes), an indication of osteoarthritis, may show up in an X-ray of an affected joint. Another clue may be Heberden's or Bouchard's nodes. These are bony lumps, not nodes, that appear over a period of years in the end and middle joints of your fingers. Blood tests may help rule out other causes of joint pain, such as rheumatoid arthritis.

How serious is osteoarthritis?

Osteoarthritis doesn't go away. The pain tends to increase over the years and may limit activity. The condition is responsible for more than seven million doctor visits a year. Eighty percent of people with osteoarthritis report some form of limitation in movement or activities.

Treatment

There's no known cure for osteoarthritis, but treatments can help reduce pain and maintain joint movement so that you can go about your daily tasks. While medications and joint replacement surgery are key components of treatment for osteoarthritis, your doctor will likely recommend you try all other possible solutions before you consider those options.

Mild osteoarthritis

For mild osteoarthritis pain that is bothersome, but not enough to have a great impact on your daily activities, your doctor may recommend that you:
- **Rest.** Find activities that don't require you to use your joint repetitively. Try taking a 10-minute break every hour.
- **Exercise.** Try to get regular exercise. Stick to gentle exercises, such as walking, biking or swimming. Exercise can increase your endurance and strengthen the muscles around your joint, making your joint more stable. If you feel new joint pain, stop. New pain that lasts more than two hours after you exercise probably means you've overdone it. If weight-bearing exercise is painful, try pool workouts, a seated elliptical machine or biking.
- **Lose weight.** Being overweight or obese increases stress on your weight-bearing joints, such as your knees and your hips. Even a small amount of weight loss can relieve some pressure and reduce your pain.
- **Use heat and cold.** Both heat and cold can relieve pain in your joint. Heat also relieves stiffness and cold can relieve muscle spasms. Soothe your painful joint with heat using a heating pad, hot water bottle or warm bath. Cool the pain in your joint with cold treatments, such as with ice packs. Don't use cold treatments if you have poor circulation or numbness.
- **Work with a physical therapist.** A physical therapist can work with you to create an individualized exercise plan that will strengthen the muscles around your joint, increase your range of motion in your joint and reduce your pain.
- **Apply over-the-counter pain creams.** Creams and gels you can buy at a drugstore may provide temporary relief from

Anatomy of a Joint

The joints in your body are made of tissues designed for a lifetime of service. Bones in your joints are capped with shock-absorbing cartilage. Cartilage is a tough, smooth, slippery material that prevents bone-against-bone contact.

The joint is surrounded and lubricated by the synovial membrane, which forms and releases lubricating fluid. The joint capsule is tough, fibrous tissue that attaches to bone on either side of a joint. It helps stabilize the joint. Ligaments — short cords of strong fiber that attach bone to bone — contribute to joint alignment and stability. Muscles end in tendons that attach to bone above or below the joint capsule.

Near many joints are small fluid-filled sacs called bursae. Bursae are located between muscles or between muscles, tendons and bone. They help reduce friction around joints.

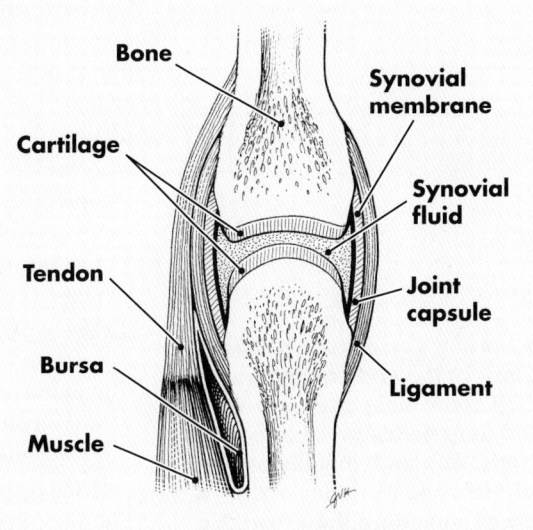

Corticosteroid Medications

Corticosteroid medications (glucocorticoids) are modified forms of two hormones — cortisone and hydrocortisone — naturally produced by your adrenal glands. This class of steroid medications is useful in treating a variety of problems.

Uses

Corticosteroids have a strong anti-inflammatory effect that can reduce swelling, pain, redness and warmth of inflamed joints.

In addition to their obvious value in treating deficiency disorders of the adrenal glands, corticosteroids can be invaluable remedies for a wide range of other ailments, including skin diseases, autoimmune diseases, allergies, certain tumors, and several types of arthritis and other musculoskeletal disorders. Corticosteroids are also used to prevent rejection of a transplanted organ.

Corticosteroids are available in tablet (oral) form, topical form, as eyedrops and as injections. The drug can be injected directly into a muscle, joint or fluid-filled sac between bone (bursa).

Corticosteroid medications aren't the same as anabolic steroid preparations (male sex hormones) that some athletes use inappropriately to increase muscle bulk.

Doses

The risk of side effects from oral corticosteroid drugs increases over time, especially with higher doses. Up to 7.5 milligrams (mg) a day of the corticosteroid prednisone is considered a low dosage, comparable to what's normally present in your body.

Some people with rheumatic diseases take corticosteroid medications for years with minimal side effects. Even so, long-term use of these drugs requires careful monitoring.

A daily dose from 7.5 to 20 mg of an oral corticosteroid is considered an intermediate-level dose and presents a moderate risk of side effects. The risk is small in the first month or so, but increases over time.

If you take 20 to 60 mg a day, your risk of side effects increases dramatically. Such a high dosage ideally should be used only for short periods, then reduced as quickly as possible.

A dosage above 100 mg a day is extremely high and should be used only in extreme circumstances.

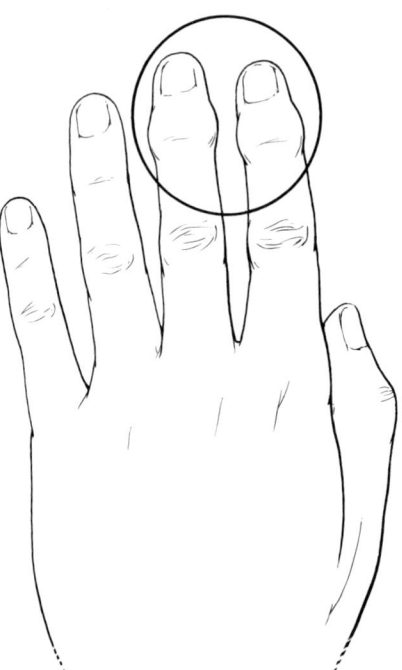

Heberden's nodes are bony lumps at the ends of fingers. They occur most often in women and may be a sign of osteoarthritis. Although initially painful, Heberden's nodes often are of little more than cosmetic concern.

osteoarthritis pain. Some creams numb the pain by creating a hot or cool sensation. Other creams contain medications, such as aspirin-like compounds, that are absorbed into your skin. Pain creams work best on joints that are close to the surface of your skin, such as your knees and fingers.

Moderate osteoarthritis

Osteoarthritis pain that persists may require medications in addition to initial treatment options. In order to get the most from your treatment, continue exercising when possible and resting when you need to. If you're overweight, continue working to lose weight.

- **Acetaminophen.** Acetaminophen (Tylenol, others) can relieve pain, but doesn't reduce inflammation. Taking more than the recommended dose can cause liver damage, especially if you consume three or more alcoholic drinks a day. Acetaminophen can also affect other medications you may be taking.

Discuss this with your doctor.
- **NSAIDs.** Nonsteroidal anti-inflammatory drugs (NSAIDs) can relieve pain and reduce inflammation. Over-the-counter NSAIDs include ibuprofen (Advil, Motrin IB, others) and naproxen sodium (Aleve, others). Stronger versions of these medications and other NSAIDs are available by prescription. An NSAID gel called diclofenac (Voltaren) you rub onto a joint is also available by prescription.

  Possible side effects may occur if NSAIDs are used at high dosages or long term. Side effects of oral medications may include ringing in the ears, gastric ulcers, cardiovascular problems, gastrointestinal bleeding, and liver and kidney damage.
- **Tramadol.** Tramadol (Ultram) is a centrally acting analgesic available only by prescription. It may provide pain relief without the side effects of NSAIDs. However, tramadol may cause nausea and constipation.

Side effects

With sustained, long-term use, the risk of side effects is high. The adrenal glands tend to shrink (atrophy). Other effects include weight gain, a loss of bone minerals (osteoporosis), muscle weakness, water retention, acne, slow healing of cuts and wounds, increased risk of infection, redistribution of body fat and a rounding of the facial features (moon face), thinning of the skin, diabetes, and cataracts. Additional side effects include high blood pressure, elevated blood sugar and stomach irritation, especially if the drug is taken with other anti-inflammatory medications.

Few, if any, people experience all of these side effects, and with short-term use and a low dosage, you have a good chance of having none. The risks with topically applied corticosteroid medications are so small you can obtain some preparations without a prescription. However, long-term use of corticosteroid creams can cause your skin to thin.

If you take enough prednisone daily for three to six months or longer, your adrenal glands atrophy. If this happens and you go off the drug abruptly, your adrenal glands can't produce the amount of cortisol your body needs to manage severe infection, injury or surgery. This can be fatal. When people whose bodies no longer produce enough cortisol have surgery or sustain an injury, doctors may prescribe prednisone or another corticosteroid drug to provide for the temporary increase in hormonal needs.

When it's time to stop taking prednisone, your doctor will work with you to slowly taper the dose so that you don't become sick. If you have taken prednisone daily or have taken it for a few months and stopped, mention this to your doctors for a year after your last dose, especially if you need surgery or invasive diagnostic tests or you become seriously ill.

Cortisone injections

Cortisone injections have remarkable effects for the treatment of acute conditions such as bursitis and tendinitis. They're also beneficial for relieving pain and swelling in individual joints affected by osteoarthritis or rheumatoid arthritis. However, as few as six injections within a 12-month period can damage bone and joint structures, so your doctor may be unwilling to administer more than three or four injections within a year. There can be a period of several days of discomfort in the joint that was injected. This occurs prior to the cortisone becoming fully active. Take a nonprescription pain reliever to control the discomfort.

Severe osteoarthritis

If you've tried other treatments but are still experiencing severe pain and disability, treatment may include:

- **Pain relievers.** Prescription pain medications may provide relief from more-severe osteoarthritis pain. These stronger medications carry a risk of dependence, though the risk is thought to be small in people with severe pain. Side effects may include nausea, constipation and sleepiness. You also can develop a tolerance to the medication, in which normal doses become less effective.
- **Cortisone shots.** Injections of corticosteroid medications may relieve pain in your joint. Your doctor may limit the number of injections you can have each year, since too many corticosteroid injections may cause joint damage.
- **Visco-supplementation.** Injections of hyaluronic acid derivatives may offer pain relief by providing some cushioning in your knee. Some of these treatments are made from bird products; others are not. These treatments are similar to a component normally found in your joint fluid. Visco-supplementation is approved only for knee osteoarthritis, though researchers are studying its use in other joints. If you're sensitive to birds, feathers or eggs, let your doctor know so that a non-bird product can be used instead.

Surgery for osteoarthritis

Surgery is generally reserved for severe osteoarthritis that isn't relieved by other treatments. You may consider surgery if your osteoarthritis makes it difficult to go about your daily tasks. Surgical treatments include:

- **Joint replacement.** In joint replacement surgery (arthroplasty), your surgeon removes your damaged joint surfaces and replaces them with plastic and metal devices called prostheses. The hip and knee joints are the most commonly replaced joints. But today implants can replace your shoulder, elbow, finger or ankle joints.

  The best results generally occur in people who: don't smoke, have a body mass index (BMI) of less than 40, stay physically active, don't take narcotics (opioids) and have their diabetes under control.
- **Cleaning up the area around the joint (debridement).** This involves removing loose pieces of cartilage and bone from around your joint to relieve your pain. Debridement is most useful if you're experiencing a locking sensation from a torn cartilage or loose debris in your knee joint.
- **Realigning bones.** Surgery to realign bones may relieve pain. These types of procedures are typically used when joint replacement surgery isn't an option.
- **Fusing bones.** Surgeons can permanently fuse bones in a joint to increase stability and reduce pain.

INTEGRATIVE MEDICINE

People with osteoarthritis spend millions of dollars each year on nontraditional therapies, including herbal preparations, acupuncture and nutritional supplements. Many turn to these treatments either because the medications they take offer little relief or because they can't tolerate the side effects of the medications. Some people use nontraditional treatments to complement a traditional treatment regimen.

There's evidence that some nontraditional treatments may be helpful:

Glucosamine and chondroitin sulfate

Two of the most popular nontraditional treatments for osteoarthritis are glucosamine and chondroitin sulfate supplements. People may take them because the supplements supposedly maintain existing cartilage and stimulate growth of new cartilage, easing symptoms and slowing progression of the disease.

Your body naturally produces glucosamine, which helps give cartilage its strength and rigidity. The supplements sold in stores are a synthetic version of this substance.

Many older studies of glucosamine and chondroitin gave very promising results. However, the results of a large trial sponsored by the National Institutes of Health was mostly negative. Only people with very severe symptoms appeared to receive some benefit.

Talk to your doctor about the supplements. While the studies may be conflicting, side effects from the supplements are few and far between. No other treatments have shown promise in increasing cartilage, and it's possible glucosamine and chondroitin may help. The supplements may be worth a try.

Relaxation techniques

Meditation, when practiced regularly, helps some people enter a deep, restful state that reduces the body's stress responses. Meditation can relax breathing, slow brain waves, and decrease muscle tension and heart rate. In these ways, it may help you manage arthritis pain.

You might also experiment with other relaxation techniques, such as guided imagery and hypnosis (see Chapter 38,"Integrative Medicine"). Another option is biofeedback, in which you learn how to control certain body functions, such as your heart rate, breathing patterns and body temperature. Managing these functions may help you cope with pain.

Acupuncture

Acupuncture is an ancient Chinese healing art that involves the insertion of thin needles into your skin at specific points in your body, called meridians. Acupuncture is based on the belief that good health is related to the free flow of qi (CHEE), the body's life force. Inserting needles into specific meridians is intended to stimulate the flow of qi. Western scientists believe the procedure may stimulate the release of endorphins, the body's natural painkillers.

Acupuncture has been shown to be effective for some conditions. The National Institutes of Health found that acupuncture may be a reasonable pain management option for osteoarthritis. More recently, however, the American College of Rheumatology reported that acupuncture works no better than a placebo. Future research may help define which individuals might benefit from acupuncture.

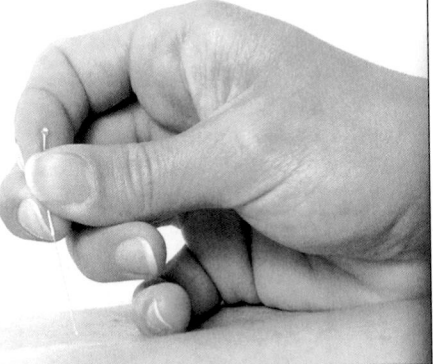

The fused joint, such as an ankle, can then bear weight without pain, but has no flexibility.

Recent studies have evaluated some types of arthroscopic procedures in people with osteoarthritis of the knees. There was no significant difference in pain relief or improved knee function two years after surgery among those who underwent arthroscopic surgery. However, carefully selected individuals who have arthritis and mechanical symptoms, such as catching or "locking" may receive some benefits from this procedure.

Additional studies are needed to better evaluate the results.

Arthritis of the thumb

Signs and symptoms

- Pain at the base of your thumb, aggravated by simple activities such as writing, opening a jar or turning a key in a lock
- Swelling and deformity
- Difficulty holding small objects due to pain

Often the first indication of osteoarthritis is pain in a thumb, which may be accompanied by swelling or limited movement. Degeneration of cartilage and bone can cause arthritis at the base of the thumb. Everyday wear and tear is the most common factor. Other contributors may be heredity and a previous injury, such as dislocation of your thumb.

Diagnosis

A diagnosis often can be made with a physical examination and X-rays.

Treatment

Avoiding or modifying certain activities may cause the swelling and pain to subside. Applying ice also may help. You can purchase splints that stabilize your thumb joint to reduce pain and stress on the joint. For a custom-fitted splint, see a physical therapist.

Ask your doctor or a therapist about tools and utensils specially designed for people with arthritis,

Baker's Cyst

Any condition that causes inflammation of the knee joint can cause the membrane lining of the joint (synovium) to produce excess lubricating (synovial) fluid. The fluid can accumulate in the popliteal bursa behind the knee, resulting in the development of a popliteal (Baker's) cyst. Other names for the condition include popliteal bursitis or synovial cyst of the popliteal space.

If the cyst is small and not painful, no treatment is needed. If the cyst is large and causes a lot of pain, your doctor may remove (aspirate) excess fluid from the knee joint with a needle. Sometimes, a doctor will inject a steroid medication, such as cortisone, into the knee to reduce the volume of fluid being produced.

If the cyst is related to an injury, such as a cartilage tear, you may need surgery to treat the torn cartilage.

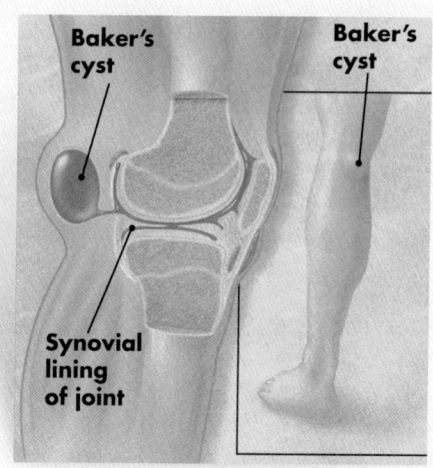

such as special scissors that close automatically and tools and utensils with large, padded handles that make them easier to grip.

Medication

To relieve pain in the joint, your doctor may recommend an over-the-counter pain reliever such as acetaminophen (Tylenol, others), aspirin or ibuprofen (Advil, Motrin IB, others). Or your doctor may prescribe a pain relief medication.

Surgery

If the pain is severe or limits mobility of your thumb, your doctor may recommend surgery. If the joint surfaces are severely damaged, a surgeon may replace the joint with an artificial joint.

Recovery typically takes several months. You won't end up with a normal thumb, but most people who have surgery are pleased with the improvement in pain and joint strength and stability.

Rheumatoid arthritis

Signs and symptoms
- Pain and swelling in the joints of the feet, wrists and hands
- Joints that are tender to the touch
- Redness and warmth over the joints
- Fatigue and malaise
- Morning stiffness
- Lumps under the skin

Unlike the more common osteoarthritis, rheumatoid arthritis isn't the result of joint wear and tear. Rather, it's an autoimmune disease in which your body's immune system triggers inflammation within the lining (synovium) of the joints and some internal organs.

Inflammation in affected joints causes pain, stiffness, warmth, redness and swelling. The inflamed lining often proliferates, invading and damaging bone and cartilage and disrupting the stability of joints. Inflammatory cells release enzymes that digest bone and cartilage and cause further damage.

Doctors don't know what causes the process that leads to rheumatoid arthritis. It's likely that rheumatoid arthritis occurs as a result of a complex combination of factors, including your genes and things in your environment, such as exposure to tobacco smoke.

Unlike osteoarthritis, which affects only the musculoskeletal system, rheumatoid arthritis is a systemic disease. In some people, it affects several organs, such as the heart, lungs, skin, nerves and eyes. It also tends to affect multiple joints, resulting in widespread stiffness and aching.

Rheumatoid arthritis tends to be symmetric, affecting, for example, both ankles or both wrists. It may also produce small lumps under the skin (rheumatoid nodules)

near the elbows, on the fingers, on the feet, along the Achilles tendons or on the buttocks. The lumps range in size from that of a pea to that of a walnut. Usually, the lumps aren't painful and present no physical problems. Occasionally, a lump can ulcerate, creating an entry point for infectious bacteria.

Rheumatoid arthritis can strike at any age, but it most often develops between ages 20 and 50. A variant of the disease called juvenile idiopathic arthritis occurs at a younger age (see page 977).

Diagnosis

Diagnosing rheumatoid arthritis usually begins with a physical exam. Your doctor will ask you about your signs and symptoms and examine your affected joints.

In addition, your doctor may recommend:
- **Blood tests.** People with rheumatoid arthritis often have an elevated erythrocyte sedimentation rate (ESR, or sed rate) or C-reactive protein (CRP), which may indicate the presence of an inflammatory process in the body. Other blood tests look for rheumatoid factor and anti-cyclic citrullinated peptide (anti-CCP) antibodies. While commonly found in the blood of people with rheumatoid arthritis, rheumatoid factor and anti-CCP antibodies aren't present in all cases.

- **Joint fluid analysis.** Your doctor may draw fluid from your joint using a needle. The fluid can be tested to help rule out other diseases and conditions.
- **X-rays.** Your doctor may recommend X-rays to help track the progression of rheumatoid arthritis in your joint over time.

How serious is rheumatoid arthritis?

Rheumatoid arthritis can be a very debilitating disease. It can damage the cartilage, bones, tendons and ligaments of affected joints. People with rheumatoid arthritis often develop joint deformity, which leads to loss of mobility. Some people also experience sweats and fever along with loss of strength in muscles attached to affected joints.

For most people, the condition is long lasting (chronic). Inflammation may fluctuate in severity but generally persists. In mild cases, periods of increased disease activity, called flares, alternate with periods of relative remission, during which symptoms such as swelling, pain, difficulty sleeping and weakness fade or disappear. For others, the disease is continuously active and progresses over time. Only 1 in 10 people with the disease has a single episode followed by long-lasting remission.

It's difficult to predict initially how severe the disease will be in any one person. People who have continuous symptoms for four or five years are likely to have a lifetime of problems with the disease.

Many people are able to live long, productive and nearly normal lives despite the disease. Proper and prompt medical care is essential for dealing effectively with the condition.

Treatment

It's important to diagnose rheumatoid arthritis early because a delay in starting treatment may reduce its effectiveness. Recent discoveries indicate that remission of symptoms is more likely when treatment begins early with strong medications known as disease-modifying antirheumatic drugs (DMARDs).

Medication

The types of medications recommended by your doctor will depend on the severity of your symptoms and how long you've had rheumatoid arthritis.

- **NSAIDs.** Nonsteroidal anti-inflammatory drugs (NSAIDs) can relieve pain and reduce inflammation. Over-the-counter NSAIDs include ibuprofen (Advil, Motrin IB, others) and naproxen sodium (Aleve, others). Stronger NSAIDs are available by prescription. Side effects may include ringing in the ears, stomach irritation, heart problems, and liver and kidney damage.
- **Steroids.** Corticosteroid medications, such as prednisone, reduce inflammation and pain and slow joint damage. Side effects may include thinning of bones, weight gain and diabetes. Doctors often prescribe a corticosteroid to relieve acute symptoms, with the goal of gradually tapering off the medication.
- **Disease-modifying antirheumatic drugs (DMARDs).** These drugs can slow the progression of rheumatoid arthritis and save the joints and other tissues from permanent damage. Common DMARDs include methotrexate (Trexall, Otrexup, Rasuvo), leflunomide (Arava), hydroxychloroquine (Plaquenil) and sulfasalazine (Azulfidine).

  Side effects vary but may include liver damage, bone marrow suppression and severe lung infections.
- **Biologic agents.** Also known as biologic response modifiers, this newer class of DMARDs includes abatacept (Orencia), adalimumab (Humira), anakinra (Kineret), certolizumab pegol (Cimzia), etanercept (Enbrel), golimumab (Simponi), infliximab (Remicade), rituximab (Rituxan), tocilizumab (Actemra) and tofacitinib (Xeljanz).

  These drugs can target parts of the immune system that trigger inflammation that causes joint and tissue damage. These types of drugs also increase the risk of infections.

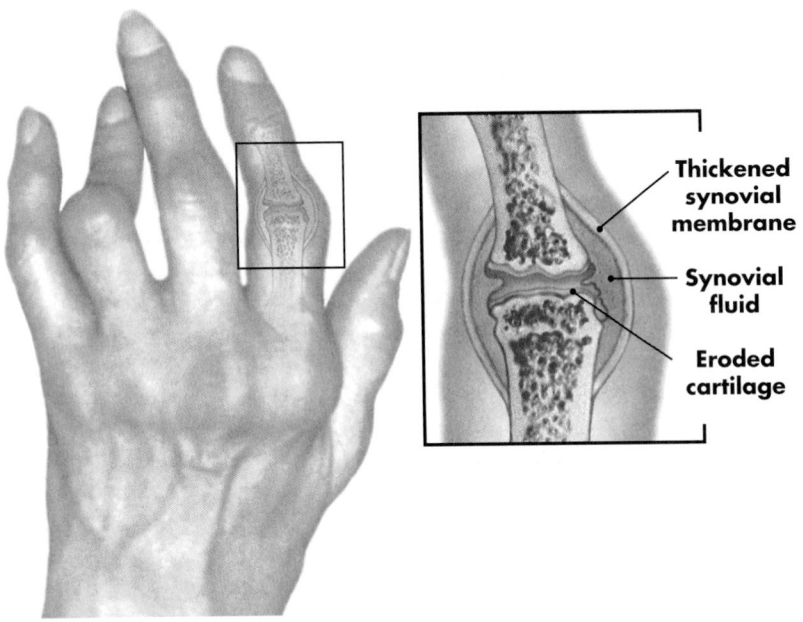

Thickened synovial membrane

Synovial fluid

Eroded cartilage

Rheumatoid arthritis can lead to deformity in the fingers. The hand may lose strength and be painful during flares of the disease.

Biologic DMARDs are usually most effective when paired with a nonbiologic DMARD, such as methotrexate.

Rest and exercise

Another key component in managing rheumatoid arthritis is to establish the optimal balance between rest and exercise. The preservation of function in affected joints requires muscle-building and range-of-motion exercises, but you also need sufficient rest.

Because of the ebb-and-flow nature of the disease, strategies used during flares and periods of remission differ. Intense disease activity during a flare puts you at risk of joint damage, so your doctor may advise a combination of rest, pain-reduction strategies and gentle activity.

During flares, refrain from exercises that strain your affected joints, but don't stop moving. During periods of remission, exercise and carry on daily activities as tolerated. It's important to recognize your limits and avoid undue fatigue.

Therapy

Your doctor may send you to a physical or occupational therapist who can teach you exercises to help keep your joints flexible. The therapist also may suggest new ways to do daily tasks, which will be easier on your joints. For example, if your fingers are sore, you may want to pick up an object using your forearms.

Assistive devices can make it easier to avoid stressing your painful joints. For instance, a kitchen knife equipped with a saw handle helps protect your finger and wrist joints. Certain tools, such as buttonhooks, can make it easier to get dressed. Catalogs and medical supply stores are good places to look for ideas.

Surgery

If other treatments aren't effective, your doctor may consider surgery, which may involve one or more of the following procedures:

- **Synovectomy.** This surgery to remove the inflamed lining of the joint (synovium) can be performed on knees, elbows, wrists, fingers and hips.
- **Tendon repair.** Inflammation and joint damage may cause tendons around your joint to loosen or rupture. Your surgeon may be able to repair the tendons around your joint.
- **Joint fusion.** Surgically fusing a joint may be recommended to stabilize or realign a joint and for pain relief when a joint replacement isn't an option.
- **Total joint replacement.** During joint replacement surgery, your surgeon removes the damaged parts of your joint and inserts a prosthesis made of metal and plastic (see page 978).

Juvenile idiopathic arthritis

Signs and symptoms

- Swelling and stiffness in the joints
- Fever
- A rash
- Fatigue and irritability
- Inflammation of the eye

Juvenile idiopathic arthritis (JIA) resembles rheumatoid arthritis in some ways but differs in others. Differences include the age of onset — juvenile idiopathic arthritis affects children and can even begin in infancy — and the long-term nature of the ailment.

There are several types of juvenile idiopathic arthritis, classified based on the joints affected, symptoms and test results. The main types are:

- **Pauciarticular.** This type affects four or fewer joints — typically larger joints, such as the knees. This is the most common form of juvenile arthritis.
- **Polyarticular.** It affects five or more joints — typically small joints, such as those in the hands and feet. Polyarticular arthritis often affects the same joint on both sides of a child's body.
- **Systemic.** Also known as Still's disease, systemic juvenile idiopathic arthritis affects many areas of the body, including joints and internal organs, often causing fevers and rashes.

The cause of juvenile idiopathic arthritis is unknown. Most likely several factors are involved, including genetics. It's possible a virus or bacterium may trigger the disease in children with a genetic predisposition.

Juvenile idiopathic arthritis most often begins during the toddler or early teenage years. Certain types and subtypes are more prevalent in one sex than the other, but in general the disease affects more girls than boys.

About half the children with short-term (acute) juvenile idiopathic arthritis recover completely, and half develop the long-lasting (chronic) form.

Diagnosis

Diagnosing the disorder generally involves a thorough physical exam and laboratory tests to measure inflammation and to detect autoantibodies — these are antibodies that attack the body's own cells.

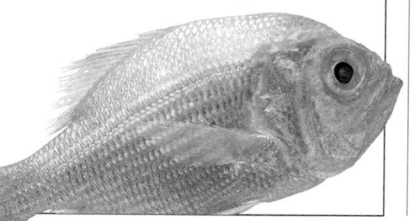

Joint Replacement

Every year, about half a million people in the United States have joint replacement surgery to regain physical function and eliminate pain in their joints caused by a joint disorder such as osteoarthritis or rheumatoid arthritis.

A surgical procedure called arthroplasty, which literally means "reforming the joint," may be the best remedy for a damaged hip or knee joint.

Replacement arthroplasty involves replacement of joint surfaces with plastic, ceramic and metal implants (prostheses). Cement is used to fasten the implants to the bone. Some prostheses are made from material that enables bone to grow into it.

The hip and knee joints are the most commonly replaced. In a hip arthroplasty, a ball on a stem replaces the top of the thighbone (femur). A metal and plastic cup typically replaces the socket of the hip. The results are often remarkable: People who were unable to walk before their hip or knee surgery are able to do so afterward.

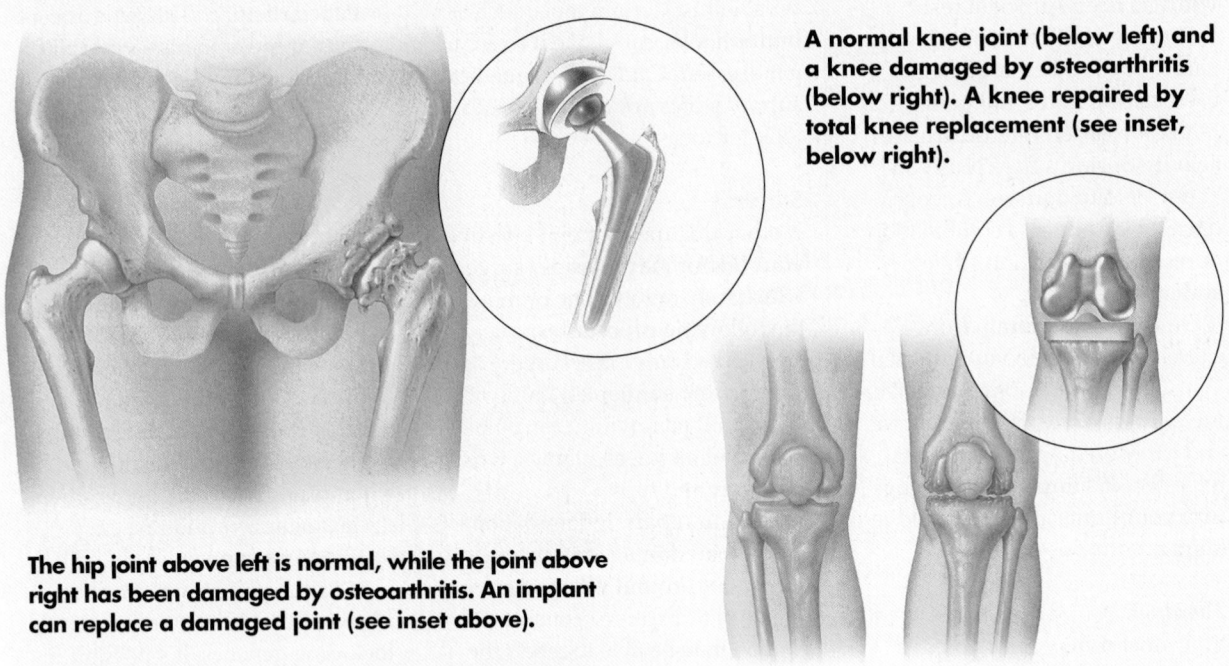

A normal knee joint (below left) and a knee damaged by osteoarthritis (below right). A knee repaired by total knee replacement (see inset, below right).

The hip joint above left is normal, while the joint above right has been damaged by osteoarthritis. An implant can replace a damaged joint (see inset above).

Children with juvenile idiopathic arthritis should have a special eye examination with a slit lamp because of the high risk of a potentially serious eye condition called uveitis (see page 605).

How serious is juvenile idiopathic arthritis?

As with adult rheumatoid arthritis, juvenile idiopathic arthritis puts the person who has it at risk of permanent joint damage. In addition, a growing child with the disease may experience abnormal bone growth. For example, the disease may accelerate growth in one leg bone but not in the other.

Another risk is that a child will refrain from moving an affected joint to avoid pain. This can result in weakened and contracted muscles and even a joint deformity.

Treatment

Treatment of juvenile idiopathic arthritis focuses on helping your child maintain a normal level of physical and social activity. To accomplish this, doctors may use a combination of strategies to relieve pain and swelling, maintain full movement and strength, and prevent complications.

Medication

For some children pain relievers may be the only medication needed. Others may need help from medications designed to limit the progression of the disease. Typical medications used include:

- **Nonsteroidal anti-inflammatory drugs (NSAIDs).** These medications, such as ibuprofen (Advil, Motrin IB, others) and naproxen sodium (Aleve, others), reduce pain and swelling. Stronger NSAIDs are available by prescription. Side effects include stomach upset and liver problems.
- **Disease-modifying antirheumatic drugs (DMARDs).** Doctors use these medications when NSAIDs alone fail to relieve symptoms of joint pain and swelling. They may be taken in combination with NSAIDs and are used to slow the progress of juvenile idiopathic arthritis. Commonly used DMARDs for children include methotrexate (Trexall)

Although the long-term durability of joint prostheses remains a concern, evidence to date suggests that replacement parts last for many years with moderate use. New developments and technologies are becoming available that provide the possibility of dramatically lowering joint-surface wear, which may further increase durability. These new technologies include metal-on-metal and ceramic-on-ceramic surfaces and a new class of polyethylenes (plastics). The goal is to eliminate friction, which may cause an artificial joint to shed particles that can irritate and destroy bone.

Other new technologies involve the way joint implants are affixed to the bone. Cement can loosen over time. Bone and soft tissue attach themselves to some new porous materials, such as tantalum and titanium, which may have an advantage over some other materials.

Prostheses can also replace ankles, elbows, shoulders, fingers, wrists and hands. Wrist and hand joint replacements are less common because the joints are small and complex and they rely heavily on soft tissue for proper function.

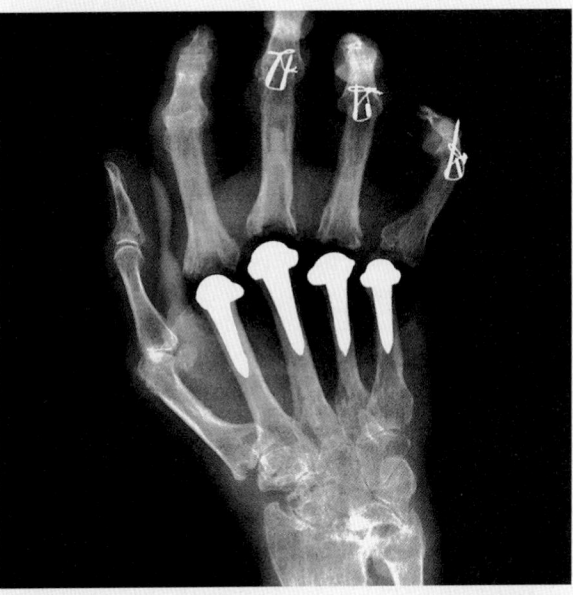

These X-rays show the deforming effects of rheumatoid arthritis on a hand (left) and the same hand following joint replacement surgery (right).

and sulfasalazine (Azulfidine). Side effects may include nausea and liver problems.

- **Tumor necrosis factor (TNF) blockers.** TNF blockers — such as etanercept (Enbrel) and adalimumab (Humira) — can help reduce pain, morning stiffness and swollen joints. But these types of drugs increase the risk of infections. There may also be a mild increase in the chance of getting some cancers, such as lymphoma.
- **Immune suppressants.** Because juvenile idiopathic arthritis is caused by an overactive immune system, medications that suppress the immune system can help. Examples include abatacept (Orencia), rituximab

(Rituxin), anakinra (Kineret) and tocilizumab (Actemra). Immune suppressants increase the risk of infections and, rarely, some types of cancer.

- **Corticosteroids.** Medications such as prednisone may be used to control symptoms until a DMARD takes effect or to prevent complications, such as inflammation of the sac around the heart (pericarditis). Corticosteroids may be administered by mouth or by injection directly into a joint. However, these drugs can interfere with normal growth and increase your susceptibility to infection. Therefore, they generally should be used for the shortest possible duration.

Other therapies
Your doctor may recommend that your child work with a physical therapist to help keep his or her joints flexible and maintain range of motion and muscle tone.

A physical therapist or an occupational therapist may make additional recommendations regarding the best forms of exercise and protective equipment for your child.

A therapist may also recommend that your child make use of joint supports or splints to help protect joints and keep them in a good functional position.

Surgery
In very severe cases of juvenile rheumatoid arthritis, surgery may

be needed to improve the position of a joint.

Other types of inflammatory arthritis

The most common form of inflammatory arthritis is rheumatoid arthritis. Other types may take one of several forms, each with somewhat different manifestations. These forms of arthritis have genetic factors. Each of them has characteristic gene markers that indicate a genetic predisposition to the disease.

A tissue-typing test can detect the presence of the marker. Having a certain gene marker doesn't mean you'll get one of these conditions, only that you're predisposed to it, which increases your risk. Why one of these disorders develops in one person and not another person remains a mystery.

Psoriatic arthritis

People with the skin condition psoriasis may develop psoriatic arthritis. Signs and symptoms include:

- Pain, swelling and decreased mobility in one or more joints, most often the small joints of the hands and feet
- Swelling of fingers or toes that gives them a sausage-like appearance
- Pitting and discoloration of the nails, which may separate from the nail beds
- Eye inflammation

Psoriasis is a common skin disease in which areas of the skin become inflamed and reddish in color (see page 1077). The skin over the elbows and knees often becomes scaly. The fingernails may become pitted and discolored. Psoriatic arthritis develops in approximately 1 in 10 people with psoriasis. More women than men have psoriatic arthritis, which typically strikes people in their 20s to 40s.

For most people, the effects of psoriatic arthritis are relatively minor, with some pain and discomfort in affected joints but little effect on overall health. In some, however, it can cause severe deformity and disability if left untreated.

Treatment

First line medications for the disease include nonsteroidal anti-inflammatory drugs (NSAIDs), such as ibuprofen (Advil, Motrin IB, others).

For persistent symptoms, your doctor may prescribe other drugs, such as the disease-modifying drugs methotrexate or sulfasalazine (Azulfidine) or tumor necrosis factor (TNF) blockers, such as etanercept (Enbrel), infliximab (Remicade) and adalimumab (Humira).

Other medications that may be used to treat the disease include apremilast (Otezla), ustekinuma (Stelara) and secukinumab (Cosentyx).

Additional treatments include range-of-motion exercises, application of heat to relax muscles around painful joints and relaxation exercises.

Reactive arthritis

Some people inherit a susceptibility to this form of arthritis, which is often precipitated by an infection, including those transmitted by sexual contact. Ingestion of contaminated food or water also can bring on the disease. Signs and symptoms include:

- Pain in joints, usually in the lower extremities, and in the heels
- Inflammation of the urethra or intestine
- Painful inflammation of the eye
- A rash

Reactive arthritis, formerly known as Reiter's syndrome, typically appears in stages. Usually, inflammation of the urethra or intestine comes first. Some time later, joint pain occurs, most often in the finger, toe, ankle, hip and knee joints. Skin lesions similar to those of psoriasis also may appear, as well as a painful eye inflammation called conjunctivitis.

Reactive arthritis may appear once or episodically. Attacks tend to last a few weeks or months. Inflammation associated with a sudden, severe attack can produce tenderness and pain and may lead to permanent joint damage.

Treatment

Treatment generally includes nonsteroidal anti-inflammatory drugs (NSAIDs) to relieve pain and inflammation. For more-severe symptoms, other medications may be prescribed.

Ankylosing spondylitis

This form of arthritis predominantly affects the sacroiliac and spinal joints. However, peripheral joints of the arms and legs and the tendons and ligaments where they attach to bones also may be affected. Signs and symptoms include:

- Pain and stiffness in the spine and perhaps other joints
- In advanced stages, a stiff, inflexible spine

Ankylosing spondylitis has no known specific cause, though genetic factors seem to be involved.

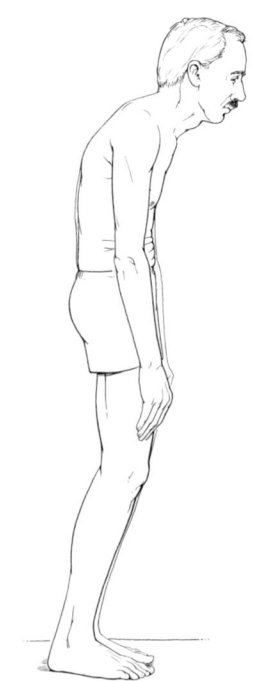

Ankylosing spondylitis can lead to a stiff, inflexible spine.

In particular, people who have a gene called HLA-B27 are at greatly increased risk of developing ankylosing spondylitis. However, only some people with the gene develop the condition. Males are affected more often than females, with onset generally before age 40.

Typically, ankylosing spondylitis begins with soreness in the sacroiliac joints and low back region. As the disease progresses, the affected bones begin to fuse together, making the joints immobile and causing a stiff, inflexible spine. Some people develop a peripheral arthritis that affects just a few joints, most often the lower extremities, and is asymmetric.

In most cases, ankylosing spondylitis is mild, so it may go undiagnosed for decades. However, once joints fuse, treatment won't help restore mobility.

Treatment
Nonsteroidal anti-inflammatory drugs (NSAIDs) — such as naproxen (Naprosyn) and indomethacin (Indocin) — are the medications doctors most commonly use to treat ankylosing spondylitis. They can relieve your inflammation, pain and stiffness. However, these medications might cause gastrointestinal bleeding.

If NSAIDs aren't helpful, your doctor might suggest starting a biologic medication, such as a tumor necrosis factor (TNF) blocker or an interleukin-17 (IL-17) inhibitor. TNF blockers target a cell protein that causes inflammation in the body. IL-17 plays a role in your body's defense against infection and also has a role in inflammation.

TNF blockers help reduce pain, stiffness, and tender or swollen joints. They're administered by injecting the medication under the skin or through an intravenous line. TNF blockers approved to treat ankylosing spondylitis are adalimumab (Humira), certolizumab pegol (Cimzia), etanercept (Enbrel), golimumab (Simponi,

Simponi Aria) and infliximab (Remicade).

Secukinumab (Cosentyx) is the first IL-17 inhibitor approved by the FDA for the treatment of ankylosing spondylitis.

TNF blockers and IL-17 inhibitors can reactivate latent tuberculosis and make you more prone to infection.

Physical therapy is also an important part of treatment and can provide a number of benefits, from pain relief to improved strength and flexibility. A physical therapist can design specific exercises for your needs.

Range-of-motion and stretching exercises can help maintain flexibility in your joints and preserve good posture. Proper sleep and walking positions and abdominal and back exercises can help maintain your upright posture.

Most people with ankylosing spondylitis don't need surgery. However, your doctor might recommend surgery if you have severe pain or joint damage, or if your hip joint is so damaged that it needs to be replaced.

Arthritis of inflammatory bowel disease
People with inflammatory bowel disease (ulcerative colitis and Crohn's disease) may develop a characteristic form of arthritis. Signs and symptoms include:
- Pain and swelling in peripheral joints, especially knees, ankles and feet
- Pain and stiffness in the spine

Joint pain and swelling — often in the large and small joints of the legs — occurs in approximately 1 in 10 people with ulcerative colitis and in 1 in 5 people with Crohn's disease. The pain and stiffness in the spine is similar to that brought on by ankylosing spondylitis.

Treatment
Symptoms are generally treated with pain relievers since nonsteroidal anti-inflammatory drugs (NSAIDs) can worsen or cause a

flare of the disease. Control of the inflammatory bowel disorder is the long-term solution.

Palindromic rheumatism
Also called palindromic rheumatoid arthritis, this disease is a rare type of inflammatory arthritis. Signs and symptoms include:
- Recurrent attacks of painful swelling, usually of one or two joints and surrounding tissues
- Attacks that start abruptly and last several hours to a few days
- Unpredictable frequency of attacks, from every few days to every few months

Attacks of palindromic rheumatism generally come and go and can recur for many years. The disease affects both men and women, typically between the ages of 20 and 50. Palindromic rheumatism usually doesn't cause joint damage, but people with the disease are at higher risk of developing rheumatoid arthritis.

Treatment
Some doctors recommend nonsteroidal anti-inflammatory drugs (NSAIDs) to relieve symptoms, but their benefit isn't clear. Corticosteroids usually aren't beneficial. Hydroxychloroquine (Plaquenil) may be helpful in some cases.

Infectious arthritis

Signs and symptoms
- Severe pain at rest and with movement in one joint, typically a knee, shoulder, hip, ankle, elbow, finger or wrist
- Warmth and redness in surrounding tissues
- Chills and fever
- Weakness

Bacteria, viruses, fungi or other infectious agents can cause a joint infection. Typically, the infecting agent enters the body and spreads to the joint via the bloodstream. In some instances, an open wound or puncture provides direct access to the joint. Unlike other joint disorders, infectious arthritis can affect anyone and anytime, regardless of age, sex or race.

Types
Here's a look at some representative types of infectious arthritis.

Gonococcal infection
Roughly one-third of individuals who contract gonorrhea, a sexually transmitted infection, experience pain in several joints. A rash also may develop. This type of infectious arthritis occurs 10 times more frequently in women than in men.

Histoplasmosis
Histoplasmosis is a fungal infection transmitted by airborne spores released from soil that contains a fungus called *Histoplasma capsulatum*. In some cases, arthritis may develop weeks or months after the initial infection. Arthritis signs and symptoms occur because your immune system responds to the fungus with an unusual amount of inflammation.

Lyme disease
Named for the town in Connecticut where it was first observed, Lyme disease is contracted from a tick bite. Usually, a disk-shaped rash will develop around the bite, and other signs and symptoms may follow, including fever, chills, sore throat, fatigue and nausea. Weeks later, you may develop stiffness and pain in your joints.

Staphylococcal infection
When a boil or other infection releases staphylococcal bacteria into your bloodstream, the infection can spread to a knee or other joint. The pain is usually intense and sudden.

Tuberculous infection
A few people with tuberculosis develop a form of arthritis caused by the bacterium that produces tuberculosis (*Mycobacterium tuberculosis*). Nontuberculosis mycobacteria also may cause infectious arthritis.

Valley fever
Valley fever is a form of coccidioidomycosis infection, caused by a fungi in the soil. Disseminated coccidioidomycosis, the most serious form of the disease, occurs when the infection spreads (disseminates) beyond the lungs to other parts of the body. Signs and symptoms depend on which parts of your body are affected and may include painful, swollen joints, especially in the knees or ankles.

Viral infections
Arthritis symptoms may occur in people who have hepatitis B, hepatitis C, human parvovirus B19, German measles (rubella), mumps and other diseases caused by viruses. In general, the arthritis resolves as the infection clears, or with viral infections such as hepatitis C, with successful treatment of the underlying disease.

Diagnosis
If your doctor suspects a form of infectious arthritis, he or she may perform a biopsy, removing fluid from an affected joint with a needle for laboratory analysis. Your doctor may also order blood tests.

How serious is infectious arthritis?
In most cases, early diagnosis and treatment of a joint infection result in rapid and complete recovery.

Treatment
Because of the risk of permanent damage to the bone or cartilage, a joint infection needs to be treated promptly. Hospitalization may be necessary.

Unless the cause of the infection is viral, your doctor will likely prescribe an antibiotic. He or she may use a needle to drain the infected joint, or a surgeon may surgically remove infected and damaged tissues. After the infection has resolved, you may need reconstructive surgery if your joint has been seriously damaged.

During recuperation from an infection, the joint may be immobilized with a splint. Physical therapy may be necessary to regain strength and mobility in the affected joint.

Gout

Signs and symptoms
- Sudden, severe pain in a single joint, often at the base of your big toe
- Swelling, redness and warmth of tissues surrounding the joint

One of humankind's oldest known diseases, gout has been recognized for more than 2,000

Rheumatic Fever

The management of rheumatic fever is one of modern medicine's success stories. It was once the cause of serious heart problems in many children. The advent of prompt antibiotic treatment of streptococcal infections, however, markedly reduced its incidence.

A common manifestation of the illness is a form of arthritis. It characteristically occurs several weeks after a streptococcal infection, usually of the throat (strep throat). Your joints may become swollen, reddened and painful to move. Typically, your joints are affected in a migratory manner — first, one joint is painful for a time, and then the pain improves and occurs in another joint.

The arthritis of rheumatic fever isn't due to joint infection. Rather it's a hypersensitivity reaction in the joints associated with a previous strep infection. In general, the treatment is the same as that for rheumatic fever, although your doctor may remove fluid from swollen joints with a needle to reduce the discomfort.

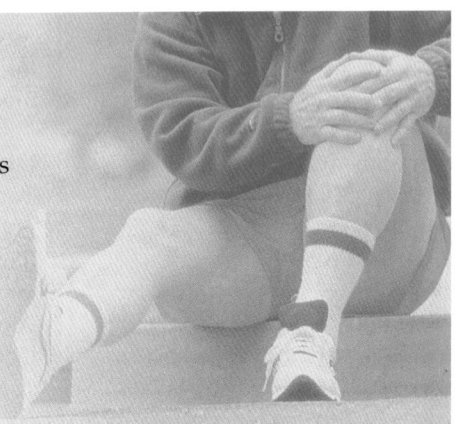

? Question and Answer

What's pseudogout?

Pseudogout is similar to gout, but it involves the deposit of crystals of a calcium salt rather than uric acid in joints. Affected joints are more likely to be knees, wrists and ankles than those of the foot. Pseudogout strikes women and men with roughly equal frequency, but the age at onset is late, typically 70 years.

Doctors usually treat pseudogout with anti-inflammatory medications, although colchicine, used for centuries to treat gout, may be effective.

years. It's caused by too much uric acid, a substance your body naturally forms from proteins called purines. When you have gout, your body either produces too much uric acid or excretes too little in the urine. In 90 percent of individuals with gout, the problem is underexcretion.

Uric acid typically dissolves in your blood and passes through your kidneys into your urine. In people with gout, the excess uric acid can build up and form sharp crystals, which deposit in a joint and surrounding tissue, causing pain, inflammation and swelling. Gout typically affects the joint of the big toe, but it can strike other joints in the feet, as well as the ankles, knees and, occasionally, the hands and elbows. Not everyone with excess uric acid develops gout symptoms.

Other factors that may contribute to gout are eating foods high in purines — organ meats, anchovies, herring and mackerel — drinking alcohol; being overweight; having high blood cholesterol, diabetes or metabolic syndrome; and taking certain medications. For instance, taking a thiazide diuretic for high blood pressure may interfere with your kidneys' abilities to remove uric acid from the body.

Daily low-dose aspirin can raise uric acid levels in the blood by decreasing excretion. The stress of an injury such as a bone fracture or a surgical procedure may provoke an attack of gout.

An episode of acute gout develops in a matter of hours. A joint suddenly becomes intensely painful, and the area around it becomes hot, red and swollen. The joint will remain very painful for several days. The discomfort generally subsides gradually over the next one to two weeks.

Gout mainly affects men older than age 40. One in 4 has a family history of the ailment. Women become increasingly susceptible after menopause.

Gout has a reputation as an illness that's caused by excessive consumption of food and drink. Although that may contribute to the problem, gout can strike at any time and for no apparent reason.

Diagnosis

To confirm the diagnosis and rule out infection as the cause, your doctor may withdraw fluid from the affected joint to look for crystals of uric acid within the white blood cells. He or she may also order blood tests to check levels of uric acid. However, blood tests can be misleading because the levels may be nearly normal during an acute attack of gout. In addition, many people with high levels of uric acid never experience gout.

A long-term accumulation of uric acid may produce lumps (tophi) just beneath the skin. The most common sites are the cartilage of the ear, elbows and Achilles tendons. Infrequently, kidney stones develop from accumulation of uric acid.

How serious is gout?

After an attack of gout has run its course — generally a matter of days and no more than a few weeks — the affected joint usually returns to normal. You may never have another attack, or you may have them several times a year. If you don't receive proper treatment, the condition can permanently damage affected joints, and uric acid deposits may cause kidney problems, including the development of kidney stones.

Treatment

An acute attack of gout is generally treated with nonsteroidal anti-inflammatory drugs (NSAIDs) and followed up with other medication to prevent a recurrence. Lifestyle changes also may help prevent a recurrence.

Medication

NSAIDs, such as ibuprofen (Advil, Motrin IB, others) and naproxen sodium (Aleve, others), are the treatments of choice for an acute gout attack. The medication colchicine has been used for centuries to relieve the pain and swelling of an acute episode. But it's more likely to cause gastrointestinal upset and toxicity than are NSAIDs. Another treatment option is cortisone, either in pill form or as an injection into the affected joint.

Once the attack is under control, your doctor may advise preventive treatment to keep uric acid levels below a target level to prevent recurrent attacks as well as joint damage. This usually involves taking medication such as allopurinol (Aloprim, Zyloprim) for months or years. Febuxostat (Uloric) recently was approved to treat high levels of uric acid in blood (hyperuricemia) in people with gout.

Self-care
Although doctors no longer consider food and drink the main causes of gout, lifestyle changes can help. If you have gout, limit or avoid alcohol, maintain a healthy weight, and avoid foods that are high in purines, including sardines, anchovies and organ meats. Diets that involve rapid weight reduction may provoke an acute attack.

If you're taking a medication such as allopurinol (Duzallo, Zyloprim) to prevent future attacks of gout, don't abruptly discontinue the drug because this may provoke an acute attack of gout. In addition, if you start taking allopurinol during an acute attack of gout, you may worsen and prolong the attack.

Bursitis

Signs and symptoms
- A dull ache or stiffness around a joint
- Worsening pain with movement or pressure
- Warmth over the joint
- Swelling and skin redness

Your body houses more than 150 bursae, tiny sacs that lubricate and cushion pressure points between your bones and the fibrous tissues of the muscles and tendons. Bursae help your joints move with ease.

Repetitive movements or pressure may cause inflammation in a bursa (bursitis). Bursitis most often affects your shoulders, elbows or hips. For example, if you spend a lot of time kneeling, such as when you garden, the pressure could cause a bursa in front of your kneecap to become inflamed. Swinging a racket or golf club can affect a bursa in your shoulder.

Bursitis may also result from an infection, arthritis or gout. Many times, the cause is unknown.

Diagnosis
Your doctor may be able to identify tenderness in a localized area. If it appears that something else may be causing the discomfort, your doctor may want an X-ray of the affected area. If bursitis is the cause, X-ray images are usually normal.

How serious is bursitis?
Bursitis often improves on its own with simple self-care remedies. If the pain is disabling or doesn't subside after a week, see your doctor. Sometimes a bursa becomes infected, especially one near the knee or elbow. If you develop increasing pain, redness or warmth over the joint, along with fever and chills, seek medical care promptly.

Treatment
Treatment of bursitis usually includes:
- Resting and immobilizing the affected area
- Applying ice to reduce swelling
- Taking nonsteroidal anti-inflammatory drugs (NSAIDs)

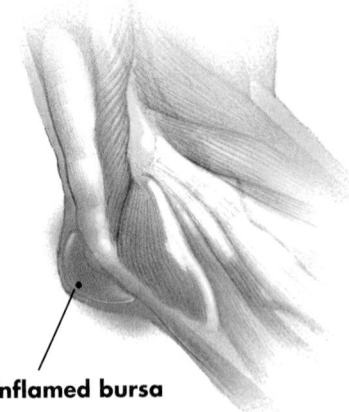

Inflamed bursa

Bursae serve as cushions between bones and fibrous tissue. Overuse of a joint — such as an elbow shown here — can lead to inflammation of a bursa (bursitis).

to relieve pain and reduce inflammation

With simple self-care and home treatment, bursitis usually disappears within a couple of weeks. Sometimes, a doctor may inject a corticosteroid drug into the bursa to relieve inflammation. This treatment generally brings immediate relief and, in many cases, one injection is all you'll need.

If your bursitis is caused by an infection, you'll need to take antibiotics. Sometimes the bursa must be surgically drained, but only rarely is surgical removal of the affected bursa necessary.

Prevention
With proper care, you may be able to keep bursitis from recurring or reduce the severity of the signs and symptoms if it does. Warm up before physical activity and stretch afterward. Strengthening exercise can help keep your muscles strong.

When doing repetitive tasks, take frequent breaks. Avoid standing or sitting for excessively long periods. Protect your joints by sitting in well-supported, cushioned chairs or using foam kneeling pads.

Frozen shoulder

Signs and symptoms
- Aching or burning pain in your shoulder
- Limited shoulder motion
- Difficulties performing activities of daily living
- Pain when trying to find a comfortable position for sleeping

As its name suggests, frozen shoulder is characterized by stiffness in the shoulder joint, along with pain. Also known as adhesive capsulitis, the condition most often affects only one shoulder.

Your shoulder is a ball-and-socket joint. The round end of your upper arm bone (humerus) fits into a shallow groove on your shoulder blade (scapula). Tough connective tissue, called the shoulder capsule, surrounds the joint and allows movement. With frozen shoulder, the shoulder capsule becomes inflamed and stiff, causing pain and loss of movement.

Frozen shoulder typically develops slowly and in three stages: painful movement, freezing and thawing. During the painful stage, which can last from two to nine months, you feel pain with shoulder movement. The pain often worsens at night.

Motion, particularly extending your arm to the side or putting on a coat, may produce or increase pain. Sometimes, people hold the affected arm close to their body and avoid moving it. Ligaments and other tissues around the joint tend to stiffen. This is the freezing stage. To prevent this, try to use your involved shoulder for activities of daily living as much as possible.

Your pain may diminish during the freezing stage, which can last from four to 12 months, but your shoulder's range of motion gradually decreases by perhaps as much as 50 to 75 percent. Movement can cause pain. During the thawing stage, which can last from one to three years, the condition may begin to improve.

No one knows what causes frozen shoulder, but it can occur after a shoulder injury or prolonged immobilization of your shoulder, such as following surgery or after a fracture of your arm. Interestingly, some people with diabetes develop the condition, which raises the possibility that frozen shoulder may have an autoimmune component, meaning that your own immune system may attack the shoulder capsule, causing the inflammation.

More women than men get frozen shoulder. The condition is most often seen in people between the ages of 40 and 65.

Diagnosis

The primary means of diagnosing frozen shoulder is by physical examination. Your doctor may ask you to raise and lower your arm to the front, side and back of your body. He or she may also move your arm to determine your passive range of motion of the shoulder joint and press on parts of your shoulder to check for tender areas.

Your doctor may order an X-ray of your shoulder and possibly a magnetic resonance imaging (MRI) scan to exclude other structural problems.

How serious is frozen shoulder?

In some cases, mobility can decrease to the point where it's difficult if not impossible to perform many everyday tasks, such as combing your hair, putting on your coat or brushing your teeth. Usually, though, the condition improves on its own over time, and most people regain nearly full range of motion and strength in the shoulder.

Treatment

Treatment for most cases of frozen shoulder involves controlling the pain and preserving as much range of motion in the shoulder as possible to permit you to perform everyday tasks.

Your doctor may recommend that you see a physical therapist. A therapist can show you how to maintain as much mobility in your shoulder as possible, without stressing your shoulder to the point of causing a lot of pain. Continue to use the involved shoulder and extremity in as many daily life activities as possible within the limits of your pain and range-of-motion constraints.

Gently and gradually moving your shoulder through range-of-motion exercises won't completely alleviate the symptoms of frozen shoulder. However, it may help restore enough shoulder motion to enable you to resume your everyday activities.

Your doctor may also recommend these treatments:

- **Nonsteroidal anti-inflammatory drugs (NSAIDs).** These medications may help relieve pain and inflammation associated with frozen shoulder. Acetaminophen (Tylenol, others) also may be effective for pain relief.
- **Heat or cold.** Applying heat or cold to your shoulder can help relieve pain.
- **Corticosteroids.** Injecting anti-inflammatory hormones into your shoulder joint may help decrease pain and shorten symptom duration during the initial painful phase. Repeated corticosteroid injections aren't recommended.
- **Joint distension.** Injecting sterile water into the joint capsule can help stretch the tissue and make it easier to move the joint.
- **Shoulder manipulation.** In some people, if severe stiffness persists, gently manipulating the shoulder after receiving a general anesthetic may help to improve range of motion.
- **Surgery.** In a small number of cases, especially if your symptoms don't improve despite other measures, surgery may be an option to remove scar tissue and adhesions from inside your shoulder joint. Doctors usually perform this surgery with a lighted, tubular instrument (arthroscope) that's inserted through an incision in your joint.
- **Electrical stimulation.** Transcutaneous electrical nerve stimulation (TENS) is a treatment that can be used to help control your pain. In this procedure, a tiny electrical current is delivered to key points on a nerve pathway. The current is delivered through electrodes taped to your skin. It isn't painful or harmful.

It's not known exactly how TENS works, but it's thought that the therapy might stimulate the release of natural pain-inhibiting molecules (endorphins) or block pain fibers that carry pain impulses.

Rotator Cuff Injuries and Exercises

Your shoulder joint has the greatest range of motion of any joint in your body, thanks largely to your rotator cuff, which is made up of four muscles and their attached tendons. The muscles connect your upper arm bone (humerus) with your shoulder blade. They also help hold the ball of your upper arm firmly in your shoulder joint socket.

A rotator cuff injury is a painful strain or tear in the tendons and muscles surrounding your shoulder joint, often caused by falling, lifting and repetitive overhead arm activities, such as throwing a ball or placing items on a shelf above your head. If you're unable to use your arm or your pain is severe or persistent, see your doctor as soon as possible.

Some rotator cuff problems result from gradual deterioration over time and not an injury. The origin of your condition — an injury or slow deterioration — will determine how it's initially treated.

For a minor symptoms, resting your shoulder, applying ice and heat, and taking an over-the-counter pain reliever may be sufficient. After a day or two, do gentle exercises to keep your shoulder muscles limber. For more significant pain, your doctor may give you a corticosteroid injection in your shoulder joint to relieve pain and inflammation. In case of an injury that produces a large tear in your rotator cuff, you may need surgery to repair the tear.

In addition, you may need shoulder exercises. Your doctor or a physical therapist will give you specific exercises designed to help heal your injury, improve flexibility of your shoulder and provide balanced shoulder muscle strength. Physical therapy may last from three weeks to several months.

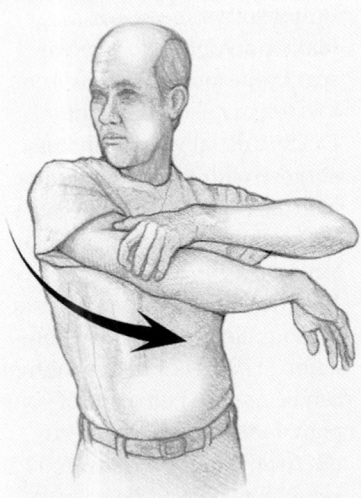

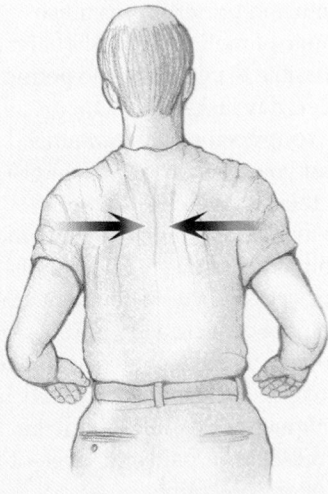

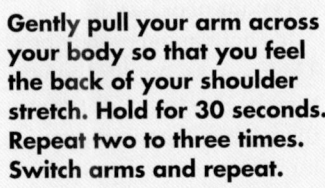

Gently pull your arm across your body so that you feel the back of your shoulder stretch. Hold for 30 seconds. Repeat two to three times. Switch arms and repeat.

With your arms bent forward at the elbows, pull your elbows back to squeeze your shoulder blades closer together. Hold for 10 seconds. Repeat three to five times.

Prevention

When your shoulder is sore from overuse or tendinitis, you may be able to avoid the freezing stage by regularly moving your shoulder through range-of-motion exercises.

Immunological Rheumatic Diseases

Immunological rheumatic diseases are sometimes called connective tissue diseases, or collagen vascular disorders. They result from alterations in your body's immune system. Common to all of them is inflammation of an unknown cause that can affect almost all tissues of the body.

Rheumatoid arthritis (see page 975) is an immunological rheumatic disease. There are several others.

Lupus

Signs and symptoms

- Fatigue
- Fever
- Joint pain, stiffness and swelling
- Butterfly-shaped rash on the face
- Sores inside the mouth or nose
- Weight loss or gain
- Skin lesions that appear or worsen with sun exposure

Lupus is a chronic disease in which an individual's immune system attacks healthy tissues, typically the joints. This causes inflammation, pain, stiffness and occasional redness in the joints. It may also produce a rash across the nose and cheeks. Both the joint discomfort and the rash tend to be episodic, with alternating periods of remission and flares.

Systemic lupus erythematosus, the most common form, affects the majority of individuals who have the disease. *Systemic* means that several body systems may be affected. The disease may also affect your kidneys, nervous system, lungs and heart. About half the people with systemic lupus erythematosus have major internal organ involvement. For the other half, skin and joints are primarily affected.

Four types of lupus exist:

- **Systemic lupus erythematosus.** This type can affect nearly any part of your body. Body systems most commonly involved include the skin, joints, lungs, kidneys and blood. When people talk about lupus, they're usually referring to systemic lupus erythematosus.
- **Discoid lupus erythematosus.** This type affects only the skin. People with discoid lupus, also called cutaneous lupus, experience a circular rash on the face, neck and scalp.
- **Drug-induced lupus erythematosus.** It occurs after you take certain prescription medications. Not everyone who takes these medications develops lupus. Drug-induced lupus affects a wide variety of body systems. Signs and symptoms usually go away when you stop taking the medication that caused your lupus.
- **Neonatal lupus.** This is a rare form of lupus that affects newborn babies. A mother with certain antibodies that are linked to autoimmune diseases can pass them to the developing fetus — even if the mother has no signs or symptoms of an autoimmune disease. A baby with neonatal lupus may experience a rash in the weeks following birth. Neonatal lupus may last about six months before disappearing.

Diagnosis

The American College of Rheumatology (ACR) has developed clinical and laboratory criteria to help physicians diagnose and classify lupus. If you have four of the 11 criteria at one time or individually over time, you probably have lupus. Your doctor may also consider the diagnosis of lupus even if you have fewer than four of these signs and symptoms.

The criteria identified by the ACR include:

- A face rash, which doctors call a malar rash, is butterfly-shaped and covers the bridge of the nose and spreads across the cheeks
- Scaly rash, called a discoid rash, which appears as raised, scaly patches
- Sun-related rash, which appears after exposure to sunlight
- Mouth sores, which are usually painless
- Joint pain and swelling that occurs in two or more joints
- Swelling of the linings around the lungs or the heart
- Kidney disease
- A neurological disorder, such as seizures or psychosis
- Low blood counts, such as a low red blood count, a low platelet count (thrombocytopenia), or a low white cell count (leukopenia)
- Positive antinuclear antibody tests, which indicate that you may have an autoimmune disease
- Other positive blood tests that may indicate an autoimmune disease, such as a positive double-stranded anti-DNA test, positive anti-Sm test, positive anti-phospholipid antibody test or false-positive syphilis test

How serious is lupus?

For many people with lupus, the disease doesn't cause serious problems. For others, it's a major illness that needs to be managed carefully to prevent or treat serious complications, especially kidney and heart disease, as well as complications of treatment. Typically, lupus is a lifelong ailment that comes and goes.

Treatment

The treatment of lupus depends on its severity and the forms it assumes.

Medication

Three types of drugs are commonly used to treat lupus when your signs and symptoms are mild or moderate. More-aggressive lupus may require more-aggressive drugs. When you receive a diagnosis of lupus, your doctor may discuss these drugs:

- **Nonsteroidal anti-inflammatory drugs.** Nonsteroidal anti-inflammatory drugs (NSAIDs), such as naproxen sodium (Aleve, others) and ibuprofen (Advil, Motrin IB, others), may be used to treat a variety of signs and symptoms associated with lupus. NSAIDs are available over-the-counter, or stronger versions can be prescribed by your doctor. Check with your doctor before taking over-the-counter NSAIDs because some have been associated with serious side effects in people with lupus. Side effects of NSAIDs include stomach bleeding and an increased risk of heart problems.
- **Antimalarial drugs.** Although there's no known relationship between lupus and malaria, these medications have proved useful in treating signs and symptoms of lupus. Antimalarials may also prevent flares of the disease. Hydroxychloroquine (Plaquenil) is the most commonly prescribed antimalarial. Side effects of antimalarial drugs include vision problems and muscle weakness.
- **Corticosteroids.** These drugs counter the inflammation of lupus, but they can have serious long-term side effects, including weight gain, easy bruising, thinning bones (osteoporosis), high blood pressure, diabetes and increased risk of infection. The risk of side effects increases with higher doses and longer term therapy. To help reduce these risks, your doctor will try to find the lowest dose that controls your symptoms and prescribe corticosteroids

for the shortest possible time. Taking the drug every other day also may help reduce side effects.

Corticosteroids are sometimes combined with another medication to help reduce the dose, and therefore the toxicity, of both drugs. Taking calcium and vitamin D supplements while using corticosteroids can reduce the risk of osteoporosis.

Life-threatening cases of lupus — those that involve kidney problems, inflammation in the blood vessels, and central nervous system problems, such as seizures — may require more-aggressive treatment.

In cases of more-severe disease, your doctor may prescribe the following medications:

- **High-dose corticosteroids.** High-dose corticosteroids can be taken orally or administered through a vein in your arm (intravenously). A high-dose regimen of corticosteroids may help control dangerous signs and symptoms quickly, but can also cause serious side effects, including infections, mood swings, high blood pressure and osteoporosis. To minimize side effects, your doctor will prescribe you the lowest dose needed to control your signs and symptoms and then reduce the dosage over time.
- **Immunosuppressants.** Drugs that suppress the immune system may be helpful in serious cases of lupus, but can cause serious side effects. Examples include azathioprine (Imuran, Azasan), mycophenolate (CellCept), leflunomide (Arava) and methotrexate (Trexall). Potential side effects may include an increased risk of infection, liver damage, decreased fertility and an increased risk of cancer. A newer medication, belimumab (Benlysta), also reduces lupus symptoms in some people. Side effects include nausea, diarrhea and fever.

Exercise

As with other conditions that affect muscles and joints, management of lupus includes daily activity to prevent muscle weakness and ease joint stiffness. You may not feel up to exercising during flares, but even then you should do gentle range-of-motion exercises such as stretching. A physical therapist can design an exercise program to suit your physical condition.

Other therapies

Your doctor may recommend that you wear sunscreen and that you limit exposure to the ultraviolet rays in sunlight and avoid tanning beds. Sunlight and ultraviolet light from the beds may help trigger the autoimmune flares of lupus. As with any chronic disease, sometimes the illness can lead to depression, which may require treatment.

Scleroderma

Signs and symptoms

- A thickening and tightening of the skin, especially on your arms, face or hands
- Change in skin color
- Puffy hands and feet, particularly in the morning
- Joint pain and stiffness
- Skin that appears shiny
- Numbness, pain or color changes in the fingers, toes, cheeks, nose or ears
- Swallowing and digestive problems
- Heart, lung or kidney problems
- Fatigue

Scleroderma, which means "hard skin," is a rare autoimmune disease that leads to an overproduction of the protein collagen. The condition causes thickening, hardening and tightness of the affected tissues. Affected skin takes on a shiny appearance. Another name for the disease is progressive systemic sclerosis.

There are several types of scleroderma. Those types that are limited and diffuse are defined by the amount of skin that's affected by the disease. Overlap syndromes refer to types that have features of both scleroderma and other connective tissue diseases, such as systemic lupus erythematosus, polymyositis and rheumatoid arthritis. Localized scleroderma includes morphea and linear scleroderma.

Raynaud's disease is a condition involving poor blood flow to the extremities and occurs more commonly in scleroderma than in any of the other connective tissue diseases.

Most people with scleroderma develop the disease in middle age, although it can occur in children and older adults. Women are about four times as likely as men to get scleroderma.

Diagnosis

Because the condition is rare and can resemble other immune system diseases, scleroderma can be difficult to diagnose.

A diagnosis typically is based on medical history, physical examination and certain laboratory tests. Your doctor may perform a biopsy, in which a tissue sample is removed for laboratory study. You may also have blood tests. People with scleroderma usually have elevated blood levels of certain antibodies produced by the immune system.

How serious is scleroderma?

Limited scleroderma may stop progressing on its own, although in rare instances the hands may be damaged permanently.

Diffuse scleroderma can severely affect internal organs and may result in high blood pressure, heart disease, lung impairments, kidney failure and intestinal tract problems that can lead to malnutrition. When there's severe internal organ involvement, the life expectancy may be shortened, especially if the heart or lungs are involved.

Treatment

There's no cure for scleroderma, but a number of medications may help to control it. Localized scleroderma may disappear or stop progressing without treatment. With systemic scleroderma, treatment generally involves medications to help control symptoms and attempt to halt progression of the disease.

Medication

Medications used to treat the disease include nonsteroidal anti-inflammatory drugs (NSAIDs) and low doses of corticosteroids to ease pain and reduce stiffness and inflammation. Your doctor may prescribe a blood vessel dilator if you have Raynaud's disease, high blood pressure medication to control high blood pressure, acid blockers or pantoprazole (Protonix) for heartburn or gastroesophageal reflux disease (GERD), and antibiotics for intestinal problems. Certain types of antihypertensive drugs called angiotensin-converting enzyme (ACE) inhibitors may have a protective effect on the kidneys. Drugs that suppress the immune system may help reduce some scleroderma symptoms.

Self-care

Exercise is an important part of treatment because it may limit stiffening of skin tissues and increase blood flow to the tissues. Your doctor may refer you to a physical or occupational therapist to help develop an exercise program.

If you smoke, quitting is important because nicotine causes blood vessels, including those in your skin, to constrict.

Using a paraffin bath — in which you dip your hands into warm, melted paraffin — can help maintain finger flexibility. Also be sure to wear mittens for protection when you're outside in cold temperatures or even when you reach into a freezer. Dress in layers for warmth. If you have heartburn, avoid eating three to four hours before bedtime.

Sjogren's syndrome

Signs and symptoms
- Dry eyes with a feeling of sandiness or grittiness
- Dry mouth

Vasculitis

Vasculitis is a general term used to describe an inflammation of the blood vessels, usually the arteries. The inflammation damages the wall of the blood vessel and may impair circulation to part of the body. Signs and symptoms of vasculitis depend on the part of the body that's affected. General symptoms may include fever, muscle weakness, loss of appetite and fatigue. If a particular organ is involved, such as the intestines, vasculitis may cause more-specific symptoms, such as abdominal pain.

Vasculitis is often associated with autoimmune disorders and is therefore treated by rheumatologists. A doctor may confirm a diagnosis of vasculitis by blood tests, an X-ray of blood vessels (angiography) or biopsy of an affected blood vessel, in which a tissue sample is removed for laboratory study.

Treatment of vasculitis depends on the type, location and severity of the problem. It often includes anti-inflammatory medications such as corticosteroids and immunosuppressant drugs.

Different types of vasculitis may include:

Polyarteritis

This serious disorder involves an inflammation of many arteries. Inflammation can result in obstruction of the vessels, reducing the supply of blood to the affected area. The skin, intestines, kidneys and heart are at greatest risk.

Typical symptoms include weight loss, fever, weakness and fatigue. If the intestines are involved, you may have abdominal pain and bloody diarrhea.

Middle-aged men are most likely to experience polyarteritis, although there's also a juvenile form of the illness. In the past, this disease often was fatal. Today, with proper treatment, many people with polyarteritis can lead normal lives.

Allergic granulomatous angiitis

Also called Churg-Strauss syndrome, this ailment may affect multiple organ systems, but it generally includes the lungs. People affected by this type of vasculitis often have asthma.

Hypersensitivity vasculitis

This form of vasculitis is the result of exposure to a drug or foreign substance. It usually involves the small blood vessels of the skin.

Giant cell arteritis

This disorder occurs almost exclusively in people older than age 50, and it affects women more often than men. Also called cranial, temporal or giant cell arteritis, it involves medium-sized arteries, especially those in the head. The condition is characterized by headache and a tender, thickened artery that can be felt at the side of the head. It's often associated with polymyalgia rheumatica.

Malaise, fatigue, loss of appetite, weight loss, fever and night sweats are common accompanying signs and symptoms. Occasionally, chewing fatigues the jaw and vision problems develop. Left untreated, it can lead to partial or total blindness.

- Fatigue
- Difficulty chewing or swallowing
- A dry nose, throat and lungs
- Muscle and joint pain

Sjogren's syndrome is an autoimmune disorder in which the immune system attacks glands that produce moisture. It causes dryness of moist mucous membranes, primarily in the eyes and mouth. Your eyes may feel as if foreign bodies have lodged in them, and you may have difficulty chewing or swallowing. It may cause vaginal dryness in women. It may also cause problems with other parts of the body, including muscles, joints, lungs, kidneys and stomach.

Sjogren's syndrome is most common in middle-aged women. The condition may develop alone or occur with other autoimmune diseases.

Diagnosis

Beyond reviewing your medical history, your doctor can use a variety of tests to diagnose Sjogren's syndrome:

- **Blood tests.** Your doctor may order blood tests to check your blood count and sedimentation rate and to check for autoantibodies, proteins formed when your immune system attacks your body's own cells. Checking your blood count lets your doctor know the proportion of the various types of blood cells in a given volume of your blood. Sedimentation rate refers to the speed at which the red blood cells settle to the bottom of a column of blood in a glass tube. Certain inflammatory conditions increase the sedimentation rate.
- **Eye tests.** Your doctor can measure the dryness of your eyes with a test called a Schirmer tear test. In this test, a small piece of filter paper is placed under your lower eyelid to measure your tears. In another version of the test, a cotton swab is used to stimulate the tear reflex in your nose.

An eye doctor (ophthalmologist) may also examine your eyes after placing a drop of liquid containing a dye in each eye. The dye stains areas of the corneas that have been damaged by dryness.
- **Imaging.** To check on the condition of your salivary glands, your doctor may order a special X-ray called a sialogram. It detects dye that's injected into your parotid glands, located behind your jaw and in front of your ears. The dye is injected through the opening of a small duct in your mouth. This procedure reveals the flow of saliva into your mouth.

Your doctor may also perform a parotid gland flow test to determine the amount of saliva that you produce over time. Another imaging test is a salivary scintigraphy, which measures your salivary gland function. Your doctor may also order a chest X-ray to check for lung inflammation.
- **Biopsy.** Your doctor may also want to do a lip biopsy to detect the presence of clusters of inflammatory cells, which can indicate Sjogren's syndrome. For this test, a small sliver of tissue is removed from salivary glands located in your lip and examined under a microscope.

- **Urine sample.** Your doctor may want you to provide a urine sample that can be analyzed in the laboratory to determine whether Sjogren's syndrome has affected your kidneys.

How serious is Sjogren's syndrome?

Sjogren's syndrome can seriously affect your quality of life, including your ability to work and to participate in day-to-day activities.

Treatment

Therapy is aimed at symptom relief. Besides taking medications, you may find it helpful to use skin moisturizers, drink plenty of fluids, use artificial saliva and get regular dental care, because reduced saliva can cause cavities.

Preservative-free artificial tears and eye ointments may help relieve the discomfort in your eyes. You can relieve your dry mouth by sucking on sugar-free lemon drops or other hard candies to stimulate the production of saliva and by sipping beverages, preferably water, throughout the day.

Medication

Your doctor will likely review the medications you're taking to be sure that they're not aggravating your dryness. He or she may

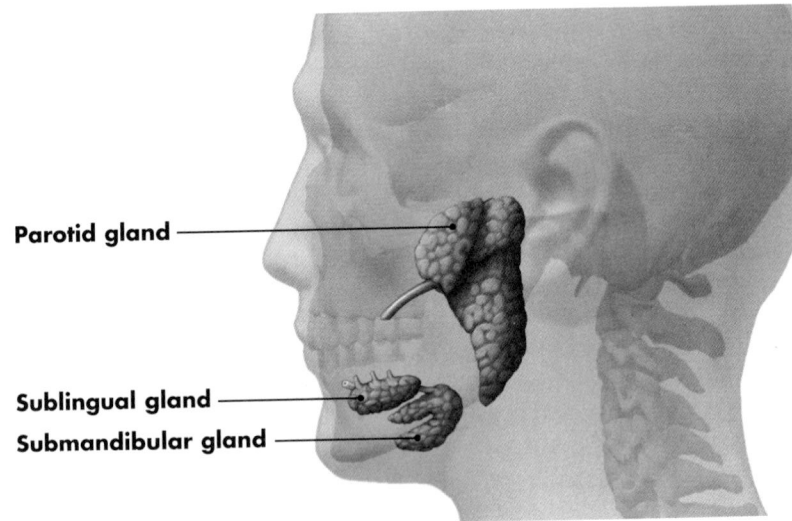

Parotid gland

Sublingual gland

Submandibular gland

The moisture-secreting glands of your mouth are among the first mucous membranes that Sjogren's syndrome attacks. The result is decreased production of saliva.

prescribe medications, such as pilocarpine (Salagen) or cevimeline (Evoxac) to stimulate the production of saliva. Cyclosporine (Restasis) may be prescribed to treat dry eyes associated with the condition.

Your doctor may also prescribe corticosteroids or immunosuppressant drugs if your case is severe and it involves kidney, lung or neurological problems. Hydroxychloroquine (Plaquenil), a drug designed to treat malaria, also may be helpful in treating some cases of Sjogren's syndrome.

Surgery

Another method to relieve dry eyes is to undergo a minor surgical procedure to seal the tear ducts that drain tears from your eyes (punctal occlusion). Collagen or silicone plugs are inserted into the ducts for a temporary closure. Collagen plugs eventually dissolve, but silicone plugs will keep ducts sealed until they fall out or are removed. Your doctor may use a laser to permanently seal your ducts.

Polymyalgia rheumatica

Signs and symptoms
- Pain and stiffness in the muscles, usually in the neck, shoulders and hips, particularly in the morning
- Fatigue
- Lack of appetite leading to weight loss
- Anemia
- A general feeling of illness
- Sometimes, a slight fever

The term *polymyalgia rheumatica* is from the Greek words that mean "pain in many muscles." Polymyalgia rheumatica typically causes pain and stiffness around the neck, shoulders and hips due to an inflammation of the joints and surrounding tissues. Most of the inflammation occurs in the hip and shoulder joints, but inflammation may occur elsewhere in the body, as well. Anemia often accompanies the disease.

Polymyalgia rheumatica usually affects adults older than age 50, and it affects women more often than men. The cause is unknown, but researchers suspect that genetic and environmental factors are involved.

Diagnosis
Information about the onset of your pain and recent changes in your health are important in making a diagnosis.

In polymyalgia rheumatica, the pain usually strikes suddenly. The discomfort is likely to be worse in the morning, but it may occur at night too. No specific tests can confirm the diagnosis, but X-ray or laboratory tests may be done to eliminate other possible causes.

With polymyalgia rheumatica, your erythrocyte sedimentation rate and C-reactive protein levels are usually elevated, indicating the presence of inflammation.

How serious is polymyalgia rheumatica?
The typical disease course is about one to two years, after which it usually disappears. However, the condition can recur.

Polymyalgia rheumatica may be associated with a disease called giant cell arteritis (temporal, or cranial, arteritis) that causes inflammation and tenderness in the arteries just under the scalp near the temples. If you have polymyalgia rheumatica and develop vision problems, scalp tenderness or headaches, call your doctor promptly.

Treatment
Medication and exercise may ease symptoms.

Medication
Corticosteroid medications often produce improvement within just a few days. You may have to take a corticosteroid until the disease runs its course. Because the medications can cause side effects, your doctor will want to give you the smallest dose possible to control the symptoms (see page 972). For a mild case, nonsteroidal anti-inflammatory drugs (NSAIDs) may provide adequate relief of symptoms without the need for corticosteroids.

Exercise
Exercise is essential to help maintain your energy and muscle strength. It can also help prevent weight gain, a possible side effect of taking corticosteroids. Your doctor may refer you to a physical therapist for suggestions on the types of exercises that will work best for you.

Polymyositis and dermatomyositis

Signs and symptoms
- Muscle weakness
- Pain and swelling in the small joints
- Reddish patches of skin on the face, knuckles, elbows, knees or ankles

Polymyositis is a disorder in which the muscles become inflamed, resulting in damage to muscle fibers. When a particular skin inflammation accompanies the muscle inflammation, the disorder is called dermatomyositis.

Adults between ages 30 and 60 are most likely to have these disorders, but they can occur at any age. Children between ages 5 and 15 may develop dermatomyositis. Women are about twice as likely as men to have polymyositis or dermatomyositis.

Diagnosis
Your doctor will likely take a medical history and perform a physical examination, focusing on your skin and testing your muscle strength. Your doctor may also order a series of blood tests to determine the presence of certain muscle enzymes. A test called electromyography can measure the electrical activity in your muscles. In addition, a biopsy, in which a tissue sample is removed

for laboratory study, may be conducted on affected muscles.

How serious are polymyositis and dermatomyositis?

Signs and symptoms of dermatomyositis and polymyositis may persist for many months or even years. A particular danger is the potential effect on the muscles of the throat, which can make swallowing difficult. Lung problems also may occur, including weakness of the muscles that help you breathe.

Treatment

The primary treatment of polymyositis and dermatomyositis is immunosuppressant medication. The corticosteroid prednisone is commonly used. Other medications that a doctor may prescribe include methotrexate (Trexall), azathioprine (Imuran, Azasan) or intravenous immunoglobulin.

Once the medication begins to take effect and the inflammation improves, your doctor may recommend an exercise program to prevent muscle wasting (atrophy) and stiffness. ■

Endocrine System

Your body's endocrine system consists of several glands that function as your body's control mechanism. Along with your nervous system, your endocrine glands coordinate how your body responds to usual and unusual events.

Endocrine glands produce hormones, the key component of the system. A hormone is a chemical messenger. Different endocrine glands secrete different types of hormones. Most of these are released into the bloodstream so that they can deliver instructions to various organs and tissues.

Although hormones circulate throughout the body, each hormone influences specific organs or tissues, so it regulates only certain body processes. The pancreas, for example, secretes the hormone insulin, which enables the body to regulate the amount of sugar in the bloodstream.

In response to physical or emotional stress, the adrenal glands secrete adrenaline (epinephrine), which can produce a sudden and remarkable burst of energy. Similarly, the pituitary, thyroid, parathyroid and sex glands each influence particular body func-

tions. Some hormones, including many produced by the pituitary gland, control the activity of other glands. Virtually every system in your body is directly or indirectly influenced by hormones.

Occasionally, the endocrine system malfunctions. Because the system is so complex, a malfunction can lead to a wide range of problems. For example, in diabetes, the most common endocrine disorder, if the pancreas doesn't secrete enough insulin too much sugar (glucose) stays in the blood. And if a child's pituitary gland malfunctions, he or she may experience growth problems.

A doctor whose special area of expertise is the endocrine system is called an endocrinologist. In the following pages, hormonal problems that endocrinologists commonly encounter are discussed.

Because hormones affect many tissues and organs throughout the body, an endocrinologist may also have expertise in areas that aren't commonly thought of as related to the endocrine system, such as bone development and blood pressure disorders.

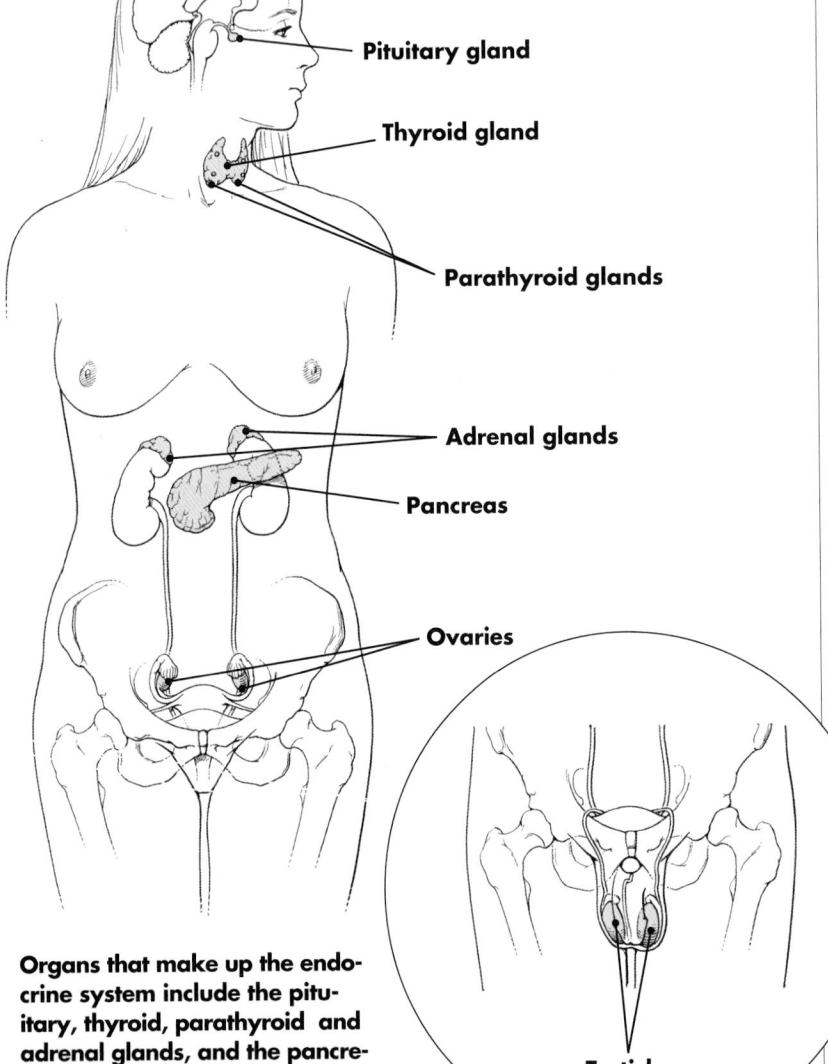

Pituitary gland

Thyroid gland

Parathyroid glands

Adrenal glands

Pancreas

Ovaries

Testicles

Organs that make up the endocrine system include the pituitary, thyroid, parathyroid and adrenal glands, and the pancreas. In women, the ovaries, and in men, the testicles, are part of the system (see inset).

Diabetes

The medical term for diabetes is *diabetes mellitus.* The origins of the term are Latin, referring to the sweetness, or honey (mellitus), that passes through to the urine as a result of the condition.

A less common form of diabetes is diabetes insipidus. It involves a different hormone that's secreted from the pituitary gland and influences the kidneys' conservation of water (see page 1015).

Diabetes mellitus, or diabetes, has become one of the most common chronic diseases in the United States, largely due to the aging of the American population and the increasing number of people who are overweight.

More than 29 million Americans, including more children and teenagers than ever before, have diabetes.

What is diabetes?

Diabetes refers to an excess amount of sugar (glucose) in your blood. The condition is often related to a malfunction of the pancreas.

Located behind your stomach, the pancreas is a long, thin organ roughly the length of your hand. It plays an important part in the digestive process, producing enzymes essential for breaking down (metabolizing) the food you eat.

The other key role of the pancreas might best be described as fuel control. The pancreas regulates your body's use of blood sugar, which provides energy for all of your cells, fueling your brain and other organs and tissues.

When your pancreas is functioning normally, the sugar concentration in your blood changes within a narrow, set range in response to a wide variety of factors, including meals, exercise, stressful situations and infections. But sometimes this precisely balanced system of control fails.

Instead of the majority of sugar being transported into your cells, significant amounts remain in your bloodstream. This excess sugar often is more than the kidneys can handle, and sugar may spill into the urine, where it can be detected by urinalysis.

Following an overnight fast, most people have blood sugar levels between 70 and 100 milligrams of glucose per deciliter of blood (mg/dL). This concentration range — equal to about 1 teaspoon of sugar in a gallon of water — is considered normal.

If your blood sugar is consistently 126 mg/dL or higher after fasting, you have diabetes. If your blood sugar measures between 101 and 125 mg/dL, you have impaired fasting glucose, which is commonly referred to as borderline diabetes or prediabetes.

Normal Metabolism

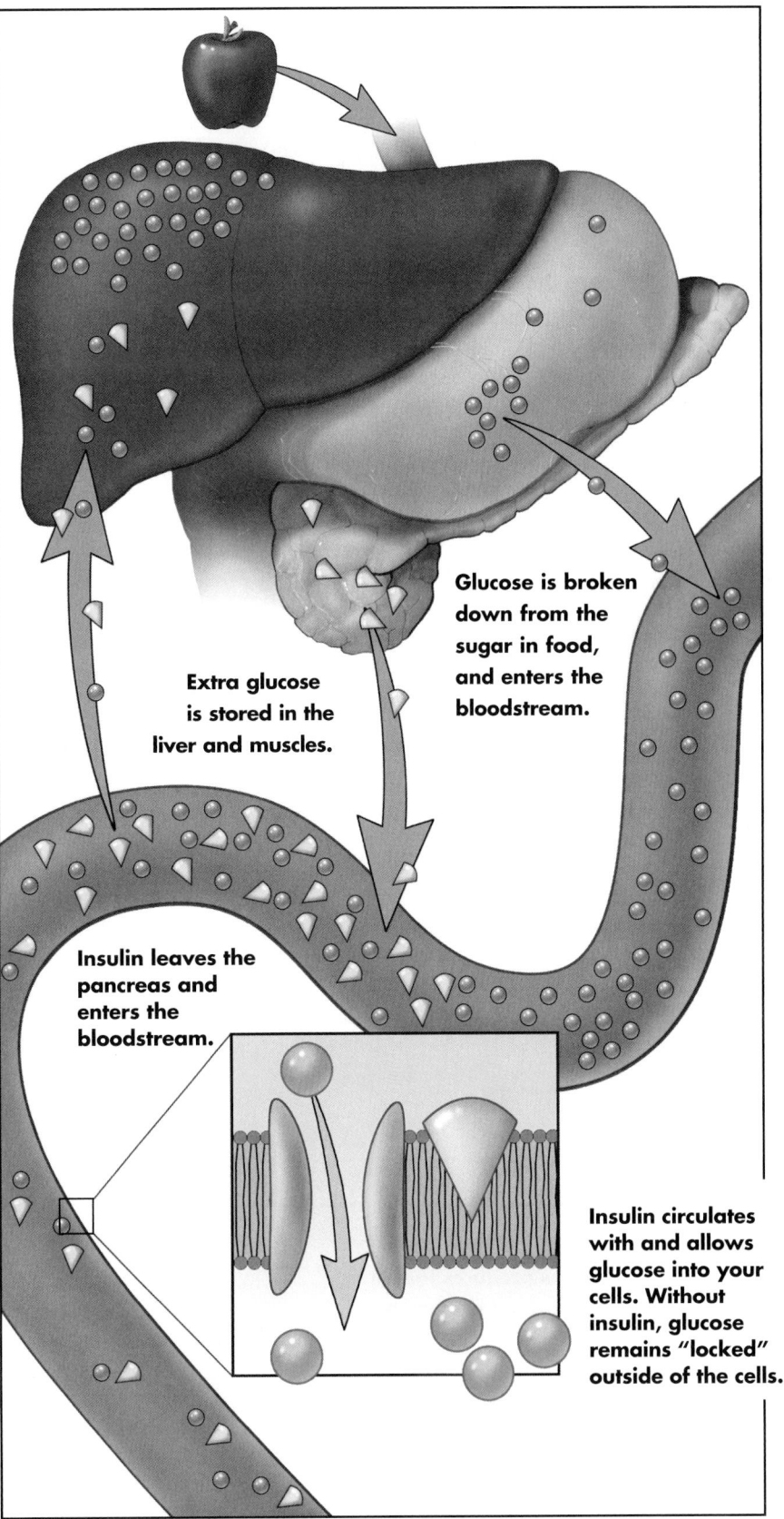

Glucose is broken down from the sugar in food, and enters the bloodstream.

Extra glucose is stored in the liver and muscles.

Insulin leaves the pancreas and enters the bloodstream.

Insulin circulates with and allows glucose into your cells. Without insulin, glucose remains "locked" outside of the cells.

Sugar (glucose) from the food you eat provides energy to fuel your body. Insulin, released from your pancreas, allows glucose to enter your cells, where it's needed for energy.

Type 1 and Type 2 Diabetes

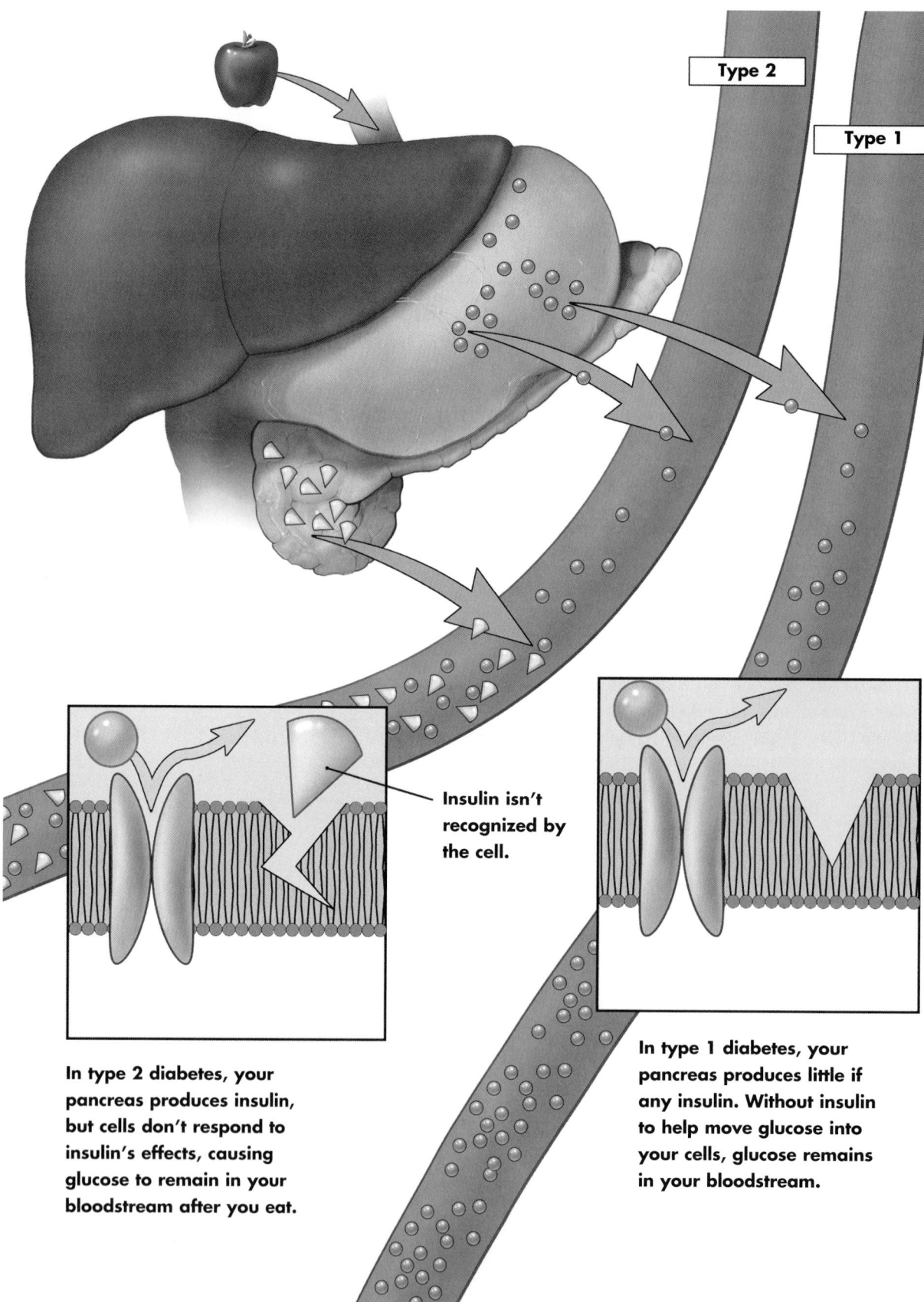

Type 2

Type 1

Insulin isn't recognized by the cell.

In type 2 diabetes, your pancreas produces insulin, but cells don't respond to insulin's effects, causing glucose to remain in your bloodstream after you eat.

In type 1 diabetes, your pancreas produces little if any insulin. Without insulin to help move glucose into your cells, glucose remains in your bloodstream.

Type 1 diabetes is a chronic condition in which your pancreas produces little or no insulin. Type 2 diabetes is a chronic condition that affects the way your body metabolizes blood sugar (glucose). Type 2 diabetes is, by far, the most common form of the disease.

Causes

Excess sugar may accumulate in your blood for a variety of reasons:

Insulin

Diabetes occurs when the pancreas is unable to produce enough of the hormone insulin or when body cells become less responsive (resistant) to insulin's effects.

Normally, when you eat, sugar is absorbed into your bloodstream from food particles in your small intestine. Cells that make up your muscles and organs rely on sugar for energy. But sugar can't enter the cells without the help of insulin.

At the same time sugar is entering your bloodstream, your pancreas is releasing insulin into your blood. The insulin circulates with the sugar and acts like a key, unlocking microscopic doors so that sugar can enter your cells. This lowers the amount of sugar in your blood. Without insulin, sugar remains in your blood and can't get into the cells where it's needed.

Liver

Your liver acts as a blood sugar storage and manufacturing center. When the level of insulin in your blood is high, such as after a meal, your liver stores extra sugar in case your cells need it later. When insulin levels are low, such as when you haven't eaten in a while, the pancreas releases a hormone called glucagon, which converts sugar stored in your liver (glycogen) into glucose and releases it into your bloodstream. This helps keep your blood sugar within a safe range.

Other hormones

In addition to insulin and glucagon, other hormones can affect your blood sugar level. In certain circumstances, hormones such as adrenaline (epinephrine) and cortisol counteract the effects of insulin, preventing sugar from entering your cells. The hormones may also encourage your liver to release its stored sugar, even if it's not needed.

Types

People often think of diabetes as one disease. But excess sugar can accumulate in your blood for various reasons, reflecting different types of diabetes.

Type 1

Type 1 diabetes develops when your pancreas makes little or no insulin. Without insulin circulating in your bloodstream, sugar can't get into your cells, so it remains in your blood.

Type 1 diabetes used to be called insulin-dependent or juvenile diabetes. *Insulin-dependent* means that you need to administer insulin medication daily to make up for the insulin that your body doesn't produce. The term *juvenile diabetes* was used because this form of diabetes most often develops in children and teenagers. Adults also can develop type 1 diabetes, although this is less common.

Type 1 diabetes is an autoimmune disease, meaning that your own immune system is the culprit. Similar to how it attacks invading viruses and bacteria, your body's infection-fighting system may attack your pancreas, zeroing in on the beta cells that produce insulin. Researchers aren't certain why this happens, but they believe that genetic factors, diet and exposure to certain viruses may be involved.

Between 5 and 10 percent of people with diabetes have type 1. Although the disease can smolder and remain undetected for several years, it usually comes on quickly, commonly following an illness.

Type 2

Type 2 diabetes is by far the most common form — 90 to 95 percent of adults with diabetes have type 2. Like type 1 diabetes, type 2 used to be called by a couple of other names: *non-insulin-dependent diabetes* and *adult-onset diabetes*. These names reflect that many people with type 2 diabetes don't need insulin shots and that the disease usually develops in adults. But as with type 1, the alternative names aren't entirely accurate.

Children and teenagers, as well as adults, can develop type 2 diabetes. In fact, the incidence of type 2 diabetes in young people is increasing. In addition, some people with type 2 diabetes need insulin to control their blood sugar.

Unlike type 1 diabetes, type 2 isn't an autoimmune disease. In type 2, your pancreas makes at least some insulin, but one or two other problems develop:
- Your pancreas doesn't make enough insulin.
- Your muscle and tissue cells become resistant to insulin.

When your cells develop a resistance to insulin, they refuse to accept it as the key that unlocks the door for sugar. As a result, sugar accumulates in your bloodstream. Exactly why the cells become insulin resistant is uncertain, although excess weight and fatty tissue seem to be important factors. Most people with type 2 diabetes are overweight.

It's unclear why excess weight is associated with an increased risk of type 2 diabetes. However, scientists have identified a protein, which they call resistin, that's produced by fat cells and appears to induce insulin resistance.

Some people with type 2 diabetes can control the disease by keeping their weight down, eating a healthy diet, exercising and, in some cases, taking medication.

Other people need more insulin than their pancreas can supply. Like people with type 1 diabetes, these individuals need insulin replacement medication to control their blood sugar.

Gestational

Gestational diabetes develops in pregnant women. This can happen temporarily when hormones secreted during pregnancy increase your body's resistance to insulin. About 2 to 5 percent of pregnant women develop

Are You at Risk?

Researchers don't fully understand why some people develop diabetes and others don't. However, they've identified a number of factors that increase your risk:

Impaired fasting glucose or impaired glucose tolerance

If blood sugar (glucose) testing shows that you have prediabetes or borderline diabetes, you're at high risk of developing diabetes.

A family history of diabetes

Your chance of developing either type 1 or type 2 diabetes increases if you have a parent, brother or sister with the disease.

Excess weight

Being overweight significantly increases your risk of getting diabetes. The majority of people with type 2 diabetes are overweight. The more fatty tissue you have, the more resistant your muscle and other tissue cells become to your own insulin, especially if your excess weight is concentrated around your abdomen.

Inactivity

The less active you are, the greater your risk of type 2 diabetes.

Age

Your risk of type 2 diabetes increases with age.

Race or ethnicity

Though it's not clear why, people of certain races or ethnic groups are more likely to develop type 2 diabetes than are others. You're at higher risk if you're Hispanic, black, Asian-American, American Indian or Pacific Islander.

In women, a history of gestational diabetes

More than half the women who experience gestational diabetes develop type 2 diabetes later in life. Women who give birth to at least one baby weighing 9 pounds or more also are at increased risk.

Polycystic ovary syndrome

Polycystic ovary syndrome (PCOS) is due to a common form of hormonal imbalance in women. It's associated with an increased risk of type 2 diabetes. Research suggests a link between PCOS and insulin. Many women with PCOS have high blood insulin levels and are less sensitive to the effects of insulin than other people are.

High blood pressure or abnormal blood fats

Because the underlying processes that put someone at risk of developing diabetes also increase the risk of high blood pressure and abnormal blood fat (lipid) levels, anyone affected by these should be screened for diabetes.

When your blood pressure is measured, it's written like a fraction. Your pressure is considered high if your systolic blood pressure (upper number) is consistently 130 millimeters of mercury (mm Hg) or higher or your diastolic blood pressure (lower number) is consistently 80 mm Hg or higher, or both. If you have diabetes, you want to keep your blood pressure below 120/80 mm Hg.

Your cholesterol and triglycerides levels are considered high, or poor, if your total cholesterol is 240 or above, your low-density lipoprotein (LDL, or "bad") cholesterol is 160 or above, your high-density lipoprotein (HDL, or "good") cholesterol is below 40, or your triglyceride level is 200 or higher. See page 701 for desirable numbers for people with diabetes.

gestational diabetes, typically during the second half of pregnancy.

Gestational diabetes often can be treated with diet alone and usually goes away after the baby is born. But more than half the women who experience gestational diabetes develop type 2 diabetes later. Type 1 diabetes also may begin during pregnancy, but this is less common.

Most pregnant women are screened for gestational diabetes to detect the condition early. If you develop this form of the disease, controlling your blood sugar level through the remainder of your pregnancy can reduce that risk of complications for you and your baby.

Other

Approximately 1 to 2 percent of the people with diabetes can trace the cause to illnesses or medications that interfere with the production of insulin or its action. These include:

- Inflammation of the pancreas (pancreatitis)
- Adrenal or pituitary gland disorders, such as acromegaly or Cushing disease
- Removal of the pancreas
- Corticosteroid medications
- Infection

Signs and symptoms

Often, diabetes develops gradually and causes few, if any, signs or symptoms. This is most common with type 2 diabetes. Other times, signs and symptoms can develop rather suddenly. These include:

- Increased thirst
- A frequent need to urinate
- Hunger
- A flu-like feeling, including weakness and fatigue
- Unexplained weight loss
- Blurred vision
- Irritability
- Slow healing of cuts and bruises
- Tingling or numbness in your hands or feet
- Red, swollen and tender gums
- Recurring infections of the gums, skin, vagina or bladder

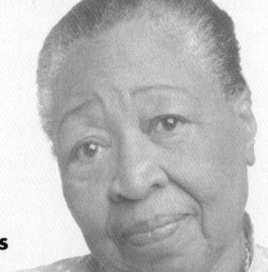

Two classic symptoms that most people with diabetes experience are increased thirst and a frequent need to urinate. When the level of sugar in your blood is high, the kidneys can't reabsorb all of the filtered sugar. The circulating sugar carries water with it, which is drawn from your tissues. As a result, you're dehydrated and feel thirsty.

To replenish the fluids being drawn out, you're almost constantly drinking water and other beverages. This water-intensive filtering process leads to more frequent urination.

Diagnosis

Often, people are shocked to learn they have diabetes because they didn't notice any symptoms. Many people with type 2 diabetes first learn they have diabetes when blood tests are done for another condition or as part of a routine physical exam. Type 1 diabetes tends to come on more suddenly, with noticeable signs and symptoms.

Sometimes, a doctor may test specifically for diabetes if he or she suspects, based on your symptoms and risk factors, that you have the disease. Individuals at high risk of developing diabetes should be tested beginning at age 30.

To determine if you have diabetes, your fasting blood sugar level will be measured. The amount of sugar in anyone's blood naturally fluctuates, but within a narrow range. Following an overnight fast, most people have blood sugar levels between 70 and 100 milligrams of glucose per deciliter of blood (mg/dL). This concentration range is considered normal.

Methods of measuring blood sugar include:

Fasting or random finger-prick screening
Finger-prick screening tests are fast, easy and inexpensive. Many health fairs offer them for free.

A drop of blood is collected from a tiny prick in your fingertip and placed on a chemically treated strip that's inserted into a small machine that displays your blood sugar level. If the result is 126 mg/dL or above, see your doctor for a more formal diagnostic test.

Random blood sugar test
A random blood sugar test is part of routine bloodwork done without prior fasting during a physical examination, when blood is drawn for a variety of laboratory tests. If the results are above 200 mg/dL, your doctor may want to do a fasting blood sugar test another day.

Fasting blood sugar test
Your blood sugar level typically is highest after a meal and lowest after an overnight fast. The preferred way to test your blood sugar is after you've fasted overnight, or for at least eight hours. A blood sample is taken and its glucose content is measured at a laboratory.

If your blood sugar measures 126 mg/dL or higher, your doctor may repeat the test. If your blood sugar is very high, a second test may not be necessary to reach a diagnosis. When a second test is ordered, if the results are again 126 mg/dL or higher, you'll likely receive a diagnosis of diabetes.

A reading of 100 to 125 mg/dL is considered prediabetes, which indicates a high risk of developing diabetes.

Glucose tolerance test
The glucose tolerance test is used less often because other tests are less expensive and easier to administer. A glucose tolerance test involves drinking about 8 ounces of a sweet liquid in the morning following an overnight fast. Your blood sugar is measured before you drink the liquid and every hour for a three-hour period afterward. If you have diabetes, this test will show your blood sugar rising higher than expected. Doctors sometimes use a modification of this test to check pregnant women for gestational diabetes.

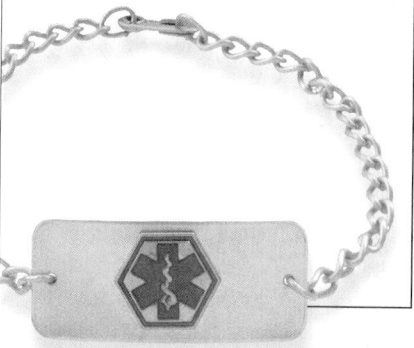

Complications of Diabetes

Excessive sugar (glucose) in your blood threatens many major organs, including your heart, nerves, eyes and kidneys. You might not feel the effects right away, but you may eventually if you don't take steps to manage and control your disease.

Researchers continue to make progress in understanding what triggers complications of diabetes and how to manage or prevent them. If you keep your blood sugar level close to normal, you can dramatically reduce your risk of complications.

Short-term complications

Diabetes can produce both short- and long-term complications. Short-term complications are medical emergencies requiring immediate attention. These include low blood sugar (hypoglycemia), high blood sugar (hyperglycemic hyperosmolar syndrome) and excessive blood acids (ketoacidosis).

Low blood sugar

Low blood sugar — generally a level below 60 milligrams of glucose per deciliter of blood (mg/dL) — results from too much insulin and too little sugar in your blood. Not enough glucose is available to enter individual cells, which become starved for energy.

Sometimes, overtreatment of diabetes with medication can cause low blood sugar (hypoglycemia). This is most common among people taking insulin. It can also occur in people taking oral medications that enhance the release or action of insulin.

Your blood sugar level can drop for many reasons. Some common reasons include skipping a meal, exercising longer or more vigorously than usual, or not adjusting your medication to accommodate changes in your blood sugar.

Signs and symptoms

Hypoglycemia symptoms vary from one person to another. Common early signs and symptoms include:

- Weakness
- Sweating, often a cold sweat
- Shakiness
- Mild confusion
- A fast heartbeat
- Dizziness
- Hunger
- Nausea
- A tingling sensation in your hands and feet

If your blood sugar continues to drop, a headache and difficulty walking may follow. In addition, you may behave unusually, appearing confused and sometimes stubborn or uncooperative.

As the condition worsens, you may seem intoxicated and feel drowsy and very confused. Your speech may be slurred. In extreme cases, unconsciousness and seizures may occur, particularly in children.

Treatment

Low blood sugar is a serious condition. But if it's recognized early, it can usually be treated easily.

When symptoms appear, stop all activity — stop the car, turn off the lawn mower, stop running — and eat or drink something that will quickly raise your blood sugar level. This might be hard candy (about five Life Savers), a regular (not sugar-free) soft drink, a half cup of fruit juice, or glucose tablets, nonprescription sugar pills made especially for treating low blood sugar. Glucose is also sold in squeeze tubes, allowing you to squirt the contents into your mouth.

Your blood sugar level should rise within 10 or 15 minutes. If the signs and symptoms continue after 15 minutes, repeat the treatment. If they still don't go away, contact your doctor.

If you lose consciousness or are unable to swallow, placing food in the mouth is no longer safe. Your blood sugar must be raised by injection. One option is injecting glucagon under your skin. Glucagon is a fast-acting hormone that stimulates the release of sugar into your blood. Friends and family members should know about this medication, including where you keep it and how to give you a shot.

Another option is administering glucose (in the form of dextrose) directly into the bloodstream. This requires emergency medical assistance.

If you ever find someone unconscious — whether or not they have diabetes — call for emergency medical assistance.

High blood sugar

Sometimes, blood sugar can reach such a high level that your cells can't absorb it all and sugar passes into your urine. This triggers a filtering process that draws tremendous amounts of fluid from your body and leads to dehydration.

Extremely high blood sugar (hyperglycemic hyperosmolar syndrome) is most common in people with type 2 diabetes, especially those who don't monitor their blood sugar or are unaware they have diabetes. It can also occur in people with diabetes who are taking high-dose steroids or drugs that increase urination.

Older people with type 2 diabetes who also have another illness and who don't drink enough water may develop a very high level of sugar in the blood. High blood sugar may be brought on by an infection, illness, stress or drinking excessive amounts of alcohol.

Signs and symptoms

- Excessive thirst
- Increased urination
- Dry mouth
- Blurred vision
- Fatigue
- Nausea
- Convulsions
- Loss of consciousness

Treatment

If your blood sugar level is persistently above 250 mg/dL, seek

Care of Your Feet

If you have diabetes, you're at increased risk of foot problems. When the network of nerves in your feet is damaged, you lose some of your ability to sense pain. You can cut your foot or develop a blister without realizing it.

Diabetes can also narrow your arteries, reducing blood flow to your feet. With less blood to nourish tissues, sores don't heal as well.

When you have diabetes, cuts, blisters, corns, calluses and other conditions that are nothing more than minor irritations to someone without diabetes can become serious medical problems. Infections and ulcers can result. In severe cases, amputation of the foot or leg may be required. Proper foot care can help you minimize this risk.

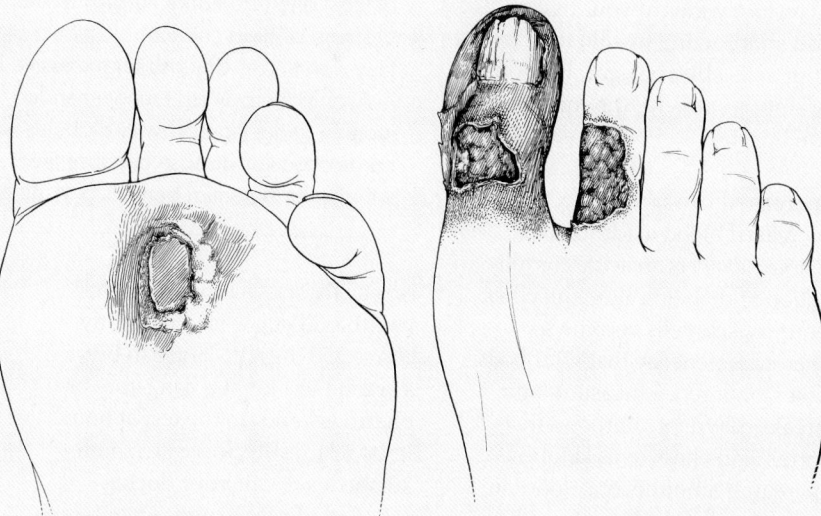

Over a period of years, diabetes can result in damage to nerves and blood vessels in your feet and other extremities. Minor wounds may lead to development of open sores (left). In some instances, the deterioration of blood vessels can severely limit blood flow, leading to gangrene (right).

Check your feet every day
Every day, examine your feet carefully, including the tops, bottoms, areas between the toes and toenails. Use a small mirror if you have difficulty seeing the bottoms of your feet.

Look for cuts and scrapes, cracks, calluses, bruises, corns, swelling, redness or other changes that may not be painful but could become more serious.

Keep your feet clean and dry
Wash your feet carefully every day, using lukewarm water and mild soap or a cleanser recommended by your doctor. To avoid burning your feet, test the water temperature with a thermometer — it should be no warmer than 90 F. Or test the water by touching a dampened washcloth to a sensitive area of your body, such as your face or wrist.

Dry your skin by blotting or patting it. Dry carefully between your toes to prevent fungal infection. Use a moisturizer regularly.

Wear clean, dry socks
Wear socks that pull (wick) sweat away from your skin. Avoid socks that are tight enough to reduce circulation or that cause your feet to sweat excessively.

Trim your toenails properly
Don't use scissors or rounded clippers on your toenails because they can cause injury to the nails and surrounding skin. Cut your toenails straight across and not too short. They should be even with the end of your toe. File rough edges so they won't cut the adjacent toe.

Use foot products cautiously
Don't use a file or scissors on calluses, corns or bunions, and don't use chemicals such as wart removers on your own. See your regular doctor or a podiatrist for treatment of warts, calluses and other problems.

Always wear shoes
Wear comfortable, safe shoes at all times to protect your feet from injury. Around the house, wear sturdy slippers. Avoid tight shoes. Run your hand around the inside of your shoes to remove debris that could irritate your feet.

Exercise carefully
Exercise increases circulation and helps maintain the health of your feet. In selecting your physical activities, however, consider the risk of injury to your feet and avoid extremes of hot and cold. When your feet or legs become tired, sit down and elevate them for a few minutes.

See your doctor if a problem develops
Consult your doctor promptly if you notice any areas of soreness or if a wound isn't healing, appears to be getting bigger or looks as if it may be infected. Your doctor should also inspect your feet at your regularly scheduled visits. He or she may recommend that you see a podiatrist, a doctor who specializes in foot care.

medical care immediately. You'll likely be given emergency treatment with intravenous (IV) fluids to restore water to your tissues and short-acting insulin to help your cells absorb sugar. Without prompt treatment, the condition can be fatal.

Increased blood acids

Increased blood acids (diabetic ketoacidosis) is an acute complication of diabetes. It occurs when your muscle cells become so starved for energy that your body takes emergency measures and breaks down fat, a process that forms acids known as ketones. Increased amounts of ketones in your blood make it more acidic.

Diabetic ketoacidosis is most common among people with type 1 diabetes and usually occurs because of insufficient insulin. This can happen when you miss or skip some of your insulin shots, are under extreme stress, or have an acute illness or injury.

Signs and symptoms

Some signs and symptoms of diabetic ketoacidosis can be confused with those of the flu. They include:

- Increased urination and an unquenchable thirst that develops over several hours, which occurs more quickly in a child
- Loss of appetite
- A sweet, fruity smell on your breath that may be confused with the smell of alcohol
- Nausea and vomiting
- Abdominal pain
- Weakness
- Drowsiness
- A flushed complexion
- Deep, rapid breathing
- Confusion

At an advanced stage, you may lose consciousness.

Treatment

Diabetic ketoacidosis demands immediate treatment because death can result. If you feel sick, check your urine for ketones. Also check for ketones if you're feeling

especially stressed or whenever your blood sugar is persistently above 250 mg/dL. You can buy a ketone test kit at a drugstore or pharmacy and do the test at home. If the test results indicate a high ketone level, call your doctor.

Ketoacidosis requires emergency medical treatment, which involves replenishing lost fluids through intravenous (IV) lines. Insulin can be combined with IV fluids.

Gradually, your blood sugar level is brought down to normal. Your blood sugar and fluid status are closely monitored. With prompt treatment, recovery is usually rapid and complete.

Long-term complications

Long-term (chronic) effects of diabetes develop slowly and generally with few early symptoms. Long-term complications involve damage to large and small blood vessels, resulting in a variety of health problems. Studies show that tight blood sugar control — keeping your blood sugar within a normal or near-normal range — can dramatically reduce your risk of long-term complications.

Nerve damage

Nerve damage (neuropathy) is a common long-term complication of diabetes. An intricate network of nerves runs throughout your body, connecting your brain to your muscles, skin and other organs. High blood sugar levels can damage these delicate nerves, affecting their ability to send messages.

Your feet and legs, and sometimes your hands and arms, might tingle, burn or feel numb, a condition called peripheral neuropathy. Over time you may lose all sense of feeling in the affected areas, leaving you more vulnerable to injury and infection.

Diabetes can also reduce blood flow to your feet. This, along with nerve damage, can lead to development of an open sore (ulcer) and possibly to gangrene. Practice good foot care to help avoid developing an infection.

Damage to nerves that control your muscles may leave you with an unsteady gait. Damage to nerves that control autonomic functions can increase your heart rate and perspiration. Such damage can also lead to problems with bladder control and diarrhea. In men it can lead to impotence.

An uncommon nerve-related problem is Charcot joint. In this condition, the small bones of the arch of your foot or ankle gradually disintegrate, and your feet become swollen, deformed and very flat. Although this condition causes little pain, it can be crippling.

Cardiovascular disease

Diabetes dramatically increases your risk of developing one of many cardiovascular problems, including chest pain (angina), a heart attack, stroke, high blood pressure and narrowing of your arteries (atherosclerosis).

Diabetes can damage your major arteries as well as your body's small blood vessels. The damage makes it easier for fatty deposits (plaques) to form in the arteries, a condition called atherosclerosis. Atherosclerosis that develops in blood vessels that supply oxygen and nutrients to the heart is called coronary artery disease.

Diabetes also increases pressure in your arteries and reduces blood circulation. High blood pressure can damage blood vessels, tissues and organs. People with diabetes are at risk of silent heart attacks, which don't cause typical symptoms.

You can reduce your risk of heart and blood vessel disease by not smoking, controlling high blood pressure, limiting fat and calories in your diet, getting more exercise, and losing weight if you're overweight.

Occasionally, people with diabetes get pain in their calves (claudication) while walking or climbing stairs. The pain eases when the activity is stopped. See your doctor if you experience such discomfort. It may be a sign of circulatory problems in the vessels that supply blood to your legs.

Kidney disease

Either type 1 or type 2 diabetes can impair your kidneys' ability to filter wastes. The longer you have diabetes, the greater your risk of kidney damage.

In its early stages, kidney disease produces few symptoms. A rise in blood pressure can be one of the first signs. Generally, signs and symptoms emerge only after extensive damage. These may include swelling of the ankles, feet and hands, shortness of breath, confusion or difficulty concentrating, poor appetite, nausea, fatigue, and itchy and dry skin.

Keeping your blood sugar levels and your blood pressure under control will help prevent or reduce kidney damage. Angiotensin-converting enzyme (ACE) inhibitors or angiotensin receptor blockers (ARBs) — medications used to treat cardiovascular problems — can help slow the progression of diabetic kidney damage.

Eye disease

Diabetic eye disease includes diabetic retinopathy (see page 620). Tiny blood vessels at the back of your eye (retina) can be damaged by high blood sugar, causing a range of effects, from mild vision problems to blindness.

Nearly everyone with type 1 diabetes and many people with type 2 diabetes develop some form of eye damage by the time they've had the disease for 20 years. If you have diabetes, you're also at increased risk of developing cataracts (see page 610) and glaucoma (see page 606).

Eye disease often produces no symptoms until it's well-advanced. For this reason, it's important to schedule yearly eye examinations with an eye specialist to identify and treat problems before permanent damage occurs.

Increased risk of infection

High blood sugar impairs the ability of your immune system cells to fight off invading germs and bacteria, putting you at higher risk of infection. High blood sugar can also damage nerves that might alert you to a potential infection. The mouth, gums, lungs, skin, feet, bladder and genital area are common infection sites.

A fever is common with many infections. Other signs and symptoms vary depending on the location of the infection. If your gums are infected, you may experience red, bleeding gums. A bladder infection typically causes frequent urination and a burning sensation while urinating. A vaginal infection commonly causes discharge and itching.

Self-care

If you have diabetes, you can do a great deal to remain healthy and reduce your risk of developing complications of the disease. In addition to keeping your blood sugar in control and seeing your doctor regularly to monitor your

diabetes, take the following self-care measures:

- Have a yearly physical in addition to your regular checkups to monitor your diabetes.
- Get a yearly eye exam.
- See your dentist regularly.
- Keep up to date on your vaccinations, especially those for the flu (influenza) and pneumonia.
- If you're a smoker, quit. Smoking is especially hazardous for people with diabetes and significantly adds to their risk of heart disease and strokes.
- Take proper care of your feet (see page 1001).
- Monitor your blood pressure and take steps to control high blood pressure through diet, exercise and medications, if needed.
- Manage stress. Stress and depression can make it more difficult to take care of yourself and your diabetes. Excessive or prolonged stress may also increase production of hormones that block the effects of insulin, causing your blood sugar to rise. Stress relaxation techniques or counseling may be helpful.

Treating Diabetes

When it comes to managing diabetes, a number of health care professionals may be involved in your care, but your role is crucial.

The single most important thing that you can do to feel your best and prevent complications is to control your blood sugar level on a daily basis. Only you can do that. The keys to managing diabetes are:

- Monitoring your blood sugar
- Eating a healthy diet
- Staying active
- Maintaining a healthy weight
- Using medications appropriately, as prescribed
- Getting regular checkups
- Adjusting your medications as instructed by your doctor

Blood sugar monitoring

Careful monitoring is the only way to make sure that your blood sugar level remains within your target range. Depending on your treatment plan, you may check and record your blood sugar as often as several times a week to as many as four to eight times a day.

Testing your blood sugar is a quick and easy process that usually takes only a couple of minutes. The tools include:

- **A lancet.** A small needle is used to prick the skin on a finger to draw a drop of blood. Spring-loaded lancets generally are less painful.
- **A test strip.** A drop of blood is placed on a chemically treated strip that's inserted into a blood glucose monitor.
- **A blood glucose monitor.** This is a small device that measures and displays glucose levels. Monitors come in many forms.

After your blood test, record the results in a logbook. Note the date and time of testing, test results, type and dosage of medication you're taking, any episodes of low blood sugar, and any circumstances that may have affected the levels, such as unusual stress or excitement, illness, travel, or an especially large meal. This information can help you and your doctor track how various factors affect your blood sugar.

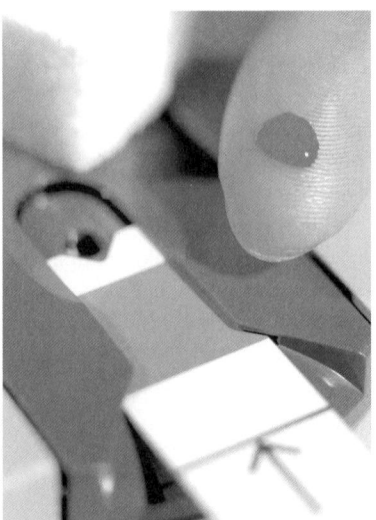

People who take insulin also may choose to monitor their blood sugar levels with a continuous glucose monitor (CGM). Although this technology doesn't yet replace the glucose meter, it can provide important information about trends in blood sugar levels.

A continuous glucose monitor uses a sensor to measure blood sugar levels in fluid under the skin. CGM readings are transmitted to a small recording device worn on your body or a compatible insulin pump. An alarm can sound if your blood sugar readings are too high or too low.

In addition to daily blood sugar monitoring, your doctor may recommend regular glycated hemoglobin (A1C) testing to measure your average blood sugar level for the past two to three months. Compared with repeated daily blood sugar tests, A1C testing better indicates how well your diabetes treatment plan is working overall. An elevated A1C level may signal the need for a change in your insulin regimen or meal plan.

Your target A1C goal may vary depending on your age and various other factors. However, for most people with diabetes, the American Diabetes Association recommends an A1C of below 7 percent. Ask your doctor what your A1C target is.

Diet

Healthy eating is a key part of managing diabetes. However, that doesn't mean that you have to buy specialized foods or follow a highly detailed and boring diet plan. For most people with diabetes, a healthy diet simply translates into variety and moderation. That means eating more of certain foods, such as fruits, vegetables and grains, which are high in nutrients and low in fat and calories — and less of others, such as animal products and sweets. It's the same eating plan recommended for all Americans.

Healthy-eating basics
Depending on your blood sugar level, whether you need to lose weight and if you have other health problems, you may need to tailor your diet to your own personal needs. But even though the details may differ, the basics remain the same. Each day you want the right balance of carbohydrates, protein and fat.

- **Carbohydrates.** They include starches (bread, cereal, rice, pasta, beans and certain vegetables, such as corn, potatoes and squash), fruits, milk products and nonstarchy vegetables. Consume about half your daily calories from carbohydrates.
- **Protein.** Foods high in protein include meat, poultry, eggs, cheese, fish, legumes and peanut butter. Most people should consume 10

Carbohydrates: Sugar and Starch

Carbohydrates are classified as either simple carbohydrates (sugar) or complex carbohydrates (starch). During digestion, your body breaks down complex carbohydrates into simple sugars. Sweets, milk, fruit and some vegetables contain simple sugars. Grain products and certain vegetables contain complex carbohydrates.

It's best to eat a mixture of complex and simple carbohydrates. The advantage of complex carbohydrates is that it takes your body longer to break them down into sugar. This means that sugar enters your bloodstream at a steadier rate. Include in your carbohydrate mix foods that are high in fiber. The more fiber a food contains, the more slowly it's digested and the more slowly your blood sugar (glucose) level rises.

For years, people with diabetes were told to avoid candy, cookies and other sugary foods because it was assumed that they would raise blood sugar faster and higher than complex carbohydrates. But studies have shown this isn't true. All carbohydrates, including table sugar, affect blood glucose about the same way. Sweets don't produce an exaggerated rise in blood sugar, provided they're eaten with your meal and counted as a carbohydrate source.

The most important thing about carbohydrates is not so much what type you eat but how much. If you eat more carbohydrates than usual, you may not have enough insulin available to transport the excess sugar into your cells, causing an increase in your blood sugar level. One way you can help control your blood sugar is by eating the same amount of carbohydrates at similar times each day.

Although sugar isn't forbidden, it's still best to limit sweets. Candy, soda pop, cookies and other sugary foods have little nutritional value. They're empty calories that can easily lead to weight gain.

to 20 percent of their daily calories from protein, or about two to three servings a day.

Select proteins that are lower in fat, such as plant products, fish, poultry without skin, lean meats, and low-fat or fat-free cheese. Limit or avoid fatty meats, eggs and high-fat cheeses.

- **Fats.** Fats are found in meat, poultry, fish, cheese, butter, margarine, oils, salad dressing, whole milk, and many desserts and snack foods. Limit total fat consumption to 25 to 35 percent of your daily calories and saturated fat to less than 10 percent of your daily calories. Saturated fat, which is found in animal products such as meat, cream and butter, raises blood cholesterol, and high blood cholesterol is a risk factor for heart disease.

Planning meals

Establish a routine of eating meals and snacks at regular times every day. Some people can keep their blood sugar in good control simply by eating three regular meals a day and avoiding too many sweets. Others need to follow a more deliberate plan, eating only the recommended number of servings from each food group, based on their individual calorie needs.

You may find it helpful to talk with a registered dietitian who can provide you with a variety of tools to help you establish an eating plan that fits your health goals and concerns, food tastes, family or cultural traditions, and lifestyle.

Aim for consistency in your eating habits. Every day try to eat about the same amount at the same time, with the same proportion of carbohydrates, protein and fats. This can help keep your blood sugar at a consistent level.

Some people use tools such as exchange lists or carbohydrate counting. Exchange lists are part of a system of grouping foods by food group and serving size. Carbohydrate counting is a way to calculate meal-related insulin doses based on the carbohydrate content of meals. Talk to a doctor or dietitian if you're interested in learning about these tools.

Physical activity

Regular physical activity is another key element in treating diabetes. Physical activity brings with it a bounty of health benefits. Even a moderate amount of exercise can improve control of diabetes.

Improves blood sugar control

As muscles contract and relax during exercise, they use sugar for energy. To meet this energy need, sugar is removed from your blood during and after exercise, lowering your blood sugar level. Exercise also reduces blood sugar by increasing your sensitivity to insulin: Your body requires less insulin to escort sugar into your cells.

Exercising on a daily basis can reduce your need for medication to lower your blood sugar level. Some people manage their diabetes through just diet and exercise.

Reduces risk of heart disease

Exercise is good for your heart and blood vessels. It improves blood flow through small blood vessels and increases your heart's pumping efficiency. In combination with a healthy diet, exercise helps lower high blood pressure and improve blood cholesterol levels.

Controls your weight

Physical activity helps you lose weight and maintain a healthy weight. Regular exercise takes off pounds by burning calories and increasing your metabolism.

Exercise can also reduce resistance to insulin that commonly occurs from being overweight.

Because physical activity usually lowers your blood sugar level, you want to be alert to signs and symptoms of low blood sugar (see page 1000) when exercising. If you're going to be active for a long period, especially if you take insulin, take a break and check your blood sugar while you're exercising.

Weight control

Being overweight is by far the greatest risk factor for type 2 diabetes — about 90 percent of people with newly diagnosed type 2 diabetes are overweight. By contrast, most people with type 1 diabetes are at or below their ideal weight.

Why is weight so important? Fat alters how your cells respond to insulin. It causes cells to become more resistant to insulin's effects, reducing the amount of sugar the hormone is able to transport from your blood to your cells.

You can reverse this process by losing weight. As you take off pounds, your cells become more responsive to insulin. For some people with type 2 diabetes, losing weight is all that's necessary to control their diabetes and return their blood sugar to normal.

The amount of weight loss doesn't have to be extreme to result in health benefits. A modest loss of 10 to 20 pounds, or 5 to 10 percent of your weight, can lower your blood sugar level, as well as reduce your blood pressure and blood cholesterol levels.

To learn about weight management strategies, see Chapter 8, "Nutrition and Weight."

With type 2 diabetes, the natural history of the disease is that it becomes more difficult to manage over time. When diet and exercise are no longer effective, the next step is generally noninsulin medications, followed by insulin. This progression may occur even if you follow lifestyle recommendations. It doesn't mean you failed in your efforts to manage the disease.

Medication

Depending on the type and severity of your diabetes, your doctor may prescribe medication. All people with type 1 diabetes need to take insulin. Most people with type 2 diabetes eventually need to take a medication — either an oral medication or insulin or other injectable drugs.

Insulin
Insulin is administered by injection with a syringe or with an in-

Exercise and Diabetes

To avoid problems with low or high blood sugar during or after physical activity, especially if you take insulin, follow these guidelines:
- Check your blood sugar approximately 30 minutes before you exercise and then again right before you start. This will help you determine if your blood sugar level is stable, rising or dropping. If your blood sugar level is under 100 milligrams per deciliter (mg/dL), eat a carbohydrate-containing snack to avoid having low blood sugar while you exercise. If your blood sugar level is more than 300 mg/dL, don't exercise. Exercise may raise your blood sugar further.
- If you have type 1 diabetes and your blood sugar level before exercising is 250 mg/dL or higher, test your urine for ketones (see page 1002). If the result indicates a moderate or high ketone level, don't exercise.
- Check your blood sugar during and after exercise. This is especially important when trying a new activity or sport or if you're increasing the intensity or duration of your activity. If you exercise for more than an hour, especially if you have type 1 diabetes, stop and test your blood sugar every 30 minutes. If it starts to fall, have a snack. Until you have a good idea of how your body reacts to exercise, check your blood sugar frequently after your activity. Hypoglycemia can occur hours after exercise.
- If you start to experience signs and symptoms of low blood sugar while exercising, stop immediately and — if possible — test your blood sugar. If your test is low, eat something with sugar. Treat yourself for low blood sugar even if you don't have your testing equipment with you.
- If you take insulin, adjust your dose for planned exercise. Avoid exercise within three hours after injecting short-acting insulin due to the potential risk of low blood sugar. Ask your doctor when would be the best time to exercise and follow the basic precautions.
- People with type 1 diabetes who exercise for more than an hour or do strenuous activities may benefit from eating a snack before or while exercising. For most people with type 2 diabetes, a snack before exercise generally isn't necessary.

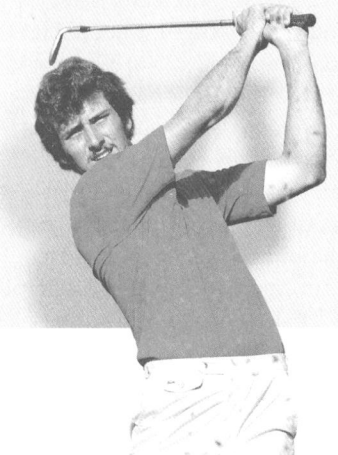

sulin pen, a device that looks like a large ink pen. Another form of administration is through constant infusion with an insulin pump.

Insulin isn't available in pill form because its chemical structure is destroyed during digestion, making the hormone ineffective by the time it gets to your bloodstream. An inhaled form of insulin was developed a few years ago but was removed from the market due to poor acceptance.

Many types of insulin are available. They differ in the time it takes for them to begin working and in their duration. Short-acting insulin works quickly but only for a short time. Intermediate-acting insulin starts working later but lasts longer. Long-acting insulin keeps a steady level of insulin in blood, without peaks and valleys, for 12 to 24 hours.

The type and dose of insulin you take depend on your specific needs. Some people take more than one type of insulin. For example, some people mix short-acting and intermediate-acting insulin. Your doctor may prescribe a mixture of insulin types to use throughout the day and night.

For many people, the best blood sugar control is achieved by taking a daily dose of long-acting insulin along with an injection of short-acting insulin before each meal. Your doctor will help you decide which approach best suits your needs.

Injections
You can use a fine needle and syringe or an insulin pen to inject insulin under your skin. Insulin pens look similar to ink pens, and are available in disposable or refillable varieties. Needles are available in a variety of sizes, so you can find one that's most comfortable for you.

If you choose injections, you'll likely need a mixture of insulin types. Multiple daily injections that include a combination of a long-acting insulin, such as Lantus or Levemir, combined with a rapid-acting insulin, such as Apidra, or Novolog, more closely mimic the body's normal use of insulin than older regimens that only required one or two shots a day. Three or more insulin injections a day has been shown to improve blood sugar levels.

Insulin pump
This device is about the size of a cellphone and is worn on the outside of your body. A tube connects a reservoir of insulin to a catheter that's inserted under the skin of your abdomen. The pump can be worn in a variety of ways: on your waistband, in your pocket, with specially designed pump belts.

There's also a wireless pump option. You wear a pod that houses the insulin reservoir on your body that has a tiny catheter that's inserted under your skin. The insulin pod can be worn on your abdomen, lower back, or on a

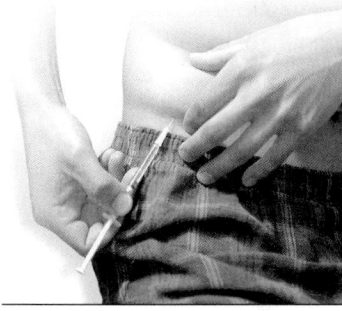

leg or an arm. The programming is done with a wireless device that communicates with the pod.

Pumps are programmed to dispense specific amounts of rapid-acting insulin automatically. This steady dose of insulin is known as your basal rate. It replaces your long-acting insulin.

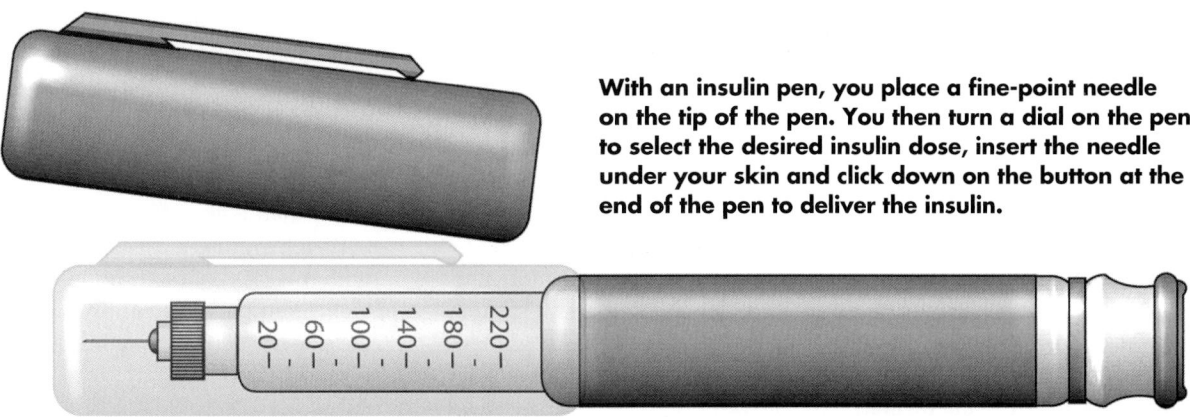

With an insulin pen, you place a fine-point needle on the tip of the pen. You then turn a dial on the pen to select the desired insulin dose, insert the needle under your skin and click down on the button at the end of the pen to deliver the insulin.

When you eat, you program the pump with the amount of carbohydrates you're eating and your current blood sugar, and it will give you what's called a "bolus" dose of insulin to cover your meal and to correct your blood sugar if it's elevated. In some people an insulin pump may be more effective at controlling blood sugar levels than injections. Many people achieve good blood sugar levels with injections, too.

Artificial pancreas

An emerging treatment approach is known as closed-loop insulin delivery. It's also called the artificial pancreas. It links a continuous glucose monitor to an insulin pump. The device automatically delivers the correct amount of insulin when the monitor indicates the need for it. There are a number of different versions of the artificial pancreas, and clinical trials have had encouraging results.

The first step toward an artificial pancreas was approved in 2013. Combining a continuous glucose monitor with an insulin pump, this system stops insulin delivery when blood sugar levels drop too low. Studies found that it could prevent low blood sugar levels overnight without significantly increasing morning blood sugar levels.

Oral medications

In addition to insulin, a variety of oral medications are used to treat type 2 diabetes. Each has its own method for lowering blood sugar.

To effectively control your blood sugar, you may need a combination of more than one oral medication or an oral medication plus insulin. Your doctor can determine if you need medication and which type. Let your doctor know if you're taking other medications or using alcohol while taking diabetes drugs so that he or she can alert you to possible drug interactions.

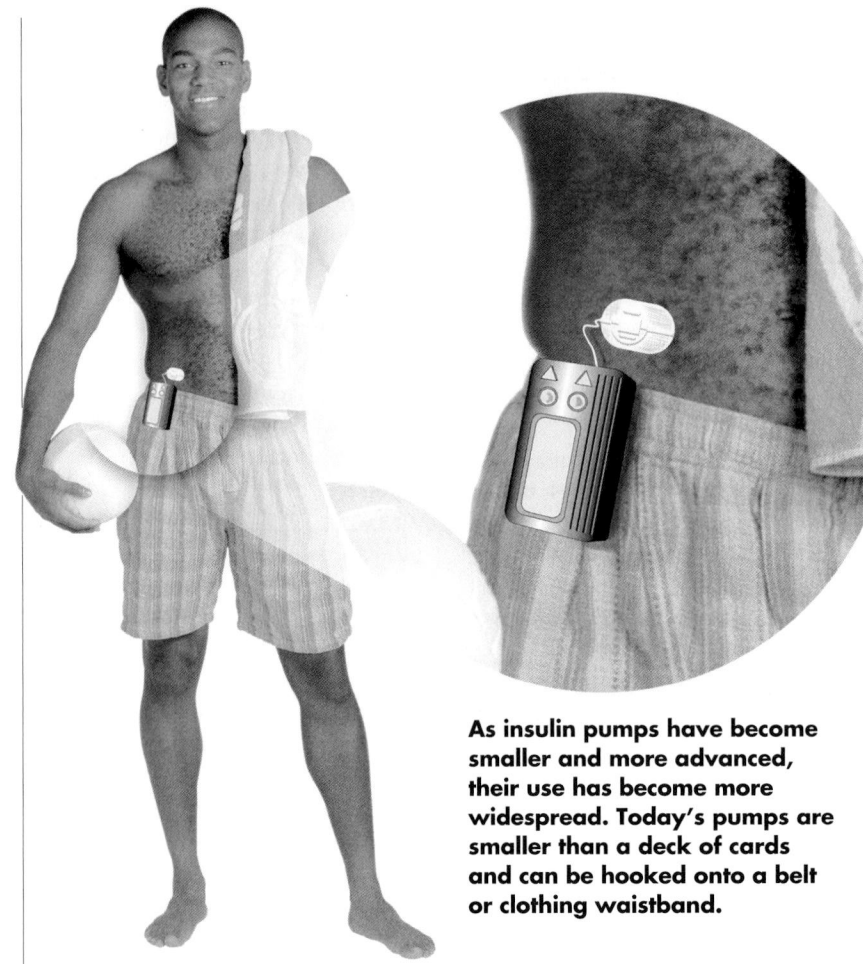

As insulin pumps have become smaller and more advanced, their use has become more widespread. Today's pumps are smaller than a deck of cards and can be hooked onto a belt or clothing waistband.

Metformin

Generally, metformin (Glucophage, Glumetza, others) is the first medication prescribed for type 2 diabetes. It works by improving the sensitivity of your body tissues to insulin so that your body uses insulin more effectively.

Metformin also lowers glucose production in the liver. Metformin may not lower blood sugar enough on its own. Your doctor will also recommend lifestyle changes, such as losing weight and becoming more active.

Nausea and diarrhea are possible side effects of metformin. These side effects usually go away as your body gets used to the medicine. If metformin and lifestyles changes aren't enough to control your blood sugar level, other oral or injected medications can be added.

Sulfonylureas

These medications help your body secrete more insulin. Examples of medications in this class include glyburide (DiaBeta, Glynase), glipizide (Glucotrol) and glimepiride (Amaryl). Possible side effects include low blood sugar and weight gain.

Meglitinides

Like sulfonylureas, meglitinides stimulate the pancreas to secrete more insulin, but they're faster acting, and the duration of their effect in the body is shorter. Meglitinides do carry a risk of causing low blood sugar, but this risk is lower than with sulfonylureas.

Weight gain is a possibility with this class of medications as well. Examples of meglitinides include the drugs repaglinide (Prandin) and nateglinide (Starlix).

DPP-4 inhibitors

These medications help reduce blood sugar levels, but tend to have a modest effect. They don't cause weight gain. Examples of these medications are sitagliptin (Januvia), saxagliptin (Onglyza) and linagliptin (Tradjenta).

Thiazolidinediones

Like metformin, these medications make the body's tissues more sensitive to insulin. This class of medications (also called glitazones) has been linked to weight gain and other side effects, such as an increased risk of heart failure and fractures. Because of these risks, these medications generally aren't a first-choice treatment.

SGLT2 inhibitors

The newest diabetes drugs on the market, they work by preventing the kidneys from reabsorbing sugar into the blood. Instead, the sugar is excreted in the urine.

Examples include canagliflozin (Invokana) and dapagliflozin (Farxiga). Side effects may include yeast infections and urinary tract infections, increased urination, and hypotension.

Alpha-glucosidase inhibitors

Alpha-glucosidase inhibitors delay digestion of carbohydrates, slowing the rise in blood sugar after eating. These drugs are taken with each meal and may be prescribed if your blood sugar reaches its highest levels right after eating. Alpha-glucosidase inhibitors include the medications acarbose (Precose) and miglitol (Glyset).

Possible side effects include abdominal bloating or discomfort, gas, and diarrhea. When taken with another diabetes medication, the risk of low blood sugar is increased. People with certain medical conditions — including irritable bowel syndrome, ulcerative colitis and Crohn's disease — or a chronic malabsorption disorder such as celiac disease shouldn't take these drugs.

Transplantation

Medication and lifestyle changes can effectively control diabetes, but a common question remains: What about a cure?

Presently, there is no cure for diabetes. Researchers continue to explore therapies that they hope will one day bring about a cure. One area of study is transplantation. Since the late 1970s, doctors have performed pancreas transplants to halt or reverse complications of diabetes, and the procedure has met with some success. Researchers are also experimenting with transplanting islet cells — the cells in the pancreas that produce insulin.

Pancreas transplantation

Pancreas transplants are often done in conjunction with or following a kidney transplant. Kidney failure is one of the most common complications of diabetes. A kidney transplant can restore a number of crucial functions. Receiving a new pancreas at the same time doesn't jeopardize — and may actually improve — kidney survival. Unlike kidney transplants, in which a living person donates a kidney, a pancreas used for transplantation usually comes from a person who has just died.

After a successful pancreas transplant, many people with diabetes no longer need insulin or to measure their blood sugar as frequently.

However, transplantation isn't always successful. In addition to the risks inherent in any major surgery, the body can reject the new organ days or years after the transplant. Transplant recipients generally need to take immunosuppressant medications for the rest of their lives to prevent organ rejection. Such medications carry significant health risks.

Islet cell transplantation

A human pancreas contains about 1 million islets, which make up about 2 percent of the gland. Beta cells within these small islets produce insulin. In people with type 1 diabetes, their immune system has attacked and destroyed their islet cells, so their pancreas is unable to produce insulin.

Researchers are studying the possibility of transplanting islet cells and potential long-term complications. Several institutions may offer islet cell transplantation to select patients in a few years. Presently, the procedure is still considered experimental.

Noninsulin injectable medications

Medications called glucagon-like peptide-1 (GLP-1) receptor agonists slow digestion and help lower blood sugar levels. Their use is often associated with some weight loss. This class of medications isn't recommended for use by itself.

Exenatide (Byetta, Bydureon), liraglutide (Victoza), albiglutide (Tanzeum) are examples of GLP-1 receptor agonists. Possible side effects include nausea and an increased risk of pancreatitis.

The drug pramlintide (Symlin) is a man-made version of a hormone called amylin, which your pancreas makes along with insulin when your blood sugar levels rise. An injection of this medication before you eat can slow the movement of food through your stomach to curb the sharp increase in blood sugar that occurs after meals. This medication may be used in the treatment of both type 1 and type 2 diabetes.

Regular checkups

Another important part of diabetes treatment is staying in regular contact with your health care team and making sure that you receive appropriate tests to evaluate how well you're controlling your blood sugar. Regular checkups give your doctor an opportunity to look for early evidence of diabetes complications. Checkups also give you a chance to review with your doctor your successes and difficulties in meeting your blood sugar goals.

How often you see your doctor or a member of your care team depends on your health. In general, if you're feeling good and keeping your blood sugar within your target range, you probably only need a checkup once every three to six months.

If you're having trouble keeping your blood sugar levels in the target range or you're changing medication, you may need to see your doctor more often.

During a checkup, you may have one or more of these tests:

Glycated hemoglobin test

A glycated hemoglobin test measures hemoglobin A1C, which indicates how well you've controlled your blood sugar over the past two to three months. It can alert you to potential problems. If you take insulin, you'll probably have this test three or four times a year. If you have type 2 diabetes and your blood sugar is in good control, you may not need it as often.

Lipids test

A lipids test measures the level of fats (lipids) in your blood. After a meal, your body digests fat in the food you eat and releases it into your bloodstream in two forms: cholesterol and triglycerides.

People with diabetes should have a lipids screening at least once a year. A rising level of blood fats can alert your doctor to an increased risk of blood vessel damage. Diabetes can accelerate the development of clogged and hardened arteries, which increases your risk of a heart attack, stroke, and poor circulation in your feet and legs. You may need to take medication to lower your cholesterol or triglyceride levels.

Serum creatinine test

The serum creatinine test is a blood test that can warn of kidney problems. It measures the level of creatinine in your blood. Creatinine is a chemical waste product that's produced when you use your muscles.

If your kidneys aren't functioning properly, they aren't able to remove as much creatinine from your blood. People with diabetes should have this test at least once a year.

Urine microalbumin test

A urine microalbumin test assesses the health of your kidneys. When your kidneys are functioning normally, they filter out blood waste products pumped through them. The waste is excreted in your urine, and protein and other helpful substances remain in the bloodstream.

When your kidneys become damaged, waste products remain in your blood, and protein (albumin) leaks into your urine. A urine microalbumin test screens for protein leakage into your urine. You should have the test every year if you have type 2 diabetes or if you've had type 1 diabetes for more than five years and you're past puberty.

Other Pancreatic Disorders

Diabetes is the most common disorder of the pancreas. Less commonly, the organ may become inflamed (pancreatitis) or it can develop tumors that may be noncancerous (benign) or cancerous (malignant).

Islet cell tumors

Rarely, tumors may arise from islet cells in the pancreas that secrete the hormones insulin and glucagon. These tumors often release excessive amounts of the hormones, resulting in serious metabolic effects.

Types

There are different types of islet cell tumors, each named after the hormone that it produces.

Insulinoma

An islet cell tumor that produces insulin is called an insulinoma. It causes periods of low blood sugar (hypoglycemia). Signs and symptoms may include episodes of weakness, sweating, a fast heartbeat and confusion. They're relieved by eating food.

Signs and symptoms tend to develop gradually over months to years. A diagnosis is usually made when your blood tests, obtained during a fast, show very low blood sugar associated with a high insulin level. This fasting test is generally performed in a hospital setting. If the results are positive, imaging tests are used to locate the insulinoma and it most often is surgically removed.

Gastrinoma

Another type of hormone-producing tumor is a gastrinoma. Most gastrinomas develop in the upper portion of your small intestine (duodenum), but they may also occur in the pancreas. Gastrin is a hormone that stimulates the stomach to secrete acid and digestive juices. A tumor that overproduces gastrin will cause severe ulcer symptoms that respond poorly to standard ulcer treatments.

Signs and symptoms associated with a gastrinoma include watery diarrhea and stomach pain that's relieved temporarily by food and antacids but grows more severe over weeks or months. Generally, a gastrinoma is diagnosed when blood tests show excessive gastrin. The condition associated with this type of tumor is called Zollinger-Ellison syndrome.

Glucagonoma

This type of tumor, which arises in the pancreas and secretes glucagon, is called a glucagonoma. Signs and symptoms associated with a glucagonoma include a rash on various areas of the body, a sore tongue, weight loss and an elevated blood sugar level.

A rash is important in diagnosing glucagonoma. Your doctor may conduct blood tests to determine if your blood sugar (glucose) concentration is abnormally high.

Others

Other hormone-producing tumors are extremely rare. They have a wide range of manifestations, including watery diarrhea — even while fasting — weight loss and a low blood potassium level. If you experience severe watery diarrhea accompanied by fatigue and weight loss over a period of several weeks, your doctor may want to do stool, blood and radiologic tests to rule out those rare conditions.

Treatment

Benign pancreatic tumors often can be treated successfully if diagnosed promptly. Surgical removal of the affected tissues is usually the key component of treatment. Some pancreatic tumors may be cancerous (malignant).

Pancreatic cancer

Cancer of the pancreas accounts for a small percentage of all cancers in the United States, but it's the fourth-leading cause of cancer death. The reason it's so deadly is that it typically produces no symptoms until it's incurably advanced. Because the pancreas is located deep in your abdomen behind other organs, a doctor usually can't detect a lump by feeling the area.

The cancer may grow undetected for years and in later stages may affect normal metabolism. For more information on pancreatic cancer, including risk factors and treatment, see page 872.

Pancreatitis

Inflammation of the pancreas (pancreatitis) disrupts the normal functions of the organ. Pancreatitis can result in a variety of signs and symptoms, including severe abdominal pain, nausea, vomiting, bloating and weight loss.

The condition can occur for various reasons, and in some cases the cause is unknown. The two most common causes of the disease are gallstones and excessive alcohol use. For more information on pancreatitis, see page 870.

Pituitary Gland Disorders

Located at the base of the brain, behind the nasal passages, the pituitary gland is roughly the size and shape of a hazelnut. Despite its small size, it's the most important endocrine gland. It serves as a control center for your body's long-term growth, day-to-day functioning and reproductive capabilities.

The pituitary gland consists of two parts, the front (anterior) lobe and the rear (posterior) lobe. The anterior lobe produces five distinct hormones, including prolactin to stimulate the production of breast milk and growth hormone to regulate your body's physical growth and use of fuel.

The other three hormones influence other glands of the endocrine system, stimulating activities in the thyroid gland, ovaries, testicles and adrenal glands.

The posterior lobe is responsible for the release of two hormones, oxytocin and anti-diuretic hormone. Oxytocin prompts uterine contractions during childbirth and stimulates the breasts to release milk during breast-feeding. Anti-diuretic hormone acts on the kidneys to control urine output.

Most problems with the pituitary gland are caused by benign pituitary tumors, which can be classified as either functioning or nonfunctioning. Functioning tumors release excess amounts of one of the normal pituitary hormones. Nonfunctioning tumors don't produce detectable hormone amounts.

Both types of tumors can cause problems simply because their increased size exerts pressure on neighboring vital tissues. Although the vast majority of pituitary tumors aren't cancerous and don't spread, they can lead to significant problems.

Nonfunctioning pituitary tumors

Signs and symptoms
- Loss of side (peripheral) vision
- Double vision
- Drooping of an eyelid
- Headache
- Excessive thirst and urination
- Fatigue and lightheadedness
- Intolerance to cold
- Constipation

In women
- Irregular or absent menstrual periods
- Infertility
- Discharge from the breasts

In men
- Decreased sexual interest
- Erectile dysfunction
- Decreased body hair

In children
- Slowed growth and development

Several types of nonfunctioning tumors — those that don't produce detectable amounts of a particular hormone — also can develop in the pituitary gland. Two of the most common are a pituitary adenoma and a craniopharyngioma.

Nonfunctioning tumors cause symptoms by pressing on the tissues surrounding the gland. The pituitary's own normal function also can be affected, leading to deficiencies of the thyroid and adrenal glands, growth, water balance or sex hormones.

In some instances, these tumors cause few, if any, problems. In others, they cause hormone deficiencies or serious and life-threatening pressure on the brain.

Diagnosis

A computerized tomography (CT) scan or magnetic resonance image (MRI) can confirm the presence of a nonfunctioning tumor. Many such tumors are found on scans performed for an unrelated condition. Your blood and urine may be tested for abnormal hormone levels.

Treatment

If treatment is necessary, the tumor is usually removed surgically. Radiation therapy may be required if the tumor can't be completely removed. Hormone deficiencies are generally treated with the appropriate hormone replacements.

Prolactinoma

Signs and symptoms
In women
- Irregular or absent menstrual periods
- Milky discharge from breasts when not pregnant or breast-feeding

In men
- Erectile dysfunction, decreased sexual interest and body hair
- Enlarged breasts

In both
- Hypopituitarism
- Loss of interest in sexual activity
- Infertility
- Headaches and visual disturbances

Prolactinoma is a condition in which a pituitary tumor overproduces the hormone prolactin. The tumor may be microscopic to several centimeters in diameter. The major effect of increased prolactin is a decrease in normal levels of sex hormones: estrogen in women and testosterone in men. Although such deficiencies aren't life-threatening, they can lead to long-term

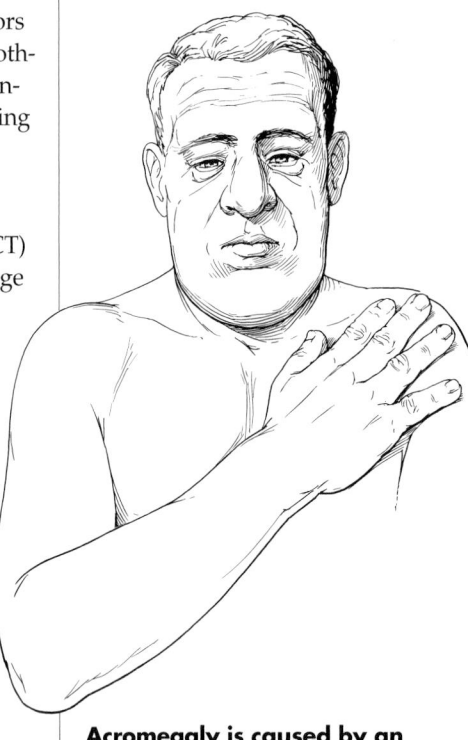

Acromegaly is caused by an excess of growth hormone in adulthood. The condition may result in enlargement of the hands, feet, jaw and forehead.

complications, such as osteoporosis, and may cause infertility and sexual dysfunction.

High prolactin levels can also result from causes other than prolactinoma, including several medications.

Diagnosis

Your doctor will likely take a careful medical history and conduct a physical examination to exclude other causes of high prolactin. Blood tests will measure your level of prolactin and other hormones. Magnetic resonance imaging (MRI) of the pituitary gland can often identify a tumor.

Treatment

Oral medications can often decrease prolactin production and eliminate symptoms. Medications also may shrink the tumor. Doctors use drugs known as dopamine agonists to treat prolactinoma. These drugs mimic the effects of dopamine, the brain chemical that normally controls prolactin

production. Long-term drug treatment is generally needed.

Surgery offers the chance of a cure with small tumors and also may be necessary to relieve pressure on the nerves controlling vision. However, many pituitary tumors recur within five years after surgical removal.

Acromegaly

Signs and symptoms
- Enlarged hands and feet
- Coarsened, enlarged facial features and enlarged tongue
- Coarse, oily, thickened skin
- Excessive perspiration
- Fatigue and muscle weakness
- Pain and limited joint mobility
- Deepened, husky voice
- Severe snoring
- Impaired vision

Acromegaly is a hormonal disorder that develops when your pituitary gland produces too much growth hormone. When this happens, your bones increase in size, including those of your hands, feet and face. Acromegaly most commonly affects middle-aged adults. In children, a tumor that produces excess growth hormone causes a condition called gigantism, characterized by significantly accelerated growth and increased height.

Excess growth hormone can also cause growth of internal organs. Other possible effects are high blood pressure, diabetes, colon polyps, arthritis and loss of vision. If acromegaly is untreated, the heart may become enlarged, leading to heart failure. These changes occur gradually, usually over several years, and often aren't apparent to the person with the disorder or to his or her family.

Diagnosis

The presence of certain physical features may suggest acromegaly. Your doctor may ask if you've had an increase in glove, shoe or hat size and whether your older rings still fit. In addition, with acromegaly, blood tests show excessive amounts of growth hormone and insulin-like growth factor-I (IGF-I).

To confirm the diagnosis, it may be necessary to measure growth hormone after you've ingested glucose. A test of your vision may be done because an enlarged pituitary gland can press on the nerves that control vision, producing a defect in your visual field.

Magnetic resonance imaging (MRI) of the head is frequently used to detect a tumor within the pituitary gland. Very rarely, a tumor located outside the pituitary can cause this syndrome.

Treatment

Surgery to remove the tumor is the most common treatment for acromegaly. Many times, it's not possible to remove the entire tumor. In this situation, radiation therapy or medications may be used. Radiation destroys the tumor and in turn stops production of growth hormone. Medications decrease growth hormone production or block growth hormone action but they don't destroy the tumor.

Conventional radiation therapy, focused radiation (stereotactic radiosurgery) or proton beam therapy may be used. Focused radiation delivers a high dose of radiation to the tumor while minimizing the amount of radiation to surrounding normal tissues.

Medications used to treat acromegaly include:

- **Somatostatin analogues.** These medications are synthetic versions of the brain hormone somatostatin. They interfere with the excess secretion of growth hormone by the pituitary gland.
- **Dopamine agonist.** This medication can lower levels of growth hormone and IGF-I.
- **Growth hormone antagonist.** This type of medication blocks the effect of growth hormone (GH) on body tissues. The medication can normalize IGF-I levels and relieve symptoms of acromegaly, but it doesn't lower GH levels or reduce the tumor size.

If the pituitary gland is damaged by the tumor or during the course of treatment, hormone replacement will be necessary. This involves taking medications that replace the hormones the pituitary gland can no longer produce.

Cushing syndrome

Signs and symptoms

- Weight gain, particularly around the midsection
- Fatigue
- Muscle weakness and wasting
- Rounding of the face (moon face) and fullness of the neck
- A flushed face
- A hump between the shoulders (buffalo hump)
- Thinning of the skin with easy bruising, slow healing and stretch marks
- Excess hair growth
- Acne
- Depression, anxiety and irritability
- Bone loss
- In men, erectile dysfunction
- In women, absence of menstrual periods

Cushing syndrome is sometimes referred to as hypercortisolism. It occurs when your body is exposed to high levels of the hormone cortisol. The condition is named for Harvey Cushing, an early 20th-century American surgeon who first described the disorder.

The most common cause of Cushing syndrome is the use of corticosteroid medication for an extended period. The condition can also occur from a tumor in the pituitary gland or overproduction of cortisol by the adrenal glands. An adrenal gland tumor, enlargement of both glands or another tumor that produces a hormone that stimulates the adrenal glands can cause this overproduction.

If you have Cushing syndrome, you're at increased risk of a heart attack or stroke because the disorder can accelerate buildup of fatty deposits (plaques) in your arteries

(atherosclerosis). Thinning of your bones (osteoporosis) and bone fractures also are common, as is impaired ability to resist or fight infections. Left untreated, Cushing syndrome can be fatal.

Diagnosis

A round, red face and extra fatty tissue above the collarbone and between the shoulder blades are physical clues to Cushing syndrome. Frequent or even spontaneous bruising on the arms and legs is another common sign.

Cushing syndrome is generally determined by measuring hormone levels in your blood, urine and saliva. Your doctor may also recommend other specialized tests that measure cortisol levels before and after stimulation or

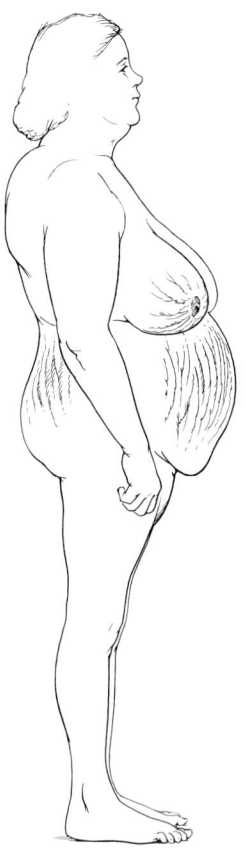

If Cushing syndrome is left untreated, it can cause an individual to develop a very round face, abdominal obesity, a characteristic hump on the back, and pink or purple stretch marks in the skin.

suppression with other hormone medications.

Magnetic resonance imaging (MRI) or a computerized tomography (CT) scan of the pituitary or adrenal glands or lungs can help determine if a tumor is present. Direct blood sampling from the veins draining the pituitary gland also may be necessary.

Treatment

Treatment depends on the cause of the excess cortisol. If your signs and symptoms are due to taking steroid medications, treatment consists of stopping their use or decreasing the dosage. Sudden discontinuation of steroid treatment can aggravate the underlying disease, such as asthma or arthritis. Your doctor will likely recommend a gradual reduction in the dosage of steroids.

In some cases, another drug may be used in place of the steroid originally prescribed. For as long as a year after steroid medication is stopped, physical stress from an injury, infection or surgery may result in a dangerous insufficiency of adrenal hormones, requiring emergency replacement treatment.

For Cushing syndrome that's caused by a tumor in the pituitary gland, adrenal gland or lung, removal of the tumor is usually the best treatment. Surgical techniques continue to evolve. Newer techniques require smaller incisions, result in shorter hospital stays, and generally produce less pain and other complications. Successful removal of a tumor is likely to result in a full recovery, although

Hormone Supplements and Aging

Because hormone levels generally decline with age, some scientists speculate that hormones may play a role in the aging process. This has led some anti-aging enthusiasts and product manufacturers to promote the use of hormone supplements as a way to set back your body's clock.

If only it were that simple. Aging is an intricate, complex process that involves many body functions and tissues. When evaluating claims about hormone supplements, some old advice remains wise — if it sounds too good to be true, it probably is. Despite tempting claims, no hormone product has been proved to prevent or reverse aging. In addition, some may have dangerous side effects.

Here's a look at some hormone supplements that are touted as anti-aging therapies:

Human growth hormone

Growth hormone, produced in the pituitary gland, fuels growth and development during childhood and adolescence. In youths and adults who have a documented deficiency of the hormone, injections of the hormone are beneficial.

Proponents of human growth hormone (HGH) supplements for healthy adults say the hormone burns fat, builds muscle and renews energy. No evidence, however, shows that taking HGH results in health or lifestyle benefits for normal, aging adults. Moreover, possible side effects include fluid retention, joint pain, diabetes, high blood pressure and colon polyps.

DHEA

Dehydroepiandrosterone (DHEA) is a precursor hormone that's converted by the body into other hormones, including the sex hormones estrogen and testosterone. Normally, DHEA levels in your body peak during early adulthood and then gradually decline. Levels are quite low in older adults.

DHEA is sold over-the-counter as a dietary supplement and is advertised as a product that can slow aging, increase muscle and bone strength, burn fat, improve cognition, strengthen the immune system, and protect against many chronic diseases. None of these claims has been proved. More troubling, DHEA may have harmful side effects. Even when taken for a short time, it may cause liver damage. Other potential problems include menstrual irregularities and unwanted facial hair in women, promotion of prostate cancer

in men, and an increased risk of heart disease.

Melatonin

Melatonin is a hormone that helps regulate your body's schedule for sleeping and waking. Claims that melatonin can slow or reverse aging and enhance sexuality remain unproved. Supplements on the market typically contain many times the amount of melatonin produced by your body. If taken improperly, melatonin can actually disrupt your sleep cycle.

Testosterone

In general, levels of the male sex hormone testosterone decline over time, although the rate of decline varies greatly among individual men. Anti-aging advocates say that increasing your level of testosterone by taking prescription supplements will improve your energy, well-being, complexion and sex drive. Such claims also remain unproved.

In high doses, testosterone can cause prostate problems, aggravate sleep apnea, stimulate excessive red blood cell production and elevate cholesterol levels. However, in men whose testosterone level is low due to testicular disease or a pituitary problem, treatment with testosterone can be beneficial.

long-term hormone replacement therapy may be required.

If surgery isn't possible or successful, treatment may include radiation. If treatment renders the adrenal glands incapable of providing the hormones your body requires, you'll need oral medications to replace the missing hormones.

In some situations when surgery and radiation don't normalize cortisol production, your doctor may prescribe medication to control excessive production of cortisol.

Hypopituitarism

Signs and symptoms
- Fatigue
- Headaches
- Low stress tolerance
- Muscle weakness
- Nausea or abdominal discomfort
- Constipation
- Weight loss or gain
- Hoarseness
- Loss of underarm and public hair
- Thirst and excess urination

In children
- Stunted growth
- Slowed sexual development

In women
- Irregular or absent menstrual periods
- Infertility
- An inability to produce milk for breast-feeding

In men
- Decreased sexual interest
- Erectile dysfunction
- Loss of facial or body hair

Hypopituitarism is a disorder in which your pituitary gland doesn't produce enough of one or more of the pituitary hormones. The name is derived in part from the Greek prefix *hypo*, which means "under." Some people inherit a tendency toward hypopituitarism. Others acquire the ailment for unknown reasons. In many instances, the cause is identifiable.

The condition is usually associated with a pituitary tumor or its treatment. Other causes include a serious head injury or inflammation of the pituitary gland

(hypophysitis). Most cases of hypophysitis are due to autoimmune damage. Hypophysitis may also occur as a side effect of certain medications used to treat some cancers. Some women experience hypopituitarism after childbirth complicated by excessive blood loss or low blood pressure, causing some or all of the pituitary tissue to die. This form of hypopituitarism is called Sheehan syndrome.

Because the pituitary gland also produces hormones that activate other glands, underproduction of those hormones can result in symptoms of other endocrine disorders.

Diagnosis
Hypopituitarism in a child results in dwarfism. The key sign is abnormally slow growth. This condition is rare — very few children who are shorter than average have such a hormone insufficiency.

If hypopituitarism is suspected, your doctor may order tests to measure hormone concentrations in your blood and urine. Subsequent testing may involve administering other hormones or medications to stimulate the pituitary gland to produce its hormones, which are then measured.

If test results indicate a shortage of pituitary hormones, further tests may be performed to try to determine the underlying cause.

Treatment
If a cause is identified, specific treatment may improve hormone levels. If not, various hormone therapies are necessary, depending on the degree of deficiency of each hormone. Thyroid hormone is replaced with oral levothyroxine taken daily. Cortisol (adrenal) deficiency is treated with oral hydrocortisone or prednisone taken once or twice daily.

In children, injections of synthetic growth hormone can stimulate growth. It restores normal body proportions of fat and muscle and can improve fatigue that occurs with hypopituitarism.

Estrogen replacement for girls and testosterone replacement for boys may be required for sexual development. Adults also may need sex hormone replacement or specific fertility treatments.

People who require hormone therapy should wear a medical alert bracelet or necklace identifying their medical condition.

Diabetes insipidus

Signs and symptoms
- Excessive thirst
- Increased urination

Emergency signs and symptoms
- Dehydration, physical collapse and low blood pressure

Despite the similarities in symptoms and name, diabetes insipidus shouldn't be confused with diabetes mellitus. Diabetes mellitus — most commonly referred to as just diabetes — stems from a deficiency of or resistance to the hormone insulin. Diabetes insipidus results from a deficiency of or resistance to anti-diuretic hormone (ADH).

When the disorder results from a deficiency of ADH, it's called central diabetes insipidus. When it results from resistance to ADH, it's termed nephrogenic diabetes insipidus. The release of ADH is controlled by the pituitary gland.

A shortage of anti-diuretic hormone or action can disturb the water balance in your body. Rather than reabsorbing enough water to maintain proper fluid levels, your kidneys simply pass the water out.

The cause of diabetes insipidus is unknown in about half the people who have it, although a pituitary disorder may become evident several years after symptoms begin.

Identifiable causes of central diabetes insipidus include damage to the pituitary gland from a head injury, surgery for a pituitary tumor and some inflammatory conditions. Identifiable causes of nephrogenic diabetes insipidus include certain medications and some types of kidney disease.

Diagnosis

The key sign of diabetes insipidus is the large volume of urine that's excreted within 24 hours. Dehydration that results from increased urination causes insatiable thirst and, sometimes, dry skin.

Your doctor may conduct a water deprivation test, in which you consume no fluid for several hours. Urine produced during that time is analyzed. If you have normal amounts of anti-diuretic hormone, the volume of urine will decrease. If you have diabetes insipidus, you'll eliminate substantial volumes of water. Your doctor may also conduct blood tests to determine the water and salt balance in your blood.

Treatment

Treatment focuses on determining the cause of diabetes insipidus, eliminating the cause, if possible, and controlling symptoms.

Diet

If you have nephrogenic diabetes, your doctor may advise that you limit consumption of salt because reducing sodium may help alleviate symptoms.

Medication

For central diabetes insipidus, you may be given an anti-diuretic hormone — taken in pill form, as a nasal spray or by injection — that usually is lifelong. If the disease resulted from an injury, the pituitary may regain its normal function over a few months to a year. In such instances, hormone medication can be discontinued.

For nephrogenic diabetes insipidus, a thiazide diuretic drug may be prescribed. Although diuretics ordinarily are used to increase urination, thiazides have been effective for treating nephrogenic diabetes insipidus.

Surgery

If a pituitary gland tumor is the cause of the disorder, surgery or radiation therapy may be necessary.

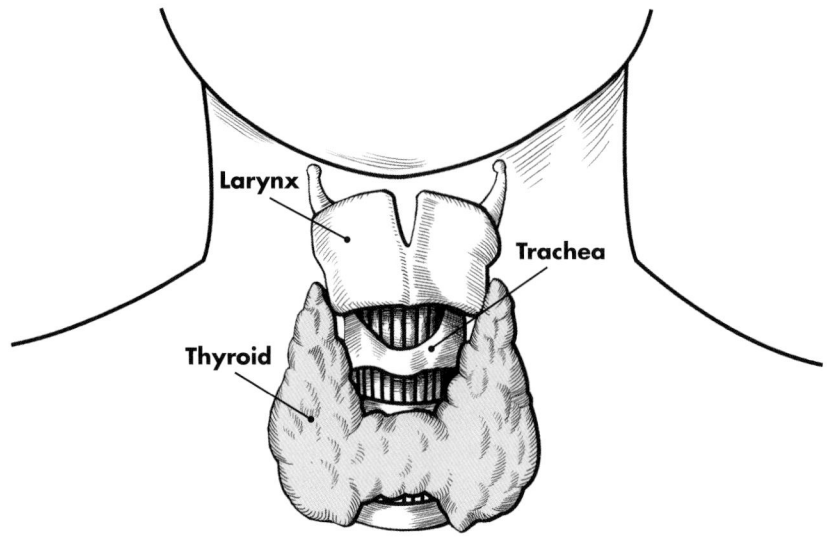

The thyroid gland consists of two lobes. It's located at the base of the throat.

Thyroid Disorders

Shaped like a bow tie or butterfly, your thyroid gland is located at the base of your throat, just below your Adam's apple. The gland wraps around your windpipe (trachea). A crossbar of tissue (isthmus) connects its two lobes.

The thyroid gland has an enormous effect on your health. It helps set the rate at which your body functions, regulating all aspects of your metabolism, from how fast your heart beats to how quickly you burn calories. In response to direction from the pituitary gland, the thyroid gland secretes the hormone thyroxine. The more thyroxine that's circulating in your bloodstream, the greater the speed at which chemical activities occur in your body. The thyroid gland also produces the hormone calcitonin.

As long as your thyroid gland produces the right amount of thyroxine, your metabolism functions normally. But sometimes the gland produces and releases too much or not enough. Disorders of the thyroid gland generally fall into two categories, one involving its function and the other involving its structure.

Overproduction of thyroxine causes hyperthyroidism (overactive thyroid disease). The opposite condition — underproduction of thyroid hormone — causes hypothyroidism (underactive thyroid disease). Both are functional disorders because they involve problems with the gland's functioning.

Hyperthyroidism

Signs and symptoms
- Weight loss despite normal or increased appetite
- A rapid or irregular heartbeat or pounding of the heart
- Nervousness, anxiety and irritability
- Sweating
- Tremor
- More frequent bowel movements, sometimes diarrhea
- Fatigue and muscle weakness
- Increased sensitivity to heat
- In women, changes in menstrual patterns
- Enlarged thyroid gland

Emergency signs and symptoms
- A very rapid pulse
- Agitation and delirium

Hyperthyroidism occurs when the thyroid gland produces or releases too much of the hormone

Hyperthyroidism (overactive thyroid disease) during pregnancy increases the risk of miscarriage, so it's best to avoid getting pregnant until your hyperthyroidism is treated. If you've been treated with radioactive iodine, avoid getting pregnant for at least six months afterward. If hyperthyroidism occurs or recurs during pregnancy, you'll be given the lowest possible dose of an anti-thyroid drug. Radioactive iodine isn't used if you're pregnant or breast-feeding.

thyroxine. Excessive thyroxine accelerates your body's metabolism.

Women are more likely to have hyperthyroidism than are men. Although it can occur at any age, it's most common in young or middle-aged adults.

Several different disease processes can cause your thyroid to release too much thyroid hormone. The most common underlying cause is an autoimmune disorder called Graves' disease. Other causes include inflammation of the thyroid gland (thyroiditis) and overactive nodules in the gland.

Hyperthyroidism can have serious consequences if untreated. Complications include heart problems, such as a rapid heart rate, an irregular heartbeat (atrial fibrillation), and congestive heart failure, as well as loss of bone mass (osteoporosis). If you have overactive thyroid disease, you're at risk of thyrotoxic crisis, a sudden intensification of signs and symptoms, leading to a fever and even delirium. This requires urgent medical care.

Manifestations of the speeded-up metabolism of hyperthyroidism include an increase in appetite, feeling warm while others may be cool or comfortable, and hands that tremble. Your skin may feel moist and sweaty. Your heart may pound forcibly at a rapid rate and occasionally develop an irregular rhythm. Sleep difficulties are common. Your thyroid gland may be enlarged, but often so slightly that it isn't noticeable. If the condition is due to Graves' disease, your eyes may be affected, causing double vision, protrusion of your eyes, dry eyes and sometimes a skin rash.

Diagnosis

Hyperthyroidism is generally diagnosed based on a medical history, physical examination and blood tests. Your doctor may try to detect a slight tremor in your fingers when they're extended. You may be asked questions about any changes in your bowel movements or sensitivity to temperature.

Blood tests can detect an increase in thyroxine concentration. They may also show low or no amounts of thyroid-stimulating hormone, which is produced by the pituitary gland and is suppressed when too much thyroid hormone is circulating.

A radioactive iodine uptake test can help establish the diagnosis. In this test, you're given a small amount of radioactive iodine that you take orally. Over several hours, the iodine collects in your thyroid gland, where it's absorbed and used to manufacture thyroxine.

A high uptake of radioactive iodine indicates that your thyroid gland is producing too much thyroxine, as occurs with Graves' disease and hyperfunctioning thyroid nodules. If the uptake is low, thyroiditis is more likely the cause, in which iodine uptake is blocked, but stored thyroid hormone in the gland is released excessively.

Your doctor may also obtain a picture of your thyroid gland (thyroid scan) to help determine the cause and possible treatment. During this test, a radioactive isotope is injected into a vein in your arm or hand. You then lie on a table while a special camera produces an image of your thyroid on a computer screen.

Treatment

Treatment for hyperthyroidism includes:

Radioactive iodine

This is the most common treatment for hyperthyroidism. Taken in liquid or capsule form, radioactive iodine is absorbed by the thyroid gland. The irradiation harmlessly and painlessly destroys thyroid tissue, causing the gland to shrink and production of thyroid hormone to slow.

The dose of radioactive iodine depends on the size of the thyroid gland and the findings on the uptake test. Production of thyroxine gradually declines over three to six months. Some people may require a second dose of radioactive iodine.

The majority of people who take radioactive iodine for hyperthyroidism are cured. However, because this treatment causes thyroid activity to slow considerably, it can result in the opposite condition — too little production of the thyroid hormone thyroxine. Many people need to take oral thyroxine every day to replace thyroxine no longer being produced.

Anti-thyroid medications

Another treatment involves taking anti-thyroid medications, such as methimazole (Tapazole). They gradually reduce symptoms of hyperthyroidism by preventing the gland from producing excess amounts of hormones.

Symptoms usually begin to improve in six to 12 weeks, but treatment with anti-thyroid medications typically continues at least a year and often longer. For some people, this clears up the problem permanently, but other people may experience a relapse. These medications can cause serious health problems.

Beta blockers

These drugs are commonly used to treat high blood pressure. They won't reduce your thyroid levels,

Are You at Risk?

Hypothyroidism occurs mainly in women age 40 or older, and the risk of developing the disorder increases with age. But it can affect either sex, from infants to older adults. You're at increased risk of hypothyroidism if you:

- Have a close relative, such as a parent or grandparent, with an autoimmune disease
- Have diabetes or an autoimmune disease and are or have been pregnant
- Have been treated with radioactive iodine or anti-thyroid medications
- Have had thyroid surgery
- Have been treated with radiation for cancer of the head or neck

but they can reduce symptoms, such as a rapid heart rate, and help prevent palpitations. For that reason, your doctor may prescribe them to help you feel better until your thyroid levels are closer to normal.

Surgery
If medications aren't able to treat the problem, you may be a candidate for surgery, although this is an option only in rare cases. During a procedure called thyroidectomy, your doctor removes part or most of the thyroid gland, reducing or stopping hormone production. If all of the gland is removed, you'll need to take medication daily to replace the hormones normally produced by the gland.

Self-care
If you've lost a great deal of weight or are experiencing muscle wasting, work with your doctor or a dietitian to plan an appropriate diet. With successful treatment, nearly everyone regains weight. It's also important to get enough calcium every day to help prevent osteoporosis. Aim for a total of 1,500 milligrams daily, either from the food you eat, calcium supplements or both.

Hypothyroidism

Signs and symptoms
- Fatigue and sluggishness
- A slow heart rate
- Increased sensitivity to cold
- Unexplained weight gain
- Constipation
- Dry skin and hair
- Elevated blood cholesterol level
- Muscle aches and weakness
- A hoarse voice
- A puffy face
- In women, heavier than normal periods

Hypothyroidism (underactive thyroid) is a condition in which the thyroid gland fails to produce and release adequate levels of the hormone thyroxine. This disease slows your body's metabolic activities.

Because thyroid hormones have such a significant effect on growth, development and daily functioning, a deficiency can lead to a wide variety of health problems. Children with the condition may experience developmental disabilities. Adults may experience a slowing of physical and mental functioning and even heart disease. An underactive thyroid can also in-crease cholesterol levels and blood pressure.

Signs and symptoms of hypothyroidism vary widely, depending on the severity of the hormone deficiency. In adults, the condition usually develops slowly over months or even years. As your metabolism continues to decrease, symptoms become more obvious.

Advanced hypothyroidism is called myxedema. It can develop if hypothyroidism goes unrecognized for several years. Symptoms of myxedema may include drowsiness, intense intolerance of cold and low body temperature, followed by profound lethargy and finally unconsciousness. A myxedema coma may be triggered by infection, use of sedatives, surgery or another stress on your body.

Hypothyroidism can occur in either sex and at any age. Middle-aged women are most commonly affected, and older adults are most likely to remain undiagnosed. The condition has various causes.

The thyroid gland may be destroyed by an autoimmune disorder, in which your own immune system attacks the gland. Hypothyroidism can result from an inflammation of the gland or from a failure of your pituitary gland to produce thyroid-stimulating hormone. This hormone signals your thyroid gland to produce thyroxine.

In addition, treatment for excess production of thyroid hormones (hyperthyroidism) can result in hypothyroidism. Some women develop hypothyroidism before or after pregnancy. In rare instances, infants are born with a defective thyroid gland or no thyroid gland.

Screening in Infants

All states in the United States require that newborns be screened with routine blood tests for hypothyroidism. That's because in an infant, untreated hypothyroidism can result in serious problems with physical and mental development. If the condition is diagnosed within the first few months of life, the chances of normal development are excellent.

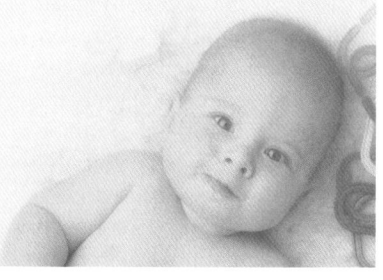

Goiter

Goiter is a general term for an enlarged thyroid gland. The word comes from the Latin word for "throat." The enlargement may be a small, localized lump or a swelling of both lobes of the thyroid gland. A goiter is usually painless.

An enlarged thyroid gland can produce normal, low or excessive amounts of hormones. In rare instances, in which the enlarged gland grows around the windpipe, the enlargement can interfere with swallowing or breathing.

Thyroid enlargement has many causes. In the past, the most common cause of a goiter was a shortage of iodine in the diet. Goiters are now rare in the United States because table salt is supplemented with iodine, and the food supply is generally rich in iodine. In some parts of the world that lack dietary iodine, goiters are still common.

Other causes of goiters include:

Simple enlargement
A soft, widespread enlargement of the thyroid gland is called simple goiter. Although infrequent, it's most common during pregnancy or adolescence. Other times, the cause is unknown, although there may be a genetic component in some instances.

Thyroiditis
Thyroiditis is an inflammation of the thyroid gland, which can cause it to enlarge. The gland may become rubbery, or it may be tender and cause pain when swallowing. Chronic lymphocytic thyroiditis, also called Hashimoto's thyroiditis, is the most common cause of thyroid enlargement in the United States. It results from an autoimmune disorder.

Graves' disease
Graves' disease causes an overactive thyroid. It usually produces a slight but generalized enlargement of the thyroid, although the gland can become quite large.

Thyroid nodules
Nodules or lumps in the thyroid gland may cause enlargement of one or both lobes. A nodule needs to be evaluated to determine if it's cancerous. Rarely, a nodule partially blocks your windpipe (trachea), causing breathing difficulties that may resemble asthma.

If your goiter isn't causing any problems, treatment may not be necessary. If the gland becomes large enough to be of cosmetic concern or interferes with eating or breathing, medication may be prescribed or all or part of the gland may be removed.

If the gland contains nodules or bumps, diagnostic tests will likely be performed to make sure the growths aren't cancerous (malignant). In case of cancer, removal of all or a portion of the gland may be necessary.

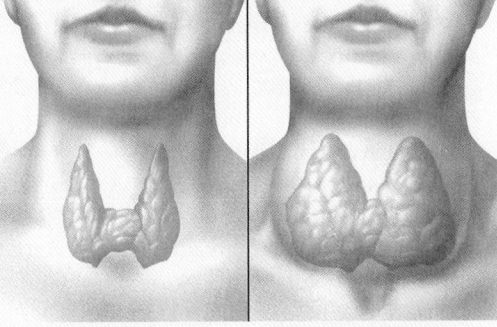

Normal thyroid   **Enlarged thyroid**

Diagnosis
Your doctor may test for an underactive thyroid if you're feeling increasingly tired or sluggish, have dry skin, constipation, and a hoarse voice or have had previous thyroid problems. Some doctors also test pregnant women for the disease.

The most effective way to diagnose hypothyroidism is with blood tests that measure levels of thyroid-stimulating hormone (TSH) and thyroxine. Low levels of thyroxine and high levels of TSH suggest hypothyroidism.

Treatment
Treatment for an underactive thyroid involves daily use of the synthetic thyroid hormone levothyroxine (Levoxyl, Synthroid). This oral medication restores adequate hormone levels.

After you start treatment, symptoms such as fatigue should start to subside, although all of your symptoms may not improve for several months. The medication may gradually lower your cholesterol level and reverse any weight gain caused by the disease.

Treatment with levothyroxine is usually lifelong and must be followed with periodic blood tests because your body's thyroid hormone requirement may change slightly over time.

Certain medications, supplements or foods may affect your ability to absorb levothyroxine. Talk to your doctor if you eat large amounts of soy products, follow a high-fiber diet, or take iron or calcium supplements.

Others

The following thyroid conditions may lead to hyperthyroidism or hypothyroidism, or pose similar signs and symptoms.

Graves' disease
Graves' disease is an autoimmune disorder named for Robert Graves, the Irish doctor who first described it. With this disease, something causes your body's immune system to produce an antibody that imitates the action of thyroid-stimulating hormone (TSH) and stimulates your thyroid gland.

Women are about seven times more likely to have Graves' disease than are men.

Graves' disease is the most common cause of hyperthyroidism. Immune system abnormalities that stimulate excess hormone production may also cause an uncommon condition called Graves' ophthalmopathy. In this disorder, the eyeballs protrude beyond their protective orbit because tissues and muscles behind the eyes swell and cause the eyeballs to move forward. Your eyes may also be red and irritated. Some people experience double vision. A small number of people with Graves' disease develop reddening and swelling of the skin, often on their shins and the top of their feet.

Treatment

No treatment exists that can stop your immune system from producing the antibodies that cause Graves' disease, but medication can control the symptoms by decreasing the production of thyroxine. Treatment for Graves' ophthalmopathy is discussed on page 622.

Thyroiditis

Thyroiditis, an inflammation of the thyroid gland, can cause enlargement of the gland. There are several types of thyroiditis. The most common is chronic lymphocytic thyroiditis, also called Hashimoto's thyroiditis. It's an autoimmune disease in which the immune system creates antibodies that damage the thyroid gland, causing underproduction of thyroid hormone. This disease is most common in older women and tends to run in families.

Thyroiditis after pregnancy is called postpartum thyroiditis. It's a painless inflammation of the thyroid gland that occurs in a small percentage of women about four to 12 months after childbirth. A short period of hyperthyroidism may occur, but thyroid function usually returns to normal after a few months. Some women, though, experience significant or long-term hypothyroidism.

Another less common condition is subacute granulomatous thyroiditis. This condition begins more suddenly than Hashimoto's thyroiditis and causes the thyroid gland to become painful and enlarged. Either hyperthyroidism or hypothyroidism may occur temporarily. This type of thyroiditis usually goes away by itself within a few months.

Treatment

Your doctor likely will examine your thyroid gland and request blood tests to measure hormone levels and antibodies.

Most people with Hashimoto's thyroiditis must take thyroid hormone replacement medication for the rest of their lives. With other forms, the thyroid gland may return to normal in a few months.

Aspirin or other nonsteroidal anti-inflammatory drugs can relieve the pain and inflammation of subacute thyroiditis. In more severe cases, a doctor may prescribe corticosteroid medications.

Thyroid nodules

A thyroid nodule is a lump within the thyroid gland. You may have several or only one. Thyroid nodules are relatively common and rarely cancerous (malignant).

One noncancerous (benign) type is an adenoma, in which a portion of the thyroid walls itself off from the rest of the gland. It forms a lump, often half an inch or more in diameter, which you can often feel and sometimes see.

Most thyroid adenomas produce little or no thyroid hormone, but occasionally an adenoma manufactures an excessive amount, a condition called hyperfunctioning thyroid nodule, causing hyperthyroidism.

Treatment

Most thyroid nodules are discovered during a routine physical exam or on an unrelated imaging test of the neck. To determine what type of nodule it is and if it's cancerous, a doctor may perform an ultrasound exam to get an image of the lump. He or she may also do a biopsy, a procedure in which a thin needle is used to take a sample of the tissue for examination. You also may have a blood test to check the level of thyroid hormones.

Often, a nodule requires no specific treatment, as most don't produce symptoms. Adenomas that produce excessive thyroid hormone are treated with surgery or radioactive iodine, which destroys the nodule.

Cancerous nodules typically require surgical removal of the thyroid gland. If the gland is removed, you'll need to take thyroid hormone replacement medication for the rest of your life.

Thyroid cancer

Cancer of the thyroid is uncommon. There are different types, based on how the cancer cells look under a microscope. The two most common types are papillary and follicular. The papillary type tends to spread to the lymph nodes in the neck. The follicular type may spread to your lungs and more distant parts of your body. Most thyroid cancers grow slowly.

In an unusual form of thyroid cancer called medullary cancer, the cancer cells secrete the hormone calcitonin. Medullary cancer frequently occurs in members of the same family. Medullary thyroid cancer is also associated with a rare hereditary disorder called multiple endocrine neoplasia (MEN) type 2 (see page 1030).

Cancer of the thyroid is more common in women than in men. You're at increased risk of developing thyroid cancer if you've been exposed to large amounts of radiation, if you've had radiation treatment to your head or neck, or if someone in your family has had medullary thyroid cancer or pheochromocytomas, rare tumors that arise from cells in the core (medulla) of the adrenal gland.

Treatment

Most thyroid cancer can be cured with treatment:

- **Surgery.** In most cases, doctors recommend removing the entire thyroid gland in order to treat thyroid cancer. The surgeon may also remove enlarged lymph nodes from your neck and test them for cancer cells. In certain situations where the thyroid cancer is very small, only one side (lobe) of your thyroid may be removed.
- **Thyroid hormone therapy.** After removal of the thyroid, you'll take the thyroid hormone medication levothyroxine (Levoxyl, Synthroid, others) for life. This medication supplies the missing hormone your thyroid would normally produce, and it suppresses the production of thyroid-stimulating hormone (TSH) from your pituitary gland. High TSH levels could conceivably stimulate any remaining cancer cells to grow.
- **Radioactive iodine.** This treatment uses large doses of a form of iodine that's radioactive. It's often used after a thyroidectomy to destroy any remaining healthy thyroid tissue, as well as microscopic areas of thyroid cancer that weren't removed during surgery. Radioactive iodine treatment may also be used to treat thyroid cancer that recurs after treatment or that spreads to other areas of the body.

    Most of the radioactive iodine leaves your body in your urine in the first few days after treatment. You'll be given instructions for precautions you need to take during that time to protect other people from the radiation.
- **External radiation therapy.** It may be an option if you can't undergo surgery and your cancer continues to grow after

radioactive iodine treatment. Radiation therapy may also be recommended after surgery if there's an increased risk that your cancer will recur.
- **Chemotherapy.** Chemotherapy may benefit some people who don't respond to other therapies. It may be combined with radiation therapy.
- **Alcohol ablation.** This treatment involves injecting small thyroid cancers with alcohol using imaging such as ultrasound to ensure precise placement of the injection. This treatment is helpful for treating cancer that occurs in areas that aren't easily accessible during surgery. Your doctor also may recommend this treatment if you have recurrent thyroid cancer limited to small areas in your neck.
- **Targeted drug therapy.** This treatment uses medications that target the signals that tell cancer cells to grow and divide. Used mainly in people with advanced thyroid cancer, targeted drugs used to treat thyroid cancer include cabozantinib (Cometriq), sorafenib (Nexavar) and vandetanib (Caprelsa).

    If you have medullary thyroid cancer, ask about genetic screening. Family members can be tested to see if they carry the genetic defect that causes inherited forms of the cancer. Thyroid surgery can prevent cancer in carriers who haven't yet developed cancer.

Parathyroid Gland Disorders

The parathyroid glands are located on the four corners of the thyroid gland, which lies at the front and base of your neck. The parathyroid glands are very small — each is about the size of a grain of rice — and they secrete parathyroid

hormone. When too much of this hormone is produced, the resulting disorder is called hyperparathyroidism. When too little of the hormone is released, the condition is called hypoparathyroidism.

The parathyroid glands maintain the level of calcium in your blood within very narrow limits by secreting more or less hormone.

Hyperparathyroidism

Signs and symptoms

- Increased thirst and urination
- Kidney stones
- Abdominal pain, nausea, vomiting or loss of appetite
- Bone thinning (osteoporosis)
- Fatigue or muscle weakness
- Confusion or poor memory

    When one or more of the parathyroid glands produce an excess of parathyroid hormone, hyperparathyroidism results. When excess parathyroid hormone circulates in your body, the calcium level in your blood becomes elevated, and the concentration of phosphorus is lowered.

    Phosphorus, like calcium, is a mineral essential to your body's functioning and is of particular importance to the development and health of your bones and teeth.

    Hyperparathyroidism can occur as one of two types:
- **Primary hyperparathyroidism.** Most of this type is caused by a noncancerous (benign) tumor on one of the parathyroid glands. The disorder can also occur when two or more glands become enlarged and produce too much hormone. In very rare cases, the cause of hyperparathyroidism may be cancer of one of the parathyroid glands.
- **Secondary hyperparathyroidism.** This less common type occurs when another medical condition causes the parathyroid glands to produce too much parathyroid hormone in response to low levels of circulating calcium. Kidney failure and malabsorption problems are

the main causes of this type of hyperparathyroidism.

Diagnosis

Most people with hyperparathyroidism have no symptoms. Often the diagnosis is made when an abnormally high calcium level is discovered by a routine blood test for some other reason. Low amounts of phosphorus in your blood also indicate you might have the disorder.

Direct measurement of the amount of parathyroid hormone in your blood and calcium in a 24-hour urine collection helps confirm the diagnosis. Your doctor may order other tests to look for the location of the enlarged gland and to check for other conditions such as kidney stones and osteoporosis.

Treatment

For some people with hyperparathyroidism, no treatment is necessary. Your doctor may simply monitor your condition. He or she may periodically order image tests of your kidneys, because of an increased risk of kidney stones, and measure your bone mineral density to assess the status of your bones, which are at risk of thinning if you have this disorder.

If your blood calcium level is very high or there's evidence of bone thinning or kidney stones, you may need treatment. Treatment usually involves surgical removal of the tumor or the glands that are overproducing parathyroid hormone. Special scans can accurately locate the tumor, which allows a surgeon to remove it with minimally invasive surgery.

In the case of secondary hyperparathyroidism, the first goal is to treat the underlying problem. The drug cinacalcet (Sensipar) can treat secondary hyperparathyroidism caused by chronic kidney disease or parathyroid cancer. Some doctors may prescribe the drug to treat primary hyperparathyroidism if surgery isn't possible.

Hypoparathyroidism

Signs and symptoms

- Tingling in fingertips, toes and lips
- Muscle aches or cramps or muscle twitching
- Fatigue and weakness
- Anxiety or nervousness
- Mood swings

When the parathyroid glands produce too little of their hormone, the disorder that results is called hypoparathyroidism. Hypoparathyroidism is far less common than hyperparathyroidism.

Without sufficient quantities of parathyroid hormone circulating in your body, the amount of calcium in your blood falls below normal levels, and the amount of phosphorus rises. A low blood calcium concentration can produce various problems, particularly muscle spasms and cramps and tingling around your fingertips and the tips of your toes.

Muscle spasms associated with hypoparathyroidism can be uncomfortable or painful, and breathing difficulties can result from spasms of the muscles controlling

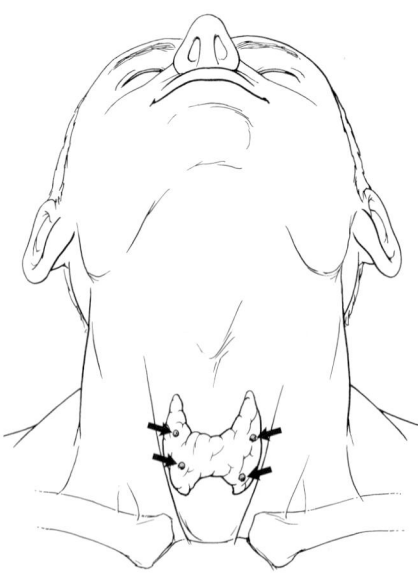

Located behind your thyroid gland, the tiny parathyroid glands (arrows) produce a hormone that controls the level of calcium in your blood.

your vocal cords. Convulsions can occur if your blood calcium is very low. If the amount of calcium in your blood has been low for many years, cataracts and brain tissue calcifications can occur.

Hypoparathyroidism is often categorized into two forms:

- **Hereditary.** Either the parathyroid glands aren't present at birth or they don't work properly. Symptoms tend to become apparent in the first 10 years of life, most often by age 2.
- **Acquired.** This form tends to develop after accidental damage to or removal of the parathyroid glands during neck or throat surgery, or during another medical procedure, such as radiation treatment. In a small number of cases, the cause is an autoimmune disorder. Your immune system rejects the glands as if they were foreign bodies.

Diagnosis

The key findings in hypoparathyroidism are an abnormally low level of calcium in the blood (hypocalcemia), an abnormally high concentration of phosphorus and an inappropriately low level of parathyroid hormone.

Treatment

Your doctor may prescribe calcium and vitamin D supplements, which you'll likely need to take for the remainder of your lifetime. You may also need to follow a diet high in calcium and low in phosphorus.

Levels of calcium in your blood must be monitored with regular blood tests to make sure you maintain normal calcium levels.

If calcium levels can't be controlled with supplements, a once-daily injection of parathyroid hormone (Natpara) may be used to treatment low blood calcium due to hyperparathyroidism.

If your muscle spasms are especially severe, you may be given an intravenous (IV) injection of calcium to provide immediate, temporary relief.

Adrenal Gland Disorders

Your adrenal glands are located on top of your kidneys. Each gland is about the size of the end of your thumb and is shaped like a boomerang. The adrenal gland consists of two portions: the inner core (medulla) and the outer layer (cortex).

The medulla produces hormones called catecholamines. The most important of these are adrenaline (epinephrine) and noradrenaline (norepinephrine). Physical and emotional stresses usually trigger their release. When secreted into the bloodstream, catecholamines increase your heart rate and blood pressure and affect several other body functions.

The cortex produces hormones called corticosteroids. An area of your brain called the hypothalamus and the pituitary gland control the production of these hormones. There are three groups of corticosteroids:

Sex hormones

Sex hormones include male androgens and female estrogens, which affect sexual development and reproduction. Sex hormones are also produced in larger amounts in the testicles and ovaries.

Glucocorticoids

The cortisol family of hormones (glucocorticoids) influence the conversion of starchy foods into glycogen, a stored form of blood sugar. One important glucocorticoid is cortisol, which has many functions. Among other tasks, it helps regulate the immune system, helps maintain proper blood pressure and blood volume, and helps your body deal with physical stress.

Mineralocorticoids

Mineralocorticoids are corticosteroids that control the body's content of the minerals sodium and potassium. Aldosterone is the main member of this group.

Unlike other corticosteroids — which are controlled by the pituitary gland hormone adrenocorticotropic hormone (ACTH) — aldosterone is mainly controlled by the hormone renin. Renin is produced by the kidneys.

Adrenal gland hormones affect virtually every system in your body to some degree. Their effects are complex, and some of their actions overlap. When problems occur in this intricate system, serious diseases and disorders can develop.

Adrenal insufficiency

Signs and symptoms
- Weakness and fatigue
- Weight loss and decreased appetite
- Darkening of the skin
- Lightheadedness when standing
- Diarrhea, nausea or vomiting
- Low blood sugar
- Joint and muscle aches
- Irritability
- Salt craving

Emergency signs and symptoms
- Severe diarrhea and vomiting
- Pain in lower back, abdomen or legs
- Loss of consciousness

There are two forms of adrenal insufficiency. Primary adrenal insufficiency — better known as Addison's disease — occurs when the outer portion (cortex) of the adrenal gland fails to produce enough steroid hormones. Addison's disease most commonly results from an autoimmune disorder, a condition in which the body's own immune system attacks itself. Other causes include infections of the adrenal glands, spread of cancer to the adrenal glands or bleeding into the glands.

Secondary adrenal insufficiency results if your pituitary gland is diseased. The pituitary gland makes the hormone ACTH, which stimulates the adrenal cortex to produce its hormones. Inadequate production of ACTH can lead to insufficient production of hormones normally produced by your adrenal glands. Darkening of the skin and salt craving are not found in this form.

Signs and symptoms of adrenal insufficiency usually develop slowly, perhaps over several months, but they may appear suddenly. In acute adrenal failure

The adrenal glands are located on the top of the kidneys. They produce corticosteroid and catecholamine hormones. Catecholamines include adrenaline and noradrenaline.

Discovery of Adrenal Tumors

Most adrenal gland tumors are discovered incidentally during imaging studies conducted for another reason. For example, you might see your doctor because of abdominal pain. An ultrasound or computerized tomography (CT) scan of the abdomen is performed, and your doctor discovers a mass on one of your adrenal glands. Typically, this tumor is small and has nothing to do with whatever is causing your symptoms.

An adrenal tumor found in this way is sometimes called an adrenal incidentaloma — meaning it's discovered incidentally in the absence of symptoms of adrenal disease. In the last 20 years, development of more-sensitive imaging equipment has greatly increased discovery of such tumors.

Once an adrenal tumor is found, two things need to be determined: Is it cancerous? Is it overproducing a hormone? A CT scan or magnetic resonance imaging (MRI) of the mass may be ordered to check for characteristics such as size and density that can help in determining whether the tumor is cancerous (malignant). The vast majority of adrenal gland tumors are noncancerous (benign). If the tumor looks benign, your doctor probably will monitor it at regular intervals to check for any changes in size. Surgery may be recommended for large or growing tumors.

To determine if the tumor is overproducing hormones, you may need to undergo urine and blood tests to check for abnormally high or low hormone and electrolyte concentrations. Electrolytes are salts in your blood that are regulated by hormones.

(addisonian crisis), signs and symptoms generally include severe diarrhea, vomiting, dehydration and loss of consciousness.

Diagnosis

If your doctor thinks that you may have adrenal insufficiency, he or she will likely request blood and urine tests to measure the amounts of corticosteroid hormones. To confirm the diagnosis, your doctor may measure your body's response to an adrenal-stimulating hormone, adrenocorticotropic hormone (ACTH), which is produced by the pituitary gland. In this procedure, you receive an injection of synthetic ACTH, and the output of hormones from your adrenal cortex is measured. If your adrenal glands are damaged, the response is blunted or nonexistent.

If the cause of the disease isn't clear, your doctor may suggest an imaging test to check the size of your adrenal glands and look for other abnormalities.

Treatment

Hospitalization is essential for treatment of acute adrenal failure, which may be provoked by physical stress, infection, injury, vomiting, diarrhea or the use of diuretic medications. Adrenal failure is a life-threatening condition that requires prompt medical care, including intravenous (IV) salt solutions and steroid hormones. Treatment for adrenal insufficiency can alleviate symptoms and allow you to live a normal life.

Medication

Because your body isn't producing sufficient steroid hormones, your doctor may prescribe one or more hormone medications to treat the deficiency. These replacement hormones may include hydrocortisone or prednisone to replace cortisol.

A second drug, fludrocortisone, is used to replace aldosterone. Aldosterone controls your body's sodium and potassium needs and keeps your blood pressure normal.

You take the hormones in daily dosages that mimic the amount your body would normally produce, thereby minimizing side effects. If you're facing a stressful situation, such as an operation, infection or illness, your doctor may instruct you to temporarily increase your dosage. If you're sick and are vomiting, you may need to take an injectable form of the hormones. If you don't take the hormones as directed, you may be at risk of acute adrenal failure.

Carrying a medical alert card and wearing an alert bracelet or necklace at all times is critical. It's also wise to carry an emergency kit that includes a needle, syringe and injectable form of a corticosteroid.

Congenital adrenal hyperplasia

Signs and symptoms
- In male infants, enlargement of the penis
- In female infants, enlargement of the clitoris
- Acute adrenal failure (occasionally)
- High blood pressure (rarely)
- Accelerated growth in early childhood that stops early, resulting in short stature

This condition is the most common adrenal gland disorder in infants and children. It's the result of a genetic abnormality that leads to an enzyme deficiency, which in turn causes the adrenal glands to produce an abnormal pattern of steroid hormones. Some women have only a partial or mild deficiency of the enzyme. They develop normally in childhood but as young adults may have problems with abnormal hairiness (hirsutism), menstrual irregularities or infertility.

Diagnosis

When congenital adrenal hyperplasia is suspected, the doctor may conduct blood and urine tests to measure the levels of hormones produced by the adrenal gland.

Hirsutism

In some women, hair may begin to grow on the face, chest, abdomen and other locations where typically only men have hair. Such excessive hair growth, called hirsutism, may stem from the use of drugs such as phenytoin (Dilantin), used to treat some seizure disorders, and from some medications used to control high blood pressure. Certain disorders of the adrenal glands and ovaries also can cause hirsutism.

If a doctor can't find an explanation for the abnormal hair growth, the condition is referred to as idiopathic hirsutism — hairiness of unknown cause. Women with idiopathic hirsutism may have a slight increase in sensitivity to, or production of, androgen hormones. These are male sex hormones that are also normally produced by women. The condition poses no health risk but is often a matter of cosmetic concern.

No oral medication has been approved specifically for treating abnormal hair growth, but several drugs may be effective for suppressing androgen levels and controlling hirsutism. These include the diuretic spironolactone, and oral contraceptives that contain the hormones estrogen and progestin. A prescription cream (eflornithine) applied twice daily may slow the growth of facial hair.

Keep in mind, however, that these are potent drugs with possible side effects. In addition, they don't work for everyone and may take several months to produce an effect. Other methods to control unwanted hair, such as laser hair removal, may be preferable.

Treatment

Once this disorder has been diagnosed, it can usually be treated with medication. For most people, treatment consists of oral corticosteroid medication on a daily basis. Some people have both adrenal glands removed, allowing for treatment with lower doses of corticosteroids.

The main long-term risk is potential side effects from the medication, so the doctor will closely monitor skeletal and other growth patterns in young people.

Pheochromocytoma

Signs and symptoms
- High blood pressure
- Excessive sweating
- Increased heart rate or the sensation of a pounding heart
- Headache
- Skin intermittently becomes pale or loses color

Pheochromocytoma is a rare tumor in the core (medulla) of the adrenal gland that can produce large amounts of the hormones adrenaline (epinephrine) and noradrenaline (norepinephrine). The high blood pressure may be constant or come in episodes associated with sweating, a headache, pallor, and a fast or pounding heartbeat.

Up to 30 percent of pheochromocytomas have a genetic cause. The most common include von Hippel-Lindau (VHL) disease, multiple endocrine neoplasia type 2 (MEN 2) and neurofibromatosis type 1 (NF1). About 10 percent of pheochromocytomas are cancerous (malignant). The tumors may be associated with malignant tumors in other endocrine glands, such as the thyroid (medullary thyroid cancer).

Pheochromocytomas can be life-threatening if untreated. They can release dangerously high levels of adrenaline into the bloodstream after an injury or during surgery.

Diagnosis

Blood or urine tests that reveal elevated levels of epinephrine and norepinephrine or their breakdown products (metanephrines) strongly suggest pheochromocytoma. Additional testing to detect a tumor may include a computerized tomography (CT) scan, magnetic resonance imaging (MRI) or a radioisotope scan.

Treatment

Surgical removal of the entire gland is the usual treatment, and in most cases the signs and symptoms disappear. Before surgery, your doctor likely will prescribe medications to block the effects of the adrenal hormones and to control blood pressure.

Primary aldosteronism

Signs and symptoms
- High blood pressure
- Muscle weakness or cramps
- Occasionally, increased urination and thirst

Primary aldosteronism is a syndrome characterized by excess production of the hormone aldosterone from the outer portion (cortex) of the adrenal gland. The condition causes your body to retain too much sodium and water and to lose potassium, resulting in high blood pressure and low blood potassium levels.

Overproduction of aldosterone may result from a noncancerous (benign) tumor in an adrenal gland (aldosterone-producing adenoma) or overactivity of both adrenal glands (idiopathic hyperaldosteronism). Very rare causes include an inherited form of the disease and cancerous (malignant) adrenal tumors.

Diagnosis

A combination of high blood pressure and low blood potassium may be clues to the condition. Further blood and urine tests indicating excess aldosterone can confirm the diagnosis. Imaging of the adrenal glands and, sometimes, direct blood sampling of the veins that drain the glands are done to help determine the underlying cause.

Treatment

The main concern of this condition are the problems that can arise from increased blood pressure. Very low potassium levels also may cause muscle weakness, cramps, fatigue and heart problems.

If a tumor is found in one adrenal gland, surgery to remove the gland often improves blood pressure and normalizes hormone and potassium levels. Some individuals may continue to need medication for high blood pressure. For idiopathic hyperaldosteronism, your doctor may recommend a medication that blocks the effects of aldosterone.

Others

Rarely, adrenal tumors can produce sex hormones of the opposite sex. Men may experience erectile dysfunction or breast enlargement. Women may experience abnormal hair growth, menstrual irregularities and deepening of the voice.

Cancers of the adrenal cortex are very rare, but are usually aggressive. They can overproduce any of the adrenal hormones. Some, however, don't produce hormones.

Several other conditions can cause enlargement of the adrenal glands, including fatty tumors, infections and the spread of cancer from another location (metastasis).

Sex Gland Disorders

The sex glands are the testicles (testes) in men and the ovaries in women. These organs, also known as gonads, produce sperm and eggs, respectively. They also produce hormones that control secondary sexual characteristics, such as facial hair and breasts, that determine the differences between men and women. Sex hormones are also important to the reproductive process.

Both men and women produce male sex hormones (androgens) and female sex hormones (estrogen and progesterone), but androgens predominate in men and estrogen and progesterone are dominant in women. Disorders of the sex glands may result in various health disorders involving the secondary sexual characteristics.

Male sex gland disorders

Testosterone is the most important of the male sex hormones (androgens). During fetal development, testosterone is needed to form male genital organs. During puberty, it's required for the development of masculine physical characteristics, and in adult men, the hormone maintains muscle mass and strength, fat distribution, bone mass, sperm production, sex drive, and erectile function.

Deficiencies or imbalances in testosterone and other sex hormones can affect sexual development, sexual characteristics and fertility.

Abnormal puberty

In boys, normal puberty begins between ages 9 and 14, often around age 12. The milestones of puberty for boys include:

- Enlargement of the testicles and penis
- Appearance of pubic and armpit hair
- Deepening of the voice
- Accelerated growth
- Increase in muscle mass
- Facial hair

Disorders of puberty may include delayed puberty, premature (precocious) puberty, and incomplete or absent puberty. Delayed puberty is the most common problem. In most children, delayed puberty is just a variation of the normal process, and no specific cause is found. In these instances, puberty just occurs late, and the child becomes a normal adult. Both early and late puberty can run in families.

Sometimes, abnormal puberty is due to a medical condition. Delayed puberty may result from conditions such as hypopituitarism, genetic abnormalities, hypogonadism and some long-term illnesses, such as asthma and kidney disease. Puberty may also be delayed in children who are involved in extensive athletic training or excessive exercise, who have an eating disorder, who are malnourished or who've had chemotherapy or radiation.

Typically, precocious puberty is caused by the abnormally early onset of the hypothalamus and pituitary changes that start puberty. The reasons for this early onset — which can occur several years earlier than usual — are usually unknown. But it can also be caused by tumors of the brain, testicles or adrenal glands.

Additional causes include congenital adrenal hyperplasia (see page 1024) or severe hypothyroidism. Precocious puberty can result in shorter adult height.

Boys whose penis and testicles haven't completely developed five years after the start of development, or who haven't experienced any testicular development by age 14, may be experiencing late puberty. On the other hand, puberty may be early if a young boy has an increase in testicle size and penis length before age 9.

Diagnosis

To evaluate the possible cause of abnormal puberty, take your child in for a physical exam. The doctor might order some tests, including:

- Hormone levels in the blood
- An X-ray of the wrist to see if bone growth is normal
- A computerized tomography (CT) scan or magnetic resonance image (MRI) of the head to look for a tumor or brain injury
- Genetic studies

Treatment

Treatment depends on the cause. Sometimes, a cause can't be found, even after several tests. Hormone replacement may be given to start development of secondary sex characteristics. Hormone treatments are also available for certain types of premature puberty.

Sometimes, children experiencing abnormal puberty need help dealing with issues related to being either less or more sexually developed than their peers. Psychological counseling may be helpful. If you think that your child could benefit from counseling, talk to your doctor.

Gynecomastia

Gynecomastia is the term for male breast enlargement. It's common during puberty. As many as two-thirds of boys experience breast tenderness and enlargement during this time. Gynecomastia occurs as a result of changes in hormones — an imbalance in the ratio of estrogen to testosterone that can normally occur at puberty or as part of aging.

It's normal for newborn boys to have enlarged breast tissue due to exposure to maternal estrogen. This typically disappears soon after birth. In adult males, the most common cause of gynecomastia is hypogonadism. It may also occur as a result of using alcohol, certain medications and some drugs, including marijuana, amphetamines and heroin. Chronic liver disease, hyperthyroidism and rare endocrine tumors can cause breast enlargement, as can breast cancer, which occurs very rarely in men.

Some men and boys have fat on their chests that makes it look as if they have breasts. This isn't the same thing as gynecomastia.

Treatment

Whether you need treatment for gynecomastia depends on your age and what the doctor learns from your medical history and exam. In teenagers, breast enlargement usually goes away on its own in two or three years, and no treatment is necessary. Younger boys and adult men with gynecomastia usually should be evaluated to find out what's causing the problem.

Treatment is necessary if the breast enlargement is caused by a disease or tumor. In men with testosterone deficiency, hormone replacement can produce a dramatic improvement. Rarely, surgery may be necessary to remove the extra breast tissue. If there's concern that it could be cancer, you may have a mammogram and a small sample of tissue may be removed (biopsied) for laboratory analysis.

Hypogonadism

Male hypogonadism, sometimes referred to as testosterone deficiency, results from an inability of the testicles to produce testosterone, sperm or both. Hypogonadism can develop at any age, even before birth. Approximately 1 in 500 men and boys is affected.

The two basic types of male hypogonadism are primary testicular failure, caused by an abnormality in the testicles, and secondary testicular failure, which stems from a problem in the hypothalamus or pituitary gland. In secondary testicular failure, the testicles are normal, but they function improperly due to lack of stimulation by pituitary hormones.

Both forms of male hypogonadism can have many causes. It's important to establish the precise cause so that appropriate treatment can be prescribed. Common causes include:
- Klinefelter's syndrome, a congenital abnormality of the sex chromosomes
- Undescended testicles
- Too much iron in the blood
- Injury to the testicles
- Mumps infection after puberty
- Prior hernia surgery
- Cancer treatment using chemotherapy or radiation
  Secondary causes include:
- Kallmann's syndrome, a hypothalamic disorder
- Pituitary tumors

- Other pituitary disorders
- Medications, including some psychiatric drugs
- Normal aging

The effects of male hypogonadism are determined primarily by the stage of life when it occurs. During fetal development, hypogonadism may affect development of the external genitalia, leading to a condition called ambiguous genitalia, in which the sex of the newborn isn't clear from external examination.

When hypogonadism occurs during puberty, it may slow growth and impair development of many secondary sex characteristics. A boy with this condition may not develop increased muscle mass, a deepened voice and body hair. The penis and testicles may not grow. Changes in skeletal development can lead to unusually long arms and legs, disproportionate to height.

In adult males, hypogonadism can cause decreased libido, erectile dysfunction and infertility. It may lead to a decrease in facial and body hair growth, thinning of the skin, development of breast tissue (gynecomastia) and loss of bone mass. Mental and emotional changes, such as mood swings, irritability, decreased sex drive and depression can accompany hypogonadism.

Diagnosis

Early diagnosis and treatment can protect men against osteoporosis and other risks of untreated hypogonadism.

A diagnosis of hypogonadism is based on symptoms and the results of blood tests that measure testosterone levels. Additional studies may be done to determine the cause. These may include hormone testing, semen analysis, pituitary imaging, genetic studies and testicular biopsy.

Treatment

Treatment depends on the cause. Testosterone replacement therapy given by injection, patch or gel is effective in restoring normal testosterone levels. In boys, it can stimulate the physical changes of puberty. No effective treatment exists to restore sperm production if you have primary hypogonadism. If a pituitary problem is the cause, pituitary hormones may stimulate sperm production and restore fertility. A pituitary tumor may require surgical removal, medication or hormone replacement.

Female sex gland disorders

In females, sex hormones work together in an intricate pattern to make the reproductive cycle function smoothly. The major female sex hormones are estrogen and progesterone, which are produced mainly by the ovaries during the reproductive years.

Besides helping control ovulation, conception and pregnancy, estrogen maintains bone strength and helps regulate cholesterol. Progesterone works with estrogen to prepare a woman's body for conception and pregnancy and helps regulate her menstrual cycle.

Problems with production and release of sex hormones can affect sexual development, sexual characteristics and fertility.

Abnormal puberty
In girls, puberty normally begins between ages 8 and 14. Milestones of puberty include:
- Development of breast buds
- Appearance of pubic and armpit hair
- Menstruation

Abnormal puberty may include delayed puberty, premature (precocious) puberty, and incomplete or absent puberty. Delayed puberty is the most common problem. In most children, delayed puberty is just a variation of the normal process, and no specific cause is found. In these instances, puberty occurs late, but the child becomes a normal adult. Both early and late puberty can run in families.

Sometimes, abnormal puberty is due to a medical condition. Delayed puberty may be caused by hypopituitarism, genetic abnormalities, hypogonadism and some long-term illnesses, such as asthma and kidney disease. Puberty may also be delayed in children who are involved in extensive athletic training or excessive exercise, who have an eating disorder, who are malnourished, or who've had chemotherapy or radiation.

Typically, precocious puberty is caused by the abnormally early onset of the hypothalamus and pituitary changes that start puberty. The reasons for this early onset — which can occur several years earlier than usual — are often unknown. Precocious puberty can also be caused by tumors of the brain or adrenal glands, or severe hypothyroidism. A potential long-term consequence of premature puberty is shorter height.

A girl may be experiencing early puberty if she develops breasts and pubic hair before age 8. Puberty may be delayed if a girl hasn't developed breast tissue by age 14 or hasn't had a menstrual period within five years of the first appearance of breast tissue.

Diagnosis
To evaluate the possible cause of abnormal puberty, a doctor will likely perform a physical examination and may order tests, including:
- Blood tests to check hormone levels
- An X-ray of the wrist to see if bone growth is normal
- Imaging tests of the head to look for a tumor or brain injury
- Ultrasound of the ovaries
- Genetic studies

Treatment
Treatment depends on what's causing the problems. Sometimes the cause can't be found. Hormone therapy may initiate the development of secondary sex characteristics. It also may be used for certain types of premature puberty.

Some children need help dealing with issues related to being either less or more sexually developed than their peers. Psychological counseling may be helpful. If you think your child could benefit from counseling, talk to your doctor.

Hypogonadism
Female hypogonadism occurs when the ovaries produce inadequate quantities of sex hormones. Primary hypogonadism originates from an abnormality in the ovaries, and secondary hypogonadism stems from a problem in the hypothalamus or pituitary gland. In secondary hypogonadism, the ovaries function improperly due to lack of stimulation by pituitary hormones.

Primary hypogonadism may be caused by Turner syndrome, a congenital abnormality of the sex chromosomes, by other genetic disorders or by an autoimmune disease that causes ovarian failure.

Causes of secondary hypogonadism include hypopituitarism, disorders involving the hypothalamus, polycystic ovary syndrome, severe stress, anorexia nervosa and excessive exercise. Many times, no clear cause can be found.

Except in Turner's syndrome, symptoms of female hypogonadism usually aren't apparent until puberty. In premenopausal women, signs and symptoms include:
- Irregular or absent menstrual periods
- Infertility
- Decreased vaginal secretions
- Decreased sex drive
- A decrease in breast size

Left untreated, females with hypogonadism are at increased risk of developing osteoporosis.

Diagnosis
A diagnosis is based on symptoms and the results of blood tests that measure estrogen and other sex hormone levels. Other studies may include chromosomal (genetic) testing, a magnetic resonance

image (MRI) of the pituitary gland and an ultrasound scan of the ovaries.

Treatment
Treatment depends on the cause. Hormone replacement with estrogen and progesterone can help women maintain secondary sexual characteristics and restore a normal menstrual cycle. To treat infertility, medications that stimulate ovulation may be used.

If a pituitary problem is the cause, pituitary hormones may be prescribed. A pituitary tumor may require surgical removal, medication or hormone therapy.

Virilization
Normally, a woman's ovaries and adrenal glands secrete some male hormones (androgens) such as testosterone. Virilization is a rare condition in which excess androgens circulate in your body, most often because your ovaries or adrenal glands are overproducing these hormones. Excess androgens may also come from taking androgen hormones, such as dehydroepiandrosterone (DHEA).

An excess of male hormones in a woman leads to development of masculine physical characteristics such as excessive hair growth, increased muscle bulk, deepening of the voice and irregular menstrual periods.

Diagnosis
If you have signs of virilization, seek prompt medical attention because a cancerous (malignant) tumor is possible. Your doctor will likely perform a physical exam and request blood tests to measure the levels of male hormones. You may also have imaging tests of your ovaries or adrenal glands to detect the presence of a tumor or identify polycystic ovaries.

Treatment
Once the underlying cause of the condition is identified, treatment may include surgery to remove a tumor or medication to reduce androgen production.

Endocrine Syndromes

Some disorders of the endocrine system affect more than one gland. An individual may have symptoms of several endocrine problems.

Two main groups of disorders affect multiple endocrine glands. In polyglandular autoimmune (PGA) syndromes, several endocrine glands become underactive and produce lower than normal amounts of hormones. In multiple endocrine neoplasia (MEN) syndromes, tumors develop in more than one of the endocrine glands.

Polyglandular autoimmune syndromes and MEN syndromes are inherited. For that reason, family members of a person with an endocrine syndrome are usually screened for a possible genetic defect or to detect signs of a disorder before serious problems appear.

Polyglandular autoimmune syndromes

Polyglandular autoimmune (PGA) syndromes cause several endocrine glands to underproduce hormones. A person with such a syndrome has an inherited tendency to develop antibodies that react to cells in the endocrine glands. This can cause inflammation of endocrine glands and, eventually, destruction of the glands. As the glands are destroyed, they stop producing hormones, leading to various disorders.

Types
There are two PGA syndromes — type 1 and type 2:

PGA 1
Type 1 is a rare inherited disorder that usually develops in early childhood and is equally prevalent among girls and boys. Frequent yeast infections in childhood are often the first sign of the syndrome. Two other features are an underactive parathyroid gland (hypoparathyroidism) and underactive adrenal glands. These problems may not develop until middle age. People with PGA 1 may also have hypogonadism, hepatitis, gallstones, difficulty in absorbing food, loss of skin pigmentation and type 1 diabetes.

PGA 2
Type 2 is more common. It also runs in families, and is seen more often in women than in men, with symptoms often beginning in young adulthood. In this disorder, the adrenal glands are underactive, and the thyroid gland may be underactive or overactive. A person with PGA 2 may have primary adrenal insufficiency, Graves' disease or autoimmune (Hashimoto's) thyroiditis, type 1 diabetes, hypogonadism, myasthenia gravis, and celiac disease. Type 2 doesn't involve recurrent yeast infections or hypoparathyroidism.

Treatment
Treatment depends on the type you have and your symptoms. If you have a hormone deficiency, you may need to take hormone therapy. This may include thyroid hormone, corticosteroids and insulin. Screening tests may detect problems before serious signs and symptoms develop.

Multiple endocrine neoplasia syndromes

Multiple endocrine neoplasia (MEN) syndromes are rare inherited diseases in which tumors develop in several endocrine glands. The syndromes are generally inherited, but there's variability, even within the same family, of which glands will develop tumors. The tumors may appear as early as infancy or as late as age 70. They may be noncancerous (benign) or cancerous (malignant). Signs and symptoms result mostly from production of excess hormones.

Types

There are two main types of MEN, based on which glands develop tumors.

MEN 1

People with MEN type 1 (MEN 1) have tumors of the parathyroid gland, the islet cells of the pancreas, the pituitary gland or all three. This type involves a genetic abnormality on chromosome 11.

MEN 2

MEN type 2 has two subtypes, MEN 2A and MEN 2B. Both are associated with genetic defects on chromosome 10 and include a rare type of thyroid cancer (medullary thyroid cancer) and adrenal gland tumors called pheochromocytomas. Parathyroid tumors can occur in MEN 2A but are rare in MEN 2B.

Individuals with MEN 2B typically have long limbs and loose joints, as well as growths or nodules around the nerves (ganglioneuromas) that may be noticeable on the eyes, lips and tongue. The nodules are also found in the gastrointestinal tract.

Treatment

Doctors generally treat each tumor individually, either by removing it or by correcting the hormone imbalance. Some people need multiple surgical procedures on two or more endocrine glands.

Several different mutations can cause MEN 2, and the specific mutation can indicate the age the individual will get medullary thyroid cancer. The results of genetic testing allow doctors to determine the best time to have the thyroid gland removed in a child who has inherited the disease. Often, such surgery occurs in early infancy to young adulthood.

If you receive a diagnosis of MEN, screening of your immedi-ate blood relatives is very important. Early detection and treatment can be lifesaving. Genetic testing along with blood and urine tests to measure hormone levels can detect early stages of the tumors. When detected early, these tumors have a much greater chance of being removed with a favorable outcome.

Obesity

It's common to hear people attribute their weight gain or being overweight to "low metabolism," heredity or a medical problem. This is rarely the case.

Genes and metabolism do play a role in your weight, but in most cases, the amount you weigh is determined by your diet and physical activity. Consuming too many calories, being physically inactive or both lead to obesity.

Genetics

A family history of obesity increases your chance of becoming obese by about 30 percent. Your genes affect the rate at which your body accumulates fat and where that fat is stored. By influencing the amount of body fat and fat distribution, genes can make you more susceptible to gaining weight.

Researchers have identified several genes known to contribute to obesity. In most cases, multiple genes interact in complex ways to cause obesity. These mechanisms aren't fully understood. A few rare inherited diseases, such as Prader-Willi syndrome and Cohen syndrome, are known to cause obesity.

In most cases of obesity, environmental factors exert an enormous influence. It's easy to eat too much in a society where large portions of high-fat foods are the norm. Plus, many people aren't physically active.

Metabolic and endocrine disorders

Some people have a naturally high metabolic thermostat — they tend to burn more calories than average even when they're asleep. Other individuals need fewer calories for the same physical activity. A low metabolic rate is rarely a cause of obesity, however.

Some endocrine disorders can cause weight gain. However, less than 5 percent of all cases of obesity can be traced to a metabolic disorder or hormonal imbalance. Endocrine disorders that may lead to obesity include:
- Cushing syndrome
- Hypothyroidism
- Insulinoma
- Tumors, injury or inflammation of the hypothalamus
- Polycystic ovary syndrome

For information on how to lose weight, see Chapter 8, "Nutrition and Weight." ■

Blood and Lymphatic System

Your blood performs a remarkable number of vital functions as it circulates throughout your body. In the tissues of your lungs, it picks up inhaled oxygen and delivers it via your arteries to tissues throughout your body. Simultaneously, your blood removes carbon dioxide from these tissues and returns it via your veins to your lungs, where it's exhaled.

Your blood carries life-sustaining nutrients from your intestines to cells throughout your body. When waste products from these cells need to be removed, your blood transports them to your kidneys, where they're filtered out, channeled into your urinary tract and excreted via your urine. Blood also transports chemicals such as hormones, helping various body parts communicate with one another and coordinate their functions.

Blood acts as a medium for your immune system by carrying cells that fight infections, as well as proteins (antibodies) that help protect your body against foreign substances. And it even helps to regulate your body temperature by dissipating heat produced in your muscles.

Understanding Your Blood

All of the crucial functions of your blood are performed by blood cells and the liquid part of your blood, called plasma. Most blood cells are produced in bone marrow located in cavities of certain bones. The majority of these cells mature and develop into specific types of blood cells within the bone marrow, but some complete the maturation process in the spleen or lymph nodes.

Blood composition

Your blood includes the following components:

Red blood cells

Red blood cells (erythrocytes) are the most abundant cells in your blood. They contain hemoglobin, a red, iron-rich, complex substance. Hemoglobin binds to oxygen in your lungs and is carried through the bloodstream to tiny blood vessels (capillaries). There the hemoglobin releases the oxygen so that it can move out of the bloodstream to cells in tissues and organs.

White blood cells

White blood cells (leukocytes) defend your body against foreign invaders, including infection-causing bacteria, viruses, fungi and parasites. The three main types of white blood cells are:
- Granulocytes, which include neutrophils, eosinophils and basophils
- Monocytes
- Lymphocytes, which include B cells and T cells
Granulocytes and monocytes respond to many different types of infection and defend your body

An Enlarged Spleen

Your spleen is located in the upper left part of your abdomen, protected by your rib cage. It has at least four major functions.
- As part of the immune system, it clears foreign organisms and antigens from the bloodstream. It also generates part of the antibody response to foreign invaders.
- It helps remove abnormal blood cells from the bloodstream.
- It helps regulate blood flow to the liver.
- Under some conditions, it may become a major site for producing blood cells.
Normally, a doctor can't feel your spleen because it's located under your rib cage. In some situations, though, the spleen enlarges (splenomegaly) and can be felt. This enlargement may occur without symptoms, or it may be accompanied by pain.

Acute enlargement of the spleen may be caused by bleeding within the organ. The bleeding may be the result of trauma to the left rib cage or upper abdomen. Enlargement can also occur with the following:

- Diseases resulting from immune system dysfunction, such as rheumatoid arthritis, systemic lupus erythematosus and immunohemolytic anemia.
- Diseases that obstruct the flow of blood to the liver, such as cirrhosis, obstruction of the major vein to the liver (portal vein) and congestive heart failure with backup of blood into the liver.
- Diseases in which abnormal red blood cells are present, such as thalassemia and sickle cell disease.
- Diseases that cause infiltration of abnormal cells into the spleen, including cancers such as leukemia and lymphoma and the noncancerous condition amyloidosis.
- Diseases such as infectious mononucleosis, tuberculosis, histoplasmosis, bacterial endocarditis and malaria. With these diseases, spleen enlargement is typically accompanied by a fever.

To further evaluate an enlarged spleen, a doctor may order tests such as an ultrasound or a computerized tomography (CT) scan, and treatment will be directed at the underlying cause. Sometimes, to make the correct diagnosis, the spleen needs to be surgically removed.

by engulfing foreign substances. Lymphocytes react to specific infectious agents.

Platelets

Platelets (thrombocytes) are colorless blood cells that repair injured blood vessels. They stop blood loss by gathering at the site of the injury and forming plugs in vessel holes. This is the first step in clot formation (coagulation), a process that's completed by proteins called clotting factors, which travel in the plasma.

Plasma

Plasma is a yellowish liquid that carries clotting factors and other proteins. It's basically what's left after the cells are removed from your blood. Serum is plasma from which the clotting factors also have been removed.

Lymph

Lymph is a nearly colorless fluid that's collected in the channels of your lymphatic system throughout your body and ultimately enters your bloodstream. Lymph helps return water and proteins from tissues to your blood.

Blood tests

When a blood disorder is suspected, often one of the first steps is to order blood tests. For these tests, blood is drawn from a vein in your arm or from capillaries in your fingertip and taken to a laboratory for analysis. Blood tests are also often part of a routine physical examination. Among blood tests are:

Complete blood count

The most common blood test is a complete blood count (CBC). It involves counting the number of each type of blood cell in a given volume of your blood and examining the cells under a microscope to check for any abnormalities in their size or shape.

A CBC includes the following blood tests:

Red blood cell count
This test counts the number of red blood cells in a microliter of blood.

Hemoglobin
This test measures the grams of hemoglobin in a deciliter of blood. A woman's hemoglobin is considered low if it's less than 10 grams per deciliter (g/dL), and a man's if it's less than 12 g/dL.

Hematocrit
This test measures the percentage of your blood volume made up of red blood cells. The normal hematocrit value in women is about 42 percent, and in men, about 47 percent.

Red blood cell size and shape
Several tests are used to measure the size and the shape (morphology and indices) of red blood cells and the amount of hemoglobin in each cell. A blood smear — a small drop of blood spread on a microscope slide — is examined under a microscope to determine the shape and appearance of red blood cells and provide clues about illnesses, such as the specific type of anemia.

Reticulocyte count
This test involves counting the immature red blood cells called reticulocytes. The count gives an indication of whether your bone marrow is functioning adequately.

Other tests

If your doctor wants to check for a disorder that involves a specific type of white blood cell, he or she will do a differential count. This determines the relative amounts of each type of white blood cell. Other blood tests measure the number of platelets and the bleeding time, an indication of how well your platelets are functioning.

To study how well your body is making new blood cells, your doctor may examine a sample of your bone marrow under a microscope. The marrow usually is taken from the back of the large pelvic bone.

Red Blood Cells

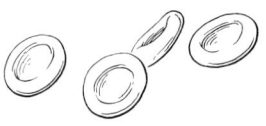

White Blood Cells

Granulocytes   **Monocytes**

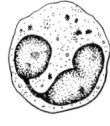 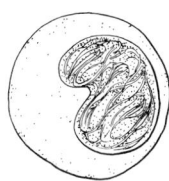

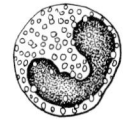

Lymphocytes

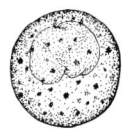 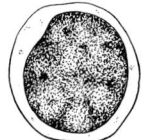

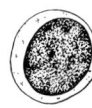

Platelets

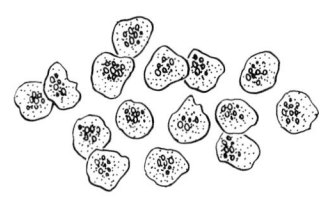

Red blood cells (erythrocytes) contain hemoglobin. White blood cells (leukocytes) defend your body against foreign invaders and are made of three types: granulocytes, monocytes and lymphocytes. Platelets (thrombocytes) help stop bleeding from injured blood vessels.

Blood disorders

Many blood-related problems can be treated by your personal physician. For more-serious blood conditions, you may be referred to a specialist in blood disorders (hematologist).

There are many blood disorders, each caused by a malfunction of a certain component of your blood. For example, anemias are characterized by too few red blood cells. Leukemias usually result from too many white blood cells, and bleeding disorders are often caused by defects in platelets, platelet numbers or clotting factors.

Bone Marrow Disorders

Bone marrow lies in spaces within the center of your bones and is the manufacturing plant responsible for making blood cells. Normally, it produces all of your red blood cells and platelets and most of your white blood cells.

When something goes wrong with your bone marrow, the consequences are often serious. Production of cells may no longer be orderly, and deficiencies may occur, leading to anemia, bleeding disorders and a vulnerability to infections.

In a young child, all of the bones contain active marrow that forms blood cells. As the body matures, active blood-forming marrow is found only in the bones of the spine, skull, ribs and pelvis. However, if the body requires extra blood cells, bone marrow in the arms and legs may be stimulated to again revert to active production.

If your doctor thinks that you may have a bone marrow disorder, a sample of your bone marrow will likely be removed by way of a thin needle inserted into bone (biopsy). The sample is then studied under a microscope.

Bone Marrow Biopsy

A bone marrow biopsy is sometimes needed to diagnose a bone marrow disorder or lymphoma. A local anesthetic is generally given at the site of the biopsy, or you may be given a light general anesthetic. In a process called aspiration, a special needle is inserted into a pelvic bone or breastbone, and a small sample of the marrow is withdrawn through the needle using suction. The sample is removed from the needle and examined under a microscope.

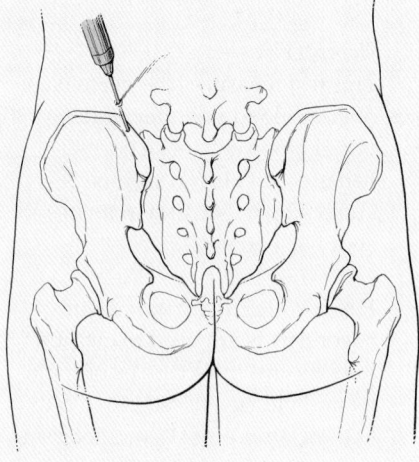

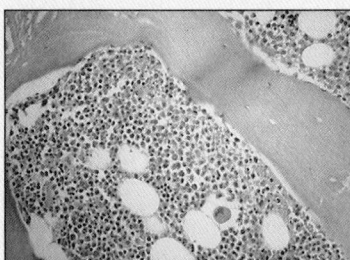

In a bone marrow biopsy, a needle is used to remove a sample of bone marrow for examination under a microscope.

Myelodysplastic syndrome

Signs and symptoms
- Fatigue
- Shortness of breath
- Paleness due to anemia
- Easy or unusual bruising or bleeding
- Frequent infections

Within your bone marrow, stem cells — master cells from which all specialized blood cells are formed — develop into mature blood cells. In people with myelodysplastic syndrome (MDS), the stem cells don't mature or function properly, leading to a lack of red blood cells, white blood cells and platelets.

In the United States, each year approximately 13,000 people receive a diagnosis of MDS. The disorder can occur at any age, but it's more likely to develop in people age 60 and older.

Because close to 1 in 3 people with myelodysplastic syndrome eventually develops acute myelogenous leukemia, the condition is sometimes referred to as a precancer.

Causes
Often, this syndrome develops for no apparent reason. In some people, it may develop after treatment with certain chemotherapy drugs or after radiation therapy. In addition, exposure to toxic chemicals — benzene in particular — is thought to increase the risk of MDS. The condition usually doesn't run in families.

Diagnosis
MDS is generally suspected through blood tests to check the number of red and white blood cells and platelets and to determine if any of the blood cells have an abnormal size, shape or appearance. Bone marrow tests are needed to confirm the diagnosis. MDS occurs in several forms, each distinguished by the number and appearance of immature cells (blasts) in the bone marrow.

How serious is myelodysplastic syndrome?
Myelodysplastic syndrome may

be mild and take a chronic, painless course. On the other hand, some types are aggressive and may progress to acute myelogenous leukemia (see page 1049). For most people with this syndrome, a cure remains elusive. Treatment is primarily focused on controlling symptoms and improving quality of life.

Treatment
The mainstay of treatment is supportive care with transfusions of red blood cells to manage anemia and platelets to control bleeding.

Medication
Antibiotics may be given to help control infections associated with low white blood cell counts. Treatment may also include the use of growth factors. These natural protein substances found in the body may help stimulate the production of healthy blood cells.

Chemotherapy
Some forms of MDS respond very well to a new medication called lenalidomide (Revlimid), a drug that's chemically similar to thalidomide (Thalomid). Other new drugs such as azacitidine (Vidaza) and decitabine (Dacogen) have shown promise in selected individuals.

Conventional chemotherapy drugs commonly used to treat acute leukemia may be used in younger people with MDS. Although not a cure, chemotherapy may put the disease in remission for a short time. Older adults generally don't tolerate chemotherapy as well.

Stem cell transplantation
The only real chance for a cure depends on a successful stem cell transplant (see page 1062). These transplants generally aren't tolerated well by older adults and carry a risk of side effects. For this reason, few people with myelodysplastic syndrome are candidates for bone marrow stem cell transplant.

Polycythemia vera

Signs and symptoms
- Headache
- Dizziness
- Itching, especially after a warm bath or shower
- Redness of your skin
- Shortness of breath
- A feeling of fullness or bloating in left upper abdomen
- Fatigue

Polycythemia vera occurs when bone marrow produces too many red blood cells. The condition may also result in production of too many white blood cells and platelets, but it's the excess of red blood cells that thickens your blood and causes most of the health concerns associated with the disease.

Because polycythemia vera causes your blood to thicken and slows blood flow, it increases your risk of developing blood clots, which can lead to a stroke or heart attack.

Polycythemia vera generally appears in late middle age. It's extremely rare in children. Almost all individuals with polycythemia vera have a mutation in the gene JAK2. This mutation doesn't run in families, but appears to be acquired during a person's lifetime. Signs and symptoms associated with the disease develop gradually.

Diagnosis
The first step in a diagnosis is usually blood tests. Your doctor may also request a measurement of vitamin B-12 and certain other substances, such as leukocyte alkaline phosphatase, in your blood. Often, these values are unusually high in this disorder. Uric acid levels also are increased, which may cause attacks of gout.

Another sign is an increase in the volume of blood without much of an increase in its plasma component. Your doctor can determine this with special blood tests.

Additional tests are used to differentiate polycythemia vera from secondary polycythemia, in which too many red blood cells result from other causes, such as heavy cigarette smoking, severe lung disease or living at high altitudes.

In polycythemia vera, blood and bone marrow can be evaluated for the presence of the JAK2 mutation. Additionally, the level of the hormone (erythropoietin) that stimulates red blood cell production is abnormally low. In contrast, in secondary polycythemia, the blood's high content of red blood cells is a response to the low oxygen concentration in the air and therefore in the blood. Because there's less oxygen in the blood, the body attempts to overcome the deficiency by making more red blood cells until there are too many.

A blood test to determine the oxygen content of the blood is helpful in the evaluation. Another helpful blood test is one that checks the level of erythropoietin, a hormone naturally produced by the kidneys to stimulate blood cell production. In polycythemia vera, the erythropoietin level is generally suppressed, but it's often increased in secondary polycythemia.

How serious is polycythemia vera?
Without treatment, signs and symptoms of polycythemia vera generally worsen, and your risk of death from a stroke or heart attack increases. With proper treatment, the risk of a stroke or heart attack lessens, but there's no cure. Most people live for more than 10 years with the disease. After many years, scarring (fibrosis) of bone marrow may occur. In a small percentage of people with polycythemia vera, acute leukemia eventually develops.

Treatment
To decrease the volume of circulating blood, blood is withdrawn from a vein (phlebotomy). This also helps decrease blood thickening and lessens the danger of a stroke. The schedule of withdrawal is about a pint of blood every few days to weeks or months.

Medication

To help suppress your bone marrow's ability to produce blood cells, your doctor may prescribe medication, such as hydroxyurea (Droxia). The use of hydroxyurea may be associated with an increased risk of developing acute leukemia at a later date. However, this remains unproved, and in general, the benefits of the medication appear to outweigh the possible risks of leukemia.

Interferon-alfa may be used to treat polycythemia vera in individuals who don't respond to other treatments. In addition, aspirin is usually recommended for people with this condition to reduce the risk of blood clots.

Surgery

The increased number of blood cells forces your spleen to work harder than normal, which causes it to increase in size. If your spleen becomes extremely enlarged, which is rare, your doctor may surgically remove your spleen.

Primary myelofibrosis

Signs and symptoms
- Breathlessness on exertion
- A rapid heartbeat
- Paleness
- A feeling of fullness or bloating in left upper abdomen
- Night sweats
- Weight loss
- A stuffed feeling after eating

In primary myelofibrosis, bone marrow gradually becomes scarred, making it less able to manufacture blood cells. Blood cells may be produced outside of the marrow, in the spleen and liver, sometimes causing these organs to become enlarged. Another name for this disorder is agnogenic myeloid metaplasia.

Treatment

For individuals with low-risk myelofibrosis, the medication most commonly used is hydroxyurea (Droxia). For individuals with debilitating symptoms and a large spleen, a drug called ruxolitinib (Jakafi) that blocks a mutation in the gene JAK2 may be prescribed.

Allogeneic stem cell transplantation may help cure the disease but it has substantial risks and is usually an option only for younger individuals with high-risk features.

Most people with this disease become dependent on blood transfusions for survival (see page 1060). Enlargement of the spleen may cause pain or reduce the number of platelets in your blood by trapping them in the spleen. On occasion, a doctor may advise surgical removal of the spleen if other treatments fail.

Plasma Cell Disorders

Plasma cells secrete antibodies called immunoglobulins (Ig) to help your body fight infections and other foreign antigens. The five classes of immunoglobulins in the body are IgA, IgD, IgE, IgG and IgM. This section discusses important plasma cell disorders.

Multiple myeloma

Signs and symptoms
- Bone pain
- Unexplained bone fractures
- Excessive thirst and urination
- Constipation
- Nausea and lack of appetite
- Weight loss
- Mental confusion
- Repeat infections
- Leg weakness and numbness

Multiple myeloma is a cancer in your plasma cells. Plasma cells are a type of white blood cell present in your bone marrow.

In multiple myeloma, abnormal plasma cells grow and take up more space in the marrow. This leads to erosion of bone, causing bone pain and bone weakening, particularly in the back and ribs.

Calcium may leach out of eroded bones, causing elevated calcium levels in your blood. This can cause symptoms such as nausea, constipation and dehydration.

The disease also interferes with the function of your bone marrow and immune system, which can lead to anemia and infection. Multiple myeloma may also cause kidney problems, including those resulting from elevated blood calcium levels.

The disease primarily affects people older than 40, with the average age at diagnosis between 65 and 70. It's almost twice as common among blacks as whites. Native Pacific Islanders also are at increased risk.

Causes

While the exact cause of the disease isn't known, doctors do know that multiple myeloma begins with an abnormal plasma cell in your bone marrow, which begins to multiply. Researchers are studying the DNA of plasma cells to understand what changes cause the cells to become cancerous. About 50 percent of people with the disease have chromosome 14 abnormalities. Of the remaining group, most have extra copies of certain chromosomes (trisomies).

Diagnosis

If your doctor suspects multiple myeloma, he or she may request blood and urine tests to look for abnormalities. Cancerous plasma cells (myeloma cells) produce abnormal proteins called M proteins. Your doctor may check samples of your blood and urine for the presence of such proteins. When a portion of the M protein is excreted in the urine, it's called the Bence Jones protein, after the doctor who discovered the substance.

Your doctor likely will also take a sample of your bone marrow for analysis. X-rays will show if your bones have any of the lesions — punched-out areas of bone — that characterize the disease.

How serious is multiple myeloma?

Although there's no cure for this disease, treatment can control the disease for many years and relieve symptoms. Your doctor will monitor your progress and response to treatment and will watch for complications such as osteoporosis, decreased kidney function and infections.

Treatment

If you have multiple myeloma and you aren't experiencing symptoms, you may not need any treatment. However, your doctor will likely monitor your condition at variable intervals, checking for evidence to indicate the disease is progressing, such as increasing levels of M protein in your blood or urine.

If you're experiencing symptoms, treatment can help relieve pain, control complications, stabilize your condition and slow the progress of the disease.

Medication

The treatment of myeloma has improved greatly in recent years. Drugs used to treat the disease include thalidomide (Thalomid), lenalidomide (Revlimid), pomalidomide (Pomalyst), bortezomib (Velcade), carfilzomib (Kyprolis), ixazomib (Ninlaro), daratumumab (Darzalex), Elotuzumab (Empliciti) and panobinostat (Farydak). Other drugs to treat myeloma include chemotherapy, as well as corticosteroids (prednisone or dexamethasone). These medications may be used alone or in combination to help kill myeloma cancer cells. Analgesics can alleviate bone pain.

Treatment for multiple myeloma is often given in cycles over a period of months, followed by a rest period. Treatment may be discontinued during a plateau phase, or remission, when your M protein level remains stable, and resumed if the level begins to rise.

When taken by pregnant women, medications such as thalidomide, lenalidomide and pomalidomide can cause severe birth defects, such as malformations of the arms, legs and organs. Therefore, the Food and Drug Administration has put in place stringent prescribing regulations.

Many multiple myeloma treatments are designed to help your body's immune system recognize and eliminate myeloma cells. Your doctor may be aware of clinical trials available to you.

Radiation

Sometimes, high-energy radiation may be directed at specific sites to destroy myeloma cells or stop their growth. The treatment, usually aimed at the spine and affected bones, can help control severe pain.

Stem cell transplantation

For people who are generally healthy, an autologous stem cell transplant is often recommended as part of the initial treatment (see page 1063).

Surgery

If your bones become unstable, surgery may be of benefit.

Other therapies

Staying active helps to retain the calcium in your bones and keep them strong. Some restrictions, such as avoiding heavy lifting, may be necessary. If pain is disabling, a back brace, cane or other support device might help you.

Amyloidosis

Signs and symptoms

Signs and symptoms of amyloidosis depend on the organs affected. The wide range of symptoms often makes this disease difficult to diagnose. Some people have no symptoms.

Signs and symptoms include:
- Swelling of your ankles and legs
- Weakness
- Weight loss
- Shortness of breath
- Numbness or tingling in your hands or feet
- Diarrhea
- Severe fatigue
- An enlarged tongue
- Skin changes
- An irregular heartbeat
- Difficulty swallowing

In addition to producing red and white blood cells and platelets, your bone marrow makes antibodies, proteins that protect you against infection and disease. After antibodies serve their purpose, your body breaks them down and recycles them.

Amyloidosis is a rare disease that occurs when cells in the bone marrow produce antibodies that can't be broken down. These antibodies build up in the bloodstream and may be deposited in your tissues or organs, interfering with their normal function. Amyloidosis most often affects the heart, kidneys, liver, spleen, nervous system and gastrointestinal tract.

Amyloidosis is classified into four major forms:
- **AL amyloidosis.** This type is referred to as light chain amyloidosis or primary amyloidosis. It's caused by multiplication of certain cells in the bone marrow called plasma cells. It primarily affects your heart, lungs, skin, tongue, nerves and intestines. AL amyloidosis results from deposits of portions of the proteins produced by plasma cells. Because the abnormal multiplication of plasma cells responsible for AL amyloidosis is also the cause of multiple myeloma (see opposite page), the two disorders sometimes coexist.
- **AA amyloidosis.** This form, also known as secondary amyloidosis, occurs in association with chronic infectious or inflammatory diseases such as rheumatoid arthritis, tuberculosis and bone infection (osteomyelitis). AA amyloidosis primarily affects your kidneys, spleen, liver and intestines, although other organs may be involved.

- **Hereditary amyloidosis.** As the name implies, this form of amyloidosis is inherited. It affects the nerves, heart and kidneys.
- **Senile amyloidosis.** This form of amyloidosis occurs in older adults, most commonly causing heart failure. Senile amyloidosis requires no specific therapy.

Diagnosis

Blood and urine tests may detect an abnormal protein that may indicate amyloidosis, but the definitive test is a tissue biopsy. If your doctor suspects that you have systemic amyloidosis — meaning that it affects several parts of your body rather than just one organ — the biopsy may be taken from your abdominal fat, bone marrow or other involved organs in the body. The tissue is examined under a microscope. These biopsies are relatively minor procedures conducted in an outpatient setting using a local anesthetic.

Occasionally, samples are taken from the liver, nerves, heart or kidney to help determine if a specific organ is affected. These procedures may require hospitalization.

How serious is amyloidosis?

The severity of the disorder depends on the type of amyloidosis and the number and extent of the organs affected. Potentially life-threatening situations include kidney failure and congestive heart failure. If the amyloid accumulations are limited to less crucial sites, you may experience no symptoms. Most cases fall between these two extremes.

Treatment

There's no cure for amyloidosis, but treatment may help control symptoms and limit the production of amyloid protein. Treatment varies greatly depending on the specific type of amyloidosis. Managing the disease is primarily done with diet and many types of medication.

Granulocytopenia and Agranulocytosis

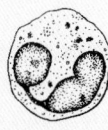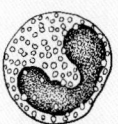

Tests of your blood may reveal a wide variety of findings. Among the more unusual disorders may be granulocytopenia or agranulocytosis.

Granulocytopenia

When your blood contains less than the normal number of white blood cells called granulocytes — a name given for their grainy appearance under the microscope — the condition is called granulocytopenia. Either the bone marrow doesn't produce enough of these cells, or they're destroyed at a rate that's higher than usual.

This condition is also known as neutropenia because the granulocytes most often affected are neutrophils. Neutrophils are your body's first line of defense against bacterial or fungal infection. Therefore, granulocytopenia increases your susceptibility to many infections.

Granulocytopenia can be the first sign of leukemia or aplastic anemia. But granulocytopenia more commonly results from another disorder or use of medication, such as chemotherapy.

Agranulocytosis

Agranulocytosis is a rare condition involving an extreme decrease in granulocytes. Almost all of the neutrophils are destroyed, leaving you particularly prone to infection.

Most often, this disorder occurs as a rare, acute response to exposure to certain chemicals, solvents or hydrocarbons or to certain medications, including penicillins, phenothiazines and anti-inflammatory agents.

The usual treatment is to avoid additional exposure to the chemicals and to protect against serious infection until the bone marrow can recover.

Because amyloidosis can cause a number of complications, you may also need treatment for specific conditions. For example, if amyloidosis affects your heart or kidneys, you may need to follow a low-salt diet to limit fluid retention. Your doctor may also prescribe diuretics and other medications.

If you have secondary amyloidosis, the primary goal of therapy is to treat the underlying condition when possible.

Stem cell transplantation

Peripheral blood stem cell transplantation involves using high-dose chemotherapy and transfusion of previously collected immature blood cells (stem cells) to replace diseased or damaged bone marrow. These cells may be your own (autologous transplant) or they may come from a donor (allogeneic transplant). Stem cell transplantation may help select individuals with AL amyloidosis.

Liver transplantation

Studies indicate that in some people with hereditary amyloidosis, a liver transplant may be a very effective treatment.

Medication

Medications used to treat AL amyloidosis include the drugs bortezomib (Velcade), cyclophosphamide and dexamethasone, a corticosteroid medication. Several other medications also are being tested for their ability to control the disease.

Anemias

Anemia results from too few healthy red blood cells to carry adequate oxygen to your tissues. It's the most common blood disorder in the United States. Women and individuals with chronic diseases are at increased risk of the condition.

Red blood cells carry, via your bloodstream, oxygen from your lungs to your brain and the other organs and tissues in your body. Oxygen helps give your body its energy and your skin a healthy glow. Hemoglobin, the red, iron-rich protein in your red blood cells, enables the cells to transport oxygen from your lungs to all parts of your body.

Anemia is a state in which the number of red blood cells or the amount of hemoglobin in them is below normal (see the illustration on page 381). When you're anemic, your body produces too few healthy red blood cells, loses too many of them or destroys them faster than they can be replaced. Your body's cells aren't adequately supplied with oxygen, leaving you fatigued.

Initially, the signs and symptoms of anemia tend to be so mild that they often go unnoticed, but their severity increases as the condition progresses. At first, you may be more tired and your skin may appear pale. The best places to check for pallor are your nail beds, your palms and the inside of your eyelids and lips. The creases in your palms may be as pale as the surrounding skin. When you exercise, you may feel more out of breath than usual and your heart may beat faster than normal. Anemia can also cause lightheadedness and cold hands and feet.

Many types of anemia exist, each with its own cause. Anemia may result from an iron or vitamin deficiency, blood loss, a chronic illness, or a genetic or acquired disorder. It may also be a side effect of a medication. Anemia can be temporary or chronic, and its symptoms may range from mild to severe.

Iron deficiency anemia

Signs and symptoms
- Fatigue and weakness
- Pale skin
- Shortness of breath
- Headache
- Lightheadedness
- Cold hands and feet
- Inflamed or sore tongue
- Brittle nails
- Unusual cravings for non-nutritive substances such as ice, dirt or pure starch
- Poor appetite, especially in infants and children

A deficiency of iron is the most common type of anemia. Your body needs iron to make hemoglobin, a substance that enables red blood cells to carry oxygen to your tissues. Oxygenated blood gives your body energy and your skin a healthy color. In iron deficiency anemia, your blood lacks adequate healthy red blood cells, due to insufficient iron.

Signs and symptoms of iron deficiency anemia tend to appear so gradually that they're often hard to notice. You may feel tired and less tolerant of exercise. Your skin, gums, nail beds and eyelid linings may be pale. Eventually, the anemia may become severe enough that your heartbeat seems more rapid and noticeable.

On rare occasions, people with the condition develop a craving for substances that aren't foods, such as ice or soil. This craving is called pica.

Causes
Iron deficiency anemia may result from too little iron in the diet, inadequate absorption of iron or blood loss, such as from heavy menstruation or other bleeding.

This type of anemia occurs most frequently among women of childbearing age. In nonpregnant women, the cause often is monthly loss of blood due to menstruation.

Virtually all pregnant women experience iron deficiency anemia if they don't take iron supplements, because their iron stores have to serve the increased blood volume of the mother during pregnancy as well as be a source of hemoglobin for the growing fetus.

Another cause of iron deficiency anemia is slow, chronic blood loss from a source within the body, such as an ulcer, a colon polyp, colon cancer or a hiatal hernia.

Iron in the food you eat is absorbed by your small intestine and enters your bloodstream. An intestinal disorder such as Crohn's disease or celiac disease can affect your intestine's ability to absorb nutrients and can lead to iron deficiency anemia. In addition, anemia can result if part of your small intestine has been bypassed or surgically removed.

Some medications can interfere with iron absorption. For example, regular use of prescription-strength medications that block production of stomach acid, called proton pump inhibitors (Aciphex, Prilosec), may lead to iron deficiency anemia. Stomach acid is needed to convert dietary iron into a form that can be readily absorbed.

Diagnosis
Blood tests are generally used to diagnose iron deficiency anemia. These tests may include a blood smear to examine the size and color of your red blood cells (see the illustration on page 381), a check of the proportion of your blood volume that's made up of red blood cells (hematocrit), and a measurement of hemoglobin and ferritin. A low level of ferritin — a protein that helps store iron in the body — usually indicates a low level of iron.

If your blood tests indicate iron deficiency anemia, your doctor may order additional tests to search for an underlying cause. If he or she suspects bleeding from the intestinal tract, the tests may include an upper endoscopy or colonoscopy.

An upper endoscopy is a procedure in which a thin, flexible tube with a light and scope is inserted down your esophagus into your stomach. In a colonoscopy, an endoscope is inserted into your rectum and threaded through your colon. Your doctor may also have your stools tested for traces of blood.

How serious is iron deficiency anemia?

Moderate to severe symptoms of iron deficiency anemia may interfere with work or school performance. Left untreated, the condition may lead to a rapid or irregular heartbeat (arrhythmia). In people who have narrowed arteries that feed the heart (coronary artery disease), untreated anemia can lead to chest pain (angina). In severe cases, anemia can precipitate a heart attack.

In pregnant women, severe iron deficiency anemia has been linked to premature births and low birth-weight babies. In infants and children, severe anemia can result in delayed growth.

Treatment

The first step in treating iron deficiency anemia is to identify and treat the underlying cause. If you become deficient in iron to the point that you develop anemia, eating more iron-rich foods is beneficial but isn't enough to correct your illness.

Supplements

For mild iron deficiency anemia, a daily multivitamin with iron may be adequate. However, iron supplementation is often necessary to restore your iron reserves and meet your body's daily iron requirements. Your doctor will likely prescribe oral iron supplements that you take daily. Because the supplements can cause constipation, your doctor may also recommend a stool softener or laxative. Iron almost always turns

stools a charcoal black color. This is a harmless side effect.

Iron deficiency can't be cured overnight. You may need to take iron supplements for several months or longer to replenish your body's reserves. Pregnant women are usually prescribed iron supplements for the duration of their pregnancy to prevent or treat iron deficiency anemia.

In adults, if iron supplements alone don't increase blood iron levels, the illness may be due to a source of bleeding or an iron absorption problem. In either case, the condition needs to be identified and treated.

Medication

Oral contraceptives can help treat iron deficiency anemia by decreasing heavy menstrual flow. For individuals with blood loss due to an ulcer, antibiotics are often prescribed to treat the ulcer.

Malabsorption problems also may be treated with medications.

Surgery

Surgery may be necessary if the cause of iron deficiency anemia is blood loss due to a tumor or bleeding polyp.

Other therapies

If you have severe anemia and immediate correction is needed, your doctor may give you a transfusion of packed red blood cells.

Prevention

Adequate nutrition is the key to preventing iron deficiency anemia that isn't the result of an underlying disease. Foods rich in iron include meat, fish, poultry, eggs, legumes (peas and beans), potatoes and rice. Many wheat products receive added iron when they're processed, but this iron isn't in a form that your body can

Getting the Most From Iron Supplements

Not all iron supplements are created equal, and not all types of anemia should be treated with iron. Your doctor will prescribe the treatment best suited to your particular needs.

Oral iron supplements are usually best absorbed if taken on an empty stomach, but they can cause indigestion, abdominal pain, nausea and constipation. The supplements can also interact with certain foods and medications. Follow these tips for safe and effective use:

- If you develop nausea or stomach pain, take your iron supplement with food.
- If side effects persist, ask your doctor about switching to a different iron preparation.
- Take your iron tablets with a source of vitamin C, such as orange juice. Vitamin C may enhance absorption.
- Don't take iron with tea. Tea reduces iron absorption.
- If possible, avoid medications that reduce iron absorption. These include antacids, acid blockers (H-2-receptor blockers), proton pump inhibitors and tetracycline.

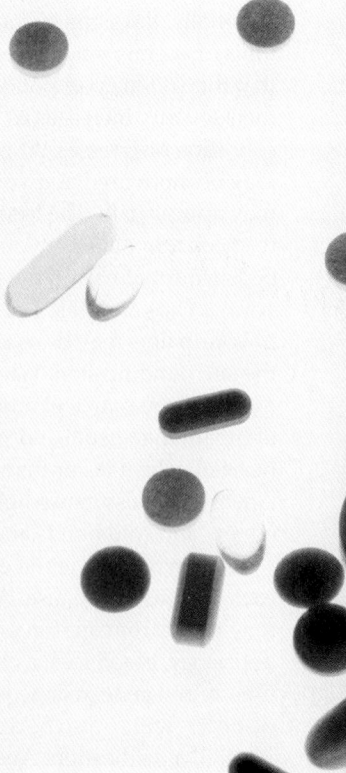

easily use. Iron in many vegetables is poorly absorbed.

Eating plenty of iron-containing foods is particularly important for people who have high iron requirements, such as children and pregnant or menstruating women. It's also crucial for individuals whose diets may not be abundant in iron, such as strict vegetarians, people on weight-loss diets and infants.

Pernicious anemia

Signs and symptoms
- Weakness
- Pale skin
- Lightheadedness
- Reduced exercise endurance
- A sore mouth or tongue
- Poor appetite
- Weight loss
- Disturbed gait and balance
- Mental confusion or forgetfulness

- Numbness or coldness in your hands and feet
- Yellowing or darkening of the skin

Anemia that's caused by an inability of your body to absorb vitamin B-12 is called pernicious anemia. Vitamin B-12 is a building block of red blood cells. Lack of a protein called intrinsic factor can lead to difficulty absorbing this vitamin.

Pernicious anemia is uncommon and occurs most often in older adults. This form of anemia is often hereditary and frequently was fatal before the availability of vitamin B-12 by injection. The term *pernicious* means "deadly."

Vitamin B-12 is broken down from food you eat. Intrinsic factor is a protein secreted by the stomach. It joins with vitamin B-12 and then escorts the vitamin through the small intestine, where the vitamin is absorbed into your blood-

stream. Without intrinsic factor, vitamin B-12 can't be absorbed and is excreted from the body as waste.

Lack of intrinsic factor may be due to an autoimmune reaction, in which your immune system attacks the stomach cells that produce intrinsic factor. Or it may be due to a genetic defect that halts production of the protein.

Only rarely does pernicious anemia result from a diet lacking in vitamin B-12, which is found mainly in meat, eggs and milk. You may be at risk if you're a strict vegetarian. Sometimes, a problem absorbing vitamin B-12 is caused by surgery to the stomach or small intestine, abnormal bacterial growth in the small intestine, or an intestinal disease, such as Crohn's disease or celiac disease.

Diagnosis
A diagnosis of pernicious anemia often results after various blood tests. One test measures the amount of vitamin B-12 in your blood, and another assesses the size, shape and number of red blood cells. If you have pernicious anemia, your red blood cells will be enlarged and there will be fewer of them.

Your doctor may order a test to check for antibodies to intrinsic factor, an indirect way of telling if you have pernicious anemia. A blood and urine test can measure the amount of a substance called methylmalonic acid. This substance is increased in people with a vitamin B-12 deficiency.

How serious is pernicious anemia?
In the past, pernicious anemia eventually caused death. Now, replacement therapy with adequate amounts of vitamin B-12 corrects the deficiency and allows for a normal life.

If the condition progresses for a long time before detection, it can lead to neurological problems that cause persistent tingling in your

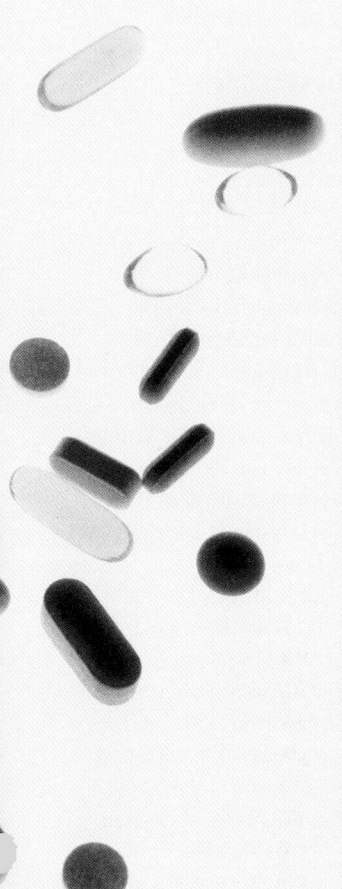

The Dangers of Too Much Iron

Too much of a good thing — in this case, iron — may be dangerous. If you take supplemental iron, make sure not to take too much.

Iron supplements are appropriate only when you need more iron than your diet can provide. If you think you need an iron supplement, check with your doctor first because overloading your body with iron can be even more serious than iron deficiency anemia.

Excess iron accumulation that leads to hemochromatosis can damage your liver or heart. Accumulation in your joints can cause conditions such as arthritis. Injury to the testicles by iron accumulation can lead to impotence and sterility.

In addition, if you're losing blood because of a serious condition such as colon cancer, taking an iron supplement may cover up the problem and delay the diagnosis. Iron deficiency anemia can be an important diagnostic clue that your doctor should investigate.

hands and feet (peripheral neuropathy). It can also lead to mental confusion and forgetfulness. A vitamin B-12 deficiency can cause these and other health problems even before it leads to anemia.

Treatment

Vitamin B-12, which may be given as an injection or orally, is used to treat pernicious anemia. This treatment is needed for life.

Vitamin B-12 deficiency that's related to a poor diet can be treated with changes to your diet, along with vitamin B-12 supplementation.

Folic acid deficiency anemia

Signs and symptoms
- Weakness and fatigue
- Pale skin
- Lightheadedness
- Low exercise endurance
- Weight loss
- Diarrhea

Folic acid deficiency anemia results from interference with the production of red blood cells, similar to pernicious anemia. Folic acid (folate) is a member of the vitamin B group. It's found mainly in fresh fruits and leafy green vegetables.

Lack of folate causes an anemia that's characterized by large, abnormal red blood cells that are few in number. Deficiency of folic acid can result if you don't get enough of it in your diet to meet your body's demands, or if your intestines aren't able to absorb it.

People with diseases of the small intestine, such as Crohn's disease or celiac disease, or who've had a large part of their small intestine removed or bypassed, may have difficulty absorbing folic acid.

Because alcohol also decreases absorption of folic acid, drinking excessive amounts of alcohol can lead to a deficiency. Certain prescription medications, such as some anti-seizure or tuberculosis medications, also may interfere with absorption.

Pregnant women and women who are breast-feeding have an increased demand for folic acid, as do people undergoing hemodialysis for kidney disease. Your doctor may also consider other causes of folate deficiency, such as the effect of certain agents used to treat cancer, bone marrow disorders, liver disease, thyroid disease or smoking.

Diagnosis

The symptoms of folic acid deficiency anemia are similar to those of pernicious anemia, except that neurological symptoms don't occur. Your doctor likely will request that you undergo various blood tests to distinguish between the two disorders.

The blood tests include examining the cells under a microscope and measuring the amount of folate in your blood. If folic acid deficiency anemia is present, your doctor may perform more tests to establish the cause.

How serious is folic acid deficiency anemia?

It's especially important to take folic acid supplements if you're pregnant or you're planning to become pregnant. A deficiency of folic acid is associated with serious neural tube birth defects, such as spina bifida, anencephaly and encephalocele.

A daily intake of at least 400 micrograms (mcg) of folic acid — up to 800 mcg if you're trying to conceive — can reduce your baby's risk of neural tube defects by 50 percent and may reduce your chance of miscarriage.

Treatment

Depending on its underlying cause, a folic acid deficiency may be chronic or acute. In either case, it's important to eliminate the underlying cause. For instance, if excessive alcohol consumption is the reason for the deficiency, successful treatment depends on your stopping drinking.

Medication

In almost all cases of folic acid deficiency anemia, supplemental folic acid is given orally every day. It's injected only if the underlying problem is a disorder of the intestinal tract that severely interferes with absorption. It usually takes a month or longer to correct folic acid deficiency anemia.

Nutrition

In some cases, adequate nutrition is the remedy. Folate is found in a wide variety of foods, but it can be destroyed by excessive cooking. The main food sources of folate are raw fruits and vegetables and organ meats, such as liver and kidney. However, if you're pregnant or may become pregnant, be careful to avoid overconsumption of liver. It also contains high levels of preformed vitamin A. Consuming vitamin A above 200 percent of the Daily Value may be related to some types of birth defects.

Sickle cell anemia

Signs and symptoms
- Fatigue
- Breathlessness
- A rapid heartbeat
- Susceptibility to infections
- Skin ulcers on the lower legs
- Yellowing of the skin

Sickle cell anemia is an inherited form of anemia. In this condition, red blood cells become rigid and shaped like crescents (sickles) rather than being round and flexible. These irregular red blood cells wear out prematurely, resulting in a chronic shortage of red blood cells.

In addition to typical signs of anemia, sickle cell disease can cause the following:
- **Episodes of pain.** Pain develops when sickled red blood cells block blood flow through tiny blood vessels. Usually, blood vessels in the chest, abdomen and joints are affected. Pain also may be felt in bones. The pain may vary in intensity and can

Porphyrias

The group of diseases called the porphyrias encompasses several rare blood disorders. They result from the body's inability to properly manufacture heme, the pigmented, iron-containing part of hemoglobin that carries oxygen throughout the body.

Heme is made in both the liver and bone marrow through seven steps of chemical reactions. Porphyria occurs when a defective enzyme blocks one of the steps. Each of the seven types of porphyria corresponds to a particular enzyme defect.

In some people with porphyria, concentrations of chemicals can build up under the surface of the skin. Exposure to sunlight may produce a toxic reaction that causes painful skin lesions. These can lead to permanent scarring and disfigurement, such as loss of an ear or nose. The skin damage can begin in childhood. If the toxins accumulate to high levels in other organs, such as the brain, the individual may survive only a few years. Occasionally, porphyrias begin in adulthood. People with these forms usually are able to lead long, relatively normal lives.

Some people with porphyria develop excessive hair growth on the face, arms, hands and legs. In some people, porphyria can cause teeth to develop a reddish hue. Fingernails and toenails may become claw-like.

Some types of porphyria can cause acute attacks of abdominal pain. However, porphyria is very rare, and most abdominal pain isn't related to porphyria. Other signs and symptoms may include pain in your limbs, muscles or back, red urine, and neurological symptoms such as personality changes or seizures. Acute attacks are generally followed by periods of remission.

No treatment exists to correct the enzyme defect responsible for porphyria. Pain medications and other drugs may provide relief. Other treatments include frequent removal of blood (phlebotomy) and, in some cases, surgical removal of the spleen.

Porphyria attacks can be extremely painful and life-threatening and require medical attention. Symptoms can be triggered by sunlight, diet or medications, so treatment often involves avoiding such triggers. Good nutrition and avoidance of alcohol also can play a role in preventing attacks.

Porphyrias usually are inherited. If porphyria exists in your or your partner's family, seek genetic counseling before having children so that you know the potential risk to any offspring.

last for a few hours to a few weeks. Some people experience few episodes of pain, and others experience a dozen or more sickling crises a year, for reasons that are unclear.

- **Hand-foot syndrome.** Swollen hands and feet are often the first signs of sickle cell anemia in babies. The swelling is caused by sickled red blood cells blocking blood flow out of the hands and feet. Pain and fever often accompany this condition, called hand-foot syndrome.
- **Frequent infections.** Sickle cell anemia makes you vulnerable to infections because sickle cells damage the spleen, which filters germs from the blood and makes antibodies. Doctors commonly prescribe daily doses of antibiotics for infants and children with sickle cell anemia to prevent potentially life-threatening infections, such as pneumonia.
- **Impaired growth.** Red blood cells provide your body with oxygen and nutrients needed for growth. A shortage of healthy red blood cells in sickle cell anemia can slow growth in infants and children and delay puberty in teenagers.
- **Vision problems.** Tiny blood vessels in the eye may become plugged with sickle cells, which can damage the retina, the portion of the eye that processes visual images.

Causes

Sickle cell anemia results from a defective gene that causes your body to make abnormal hemoglobin. Normal adult red blood cells contain hemoglobin A. People with sickle cell anemia make hemoglobin S (for sickle).

Red blood cells that contain normal hemoglobin are soft and round (doughnut-like) and can squeeze through tiny blood vessels to deliver oxygen. Red blood cells that contain sickle hemoglobin start off soft and round, but once they deliver oxygen, the defective hemoglobin causes many of them to change shape and stiffen.

Sickled red blood cells are sticky and clump together more easily, forming temporary plugs in small blood vessels, stopping blood flow. These cells also are fragile, living only 10 to 20 days, and can obstruct blood vessels as they break apart.

The sickling of red blood cells causes the symptoms and complications of the disease. Sometimes, sickling is worse than at other times. Sickling crises can occur spontaneously, or they may be triggered by factors such as stress, an infection, dehydration, temperature extremes and decreased oxygen, such as at high altitudes in an airplane.

The sickle cell gene is particularly common among people of African,

Spanish, Mediterranean, Middle Eastern and Indian ancestry. In the United States, the disease most commonly affects blacks and Hispanics.

To acquire sickle cell anemia, you must inherit the gene for hemoglobin S from both parents. This gene is recessive, so if you inherit the gene from only one parent, you won't have the disease but will carry the sickle cell trait. As a carrier, you can pass the disease on to your children.

If you're a carrier, your red blood cells may be deformed, but no symptoms occur unless you're at high altitude. The decreased level of oxygen renders the red blood cells more fragile and deformed, thus increasing their tendency to sickle and break up (hemolysis).

Diagnosis

People who have sickle cell anemia usually receive the diagnosis as a newborn. A blood test that can check for the disease is part of routine newborn screenings performed after birth. The diagnosis is confirmed by further tests, including a laboratory procedure that can isolate and identify hemoglobin S.

How serious is sickle cell anemia?

There's no known cure for sickle cell anemia, a potentially fatal disease. However, treatments can relieve symptoms and prolong life. Many people with sickle cell anemia lead fairly normal lives and enjoy reasonably good health into their 40s and beyond.

Serious complications of the disease include:

Stroke

A stroke can occur if sickled red blood cells block blood flow to an area of the brain. A stroke is one of the most serious complications of the disease. Roughly 10 percent of children with sickle cell anemia experience a stroke.

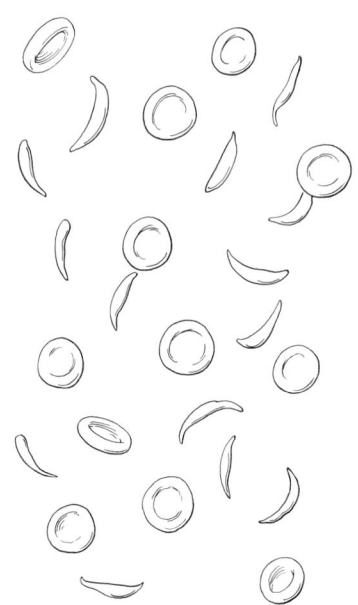

This illustration shows normal and sickled red blood cells. The sickled cells assume a crescent shape.

Acute chest syndrome

Acute chest syndrome is a life-threatening complication of sickle cell anemia caused by a lung infection or trapped sickled blood cells in the lung. It causes chest pain, a cough, fever and difficulty breathing and requires emergency treatment with antibiotics, blood transfusions and drugs that open up lung airways. Recurrent attacks can damage the lungs.

Organ damage

Sickled red blood cells can block blood flow through blood vessels, depriving an organ of blood and oxygen. Chronic deprivation of oxygen-rich blood can damage nerves and organs, including the kidneys, liver and spleen.

Blindness

Tiny blood vessels in the eye may become plugged with sickle cells. Over time, this can damage the retina, the portion of the eye that processes visual images, and lead to blindness.

Other conditions

Sickle cell anemia can lead to leg ulcers, caused by sickled red cells obstructing blood vessels that nourish the skin. When red blood cells are destroyed, a substance called bilirubin is produced, which can cause yellowing of the skin and eyes (jaundice) and lead to gallstones.

Men with sickle cell anemia may experience painful and prolonged erections when sickled red blood cells prevent blood flow out of an erect penis (priapism). Over time, priapism can damage the penis and lead to impotence.

Treatment

Although there's no cure for sickle cell anemia, your doctor can do a great deal to help you or your child live with the disease. In addition, treatments are continually improving. People with sickle cell anemia may benefit from treatment by specialists at a hospital or a sickle cell anemia clinic. Regular visits to the doctor are important.

Medication

Medications used to treat sickle cell anemia include:

- **Antibiotics.** Children with sickle cell anemia usually begin taking the antibiotic penicillin when they're about 2 months old and continue taking it until they're 5 years old. It helps prevent infections that can be life-threatening to an infant or child with sickle cell anemia. Antibiotics may also help adults with sickle cell anemia fight infections.
- **Pain-relieving medications.** To relieve pain during a sickling attack, your doctor may advise over-the-counter pain relievers and application of warm heat to the affected area. Sometimes, stronger prescription pain medications are necessary.
- **Hydroxyurea.** This prescription drug, usually used to treat leukemia, has been shown to reduce the number of painful sickling crises and reduce the need for blood transfusions. Hydroxyurea (Droxia) appears

to stimulate production of fetal hemoglobin, a type of hemoglobin found in newborns, which helps prevent sickling of red blood cells.

There's some concern about the possibility that long-term use of this drug may cause tumors or leukemia in certain people. Your doctor can help you determine if this drug may be beneficial for you.

- **Folic acid.** Your doctor likely will prescribe a daily oral supplement of folic acid because the disease increases your body's need for this vitamin.

Blood transfusions

Blood transfusions can increase the number of normal red blood cells in circulation to relieve anemia. In children with sickle cell anemia at high risk of a stroke, periodic blood transfusions can decrease their risk of a stroke.

Blood transfusions carry some risk. Blood contains iron and regular transfusions can cause an excess amount of iron to build up in your body, which can damage your organs. Your doctor may prescribe a medication called deferasirox (Exjade) to reduce excess iron levels.

Supplemental oxygen

You may be given oxygen through a breathing mask during a sickling crisis or with acute chest syndrome to add oxygen to your blood and help you breathe easier.

Bone marrow transplantation

This procedure allows people with sickle cell anemia to replace their bone marrow — and its sickle-shaped red blood cells — with healthy bone marrow from a donor who doesn't have the disease. It can be a cure, but the procedure is risky, and it's difficult to find suitable donors.

Currently, the procedure is recommended only for people who have significant symptoms and problems from the disease.

Experimental treatments

Among the new treatments researchers are studying is gene therapy. Researchers are exploring whether inserting a corrected gene to control production of hemoglobin into the bone marrow of people with sickle cell anemia will result in the production of normal hemoglobin.

Scientists are also exploring the possibility of turning off the defective gene while reactivating another gene responsible for the production of fetal hemoglobin, which would prevent sickling.

Prevention

If you carry the sickle cell trait, you may wish to see a genetic counselor before trying to conceive a child. A genetic counselor can help you understand the risk of having a child with sickle cell anemia. He or she can also explain possible treatments, preventive measures and reproductive options.

Hemolytic anemias

Signs and symptoms

- Fatigue
- Pale skin
- Breathlessness
- A faster and more noticeable heartbeat during exertion
- Yellowing of the skin
- Dark urine
- Pressure or fullness under the left ribs
- Sudden onset of pain in the upper abdomen

Hemolytic anemias refer to those anemias in which red blood cells are broken down (hemolyzed) faster than your bone marrow can produce new ones to replace them. The word *hemolytic* comes from Greek roots meaning "destruction of blood."

Hemolytic anemias can be inherited or acquired. Inherited hemolytic anemias generally result from abnormalities in the red blood cell membrane or from red blood cell enzyme deficiencies. In one inherited type, called spherocytosis, red

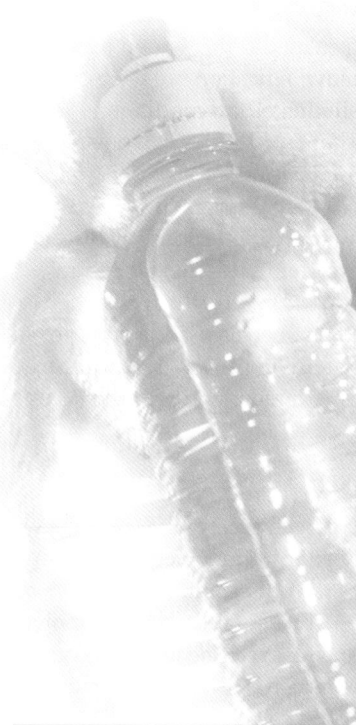

blood cells are small, round and fragile. Another inherited type, called glucose-6-phosphate dehydrogenase deficiency, results from an enzyme deficiency.

Acquired forms may result from medications taken for other conditions, such as infections or high blood pressure. Hemolytic anemia may also develop from an immune response in which your immune system attacks your own red blood cells.

Diagnosis

If your doctor thinks that you may have a hemolytic anemia, he or she will likely have your blood examined to count the number of young red blood cells (reticulocytes) and to see if the cells are deformed. The number of young red cells is increased in hemolytic anemia. Your doctor may examine your upper abdomen to see if your spleen or liver is enlarged.

How serious is hemolytic anemia?

Some forms of hemolytic anemia are hard to treat, but these types of anemia are seldom fatal.

Treatment

When hemolytic anemia is caused by a medication, stopping use of that medication often improves or eliminates the condition.

Medication

For hemolytic anemia caused by an immune response, medications are often prescribed to treat the condition. Corticosteroid medications, such as prednisone, are often helpful in preventing the destruction of red blood cells (hemolysis).

Surgery

If the condition has caused an enlarged spleen, the spleen may need to be removed. The spleen filters out and stores defective red blood cells, and certain hemolytic anemias can cause it to become enlarged with damaged red blood cells.

Other anemias

In addition to the more common types of anemias, other, more rare forms exist. Some uncommon anemias include:

Glucose-6-phosphate dehydrogenase deficiency

This type of anemia is the result of an inherited defect in an enzyme, glucose-6-phosphate dehydrogenase, in red blood cells. Like hemolytic anemia, this disorder causes the premature breakdown of red blood cells. It occurs commonly in people of Mediterranean and African ancestry.

Symptoms range from mild to severe, depending on which form of defective gene is present. Symptoms tend to be less severe in people of African ancestry than in those of Mediterranean ancestry.

The gene for the glucose-6-phosphate dehydrogenase enzyme is carried on the X chromosome. Like the blood disorder hemophilia, this disease almost always affects boys and men — who have only one X chromosome — rather than girls and women — who have two X chromosomes. If you have two X chromosomes, then you're likely to have one without the defect.

Thalassemia

Thalassemia is a disease that has two forms. Both are based on inherited defects in hemoglobin. In alpha-thalassemia, not enough of the portion of hemoglobin called alpha-globin is produced. In beta-thalassemia, beta-globin is lacking.

Alpha-thalassemia occurs most often in people of Southeast Asian descent. Beta-thalassemia, also called Cooley's anemia or Mediterranean anemia, is common in the Mediterranean region.

The thalassemia genes are recessive, so you have to inherit them from both parents to get the disease. If you have only one defective gene, you carry the trait but have no symptoms. Thalassemia frequently causes severe chronic anemia with poor growth, an enlarged spleen and, sometimes, heart failure.

Without treatment, death occurs in early childhood. There's no cure, but therapy can often prolong life into the 20s or 30s. Treatment involves repeated transfusions of red blood cells. These cells carry a great deal of iron, which can overload the body's vital organs. To lessen this effect, medication may be given that causes extra iron to be excreted in the urine. Stem cell transplantation is another possible treatment. Genetic counseling can help individuals avoid passing the disorder on to their children.

A milder form of thalassemia, called thalassemia minor or thalassemia trait, is common. It is caused by inheriting one defective gene from either your mother or father. This disorder produces blood cells that look like those present in iron deficient blood, but they produce no symptoms. By itself, the disorder doesn't cause problems.

Anemia of chronic disease

Some chronic diseases interfere with the production of red blood cells, resulting in chronic anemia. Kidney failure is one example. Your kidneys produce a hormone called erythropoietin, which stimulates your bone marrow to produce red blood cells. A shortage of erythropoietin can result in a shortage of red blood cells. The bone marrow of some people with rheumatoid arthritis doesn't use erythropoietin efficiently, resulting in anemia. A shortage of erythropoietin can also be caused by chemotherapy.

Other chronic diseases associated with anemia include AIDS, cancer, chronic liver disease, acute and chronic infections, and certain types of ulcers.

Anemia of chronic disease is curable only if the underlying disorder causing it can be cured or improved with treatment. If you have severe anemia of chronic disease,

Rare Hemoglobin Diseases

Rare hemoglobin diseases, called hemoglobinopathies, result from variant forms of hemoglobin. Over 400 variants have been identified. These abnormal hemoglobins tend to be less efficient at transporting oxygen to tissue cells.

One example is hemoglobin SC disease. People with this disease have inherited the sickle cell trait (hemoglobin S) from one parent and another variant (hemoglobin C) from the other parent. Their life span is slightly decreased, and they experience persistent mild to moderate anemia. Individuals with hemoglobin SC can have attacks of pain similar to those experienced by people with sickle cell anemia.

treatment consists of red blood cell transfusions and, in some cases, erythropoietin injections.

Aplastic anemia

Aplastic means "failure in development." This form of anemia is caused by a drastic decrease in the bone marrow's production of all types of blood cells, including white blood cells that fight germs and platelets that help your blood to clot. This condition puts you at risk of infections and uncontrolled bleeding.

This uncommon and life-threatening illness can be inherited — Fanconi's anemia — or triggered by a serious infection such as hepatitis, a bone marrow disorder such as leukemia, high-dose radiation, chemotherapy, exposure to toxic chemicals or use of certain medications. It results from damage to your bone marrow.

Aplastic anemia can come on suddenly and last only a short while, or it can persist. Without treatment, it may progress and become fatal.

Treatment generally begins with eliminating the cause, if it's known. For example, aplastic anemia that's caused by radiation, chemotherapy or other drug treatment usually improves once the treatment is stopped.

Your doctor will try to protect you from infections and will likely aggressively treat any that do occur with antibiotics. Other treatment options include trans-fusions of red blood cells and platelets and, if your case is severe and a suitable donor is available, stem cell transplantation.

In adults, aplastic anemia occurring without an obvious cause is usually autoimmune and requires treatment with allogeneic stem cell transplantation, in which normal bone marrow stem cells from a matched donor are used. Among individuals who aren't candidates for stem cell transplantation, treatment generally involves the medications such as cyclosporine to suppress the immune system.

Sideroblastic anemia

Sideroblasts are young red blood cells that contain excess iron. Sideroblastic anemias are rare disorders in which the red blood cells contain a high concentration of iron and hemoglobin production is defective.

Treatment depends on the cause. You can acquire this anemia as a result of certain medications or exposure to toxins, such as ethanol and lead. When the offending agent is removed, the anemia may disappear. Sideroblastic anemia is also associated with certain cancers, such as leukemia, lymphoma and myeloma, and with inflammatory diseases, such as rheumatoid arthritis. As the underlying condition is treated, the anemia may improve.

There's also an inherited form of sideroblastic anemia. In some cases, no cause can be identified.

For these forms, blood transfusions may be needed, along with a medication to remove extra iron via your urine.

Leukemias

Leukemia is cancer of your body's blood-forming tissues, including your bone marrow and lymphatic system. It usually starts in your white blood cells.

Your white blood cells are potent infection fighters — they normally grow and divide in an orderly way, as your body needs them. In leukemia, your bone marrow produces a large number of abnormal white blood cells, which don't function properly.

These abnormal cells remain immature in what's known as blast form, but they maintain the ability to multiply, causing the formation of excessive numbers of abnormal white blood cells. These abnormal cells reach high concentrations in bone marrow, the lymphatic system and bloodstream and begin to interfere with the functions of vital organs.

Normal white blood cells are potent infection fighters. The abnormal white blood cells decrease production of normal white blood cells, impairing your ability to fight off infection.

Abnormal white blood cell production that takes control of the bone marrow interferes with the production of red blood cells and platelets in the bone marrow.

A deficiency in red blood cells means that your body's organs don't receive enough oxygen. A shortage of platelets makes the blood-clotting process less effective, leaving your body more vulnerable to bleeding and bruising.

Risk factors

Experts aren't sure what causes abnormal cells to develop and multiply, but they've identified

Enlarged Lymph Nodes

Lymph nodes are distributed throughout the body, in the neck, armpits, chest, abdomen and groin. They serve an immune function similar to that of the spleen, filtering out foreign substances (antigens) from lymph fluids.

Enlarged lymph nodes (lymphadenopathy) commonly occur with infections. They're due to an increase in certain white blood cells (lymphocytes) needed to fight the infection. Other causes of lymph node enlargement include autoimmune disorders, such as lupus, and certain cancers, such as leukemias and lymphomas. If cancer is suspected, a lymph node biopsy may be analyzed for cancerous cells. When cancer is the cause of lymph node enlargement, the nodes typically aren't painful. In other conditions, they may be.

certain factors that place you at increased risk of leukemia:

- **Age.** The risk of genetic mutations increases with age. More than half the people who develop leukemia are older than age 60.
- **Cancer therapy.** People who've had certain types of chemotherapy and radiation therapy for other cancers have a slightly elevated risk of developing leukemia.
- **Genetics.** At least part of the risk of leukemia may be inherited. Some genetic disorders, such as Down syndrome, are associated with an increased risk.
- **Environmental hazards.** Smoking, exposure to intense radiation and long-term exposure to benzene, a chemical found in unleaded gasoline, may mutate genes. These hazards are linked to greater risk.

Types

Leukemia has four main types and many subtypes. The four main types are:

- Chronic myelogenous leukemia
- Acute myelogenous leukemia
- Acute lymphocytic leukemia
- Chronic lymphocytic leukemia

Myelogenous leukemia is a cancer of the granulocytes, a type of white blood cell formed in the bone marrow. Lymphocytic leukemia involves the lymphocytes, a type of white blood cell produced in the lymph system and bone marrow.

Types of leukemia are further divided according to how quickly they progress. In acute leukemia, leukemia cells multiply rapidly, and the disease worsens in weeks or months. In chronic leukemia, abnormal blood cells replicate or accumulate more slowly and can function normally for a period of time.

Other, rarer types of leukemia include hairy cell leukemia and chronic myelomonocytic leukemia.

Chronic myelogenous leukemia

Signs and symptoms

- Easy bleeding
- Fatigue
- Fever
- Frequent infections
- Weight loss
- Loss of appetite
- Pain or fullness below the ribs on the left side
- Pale skin
- Night sweats

Chronic myelogenous leukemia (CML) is an uncommon type of cancer of the blood cells. It results from production of cancerous versions of granulocytes. Granulocytes are a type of white blood cell formed in bone marrow. This type of leukemia may also be called myeloid, myelocytic or granulocytic.

The disease occurs when something goes awry in the genes of your blood. In people with CML, chromosomes in blood cells swap sections with each other. A section of chromosome 9 fuses with a section of chromosome 22 (t9;22 translocation), creating an extra-short chromosome 22 and an extra-long chromosome 9. The extra-short chromosome 22 is called the Philadelphia chromosome, named for the city where it was discovered.

The Philadelphia chromosome or the genetic abnormality associated with it (termed bcr-abl) is present in all people with CML. It produces an abnormal protein (bcr-abl protein) that eventually results in the creation of diseased white blood cells that build up in huge numbers, crowding out healthy blood cells and damaging bone marrow.

Diagnosis

Often, people receive a diagnosis of the disease before symptoms develop, when routine blood tests reveal abnormal results.

Further tests are used to determine if you have chronic myelogenous leukemia. These include a complete blood count, a differential count of the various types of white blood cells and measurement of an enzyme called leukocyte alkaline phosphatase. Your bone marrow also may be examined.

Specialized tests, such as fluorescence in situ hybridization (FISH) analysis and the polymerase chain reaction (PCR) test, analyze blood or bone marrow samples for the presence of the Philadelphia chromosome or specific gene abnormalities.

How serious is chronic myelogenous leukemia?

Chronic myelogenous leukemia is a progressive disease. In most people with the disorder, an acute phase, called a blast crisis or blastic phase, develops within three to five years.

The blast phase is characterized by a high concentration of immature white blood cells (blasts) in the blood and by red pinpoints (petechiae) on the skin that result from bleeding due to lack of platelets. A blast crisis is a form of acute leukemia that's particularly resistant to treatment and may be fatal.

Treatment

For most people, it's not possible to eliminate all diseased blood cells, but treatment can help achieve a long-term remission.

Medication

The drug treatment of choice for chronic myelogenous leukemia is the oral medication imatinib (Gleevec), which stops the growth of abnormal white blood cells by blocking the increased enzyme activity resulting from the gene fusion. It can produce complete eradication of all of the cells with the abnormal Philadelphia chromosome. Imatinib can be used to treat both the chronic phase and the blastic phase. Remission rates are very high, especially in the chronic phase of the disease.

Other drugs similar to imatinib also available include nilotinib (Tasigna), dasatinib (Sprycel), bosutinib (Bosulif) and ponatinib. The role of these newer more active agents is evolving. Some of the drugs are reserved for people who don't respond well to imatinib; however, some people may start on a newer medication such as nilotinib.

Stem cell transplant

Another option for this chronic form is a stem cell transplant, also called a bone marrow transplant. This procedure may be used in people younger than age 65, who have not responded to imatinib.

During a blood stem cell transplant, high doses of chemotherapy drugs are used to kill the blood-forming cells in your bone marrow. Then blood stem cells from a donor or your own cells that were previously collected and stored are infused into your bloodstream. The hope is that the new cells will form new, healthy blood cells to replace the diseased cells.

Other therapies

Chemotherapy drugs may be combined with other treatments to treat CML. Other options under study include biological therapies that harness your body's immune system to help fight the cancer.

Acute myelogenous leukemia

Signs and symptoms

- Fever
- Weight loss
- Bone pain
- Fatigue and weakness
- Shortness of breath
- Pale skin
- Frequent infections
- Easy bruising
- Unusual bleeding
- Feeling of fullness under your left ribs

Acute myelogenous leukemia (AML) is a cancer of the blood and bone marrow. It results from damage to the DNA of a group of immature white blood cells called myeloid cells. Myeloid cells normally develop into various types of mature blood cells, such as white blood cells, red blood cells and platelets. The abnormal myeloid cells are unable to function properly, and they build up and crowd out healthy cells.

It's not clear what causes the DNA mutations that lead to the leukemia. Radiation, exposure to certain chemicals and some chemotherapy drugs may play a role.

AML is the most common type of acute leukemia in adults. The disease is also referred to as non-lymphocytic, myeloid, monocytic, myelogenic or myelocytic leukemia.

Diagnosis

Diagnosis of acute myelogenous leukemia is generally based on

Treating Leukemia

Various therapies are used to treat leukemia. The form of treatment your doctor recommends is based on a number of factors, including the type of leukemia you have.

- *Chemotherapy.* Chemotherapy, which uses chemical agents to kill cancer cells, is the major form of treatment for leukemia. Depending on the type of leukemia that you have, you may receive a single chemical agent or a combination of agents. Rapidly multiplying cells are often more sensitive to the effects of chemotherapy. For this reason, acute leukemia is usually quite responsive to chemotherapy.
- *Radiation.* Radiation therapy uses X-rays or other high-energy rays to damage leukemic cells and stop their growth.
- *Stem cell transplantation (bone marrow transplant).* Chemotherapy or radiation therapy destroys your body's bone marrow, affecting its ability to produce healthy new blood cells. Your doctor may use a stem cell transplant to repopulate your blood with healthy cells.
- *Interferon-alfa.* Interferon is an antiviral agent that works to stop the spread of leukemic cells and helps bolster your immune system.
- *Cell-specific antibodies.* Antibodies that can destroy leukemic cells can be removed from your body, and their number can be greatly increased in a laboratory. This larger number of antibodies then can be put back in your body to help destroy more cancer cells.
- *Retinoic acid.* A problem associated with leukemia is that the abnormal white blood cells produced don't mature as normal cells do. They multiply, but they don't mature and die off. All-trans retinoic acid (ATRA) causes leukemic cells to mature and die.

Superficial Bleeding

Petechiae are round, pinpoint-sized spots caused by superficial bleeding into the skin. The spots aren't raised and initially are red but turn bluish-purple with time. Petechiae commonly appear on the lower legs but may appear over the whole body. A petechial rash isn't a disease but a sign of an underlying blood problem.

A common cause of petechiae is a marked decrease in the number of platelets in the blood. Platelets play an important role in controlling bleeding. A low platelet count (thrombocytopenia) can have many causes, including:

- Bone marrow disorders, such as leukemia
- Autoimmune diseases, such immune thrombocytopenia or lupus
- Viral infections, such as mononucleosis and German measles (rubella)
- Drug reactions

Petechiae usually go away upon successful treatment of the underlying problem. Because of the seriousness of some causes of petechiae, it's important to determine the cause. If you develop a petechial rash, see your doctor promptly.

the results of various blood tests and examination of bone marrow. Your doctor may also look for certain chromosome abnormalities that can help establish the diagnosis or indicate how your body may respond to the disease. In some cases, spinal fluid is taken for analysis. The fluid is generally collected by inserting a small needle into the spinal canal in the lower back.

How serious is acute myelogenous leukemia?

The course of acute myelogenous leukemia can be extremely rapid. Without treatment, death can occur within weeks. Treatment with combinations of certain chemotherapy medications can produce remission in about 2 out of 3 people who seek treatment.

Younger individuals generally respond better to treatment than do older adults. However, recurrences develop in the majority of people who enter remission.

Treatment

Treatment generally falls into two phases. The purpose of the first phase — remission induction therapy — is to kill the leukemia cells in your blood and bone marrow. The purpose of the second phase — consolidation therapy — is to destroy any remaining leukemia cells and help develop healthy cells.

Therapies used in these stages include:

- **Chemotherapy.** Chemotherapy that includes the drugs daunorubicin (Cerubidine) and cytarabine (Depocyt) is the standard form of remission induction therapy, though it can also be used for consolidation therapy. Chemotherapy uses chemicals to kill cancer cells in your body. If the first cycle of chemotherapy doesn't cause remission, you may need it repeated one or two more times.
- **Other drug therapy.** Arsenic trioxide (Trisenox) and all-trans retinoic acid are chemotherapy drugs that may be used alone or in combination with chemotherapy agents for remission induction. These drugs cause leukemia cells with a specific gene mutation to mature and die, or to stop dividing.
- **Biological therapy.** Also known as immunotherapy, biological therapy uses substances that bolster your immune system's response to cancer. Monoclonal antibodies are one form of biological therapy. The antibodies are produced in a laboratory, but they mimic proteins in your immune system (antibodies) that attack foreign substances on leukemic cells. One monoclonal antibody used as a biological therapy in AML is gemtuzumab ozogamicin (Mylotarg). The drug carries a chemical toxin that's released when it attaches to AML cells.
- **Bone marrow stem cell transplant.** This procedure may be used for consolidation therapy. Bone marrow stem cell transplant helps re-establish healthy stem cells by replacing unhealthy bone marrow with leukemia-free stem cells that will regenerate healthy bone marrow. Prior to a stem cell transplant, you receive very high doses of chemotherapy or radiation therapy to destroy your leukemia-producing bone marrow. Then you receive infusions of stem cells from a compatible donor (allogeneic transplant). You can also receive your own stem cells (autologous transplant) if you were previously in remission and had your healthy stem cells removed and stored for a future transplant.

Acute lymphocytic leukemia

Signs and symptoms

- Bleeding from gums
- Fever
- Frequent infections
- Frequent or severe nosebleeds
- Loss of appetite and weight loss
- Enlarged lymph nodes in and around the neck, underarm and groin
- Pale skin
- Fatigue and weakness

Acute lymphocytic leukemia (ALL) is a type of cancer that affects white blood cells called lymphocytes. The disease is also known as acute lymphoblastic leukemia and acute childhood leukemia.

Although it occurs in both adults and children, it most commonly affects children.

It's not clear what causes the abnormalities that can lead to ALL, but certain factors may put you at increased risk. These include previous cancer therapy, exposure to radiation, having Down syndrome, or having a brother or sister with the disease. However, most people with ALL have no known risk factors.

Diagnosis

Your doctor will likely perform blood tests, including a complete blood count with a differential count of the various types of white blood cells. If the results of these tests suggest acute lymphocytic leukemia, a sample of your bone marrow will likely be examined for cell abnormalities. These and other tests help characterize the disease and indicate the best treatment.

How serious is acute lymphocytic leukemia?

Without treatment, bleeding and infection can lead to death within months. Before current treatments were developed, this was the inevitable outcome of the disease. Fortunately, one of medicine's great success stories is the treatment of this leukemia in children.

The younger an individual is and the lower his or her white blood cell count at the time the disease is diagnosed, the better the chances of a cure. The prognosis isn't as good for older children and adults.

Treatment

Treatment of acute lymphocytic leukemia has two phases. The first, called induction therapy, is intended to kill as many leukemia cells as possible. The goal of the second phase is to kill any remaining leukemia cells and help develop healthy cells.

Therapies used in these stages include:

- **Chemotherapy.** Chemotherapy, which uses drugs to kill cancer cells, is the most common form of induction therapy for children and adults with acute lymphocytic leukemia. Chemotherapy drugs can also be used in the consolidation and maintenance phases.
- **Targeted drug therapy.** Targeted drugs attack specific abnormalities present in cancer cells that help them grow and thrive. One targeted drug, imatinib (Gleevec), specifically attacks cancer cells that have a certain abnormality called the Philadelphia chromosome. The drug dasatinib (Sprycel) works in a similar way. These drugs are only approved for people with the Philadelphia chromosome-positive form of ALL. Another drug, rituximab (Rituxan), targets cancer cells that have an overabundance of a certain protein. Targeted drug treatments may be combined with chemotherapy drugs.
- **Radiation therapy.** Radiation therapy uses high-powered beams, such as X-rays, to kill cancer cells. If the cancer cells have spread to the central nervous system, your doctor may recommend radiation therapy.
- **Bone marrow stem cell transplant.** A bone marrow stem cell transplant may be used as consolidation therapy in people at high risk of relapse or for treating relapse when it occurs. This procedure allows someone with leukemia to re-establish healthy stem cells by replacing leukemic bone marrow with leukemia-free marrow.

A bone marrow stem cell transplant begins with high doses of chemotherapy or radiation to destroy any leukemia-producing bone marrow. The marrow is then replaced by bone marrow from a compatible donor (allogeneic transplant). In some cases, people are able to use their own bone marrow for transplantation (autologous transplant). This may be possible if you or your child goes into remission and healthy bone marrow is then harvested for a future transplant.

Chronic lymphocytic leukemia

Signs and symptoms
- Swollen lymph nodes
- Fatigue and weakness
- Fever
- Night sweats
- Weight loss
- Frequent infections

Chronic lymphocytic leukemia (CLL) is a cancer of the bone marrow that causes a slow increase in the number of white blood cells known as lymphocytes (see the illustration on page 381). It most often affects older adults, though it may occur at any age.

With CLL, a genetic mutation occurs that causes your blood cells to produce abnormal, ineffective lymphocytes, a type of white blood cell that helps your body fight infection.

The abnormal lymphocytes begin accumulating in your blood and certain organs, where they cause complications. They may crowd healthy cells out of bone marrow and interfere with normal blood cell production.

Diagnosis

Most cases are detected by routine blood tests performed for another reason. Your doctor may then conduct further tests to establish what subtypes of lymphocytes are affected. The results of these tests can help predict how rapidly or slowly the disorder will advance, and they'll help you and your doctor determine how to proceed with treatment.

How serious is chronic lymphocytic leukemia?

The course of chronic lymphocytic leukemia varies widely. Because the lymphocytes are mature and functional, people with this disorder may survive for many years without treatment. In some people, the disorder progresses more rapidly, requiring earlier treatment.

Treatment

People with early-stage chronic lymphocytic leukemia typically don't receive treatment, though clinical trials are evaluating whether early treatment may be helpful. To date, studies have suggested that early treatment doesn't extend lives for people with early-stage chronic lymphocytic leukemia. Rather than put you through the potential side effects and complications of treatment before you need it, doctors monitor your condition and reserve treatment for when your leukemia progresses.

About 1 out of every 3 people with chronic lymphocytic leukemia diagnosed at the earliest stages will never need treatment.

If your doctor determines your chronic lymphocytic leukemia is progressing or is in the intermediate or advanced stages, your treatment options may include:

- **Chemotherapy.** Chemotherapy drugs most commonly used to treat CLL include fludarabine or pentostatin (Nipent) combined with cyclophosphamide and a targeted agent such as rituximab (Rituxan).
- **Immunotherapy.** This newer form of treatment involves harnessing your immune system to fight the cancer. Chimeric antigen receptor engineered T (CAR-T) cell therapy involves immune cells that are engineered to target specific antigens found on cancer cells, helping to destroy the cancer. The therapy has produced very positive responses in the treatment of acute lymphocytic leukemia.
- **Targeted drug therapy.** These drugs are designed to take advantage of the specific vul-

nerabilities of your cancer cells. Chronic lymphocytic leukemia cells have a variety of proteins on their surfaces. Targeted therapy drugs are designed to bind to a specific protein as a way to target and kill leukemia cells.

Two targeted drug therapies used in treating chronic lymphocytic leukemia are rituximab (Rituxan), which is used in combination with chemotherapy, and alemtuzumab (Campath), which may be used alone or in combination with other drugs. Other targeted drugs that may be used to treat CLL include obinutuzumab (Gazyva) and idelalisib (Zydelig).

- **Bone marrow stem cell transplant.** Bone marrow stem cell transplants use strong chemotherapy drugs to kill the stem cells in your bone marrow that are creating diseased lymphocytes. Healthy adult blood stem cells are then infused into your blood, where they travel to your bone marrow and begin making healthy blood cells.

Stem cell transplantation may be a treatment option for people who aren't helped by other therapies. For certain individuals with very aggressive chronic lymphocytic leukemia, bone marrow stem cell transplantation is an important treatment option.

Lymphocytosis

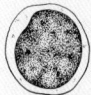

Lymphocytosis is the term for an increase in the percentage of lymphocytes — a type of white blood cell — in your blood. The condition generally causes no symptoms and may be discovered during a routine blood test for some other purpose.

Your bone marrow produces lymphocytes in great quantities. These white blood cells play an important role in your immune system response, defending against infection.

A marked increase in lymphocytes commonly occurs in response to a viral infection, but it may also be due to chronic lymphocytic leukemia. Sometimes, the percentage of lymphocytes increases because of a decrease in the number of other white blood cells. Doctors refer to this as relative lymphocytosis.

Hairy cell leukemia

Signs and symptoms
- Fatigue and weakness
- Feeling of fullness in abdomen
- Easy bruising
- Recurring infections
- Weight loss

Hairy cell leukemia is a rare, slow-growing cancer of the blood in which your bone marrow makes too many B cells (lymphocytes), a type of white blood cell. These excess B cells are abnormal and look "hairy" under a microscope because of fine projections (villi) from their surface.

This type of cancer occurs most commonly in middle-aged or older adults. Children and teenagers don't get hairy cell leukemia. The cancerous cells generally collect in the spleen, causing it to swell. The cause of this type of leukemia is unknown.

Diagnosis
Hairy cell leukemia is generally diagnosed based on results from a physical examination, blood tests and a bone marrow sample. People with hairy cell leukemia have low levels of all three types of blood cells — red blood cells, white blood cells and platelets.

How serious is hairy cell leukemia?
Hairy cell leukemia progresses very slowly and sometimes

remains stable for many years. Untreated hairy cell leukemia that progresses can lead to serious complications such as infections, bleeding and a ruptured spleen. People with hairy cell leukemia are also at increased risk of developing a second cancer.

Treatment

If you aren't experiencing signs or symptoms, treatment may not be necessary. The first line of treatment for the disease is chemotherapy. The drug cladribine — also known as 2-chlorodeoxy-adenosine and 2-CdA — is used to treat hairy cell leukemia. Most people who receive cladribine experience a complete remission that can last for several years. Another drug used to treat the disease is pentostatin (Nipent). It also can produce remission rates similar to cladribine. Interferon also may be used if you can't take chemotherapy.

Lymphomas

Lymphomas are cancers of the lymphatic system, the disease-fighting network spread throughout your body. The lymph system includes the lymph nodes, which are located throughout the body and are connected by small vessels called lymphatics. The tonsils, adenoids, spleen, thymus and bone marrow also are part of the lymphatic system.

Often, the first symptom of lymphoma is enlargement of lymph nodes with no other obvious symptoms. However, lymphomas may also occur outside the lymph nodes in other parts of the body.

Hodgkin lymphoma

Signs and symptoms
- Painless swelling of lymph nodes in the neck, armpits or groin
- Fatigue
- Fever and chills
- Night sweats
- Weight loss and loss of appetite
- Itching

Hodgkin lymphoma (Hodgkin's disease) is a cancer of the lymphatic system. It's named after the 19th-century English doctor Thomas Hodgkin who first described it in 1832. It's an uncommon cancer with several characteristics that distinguish it from other lymphomas.

Hodgkin lymphoma causes the development of abnormal B cells, which originate in bone marrow and are an important component of the immune system response. B cells normally work with T cells, derived from the thymus, to fight infection. T cells kill foreign invaders directly. B cells become plasma cells, which produce antibodies that neutralize foreign invaders.

In most cases of Hodgkin lymphoma, B cells develop into large, abnormal cells called Reed-

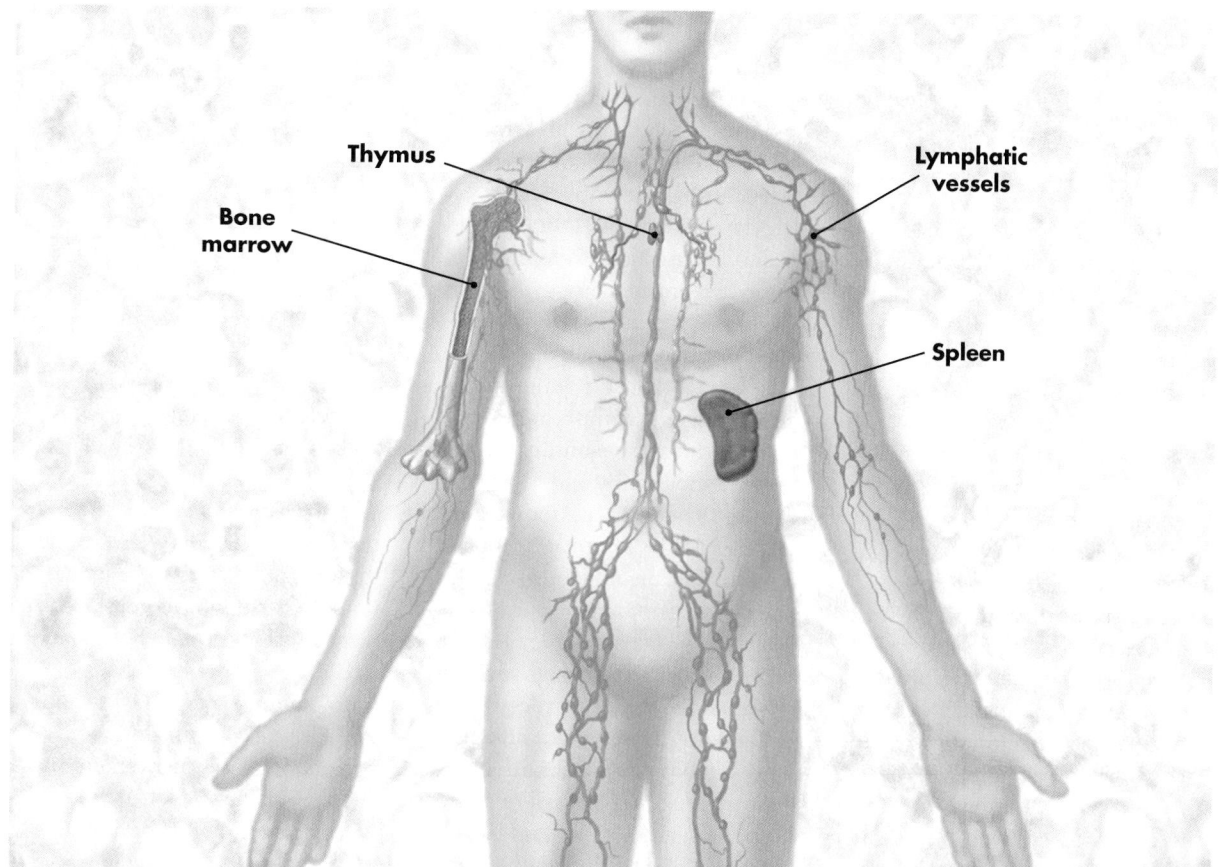

Your lymphatic system is a complex network of thin-walled vessels. It includes the spleen, thymus, bone marrow, lymphatic vessels and, not shown here, the tonsils and adenoids.

Sternberg cells. Instead of undergoing the normal life-and-death cycle of cells, Reed-Sternberg cells continue to live and to produce more cancerous (malignant) B cells. What causes these changes is unknown. In about 50 percent of the individuals with Hodgkin lymphoma, the Epstein-Barr virus is contained in malignant cells. Whether this is the cause of the disease isn't known.

Hodgkin lymphoma normally begins in lymph nodes in your neck, above your collarbone, under your arms or in your groin area. As the abnormal B cells continue to multiply, they may spread beyond the lymphatic system and compromise your body's ability to prevent or fight infection.

Diagnosis

Diagnosis of Hodgkin lymphoma usually involves a medical history, a thorough physical examination, a chest X-ray, and blood and urine tests. A lymph node biopsy, in which lymph node tissue is removed and studied for the presence of the patterns typical of Hodgkin lymphoma, may confirm the diagnosis.

Your doctor may conduct more tests to find out how advanced the cancer is and to determine how best to treat it. These may include a computerized tomography (CT) scan or magnetic resonance imaging (MRI). Other tests, such as a gallium scan, which uses a radioactive substance to indicate where Hodgkin lymphoma may be present, also may be used.

How serious is Hodgkin lymphoma?

Fifty years ago, the disease was almost always fatal but today it's highly treatable. When Hodgkin lymphoma is detected and treated early, the five-year survival rate is greater than 90 percent. Many individuals who die within 15 years after treatment do so because of complications of the treatment, such as secondary cancers or heart failure, rather than of the disease itself.

Treatment

Your treatment depends on several criteria, including the type and stage of the disease, the number and regions of lymph nodes affected, your age, and your overall health. Options include:

Radiation

When the disease is limited to one or two areas, radiation therapy is often used in combination with chemotherapy. It's typical to radiate the affected nodes and the next area of nodes where the disease might progress. Some forms of radiation therapy may increase your risk of other cancers, such as breast or lung cancer.

Chemotherapy

When the disease progresses and involves more lymph nodes or other organs, chemotherapy is often the preferred treatment. Chemotherapy uses specific drug preparations to kill cancer cells.

Currently, the greatest concerns about using chemotherapy for Hodgkin lymphoma are long-term side effects and complications, which include heart, kidney and liver damage and development of secondary cancers.

Drug regimens have been developed that substantially diminish the likelihood of such long-range, life-threatening complications in people who receive multiple courses of chemotherapy and radiation therapy. The most common drug regimen is ABVD. It stands for doxorubicin, bleomycin, vinblastine and dacarbazine.

For individuals in which ABVD isn't effective, other drugs such as brentuximab vedotin (Adcetris) and nivolumab (Opdivo) may be used. Nivolumab is an immunotherapy drug that basically releases the brakes (checkpoints) on your immune cells so that your body can attack the cancer. (See "Checkpoint inhibitors," page 426)

Bone marrow transplant

If the disease recurs after an initial chemotherapy-induced remission, transplantation of your own (autologous) bone marrow or peripheral stem cells may be considered. Peripheral stem cells are bone marrow cells mobilized from the bone marrow into the bloodstream.

Non-Hodgkin lymphoma

Signs and symptoms
- Fever
- Night sweats
- Fatigue
- Weight loss
- Abdominal pain or swelling
- Chest pain, coughing or trouble breathing
- Itchy skin

Non-Hodgkin lymphoma is a cancer that develops from a type of white blood cell (lymphocyte) in your lymphatic system. Non-Hodgkin lymphoma is more than five times as common as the other general type of lymphoma — Hodgkin lymphoma.

Normally, lymphocytes go through a predictable life cycle. Old lymphocytes die, and your body creates new ones to replace them. But in non-Hodgkin lymphoma, your body produces abnormal lymphocytes that continue to divide and grow without control. This oversupply of lymphocytes crowds into your lymph nodes, causing them to swell. Lymphocytes occur either as B cells that originate in bone marrow or T cells, which derive from the thymus gland. About 85 percent of non-Hodgkin lymphomas occur in B cells and the rest in T cells.

There are more than 20 different types of non-Hodgkin lymphoma. The disease accounts for about 4 percent of all new cancers in the United States.

Non-Hodgkin's lymphoma occurs more frequently among people who have received organ transplants, because their immune systems are inhibited by immuno-suppressant therapy. Individuals with AIDS also are at higher risk of developing this disorder. The disease is most common in people in their 60s or older.

Diagnosis

Your doctor may use these procedures to help diagnose non-Hodgkin lymphoma:

- **Physical examination.** Your doctor may examine not only your swollen lymph nodes but also other lymph nodes to determine their size and consistency.
- **Blood and urine tests.** Much of the time, having swollen lymph nodes means you're fighting an infection. Blood and urine tests may help your doctor rule out an infection or other disease, or they may help identify the particular type of non-Hodgkin lymphoma you have.
- **Imaging techniques.** An X-ray or computerized tomography (CT) scan of your chest, neck, abdomen and pelvis may detect the presence and size of tumors. Doctors also use positron emission tomography (PET) scanning to detect non-Hodgkin lymphoma. For a PET scan, a small amount of a radioactive tracer is injected into your body. Tumors absorb more of the tracer than other tissues, making them more noticeable during imaging.
- **Lymph node biopsy.** Taking a sample of lymph node tissue for examination in the laboratory may reveal whether you have non-Hodgkin lymphoma and, if so, which type.
- **Bone marrow biopsy.** To find out if the disease has spread, your doctor may request a biopsy of your bone marrow.

How serious is non-Hodgkin lymphoma?

Less aggressive disease is typically very responsive to initial therapy and the survival rate is good. Aggressive non-Hodgkin lympho-mas, meanwhile, require aggressive treatments in an attempt to produce a complete remission. Still, more than half of affected individuals enter a complete remission with chemotherapy.

Treatment

Several factors, including the type of lymphoma you have, how aggressive it is, your age and your overall health, affect your choice of treatment.

Medications

Different types of drugs may be used to treat non-Hodgkin lymphoma. This includes the drugs cyclophosphamide, doxorubicin, vincristine and prednisone. These medications are often combined for maximum benefit.

Other treatments include antibody and vaccine therapies. Rituximab (Rituxan) is a monoclonal antibody that responds to a special antigen found on lymphoma cells. The medication ibritumomab tiuxetan (Zevalin), consists of a monoclonal antibody joined to a radioactive isotope, as part of a treatment regimen for one type of low-grade non-Hodgkin lymphoma.

Both Rituxan and Zevalin are designed to help your immune system target and destroy cancer cells. Zevalin produces serious side effects, including reduced blood cell counts, and the FDA has approved its use only for people who've had no success with other treatments.

Chimeric antigen receptor engineered T (CAR-T) cell therapy is being studied for treatment of non-Hodgkin lymphoma. It involves immune cells that are engineered to target specific antigens found on cancer cells, helping to destroy the cancer. The drug idelalisib (Zydelig) also may be used to treat the disease.

Radiation

For some types of non-Hodgkin lymphoma, high doses of radia-tion are used to kill cancerous cells and shrink tumors. Sometimes, radiation is used along with chemotherapy to treat specific sites, such as the brain.

Stem cell transplantation

If the cancer relapses after initial, successful treatment, your doctor may recommend an autologous stem cell transplant (see page 1063).

Bleeding Disorders

Bleeding disorders result from a disruption in the complex process by which blood clots form. The clotting process (coagulation) involves blood platelets as well as plasma proteins involved in coagulation (clotting factors).

The process begins when platelets stick to a blood vessel at the site of an injury. An intricate cascade of enzyme reactions occurs to produce a web-like protein network that encircles the platelets and holds them in place (platelet phase) to form a clot (coagulation phase). In this cascade, each clotting factor is transformed, in turn, from an inactive to an active form. Specialized laboratories can study the coagulation mechanism in an affected person's blood to pinpoint the place in the cascade at which the fault lies.

Problems with clotting factors cause bleeding disorders such as hemophilia, von Willebrand disease and disseminated intravascular coagulation. Bleeding disorders based on clotting factor problems tend to cause bleeding in deep tissues and joints, although excessive bruising, severe nosebleeds and other types of bleeding can occur as well.

When platelets are too few (thrombocytopenia) or fail to function, one result is reddish-purple pinpoint hemorrhages seen in the skin (petechiae).

Hemophilia

Signs and symptoms
- Many large or deep bruises
- Joint pain and swelling
- Unexplained bleeding or bruising
- Blood in your urine or stool
- Prolonged bleeding from cuts or injuries
- Nosebleeds with no obvious cause
- Tightness in your joints

Hemophilia is a disorder of your blood-clotting system that causes prolonged bleeding. Small cuts aren't usually much of a problem. The greater concern is deep internal bleeding and bleeding into joints.

The severity of bleeding varies from person to person. The more-severe forms of hemophilia typically become apparent early in life. Excessive bleeding happens often and even spontaneously without any apparent cause. In its mild forms, hemophilia may not become apparent until later in life, and troublesome bleeding episodes may happen only after medical events such as surgery, tooth extraction or a major injury.

The clotting (coagulation) process involves blood particles called platelets and procoagulant plasma proteins called clotting factors. Your blood has 20 clotting factors that are involved in the clotting process. The cause of hemophilia is a deficiency of one of your body's clotting factors. Which type of hemophilia you have depends on which clotting factor is deficient.

- **Hemophilia A.** The most common type, hemophilia A is caused by lack of enough clotting factor VIII.
- **Hemophilia B.** This second most common type is caused by lack of enough clotting factor IX.
- **Hemophilia C.** This type is rare in the United States. Its cause is a lack of clotting factor XI, and symptoms are generally mild with this type of hemophilia.

Hemophilia A and B
Hemophilia A and B almost always occur in boys. Generally, hemophilia A and B pass from mother to son through one of the mother's genes.

With some rare exceptions, everyone has two sex chromosomes, one from each parent. Females inherit an X chromosome from their mother and an X chromosome from their father. Males inherit an X chromosome from their mother and a Y chromosome from their father. The gene that causes hemophilia A or B is located on the X chromosome. This is why men can't pass along the gene that causes hemophilia to their sons.

Most women who have the defective gene are simply carriers and exhibit no signs or symptoms of hemophilia. It's also possible for hemophilia A or B to occur through spontaneous gene mutation.

Hemophilia C
Hemophilia C can occur in both boys and girls. The defective gene that causes hemophilia C can be passed on to children by mothers and fathers, but it follows an inheritance pattern different from that which occurs with hemophilia A and B.

Diagnosis
Analysis of a blood sample from either a child or an adult can show a deficiency of a clotting factor. For people with a family history of the disease, it's possible to test the fetus to determine if the child is affected.

How serious is hemophilia?
Hemophilia is a lifelong disease, but with medication, replacement of deficient clotting factors and proper self-care, most people with the disease lead active, productive lives.

Without treatment, recurrent bleeding into the joints can cause chronic pain and weakness and may even destroy the joints. Bleeding into muscle and soft tissue may put pressure on nerves, producing pain, stiffness and numbness. Permanent nerve damage and muscle wasting eventually may occur. If bleeding occurs in your head, neck or digestive system, the condition is considered extremely serious.

Treatment
Treatment varies with the severity of the disorder. If you have mild hemophilia A, a bleeding episode may be treated with slow injection into a vein of the medication desmopressin (DDAVP). This drug helps stop bleeding by stimulating the release of factor VIII and making blood vessels contract. Occasionally, desmopressin (Stimate) is given by nasal inhalation.

If you have hemophilia B or more-severe hemophilia A, bleeding episodes may stop only after an infusion of clotting factors derived from donated human blood or genetically engineered products called recombinant clotting factors. For factor XI deficiency, plasma infusions are used to stop the bleeding episodes.

Infusion of a clotting factor two or three times a week may help prevent bleeds in hemophilia A and B. This approach may be a way to reduce time spent in the hospital and away from home, work or school and to limit side effects such as damage to joints. Your doctor may train you to do your own infusions of desmopressin or of clotting factor at home, work or school.

Wear a medical alert bracelet so that emergency medical personnel will be alerted to your condition and the type of clotting factor that's best for you. Don't use medications that might worsen bleeding, such as aspirin.

Surgery
When recurrent internal bleeding destroys a joint, your doctor may

Physical therapy and daily physical activity can help joints damaged by hemophilia function better. Swimming, bicycle riding and walking can build up your muscles to help protect your joints. Regular physical activity may help you avoid surgery to replace a severely damaged joint. But don't engage in contact sports.

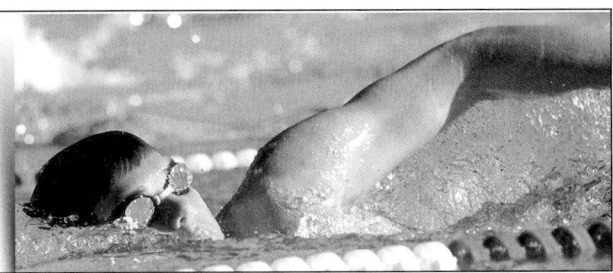

recommend replacing the joint with an artificial joint.

Von Willebrand disease

Signs and symptoms

- Recurrent and prolonged nosebleeds
- Bleeding from the gums
- Increased menstrual flow in women
- Excessive bleeding from a cut or dental procedure
- Blood in stool or urine

Von Willebrand disease is the most common inherited bleeding condition. This chronic disorder is caused by a defect in a clotting factor called von Willebrand factor. The disease is named for the Finnish doctor who described it in 1926. It's also referred to as pseudohemophilia or vascular hemophilia.

In general, it takes longer for people with von Willebrand disease to form clots and stop bleeding when they're cut. The cause of the disease is a defect in the gene that controls von Willebrand factor. When this factor is scarce, or not functioning properly, small blood cells called platelets cannot stick together as they normally do, resulting in uncontrolled bleeding.

In the majority of cases, von Willebrand disease is a mild disorder, called type 1. Type 2 produces mild to moderate symptoms. Type 3, which is rare, is the most severe.

A family history of von Willebrand disease is the leading risk factor. A parent can pass the abnormal gene for the disease to his or her child.

Diagnosis

Specialized blood tests are needed to diagnose the disease. Tests include bleeding time, platelet aggregation, and the level and function of active von Willebrand factor.

Treatment

Type 1 is treated with the medication desmopressin in a nasal spray form (Stimate), typically taken before surgery or menstruation. The medication stimulates your body to release more von Willebrand factor stored in the lining of your blood vessel walls.

Types 2 and 3 require more-complicated treatments. Transfusion of clotting factor concentrates (cryoprecipitate) or plasma may be used. Cryoprecipitate is a clotting factor concentrate derived from donated human blood.

If you have von Willebrand disease, avoid medications that might worsen bleeding, such as aspirin and other nonsteroidal anti-inflammatory drugs (NSAIDs), which interfere with clotting. Also avoid antihistamines, because they can affect platelet functioning.

Disseminated intravascular coagulation

Signs and symptoms

- Bleeding from many sites in the body

Disseminated intravascular coagulation is a nonhereditary bleeding disorder that results paradoxically from excessive coagulation. It occurs when activated clotting factors are present throughout the bloodstream instead of being limited to sites of injury. These

factors can cause blood to clot (coagulate) in small blood vessels all over the body.

Because so much of the body's supply of clotting factors and platelets is used up by this inappropriate coagulation, not enough is available for the formation of clots at injury sites. The body also reacts by stepping up the system that dissolves clots, promoting generalized bleeding.

This rare disorder almost always occurs as a complication of a serious underlying disease, including infection and malignancy, or following trauma or surgery.

Diagnosis

Your doctor will likely request a variety of blood tests to establish the diagnosis.

How serious is disseminated intravascular coagulation?

The severity of this disorder varies. When disseminated intravascular coagulation occurs with cancer or some other disorder, it may be chronic. In such instances, you may not experience spontaneous bleeding and the condition might be detected by blood tests done for other reasons.

More often, the disorder is acute, causing severe bleeding from multiple sites, such as surgical incisions. Clots may form in the legs, or a stroke may occur.

If the conditions that cause the disorder can be successfully treated, disseminated intravascular coagulation will often stop.

Treatment

The only effective approach is to treat the underlying condition.

Transfusion of various blood products also may be necessary to replace the clotting factors depleted by the widespread coagulation. Treatment with heparin, a medication that prevents clotting, may be necessary if there's evidence of clotting or if there's continued bleeding despite blood product transfusions.

Thrombocytopenia

Signs and symptoms
- Easy or excessive bruising
- A reddish-purple skin rash, usually on the lower legs
- Prolonged bleeding from cuts
- Spontaneous bleeding from your gums or nose
- Blood in urine or stools
- Heavy menstrual flow in women
- Profuse bleeding during surgery

Thrombocytopenia is the medical term for a low blood platelet count. Platelets are colorless blood cells that stop blood loss by clumping together and forming plugs in blood vessel holes.

At any given time, you have anywhere from 150,000 to 450,000 platelets per cubic millimeter of circulating blood. Because each platelet lives only about 10 days, your bone marrow makes new platelets daily. When, for any reason, your blood platelet count falls below normal, the condition is called thrombocytopenia.

Causes of thrombocytopenia include:
- Reduced production of platelets by bone marrow
- Early destruction of platelets by the immune system
- Trapping of platelets in the spleen, which filters blood

Sometimes, mild thrombocytopenia is a temporary problem that's self-correcting. Other more serious forms of the condition require treatment.

One form that requires treatment is idiopathic thrombocytopenic purpura (ITP). This condition results when your immune system malfunctions and forms antibod-

ies to attack healthy platelets. It may be related to an autoimmune disease, follow a recent infection or result from certain medications. ITP occurs most often in children and young adults.

Thrombotic thrombocytopenic purpura (TTP) is a rare, life-threatening condition that causes a sudden, sharp drop in blood platelets. The drop occurs when the platelets are drawn into small blood clots that suddenly form throughout the body. The clots can put you at risk of stroke-like symptoms.

Thrombocytopenia may also be caused by a number of disorders or medications. The disorders include systemic lupus erythematosus, lymphoma, chronic lymphocytic leukemia, sarcoidosis, ovarian cancer and viral infections. Medications that can cause thrombocytopenia include heparin, quinidine, sulfonamides, rifampin and many chemotherapy drugs.

Diagnosis
To confirm a diagnosis of thrombocytopenia, your doctor likely will order blood tests to obtain a platelet count and examine your blood under a microscope. He or she may order special blood tests and a bone marrow examination to help determine the cause.

How serious is thrombocytopenia?
The seriousness of thrombocytopenia depends on its cause. Thrombocytopenia may occasionally resolve without any treatment, particularly in children. In these cases, the bone marrow may make up for the shortened life span of platelets by producing large numbers of new ones until the initiating cause subsides.

ITP in adults is often chronic. It may vary in severity over time, and it can even recur after an apparent complete remission. Fortunately, the most serious complications, such as bleeding into the brain and digestive tract, occur only rarely.

Treatment
Sometimes, treatment isn't necessary. If the cause of thrombocytopenia is apparent, treating the underlying condition or stopping use of the offending medication may be sufficient.

Medication
For idiopathic thrombocytopenic purpura, treatment may include medications that block the antibodies that attack platelets, such as a corticosteroid or intravenous immunoglobulin therapy. If these don't help, your doctor may recommend medications that suppress your immune system to reduce antibody formation, such as cyclophosphamide or azathioprine (Imuran).

Surgery
Sometimes, the spleen is removed (splenectomy) to relieve symptoms or to help cure chronic ITP that doesn't respond to corticosteroids. The spleen destroys platelets that are attacked by antibodies.

Blood transfusion
For severe bleeding, lost blood is replaced with transfusions of packed red blood cells. Platelet concentrates are given to treat severe thrombocytopenia, particularly that related to cancer or chemotherapy.

Thrombosis

Thrombosis is the medical term for the condition that occurs when a blood clot (thrombus) forms in a vein or artery. Most often these unwanted clots originate in a deep vein in your leg or pelvis — what is known as deep vein thrombosis. When clots develop in a vein near the surface of your skin, the condition is called superficial thrombosis.

Clots in superficial veins rarely present a serious problem and often clear on their own. But clots in deep veins may detach and travel in the blood to another part of your body. A clot that travels to another part of your body is called an embolus. A clot can migrate to your lungs, causing a pulmonary embolism, or to the brain, causing a stroke.

A blood clot is made up of a plug of platelets, colorless blood cells that repair injured blood vessels, enmeshed in a network of red blood cells and a protein called fibrin. Clots are the end result of a complex process that helps stop bleeding after you've been injured. Sometimes, though, clots form for no purpose.

Those clots that remain localized may not cause symptoms. Often, though, they produce localized pain and swelling. You may also experience redness and warmth over the affected area.

Risk factors

Factors that increase your risk of deep vein thrombosis include:

- **Inherited blood-clotting disorder.** Some people inherit a disorder that makes their blood clot more easily. This inherited condition may not cause problems unless combined with one or more other risk factors.
- **Long periods of inactivity.** Inactivity during prolonged bed rest or a long plane or car trip can decrease blood flow, causing pooling of blood in leg veins and increasing the risk of clotting. Cramped airline seats with little legroom likely have contributed to an increase in deep vein thrombosis. In addition, people who are immobilized after surgery, a heart attack or serious injury are more likely to develop blood clots than individuals who are able to get up and walk around.
- **Pregnancy.** Women are at increased risk during pregnancy and the period immediately after delivery, possibly due to extra pressure on veins in the legs and pelvis. A blood clot traveling to a lung artery (pulmonary embolism) is the most frequent cause of maternal death associated with childbirth. Many women who have pregnancy-related venous thromboembolism also have an inherited clotting disorder.
- **Certain medical conditions.** People with certain forms of cardiovascular disease, a heart attack, stroke or heart failure are more likely to develop blood clots in their veins.
- **Injury to veins.** This may occur during certain surgical procedures, especially hip surgery or knee replacement. It may also result from leg or pelvic fractures. Finally, a direct traumatic injury to the leg may injure the veins and cause a subsequent clot.
- **Certain types of cancer.** Pancreatic, ovarian and lung cancers, in particular, are known to increase levels of clotting factors. Some studies indicate that menopausal women with a history of breast cancer taking tamoxifen also have an increased risk.
- **Estrogen use.** The female hormone estrogen found in birth control pills and estrogen replacement therapy may increase clotting factors in the blood, especially when the medications are combined with tobacco use.
- **Being overweight.** Researchers aren't certain why excess body weight increases the risk of blood clots. One theory is that increased levels of estrogen stored in fatty tissue may contribute to blood clots in some women.
- **Personal or family history.** If you've had deep vein thrombosis before, you're more likely to experience the condition again in the future. If someone in your family has had deep vein thrombosis or a pulmonary embolism, your risk of developing thrombosis is increased.

Diagnosis

To diagnose thrombosis, your doctor will likely ask you a series of questions about your symptoms. He or she may also perform a physical exam to check for areas of swelling, tenderness or discoloration of your skin.

An ultrasound exam, computerized tomography (CT) scan or magnetic resonance imaging (MRI) may be used to identify a clot. Blood tests may also be ordered to check for blood-clotting disorders.

Treatment

People with thrombosis are generally treated with blood thinners (anticoagulants) such as heparin or warfarin (Coumadin) to help stop clot formation. Treatment may also include a newer class of targeted drugs, including the medications dabigatran (Pradaxa), rivaroxaban (Xarelto), apixaban (Eliquis) and edoxaban (Savaysa).

The exact duration of the treatment depends on your particular situation. If you have a chronic disorder that puts you at high risk of recurrent clot formation and pulmonary embolism, you may need to stay on these medications indefinitely. In general, though, you take the medication only for a limited time, usually three to six months, for deep blood clot treatment.

As with all medications, the benefits of anticoagulants in preventing clots needs to be weighed against the risks. Anticoagulants increase your risk of bleeding complications. Many of these complications are minor, such as bleeding from your gums, but some bleeding may be severe and life-threatening.

People taking warfarin need periodic blood tests to check whether their dosage is appropriate: Too high a dose can lead to bleeding, and too low a dose isn't effective in preventing clot formation.

If you have a more serious type of thrombosis or pulmonary embolism, or if other medications aren't working, your doctor may prescribe a type of medication called thrombolytics. These drugs, such as tissue plasminogen activator (TPA), are given intravenously to break up blood clots. Because they can cause serious bleeding, they're used on a limited basis.

During anticoagulant therapy, avoid use of aspirin and other nonsteroidal anti-inflammatory drugs (NSAIDs), such as ibuprofen (Advil, Motrin IB, others). These medications also affect your platelets' ability to form clots, and when combined with warfarin or heparin, may increase your risk of bleeding.

Your doctor may also recommend that you wear compression stockings, which help prevent swelling associated with deep vein thrombosis. The stockings are worn on the leg from your foot to about the level of your knee. The pressure they apply helps reduce the chances that your blood will pool and clot.

Transfusions and Transplants

A variety of treatments are used to treat blood disorders. Two of the most common forms of treatment are blood transfusions and stem cell transplants.

Blood transfusions

Blood transfusions are often a necessary component of treatment for people with certain blood disorders. Blood transfusions increase the blood's ability to transport oxygen, boost immunity and speed clotting time. Transfusions are also used to replace lost blood after an accident or surgery. More than 4 million Americans receive blood transfusions each year.

During a blood transfusion, either whole blood (blood cells plus plasma) or a component of blood is infused into your bloodstream. The blood used in a transfusion is compatible with your blood type and enters your bloodstream through an intravenous (IV) line.

Types

Various components of blood may be transfused. These include packed red blood cells, fresh-frozen plasma, cryoprecipitate, coagulation factor concentrate, granulocytes (a type of white blood cell) and platelets.

When donated blood stored as collected is infused, this is known as whole blood transfusion. The type of transfusion given usually depends on the condition being treated.

Red blood cells
If you're deficient in red blood cells but not in the other components of blood, a transfusion of packed red blood cells is often best. This provides only the red blood cells that you need, without extra blood volume from other blood components. Too much blood circulating in your blood vessels can cause complications such as congestive heart failure.

Transfusions of red blood cells are often used to treat various types of anemia. Red blood cells may also be infused during an acute crisis of inherited anemias such as sickle cell disease, thalassemia or glucose-6-phosphate dehydrogenase deficiency.

Red blood cells can be kept in storage in a liquid form for a maximum of six weeks. Frozen red blood cells may be stored for up to 10 years.

Fresh-frozen plasma
Fresh-frozen plasma is used to treat clotting disorders, including mild forms of hemophilia and von Willebrand disease, as well as serious burns. This blood product can be stored frozen for a year.

Cryoprecipitate
People who are missing certain blood-clotting factors sometimes receive cryoprecipitate, a component of plasma containing certain blood-clotting factors. It's used to treat hemophilia, von Willebrand disease and other clotting disorders.

Coagulation factor concentrate
Coagulation factor concentrates are freeze-dried preparations of specific clotting factors from plasma. Before being transfused, the concentrate must be reconstituted. It's used to treat certain disorders, such as hemophilia.

Granulocytes
Transfusions of granulocytes may be used to treat severe neonatal sepsis, a widespread infection in the body. However, these transfusions are rarely needed today because of the availability of antibiotics. Granulocytes can be stored for only a few hours.

Platelets
Platelet transfusions are used to control bleeding in people who have conditions with certain blood abnormalities. Among people who have undergone chemotherapy or radiation to treat diseases such as leukemia, lymphoma or thrombocytopenia, production of platelets may be suppressed. These individuals are sometimes given transfusions of platelets. Platelets can be stored for only about five days before they become inactive.

Blood groups

When a transfusion is necessary, not just any blood will do. Your blood type dictates the type of blood you can receive.

Blood groups were discovered around 1900, when it was observed that blood collected for transfusions was compatible in some recipients

Blood Safety

Which is safer? Getting in your car and driving to the grocery store or receiving a blood transfusion? A blood transfusion is far safer.

Emergence of the AIDS epidemic prompted significant changes in the way blood is donated, tested and transfused. As a result, the nation's blood supply is safer than at any time in the past.

- *Blood banks are carefully regulated.* All blood banks in this country are federally regulated by the Food and Drug Administration (FDA).
- *Potential donors are carefully screened.* Donors must fill out a written medical history that includes direct questions about behaviors that may lead to a higher risk of transmitting blood-borne infection. They're also interviewed by a trained health care professional who reinforces the importance of a safe blood supply and risk factors that compromise that goal.
- *All donated blood is thoroughly tested.* A highly sensitive test for human immunodeficiency virus (HIV) is used to screen all donated blood. Screening tests also are done to check for hepatitis viruses, human T-lymphotropic viruses and syphilis.

Researchers continue to investigate methods for sterilizing various blood components. Certain techniques are in clinical trials but have yet to receive FDA approval.

Donating Blood

Individuals 18 years of age or older and who weigh at least 110 pounds are eligible to donate blood. However, having certain communicable diseases may preclude you from giving blood. These include hepatitis and the human immunodeficiency virus (HIV). In addition, don't donate blood if you think that you may have an infection. Instead, see your doctor.

When you agree to give blood, trained staff will take a small sample of your blood to check if it contains adequate hemoglobin, the oxygen-carrying component of your blood. They'll also ask you some questions about your health and check your heart rate, blood pressure and temperature. If your health is good and your hemoglobin concentration is normal, staff will draw a pint of blood from a vein in your arm.

Giving blood is quick and generally causes little, if any, pain. It's also safe. New, sterile, disposable equipment is used for each donor. Therefore, there's no risk of contracting a blood-borne disease by donating blood.

The average volume of blood in the body is 10 to 12 pints in men and 8 to 9 pints in women. The usual amount of blood taken during donation is 1 pint. If you're a healthy adult, you can spare this amount without affecting your well-being. Within a few hours, your body will have replaced the fluid you've lost. Your red blood cells will have returned to their usual numbers well before you're eligible to donate again.

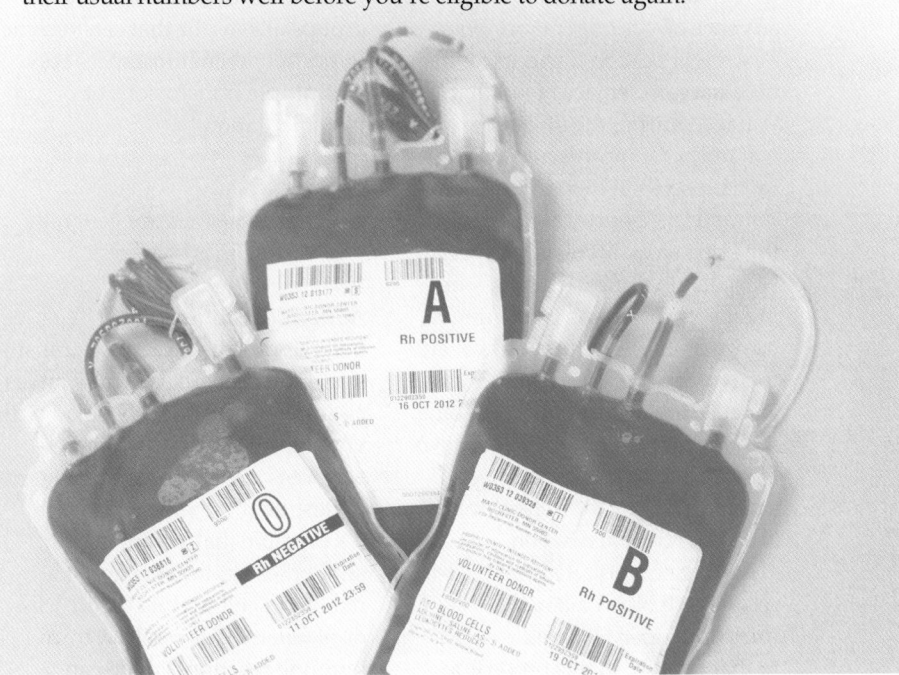

but not in others. It was determined that each person spontaneously forms antibodies against specific proteins (antigens) that his or her own red blood cells lack. If you receive blood that contains proteins different from those in your own blood, your antibodies attack the cells in the transfused blood that carry them.

Blood groups are based on the proteins (antigens) carried on your red blood cells. Like other physical characteristics, the specific antigens in your blood are determined by genes inherited from your parents.

There are four major blood groups: A, B, AB and O. Each of these is divided into two rhesus (Rh) types, positive and negative. The most common blood group in the United States is O positive, followed by A positive, B positive, O negative, A negative, AB positive, B negative and AB negative.

If your blood group is A, your red blood cells are coated with A antigens, and your plasma develops antibodies against B. If your blood group is B, you have B antigens and your plasma develops antibodies against A. Type AB blood has both A antigens and B antigens, and type O has neither.

Autologous Transfusions

The safest blood for you to receive is your own. Your immune system won't consider your blood foreign, and you can't give yourself any infections that you don't already have. Transfusing one's own blood, known as autologous transfusion, is becoming more popular.

In an emergency, you may have to rely on transfusions from random donors unless you're at a medical center that can salvage blood otherwise lost during surgery. However, if your doctor is planning elective surgery, ask if you can donate your own blood ahead of time. Usually, you give it over a period of a few weeks in advance of your operation. Your blood will be stored and used, if necessary, to replace blood that you lose during the operation.

It may cost more to receive your own blood than to get a random donor transfusion. The reason is the extra work involved in specially labeling your own blood, storing it separately and delivering it to you at the right time. However, many people consider the added expense to be worth it. If, for some reason, you can't donate your own blood, a blood bank will select a donor whose blood shouldn't cause an adverse reaction.

During surgery, it's possible to recover the blood a patient loses during an operation and return it to that person. In this procedure, known as intraoperative autologous transfusion, surgeons salvage blood cells from the wound while they're operating. The cells are washed free of debris from the wound and then returned to the patient.

Because there will always be situations in which using your own blood is impossible, the increase in autologous transfusions doesn't eliminate the need for blood donors.

In most cases, blood that's the exact same type as yours must be used in a transfusion. For example, if you have A positive blood, you must receive A positive blood. However, type O negative can be used in emergencies for all of the blood types.

If your blood is Rh negative, your red blood cells don't carry an antigen called the rhesus (Rh) factor. If it's Rh positive, they do.

Women may develop anti-Rh antibodies after exposure to Rh positive blood at the time of their first pregnancy. If exposed again to Rh positive blood, serious complications and even death could result. To avoid risks, Rh typing is done routinely before transfusions, and blood of the same Rh type is used for transfusions.

Many other minor blood subgroups also occur that can become important in circumstances such as multiple transfusions or organ transplantation.

Risks

Blood transfusions are generally safe, but there is some risk.

Antibody reactions

Before you receive a blood transfusion, a blood bank typically mixes a sample of the donor's blood with yours to check compatibility — a process called crossmatching.

Despite these precautions, it's possible that you may carry antibodies against the donor's red blood cells, white blood cells or platelets. This can lead to an immune reaction, which can cause a variety of signs and symptoms, including shaking, chills, fever, hives, wheezing and shortness of breath, chest pain, low back pain, pink urine, nausea, and pain along the vein that received the transfusion. Shock, kidney failure or intravascular coagulation rarely ensue but may cause death.

Your risk of having such an immune reaction is increased if you've received multiple blood transfusions in the past. Exposure to blood antigens from multiple donors may lead to antibodies against obscure blood groups.

Communicable diseases

The risk of contracting a communicable disease from a blood transfusion is remote, but it's always a possibility. All blood donors are screened, and donated blood is tested for viruses such as the human immunodeficiency virus (HIV), hepatitis and human T-lymphotropic virus. Methods to sterilize blood components have been developed and are being tested in clinical trials. These methods may further improve safety in the future.

Other reactions

Other adverse reactions to transfusions are possible. For instance, if you have heart trouble, you may have difficulty handling an increase in blood volume. In addition, if you receive repeated transfusions of red blood cells — 200 transfusions or more — you may experience iron overload.

It's important to realize that most people who receive a transfusion have no adverse reactions or infections as a result. If you need a transfusion, don't let unfounded fears keep you from accepting it.

Future products

Researchers at many medical centers are working to develop synthetic substitutes for blood. There are several reasons for this effort. Synthetic substitutes could help to prevent transfusion complications, such as infections and immunological reactions, and overcome shortages of donated blood. The substances are still experimental. In addition, although they're designed to carry oxygen, they can't perform other important functions of blood.

Stem cell transplantation

Transplanting stem cells offers hope to people with certain blood and bone marrow disorders, including aplastic anemia, leukemia, lymphoma and multiple myeloma.

Stem cells produce all of the different types of cells and tissues that make up your body. When a stem cell divides, one of the resulting cells becomes specialized — it creates certain types of cells in your body, such as blood, heart or brain cells. The other cell from that division is an exact copy of the original stem cell and is available for future division when repair is needed.

Transplanting blood-producing stem cells harvested from bone marrow or blood can allow the body to replenish healthy blood cells when existing cells are damaged, either due to disease or use of medication to destroy disease. For example, high doses of chemotherapy or radiation treatments used to kill cancer cells also destroy stem cells.

Healthy blood-producing stem cells generate the 200 billion new oxygen-carrying red blood cells required by your body each day, as well as infection-fighting white blood cells and platelets that help stop bleeding. Blood-producing stem cells can be harvested from the bone marrow or blood, either from a donor or from the individual in need of them.

When treating blood disorders, bone marrow has traditionally been used as the source of blood-producing stem cells. This sponge-like material found inside certain bones produces most stem cells. After treatments such as chemotherapy and radiation to treat cancer, bone marrow is transplanted into the individual receiving treatment. Bone marrow transplants have been performed successfully for more than 30 years.

Currently, stem cell transplants commonly use blood rather than bone marrow as the source of the stem cells. In the early 1980s, researchers discovered that stem cells circulate in the bloodstream. These cells are called peripheral

blood stem cells. They're rather scarce in the bloodstream, but their numbers can be increased by medications that encourage bone marrow to release stem cells.

The use of peripheral blood stem cells instead of bone marrow makes transplants safer, particularly for older adults. This type of transplant procedure is called peripheral blood stem cell transplantation.

Types

A stem cell transplant may be performed in a variety of manners:

Syngeneic

In a syngeneic transplant, the donor is the identical twin of the stem cell recipient. Identical twins have the same genetic makeup, so the recipient isn't at risk of a severe reaction to the transplant. However, few people have identical twins.

Allogeneic

In this type of transplant, the donor is, preferably, a sibling or parent of the recipient. In order to establish the compatibility of the potential donor's stem cells, a test for human lymphocyte antigens

(HLA test) is done to determine if there's an HLA match.

This test examines six proteins found on the surface of the white blood cells and most other cells. The odds of an HLA donor match are about 25 percent with two siblings in a family, but they increase to about 75 percent with six siblings.

If no relative is found with an HLA match, an unrelated donor is selected on the basis of that person's HLA results being identical or nearly identical to the recipient's. A national bone marrow registry has been set up to help locate HLA-matched bone marrow donors.

Autologous

An autologous transplant is often used in individuals with cancer. In an autologous stem cell transplant, stem cells are collected from the person with cancer and stored for later transplant. After the individual receives treatment with high doses of chemotherapy or radiation that can destroy stem cells, the stored cells are transplanted back into the individual. Because the person's own cells are used, there's no risk of rejection.

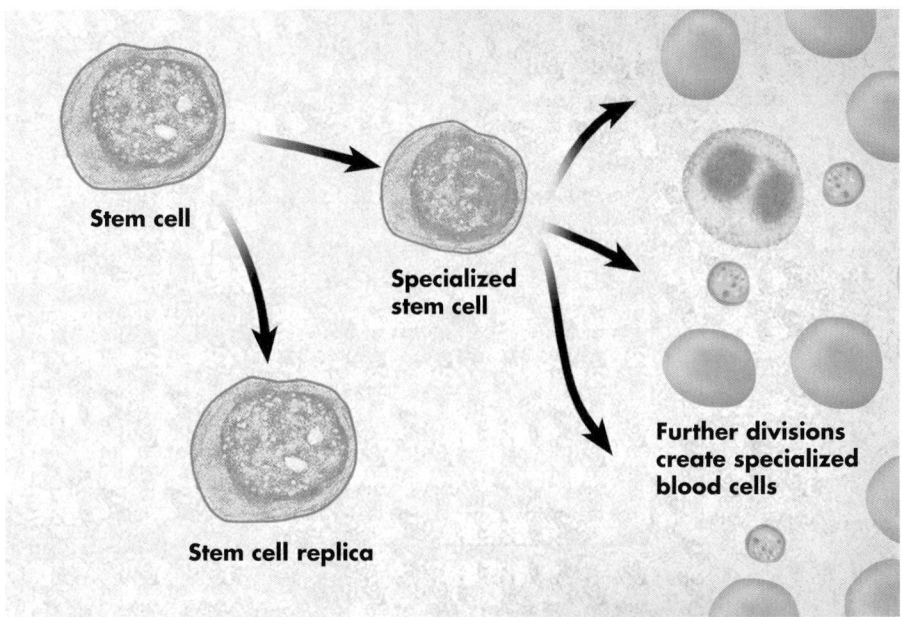

Stem cell

Specialized stem cell

Further divisions create specialized blood cells

Stem cell replica

When a stem cell divides, it creates a stem cell that's specialized — one that can create cells, such as blood cells, that perform specific functions. It also creates an exact replica of itself.

The procedure

The first step in the transplantation process is the collection (harvest) of stem cells. The procedure used depends on whether blood or bone marrow is chosen as the source of the cells. If blood is chosen, growth factor injections are administered with or without chemotherapy in an attempt to release (mobilize) stem cells from the bone marrow into the bloodstream.

Blood tests are then done to determine if sufficient stem cells have been mobilized. The cells are then collected from a vein — much like when donating blood — but using an apheresis machine. This machine separates the blood into its various components, and only those parts that are needed are saved. The other parts are returned to the body.

When bone marrow is selected as the source of the cells, the person is given general anesthesia and marrow is removed from a pelvic bone. This involves making small cuts in the skin over the pelvic bone and inserting a large needle to draw marrow from the bone. The process takes about an hour.

The next step typically is the administration of chemotherapy with or without radiation therapy to kill the cancer cells. This is followed by preparation of the recipient's bone marrow to accept the transplanted stem cells. Finally, the collected stem cells are injected into the recipient's veins. Once in the blood, the cells travel throughout the body until they reach bone marrow, where, in about two to three weeks, they produce new cells.

In syngeneic and allogeneic stem cell transplantation, the stem cells generally are removed from the donor and injected into the recipient on the same day. In autologous transplantation, the stem cells are removed and frozen. These cells can remain frozen for months to years — until the individual has completed treatment.

Diseases when transplantation is used

The best results from allogeneic and syngeneic transplantation have been obtained in cases of severe aplastic anemia, chronic myeloid leukemia and acute myelogenous leukemia. Clinical trials are evaluating the use of stem cell transplantation for treating acute nonlymphocytic leukemia in remission, acute lymphocytic leukemia in remission, lymphoma in remission and neuroblastoma in remission.

In autologous transplantation, the best results have been obtained in treating multiple myeloma, Hodgkin lymphoma and non-Hodgkin lymphoma. Studies suggest that those whose disease is responsive to chemotherapy or who achieve complete remission following the use of chemotherapy after a relapse are the best candidates for this procedure. The role of stem cell transplants in breast cancer, ovarian cancer and other solid tumors isn't well-established.

Risks

The major cause of toxicity and death in allogeneic stem cell transplantation is graft-versus-host disease (GVHD). This complication occurs when the transplanted white blood cells from the donor marrow (graft) attack the marrow recipient's (host's) own cells because they perceive the host's cells as foreign.

GVHD can affect the skin, liver, gastrointestinal tract and lungs of the transplant recipient. It's the major complication in allogeneic transplantation, but it isn't a problem in syngeneic or autologous transplantation.

The mortality rate among recipients of an allogeneic transplant ranges from about 10 to 40 percent in the first 100 days after the procedure, primarily from infection or GVHD. Another major problem is pneumonia, which can result from an infection or other complications.

Among people receiving an autologous stem cell transplant, the mortality rate in the first 100 days after the procedure is less than 5 percent.

Clinical trials are being conducted to determine methods to prevent graft-versus-host disease and to increase the safety and effectiveness of stem cell transplants. ■

Skin, Hair and Nails

Your skin is a unique and remarkable organ. The 2 square yards of skin that cover the average adult constitute approximately 15 percent of the body's total weight. Each square inch of your skin contains millions of cells and many specialized nerve endings for sensing heat, cold and pain. In addition, skin contains oil glands, hair follicles and sweat glands. An intricate network of blood vessels nourishes this complex structure.

Your skin serves many purposes. For one, it's your body's first line of defense against the environment around you. It helps protect you from injury, infection and harmful substances. By its texture, temperature, color and clarity, your skin gives information about your general health.

Your skin also serves as your body's heat regulator. Blood vessels in your skin dilate or constrict according to your body's temperature. When you're hot, you sweat and the evaporation of the sweat on your skin lowers your body's temperature. When your body is chilled, these blood vessels become narrowed, and your skin becomes

pale and cold. This constriction decreases the flow of blood through your skin, reducing heat loss and conserving heat for other organs of your body.

Your sweat glands also excrete waste products, such as urea. However, this is a minor pathway of waste disposal compared with your kidneys' production of urine.

Your skin plays a major role in your sense of touch. Sensory nerves send signals to your brain about hazards. Another group of specialized nerve endings in your skin can arouse your nervous and endocrine systems to sexual excitement.

Your nails and your hair serve important functions, too. Your nails, which are a product of your skin cells, help you pick up and handle objects and provide signs of your general health. Each individual hair on your body grows from its own follicle located in your skin. Your hair helps protect your scalp from excessive sun exposure and your head from trauma.

Over your lifetime, you may develop problems with your skin, hair and nails. Most of these conditions are best treated by a skin specialist called a dermatologist.

The Basics

Your skin, hair and nails are interrelated. Your nails, hair and outer layer of skin (epidermis) are each composed of the protein keratin. But each of these three body parts has its own unique characteristics.

Your skin

Your skin is composed of three layers — the epidermis, the dermis and the subcutaneous tissue. Your skin averages only a tenth of an inch in thickness, ranging from very thin on your eyelids and the inner folds of your elbows to very thick on the palms of your hands and soles of your feet. Housed in your skin are sweat glands, oil glands and hair follicles.

Epidermis
Your skin's outer layer, the epidermis, is as thin as a pencil line. It provides a protective layer of skin cells that you continuously shed. Squamous cells lie just below the outer surface. Basal cells, which produce new skin cells, are at the bottom of the epidermis.

It takes approximately a month for new skin cells to move from the basal cells to the outer surface. As the cells move away from their source of nourishment, they become smaller and flatter, changing into a lifeless protein called keratin. They remain on the surface only briefly as a protective cover and then flake off as a result of washing and friction. Thus, the skin is a dynamic organ that's constantly replenished.

Cells that manufacture skin constitute about 95 percent of your epidermis. The remaining cells produce a black pigment, called melanin.

Melanin provides the coloring of your skin and helps protect it from ultraviolet light. People of all races are born with the same number of pigment cells (melanocytes). The rate at which melanin granules

Your Skin

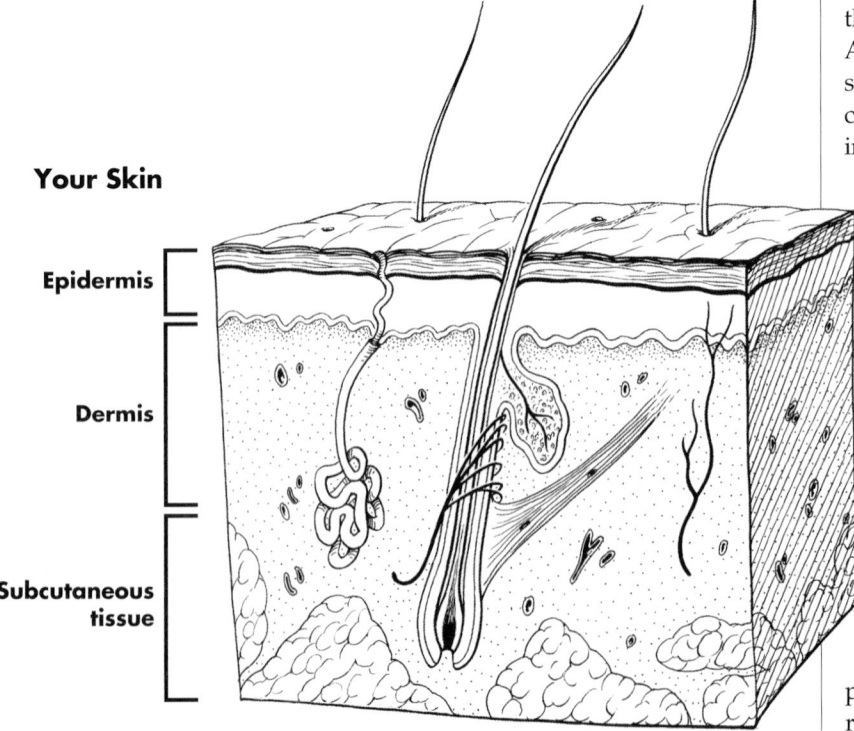

Epidermis

Dermis

Subcutaneous tissue

are formed in these cells and their concentration in the epidermis are inherited characteristics and major factors in skin color differences.

Dermis

Just below the epidermis is the dermis, which makes up 90 percent of the bulk of your skin. It's a dense bed of strong fibers (collagen) and elastic fibers (elastin) through which blood vessels, muscle cells, nerve fibers, lymph channels, hair follicles and glands are interspersed.

The dermis gives strength and elasticity to your skin. As you age, the dermis layer becomes thinner and your skin more transparent, particularly in sun-exposed areas. This accounts for the prominence of blood vessels in the skin of older adults.

Subcutaneous tissue

The deepest layer of skin is the subcutaneous tissue, through which blood vessels and nerves run. This layer, composed primarily of fat, insulates and protects your inner organs and helps keep your skin resilient. Your oil and sweat gland bases are located here. Subcutaneous tissue also thins with aging.

Oil glands

Oil glands (sebaceous glands) are distributed throughout your skin but are most concentrated in your scalp, face, midchest and genitals. They're each attached to a hair follicle and secrete an oily substance (sebum) that rises through the follicle to the surface of the skin. The oily sebum — made up of fatty acids, cholesterol, various hydrocarbons, unsaturated alcohols and waxes — lubricates and protects your skin.

Sweat glands

You have two types of sweat glands. The eccrine glands are distributed throughout your body, with the richest supply in your palms, soles, scalp and underarms

(see the illustration on page 370). The apocrine glands are specialized sweat glands that secrete sweat in times of stress or emotion. In the ear, they form a portion of the earwax. They're most abundant under your arms and around your nipples and genitals.

Your hair

The human being is a hairy animal. Only your lips, palms and soles are truly hairless. Each hair grows from a single, live follicle that has its roots in the subcutaneous tissue of your skin.

Oil from an oil gland next to the hair follicle provides gloss and, to some degree, waterproofing for the hair. Your hair follicles are nourished by minerals, proteins, vitamins, fats and carbohydrates brought to them by tiny blood vessels (capillaries).

Hair is made up of the dead protein keratin and also contains

melanin. Just as the pigment cells determine your skin color, the number and type of melanin granules in your hair determines its color.

Your fingernails and toenails

Your fingernails and toenails also are products of your epidermis and are composed of the protein keratin. Each nail grows outward from a nail root (matrix) that extends into a skin nail fold.

The structure of your nails isn't related to the structure of your bones. You can't strengthen brittle fingernails or toenails by taking extra calcium or gelatin.

Your fingernails normally grow approximately two to three times faster than your toenails, and nail growth slows in old age. Sudden or significant changes in the appearance of your nails can be an early sign of illness.

Hair Follicle

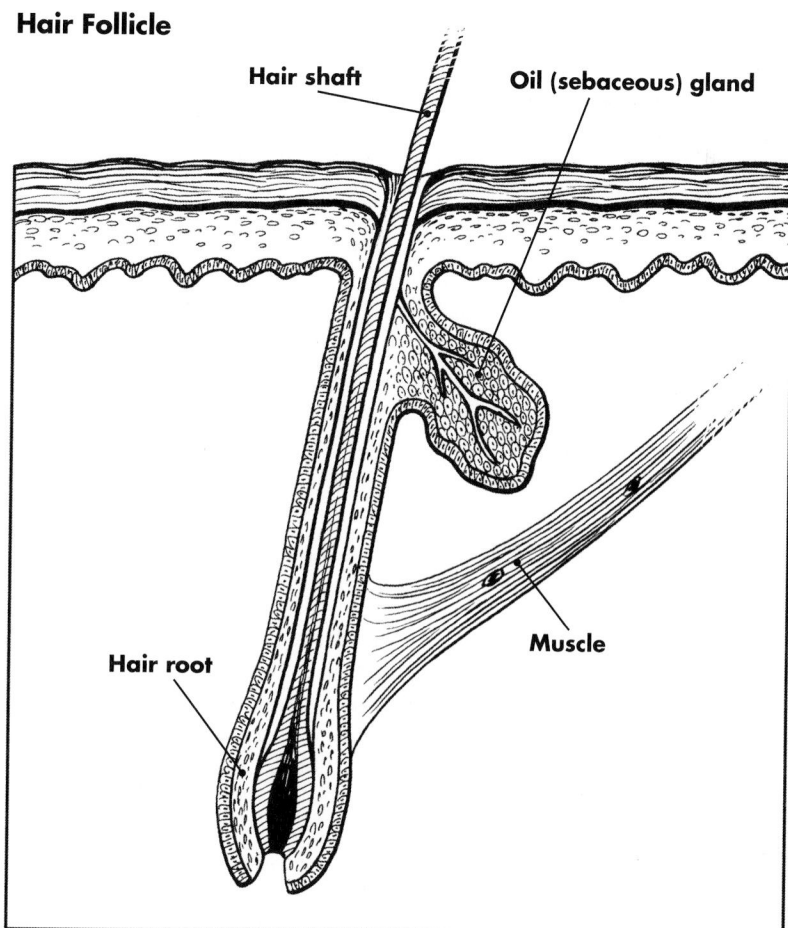

Hair shaft

Oil (sebaceous) gland

Muscle

Hair root

Your Fingernail

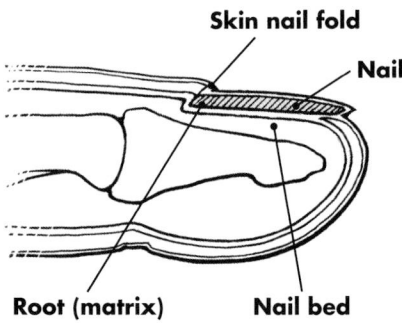

- Skin nail fold
- Nail
- Root (matrix)
- Nail bed

Proper Skin Care

Your skin isn't the baby-soft body glove you were born with. With age, your skin normally becomes thinner and finely wrinkled. Oil-producing (sebaceous) glands become less active, and your skin becomes drier. The number of blood vessels in your skin decreases, and your dermis can get thinner and more fragile, so you lose your youthful color and glow.

In addition, with aging your skin replaces old cells more slowly, and cells repair themselves less effectively. This can result in slower turnover of surface skin and slower healing of damaged skin.

Good self-care habits can help delay the natural aging process and prevent many skin problems. The single most important goal is to protect your skin from ultraviolet light, which naturally breaks down elastin and collagen in skin. Follow these tips to keep your skin healthy. The benefits of good skin care will become increasingly apparent as you grow older.

Avoid the sun
Regardless of your skin color or your age, avoiding ultraviolet rays from the sun and tanning beds can help prevent unnecessary aging as well as skin cancer.

Dark skin can tolerate more sun than can fair skin. However, any skin can become blotchy, leathery and wrinkled from long-term overexposure to the sun. Avoiding the sun — particularly during peak hours of 10 a.m. to 3 p.m. — wearing protective clothing, applying sunscreen and moisturizing your skin daily can help protect it from the sun's harmful effects.

Don't smoke
Nicotine constricts blood vessels that nourish your skin. Over time, smoking can cause your skin to become pale and sallow. It can also cause deep wrinkles to develop around your lips and slow your skin's ability to heal.

Use appropriate cosmetics
If you use cosmetics, be sure to match them to your skin type. If you have dry skin, use makeup with a heavier, creamier base. If you have skin that's oily or acne prone, use a water-based product that's labeled noncomedogenic, which means that it's less likely to clog the small pores in your skin. Preferably, choose a brand of foundation, lipstick and eyeliner that's nonallergenic. Look for a moisturizer that's fragrance-free and has the least amount of preservatives. If you're allergic to any of the ingredients in a product, avoid it.

Cleanse gently
Proper cleansing is another important strategy in protecting your skin. If you wear eye makeup, remove it first using cotton balls to avoid damaging the delicate tissue around your eyes. When washing your face, use tepid, never hot, water and a washcloth or sponge to remove dead cells. Use a mild soap for your face and skin. A mild superfatted variety of soap, such as Dove or Basis, may be better if your facial skin is dry. You may need to clean oily skin two or three times each day.

Bathing can dry your skin. Especially during dry weather, follow the anti-drying bathing basics found on page 1078.

What's Your Skin Color?

Skin color is defined by the degree to which you tan or burn when exposed to the sun. Your skin color affects your risk of skin cancer and photoaging, a term that describes damage from ultraviolet rays to the skin, including wrinkles, pigmentation and roughness.

The Fitzpatrick classification of skin type divides skin into the following six categories:
1. Always burns, never tans (pale, white skin)
2. Always burns easily, tans minimally (white skin)
3. Burns moderately, tans uniformly (light brown skin)
4. Burns minimally, always tans well (moderate brown skin)
5. Rarely burns, tans profusely (dark brown skin)
6. Never burns (deeply pigmented dark brown to black skin)

Type 1 people typically have pale, white skin, red or blond hair, blue or green eyes and Celtic (Irish, Scottish, Welsh or Breton) ancestry. People with this skin type have the greatest risk of sun-induced skin problems, including skin cancer and photoaging. Type 2 and 3 people have more pigmented shades of white skin and have a moderate to strong risk of sun-induced skin problems. Type 4 and 5 people have olive to medium brown skin color and have moderate to low risk of sun-induced skin problems. Type 6 people have dark brown to black skin color. Their risk of skin problems related to sun exposure is minimal.

Because no one is completely immune from sun damage and skin cancer, dermatologists recommend using a broad-spectrum sunscreen with a sun protection factor (SPF) of 15 or higher for all skin types.

Shave gently

Shaving can irritate your skin. If you shave with a blade razor, always use a sharp blade. Men can soften their beard before shaving by applying a warm washcloth for a few seconds and using plenty of shaving cream. Using an electric razor too vigorously also can irritate your skin. You can buy various preparations to prevent skin irritation caused by an electric razor.

Women who shave or use hair remover also need to take steps avoid skin irritation.

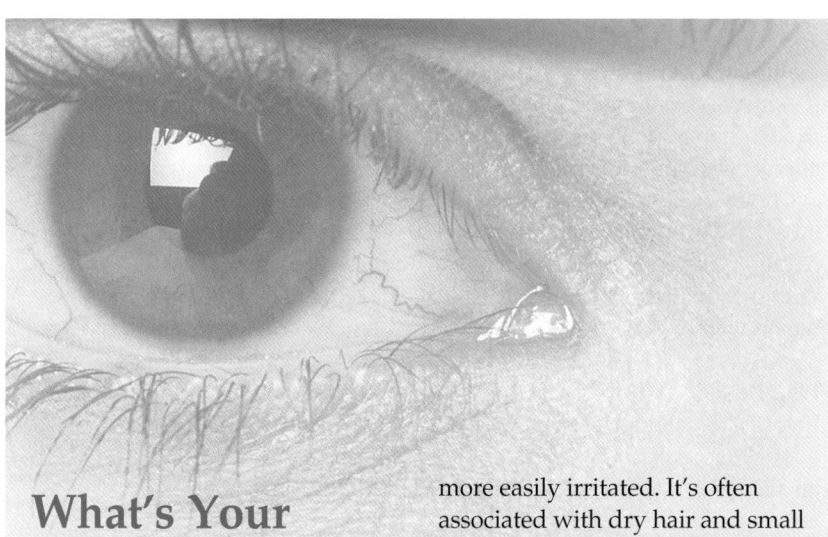

What's Your Skin Type?

The skin of your face is generally the best guide in classifying skin type. Examine your skin closely, especially the pores.

Oily skin

Oily skin is caused by overactivity of the oil-producing (sebaceous) glands. Oily skin has large pores. People with oily skin tend to develop acne, and they're less likely to develop wrinkles as early in life as people with dry skin are. Most people with oily skin also have oily hair.

Dry skin

Dry skin can be caused by underactivity of the sebaceous glands, environmental conditions or normal aging. Dry skin is usually

more easily irritated. It's often associated with dry hair and small pores. People with dry skin tend not to develop acne. As they age, their skin tends to become drier and more wrinkled than that of people with oily skin.

Balanced skin

Balanced skin is neither oily nor dry. It's smooth with fine texture and few problems. It has a tendency to become dry as a result of environmental factors and aging.

Combination skin

Combination skin consists of oily regions — often on the forehead and around the nose — and regions that are balanced or dry.

Eczema

Eczema refers to the skin conditions known as dermatitis. Most often eczema is used interchangeably with atopic dermatitis. However, there are many types of dermatitis; therefore, there are many types of eczema.

Atopic dermatitis

Signs and symptoms

- Thickened, fissured skin, most often in the folds of the elbows or backs of the knees and on the face, neck, hands and feet
- A rash
- Itching

Eczema (atopic dermatitis) is an itchy inflammation of the skin (see the illustration on page 396) that's often accompanied by asthma and allergies such as hay fever (allergic rhinitis). Frequently, it runs in families in which other family members have asthma or hay fever. The condition can cause extreme itching and great frustration.

Eczema is common. In the United States, it affects about 10 percent of infants and 3 percent of all Americans. When it occurs in infants, it's called infantile eczema. This condition typically begins in infancy and may vary in severity during childhood and adolescence. It tends to become less of a problem in adulthood, unless it's caused by allergens or irritants in the workplace.

In infants, the condition often involves an oozing, crusting rash, mainly on the face and scalp, but it can occur anywhere. The condition typically improves before age 2, and treatment can help relieve the itching until then. After infancy, the rash becomes dryer and tends to be red to brownish-gray in color. The skin may be scaly or thickened. The intense itching may continue.

In teens and young adults, the patches typically occur on the hands and feet but can occur anywhere, including the bends of the elbows, backs of the knees, ankles, wrists, face, neck and upper chest.

Treatment

Although eczema is related to allergies, eliminating allergens alone is rarely helpful in treating this condition. Occasionally, items that trap dust — such as feather pillows, down comforters, mattresses, carpeting and drapes — can worsen the condition. Allergy shots usually aren't successful in treating eczema and might even make the condition worse.

Avoid clothing that's rough, tight or scratchy or doesn't ventilate well. Temperature changes, sweating and stress also can worsen the condition. Avoid direct contact with wool products, as well as harsh soaps and detergents.

Treatment often consists of applying hydrocortisone-containing lotions or nonsteroidal creams to the affected areas. Tacrolimus (Protopic) and pimecrolimus (Elidel) are nonsteroidal creams that help suppress itching, redness and inflammation. Both are approved for short-term or long-term intermittent treatment, often when other treatments don't work or aren't well-tolerated. Tacrolimus and pimecrolimus are more commonly used for mild to moderate eczema. The medication crisaborole (Eucrisa) may be prescribed for eczema unresponsive to other treatments.

If your skin cracks open, your doctor may prescribe mildly astringent wet dressings to prevent infection. If itching is severe, oral antihistamines may help. Diphenhydramine (Benadryl, Sominex) has substantial sedative action and may be helpful at bedtime.

Contact dermatitis

Signs and symptoms
- Redness and itching
- Blisters and weeping from the involved skin in severe cases
- Skin changes limited to the area of contact with the causative agent

Contact dermatitis (see the illustration on page 392) results from direct contact with an irritant or allergen. Common irritants include laundry soap, skin soap and cleaning products. Possible allergens include rubber, metals, jewelry, perfume, cosmetics and plants such as poison ivy. If you're sensitive to an allergen, just brief exposure to a small amount of allergen can cause dermatitis.

In contact dermatitis, only the areas of skin contacted by the offending substance react. The area with the greatest exposure reacts most severely.

Diagnosis
If your dermatologist suspects your skin problem is the result of an allergic reaction, he or she may test your skin by applying small amounts of different substances and examining the site for allergic reactions 48, 72 and 96 hours later. This assessment, called patch testing, determines if you have allergic contact dermatitis, which is caused by an immune system reaction. Relatively few people have such a response. In allergic contact dermatitis, the allergen might be something that you had been in contact with for years without trouble until now.

Substances such as acids, solvents, strong soaps and detergents are usually irritants rather than allergens. When an irritant causes a skin reaction, the condition is known as irritant contact dermatitis. Some substances are both allergens and irritants.

Some hard-to-identify causes of contact dermatitis include ingredients in:
- Medicinal lotions, such as antihistamines, antibiotics or antiseptics
- Plants, ranging from trumpet creeper to mangoes
- Rubber
- Metals, such as nickel
- Dyes
- Cosmetics
- Chemicals used in manufacturing, such as those used in the production of shoes or clothing

Some substances cause dermatitis only when they contact skin exposed to sunlight (see page 1088), what's known as photosensitivity. Typical examples include shaving lotions, sunscreens, ointments containing sulfa drugs, some perfumes and coal tar products. Other causes of contact dermatitis may be airborne, such as ragweed pollen and insecticide spray.

Treatment
Treatment of contact dermatitis consists primarily of identifying the offending agent and avoiding it. Sometimes, hydrocortisone-containing creams or slightly astringent wet dressings may help relieve redness and itching. A slightly astringent dressing can be

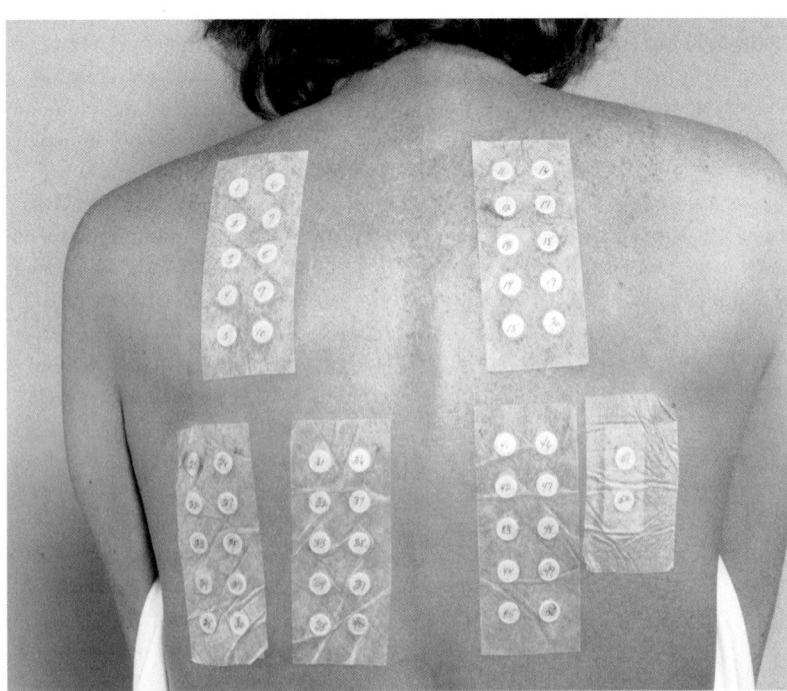

Patch testing can be helpful in determining if you're allergic to a specific substance. Small amounts of different substances are placed on your skin under an adhesive paper tape.

made by wetting a dressing with a solution of 1 ounce white vinegar to 16 to 32 ounces water.

The blisters that form from contact dermatitis contain serum from blood and they don't "spread." However, they should be left intact, if possible.

Neurodermatitis

Signs and symptoms

- Itching, aggravated by nervous tension
- Small patches of thickened, leathery skin
- Scratch marks (excoriations)

Neurodermatitis is a common skin disorder, sometimes referred to as lichen simplex chronicus, that consists of small, flat growths (plaques) of various sizes, generally 1 to 10 inches in diameter. The growths have definite margins that have become thickened and leatherlike (lichenified).

Neurodermatitis can occur when something such as a tight garment rubs or scratches your skin. This irritation may lead you to rub or scratch your skin repeatedly. Common locations for the disorder include the ankles, waist, outer forearms or arms, and the back of your neck.

Generalized neurodermatitis is a similar condition, but it tends to involve more of the body. The affected skin tends to be less leathery. Long-standing neurodermatitis may lead to brownish pigmentation. This condition is often associated with nervous tension and anxiety.

Treatment

The primary treatment for these skin problems is to stop the scratching. Scratching makes the skin itch more, creating a vicious cycle. If you have trouble ignoring the itchy area, try placing a dressing over it that's difficult to remove.

Antihistamines or anti-anxiety medications (anxiolytics) may help you stop the scratching, but your doctor will want to monitor your

use of anxiolytics because they can be addictive.

Your doctor may recommend over-the-counter hydrocortisone-containing lotions to decrease the itching and inflammation. If the inflammation is more severe, your doctor may prescribe a stronger cortisone preparation. In addition, the thickened plaques may be thinned by applying tar or salicylic acid-containing ointments, which have a soothing and peeling effect.

Stasis dermatitis

Signs and symptoms

- Thickening of the skin at your ankles and shins
- Discolored — reddish or brownish — skin
- Itching
- Varicose veins

Varicose veins and other circulatory conditions in which the return of fluids to the heart is reduced can cause an increase of fluid in tissues beneath the skin (edema). Such areas may be poorly nourished and become fragile.

Because your ankles in your lower body have less supportive tissue, they're often the site of edema. The overlying skin may inflame, itch and discolor. In severe situations, open ulcers that are hard to heal may develop in the skin around the ankles. This condition is called stasis dermatitis (see the illustration on page 392).

Although initially the skin may become thin, it later becomes irregularly thickened, perhaps in response to the itching and excessive scratching.

Treatment

Treatment of stasis dermatitis consists of correcting the condition that causes fluid to accumulate in your ankles. Options for controlling edema include frequently elevating your legs above the level of your heart. The mainstay of treatment, however, is the use of elastic support stockings that help

prevent fluid from accumulating in the ankles by exerting graduated pressure over the ankles and lower legs.

Mildly astringent dressings may be used to soften the thickened, yet fragile, skin and to control infection. Low-potency topical corticosteroids also might be helpful. In more-severe cases, surgical removal of damaged veins or skin may be necessary.

Seborrheic dermatitis

Signs and symptoms

- Greasy-appearing, scaling, itching areas in your scalp, at the sides of your nose, between your eyebrows, behind your ears or over your breastbone
- Stubborn, itchy dandruff

Seborrheic dermatitis (see the illustration on page 392) is characterized by greasy scaling and a somewhat reddened appearance of the skin. It's predominantly found in the scalp and in the folds at the sides of the lower portions of the nose, above the bridge of the nose, and over the breastbone. It also occurs beneath the breasts, in the folds of skin in the genital regions and around the bellybutton (navel) in obese people.

Seborrheic dermatitis can cause stubborn, itchy dandruff. It also may appear as cradle cap — crusty, scaly skin on your baby's scalp. Cradle cap usually doesn't appear in children older than 1 year.

Some people are born with an inherited tendency to develop seborrheic dermatitis and will never completely get rid of it, although treatment can help keep it under control. It may occur during times of stress or in people who have neurological conditions such as Parkinson's disease.

In folds of skin that are kept moist by contact with other skin, for example, beneath your breasts or around your genitals, secondary yeast infections may complicate the condition. You may be more

Infant Skin Conditions

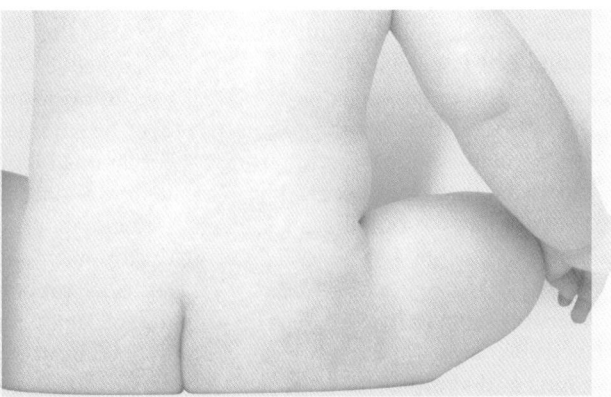

Many parents expect their newborn baby's skin to be flawless. The blemish-free babies in magazine ads may have raised your expectations, but most babies — even those who will someday be in ads — have rashes or blemishes in the early weeks. Most of the time, infant skin conditions are easily treated.

Common infant skin conditions include:

- *Cradle cap.* This crusty skin on the baby's scalp is also called seborrheic dermatitis. Shampooing your baby's hair once a week can help. If cradle cap persists, your baby's doctor may suggest a medicated lotion or another treatment.
- *Diaper rash.* This redness of the skin is caused by moisture, chafing of diapers, and the acid in urine or stool. Frequent diaper changes may prevent the rash, but most newborns have diaper rash periodically because their skin is tender. If your child has diaper rash, change your child's diaper frequently, taking care to dry his or her bottom thoroughly, and use a protective cream or ointment. If the rash is mild, you may not need to use the cream or ointment. Check with your baby's doctor if the rash persists.
- *Erythema toxicum.* This is a blotchy, red rash, sometimes with yellowish centers. Most newborns have this rash, typically on the face and torso. It generally disappears without treatment.
- *Heat rash.* In hot, humid weather, your baby may develop tiny, pink bumps on the skin — usually on the back of the neck and upper back. This condition may also be a result of your baby's being wrapped too warmly. The rash usually disappears without treatment, though giving your child cool rinses and dressing him or her in lighter clothing can help.
- *Infant acne.* Infant (newborn) acne may occur within the first six to eight weeks. Whiteheads appear on the face, neck, upper chest or back. This, too, is temporary and doesn't mean that the child will have future skin problems. Treat the condition by gently washing your baby with water daily and with mild soap and water weekly. It the acne appears severe, deep or is leaving scars, see a doctor.
- *Infantile eczema.* Infantile eczema (atopic dermatitis) is a rough, red, patchy rash usually associated with extremely dry, sensitive skin. It tends to appear on the cheeks, arms, legs, hands and feet. Avoid temperature extremes. Most babies with eczema do better in a mild climate with moderate humidity. Sweating seems to aggravate the rash. Avoid wool clothing and don't lay the baby on wool carpeting. During baths use warm water and a bland emollient to lubricate the dry skin.
- *Milia.* Milia are tiny, white spots on the nose and cheeks. More than half of all newborns have these little spots, which eventually disappear and don't require treatment.
- *Neonatal pimples.* About 20 percent of babies have pimples at birth or in the first one or two months after birth. Periodic cleaning with mild soap and water is usually adequate. Neonatal pimples don't indicate that your child will have skin blemishes later in life.
- *Peeling, dry skin.* Dry skin on the feet and hands is common in the first two weeks and will respond to over-the-counter lotions such as Nivea and Lubriderm.
- *Yeast infection.* This is a persistent, bright red rash in the diaper region, with surrounding lesions, that usually follows a diaper rash. Yeast infections are caused by a fungal organism (*Candida albicans*) that flourishes in a warm, moist environment. If your baby has such a yeast infection, an antifungal cream will help. In addition, frequent diaper changes and airing of the bottom promote dryness.

Although rashes are common and most often treatable at home, have your baby examined if you notice a rash that's purple, crusty, weepy or blistering.

Birthmarks also are common among babies. They include:

- *Café au lait spots.* As the name implies, these permanent birthmarks are the color of coffee with cream, occurring most commonly on the baby's torso, arms and legs.
- *Mongolian spots.* This is the traditional term, but you may hear them called blue-gray macule of infancy. These large, blue-gray birthmarks sometimes resemble bruises. They're more common in dark-skinned babies, appearing on the lower back and, less commonly, on the buttocks and legs. They usually disappear later in childhood.
- *Salmon patches.* Sometimes affectionately called stork bites or angel kisses, these reddish or pink patches often occur above the hairline at the back of the neck, on the eyelids or between the baby's eyes. These marks are caused by collections of tiny blood vessels (capillaries) close to the skin. They fade within a child's first two years but may not completely go away.

susceptible to these infections if you're taking antibiotics.

Treatment

For dandruff, treatment consists of frequent shampooing of your scalp, followed by careful rinsing. Your doctor may recommend that you shampoo alternately with a regular shampoo and a medicated shampoo, such as Nizoral, which contains ketoconazole and is available over-the-counter or by prescription.

Application of hydrocortisone-containing creams or solutions or ketoconazole cream may soothe your skin. You may also need treatment for a secondary infection.

Dandruff

Everyone has some degree of scaling of the skin on his or her scalp because of the normal process of shedding your outer layer of skin cells. If the flaking becomes obvious on your hair and clothing, it's commonly called dandruff. New studies suggest that a yeastlike organism may cause dandruff. The *Malassezia ovalis* fungus causes irritation and increased sloughing of the top layer of skin cells on your scalp.

If your dandruff persists or you have large flakes together with redness or scaling around your nose, ears or chest, you may have a more severe form of dandruff or perhaps even psoriasis of the scalp. If you have questions about the seriousness of your condition, consult your doctor or a dermatologist.

Treatment

Here are some steps you can take to control or prevent mild to moderate dandruff:
- Shampoo regularly. Start with a mild, nonmedicated shampoo. Gently massage your scalp to loosen flakes. Rinse thoroughly.

Overtreatment dermatitis

Signs and symptoms
- Redness and sensitivity of skin treated for another skin disorder

Overtreatment dermatitis is the result of overtreatment of a skin condition. Dermatologists often see people who have inflammation of the skin that has persisted for several weeks or months and worsened, despite frequent application of several ointments or other treatments. The inflammation resulting from the excessive treatment obscures the underlying disease, which may or may not still be present. Typically, there's no way that the underlying disorder can be identified.

- Use medicated shampoo (Head & Shoulders, Selsun Blue) for stubborn cases. Look for shampoos containing pyrithione zinc, salicylic acid, coal tar or selenium sulfide. If necessary to control flaking, use a dandruff shampoo each time you shampoo. Rotating different types of shampoo may help. For mild dandruff, alternate dandruff shampoo with your regular shampoo.
- Consider trying the antifungal shampoo Nizoral to kill dandruff-causing fungi that may live on your scalp. Nizoral is available both over-the-counter and by prescription.
- If you use tar-based shampoos, use them carefully. They can leave a brownish stain on light-colored or gray hair and make your scalp more sensitive to sunlight.
- Use a conditioner regularly.

If dandruff persists or your scalp becomes irritated or severely itchy, you may need a prescription shampoo. Dandruff isn't contagious and is rarely serious, but your skin may be more susceptible to infection. If your dandruff persists, you may have another skin condition. See your doctor.

Treatment

Your doctor may recommend that you discontinue all treatment other than the most soothing measures for a week or two. Assessing the problem is possible only after all medications are withdrawn. Meanwhile, the problem may improve considerably — or even disappear.

Other Skin Conditions

Following are other common skin conditions. These conditions aren't life-threatening, but they can cause discomfort or make you upset about your appearance.

Acne

Signs and symptoms
- Blackheads or whiteheads on the face, neck, shoulders or back
- Pimples
- Cysts

Acne, a skin disorder characterized by pimples due to clogged hair follicle openings, is a common frustration for teens. It affects about 4 of every 5 people between the ages of 12 and 24. But it can affect people of all ages. Many people continue to experience acne well into adulthood. It's estimated nearly half of all adult women experience mild to moderate acne.

Acne occurs when the hair follicles of your skin become plugged. Each follicle contains oil-producing (sebaceous) glands that secrete a fatty oil (sebum) to lubricate your hair and skin. When your body produces sebum and dead cells faster than they can exit from the opening of the hair follicle on the skin surface, the two solidify as a soft, white plug. This plug may clog the opening, causing the follicle wall to bulge, thus creating a whitehead. If the opening stays open, the top surface of the plug may darken, causing a blackhead.

A pimple is inflammation that develops when a whitehead ruptures a hair follicle wall below the skin surface. After the rupture, solidified sebum, dead cells and bacteria invade your skin. Ruptures deep within your skin form boil-like lesions called cystic acne (see the illustration on page 395).

In some situations, the sebaceous gland continues to secrete material that doesn't rupture through the skin. Instead, a flattened, pliable lump forms under the skin. This is called a sebaceous or epidermoid cyst (wen). Sometimes, the lumps can be an inch or more in diameter. Generally, there's no discoloration or pain unless the cyst becomes infected.

Acne is most prevalent in adolescence because hormonal changes stimulate the sebaceous glands to increase sebum production during these years. Acne related to hormonal changes is also common in:

- Women and adolescent girls two to seven days before their periods
- Pregnant women
- People under stress
- People using certain medications

Other risk factors for acne include:

- Exposing your skin directly to greasy or oily substances
- Having a family history of acne
- Sports equipment or clothing that rubs against your skin

Application of oil or grease to your skin can aggravate acne. This includes use of oil-based makeup, suntan oil or hairdressing solutions, as well as oils from machinery or cooking. Acne isn't caused by dirt. In fact, scrubbing the skin too hard or cleansing with harsh soaps or chemicals can cause irritation, which may make acne worse.

Diagnosis

Acne usually is easy to diagnose. Pimple-like pustules alone, with no blackheads or whiteheads, may be another skin disease or a reaction to medications such as corticosteroids.

How serious is acne?

For many people, acne is an ongoing (chronic) problem from puberty through early adulthood. It eventually clears up in most cases, but you may want to seek treatment from a dermatologist for persistent pimples or inflamed cysts to avoid scarring or other damage to your skin.

The condition can affect self-esteem, confidence and social interaction. These potential problems also are legitimate reasons to treat acne. Medical treatment usually provides visible improvement within a few months.

Sudden onset of severe acne in a mature adult may signal an underlying disease, such as a tumor that affects certain hormone production. Seek prompt medical attention.

Treatment

Acne treatments work by reducing oil production, speeding up skin cell turnover, fighting bacterial infection, reducing the inflammation or doing all four. With most prescription acne treatments, you may not see results for four to eight weeks, and your skin may get worse before it gets better.

Your doctor or dermatologist may recommend a prescription medication you apply to your skin (topical medication) or take by mouth (oral medication). Oral prescription medications for acne should not be used during pregnancy, especially during the first trimester.

Types of treatments include:

- **Topical treatments.** Acne lotions may dry up the oil, kill bacteria and promote sloughing of dead skin cells. Over-the-counter lotions are generally mild and contain benzoyl peroxide, sulfur, resorcinol, salicylic acid or lactic acid as their active ingredient. These products can be helpful for very mild acne. If your acne doesn't respond to these treatments, you may want to see your doctor or dermatologist to get a stronger prescrip-

tion lotion. Tretinoin (Retin-A, Renova, others) and adapalene (Differin) are examples of topical prescription products derived from vitamin A. They work by promoting cell turnover and preventing plugging of the hair follicles. A number of topical antibiotics also are available. They work by killing excess skin bacteria. Often, a combination of such products is required to achieve optimal results.

- **Antibiotics.** For moderate to severe acne, prescription oral antibiotics may be needed to reduce bacteria and fight inflammation. You may need to take these antibiotics for months, and you may need to use them in combination with topical products.
- **Anti-androgen agent.** The drug spironolactone (Aldactone) may be considered for women and adolescent girls if oral antibiotics aren't helpful. It blocks the effects of androgen hormones on the sebaceous glands. Possible side effects include breast tenderness, painful periods and the retention of potassium.
- **Isotretinoin.** For deep cysts, antibiotics may not be enough. Isotretinoin (Amnesteem, Claravis, Myorisan) is a powerful medication available for scarring cystic acne or acne that doesn't respond to other treatments. This medicine is reserved for the most severe forms of acne. It's very effective, but people who take it need close monitoring by a dermatologist because of the possibility of severe side effects. Isotretinoin is associated with severe birth defects, so it shouldn't be taken by pregnant women or women who may become pregnant during the course of treatment or within several weeks of concluding treatment. The drug carries such serious potential side effects that women of reproductive age must participate in a Food and Drug Administration-approved

monitoring program when taking it. In addition, isotretinoin may increase the levels of triglycerides and cholesterol in the blood and may increase liver enzyme levels. Although cause and effect hasn't been proved, studies have reported the development of inflammatory bowel disease with isotretinoin use.

- **Oral contraceptives.** Oral contraceptives, including a combination of norgestimate and ethinyl estradiol (Ortho Cyclen, Ortho Tri-Cyclen), have been shown to improve acne in women. However, oral contraceptives may cause other side effects that you'll want to discuss with your doctor.
- **Laser and light therapy.** Laser- and light-based therapies reach

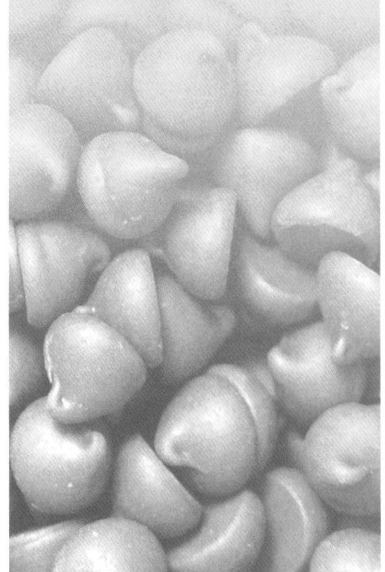

? Question and Answer

Does diet affect acne?

Contrary to what many people think, foods have little effect on acne. Neither chocolate nor greasy foods such as french fries are likely to cause or aggravate acne. However, if certain foods seem to make your acne worse, it may be best to avoid them. Discuss this with your doctor.

the deeper layers of skin without harming the skin's surface. Laser treatment is thought to damage the oil (sebaceous) glands, causing them to produce less oil. Light therapy targets the bacterium that causes acne inflammation. These therapies can also improve skin texture and lessen the appearance of scars, so they may be good treatment choices for people with both active acne and acne scars.

- **Cosmetic procedures.** Chemical peels and microdermabrasion may be helpful in controlling acne. These cosmetic procedures — which have traditionally been used to lessen the appearance of fine lines, sun damage and minor facial scars — are most effective when used in combination with other acne treatments.
- **Steroid injection.** Nodular and cystic lesions can be treated by injecting a steroid drug directly into them. This improves their appearance without the need for extraction. Side effects of this technique include thinning of the skin, lighter skin and the appearance of small blood vessels on the treated area.

Treating acne scars

Doctors may be able to use certain procedures to diminish scars left by acne. These include fillers, dermabrasion, intense light therapy and laser resurfacing.

- **Soft tissue fillers.** Collagen or fat can be injected under the skin and into scars to fill out or stretch the skin, making the scars less noticeable. Results from this acne scar treatment are temporary, so you'd need to repeat the injections periodically.
- **Dermabrasion.** Usually reserved for more severe scarring, dermabrasion involves removing the top layer of skin with a rapidly rotating wire brush. Surface scars may be completely removed, and deeper acne scars may appear less noticeable. Dermabrasion may cause pig-

mentation changes for people with darker skin.

- **Chemical peels.** High-potency acid is applied to your skin to remove the top layer and minimize deeper scars.
- **Laser, light source and radiofrequency treatments.** In laser resurfacing, a laser beam destroys the outer layer of skin (epidermis) and heats the underlying skin (dermis). As the wound heals, new skin forms. Less intense lasers (nonablative lasers), pulsed light sources and radiofrequency devices don't injure the epidermis. These treatments heat the dermis and cause new skin formation. After several treatments, acne scars may appear less noticeable. This means shorter recovery times, but treatment typically needs to be repeated more often and results are subtle.
- **Skin surgery.** A minor procedure (punch excision) cuts out individual acne scars. Stitches or a skin graft repairs the hole left at the scar site.

Rosacea

Signs and symptoms

- Red facial areas
- A tendency to flush or blush easily
- Visible small blood vessels on nose and cheeks (telangiectasia)
- Small red bumps or pustules on the nose, cheeks, forehead and chin
- Inflammation of the cheeks, nose, forehead and chin
- A burning or gritty sensation in the eyes (ocular rosacea)
- A red, bulbous nose (rhinophyma)

Rosacea is an inflammatory skin condition often resulting in redness of the face (see the illustration on page 395). Its characteristics — a red nose, flushed cheeks and small red, pus-filled bumps (pustules) — are frequently mistaken for acne. Rosacea is also sometimes referred to as adult acne or acne rosacea, but in reality it has little to do with the pimples and blackheads that commonly afflict teenagers.

The condition may be progressive, meaning it tends to worsen over time. But in most people it's cyclic. It may be active for a time, lessen in intensity, then flare.

Besides acne, rosacea can also be mistaken for other skin problems, such as a skin allergy. Once diagnosed, it's highly treatable.

Rosacea affects mostly fair-skinned adults between the ages of 30 and 60. Although rosacea is more common in women, men are more likely to have the severe form, with a bright red, bulbous nose (rhinophyma). Rosacea isn't life-threatening, but it can affect appearance — and self-esteem.

Common progression

The condition may begin as a simple tendency to flush or blush easily, then progress to a persistent redness in the central portion of your face, particularly the nose. This redness results from the dilation of blood vessels close to the skin's surface.

As symptoms worsen, vascular rosacea may develop — small blood vessels on your nose and cheeks swell and become visible (telangiectasia). Your skin may become overly dry and sensitive. However, rosacea may also be accompanied by oily skin, as well as dandruff.

Small red bumps may appear and persist, spreading across your nose, cheeks, forehead and chin. This is sometimes known as inflammatory rosacea. In severe and rare cases, the oil glands (sebaceous glands) in the nose and sometimes the cheeks become enlarged, resulting in a buildup of tissue on and around the nose (rhinophyma).

More than half the people with rosacea experience ocular rosacea at times. They may feel a burning and gritty sensation in the eyes, and the eyelids may be inflamed or appear scaly.

The cause of rosacea is unknown, but researchers believe it's likely due to a combination of genetic and environmental factors. It's not caused by alcoholism. However alcohol consumption does lead to flushing of the skin and may worsen rosacea.

These factors can aggravate rosacea by increasing blood flow to the surface of the skin:

- Hot foods or beverages
- Spicy foods
- Alcohol
- Caffeine withdrawal (caffeine itself isn't a factor)
- Temperature extremes
- Sunlight
- Stress, anger or embarrassment
- Strenuous exercise
- Hot baths, saunas
- Corticosteroids, as well as drugs that dilate blood vessels
- Skin care products that contain ingredients such as acids, alcohol and other irritants

Diagnosis

If you experience persistent redness in your face, see your doctor or a dermatologist. Because of the progressive nature of rosacea, an early diagnosis is important.

Treatment

There's no way to eliminate rosacea, but effective treatment can relieve its signs and symptoms. Your doctor also may recommend certain moisturizers, soaps, sunscreens and other products to improve the health of your skin.

Medications

You may need a combination of prescription-strength topical medication (lotion, cream or gel) and oral medication (pill, capsule or tablet) to treat rosacea.

- **Topical medications.** Medications you apply to your skin once or twice daily may help reduce inflammation and redness. They may also be used along with oral medications or as part of a maintenance program to control symptoms. Common

topical medications include antibiotics (metronidazole), tretinoin, benzoyl peroxide and azelaic acid. The medications brimonidine (Mirvaso) and oxymetazoline hydrochloride (Rhofade) may help reduce facial skin redness.
- **Oral antibiotics.** Doctors may prescribe oral antibiotics to treat rosacea, more for their anti-inflammatory properties than to kill bacteria. Oral antibiotics are also prescribed because they tend to work faster than topical ones. Common prescription oral antibiotics include tetracycline, minocycline and erythromycin.
- **Isotretinoin.** Isotretinoin (Amnesteem, Claravis, Myorisan) is a powerful oral medication sometimes used for severe cases of inflammatory rosacea if other treatment options don't help. Usually prescribed for cystic acne, isotretinoin works to inhibit the production of oil by sebaceous glands. People who take it need close monitoring by a dermatologist because of the possibility of serious side effects.

Your doctor may treat ocular rosacea with oral antibiotics or steroid eyedrops.

The duration of your treatment depends on the type and severity of your symptoms, but typically you'll notice an improvement within one to two months. Because symptoms may recur if you stop taking medications, long-term regular treatment is often necessary.

Surgery

Enlarged blood vessels, some redness and changes due to rhinophyma often become permanent. In these cases, surgical methods, such as laser surgery and electrosurgery, may reduce the visibility of blood vessels, remove tissue buildup around your nose and generally improve your appearance.

Self-care

One of the most important things that you can do is to minimize your exposure to anything that causes a flare-up. It's important to find out what factors affect you and avoid them. Other suggestions for preventing flare-ups include:

- Protect your face from the sun by wearing a broad-brimmed hat or using sunscreen with a sun protection factor (SPF) of 15 or higher.
- Protect your face in the winter with a scarf or ski mask.
- Don't irritate your facial skin by rubbing or touching it too much.
- Avoid facial products that contain alcohol or other skin irritants.
- When using a moisturizer with a topical medication, apply the moisturizer after the medication has dried.
- Use products labeled noncomedogenic to avoid clogging hair follicle openings.
- Stay cool on hot days.
- Try to avoid stressful situations.
- If you wear makeup, try green-tinted pre-foundation cream to counter skin redness.

Psoriasis

Signs and symptoms
- Dry, red patches of skin covered with silvery scales
- Small scaling spots (most commonly seen in children)
- Swollen and stiff joints

Emergency signs and symptoms
- Reddening and scaling affecting the entire skin

Psoriasis, a common skin disease, affects the life cycle of skin cells. Normally, it takes about a month for new cells to move from the lowest skin layer, where they're produced, to the outermost layer, where they die and scale off in tiny flakes. With psoriasis, the entire cycle takes only days. As a result, cells accumulate rapidly, forming thick patches with scales.

Psoriasis (see the illustration on page 392) is a persistent, long-lasting (chronic) disease that affects millions of Americans. Psoriasis can occur suddenly at any age, but the onset is usually gradual and begins between ages 15 and 35.

The inflammation can be frustrating if you have it, causing unsightly patches of skin, discomfort and even pain. The attacks can range from a few spots of dandruff-like scaling to large areas with major eruptions. Psoriasis most commonly affects the elbows, knees, trunk and scalp. Pits or ridges may develop in the nails. The eruptions take various forms, including pustules, cracking skin, itching or minor bleeding.

Sometimes arthritis accompanies psoriasis. For most individuals, the effects of psoriatic arthritis are minor. It produces some pain in affected joints but has little effect on overall health. Less commonly, joint symptoms can lead to significant disability, similar to that sometimes experienced by people with rheumatoid arthritis.

Causes
Psoriasis is related to your immune system, and more specifically, a type of white blood cell called a T cell (T lymphocyte). Normally, T cells travel throughout the body to detect and fight off foreign substances, such as viruses or bacteria. With psoriasis, the T cells attack healthy skin cells by mistake, as if to heal a wound or to fight an infection.

Overactive T cells trigger other immune responses, including dilation of blood vessels in the skin around the plaques and an increase in other white blood cells. These changes result in increased production of both healthy skin cells and more T cells and other white blood cells. What results is an ongoing cycle in which new skin cells move to the outermost layer of skin too quickly — in days rather than weeks. Dead skin and white blood cells can't slough off quickly enough and they build up as thick, scaly patches on the skin's surface. The cycle doesn't stop unless interrupted by treatment.

What causes T cells to malfunction in people with psoriasis isn't entirely clear, although researchers think genetic and environmental factors both play a role. Psoriasis typically starts or worsens because of a trigger that you may be able to identify and avoid. Factors that may trigger psoriasis include:

- Infections, such as strep throat or thrush
- Injury to the skin, such as a cut or scrape, bug bite, or a severe sunburn
- Stress
- Cold weather
- Smoking
- Heavy alcohol consumption
- Certain medications — including lithium, prescribed for bipolar disorder; high blood pressure medications such as beta blockers; antimalarial drugs; and iodides

Diagnosis
A diagnosis of psoriasis usually is based on a physical inspection. Your doctor may need to obtain a skin sample (biopsy) for microscopic analysis to rule out other disorders or a fungal infection.

How serious is psoriasis?
Psoriasis ranges from mild and short term (acute) to severe and chronic. The disease can't be cured, but treatments are usually effective. If almost all of your skin is affected, you may require prompt treatment. Acute secondary infections also can start during any flare-up.

Treatment
Psoriasis treatments can be divided into three main types: topical treatments, light therapy and oral medications.

Topical treatments
Creams and ointments that you apply to your skin can effectively treat mild to moderate psoriasis. When the disease is more severe, creams are likely to be combined with oral medications or light

therapy. Topical psoriasis treatments include:

- **Topical corticosteroids.** Anti-inflammatory drugs are the most frequently prescribed medications for treating mild to moderate psoriasis. They slow cell turnover by suppressing the immune system, which reduces inflammation and relieves associated itching. Topical corticosteroids range in strength, from mild to very strong. Low-potency corticosteroid ointments are usually recommended for sensitive areas, such as your face or skin folds, and for treating widespread patches of damaged skin. Your doctor may prescribe stronger corticosteroid ointment for small areas of your skin, for persistent plaques on your hands or feet, or when other treatments have failed. To minimize side effects and increase effectiveness, topical corticosteroids are generally used on active outbreaks until they're under control.
- **Vitamin D analogues.** These synthetic forms of vitamin D slow down the growth of skin cells. Calcipotriene (Dovonex) is a prescription cream, ointment or solution containing a vitamin D analogue that may be used alone to treat mild to moderate psoriasis or in combination with other treatments. Calcitriol (Vectical) is expensive but may be equally effective and possibly less irritating than calcipotriene.
- **Anthralin.** This medication is thought to normalize DNA activity in skin cells. Anthralin can also remove scales, making the skin smoother. However, anthralin stains virtually anything it touches, including skin, clothing, countertops and bedding. For that reason doctors often recommend short-contact treatment — allowing the cream to stay on your skin for a brief time before washing it off. Anthralin may be used in combination with ultraviolet light.
- **Topical retinoids.** Tazarotene (Tazorac, Avage) was developed specifically for the treatment of psoriasis. Like other vitamin A derivatives, it normalizes DNA activity in skin cells and may decrease inflammation. The most common side effect is skin irritation. It may also increase sensitivity to sunlight, so sunscreen should be applied while using the medication. Although the risk of birth defects is far lower for topical retinoids than for oral retinoids, your doctor needs to know if you're pregnant or intend to become pregnant if you're using tazarotene.
- **Calcineurin inhibitors.** The drugs tacrolimus (Protopic) and pimecrolimus (Elidel) reduce inflammation and plaque build-up. Calcineurin inhibitors aren't recommended for long-term or continuous use because of a potential increased risk of skin cancer and lymphoma. They may be especially helpful in areas of thin skin, such as around the eyes, where steroid creams or retinoids are too irritating or may cause harmful effects.
- **Salicylic acid.** Available over-the-counter and by prescription, salicylic acid promotes sloughing of dead skin cells and reduces scaling. Sometimes it's combined with other medications to increase its effectiveness. Salicylic acid is available in medicated shampoos and scalp solutions to treat scalp psoriasis.
- **Coal tar.** A thick, black byproduct of the manufacture of petro-

Bathing Basics

If you have dry or sensitive skin, follow these tips to minimize the drying effects of bathing:

1. Bathe less frequently. Two or three times a week is often enough for most people. Limit yourself to 15 minutes, and use warm, rather than hot, water.
2. Choose mild superfatted soaps such as Basis or Dove, which dry skin less. Add Aveeno oatmeal powder or bath oils to your bath water. Soap substitutes in bar, gel and liquid forms are less drying than are deodorant and antibacterial soaps. Use soap only on your face, underarms, genital areas, hands and feet. Use clear water elsewhere.
3. After bathing, brush your skin rapidly with the palms of your hands or gently pat your skin with a towel.
4. Apply an oil or cream to your skin immediately after drying. Use a heavy, water-in-oil moisturizer, not a light "disappearing" cream that contains mostly water. Avoid creams or lotions containing alcohol. Pay special attention to your legs, arms, back and the sides of your body.

leum products and coal, coal tar is probably the oldest treatment for psoriasis. It reduces scaling, itching and inflammation. Exactly how it works isn't known. Coal tar has few known side effects, but it's messy, stains clothing and bedding, and has a strong odor. Coal tar is available in over-the-counter shampoos, creams and oils.

- **Moisturizers.** By themselves, moisturizing creams won't heal psoriasis, but they can reduce itching and scaling and can help combat the dryness that results from other therapies. Moisturizers in an ointment base are usually more effective than are lighter creams and lotions.

Itching

The medical term for itching is pruritus. No matter what you call it, itching can be a miserable, distressing condition.

Causes
Although the most common cause of itching is dry skin, itching occurs in a variety of diseases or disorders. It can on occasion indicate a systemic condition such as liver or kidney disease and some blood disorders. Itching may also result when larvae of the hookworm family of parasites penetrate your skin. This includes swimmer's itch, eruption caused by the larvae of cat and dog hookworm, and ground itch caused by the true hookworm.

Many other skin disorders also can have itching as a major symptom, including insect bites, dermatitis, hives and skin parasites, such as scabies. Some medications, such as aspirin and codeine-related pain relievers, can cause itching, which may or may not be accompanied by a rash.

Emotional stress can contribute to or increase the sensation of itching, no matter what the underlying

Light therapy (phototherapy)
As the name suggests, this psoriasis treatment uses natural or artificial ultraviolet light. The simplest and easiest form of phototherapy involves exposing your skin to controlled amounts of natural sunlight. Other forms of light therapy include the use of artificial ultraviolet A (UVA) or ultraviolet B (UVB) light either alone or in combination with medications.

- **Sunlight.** Ultraviolet (UV) light is a wavelength of light in a range too short for the human eye to see. When exposed to UV rays in sunlight or artificial light, the activated T cells in the skin die. This slows skin cell turnover and reduces scaling

cause may be. If emotional factors are the primary cause, the condition is known as psychogenic itching.

Treatment
Antihistamines may relieve itching due to hives, certain drug rashes and some forms of dermatitis. Most antihistamines also have a mild sedative effect and may help you sleep. Creams or ointments containing hydrocortisone, menthol, camphor and other medications may help control the itch of insect bites and dermatitis.

For dry skin associated with aging, moisturizing the skin is key. For severe itching from dry skin, use oatmeal powder or bath oils in your bath water.

You can get much the same effect from an oatmeal bath or a starch-and-soda bath. For an oatmeal bath, tie a handful of oatmeal into a piece of cotton cloth. Boil it just as you would cook the oatmeal. Then use this "oatmeal sponge" while you bathe in a tub half full of lukewarm water. To prepare a starch-and-soda bath, add half of a 16-ounce box of baking soda and one 16-ounce box of laundry starch to a tub half full of lukewarm water. Mix well and bathe without using soap.

and inflammation. Brief, daily exposures to small amounts of sunlight may improve psoriasis, but intense sun exposure can worsen symptoms and cause skin damage. Before beginning a sunlight regimen, ask your doctor about the safest way to use natural sunlight for psoriasis treatment.

- **UVB phototherapy.** Controlled doses of UVB light from an artificial light source may improve mild to moderate psoriasis symptoms. UVB phototherapy, also called broadband UVB, can be used to treat single patches, widespread psoriasis and psoriasis that resists topical treatments. Short-term side effects may include redness, itching and dry skin. Using a moisturizer may help decrease these side effects.
- **Narrow band UVB therapy.** A newer type of psoriasis treatment, narrow band UVB therapy may be more effective than broadband UVB treatment. It's usually administered two or three times a week until the skin improves, then maintenance may require only weekly sessions. Narrow band UVB therapy may cause more severe and longer lasting burns, however.
- **Photochemotherapy, or psoralen plus ultraviolet A (PUVA).** Photochemotherapy involves taking a light-sensitizing medication (psoralen) before exposure to UVA light or soaking the affected area in a psoralen solution beforehand. UVA light penetrates deeper into the skin than does UVB light, and psoralen makes the skin more responsive to UVA exposure. This more aggressive treatment consistently improves skin and is often used for more-severe cases of psoriasis, and for pustular psoriasis of the hands or feet. PUVA involves two or three treatments a week for a prescribed number of weeks. Short-term side effects include

nausea and headache with oral use and burning and itching with topical or oral techniques. Long-term side effects include dry and wrinkled skin, freckles and increased risk of skin cancer, including melanoma, the most serious form of skin cancer.

- **Excimer laser.** This form of light therapy, used for mild to moderate psoriasis, treats only the involved skin. A controlled beam of UVB light of a specific wavelength is directed to the psoriasis plaques to control scaling and inflammation. Healthy skin surrounding the patches isn't harmed. Excimer laser therapy requires fewer sessions than does traditional phototherapy because more powerful UVB light is used. Side effects can include redness and blistering.

- **Combination light therapy.** Combining UV light with other treatments such as retinoids often improves effectiveness. Combination therapies are often used after other phototherapy options are ineffective. Some doctors give UVB treatment in conjunction with coal tar, called the Goeckerman treatment. The two therapies together are more effective than either alone because coal tar makes skin more receptive to UVB light.

Oral or injected medications
If you have severe psoriasis or it's resistant to other types of treatment, your doctor may prescribe oral or injected drugs. Because of severe side effects, some of these medications are used for just brief periods of time and may be alternated with other forms of treatment.

- **Retinoids.** Related to vitamin A, this group of drugs may help if you have severe psoriasis that doesn't respond to other therapies. Side effects may include lip inflammation and hair loss. Because retinoids such as acitretin (Soriatane) can cause severe birth defects, women must avoid

pregnancy for at least three years after taking the medication.

- **Methotrexate.** Taken orally, methotrexate (Trexall) helps psoriasis by decreasing the production of skin cells and suppressing inflammation. It may also slow the progression of psoriatic arthritis in some people. Methotrexate is generally well-tolerated in low doses. When used for long periods, it can cause a number of serious side effects, including severe liver damage and decreased production of red and white blood cells and platelets.

- **Cyclosporine.** Cyclosporine (Gengraf, Neoral, Sandimmune) suppresses the immune system and is similar to methotrexate in effectiveness. It's most often used for shorter periods of time or as a bridge to another form or treatment. Cyclosporine increases your risk of infection and other health problems, including cancer and kidney disease.

- **Biologics.** Several drugs that alter the immune system are approved for the treatment of moderate to severe psoriasis. They include etanercept (Enbrel), infliximab (Remicade), adalimumab (Humira), ustekinumab (Stelara), golimumab (Simponi), apremilast (Otezla), secukinumab (Cosentyx) and ixekizumab (Taltz). Most of these drugs are given by injection (apremilast is oral) and are usually used for people who have failed to respond to traditional therapy or who have associated psoriatic arthritis. Biologics must be used with caution because they have strong effects on the immune system and may permit life-threatening infections. In particular, people taking these treatments must be screened for tuberculosis.

- **Others.** Thioguanine and hydroxyurea (Droxia, Hydrea) are medications that can be used when other drugs can't be given.

Self-care
You can take a number of steps to control your psoriasis:

- Eat a nutritious diet, get adequate rest and exercise regularly.
- Maintain a healthy weight. Psoriasis often occurs in skin creases or folds.
- Avoid scratching, rubbing or picking at patches of psoriasis.
- Bathe daily to soak off the scales. Avoid hot water or harsh soap.
- Keep your skin moist. Pat rather than rub dry after bathing, apply a heavy, water-in-oil moisturizing cream immediately after bathing while your skin is still moist, avoid creams or lotions containing alcohol, use a humidifier, and keep room temperatures cool.
- Use soaps, shampoos, cleansers or ointments containing coal tar or salicylic acid.
- Expose your skin to moderate sunlight, but avoid sunburn.
- Apply an over-the-counter cortisone cream for a few weeks when symptoms are especially bad.

Lichen planus

Signs and symptoms
- A rash that appears as raised, flat areas that may vary in color from violet to pink to red
- A rash that typically appears on the arms and legs but sometimes involves the scalp or mucous membranes that line the mouth, gums, tongue, nose, vagina and anus
- Itching
- Soreness or a burning sensation involving the mucous membranes

Lichen planus is a rare, persistent, itchy rash characterized by shiny, reddish purple spots on the skin and gray-white ones in the mouth. Most commonly, lichen planus appears in midlife, between the ages of 45 and 60. The initial attack may persist for weeks or months, and recurrences can continue over many years. Oral symptoms often consist of a dry mouth and a metallic taste

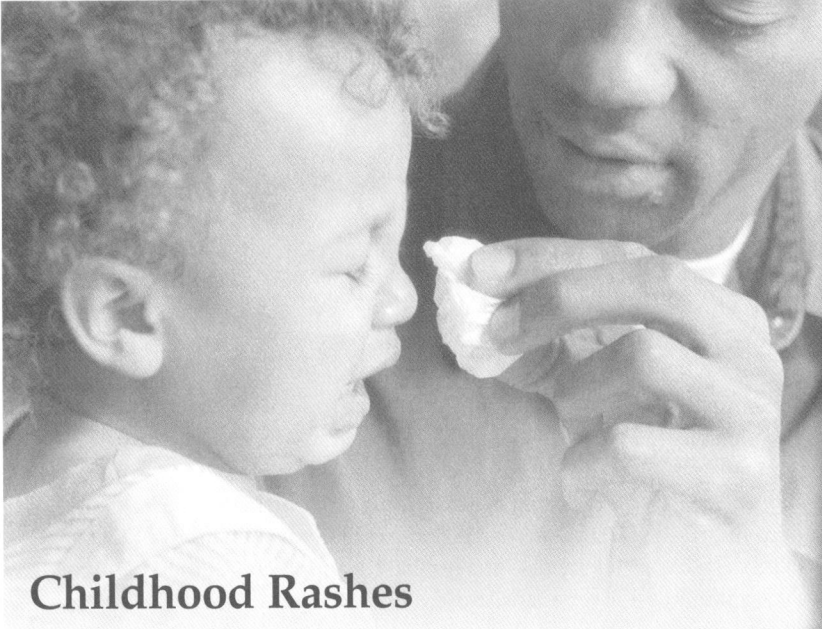

Childhood Rashes

Sometimes it can be difficult to determine the cause of a rash. Here are four childhood illnesses that can cause a rash:

Chickenpox
Chickenpox (varicella) causes itchy, red spots on the face or chest that spread to the arms and legs. These spots quickly fill with a clear fluid to form blisters that rupture and turn crusty. New spots generally continue appearing over four to five days. Fever, runny nose or cough often accompanies chickenpox, which is contagious until the rash crusts.

Seek medical help if the rash involves the eyes or is accompanied by a cough or shortness of breath. In addition, seek medical help if chickenpox develops twice in the same person or occurs after vaccination.

Fifth disease
With fifth disease, bright red, raised patches appear on both cheeks, giving a slapped-cheek appearance. During the next few days, a pink, lacy, slightly raised rash may also develop on the arms, trunk, thighs and buttocks. The rash may come and go for up to three weeks. Some children develop a slight fever and other mild, cold-like symptoms.

Measles
Measles (rubeola) typically begins with a fever, often as high as 104 to 105 F, a cough, sneezing, a sore throat and inflamed, watery eyes. A rash appears two to four days later. It often begins as fine, red spots on the face and spreads to the trunk, arms and legs. Spots may become larger and usually last about a week. Small, white spots may appear on the inside lining of the cheek.

See a doctor if you suspect that your child may have the measles. It may lead to uncommon but potentially serious complications, such as pneumonia, encephalitis or a bacterial infection.

Roseola
Roseola often begins with a high fever lasting about three days. When it subsides, a rash appears on the trunk and neck and lasts a few hours to a few days. The virus most often affects children between ages 6 months and 3 years. See a doctor if the rash lasts longer than three days.

or blunted taste sensation, or burning in the mouth. They may appear before the rash and be the only evidence of the disease.

Lichen planus can also appear in the lining of your mouth. For more information on oral lichen planus see page 686.

The cause of this disorder usually can't be determined. In some cases, it may represent a reaction to medication or stress. Some cases have been linked to infections, such as hepatitis.

How serious is lichen planus?
Lichen planus of the skin is generally noncancerous (benign). It may clear up with treatment but can persist for months to years.

People with long-term lesions of the mucous membranes are at greater risk of squamous cell carcinoma — a form of skin cancer. In these cases, a doctor may advise regular examinations to monitor any changes in the lesions. It's also important to stop any tobacco use, which raises your risk of squamous cell carcinoma.

Diagnosis
A diagnosis of lichen planus is generally made by inspection or laboratory examination of a tissue sample (biopsy).

Treatment
Treatment usually focuses on relieving the itching and may include:
- An ointment or cream containing a corticosteroid medication or a calcineurin inhibitor (Elidel, Protopic)
- Phototherapy with ultraviolet light
- Oral corticosteroid medications, in severe cases
- Immune-modulating therapy, in severe cases

Lichen sclerosis

Signs and symptoms
- Itching (pruritus), which can be severe
- Smooth white spots on your skin

Protecting Your Skin From the Sun

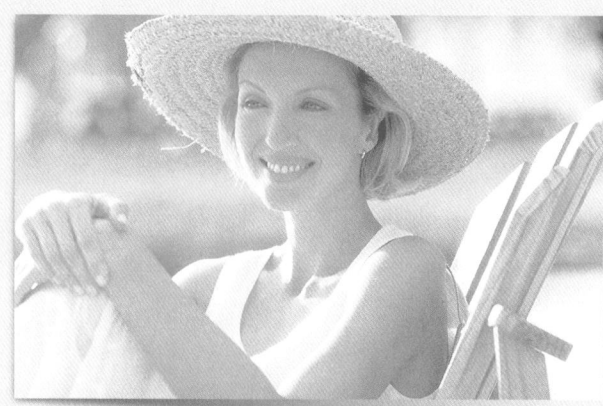

It's the first warm, sunny day after a long winter. You step outside for a deep breath of fresh air, close your eyes and turn your face to the sun. The soothing warmth of the sun on your skin feels so good. You imagine the look of a nice suntan, but what you may be getting instead are wrinkles and liver spots.

Despite the still-prevalent image of a tan being healthy, excessive exposure to the sun is responsible for much of the skin damage associated with aging. It's a lifelong process, as over time your skin slowly accumulates the damaging effects of the sun.

Accumulated exposure to the ultraviolet (UV) radiation in sunlight and tanning beds causes your skin to age prematurely and leads to wrinkles and skin discoloration. Often, much of the damage is cosmetic, but some effects can be deadly. Excessive sun exposure is the leading cause of skin cancer, by far the most common form of cancer diagnosed today. It's estimated 1 in 5 Americans will develop skin cancer at some point in life.

Sun sense

Armed with adequate sunscreen and protective clothing, you can — at any age — prevent damage to your skin.

Avoidance
When possible, avoid overexposure to the sun by planning outdoor activities for early morning or late afternoon. UV radiation is most intense from 10 a.m. to 3 p.m.

Tanning beds also damage skin. They emit ultraviolet A (UVA) rays, which are often touted as less dangerous than are ultraviolet B (UVB) rays. But UVA light penetrates even deeper into your skin, causes precancerous skin lesions and increases your risk of skin cancer.

Proper clothing
If you expect to be in sunlight for lengthy periods, protect yourself. Wear a hat, a shirt with long sleeves and avoid shorts. Several clothing manufacturers market items designed to provide protection from the sun while you're outdoors.

Sunscreen
Use a premium-quality sunscreen whenever you're outdoors for sustained periods. A sunscreen can protect you from burning and allow some tanning. Avoid lotions touted as tan accelerators, such as cocoa butter or baby oil. These products don't make you tan faster, and they provide very little protection from UV radiation.

Good sunscreens contain derivatives of p-aminobenzoic acid (PABA), cinoxate, oxybenzone, homosalate or avobenzone. Some contain combinations of these elements. Alcohol-based sunscreens seem to penetrate deeper and are less likely to aggravate acne. Some sunscreens also contain physical blockers such as zinc oxide or titanium dioxide, which provide even better protection and are more resistant to water and perspiration.

Sunscreens are rated by their sun protection factor (SPF). SPFs range from 2 to more than 100, with higher numbers offering the most protection. Sunscreen SPFs mainly relate to the ability of the sunscreen to block UVB, not UVA. It's best to use a sunscreen with an SPF rating of at least 30 that blocks both UVA and UVB rays.

Apply it at least half an hour before exposure. Reapply your sunscreen frequently because protection diminishes as the sunscreen evaporates. Swimming and perspiration can wash it away as well.

Also be sure to use a sunscreen for winter sun exposure. The greatest hazard in winter months is on cloudy days after a fresh snow, especially at higher altitudes, where UV radiation is greater.

The delicate skin around your eyes, nose and lips needs extra protection. Some people prefer to use a sunblock, such as zinc oxide or titanium dioxide, which stops all radiation from reaching the skin. Many people use a special lip sunscreen with an SPF rating of 30 or higher.

Sun sensitizers
Certain medications and skin products may make you more sensitive to the sun, including some antibiotics and antihistamines. Be especially careful to avoid the sun and tanning beds when using these substances. Avoid perfumes and after-shave lotion before sun exposure because such preparations may produce discolored patches on your skin.

Cleansing
After sun exposure, bathe or shower away perspiration, salt, pool chemicals and sunscreen products. Then apply a lubricant to your skin.

- Blotchy, wrinkled patches
- Easy bruising or tearing
- Bleeding, blistering or ulcerated lesions
- Painful intercourse

Lichen sclerosus is an uncommon condition that creates patchy, white skin that's thinner than normal. It can affect skin anywhere on your body, but it most often involves skin of the vulva, foreskin of the penis or skin around the anus.

The exact cause of lichen sclerosus isn't known. An overactive immune system or an imbalance of hormones may play a role. Previous skin damage at a particular site on your skin may increase the likelihood of lichen sclerosus at that location. Anyone can get lichen sclerosus but postmenopausal women have a high risk.

How serious is lichen sclerosis?

Skin cancer may rarely develop in areas affected by lichen sclerosus, though lichen sclerosus doesn't cause skin cancer. Women with lichen sclerosus on the vulva are more likely to develop vulvar cancer. Severe lichen sclerosus can make sex extremely painful for women because itching and scarring may narrow the vaginal opening and affect the ability or desire to have sexual intercourse.

Lichen sclerosus may rarely cause tightening and thinning of the foreskin in uncircumcised men. This can cause problems during an erection or when urinating.

Diagnosis

Your doctor may diagnose lichen sclerosis based on a physical examination and removal of a small piece of tissue for examination (biopsy).

Treatment

Corticosteroid ointments or creams are commonly prescribed for lichen sclerosus. Initially, you apply the medication daily. Later, your doctor may recommend that you use these medications twice a week to prevent a recurrence. If corticosteroid treatment doesn't work, other treatments include immune-modulating medications, such as tacrolimus (Protopic) and pimecrolimus (Elidel), and ultraviolet light treatment for nongenital areas.

Pityriasis rosea

Signs and symptoms

- A mild, itchy rash, ranging from pink to tan
- A rash that starts as one large spot on an arm, a leg or the trunk

Pityriasis rosea is a skin condition that causes a fine, scaly rash ranging in color from pink to tan. The itchy rash may start as one large spot, called a herald patch, on an arm, a leg or your trunk. After several days, the rash may spread to other parts of the body. The rash may peel.

The cause of pityriasis rosea isn't clear. It may be due to a viral infection. Pityriasis rosea usually affects children and young adults. The rash may last for three to 12 weeks. It rarely recurs.

Treatment

There's no specific treatment for pityriasis rosea. The rash usually disappears without treatment. Exposure to sunlight may help reduce the rash — but avoid sunburn. You may relieve the itching by applying a moisturizing cream or an over-the-counter hydrocortisone cream.

Dry skin

Signs and symptoms

- Itching
- Flaking, scaly skin
- Skin feels tight

Dry, itchy skin, also known as asteatosis, is a common problem, especially in older adults. Cold air and low humidity can be especially tough on your skin.

Symptoms of dry skin result from the loss of natural moisture and oil from the skin. Your skin may become cracked. Round patches of irritated skin may develop, resembling ringworm. The most common sites are the lower legs, upper arms, sides (flanks) and thighs.

Though most cases of dry skin are caused by environmental exposures, certain diseases also can significantly alter the function and appearance of your skin. Potential causes of dry skin include:

- **Weather.** In general, your skin is driest in winter, when temperatures and humidity levels plummet. Winter conditions also tend to make many existing skin conditions worse. The reverse may be true if you live in desert regions, where temperatures can soar but humidity levels remain low.
- **Central heating and air conditioning.** Central air and heating, wood-burning stoves, space heaters and fireplaces all reduce humidity and dry your skin.
- **Hot baths and showers.** Frequent showering or bathing, especially if you like the water hot and your baths long, breaks down the lipid barriers in your skin. So does frequent swimming.
- **Harsh soaps and detergents.** Many soaps and detergents strip lipids and water from your skin. Deodorant and antibacterial soaps are usually the most damaging, as are many shampoos, which dry out your scalp.
- **Sun exposure.** Like all types of heat, the sun dries your skin. Yet damage from ultraviolet (UV) radiation penetrates far beyond the top layer of skin (epidermis). The most significant damage occurs deep in the dermis, where collagen and elastin fibers break down much more quickly than they should, leading to deep wrinkles and loose, sagging skin (solar elastosis). Sun-damaged skin may have the appearance of dry skin.
- **Psoriasis.** This skin condition is marked by a rapid buildup of rough, dry, dead skin cells that form thick scales.

- **Thyroid disorders.** Hypothyroidism, which occurs when your thyroid produces too little thyroid hormone, reduces sweat and oil gland activity, leading to rough, dry skin.

Treatment

In most cases, dry skin problems respond well to home and lifestyle measures, such as using moisturizers and avoiding long, hot showers and baths. If you have very dry and scaly skin, your doctor may recommend you use an over-the-counter (nonprescription) cream that contains lactic acid or lactic acid and urea.

If you have a more serious skin disease, such as ichthyosis or psoriasis, your doctor may prescribe prescription creams and ointments or other treatments in addition to home care.

Ichthyosis

Signs and symptoms

- Severely dry, scaly skin starting in early childhood

Ichthyosis is a group of inherited skin disorders. *Ichthy* is taken from the Greek root for "fish" and refers to the dry, scaly appearance of skin associated with the disease. Ichthyosis occurs when the skin's natural shedding process is too slow or the production of skin cells is too fast.

Most cases of ichthyosis are mild, but some can be severe. The disorder occasionally is seen at birth, but often appears between ages 1 and 4. Sometimes it disappears entirely for most of the adult years, only to return later on. The rash tends to be most predominant on the elbows, knees and hands. It usually worsens in the winter. Ichthyosis may be associated with eczema.

Treatment

The goal of treatment is to manage symptoms by moisturizing the

Care for Wrinkled Skin

Wrinkling is a natural part of aging. As you grow older, your skin gets thinner, drier, less elastic and more wrinkled. And it tends to lose its youthful color and glow.

Dryness is a result of decreased oil production within your skin and loss of the skin's ability to retain moisture within its top layer. Deterioration in the connective tissues (elastin and collagen) in your dermal layer causes sagging, wrinkling and thinning. Finally, as your blood supply slows, your rosy glow begins to fade. Although aging of your skin is inevitable, it can be slowed by consistently using sunscreen whenever you're outdoors and by not smoking.

To treat wrinkled skin, you have several options:

Medications
- *Topical retinoids.* Derived from vitamin A, retinoids that you apply to your skin may be able to reduce fine wrinkles, splotchy pigmentation and skin roughness. Retinoids must be used with a skin care program that includes sunscreen and protective clothing because the medication can make your skin burn more easily. It may also cause redness, dryness, itching, and a burning or tingling sensation. Tretinoin (Renova, Retin-A, others) and tazarotene (Avage, Tazorac) are examples of topical retinoids.
- *Nonprescription wrinkle creams.* The effectiveness of anti-wrinkle creams depends in part on the active ingredient or ingredients. Retinol, alpha hydroxy acids, kinetin, coenzyme Q10, copper peptides and antioxidants may result in slight to modest improvements in wrinkles. However, nonprescription wrinkle creams contain lower concentrations of active ingredients than do prescription creams. Therefore results, if any, are limited and usually short-lived.

Other techniques
- *Skin resurfacing.* A number of techniques — from chemical peels to lasers — may be used to remove the outer layer of your skin, causing new, smoother skin to regenerate. For more information on these procedures, which may be used to reduce wrinkles, see page 1118.
- *Botulinum toxin type A (Botox).* When injected in small doses into specific muscles, Botox blocks the chemical signals that cause muscles to contract. When the muscles can't tighten, the skin flattens and appears smoother and less wrinkled. Botox works well on frown lines between the eyebrows and across the forehead, and crow's-feet at the corners of the eyes. Results typically last about three to four months. Repeat injections are needed to maintain results.
- *Soft tissue fillers.* Soft tissue fillers, which include fat, collagen and hyaluronic acid (Restylane, Juvéderm), can be injected into deeper wrinkles on your face. They plump and smooth out wrinkles and furrows and give your skin more volume. You may experience temporary swelling, redness and bruising in the treated area. The procedure may need to be repeated every few months.
- *Face-lift.* The face-lift procedure involves removing excess skin and fat in your lower face and neck and tightening the underlying muscle and connective tissue. The results typically last five to 10 years. Healing times can be lengthy after a face-lift. Bruising and swelling are evident for several weeks after surgery.

Keep in mind that results vary depending on the location of your wrinkles and how deep your wrinkles are. However, nothing stops the aging process of skin, so you'll likely need the treatments repeated to maintain benefits.

skin. The simplest treatment may consist of petroleum jelly applied to the affected areas, sometimes with a plastic wrap to keep the petroleum jelly from staining clothes or furniture. Twice daily applications of a lactic acid, urea or other creams also may help.

In severe cases, your doctor might prescribe retinoids — medications derived from vitamin A. They reduce the proliferation of skin cells. Side effects from the medication may include eye and lip inflammation, bone spurs and hair loss, as well as birth defects if taken during pregnancy.

Hives

Signs and symptoms
- Raised, red, often itchy welts of various sizes that appear and disappear at random on the surface of the skin
- The development of welts where the skin is scratched (dermatographism)

Hives is common. Typically, the condition appears as a reaction to internal or external allergens. A rare form of hives, called angioedema, can be life-threatening. Therefore, it's important to avoid substances that trigger hives, if possible. For a discussion of hives and angioedema, see page 505.

Treatment
The typical treatment for hives is with an antihistamine. For more-severe cases, other drugs may be used, such as an injection of adrenaline (epinephrine). Occasionally, hives is treated with a prescription corticosteroid medication.

Pigmentary changes

Signs and symptoms
- Slowly growing white patches of skin
- Dark brown patches of skin
  Skin color is the result of the melanin pigment created by certain cells (melanocytes) in skin.

Occasionally, something happens to this mechanism.

Melasma
When an area of skin produces too much melanin and becomes darker, it's called melasma (see the illustration on page 393). Melasma patches are most common on the face. They seldom spread far. In women, they're often associated with pregnancy or use of birth control pills, but both men and women can get them for no known reason.

Vitiligo
Vitiligo is a condition in which your skin loses melanin, the pigment that determines the color of your skin, hair and eyes. Vitiligo occurs when the cells that produce melanin die or no longer form melanin, triggering the development of slowly enlarging white patches of irregular shapes to appear on your skin (see the illustration on page 393).

The condition affects both sexes and all races, but is often more noticeable and more disfiguring in people with darker skin. Vitiligo usually starts as small areas of pigment loss that spread and become larger with time. These changes in your skin can result in stress and worries about your appearance.

Although any part of your body may be affected by vitiligo, depigmentation usually develops first on sun-exposed areas of your skin, such as your hands, feet, arms, face and lips. Although it can start at any age, vitiligo often first appears between the ages of 20 and 30.

Vitiligo generally appears in one of three patterns:
- **Focal.** Depigmentation is limited to one or a few areas of your body.
- **Segmental.** Loss of skin color occurs on only one side of your body.
- **Generalized.** Pigment loss is widespread across many parts of your body.

The natural course of vitiligo is difficult to predict. Sometimes the patches stop forming without treatment. In other cases, pigment loss can involve most of the surface of your skin.

How serious are pigmentary changes?
Neither vitiligo nor melasma is life-threatening. Cosmetics or skin dyes often are used to hide the

Spider Veins

Spider veins really have nothing to do with spiders, although the pattern of bluish veins seen through your skin may look a bit like a spider. Spider veins result when blood vessels close to the skin's surface widen (dilate). Spider veins are most common on the legs and face. They're not dangerous, but if associated with varicose veins, they can on occasion cause your legs to ache after extended time on your feet.

The cause of spider veins is unknown and nothing can be done to prevent them from appearing. Unlike varicose veins, spider veins are primarily painful to your vanity. For some people, wearing a skirt or shorts is no longer an option because of worries about the appearance of the purple-blue veins on their legs.

Treatment
The easiest course is to ignore the veins. They're a common, mild and medically insignificant variety of varicose veins. If the unsightly blood vessels concern you or, more importantly, if they prevent you from taking part in activities you would otherwise enjoy, ask your doctor about treating them with sclerotherapy, laser surgery or other options (see page 757).

patches. Because vitiligo patches sunburn easily, you'll need to use skin protection — clothing, sunscreen, sun avoidance or all three.

Treatment

Repigmentation and depigmentation treatments are used to restore uniform skin color. They include:

- **Tretinoin (Avita, Retin-A, others).** Applied nightly, it may help to lighten the dark patches of melasma. So-called "bleaching" creams also may be helpful. They contain a low concentration of hydroquinone, which reduces the pigmentation of the affected skin but does not contain bleach. Sun protection is a must to avoid rapid repigmentation of melasma.
- **Topical corticosteroid therapy.** Applying a corticosteroid cream to affected skin may help return color, particularly if you start using it early in the disease. You may not see a change in your skin's color for several months.

  This type of cream is effective and easy to use, but it can cause side effects, such as skin thinning or the appearance of streaks or lines on your skin.

  Milder forms may be prescribed for children and for people who have large areas of discolored skin.
- **Topical psoralen plus ultraviolet A (PUVA).** Topical PUVA may be a treatment option if you have a small number of depigmented patches (affecting less than 20 percent of your body). PUVA, also called photochemotherapy, is performed under artificial UVA light once or twice a week in your doctor's office. A thin coating of psoralen is applied to the depigmented patches of your skin about 30 minutes before UVA light exposure. You're then exposed to an amount of UVA light that turns the affected area of your skin pink. Your doctor may slowly increase the dose of UVA light over many weeks. Eventually, the pink areas

of your skin fade and a more normal skin color appears.

Potential side effects of topical PUVA therapy include severe sunburn and blistering and too much repigmentation or darkening of the treated patches or the normal surrounding skin (hyperpigmentation). Hyperpigmentation is usually a temporary problem and eventually disappears when treatment stops.
- **Oral psoralen plus ultraviolet A, or oral PUVA.** Oral PUVA therapy may be used if you have extensive vitiligo (affecting more than 20 percent of your body) or if you haven't responded to topical PUVA therapy. Oral PUVA isn't recommended for children younger than 10 years of age because of an increased risk of damage to the eyes, such as cataracts. For oral PUVA therapy, you take a prescribed dose of psoralen by mouth about two hours before exposure to artificial UVA light or sunlight. Your doctor adjusts the dose of light until the skin areas being treated become pink. Treatments are usually given two or three times a week, with at least one day in between.

Side effects of oral PUVA may include sunburn, nausea and vomiting, itching, abnormal hair growth, and too much repigmentation or darkening of the treated patches or the normal surrounding skin (hyperpigmentation). If used for longer periods of time, this type of treatment may increase your risk of skin cancer. To avoid sunburn and reduce your risk of skin cancer, apply sunscreen and avoid direct sunlight for 24 to 48 hours after each treatment. Wear protective UVA sunglasses for 18 to 24 hours after each treatment to avoid eye damage.
- **Narrow band ultraviolet B (UVB) therapy.** Narrow band UVB, a special form of UVB light, may be used as an alternative to PUVA. This type of therapy can

be administered like PUVA and given up to three times a week. No pre-application of psoralen is required, simplifying the treatment process. Narrow band UVB may be a safer long-term alternative to PUVA. Because it's simpler to administer, it's gaining wide acceptance.
- **Depigmentation.** Depigmentation involves fading the rest of the skin on your body to match the already-white areas. If you have vitiligo on more than 50 percent of your body, depigmentation may be the best treatment option. The drug monobenzone is applied twice a day to the pigmented areas of your skin until they match the already-depigmented areas. Avoid direct skin-to-skin contact with others for at least two hours after applying the drug.

A major side effect is redness and swelling (inflammation) of the skin. You may experience itching, dry skin or abnormal darkening of the membrane that covers the white of your eyes. Depigmentation is permanent and cannot be reversed. If you undergo depigmentation you will always be extremely sensitive to sunlight.

Surgical therapies

Surgical therapies include:
- **Autologous skin grafts or 'minipunch' skin transfer.** This type of skin grafting uses your own tissues (autologous). Your doctor removes tiny pieces of skin from one area of your body and attaches them to another. This procedure is sometimes used if you have small patches of vitiligo. Your doctor removes very small sections of your normal, pigmented skin (donor sites), often containing a small hair and places them on the depigmented areas (recipient sites). Possible complications of this procedure include infection at the donor or recipient site, but this is rare. The recipient and

donor sites may develop scarring, a cobblestone appearance, spotty pigmentation, or may fail to repigment at all.

- **Blister grafting.** In this procedure, your doctor creates blisters on your pigmented skin primarily by using suction. The tops of the blisters are then cut out and transplanted to a depigmented skin area where a blister of equal size has been created and removed. The risks of blister grafting include the development of a cobblestone appearance, scarring and lack of repigmentation. However, there's less risk of scarring with this procedure than with other types of skin grafting.

- **Tattooing (micropigmentation).** Tattooing implants pigment into your skin with a special surgical instrument. For treatment of vitiligo, tattooing works best for the lip area, particularly if you have dark skin. However, it may be difficult for your doctor to match your natural skin color. Tattooing tends to fade over time, and when used on the lips it may lead to episodes of blisters caused by the herpes simplex virus.

Bullous pemphigoid

Signs and symptoms
- Large, fluid-filled blisters
- Itchy skin around the blisters
- Skin around blisters may be reddish or darker than normal

Bullous pemphigoid is a rare skin condition that causes large, fluid-filled blisters. The blisters develop on areas of skin that often flex — such as the lower abdomen, upper thighs or armpits. The condition is most common in people older than age 60.

Bullous pemphigoid occurs when your immune system attacks a thin layer of tissue below your outer layer of skin. The reason for this abnormal immune response is unknown, although it sometimes can be triggered by taking certain medications.

Treatment
Your doctor will likely prescribe a combination of drugs that inhibit immune system activities that cause inflammation. These drugs may include:

- **Corticosteroids.** The most common treatment is prednisone, which comes in pill form. Corticosteroid ointment can be rubbed on your affected skin and causes fewer side effects.

- **Drugs that suppress the immune system.** They inhibit the production of your body's disease-fighting white blood cells. Examples include azathioprine (Azasan, Imuran) and mycophenolate mofetil (CellCept).

- **Other drugs that fight inflammation.** Other drugs with anti-inflammatory properties may be used alone or with corticosteroids. Examples include methotrexate (Trexall), tetracycline and dapsone (Aczone).

Drug rashes

Signs and symptoms
- Skin changes, including redness, hives, blisters and bleeding into the skin
- Itching

Drug rashes are a result of an allergic reaction to either an over-the-counter medication or one prescribed by your doctor. If a rash develops while you're taking any kind of drug, the medication may be the cause.

Drug reactions can involve more than an itch or rash. Signs and symptoms of a drug reaction may be extremely varied. In addition to the rash, you might experience fever, seizures, nausea, vomiting, diarrhea, heartbeat irregularities, difficulty breathing, asthma or decreased urine flow. In addition, laboratory tests may demonstrate an effect on your hemoglobin value or white blood cell count.

Fever is often the earliest sign of a drug reaction. Fortunately, rashes usually appear early during the course of a drug reaction and warn you that you may be experiencing a drug reaction. If you take one or more medications, a persistent rash is a warning to seek medical advice.

Treatment
If your rash is caused by a medication, the signs and symptoms should improve when you stop taking the drug. If the drug is a

Prickly Heat Rash

For some people, hot weather means the arrival of prickly heat rash. The condition is characterized by a rash of pinhead-sized bumps surrounded by a zone of red skin. Prickly heat rash itches intensely. Often, there's an accompanying prickling, stinging sensation. Typically, it occurs on the neck, upper chest, groin and armpits. The medical name for the most common variety of prickly heat is miliaria rubra.

Excessive perspiration produces prickly heat because the moisture damages cells on the surface of your skin. These damaged cells form a barrier that blocks the free flow of sweat out to the surface of your skin. Instead, the sweat accumulates beneath your skin.

The best treatment for prickly heat rash is prevention. Avoid situations that lead to excessive perspiration. If you already have a prickly heat rash, keep the affected area cool and dry, and the problem will likely clear up spontaneously within a few days.

An air-conditioned environment can be helpful. In addition, avoid antiperspirants, lotions, insect repellents or powders if you're still perspiring. After your skin is cool and dry, use a calamine-type lotion to help relieve the symptoms.

prescription medication, consult your doctor before discontinuing its use.

If your rash is itchy, oatmeal baths or wet dressings may soothe it (see page 1079). Topical hydrocortisone cream also may help. Antihistamines sometimes relieve the itch and diminish the rash of certain types of drug rashes.

Sunburn

Signs and symptoms
- Red, tender, swollen skin
- Water blisters
- Peeling skin

Emergency signs and symptoms
- Fever and chills
- Nausea
- Delirium

Sunburn is the result of the skin's overexposure to ultraviolet (UV) radiation from the sun or tanning beds. Congestion in the capillaries that supply blood to your skin causes the swollen, red skin of a sunburn.

Sunburn is thought to play a role in the dramatic increase in malignant melanoma, the most lethal form of skin cancer. A history of painful, blistering sunburns, especially in childhood, increases your risk of developing melanoma later in life (see page 1109). Intense, brief exposure to the sun is also a hazard. Whatever your age, there's no such thing as a healthy tan.

Mild sunburn or exposure to sun may stimulate your skin to produce extra melanin as protection against further ultraviolet penetration. More melanin means a deeper tan, if the additional pigment is distributed evenly. Otherwise, it forms freckles, liver spots or discolored splotches. Melanin production and dispersal are under genetic control. There's nothing you can do to change your tanning capacity.

Your skin, eye and hair color are good predictors of how much sun you can tolerate before you suffer a sunburn (see page 1068). You're most likely to sunburn without tanning if you have fair skin, blue or green eyes, and blond or red hair. Tanning is more likely if you have dark brown eyes, brown or black hair, and brown or black skin.

Diagnosis
Symptoms of sunburn may not appear until a few hours after exposure.

How serious is sunburn?
If the sunburn is severe, skin cells die and blisters form. The skin then heals in a period of one to two weeks. During the healing process, skin damaged by sunburn may peel off in patches.

Damage to your skin cells from recurrent sunburn is cumulative, and continued overexposure to UV radiation produces long-term effects. These can include skin discolorations, actinic keratosis and skin cancer. Most skin cancer results from irreversible skin damage.

Treatment
Treat your sunburn with cool tap water compresses and, if the burn is severe, hydrocortisone cream several times daily. Soaking in cool tub water with or without oatmeal may help. Leave water blisters intact to speed healing. If they break open on their own, remove the skin fragments and apply an antibacterial ointment on the open areas to help prevent infections. Keep the wounds clean.

For a severe sunburn, contact your doctor before signs and symptoms fully develop. Your doctor may prescribe an oral corticosteroid to decrease the reaction.

Photosensitivity

Signs and symptoms
- Redness
- A rash
- Blistering or swelling

Photosensitivity is a heightened reaction of skin to ultraviolet (UV) rays from the sun or tanning beds, usually after consuming certain medications or touching certain substances or plants. When skin products cause a sunlight allergic reaction, the condition is called photocontact dermatitis.

Medications that can cause photosensitive reactions include:
- Antibiotics
- Anticonvulsants
- Antidepressants
- Antihistamines
- Birth control pills
- Chemotherapy medications
- Diuretics
- High blood pressure medications
- Nonsteroidal anti-inflammatory drugs (NSAIDs)
- Oral diabetes medications
- Topical antiseptic creams
- Tranquilizers

Some substances and plants can cause photosensitivity when they come in contact with your skin. These include:
- Artificial sweeteners (cyclamates)
- Perfumes containing bergamot, sandalwood, lavender or citron oils
- After-shave lotions
- Antibacterial deodorant soaps
- Detergents
- Medicated cosmetics
- Shampoos or soaps with coal tar ingredients
- Sunscreens with para-aminobenzoic acid (PABA)
- Skin-bleaching creams
- Certain fruits and plants, such as limes, parsley, celery, parsnips, carrots and figs

Types
There are two categories of photosensitive reactions: photoallergic and phototoxic.

Photoallergic
A photoallergic reaction is a result of changes in your immune system. When this occurs, your skin reacts each time it's exposed to sunlight after exposure to or contact with a particular sensitizing drug, chemical or plant.

Your skin becomes red, although not necessarily sunburned, and develops a bumpy rash, similar to that caused by poison ivy. Discolored patches, blisters or swelling also can occur. Symptoms can extend to areas not exposed to the light.

Phototoxic

A phototoxic reaction looks and feels like an exaggerated sunburn with inflammation, redness, blisters and the characteristic discomfort. You may have this reaction any time a sufficient amount of the sensitizing chemical is present in your body or on your skin and you're exposed to the activating wavelength of light.

Treatment

A photosensitive reaction usually disappears within a week after you take steps to protect your skin from UV exposure and avoid the sensitizing substance.

If you've had a photoallergic reaction, it's especially important to wear protective clothing and use a broad-spectrum sunscreen that blocks both ultraviolet A and ultraviolet B rays when you're outdoors.

For a severe reaction, your doctor may prescribe a corticosteroid ointment or cream or hydroxychloroquine tablets to help suppress photoallergic reactions.

Sun-damaged skin

Signs and symptoms

- Loose, sagging or wrinkled skin
- Dry, tough, leathery skin

Excessive exposure to sunlight over many years damages collagen and elastin fibers that help support skin. This can lead to loose, sagging, tough and wrinkled skin that can look 15 to 20 years older than normal.

Your skin is composed of two types of connective tissue. One type is a strong fiber (collagen). The other is an elastic fiber (elastin). Ultraviolet radiation penetrates skin and can damage these tissues. Orderly structural arrangement of skin cells and connective

tissues deteriorates, and abnormal cell growth begins.

Each exposure to ultraviolet light causes slight but irreversible changes, so the damage accumulates over the years. Signs and symptoms appear gradually as the skin loses its resilience, flexibility and water-holding capacity.

If you sunburn easily and tan poorly, you're most susceptible to a condition called solar elastosis. It usually occurs in fair-skinned, blue- or green-eyed people with blond or red hair who are frequently exposed to intense sunlight without protection. The risk is highest for individuals who are often outdoors. Those who live in regions with intense sunlight are more at risk. Such areas include higher elevations and the Western plains.

Diagnosis

You can see the effects of solar elastosis by comparing your protected skin with overexposed skin — the skin on your face, hands and legs. Your dermatologist can establish the diagnosis by examination.

How serious is sun-damaged skin?

No medical treatment can reverse the damage to your skin or rejuvenate your skin. If your skin has been damaged enough to cause solar elastosis, your risk of acquiring skin cancer is increased. Make sure to see your doctor whenever you have a new growth or a change in an existing growth such as a mole.

Treatment

To prevent further damage, avoid sunlight whenever you can. If you can't, protect your skin with sunscreen and proper clothing.

Your dermatologist may recommend lubricating creams to reduce dryness and soften your skin. Facial massages and masks can make your face feel better for a while by toning muscles and stimulating blood circulation.

Senile skin

Signs and symptoms

- Skin discolorations, including liver spots, freckles and red, yellow, gray or brown blotches
- Skin texture changes, including coarse wrinkles, sagging folds, sallowness, roughness, excessive dryness or leathery toughness
- Skin growths, including scaly patches

The effects of aging on the skin are generally gradual. However, signs of aging may appear more quickly and at a younger age if you're susceptible to sun damage and your skin has had considerable sun exposure.

Treatment

There's no way to reverse the effects of aging skin, but you can take steps to prevent further changes. For more information on common skin conditions related to aging, see sun-damaged skin on this page, liver spots (page 1102) and actinic keratosis (page 1101).

Xanthelasma and xanthoma

Signs and symptoms

- Soft, fatty, yellowish bumps beneath the surface of your skin

Both xanthelasma and xanthoma are yellowish bumps that appear beneath the skin and that have sharply defined margins. The bumps can be removed, but they may reappear.

Xanthelasmas

Xanthelasmas are flat and they appear in the skin above your eyelids near your nose. They don't hurt, and they may be harmless. However, they're associated with high levels of fat (lipids) in the blood (hyperlipidemia) in at least half of all people who have them. Therefore, you'll probably want to have your blood tested to determine your levels of cholesterol and triglycerides.

Xanthomas

Xanthomas are a symptom of an underlying metabolic disorder that increases the fat (lipid) concentration in the blood. Xanthomas can appear anywhere on your body but most commonly occur over joints or tendons. With certain disorders, they tend to appear where your skin receives persistent pressure, such as on your knees, elbows, hands, feet or buttocks. The bumps are flat and can vary from less than 1 inch to more than 3 inches across.

In addition to hyperlipidemia, xanthomas may also be associated with diabetes, primary biliary cirrhosis, some cancers and several inherited metabolic disorders.

Corns and calluses

Signs and symptoms
• Thickened, hardened layers of skin or raised bumps of hardened skin on your hands and feet
Corns often appear as raised bumps of hardened skin less than $1/4$ inch long. Calluses vary in size and shape. Corns and calluses are your skin's attempt to protect itself. Although they can be unsightly, treatment generally is necessary only if they cause discomfort. For most people, eliminating the source of friction or pressure helps corns and calluses disappear.

Treatment
In most cases, you can treat your corn or callous on your own at home. If it becomes painful or inflamed, contact your doctor. Try the following self-care tips:
• Wear properly fitted shoes with adequate toe room. Have your shoes stretched at any point that rubs or pinches. Place pads under your heels if your shoes rub. Try over-the-counter remedies to cushion or soften the corn while wearing shoes.
• Wear padded gloves when using hand tools or try padding your tool handles with cloth tape or covers.

• Rub your skin with a pumice stone or a washcloth during or after bathing to gradually thin some of the thickened skin. Do not perform this method if you have diabetes or poor circulation.
• Try over-the-counter corn dissolvers containing salicylic acid.
• Don't cut or shave corns or calluses with a sharp instrument.

Perspiration Disorders

Sitting in the heat of the sun, working out at the gym, giving a presentation at work — all of these things can make you sweat. It's natural to sweat under these conditions. In fact, when you exercise strenuously, are exposed to heat or are under extreme emotional stress, you may lose several quarts of fluid in perspiration.

Sometimes the complex mechanism of perspiration goes awry, resulting in either excessive perspiration (hyperhidrosis) or little or no perspiration (anhidrosis). Excessive sweating can be embarrassing and may sometimes signal a more serious health problem. Anhidrosis is potentially life-threatening.

For most people, sweating is simply a minor nuisance. Although perspiration is basically odorless, it can take on an unpleasant smell when it comes into contact with bacteria on your skin.

How much you sweat and even the way your sweat smells can be influenced by your mood, certain foods and beverages, some drugs and medical conditions and even your hormones.

Anhidrosis

Signs and symptoms
• Lack of perspiration in hot weather and when exercising
Many people worry about excessive sweating. But some people

sweat very little or not at all — a condition that can be potentially life-threatening. Factors that may affect your ability to perspire normally include:
• Certain drugs, including some antipsychotic medications
• Hypohidrotic ectodermal dysplasia, a rare disorder in which children are born without sweat glands or with underdeveloped sweat glands
• Autonomic neuropathy, a disorder of nerves
• Infections of the sweat glands
• Burns
• Dehydration
• Heatstroke
• Diabetes, which can cause autonomic neuropathy

How serious is anhidrosis?
When you stop sweating or don't perspire enough to cool your body, the results can be serious or even fatal. Complications of too little perspiration include heat exhaustion and heatstroke. The main sign of heatstroke is a high temperature — generally greater than 104 F — with hot, dry skin and confusion. Early signs and symptoms may include abnormal irritability, headache and nausea. Coma can result from unrecognized and untreated heat exhaustion.

Treatment
Treating anhidrosis involves treating the underlying condition, if possible. In some instances, this may mean changing medications. It's also important to take steps to prevent heat exhaustion, heatstroke and dehydration.

Hyperhidrosis

Signs and symptoms
• Abnormally excessive and bothersome perspiration during exercise or in hot weather
• Excessive and bothersome perspiration on your face, underarms, palms and the soles of your feet that's triggered by nervousness, anxiety or stress

You have two types of sweat glands in your skin: eccrine glands and apocrine glands. Eccrine glands occur over most of your body and open directly onto the surface of your skin. Apocrine glands develop in association with hair follicles on your scalp, underarms, nipples and genitals.

You have between 2 million and 5 million eccrine sweat glands. When your body temperature rises, your autonomic nervous system stimulates these glands to secrete fluid onto the surface of your skin, where it cools your body by evaporation. This fluid (perspiration) is composed of water, salt (sodium chloride), urea and trace amounts of other electrolytes — substances that help regulate the balance of fluids in your body.

Apocrine glands, on the other hand, secrete a fatty sweat directly into the tubule of the gland. When you're under emotional stress, the wall of the tubule contracts, and the sweat is pushed to the surface of your skin where bacteria begin breaking it down. Most often, it's the bacterial breakdown of apocrine sweat that causes the strong odor.

Some people simply sweat more than others for no apparent reason. But certain factors may make you sweat heavily. These include:

- Certain foods and beverages, including caffeine, alcohol and spicy foods
- Certain drugs, including some antipsychotic medications, morphine, certain painkillers and excess doses of the thyroid hormone thyroxine
- Fever
- Menopause
- Low blood sugar (hypoglycemia)
- Overactive thyroid (hyperthyroidism)
- A heart attack
- Tuberculosis
- Malaria

Complications

Common skin disorders associated with excessive sweating include:

- Fungal nail infections
- Athlete's foot and jock itch
- Bacterial infections and warts

Diagnosis

See your doctor if you suddenly begin to sweat more than usual or experience night sweats for no apparent reason. Infections, thyroid gland problems, menopause and certain types of cancer, such as leukemia and lymphoma, can produce unusual sweating patterns.

A cold sweat is usually your body's response to a serious illness, anxiety or severe pain. Seek immediate medical attention for a cold sweat if you have signs of lightheadedness or chest and stomach pains. Also talk to your doctor if you notice a change in body odor. A fruity smell, for example, may be a sign of diabetes, while an ammonia-like smell could indicate liver or kidney disease.

In addition, a rare condition known as fish-odor syndrome (trimethylaminuria) causes an odor similar to rotting fish. People with fish-odor syndrome have a defective gene that prevents them from metabolizing trimethylamine — a natural byproduct in the digestion of foods such as saltwater fish, eggs and liver.

Treatment

For some people who sweat excessively, the answer may be simple: an over-the-counter antiperspirant used on the hands and feet as well as the underarms. Antiperspirants inhibit the action of your sweat ducts with aluminum salts, reducing the amount of perspiration that reaches your skin. Deodorants, which can eliminate odor but not perspiration, turn your skin acidic, which makes it less attractive to bacteria. Although you may have heard stories linking antiperspirants and breast cancer, there's no evidence of such a link.

If over-the-counter products aren't strong enough, your doctor may suggest a prescription antiperspirant. For more-severe problems with sweating, your doctor may recommend other treatments.

Iontophoresis

In this procedure a dermatologist uses a battery-powered device to deliver a low current of electricity to the affected area. The instrument introduces ions into the skin, which prevent the sweat glands from working. Although iontophoresis is painless and quite safe, it may be no more effective than a topical antiperspirant.

Botulinum toxin injections

Researchers have discovered that botulinum toxin type A (Botox) injections are an effective way to treat severe hyperhidrosis. The Botox blocks the nerves that control the sweat glands. It's used mainly in the armpits.

Careful application is required, as in some situations it can cause muscle atrophy. This procedure isn't a cure-all. It may take several injections to achieve the desired results, the treatment can be painful and the results only last a few months.

Surgery

In rare cases, surgery may be an option. If excess sweating occurs just in your armpits, removing the sweat glands there may help.

If excess sweating occurs on your hands, one possible treatment is to cut the nerves that carry messages from the sympathetic nerves to the sweat glands. The surgery, which generally requires only a day in the hospital and produces minimal scarring, typically doesn't reduce sweating of the underarms, feet or body, but it can permanently stop sweating on the hands. As a side effect of surgery, increased sweating can occur elsewhere on your body.

Self-care

You can do a number of things to reduce sweating and body odor. The following steps may help:

- **Bathe daily.** This helps keep the number of bacteria on your skin in check.
- **Dry your feet thoroughly after you bathe.** Microorganisms thrive in the damp spaces between your toes. Use over-the-counter foot powders to help absorb sweat.
- **Apply antiperspirants nightly.** At bedtime, apply antiperspirants to sweaty palms or soles of the feet. Try perfume-free antiperspirants.
- **Choose shoes and socks made of natural materials.** Shoes made of natural materials, such as leather, can help prevent sweaty feet by allowing your feet to breathe. In addition, wear the right socks. Cotton and wool socks help keep your feet dry because they absorb moisture. When you're active, moisture-wicking athletic socks are a good choice.
- **Change your socks often.** Change your socks or pantyhose once or twice a day, drying your feet thoroughly each time. Women who wear pantyhose may want to try those with cotton soles.
- **Rotate your shoes.** Shoes won't completely dry overnight, so if you have trouble with sweaty feet, try not to wear the same pair two days in a row.
- **Air your feet.** Go barefoot when you can or at least slip out of your shoes now and then.
- **Choose natural-fiber clothing.** Wear natural fabrics, such as cotton, wool and silk, that allow your skin to breathe. When you exercise, you might prefer high-tech fabrics that wick moisture away from your skin, such as Coolmax.
- **Try relaxation techniques.** Consider relaxation techniques such as yoga, meditation or biofeedback. If your perspiration problem is related to stress, these techniques may help you learn to control the stress that can trigger your sweating.

Skin Infections

Because your skin is your first line of defense, it often must deal with attacks from bacteria, viruses, fungi and insects. Skin infections range from localized, superficial infections to widespread, life-threatening infections. The signs and symptoms depend on where the infection develops and the organism causing it.

Impetigo

Signs and symptoms
- Itchy, red sores with yellow or gray crusts, on the face, legs or arms

Impetigo is a fairly common superficial skin infection caused by bacteria — staphylococci (staph), streptococci (strep) or both. It may occur on normal skin, but the bacteria usually invade through a crack, abrasion, insect bite or an area of dry or inflamed skin.

The infection starts as a red sore that blisters briefly and then oozes during the next few days to form a sticky crust (see the illustration on page 396). The sore tends to grow and is contagious through contact with bacteria in the blister's fluid. Physical contact — including scratching — can spread the infection to other parts of the body or even to other people.

An ulcerating form of impetigo (ecthyma) appears as itchy, thick, brown-black crusts ringed by red skin. In rare instances, the bacteria may infect the bloodstream and, in children, lead to kidney disease. The incidence of impetigo is highest among children with poor hygiene. In adults, it appears mostly as a complication of an underlying skin problem.

Diagnosis
A diagnosis of impetigo may be made after examination of the skin and a lab analysis of the bacteria causing your infection.

Treatment
Topical medications are often effective for limited and minor infections. It may also help to apply a diluted vinegar compress. Fold a clean cloth and moisten it with a solution of 1 ounce white vinegar to 16 to 32 ounces water. For more extensive infections, your doctor may prescribe an oral antibiotic.

Wash the area several times each day with antibacterial soap or cleanser to soften the crusts, and then gently remove them. To avoid spreading the infection, don't share towels, clothing and razors. Avoid skin contact until the condition clears. The sores heal slowly, but the rate of successful treatment is very high.

Folliculitis

Signs and symptoms
- Clusters of small red bumps that develop around hair follicles
- Pus-filled blisters that break open and crust over
- Itchiness or tenderness
- A large swollen bump or mass
- Pain

Folliculitis is a superficial infection of the hair follicles (see the illustration on page 398). This type of infection is common and is usually caused by staphylococci (staph) bacteria, yeast or fungi.

It can occur anywhere on your skin as a result of clothing friction, hair follicle blockage or injury. For example, shaving your neck or underarms can produce a rash that becomes long lasting (chronic) unless treated.

There are two main forms of folliculitis. That which affects the upper part of the hair follicle is known as superficial folliculitis. Deep folliculitis starts deeper in the surrounding skin and affects the entire hair follicle.

Superficial folliculitis
It includes the following:
- **Staphylococcal folliculitis.** This common type of folliculitis is marked by itchy, white,

pus-filled bumps that can occur anywhere on your body. When it affects the beard area of men, it's called barber's itch. It occurs when hair follicles become infected with *Staphylococcus aureus* (staph) bacteria. Although staph bacteria live on your skin all the time, they generally cause problems only when they enter your body through a cut or other skin injury.

- **Hot tub folliculitis (pseudomonas folliculitis).** The pseudomonas bacteria that cause this form of folliculitis thrive in a wide range of environments, including hot tubs whose chlorine and pH levels aren't well-regulated. Within eight hours to five days of exposure to the bacteria, a rash of red, round, itchy bumps will appear that later may develop into small pus-filled blisters (pustules). The rash is likely to be worse in areas covered by your swimsuit.
- **Tinea barbae.** Caused by a fungus rather than a bacterium, this type of folliculitis develops in the beard area in men, causing itchy, white bumps. The surrounding skin also may become reddened. A more serious, inflammatory form of the infection appears as pus-filled nodules that eventually form a crust and that may occur along with swollen lymph nodes and fever.
- **Pseudofolliculitis barbae.** An inflammation of the hair follicles in the beard area, pseudofolliculitis barbae affects men with curly beards. It develops when shaved hairs curve back into the skin, leading to inflammation and, in rare cases, to dark raised scars (keloid scars) on the face and neck.
- **Pityrosporum folliculitis.** Most common in young and middle-aged adults, this form produces chronic, red, itchy pustules on the back and chest and sometimes on the neck, shoulders, upper arms and face. It's caused by the yeastlike fungus.

Blister Basics

Friction blisters develop when pressure or friction causes fluid to accumulate between layers of your skin. If you feel a hot spot developing, stop what you're doing and cover the affected area with an adhesive bandage.

Don't puncture a blister unless it's painful or prevents you from walking or using one of your hands. Cover a small blister with an adhesive bandage and cover a large one with a porous, plastic-coated gauze pad that absorbs moisture and allows the wound to breathe.

If you must open the blister, first wash your hands and the blister area with soap and warm water. Swab the blister with iodine or 70 percent alcohol. Then puncture the blister at several points along the base with a sterile needle. Drain the fluid, but leave the overlying skin intact. Apply antibiotic ointment to the site and cover it with a gauze pad. After a few days, use a tweezers to lift any dead skin and a scissors to cut it away. Reapply ointment and gauze and check for signs of infection (redness or pus). See a doctor if the blister appears to be infected.

- **Herpetic folliculitis.** Shaving through a cold sore — a small, fluid-filled blister caused by the herpes simplex virus — may spread the herpes infection to neighboring hair follicles.

Deep folliculitis
Types of deep folliculitis include:
- **Gram-negative folliculitis.** It can develop in people receiving long-term antibiotic treatment for acne. Antibiotics alter the normal balance of bacteria in the nose, leading to an overgrowth of harmful organisms (gram-negative bacteria). In most people, this doesn't cause problems, and the flora in the nose returns to normal once antibiotics are stopped. In a few people, however, gram-negative bacteria spread to the cheeks, chin and jaw line, where they cause new, sometimes-severe acne lesions.
- **Boils and carbuncles.** These occur when hair follicles become deeply infected with staph bacteria. See page 1094 for more information.
- **Eosinophilic folliculitis.** Seen primarily in HIV-positive people, this type of folliculitis is characterized by recurring patches of inflamed, pus-filled sores, primarily on the face and sometimes on the back or upper arms. The sores usually spread, may itch intensely and often leave areas of darker than normal skin when they heal. The exact cause of eosinophilic folliculitis isn't known, but it may involve the same yeastlike fungus responsible for pityrosporum folliculitis.

Treatment
For some, folliculitis goes away without medical treatment within two to three days. During that time, self-care measures, such as warm compresses and anti-itch creams, can help relieve your symptoms.

Persistent or recurring cases are likely to require treatment. The therapy your doctor recommends will depend on the type and severity of your infection.
- **Staphylococcal folliculitis.** Your doctor may prescribe an antibiotic that you apply to your skin (topical) or that you take by mouth (oral). Your doctor may also recommend that you avoid shaving the affected area until the infection heals. If you must shave, use an electric razor or clean razor blade every time.
- **Hot tub folliculitis (pseudomonas folliculitis).** Hot tub folliculitis rarely requires specific treatment, although your doctor

may prescribe an oral or topical medication to help relieve itching (anti-pruritic). More-severe cases may require an oral antibiotic.

- **Tinea barbae.** This infection — especially the inflammatory form — can be treated with oral antifungal medications.
- **Pseudofolliculitis barbae.** Self-care measures are the best treatments for this condition. Shaving with an electric razor, which doesn't cut as closely as a razor blade does, can help. If you do use a blade, massage your beard area with a warm, moist washcloth or facial sponge to lift the hairs so that they can be cut more easily. Use a shaving gel instead of cream, and shave in the direction of the hair growth. When you're finished, rinse thoroughly with warm water and apply a moisturizing after-shave. If these measures don't help, your doctor may prescribe the acne medication tretinoin (Retin-A, Avita, others).
- **Pityrosporum folliculitis.** Topical or oral antifungals are the most effective treatments for this type of folliculitis. Because the condition often returns once you've finished the course of oral medication, your doctor may recommend using topical ointments indefinitely. Antibiotics aren't helpful in treating pityrosporum folliculitis and may make the infection worse by upsetting the normal balance of bacteria on your skin.
- **Herpetic folliculitis.** If you're a healthy adult, herpetic folliculitis may clear without treatment in seven to 10 days. But if you're living with HIV/AIDS or you experience frequent cold sores, your doctor may prescribe an oral antiviral medication such as acyclovir, famciclovir or valacyclovir. Although these drugs can clear the infection, they won't necessarily prevent it from recurring, and they may also cause side effects such as headache, diarrhea, nausea and abdominal pain.
- **Gram-negative folliculitis.** This type of folliculitis results from long-term antibiotic therapy for acne. It's usually treated with certain antibiotics or with isotretinoin (Claravis, Myorisan).
- **Boils and carbuncles.** Your doctor may drain a large boil or carbuncle by making a small incision in the tip. This relieves pain, speeds recovery and helps lessen scarring. Deep infections that can't be completely cleared may be covered with sterile gauze so that pus can continue to drain. Sometimes your doctor may prescribe antibiotics to help heal severe or recurrent infections.
- **Eosinophilic folliculitis.** A number of therapies are effective against eosinophilic folliculitis, but topical corticosteroids are often the treatment of choice. Your doctor may prescribe a short course of oral corticosteroids if you have a severe infection. All steroids can have serious side effects and should be used for as brief a time as possible. If you're living with HIV/AIDS and have mild eosinophilic folliculitis, your doctor may prescribe topical steroids in conjunction with oral antihistamines. Severe cases may require treatment with isotretinoin (Claravis, Myorisan) for several months.

Boils and carbuncles

Signs and symptoms

- A swollen, tender nodule on your skin, usually pink or red, that often eventually drains pus
- A spreading area of swelling, redness and pain in the skin
- Fever
- Exhaustion

A boil (furuncle) is a local infection in one or more hair follicles and is usually caused by staphylococci (staph) bacteria. When multiple boils appear anywhere on the body, the condition is called furunculosis. In contrast, a carbuncle is a cluster of boils that forms a connected area of infection under the skin. Contact with other parts of the body and other people can easily spread these infections.

Sometimes a boil will go away after the initial stage of itching or mild pain. More often, it grows rapidly over a few days. As pus collects within the lesion, pressure and pain increase. It comes to a head with a white or yellow center in the nodule and then bursts, drains and heals. It may recur later near the same site and go through the same cycle.

Boils are common. A boil can occur anywhere on your skin but is most likely to appear on your face, neck, armpits, buttocks or thighs. Poor health, clothing that binds or

---

PREVENTION TIP

To prevent wound infections, follow these basic self-care measures:
- Keep skin wounds clean.
- Apply an antibiotic cream or ointment. If a rash develops, stop using the ointment and talk to your doctor or pharmacist. Ingredients in such ointments can cause a mild rash in some people.
- Cover the area with a bandage to help keep it clean and keep harmful bacteria out. Repeatedly drain covered blisters until a scab forms.
- Change the bandage daily or whenever it becomes wet or dirty.

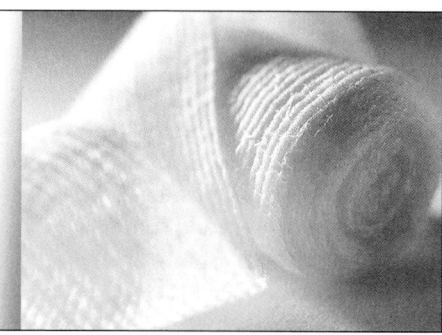

chafes, and disorders such as acne, dermatitis, diabetes and anemia can increase your risk of infection.

Carbuncles commonly appear on the upper back and on the nape of your neck. They're less common than boils. Men are more prone to have them than are women. Carbuncles develop slowly and may not reach your skin's surface to drain on their own.

Diagnosis

A boil or carbuncle can usually be identified by a visual inspection of the affected area. A culture of the pus may be necessary to determine the specific bacteria involved. Blood and urine tests may be necessary if your doctor suspects an underlying disorder.

How serious are boils and carbuncles?

A boil usually will burst within two weeks. A carbuncle or boil that persists longer might spread the infection to your bloodstream. Internal staph infections, which can be life-threatening, often start as skin infections.

A boil or carbuncle on or near your nose, cheeks, forehead or spine can spread rapidly to become a brain abscess or spinal abscess. Prompt medical treatment can help prevent these serious complications.

A frequent occurrence of boils may indicate an underlying disorder that needs medical attention.

Treatment

To avoid spreading the infection and to minimize discomfort, follow these self-care measures:

- For about 30 minutes every few hours, apply a washcloth or compress moistened with warm salt water. This may help the boil burst and drain much sooner. To prepare warm salt water, add 1 teaspoon of salt to 1 quart of boiling water and let it cool. Prevent the drained matter from contacting other skin areas.
- Gently wash the sore twice a day with antibacterial soap. Cover the sore with a bandage to prevent the infection from spreading.
- Apply an over-the-counter antibiotic ointment.
- Never squeeze or lance a boil because you might spread the infection.
- Launder towels, compresses and clothing that have touched the area.

Contact your doctor if the infection is located over your spine or on your face, if it worsens rapidly, causes severe pain, hasn't disappeared within two weeks or is accompanied by fever or reddish lines radiating from the boil. In some cases, antibiotics or surgical drainage may be necessary to clear your infection.

Cellulitis and erysipelas

Signs and symptoms

- Painful area of hot, red, swollen skin, sometimes accompanied by red streaks

Cellulitis is an acute inflammation of the connective tissue of your skin that results from a bacterial or fungal infection. It may appear gradually over a couple of days or rapidly over a few hours. It begins as a localized area of red, painful, warm skin, and it may be accompanied by fever and swelling (see the illustration on page 398).

Cellulitis occurs when one or more types of bacteria enter through a crack or break in your skin, most commonly streptococcus and staphylococcus. The incidence of a more serious staphylococcus infection called methicillin-resistant *Staphylococcus aureus* (MRSA) is increasing. People with chronic leg or foot swelling, immune deficits or circulatory deficiencies, such as those related to diabetes, are more prone to developing cellulitis.

Erysipelas is a severe form of cellulitis caused by streptococci (strep) bacteria, in which the infected area is shiny and sharply defined. It's characterized by high fever and recurrences. Gangrene is a rare complication of these infections.

Treatment

After an examination, your doctor may prescribe an antibiotic, which usually stops the infection within a week. Elevating the infected area and applying hot, moist compresses to the site also may help. If the infection spreads, you may require intravenous antibiotics and possibly surgery to control the infection.

Methicillin-resistant *Staphylococcus aureus*

Signs and symptoms

- A red or swollen bump or infected area
- Painful
- Warm to the touch
- Full of pus or other drainage
- Fever
  Methicillin-resistant *Staphylococcus aureus* (MRSA) is a potentially dangerous type of staph bacteria that's resistant to certain antibiotics and may cause skin and other infections. MRSA is spread through direct contact with an infected person or by sharing personal items, such as towels or razors that have touched infected skin.

How serious is methicillin-resistant *Staphylococcus aureus*?

The infections are difficult to treat and can be potentially dangerous. Recognizing the signs and symptoms and receiving treatment in the early stages reduces the chances of the infection becoming severe.

Treatment

Treatment of MRSA skin infections may include having your doctor or a health care professional drain the infection and, in some cases, prescribe an antibiotic. Don't attempt to drain the infection yourself, doing so could worsen the infection or spread it to others.

Lymphadenitis and lymphangitis

Signs and symptoms

Lymphangitis
- Swollen areas of skin, sometimes with redness and pain
- Throbbing pain in the wound area
- Malaise
- Fever, sweating and chills
- Loss of appetite

Emergency signs and symptoms
- A red streak running from the site of the infection up the extremity, or running to the armpit or groin

Lymphadenitis
- Enlarged lymph nodes, such as in the neck, armpits and groin
- Tender or painful lymph nodes
- A smooth, irregular, soft or rubbery feel to the lymph nodes, which indicates an abscess may have formed
- Reddened, hot skin over the lymph nodes

Lymphadenitis is an inflammation of lymph nodes caused by infection from bacteria, viruses, fungi or other microorganisms. Areas where you can easily feel lymph nodes, especially if they're enlarged, are the groin, armpits and neck. Lymphangitis is a similar infection of the lymphatic channels. Both may be associated with pus-filled abscesses and cellulitis.

Lymphangitis occurs after an acute infection of the skin, such as cellulitis, or an abscess in the skin or soft tissues. It causes a throbbing pain, malaise, fever and loss of appetite. If you develop a red streak running from the site of the infection up the extremity or to the armpit or groin, immediate treatment is essential. The infection can spread rapidly to the bloodstream and may be fatal if untreated.

Lymphadenitis causes enlargement of the lymph nodes, which may be tender or painful. It often results from cellulitis or a bacterial infection by streptococci (strep) or staphylococci (staph), but it can result from any bacterial, fungal, viral or other infection. Sometimes an abscess occurs.

Diagnosis
Tests may include blood cultures, a white blood cell count, and a lymph node culture or biopsy.

Treatment
Treatment varies, depending on the source of the infection. Antibiotic treatment, begun immediately, usually brings the disease under control in a few days with a complete recovery. Aspirin can help relieve the pain, inflammation and swelling. Abscesses may need to be surgically drained.

Cold sores

Signs and symptoms
- Small, fluid-filled blisters on a raised, red, painful area of skin, usually located on the lips but sometimes on your nostrils, cheeks or fingers
- Pain or tingling, often preceding the blisters by one or two days

The scenario is all too familiar: You feel a tingling on your lip and a small, hard spot that you can't see. Sure enough, in a day or two, a red blister appears on your lip (see the illustration on page 400). It's another cold sore, probably happening at a bad time, and there's no way to hide it or make it go away quickly.

Cold sores — also called fever blisters — affect millions of Americans, perhaps more than half the population.

Cold sores are quite different from canker sores, a condition people sometimes associate them with. Cold sores are caused by a form of the herpes simplex virus, and they're contagious. Canker sores, which aren't contagious, are ulcers that occur in soft tissues inside the mouth, whereas cold sores may appear on the gums or the roof of your mouth (hard palate). Cold sores usually appear on your lip, but occasionally they occur on your nostrils, cheeks or fingers.

Herpes simplex virus type 1 usually causes cold sores. Herpes simplex virus type 2 is usually responsible for genital herpes. However, either form of the virus can cause sores in the facial area or on the genitals.

You get cold sores from another person who has an active lesion. Shared eating utensils, razors and towels may spread this infection. The greatest risk of infection is

---

from the time the blisters appear until they've completely dried and crusted over. Cold sores seem to run in families. You may have a greater tendency to get cold sores if an immediate family member also experiences them. This may be due to the contagious aspect of cold sores, but it's more likely due to genetic susceptibility.

Symptoms of your first cold sore may start as long as 20 days after exposure to the virus and may last for seven to 10 days. The blisters form, break and ooze. A yellow crust forms and finally sloughs off to uncover pinkish, healing skin. The virus then reverts to a latent form within your nerve cells.

The herpes virus may emerge again as an active infection on or near the original site causing another cold sore. You may experience an itch or heightened sensitivity at the site preceding each attack. Recurrences are generally milder than the initial infection and may be triggered by menstruation, sun exposure, stress or any illness accompanied by a fever.

Diagnosis

Your doctor can diagnose cold sores by physical examination. A culture or smear of material from your sore can confirm the presence of herpes simplex virus but is rarely necessary.

How serious are cold sores?

Cold sores rarely cause problems, but the infection can cause some potentially serious complications.

If you have a cold sore, avoid contact with infants, anyone who has eczema (atopic dermatitis) and individuals with a suppressed immune system, such as people with cancer or AIDS or those who have received an organ transplant. The herpes virus can be life-threatening for these individuals.

Treatment

For most adults and especially children, cold sores generally clear up without treatment in seven to 10 days. In the meantime, the following may provide relief:

- Apply rubbing alcohol or diluted white vinegar to help dry up the sore.
- Try over-the-counter anesthetics containing benzocaine (Anbesol, Orajel). They provide comfort, but they don't speed healing.
- Apply ice to the blisters to ease the pain.
- Take a pain reliever if the sore is still painful after it has dried up and anesthetics and ice aren't helpful.
- Avoid squeezing, pinching or picking at any blister.

If you experience frequent or severe cold sores, your doctor may prescribe an antiviral medication. Commonly used antivirals include acyclovir (Zovirax), available in both pill and ointment forms, the oral drugs famciclovir and valacyclovir (Valtrex), and the ointment penciclovir (Denavir). Medication may shorten the duration of cold sores, but it won't prevent recurrences.

Shingles

Signs and symptoms

- Pain, burning, tingling or itching in a localized area
- A red rash characterized by small, fluid-filled blisters
- Fever
- Headache

The same virus that causes chickenpox (varicella) causes shingles (herpes zoster). After you've had chickenpox, the virus may remain dormant within your nerve cells. It can re-emerge years later as shingles, a localized infection.

Symptoms generally occur in a sequence as the virus reactivates. The initial sensation is pain, burning, tingling or itching as the virus proliferates along a peripheral nerve that spreads outward from your spinal cord. Shingles affects only the area of your body served by that nerve. A rash of small, fluid-filled blisters appears two or three days later, after the virus reaches the nerve endings in your skin (see the illustration on page 398).

Over the next three to five days, the rash reaches its maximum extent. It may appear as a rectangular strip or belt (*zoster* is Latin for "belt") on one side of your body running from your spine to your breastbone. Or it may appear over an extremity, such as an arm, or on one side of your face or head. The blisters dry up in a few days, forming crusts that fall off two or three weeks after your initial symptoms.

Shingles is more common in adults than in children. About 1 in 5 adults experiences shingles, usually after age 50. You can develop shingles more than once, although that's uncommon.

Because your immune system protects you from a new invasion by the virus that causes chickenpox, you can't get shingles from someone else if you've already had chickenpox. However, shingles is contagious for anyone who hasn't had chickenpox and can be debilitating for those with a weakened immune system.

If you have blisters, avoid physical contact with the following individuals. Once your blisters scab over, there's less chance of you spreading the infection to another person.

- Anyone who has never had chickenpox
- Pregnant women, because the infection is dangerous to fetuses
- Newborns, because their immune systems are still forming
- People who are immune compromised, such as those with cancer or AIDS or those who have had an organ transplant

Diagnosis

A diagnosis of shingles is generally made based on your symptoms and the characteristic appearance of the rash.

How serious is shingles?

Shingles normally isn't a serious condition and usually resolves in two or three weeks. However, some people may have continuing pain for months or even years along the involved nerve. This painful condition is called postherpetic neuralgia. It occurs more often in people who've had shingles after age 70. Most often, postherpetic neuralgia clears up in less than a year, even in people older than age 70.

Shingles damages nerve fibers. The ability of your nerves to send messages from your skin becomes confused and exaggerated. People with postherpetic neuralgia often say they have multiple types of pain, sometimes at the same time.

When shingles affects a major facial nerve, such as the trigeminal nerve, the rash can occur on your face, inside of your mouth, or in or near an eye. Any pain or rash in or near your eye requires prompt medical attention by an ophthalmologist. An eye infection can lead to permanent vision damage.

Treatment

Early treatment of shingles is important. Prompt intervention can shorten the duration of infection and possibly decrease your risk of persistent pain due to neuralgia.

See your doctor as soon as symptoms occur, especially if you're older than age 60. Be sure to see an ophthalmologist if the pain or rash occurs near your eyes or on your nose because the cornea could become involved. You'll need special treatment to avoid visual complications.

Medication

Your doctor will probably take a three-pronged treatment approach:
- High doses of an antiviral drug to reduce the duration and severity of symptoms.
- An anti-inflammatory drug to ease inflammation.
- Pain relievers to control pain.

Self-care

Your doctor may also recommend that you take these self-care steps:

- Wash the blisters twice a day with regular soap and water, but don't bandage them.
- To help relieve the pain, apply cool, wet compresses of water or water mixed with white vinegar — 1 ounce vinegar to 32 ounces water — to the blisters. Do this one to three times a day.
- Soak in a tub of lukewarm water, with or without an oat-bath additive (Aveeno).
- Apply a soothing calamine-type lotion.

Prevention

The varicella-zoster vaccine can help prevent shingles in adults who've had chickenpox. Like the chickenpox vaccine, the shingles vaccine doesn't guarantee that you won't get shingles. But it should lessen the course and severity of the disease and reduce your risk of postherpetic neuralgia.

There are two vaccines — Zostavax and Shingrix, a new vaccine awaiting official CDC approval at the time this book went to press. Shingrix, which is more effective, is recommended for all adults age 50 and older. It's administered in two separate shots two months apart. People who received the Zostavax vaccine should also be vaccinated with Shingrix.

Molluscum contagiosum

Signs and symptoms
- Tiny, pearl-like papules on the skin with a core of white, cheesy matter

Molluscum contagiosum is a relatively common viral infection of the skin. Each small, globular papule characteristically has a small indentation or dot on its summit (see the illustration on page 396).

In children, nodules usually appear on the face, trunk or limbs. In adults, common sites for the nodules are the genitals, abdomen and inner thighs. The infection is contagious by contact.

In adults, it's often spread through sexual contact. Adults

with reduced immunity sometimes experience multiple molluscum lesions on the face.

The firm nodules are often painless and disappear within a year. If the nodules and surrounding skin are injured, local spreading can occur.

Treatment

Left untreated, more lesions may occur as the virus sheds from lesions to normal skin. Your doctor can remove the nodules by freezing them, surgical scraping or squeezing out the core matter.

Fungal infections

Signs and symptoms
- Itching, stinging or burning skin
- Cracking and peeling skin
- Extremely dry skin with small, white scales
- Itchy, red or grayish, scaly patches on the scalp
- Itchy, red, scaly, slightly raised rings
- Moist, well-marked, reddened patches rimmed with small, red bumps
- Reddened areas with white patches inside

Fungal skin infections are caused by microscopic fungal organisms that become parasites on your skin. Your body hosts a great variety of microorganisms including mold-like and yeast-like fungi. Some serve useful purposes and cause no problems. Others can proliferate as infectious colonies.

Athlete's foot, jock itch and ringworm

Mold-like fungi (dermatophytes) cause athlete's foot and jock itch, as well as ringworm of the skin or scalp. These fungi live on dead tissues of your hair, nails and the outer layer of your skin. Poor hygiene, continuously moist skin, and minor skin or nail injuries increase your susceptibility to infection by these fungi.

The primary signs and symptoms of jock itch and athlete's foot are itching and a rash. Jock itch affects the groin and anal areas. Athlete's foot can affect the soles of the feet, the palms, and between the toes and fingers.

Ringworm most often affects children. The characteristic rings may be irregular. They start on the scalp but can expand beyond it. The ring grows outward as the infection spreads, and the central area becomes less actively infected (see the illustration on page 398).

This type of infection is very contagious and can be passed from shared hats, combs, brushes and barber tools. It's also possible to be infected with ringworm from pets or domestic animals.

Candida albicans
A persistent, bright red rash in the diaper region may indicate a yeast infection caused by *Candida albicans,* which flourishes in a warm, moist environment. Other candida infections include oral thrush and rubbing or chafing infections, which can occur in the folds of skin of overweight people. Pregnancy, obesity, diabetes, cancer, AIDS, and use of certain medications, such as antibiotics and corticosteroids, can increase your susceptibility to a candida infection.

Tinea versicolor
Tinea versicolor is a type of yeast infection that appears as a tissue-thin coating of fungus on your skin (see the illustration on page 398). The only symptoms are patches of discolored skin that slowly grow. Tinea versicolor is common among teenagers and young adults.

Diagnosis
Your doctor may only need to examine your skin to make the diagnosis of a fungal skin infection. Other times, he or she may need to obtain material from the lesion for laboratory analysis.

How serious are fungal infections?
Fungal infections are rarely life-threatening. They can range from mild to severe and often persist or recur. Treatment is generally successful, but in some cases it may include long-term medication use and continued measures to prevent recurrence.

Rarely, a skin infection by candida yeast can spread through your bloodstream to internal organs.

Treatment
The appropriate treatment depends on the type of fungal infection.

Athlete's foot, jock itch and ringworm
For these conditions, apply an over-the-counter antifungal ointment, lotion, powder or spray. Most infections respond well to these topical agents.

Your doctor may prescribe an oral antifungal medication if the infection is persistent (chronic) or severe. Side effects from oral antifungal medications can be severe and include gastrointestinal upset, rash and liver failure. They may also interfere with the effects of certain medications, including warfarin (Coumadin, Jantoven).

The Food and Drug Administration issued a public health advisory regarding two antifungal medications, itraconazole (Sporanox) and terbinafine (Lamisil), because of concerns they may

---

PREVENTION TIP

Preventing jock itch and athlete's foot requires good personal hygiene. Follow these suggestions:

Jock itch
- Keep the affected area clean and dry.
- Avoid clothes that chafe.
- If you use athletic supporters, launder them frequently.
- Shower and change clothes after exercise.

Athlete's foot
- Keep your feet dry, especially between the toes.
- Wear socks made of natural material, such as cotton or wool.
- Change socks and stockings regularly — twice a day if your feet sweat a lot.
- Wear light, well-ventilated shoes made of natural, not synthetic, materials.
- Alternate the pairs of shoes that you wear so that they can dry between wearings.
- Wear waterproof sandals or shower shoes in communal showers, pools, fitness centers and other public areas.
- Use an antifungal foot powder or spray daily.
- Don't borrow shoes.

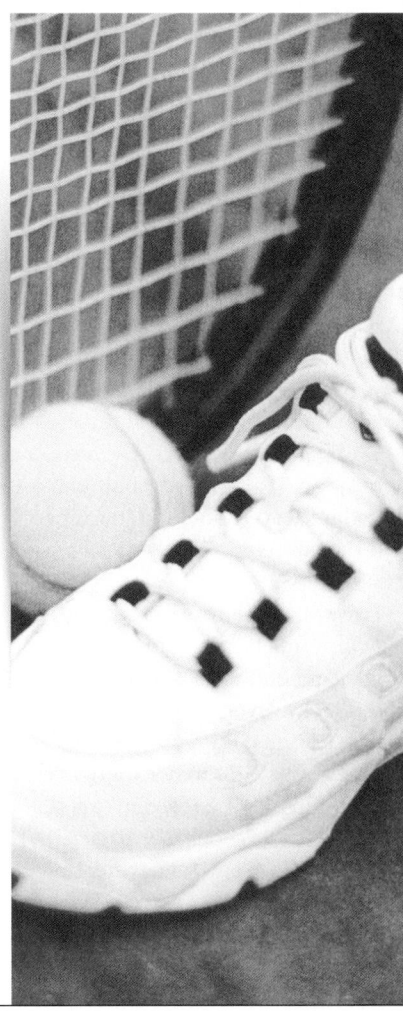

cause congestive heart failure. This medication-induced effect stopped when use of the drug was discontinued. The warning doesn't apply to cream and solution forms of Lamisil, which are applied topically.

Candida infections
Diaper rash and chafing can be treated using an antifungal cream and by keeping the affected area clean and dry. Frequent diaper changes will help promote dryness. For other candida infections that are severe or persistent, your doctor may prescribe an oral antifungal medication. It's important that your doctor supervise this treatment because long-term use of this type of drug can have serious side effects.

Tinea versicolor
For tinea versicolor, frequent showering can help. In addition, apply topical agents such as selenium sulfide (Selsun) or antifungal creams such as ciclopirox (Loprox).

Insect bites

Signs and symptoms
- Itchy, red bumps
- A red, painful, ulcerating sore
- Local numbness or a pins-and-needles sensation

Emergency signs and symptoms
- A swollen face
- Widespread numbness
- Muscle cramping
- Difficulty breathing
- Headache
- Nausea
- Fever
- Coma

The injection of venom or other agents into your skin causes the symptoms from insect bites. Most often the reaction is local and temporary, but the venom can affect your entire body if you're hypersensitive to the venom or if it's exceptionally potent.

The bite of a black widow spider feels like a pinprick. Some people aren't aware they've been bitten. At first, they may experience only slight swelling and faint red marks in the area of the bite. Within a few hours, intense pain and stiffness begin. Other signs and symptoms may include chills, fever, nausea and severe abdominal pain. Generally, the pain lessens after a few hours but may return over the next two to three days.

Bites by the brown recluse and other spiders cause a mild stinging followed by local redness and intense pain within eight hours. A fluid-filled bump forms at the site and then sloughs off, sometimes leaving a large, deep, growing ulcer. Signs and symptoms can vary from a mild fever and rash to nausea and listlessness.

Most ant bites cause only local redness and swelling. Fire ants, however, can produce many small, fluid-filled bumps that ulcerate like spider bites. Other biting insects inject chemicals as they feed on you. These insects include mosquitoes, fleas, flies, bedbugs and chiggers.

Stings by bees, wasps and hornets inject venom that causes immediate pain and rapidly enlarging red bumps. A few hours after a sting, the pain generally subsides, and the affected area turns itchy.

Diagnosis
Sometimes you can recognize an insect bite or sting easily because you feel the sting when it happens. At other times, bites just seem to appear. If you have a severe reaction, knowing what bit you will help your doctor determine the treatment.

How serious are insect bites?
Symptoms from a typical bite or sting generally last a few hours or days. However, if you're allergic to bee stings or if you receive multiple stings, you may experience a life-threatening reaction called anaphylactic shock (see page 47). This requires emergency treatment.

Bee stings cause more deaths than do snakebites. Poisonous spider bites are rarely fatal. However, small children and older adults are especially vulnerable to the effects of spider bites.

Treatment
Mild insect bites may be treated by applying ice cubes to the affected area to decrease pain. In addition, applying over-the-counter hydrocortisone cream or calamine-type lotion may help relieve itching or inflammation. For a more severe reaction, your doctor may prescribe a corticosteroid cream.

An individual who's allergic to the venom of a particular insect, such as a bee or hornet, may require an immediate injection of adrenaline (epinephrine) if stung. A doctor can prescribe an emergency medical kit to keep handy that includes emergency medication. If faintness, listlessness or shortness of breath occurs, seek emergency medical care immediately.

If you're bitten by a black widow spider, you may need to be hospitalized. Treatment may include hot soaks, injections of antivenom and intravenous infusion of calcium gluconate to relieve cramps.

Treatment for a brown recluse spider bite often involves corticosteroid injections and surgical removal of the ulcer.

Portuguese man-of-war stings

Signs and symptoms
- Stinging and pain
- Red, hive-like lesions in a line
- Shortness of breath
- Nausea and stomach cramps
- Emotional upset

The Portuguese man-of-war is a jellylike marine animal that has no backbone (invertebrate). It's easy to recognize on account of the highly characteristic blue or red bell-shaped body that floats at the surface of the water and ranges from less than an inch to more than a foot in diameter.

A cluster of tentacles hangs beneath the body of the man-of-war. Most are short and frilly, but one or more can be many feet long.

These long fishing tentacles are responsible for the stings.

If you touch one of these tentacles, it will whip around the contact area and inject a toxic venom into your skin. Because the venom (a neurotoxin) remains potent long after the man-of-war is dead, wading in shallow water or walking along the beach can be hazardous. The tentacles discharge their venom for long periods, even after they're separated from the main body of the man-of-war. The venom is carried into a person by tiny barbs on the tentacles.

Diagnosis

Common symptoms range from mild prickling to severe burning and numbness. A red line develops on the area of the skin exposed to the tentacles. Sometimes a line of welts or blisters develops.

How serious are Portuguese man-of-war stings?

Death from Portuguese man-of-war stings is unusual, but the stings can be painful. Severe stings can lead to muscle cramping, fainting, coughing, vomiting and difficulty breathing. In rare cases, a potentially fatal reaction called anaphylactic shock (see page 47) may occur.

Treatment

Here are some tips for coping with Portuguese man-of-war stings:

- **Get out of the water.** The pain and cramps can be disabling and cause you to drown.
- **Deactivate the stinging.** Sprinkle the affected area with vinegar, salt, sugar or even dry sand. This often offers quick relief.
- **Cleanse the wound.** Approximately 15 minutes after deactivating the wound, gently wash the area with seawater. Don't use fresh water and don't rub the skin because either action could trigger discharge of more venom.
- **Remove the stinging tentacles.** Apply a paste made of seawater

and sand, baking soda, talcum powder or flour. Scrape the residue with a knife or other suitable object, such as a clamshell. It's best to wear gloves or use a towel while removing the residue.

- **Apply medication.** Use a nonprescription hydrocortisone cream to relieve redness and swelling. A local anesthetic ointment, such as those containing benzocaine, can help relieve pain, and a calamine-type lotion reduces itching.

If you have a significant reaction to a sting, see a doctor.

Prevention

Extra clothing, particularly a wet suit or body stocking, is your best protection from Portuguese man-of-wars if you're swimming in waters where they live. In addition, wear sneakers or beach shoes while walking along the beach. And watch where you step.

Noncancerous Skin Tumors

Noncancerous (benign) skin tumors are common and usually harmless. As you grow older, you're likely to have a number of them. With the exception of actinic keratoses and certain moles, benign tumors don't require removal unless they're irritating or cosmetically displeasing. As a precaution, however, consult your doctor about any new growth or changes in old growths.

Actinic keratoses

Signs and symptoms

- Gritty, scaly, pale gray to dark pink patches on the face, scalp and back of hands

Actinic keratoses (solar keratoses) occur mostly in fair-skinned people with sun-damaged skin. Initially, the keratoses are flat and scaly. Later, they have a hard, wart-

like surface (see the illustration on page 393). Their sandpaper-like surface is more easily felt than seen. Actinic keratoses are considered noncancerous (benign) tumors, but they may represent precancerous changes in your skin.

Treatment

Medical attention is needed for an actinic keratosis because left untreated it may develop into squamous cell skin cancer. Your doctor can remove it by freezing it with liquid nitrogen, using topical medication, scraping off the damaged cells, or using photodynamic or laser therapy. A sample of the tissue may be examined for signs of cancer.

Cherry angiomas

Signs and symptoms

- A small, smooth, cherry red spot on the skin

Cherry angiomas are noncancerous (benign) skin tumors of unknown origin that appear most frequently after age 40. They can occur almost anywhere on your skin but most commonly are found on the torso. Cherry angiomas range from pinhead size to $1/4$ inch across (see the illustration on page 393). Large angiomas can bleed profusely when they're injured.

Treatment

A cherry angioma is painless and harmless, but you may want it removed for cosmetic reasons. Your doctor can remove it easily by freezing the angioma with liquid nitrogen, using laser treatment or destroying it by a minor electrosurgical procedure.

Keloids

Signs and symptoms

- Light-colored nodular or ridged growths over scars on the skin

A keloid is an overproduction of scar tissue. It's sometimes called hypertrophic scarring.

A keloid occurs at the site of a skin injury resulting from, for example, an operation, a vaccination, severe acne, a burn or even a minor scratch. It's fairly common on black skin and much less common on white skin.

A keloid is harmless, but it may be tender, itchy or disfiguring. Some keloids stop growing or even disappear without treatment.

Treatment

Surgical removal of a keloid often causes further scarring unless it's followed by X-ray treatment or injection of steroids at the site. Small keloids may be removed by freezing them with liquid nitrogen.

Liver spots (age spots)

Signs and symptoms

• Flat spots of increased pigmentation — usually brown, black or gray — on your face or the backs of your hands

Liver spots (senile lentigines) are harmless flat patches of increased pigmentation that range from freckle-sized to a few inches across. These flat, gray, brown or black spots affect more than 90 percent of fair-skinned people age 50 and older.

Liver spots are most common on areas most exposed to the sun — your face and the backs of your hands (see the illustration on page 393). They tend to darken with sun exposure. Despite the name, they're unrelated to the liver.

How serious are liver spots?

True liver spots hardly ever become cancerous, although they can look like some cancerous growths. In rare circumstances they may turn into lentigo maligna, a slow-growing, nonaggressive form of skin cancer.

Treatment

For cosmetic reasons, liver spots can be lightened with skin-bleaching products or removed by freezing or laser therapy. You can help

prevent new spots by avoiding the sun and using sunscreen.

Moles

Signs and symptoms

• Flesh-colored, brown, blue or black spots on the skin

Nearly everyone has moles. These noncancerous (benign) tumors are nests of pigment cells. They may be smooth, contain hairs, and become raised or wrinkled (see the illustrations on page 394). New moles may appear up until age 40, but most appear by age 20. Some moles disappear with advancing age.

Moles are usually harmless, but they can become cancerous (see page 1105). Consult your doctor if a mole changes in color or size or if it develops itching, pain, bleeding or inflammation. Certain moles — such as those that are

irregular in shape and are located around or under your nails or near your genitals — should be monitored by a doctor for evidence of melanoma. Some moles have a higher than average risk of becoming cancerous. They include:

• **Large moles present at birth.** Large moles present at birth are called congenital nevi and may increase your risk of malignant melanoma, a form of skin cancer. Moles that are more than 8 inches in diameter pose the greatest risk. Any mole that has been present since birth and is the size of a credit card or larger should be examined by a doctor.

• **Moles that run in families.** Moles that are larger than average — about the diameter of a pencil eraser — and irregular in shape are known as atypical or dysplastic nevi. These moles tend to be hereditary

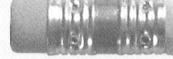

Monitor That Mole

Moles have no known purpose, and no one knows why they develop. Most moles are harmless, but you do need to monitor them for changes that may signal melanoma, a serious form of skin cancer.

The best way to catch potential problems at an early stage is to become familiar with the location and pattern of your moles. Remember to check areas that aren't exposed to sunlight, including your scalp, armpits, feet (between the toes) and genital area.

Examine your skin carefully on a regular basis. If necessary, use a hand-held mirror along with a wall mirror to scan hard-to-see places like your back. If your moles are larger than average — about the diameter of a pencil eraser — and irregular in shape, you're at greater risk of developing malignant melanoma and may want to consider having a dermatologist check your moles on a regular basis.

When checking your moles to determine if they may be cancerous, follow the ABCDE guide from the American Academy of Dermatology (see page 1105). Watch for irregular borders, changes in color and an increasing diameter. Other factors to watch for include:

• *Texture.* Scales, shedding of skin, oozing or mild bleeding can signal melanoma. So can hardening or softening of the colored area.

• *Sensation.* Is there itching, tenderness or pain?

• *Nearby skin.* Pay attention to swelling, redness or other coloring that spreads into skin near the pigmented area.

and usually have dark brown centers and lighter, uneven borders. Overall, they may look red or tan. If you have dysplastic nevi, you have a greater risk of developing malignant melanoma.

- **Numerous moles.** If you have many moles larger than 6 millimeters across — about the diameter of a pencil eraser — you may be at greater risk of developing melanoma.

Other important factors that increase your risk of melanoma include family history, a history of severe sunburns, and a fair complexion with reddish hair and blue eyes. Not all melanomas arise from pre-existing nevi.

Diagnosis

If your doctor suspects that a mole may be cancerous, he or she may take a sample of the tissue to be examined under a microscope.

Treatment

If your doctor finds that your mole is cancerous, the entire mole and a margin around it will be removed. Usually, a mole that has been removed won't reappear. If it does, see your doctor promptly.

Most moles don't require treatment, but if you want one removed for cosmetic reasons, it can be done in several ways. Your doctor may use a method known as shave excision in which the area around the mole is numbed and the mole is removed close to the skin. Moles may also be removed with a small incision or punch biopsy technique. The procedure is usually performed in a doctor's or dermatologist's office and takes only a short time.

Seborrheic keratoses

Signs and symptoms

- Brown, black or pale growths on the face, chest, shoulders and back that look waxy, as if they were dripped on the skin by a candle

Seborrheic keratoses are noncancerous (benign) skin tumors of unknown origin that commonly appear after age 40. The oval growths have a waxy, wartlike, scaly, slightly elevated surface and range from $1/3$ to 1 inch or more across (see the illustration on page 393). Their color varies from pale yellow to dark brown or black, and they have a pasted-on appearance. Occasionally, they appear singly but most often are multiple.

Treatment

A seborrheic keratosis is normally painless and requires no treatment unless it itches, irritates or detracts from your appearance. This type of growth is never deeply rooted, so removal is simple and nonscarring. Your doctor can remove it with a simple surgical procedure or freeze it off with liquid nitrogen. Sometimes it recurs.

Skin tags

Signs and symptoms

- Small tags of skin on your neck, armpits, upper trunk and body folds

Skin tags (acrochordons) are tiny, noncancerous (benign) tumors of unknown origin that protrude from your skin on a narrow stalk (see the illustration on page 394). They're soft and normally skin-colored but may appear darker. Skin tags are common, especially after middle life. They're usually painless but can become irritated by friction with clothing.

Treatment

Treatment of a skin tag is unnecessary unless it's bothersome. Your doctor can remove it by freezing it with liquid nitrogen, cutting it off or burning it off with electricity.

Warts

Signs and symptoms

- Small, fleshy, grainy bumps that may be skin-colored, white, pink or tan

Warts are skin growths caused by the human papillomavirus (HPV), which stimulates the rapid growth of cells on the outer layer of your skin. More than 50 types of warts occur and can affect any part of your body, most often the hands and feet. Warts may disappear in a few weeks, or they may last a long time.

Types

The two kinds of warts most often seen by doctors are common warts and plantar warts.

Common warts
Common warts appear as skin growths near the fingernails but can also appear on any part of the hand (see the illustration on page 394). Young adults and children are affected most often. Common warts are typically painless.

Plantar warts
Plantar warts appear on the feet and may appear to have tiny black dots in them. The dots are small, clotted blood vessels. Plantar warts can be painful because they press inward when you stand on them.

Causes

You can acquire warts through direct contact with an infected person or surface, such as a shower floor. Warts usually spread through breaks in your skin.

Each person's immune system responds differently, meaning that not everyone who comes in contact with HPV will develop warts. Generally, the incubation period — the time from when you're initially infected until warts appear — is about three months, but the virus can lie dormant for years. Because warts are more common in children, some experts believe that adults may develop an immunity to HPV.

How serious are warts?

Common warts and plantar warts aren't usually a serious health concern, and many disappear on their own within two years. But they may be bothersome, requiring medical treatment to remove them. Warts may also recur after treatment and become a persistent problem.

Warts that don't occur in your genital areas are neither a sign of cancer nor a precursor to it. Because warts shed HPV, new warts can appear nearby. There's also a potential to infect others, such as family members who might share bathing facilities.

Warts that occur on the sexual organs are called genital warts and are considered a sexually transmitted infection. They can be a serious health concern because they may increase the risk of cervical cancer in women. Virtually all cases of cervical cancer are caused by HPV. In addition, pregnant women infected with HPV can pass on the virus to their babies during childbirth.

Treatment

For warts that aren't located on your genitals, home treatment may be possible. Don't try to treat genital warts with over-the-counter medications, which are not intended for use in the moist tissues of the genital areas. Doing so can cause pain and soreness in the treated areas. See your doctor if warts occur on your genitals.

Over-the-counter wart medications are available at drugstores and discount and grocery stores. Unless you have an impaired immune system, there's generally no reason you shouldn't try a self-care approach. Look for products containing salicylic acid, which peels off the infected skin. These products require twice-daily use, often for a few weeks.

One caution about over-the-counter products is that the acid in them can irritate or damage normal skin. It's common to use a 17 percent acid solution on your hands and a 40 percent acid solution on your feet. If you're pregnant, talk

with your doctor before using an acid solution.

See your doctor if, despite home treatment, the warts persist or spread. Warts, especially plantar warts, can be difficult to eradicate completely. New ones may appear after treatment. More than one treatment or more than one treatment approach may be needed to achieve success. Your doctor may suggest one or more of the following approaches:

Freezing
Your doctor may destroy a wart by freezing it with liquid nitrogen. The dead tissue later sloughs off. This method may be effective, but you may need repeated treatments.

Minor surgery
The surgical method involves cutting away the wart or destroying it by using an electric needle in a process called electrodesiccation and curettage.

Laser surgery
One type of laser emits a narrow beam of intense light that cuts away or vaporizes growths. Another type of laser emits a beam that vaporizes the blood vessels supplying the wart so that the wart dies.

Injection
Your doctor may inject medications such as interferon alfa or bleomycin into the wart to kill the HPV virus.

Skin Cancer

Skin cancer — the abnormal growth of skin cells — is by far the most common form of cancer. Current estimates are that 1 in 5 Americans will develop skin cancer in his or her lifetime.

Basal cell cancer and squamous cell cancer are the two most common forms of skin cancer. Both are superficial, slow growing

and highly treatable, especially if found early. Melanoma is a more serious form of skin cancer. It can affect deeper layers of the skin and has the greatest potential to spread to other tissues in the body.

Skin cancer is on the rise. Fair-skinned people who live in areas with a lot of sunlight are at greatest risk. But anyone can develop skin cancer, which is most commonly caused by overexposure to ultraviolet (UV) radiation. The good news is that the vast majority of skin cancers are preventable. If caught early, most are also highly curable.

It's important to protect your skin from UV radiation and to check your skin regularly for signs of cancer. Left undetected or untreated, skin cancer can be damaging and even deadly. Skin cancer claims approximately 10,000 lives a year in the United States.

Risk factors

Generally, your risk of developing skin cancer increases with age. But skin cancer isn't limited to middle-aged and older people. People in their 20s and 30s can develop skin cancer. Half of all melanomas occur in people under age 50.

Although overexposure to UV radiation is the most common cause of skin cancer, several factors may increase your risk of developing skin cancer:

Fair skin
Having less pigment (melanin) in your skin provides less protection from damaging UV radiation from the sun or tanning beds. If you have blond or red hair, light-colored eyes and you freckle or sunburn easily, you're 20 to 30 times more likely to develop skin cancer in your lifetime than is a person who doesn't have these traits.

Sunny or high-altitude climates
People who live in sunny, warm climates are exposed to more

sunlight than are people who live in colder climates. In the United States, for example, skin cancer is much more prevalent in Arizona than it is in Minnesota.

In addition, people who live at higher elevations are exposed to more UV radiation than are people who live at lower elevations.

Excessive sun exposure
Individuals who spend considerable time in the sun, including those who tan, may develop skin cancer. This is especially true if the skin is unprotected by sunscreen or clothing.

A history of sunburns
Sunburn is the result of over-exposure to the sun's UV radiation. Every time you sunburn your skin, you increase your risk of developing skin cancer. People who've had one or more severe, blistering sunburns as a child or teenager are at increased risk of skin cancer as an adult. Sunburns in adulthood also are a risk factor.

Genetics
Chronic sun exposure doesn't explain melanomas or other skin cancers that develop on skin not exposed to sunlight, such as the soles of the feet. But genetics seem to play a role. If your parent or a brother or sister has had skin cancer, you may be at higher risk of the disease.

Personal history of skin cancer
If you develop skin cancer once, you're at risk of getting it again.

Moles
People who have multiple moles called dysplastic nevi are at increased risk of skin cancer (see page 1102).

Precancerous skin lesions
Many doctors consider skin lesions known as actinic keratoses to be precancerous conditions because they can develop into skin cancer (see page 1101).

A weakened immune system
People with impaired immune systems are at greater risk of

The ABCDEs of Melanoma

Melanoma is often curable if you find it early. Follow this self-examination guide, adapted from the American Academy of Dermatology's ABCDE guide, to determine if an unusual mole or suspicious spot on your skin may be melanoma.

A is for asymmetry
Symmetrical round or oval growths are usually non-cancerous (benign). Look for irregular shapes where one half is a different shape from the other half.

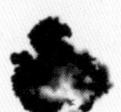

B is for border
Growths with irregular, notched, scalloped or vaguely defined borders need to be checked out.

C is for color
Look for growths that have many colors or an uneven distribution of color. Often, growths that are the same color all over are benign.

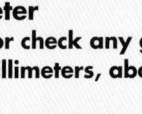

D is for diameter
Have your doctor check any growths that are larger than 6 millimeters, about the diameter of a pencil eraser.

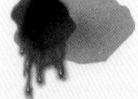

E is for evolving
Look for changes over time, such as a mole that grows in size or that changes color or shape. Moles may also evolve to develop new signs and symptoms, such as new itchiness or bleeding.

Laser Surgery

Laser beams are strong enough to cut through diamonds, yet they can be gentle enough to sculpt your skin. In the medical world, these scalpels of light are helpful in many procedures. But as high-tech as these devices are, they can't zap away every problem. They may be the right tool for some procedures but not the best choice for others.

In addition, as with any operation, the success of laser surgery depends largely on the surgeon's skill and on whether the procedure is appropriate for you.

Intense light

The word *laser* stands for light amplification by stimulated emission of radiation. Laser beams are strong beams of light produced by electrically stimulating a particular material. A solid, liquid or gas is used. Generally, lasers are named for the substances that produce them and vary from carbon dioxide and argon to ruby.

The combination of light intensity and the ability to focus it on a small area gives lasers their unique role in medicine. Lasers can be used to:
- Cut or destroy tissue that's abnormal or diseased
- Shrink or destroy tumors or lesions
- Burn off or vaporize tissue
- Seal blood or lymph vessels
- Close nerve endings to reduce pain

Different types of lasers do different things. Some lasers cut tissue. Some heat up tissue. Others vaporize tissue. Some lasers target a specific skin component, such as blood vessels or hair.

Distinct advantages

Lasers haven't replaced scalpels, but they do help doctors perform some procedures more effectively than with traditional methods. Lasers cause minimal bleeding, providing surgeons a clear view of the area of surgery. Because of their precision, lasers allow doctors to work on small and hard-to-reach parts of the body. Doctors can also vary how deeply the laser penetrates tissue by adjusting the light's intensity.

In addition, laser surgery may pose less risk of infection and scarring. In some cases, laser surgery is faster than traditional surgery, shortening recovery time. Some laser surgeries are performed under a local anesthetic in a doctor's office. Others require general anesthesia and hospitalization.

Versatile tool

Laser therapy is used in many dermatological procedures. It can remove, lighten or improve:
- Birthmarks such as port-wine stains

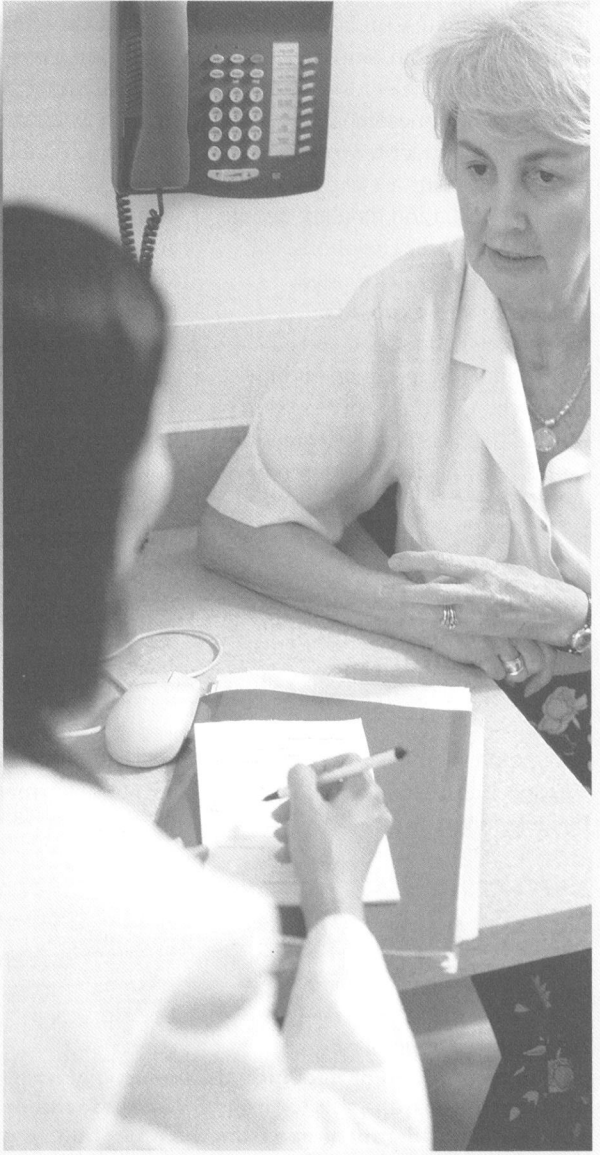

- Fine wrinkles
- Pigmentation disorders, such as freckles or liver spots
- Tattoos
- Acne
- Spider veins
- Noncancerous (benign) skin growths
- Some skin cancers
- Unwanted hair
- Cellulite

Precautions

Despite what advertisements might suggest, lasers aren't magical, fix-all tools. Risks associated with using a laser are similar to those of using a more conventional procedure. They include pain, infection and, rarely, scarring. Imprecisely aimed lasers can burn or destroy healthy tissue. Although lasers can remove marks on skin, they can also change skin pigmentation and, therefore, coloring.

many diseases, including skin cancer. This may include individuals who've undergone an organ transplant, people receiving cancer treatment, or individuals with human immunodeficiency virus (HIV) or AIDS.

Fragile skin

Skin that has been burned or injured from disease is more susceptible to sun damage and skin cancer. Certain psoriasis treatments also can increase the risk of skin cancer.

Exposure to environmental hazards

Exposure to environmental chemicals, including some herbicides, may increase the risk of skin cancer.

Detection and diagnosis

A skin change is the most common warning sign of skin cancer. You may notice the appearance of a small growth or a sore that bleeds, crusts over, heals and then reopens. The first sign of melanoma may be a change in an existing mole or the development of a new, suspicious-looking mole.

Skin cancer develops mainly on areas of skin that are exposed to a lot of sun — the scalp, face, lips, ears, neck, chest, arms and hands. But skin cancer can also develop on unexposed areas, such as the palms, the spaces between toes and the genital area. A cancerous skin lesion can appear suddenly, or it can develop slowly.

Check your skin regularly and report changes to your doctor. Examine your skin at least every three months for the development of new skin growths or changes in existing moles, freckles, bumps and birthmarks. With the help of mirrors, check your face, neck, ears and scalp. Examine your chest and trunk and the tops and undersides of your arms and hands. Examine the front and back of your legs, your feet, including the soles and between your toes, your

genital area, and between your buttocks.

Although skin cancers don't all look the same, they all involve a change in the skin's appearance in a localized area. If you notice any change in your skin, consult your doctor right away. Don't wait for the area to start hurting because skin cancer seldom causes pain.

If your doctor suspects skin cancer after a visual inspection of your skin, he or she may want to take a small sample of your skin (biopsy) for analysis in a laboratory to confirm the diagnosis. A biopsy can usually be performed in a doctor's office after administering a local anesthetic.

Doctors generally divide skin cancer into two stages: local, affecting only the skin, or metastatic, spreading beyond the skin. Because superficial skin cancers such as basal cell cancer or squamous cell cancer rarely spread, a biopsy often is the only test needed to determine the cancer stage.

In cases where a growth is very large or has existed for a while, your doctor may check your lymph nodes in the area. You may also need additional tests, such as special X-rays, to determine whether the cancer has spread to other parts of the body. Knowing the stage of a skin cancer helps your doctor plan the best treatment.

Basal cell cancer

Signs and symptoms
- A pearly or waxy bump on the face, ear or neck
- A flat, flesh-colored or brown scar-like lesion on the chest or back

Basal cell cancer is a common form of skin cancer. When basal cells in your epidermis become cancerous, they form a pearl-like or waxy bump or a flat lesion. The lesion may ulcerate, slowly enlarge and never heal completely (see the illustration on page 394).

Basal cell skin cancers usually occur on unprotected areas of skin.

The primary cause of this type of skin cancer is repeated overexposure to ultraviolet radiation from the sun, or from tanning beds or sunlamps.

Basal cell cancer most commonly occurs after age 40. The cancer generally remains a local growth and only rarely spreads to other parts of the body. However, lack of medical attention can allow the growth to invade nearby tissues and underlying structures, including your nerves, bones or brain.

Treatment

In order to make a diagnosis of basal cell cancer, your doctor will need a sample of the lump or lesion to be examined in a laboratory (biopsied). Treatment depends on the cancer's size, depth and location and may include scraping and cauterization of the cancer, freezing (cryosurgery), radiation, surgical excision or a series of microscopically controlled shaved excisions, called the Mohs procedure (see page 1108).

Because many skin cancers are on the face, a surgeon may also perform a reconstructive procedure, such as a skin graft, if necessary.

With early treatment, basal cell cancer has a very high cure rate. You'll need to diligently practice good sun protection techniques to avoid further growths. Avoid the midday sun, wear protective clothing and use sunscreen on exposed skin. In addition, have regular medical examinations.

Squamous cell cancer

Signs and symptoms
- A firm, red nodule on the face, lip, ear, neck, hand or arm
- A flat lesion with a scaly, crusted surface on the face, ear, neck, hand or arm

Squamous cell cancer is a cancerous (malignant) tumor that arises from the midportion of the epidermal layer of the skin. It is more aggressive than basal cell cancer and can spread (metastasize)

Skin Cancer Treatments

The appropriate treatment for skin cancer depends on the size, type, depth and location of a lump or lesion. Most treatments use a local anesthetic and can be performed in an outpatient setting.

Standard therapies

Treatment for skin cancer includes:

Freezing
To prevent skin cancer, a doctor may destroy precancerous skin lesions that increase the risk of skin cancer, such as actinic keratoses, by freezing them with liquid nitrogen (cryosurgery). This procedure may also be used on some small, early skin cancers. The dead tissue later sloughs off. The treatment may leave a small, white scar. You may need a repeat treatment to remove the growth completely.

Laser therapy
Laser therapy involves a precise, intense beam of light that vaporizes growths, generally with little damage to surrounding tissue and with minimal bleeding, swelling and scarring. A doctor may use this therapy to treat superficial skin cancers or precancerous growths on the lips.

Excisional surgery
Excisional surgery may be appropriate for any type of skin cancer. A doctor cuts out (excises) the cancerous tissue and a margin of healthy skin around it. A wide excision — removing extra normal skin around the tumor — may be best for melanoma. To minimize or avoid scarring, especially on the face, skin reconstruction may be needed.

Mohs surgery
Mohs surgery is a technique used for larger, recurring or difficult-to-treat skin cancers, which may include both basal cell and squamous cell types. A doctor removes the skin growth layer by layer, examining each layer under the microscope, until no abnormal cells remain. Mohs surgery is the treatment of choice to remove skin cancer without taking an excessive amount of surrounding healthy skin.

Curettage and electrodesiccation
With this procedure, a doctor scrapes away layers of cancer cells using a circular blade (curet). An electric needle destroys any remaining cancer cells. This simple, quick procedure is common in treating small or thin basal cell cancers. It leaves a small, flat, white scar.

Radiation therapy
If surgery isn't an option, your doctor may recommend daily radiation treatments, usually for one to four weeks, to destroy basal cell and squamous cell skin cancers.

Chemotherapy
Chemotherapy uses drugs to destroy cancer cells. Chemotherapy can be given intravenously, in pill form or both so that it travels throughout your body.

Chemotherapy can also be given in a vein in your arm or leg in a procedure called isolated limb perfusion. During this procedure, blood in your arm or leg isn't allowed to travel to other areas of your body for a short time so that the chemotherapy drugs travel directly to the area around the melanoma and don't affect other parts of your body.

Biological therapy
Biological therapy boosts your immune system to help your body fight cancer. These treatments are made of substances produced by the body or similar substances produced in a laboratory. Side effects of these treatments are similar to those of the flu, including chills, fatigue, fever, headache and muscle aches.

Biological therapies used to treat melanoma include interferon and interleukin-2, ipilimumab (Yervoy), nivolumab (Opdivo), and pembrolizumab (Keytruda).

Targeted therapy
Targeted therapy uses medications designed to target specific vulnerabilities in cancer cells. Side effects of targeted therapies vary, but tend to include skin problems, fever, chills and dehydration.

Vemurafenib (Zelboraf), dabrafenib (Tafinlar) and trametinib (Mekinist) are targeted therapy drugs used to treat advanced melanoma. These drugs are only effective if your cancer cells have a certain genetic mutation. Cells from your melanoma can be tested to see whether these medications may help you.

to other locations, including lymph nodes or internal organs. However, spread to other parts of the body is unusual if the cancer is treated early.

The tumor initially is painless, although pain may develop if it ulcerates and never completely heals (see the illustration on page 394). It may begin in normal skin, in a burn or scar or at a site of chronic inflammation. Squamous cell cancer also may originate from precancerous skin tumors such as actinic keratoses (see page 1101).

Ultraviolet radiation is usually the main cause of this type of cancer, but genetic predisposition may be a contributing factor. Fair-skinned, blue-eyed, blond or red-haired people are the most vulnerable. The onset most commonly occurs after age 50.

Treatment
Treatment depends on the cancer's size, depth, location and evidence

of spread (metastasis). The tumor and the skin around it will likely be removed through surgery. In some cases, radiation may be necessary. Some individuals also need a skin graft to replace excised skin. For cancers that recur after surgical removal, the Mohs procedure may be necessary, followed by a reconstructive procedure.

With early treatment, the cure rate for squamous cell cancer is very high. Use of high-protection sunscreens and other sun protection techniques can help minimize further development of skin lesions. Be sure to follow up with regular medical examinations to detect possible recurrence.

Melanoma

Signs and symptoms
- A mole that changes in color, size or consistency
- A mole that bleeds or has new hair growth
- A small lesion with an irregular border
- Red, white, blue or blue-black spots on your trunk or limbs
- Shiny, firm, dome-shaped bumps anywhere on the skin
- Dark lesions on the palms, soles of the feet, tips of the fingers and toe, or mucous membranes
- A large brownish spot with darker speckles

Melanoma is the most deadly skin cancer. It's less common than basal and squamous cell cancers, but incidence is on the rise, with the number of new cases of melanoma doubling in the past 20 years. An estimated 162,000 Americans are diagnosed with melanoma annually. Young men who are diagnosed with this disease have a higher mortality rate than do young women with the disease.

Melanoma typically arises painlessly from cells that produce the skin's pigment (melanin). Approximately 70 percent of melanomas appear on normal skin, and 30 percent arise from an existing mole that undergoes changes in color

or size or that becomes painful, itches, bleeds or swells (see the illustration on page 394).

The cancer first spreads to the surrounding skin and is highly curable at this phase. If not treated, the tumor begins to spread downward into other areas of the skin or to lymph nodes or internal organs.

Ultraviolet radiation is considered the chief cause of melanoma. Certain moles also tend to transform into melanoma. Other risk factors include your skin type, a history of sunburns, your health status and genetics.

Melanomas are divided into four types:
- **Superficial spreading melanoma.** Superficial spreading melanoma accounts for 70 percent of melanoma cases and strikes at any age. It appears as a small lesion with an irregular border. The color of the lesion may be red, white, blue or blue-black. It can occur anywhere on the body but most commonly appears on the trunk or limbs.
- **Nodular melanoma.** Nodular melanoma is the most aggressive type of melanoma. It appears as a shiny, firm, dome-shaped bump anywhere on the skin. It's usually black, but it can be blue, gray, white, brown, tan, red or the color of your skin. It may ulcerate and fail to heal completely. Nodular melanomas account for 10 to 15 percent of melanoma cases.
- **Acral-lentiginous melanoma.** Acral-lentiginous melanoma appears as dark lesions on the palms, soles, tips of fingers and toes, or the mucous membranes. It accounts for 10 percent of melanoma cases and is more common in non-Caucasians.
- **Lentigo maligna melanoma.** Lentigo maligna melanoma appears as a large, brownish spot with darker speckles on skin that has been overexposed to the sun, such as that on the face, ears, arms and upper trunk. It accounts for about 5 percent of

melanoma cases. It frequently afflicts older adults and is associated with senile skin (see page 1089). A noncancerous (benign) brownish spot may appear several years before turning cancerous.

Diagnosis
Your doctor may suspect a melanoma from visual inspection. To confirm the diagnosis, he or she will take a sample of skin tissue to be examined in a laboratory (biopsied). If your doctor thinks that the melanoma may spread to other locations, he or she may order further testing, including a chest X-ray and computerized tomography (CT) scan. A procedure to determine if the cancer has entered the lymph system may be performed.

How serious is melanoma?
The five-year survival rate for people whose melanoma is detected and treated before it spreads to the lymph nodes is 98 percent. Five-year survival rates for regional and distant stage melanomas are 62 percent and 18 percent, respectively.

Treatment
The usual treatment for melanoma is surgical removal of the tumor along with a wide margin of normal skin (see opposite page). Sometimes, nearby lymph nodes are removed. This may be followed by a skin graft at the site of the operation. If the cancer has spread to other organs, additional treatment may include chemotherapy or radiation therapy.

Long-term management of melanoma includes periodic medical examinations for evidence of recurring cancer.

Kaposi's sarcoma

Signs and symptoms
- Red to purple nodules anywhere on the skin or mucous membranes
- Dark blue or purple-brown

nodules on the toe or leg
- Swelling of the legs, groin or skin around the eyes

Kaposi's sarcoma is a cancer that starts in connective tissues, such as the dermis — the layer of skin just beneath the surface layer — cartilage, bone, fat, muscle, blood vessels or fibrous tissue. It typically appears as a nodule on the skin or the mucous membranes. Early lesions are red to purple and resemble a birthmark, and older lesions become brown to black and tend to be flatter.

The disease can cause blockage of lymph nodes or lymph vessels, leading to painful swelling (lymphedema) that usually affects the legs, groin or the skin around the eyes. Kaposi's sarcoma is sometimes associated with other cancers, including leukemia or lymphoma, as well as immune deficiency disorders, including human immunodeficiency virus (HIV) and AIDS.

The disease appears in two forms: aggressive and indolent. The aggressive form occurs both internally and externally. It's now occurring with greater frequency because of its association with HIV and AIDS. Before AIDS, Kaposi's sarcoma was a rare disease that appeared primarily in older Italian and Jewish men.

The indolent form, which is generally marked by darker tumors, is caused by blood vessel involvement. It can spread to the hands and arms or produce funguslike growths or both. This cancer may penetrate underlying tissue and invade bone, lymph nodes and internal organs.

Treatment

Treatment for Kaposi's sarcoma may include local procedures such as freezing therapy (cryotherapy) or surgery, radiation, chemotherapy or therapies that affect the immune system. Elastic support hose may provide some relief by reducing swelling.

Hair

Your hair is composed of keratin, the same protein that makes up nails and the outer layer of your skin. The part of the hair that rises out of your skin is the hair shaft. An average head has about 100,000 of them. Below your skin is the hair root, enclosed by a sac-like structure called the hair follicle. Tiny blood vessels at the base of the follicle provide nourishment to your hair. Nearby oil-producing glands keep your hair shiny and somewhat waterproof.

Each hair shaft consists of three layers. The outermost layer (cuticle) is thin and colorless. The middle layer (cortex) is the thickest. It determines your hair color and whether your hair is straight or curly. Your hair color results from melanin from your pigment cells. Blond hair has few melanin granules in the cortex layer, and dark hair has many. The innermost layer (medulla) is nearly colorless and doesn't extend all the way to the tip of the hair shaft. Light reflected from the medulla creates sheen and the variations in color tone.

Like skin cells, hair grows and is shed regularly. Most people lose 50 to 100 hairs a day. This hair is usually replaced by new hair, which grows at a rate of approximately $\frac{1}{2}$ inch each month. When the rate of shedding exceeds the rate of regrowth, hair loss results. The new hair may be thinner than the hair shed, or it may not come back, leading to baldness.

Hair loss

Your hair loss may have started with a few extra hairs in the sink or in your comb. But now you can't look in the mirror without seeing more of your scalp.

Baldness typically refers to excessive hair loss from your scalp and can be the result of heredity, certain medications or an underlying medical condition. Anyone —

men, women and children — can experience hair loss.

Some people prefer to let their baldness run its course untreated and unhidden. Others may cover it up with hairstyles, makeup, hats or scarves. And still others choose one of the medications and surgical procedures that are available to treat hair loss. Before pursuing any of these treatment options, talk with your doctor about the cause of and best possible treatments for your hair loss.

The medical term for hair loss is alopecia. Pattern baldness (androgenetic alopecia), the most common type of alopecia, affects roughly one-third of men and women. It's typically permanent. Other types of alopecia are temporary, including alopecia areata. It can involve hair loss on your scalp or other parts of your body.

Permanent hair loss

Types include:
- **Male-pattern baldness (androgenetic alopecia).** For men, pattern baldness can begin very early, even in the teens or early 20s. It's typically characterized by a receding hairline at the temples and balding at the top of the head. The end result may be partial or complete baldness.
- **Female-pattern baldness (androgenetic alopecia).** Women with permanent hair loss usually have hair loss limited to thinning at the front, sides or crown. Women usually maintain their frontal hairline and rarely experience complete baldness.
- **Scarring (cicatricial) alopecia.** This rare condition occurs when inflammation damages and scars the hair follicle, causing permanent hair loss. Sometimes the patchy hair loss is associated with slight itching or pain.

Temporary hair loss

Types include:
- **Alopecia areata.** Hair loss usually occurs in small, round, smooth patches about the size

Caring for Your Hair

Healthy, lustrous hair is a sought-after symbol of beauty as evidenced by the millions of dollars spent on hair care products each year. Use the following tips to help keep your hair healthy:

Handle your hair gently
Wet hair is especially fragile because it might become stretched. When possible, allow your hair to air-dry. A natural-bristle brush is preferable to a synthetic one because the synthetic material may cut your hair. Brush your hair gently from your scalp to disperse scalp oil over your hair. If you prefer a comb, use a wide-toothed comb to avoid injury to your hair. If you must use a blow-dryer, use it on a low setting and leave your hair slightly damp.

Shampoo your hair as needed
The amount of washing that your hair needs depends on your hair type, the weather, your physical activities and perhaps even your occupation. Daily shampooing won't damage your hair if you do it gently.

Buy shampoos tailored to your hair type — oily, dry or normal. Protein shampoos don't penetrate your hair, but they do coat it, temporarily giving your hair more bulk. A protein shampoo acts as a shampoo and conditioner in one. Permanent-waved, straightened or dyed hair needs a low-pH shampoo. If your hair is longer or has a tendency to be dry, follow your shampoo with a cream rinse or conditioner. These products lubricate your hair between washings and help minimize damage from brushing or combing.

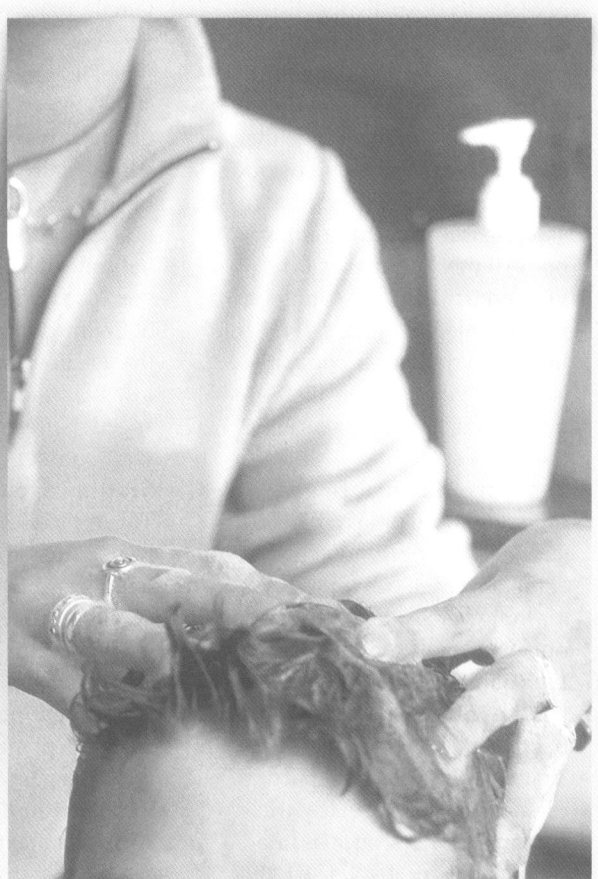

Choose a hair-healthy style
Certain hairstyles and treatments can cause breakage or root damage. Avoid excessively tight braiding, buns or ponytails and don't roll your hair too tightly in curlers. Curling is safest if you twist your hair into pin curls overnight. For safe curling of fine hair, wind slightly dampened hair around sponge rollers and let it air-dry. Use of excessively hot rollers or curling irons may damage even coarse hair. Use these devices cautiously. Teasing and back-combing should be done gently or not at all.

A styling gel or mousse can give your hair more body or thickness. These products don't necessarily damage your hair, but they might make it extra dry, especially at the ends. Permanent waving (a perm) is safe for healthy hair, but you may find that it results in increased dryness and splitting. Straightening and permanent waving use the same chemicals to change the properties of hair strands. The initial (waving) solution dissolves a chemical linkage in the hair. After the hair is arranged in its new, curly configuration, application of the second solution, the neutralizer, restores the linkage. Like other aggressive cosmetic treatments, permanent waving can be damaging when done to excess.

Be careful with coloring
Hair bleaches chemically alter the melanin granule in the middle layer of each hair strand. Despite careful treatment, persistent bleaching eventually damages even healthy, strong hair shafts, but it doesn't injure the roots from which future hair growth takes place.

Hair dyes work more like paint by covering hair strands with color or by mixing with the melanin granules without altering them. Dyes come in temporary form, which eventually washes out, and semipermanent and permanent forms, which penetrate your hair.

Avoid chemical and sun damage
Too much exposure to sun, wind and swimming pool chemicals will dry out your hair.

Eat a balanced diet
The quality of your hair reflects, in part, the adequacy of your diet. Contrary to what you may have heard or read, consuming extra protein or amino acid preparations won't promote hair growth. However, crash diets and eating disorders such as anorexia nervosa can damage hair dramatically and cause rapid hair loss.

of a quarter. Usually the disease doesn't extend beyond a few bare patches on the scalp, but it can cause patchy hair loss on any area that has hair, including eyebrows, eyelashes and beard. In rare cases, it can progress to cause hair loss over the entire body. If the hair loss includes your entire scalp, the condition is called alopecia totalis. If it involves your whole body, it's called alopecia universalis. Soreness and itching may precede the hair loss.

- **Telogen effluvium.** This type of temporary hair loss occurs suddenly. Handfuls of hair may come out when combing or washing your hair or may fall out after gentle tugging. This type of hair loss usually causes overall hair thinning and not bald patches.
- **Traction alopecia.** Bald patches can occur if you regularly wear certain hairstyles, such as braids or cornrows, or if you use tight rollers. Hair loss typically occurs between the rows or at the part where hair is pulled tightly.

Causes

Your hair goes through a cycle of growth and rest. The course of each cycle varies by individual. But in general, the growth phase of scalp hair, known as anagen, typically lasts two to three years. The resting phase is called telogen. This phase typically lasts three to four months. At the end of the resting phase, the hair strand falls out and a new one begins to grow in its place. Once a hair is shed, the growth stage begins again.

Gradual thinning is a normal part of aging. However, hair loss may lead to baldness when the rate of shedding exceeds the rate of regrowth, when new hair is thinner than the hair shed or when hair comes out in patches.

Causes of specific types of hair loss
- **Pattern baldness (androge-netic alopecia).** In male- and female-pattern baldness, the time of growth shortens, and the hairs are not as thick or sturdy. With each growth cycle, the hairs become rooted more superficially and more easily fall out. Heredity likely plays a key role. A history of androge-netic alopecia on either side of your family increases your risk of balding. Heredity also affects the age at which you begin to lose hair and the developmental speed, pattern and extent of your baldness.
- **Scarring (cicatricial) alopecia.** This type of permanent hair loss occurs when inflammation damages and scars the hair folli-cle. This prevents new hair from growing. This condition can be seen in several skin conditions, including lupus erythematosus or lichen planus. It's not known what triggers or causes this inflammation.
- **Alopecia areata.** This is classi-fied as an autoimmune disease, but the cause is unknown. People who develop alopecia areata are generally in good health. A few people may have other autoimmune disorders including thyroid disease. Some scientists believe that some peo-ple are genetically predisposed to develop alopecia areata and that a trigger, such as a virus or something else in the environ-ment, sets off the condition. A family history of alopecia areata makes you more likely to devel-op it. With alopecia areata, your hair generally grows back, but you may lose and regrow your hair a number of times.
- **Telogen effluvium.** This type of hair loss is usually due to a change in your normal hair cycle. It may occur when some type of shock to your system — emotional or physical — causes hair roots to be pushed prema-turely into the resting state. The affected growing hairs from these hair roots fall out. In a month or two, the hair follicles become active again and new hair starts to grow. Telogen effluvium may follow emotional distress, such as a death in the family, or after a physiological stress, such as a high fever, sudden or excessive weight loss, nutritional deficiencies, surgery, or metabolic disturbances. Hair typically grows back once the condition that caused it cor-rects itself, but it usually takes months.
- **Traction alopecia.** Excessive hairstyling or hairstyles that pull your hair too tightly cause traction alopecia. If the pulling is stopped before there's scar-ring of your scalp and perma-nent damage to the root, hair usually grows back normally.

Hair loss may also result for other reasons such as disease, poor nutrition, use of certain medications, hormonal changes or scalp infections.

Diagnosis

Tests may be necessary if the cause isn't apparent after the examination. These include:
- **Pull test.** This is when several dozen hairs are gently pulled to see how many come out. This helps determine the stage of the shedding process and can help diagnose or rule out telogen effluvium.
- **Skin scrapings.** Samples taken from the skin or from a few hairs plucked from the scalp can help verify whether an infection is causing hair loss.
- **Punch biopsy.** When a diag-nosis is difficult to confirm, especially in the case of alopecia areata or scarring alopecia, your doctor may perform a punch biopsy. During this test, the doctor uses a circular tool to remove a small section of your skin's deeper layers.
- **Screening tests for related diseases.** Your doctor may per-form tests to determine if you have a medical condition that causes hair loss, such as thyroid

disease, diabetes or lupus. Your doctor may also ask questions about the types of medications you're taking. Sometimes hair loss is a side effect of certain drugs, such as those used to treat gout, arthritis, depression, heart problems and high blood pressure.

Treatment

Baldness, whether permanent or temporary, can't be cured. But hair loss treatments are available to help promote hair growth or hide hair loss. For some types of alopecia, hair may resume growth without any treatment.

Medication

The effectiveness of medications used to treat alopecia depends on the cause of hair loss, extent of the loss and individual response. Generally, treatment is less effective for more-extensive cases of hair loss. Medications include:

- **Minoxidil (Rogaine).** This over-the-counter (nonprescription) medication is approved for the treatment of androgenetic alopecia and alopecia areata. Minoxidil is a liquid or foam that you rub into your scalp twice daily to grow hair and to prevent further loss. Some people experience some hair regrowth or a slower rate of hair loss or both. New hair resulting from minoxidil use may be thinner and shorter than previous hair. But there can be enough hair growth for some people to hide their bald spots and have them blend with existing hair. New hair stops growing soon after you discontinue the use of minoxidil.
- **Finasteride (Propecia).** This prescription medication to treat male-pattern baldness is taken daily in pill form. Many men taking finasteride experience a slowing of hair loss, and some may show some new hair growth. Positive results may take several months. Finas-

teride works by stopping the conversion of testosterone into dihydrotestosterone (DHT), a hormone that shrinks hair follicles and is an important factor in male hair loss. Rare side effects of finasteride include diminished sex drive and sexual function. As with minoxidil, the benefits of finasteride stop if you stop using it. Finasteride is not approved for use by women. In fact, it poses significant danger to women of childbearing age. If you're pregnant, don't even handle crushed or broken finasteride tablets because absorption of the drug may cause serious birth defects in male fetuses.

- **Corticosteroids.** Injections of cortisone into the scalp can treat alopecia areata. Treatment is usually repeated monthly. Doctors sometimes prescribe corticosteroid pills for extensive hair loss due to alopecia areata. New hair may be visible four weeks after the injection. Ointments and creams also can be used, but they may be less effective than injections.
- **Anthralin.** Available as either a cream or an ointment, anthralin is a synthetic, tarry substance that you apply to your scalp and wash off daily. It's typically used to treat psoriasis, but doctors can prescribe it to treat other skin conditions. Anthralin may stimulate new hair growth for cases of alopecia areata. It may take up to 12 weeks for new hair to appear.
- **Immunotherapy.** Immunomodulatory drugs, specifically, Janus kinase (JAK) inhibitors — such as tofacitinib (Xeljanz) and ruxolitinib (Jakafi) — are a new type of therapy being tested for alopecia areata. The medications were originally approved to treat certain blood disorders and rheumatoid arthritis. A topical formulation is currently in clinical trials in the United States.

Surgery

Hair transplants and scalp reduction surgery are available to treat androgenetic alopecia when more conservative measures have failed. During transplantation a dermatologist or cosmetic surgeon takes tiny plugs of skin, each containing one to several hairs, from the back or side of your scalp. The plugs are then implanted into the bald sections. Several transplant sessions may be needed, as hereditary hair loss progresses with time.

Scalp reduction, as the name implies, means decreasing the area of bald skin on your head. Your scalp and the top part of your head may seem to have a snug fit. But the skin can become flexible and stretched enough for some of it to be surgically removed. After hairless scalp is removed, the space is closed with hair-covered scalp. Doctors can also fold hair-bearing skin over an area of bald skin in a scalp-reduction technique called a flap. Scalp reduction can be combined with hair transplantation to fashion a natural-looking hairline in those with more extensive hair loss.

Surgical procedures to treat baldness are expensive and can be painful. Possible risks include infection and scarring. It will take six to eight months before the quality of the new hair can be properly evaluated.

Wigs and hairpieces

If you would like an alternative to medical treatment for your baldness or if you don't respond to treatment, you may want to consider wearing a wig or hairpiece. They can be used to cover either permanent or temporary hair loss. Quality, natural-looking wigs and hairpieces are available.

Hirsutism

Signs and symptoms

- Growth of hair in unwanted locations, such as on the face in women

There's a paradox about hair. People generally regard an ample and healthy head of it as beautiful. But the presence of hair in other locations, especially in women, may be considered anything but beautiful.

Amounts of facial and body hair vary greatly from one person to another. Many women develop considerable amounts of body and facial hair during puberty. In some cases, even faint mustaches appear. The normal secretion of androgen hormones produces many changes in a young girls' bodies, including hair growth in the pubic and underarm regions.

In women, facial and body hair usually increases slowly with age, even past menopause. Similarly, men may develop considerably more body hair as they age.

Too much hair is called hirsutism. How much is too much is largely a matter of personal perception. Part of the solution to a cosmetic problem of excessive hair is the simple acceptance that the amount you have is right for you. On the other hand, if you have a sudden increase in hair — for example, over a period of a few months — consult your doctor. This type of hair growth may have a medical cause, such as a tumor of the ovary or adrenal gland or a side effect of a medication.

Treatment

If you feel that you have too much facial or body hair and would like to get rid of it, you have several treatment options.

- **Plucking.** This is the most common cosmetic method, if your problem is a few scattered hairs. Wash the area first and dab on a little alcohol with a cotton ball to help prevent an infection in the hair follicle. Use good tweezers to remove the hair by pulling it out in the direction it's growing. Plucking is a temporary solution. The hair will likely grow back.
- **Shaving.** This popular but temporary method can be irritating to your skin if you do it haphazardly. The underarms, lower legs and face are common and safe areas for shaving. Similar to plucking, shaving doesn't make your hair grow faster or become darker or coarser.
- **Wax removal.** This method is popular for removing hair on the eyebrows, upper lip, chin and legs. Waxing can be painful and may irritate your skin. Seek the services of a trained cosmetician. First, the cosmetician applies melted wax to the area, then, after it cools and sets, quickly strips it off in the direction of the hair growth. The results last longer than shaving because the hair is pulled out below your skin's surface. New hairs generally appear after a month. As with plucking, infection of the hair follicles may occur.
- **Abrasive agents.** The use of pumice and other abrasive agents is the oldest method of hair removal. The process is slow and tedious, and the vigorous rubbing can irritate your skin. You may find it useful for scattered hairs, but it's not practical for large areas.
- **Bleaching.** Bleaching is useful for large areas, such as forearms or thighs, to make unwanted hair less conspicuous. Use a product specially designed for this purpose and follow the directions. Be sure to do a test on a small area to check for possible irritation before applying the product over a large area.
- **Depilatories.** Chemical agents called depilatories dissolve hair protein. You can buy them in foam, cream or lotion form. Follow the directions and test the product on a small area of your skin for possible irritation. Some people find depilatories inconvenient because they must stay on for 10 to 15 minutes. Don't use these products on injured or inflamed skin.
- **Eflornithine.** This prescription topical cream (Vaniqa) reduces the rate of facial hair growth in some women by blocking an enzyme that stimulates growth. It may take up to two months to work. The possible side effects include stinging, tingling, ingrown hairs and acne.
- **Electrolysis.** In this procedure, an electrologist inserts a very fine needle into each hair follicle, and a burst of electric current is delivered through the needle to destroy the hair root. The hair grows back about 30 percent of the time. Infections, scarring or discoloration around the follicle may occur. It's wise to have the electrologist do a few hairs and observe the results before embarking on an extensive program of hair removal. You may need several sessions because the maximum removal rate is about 100 hairs a visit. Electrolysis treatment can be long, tedious and expensive, but it might be a permanent solution to unwanted hair.
- **Lasers.** Lasers use light energy to destroy hair follicles. Significant improvements have been made in the multiple laser systems available to reduce unwanted hair and the technique has been gaining in popularity as an option for hair removal. Multiple treatments are required. Lasers can only be used to treat dark hair. Blond or gray hair isn't affected.

Fingernails and Toenails

Cells at the base of your nail beds produce your fingernails and toenails. Your nails are composed of laminated layers of a protein called keratin. Each nail grows toward the end of your finger or toe from a nail root that extends into a groove of skin. Just in front of your nail root is your cuticle skin, which is attached to the nail surface and helps protect new keratin cells that slowly emerge from below.

Your nails may give the first signal of an illness. Occasionally they provide clues for diagnosis as well as information about your age and diet. In addition, your fingernails assist you with the tasks of daily living, although you may not be conscious of how much you use them until an injury, infection or other disorder limits their use.

Healthy nails are smooth, without ridges or grooves. They're uniform in color and consistency and free of spots or discoloration. Remember that no nail care product can give you healthy nails. The only way you can help your nails to look their best is to protect them from damage and irritants such as chemicals and detergents and trim them regularly.

Paronychia

Signs and symptoms
- A red, swollen, painful area on the skin next to a nail
- Blisters, which may ooze pus

Signs and symptoms of a severe infection
- A raised cuticle
- A detached nail
- Nail distortion or discoloration
- Red lines along your skin

Paronychia is a superficial infection of the skin around the nail. The most common cause of paronychia is either staphylococci (staph) bacteria or yeast. The infection is usually the result of an injury, such as biting off a hangnail, or is caused by manipulating or pushing back the cuticle.

Bacterial paronychia is usually a sudden and painful infection. Superficial pus-filled blisters may appear. Pressing the affected area can produce oozing pus.

Another form of paronychia is caused by fungal infections and is common among people with diabetes and individuals who have their hands in water for long

Nail Discoloration or Deformity

Your nails can tell you a lot about your general health. Take a look at your fingernails. Are they strong and healthy looking? Or do you see ridges or areas of unusual color or shape?

Many less than desirable nail conditions can be avoided through proper nail care, but some conditions may be indications of an illness that requires attention.

Some nail conditions are harmless. These include vertical ridges, which tend to increase as you age. A minor injury can cause nail discoloration. The black spot under your thumbnail after a hammer blow is blood. White, cloud-like marks on the tips of your nails are the result of minor trauma.

Overexposure to strong soaps or chemicals can cause splitting, peeling or brittleness, and tight or ill-fitting shoes can cause ingrown or thickened toenails.

Other nail conditions may indicate disease, so remove your nail polish when you see your doctor. Here are some conditions that might require medical attention:

Separation of a nail from its bed
Separation of a nail from its bed (onycholysis) may be associated with injury, psoriasis, drug reactions, fungal disease or a reaction to nail hardeners or acrylic nails.

Yellow nail syndrome
Swelling in the hands or a respiratory condition, such as chronic bronchitis, can cause one or more of your nails to turn yellow or green. The condition is associated with very slow nail growth — your nails may need clipping only once every several months.

Pitting
Small depressions in the nail are common in people with psoriasis or nail injuries.

Terry's nails
Terry's nails is a condition in which your nails look opaque, but the tips each have a dark band. This may be a sign of serious illness, such as cancer, congestive heart failure or diabetes, or it may just be a sign of aging.

Clubbing
Nails that curve around the fingertips or toes, along with broadening of the fingers or toes, may be a sign of lack of oxygen. It's associated with a number of diseases, including heart disease and emphysema.

Beau's lines
Beau's lines are indentations that run across the nail. They can appear when growth at the nail bed is interrupted by severe illness, such as a heart attack or pneumonia, or by high fever.

Mees' lines
Mees' lines are caused by arsenic poisoning. They're white lines that run across the nail.

Spoon nails
Spoon nails — soft nails that look scooped out — may be a sign of iron deficiency anemia. The depression is usually large enough to hold a drop of liquid.

It's not unusual for your nails to be affected during an illness and to recover afterward. Damage can be repaired only by the slow process of new growth, about $1/8$ inch a month for fingernails and $1/24$ inch for toenails. After your underlying disorder is under control or cured, your nails will gradually return to normal. But report any new changes in color or markings to your doctor.

periods of time. Fungal infections develop slowly but tend to persist. Sometimes, both bacteria and fungi are present.

A severe (acute) infection, which usually affects the fingers, can extend around your nail and cuticle to invade beneath them. Your cuticle becomes raised. The nail may become detached. Nail distortion or discoloration might occur. Red lines along your skin are a signal that bacteria have entered your bloodstream. If this occurs, see your doctor. The diagnosis may require a culture to determine which type of microorganism is causing your paronychia.

Treatment

Soaking the affected area in warm water should help decrease inflammation of the tissues. Topical application of an antibacterial agent will help fight a bacterial infection. If a fungal infection is present, you might try soaking the nail in a dilute vinegar solution of 1 ounce white vinegar to 16 ounces water.

Fungal infection

Signs and symptoms

- Thickened, lusterless fingernails or toenails
- Nail discoloration, usually yellow or brown
- Crumbling nail edges
- A detached nail

Fungus spores may attach themselves to the dense bed of keratin cells that make up your nails. These microscopic plants can digest the keratin and live within it. The resulting infection, called onychomycosis, can persist indefinitely.

When infected by a fungus, your nails may thicken, detach and shed (see the illustration on page 398). There's usually an accumulation of keratinous debris beneath the free edge of an infected nail. You may feel some pain in the nail and detect a slight odor. In some cases, the nail is destroyed.

You can contract fungal infections in several ways, including walking barefoot in public places or as a complication of athlete's foot or paronychia. People with decreased blood circulation or diabetes are more prone to infection. Your risk of fungal infection of a toenail is greater if your feet perspire heavily and if you wear socks and shoes that hinder ventilation and don't absorb perspiration.

Fingernail fungal infections often result from overexposure to water and detergents. Moisture caught under artificial nails also can encourage fungal growth.

Fungal infections are more common among older adults. After age 40, your nails grow more slowly and begin to thicken, making them more susceptible to infection. Once a fungal nail infection begins, it can persist indefinitely if not treated. See your doctor at the first sign of infection. Fungal nail infections usually begin as a tiny white or yellow spot on your nail that spreads.

Diagnosis

Diagnostic tests may include scraping up some of the debris beneath the nail edge for microscopic examination to identify the fungus. Presence of a fungus rules out other diseases of the nails.

Treatment

Fungal nail infections can be difficult to treat, and repeated infections are common. If you have a fungal infection, your doctor may prescribe an oral antifungal medication. These drugs, which are effective most of the time, include itraconazole (Sporanox), fluconazole (Diflucan) and terbinafine (Lamisil). The drugs help a new, infection-free nail grow out while the older, infected portion of your nail is slowly replaced. Although the drugs can usually eliminate an infection in six to 12 months, recurrent infections are possible.

These oral medications, however, may cause side effects ranging from skin rashes to liver damage. Itraconazole and fluconazole also can cause adverse interactions with other drugs, including some anticoagulant and allergy medications. Several years ago, the Food and Drug Administration issued a public health advisory regarding itraconazole and terbinafine over concerns that they may cause congestive heart failure. The warning doesn't apply to the cream and solution forms of Lamisil, which are applied topically.

Before you and your doctor decide to use oral medications, discuss and consider the possible side effects.

Over-the-counter antifungal nail creams may help soften your nail and keep a fungal infection from spreading while a new nail grows. Other antifungal creams or lotions are available by prescription.

Another option is a topical antifungal lacquer. You paint the lacquer onto infected nails and surrounding skin once daily. After seven days, you remove the layers and start with a fresh application. Daily use for up to one year or longer has been shown to help clear up some fungal nail infections.

If your nail infection is severe or extremely painful, your doctor may suggest removing your nail. A new nail will usually grow in its place.

Care of your nails

Perhaps the single most important element in taking care of your nails is to avoid abusing them. Don't use them as tools and don't bite them or pick your cuticles. Even a minor cut alongside your nail can allow bacteria or fungi to enter and cause an infection. Because your nails grow slowly, an injured nail retains signs of its injury for several months.

Regular fingernail trimming is important because nails that are smooth and cared for are less likely to become damaged. Use sharp manicure scissors or clippers to trim your fingernails and use an emery board. Trim your toenails straight across and not too short.

Toenails grow more slowly than fingernails. They also tend to be thicker, especially on your big toe, so the best time for a trim is after bathing when your nails are softer.

If you have a hangnail, don't attempt to pull it off. Pulling almost always rips into living tissue.

Instead, clip it off neatly, leaving a slight angle outward. This may help prevent recurrence. Using hand lotion regularly can help prevent hangnails.

Use nail products cautiously

Some nail products can be hard on your nails. Cuticle removers are corrosive alkali-based products that destroy these naturally protective bands. Some nail strengtheners can discolor or break your nails. Polish removers dry and weaken your nails.

Despite advertising claims, most polishes are chemically similar. They make your nails stronger only in the sense that the polish coats and thus protects the nail.

Keep them tough

Here are some tips to toughen or protect weak fingernails:

- Apply a nail hardener, but avoid products containing toluene sulfonamide/formaldehyde resin or formaldehyde, which can cause itchiness, redness or irritation of the skin.
- Apply a moisturizer each time you wash your hands. At bedtime, moisturize your nails and cuticles and wear cotton gloves.
- Wear cotton-lined rubber gloves when exposing your hands to water or household chemicals. Between uses, turn rubber gloves inside out to dry to prevent microorganisms from growing inside them.
- Don't use nail polish remover more than twice a month. Instead, touch up the polish. When you do need a remover, avoid those that contain acetone.
- Repair splits or tears with nail glue or clear polish.
- Avoid dietary practices that supposedly strengthen nails. They won't work. Unless you're deficient in protein, which is uncommon among people in the United States, adding protein to your diet won't strengthen your nails. Soaking your nails in gelatin won't help either.

Ingrown Toenails

Ingrown toenails usually occur on the big toe. They form when the edge of your nail curls and grows into the soft underlying tissue. Ingrown toenails are caused by:
- Improper cutting of nails
- Faster nail growth at the edge than at the center
- Pressure from poorly fitting shoes

If you experience severe discomfort, pus or redness that seems to be spreading from the side of the toe, seek medical attention. Your doctor may need to remove the ingrown portion of the nail and prescribe antibiotics.

You can do several things to prevent and treat ingrown toenails at home. Follow these self-care tips:
- Trim your toenails straight across and not too short.
- Wear socks and shoes that fit properly and don't place excessive pressure on your toes.
- Wear open-toe shoes or sandals, if appropriate.

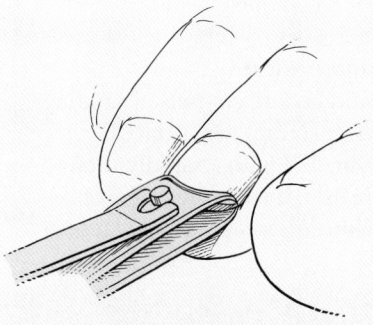

To avoid ingrown toenails, cut your nails straight across and not too short.

- Soak your feet in warm salt water — 1 tablespoon of salt per quart of water — two to four times a day to reduce swelling and relieve tenderness.
- After soaking, put tiny bits of sterile cotton under the ingrown edge. This will help the nail eventually grow above the skin edge. Change the cotton daily until the pain and redness subside.
- Apply an antibiotic ointment to the tender area.

Cosmetic Procedures

As you grow older, you'll no doubt see the effects of time and aging when you look in the mirror. You may be perfectly happy to proudly wear evidence of your life's ups and downs. But if you find these signs distressful and have money to spend, consider cosmetic procedures, which can markedly diminish many signs of aging. You can meet with a dermatologist or plastic surgeon to discuss the limitations, benefits, risks and side effects of available procedures.

Keep in mind that cosmetic procedures usually aren't covered by health insurance, and they may have to be repeated to maintain benefits.

Common cosmetic concerns

Cosmetic procedures are used to treat a number of skin-related conditions. Some of the most common cosmetic concerns include:

Aging and sun-exposed skin
Skin resurfacing techniques, such as chemical peels, dermabrasion or laser resurfacing, can help get rid of wrinkles, sags and bags, as well as scars resulting from acne. Other procedures to reduce wrinkles include soft tissue fillers and face-lifts.

Varicose and spider veins
Some people are so embarrassed by varicose or spider veins that they refuse to wear clothes that show their legs. However, several treatments are available that can get rid of these unwanted veins.

Fat
Liposuction may be an option for men or women who aren't happy with the shape of their thighs or who want to get rid of those love handles that never seem to disappear.

Selecting a surgeon

No cosmetic procedure is without risks. That's why it's crucial to find the right doctor if you're considering cosmetic surgery. Be sure the person is properly trained and board certified in a specialty dealing with cosmetic surgery: a plastic surgeon, dermatologic surgeon or an ear, nose and throat (ENT) surgeon. If you're considering laser surgery, make sure the doctor has experience working with lasers.

Skin resurfacing techniques

Skin resurfacing techniques can be used to reduce fine wrinkles, scars such as those left by acne and pigmentation problems such as liver spots. This is done by removing the outer layer of skin (epidermis) to let smoother, younger looking skin grow back in its place. Resurfacing techniques include:

Dermabrasion
This procedure consists of sanding down (planing) the surface layer of your skin with a rapidly rotating brush. The planing removes the skin surface and a new layer of skin grows in its place. Redness, scabbing and swelling generally last a couple of weeks. It may take several months for the pinkness to fade and to see the desired results.

Microdermabrasion
This technique is similar to dermabrasion, but less surface skin is removed. It's done using a vacuum suction over your face while aluminum oxide crystals essentially sandblast your skin. Only a fine layer of skin is removed. You may notice a slight redness to the treated areas. Microdermabrasion usually requires repeated treatments to maintain the subtle, temporary results.

Laser, light source and radio-frequency treatments
In ablative (wounding) laser resurfacing, a laser beam destroys the outer layer of skin (epidermis) and heats the underlying skin (dermis), which stimulates the growth of new collagen fibers. As the wound heals, new skin forms that's smoother and tighter. It can take up to several months to fully heal from ablative laser resurfacing. Newer developments in laser technology have decreased the healing time. Less intense lasers (nonab-

Vein Surgery

Millions of Americans, mostly women, are bothered by varicose veins or spider veins, a mild variation of varicose veins. Varicose veins are gnarled, enlarged veins close to your skin. The name *varicose* comes from the Latin root *varix*, which means "twisted." Any vein may become varicose, but the most commonly affected areas are the legs and ankles. Spider veins result when small veins close to the skin's surface dilate. They're most common on the legs and face.

For many people, varicose veins and spider veins are simply a cosmetic concern. For other people, they can cause aching pain and discomfort. Sometimes varicose veins lead to more-serious problems such as leg ulcers.

Self-care measures — such as exercising, losing weight, not wearing tight clothes, elevating your legs, and avoiding long periods of standing or sitting — can ease the pain and prevent varicose veins from getting worse. If your varicose veins don't respond to self-help or if they're more severe, your doctor may advise surgery — including removal of the enlarged vein or another type of procedure to seal off the vein. For information on treatment of varicose and spider veins, see page 757.

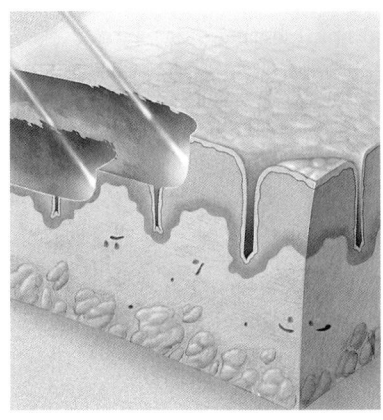

With laser resurfacing, an intense, pulsating beam of light vaporizes outer skin tissues. Underlying skin eventually heals more tightly and smoothly.

lative lasers), pulsed light sources and radiofrequency devices don't injure the epidermis. These treatments heat the dermis and cause new collagen and elastin formation. After several treatments, skin feels firmer and appears refreshed. This means shorter recovery times, but treatment typically needs to be repeated more often and results are subtle.

Chemical peel

Your doctor applies an acid to the affected areas, which burns the outer layer of your skin. With medium-depth peels, the entire epidermis and a small portion of the dermis are removed. New skin forms to take its place. The new skin is usually smoother and less wrinkled than your old skin. Redness lasts up to several weeks. With superficial peels, only a portion of the epidermis is removed. With a deep peel your skin will develop a scab for about seven to 10 days and will be pink for about three months. After a series of peels, you may notice less fine wrinkling in your skin and a fading of brown spots.

Botulinum toxin type A (Botox)

When injected in small doses into specific muscles, Botox blocks the chemical signals that cause muscles to contract. When the muscles can't tighten, the skin flattens and appears smoother and less wrinkled. Botox works well on frown lines between the eyebrows and across the forehead, and crow's-feet at the corners of the eyes. Results typically last about three to four months. Repeat injections are needed to maintain results.

Soft tissue fillers

Collagen from humans or animals, fat from your thigh or abdomen, or newer fillers derived from human substances can be injected into wrinkles on your face. The injected collagen plumps up your skin, smoothing out the wrinkles and filling in furrows, such as those around your nose and mouth and between your eyebrows. The collagen gradually degrades over several months but it may trigger your body to produce new collagen. To maintain the effect, you may need to have the procedure repeated every few months.

Some people are allergic to collagen from cattle, so prior testing is necessary.

Face-lift

A face-lift requires more extensive surgery to remove drooping skin and jowls and smooth out wrinkles. It involves removing excess skin and fat, tightening the underlying muscle and connective tissue, and doing it all without leaving prominent, visible traces. Each operation varies, depending on what your surgeon thinks is appropriate for you.

Not everyone is a good candidate for a face-lift. You have the best chance of good results if your skin still has some elasticity, if you have a strong and well-defined bone structure, and if you're not overweight. Most people who have a face-lift are between the ages of 40 and 70, but if you're in your 70s or even 80s, you can still have good results.

Surgeons can also perform eyelid surgery to correct droopy eyelids, a procedure called blepharoplasty. This can be done alone or at the same time as a face-lift.

After surgery

Although it's elective and cosmetic, a face-lift is no walk in the park. The first time you look in the mirror, expect to see a pale, puffy and bruised face staring back at you.

Levels of discomfort vary, but usually can be managed with pain medication. Parts of your face may feel numb for a few weeks or even months. This is normal and eventually disappears, although some tingling sensations may persist for a while longer. Scars take longer to fade, but because they're hidden in hairlines, behind the ears and in natural folds, they're barely noticeable.

Risks

Although complications are uncommon, when they occur they can be serious. They include:

- **Hematoma.** This is a collection of blood under the skin. The excess blood can be removed by your surgeon. Small hematomas may resolve on their own.
- **Weakness of your facial muscles.** This is usually temporary, but until the nerves heal, parts of your face may not move normally.
- **Poor healing.** Smokers are more likely to be affected by poor healing, because substances in cigarettes constrict the small blood vessels of the skin.
- **Infection.** Incisions can become infected.

Liposuction

The concept behind liposuction seems almost too good to be true: Unwanted fat deposits can simply be sucked away with a tiny vacuum. However, the problem isn't that easy to fix.

Liposuction is a serious surgical procedure in which the recovery can be painful. Although rare, the surgery can also cause serious complications. A decision about whether to undergo liposuction should be considered very carefully.

A popular treatment

Instant fat reduction holds great appeal to many, making liposuction one of the most common cosmetic procedures performed in the United States. The areas most commonly treated are the outer thighs and abdomen in women and the flanks, or love handles, in men. Liposuction can also remove unwanted fat from your hips, buttocks, knees, upper arms, chin, cheeks, neck and other areas.

Liposuction is most effective for removing localized fat deposits in parts of your body that don't respond to dieting or exercising. After the procedure, it's important to continue with an exercise and weight management program for best results.

Liposuction techniques

Two basic techniques are used in liposuction: tumescent, developed by dermatologic surgeons, and ultrasonic, developed by plastic surgeons. Both share core surgical elements. In fact, even if ultrasound is used, it will be followed by tumescent liposuction. Whether you use tumescent or ultrasonic liposuction depends on a number of individual factors that your surgeon will discuss with you.

Some new devices have been developed that liquefy fat when applied externally — so-called noninvasive liposuction. However, their effectiveness hasn't been established.

Tumescent liposuction

In tumescent liposuction, your surgeon pre-injects your fat deposits with a saltwater solution containing the hormone adrenaline (epinephrine). The solution might also contain a local anesthetic.

Your surgeon will decide whether to use additional anesthetics — local, regional or general — or use only the saltwater solution with a local anesthetic. The decision on what type of anesthetic to administer is based largely on the amount of fat to be suctioned and whether ultrasound will be used.

To begin the procedure, a surgeon typically makes one or more small incisions near the area to be suctioned. Whenever possible, the incisions will be placed within the natural folds or contour lines of your skin so that they aren't highly noticeable.

A slim, hollow tube called a cannula is then inserted into your skin through the incision so that its tip penetrates the underlying fat. After the cannula is connected by flexible tubing to a suction pump, your surgeon moves the cannula back and forth through the fat. The fat is then vacuumed into the tube. Minimal bleeding, bruising and swelling result from tumescent liposuction.

Ultrasonic liposuction

Ultrasound-assisted liposuction (UAL) is a two-step technique that uses the energy from sound waves to liquefy fat deposits before they're suctioned. In UAL, a surgeon inserts a small, heated probe that produces vibrations at frequencies above what your ear can hear (ultrasonic). This energy causes your fat cells to rupture, releasing their oily contents. These oily contents are then suctioned out using the tumescent technique.

Potential advantages to UAL include the ability to remove fat in difficult areas, such as the upper abdomen, the flanks, the back and the male chest. However, UAL is associated with significantly greater complications than is tumescent liposuction, such as more pain, swelling and other complications.

After surgery

Recovery from liposuction can be uncomfortable, but most people

are back to their normal routine within three to 10 days. During the first few weeks, most people experience varying degrees of pain, burning, swelling and temporary areas of numbness.

Pain medications can offer some relief, and special compression garments can reduce swelling. You may be advised to refrain from strenuous physical activity other than walking for about a week after the procedure.

Although your new body contour usually begins to emerge in the first couple of weeks, some swelling may remain for several months. Major weight gain or loss after liposuction can produce unwanted skin surface irregularities.

Many people assume that because liposuction removes fat cells, it's impossible to regain weight in the treated areas. However, remaining fat cells may grow larger, especially if you abandon exercise and a healthy diet. This means problem spots can return. It's more likely, though, that weight gain after liposuction will be distributed to other parts of your body.

Risks

Liposuction isn't without risks. In general, the larger the volume of fat removed, the higher the potential for complications. Some surgeons will suction a greater amount of fat at one time and complete the job in one procedure, whereas others will suction smaller volumes over the course of multiple procedures.

People with certain medical conditions, such as diabetes, heart disease, lung disease and poor circulation, as well as individuals who smoke or are subject to blood clots, are at increased risk of complications from liposuction, just as they are for any surgical procedure.

Rare but serious complications include blood clots, which can migrate to the lungs and cause death, infection and allergic reactions. ■

Mental Illness

Mental illness is mysterious and confusing to many people. Is a stretch of sleepless nights the result of depression? Are your worries typical, or do you have an anxiety disorder?

Part of the challenge is that there's no clear dividing line between mental health and mental illness. A recent report by the Surgeon General views mental health and mental illness as points on a continuum. To some extent, any definition of mental health reflects culture and circumstances. Different cultures have different ways of coping with stress and adversity. Behavior that's considered abnormal in one culture may be perfectly acceptable in another.

In general, mental health refers to normal mental functioning that allows a person to be productive, develop fulfilling relationships, adapt to change and cope with adversity. Mental illness refers to changes in thinking, mood or behavior that cause distress and interfere with a person's ability to function in a variety of ways. A person with a mental illness has trouble — to a lesser or greater degree — with daily activities, family responsibilities, relationships, work or school.

Like other illnesses, mental disorders range in severity from mild to severe. Some mental disorders last a short time and gradually improve. Others are lifelong, requiring ongoing treatment.

A Common Problem

Mental illnesses are common. According to the National Institute of Mental Health, close to 18 percent of U.S. adults experience a mental illness in a given year.

Mental illness can take a great toll on your quality of life and the lives of those with whom you interact — family, friends, employ-ers and co-workers. Many people with unrecognized, untreated or inadequately treated mental illness endure lives that are sapped of vitality or undermined by tension and conflict.

Fortunately, most mental illnesses are treatable. Many people can recover, and others with more long-term (chronic) disorders can learn to manage their symptoms, much as people learn to manage and live with diabetes or arthritis. A growing body of research is helping to identify effective therapies and new medications that cause fewer or less severe side effects.

Despite such significant advances, too many people don't recognize or acknowledge mental illness, and many don't receive care until a crisis occurs. Unfortunately, despite growing awareness of mental illness, a societal stigma is still attached to mental disorders.

Mental illnesses don't involve lack of willpower and self-discipline. As with cancer and heart disease, they arise from a mixture of influences — the complex interplay of heredity, biology and environmental factors.

Life Issues and Mental Illness

After years of research on brain function and human behavior, the artificial split between illnesses of the mind and of the body is disappearing. Mental disorders are now recognized as illnesses with a biological basis that are often influenced by psychological and social stress. Even in the womb, experience shapes brain development, influencing the types and amounts of chemicals that convey messages throughout the nervous system. Changes in these pathways may even set the stage for some mental disorders.

Although many mental illnesses have a strong biological or genetic basis, that's not the entire story. Many factors can play a role in the development of signs and symptoms related to mental illness. A mental disorder can occur as a manifestation of another illness, as a reaction to a medication or to drug or alcohol abuse, or as a result of a stressful or emotionally difficult life experience.

One person may have mental illness due to nature — a specific genetic defect that alters brain circuitry. Another may have mental illness caused by nurture — one or more environmental factors that alter natural brain chemistry. Mental illness is usually a complex interaction of both nature and nurture.

Risk factors

Some of the factors that can contribute to mental illness are as follows:

Genetics
Hereditary traits are conveyed through individual genes, which carry instructions that direct the formation and guide the function of every structure of the human body. Some genes are actively expressed throughout an individual's life, and others lie dormant unless stimulated.

Genetic factors play a role in many human diseases. An inherited susceptibility to a disease occurs when one or more genes fail to give correct instructions for the manufacturing or functioning of cells. This failure may make you more vulnerable to disease. Genes can also influence the severity or progression of a disease.

It's unlikely that a single genetic abnormality can cause mental illness, but a composite of genetic abnormalities may increase susceptibility to some mental illnesses. Genetic factors alone probably aren't enough to trigger the illness. Other factors also come into play.

Sex and stress hormones are among the substances produced

by the body that may play a role. External factors, such as stress, drugs or alcohol, may activate a genetic susceptibility to mental illness.

If someone in your family has or had a mental illness, such as depression, it doesn't necessarily mean that you'll develop it too. But a family history of mental illness does increase your risk.

Stress and grief

Stressful life events can unmask vulnerability to mental illness. For example, if you have a major crisis in your life, such as a divorce or the death of a loved one, you may become sad and depressed. Even after your life situation has improved, these symptoms may persist. Stress or grief can trigger an illness that needs professional treatment.

The death of a loved one is a common trigger of mental disorders. Grief is a normal and necessary response to such a loss, but grief that's especially disproportionate to what would be considered normal or that lasts longer than a year may be complicated by a mental disorder, such as depression.

Stress can result from many other situations, such as relationship or work troubles, major life changes, and illness.

Past experiences

People who have experienced deeply upsetting events — for example, childhood abuse or wartime combat — are at higher risk of developing mental disorders such as depression or post-traumatic stress disorder.

Any form of abuse during childhood — sexual, physical or emotional — can make a person more vulnerable to mental disorders. Other aspects of family environment that may contribute to mental disorders include a high level of conflict between parents, family violence, substance abuse or loss of a parent due to death.

The connection between past traumas and mental illness is partly related to the way the human body responds to danger and stress. When confronted with real or perceived danger, your body gears up to face the challenge (fight) or to move out of harm's way (flight). This fight-or-flight response results from the release of hormones that cause your body to shift into overdrive. Severe or ongoing stressful experiences trigger stress responses in your brain circuits, and hormonal systems may become chronically hyperactive.

In addition, children who don't acquire good coping skills when growing up may be less able to cope when they're faced with a stressful situation during adulthood. Consequently, they may be more adversely affected by stress than are people with better coping skills.

Substance use

Some people with mood or anxiety disorders have substance abuse problems. Evidence suggests that addictive substances such as alcohol, some prescription medications, nicotine and cocaine affect levels of dopamine, a brain chemical (neurotransmitter) associated with feelings of pleasure.

Other medical conditions

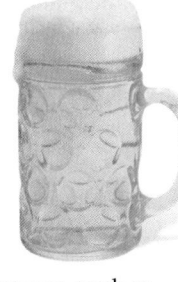

Other physical illnesses and medical conditions may trigger what appears to be a mental illness. For example, some hormone-related diseases, such as an underactive thyroid (hypothyroidism), have a direct link to the development of depression. Some medical conditions such as stroke, cancer, Alzheimer's disease, Parkinson's disease, obstructive sleep apnea, epilepsy and chronic pain are associated with an increased risk of depression.

Children and mental illness

Despite its image as a carefree time of life, childhood is far from easy. Many children and adolescents experience emotional difficulties as they deal with a wide range of issues — self-control, learning to socialize with peers, separation from parents, and so on. Adolescence is a time of tumultuous physical and emotional changes, including increasingly intense self-awareness and developing sexuality, which can make for a traumatic and rocky road.

For some children and adolescents, these normal developmental struggles are compounded by a mental illness. Some of the disorders that may develop during childhood or adolescence are depression, anxiety disorders, eating disorders and substance abuse. Depression and anxiety disorders, in particular, are common among children and teens. Less commonly, bipolar disorder and schizophrenia may first appear during the teenage years. In addition to these mental conditions, a number of disorders involving learning and development are typically first diagnosed during childhood or adolescence.

When children and teenagers have untreated mental illness, their family relationships can suffer, their social development may be affected, they may do poorly in school, they may abuse alcohol or drugs, and they may be at risk of suicide. Suicide is the third-leading cause of death for 15- to 24-year-olds and the sixth-leading cause of death for 5- to 15-year-olds. These rates have tripled since 1960 and continue to rise.

Prompt identification and treatment of mental disorders in children and teenagers can reduce the severity and duration of illness and the risk of complications. During the last two decades, health care professionals have improved efforts to better understand,

Is Your Child at Risk?

The American Psychiatric Association lists the following warning signs of possible mental illness in children:

- Frequent crying
- Frequent requests or hints for help
- Constant anxiety, worry or preoccupation
- Fears or phobias that are unreasonable or interfere with routine activities
- An inability to concentrate on schoolwork and other age-appropriate tasks
- A decline in school performance that doesn't improve
- A loss of interest in playing
- Isolation from other children
- Fighting with other children
- Low self-esteem and little self-confidence
- Setting fires

If your child is experiencing any of these signs or symptoms, it may be appropriate to consult your child's pediatrician, your family doctor or a mental health professional.

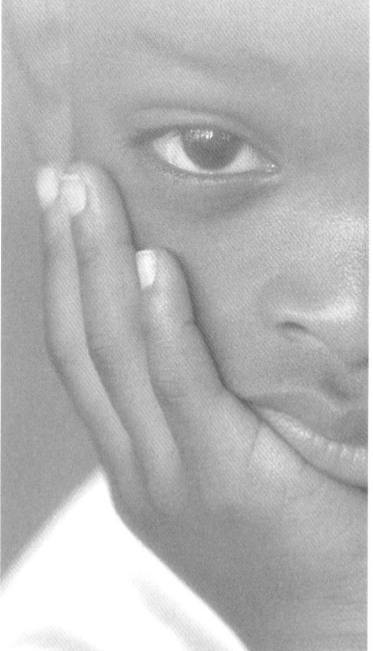

recognize and treat mental illness in children and adolescents.

In response to the increasing rate of depression in children and teens, more efforts are being made to recognize and treat depression in this age group. Studies show that early treatment of mild to moderate depression may help prevent severe depression and related disorders, such as substance abuse and eating disorders. For children and teens at high risk of mental illness due to family history, short-term, family-based educational intervention seems to help reduce the risk of a first episode of illness.

For more about specific conditions in children and adolescents, see Chapter 5, "Preschool and Early School Years," and Chapter 6, "Preteen and Teenage Years."

Older adults and mental illness

Just as young people struggle to adjust to the changes that occur in their lives, so do older adults. The aging process may bring a number of physical and mental changes that can contribute to mental illness, especially depression. Increased health problems, a change in normal routine, financial stress, overmedication, substance abuse, loss of independence or mobility, and the death of family and friends can increase the risk of depression. Many adults age 65 and older experience depression, and many don't receive treatment.

Depression can occur with illnesses that are more common later in life, such as Alzheimer's disease, Parkinson's disease, stroke, heart disease and cancer. Because signs and symptoms of these diseases may overlap with those of depression, depression may be underdiagnosed or overdiagnosed in people with these health conditions. Dementia may be confused with depression, as well as failing senses, such as hearing and eyesight.

Undiagnosed and untreated mental illness in older adults can diminish their quality of life. It can lead to decreased physical functioning and an increased reliance on others. Untreated depression may even be associated with an increased risk of early death among people with certain forms of heart disease. Fortunately, treatment for depression is generally as effective in older adults as it is in younger people.

Depression

Depression is one of the most common health conditions in the world. Depression isn't a weakness, nor is it something that you can simply "snap out of." Depression, formally called major depression or major depressive disorder, is a medical illness that involves the mind and body. It affects how you think and behave and can cause a variety of emotional and physical problems. You may not be able to go about your usual daily activities, and depression may make you feel as if life just isn't worth living anymore.

Most health professionals today consider depression a chronic illness that requires long-term treatment, much like diabetes or high blood pressure. Although some people experience only one episode of depression, most have repeated episodes of depression symptoms throughout life.

Effective diagnosis and treatment can help reduce even severe depression symptoms. With effective treatment, many people with depression feel better, often within weeks, and can return to the daily activities they previously enjoyed.

Signs and symptoms

The hallmark symptoms of depression are a depressed mood and loss of pleasure. You may feel sad, helpless and hopeless. Your self-esteem and self-confidence may plummet, and you may feel guilty or worthless. Interestingly, some people experience depression without feeling depressed.

Depression can affect more than just your mood. It can also cause physical changes and changes in thinking and behavior. It can disrupt your sleeping and eating patterns and reduce your sexual drive. It affects how you think about things, making your thoughts more negative and pessimistic and hampering your ability to concentrate or make a decision. It also impacts how you act. You may be more irritable, withdrawn or ambivalent.

Signs and symptoms of depression include:

- Loss of interest in routine daily activities
- Feeling sad or down
- Feeling hopeless
- Crying spells for no apparent reason
- Problems sleeping
- Trouble focusing or concentrating
- Difficulty making decisions
- Unintentional weight gain or loss
- Feelings of guilt
- Irritability
- Restlessness
- Being easily annoyed
- Feeling fatigued or weak
- Feeling worthless
- Loss of interest in sex
- Thoughts of suicide or suicidal behavior
- Unexplained physical problems, such as back pain or headaches

Depression symptoms can vary greatly because different people experience depression in different ways. A 25-year-old with depression, for example, may not have the same symptoms as a 70-year-old who is depressed.

For some people, depression symptoms are so severe that it's obvious something isn't right — both to the person experiencing the depression and to friends and family. Others with depression may feel generally unhappy without really knowing why.

Causes

It's not known specifically what causes depression. As with many mental illnesses, a variety of biochemical, genetic and environmental factors are likely involved:

- **Biochemical.** Some evidence from high-tech imaging studies indicates that people with depression have physical changes in their brains. The significance of these changes is still uncertain but may eventually help pinpoint causes. The naturally occurring brain chemicals called neurotransmitters, which are linked to mood, also may play a role in depression. Hormonal imbalances also could be a culprit.
- **Genes.** Some studies show that depression is more common in people whose biological family members also have the condition. Researchers are trying to find genes that may be involved in causing depression.
- **Environment.** Environment is also thought to play a causal role in some way. Environmental causes are situations in your life that are difficult to cope with, such as the loss of a loved one, financial problems and high stress.

Depression typically begins in the late 20s, but it can arise at any age, affecting everyone from young children to older adults. Depression can occur by itself, or it can be a complication of another illness. Sometimes depression just happens, with no apparent trigger but is likely associated with alterations in brain neurotransmitter levels or brain function.

Types

Depression can take many forms, differentiated by the symptoms and circumstances associated with each form and the duration and severity of symptoms. Often, though, different types of depression have no clear-cut distinctions, and they share many characteristics. People

Brain Communication

Brain cells communicate by sending messages along a complex system of nerve bundles that connect different regions of the brain. The ends of brain cells contain chemical messengers (neurotransmitters) that serve as communication links between nerve cells (neurons). It's thought that neurotransmitters play a key role in depression and other mental disorders.

Nerve cells release neurotransmitters into a small gap (synapse) between a sending nerve cell and a receiving nerve cell (see the illustration on page 366). The neurotransmitter binds to a receptor on the receiving nerve cell. During the transfer of information, electric signals from the sending nerve cell are changed into chemical signals that communicate the message to the receiving nerve cell. When the transfer is complete, the receiving cell changes the chemical signals back to electric signals. Communication from one cell to another occurs very rapidly.

People who are depressed may have reduced activity of certain neurotransmitters, such as serotonin and norepinephrine, in the synapse between nerve cells compared with people who aren't depressed. Antidepressant medications increase the amount and activity of neurotransmitters in the synapse. This allows nerve cells in the treated individual to get messages in a way similar to that of people who aren't depressed.

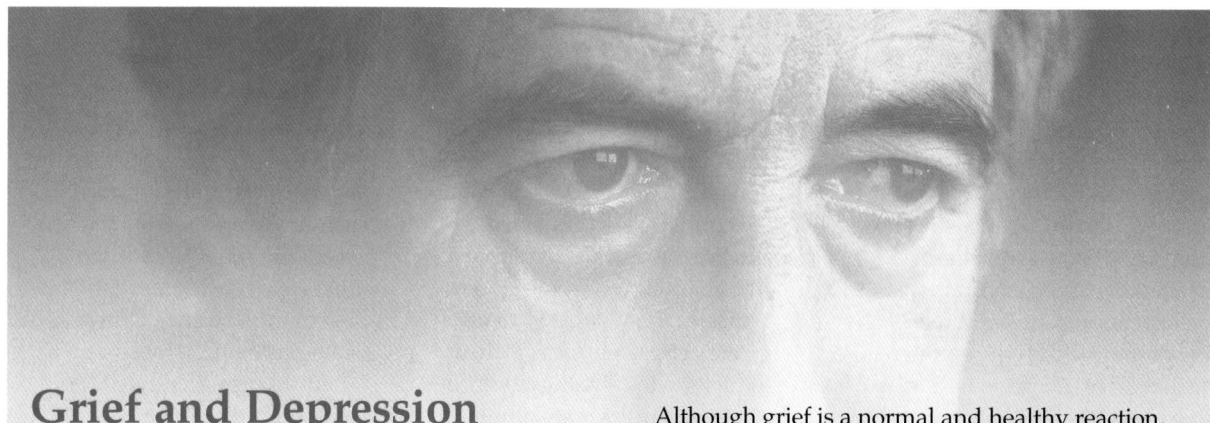

Grief and Depression

Grief is the emotional and physical response to a significant loss, such as the death of a loved one, the end of a relationship, a move to a new town, a change in health or the death of a pet. Grieving is a process of coming to terms with the loss and letting go. It takes a long time, and it's hard work. Grieving is a private journey that's different for each person.

In many ways, grief and depression are similar. They share many signs and symptoms, including feelings of sadness, lack of interest in usually pleasurable activities, problems with sleeping and eating, irritability, sexual difficulties, and difficulty concentrating. Other symptoms you may experience if you're grieving are a sense of confusion or disorientation, headaches or other physical complaints, anger, resentment or bitterness, and withdrawal from social activities.

Although grief is a normal and healthy reaction, depression isn't. The differences between grief and depression are in how long the feelings last and to what extent your daily activities are impaired. Depression can complicate grief in two ways: It can produce short-term symptoms that are more severe than those typically associated with grief, and it can cause symptoms of grief to be more intense and to persist longer than normal.

There's no specific treatment for grief, other than time. The grief process can take a year or more. During this time it's important to surround yourself with people who are supportive. If your grief is severe or lasts longer, it may be complicated by depression. Studies suggest that another difference between grief and depression is self-denigration. People who are depressed often have feelings of worthlessness, but people who are grieving usually don't have such feelings.

may have more than one type of depression.

Major depression

Major depression is the most common form of the illness. It's characterized by a mood change that lasts more than two weeks and includes one or both of the primary signs of depression — overwhelming feelings of sadness or grief and loss of interest in usually pleasurable activities. People with major depression also experience at least five of the following signs and symptoms regularly, if not daily:
• Sleep disturbance
• Slowed or restless movement
• Fatigue or loss of energy
• Low self-esteem or inappropriate guilt
• Feelings of worthlessness, helplessness or hopelessness
• Impaired thinking or concentration

• Significant weight loss or gain
• Loss of sexual desire
• Recurrent thoughts of death or suicide

You may experience major depression only once, or it may return. After your first bout of major depression, you have more than a 50 percent chance of having it again, and the odds of recurrence increase with each episode.

If not treated, episodes typically last from six to 18 months. Early treatment may keep depression from becoming more severe. Continued treatment can keep it from coming back.

Seasonal affective disorder

Seasonal affective disorder (SAD) is the term for depressive periods that correspond with the change of seasons. This disorder is more than simply cabin fever.

No one knows for certain what causes SAD. Some researchers believe that a lack of daylight disrupts your circadian rhythms, which regulate your body's internal clock. SAD is more common in places where daylight hours are seasonally limited. People with SAD usually notice mood changes starting in late fall, with improvement in spring. But some people experience summer depression.

SAD usually begins in adolescence or young adulthood and is more common in women than in men. You may have the condition if you've experienced depression and related symptoms during at least two consecutive winters, followed by non-depressed periods in the spring and summer.

Individuals with SAD generally sleep more in the winter and gain some weight. Some may become irritable and feel low on energy.

Persistent depressive disorder
Persistent depressive disorder (PDO) is a less severe but a more chronic form of depression. While it's usually not disabling, PDO can prevent normal daily functioning and living life to its fullest. PDO is characterized by a persistently gloomy outlook as well as overwhelming feelings of sadness or grief and loss of interest in usually enjoyable activities.

PDO generally lasts for at least two years and sometimes more than five years. Depressive periods may alternate with brief intervals of feeling normal. The condition can interfere with work and social life. Many people with PDO become socially withdrawn and less productive. Individuals with this condition also have a greater risk of developing major depression.

Signs and symptoms of PDO are like those of major depression but not as intense, and you may not experience as many of them. They may include:
- Social withdrawal
- Difficulty concentrating or making decisions
- Irritability
- Restlessness or sluggishness
- Problems sleeping
- Weight gain or loss

Some people with PDO first experience feelings of depression in childhood or adolescence. Others develop the disorder later in life, often after a medical illness.

Adjustment disorder
An adjustment disorder is a severe emotional reaction to a difficult event in your life — a response that may be out of proportion to what's considered normal but less than an episode of major depression. It's a type of stress-related mental illness that may affect your feelings, thoughts and behavior.

Postpartum Depression

Many women experience temporary feelings of sadness after childbirth. These so-called baby blues tend to gradually diminish and usually don't require treatment. Some women, though, experience a form of major depression after childbirth called postpartum depression. Compared with those of the baby blues, the signs and symptoms of this type of depression are more severe and persistent. An episode of postpartum depression increases the likelihood that you'll have recurrent bouts of major depression or another mental illness after subsequent births or at other times.

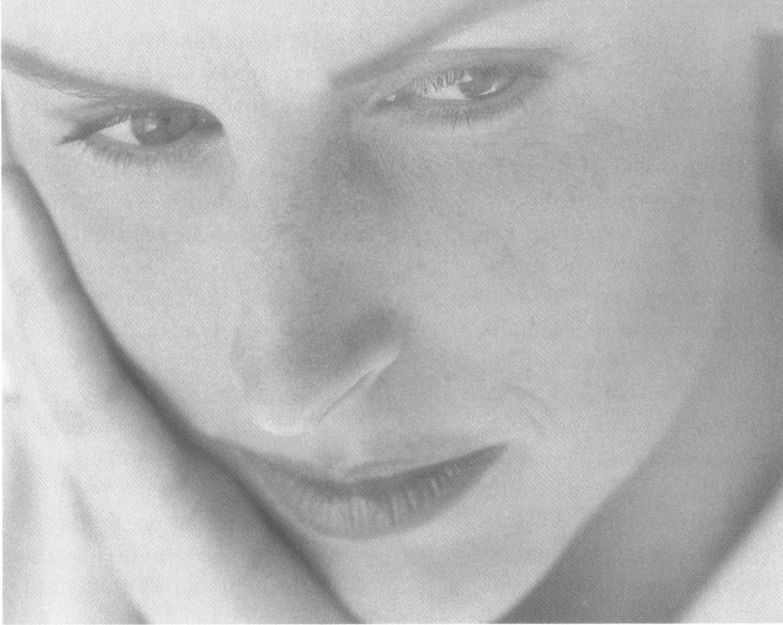

One or more stressful life events may put you at risk of developing adjustment disorder. Some common examples include a serious illness, divorce, job loss or financial problems. Sometimes the stressful change in your life goes away, and symptoms of adjustment disorder get better on their own. But often, the stressful event remains part of your life. Or a new stressor arises, and you face the same emotional struggles all over again.

There are six main types of adjustment disorders. Although they're all related, each type has certain signs and symptoms.
- **Adjustment disorder with depressed mood.** Symptoms mainly include feeling sad, tearful and hopeless and having a lack of pleasure in the things you used to enjoy.
- **Adjustment disorder with anxiety.** Symptoms mainly include nervousness, worry, difficulty concentrating or remembering things, and feeling overwhelmed. Children who have adjustment disorder with anxiety may strongly fear being separated from their parents and loved ones.
- **Adjustment disorder with mixed anxiety and depressed mood.** Symptoms include a mix of depression and anxiety.
- **Adjustment disorder with disturbance of conduct.** Symptoms mainly involve behavioral problems, such as fighting, reckless driving or ignoring your bills. Youngsters may skip school or vandalize property.
- **Adjustment disorder with mixed disturbance of emotions and conduct.** Symptoms include

Depression and Other Mental Illnesses

Depression often accompanies other mental illnesses, most commonly anxiety disorders, eating disorders and substance abuse. For example, up to 50 percent of individuals who are depressed experience anxiety, and 50 to 75 percent of people with an eating disorder have a history of depression.

Of people who abuse alcohol, about 30 percent meet the criteria for depression. Experts speculate that some people who abuse alcohol or drugs may be trying to self-medicate or "normalize" their neurotransmitters in an attempt to feel better. But even moderate amounts of alcohol or other substances can cause depression or increase its severity.

The intermingling and intensity of symptoms in combined mental disorders can present challenges and obstacles to diagnosis and treatment. The only way to untangle the interdependence of combined disorders is to recognize and treat both conditions. One way you can help yourself is to be honest and forthcoming when you discuss your symptoms with your doctor or a mental health professional. This can help greatly in recognizing combined disorders and determining the best treatment approach.

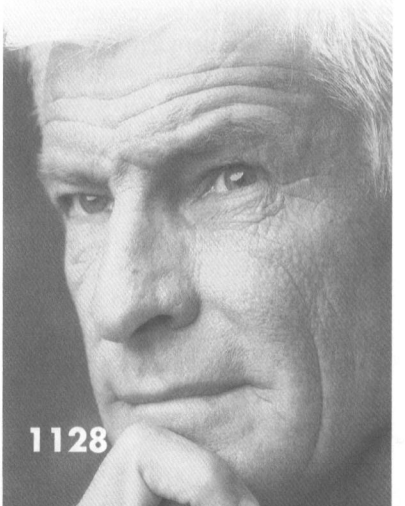

a mix of depression and anxiety as well as behavioral problems.

- **Adjustment disorder unspecified.** Symptoms don't fit the other types of adjustment disorders but often include physical problems, problems with family or friends, or work or school problems.

The main type of treatment for an adjustment disorder is psychotherapy (see page 1151).

Bipolar disorder

Bipolar disorder is a mental health condition that causes extreme mood changes that include emotional highs (mania or hypomania) and lows (depression). The disorder can affect sleep, energy, activity, judgment, behavior and the ability to think clearly.

Episodes — extreme highs or extreme lows — may occur rarely or several times a year.

Bipolar disorder isn't as common as major depression or dysthymia. The illness typically emerges in adolescence or young adulthood and continues intermittently throughout life. It often runs in families. Both men and women are equally at risk.

There are degrees of mania. During a manic phase, you may feel unstoppable. You might spend money recklessly or make unwise decisions, which may include promiscuous or reckless behavior. Some people experience bursts of increased creativity and productivity during a manic phase.

Signs and symptoms include:
- Abnormal or excessive elation
- Markedly increased energy
- A decreased need for sleep
- Unusual irritability
- Unrealistic beliefs in one's abilities and powers
- Increased talkativeness
- Racing thoughts
- Poor judgment
- Increased sexual desire
- Provocative, intrusive or aggressive social behavior
- Abuse of alcohol or other substances

Your manic or hypomanic state might not be obvious to those who don't know you well, but friends and loved ones may come to recognize it as typical of the manic phase. Your speech and thoughts seem to run at high speed and things you say may make little sense to anyone but you.

A major depressive episode, on the other hand, includes symptoms that are severe enough to cause noticeable difficulty in day-to-day activities, such as work, school, social activities or relationships.

Signs and symptoms of bipolar disorder tend to become more severe over time, if the disease goes untreated. You may start out with episodes of depression, mania or a mixture of both moods, separated by periods with no symptoms. Over time, episodes of mania and depression become more frequent, with shorter normal periods. Severe depression or elation may be accompanied by psychosis, including hallucinations and delusions.

The different forms of bipolar disorder are classified by their severity and symptom patterns. As with other forms of depression, it's critical to get treatment early to prevent the illness from progressing and to decrease the risk of suicide.

Others

Other forms of depression include:
- **Cyclothymia.** Cyclothymia (cyclothymic disorder) is a milder form of bipolar disorder.
- **Postpartum depression.** It occurs in a new mother, usually within a month of having a baby (see page 130).
- **Psychotic depression.** This is severe depression accompanied by psychosis, such as delusions or hallucinations.
- **Schizoaffective disorder.** Schizoaffective disorder is a condition in which a person meets the criteria for both schizophrenia and a mood disorder.

Light Therapy for SAD

Light therapy (phototherapy) is a common treatment for seasonal affective disorder (SAD). The therapy consists of exposure to intense light under specified conditions. The lighting system most often used is a box that you set on a table or desktop. The box contains a set of special fluorescent bulbs with a diffusing screen to help block out ultraviolet rays, which can cause cataracts and skin problems.

Treatment involves sitting near the light box with the lights on and your eyes open. You shouldn't look directly at the light, but you want your head and body oriented so that the light can enter your eyes. Researchers believe that when bright light enters your eyes, it has antidepressant-like effects, causing changes in brain chemical activity in certain areas of the brain.

Light therapy improves symptoms in about 3 out of 4 people with SAD. Many people begin to feel better in a few days, but symptoms often reappear if therapy is stopped. It's important that light therapy be monitored by a health care professional.

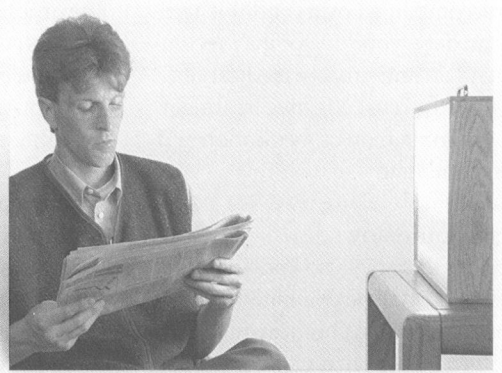

Phototherapy for seasonal affective disorder involves sitting near a bright light for a specified period each day. You shouldn't stare at the light, but you want the light to enter your eyes.

Diagnosis

When doctors suspect depression, they typically run a battery of medical and psychological tests and exams. These can help rule out other problems that could be causing your symptoms, pinpoint a diagnosis and also check for any related complications. These exams and tests generally include:

- **Physical exam.** This may include measuring height and weight; checking vital signs, such as heart rate, blood pressure and temperature; listening to the heart and lungs; and examining the abdomen.
- **Laboratory tests.** These may include a complete blood count (CBC), screening for alcohol and drugs, and a check of your thyroid function.
- **Psychological evaluation.** A doctor or mental health provider will talk to you about your thoughts, feelings and behavior patterns. He or she will ask about your symptoms, including when they started, how severe they are, how they affect your daily life and whether you've had similar episodes in the past. It's important to discuss any thoughts you may have of suicide or self-harm. You also may be asked to fill out a questionnaire.

Treatment

Once depression is diagnosed, it's crucial that you seek treatment. Untreated depression can raise your risk of a number of other health conditions. Studies show that even mild depression may be associated with poor physical and social functioning, increased risk of future depression, and suicide attempts.

From medications to psychotherapy, many options are available for treating depression, and each can play an important role. Just as the cause of depression may be a complex interplay of factors, finding the most effective treatment for your illness can be a complex process that takes time and professional guidance.

Medication

Antidepressant medications are often the first line of treatment for depression (see page 1149). Antidepressants can relieve symptoms, but they can cause side effects. Many types are available. If one doesn't work for you, another may.

The initial goal of treatment is to relieve signs and symptoms. When you start taking an antidepressant, you may not notice a change for three weeks or longer. It's important not to feel discouraged and to keep taking the medication even if it seems to be having no effect. Once your signs and symptoms have eased — often not all at once — use of medication (maintenance treatment) typically continues for nine to 12 months to prevent a relapse. Even though you may feel fine, it's important to keep taking your medication as prescribed. If you've had recurrent episodes of depression, your doctor may recommend that you continue taking medication longer — perhaps for years. Episodes of depression recur in more than 50 percent of people who've had one episode. The longer you stay on medication, the less likely it is that depression will recur.

Depending on the type of depression you have, your doctor may recommend a second medication in addition to an antidepressant. Mood stabilizers are used to treat bipolar disorder. If your depression is accompanied by a condition such as anxiety, your doctor may recommend an anti-anxiety medication. Often, the most effective treatment is a combination of medication and psychotherapy.

Psychotherapy

Psychotherapy, also known as talk therapy, may be combined with medication. Psychotherapy involves help from a mental health professional through a combination of talking and listening. Psychotherapy can help you understand the source of your feelings and find better ways of coping with problems and conflicts.

When you're acutely depressed, psychotherapy can provide support during the time needed for your medication to take effect. As symptoms improve, psychotherapy can help you understand why the depression occurred and what you can do to prevent a recurrence.

Several different types of psychotherapy are used to treat depression. For more information, see page 1151.

Others

Other treatments for depression are discussed beginning on page 1152. They include:
- Electroconvulsive therapy (ECT)
- Transcranial magnetic stimulation (TMS)
- Vagus nerve stimulation

Depression and suicide

More than 40,000 Americans die by suicide each year. Many more people attempt to kill themselves.

Most individuals who die by suicide have one or more mental illnesses, most commonly depression. The more severe the depression — especially if it's untreated or inadequately treated — the greater the suicide risk.

Several warning signs indicate that someone may be at risk of suicide. Many of the warning signs are also features of depression, and it can be difficult to determine if they represent suicidal intentions or are symptoms of depression.

If you or someone you know displays any of the following warning signs of potential suicide, seek professional help:
- **Suicidal threats.** Sometimes, an individual will tell others outright that he or she is thinking of committing suicide. The person may say things such as, "I wish I'd never been born," "I'd be better off dead," or "You'll be better off when I'm gone." The common assumption that people who threaten suicide don't do it isn't true.
- **Withdrawing from others.** People at risk of suicide often are less willing to communicate with others or may want to be left alone. Trouble at work or poor grades also can be signs of withdrawal.
- **Moodiness.** We all have our ups and downs. But drastic mood swings — an emotional high one day and deep discouragement the next — aren't typical.
- **Difficulty with a personal crisis.** A major life crisis, such as a divorce, a job loss or the death of a loved one, can be difficult for anyone to manage. Among people who are depressed, such a crisis can push them over the edge, triggering a suicide attempt.
- **Personality changes.** Before someone attempts suicide, he or she may exhibit marked changes in personality and routines, such as eating or sleeping patterns. For example, an outgoing person may become withdrawn. You might notice a change in his or her energy level or attitude toward personal appearance.
- **Displays of risky behavior.** Uncharacteristically dangerous activities, such as high-speed driving, unsafe sex or drug abuse, can be signs of a desire to die.
- **Giving away possessions.** Sometimes, a person who is considering suicide begins to give away cherished belongings, believing they won't be needed any longer.

If someone has been struggling with depression for a long period, the start of treatment may be the first time that he or she sees the problems his or her depression has caused. However, starting treatment doesn't necessarily mean suicidal worries are over.

Anxiety Disorders

Everyone has moments of anxiety, worry and fear. It's common to feel your stomach churn after a disagreement with your boss or if your child is late getting home. Feeling anxious about the future during a recession is a common reaction.

A moderate amount of anxiety is essential for human survival. It helps you respond appropriately to real danger, and it may help motivate you to excel at work and at home. But when worries or fears center on events that are unlikely to occur and when they consume your life and dictate your actions, you've moved beyond reasonable levels of anxiety. You may not even know what's causing your distress, or the source of your anxiety may seem minor compared with the intensity of your reaction. Severe anxiety can be a symptom of or a form of mental illness. Anxiety that affects your daily life is called an anxiety disorder.

Anxiety disorders are some of the most common mental health disorders, affecting a number of U.S. adults. About twice as many women as men are affected. Some personality types are more prone to anxiety disorders, and the disorders tend to run in families.

Anxiety may be associated with another medical illness, such as a thyroid condition or cardiovas-

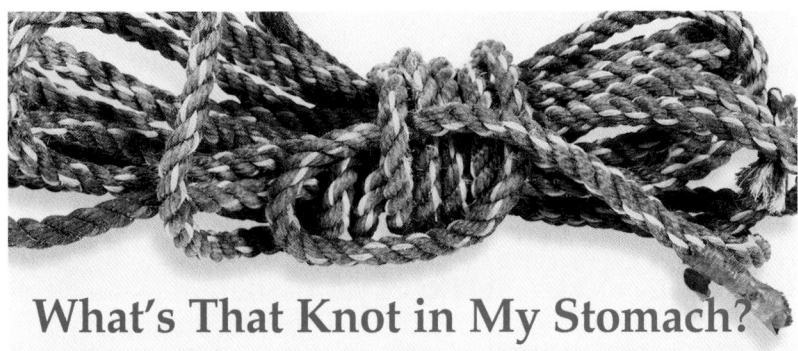

What's That Knot in My Stomach?

Stress or anxiety can bring on not only a tension headache but also tension in your gut. Muscles in the wall of your stomach and intestines may suddenly contract, giving you the feeling of a knot, much like a muscle cramp in your leg.

This may cause discomfort or pain, but it isn't serious. As your anxiety lessens, the feeling usually goes away. If the knot is persistent or intense or if you also have nausea, vomiting, diarrhea or difficulty swallowing, see your doctor. These signs and symptoms could indicate some other problem.

- Gastrointestinal distress, such as diarrhea
- Sweating
- Dry mouth
- Dizziness
- Restlessness or an inability to relax
- Irritability or impatience
- Problems sleeping
- Difficulty concentrating

Your signs and symptoms may become long term (chronic) and progressively worse if you don't receive appropriate help. Treatment for an anxiety disorder — which may include cognitive behavioral therapy, exercise, meditation and other relaxation techniques — can be highly effective at calming or eliminating many of your signs and symptoms.

cular disease. Anxiety disorders frequently occur in combination with depression. About half of all people with depression experience anxiety. When their depression is treated, their anxiety often improves as well.

The stress response

Scientists are mapping circuits and structures of the nervous system that are prominent in mental disorders such as anxiety. They believe that the almond-shaped structure in the temporal lobe of the brain (amygdala) may transmit emotions and sensations that constitute anxiety. The amygdala picks up and processes signals from areas of the brain that sense danger.

Evidence suggests that the amygdala sends signals to parts of the nervous system that perceive fear and prompt the stress (fight-or-flight) response. Nerve cells (neurons) in the amygdala and other regions of the brain secrete a hormone known as corticotropin-releasing factor (CRF). CRF turns on a cascade of other hormones that cause signs and symptoms often associated with the stress response, such as a

pounding heart, rapid breathing, increased sweating, a dry mouth, increased blood pressure and tense muscles. You may also experience nausea or diarrhea.

When anxiety gets out of control, this response can occur almost continuously or even during low levels of stress. It can also occur during periods of calm. Why this happens isn't fully understood. One theory is that an anxiety disorder may develop after you experience one or more very fearful events that trigger the fight-or-flight response. The deeply etched memory of the event may prime you to become hypervigilant and to overreact to everyday situations.

Signs and symptoms

Signs and symptoms vary depending on the type of anxiety disorder you have. Physical signs and symptoms triggered by the stress response are common in many anxiety disorders. These include:
- Muscle tension
- A rapid heartbeat
- Rapid breathing or the feeling that you can't get enough air
- Tremors

Types

Anxiety may accompany depression, or it may develop as a separate disorder.

Generalized anxiety disorder

One of the most common anxiety disorders is generalized anxiety disorder. With this condition, your general approach to life is an anxious one. You may be high-strung or nervous and feel anxious most of the time, usually without a readily identifiable cause. You may be plagued by a sense of self-doubt and indecisiveness and have a nagging feeling that something bad is about to happen. You worry about your kids, your job or your health for no apparent reason. You may feel tense all of the time, making it difficult to function at home or at work. While you may feel anxious all or most of the time, stress tends to make your symptoms worse.

If you have this condition, you may have trouble sleeping and wake up feeling wired. You may experience fatigue, exhaustion, muscle tension, irritability, chest pain, a lump in your throat, fast breathing, stomachache, diarrhea, headaches, dry mouth or sweaty palms.

Generalized anxiety disorder can begin at any age and may continue throughout your life. In children and adolescents with the disorder, their worries often center on their performance at school or in sports. In older adults, generalized anxiety often coincides with depression.

Adjustment disorder with anxiety

An adjustment disorder with anxiety occurs when your response to a stressful situation causes signs and symptoms of anxiety, such as nervousness, worry or jitteriness. The stressor may be a single event, such as the end of a romantic relationship, or multiple events. Most people eventually come to terms with the consequences of such stress, but the process takes longer for people with an adjustment disorder.

Adjustment disorders can affect anybody. They often occur at a time in your life when you're more vulnerable — when you move away from your parents or at the end of your career, for instance.

Panic disorder

A panic disorder typically includes recurrent episodes of terror that strike suddenly and repeatedly with no warning and often for no reason. During a panic attack your heart may race, you may sweat or hyperventilate, and you may feel weak, faint or dizzy. The physical symptoms are so intense that you may think you're dying or losing your mind. Symptoms can mimic a heart attack. You may have chest pain, shortness of breath or a feeling that you're being smothered. You may experience a sense of unreality or of losing control.

Attacks can occur at home or in public, and they can even awaken you from a deep sleep. An attack typically lasts only a few minutes but may go on for up to 10 minutes or longer. You may feel fatigued and worn out after it subsides.

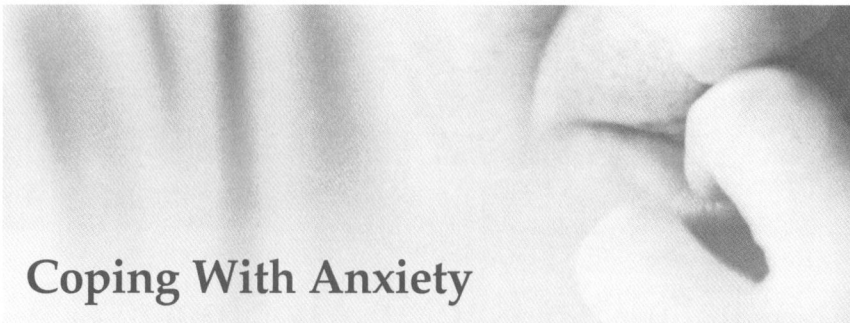

Coping With Anxiety

To deal with everyday anxiety, whatever the cause, try these strategies:
- *Take action.* Determine what's making you anxious and address it. For example, if you're worried about finances, draw up a budget.
- *Let it go.* Try not to dwell on past concerns. Change what you can and let the rest take its course.
- *Break the cycle.* When you feel anxious, take a brisk walk or delve into a hobby.
- *Take care of yourself.* Get enough rest, eat a balanced diet, exercise and take time to relax. Avoid caffeine and nicotine, which can worsen anxiety. Don't turn to alcohol or unprescribed drugs.
- *Talk to someone.* Share your problems with a friend or counselor who can help you gain perspective.

Because the attacks are unpredictable, people with a panic disorder often develop intense anxiety or lingering worry about the possibility of having another attack at any time. About half the people with panic disorder develop condition in which you become afraid to leave your home or visit the place where the spells first occurred (agoraphobia). In addition, about half the people who experience panic attacks experience at least one episode of depression.

Many people experience a panic attack at some time in life, but a much smaller number of people have true panic disorder. Panic disorder tends to run in families.

Without treatment, panic disorder can become debilitating and destructive. Fear of recurrent attacks can cause you to adopt avoidance behavior, such as refusing to go shopping or to leave the house by yourself.

Phobias

A phobia is a persistent, irrational fear of an object or a situation. You may be afraid of enclosed spaces, bridges, heights, flying, or creatures such as snakes or spiders. Even though you understand that your fear is excessive or unwarranted, you try to avoid the object of your phobia at all costs.

It's normal to feel some discomfort about certain objects or situations. But if your fears become irrational and uncontrollable and your avoidance of the feared object affects your social interactions and daily activities, you may have a phobia.

Fears of animals and other objects are common in childhood but usually pass. Such fears aren't categorized as phobias unless they impair the child's functioning — for example, if the child refuses to go to school for fear of encountering a dog on the street.

When exposed to the feared object or situation, a person with a phobia becomes panicky and has signs and symptoms similar to those experienced with panic disorder. Just anticipating an encounter with the feared object may provoke feelings of intense anxiety, so you go out of your way to avoid what you fear.

Social anxiety disorder

Everyone feels nervous from time to time. Going on a first date or giving a speech often prompts a queasy stomach. But for some people, nervousness mushrooms into extreme fear. Everyday activities such as starting a conversation, eating with others or attending a party become impossible. This condition is known as social anxiety disorder (social phobia).

You may receive a diagnosis of social anxiety disorder if your fears significantly interfere with your day-to-day life or cause significant distress. You may become anxious when you're around people you don't know, or you may fear a particular situation, such as talking in front of others.

Common, everyday experiences such as using a public restroom or telephone, returning items to a store, writing in front of others, making eye contact, or ordering food in a restaurant can cause severe anxiety.

Social anxiety disorder typically starts in the teenage years or after a stressful or humiliating experience. It can vary in intensity over the course of a person's life but generally is lifelong. As with other anxiety disorders, it appears to have a hereditary component.

Obsessive-compulsive disorder

No longer classified as an anxiety disorder, obsessive-compulsive disorder (OCD) is a disorder in which you have unreasonable thoughts and fears (obsessions) that lead you to engage in repetitive behaviors (compulsions). With obsessive-compulsive disorder, you may realize that your obsessions aren't reasonable, and you may try to ignore them or stop them. But that only increases your distress and anxiety. Ultimately, you feel driven to perform compulsive acts in an effort to ease your distress.

Obsessive-compulsive disorder often centers around a theme, such as a fear of getting contaminated by germs. To ease your contamination fears, you may compulsively wash your hands until they're sore and chapped. Despite your efforts, the distressing thoughts of obsessive-compulsive disorder keep coming back. This leads to more ritualistic behavior — and a vicious cycle that's characteristic of obsessive-compulsive disorder.

Common obsessions include:
- Fear of dirt or contamination
- Concern with order, symmetry and exactness
- Constant thoughts about certain sounds, images, words or numbers
- Fear of harming a family member or friend
- Fear of thinking thoughts you consider evil or sinful
- Worry about making a mistake

Compulsions are repetitive behaviors that you're driven to perform regularly to combat your obsessions. Typical compulsions include:
- Washing hands excessively
- Checking repeatedly that doors are locked and appliances are turned off
- Arranging items in a precise order
- Counting over and over to a certain number
- Touching certain objects several times

If you have obsessive-compulsive disorder, you may do everything

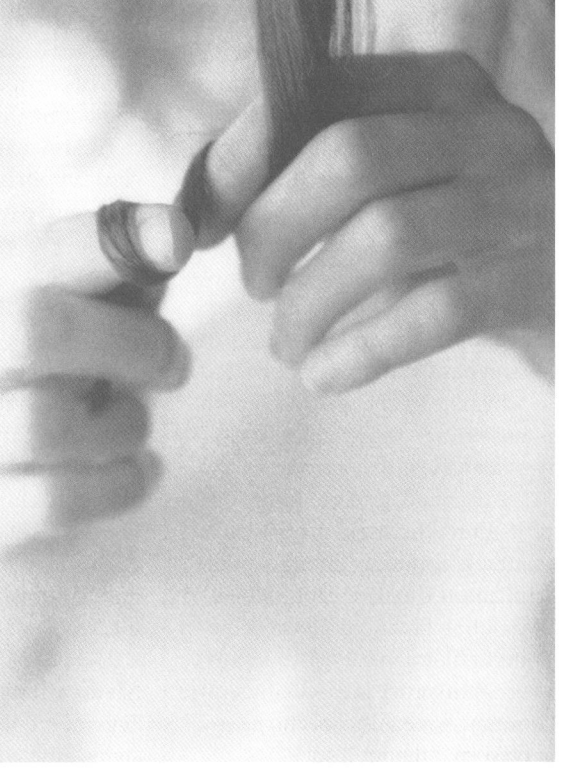

Perfectionism or Obsessive-Compulsive Disorder?

There's a difference between being a perfectionist and having obsessive-compulsive disorder. Perhaps you get your work done ahead of schedule, your hair is never out of place, and the floors in your house are so clean that you could eat off them. That doesn't mean you have obsessive-compulsive disorder. Instead, you may belong to the group of people who hold themselves to a very high standard in all that they do. This behavior can build self-esteem and success. In contrast, behaviors associated with obsessive-compulsive disorder interfere with normal functioning, such as repeatedly checking that the doors are locked and appliances turned off before you leave the house.

Sometimes the distinction isn't so clear. You may feel that your perfectionism isn't extreme, but family members disagree. They claim that your behavior is excessive. In such cases, it may be useful to get an evaluation from a mental health professional.

in a meticulous, precise, orderly fashion. If the compulsive need isn't fulfilled, you may experience over-whelming anxiety. When you perform these rituals, you may feel some relief from anxiety, but not for long. Your discomfort soon returns, and you feel compelled to repeat the behaviors.

You realize that your repetitive thoughts and behaviors are irrational and senseless, but you can't free yourself from them. You may be able to control the unwanted behaviors for a while, but your resistance may weaken after months or years of struggle. Eventually, your rituals may take up more of your time, making it difficult to lead a typical life.

OCD treatment can help you bring symptoms under control so that they don't rule your daily life. The two main treatments for obsessive-compulsive disorder are psychotherapy (see page 1151) and medication (see page 1149).

Post-traumatic stress disorder

As the name implies, post-traumatic stress disorder (PTSD) is a form of anxiety disorder triggered by a traumatic experience that you lived through or witnessed.

The disorder may affect survivors of sexual assault, physical abuse, war, torture, natural disasters, automobile accidents, airplane crashes, hostage situations or death camps. It can also affect rescue workers at an airplane crash or mass shooting or someone who witnessed a traumatic accident. Whatever the trauma, the person has lived through a period in which he or she was faced with intense fear, a sense of helplessness and a loss of control.

People of all ages can have post-traumatic stress disorder. It's relatively common among adults, with about 7 to 8 percent of the population having PTSD at some point in their lives. Post-traumatic stress disorder is especially common among those who have served in combat.

Post-traumatic stress disorder shares many of the same signs and symptoms of depression. The major difference is that with post-traumatic stress disorder, you continue to have prominent memories and intrusive thoughts of the event or events that initially triggered the disorder.

Signs and symptoms typically appear within three months of the traumatic event. In some instances, they may not occur until years later and may include:

- Flashbacks, disturbing dreams and hallucinations
- Shame or guilt
- Upsetting dreams about the traumatic event
- Trouble sleeping
- Trying to avoid thinking or talking about the traumatic event
- Feeling emotionally numb
- Irritability or anger
- Poor relationships
- Hopelessness about the future
- Trouble concentrating
- Being easily startled or frightened
- Hearing or seeing things that aren't there

Having post-traumatic stress disorder may also place you at a higher risk of other conditions such as drug abuse, alcohol abuse and eating disorders.

Treatment for PTSD often includes both medication (see page 1149) and psychotherapy (see page 1151).

Treatment

Treatment for an anxiety disorder depends on the type of disorder you have. With treatment most people with anxiety disorders are able to resume everyday activities. For the most effective results, your doctor may recommend a combination of medication and psychotherapy.

Medications

Several medications may relieve signs and symptoms of anxiety:

Antidepressants

Many drugs used to treat depression also have anti-anxiety effects. In fact, antidepressants are the treatment of choice for some anxiety disorders. Examples of antidepressant drugs used to treat anxiety include fluoxetine (Prozac, Sarafem), paroxetine (Paxil, Brisdelle) and imipramine (Tofranil). For more on these medications, see page 1149.

Anti-anxiety medications

Anti-anxiety medications include a class of tranquilizing drugs called benzodiazepines, as well as the medication buspirone (BuSpar, Vanspar). See page 1151 for more information.

Beta blockers

These medications work by blocking the stimulating effect of adrenaline (epinephrine). They may reduce heart rate, blood pressure, pounding of the heart, and shaking voice and limbs. Because of that, they may be used infrequently to control symptoms for a particular situation, such as giving a speech. They're not recommended for general treatment of anxiety disorder.

Psychotherapy

Types of psychotherapy that are especially effective in treating anxiety disorders are cognitive behavioral therapy, relaxation therapy, and desensitization and exposure therapy. These therapies are discussed on page 1151.

Adult ADHD

Adult attention-deficit/hyperactivity disorder (ADHD) is a mental health disorder that includes a combination of persistent problems, such as difficulty paying attention, hyperactivity and impulsive behavior. Adult ADHD can lead to unstable relationships, poor work or school performance, low self-esteem, and other problems.

Signs and symptoms

Adult ADHD symptoms include:
- Impulsiveness
- Disorganization and problems prioritizing
- Poor time management skills
- Problems focusing on a task
- Trouble multitasking
- Excessive activity or restlessness
- Poor planning
- Low frustration tolerance
- Frequent mood swings
- Problems following through and completing tasks
- Hot temper
- Trouble coping with stress

Though it's called adult ADHD, symptoms start in early childhood and continue into adulthood. In some people, ADHD isn't recognized or diagnosed until the person is an adult. Adult ADHD symptoms may not be as clear as ADHD symptoms in children. In adults, hyperactivity may decrease, but struggles with impulsiveness, restlessness and difficulty paying attention may continue.

Many adults with ADHD aren't aware they have it — they just know that everyday tasks can be a challenge. Adults with ADHD may find it difficult to focus and prioritize, leading to missed deadlines and forgotten meetings or social plans. The inability to control impulses can range from impatience waiting in line or driving in traffic to mood swings and outbursts of anger.

Treatment

Standard treatments for ADHD in adults typically involve medication, education, training and psychological counseling. A combination of these is often the most effective treatment. These treatments can relieve many symptoms of ADHD, but they don't cure it. It may take some time to determine what works best for you.

Medications

Stimulant medications that include methylphenidate (Ritalin, Concerta) or amphetamine are commonly prescribed to treat adult ADHD. Stimulants appear to boost and balance levels of brain chemicals called neurotransmitters.

Other medications used to treat ADHD include the nonstimulant atomoxetine (Strattera) and certain antidepressants such as bupropion (Wellbutrin XL, Wellbutrin SR). Atomoxetine and antidepressants work slower than stimulants do, but these may be good options if you can't take stimulants because of health problems or a history of substance abuse or if stimulants cause severe side effects.

Psychotherapy

Types of psychotherapy include:
- **Cognitive behavioral therapy.** This structured type of counseling teaches specific skills to manage your behaviors and thinking patterns. It can help you deal with life challenges, such as work, school or relationship problems.
- **Marital counseling and family therapy.** This type of therapy can help loved ones cope with the stress of living with someone who has ADHD and learn what they can do to help. Such counseling can improve communication and problem-solving skills.

Psychotherapy may help you improve your time management and organizational skills, develop better problem-solving skills, and improve your self-esteem.

Substance and Nonsubstance Use Disorders

Substance use and nonsubstance use disorders involve behavioral patterns in which people continue to use a substance or take part in

an activity despite experiencing problems from its use or involvement. The disorders can result in health problems, financial problems, disability, and failure to meet responsibilities at work, school or home. Substance use and nonsubstance use disorders are often referred to in the general public as addictive behaviors.

Substance and nonsubstance use disorders — which may be mild, moderate or severe — are based on evidence of impaired control, social impairment, risky use and pharmacological criteria.

Substance and nonsubstance use disorders can occur in combination with other mental illnesses. Studies indicate that more than half the people who abuse alcohol or drugs have another mental illness or have experienced one in the past. Contrary to that, depression may be the result of several years of addiction.

Substance use disorders

Following are some of the most common substance use disorders.

Alcohol use disorder
Alcohol use disorder (which includes a level often called alcoholism) is a pattern of alcohol use that involves problems controlling your drinking, being preoccupied with alcohol, continuing to use alcohol even when it causes problems, having to drink more to get the same effect, or having withdrawal symptoms when you rapidly decrease or stop drinking.

Alcohol use disorder can be mild, moderate or severe, based on the number of symptoms you experience. Signs and symptoms may include:
- Being unable to limit the amount of alcohol you drink
- Wanting to cut down on how much you drink or making unsuccessful attempts to do so
- Spending a lot of time drinking, getting alcohol or recovering from alcohol use

Alcohol Intoxication

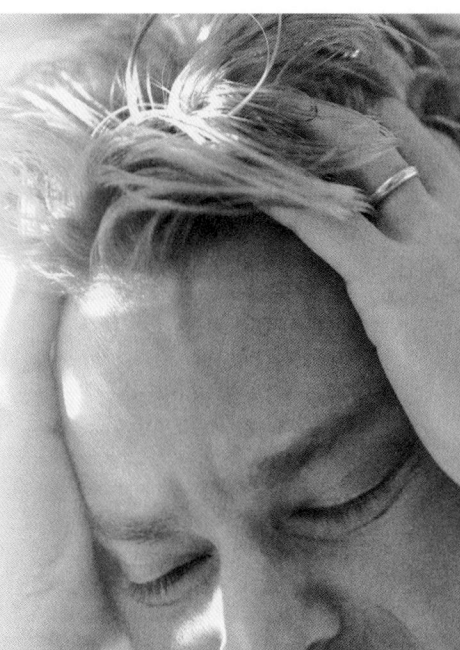

The form of alcohol in the beverages people drink is ethyl alcohol (ethanol). Ethanol is produced by the fermentation of sugars in grains and fruits such as barley and grapes.

The intoxicating effects of alcohol relate to the concentration of alcohol in the blood. For example, if you're not a regular drinker and your blood alcohol concentration is more than 100 milligrams of alcohol per deciliter of blood (100 mg/dL), you may be quite intoxicated and have difficulty speaking, thinking and moving around. Most states define legal intoxication as a blood alcohol concentration of at least 70 to 100 mg/dL — 0.07 to 0.10 percent.

Your response to alcohol is affected by how much food you've eaten and how recently you ate before drinking. Size, body fat and tolerance to the effects of alcohol also play significant roles. Women generally achieve a higher blood alcohol concentration per drink than men do because they tend to be smaller and experience quicker uptake of alcohol into the bloodstream, resulting in the alcohol being less diluted in their bodies. In addition, they may metabolize alcohol more slowly than do men.

- Feeling a strong craving or urge to drink alcohol
- Failing to fulfill major obligations at work, school or home due to repeated alcohol use
- Continuing to drink alcohol even though you know it's causing physical, social or interpersonal problems
- Giving up or reducing social and work activities and hobbies
- Using alcohol in situations where it's not safe, such as when driving or swimming
- Developing a tolerance to alcohol so you need more to feel its effect or you have a reduced effect from the same amount
- Experiencing withdrawal symptoms — such as nausea, sweating and shaking — when you don't drink, or drinking again to avoid these symptoms

Genetic, psychological, social and environmental factors can impact how drinking alcohol affects your body and behavior. Theories suggest that for certain people consuming alcohol has a different and stronger impact that can lead to alcohol use disorder.

Over time, drinking too much alcohol may change the function of the areas of your brain associated with the experience of pleasure, judgment and the ability to exercise control over your behavior.

This may result in craving alcohol to try to restore good feelings or reduce negative ones.

Treatment for alcohol use disorder can vary, depending on your needs. Treatment may involve a brief intervention, individual or group counseling, an outpatient program, or a residential inpatient stay. For more information on alcohol use disorder and treatment, see Chapter 11, "Unhealthy Behaviors."

Stimulant use disorder

Stimulants increase alertness, attention and energy, as well as elevate blood pressure, heart rate and respiration. Stimulants include both prescription medications and illegal substances. They can be manufactured synthetically, such as amphetamines, or plant-derived, such as cocaine.

Symptoms of stimulant use disorder include a craving for stimulants, failure to control their use, continued use despite interference with daily and social functioning, use of larger amounts over time, development of a tolerance to the substances, and withdrawal symptoms after stopping or reducing their use.

Continued use of stimulants appears to result from alteration in the reward pathways in the brain.

The drugs change the process by which nerve cells (neurons) in the brain use brain chemicals (neurotransmitters) to communicate. The changes vary with the type of drug that's used.

For more information on stimulant use and treatment, see Chapter 11, "Unhealthy Behaviors."

Opioid use disorder

Opioids reduce the perception of pain, but they can also produce several other effects within your body. Some people experience a euphoric response with opioid use. Opioids include illegal drugs such as heroin and legally available pain relievers such as oxycodone and hydrocodone. In individuals who misuse them, they can produce serious health problems.

Signs and symptoms of opioid use disorder include a strong desire for opioids, an inability to control their use, continued use despite interference with daily and social functioning, use of larger amounts over time, development of a tolerance to the substance, and withdrawal symptoms after stopping or reducing their use.

For more information on opioid use and treatment, see Chapter 11, "Unhealthy Behaviors" and Chapter 37, "Pain Management."

Tobacco use disorder

Nicotine, one of the key ingredients in tobacco products, can be as stimulating as cocaine. Nicotine — like cocaine — increases the amount of the brain chemical dopamine, which makes you feel good. Getting that dopamine boost is part of the addiction process.

Misuse of nicotine alters your mood. When you try to stop using nicotine, you may develop withdrawal signs and symptoms — irritability, a depressed mood, insomnia, restlessness, anxiety and a decreased ability to concentrate.

Indications that you may have a tobacco use disorder include:

- An inability to quit smoking or using products such as spit tobacco, despite a desire to stop
- Withdrawal symptoms if you stop smoking
- Smoking to avoid withdrawal symptoms
- Using up your supply of cigarettes or other nicotine-containing products faster than you expected
- Forgoing an activity because it takes place in an area where smoking is prohibited
- Continuing to smoke or use any nicotine-containing product despite having medical problems related to tobacco use

For more information on tobacco use disorder and treatment, see Chapter 11, "Unhealthy Behaviors."

Other substance use disorders

Other substances that can cause substance-related disorders include marijuana (cannabis); hallucinogens, such as LSD; sedatives, such as diazepam (Valium); inhalants, such as paint thinners and certain glues; and anabolic steroids.

Nonsubstance use disorders

Nonsubstance disorders include harmful activities that do not involve the use of a drug or other substance. These conditions are sometimes referred to as behavioral addictions.

Gambling disorder

Gambling disorder is the uncontrollable urge to keep gambling despite the toll it takes on your life. Gambling can stimulate the brain's reward system much like drugs or alcohol can, leading to misuse. If you have a problem with compulsive gambling, you may continually chase bets that lead to losses, hide your behavior, deplete savings, accumulate debt, or even resort to theft or fraud to support your disorder.

Gambling disorder is an impulse control disorder, meaning that you're unable to resist engaging in a behavior that's harmful to you or to someone else. People with impulse control disorders usually feel a sense of emotional arousal or excitement before engaging in the behavior, followed by initial pleasure and gratification, and then guilt or remorse.

Indications that you or someone you know may have a gambling disorder include:

- A preoccupation with gambling and constantly planning how to get more gambling money
- Needing to gamble with increasing amounts of money to get the same thrill
- Trying to control, cut back or stop gambling, without success
- Feeling restless or irritable when trying to cut down on gambling
- Gambling to escape problems or relieve feelings of helplessness, guilt, anxiety or depression

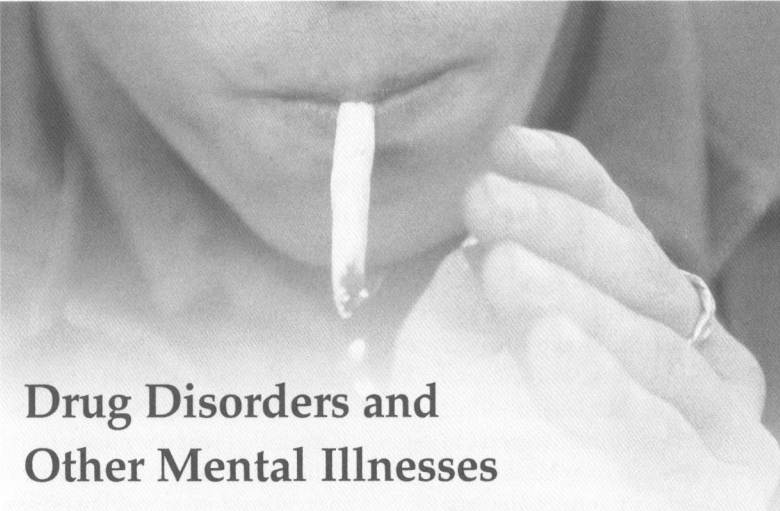

Drug Disorders and Other Mental Illnesses

A drug disorder may occur in conjunction with another mental illness, such as depression or schizophrenia. For successful recovery, it's critical that you receive an accurate diagnosis of and treatment for all relevant disorders.

It can be difficult to determine whether drug misuse is causing symptoms of mental illness or if the mental illness is prompting the drug disorder. Either way, drug disorders can worsen the symptoms of other mental illnesses and complicate treatment.

If symptoms of mental illness are strictly due to a substance misuse, they usually diminish within weeks after the person stops taking the substance. But it may take four to six months for the effects of a drug to resolve. Sometimes, the effects never fully disappear. People who've taken LSD, for example, may experience flashbacks for the rest of their lives. Ecstasy is another drug that may cause long-term mental effects.

It's helpful to work with a professional who has expertise in treating both substance misuse and mental illness.

Are You at Risk?

The following factors increase your risk of developing an eating disorder:

- *Gender.* Teenage girls and young women are more likely to develop eating disorders than are teenage boys and young men.
- *Age.* Although eating disorders can occur in midlife, they're most common among people in their teens and 20s.
- *Family influences.* People who feel less secure in their families — whose parents and siblings may be overly critical — are at higher risk.
- *Heredity.* Eating disorders are more common in people who have close family members with eating disorders.
- *Emotional disorders.* People with depression, anxiety disorders and obsessive-compulsive disorder are more likely to have an eating disorder.
- *Athletics.* People who participate in some athletic activities may be at greater risk of developing an eating disorder. Young women in sports such as gymnastics, ballet and figure skating are at particular risk of developing anorexia nervosa.

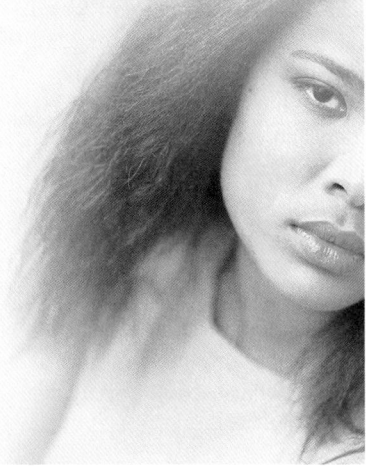

- Trying to get back lost money by gambling more (chasing losses)
- Lying to family members or others to hide the extent of gambling losses
- Jeopardizing or losing important relationships, a job, or school or work opportunities because of gambling
- Resorting to theft or fraud to get gambling money
- Asking others to bail you out of financial trouble because you gambled money away

Treatment

Treatment for compulsive gambling typically involves a combination of approaches:

- **Therapy.** Behavioral therapy or cognitive behavioral therapy may be beneficial. Behavior therapy uses systematic exposure to the behavior you want to unlearn and teaches you skills to reduce your urge to gamble. Cognitive behavioral therapy focuses on identifying unhealthy, irrational and negative beliefs and replacing them with healthy, positive ones.
- **Medications.** Antidepressants and mood stabilizers may help emotional issues that often go along with compulsive gambling, but not necessarily compulsive gambling itself. Medications called narcotic antagonists, which have been found useful in treating substance abuse, may help treat compulsive gambling.
- **Self-help groups.** Some people find that talking with others who have gambling problems is helpful in learning how to manage and live with the disorder. For many individuals, organizations such as Gamblers Anonymous are a key part of their treatment.

Other nonsubstance use disorders

Other disorders that fall under this classification include addictions to pornography, sex, shopping, technology and exercise.

Eating Disorders

Eating disorders are characterized by a preoccupation with weight that results in severe disturbances in eating behavior. In general, eating disorders, like other forms of mental illness, often involve a complex interplay of medical, psychological and social factors.

It's not easy to distinguish between an eating disorder and the whims and fads of adolescence. Most teenage girls, and some teenage boys, go on diets to lose weight and then stop dieting after two or three weeks. Binge eating and dieting aren't uncommon among teenage girls. These behaviors also occur, though not as frequently, among teenage boys.

General indications of an eating disorder include:

- Not wanting to eat meals with the family
- Frequent, lengthy visits to the bathroom during or just after meals — especially if running water is used to obscure the sound of induced vomiting
- Skipping meals
- Excessive exercise or preoccupation with weight and body image
- Weight loss or failure to gain weight

Types

The most common eating disorders are anorexia nervosa, bulimia nervosa and binge-eating disorder.

Anorexia nervosa

People with anorexia nervosa have a distorted body image and view themselves as fat even when they're underweight. They go to great lengths to keep a low body weight. They eat very little, often to the point of starvation, and may compulsively exercise. Individuals with anorexia nervosa often tend to be perfectionists.

Anorexia nervosa is most common in teenage girls and young women. The disorder occurs infrequently in adult women and males.

Left untreated, anorexia nervosa may result in serious medical complications or death. Signs and symptoms of anorexia nervosa include the following:

- Resistance to maintaining a healthy body weight
- An irrational fear of gaining weight
- An unrealistic view of body shape and size

Bulimia nervosa
Bulimia nervosa involves eating large amounts of food within a short period (bingeing) and then purging the food by vomiting or using enemas, laxatives or diuretics. Many people with this disorder also exercise compulsively. Between the bingeing and purging episodes, people with bulimia nervosa may restrict how much they eat.

Teenage girls and young women account for most instances of bulimia nervosa. Individuals with the disorder are more likely to act compulsively, and similar to individuals affected by anorexia nervosa, they tend to be preoccupied with weight and body image. Feelings of disgust or shame related to the illness can trigger further bulimic episodes, leading to the development of a vicious cycle. People with bulimia may be of normal weight or even obese. Excessive purging can cause potentially serious changes in body chemistry.

Binge-eating disorder
Binge eating involves a loss of control over eating behavior and the consumption of excessive amounts of food within a short time. The disorder is defined as having binge-eating episodes at least two days a week for at least six months. Unlike the bingeing associated with bulimia nervosa, the eating episodes in binge-eating

disorder aren't followed by purging or excessive exercise.

As with other eating disorders, people with binge-eating disorder are usually preoccupied with weight and food. The disorder is most common in adult, overweight women.

Causes

It's not known with certainty what causes eating disorders. As with other mental illnesses, the possible causes are complex, and they may result from an interaction of biological, psychological, family, genetic, environmental and social factors.

Possible causes of eating disorders include:

- **Biology.** Some people may be genetically vulnerable to developing eating disorders. Some studies show that people with biological siblings or parents with an eating disorder may develop one too, suggesting a possible genetic link. In addition, there's some evidence that serotonin, a naturally occurring brain chemical, may influence eating behaviors because of its connection to the regulation of food intake.
- **Psychological and emotional health.** People with eating disorders may have psychological and emotional characteristics that contribute to the disorder, such as perfectionism, impulsive behavior, low self-esteem, family conflicts and troubled relationships. These may vary from one eating disorder to another.
- **Socio-cultural issues.** Modern Western culture often cultivates and reinforces a desire for thinness. Success and worth are often equated with being thin. The media and entertainment industries often focus on appearance and body shape. Peer pressure may fuel this desire to be thin, particularly among young girls.

Complications

People with anorexia nervosa have a greater variety of health complications and a greater risk of death than do people with other eating disorders. However, any eating disorder can result in serious health problems. Possible complications include:

- **Heart disease.** Anorexia nervosa and bulimia nervosa can cause irregular heart rhythms. Heart complications are a common cause of death for people with anorexia.
- **Hormonal changes.** Changes in sex hormones and thyroid hormones can cause absence of menstruation (amenorrhea), infertility, bone loss and retarded growth.
- **Imbalance of minerals and electrolytes.** Your body needs adequate levels of minerals, particularly calcium and potassium, to maintain normal function of organs. Disruption of your body's fluid and mineral content can create an electrolyte imbalance that can be life-threatening.
- **Nerve damage.** Anorexia nervosa may cause brain and nerve damage, seizures, and loss of feeling in hands and feet.
- **Blood disorders.** Lack of nutrition can deplete your body's vitamin B-12, causing anemia.
- **Digestive problems.** Anorexia nervosa can cause constipation and bloating. Vomiting and purging may cause irritation of the walls of your esophagus and rectum.
- **Teeth and gum disease.** Gastric acid in your mouth from induced vomiting can damage your teeth and gums.
- **Drug dependence.** Over-the-counter drugs used during purge cycles may result in dependence on the drugs to keep the bowels working. These include laxatives, diuretics, appetite suppressants and ipecac syrup, a drug that induces vomiting.

- **Weight gain.** People with binge-eating disorder often are overweight, which raises the risk of diabetes, heart disease and other conditions.
- **Lowered self-esteem.** Binge eaters may feel self-loathing, shame or disgust about their eating pattern, leading to poor self-esteem.

Treatment

Treatment depends on the specific type of eating disorder. In general, treatment typically includes psychotherapy, nutrition education and medication. If your life is at risk due to lack of essential nutrients, you may need to be hospitalized to stabilize your health. Your treatment team may include medical doctors, mental health providers and dietitians.

Psychotherapy
Individual psychotherapy can help you learn how to exchange unhealthy habits for healthy ones. You learn how to monitor your eating and your moods, develop problem-solving skills, and explore healthy ways to cope with stressful situations. Psychotherapy can also help improve your relationships and your mood. A type of psychotherapy called cognitive behavioral therapy is commonly used in eating disorder treatment. Family therapy and group therapy is also helpful for many people.

Nutrition education
Dietitians and other medical providers can offer information about a healthy diet and help design an eating plan to achieve a healthy weight and healthy-eating habits. If you have binge-eating disorder, you may benefit from medically supervised weight-loss programs.

Hospitalization
If you have serious health problems or if you have anorexia and refuse to eat or gain weight, your doctor may recommend hospitalization. Hospitalization may be on a medical or psychiatric ward. Some clinics specialize in treating people with eating disorders. Some may offer day programs, rather than full hospitalization.

Medications
Medication can't cure an eating disorder. However, medications may help you control urges to binge or purge or to manage excessive preoccupations with food and diet. While medications such as antidepressants and anti-anxiety medications may help with symptoms of depression or anxiety, attaining and maintaining a healthy weight is the best way to manage mood symptoms in people with eating disorders.

Personality Disorders

Personality disorder is a general term for a type of mental illness in which your ways of thinking, perceiving situations and relating to others are dysfunctional. There are many specific types of personality disorders.

In general, having a personality disorder means you have a rigid and potentially self-destructive or self-denigrating pattern of thinking and behaving no matter what the situation. This leads to distress in your life or impairment of your ability to go about routine functions at work, at school or in social situations. In some cases, you may not realize that you have a problem because your way of thinking and behaving seems natural to you, and you may blame others for your circumstances.

Types

The specific types of personality disorders are grouped into three clusters based on similar characteristics and symptoms.

Cluster A
These are personality disorders characterized by odd, eccentric thinking or behavior and include:

Paranoid personality disorder
- Believing that others are trying to harm you
- Distrust and suspicion of others
- Emotional detachment
- Hostility

Schizoid personality disorder
- Lack of interest in social relationships
- Limited range of emotional expression
- Inability to pick up normal social cues
- Appearing dull or indifferent to others

Schizotypal personality disorder
- Peculiar dress, thinking, beliefs or behavior
- Perceptual alterations, such as those affecting touch
- Discomfort in close relationships
- Flat emotions or inappropriate emotional responses
- Indifference to others
- "Magical thinking" — believing you can influence people and events with your thoughts
- Believing that messages are hidden for you in public speeches or displays

Cluster B
These are personality disorders characterized by dramatic, overly emotional thinking or behavior and include:

Antisocial (formerly sociopathic) personality disorder
- Disregard for others
- Persistent lying or stealing
- Recurring difficulties with the law
- Repeatedly violating the rights of others
- Aggressive, often violent behavior
- Disregard for the safety of self or others

Borderline personality disorder
- Impulsive and risky behavior
- Volatile relationships
- Unstable mood
- Suicidal behavior
- Fear of being abandoned

Histrionic personality disorder
- Constantly seeking attention
- Excessively emotional
- Extreme sensitivity to others' approval
- Unstable mood
- Excessive concern with physical appearance

Narcissistic personality disorder
- Believing that you're better than others
- Fantasizing about power, success and attractiveness
- Exaggerating your achievements or talents
- Expecting constant praise and admiration
- Failing to recognize other people's emotions and feelings

Cluster C

These are specific personality disorders characterized by anxious, fearful thinking or behavior. They include:

Avoidant personality disorder
- Hypersensitivity to criticism or rejection
- Feeling inadequate
- Social isolation
- Extreme shyness in social situations
- Timidity

Dependent personality disorder
- Excessive dependence on others
- Submissiveness toward others
- A desire to be taken care of
- Tolerance of poor or abusive treatment
- Urgent need to start a new relationship as soon as one has ended

Obsessive-compulsive personality disorder
- Preoccupation with orderliness and rules

- Extreme perfectionism
- Desire to be in control of situations and events
- Inability to discard broken or worthless objects
- Inflexibility

Obsessive-compulsive personality disorder isn't the same as obsessive-compulsive disorder, a type of anxiety disorder.

Treatment

The treatment that's best for you depends on your particular personality disorder, its severity and your life situation. Often, a team approach is appropriate to make sure all of your psychiatric, medical and social needs are met. Because personality disorders tend to be chronic and can sometimes last much of your adult life, you may need long-term treatment.

If you have mild symptoms that are well-controlled, you may not need treatment. For moderate to severe symptoms, find a medical or mental health provider with experience in treating personality disorders.

Treatment options
Several treatments are available for personality disorders. They include:
- Psychotherapy
- Medications
- Hospitalization

Psychotherapy
Psychotherapy is the main way to treat personality disorders. *Psychotherapy* is a general term for the process of treating personality disorders by talking about your condition and related issues with a mental health provider.

During psychotherapy, you learn about your condition and your mood, feelings, thoughts, and behavior. Using the insights and knowledge you gain in psychotherapy, you can learn healthy ways to manage your symptoms.

Types used to treat personality disorders may include:

- **Cognitive behavioral therapy.** This combines features of both cognitive and behavioral therapies to help you identify unhealthy, negative beliefs and behaviors and replace them with healthy, positive ones.
- **Dialectical behavior therapy.** This is a type of cognitive behavioral therapy whose primary objective is to teach behavioral skills to help you tolerate stress, regulate your emotions and improve your relationships with others.
- **Psychodynamic psychotherapy.** This therapy is based on the theories of psychoanalysis and focuses on increasing your awareness of unconscious thoughts and behaviors, developing new insights into your motivations, and resolving conflicts to live a happier life.
- **Psychoeducation.** This teaches you — and sometimes family and friends — about your illness, including treatments, coping strategies and problem-solving skills.

Psychotherapy may be provided in individual sessions, as a part of group therapy, or in sessions that include family or friends. The type of psychotherapy that's right for you depends on your individual situation. Group therapy tends to be highly effective.

Medications
There are no medications specifically approved by the Food and Drug Administration to treat personality disorders. However, several types of psychiatric medications may help with various personality disorder symptoms, particularly when other disorders are present.
- **Antidepressant medications.** Antidepressants may be useful if you have a depressed mood, anger, impulsiveness, irritability or hopelessness, which may be associated with personality disorders.
- **Mood-stabilizing medications.** As their name suggests, mood

stabilizers can help even out mood swings or reduce irritability, impulsiveness and aggression.

- **Anti-anxiety medications.** These may help if you have anxiety, agitation or insomnia. But in some people, they can increase impulsive behavior.
- **Antipsychotic medications.** Also called neuroleptics, these medications may be helpful if your symptoms include losing touch with reality (psychosis) or in some cases if you have anxiety or anger problems.

Hospitalization and residential treatment programs
In some instances, a personality disorder may be so severe that you require psychiatric hospitalization. Psychiatric hospitalization is generally recommended only when you aren't able to care for yourself properly or when you're in immediate danger of harming yourself or someone else. Psychiatric hospitalization options include 24-hour inpatient care, partial or day hospitalization, or residential treatment, which offers a supportive place to live.

Psychotic Disorders

Over the years, the word *psychotic* has been used in several different ways, and it still has no universally accepted definition. People sometimes use the term in everyday speech to mean insane or dangerous. The American Psychiatric Association defines psychotic as referring to the presence of certain signs and symptoms — hallucinations, delusions and, to a lesser extent, bizarre speech or behavior.

Psychosis refers to an impairment of thinking in which your interpretation of reality is severely abnormal. Although psychosis is often associated with other mental illnesses, psychotic symptoms may also result from physical illnesses, including some infections, cancer, nervous system disorders, thyroid disorders and immune system disorders. Psychotic signs and symptoms can also be a complication of Parkinson's disease, Alzheimer's disease and other dementias. Psychosis may also represent a distinct type of mental disorder that can occur by itself.

Signs and symptoms

Psychotic disorders typically have one and, often, two hallmark

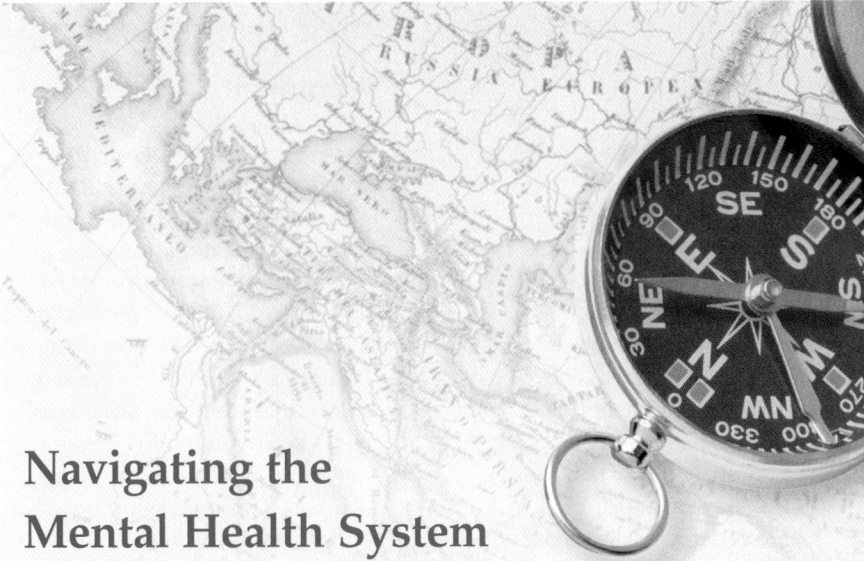

Navigating the Mental Health System

Millions of adults, children and adolescents in the United States use mental health services. Because services are spread across many professions and agencies, deciding where or how to get help may be a challenge. The following overview of resources may help you find the help that's best for you:

Primary care doctor
Your primary care doctor may be able to help determine the nature of your problem and the type of help best suited to your circumstances. If your symptoms are mild, he or she may provide the treatment. Or your primary care doctor may refer you to a psychiatrist, psychologist or other mental health professional.

Hospitals and medical schools
A hospital in your area may be staffed with mental health professionals. The psychiatry department of the medical school in your area may provide treatment or referrals.

Advocacy groups
Local branches of organizations such as the National Alliance on Mental Illness (NAMI) often supply contact information. NAMI distributes brochures, books and videos about mental illness and offers advice on talking to mental health professionals.

Professional societies
Local or state branches of professional organizations such as the American Psychiatric Association or the American Psychological Association can help you find local mental health providers.

symptoms. One is hallucinations and the other is delusions.

Hallucinations

Hallucinations occur when you sense things that don't exist. A common hallucination is hearing voices. A person experiencing hallucinations may carry on a conversation with voices that no one else can hear. Or the individual may perceive voices telling him or her what to do.

Delusions

Delusions are firmly held personal beliefs that have no basis in reality. For example, individuals with paranoid schizophrenia hold irrational beliefs that others are persecuting them or conspiring against them. For instance, a delusional person may believe her noisy neighbors are purposely trying to keep her awake at night.

Types

Some examples of psychotic disorders are schizophrenia, brief psychotic disorder and substance-induced psychotic disorder.

Schizophrenia

Schizophrenia is a serious brain disorder in which reality is interpreted abnormally. Schizophrenia results in hallucinations, delusions, and disordered thinking and behavior. People with schizophrenia may withdraw from people and activities in the world around them and retreat into an inner world marked by psychosis.

Contrary to popular belief, schizophrenia isn't the same as having multiple personalities. While the word *schizophrenia* does mean "split mind," it refers to a disruption of the usual balance of emotions and thinking.

Schizophrenia generally causes progressive deterioration in a person's ability to function in various roles, especially in a job and personal relationships. Schizophrenia is rare in children. In men, the disease typically emerges in the teens or 20s. In women, onset typically is in the 20s or early 30s. Schizophrenia may exist alone or in combination with other psychiatric conditions.

Signs and symptoms

There are several types of schizophrenia, so signs and symptoms of the condition vary. In general, schizophrenia signs and symptoms may include:
- Beliefs not based on reality (delusions), such as the belief

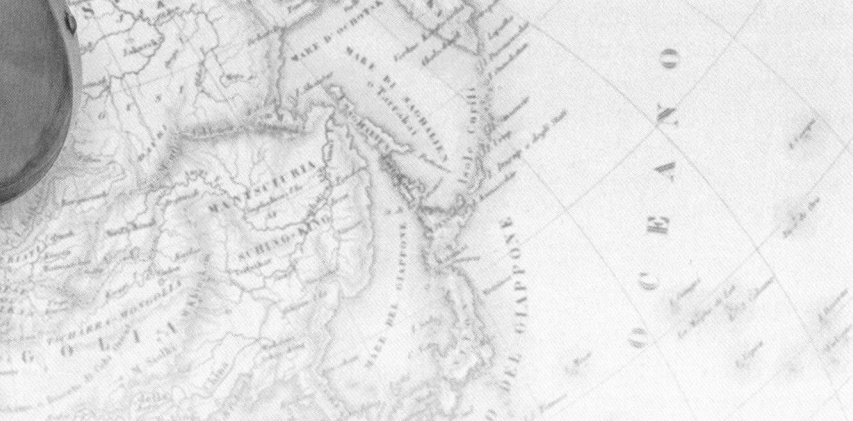

Community mental health centers

Community mental health centers were established on a national scale in the 1960s in an effort to allow individuals with severe mental illness to move from psychiatric hospitals into local neighborhoods. Today, these centers help people with mild and severe illness. Services include psychotherapy, management of medication, crisis intervention and substance abuse treatment.

Insurance companies

Often third-party payers have lists of health care workers, but they may include — and pay for services performed by — only mental health professionals within their own network.

Employee assistance programs

Many employers provide referrals to workers for problems that can affect work performance, such as substance abuse, family and relationship problems, and mental and emotional difficulties.

Hotlines and help lines

Many communities have telephone lines that provide referrals for mental health problems. Check the telephone directory.

Social service organizations

Agencies such as the United Way can supply information about community resources, including mental health providers.

Clergy

Religious leaders often are sources of comfort and advice. A clergy member at your place of worship may be able to provide assistance.

School districts

Your child's teachers, school principal, counselor or school nurse may be a good resource.

Schizophrenia: What It Is and Isn't

People hold many misconceptions about schizophrenia and its relation to other mental illnesses.

- Schizophrenia isn't the same as multiple personality disorder, which is a separate, rare condition.
- Although some people with schizophrenia become violent, most don't. Many withdraw into themselves rather than interact with others.
- Not everyone who is paranoid or distrustful has schizophrenia. People who have paranoid personality disorder or some forms of bipolar disorder are suspicious or distrustful of others, but these disorders don't include other features of schizophrenia.
- Not everyone who hears voices is schizophrenic. Some people with severe depression may hear voices. Hearing voices may also occur with a serious medical illness or from side effects of medication or drug abuse.

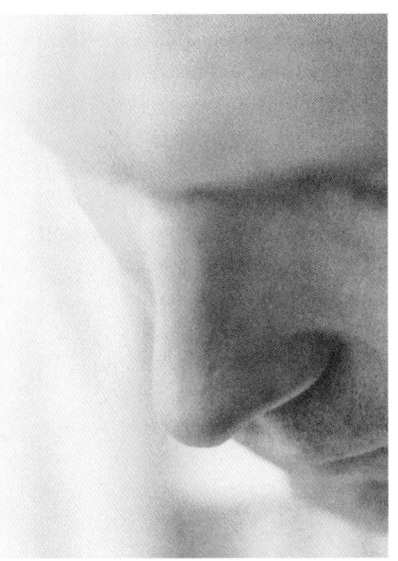

that there's a conspiracy against you
- Seeing or hearing things that don't exist (hallucinations), especially voices
- Incoherent speech
- Neglect of personal hygiene
- Lack of emotions
- Emotions inappropriate to the situation
- Angry outbursts
- Catatonic behavior
- A persistent feeling of being watched
- Trouble functioning at school and work
- Social isolation

Schizophrenia ranges from mild to severe. Some people may be able to function well in daily life, while others need specialized, intensive care. In some instances, schizophrenia symptoms seem to appear suddenly. Other times, schizophrenia symptoms seem to develop gradually over months or years, and they may not be noticeable at first.

Over time, it can become difficult to function in daily life. You may not be able to go to work or school. You may have troubled relationships, partly because of difficulty reading social cues or others' emotions. You may lose interest in activities you once enjoyed. You may be distressed or agitated or fall into a trancelike state, becoming unresponsive to others.

Medications

Schizophrenia is a chronic condition that requires lifelong treatment, even during periods when you feel better and your symptoms have subsided.

Medications are the cornerstone of schizophrenia treatment. But because medications for schizophrenia can cause serious but rare side effects, you may be reluctant to take them. Work with your psychiatrist and other medical professionals to find a medication regimen that works for you, with the fewest side effects.

Antipsychotic medications are the most commonly prescribed medications to treat schizophrenia. They're thought to control symptoms by affecting the brain neurotransmitters dopamine and serotonin. There are two main types of antipsychotic medications:

- **First-generation antipsychotics.** This group of medications includes haloperidol (Haldol), chlorpromazine and fluphenazine. These medications have traditionally been very effective in managing symptoms of schizophrenia. The medications have frequent and potentially severe neurological side effects, including the possibility of tardive dyskinesia or involuntary jerking movements.

First-generation antipsychotics are often cheaper than their newer counterparts, especially the generic versions, which can be an important consideration when long-term treatment is necessary.

- **Second-generation antipsychotics.** Second-generation medications are effective at managing both positive and negative symptoms. They include clozapine (Clozaril), risperidone (Risperdal), olanzapine (Zyprexa), quetiapine (Seroquel), ziprasidone (Geodon), aripiprazole (Abilify), paliperidone (Invega), asenapine (Saphris), brexpiprazole (Rexulti), cariprazine (Vraylar), iloperidone (Fanapt) and lurasidone (Latuda).

Second-generation antipsychotic medications pose a risk of metabolic side effects, including weight gain, diabetes and high cholesterol.

Which medication is best for you depends on your individual situation. It can take several weeks after first starting a medication to notice an improvement in your symptoms. In general, the goal of treatment with antipsychotic medications is to effectively control signs and symptoms at the lowest possible dosage. Other medications also may be helpful, such as antidepressants or anti-anxiety medications.

Be aware that all antipsychotic medications have side effects and possible health risks. Certain antipsychotic medications, for instance, may increase the risk of diabetes, weight gain, high cholesterol and high blood pressure. Clozaril can cause dangerous changes in your white blood cell count. Certain antipsychotic medications can cause serious health problems in some older adults and should be avoided. Antipsychotic medications can also have dangerous interactions with other substances. Your doctor should know about all medications and over-the-counter substances you take, including vitamins, minerals and herbal supplements.

Psychosocial treatments
Although medications are the cornerstone of schizophrenia treatment, psychotherapy and other psychosocial treatments also are important. These treatments may include:

- **Individual therapy.** Psychotherapy with a skilled mental health provider can help you learn ways to cope with the daily life challenges brought on by schizophrenia. Therapy can help you improve communication skills, relationships, your ability to work and your motivation to stick to your treatment plan. Learning about schizophrenia can help you understand it better, cope with lingering symptoms and understand the importance of taking your medications. Therapy can also help you cope with the stigma surrounding schizophrenia.
- **Social skills training.** This focuses on improving communication and social interactions and improving the ability to participate in daily activities.
- **Family therapy.** Both you and your family may benefit from therapy that provides support and education to families. You have a better chance of improving if your family members

understand your illness, can recognize stressful situations that might trigger a relapse and can help you stick to your treatment plan. Family therapy can also help you and your family communicate better with each other and understand family conflicts. Family therapy can also help family members cope and reduce their distress about your condition.

- **Rehabilitation.** Training in social and vocational skills to live independently is an important part of recovery from schizophrenia. With the help of a therapist, you can learn such skills as good hygiene, cooking and better communication. Many communities have self-help groups and programs to help people with schizophrenia find jobs and housing and deal with crisis situations. If you don't have a case manager to help you with these services, ask your doctor about getting one. Today, fewer people with schizophrenia require long-term hospitalization because effective treatments are available.

Electroconvulsive therapy
For adults with schizophrenia who don't respond to drug therapy, electroconvulsive therapy (ECT) may be considered. ECT also may be helpful for someone with severe depression who doesn't respond to the usual medications.

Hospitalization
During crisis periods or times of severe symptoms, hospitalization may be necessary to ensure safety, proper nutrition, adequate sleep and basic hygiene.

Brief psychotic disorder
Brief psychotic disorder involves the sudden onset of at least one type of psychotic sign or symptom — delusions, hallucinations, speech that makes no sense or wanders, or disturbed or catatonic

behavior. The main difference is the time factor. The disturbance lasts less than a month — compared with at least six months of symptoms for schizophrenia.

The signs and symptoms often appear after an extremely stressful event, such as military combat or the loss of a loved one. A person with this disorder may experience overwhelming confusion or a rapid fluctuation of emotions.

Behavior and dress may be bizarre, and the individual may adopt peculiar postures and scream or become mute. Speech may sound foolish, often involving the repetition of nonsense phrases. Disorientation and memory impairment may occur. After the symptoms subside, the individual may continue to feel a loss of self-esteem or be mildly depressed for a while.

Treatment may include antipsychotic medications and psychotherapy (see page 1151).

Substance-induced psychotic disorder
Substance-induced psychotic disorder is a psychosis caused by an overdose of certain drugs — prescribed medications as well as hallucinogens or amphetamines — or by drug or alcohol withdrawal.

Use of cocaine, amphetamines, over-the-counter sleeping pills and antihistamines, antidepressants, and medications used for Parkinson's disease can cause psychotic symptoms. A psychotic reaction after use of hallucinogenic drugs such as LSD or phencyclidine (PCP, or angel dust) and occasionally marijuana or hashish is often referred to as a bad trip.

Signs and symptoms may include anxiety or panic as well as delusions and hallucinations.

Treatment generally addresses the drug addiction and may involve antipsychotic drugs and psychotherapy — or withdrawal of the prescription medication that prompted the disorder.

Somatic Symptom Disorder

Somatic symptom disorder involves having a significant focus on physical symptoms — such as pain or fatigue — to the point that it causes major emotional distress and problems functioning. You may or may not have another diagnosed medical condition associated with these symptoms.

Excessive thoughts, feelings and behaviors in response to physical symptoms may lead to frequent doctor visits. You often think the worst about your symptoms and continue to search for an explanation, even when other serious conditions have been excluded. Health concerns may become such a central focus of your life that it's hard to function, sometimes leading to disability.

Signs and symptoms

Symptoms of somatic symptom disorder may include specific sensations, such as pain or shortness of breath, or more general symptoms, such as fatigue or weakness. Pain is the most common symptom.

Your symptoms may not be associated with an identifiable medical cause. This doesn't mean the symptoms are imagined. It simply means that they may be associated with factors that are difficult to diagnose or may be due to physical processes not yet understood.

Or your symptoms may be related to a medical condition such as arthritis or heart disease, but they're more significant than what's usually expected.

You may have a single symptom, multiple symptoms or varying symptoms, which may be mild, moderate or severe.

For somatic symptom disorder, more important than the specific physical symptoms you experience is the way you interpret and react to the symptoms and how they impact your daily life.

Diagnosis

To determine a diagnosis, you'll likely have a physical exam and any tests your doctor recommends. Your doctor also may have you fill out a psychological self-assessment or questionnaire.

The Diagnostic and Statistical Manual of Mental Disorders (DSM-5), published by the American Psychiatric Association, emphasizes these points in the diagnosis of somatic symptom disorder:

- You have one or more somatic symptoms that are distressing or result in problems with your daily life.
- You have excessive and persistent thoughts about the seriousness of your symptoms; you have a persistently high level of anxiety about your health or symptoms; or you devote too much time and energy to your symptoms or health concerns.
- You continue to have symptoms that concern you — typically for more than six months — even though the symptoms may vary.

Treatment

The goal of treatment for somatic symptom disorder is to improve your symptoms, making you better able to function in daily life. Psychotherapy, specifically cognitive behavioral therapy, can be helpful for somatic symptom disorder. Sometimes psychotherapy may be combined with medications.

Psychotherapy

Physical symptoms may be associated with psychological distress and a high level of health anxiety. Psychotherapy — also called talk therapy — can help improve physical symptoms.

A form of psychotherapy known as cognitive behavioral therapy is often most effective. It's designed to help you:

- Examine and adapt your beliefs and expectations about health and physical symptoms
- Learn how to reduce stress
- Learn how to cope with physical symptoms
- Reduce your preoccupation with symptoms
- Find ways to cope with or avoid situations and activities that produce uncomfortable physical sensations

---

? Question and Answer

Since I started taking an antidepressant, I've developed sexual difficulties. Is there anything I can do?

Selective serotonin reuptake inhibitors (SSRIs) are among the medications most frequently prescribed for treating depression and anxiety, but these drugs can cause sexual side effects, such as delayed ejaculation, inability to achieve orgasm and loss of interest in sex. Men and women experience sexual side effects in similar numbers. People who are affected usually experience problems within weeks of starting the medication or after increasing the dosage.

Sometimes, the problem improves over time or if your doctor reduces your dosage. Switching to a drug in a different class of antidepressant, such as bupropion (Wellbutrin SR, Wellbutrin XL) or mirtazapine (Remeron) also may help. In addition, certain medications may counter the side effects of SSRIs.

Talk with your doctor about possible ways to overcome sexual difficulties associated with your medication.

Mental Health Professionals

Professionals who provide mental health care include the following:

Psychiatrists

A psychiatrist is a medical doctor who has had at least four years of specialty training after earning a doctor of medicine (M.D.) degree. Psychiatrists must be licensed to practice medicine in the state in which they work, and most are certified by the American Board of Psychiatry and Neurology. Psychiatrists are qualified to carry out many aspects of treatment, including prescribing medication and doing psychotherapy. They also lead treatment teams in hospitals.

Psychologists

A psychologist usually has a doctoral degree (Ph.D., Ed.D. or Psy.D.) in psychology or counseling, although many states allow providers with master's degrees to provide mental health care. A period of supervised training is required after completion of the doctorate. All states license psychologists, who may also be certified by the American Board of Professional Psychology.

Psychologists use testing and other methods to help diagnose, evaluate and treat individuals with psychological problems. They use various forms of psychotherapy, but in most states they can't prescribe medications.

Social workers

A clinical social worker must have a master's degree in social work and be licensed or certified by the state in which he or she practices.

To be designated a licensed clinical social worker (L.C.S.W.) or licensed independent clinical social worker (L.I.C.S.W.), candidates usually undergo supervised training in psychotherapy. A clinical social worker may work for a social service agency, in a private practice, or as part of a hospital- or clinic-based multidisciplinary treatment team that includes a psychiatrist, a psychologist, nurses, and recreational and vocational therapists. Social workers can't prescribe medications.

Advanced practice prescribers

Advanced practice prescribers include individuals who have advanced training in medical care. This includes nurses and midlevel providers such as physician assistants.

A psychiatric nurse has a degree in nursing, is licensed as a registered nurse (R.N.) and has additional experience in psychiatry. A clinical nurse specialist (C.N.S.) has a bachelor's degree in nursing, is licensed as an R.N., and holds a master's degree in psychiatric and mental health nursing or a related field. A nurse practitioner (N.P.) or physician assistant (P.A.) also may work in psychiatry. They have advanced training in physical assessment, physiology, pharmacology and physical diagnosis, and they may prescribe medications.

Others

Other types of mental health professionals include couples and family therapists and pastoral counselors. Couples and family therapists may be psychiatrists, psychologists, social workers or nurses, or they may have other training. They diagnose and treat mental illness within the context of relationships. Those who are members of the American Association for Marriage and Family Therapy have at least a master's degree and two years of supervised practice with couples and families.

A pastoral counselor is a member of the clergy who integrates religious concepts with training in the behavioral sciences, according to the American Association of Pastoral Counselors (AAPC). Licensure isn't required, but counselors can seek certification with the AAPC.

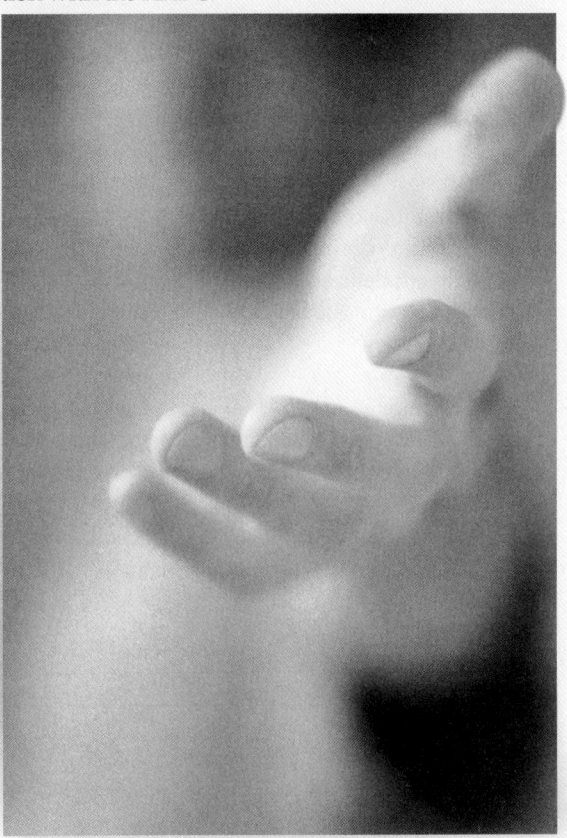

According to one study, more than 1 in 3 people with severe depression or anxiety uses some form of integrative or alternative care to treat an illness. This includes herbal and dietary supplements sold without a prescription. Some of the more popular supplements marketed or taken for treatment of depression include:

St. John's wort

An herbal preparation from the plant *Hypericum perforatum,* St. John's wort has long been used in folk medicine and is widely used in Europe to treat anxiety, depression and sleep disorders. In the United States, it's sold in the form of tablets or a tea.

Some studies have suggested that St. John's wort may work as well as a prescription antidepressant for mild to moderate depression. But a large clinical trial found it ineffective for treatment of major depression.

Adverse reactions to this herbal preparation can include dry mouth, dizziness, digestive problems, fatigue, confusion and sensitivity to sunlight. St. John's wort can interfere with the effectiveness of certain prescription medications, including antidepressants and drugs used to treat human immunodeficiency virus (HIV) infection and AIDS.

SAMe

S-adenosyl-L-methionine (SAMe) is a chemical substance that's available in Europe as a prescription drug for the treatment of depression. In the United States, it's sold as an over-the-counter supplement. SAMe is found in human cells and plays a role in many body functions. In supplement form, it's thought to increase levels of serotonin and dopamine, though this has not been confirmed in larger studies. Taken in large quantities, SAMe can be harmful.

Omega-3 fatty acids

Omega-3 fatty acids, a kind of nutrient found in fish oils and certain plants, are being investigated as a possible mood stabilizer for people with bipolar disorder. Fish oil capsules containing omega-3 fatty acids are sold in many stores. The capsules are high in fat and calories and may produce gastrointestinal problems. A better way to get more of these fatty acids is simply to eat more cold-water fish, such as salmon, mackerel and herring.

5-HTP

One of the raw materials that your body needs to make the neurotransmitter serotonin is a chemical called 5-hydroxytryptophan (5-HTP). It's prescribed in Europe to treat depression and is available over-the-counter in the United States. Although it's possible that 5-HTP may help some individuals with depression, more research on safety and effectiveness is needed before it can be recommended.

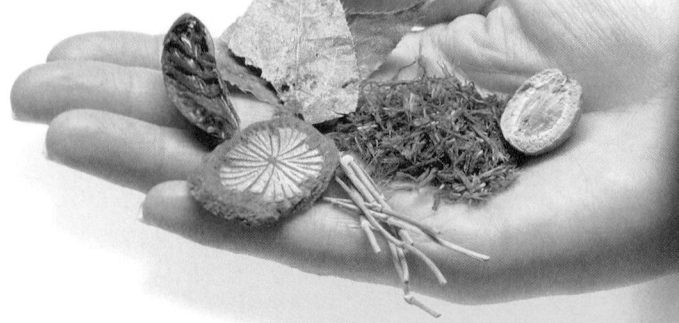

- Improve daily functioning at home, at work, in relationships and in social situations
- Address depression and other mental health disorders

In addition, family therapy can help examine family relationships and improve family support.

Medications

Antidepressant medications may help reduce symptoms associated with depression, including pain that often occurs with somatic symptom disorder.

If one medication doesn't work well for you, your doctor may recommend switching to another or combining certain medications to boost effectiveness. Keep in mind that it can take several weeks after first starting a medication to notice an improvement in symptoms.

Talk with your doctor about medication options and the possible side effects and risks.

Self-care

These practical steps can be beneficial in treating somatic symptom disorder.

- **Practice stress management and relaxation techniques.** Learning stress management and relaxation techniques, such as progressive muscle relaxation and deep breathing, may help improve symptoms.
- **Get physically active.** A graduated activity program may have a calming effect on your mood, improve your physical symptoms and help improve your physical function.
- **Participate in activities.** Stay involved in work, social and family activities. Don't wait until your symptoms are resolved to participate.
- **Avoid alcohol and recreational drugs.** Substance use can make your care more difficult. Talk to your doctor if you believe you may have a problem with drug use or alcohol use.

Common Treatments

Mental illness may seem like an unbearable burden, but in reality most forms are treatable. Three general approaches to treating mental illness are medication, psychotherapy and other medical therapies, which include electroconvulsive therapy (ECT). Frequently, a combination of approaches is most effective.

Treatment for any mental illness must be tailored to the individual. No single treatment regimen will work for everyone. Although most treatment occurs in an outpatient setting, some people receive care in a hospital or residential setting, such as a halfway house.

Medication

Dozens of medications are available to treat mental health disorders. Most people find the best relief of symptoms by combining medications and psychotherapy.

Some medications used to treat mental health disorders have been specifically approved by the Food and Drug Administration (FDA). Doctors also can use their medical judgment to prescribe other medications that haven't been FDA approved to treat mental health disorders but that may be effective anyway — a common and perfectly legal practice called off-label use.

Antidepressants

There are several different types of antidepressants. Antidepressants are generally categorized by how they affect the naturally occurring chemicals in your brain to change your mood. To determine which antidepressant may be most effective, doctors typically follow general practice guidelines.

Other factors your doctor will consider when prescribing an antidepressant are your symptoms, your family history of de-

Use of Stimulants

When an individual is severely depressed, a doctor may prescribe both a stimulant and an antidepressant. Stimulants include methylphenidate (Ritalin, Concerta) and dextroamphetamine and amphetamine (Adderall). They help boost your mood and energy level during the time before an antidepressant becomes fully effective. Typically, after a few weeks you stop taking the stimulant and remain on the antidepressant.

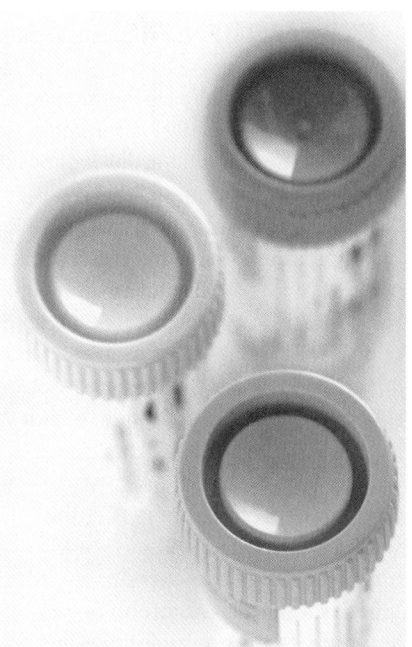

pression and other conditions you may have. Don't give up until you find an antidepressant or medication that's suitable for you — you have a good chance of finding one that works and that doesn't have intolerable side effects, even if it takes a few tries. Most antidepressants are equally effective. But some pose a higher risk of serious side effects than do others.

It can take as long as eight to 12 weeks to gain the full benefits of an antidepressant, although you may notice some improvements in your mood or related symptoms before that. Certain genetic factors may influence whether or not an antidepressant works for you and how long it takes for symptoms to improve. If you don't experience improvements in your mood and thoughts, your doctor may suggest either increasing your dose, combining medications or switching to a new medication.

Selective serotonin reuptake inhibitors (SSRIs)

This group of antidepressants influences the activity of the neurotransmitter serotonin, which is thought to play a crucial role in depression and other mood disorders.

Selective serotonin reuptake inhibitors (SSRIs) include fluox-

etine (Prozac, Sarafem), paroxetine (Paxil, Brisdelle), sertraline (Zoloft), citalopram (Celexa) and escitalopram (Lexapro). These medications aren't necessarily more effective than first-generation antidepressants, but they're safer to use and produce milder, more tolerable side effects.

If you take an SSRI for depression, it's often effective in improving your mood and eliminating other signs and symptoms of depression. If you take an SSRI for an anxiety disorder, it may help you become less tense and anxious.

Side effects of SSRIs include gastrointestinal problems and drowsiness, which often decrease or disappear over time. SSRIs may reduce sexual desire or prevent orgasm. In men, they can cause inability to achieve an erection.

Serotonin and norepinephrine reuptake inhibitors (SNRIs)

Serotonin and norepinephrine reuptake inhibitors are a type of antidepressant medication that increases the levels of both the neurotrasmitters serotonin and norepinephrine by inhibiting their reabsorption (reuptake) into brain cells. Although the precise mechanism of action isn't clear, it's thought that these higher levels

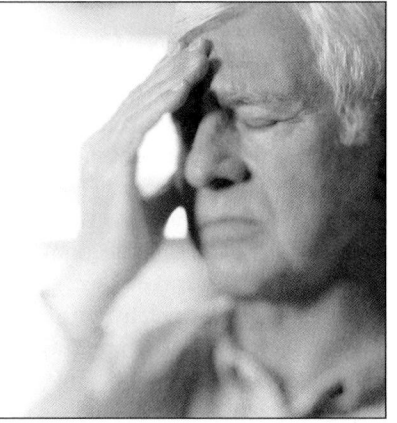

A rare but potentially life-threatening side effect of selective serotonin reuptake inhibitors (SSRIs) is serotonin syndrome. Signs and symptoms include confusion, hallucinations, fluctuations in blood pressure and heart rhythm, fever, seizures, and possibly coma.

Serotonin syndrome most often develops when an SSRI interacts with other antidepressants, usually a monoamine oxidase inhibitor. But it can also occur when an SSRI is taken with other medications that influence serotonin. For this reason you shouldn't take an SSRI with St. John's wort, which is a nonprescription herbal supplement that affects serotonin activity. It's also important to always inform your doctors of all of the medications — prescription and nonprescription — that you take.

enhance neurotransmission — the sending of nerve impulses — and improve and elevate mood.

Medications in this group of antidepressants are sometimes called dual reuptake inhibitors. They include the drugs duloxetine (Cymbalta), venlafaxine (Effexor XR), desvenlafaxine (Pristiq, Khedezla) and levomilnacipran (Fetzima).

Atypical antidepessants

These medications don't fit neatly into any of the other antidepressant categories. They include bupropion (Wellbutrin XL, Wellbutrin SR, Aplenzin, Forfivo XL), mirtazapine (Remeron), nefazodone, trazodone, vortioxetine (Trintellix) and vilazodone (Viibryd).

Tricyclic antidepressants

These older antidepressants have been used since the 1950s. Tricyclic antidepressants include the medications amitriptyline, desipramine (Norpramin), imipramine (Tofranil), nortriptyline (Pamelor), protriptyline (Vivactil) and trimipramine (Surmontil).

Tricyclic antidepressants can cause more-bothersome side effects than newer antidepressants, but many people tolerate them well. Side effects may include dry mouth, blurred vision, dizziness, drowsiness, weight gain, constipation and difficulty urinating. Tricyclics may trigger or worsen certain medical conditions, including an enlarged prostate, some forms of glaucoma and some types of heart disease.

Monoamine oxidase inhibitors

Monoamine oxidase inhibitors (MAOIs) — such as tranylcypromine (Parnate), phenelzine (Nardil) and isocarboxazid (Marplan) — can have serious side effects and are most often prescribed when other drugs haven't worked. Using MAOIs requires a strict diet because of dangerous (or even deadly) interactions with foods — such as certain cheeses, pickles and wines — and some medications and herbal supplements.

Selegiline (Emsam), a newer MAOI that sticks on the skin as a patch, may cause fewer side effects than other MAOIs do. These medications can't be combined with SSRIs.

Side effects of antidepressants

All antidepressants can cause unwanted side effects. Not everyone experiences the same number or intensity of side effects, though. You may find that your side effects are so mild that you don't need to stop taking the antidepressant. Coping strategies can help you manage side effects. In addition, side effects often go away or lessen within several weeks of starting an antidepressant.

If you experience unpleasant or intolerable side effects, don't just stop taking an antidepressant without consulting your doctor first. Some antidepressants can cause withdrawal-like symptoms unless you slowly taper off your dose.

Precautions when taking antidepressants

Although studies have shown that antidepressants are generally safe, some precautions are in order when taking them. All antidepressant medications carry black box warnings. These are the strictest warnings that the FDA can issue for prescription medications.

The antidepressant warnings note that in some cases, children, adolescents and young adults ages 18 to 24 may have an increase in suicidal thoughts or behavior when taking antidepressants, especially in the first few weeks after starting antidepressant therapy or when the dose is changed. Because of this risk, people in these age groups must be closely monitored by loved ones, caregivers and doctors.

Make sure you understand the risks of the medications you're taking and that you're being properly monitored. In addition, if you're pregnant or breastfeeding, some antidepressants may pose an increased health risk to your unborn child or nursing child. Talk to your doctor about any concerns you have. Again, make sure you understand the risks of the various antidepressants. Working together, you and your doctor can explore options to get your depression symptoms under control.

Mood stabilizers

Mood stabilizers are taken for bipolar disorder. The two main types of mood stabilizers are lithium and anticonvulsants. Lithium curbs mania, helps prevent extreme mood swings and, in some people, can ease sadness. It's sold by prescription under the brand name Lithobid and as the generic drug lithium carbonate.

If you take lithium, your doctor will measure lithium levels in your blood to adjust the dose. He or she will also need to know what other medications you take, including over-the-counter medications, to avoid drug interactions. The most common side effects of lithium are nausea, diarrhea, fatigue, confusion and trembling hands. Lithium can also affect kidney and thyroid function.

Divalproex (Depakote), carbamazepine (Carbatrol, Tegretol) and lamotrigine (Lamictal) are prescribed primarily for seizure disorders, but they're also used to treat bipolar disorder. It's uncertain exactly how these anticonvulsant drugs help the disorder. An anticonvulsant may be taken in combination with lithium.

Side effects of divalproex include drowsiness, increased appetite, weight gain and digestive problems. Carbamazepine may cause drowsiness, dizziness, confusion, headaches, nausea, a skin rash and a lowered white blood cell count. Both medications can cause liver problems in some people.

Anti-anxiety medications

Antidepressants, particularly the selective serotonin reuptake inhibitors (SSRIs), are widely used to treat and prevent a variety of anxiety disorders.

In limited circumstances, your doctor may prescribe a sedative for short-term relief of anxiety symptoms. Sedatives called benzodiazepines ease anxiety — often within 30 to 90 minutes. But these drugs can be habit-forming if taken for more than a few weeks. For this reason, doctors usually prescribe them for only a short time to help with getting through a particularly anxious period.

Sedatives taken to control anxiety include alprazolam (Xanax), clonazepam (Klonopin), diazepam (Valium) and lorazepam (Ativan). These medications may cause dizziness, drowsiness, imbalance and reduced muscle coordination. You shouldn't drive, use alcohol or operate heavy machinery while taking them.

When discontinuing a sedative, you want to reduce the dose gradually over several days or weeks, with the advice of your doctor. This can help prevent withdrawal symptoms, such as nausea, loss of appetite, irritability, insomnia, headaches, dizziness and trembling.

Another medication prescribed for anxiety is buspirone. It influences the activity of serotonin but in a different way than SSRI antidepressants do. Buspirone often doesn't work as well if you've taken benzodiazepines in the past. A common side effect of buspirone is a brief feeling of lightheadedness shortly after taking the medicine. Less common side effects include headaches, nausea, nervousness and insomnia.

Antipsychotic medications

Available since the 1950s, antipsychotic medications are typically prescribed to treat symptoms of psychosis, including hallucinations and delusions. Some of the more commonly used medications include haloperidol (Haldol), olanzapine (Zyprexa), quetiapine (Seroquel), risperidone (Risperdal), thioridazine, trifluoperazine and ziprasidone (Geodon).

Antipsychotics block the effects of the neurotransmitter dopamine, which is associated with psychosis. The medications are often effective but may cause side effects, including weight gain, dry mouth, blurred vision, constipation, drowsiness, tardive dyskenasis and increased tendency to sunburn (photosensitivity).

Psychotherapy

Psychotherapy is another key treatment for depression and other mental illnesses. It's often used along with medication treatment. *Psychotherapy* is a general term for a way of treating a condition by talking about it and related issues with a mental health provider. Psychotherapy is also known as therapy, talk therapy, counseling or psychosocial therapy.

Through these talk sessions, you learn about the causes of your condition so that you can better understand it. You also learn how to identify and make changes in unhealthy behavior or thoughts, explore relationships and experiences, find better ways to cope and solve problems, and set realistic goals for your life.

Psychotherapy can help you regain a sense of happiness and control in your life and help alleviate depression symptoms, such as hopelessness and anger. It may also help you adjust to a crisis or other current difficulty.

Depending on how severe your disorder is and the type of psychotherapy you receive, your treatment may last just a few sessions or it may continue for several months or longer. In general, the more severe or complicated the disorder, the longer the time needed to treat it.

There are several types of psychotherapy that are effective.

Cognitive behavioral therapy

Cognitive behavioral therapy, also called cognitive therapy, examines distortions in thinking that lead to psychological problems. It's the most studied therapy and is highly effective in treating mental illness. Brain imaging research shows that cognitive therapy can produce changes in brain activity in regions associated with depression.

This type of therapy is based on the foundation that how you think influences how you feel. You identify — with your therapist's help — distorted thoughts and beliefs that trigger psychological stress, fears or depression. You learn to replace negative thoughts with more-positive, realistic perceptions, and you learn ways you can view and cope with life events differently.

The treatment emphasizes learning to develop a sense of mastery and control of your thoughts and feelings. Cognitive therapy is generally a short-term treatment.

Interpersonal therapy

Interpersonal therapy focuses on relationships as the key to understanding and overcoming signs and symptoms of mental illness. The goal is to improve your relationship and communication skills and boost your self-esteem. Interpersonal therapy typically explores four major areas: unresolved grief, conflicts with others, transitions from one social or occupational goal to another, and difficulties with interpersonal or people skills.

Like cognitive behavioral therapy, interpersonal therapy is usually short term. It can help improve your ability to form relationships and function in social settings.

Desensitization and exposure therapy

Desensitization and exposure therapy is a therapy that's especially helpful for treating phobias, post-traumatic stress disorder and obsessive-compulsive disorder.

Treatment focuses on changing your response to a particular object or situation. For example, repeated exposure to a feared object or obsession may help you conquer your fear. You gradually increase your exposure to more anxiety-provoking thoughts and situations while learning how to

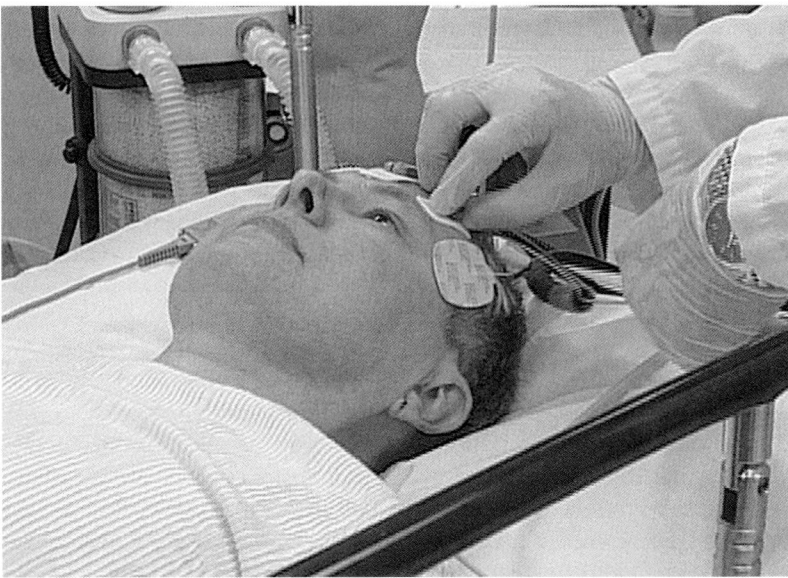

During electroconvulsive therapy (ECT), a doctor places small pads with attached wires (electrodes) on your scalp. The electrodes are connected to the ECT machine. Pads that measure brain activity are also placed on your scalp.

remain calm. Eventually, your fear and anxiety diminish so that you no longer need to avoid certain situations and thoughts.

Psychodynamic psychotherapies

Psychodynamic psychotherapies are intended to help people understand and change behaviors or interactions that have become outdated, ineffective or destructive. Using concepts related to unconscious mental processes, these therapies evolved from principles developed by Sigmund Freud.

Psychodynamic psychotherapies generally take longer than six months and may continue for several years. Individuals most likely to benefit from long-term therapy are those who have more than one mental disorder or who have persistently painful or costly patterns of behavior, such as fear of commitment or difficulty maintaining good relationships with others.

Group therapy

Group therapy involves a group of unrelated people and one or more mental health professionals who help facilitate the therapy

sessions. It isn't the same as a support group, which may be led by peers or lay people rather than professionals. The group may be formed on the basis of diagnosis, sex, age or other characteristics.

Group therapy strives toward many of the same goals as individual therapy but relies in part on advice, feedback and support from group participants. This type of therapy can be useful in treating social phobia, eating disorders, and addictions to drugs, alcohol and gambling.

Couples and family therapy

Couples and family therapy can be useful in helping spouses, partners and families work together to deal with the emotional turmoil and stress that mental illness can cause. Instead of focusing on the individual, couples and family therapy focuses on the interaction between the couple or family members.

Electroconvulsive therapy

In electroconvulsive therapy (ECT), electrical currents are passed through the brain to trigger a seizure. Although many

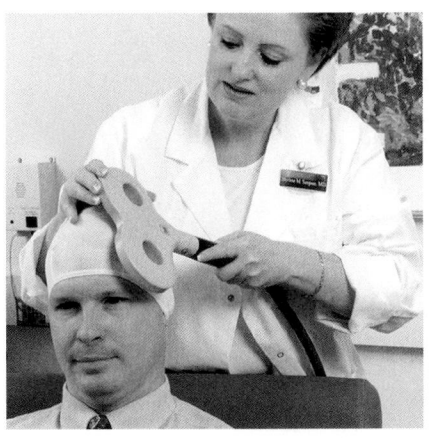

During transcranial magnetic stimulation, a device that emits a strong magnetic pulse is held to your scalp. The magnetic energy passes through your skull and stimulates nerve cells in your brain.

people are leery of ECT and its side effects, it typically offers fast, effective relief of depression symptoms. Experts aren't sure how this therapy relieves the symptoms of depression. The procedure may affect levels of neurotransmitters in the brain.

ECT is usually used in people who don't get better with medications, who are at high risk of suicide, and who have more-severe symptoms of depression.

How it works

During this procedure a doctor places small electrodes, each about the size of a silver dollar, on your head. While the electrodes are being positioned, you're given intravenous (IV) injections of a short-acting anesthetic to make you go to sleep and a muscle relaxant to prevent strong muscle contractions that can occur during the procedure.

A doctor then presses a button on the ECT machine that causes a small electric current to pass through your brain, producing a seizure that usually lasts 30 to 60 seconds. After the seizure, you're taken to a recovery room, where a nurse monitors you while the effects of the anesthetic and muscle relaxant wear off. The total duration of anesthesia is about

10 minutes, followed by 30 to 45 minutes in the recovery room.

Doctors consider ECT one of the most effective treatments for major depression and some other types of severe mental illness. Unlike antidepressant medications or psychotherapy, which can take weeks to show an effect, ECT often begins to work within a few days, although a series of treatments is often necessary. In people who complete the course of treatment, ECT is effective in approximately 80 percent of people.

After a successful course of ECT treatment, it's important to follow through with some form of ongoing treatment to prevent a relapse. Ongoing treatment may include medication or maintenance ECT.

Side effects

A major side effect of ECT is memory impairment. Immediately after an ECT treatment, you're likely to experience a period of confusion. You may not know where you are or why you're there. This period generally lasts from a few minutes to several hours and may get longer with each successive treatment. Rarely, the confusion may last several days.

After the course of treatment is over, the confusion gradually clears up. New memories that may have formed during your treatment may be lost. In rare instances, people have trouble remembering life events going back several years. Sometimes, these long-term memories return after the ECT treatments are done. Other times they remain permanently forgotten.

After an ECT treatment, you may experience some side effects including nausea, headache, muscle ache or jaw pain. These minor side effects are common and can be treated with medications. They may be distressing, but they're not serious.

Transcranial magnetic stimulation

In some ways, transcranial magnetic stimulation (TMS) is similar to electroconvulsive therapy (ECT). With TMS, electric current passes through a wire coil inside a hand-held device. The electric current creates a strong magnetic pulse that passes through your scalp and skull to stimulate nerve cells in the brain.

TMS doesn't require anesthesia and doesn't intentionally cause a seizure. However, on rare occasions, a seizure may occur. Another advantage of TMS is that it doesn't cause memory difficulties such as those associated with ECT.

Vagus nerve stimulation

Vagus nerve stimulation (VNS) uses electrical impulses with a surgically implanted pulse generator to affect mood centers of the brain. The FDA has approved this treatment for some forms of severe or chronic, treatment-resistant depression. For more information on the procedure see page 531.

Hospitalization and residential treatment programs

It's not often that depression becomes so severe that someone require psychiatric hospitalization. And even when depression is severe, it still may not be easy to decide if hospitalization is appropriate. If you can be treated just as effectively or better outside of the hospital, your doctor probably won't recommend hospitalization.

Psychiatric hospitalization is generally recommended only when you aren't able to care for yourself properly or when you're in immediate danger of harming yourself or someone else. You may also need to be hospitalized to receive ECT. Psychiatric hospitalization options include 24-hour inpatient care, partial or day hospitalization, or residential treatment, which offers a supportive place to live.

Self-care

After professional treatment brings your mental disorder under control and helps you feel better, you still have to cope on a day-to-day basis. Life inevitably presents challenges and frustrations. In addition to the help you get from a mental health professional, it's up to you to look for ways to enhance your overall well-being. Adopting healthy habits can help you recover from a mental illness and reduce your risk of a recurrence. These healthy living strategies are grounded in the importance of taking good care of your whole being:

Keep active
Research shows that regular exercise can help manage mild to moderate depression, anxiety and possibly other psychiatric disorders. One study, for example, found that individuals with depression who exercised for 20 to 60 minutes three times a week experienced noticeable improvements in their mental health. Exercise stimulates the production of brain chemicals that produce feelings of satisfaction and wellness (endorphins). Exercise also provides many other health benefits and generally improves quality of life.

Eat well
A balanced diet can improve the way you feel on many levels. Both your body and your brain need good nutrition to function efficiently.

Get adequate sleep
Sleep refreshes you. It improves your attitude and gives you energy for physical activity and coping with stress.

Get involved
A strong social network is an important component of overall health, including your mental health. Good friends and a supportive family can provide a sense of purpose or meaning, encouragement, and feedback, and they can lend a hand when you need help.

Control stress and practice relaxation techniques
Relaxation helps produce a physical and mental state of calm that's the opposite of the fight-or-flight response triggered by stress. Leisure and recreational activities also may help reduce stress. See Chapter 10, "Stress," for information on relaxation techniques and managing stress.

Attend to your spiritual needs
Spiritual practices — whether they involve meditation, religious services, nature or something else — have a beneficial effect on health. Your spirituality can help you live more fully despite your symptoms.

Consider a support group
Self-help organizations can be potent allies for many people who are coping with mental illness or who care about someone with such an illness. These groups include Alcoholics Anonymous and similar groups for people with other types of addictions. In many communities, self-help groups are available for people with depression, anxiety, schizophrenia and other mental illnesses. ■

Sleep Disorders

Sleep is a basic necessity, as fundamental to your health and well-being as fresh air, clean water and nutritious food. Humans spend about a third of their life sleeping. Sleep is more than just a timeout from daily life or a passive retreat. It's an active state that renews mental and physical health. After a good night's sleep, you wake up feeling refreshed, alert and ready to tackle the day's tasks.

When you don't get enough sleep, you may feel less alert and less vigorous and, perhaps, more confused, irritable and fatigued. Lack of sleep affects not only your energy level but also your mental and social functioning. It can make it more difficult for you to concentrate, and you may be impatient with others, less interactive in your relationships and less productive at work. Insufficient sleep also can be downright dangerous. According to the National Highway Traffic Safety Administration, more than 100,000 crashes each year are due to drivers falling asleep at the wheel. Recent data also indicates that insufficient sleep can increase death from other causes too — not just accidents.

So how much sleep is enough? The amount needed each night varies from person to person. Although some people claim to feel fine with only five to six hours of sleep a night, most people need at least seven hours of sleep a night on a consistent basis to feel rested the next day.

More important than counting hours is assessing how you feel during the day. If you are functioning well and feel alert, even when you sit down and relax for a few minutes, you're probably getting enough sleep.

Unfortunately, about 1 in 3 adults has occasional sleep problems. For many people, a hectic lifestyle and increased work demands put time at a premium, and sleep often takes a back seat.

Various sleep disorders also deprive people of their needed slumber. Insomnia, characterized by difficulty falling or staying asleep, in addition to daytime symptoms or impairment, is the most common sleep problem. Insomnia and other sleep disorders are discussed in this chapter, along with normal sleeping patterns.

Fortunately, most sleep difficulties are treatable, and addressing them often leads to a better night's sleep.

Sleep Stages and Patterns

While you're sleeping, many things are happening within your body. Sleep is a dynamic process, and not all sleep is the same. By measuring brain waves, sleep researchers have identified several stages of sleep that recur in fairly regular cycles throughout the night.

Are You Getting Enough Sleep?

Many people think they're getting adequate sleep but really aren't. You may not be getting the right amount and quality of sleep if:
- You routinely ignore your alarm clock or snatch a few extra minutes to snooze before getting up.
- You look forward to catching up on your sleep on the weekends.
- You have to fight to stay awake during long meetings or after a heavy meal.
- You're irritable with co-workers, family and friends.
- You have difficulty concentrating or remembering.
- It takes you a long time to fall asleep at night.
- You wake repeatedly throughout the night.
- You wake up groggy and not refreshed.
- Your spouse or partner complains about your snoring or fitful sleeping.

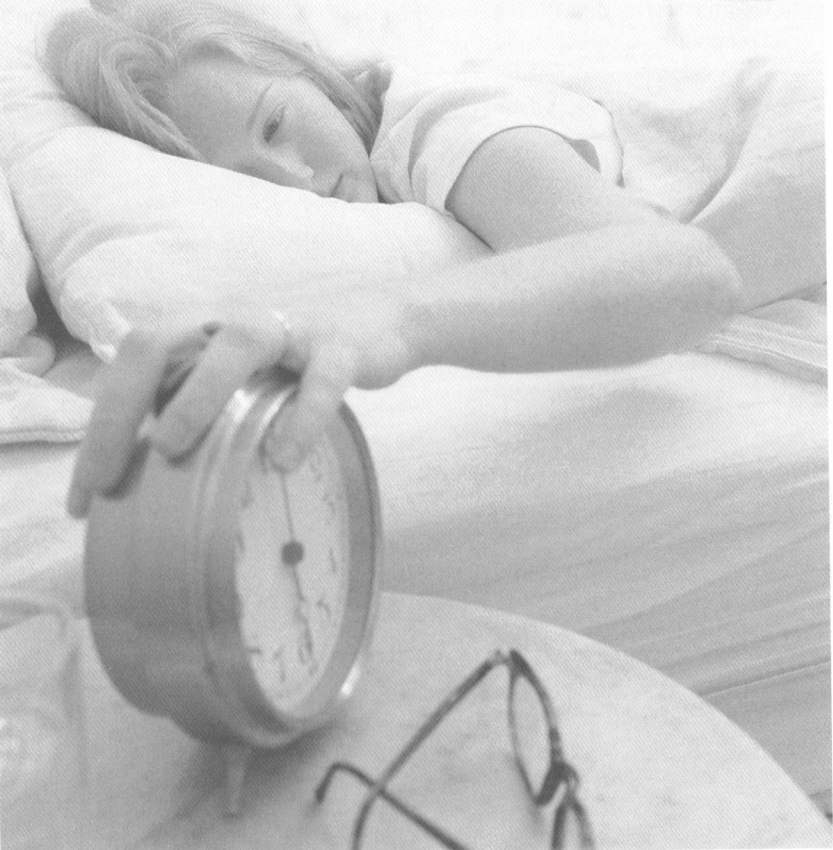

Sleep types and stages

The two types of sleep are non-rapid eye movement (NREM) and rapid eye movement (REM).

NREM sleep

The first stage of NREM sleep is called stage N1. This is a light stage of sleep during which your brain activity and body functions slow. Stage N2, an intermediate sleep stage, is the one in which you spend the most time. During this stage, your brain waves become larger, with bursts of electrical activity. Stage N3 is a deep sleep, and the most restful. In this stage, brain waves are large and slow, and you're more difficult to awaken.

REM sleep

Dream sleep (REM sleep) occurs about an hour and a half to two hours after you fall asleep. During REM sleep, your eyes move rapidly behind your closed lids, hence the name. This is a period of increased activity during which your dreams are more vivid and your body functions speed up.

During REM sleep, your brain waves show faster electrical activity at lower amplitude than at other sleep stages, a pattern that's similar to the brain waves of wakefulness. This suggests that you do more thinking, in the form of dreaming, in this stage than in the other sleep stages. People awakened during REM sleep may recall their dreams.

Even though some body functions speed up, most of your muscles are paralyzed — probably to keep you from acting out your dreams.

Sleep patterns

Your sleep patterns and needs are regulated by a biological clock in your brain.

The natural pattern of waking and sleeping that occurs within a 24-hour day is called the circadian rhythm. The word *circadian* comes from two Latin words, *circa*

Sleep Cycles

Throughout the night, you continuously move from one stage or type of sleep to another in cycles that can last from 70 to 90 minutes each. Early REM periods are usually short. You may experience several longer REM periods as the night progresses. Because REM sleep is more active, people often feel that sleep during the second half of the night is much shallower than that of the first half.

Light sleep
Body movement decreases. Spontaneous awakening may occur.

Your Natural Sleep Cycle

REM (rapid eye movement)
Dreaming occurs. Heart rate increases. Lasts about 10 minutes in first cycle, 20-30 minutes in later cycles.

Typically, you have four to six sleep cycles a night. Each cycle lasts 70 to 90 minutes.

Intermediate sleep
Most of the night is spent in this stage.

Deep sleep
Difficult to arouse. Most restorative stage, lasting 30-40 minutes in first few cycles, less in later cycles.

for "around" and *dia* for "day." Circadian rhythms guide not only your wake and sleep cycle but also your metabolism and your body temperature.

This internal clock usually makes you sleepy at night and ready to wake up in the morning. Most people's clocks run on a cycle of about 24 hours, but individual clocks vary. Some people are morning people and find that they have more energy and are more alert in the morning. Others, commonly referred to as night owls, are more alert late in the day. However, most people need to sleep between midnight and dawn. Many people are also somewhat sleepy in the early afternoon.

When your natural circadian rhythm is upset, sleep can become difficult. This can happen if you spend prolonged periods in bed, you're in an area with little natural light for an extended period, or you go to bed or wake at random times. Crossing several time zones during air travel can interrupt your circadian rhythm, causing jet lag. People who change work shifts often experience sleep difficulties. Temperature, metabolism and your mood also can affect your sleep pattern.

Changing sleep patterns with age

Sleep patterns vary according to age. During the first few weeks of life, most babies spend at least half their time sleeping. When they're born, infants seem unaware of the difference between night and day, but eventually they establish their own circadian rhythms, adapting their habits to fit a 24-hour day.

Babies spend about half their sleep time in rapid eye movement sleep, compared with about 20 percent for adults. Younger infants sometimes fall into REM sleep immediately, but adults usually pass through other sleep stages first. Scientists believe that REM sleep activates the learning areas of the brain.

As children grow, their sleeping habits become more organized. Frequent, unpredictable periods of sleep give way to about 11 hours of sleep at night, often in addition to a nap during the day. By about age 5, most children stop napping, and the number of hours of sleep they need gradually decreases. Although eight hours of sleep a night is often sufficient for children, many adolescents need a bit more — eight to 11 hours each night. During adolescence, the biological

Sleep and Aging

Some people have more trouble sleeping as they get older. In a study of more than 9,000 people age 65 and older, as many as 1 in 3 reported having trouble sleeping. Older adults often have trouble falling asleep at night, or they may wake up very early in the morning and not be able to go back to sleep.

Many factors conspire to make it more difficult to get a good night's sleep with age. These include:

Changes in sleep-wake pattern
As you age, your circadian rhythm typically changes. Older adults often get sleepy earlier in the evening and wake up earlier in the morning.

Lifestyle changes
You may be less physically or socially active. Activity helps promote good sleep. You may have more free time and, as a result, drink more caffeine or alcohol or take a daily nap. These things can interfere with nighttime sleep.

Medical conditions and life changes
Chronic pain from conditions such as arthritis or back problems can disrupt sleep. Other illnesses that can interfere with your sleep include arthritis, acid reflux, Parkinson's disease, dementia, Alzheimer's disease and lung disease.

Older men often develop noncancerous enlargement of the prostate gland (benign prostatic hyperplasia, or BPH). This can lead to more frequent urination at night. In women, hot flashes associated with menopause can disrupt sleep.

Mental health issues
Depression, stress and bereavement are common in older adults as they cope with life changes such as physical limitations, loss of loved ones and leaving their homes. These conditions often cause sleep difficulties.

Medications
Many medications have stimulating effects and can cause sleep difficulties. Medications that can interfere with sleep include some antidepressants, decongestants, bronchodilators, corticosteroids and high blood pressure drugs.

Sleep disorders
Several sleep disorders become more common with age. These include sleep apnea, restless legs syndrome, periodic limb movement disorder and rapid eye movement (REM) sleep behavior disorder.

Despite all of these changes, however, poor sleep isn't inevitable with age. You can do many things to improve the quality of your sleep. For example, daily exercise or more exposure to sunlight can help reinforce your sleep-wake cycle.

Women and Sleep

Menstruation, pregnancy and menopause all can affect how well women sleep. That's because changing levels of the female sex hormones estrogen and progesterone affect sleep.

During your menstrual cycle, the hormone progesterone rises after ovulation and may cause you to feel more sleepy or tired. Progesterone levels peak around days 19 to 21 of the cycle and then begin to fall. During this low point, you may find it more difficult to fall asleep. During the week before menstruation, some women who experience premenstrual syndrome (PMS) commonly report insomnia and daytime sleepiness.

Sleep disturbances during pregnancy are also common, especially as the pregnancy progresses. During the first trimester, daytime sleepiness may occur as a result of high progesterone levels. In the last trimester of pregnancy, physical discomfort, leg cramps, heartburn and an increased need to urinate may

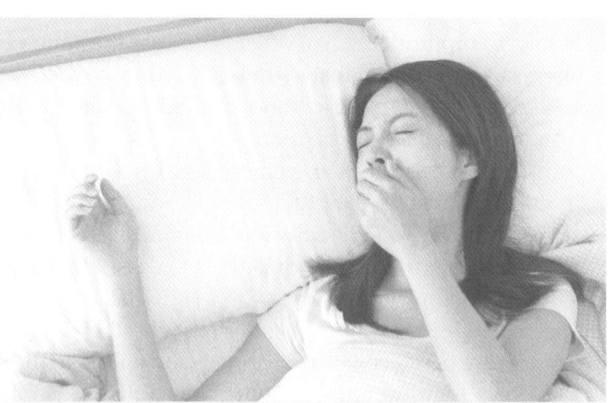

disturb sleep. Some pregnant women develop restless legs syndrome, which usually resolves after the baby is born. Sleep often continues to be interrupted after delivery because of the necessity to tend to the baby's needs during the night.

Women report the most sleep problems during menopause. Changing and decreasing levels of estrogen can cause symptoms that can disrupt sleep, such as hot flashes. Snoring is more common and more severe in postmenopausal women.

clock also changes. Teens start to stay up later and have a harder time waking up early. Studies suggest this change is partly due to a delay in the secretion of a hormone that induces sleepiness and helps set a person's circadian rhythm (melatonin). Sleep patterns are also influenced by social factors, such as time spent in front of video or TV screens, on the telephone, or with friends.

Sleep needs generally remain constant throughout adulthood. Despite the popular notion you need less sleep as you age, the amount of sleep your body and brain require changes little. However, sleep patterns change with age and sleep becomes less restful. You not only get less restorative sleep but also sleep more lightly and awaken more easily.

Insomnia

Insomnia is the most common sleep disorder. Insomnia refers to difficulty getting to sleep or staying asleep to the point where daytime functioning seems affected. Everyone experiences insomnia occasionally, but when it occurs on a regular or frequent basis, it can affect your quality of life.

Signs and symptoms
- Difficulty falling asleep at night
- Waking up often or for a prolonged period during the night
- Waking too early in the morning
- Daytime fatigue or sleepiness
- Daytime irritability or mood disturbance
- Difficulty with attention, concentration or memory

About a third of all people experience insomnia at some point.

Consequences

For most people, a night or two of poor sleep, or even a night of no sleep, isn't that bad. Lost sleep may sap your motivation and make it difficult to concentrate, but

as long as you get back to a normal sleep schedule within a few days, you'll experience no lasting consequences. One good night of sleep after a few poor ones usually is enough to catch up.

However, chronically losing sleep can result in sleep debt, which can lead to serious consequences. Sleep debt is cumulative, and even small nightly sleep losses can add up to affect daytime function. Possible consequences include increased accidents and poor performance on the job or in school. Researchers also have found that people who get significantly more or less than seven hours of sleep each night have a shorter life span.

Long-term sleep deprivation, from any cause, can affect your physical and mental health. Sleep helps bolster your immune system so that you can fight off viruses and bacteria.

Causes

The causes of insomnia are many and varied. They include:

Stress and anxiety
Concerns about work, school, health or family can keep your

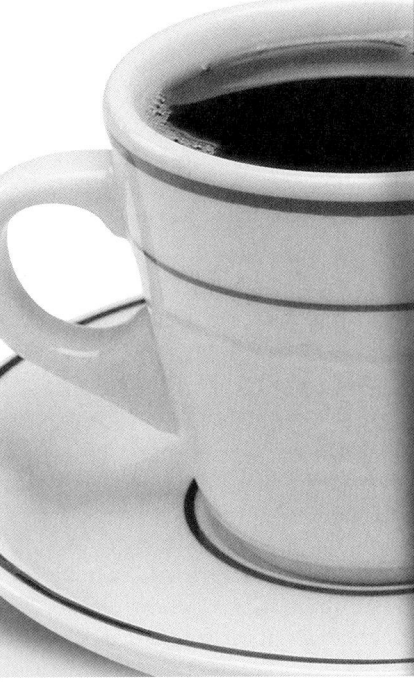

mind too active and unable to relax for sleep. Excessive inactivity or stress from a long illness can keep you awake. Everyday anxieties as well as severe anxiety disorders may keep your mind too alert to sleep.

Depression
People who are depressed often either sleep too much or have trouble falling or staying asleep. This may be due to chemical imbalances in the brain or because anxiety that can accompany depression prevents relaxation.

Environment or work changes
Long-distance air travel or having to work a late or early shift can disrupt your body's circadian rhythms.

Age
Insomnia becomes more prevalent with age.

Stimulants and medications
Drinking coffee, tea or colas can trigger insomnia. If you're especially sensitive to caffeine, more than two servings a day or even one serving after noon can keep you awake at night.

Smoking can also contribute to insomnia. Nicotine is an addictive stimulant that can keep you awake. In addition, smokers experience withdrawal symptoms at night, making it harder both to fall asleep at night and to wake up in the morning.

Some prescription medications, including steroids, some high blood pressure medications and antidepressants, can interfere with sleep. Many over-the-counter medications, including some pain medications, decongestants and weight-loss products, contain caffeine and other stimulants.

Alcohol
Although a drink or two of an alcoholic beverage seems to help some people relax enough to fall asleep, even moderate amounts can distort normal sleeping patterns. Alcohol

may help you get to sleep, but it also frequently wakes you up in the middle of the night. It can also cause long-term sleep problems even if you quit drinking altogether.

Learned insomnia

After a few nights of poor sleep, you may start worrying about sleep. The more you worry, the less you sleep. You may come to associate being in your bedroom with being awake. Most people who have this type of insomnia sleep better when they're away from their usual sleep environment or when they're not trying to sleep, such as when they're watching television.

Medical conditions and life changes

Diseases or disorders that cause pain, such as arthritis, fibromyalgia or a nerve disorder (neuropathy), can interfere with sleep. Allergies, thyroid problems and menopause also can affect your sleep.

Eating too much too late

Eating too much before bedtime may cause you to feel physically uncomfortable while lying down, making it difficult to sleep. You may experience heartburn, a reflux of food from the stomach into the esophagus. This uncomfortable feeling may keep you awake.

Poor sleep environment

A bed partner's snoring, a barking dog and an overheated room are some environmental conditions that can make it difficult to sleep.

Diagnosis

If you're more tired than usual and you haven't been able to sleep well at least three times a week for three months or more, you may have chronic insomnia. See your doctor. Your doctor may ask you about your sleep patterns, such as how long you've experienced troublesome symptoms and

whether they occur every night. He or she may also ask about your mood, your work schedule, whether you snore, how well you function during the day, and if you take any medications or have other health disorders. You may also be asked to complete a questionnaire to determine your level of daytime sleepiness.

? Question and Answer

I work the night shift and have trouble sleeping during the day. Is there anything I can do?

For many shift workers, sleep is particularly elusive. Shift work forces you to try to sleep when activities around you and your own biological rhythms signal you to remain awake — and vice versa.

To promote better sleep, keep your bedroom as quiet and dark as possible and stick to a sleep schedule. If possible, remain "shifted" on the days that you're not working, that is, follow the same sleep-wake pattern as you would on a workday.

Using caffeine to keep awake while you're working also may make it more difficult to sleep once you get home. Try to limit caffeine consumption to the beginning of your shift.

If it's daylight when you're on your way home from work, try wearing sunglasses to prevent confusing your internal clock.

Some people's sleep problems are a result of frequent changes in their work shifts. Try to stay on a specific shift, such as the night shift. If that's not possible, try rotating from morning to evening shifts rather than working shifts in random order.

Your doctor may have you keep a sleep diary for a couple of weeks, with observations about when you went to bed, when you got up, how long it took to fall asleep, how much you think you slept during the night, how much caffeine or alcohol you consumed, and how rested you felt the next morning. He or she may also suggest that you spend a night at a sleep disorders center so your sleep can be monitored and studied.

Treatment

Insomnia is usually temporary. If self-help measures don't work, your doctor may recommend other approaches.

Cognitive behavioral therapy

Cognitive behavioral therapy for insomnia (CBT-I) tends to be more effective than medications are for long-term treatment of insomnia. This type of treatment can educate you about sleep and help you try to adjust your sleep behaviors and how you think about sleep. CBT-I may include:

Relaxation training
Relaxation training, in which you learn different physical and mental relaxation techniques, is a useful part of CBT-I for most people with insomnia.

Stimulus control
Stimulus control trains you to associate your bedroom with sleep. You may be asked to limit activities in your bedroom to sleep and sex, to go to bed only when you're sleepy, and to leave the bedroom if you don't fall asleep quickly.

Sleep restriction
Your doctor may ask you to reduce the time you spend in bed to as few as five hours a night, then gradually increase the time until the desired quality and duration of sleep are achieved. The idea is to reduce the amount of time spent in bed without sleeping.

Medication

To help you sleep, your doctor may prescribe medications, often as a short-term treatment until other therapies begin to work.

Prescription sleeping pills

Depending on your diagnosis, you may take a prescription sleep aid for a couple of weeks until you have less stress in your life or until you notice benefits from lifestyle changes or cognitive behavioral therapy for insomnia. When your sleep seems to be improving, your doctor may gradually lower the dose of the medication.

Benzodiazepines such as triazolam (Halcion) are older types of sleeping pills that slow down your central nervous system. This type of medication may lose its effectiveness after a few months of use and can worsen insomnia when you stop using it.

Some of the newer sleeping pills zolpidem (Ambien) and zaleplon (Sonata) tend to be less habit-forming than the older ones, but they can be associated with other side effects, such as sleepwalking. They're usually not recommended for long-term use.

Tips for Better Sleep

If you're experiencing insomnia, the first thing to consider is whether simple changes in your daily routine may help you sleep. Here are some ways to improve your sleep:

- *Stick to a sleep schedule.* Go to bed and get up at about the same time every day, including on weekends.
- *Establish and follow a bedtime ritual.* In the evening, slow the pace of your activities and avoid activities that keep you mentally alert or require the use of electronic devices close to bedtime.
- *Limit your time in bed to no more than 8 hours.* Spending too much time in bed may disrupt sleep.
- *Don't eat or drink a lot before bed.* A light snack may help you sleep, but avoid heavy meals and fluids or foods that stimulate stomach acid production, which could cause heartburn. Drink less liquid before bedtime so that you won't have to go to the bathroom as often.
- *Avoid or limit naps.* Regular daytime naps may contribute to insomnia. If you can't get by without one, keep it to less than 30 minutes and don't nap in the late afternoon or evening.
- *Schedule worry time.* If worries keep you awake, attempt to deal with them before bedtime. Set aside a worry time during the day. Make a list of problems and identify possible solutions.
- *Avoid or limit caffeine, nicotine and alcohol.* Don't drink caffeinated coffee, tea, cocoa or cola after lunchtime. If you drink more than 4 cups of caffeinated coffee a day (or the equivalent) and are experiencing insomnia, you may want to cut back.
- *Don't watch the clock.* Place your bedside clock in a dresser drawer or under the bed.
- *Exercise and stay active.* Regular activity helps promote a good night's sleep. Aim for at least 150 minutes of moderate aerobic activity or 75 minutes of vigorous aerobic activity a week and strength training exercises at least twice a week. Schedule exercise at least a few hours before bedtime.
- *Find ways to relax.* Taking a warm bath or drinking a cup of warm milk may help. Try relaxation exercises.

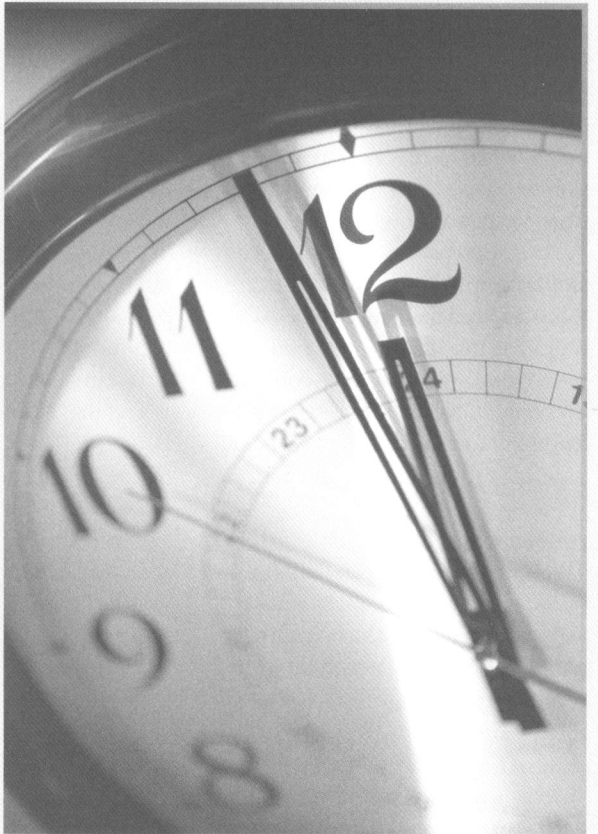

- *Create a comfortable sleep environment.* Keep your sleeping environment quiet, dark and comfortably cool. Make sure your bed is comfortable.
- *Don't rely on sleeping pills.* If you do take a sleep medication for a few days, ask your doctor how to reduce the dosage gradually when you want to discontinue using it.
- *Check your medications.* Ask your doctor if your prescription medications may be contributing to your insomnia. Check over-the-counter products to see if they contain caffeine or other stimulants, as well.
- *If sleep doesn't come naturally, get up.* Read a book, listen to music or watch television until you feel drowsy. Then go to your bedroom to fall asleep. But don't change your rising time in the morning. Keep the time you get up each day consistent.

Sleep medications should only be used if you spend enough time in bed, because they can cause sedation and impair your ability to drive or operate heavy machinery. Alcohol, which is also a sedative, exaggerates the effects of sleep medications and should not be used along with sleeping pills. If you're over age 65, some sleeping pills may not be appropriate because their sedating effects can increase your risk of falling.

Over-the-counter sleeping pills
Over-the-counter sleeping pills are less effective than prescription medications. Many nonprescription sleep medications contain antihistamines to induce drowsiness.

These products are OK for occasional sleepless nights, but they, too, often lose their effectiveness the more you take them. Many nonprescription sleeping pills contain diphenhydramine, which can cause difficulty urinating and may make you feel drowsy during the day.

Antidepressants
Treating depression can help improve sleep, but most antidepressants don't improve sleep right away, and some can even interfere with sleep.

Your doctor may prescribe a low dose of a sedating antidepressant, such as the drug trazodone, to help you sleep.

Sleep Apnea

Sleep apnea occurs in two main types. Obstructive sleep apnea, the more common form, occurs when your throat muscles relax and obstruct breathing. Central sleep apnea occurs when your brain doesn't send proper signals to the muscles that control breathing or when the muscles and nerves of the chest that control breathing aren't working well.

Some people have complex sleep apnea syndrome, also known as treatment-emergent central sleep

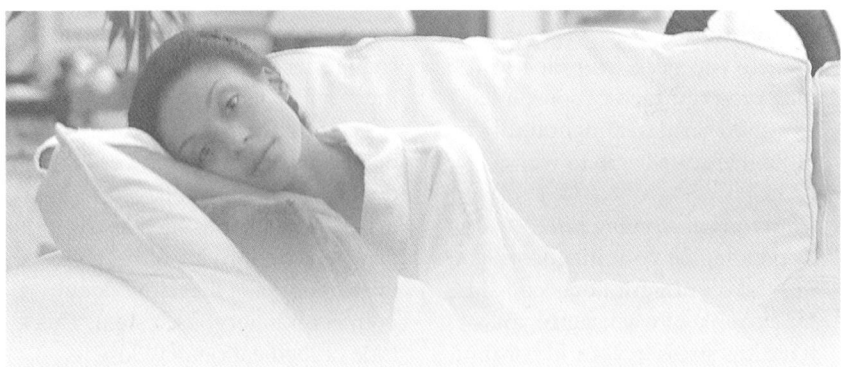

To Nap or Not to Nap?

It's afternoon and your eyelids are getting heavy. You try to ignore the feeling, but you have to fight to stay awake. Should you follow the irresistible urge to snooze, or will taking a nap keep you from sleeping well at night?

It depends. If you're not getting enough sleep, napping may or may not help. The best solution is to try to go to bed earlier. If that's not possible, a daytime nap may give you the boost you need, helping you feel more energized and alert. For people who have insomnia, however, a daytime nap can make sleeping at night more difficult.

The urge for a midday nap is built into your body's biological clock. Between 1 and 3 p.m., most people experience a slight drop in body temperature and a possible lull in alertness. For this reason, some cultures incorporate an afternoon nap into their lifestyle.

If you do nap, keep it short — limit it to 20 or 30 minutes late in the morning or in the early afternoon. But don't rely on naps to keep you going. Try to get enough sleep each night to avoid accumulating a sleep deficit.

INTEGRATIVE MEDICINE

Melatonin is a hormone that occurs naturally in the human body and that helps establish your sleep-wake rhythm. Melatonin supplements sold in stores are a synthetic or animal form of the hormone.

Some research suggests that over-the-counter melatonin supplements taken at the right time might be helpful in treating jet lag or other sleep disorders that involve poor alignment of your natural biological clock with the night-day pattern around you. Melatonin might also reduce the time it takes to fall asleep — although this effect is typically mild. Avoid activities that require alertness, such as driving or operating heavy machinery, for four to five hours after taking melatonin.

In addition to melatonin, the herbal supplement valerian has been shown to be effective as a sleep aid in a small number of studies. Valerian may help some people fall asleep more quickly and improve sleep quality. Some people find drinking chamomile tea helpful.

If you're considering taking melatonin supplements or valerian, check with your doctor first — especially if you have any health conditions. Supplements are less regulated than are medications. Your doctor can help determine if the product is safe for you and the correct dosage to take.

apnea. This occurs when someone has obstructive sleep apnea and central sleep apnea.

Signs and symptoms

Signs and symptoms of sleep apnea may include:

- Excessive daytime sleepiness
- Frequent loud snoring
- Waking with a snorting, choking or gasping sensation
- Observed episodes of stopping breathing during sleep
- Multiple nighttime awakenings
- Feeling unrefreshed when you wake up
- Morning headache
- Elevated blood pressure

Other signs and symptoms include irritability, low mood, difficulty concentrating, impotence, decreased sex drive, dry mouth and sore throat.

During sleep, the muscles in the back of your throat (pharynx) relax. These muscles normally keep your airway open, and they support structures in your mouth and throat, such as the small, teardrop-shaped tissue at the back of your throat (uvula), the soft palate, your tonsils and your tongue.

With obstructive sleep apnea, the muscles collapse on themselves and obstruct airflow. Obstruction of airflow lowers the level of oxygen in your blood. After 10 to 20 seconds or more of an insufficient exchange of air, your brain senses the problem and rouses you to a lighter level of sleep or brief wakefulness. The muscles then regain their normal tone (tenseness), the obstruction is relieved, and you resume breathing, possibly with a snort.

This pattern can repeat itself several times an hour, all night long. You may not be aware of these interruptions of your sleep. In fact, many people with sleep apnea think they sleep well. But the repetitive obstructions prevent them from reaching the deep, restorative phases of sleep.

Central sleep apnea has a different cause. In this form, the airway

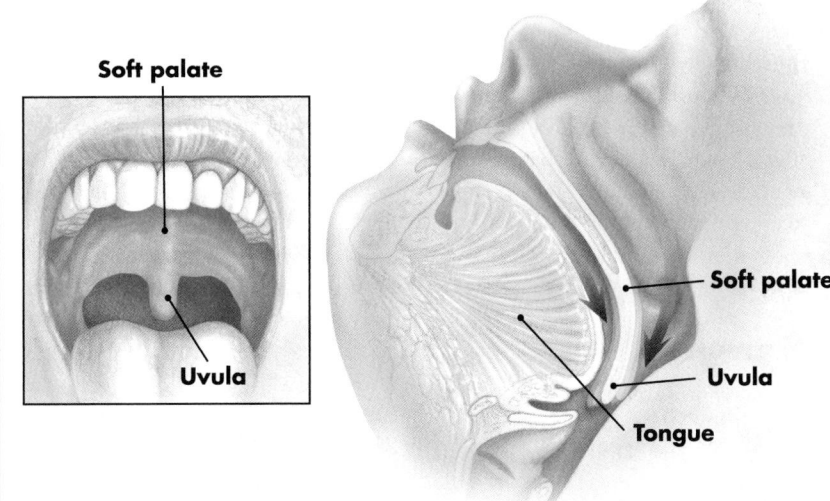

Soft palate

Uvula

Soft palate

Uvula

Tongue

In obstructive sleep apnea, the muscles that normally keep your airway open relax and sag during sleep, causing your tongue, tonsils, soft palate or uvula to repeatedly block your breathing.

stays open, but the diaphragm or chest muscles stop working, resulting in an interruption in breathing. The level of carbon dioxide in the blood rises, which may cause you to wake up.

Sleep apnea is most common in middle-aged, overweight men, although women, young people and people who aren't overweight also may have it.

Dangers

Sleep apnea is considered a serious medical condition because sudden drops in blood oxygen levels strain the cardiovascular system. The pauses in breathing (apneas) force your heart to pump harder every time it's deprived of oxygen. Untreated sleep apnea is associated with an increased risk of heart attack, coronary artery disease, stroke, heart rhythm problems and congestive heart failure.

In addition, more than half the people with obstructive sleep apnea have high blood pressure, which also raises the risk of stroke and heart failure. Treating sleep apnea may lower blood pressure.

The repeated awakenings associated with sleep apnea make

Are You at Risk?

Certain factors may put you more at risk of having obstructive sleep apnea. They include:

- *Excess weight, especially around the neck.* A fat or thick neck tends to narrow the airway in your throat.
- *A narrow airway, enlarged tonsils or adenoids, and certain facial features.* They can narrow your airway.
- *Being male.* Men are more likely than women to suffer from sleep apnea.
- *Being older.* Your risk of sleep apnea increases as you get older.
- *High blood pressure.* Sleep apnea is common in people with hypertension.
- *Family history.* Family members with the disorder increase your risk.
- *Smoking.* People who smoke are more likely to have obstructive sleep apnea.

normal, restorative sleep impossible. They can also keep a roommate or bed partner from sleeping well. People with sleep apnea may have difficulty concentrating and may find themselves falling asleep at work, while watching television or even when driving. People with sleep apnea are much more likely to have motor vehicle accidents than people without the disorder.

Diagnosis

See your doctor if:
- Your breathing pauses during sleep.
- You or others have noticed that you awaken at night snorting, choking or gasping.
- You snore frequently or loudly enough to disturb another person's sleep.
- You experience excessive daytime drowsiness that may cause you to fall asleep while you're working, driving or inactive.

Your doctor may ask you and your partner questions about your snoring, any pauses in breathing and other sleep behaviors. Excess weight or high blood pressure also suggest possible sleep apnea.

Your doctor may refer you to a sleep disorders clinic for a sleep evaluation to confirm the diagnosis. A sleep evaluation usually involves an overnight stay at the facility during which staff monitor your breathing and other body functions during sleep.

In a test called polysomnography, sensors (electrodes) are placed at various locations on your body and are attached to equipment that monitors your heart, lung and brain activity, breathing patterns, arm and leg movements, and blood oxygen levels. In some circumstances, a sleep test may be done at home using a portable monitoring device. Because treatments for sleep disorders differ, it's important to get an accurate diagnosis and determine exactly what's causing your sleeping problem.

Treatment

Sleep apnea rarely goes away on its own, but it can be treated. If you have mild sleep apnea, your doctor may recommend self-care measures such as losing weight and avoiding sleeping on your back. For most people with moderate to severe sleep apnea, the best treatment is continuous positive airway pressure (CPAP). For some people, surgery may be necessary.

Self-care
A number of steps can help treat obstructive sleep apnea or keep it from getting worse. These include:
- *Losing excess weight.* Even small reductions in weight can produce major improvements in sleep apnea.
- *Sleeping on your side or stomach.* Sleeping on your back can cause your tongue and soft palate to rest against the back of your throat and block your airway. If your sleep apnea occurs because you sleep mostly on your back or if you have a mild case of sleep apnea, sewing a pocket or an athletic stocking on the back of your pajamas and placing a tennis ball inside the pocket or stocking is a trick that may keep you from sleeping on your back.
- *Avoiding alcohol and certain medications.* Alcohol, tranquilizers and sleeping pills relax the muscles in the back of the throat, interfering with your breathing.

CPAP
With a CPAP device, you usually place a mask over your nose. The mask is connected to a small machine that gently increases the pressure of the air you breathe. The pressure keeps your upper airway passages open, preventing apnea and snoring. This form of treatment is extremely effective. It can eliminate snoring, dramatically improve the quality of your sleep, eliminate excessive daytime sleepiness and lower your blood pressure. In some individuals, a full mask, which covers both the nose and mouth, just the mouth, or inside or over the nostrils, may be used.

CPAP isn't a permanent cure — when you stop using the machine, sleep apnea returns. In addition, some people won't use the machine. They don't like the feel of the mask, or may be self-conscious about wearing it.

Oral appliance therapy
Your doctor may recommend a dental device designed to open your throat by bringing your jaw forward or holding your tongue forward. You wear the device at night. It may relieve snoring and mild to moderate sleep apnea.

Surgery
If you can't tolerate a CPAP machine and don't benefit from other treatments, your doctor may recommend surgery to increase the size of your airway. Here are several common types of surgical procedures.

During a uvulopalatopharyngoplasty (UPPP), tissue from the back of your mouth and top of your throat is removed. Tonsils and adenoids are usually removed as well. UPPP can decrease or eliminate snoring. It's less effective than CPAP, and it isn't considered a reliable treatment for obstructive sleep apnea.

Another surgical procedure is laser-assisted uvulopalatoplasty (LAUPP), in which a laser is used to remove tissue from the back of your throat. This method has been effective in reducing snoring but has shown minimal success in treating obstructive sleep apnea.

If your jaw or nasal structures are contributing to a blocked airway, your doctor may recommend surgery to remove polyps, straighten a deviated septum, remove enlarged tonsils or adenoids, or move the jaw and tongue forward.

In carefully selected individuals, a nerve stimulator that's surgically

able as well as different devices to deliver the oxygen to your lungs.

Treating associated problems
Possible causes of central sleep apnea (see page 1162) include heart or neuromuscular disorders or opioid pain medications. Treating the conditions or discontinuing the medications may improve sleep apnea.

Narcolepsy

Narcolepsy is a disease in which people feel excessively sleepy during the day. The term comes from the Greek word *narke,* meaning "stupor." This sleep disorder is a neurological problem involving sleep-wake mechanisms in the brain and abnormalities of rapid eye movement (REM) sleep.

Signs and symptoms
Signs and symptoms of narcolepsy may include:
- Excessive daytime sleepiness
- Sudden loss of muscle tone (cataplexy)
- A feeling of paralysis when going to sleep or waking up
- Dreamlike hallucinations

People with narcolepsy may at any time begin to feel drowsy and

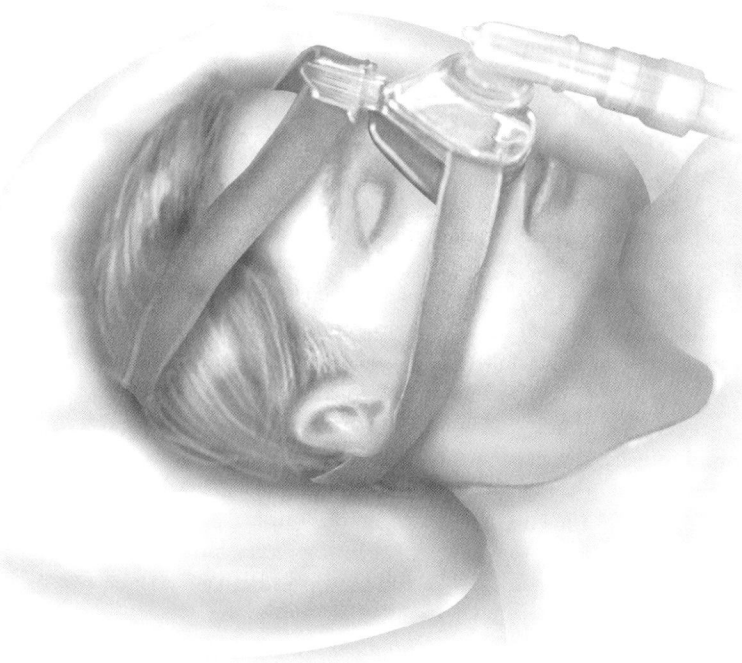

A continuous positive airway pressure (CPAP) nasal device delivers air pressure to keep your upper airway passages open, preventing apnea and snoring.

implanted may be used to treat obstructive sleep apnea. This is called maxillomandibular advancement surgery.

Another surgery called tracheotomy is recommended only if all other treatments have failed and you have severe, life-threatening sleep apnea. An opening is made in the windpipe (trachea). During the day, the opening is covered, but at night it's uncovered to allow air to pass in and out of the lungs, bypassing the blockage in your throat.

Supplemental oxygen
In some cases, using supplemental oxygen while you sleep may help. Various forms of oxygen are avail-

Snoring

Snoring is very common. As many as half of adults snore. It results when air flows past relaxed tissues in your throat, causing the tissues to vibrate. You hear this vibration as snoring.

If your snoring is frequent, loud, or associated with snorting, choking, gasping, pauses in your breathing or daytime drowsiness, you may have sleep apnea, and a sleep study may be necessary. Even if your snoring isn't associated with sleep apnea, it can be disruptive to your partner's sleep.

There are many steps you can take to treat snoring. Losing weight, sleeping on your side, treating nasal congestion or obstruction, and avoiding alcohol and sedating medications may help. Nasal strips are another remedy to try. They may help increase the area of

your nasal passages, enhancing your breathing. A customized dental device also may help reduce or eliminate snoring.

In addition to traditional uvulopalatopharyngoplasty (UPPP), laser-assisted uvulopalatoplasty (LAUPP) and somnoplasty are used at some medical centers to treat snoring. During somnoplasty, high-frequency sound waves heat throat tissue and shrink part of the tongue and soft palate. In LAUPP, the surgeon uses a laser to remove the uvula and a small portion of the soft palate. These treatments aren't advised for occasional or light snoring, but may be an option if your snoring is frequent, loud and disruptive. The long-term effectiveness of either of these procedures isn't known.

instantly enter REM sleep, without first passing through the non-rapid eye movement (NREM) sleep stages. Researchers believe that genetics, brain chemicals called neurotransmitters and some sort of trigger, such as a virus, all may play a role in causing narcolepsy.

Narcolepsy is an underrecognized and underdiagnosed condition that affects about 1 in every 2,000 Americans. Narcolepsy is often mistaken for depression, lack of sleep or other conditions that may cause daytime sleepiness. The primary symptom of narcolepsy is an overwhelming feeling of drowsiness and uncontrollable need to sleep during the day. These sleep attacks often occur after lunch and during sedentary situations, but they may also happen during active times — for example, while you're driving or having a conversation. Extreme sleepiness may cause low sex drive or impotence.

Cataplexy occurs in people who have narcolepsy type 1. This loss of muscle tone can cause a range of physical changes, from slurred speech to total physical collapse, lasting for a few seconds to a few minutes. Cataplexy is often triggered by strong emotions, such as laughter, anger, embarrassment, excitement, surprise or joy. People have narcolepsy type 2 if they have narcolepsy but not cataplexy.

Some people with narcolepsy experience a temporary inability to move or talk while falling asleep or waking (sleep paralysis). People often feel awake or half-awake during this paralysis, which may last a few seconds to a few minutes.

Hallucinations can take place if you fall quickly into REM sleep. Because you may be semiawake when you begin dreaming, you interpret the dreams as reality, and they may be vivid and frightening.

Other signs and symptoms include restless nighttime sleep and sleep talking. Some people perform routine tasks but aren't aware of and don't remember doing them.

Diagnosis

Your doctor may suspect that you have narcolepsy based on your symptoms and age. Most people who have narcolepsy develop symptoms between 10 and 30 years of age. You may be referred to a sleep specialist for additional studies and evaluation.

Methods of diagnosing narcolepsy and determining its severity include polysomnogram tests taken while you're asleep to measure brain waves, body movements, and nerve and muscle functions. A multiple sleep latency test measures how long it takes for you to fall asleep during the day.

Treatment

A combination of medications and lifestyle adjustments are generally used to manage narcolepsy. The goal is to improve your alertness during critical times of the day,

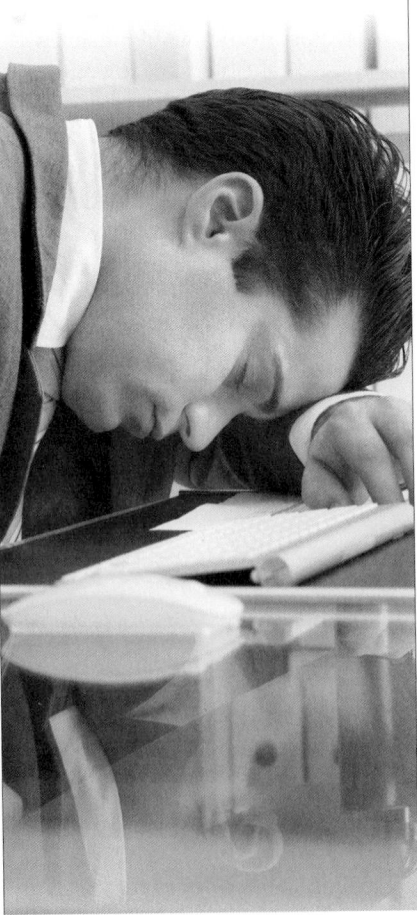

such as at work and school and while driving.

Medication

Medical treatment of narcolepsy includes the following medications:

Stimulants

Medications that stimulate the central nervous system have long been the primary treatment to help people with narcolepsy stay awake during the day. These drugs include amphetamines and the drug methylphenidate (Aptensio XR, Concerta, Ritalin).

Although these medications improve symptoms in many people, they may cause side effects and can be addictive.

Modafinil and armodafinil

The medications modafinil (Provigil) and armodafinil (Nuvigil) also improve alertness in people with narcolepsy. How these medications work isn't clearly understood. Research results so far show that they are less addictive and have fewer side effects when compared with traditional stimulants.

Antidepressants

Doctors often prescribe antidepressant medications, which suppress REM sleep, to help alleviate the signs and symptoms of cataplexy, hallucinations and sleep paralysis. These medications affect levels of neurotransmitters — brain chemicals that may play a role in narcolepsy.

Antidepressants used to treat narcolepsy include tricyclic antidepressants, such as protriptyline (Vivactil) and imipramine (Tofranil), as well as selective serotonin reuptake inhibitors (SSRIs), such as fluoxetine (Prozac, Sarafem, Selfemra). Venlafaxine (Effexor XR) is also commonly used.

Sodium oxybate (Xyrem) is another drug used to treat cataplexy, as well as daytime sleepiness. This potent medication requires special education and a specific dosing schedule.

Self-care

Lifestyle modifications are important in managing the symptoms of narcolepsy. Self-care measures include:

- Going to sleep and waking up at the same time every day, including weekends
- Making sure you get seven to eight hours of sleep at night
- Scheduling 20-minute naps each day
- Stopping for naps and exercise breaks when you feel drowsy
- Avoiding nicotine and alcohol, which can worsen signs and symptoms, especially when used at night

- Working with your doctor to establish a medication schedule that ensures the greatest likelihood of wakefulness when you drive
- Telling your employer, co-workers or teachers about your condition and working to find ways to accommodate your needs — including napping during the day, breaking up monotonous tasks and taking occasional walks

Having narcolepsy can be a challenge to your personal and professional life. Others may perceive people with narcolepsy as being lazy, lethargic or rude. Narcolepsy can affect intimate relationships because of sexual dysfunction and emotional difficulties. Support groups and counseling can help people with narcolepsy and their loved ones cope with the disorder.

Sleep Centers

Many hospitals and medical centers operate sleep clinics to diagnose sleep disorders. These centers are accredited by the American Academy of Sleep Medicine. More than 2,500 sleep centers are accredited nationwide.

If you have a sleep problem, you may be referred to a sleep center. During your first visit, a sleep history will likely be assembled based on questions about your sleep and daytime habits. Family members also may be asked to provide information about your sleep habits.

After the initial consultation, you may spend a night at the center so that your sleep can be monitored. Before you go to sleep, small sensors (electrodes) and other types of monitoring equipment are placed on your head and body to record a variety of bodily activities during the night, including brain wave patterns, breathing and heart rate, muscle activity, and eye and body movements. This monitoring, called a polysomnography, isn't painful. Other tests may be conducted.

The results of these studies help sleep disorder specialists identify your condition so that it can be treated appropriately.

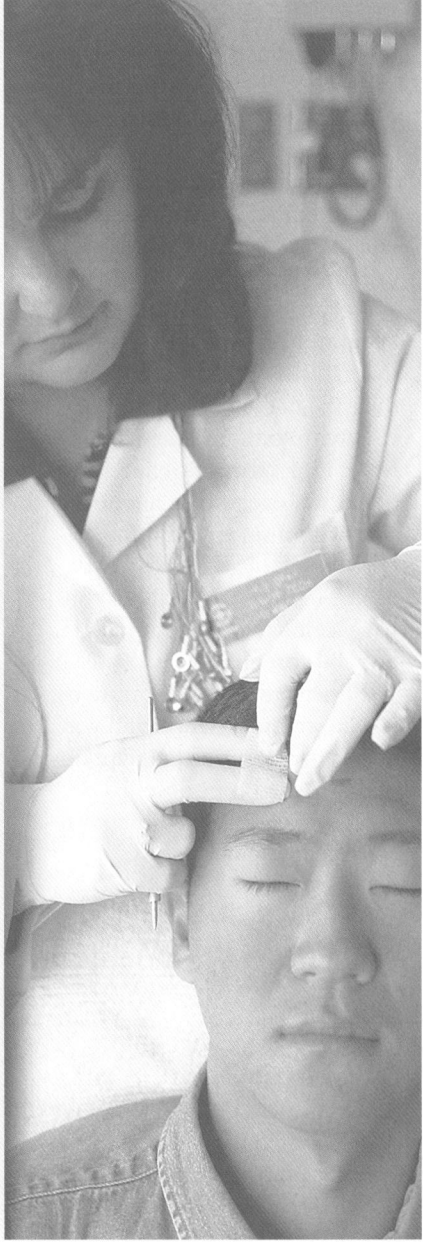

Restless Legs Syndrome

Restless legs syndrome (RLS), also known as Willis-Ekbom disease, is a condition in which you feel a strong urge to move your legs when you're resting or sitting still in the evening. You may also feel other sensations, including creeping, crawling, jittery, tingling, burning or aching — or it may feel like insects crawling inside your legs. The feelings are unpleasant but usually not painful.

To combat the sensations, people stretch or jiggle their legs, pace the floor, or exercise. These activities may relieve the symptoms only briefly.

Signs and symptoms

- An irresistible urge to move your legs when you're sitting or lying down. This sensation is at least temporarily relieved by moving your legs or walking.
- Symptoms that worsen during the evening and nighttime hours and are better during the day.
- Unpleasant sensations in the legs and occasionally other areas of the body.

The sensations associated with this condition may begin shortly after you go to bed. That's why some people with restless legs syndrome find it difficult to get to sleep or stay asleep, resulting in daytime sleepiness.

The disorder isn't dangerous, but it can be intensely uncomfortable and disruptive to sleep. Many people with RLS also experience involuntary leg twitches and jerks during sleep, called periodic limb movements of sleep.

RLS affects 7 to 10 percent of Americans, although the condition is thought to be underdiagnosed. It can develop at any age, even during childhood. It's more common with increasing age and more common in women than in men.

The cause of RLS is unknown, but it sometimes runs in families, especially if the condition starts before age 50. Some people with RLS have anemia or iron deficiency. Chronic diseases such as kidney failure, diabetes and Parkinson's disease are associated with RLS. Certain medications can cause RLS or make its symptoms worse. Some pregnant women develop RLS, especially in the last trimester. For most, symptoms disappear within a month after delivery.

Diagnosis

Your doctor may diagnose RLS by evaluating your symptoms and asking questions about your sleep habits. Blood tests may be done to check your iron levels and look for other conditions, such as anemia or diabetes.

If an underlying condition is causing your symptoms, treating that condition often alleviates many symptoms. In people with iron deficiency, iron replacement may help. But iron should only be taken under your doctor's supervision after a blood test has confirmed an iron deficiency, because iron overload can be harmful to your health.

Treatment

For people with mild to moderate symptoms of RLS, lifestyle changes can often reduce or eliminate symptoms.

Self-care
To help prevent or ease symptoms:
- **Try baths and massages.** Taking warm baths and massaging your legs before bed can relax your muscles.

- **Exercise.** Moderate, regular exercise may relieve symptoms of RLS, but overdoing it at the gym or working out too late in the evening may intensify symptoms.
- **Stretch before bedtime.** See the illustrations on page 939.
- **Avoid caffeine, alcohol and tobacco.** These substances may aggravate or trigger symptoms in people who are predisposed to develop RLS.
- **Distract yourself.** When you begin to notice symptoms of RLS, try to distract yourself by doing something interesting.
- **Eat a balanced diet.** Include foods that contain iron.

Medication
If self-care measures don't help, a prescription medication may be used to help treat symptoms of RLS. The most commonly used medications are those that increase the amount of dopamine in your body. These include pramipexole (Mirapex) and ropinirole (Requip).

Pregabalin (Lyrica) and gabapentin (Neurontin) are also used to treat RLS. These medications reduce the nerve activity that causes RLS symptoms and seem to have fewer long-term side effects compared with dopamine agonists.

For more-severe symptoms, opioids such as codeine may be used, but these medications can have serious side effects and may be habit-forming.

With any of these medications, it is important to work with your doctor to determine the right time of day to take your dose. To get the most benefit, take medications in a consistent manner.

Periodic Limb Movement Disorder

Periodic limb movement disorder (PLMD) is an uncommon disease.

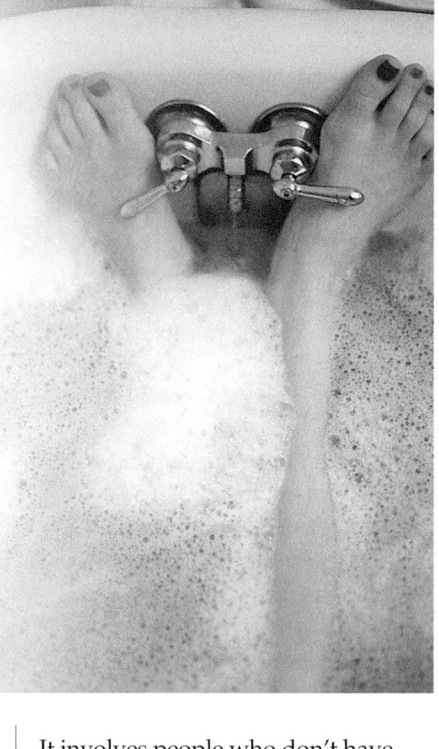

It involves people who don't have RLS but experience involuntary leg twitches or jerking prior to or during sleep. These movements disrupt sleep and can cause you to feel tired during the day.

Signs and symptoms
- Twitches, jerks or kicks of the legs or flexing of the feet that disrupt sleep
- Daytime sleepiness or tiredness caused by involuntary leg movements during sleep
- Trouble getting back to sleep after being awakened by leg movements
- Not having the typical signs or symptoms of restless legs syndrome

The involuntary movements typical of this disorder last one to three seconds and are spaced 20 to 40 seconds apart. The movements aren't harmful, but they can wake you from sleep and disturb your bed partner.

Many people with PLMD are not aware of their leg movements, but their bed partners report getting kicked at night. People with the condition feel tired during the day because the leg movements disrupt their sleep.

Periodic limb movement disorder is rare. Women and men seem to be equally affected. As with restless legs syndrome, iron deficiency anemia and kidney failure increase the risk of developing this condition.

Diagnosis

Your doctor will talk to you about your symptoms and may ask for information from your bed partner. Diagnosing PLMD involves an overnight evaluation at a sleep clinic. This testing will help rule out other possible sleep disorders that also can cause restless sleep, including sleep apnea.

Treatment

Whether to treat PLMD must be decided on an individual basis. Avoiding caffeine, nicotine and alcohol may be beneficial in limiting the symptoms.

Some people may need medication. Your doctor may recommend a low dose of a medication used to treat Parkinson's disease, such as pramipexole (Mirapex) or ropinirole (Requip).

Your doctor may measure the amount of iron in your body and suggest iron supplements if you have an iron deficiency.

Other Sleep Disorders

Other types of sleep disorders that involve unusual physical behaviors, such as walking during sleep, are called parasomnias.

Nightmares and sleep terrors

Signs and symptoms
Nightmares
- Unpleasant or frightening dreams that take place during rapid eye movement (REM) sleep

Sleep terrors
- Arousal from sleep accompanied by extreme fear, screaming or crying, usually with no memory of a frightening dream

A nightmare is a scary dream from which you may awaken in fright. When they recur, nightmares may suggest a psychological disturbance or stress brought on by a difficult life situation. However, most people have nightmares from time to time throughout life.

Sleep terrors are most common in children between the ages of 4 and 12. They're infrequent after that. During deep, non-rapid eye movement (NREM) sleep, the child may wake up screaming, terrified and unable to explain what happened. He or she can't be comforted or fully awakened.

Although the terror may last for several minutes, the child usually doesn't remember the episode the next morning. Unless awakened, the child typically returns to peaceful sleep.

Sleep terrors are often more distressing for parents than the child. The best response to your child's sleep terror is usually to just let it run its course without waking the child.

Sleep terrors usually happen during the first third of the night, while nightmares tend to occur closer to morning. Individuals generally don't remember sleep terrors, but they may recall a nightmare vividly.

Sleep terrors seem to run in families. In adults, they can worsen with the use of alcohol. Emotional stress also can make them more likely to occur.

Treatment
Children usually outgrow sleep terrors. In adults, meeting with a psychiatrist or psychologist may be recommended. Medication is rarely used to treat sleep terrors, particularly for children. If necessary, however, use of benzodiazepines may be effective.

Sometimes further sleep tests are recommended to see if any other sleep disorders might be waking you up, such as sleep apnea.

If stress or anxiety seems to be contributing to the sleep terrors, your doctor may suggest meeting with a therapist or counselor. Cognitive behavioral therapy, hypnosis, biofeedback and relaxation therapy may help.

Sleepwalking

Signs and symptoms
- Walking or doing other activities during sleep
- Eyes are open
- Blank or dazed facial expression
- Confusion or disorientation if awakened

Sleepwalking involves not only walking but also other activities performed during sleep, such as rearranging furniture, dressing or undressing, and even getting into a car and driving, although this is rare.

Sleepwalking usually occurs during the first third of the night and typically lasts a few minutes. Many people believe that sleepwalkers don't get hurt during their travels. This is a misconception. Sleepwalkers commonly are injured by tripping or losing their balance.

Sleepwalking is common in children. Fatigue and prior sleep loss increase the frequency of sleepwalking in children. Sleepwalking also tends to run in families. Lack of sleep can increase the risk of sleepwalking.

Treatment
To prevent injury, it's a good idea to make your bedroom and house safe for the sleepwalker. Avoid leaving small objects, electrical cords and furniture in the middle of rooms. Block the top of staircases with gates, and lock outside doors and windows.

Sometimes, a doctor will prescribe benzodiazepines or certain antidepressants if the sleepwalking leads to the potential for injury, is disruptive to family members, or results in embarrassment or sleep disruption for the person who sleepwalks. Hypnosis also may be helpful. Avoiding alcohol and other central nervous system depressants also might help. Sometimes, sleep studies can pinpoint other sleep disorders that might increase the chances of sleepwalking.

REM sleep behavior disorder

Signs and symptoms

- Excessive physical movements while dreaming — such as thrashing, flailing, punching, kicking, falling or leaping from bed
- Waking up with unexplained injuries or falling out of bed

Most people experience a type of paralysis as they begin dreaming in the rapid eye movement (REM) phase of sleep. Usually this paralysis keeps you from acting out your dreams.

In REM sleep behavior disorder, the paralysis is incomplete or missing. As a result, dramatic, often violent behaviors occur during REM sleep, usually accompanied by vivid dreams.

People with this disorder may thrash about in bed, sometimes falling or leaping out of bed. They may yell, punch or kick, injuring themselves or their bed partners.

These episodes may occur once every few weeks or months or up to several times a night. Most people with the disorder say their dreams have become more vivid, action packed and violent over the years. Some people feel sleepy during the day as a result of the disruption of their sleep at night.

The disorder is most common in older men. It can be associated with neurological disorders, such as Lewy body dementia, Parkinson's disease or multiple system atrophy. REM sleep behavior disorder may be the first manifes-

tation of these conditions, so be sure to inform your doctor of your symptoms.

Certain drugs may cause REM sleep behavior disorder, including antidepressants. People with untreated sleep apnea also can move around similarly in their sleep, mimicking a REM sleep behavior disorder. Nighttime seizures also can have similar signs and symptoms. A sleep study is required to find the exact cause.

Treatment

The first step is to make your sleep environment safer by removing dangerous objects from the bedroom and moving furniture away from the bed. Some people even place the mattress directly on the floor. Your bed partner may need to move to a separate bed to prevent risk of injury.

Supplements such as melatonin and medications such as clonazepam (Klonopin) may be prescribed to reduce nighttime movements and risk of injury.

Teeth grinding

Signs and symptoms

- Grinding, gnashing or clenching of the teeth during sleep
- The tips of teeth worn down, flattened or chipped
- Worn tooth enamel
- Increased tooth sensitivity
- Jaw pain or tightness in the jaw muscles
- Popping, clicking or locking of jaw joint
- Dull morning headache
- Earache due to jaw muscle contractions
- Chronic facial pain

Teeth grinding (bruxism) is a condition in which you grind, gnash or clench your teeth during sleep. It affects about 15 to 40 percent of children and 8 to 10 percent of adults.

Bruxism can be mild and occasional or frequent and violent. It usually occurs in the early part of the night and may disturb your bed partner. Some people grind

(brux) so loudly that they can't duplicate the sound while awake.

Severe bruxism can damage your teeth and cause tension headaches, facial pain and temporomandibular disorders. Temporomandibular disorders occur in the temporomandibular joint (TMJ) located just in front of your ear.

Sometimes, bruxism is caused by a problem in the way your upper and lower teeth fit together when your jaws are closed. Reflux or psychological factors also may be involved. People with bruxism may have undiagnosed sleep apnea. Bruxism can be an uncommon side effect of some psychiatric medications and stimulants.

Treatment

Treatment for bruxism varies, depending on the cause. If it's stress related, your doctor may recommend strategies to help you relax and may recommend that you see a psychiatrist or psychologist. Muscle relaxation medications or injections of a form of botulinum toxin (Botox), may help some people with severe bruxism who don't respond to other treatments. Cutting back on caffeine and alcohol also may help. Bruxism is often made worse by alcohol.

If your bruxism is related to dental problems, your dentist may treat it by adjusting your bite pattern to correct any misalignment. Wearing a mouth guard or bite plate can prevent tooth damage from bruxism.

If you develop bruxism as a side effect of a medication, your doctor may change your medication or prescribe another medication to counteract the bruxism. ■

Women's Health

The primary biological function of the female reproductive system is the creation of offspring. But the sex organs also play a crucial role in your overall health and well-being. Maintaining good reproductive health is important. Doing so involves having regular checkups and tests. Understanding how the female reproductive system functions also can help you understand natural changes that take place during life.

Reproductive Organs

The female reproductive system is made up of the organs associated with childbearing — two ovaries, the fallopian tubes, the uterus and the external genitalia.

Ovaries

The ovaries are situated in the lower part of the female pelvis, about 4 or 5 inches below the waist. Before birth, a female fetus contains more than a million eggs (ova), many of which disappear before birth. By the time a baby girl is born, her ovaries contain all the eggs she'll need throughout her lifetime. Beginning in puberty, the ovaries regularly release an egg into the fallopian tubes in a process called ovulation.

The ovaries also produce the female sex hormones estrogen and progesterone, which are important in the development and maintenance of feminine physical characteristics. The ovaries change in size during the reproductive years, the normal range varying from the size of an almond to the size of a walnut.

Fallopian tubes

Between each ovary and the uterus lies a thin, 4- or 5-inch-long

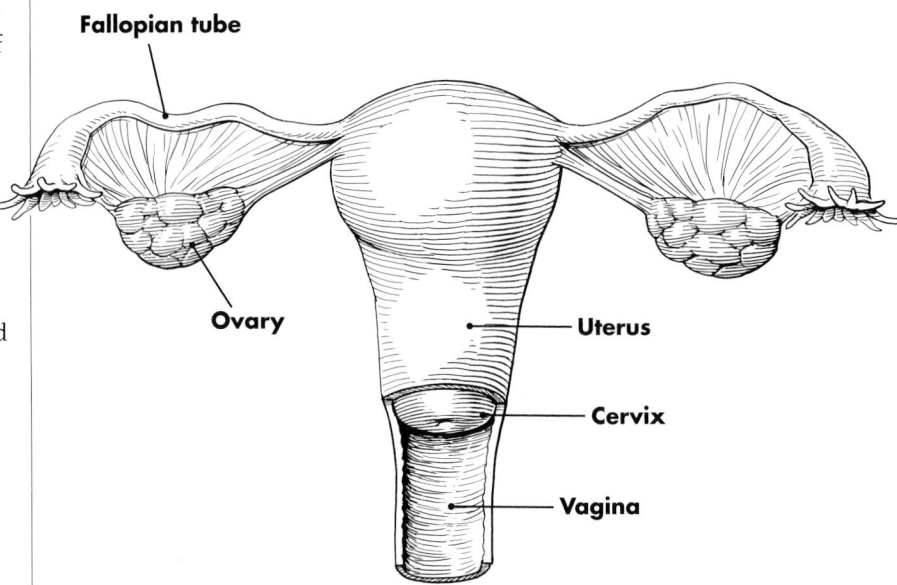

Female Reproductive Organs

Fallopian tube

Ovary

Uterus

Cervix

Vagina

passageway called a fallopian tube. Each tube is no wider than a needle. Fertilization takes place within a fallopian tube when a sperm penetrates an egg that has been released from one of the ovaries. The fertilized egg then travels down the tube and into the uterus.

Uterus

The uterus is a pear-shaped organ, about 3 inches long in a nonpregnant woman. The walls of the uterus are thick and made up primarily of powerful muscles.

When a fertilized egg reaches the uterus, it implants itself within the uterine wall, where it begins to develop into a baby. If the egg isn't fertilized, it degenerates along with the lining of the uterus, which is shed during menstruation.

The narrow neck of the uterus (cervix) also has thick walls. Ordinarily, the opening of the cervix is very small — big enough for menstrual fluids to pass through but not large enough, for example, that you could accidentally insert a tampon into it. During labor, the cervical opening expands (dilates) to allow passage of the baby, and the muscles of the uterine wall contract to push the baby out.

The cervix extends into the vagina, a muscular tube about 6 inches long. Most of the time, the walls of the vagina touch, but they can expand to accommodate something as small as a tampon or as large as a full-term baby. Cells in the vaginal walls secrete lubricants. In girls, the hymen — a thin membrane — partly blocks the opening of the vaginal canal. It may remain intact until first sexual intercourse; however it's common for the hymen to break with vigorous exercise, such as horseback riding, or after the insertion of a tampon. In rare cases, a doctor has to make an incision in the hymen before a girl can menstruate.

External genitals

The female external genitals — the mons pubis, the labia, the clitoris and the opening (vestibule) of your vagina — are called the vulva. The mons pubis is the pad of fatty tissue at the base of the abdomen that becomes covered with hair at puberty. The labia are double folds of tissue that extend downward on each side of your vagina — the outer folds are the labia majora and the inner folds are the labia minora. *Labia* is the Latin word for "lips."

Successful Reproduction

During sexual intercourse — when a man inserts his erect penis into a woman's vagina and ejaculates sperm-saturated semen — the vagina is flooded with millions of sperm swimming in all directions in search of an egg to fertilize. Most sperm die within the vagina and never even reach the cervical canal, the opening between the vagina and the uterus. Of those that make it to the 1-inch cervical canal, most never make it any farther.

Only a few sperm reach the uterus and successfully make the journey midway down one of the fallopian tubes where an egg is located, provided it's the time of the month when the female has released an egg from an ovary (ovulated). When a sperm finds and penetrates an egg, fertilization has occurred and a pregnancy has begun. The sperm that fertilizes an egg has overcome enormous odds.

To result in pregnancy, sexual intercourse usually must take place within the 72 hours before an egg (ovum) enters a fallopian tube. Some of these sperm are stored in the female cervical mucus and released over time into the uterus and fallopian tubes. If some of these sperm stay viable for up to a few hours after an egg is released from an ovary, one of them may find and fertilize the egg. The best chance of becoming pregnant is just before the release of an egg (ovulation). Ovulation usually occurs once every menstrual cycle, about 14 days before the start of a woman's next period.

Even perfect timing, though, doesn't guarantee a pregnancy. To become pregnant through sexual intercourse requires both a healthy female and a healthy male reproductive system.

In a woman, an irregular ovulation pattern can make fertilization of an egg more difficult. The fallopian tubes must be open and receptive to the egg and sperm. Women whose tubes contain scar tissue from a previous infection or surgery may not be able to get pregnant without surgery or reproductive assistance. Even cervical mucus must have just the right characteristics to allow sperm entry. Mucus that's too thick or acidic can prevent fertilization. Acidic mucus can make the vagina hostile to sperm, which thrive in alkaline surroundings.

As for the man, he must produce not only an adequate number of sperm but sperm that are active and healthy (see Chapter 34, "Men's Health").

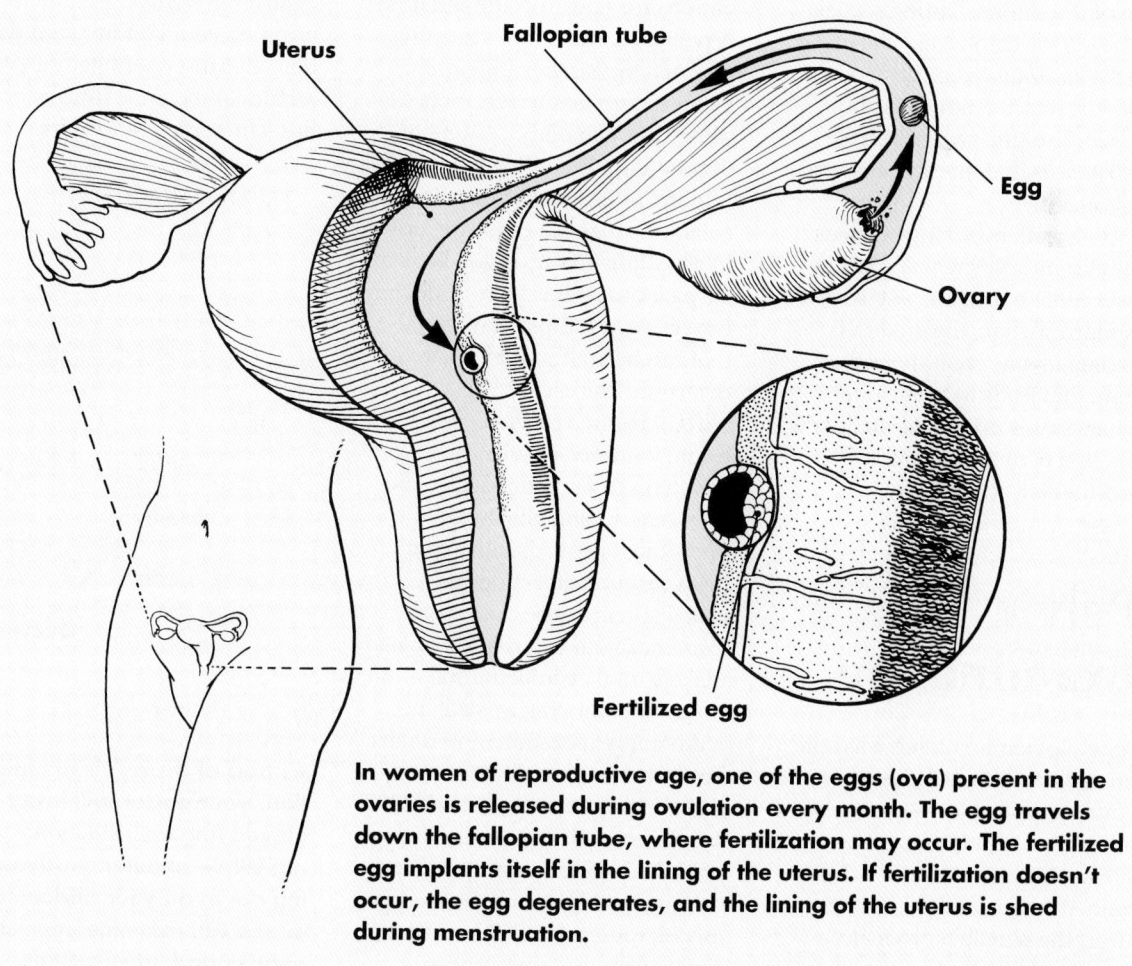

Uterus **Fallopian tube** **Egg** **Ovary** **Fertilized egg**

In women of reproductive age, one of the eggs (ova) present in the ovaries is released during ovulation every month. The egg travels down the fallopian tube, where fertilization may occur. The fertilized egg implants itself in the lining of the uterus. If fertilization doesn't occur, the egg degenerates, and the lining of the uterus is shed during menstruation.

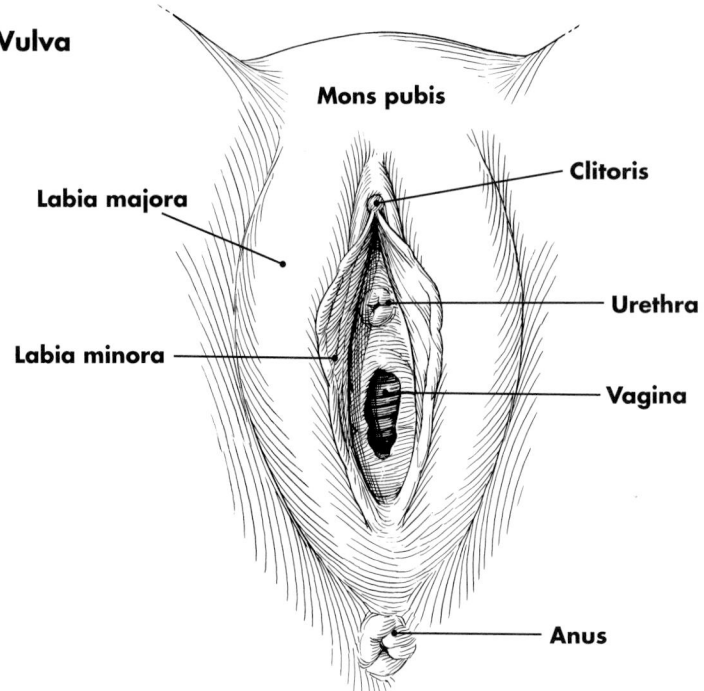

Vulva

Mons pubis

Clitoris

Labia majora

Urethra

Labia minora

Vagina

Anus

Where the labia meet near the front of the body, they cover a small protrusion, which is the tip of the clitoris. During sexual arousal, the clitoris, like the male penis, becomes erect. Bartholin's glands, which empty into the vestibule of the vagina, secrete substances that lubricate the vaginal opening.

The smaller opening between the clitoris and vagina is the entrance to the urethra. Not involved in reproduction, the urethra is a passageway, about 1½ inches long, that leads to the bladder, which stores urine. The bladder is situated between the pubic bone and uterus.

Pelvic Examination

A pelvic examination is a simple procedure that can be done by your family doctor, a gynecologist or another health care professional. A gynecologist is a doctor trained to treat disorders that affect the female reproductive system. How often pelvic exam-

inations are done and when you should begin having them varies. Talk to your doctor for recommendations for your specific situation. A pelvic examination is usually part of a physical examination. Pelvic exams are important because they can detect a number of problems, including cysts, tumors, infection and muscle weakness that can cause the uterus or vagina to sag. If you have a suspicious discharge, your doctor can obtain a sample of material that can be analyzed to determine the cause.

To perform a pelvic exam, your doctor will have you lie on your back on an examining table with your knees bent. Usually, your heels rest in metal supports called stirrups. The doctor first examines your external genitals to make sure they look normal — no sores, discoloration or swelling.

An internal examination is next. To see the inner walls of the vagina and the cervix, an instrument called a speculum is inserted to hold the vaginal walls apart. Your doctor then shines a light inside to look for lesions, inflammation, signs of abnormal discharge or

anything else that's unusual. Generally, the next step is to take a sample of cells from the cervix. With the speculum in place, your doctor scrapes the cervix gently with a small spatula or brush. The sample is sent to a laboratory to screen for cancer of the cervix.

Your doctor can't see your internal organs, such as your uterus and ovaries, but can examine them by touch (palpation) after removing the speculum. To do this, your doctor inserts two lubricated, gloved fingers into your vagina. With his or her fingers inside your vagina and by pressing down on your abdomen with the other hand, he or she can locate your uterus, ovaries and other organs, judge their size, and confirm that they're in the proper positions. By touching the contours of these organs, your doctor sometimes can detect tumors or cysts.

To palpate the same organs from a different angle, and to examine your rectum, your doctor may also insert a finger into your rectum at the same time he or she has a finger in your vagina.

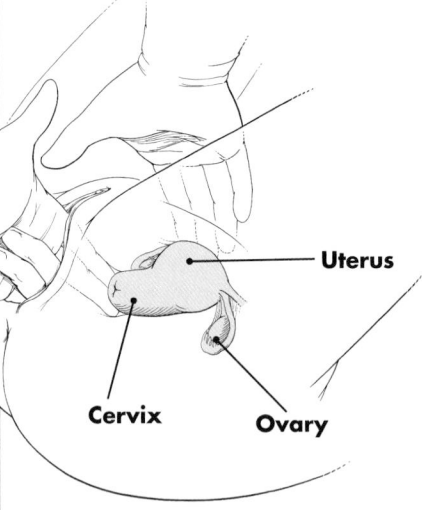

Uterus

Cervix

Ovary

As part of the pelvic examination, your doctor will insert two gloved fingers inside your vagina. While simultaneously pressing down on your abdomen, he or she can examine your uterus, ovaries and other organs.

As your doctor palpates your internal organs, you may feel somewhat uncomfortable. However, the experience shouldn't be painful. If you do experience pain or tenderness, say so immediately. You'll feel less discomfort if you can relax the muscles in your pelvic area. It often helps to take slow, deep breaths.

A gynecological exam also includes a medical history and an examination of your breasts. If you've begun menstruating, your doctor will want to know the date of your last menstrual period. You'll likely be asked about past pregnancies and their outcomes and about what form of birth control you're using, if any. You may be weighed and have your blood pressure measured, and you may be asked for urine and blood samples to be analyzed in the laboratory.

The American College of Obstetricians and Gynecologists recommends a girl's first visit to a gynecologist take place between ages 13 and 15, focusing on health guidance and disease prevention. The visit may not include a pelvic exam. It's recommended females have their first cervical cancer screens at age 21.

Menstrual Cycle

From puberty through menopause, most women cycle through an intricate monthly process of hormonal fluctuations and changes. Designed to enable them to bear children, the process most often ends in the shedding of the uterine lining known as menstruation.

Puberty and menarche

At birth, your ovaries contain all the eggs (ova) they'll ever have. However, the eggs remain almost dormant until stimulated by a surge of pituitary hormones. That begins at puberty, which normally takes place between ages 7 and 16 in girls. At that time, a few eggs each month begin to enlarge and to develop additional layers of outer cells. The cells form a capsule (follicle) around the egg, and they begin to produce the hormone estrogen.

During childhood, a girl's body produces estrogen in very small quantities, but at puberty her estrogen level increases about twentyfold. Meanwhile, the ovaries themselves grow larger as the eggs develop, and other internal reproductive organs also grow and mature.

The first visible sign of puberty is usually the development of breast buds, which generally occurs between ages 7 and 13. One breast may start to grow before the other, and the two may develop at different rates, but they usually end up approximately the same size. Next, the girl develops pubic hair and, later, underarm hair. She experiences a growth spurt, and as her hips and breasts become more rounded, she begins to look more like an adult.

About two years after a girl's breasts begin to bud, she reaches menarche — that is, she menstruates for the first time. Menarche marks the beginning of her

Seeing a Gynecologist

Gynecology is the branch of medicine concerned with the health and study of the female organs of reproduction. The term originates from the Greek words *gyne*, meaning "woman," and *logos*, meaning "study." Gynecologists are medical doctors trained to treat disorders affecting female reproductive organs. You might consult a gynecologist for any of the following:
- Menstrual problems
- Breast problems
- Advice on birth control
- Sexual health concerns
- Treatment of infertility or sexually transmitted infections (STIs)
- Questions or concerns about menopause
- Cancer that develops in any of your reproductive organs

Because gynecologists are also trained as obstetricians, many also see women through pregnancy and childbirth. Many women choose a gynecologist as their primary care doctor during their reproductive years. Family physicians, internists, and some nurse practitioners and physician assistants also can provide routine gynecologic care.

Another alternative is a nurse who has had specialized training in obstetrics and gynecology (certified nurse-midwife). Certified nurse-midwives may deliver babies and provide well-woman care, including routine breast examinations and pelvic examinations with cervical cancer screens. They generally work with at least one doctor who's available for consultations and in emergencies.

To find a gynecologist, you can ask another doctor to recommend one, call a local medical clinic or hospital for suggestions, or ask female friends for recommendations.

During your first visit to a gynecologist or to a primary care provider for a gynecologic exam, you may be looking for answers to important questions: Is the doctor willing to take time to explain things in language you can understand? Are you comfortable with this person? If you're not, you may want to consult other providers before making a final choice.

reproductive life, just as menopause — the cessation of ovarian functioning — marks the end of it.

In addition, during puberty a girl's pituitary gland begins to secrete increasing amounts of two key hormones: follicle-stimulating hormone (FSH) and luteinizing hormone (LH). As a result of FSH secretion, fluid develops within some of the follicles that surround the eggs. Some grow larger and bulge, while others shrivel and die. Every month after puberty, one — or sometimes two — of these fluid-filled follicles reaches full development.

A surge of LH stimulates the follicle to release an egg, which then bursts through the surface of the ovary and into the adherent fallopian tube. This process is called ovulation, which generally occurs at the midpoint of the menstrual cycle. In any given cycle, ovulation usually occurs from one ovary.

Males have no counterpart to menarche, which marks a dramatic change in a female's biological status. A girl's attitude toward menstruation and her feelings about what it means to be female may be influenced by the way her family and friends respond to her menses.

Menarche typically happens between the ages of 7 and 16. On average, girls in the United States begin menstruating at age 12, which is younger than in previous generations. For the past 100 years, the average age at menarche in the U.S. has been dropping at a rate of three or four months every decade. Medical experts attribute the change to better nourishment and healthier living conditions. However, increasing obesity among young children and teens also may be a factor.

Girls who are overweight commonly have their first menstrual period earlier than do those who aren't. Very athletic girls or those who are malnourished or have a chronic disease, often begin menstruating later.

If a girl's breasts begin to bud before she's 7 years old or if she has her first period before age 8, she may have precocious puberty, which needs to be evaluated to look for underlying causes. It's also a good idea to consult a doctor if a girl has no breast development by age 14 or if she hasn't begun to menstruate by the time she's 16.

For the first few years after menarche, it's normal for a girl's menstrual cycle to be irregular and for her to skip a period at times. Her ovaries probably aren't yet releasing an egg every month. However, young women need to be aware that they can become pregnant even before their first period, because the first egg may be released before menstruation begins.

In medical terms, puberty ends only after menstruation is established and is regular.

Normal menstrual cycle

Your menstrual cycle begins on the first day of flow of one menstrual period and ends on the first day of flow of the next. The release of an egg — a single cell barely visible to the naked eye — occurs approximately in the middle of the normal menstrual cycle.

Each month, as you menstruate, several follicles begin to develop in one of your ovaries, getting your next cycle under way. After a week or so, one follicle begins to outgrow the others, which shrink to normal size. Meanwhile, your ovaries secrete more estrogen, much of it produced by the outer cells of that single, dominant follicle. The estrogen acts on the lining of the uterus (endometrium), causing it to grow and thicken.

A day or two before ovulation, estrogen levels peak. They then start to decrease, and the dominant follicle begins to produce tiny amounts of the hormone progesterone. The follicle swells, ruptures and releases its egg, while the oth-

er follicles that were in the race for ovulation disappear. Other bodily changes include a slight increase in body temperature and a change in secretions from the glands in your cervix.

After its release from the follicle, the egg is picked up by one of the fallopian tubes and begins a journey to your uterus that generally takes about six days. While the egg is in transit, a sperm may fertilize it if you've recently had sexual intercourse. Fertilization generally takes place within a few hours after ovulation, before the egg has traveled more than a third of the way down the tube.

Even as the egg travels toward your uterus, its empty follicle in your ovary changes. Once again, it enlarges rapidly — at this stage it's called the corpus luteum — and begins to secrete large quantities of progesterone and estrogen. Under the impact of these hormones, your endometrium begins to function. Its glands secrete substances and release nutrients, and its blood supply and number of tiny blood vessels in the tissue increase. By the end of your menstrual cycle, the uterine lining has doubled in thickness, and large amounts of nutrients have been stored there, ready to nourish a fertilized egg.

If you become pregnant — meaning that a fertilized egg has become implanted in your endometrium — the hormones secreted by the corpus luteum will help to sustain the pregnancy. If you don't become pregnant, the egg disintegrates or leaves your body in vaginal secretions, usually before menstruation begins.

About two weeks after ovulation, the corpus luteum begins to shrink, and levels of estrogen and progesterone decrease. Your uterus starts to shed its lining, and menstrual bleeding (menses) begins.

Menstrual flow contains blood, vaginal and cervical secretions, and tissue sloughed from the lining of your uterus. By the fourth or fifth day of your period, the

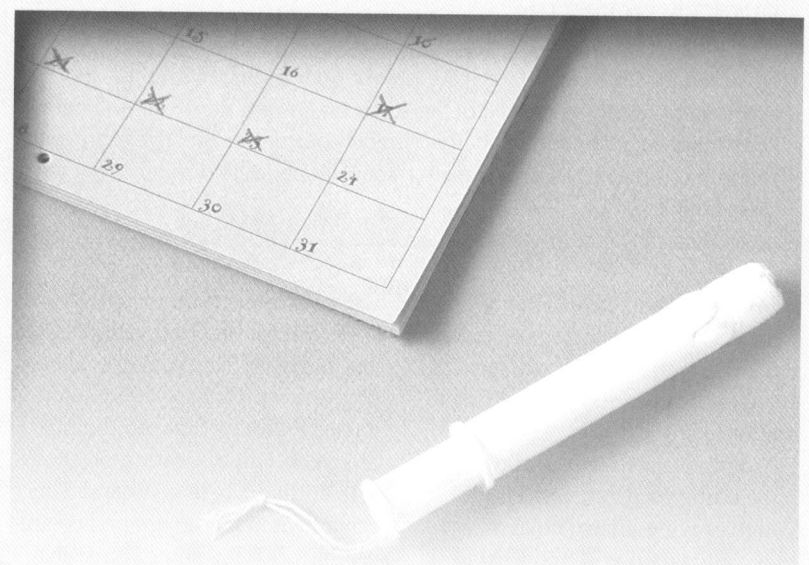

Menstrual Products

Years ago, women who were menstruating used cloths to catch their menstrual flow, rinsing them out and reusing them. Today, commercially made sanitary napkins are available, as are tampons and menstrual sponges that women insert into the vagina to absorb menstrual fluids.

Napkins and tampons are often labeled "regular" or "super." These terms refer to the product's ability to absorb, rather than to its physical size. Because there are no common standards and one brand's "regular" may be as absorbent as another brand's "super," you'll have to find out by trial and error what works best for you.

Change the tampon every few hours, and consider using a pad instead of a tampon at night. One reason for such precautions is toxic shock syndrome, a rare disorder that's associated with tampons and occasionally with extended use of contraceptive sponges, especially among women younger than age 30.

In the early 1980s, there was a small epidemic of toxic shock syndrome, for the most part involving young, menstruating women who had been using a particular brand of superabsorbent tampons. Researchers reported that the syndrome appeared to be caused by toxins produced by a type of bacteria called *Staphylococcus aureus.*

Researchers theorized that when the women left superabsorbent tampons in place for a long time, the tampons became a breeding ground for these bacteria. Others suggested that the fibers in the tampons scratched the surface of the vagina, making it possible for the bacteria or their toxins to enter the bloodstream.

The brand of tampons associated with the original epidemic was taken off the market, and cases of toxic shock syndrome have generally declined. There continues to be some controversy about the relationship of tampons to this condition, but in general, it's recommended that if you use tampons you change them every four to six hours.

If you use a napkin or tampon that's scented or deodorized, your vagina or vulva may begin to itch or become irritated during your period. Some women are allergic to the chemicals used in these products. Menstrual fluid is actually odorless until it comes into contact with bacteria and air. In general, if you bathe regularly and change napkins or tampons often, you won't have a problem with odor.

endometrium has become thin, and the process of rebuilding it has already begun.

On average, a menstrual cycle is 28 days long, although cycles normally range anywhere from 23 to 35 days. If your cycle doesn't fall within this range, it may not be a problem. However, extremely long or extremely short cycles should be evaluated by a doctor. On average, menstrual bleeding lasts four to five days, but periods as short as two days or as long as seven aren't unusual.

At times, your period may become temporarily irregular for no obvious reason. You may skip a period or have one that's much longer, shorter or heavier than usual. Sometimes this change simply reflects your age. Menstrual cycles are apt to last longer both at menarche and as you approach menopause. At other times, stress may play a role.

Preventing Pregnancy

Most unintended pregnancies result from a lack of contraception or contraception that's used incorrectly or inconsistently. Choosing the right method of contraception for you is a very important decision.

The best method of contraception varies. Individuals and couples need to choose a method that best fits their lifestyles, beliefs and health goals. And most importantly, they need to choose a method they'll use correctly and consistently. For methods that rely primarily on actions taken by the male, see page 1231. Information on other contraceptive choices follows.

Birth control pills

Women who take birth control pills correctly and consistently have about a 1 percent chance of becoming pregnant within a year. Among women who sometimes miss taking a pill, about 8 percent become pregnant within a year.

Today's birth control pills are lower in hormone content, especially in estrogen. When oral contraceptives contained high levels of estrogen, they carried a greater risk of blood clots. You still face some risk of blood clots if you take the newer pills, but the danger is reduced. Smoking greatly increases the risk of side effects from birth control pills. Smokers older than age 35 shouldn't use birth control pills.

Two families of oral contraceptives are available. The most commonly prescribed pill combines estrogen and progestin. Women who cannot take or don't want an estrogen-containing pill may take a progestin-only pill. The progestin-only pill is less effective in preventing pregnancy than the combination pill, but when combined with breast-feeding — which suppresses ovulation — this pill is usually adequate. Breast-feeding alone doesn't eliminate the possibility of getting pregnant.

How they work

Birth control pills prevent the hormone control center in the brain (hypothalamus) from instructing the pituitary gland to mobilize follicle-stimulating hormone and luteinizing hormone. With these hormones suppressed, you don't release an egg (ovulate).

In addition, the pill prevents the cervical mucus from becoming watery, as it normally does during ovulation. Instead, the mucus remains thick throughout your cycle, making it difficult for sperm to reach the fallopian tubes.

The pill results in a lighter and shorter period and also decreases menstrual cramps and pain.

Side effects

Although effective and easy to use, birth control pills may have

side effects, most of which are minor. They include nausea, breast tenderness, fluid retention, mood changes, headaches and decreased libido.

You may also have spotting or bleeding between periods, or you may not menstruate at all, especially when you first start to take the pill. If you are having these problems, often your doctor can prescribe a different type or regimen of birth control pill to eliminate the problem.

Some women bleed regularly while they're taking the pill but stop having periods after they discontinue using it. This effect is usually temporary.

Because there's still a small risk that the pill will cause serious side effects, watch for danger signs if you're taking it. If you have pain or swelling in your legs or severe headaches, contact your doctor.

One of the most serious side effects is development of blood clots in your veins, which can be fatal if they travel to your lungs. The frequency of blood clots associated

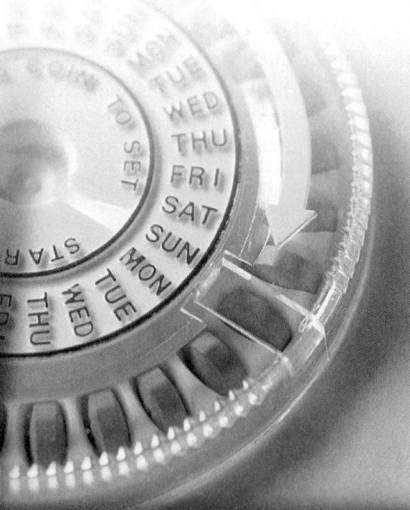

with pill use is rare. In general, it's greater in the first year of use and is greatest in women who are obese or who have certain hereditary conditions that put them at increased risk of clotting problems.

In addition, between 1 and 5 percent of women who use oral contraceptives develop some increase in blood pressure. In most cases, their blood pressure returns to normal if they stop taking the pill.

The combination pill doesn't appear to increase the incidence of cancer in the reproductive organs. In fact, there's good evidence that oral contraceptives decrease the risk of ovarian and endometrial (uterine) cancers. In addition, the pill is beneficial for reducing acne, painful periods, menstrual blood loss, premenstrual syndrome (PMS), endometriosis symptoms, fibroids, ovarian and breast cysts, and pelvic infections. For many of these conditions, it's especially helpful to take the pill in an extended or continuous way because doing so eliminates menses. Not having a period is not unhealthy in these circumstances and may be quite helpful and more convenient.

Shots, patches, implants and rings

The first hormonal contraceptive was the combination birth control pill, which appeared on the U.S. market in the early 1960s. Since then, hormonal contraceptive options have expanded to include the following:

- Shots (injections)
- Skin patch
- Vaginal ring
- Implant

Birth Control Pills: Common Questions

How do pills that eliminate some or all your periods differ from other birth control pills?

Traditional birth control pills make your reproductive system mimic a regular 28-day monthly cycle. For the first 21 days, you take active pills containing reproductive hormones. For the last seven days, you take a placebo. While you're taking the placebo pills, you bleed vaginally, as if you were having a regular menstrual period. By contrast, some pills now contain 24 days, three months or even one year of active hormones, which suppress all menstrual bleeding. Extending the time between periods may be appropriate for women with heavy, prolonged, frequent or painful periods, or women with menstrual migraines, endometriosis or other conditions worsened by menstruation.

If you plan to have a baby, how soon after stopping the birth control pill can you conceive?

One of the advantages of the birth control pill is that it's quickly reversible. After you stop taking the pill, you may have only a two-week delay before you ovulate again. Your period would follow about four to six weeks after you take the last pill. Once ovulation resumes, you can become pregnant. If this happens during your first cycle off the pill, you may not have a period at all. However, although possible, this scenario isn't likely.

Is there an advantage to waiting a few months after stopping the pill before trying to conceive?

For the purpose of dating the pregnancy — estimating when you ovulated and when your baby is due — it's somewhat advantageous to have at least one normal period before conceiving. In the past, doctors had concerns that if you conceived immediately after stopping the pill, you had a higher risk of miscarriage. However, these concerns have proved to be largely unfounded. If you plan to wait a few months, use a backup form of birth control while your menstrual cycles get back to normal.

What happens if you take birth control pills while you're pregnant?

If you continued taking your birth control pill because you didn't realize you were pregnant, don't be alarmed. Despite years of this accident happening, there's very little evidence that exposure to the hormones in birth control pills causes birth defects. Still, the birth control pill is a potent estrogen. Lessons learned from women who took diethylstilbestrol — a synthetic estrogen that was later linked with cancer — to prevent miscarriage in early pregnancy suggest that such exposure should be minimized. Once you learn that you're pregnant, stop taking the birth control pill.

Do birth control pills cause weight gain?

Women often blame the birth control pill for weight gain. But studies have shown that the effect of the birth control pill on weight is small — if it exists at all. However, the way the hormones in birth control pills act on tissues in your breasts, hips and thighs can make you feel as if you've gained weight. This is usually due to fluid retention and not increased body mass or fat. Estrogen in birth control pills directly affects fat (adipose) cells, making them larger, but not greater in number. In very rare circumstances women may add muscle, which can add weight, when taking the pill. This is due to the slight male sex hormone effect that the pill may have on some women. But no matter if pill-related weight gain is perceived or real, many women find this side effect undesirable. Taking pills with a low dose of estrogen may diminish these effects, but you may also experience a greater risk of spotting between periods.

How do birth control pills affect your risk of cancer?

Scientific evidence suggests using birth control pills for long periods of time increases your risk of certain cancers, such as cervical cancer and liver cancer, but it also decreases your risk of other types of cancer, including ovarian cancer and endometrial cancer. The effect of birth control pills on breast cancer risk isn't quite clear. In one study, use of birth control pills led to a higher risk of premenopausal breast cancer in women who took the pill for four or more years before having a baby. Other evidence suggests that 10 or more years after you stop taking the pill, your breast cancer risk returns to the same level as if you had never taken birth control.

All of these options provide comparable effectiveness in preventing pregnancy. So how do you decide which of these methods to use? The key to making this decision is deciding which method best suits your lifestyle.

Shots

Medroxyprogesterone (Depo-Provera) is the only injectable contraceptive currently available in the United States. Each injection contains high doses of the hormone progestin, which prevents pregnancy for up to three months.

Depo-Provera is highly effective in preventing pregnancy, even if you are a few days late in receiving a scheduled dose. It's also ideal for women who aren't likely to, or don't want to, take a pill every day. The typical effectiveness rate among users is 96 percent, meaning that 4 out of 100 women using the injection for one year will get pregnant. If injections are received every three months, Depo-Provera can be more than 99 percent effective, meaning that fewer than 1 in 100 women will get pregnant in a year. The injection may be especially beneficial for women who have a seizure disorder or sickle cell disease, as the drug tends to lessen the risk of seizures and sickle cell crises.

If you decide on Depo-Provera, you receive an injection in your upper arm or buttock every three months. You should get the first injection within the first five days of your menstrual period for immediate effectiveness. If you get the first injection later than that, use a backup method of birth control for two weeks.

Side effects

You'll experience changes in your menstrual periods while using Depo-Provera. Periods may become irregular or unpredictable, or you may not bleed at all. The absence of periods isn't harmful, and periods typically return to normal after you stop using Depo-Provera. Other side effects may include weight gain, breast tenderness and mood changes. Women who take Depo-Provera don't experience the side effects of estrogen exposure, such as an increased risk of blood clots and cardiovascular disease. The injection doesn't protect against sexually transmitted infections (STIs).

Prolonged use of Depo-Provera may result in bone loss, but bone density returns to normal when you stop using Depo-Provera.

The return of normal menstrual periods after Depo-Provera can be delayed, sometimes for months. As a result, you may not experience a prompt return to fertility after stopping the injections.

Skin patch

The only skin patch currently available in the United States goes by the brand name Xulane. It's a nearly 2-inch adhesive square that slowly releases the hormones estrogen and progestin through the skin and into the bloodstream.

The effectiveness rate of the patch is the same as combined estrogen-progestin oral contraception. This means that 1 out of 100 women using the patch over one year will get pregnant if the patch is used correctly. Effectiveness among typical users of the patch is closer to 91 percent, meaning that 9 out of 100 women using it for one year will get pregnant. There's some evidence to suggest that the patch may be less reliable in women who weigh more than 198 pounds.

To use the patch, you apply a new patch weekly for three consecutive weeks. The fourth week is patch-free, which allows you to have your menstrual period. Place the patch on your buttocks, lower abdomen or upper body, but not on your breasts. Here are a few additional tips for patch use:
- Don't apply oils, creams or cosmetics near the patch.
- If your patch becomes detached, replace it with a new patch immediately. Review your package insert for information on whether you need to use a backup method of birth control.

Side effects

The most common side effects are skin irritation, headaches, breast tenderness, nausea, vomiting, bloating, decreased sex drive and depression. Women who use the patch may be at a slightly increased risk of heart attack, stroke and blood clots. Users of the patch are exposed to higher levels of estrogen — about 60 percent greater — than are users of contemporary birth control pills. Increased exposure to estrogen may increase the risk of side effects, but that hasn't yet been demonstrated.

Vaginal ring

The vaginal ring (NuvaRing) is a flexible, transparent plastic device that slowly releases the hormones estrogen and progestin. This device, which measures 2 inches in diameter, is inserted into the vagina to prevent pregnancy. Each ring provides pregnancy protection for one month.

The effectiveness rate with perfect use is 99 percent. Among typical vaginal ring users, it's about 91 percent effective, meaning that 9 out of 100 women using it for one year will get pregnant.

To use this method, you insert the ring in your vagina and leave it in place for three weeks. Here are some additional tips for ring use:
- You may insert the vaginal ring anywhere in your vagina, but placing it deeply makes you less likely to feel it once inserted.
- An additional method of birth control must be used during the first week of use.
- If the ring falls out, it should be rinsed with warm water and reinserted within three hours.
- If the ring is out of the vagina for more than three hours during the first three weeks of the cycle, pregnancy prevention is compromised, and you must

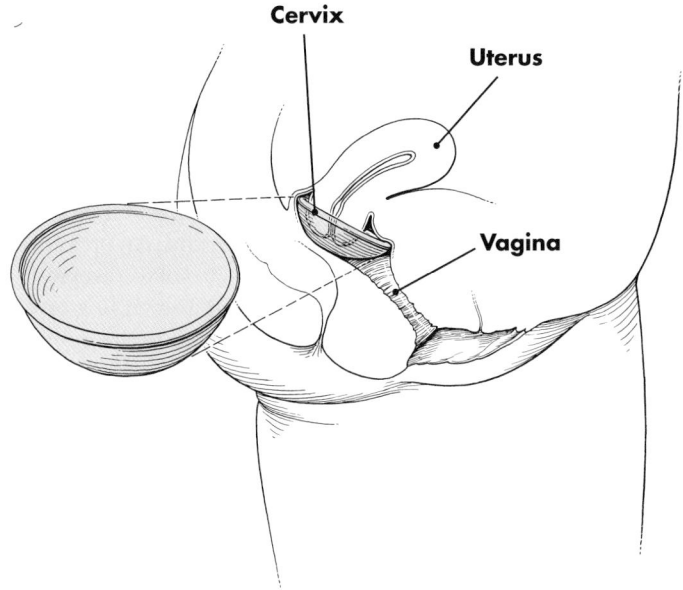

The contraceptive device known as a diaphragm is a rubber cup that's inserted into the vagina to cover the opening to the uterus (cervix).

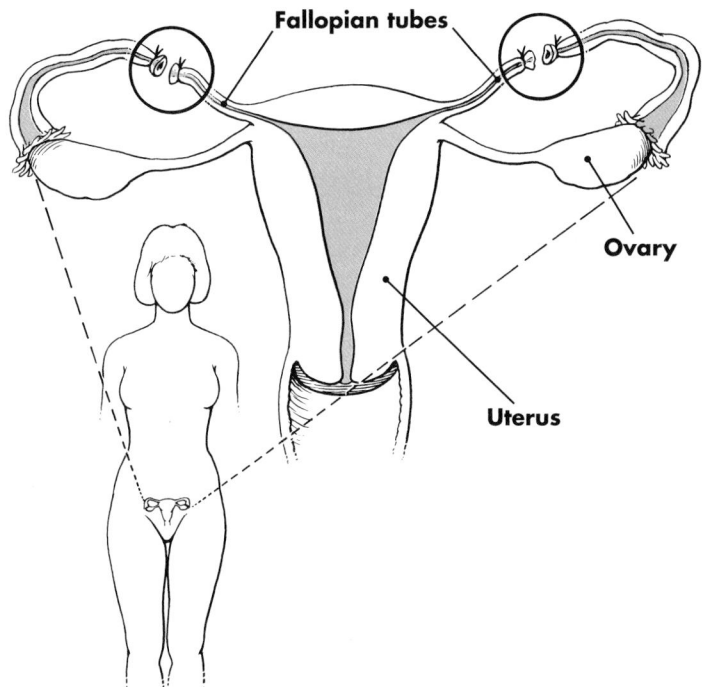

In a tubal ligation, the most common surgical procedure to sterilize a female, the path normally taken by eggs (ova) is interrupted by cutting and sealing off the fallopian tubes.

use a backup method of birth control for one week. The fourth week should be ring-free, which allows you to have your menstrual period.

Side effects
Side effects of the vaginal ring may include vaginal infections and irritation, irregular vaginal bleeding, headaches, breast ten-

derness, weight gain or loss, nausea, vomiting, bloating, decreased sex drive, and depression. Women who use the vaginal ring may be at a slightly increased risk of heart attack, stroke and blood clots.

Implant

Etonogestrel (Nexplanon) is an implantable contraceptive device. The matchstick-sized device releases a low, steady dose of progestin to prevent pregnancy. The implant can be left in place for up to three years and removed by your doctor at any time.

Nexplanon is 99 percent effective in preventing pregnancy when the device is implanted properly, which means that 1 out of 100 women using Nexplanon for one year will get pregnant.

If you decide on Nexplanon, a doctor will place the implant under the skin of your inner, upper arm. The implant is effective for up to three years, at which time you can get it removed and have a new one implanted.

Side effects
Nexplanon can cause irregular menstrual bleeding and spotting. For some women, Nexplanon stops menstruation entirely. Other side effects may include mood changes, headaches, breast tenderness and weight changes.

Intrauterine devices

Intrauterine devices (IUDs) are among the safest contraceptive devices, and are commonly used worldwide. In recent years, IUDs have become a popular method of birth control in the United States.

Intrauterine devices (IUDs) are about 98 to 99 percent effective for preventing pregnancy. An IUD is a small piece of plastic inserted into your uterus by your doctor, usually during your menstrual period when the cervix is more open. IUDs prevent pregnancy in several ways, but primarily they keep sperm from reaching an egg located in the fallopian tubes.

Currently available IUDs include one that contains copper and four others that contain progestin hormone. The copper IUD lasts 10 years and the progestin-containing IUDs last either three or five years depending on the type.

Side effects
Common side effects are changes in bleeding that may be heavy, prolonged, irregular or absent. Less common side effects include weight gain, ovarian cysts, headache, mood changes, nausea, abdominal pain, vaginal dryness or decreased libido.

Barrier methods

Barrier methods of contraception block the sperm from getting to the egg. There are physical barriers, such as the diaphragm and cervical cap, and chemical barriers (spermicides) that come in the form of creams, gels, foams and suppositories. If used perfectly, barrier methods can be up to 95 percent effective. The effectiveness among typical users is closer to about 80 to 85 percent. You can enhance the effectiveness of these methods by combining a physical barrier with a spermicide.

Diaphragm
The diaphragm is an effective barrier method for women when it's used consistently and correctly. Developed more than 100 years ago, the diaphragm is a rubber cup that you insert into your vagina to cover your cervix. The device needs to be fitted by a doctor. Proper fit is essential because the diaphragm must cover the cervix and fit snugly in the vagina to be effective. If you gain or lose a large amount of weight or deliver a baby, you may require a diaphragm of a different size.

Before intercourse, insert your diaphragm with about a teaspoon of spermicidal cream or jelly spread around the edge and in the center of the device. After intercourse, wait at least six hours to remove the diaphragm. Always use spermicide with a diaphragm. If you have intercourse again within the six hours, you must apply more spermicide without removing the diaphragm. Try not to leave it in place for more than 24 hours.

Clean your diaphragm with soap and water. Periodically check for holes or thinning of the rubber. If you find either, you need a new diaphragm.

Side effects with a diaphragm are rare as long as you're not allergic to the spermicide or latex or at increased risk of urinary tract infections. The most common complaint among women who use a diaphragm is having to interrupt sex to insert it.

Cervical cap
The cervical cap is a plastic cap designed to fit snugly over the cervix. It's similar to the diaphragm in that a doctor must fit it. Unlike the diaphragm, however, the cap may be difficult to insert because it needs to be placed deep within the vagina. As a result, women may be tempted to leave the cap in for extended periods. That can cause problems because the cap becomes a breeding ground for bacteria.

With perfect use, the effectiveness rate of the cervical cap can be up to 94 percent. In typical users, it's about 85 percent effective for preventing pregnancy but is less effective among women who have given birth.

Female condom
The female condom, a type of condom worn by women, comes in several forms. Many are made of thicker latex than typical male condoms. All extend to the outside of the vagina, and several have a diaphragm-like end that fits over the cervix. Insertion methods vary. With perfect use, female condoms can be up to 95 percent effective, but the effectiveness rate among typical users is closer to 80 percent.

Permanent birth control

There are two forms of permanent birth control.

Tubal ligation
Tubal ligation works by keeping the egg and the sperm from meeting. To perform a tubal ligation — the most common method of female sterilization — a surgeon cuts and seals off the fallopian tubes so that eggs (ova) can't travel down the tubes and sperm can't move up. The risk of tubal ligation failure is low.

Some women opt to be sterilized immediately or shortly after giving birth. The procedure doesn't lengthen a postpartum hospital stay. In case of a cesarean delivery,

Reversing a Tubal Ligation

Some women who've been sterilized decide later that they want to become pregnant. An operation can be done to try to reverse tubal ligation. Depending on certain factors, such as the individual's age, about 40 to 80 percent of women who have a reverse procedure are eventually able to conceive. However, the risk of tubal (ectopic) pregnancy increases. For these reasons, doctors stress that before you undergo sterilization, be very sure you won't want to become pregnant.

Another possibility for women who want to conceive after tubal ligation is in vitro fertilization, a procedure in which mature eggs are removed from the ovary, fertilized with sperm in a laboratory and implanted into her uterus. This procedure is more common today than is tubal reversal surgery.

a doctor can perform a tubal ligation in a matter of minutes.

Among women who've recently had a vaginal delivery, a common method for performing a tubal ligation is minilaparotomy. The doctor makes a small incision below the navel through which he or she raises a "knuckle" of each tube, ties the base, cuts the tube, then ties the two separated ends.

For sterilizations done weeks or months after delivery, a laparoscope is most often used. It isn't used for procedures performed soon after delivery because of the size of the uterus. A laparoscope is a thin instrument that's inserted through a small incision below the navel. The instrument has a viewing scope through which a doctor can see the reproductive organs. Using operating instruments through either the same incision or a second one, the doctor locates the tubes and either cauterizes them or attaches plastic clips or rings to them.

As with any operation, tubal ligation carries risk. About 1 in 1,000 women develops a complication. This may include reactions to the anesthetic, a pelvic infection, injury to blood vessels in the abdomen, or bowel or bladder injuries.

If you're pregnant and considering sterilization, discuss options with your doctor. Some doctors perform the tubal ligation immediately after childbirth, while others prefer to wait three to six months. Before doctors perform tubal ligations, they often recommend that the parents wait to be sure their last child is healthy. If there's a problem, the parents may decide they want another child.

Hysteroscopic tubal sterilization

Hysteroscopic tubal sterilization (Essure) is a permanent birth control method in which tiny metal coils are placed in the fallopian tubes. The procedure is done using a local anesthetic and a narrow instrument that's inserted into the vagina, through the cervix and into the uterus, where the doctor can see the fallopian tube openings. Over time, scar tissue grows in and around these coils, which block the tubes so that sperm can't reach the female eggs. It's unlike other sterilization procedures because it doesn't require incisions.

During the three months after the procedure, you must use another type of birth control. After three months, you'll have an X-ray to confirm that your fallopian tubes are blocked. If the procedure is successful, you can stop using backup birth control.

According to one study, Essure is not as effective as tubal ligation, with a failure rate of about 10 percent over 10 years. Essure isn't intended for women who might wish to become pregnant in the future.

The most commonly reported side effects in the clinical studies included mild to moderate pain during the procedure and vaginal bleeding for a few days afterward. Essure doesn't protect against sexually transmitted infections (STIs).

Natural family planning

Natural family planning (fertility awareness) encompasses several methods that rely on the female menstrual cycle to determine what days may be safe for intercourse. They're variations of the so-called rhythm method.

Each of the approaches in natural family planning involves a conscientious awareness of when you can become pregnant — from about 72 hours before ovulation to about 24 hours after ovulation. The key is to determine when these days occur in your cycle and to avoid having intercourse at that time.

Highly motivated couples can use natural family planning effectively. Natural family planning has a failure rate of about 25 percent over one year. Predicting ovulation is difficult because a woman's cycle may vary from month to month. If you decide to try natural family planning, keep records for several months to establish a pattern for your menstrual cycle. There are four ways to calculate the time of ovulation: the temperature method, the calendar method, the cervical mucus inspection method and the mucothermal method. Effective natural family planning requires using all of these techniques.

Temperature method

Most women have a slight rise in body temperature just after ovulation. To detect a temperature change, take and record your temperature every day when you wake up. You'll need to use a basal thermometer — a special thermometer designed to detect the post-ovulatory rise in temperature. Basal thermometers are available in most pharmacies. This technique can be helpful in recognizing patterns, but since temperatures change only after ovulation, it's not effective alone.

Calendar method

To use this method, you need to keep a record of your cycles for a year. Then take the number of days in your shortest cycle and subtract 18 (18 is used because it equals 14 days from ovulation to the first day of your period plus 4 days for the average life span of a sperm). Subtract 10 from the number of days in your longest cycle (10 equals 14 days from ovulation to the first day of your period minus one day for the life span of an egg and minus three more days for a margin of error). The results of your calculations are the first and last days of your cycle during which you can become pregnant.

For example, if your shortest cycle is 24 days and the longest is 35 days, then the time during which you can become pregnant is between 24 days minus 18 days (the sixth day) and 35 days minus

10 days (the 25th day). So, potentially, you could become pregnant from the sixth through the 25th days of each cycle.

This method requires that menstrual cycles be very regular, and it demands long periods of abstinence.

Cervical mucus inspection method

About four days before the release of an egg, your vaginal mucus becomes thin, clear, runnier and profuse. To prevent pregnancy, avoid intercourse from the time such mucus appears until four days after it becomes thicker and drier. This method is somewhat more complex, but it can be effective.

Mucothermal method

A combination of the temperature and mucus inspection methods — the mucothermal method — generally is the most reliable natural method. Use both your basal temperature and your cervical mucus to determine when you have the potential to become pregnant.

Infertility

An estimated 10 to 18 percent of couples experience difficulty becoming pregnant. Issues may include problems with the sperm or the egg or difficulties encountered in their union. Abnormal function of the fallopian tubes or uterus, infections, immunological issues, and other factors may cause infertility.

To doctors, the term infertility usually means the inability to achieve pregnancy after one year of sexual intercourse without using contraception. Infertility often can be overcome, but for many couples pregnancy may not occur for more than a year after starting treatment.

Note that infertility is not the same thing as sterility, which means the inability to conceive a child under any circumstances.

With infertility, conceiving a child may be possible.

In about one-third of cases, the male is the infertile partner. The female also is infertile about one-third of the time. In the remaining cases, both partners contribute to infertility, or the cause can't be determined.

Infertility doesn't mean anyone is incomplete or defective. It has nothing to do with attractiveness or sexual prowess. Moreover, it's not a comment on a couple's relationship.

Medically speaking, infertility is simply the existence of some obstacle in the long and exceedingly complex chain of events that leads to pregnancy. Infertility can be frustrating and disappointing and a source of great sorrow for couples experiencing it.

Evaluation

When should you seek a medical evaluation for problems with conceiving? If you're under age 35, most doctors recommend trying to get pregnant for at least a year before testing or treatment. If you're between the ages of 35 and 40, your doctor may recommending trying for six months. If you're older than 40 years of age, your doctor may want to begin testing or treatment right away.

Your doctor also may want to begin an evaluation right away if you or your partner has known fertility problems, or if you have a history of irregular periods, pelvic inflammatory disease, repeated miscarriages, prior cancer treatment or endometriosis. A gynecologist or family doctor can determine if there's a fertility problem that may require the services of an infertility specialist.

Before deciding to undergo infertility testing, be aware that the process requires commitment. The doctor will need to know your sexual habits and may make recommendations about how to change those habits. Tests and pe-

riods of trial and error may extend over several months, and, in some cases, may include operations or uncomfortable procedures.

Evaluation is expensive and may not be covered by your medical insurance. Finally, there's no guarantee, even after all the tests and procedures, that you'll be able to conceive. However, if you're determined to try to have your own child, infertility evaluation is the route to take, and it often results in a successful pregnancy.

Male tests

For a man to be fertile, his testicles must produce enough sperm, the sperm must be able to reach the seminal vesicles, and the sperm must be ejaculated effectively into a woman's vagina. Male fertility tests attempt to determine if any of these steps are impeded.

A doctor will likely begin with a medical history, including illnesses, disabilities and medications. You may then have a physical examination, including examination of your genitals.

The doctor will likely ask for a specimen of ejaculated semen. You provide the sample by masturbating and ejaculating the semen into a clean container. You may need to provide more than one specimen during the fertility testing process. A laboratory analysis of the semen notes its quantity and color as well as the number of sperm and the presence of infections or blood. Laboratory analysis also determines the concentration of sperm present in the ejaculate, their shape and their activity (motility).

You may be asked to take a blood test to determine your level of testosterone or other hormones. A post-ejaculatory urinalysis can indicate that your sperm are traveling backward into the bladder instead of out your penis during ejaculation (retrograde ejaculation). Ultrasound, genetic tests or specialized sperm function tests may also be used to detect possible causes of infertility.

Female tests

For a woman to be fertile, her ovaries must release healthy eggs regularly, and her reproductive tract must allow the eggs and sperm unobstructed passage for a possible union in the fallopian tubes. Your doctor will likely start with a medical history, followed by a general physical examination, including a gynecologic examination. He or she may also ask you questions about medications you take and about your menstrual cycle.

The following tests are used to determine possible causes of female infertility. Not everyone needs to undergo all, or even many, of the tests before the cause is found. Your doctor will discuss the tests with you and, with your agreement, determine which ones to use. In some cases, despite careful testing, no cause for infertility can be found.

Hormone testing

An at-home, over-the-counter ovulation prediction kit detects the surge in luteinizing hormone (LH) that occurs before ovulation. You may be asked for a blood sample to test for levels of hormones involved in successful ovulation and other reproductive processes. After receiving the results of one or more of these tests, your doctor can assess whether your ovaries are functioning.

Hysterosalpingography

This procedure may be used to evaluate the condition of the uterus as well as the fallopian tubes. After a contrast fluid is injected into the uterus, an X-ray determines if the fluid travels out of the uterus and up the fallopian tubes. This test often can locate blockages or find other problems.

Ovarian reserve testing

This testing helps determine the quality and quantity of eggs available for ovulation. Women at risk of a depleted egg supply —

including women older than 35 — may have this series of blood and imaging tests.

Ultrasound

A doctor may use ultrasound to examine the pelvic area and look for abnormalities in your ovaries and uterus. Sometimes a hysterosonography is used to see details inside the uterus that are not seen on a regular ultrasound.

Hysteroscopy

Hysteroscopy is a procedure in which your doctor uses a small instrument to examine the interior of your cervix and uterus for irregularities that might lead to infertility.

Laparoscopy

Rarely, a doctor will perform a minimally invasive operation — in either a hospital or outpatient surgical center — with general anesthesia. During the procedure, a doctor inserts a thin, illuminated viewing device (laparoscope) into your abdomen and pelvis to examine your fallopian tubes, ovaries and uterus.

Causes of infertility most commonly identified with laparoscopy are fallopian tube or ovarian adhesions or endometriosis. Endometriosis is a condition in which the tissue that lines the uterus (endometrial tissue) is found outside the uterus. Through the laparoscope, a doctor can identify and may be able to treat blockages or scarring of the fallopian tubes and uterus that may prevent fertilization.

Causes

The causes of infertility can involve one or both partners.

Female causes

Ovulation disorders, meaning you ovulate infrequently or not at all, account for infertility in about 25 percent of couples who are infertile. Problems with the regulation of reproductive hormones by the

hypothalamus or the pituitary gland or problems in the ovary, can cause ovulation disorders.

Hypothalamic dysfunction is a condition that disrupts the production of one or more hormones responsible for stimulating ovulation each month. Excess physical or emotional stress, a very high or very low body weight, or a recent substantial weight gain or loss can cause this problem. Irregular or absent periods are the most common signs.

Polycystic ovary syndrome may also result in infertility. With this condition, the female body produces an excess of male hormones. The ovaries may become large and studded with small follicles. Many women who experience this condition never establish a normal menstrual rhythm. Some never start menstruating. Additional causes of anovulation include diseases such as diabetes and thyroid disease.

Problems with ovulation can also be caused by primary ovarian insufficiency or excess production of the hormone prolactin (hyperprolactinemia), which reduces estrogen production.

If ovulation is normal, the problem lies elsewhere. Abnormalities of the fallopian tubes can sometimes be the problem, or contribute to it. Damaged or blocked fallopian tubes keep sperm from getting to the egg or block the passage of the fertilized egg into the uterus. As mentioned, with endometriosis, some of the tissue that lines the uterus and is shed each month during the menstrual cycle grows outside the uterus. This tissue can interfere with fertility.

Sometimes the cause of infertility stems from the uterus. An irregular-shaped uterus or tumors (fibroids) in the uterine cavity can cause problems. Surgical correction may or may not restore fertility. Problems of the cervix that can cause infertility include cervical narrowing (stenosis). Sometimes the cervix isn't able to produce the best type of mucus to allow the sperm to travel through the cervix into the uterus.

Age also plays an important role in female infertility. Infertility rates increase more significantly after age 35.

Male causes

The prime cause of male infertility is impaired sperm production. The absence of sperm in the semen (azoospermia) generally is due to a disorder of the testicles or, rarely, a blockage in the passageways leading from the testicles. With oligospermia, sperm are present in the semen but not in enough quantity to readily fertilize an egg.

One potential cause of male infertility is a varicocele, a condition in which varicose veins surrounding the testicles prevent normal cooling of the testicles. An increase in testicular temperature impairs sperm production. Other problems with the testicles also may be responsible for infertility.

A blood test can often identify hormonal disorders that may be the underlying cause of testicular problems. Sexually transmitted infections (STIs) or other infections can block the passageways through which sperm travel, or they can injure or kill sperm, causing infertility. Mumps and some other infections sometimes cause an inflammation of one or both testicles (orchitis) that can permanently impair or prevent sperm production in the affected testicle. Injuries and prior surgeries also can affect sperm production.

Some men have a condition called retrograde ejaculation, in which they produce sperm normally but ejaculate into the bladder rather than out the penis. This is most frequently seen in men with diabetes.

Male and female causes

Immunological factors may cause infertility. A few women produce antibodies that kill sperm before

Factors to Consider

Determining the cause of infertility and treating it can be demanding for both the couple and the doctor. It requires energy and commitment for what may be a prolonged period.

Personal attitudes

It's important for a couple considering fertility therapy to take into account their attitudes about the process. Just because something is possible doesn't mean that it should be done. Attitudes toward conception vary greatly. Some couples believe that if sexual intercourse doesn't produce a child, they should accept the situation and not take further steps toward possible pregnancy. Conversely, other couples are so eager to have their own biological child that they believe no procedure is too much, no therapy too complicated, and no expense or hardship too great.

Most couples find themselves somewhere between these two positions. Doctors who specialize in fertility problems are often prepared to discuss these issues with you. They can help you to examine your attitudes and to keep your

expectations realistic. Even though medical science has provided many new techniques, they all have limitations, and none is 100 percent successful.

Ethical considerations

When fertilization is possible only through medical intervention, some couples believe that taking advantage of the latest technology crosses a line. It raises questions and ethical considerations for them.

A significant issue for many people is using donor sperm or donor eggs from someone other than their own partner. Using sperm or eggs from a stranger raises many questions: Does the donor have any rights concerning the child? Might future court decisions award donors visitation rights? Should I use an anonymous or a known donor?

Other ethical considerations concern issues of selective reduction in the number of embryos in case of a multifetal pregnancy.

In the end, only you and your partner can decide how far you should go and whether you can deal with issues that may arise. The time to consider your ethical positions on fertility therapy is before you embark upon these treatments.

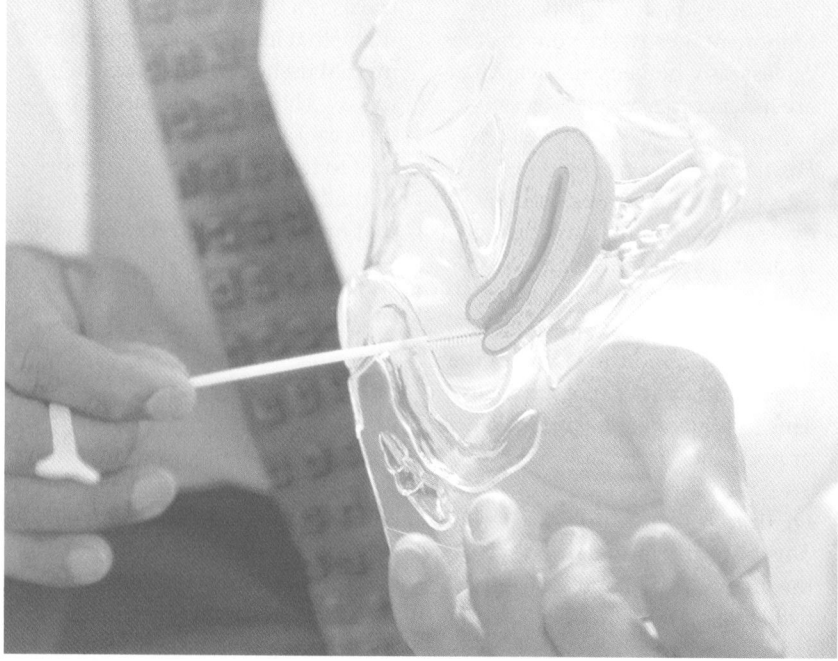

one can penetrate an egg. Similarly, some men produce antibodies that are meant to fight an infection but inadvertently attack sperm instead. Clearing up an infection may eradicate this problem.

In men as well as women, numerous diseases that can affect the genitourinary tract can cause infertility. These include sexually transmitted infections. Pelvic inflammatory disease commonly is caused by sexually transmitted infections such as gonorrhea, chlamydia and vaginitis and, less commonly, by tuberculosis and anaerobic streptococcal infection.

In women with pelvic inflammatory disease, aggressive treatment with antibiotics can clear up the infection and re-establish fertility. Even with treatment, pelvic inflammatory disease may result in tubal obstruction (occlusion) and infertility.

Treatable problems with sexual intercourse may also affect fertility. Erectile dysfunction, premature ejaculation, painful intercourse, or psychological and relationship problems can contribute. Use of lubricants such as oils or petroleum jelly can be toxic to sperm and impair fertility.

Treatment

Treatments for infertility are numerous, and recent developments have increased the number of couples who were once infertile and can achieve pregnancy. The method that may work best for you depends on the cause of your infertility. Some causes of infertility can't be corrected. However, even in those cases, various means of insemination or embryo transfer may be possible so that a woman can still become pregnant.

Restoring fertility
Sperm survive in the female reproductive tract for up to 72 hours, and an egg can be fertilized for a few hours after its release. Therefore, by having intercourse every

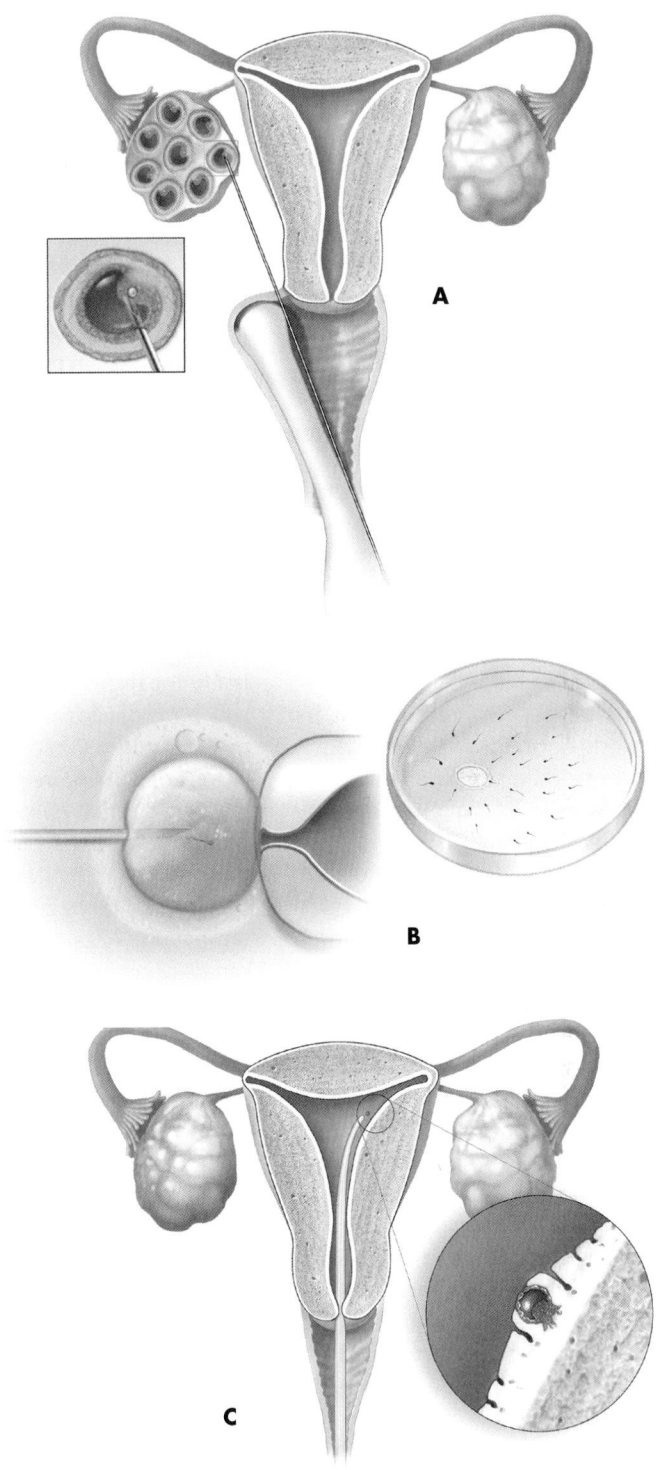

In vitro fertilization: Figure A shows eggs being removed from mature follicles within an ovary. Figure B shows healthy eggs being fertilized. This is done in one of two ways. On the left, a single sperm is injected into an egg (intracytoplasmic sperm injection). On the right, an egg is mixed with sperm in a petri dish. Figure C shows fertilized eggs (embryos) being transferred into the uterus, with the hope that at least one will implant itself in the uterine lining.

two to three days at midcycle, couples can effectively eliminate faulty timing as a factor contributing to infertility. Sexual problems, such as impotence or premature ejaculation, also can be treated to improve fertility.

When the source of infertility is the male sperm, restoring or initiating fertility is sometimes possible. For example, surgically correcting a varicocele appears to restore fertility in some cases. Some problems with the testicles, prostate gland, seminal vesicles and urethra also may be corrected.

When sperm production is impaired because of damage to the sperm-producing cells of the testicle, drug treatment has proved to be of little benefit. In rare cases where infertility is caused by abnormal hormone production, your doctor might recommend hormone therapy. When infections hamper sperm production, treating the infection may improve fertility. This is particularly true of sexually transmitted infections, for which both partners must be treated.

In women, treatment also depends on the results of examinations and tests. If the fertility problem is related to failure to release an egg (anovulation), a doctor can attempt to bring about ovulation by administering treatments that promote or regulate ovulation, such as clomiphene citrate or gonadotropins. In certain circumstances, other drugs such as metformin, letrozole or bromocriptine may be used to improve fertility.

Surgery sometimes is used to improve female fertility. Certain procedures can correct problems in the fallopian tubes or abnormalities of the uterus or remove endometrial polyps. Microsurgical techniques make such delicate operations possible. Surgical repair offers a chance of pregnancy. Today, however, assisted reproductive technology is often used instead of an operation.

Assisted reproductive technology

Assisted reproductive technology (ART) refers to medical procedures that enable many couples to have children when fertility can't be restored. In vitro fertilization is the most commonly used and most effective ART technique. It involves retrieving mature female eggs, fertilizing them with sperm in a laboratory and implanting the fertilized eggs in the uterus.

If you're using your own eggs, you'll begin the process by taking medications that stimulate your ovaries to produce more eggs than usual. The period of ovarian stimulation typically lasts one to two weeks. You'll then undergo a vaginal ultrasound and blood test to determine if your follicles are ready for retrieval.

If your follicles are ready, you'll receive an injection of human chorionic gonadotropin (HCG) to help the eggs mature. Eggs are retrieved 34 to 36 hours after the HCG injection and before ovulation.

It usually takes 20 minutes to retrieve the eggs. The procedure can be done in a doctor's office or a clinic. You'll be sedated and given pain medication to help keep you comfortable and relaxed throughout the procedure. Using transvaginal ultrasound, your doctor guides a needle through the vagina to an ovary. Eggs are then recovered from mature follicles. If your ovaries aren't accessible through transvaginal ultrasound, an abdominal surgery or laparoscopy may be used to guide the needle.

After being removed from the follicles, the fluid that contains the eggs is taken immediately to a laboratory, where the eggs are immersed in a special solution and placed in an incubator. How long the eggs remain in the incubator depends on their maturity.

One of the most common methods of fertilization is insemination. During insemination, healthy sperm and mature eggs are mixed and incubated overnight. In anoth-

er common technique, known as intracytoplasmic sperm injection, a single healthy sperm is injected directly into each mature egg.

Usually, embryo transfer takes place two to six days after the eggs have been retrieved. The number of embryos implanted is typically based on the age and number of eggs retrieved. Make sure you and your doctor agree on the number of embryos that will be implanted before they're transferred.

Embryo transfer is a brief procedure in which your doctor threads a soft, flexible catheter (cannula) through your cervix into your uterus. Extra embryos can be cryopreserved (frozen) so that you don't have to repeat the ovarian stimulation and retrieval process. If conception doesn't occur after the embryo transfer or if you want more children, the frozen embryos may be used at a later date. You'll have a pregnancy test, usually two weeks after the procedure.

The success rate for in vitro fertilization — that is, the percentage of ART cycles started that resulted in a live birth — is approximately 50 percent for women under age 35 who are undergoing a fresh embryo transfer. Success rates decrease with age. In vitro fertilization is generally the treatment of choice when both fallopian tubes are blocked. It's also used widely for a number of other infertility conditions, including endometriosis, unexplained infertility, male factor infertility and ovulation disorders.

ART works best when a woman has a healthy uterus, responds well to fertility drugs and ovulates naturally. The success rate is lower in women older than age 40 and women with untreated conditions of the uterus, such as scar tissue, fibroids and polyps. The success rate is also lower in men with low sperm counts, low sperm motility or abnormal sperm function.

Other techniques are sometimes used to aid an in vitro fertilization cycle. One of these techniques is a method called intracytoplasmic sperm injection (ICSI). It involves the injection of a single sperm into an egg to achieve fertilization. This procedure is especially helpful for couples who haven't been able to achieve fertilization with standard techniques and for men with low sperm concentrations.

Depending on the situation, another aid to in vitro fertilization may be assisted hatching. During this laboratory procedure, the shell-like protein that surrounds the egg is mechanically or chemically opened before embryo transfer to help the embryo hatch.

The risks associated with ART involve the medications and procedures used to remove the eggs. These risks include hemorrhage, infection, damage to adjacent organs and overstimulation of ovaries, which causes ovarian enlargement and abdominal discomfort. The greatest risk is an increased chance of a multiple pregnancy.

Intrauterine insemination
Intrauterine insemination takes just a minute or two and is usually done in a doctor's office or clinic. It requires no medications or pain relievers. Your doctor or a specially trained nurse performs the procedure.

During the procedure, a speculum will be inserted into your vagina — similar to what you experience during a pelvic examination. A syringe containing a small sample of healthy sperm is attached to the end of a long, thin, flexible tube (catheter). A catheter is then inserted through the cervical opening of your vagina in order to deposit the sperm into your uterus.

Your doctor will likely instruct you to wait two weeks before taking an at-home pregnancy test. Your doctor may also ask you to return about two weeks after your home kit results for a blood test, which is more sensitive in detecting pregnancy hormones after fertilization.

Sexual Function and Dysfunction

Sexuality is an important aspect of the human experience, evolving across a woman's lifetime. Sexual health is an important part of overall health, but it varies in significance for each woman and each couple. Sex can be a source of pleasure or pain. It can offer health benefits or it can be affected negatively by health conditions.

If you have questions or concerns about your sexual function or sexual enjoyment, bring those questions and concerns to the attention of your doctor.

An older model of female sexual response that is still endorsed by some women is that there is a four-stage sexual response cycle:

- **Desire.** Feelings for your partner, fantasies or thoughts about sex, desire for sexual activity.
- **Excitement or arousal.** Vaginal lubrication and increased blood flow to the genitals resulting in genital swelling and feelings of pleasure.
- **Orgasm.** Building of excitement and pleasure, which can lead to a release of sexual tension and pleasurable rhythmic contractions of the pelvic muscles and uterus or vagina. Orgasms are unique to each woman — some have a single orgasm and others have multiple orgasms.
- **Resolution.** A relaxed, pleasurable stage of enjoyment after sexual activity, leading to a return to a nonaroused state.

For women, sexual response is complex. It often has as much to do with a woman's feelings for her partner as it does with sexual stimuli. Beyond having a desire or drive for sex, many women are sexual because they want to feel close to their partner. This aspect of sexuality is incorporated into a newer model of female sexual response

that depicts emotional intimacy as an important motivation for women to engage in sexual activity.

If emotional intimacy is present, then a woman may seek out and be receptive to sexual activity. If biological and psychological factors are in order, then sexual arousal can proceed, which may then lead to emotional and physical satisfaction, closeness to her partner, and a desire for more intimacy. Understanding this helps to understand the different factors that may need to be addressed to treat sexual dysfunction.

Sexual problems are common in women as well as in men. But not all people who experience sexual concerns have sexual dysfunction. Sexual dysfunction is defined as a problem with a stage of sexual function that's associated with personal distress. Among women, an estimated 40 to 50 percent report some form of sexual dysfunction in their lifetime.

Common sexual concerns in women include lack of desire or drive for sex, difficulty becoming aroused, difficulty with or an inability to reach orgasm, and painful sex.

Some instances of sexual dysfunction are due to a lack of basic sex education. It's important to understand your anatomy and your body's normal physiological response to sexual stimulation. It can be hard for you to achieve orgasm if you've never had one, don't know what it feels like or what stimulation your body requires to get there. Also, many people are unaware that it often takes a woman longer to become sexually aroused than it does a man.

A common problem for women is fatigue and the various stressors and demands on them as they try to meet myriad needs and fill multiple roles. For women as well as men, factors that can lead to sexual dysfunction include high blood pressure, heart disease, depression or anxiety, diabetes, neurological conditions, certain medications, and substance abuse.

Sexual dysfunction in women is generally divided into four categories: hypoactive sexual desire disorder, sexual arousal disorder, orgasmic disorder and sexual pain disorder.

Keep in mind that these are categories, not causes. The categories have many commonalties. Hormonal changes, such as those experienced during pregnancy or menopause, can affect sexual response. So can breaches in your relationship, or negative feelings toward your partner. Emotional problems, such as anxiety or depression, can contribute to any of the sexual disorders. Sexual dysfunction can affect your self-esteem or that of your partner.

Hypoactive sexual desire disorder

Signs and symptoms
- Diminished or absent sexual desire, including recurrent or long-lasting lack of sexual thoughts and fantasies
- Insufficient sexual desire to sustain interest in sexual activity
- Distress over the lack of desire

Possibly the most common type of sexual disorder among women, hypoactive sexual desire disorder means a woman has a low libido, or lack of sex drive. She doesn't think about or fantasize about sex. She may even be having sex and experiencing orgasm, but may lack desire to be sexually active. This condition is considered a sexual disorder only if the individual is distressed by it.

Over a lifetime, most couples experience a mismatch in sexual desire at one time or another. Women, in particular, commonly experience low interest in sex at times of stress, medical illness, after childbirth and when taking certain medications. How couples negotiate a mismatch in sexual interest often follows a pattern similar to how they negotiate other differences in their relationship.

If you experience a persistent lack of sexual thoughts and desire to be sexually active, if it bothers you, and if it persists, seek help. Problems with reduced sex drive can be related to changes in your body at different life stages, as well as relationship issues, emotional and physical health problems, medication side effects, and other causes.

Finding the cause and exploring approaches to enhance or restore your interest and enjoyment in sexual activity can be helpful to you and the health of your relationship.

Treatment of hypoactive sexual desire disorder depends on the underlying cause.

Sexual arousal disorder

Signs and symptoms
- Diminished arousal during desired sexual activity
- Vaginal dryness during sexual intercourse
- Distress over the lack of arousal

With sexual arousal disorder, your desire for sex may be intact, but you're unable to maintain your arousal during sexual activity.

As with other sexual problems, an occasional lack of arousal doesn't mean you have a disorder. It's only considered dysfunctional if it persists and causes you distress. A lack of sexual response when you haven't had enough time with foreplay or adequate stimulation isn't a disorder. That is normal.

Many things can affect sexual arousal. Impaired sexual arousal may be due to estrogen deficiency, use of certain medications such as some antidepressants, and a variety of other conditions that affect nerve sensation or blood flow to the genitals.

Other possibilities include radiation or surgery to the pelvis, diabetes, cardiovascular disease and neurological diseases.

Lubricants to Treat Dryness

Couples shouldn't think that using a lubricant is a sign of failure. If there's dryness, a lubricant can make sexual touch and intercourse more pleasurable. Many couples use a lubricant during sexual activity, particularly at midlife and beyond for women. Lubricants come in water-based or silicone-based formulas.

Water-based lubricants
These lubricants are the ones most widely available in drugstores and grocery stores. They're available in a variety of brands. Water-based lubricants work well for lubricating the vagina or penis. They have two potential disadvantages, however. They tend to dry quickly, and they may need to be reapplied during sexual activity. Secondly, some of them contain glycerin, which may provide a favorable environment for yeast growth. If you have problems with yeast infections, consider getting a glycerin-free water-based lubricant.

Silicone-based lubricants
These lubricants require only a very small amount on application and are very slippery. They, too, are sold in a variety of brands. Silicone-based lubricants are long lasting, but they have two potential disadvantages. They don't wash off well with soap and water, and they can make the floor of the bath or shower very slippery. In addition, for men with erectile dysfunction, silicone lubricants may result in too much slipperiness, decreasing friction during intercourse and making it more difficult to achieve or maintain an erection.

Vaginismus

An important and treatable cause of painful intercourse is vaginismus. If you have vaginismus, the muscles surrounding the entrance to the vagina contract, making intercourse difficult, if not impossible. Women affected by this condition may be unable to use a tampon or have a pelvic exam. It's common to be embarrassed by this condition and be hesitant about seeking help. But it's important that you consult a doctor trained in treating sexual disorders.

Treatment often combines progressive vaginal enlargement (dilation) with pelvic floor physical therapy, counseling and education by a sex therapist to help you learn how to bring your vaginal and pelvic floor muscles under control. You learn how to relax and tighten the muscles. Then you begin use of progressive vaginal dilators and eventually proceed to vaginal penetration.

Orgasmic disorder

Signs and symptoms
- An inability to reach orgasm during sex after sufficient stimulation
- Delay in reaching orgasm despite sufficient stimulation
- Distress over the lack of orgasm

Although most women are biologically able to have an orgasm, some women never experience an orgasm, some attain orgasm only sometimes, and some lose the ability to experience orgasm when earlier in life they were easily able to experience it. A change in your normal pattern that causes you stress and leads to dissatisfaction with sexual activity merits further evaluation.

Orgasmic disorder is defined as persistent or recurrent difficulty or delay in achieving orgasm after sufficient sexual stimulation

and arousal. Orgasmic disorder is often intertwined with sexual arousal disorder. In some cases of orgasmic disorder, a woman does experience orgasm, but has to work unreasonably hard or long to attain it.

Female sexual response is complex, involving sexual desire, sexual stimulation and the ability to be present during the sexual experience — letting go of distracting thoughts or worries.

Understanding how your body responds to sexual stimulation, knowing what gives you pleasure and communicating your sexual needs to a responsive partner is important for experiencing orgasm.

Most women don't have orgasm with vaginal penetration and normally need to experience stimulation of the clitoris to reach orgasm.

Causes of orgasmic disorder are similar to some of the causes of arousal disorder, including problems with blood flow, nerve sensation, medication side effects and hormone deficiency. Another important cause is lack of understanding of the normal sexual response. Some women are distracted or anxious during sexual activity. In addition, focusing too hard on trying to have an orgasm can impair your ability to experience one.

Sexual pain disorder

Signs and symptoms
- Pain during sexual stimulation
- Pain upon vaginal penetration
- Distress over the pain

Painful sexual intercourse, also called dyspareunia, occurs more commonly early in a woman's sexual life when she is sexually inexperienced, or after childbirth, particularly if the birth was traumatic with injury to the perineum. Painful sex can also occur after menopause when genital and vaginal tissues become more dry and fragile. However, discomfort during sex can occur at any age and stage of life.

The tendency is often for women to go ahead with sex even when there's discomfort, thinking they should just bear the pain. But it's important to determine what's causing the pain and get medical help, if needed.

Consider whether the pain occurs at the vaginal opening or deeper inside. A common cause of what's known as insertional dyspareunia is lack of lubrication or lack of time for sufficient arousal. For this, you want to take more time for foreplay and arousal, and use a lubricant. If you still have pain on insertion, see your doctor. Potential causes include infection, skin conditions, vulvar vestibulitis, vaginismus or other conditions that may require medical treatment.

Deep dyspareunia may result from pelvic floor muscle tightness, endometriosis, fibroids, bowel conditions, tumors, cysts or many other possible causes. Sometimes adjusting your position during intercourse can help. If it doesn't, see your doctor.

Seeking help

If your sexual disorder causes you distress, it's important that you seek help. Sexual disorders are common, and effective treatment is available. In addition, doctors are becoming more sensitive to sexual problems and are more knowledgeable about treatment options. If your doctor is unable to address your concerns or your problem doesn't seem to be improving, ask for a referral to a health care professional with expertise in the treatment of sexual dysfunction.

Menstrual Disorders

Your menstrual cycle is regulated by hormones that are ultimately controlled by your hypothalamus, an area at the base of your brain that acts as a kind of regulator for your whole reproductive system. Your hypothalamus interacts with your pituitary gland, and some of the gland's hormones regulate the hormone action of your ovaries. It's primarily the ovarian hormones that affect the uterus.

Given the complexity of this system and given that both physical and mental stress can affect the hypothalamus, it's remarkable that women's menstrual cycles are as regular as they are. Sometimes, though, irregularities in the cycle can occur. A variety of factors can cause menstrual disorders.

Absence of periods

Signs and symptoms
- No menstruation by age 16
- A three-month absence of menstruation in women who aren't pregnant or menopausal Inability to menstruate is called amenorrhea. Amenorrhea can happen during puberty or later in life.
- Primary amenorrhea describes a condition in which you haven't had any menstrual periods by age 16.
- Secondary amenorrhea occurs when you were previously menstruating, but then stopped having periods.
Pregnancy may be your first thought if you miss a period, but there are many possible explanations for absence of menstruation. Depending on the cause of amenorrhea, you might experience other signs or symptoms along with the absence of periods, such as milky nipple discharge, headache, vision changes, or excessive hair growth on your face and torso (hirsutism).

A sign, not a disease, amenorrhea seldom results from a serious condition.

Causes of primary amenorrhea
Primary amenorrhea is a rare condition in adolescent girls in the United States. The most common causes of primary amenorrhea include:

- **Chromosomal abnormalities.** Certain chromosomal abnormalities can cause a premature depletion of the eggs and follicles involved in ovulation and menstruation.
- **Problems with the hypothalamus.** Functional hypothalamic amenorrhea is a disorder of the hypothalamus — an area at the base of your brain that acts as a control center for your body and regulates your menstrual cycle. Excessive exercise, eating disorders, such as anorexia, and physical or psychological stress can all contribute to a disruption in the normal function of the hypothalamus. Less commonly, a tumor may prevent your hypothalamus from functioning normally.

- **Pituitary disease.** The pituitary is another gland in the brain that's involved in regulating the menstrual cycle. A tumor or other invasive growth may disrupt the pituitary gland's ability to perform this function.
- **Lack of reproductive organs.** Sometimes problems arise during fetal development that lead to a baby girl being born without some major part of her reproductive system, such as her uterus, cervix or vagina. Because her reproductive system didn't develop normally, she won't have menstrual cycles.
- **Structural abnormality of the vagina.** An obstruction of the vagina may prevent visible menstrual bleeding. A membrane or wall may be present in the

Sports and Menses

Female dancers, runners and women involved in vigorous sports frequently find that they skip menstrual periods or stop menstruating (amenorrhea). This is more likely to happen if you're young, especially if your menstrual cycle tends to be irregular. In fact, some teenagers who train heavily for an athletic event reach their late teens before they start menstruating.

Medical experts believe that several factors are involved, including stress and perhaps the ratio of fat cells to other cells in your body. In either case, you stop menstruating because your ovaries don't produce hormones in the cyclic manner that causes the uterine lining to thicken and then shed.

Reducing your exercise schedule or gaining weight may cause you to begin menstruating again. If that doesn't work, or if you don't want to exercise less or gain weight, your doctor may suggest hormone

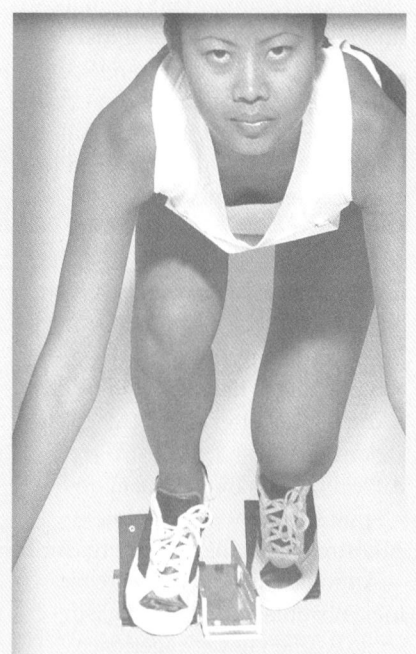

therapy, often in the form of oral contraceptives.

Spontaneous recovery is common, although it may occur many months after the underlying cause is resolved. You could ovulate at any time and be at risk of pregnancy, so don't forget about birth control if you don't want to become pregnant.

vagina that blocks the outflow of blood from the uterus and cervix.

Causes of secondary amenorrhea

Secondary amenorrhea is much more common than primary amenorrhea. Many possible causes of secondary amenorrhea exist:

- **Pregnancy.** In women of reproductive age, pregnancy is the most common cause of amenorrhea.
- **Contraceptives.** Some women who take birth control pills may not have periods. When oral contraceptives are stopped, it may take several months to resume regular ovulation and menstruation. Contraceptives that are implanted or injected, such as Depo-Provera, also may cause amenorrhea, as can progesterone-containing intrauterine devices, such as levonorgestrel (Mirena).
- **Breast-feeding.** Mothers who breast-feed often experience amenorrhea. Although ovulation may occur, menstruation may not. Pregnancy can result despite the lack of menstruation.
- **Stress.** Mental stress can temporarily alter the functioning of your hypothalamus — an area of your brain that controls the hormones that regulate your menstrual cycle. Ovulation and menstruation may stop as a result. Regular menstrual periods usually resume after your stress decreases.
- **Medication.** Certain medications can cause menstrual periods to stop. For example, antipsychotics, oral corticosteroids, and some chemotherapy drugs and hormonal treatments can cause amenorrhea.
- **Illness.** Chronic illness may postpone menstrual periods. As you recover, menstruation typically resumes.
- **Hormonal imbalance.** A common cause of amenorrhea or irregular periods is polycystic ovary syndrome (PCOS). This condition causes relatively high and sustained levels of estrogen

and androgen, a male hormone, rather than the fluctuating levels seen in the normal menstrual cycle. This results in a decrease in the pituitary hormones that lead to ovulation and menstruation. PCOS is associated with obesity; amenorrhea or abnormal, often heavy uterine bleeding; acne; and sometimes excess facial hair.
- **Low body fat.** An excessively low percentage of body fat interrupts many hormonal functions in your body, potentially halting ovulation. Women who have an eating disorder, such as anorexia or bulimia, often stop having periods because of these abnormal hormonal changes.
- **Excessive exercise.** Women who participate in activities that require rigorous training, such as ballet, long-distance running or gymnastics, may find their menstrual cycle interrupted. Several factors combine to contribute to the loss of periods in athletes, including low body fat, stress and high energy expenditure.
- **Thyroid malfunction.** An underactive thyroid gland (hypothyroidism) commonly causes menstrual irregularities, including amenorrhea.
- **Pituitary tumor.** A noncancerous (benign) tumor in your pituitary gland (adenoma or prolactinoma) can cause an overproduction of prolactin. Excess prolactin can interfere with the regulation of menstruation. This type of tumor is treatable with medication, but it sometimes requires surgery.
- **Uterine scarring.** Asherman's syndrome, a condition in which scar tissue builds up in the lining of the uterus, can sometimes occur after uterine procedures, such as a dilation and curettage (D&C), cesarean section, or treatment for uterine fibroids. Uterine scarring prevents the normal buildup and shedding of the uterine lining, and can result in very light menstrual bleeding or no periods at all.

- **Primary ovarian insufficiency.** Primary ovarian insufficiency is the loss of normal function of your ovaries before age 40. If your ovaries fail, they don't produce normal amounts of the hormone estrogen or release eggs regularly. Infertility is a common result. The lack of ovarian function decreases the amount of circulating estrogen in your body, which can increase your risk of heart disease, osteoporosis, sexual dysfunction and mental health concerns.

Primary ovarian insufficiency can result from genetic factors, autoimmune disease or cancer treatment. Sometimes, no cause can be found. Your doctor may recommend that you take menopausal hormone therapy until the natural age of menopause in order to lower your risk of certain conditions associated with primary ovarian insufficiency, including dementia, parkinsonism, heart disease, osteoporosis, mood disorders, sexual dysfunction and early death.

Diagnosis

Although amenorrhea rarely results from a life-threatening condition, it can encompass a complex set of hormonal problems. Finding the underlying cause of amenorrhea can take time and may require several types of testing.

First, your doctor may have you take a pregnancy test. Your doctor may also perform a pelvic exam to check for problems with your reproductive organs. Your doctor will also perform a physical examination and ask about your medical history. In young women, this exam will include checking for signs and symptoms of changes that are normal to puberty.

The next step may include blood tests to check your hormone levels, for instance a thyroid function test. A progestin challenge test — in which you take a hormonal medication (progestogen) for seven to

10 days to trigger bleeding — may be another kind of test your doctor administers. Results from this test can tell your doctor whether your periods have stopped due to a lack of ovulation.

Depending on your signs and symptoms and the result of any blood tests you've had, further testing may be needed. Imaging tests, such as computerized tomography, magnetic resonance imaging or ultrasound, can reveal pituitary tumors or structural abnormalities of your reproductive organs. Finally, laparoscopy or hysteroscopy — minimally invasive surgical techniques to view your internal organs — may sometimes be recommended.

How serious is absence of periods?

Amenorrhea often indicates that something isn't working properly and should be treated. If you're not menstruating, you may find it difficult to become pregnant, although a lack of menstruation isn't a reliable protection against pregnancy. Amenorrhea can be the result of conditions that could cause you medical problems later in life. If you're producing estrogen but not having periods, you could be at a greater long-term risk of endometrial (uterine) cancer.

Treatment

What type of treatment you need depends on what's causing the amenorrhea. Your doctor may suggest that you make changes to your lifestyle related to your weight, physical activity or stress level. If you have PCOS or athletic amenorrhea, your doctor may try hormonal treatment to manage the problem. Amenorrhea caused by thyroid or pituitary disorders may be treated with medications.

Polycystic ovary syndrome

Signs and symptoms
- Unpredictable, or irregular, menstruation, or failure to menstruate

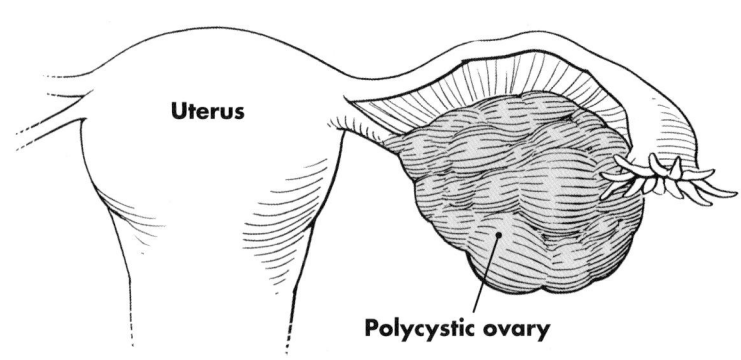

Polycystic ovary syndrome is a disorder involving irregular menstrual periods and occasionally an excess of facial and body hair. The ovaries develop multiple cysts and fail to release eggs.

- Reduced fertility
- An increased amount of facial and body hair
- Acne
- Tiny ovarian cysts

Polycystic ovary syndrome (PCOS) is a common hormonal disorder among women of reproductive age in the United States, affecting approximately 1 in 10 women. Most women with PCOS never establish a normal menstrual rhythm in their teens and eventually stop menstruating altogether. Some never start. Many women with PCOS ovulate less often and have decreased menstrual frequency, variable amounts of bleeding from cycle to cycle, and unpredictable menstrual symptoms.

With PCOS, the female body can produce an excess of male hormones (androgens), which may lead to excess facial hair and acne. Women with this condition may also be overweight.

The name of the condition comes from the appearance of the ovaries in some women with the disorder. The ovaries may be large and studded with numerous tiny (poly) cysts. These cysts are follicles — fluid-filled sacs that contain immature eggs. The condition may delay conception or require fertility therapy but is usually treatable.

Doctors don't know the cause of PCOS, but research suggests a link to insulin, the hormone produced in the pancreas that facilitates transport of sugar (glucose) from blood to individual cells. Usually, the condition is lifelong and requires close supervision and management to prevent endometrial cancer, as well as increased risk of diabetes, high blood pressure and heart disease.

Diagnosis

Blood tests may reveal a typical pattern of hormone level abnormalities. Your doctor may request an ultrasound exam to examine your ovaries for ovarian volume, which may be painlessly increased due to tiny cysts. You may also undergo an endometrial biopsy, in which a tissue sample is taken from the uterine lining to detect any precancerous conditions.

How serious is polycystic ovary syndrome?

Women with PCOS are at increased risk of conditions such as diabetes, high blood pressure, abnormal cholesterol and triglyceride levels, and coronary artery disease. Women with PCOS are also at increased risk of abnormal uterine bleeding and uterine and ovarian cancer.

Treatment

Polycystic ovary syndrome treatment generally focuses on management of your main concerns, such as infertility, increased body hair, acne or abnormal menses.

Long term, the most important aspect of treatment is managing cardiovascular risks, such as obesity, high blood cholesterol, diabetes and high blood pressure. To help guide ongoing treatment decisions, your doctor will likely want to see you for regular visits to perform a physical examination, measure your blood pressure, and obtain fasting glucose and lipid levels.

You can benefit from counseling about healthy-eating choices and regular exercise. This is particularly important if you're overweight. Obesity makes insulin resistance worse. Weight loss and exercise can reduce both insulin and androgen levels, and may restore ovulation. Ask your doctor to recommend a weight-loss program.

Your doctor may prescribe one or more medications to help manage the symptoms and risks associated with PCOS.

Medications for regulating your menstrual cycle

If you're not trying to become pregnant, your doctor may prescribe low-dose oral contraceptives that combine synthetic estrogen and progestin, which decrease androgen production. Progestin contraceptives, including pills, rings and intrauterine devices (IUDs) reduce your risk of endometrial cancer and correct abnormal bleeding.

An alternative approach is taking progestin tablets for part of each month. This regulates your menstrual cycle and offers protection against endometrial cancer, but it doesn't improve androgen levels.

Your doctor may also prescribe metformin (Glucophage, Fortamet, others), an oral medication for type 2 diabetes that treats insulin resistance. This drug is still being studied as a treatment for polycystic ovary syndrome, but research has demonstrated that it improves ovulation and may reduce androgen levels. However, doctors don't

yet know if metformin offers the same protection against endometrial cancer as does treatment with oral contraceptives or with progestin alone.

Medications for reducing excessive hair growth

Your doctor may add a medication specifically targeted at countering the effects of excess androgen. Spironolactone (Aldactone) blocks the effects of androgen and reduces new androgen production. For those reasons, the drug isn't recommended if you're pregnant or not using contraception. Spironolactone is also a diuretic and may cause you to urinate more frequently.

Your doctor might also prescribe eflornithine (Vaniqa), a prescription cream that slows facial hair growth in women. Avoid using this medication during pregnancy.

Medications for achieving pregnancy

To become pregnant, you may need a medication to trigger ovulation. Clomiphene (Clomid) is an oral anti-estrogen medication that you take in the first part of your menstrual cycle. If clomiphene alone isn't effective, your doctor may add metformin to help trigger ovulation.

If you don't become pregnant using clomiphene and metformin, your doctor may recommend using gonadotropins — follicle-stimulating hormone (FSH) and luteinizing hormone (LH) medications that are administered by injection.

With clomiphene or gonadotropins, the risk of multiple births is increased.

Other treatments for excessive hair growth

Several options exist for hair removal. They include shaving, plucking and over-the-counter remedies such as waxes, gels, creams and lotions (depilatories). However, depilatories may irritate your skin, so follow package directions, and on first use,

apply the product to an inconspicuous area to determine if it's suitable for you. The results may last several weeks, and then you must repeat treatment.

Surgical options for longer lasting hair removal include:

- **Electrolysis.** To permanently remove excess hair, some women undergo electrolysis in addition to medical therapy. A fine needle is inserted into the hair follicle, and electric current is applied to kill the follicle. Because only one follicle can be treated at a time, this method isn't useful for large areas of the body. Several treatments are usually necessary.
- **Laser therapy.** Laser hair removal systems use laser light — an intense, pulsating beam of light — to remove unwanted hair. Laser hair removal can be effective on short, visible hair. Before the procedure, you shave the area to be treated, and allow it to grow to a stubble. Your doctor may use multiple treatments to target the affected areas. After several months, laser procedures permanently reduce one-third or more of the hair in the targeted area.

Premenstrual syndrome

Signs and symptoms

- Bloating, fluid retention, abdominal swelling, swollen hands and feet, and weight gain
- Breast soreness
- Fatigue
- Headache
- Gastrointestinal upset, including nausea, vomiting, diarrhea and constipation
- Mood swings, difficulty concentrating and lethargy
- Irritability, anxiety and tension

Premenstrual syndrome (PMS) is a predictable pattern of physical or emotional changes that occur just before menstruation. Estimates of menstruating women who experience at least one PMS symptom range widely from around 45 to 85 percent. For about 3 to 8 percent of these women, the symptoms may be severe. Symptoms can develop anytime after the midpoint in your menstrual cycle, and they disappear when your period starts.

No one knows exactly what causes PMS. It's presumed to be related to cyclic changes in hormone levels because symptoms disappear during pregnancy and after menopause. Stress can aggravate the problem, but it's not the cause. Occasionally, some women with severe PMS may have undiagnosed depression, though depression alone doesn't explain all of the symptoms of PMS. Caution should be used in blaming PMS for mood problems that occur at various times during the menstrual cycle.

Diagnosis

A doctor will attribute a particular symptom to PMS only if it's part of a predictable premenstrual pattern. To determine if there's a pattern, your doctor may ask you to keep a record of your symptoms over several menstrual cycles. On a calendar or in a diary, you record all of your symptoms, the day you first noticed them and the day they disappeared. Note, too, the day your period began.

How serious is premenstrual syndrome?

PMS can be hard to tolerate, but it's not associated with a serious underlying disease. If you find your PMS symptoms hard to live with, there a number of management options.

Treatment

Treatment often includes these strategies.

Self-care

Follow these tips to reduce the effects of PMS symptoms:
- Limit consumption of caffeine, salt and alcohol.
- Stay adequately hydrated.
- Increase complex carbohydrates, including foods with whole grains, fruits, vegetables, beans and legumes.
- Consider taking supplements, including 1,000 to 1,200 milligrams (mg) of calcium daily and 400 mg of magnesium.
- Exercise for at least 30 minutes most days of the week, if possible.
- Use relaxation techniques such as mindfulness, meditation and yoga.

Medication

Commonly prescribed medications for premenstrual symptoms include:
- **Nonsteroidal anti-inflammatory drugs (NSAIDs).** Taken before or at the onset of your period, NSAIDs such as ibuprofen (Advil, Motrin IB, others) or naproxen sodium (Aleve) can ease cramping and breast discomfort and headache.
- **Oral contraceptives.** These prescription medications stop ovulation and stabilize hormonal swings, thereby offering relief from PMS symptoms. Contraceptive pills containing the progestin drospirenone are often helpful when used, to limit the number of menses.
- **Antidepressants.** Selective serotonin reuptake inhibitors (SSRIs), which include fluoxetine (Prozac, Sarafem), paroxetine (Paxil, Pexeva, others), sertraline (Zoloft) and others, have been successful in reducing symptoms such as moodiness, irritability, sleep problems, abdominal bloating and breast tenderness, and are the first line agents for treatment of severe PMS or PMDD. These drugs are generally taken daily. But for some women with PMS, use of antidepressants may be limited to the two weeks before menstruation begins.

Mittelschmerz

Signs and symptoms
- Pain in the lower abdomen at the time of ovulation
- Slight vaginal bleeding accompanying the pain

Mittelschmerz is a German word meaning "middle pain." The condition occurs at the midpoint in the menstrual cycle, around the time of ovulation. Typically, the pain is a dull ache that lasts from a

Hormone Abnormalities and Menstruation

A complex cascade of hormones governs the menstrual cycle. The hypothalamus in your brain sends chemicals called releasing factors to your pituitary gland. Your pituitary then releases pituitary hormones (gonadotropins) that travel through your bloodstream to your ovaries. These hormones cause ovarian follicles to produce estrogen and progesterone. Estrogen and progesterone prepare your uterus for a possible pregnancy. At any stage in this process, things can go wrong.

Many hormone-related disorders can cause menstrual irregularity. The hypothalamus may be affected by illness, stress or drugs. More rarely, your hypothalamus develops a disorder such as a tumor or infection, which can affect menstruation.

If the hypothalamus fails to stimulate the pituitary gland, estrogen production and menstruation will cease. Sometimes, the pituitary gland produces too much of the hormone prolactin. Prolactin stimulates milk production when a mother is breast-feeding. Released in excess at other times, it can prevent ovulation and menstruation.

few minutes to a few hours. It may be accompanied by spotting.

During your menstrual cycle, the female sex hormone estrogen causes your uterine lining (endometrium) to thicken every month to create a nourishing environment for a fertilized egg. Soon afterward, a follicle — a tiny sac in your ovary that contains a single egg (ovum) — ruptures and releases its egg (ovulation).

Mittelschmerz occurs during ovulation, when the follicle ruptures and releases its egg. While the exact cause of mittelschmerz is unknown, here are possible reasons you may feel pain:

- Just before an egg is released with ovulation, follicle growth stretches the surface of your ovary, causing pain.
- Blood or fluid released from the ruptured follicle irritates the lining of your abdomen (peritoneum), leading to pain.

Pain at any other point in your menstrual cycle isn't mittelschmerz. It may be normal menstrual cramping, if it occurs during your period, or it may be from other abdominal or pelvic problems.

Treatment

Treatment varies depending on how often you experience mittelschmerz and how painful it is. You can take a mild analgesic such as acetaminophen, aspirin or ibuprofen to ease the pain. If it's severe and occurs most months, your doctor may recommend that you take birth control pills to prevent ovulation.

Painful periods

Signs and symptoms
- Pain in the lower abdomen during menstruation, possibly extending to the hips, lower back or thighs

The majority of women have mild abdominal cramps on the first day or two of their periods. For some women, though, menstrual pain (dysmenorrhea) is so severe that they require medication to function normally.

If the pain isn't a symptom of an underlying gynecologic disorder and begins with the onset of regular menses in young women, the problem is called primary dysmenorrhea. The prefix *dys* means "difficult," *men* signifies "month," and *rhoia* means "a flow." Medical experts believe that production of prostaglandins, substances that make the uterus contract, cause primary dysmenorrhea.

When a gynecologic disorder causes painful menstruation, it's known as secondary dysmenorrhea. In general, there's likely to be a secondary cause when the pain lasts longer than the first one to three days of the menstrual period and is worse than the menstrual pain experienced in the past. The underlying cause could be fibroids, adenomyosis or endometriosis.

Diagnosis
Your doctor's first concern is to check for the underlying disorders that cause secondary dysmenorrhea. You'll likely have a pelvic examination and perhaps blood tests and a urinalysis. Your doctor also may order diagnostic tests, such as ultrasound, to get images of your pelvic organs.

How serious are painful periods?
Primary dysmenorrhea can be extremely painful, but it's not harmful. More common during adolescence, it's likely to ease or disappear over the years or after you've had your first baby. Secondary dysmenorrhea is more serious, but most of the disorders that underlie it are treatable.

Treatment
Treatment depends on the type of dysmenorrhea you have. For primary dysmenorrhea, your doctor may prescribe a nonsteroidal anti-inflammatory drug (NSAID) such as ibuprofen (Advil, Motrin IB, others) or naproxen sodium (Aleve, others) to help relieve or prevent the pain. These medications, which block prostaglandin formation, can relieve the symptoms of primary dysmenorrhea. They work best when they're started with the onset of menstrual pain and are continued on a scheduled basis as long as the pain lasts. Oral contraceptives and other hormonal contraception generally improve menstrual pain for both primary and secondary dysmenorrhea.

Abnormal uterine bleeding

Signs and symptoms
- Vaginal bleeding that occurs at irregular intervals
- Vaginal bleeding that's unpredictable in amount or duration

The menstrual cycle varies from woman to woman, but menstrual flow generally occurs about every 28 days, lasts four to five days and produces blood loss of around 80 milliliters.

Abnormal uterine bleeding refers to irregular bleeding that's not caused by an anatomic abnormality. Common and usually painless, it occurs most often in girls who have just begun to menstruate, in women approaching menopause or as a consequence of other factors that can alter the normal hormonal cycle. In most cases, the uterine lining isn't shed completely each month because the ovaries aren't producing hormones normally. Abnormal uterine bleeding can take a number of forms, including heavy periods (menorrhagia), infrequent periods (oligomenorrhea), abnormally frequent periods (polymenorrhea) and irregular, heavy periods (metrorrhagia).

When not due to a life stage or stress, abnormal uterine bleeding is most commonly due to anovulation associated with polycystic ovary syndrome. Less frequently, the problem is an estrogen-producing ovarian tumor or abnormal estrogen metabolism due to liver disease.

Rarely, a female who's not nearing menopause may begin to menstruate infrequently and develop acne and an unusual amount of hair on her face and body. In this case, the problem may be an excess of androgen, produced either by her adrenal glands or by an ovarian tumor.

Diagnosis

Your doctor will most likely ask you about your medical history and menstrual cycles and do a pelvic examination to make sure the source of the bleeding is your uterus and not your bladder, vagina or cervix. Your doctor may also try to determine if a tubal (ectopic) pregnancy or an early miscarriage could be the cause of your bleeding. Associated symptoms that may be cause for concern are excessive facial hair, breast discharge, thyroid problems or abnormal blood clotting.

Your doctor may recommend a hysteroscopy to determine the cause of bleeding. Hysteroscopy is a procedure in which your doctor uses a small instrument to examine the interior of your cervix and uterus.

How serious is abnormal uterine bleeding?

If the bleeding is outside of what's normal for your periods, see your doctor. Abnormal uterine bleeding usually requires treatment. If you menstruate infrequently and can't achieve a desired pregnancy, you may need to see a fertility specialist. Women with chronic irregular bleeding are sometimes infertile.

Treatment

Treatment depends on the cause of the condition. Once the cause is defined, oral contraceptives can be very useful in promoting regular menstrual cycles. If the bleeding is heavy, you may require urgent evaluation. If you've become anemic, you may need iron supplements. In rare cases, a surgical procedure is performed to control heavy bleeding.

If your ovaries are producing too little estrogen, your doctor may prescribe hormone therapy to help prevent osteoporosis. Estrogen helps protect against bone loss and other conditions associated with low estrogen levels. If the cause of your problem is excessive male hormones (androgens), treatment will likely focus on correcting the underlying cause.

Heavy menstrual bleeding

Signs and symptoms

- Menstrual flow that soaks through one or more sanitary pads or tampons every hour for several consecutive hours
- The need to use double sanitary protection to control your menstrual flow
- The need to change sanitary protection during the night
- Menstrual periods lasting longer than seven days
- Menstrual flow that includes large blood clots
- Heavy menstrual flow that interferes with your regular lifestyle
- Constant pain in your lower abdomen during menstruation
- Tiredness, fatigue or shortness of breath (symptoms of anemia)

Menorrhagia is the medical term for excessive or prolonged menstrual bleeding — and for periods that are both heavy and prolonged. The condition is also known as hypermenorrhea.

Heavy periods are common, especially in young women who aren't ovulating regularly and in women approaching menopause. However, any woman in her reproductive years may experience heavy bleeding. Some women have heavy periods almost every cycle.

Some women experience blood loss severe enough to be defined as menorrhagia. In certain cases, the cause of heavy menstrual bleeding is unknown, but a number of conditions may cause menorrhagia. Causes include:

- **Ovulatory dysfunction.** In a normal menstrual cycle, a balance between the hormones estrogen and progesterone regulates the buildup of the lining of the uterus (endometrium), which is shed during menstruation. Dysfunction of the ovaries may cause a hormonal imbalance. If a hormonal imbalance occurs, the endometrium develops in excess and sheds by way of heavy menstrual bleeding. Hormonal imbalance occurs most often in adolescent girls and in women approaching menopause. If menorrhagia is caused by a specific hormonal imbalance, such as thyroid disease, the heavy menstrual flow often can be controlled with hormone medications. However, improper use of hormone medications can also be a direct cause of menorrhagia.
- **Uterine fibroids.** These noncancerous (benign) tumors of the uterus appear during your childbearing years. Uterine fibroids may cause heavier than normal or prolonged menstrual bleeding.
- **Polyps.** Small, benign growths on the lining of the uterine wall (uterine polyps) may cause heavy or prolonged menstrual bleeding. Polyps of the uterus most commonly occur in women of late reproductive and early menopausal years.
- **Adenomyosis.** This condition occurs when glands from the endometrium become embedded in the uterine muscle, often causing heavy bleeding and pain. Adenomyosis is most likely to develop in middle-aged women after childbearing.
- **Pregnancy complications.** A single, heavy, late period may be due to a miscarriage. If bleeding occurs at the usual time of menstruation, however, miscarriage is unlikely the cause. An ectopic pregnancy — implantation of a

Endometrial Ablation

Newer, minimally invasive surgical procedures and progestin-releasing intrauterine devices are making hysterectomy unnecessary for many women with heavy menstrual periods. The procedures are typically done in outpatient settings, and you usually can return to full activity within 48 hours. However, you're only eligible for these procedures if you have no desire to become pregnant. A pregnancy can't progress normally after the uterine lining (endometrium) has been surgically removed or destroyed. Failure rates for these procedures are higher in women under age 40.

The surgical alternatives involve removing or destroying (ablating) the uterine lining. The most common techniques involve freezing the tissue (cryoablation) or destroying it with radiofrequency energy (radiofrequency ablation) or thermal heat (thermal balloon ablation). You may be a candidate for one of these treatments if:
- You often need to change your pad or tampon more than every hour
- You develop iron deficiency anemia as a result of your blood loss
- Excessive bleeding interferes with your normal activities
- Hormonal or other treatments fail
- The cause of your bleeding is noncancerous (benign)
- You wish to avoid a hysterectomy

Be aware that a small percentage of women who undergo ablation still may need a hysterectomy later to control bleeding or for other reasons.

Thermal balloon ablation
This procedure uses a fluid-filled balloon that's inflated inside the uterus. After a probe inside the balloon heats the fluid, the balloon is left in place for about eight minutes. The heat destroys cells in the uterine lining, and the lining eventually sloughs off. The whole procedure takes about 30 minutes. Most balloons used are latex-free, so women with latex allergies can be treated with this procedure.

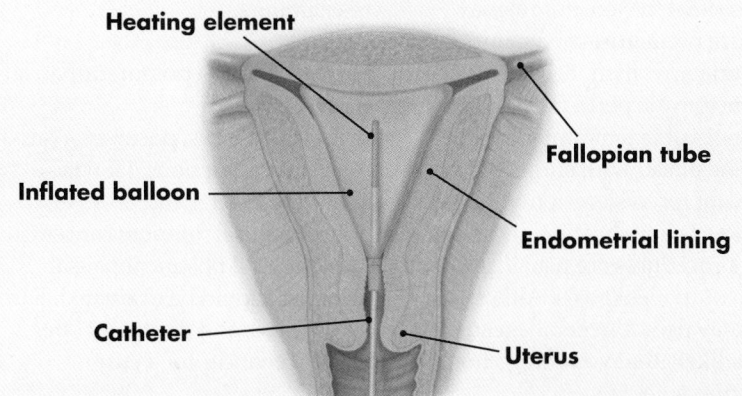

Heating element

Inflated balloon

Catheter

Fallopian tube

Endometrial lining

Uterus

A doctor inserts a fluid-filled thermal balloon and inflates it. A heated probe inside the balloon heats the fluid. The balloon is left in place for about eight minutes. The heat destroys cells in the uterine lining.

fertilized egg within the fallopian tube instead of the uterus — also may cause menorrhagia.
- **Cancer.** Rarely, uterine cancer or cervical cancer can cause excessive menstrual bleeding.
- **Abnormal clotting.** Hereditary problems that cause reduced clotting and certain drugs, including anticoagulants, can contribute to heavy or prolonged menstrual bleeding.

- **Other medical conditions.** A number of other medical conditions, including pelvic inflammatory disease (PID), thyroid problems, endometriosis, and liver or kidney disease, may cause menorrhagia.

You probably don't need medical attention if you have a single heavy period. If the bleeding doesn't stop or slow significantly within 24 hours, call your doctor. If you have several heavy periods, see a doctor to make sure that you're not developing iron deficiency anemia, a condition that results from the loss of blood.

Diagnosis
Your doctor will most likely ask about your medical history and menstrual cycles. You may be asked to keep a diary of bleeding and nonbleeding days, including notes on how heavy your flow was and how much sanitary protection you needed to control it. Your doctor may do a physical exam and recommend one or more tests or procedures such as:
- **Blood tests.** A sample of your blood is evaluated in case excessive blood loss during menstruation has made you anemic. Tests may also be done to check for thyroid disorders or blood-clotting abnormalities.
- **Cervical cancer screen.** Your doctor collects cells from your cervix for microscopic examination to detect changes that may be cancerous or precancerous.
- **Endometrial biopsy.** Your doctor takes a sample of tissue from the inside of your uterus to be examined under a microscope.
- **Ultrasound scan.** This imaging method uses sound waves to produce images of your uterus, ovaries and pelvis.

Based on the results of your initial tests, your doctor may recommend further testing. This may include:
- **Sonohysterogram.** This ultrasound scan is done after fluid is injected through a tube into the

uterus by way of your vagina and cervix. This allows your doctor to look for problems in the lining of your uterus.

- **Hysteroscopy.** A tiny tube with a light is inserted through your vagina and cervix into the uterus, which allows your doctor to see the inside of your uterus.
- **Dilation and curettage (D&C).** In this procedure, your doctor opens (dilates) your cervix and then inserts an instrument (curet) into your uterus to collect tissue from the uterine lining. This tissue is examined in the laboratory.

How serious are heavy periods?

Menorrhagia is inconvenient, and it can be distressing. However, most of the time it doesn't indicate a serious underlying disorder.

Treatment

Drug therapy for menorrhagia may include the following:

- **Iron supplements.** If the condition is accompanied by anemia, your doctor may recommend that you take iron supplements regularly. If your iron levels are low but you're not yet anemic, you may be started on iron supplements rather than waiting until you become anemic.
- **Nonsteroidal anti-inflammatory drugs (NSAIDs).** NSAIDs such as ibuprofen (Advil, Motrin IB, others) can help reduce menstrual blood loss. NSAIDs have the added benefit of relieving painful menstrual cramps (dysmenorrhea).
- **Oral contraceptives.** Aside from providing effective birth control, oral contraceptives can help regulate ovulation and reduce episodes of excessive or prolonged menstrual bleeding.
- **Progesterone.** The hormone progesterone can help correct hormonal imbalance and reduce menorrhagia. Often the progesterone is delivered directly to the uterus with an intrauterine contraceptive (IUD). If you

have menorrhagia from taking hormone medication, you and your doctor may be able to treat the condition by changing or stopping your medication.

You may need surgical treatment for menorrhagia if drug therapy is unsuccessful. Treatment options include:

- **Endometrial ablation.** Using ultrasonic energy, your doctor permanently destroys the entire lining of your uterus (endometrium). After endometrial ablation, most women have normal menstrual flow. However, some women have little or no menstrual flow after the procedure. Endometrial ablation reduces your ability to become pregnant.
- **Hysteroscopic resection of fibroids.** Heavy periods can be caused by noncancerous growths of the uterus (uterine fibroids) located just under the endometrial lining. Removal of the fibroids helps the endometrium function normally.
- **Hysterectomy.** Surgical removal of the uterus is a permanent procedure that causes sterility and cessation of menstrual periods. Additional removal of the ovaries (total hysterectomy) may cause premature menopause in younger women. Because hysterectomy is permanent, be sure you want this treatment before going ahead with surgery.

Except for hysterectomy, which requires hospitalization, these surgical procedures are usually done on an outpatient basis. Although you may need a general anesthetic, it's likely that you can go home later the same day.

When menorrhagia is a sign of another condition, such as thyroid disease, treating that condition usually results in lighter periods.

Postmenopausal bleeding

Signs and symptoms
- Vaginal bleeding a year or more after your last menstrual period
- Bleeding after intercourse

Vaginal bleeding after menopause has a number of possible explanations. It may stem from vaginal atrophy, in which the walls of your vagina become thinner and more fragile. Bleeding due to vaginal atrophy commonly occurs with sexual intercourse. Menopausal hormone therapy can cause bleeding. Vaginal bleeding after menopause can also be the result of a precancerous change or an early sign of uterine cancer.

Diagnosis

See your doctor if you experience vaginal bleeding and are in menopause. Your doctor will likely perform a pelvic examination. The first concern will be to establish the source and cause of the bleeding.

This may involve a cervical cancer screen, a vaginal ultrasound exam or an endometrial biopsy. If any of the tests are abnormal, the next step may be a hysteroscopy or a uterine dilation and curettage (D&C) for further evaluation.

Sometimes, exhaustive study fails to reveal the cause of postmenopausal bleeding. However, even if a cause isn't found, if the bleeding recurs, you should be re-examined.

How serious is postmenopausal bleeding?

In most instances, postmenopausal bleeding isn't serious. However, it's the most common sign of endometrial (uterine) cancer. Therefore, all postmenopausal bleeding should be evaluated. Early diagnosis and treatment offer the best chances for a cure.

Treatment

Treatment depends on the underlying cause. If the tissue lining your vagina has become fragile, your doctor may prescribe estrogen. Estrogen helps protect against thinning of vaginal tissue. If the bleeding is a result of a precancerous change or cancer, surgery and other treatments may be needed.

Menopause

Signs and symptoms

- No menstrual cycle for 12 months
- Hot flashes and night sweats
- Loss of fertility
- Vaginal dryness or irritation
- Insomnia
- Anxiety symptoms or depressed mood
- Joint aches

Menopause, the permanent end of menstruation and fertility, is a natural biological process, not a medical illness. It's defined as occurring 12 months after your last menstrual period. Menopause can happen in your 40s or 50s, but the average age is 51 in the United States. Women experiences menopause differently. Some women have no physical symptoms other than loss of menstrual periods. Others are troubled by hot flashes, night sweats and difficulty sleeping that may last for years. Medical treatments are available when needed for symptom relief.

Perimenopause

Also known as the menopausal transition, perimenopause refers to the time when menopausal symptoms start, while periods haven't stopped. During this phase, which may last for six years or longer, ovulation becomes less predictable and the production of the hormones, estrogen and progesterone, is more erratic.

Periods may become longer or shorter, heavier or lighter, and more or less frequent. Commonly, cycles get shorter, with periods occurring more often than monthly. Late in perimenopause, it's more common to skip periods. There's no way to know in advance exactly which period will be your last.

It can be difficult to know when you should be concerned about changes in menstrual bleeding during perimenopause. If the bleeding becomes extremely heavy, lasts more than seven days, occurs more frequently than at 21-day intervals or if spotting or bleeding between periods occurs, seek medical evaluation.

Even in the absence of abnormal bleeding or troublesome menopausal symptoms such as hot flashes or night sweats, it's important to continue regular preventive health checks with your doctor during perimenopause. At these visits, make sure to ask your doctor any questions you have. The better informed you are about what to expect over the menopausal transition, the more smoothly you may be able to adjust to the changes in your body.

During perimenopause it's still possible to get pregnant, and those who don't want to become pregnant need to continue with contraception. If you're taking hormonal contraception, symptoms of menopause may be masked, so you will need to check with your doctor about when to stop.

Natural menopause

Natural menopause is defined as the time after 12 months have passed since your last period. Menopause typically occurs between ages 46 and 56, with the average age being 51 years. In most cases, hormone testing is not helpful or needed to tell if you are in menopause. Menopause is confirmed when you have had no menstrual bleeding for 12 months in a row.

The years that occur after menopause, called postmenopause, are often times of greater hormonal stability and sometimes less troublesome symptoms than during perimenopause.

Early and premature menopause

Menopause that occurs between the ages of 40 and 45 is considered early, while menopause that happens before 40 is considered premature. Women affected by early and premature menopause are at greater risk of certain conditions later in life, including heart disease, osteoporosis, dementia, neurological diseases, sexual dysfunction, mental health issues and early mortality. This is due to experiencing reduced estrogen levels for many years.

If your periods stop before age 40 or 45, it's important to have a complete medical evaluation to check for underlying causes and identify reversible or treatable conditions. For women found to have early or premature menopause, it's important to take hormone replacements or hormonal contraceptives until the natural age of menopause, unless there's a medical reason not to do so. Menopausal hormone therapy can reduce the risks of conditions associated with early and premature menopause.

Induced menopause

Menopause that's caused by surgery or medical interventions can occur at any age. Surgery causes an abrupt onset of menopause when both ovaries are removed (bilateral oophorectomy). Women who undergo surgical menopause tend to experience more abrupt and intense menopausal symptoms and need estrogen therapy more frequently than do women experiencing natural menopause. In this case, estrogen therapy is typically continued until at least the age of natural menopause, and sometimes longer.

Induced menopause can occur as a result of cancer treatments, including chemotherapy or radiation to the abdomen and pelvis. In advance of planned surgery or treatment that might bring on menopause, women who may not have completed their desired childbearing should address this with their medical team. Options are often available for harvesting eggs and freezing the eggs or fertilized embryos for later use.

Dealing with symptoms

Menopause may be associated with a number of signs and symptoms.

Hot flashes

The majority of women going through menopause experience hot flashes or night sweats. You may experience redness, or flushing, of your face and neck, perspiration, awakening during the night, followed by a chilled feeling. Some women experience palpitations and a feeling of anxiety with or before hot flashes.

Reducing triggers to hot flashes — such as stress, hot or spicy foods, alcohol, or caffeine — can be helpful for some women, but it's insufficient for most. For those women whose hot flashes are more severe, interfere with daily life or don't resolve on their own, the following are some helpful strategies:

- **Lifestyle changes.** Identify and reduce triggers. Try meditation, yoga, tai chi, biofeedback, acupuncture or massage. Dress in layers. Use a fan or cold pack to cool down.
- **Menopausal hormone therapy.** Menopausal hormone therapy may help relieve symptoms. For more information on menopausal hormone therapy, see page 1204.
- **Other prescription medications.** Low-dose paroxetine mesylate (Brisdelle) is the only non-hormonal medication that is FDA-approved to treat hot flashes. In addition, antidepressants such as venlafaxine (Effexor XR), paroxetine (Paxil, Pexeva), citalopram (Celexa) and sertraline (Zoloft) may be used to relieve hot flashes for women who can't take estrogen or choose not to take menopausal hormone therapy. Another medicine sometimes used is gabapentin (Neurontin, Gralise, others). This medication is approved to treat seizures and some pain conditions, but has also been found to reduce hot flashes. However, antidepressants and gabapentin are less effective than menopausal hormone therapy for treating hot flashes.

Sleep disturbances

Easy awakenings, with trouble falling back to sleep, are common with menopause and in the years after menopause (postmenopause). Strategies to improve sleep routines are most important to start with. Avoid heavy meals before bedtime. Adjust light, noise and temperature in the bedroom. Avoid alcohol, caffeine and nicotine all day. Try keeping a regular sleep schedule. Sleeping pills may be helpful to break a cycle of insomnia but should be limited to short-term use. An herbal supplement with valerian is sometimes helpful. Estrogen therapy is helpful if sleep problems are related to menopause and not due to other causes.

In postmenopausal women, obstructive sleep apnea and restless legs syndrome are more common and can contribute to sleep disturbances. Many postmenopausal women with sleep concerns have underlying causes such as obstructive sleep apnea, restless legs syndrome or both. So if sleep problems persist despite lifestyle changes, see your doctor to evaluate for more serious sleep problems.

Headaches

During perimenopause when hormone levels are erratic, headaches may start or worsen, particularly for women with a history of hormonally influenced headaches, such as menstrual migraine headaches. Hormonally related headaches usually get better after menopause. If treatment is needed sooner and usual headache prevention or treatment strategies aren't working, hormonal interventions to stabilize fluctuating hormone levels may be an option.

Genitourinary symptoms

The genitourinary system includes the genital and urinary organs. Thinning of genital and urinary tissues occurs when estrogen levels are low. Reduced lubrication and fragile vaginal and vulvar tissue may make intercourse painful. Symptoms of vaginal irritation and urinary frequency or burning can occur outside of intercourse. Vaginal lubricants and moisturizers are available over-the-counter and may reduce discomfort. Vaginal estrogen is most effective for these symptoms and minimizes the risks associated with systemic estrogen therapy.

Memory or concentration changes

Difficulty with memory or concentration is commonly reported by women in perimenopause and early menopause. While women commonly worry about these symptoms representing the start of dementia, they usually are not. A helpful strategy is to focus on getting restful sleep and managing an anxious or a depressed mood.

Mood swings, depression and anxiety

Some perimenopausal women experience troublesome mood irritability, tearfulness, fatigue, feeling discouraged or overwhelmed more easily. Generally these symptoms are thought to be related more to disrupted sleep or other life factors than menopause itself. But for women with a history of depression or anxiety at other times of hormonal fluctuation, and women who experience a longer menopausal transition or more-severe menopausal symptoms, perimenopause may be an emotionally vulnerable time. In this case, you'll want to take a proactive approach to managing mood changes over the menopausal transition. Exercise regularly, eat a healthy diet, take time for yourself, manage stress, and try to get adequate sleep. Work with a mental health professional if self-care strategies aren't working.

Sexual function

Sexual drive may decline gradually with age for both women and men. While your sex drive may change, the desire for intimacy tends to be ageless.

Changes in sexual desire sometimes attributed to menopause are more commonly related to other factors, such as fatigue, stress, body image, availability of a partner, relationship factors, medications or medical conditions that interfere with sexual arousal or enjoyment.

For some women, sex drive decreases, and for others it increases with menopause. Most women who enjoyed sex earlier in life continue to do so over the menopausal transition and beyond. Women who undergo surgical menopause at a young age, however, may be more vulnerable to sexual function changes due to accelerated loss of certain hormones.

If you're experiencing sexual function changes that concern you, work with your doctor to identify strategies or treatments to help. Sexual function changes in women are usually multifaceted, often involving physical, hormonal, social and psychological factors.

Possible complications

Several chronic medical conditions tend to appear after menopause. By becoming aware of them, you can take steps to help reduce your risk:

- **Cardiovascular disease.** Once your estrogen levels decline, your risk of cardiovascular disease increases. Heart disease is the leading cause of death in women as well as in men. Yet you can do a great deal to reduce your risk of heart disease. These risk reduction steps include stopping smoking, reducing blood pressure and cholesterol levels, getting regular aerobic exercise, and eating a diet low in saturated fats and plentiful in whole grains, fruits and vegetables.
- **Osteoporosis.** During the first few years after menopause, you tend to lose bone density at a rapid rate, increasing your

risk of osteoporosis. Osteoporosis causes bones to become brittle and weak, leading to an increased risk of fractures. Postmenopausal women are especially susceptible to fractures of the hip, wrist and spine. That's why it's important during this time to get adequate calcium and vitamin D — about 1,200 milligrams of calcium and at least 800 to 1,000 international units of vitamin D daily. It's also important to exercise regularly. Strength training and weight-bearing activities such as walking and dancing are especially beneficial in keeping your bones strong.
- **Urinary incontinence.** Urinary signs symptoms become more common with age. You may experience frequent, sudden, strong urges to urinate, followed by an involuntary loss of urine (urge incontinence) or the loss of urine with coughing, laughing or lifting (stress incontinence). While urge incontinence is likely related to loss of estrogen, stress incontinence is related to structural changes in the pelvis and muscle weakness. Both of these conditions are treatable, but many women avoid seeking help due to embarrassment.
- **Bowel control problems.** Bowel control problems (fecal incontinence) are more common in older adults, and more common in women than in men. A number of treatment options are available, including changes in nutrition, medications, bowel training and surgery.
- **Weight gain.** Many women gain weight during the menopausal transition, though aging more than menopause is primarily responsible for the extra pounds. Changes in lifestyle and genetic factors also may play a roll. Loss of estrogen can result in changes in your body composition and a shift in weight to the midsection. Focus on maintaining a healthy weight by eating a healthy diet

and exercising regularly. Exercise is particularly important to avoid weight gain after menopause and to maintain your weight after weight loss, but to lose weight, calorie restriction is necessary.

Treatment

Menopause itself requires no medical treatment. Instead, treatments focus on relieving your symptoms and on preventing or lessening chronic conditions that may occur with aging.

Medications

Treatments include:
- **Menopausal hormone therapy.** Estrogen-based hormone therapy remains, by far, the most effective treatment option for relieving menopausal hot flashes. Depending on your personal and family medical history, your doctor may recommend menopausal hormone therapy to provide symptom relief for you. For more information, see "Menopausal hormone therapy," on page 1204.
- **Low-dose antidepressants.** Antidepressants related to the class of drugs called selective serotonin reuptake inhibitors (SSRIs) have been shown to decrease menopausal hot flashes. SSRIs that can be helpful include venlafaxine (Effexor XR), fluoxetine (Prozac, Sarafem), paroxetine (Paxil, Pexeva), citalopram (Celexa) and sertraline (Zoloft).
- **Low-dose paroxetine mesylate (Brisdelle).** This medication is currently the only nonhormonal therapy for hot flashes that's FDA approved.
- **Gabapentin.** Gabapentin (Neurontin, Gralise) is approved to treat seizures, but it may also reduce hot flashes.
- **Bisphosphonates.** Doctors may recommend these nonhormonal medications, which include alendronate (Fosamax),

risedronate (Actonel) and ibandronate (Boniva), to prevent or treat osteoporosis. The medications reduce bone loss and your risk of fractures.

- **Menopausal hormone therapy.** Another option for bone protection is menopausal hormone therapy. It's often used when other therapies aren't tolerated or are ineffective, as well as when women are also experiencing bothersome hot flashes.
- **Selective estrogen receptor modulators (SERMs).** SERMs are a group of drugs that includes raloxifene (Evista). Raloxifene mimics estrogen's beneficial effects on bone density in postmenopausal women. But unlike menopausal hormone therapy, it reduces the risk of breast cancer.
- **Vaginal estrogen.** To help relieve vaginal dryness, discomfort with intercourse, and urinary urgency and frequency, estrogen can be administered locally using a vaginal cream, tablet or ring. This treatment releases just a small amount of estrogen, which is absorbed by the vulvar and vaginal tissues.

  Before deciding on any form of treatment, talk with your doctor about your options and the risks and benefits involved with each.

Lifestyle and home remedies

Many of the signs and symptoms associated with menopause resolve with time. For example, hot flashes typically resolve after seven to nine years. Take these steps to help reduce or prevent the effects of menopause symptoms:

- **Cool hot flashes.** Some women may find it helpful to dress in layers and reduce triggers such as hot beverages, spicy foods, alcohol and warm temperatures.
- **Decrease vaginal discomfort.** Use over-the-counter water-based vaginal lubricants or moisturizers that are free of potential irritants such as glycerin, parabens, warming or tingling properties, and flavors. Staying sexually active also helps.
- **Optimize your sleep.** Avoid caffeine, and plan to exercise during the day, although not right before bedtime. Relaxation techniques, such as deep breathing, guided imagery and progressive muscle relaxation, can be very helpful. You can find a number of books and tapes on different relaxation exercises. If hot flashes disturb your sleep, you may need to find a way to manage them before you can get adequate rest.
- **Strengthen your pelvic floor.** Pelvic floor muscle exercises, called Kegel exercises, can improve some forms of urinary incontinence (see page 913).
- **Eat well.** Eat a balanced diet that includes a variety of fruits, vegetables and whole grains and that limits saturated fats and sugars. Aim for 1,200 milligrams of calcium and at least 800 to 1,000 international units of vitamin D a day. Ask your doctor about supplements to help you meet these requirements, if necessary.
- **Quit smoking.** Smoking increases your risk of heart disease, stroke, osteoporosis, cancer and a range of other health problems. It may also increase hot flashes and bring on earlier menopause. It's never too late to benefit from stopping smoking.
- **Exercise regularly.** Get at least 30 minutes of moderate-intensity physical activity most days of the week to protect against cardiovascular disease, diabetes, osteoporosis and other conditions. More-vigorous exercise for longer periods may provide further benefit and is particularly important if you are trying to avoid weight gain. Exercise can also help reduce stress.

Menopausal hormone therapy

During menopause, your ovaries stop producing the female hormones estrogen and progesterone. This decline in hormones puts a permanent end to menstruation and fertility, but it can also cause hot flashes, mood swings, vaginal dryness and urinary problems.

While menopausal hormone therapy is not a magical cure for aging, it's considered to be the most effective treatment for unpleasant menopausal symptoms for most women. If you're facing menopause, learn more about the benefits and the risks of hormone therapy.

What are the benefits of menopausal hormone therapy?

Estrogen remains the most effective treatment for relief of troublesome menopausal hot flashes and night sweats. It can also ease vaginal symptoms of menopause, such as dryness, itching, burning and discomfort with intercourse, and help treat urinary frequency, urgency and urge incontinence.

Long-term menopausal hormone therapy for the prevention of postmenopausal conditions is no longer routinely recommended. But women who take estrogen for short-term relief of menopausal symptoms may gain some protection against the following conditions:

- **Osteoporosis.** Studies show that menopausal hormone therapy can prevent the bone loss that occurs after menopause, which decreases the risk of osteoporosis-related hip fractures.
- **Heart disease.** Some data suggest that estrogen can decrease the risk of heart disease when it's taken early in your postmenopausal years.

For women who undergo menopause naturally, estrogen is typically prescribed as part of a combination therapy of estrogen and progestin. This is because estrogen without progestin can increase the risk of uterine cancer. Women who undergo menopause as the result of a hysterectomy can take estrogen alone.

What are the risks of menopausal hormone therapy?

Much has been written about the risks of hormone therapy. Given the available information, experts agree that the benefits of hormone therapy outweigh the risks for healthy women younger than age 60 and within 10 years of their last period who are seeking relief for moderate to severe symptoms of menopause. The benefits are also significant for women who have early or premature menopause .

But as with any medication, the risks should be considered. There are different treatments available that vary in terms of the hormones used and their dosages, as well as the delivery methods. Each type carries its own benefits and risks. Regardless of the type of hormone therapy, the dosage and duration of treatment should be individualized to your preferences and treatment goals. Although it's not recommended that you start hormone therapy after age 60, continuing treatment past this age may be considered based on your symptoms and risk factors.

Who should consider menopausal hormone therapy?

Despite the potential health risks, estrogen is still the gold standard for treating menopausal symptoms. Your doctor may recommend menopausal hormone therapy to treat troublesome hot flashes or other menopausal symptoms if you're younger than 60 and within 10 years of the start of menopause.

Data surrounding menopausal hormone therapy can be scary and confusing. But the absolute risk to a woman taking menopausal hormone therapy is quite low. Talk with your doctor about your personal risks.

Who should avoid menopausal hormone therapy?

Women with breast cancer, heart disease or a history of blood clots should not take menopausal hormone therapy for relief of

Vaginal Pain

When vaginal pain occurs during intercourse, it's called dyspareunia. A frequent cause is genitourinary syndrome of menopause. The symptoms are vaginal soreness or persistent or recurrent pain during intercourse. Sometimes your vagina may simply be irritated by a feminine hygiene spray or contraceptive cream or jelly.

Rarely, dyspareunia can result from pelvic floor muscle dysfunction or bladder problems such as cystitis or urethritis. If intercourse causes deep internal pain, you may have endometriosis, or you could have some other disorder of your cervix, uterus, fallopian tubes or ovaries.

If you're breast-feeding or you're past menopause, your vaginal lining may have thinned because you're producing less estrogen. Some women also have a problem called vaginismus — involuntary contractions of muscles at the opening to the vagina.

To determine the causes of vaginal pain, your doctor will likely do a pelvic examination, and possibly order imaging tests. Treatment depends on what's causing your pain.

menopause symptoms. Women who don't experience menopause symptoms should not take menopausal hormone therapy for preventing heart disease, memory loss or strokes. Instead, talk to your doctor about lifestyle changes you can make or other medications you can take for long-term protection from these conditions.

Protecting yourself from the added risks

Analysis of the Women's Health Initiative data and other trials suggest there are several ways to reduce the potential risks of menopausal hormone therapy. Talk to your doctor about these strategies:

- **Time it right.** The risk of menopausal hormone therapy causing heart disease is not significantly raised in women under age 60. In fact, some studies suggest that estrogen may protect the heart when taken early in your menopausal years.
- **Take the appropriate amount of medication for you.** Work with your doctor to determine the dose and duration of menopausal hormone therapy that's right for you. Women who experience premature menopause should generally take estrogen until at least the age of natural menopause.

- **Find the best delivery method for you.** You can take estrogen in the form of a pill, patch, gel, vaginal cream, or slow-releasing suppository or ring that you place in your vagina. If you experience only isolated vaginal symptoms, estrogen in a vaginal cream, tablet or ring is usually a better choice than a pill or a skin patch. That's because estrogen applied directly to your vagina is more effective at a lower dose than is estrogen given in pill or skin patch form.

  If you haven't had a hysterectomy and are using oral or skin patch estrogen therapy, you'll also need progestogen, which is available in a pill, combination pill, intrauterine device or combination skin patch. Your doctor can help you find the delivery method that offers the most benefit and convenience with the least risk and cost.

If you can't take menopausal hormone therapy

There are many treatments besides menopausal hormone therapy that may relieve certain symptoms. These include nonhormonal medications as well as integrative and complementary treatments such as mind-body practices, cognitive behavioral therapy and hypnosis.

The bottom line

The only way to determine if menopausal hormone therapy is the best treatment for you is to talk to your doctor about your individual symptoms and health risks. Be sure to keep the conversation going throughout your menopausal years.

As researchers learn more about menopausal hormone therapy and other menopausal treatments, recommendations may change. Review your current treatments with your doctor to make sure they're your best option.

Vaginal and Vulvar Disorders

Your vagina is the passageway that connects your uterus to your external genitals. Beneath the vagina are strong muscles. Most of the time your vagina is so narrow that its walls touch, but it can expand dramatically. The neck of your uterus (cervix) extends into your vagina at the upper end.

In girls, the outer end of the vagina is partially blocked by a thin membrane called the hymen. In very rare cases, the hymen may close off the vagina altogether.

The area of the external genitals is called the vulva. It includes the liplike folds of tissue — labia majora and labia minora — that shield your vagina and urethra. Just below the mons pubis, where the labia come together, is the clitoris. The clitoris is a small organ that becomes distended during sexual arousal.

Your urethra, which opens just below your clitoris, leads to your bladder. Below your urethra is your vaginal opening. Glands located in the vulva and vagina lubricate this area during sexual arousal.

Vaginal Hygiene

Normally, your vagina is self-cleansing. Your vaginal walls produce their own fluid, which carries away dead cells and organisms as it flows downward. This healthy discharge is either clear or milky, becoming yellowish when it dries. It's somewhat slippery and has a mild, not unpleasant odor. It increases in amount at about the time you ovulate and during sexual arousal. If you have a vaginal discharge that's a different color or has a strong smell, you may have a vaginal infection and should see a doctor.

Washing your genitals once a day with water is sufficient. A mild soap without perfumes or dyes also can be used when necessary. Douches and feminine hygiene sprays are unnecessary, and at times they can be harmful. Some commercial douches contain irritating chemicals. Douching can change the normally acidic vaginal environment that discourages the growth of yeast and other organisms that can cause infections.

Bacteria and fungi that cause vaginal infections tend to thrive in warm, moist conditions. For that reason, it's a good idea to wear cotton underpants or synthetic underpants with a cotton lining and to avoid tight pantyhose. Tight, nylon underpants and pantyhose trap heat and moisture in the genital area. Sleeping without underpants — except, perhaps, during your period — can be helpful.

Developmental disorders

Signs and symptoms

- Undersized or absent vagina, or a very short vagina and no cervix
- Absent uterus
- Malformed uterus
- Abnormally formed ovaries (ovarian dysgenesis)
- Genitals in a female that partly resemble male genitals

At conception, the embryo acquires either male (XY) or female (XX) chromosomes. For the next 40 days, males and females are indistinguishable. After that time, if the fetus has a Y chromosome, testicles begin to develop. In the absence of a Y chromosome and the presence of two X chromosomes, ovaries develop. These organs secrete male or female hormones, respectively, that cause the fetus to develop either a male or a female urogenital tract.

Sometimes, a female is born with sexually ambiguous genitals. She may have an unusually large clitoris, or the labia majora may be partially fused together and resemble a scrotum. The most common cause for ambiguous genitals is congenital adrenal hyperplasia, sometimes called pseudohermaphroditism. When this happens, the body doesn't produce enough of certain enzymes at a crucial time in fetal development. The internal organs of a female born with this condition are usually normal.

Early surgery can alter the genitals, if necessary. If the genital ambiguity is due to congenital adrenal hyperplasia, a potentially fatal complication (addisonian crisis) could develop unless your doctor is on the alert to prevent it.

Diagnosis

A doctor will do a physical examination and, because developmental disorders occasionally run in families, may take a family history. Laboratory tests on blood or skin cells can establish if a chromosomal problem caused the condition. Laboratory tests can also identify hormonal problems.

How serious are developmental disorders?

Girls with congenital adrenal hyperplasia have normal internal organs. Given surgical correction of abnormalities in the vulva and proper medication, they may be able to have children. Women with an absent uterus may require a surrogate to carry a pregnancy. A malformed uterus may have no impact or may cause pregnancy complications, depending on the degree of malformation. Ovarian dysgenesis may be associated with other developmental abnormalities.

Treatment

Depending on the cause of the disorder, treatment may involve medication or surgery or both. For congenital adrenal hyperplasia, doctors often prescribe corticosteroids to prevent a buildup of undesirable hormones. For girls born without a normal vagina, surgeons can create an artificial one, or a vagina can be formed with the use of a dilator. Surgery can also fix certain structural problems of the uterus.

Vulvitis

Signs and symptoms

- Swelling of the vulva, with redness and itching
- Blisters that may ooze or crust over
- White or thickened areas of the vulva

Vulvitis is an inflammation of your external genitals (vulva). It can be caused by a reaction to a vaginal spray, to the detergent with which you wash your underwear or to a medication. Or it could stem from excess moisture or a bacterial, viral or fungal infection.

Diagnosis

Your doctor will likely do a pelvic examination and possibly order blood tests, a urinalysis or other laboratory tests. If there's a possibility you have a sexually transmitted infection (STI), he or she will likely test for that. If the inflammation persists, you may need a biopsy to make sure of the cause.

Treatment

Treatment varies depending on the cause of the problem. To help reduce symptoms and prevent a recurrence, keep the area clean and dry and wear loose, absorbent clothing and cotton underpants. If the vulvitis consistently develops after you use a specific product such as a spray or deodorant, stop using the product. The vulvitis may be a reaction to what you're using.

Vulvar dystrophy

Signs and symptoms

- Dry, reddened areas in the vulva
- Itching in the affected area
- White or thickened areas of the vulva
- Papery or shiny skin around the vulva and anus
- A shrinking of the labia minora and vaginal opening

Dystrophy is a kind of degeneration of tissue. The word is derived from the Greek words for poor nutrition. Vulvar dystrophy tends to occur in women who are past menopause. It can cause patchy white and thickened areas of the vulva (hypertrophic vulvar dystrophy) or thin, whitish skin around the vulva and anus (lichen sclerosus).

Diagnosis

To aid in diagnosis or make sure that you don't have cancer, your doctor may remove a small piece of tissue for microscopic analysis (biopsy). He or she may also check for signs of an underlying infection.

Treatment

Treatment depends on the source of the problem. Your doctor may prescribe a topical steroid cream to relieve symptoms, including itching. It's important to have periodic examinations to determine whether precancerous changes have developed.

Vulvodynia

Signs and symptoms

- Burning or stinging, irritation, itching of the vulva
- Stabbing pain in the vulvar area
- Rawness in the vulvar area

Vulvodynia means "painful vulva." Your vulva is the area around the opening to your vagina. It consists of the labia, the clitoris and the opening of your vagina.

The pain of vulvodynia may be constant or intermittent and localized or widespread and can last for months or even years. In a type of vulvodynia known as provoked vestibulodynia, you may experience pain when there's pressure on the vulvar area, such as with bicycle riding, tampon use or sexual intercourse. With unprovoked vestibulodynia, there may be discomfort even without pressure or touch.

Diagnosis

Vulvodynia can be difficult to diagnose because it may have no visible signs, and the pain may come and go. The discomfort can be serious enough to interfere with your lifestyle, but the condition itself isn't life-threatening.

Treatment

Vulvodynia treatments are directed at addressing the cause of the pain. No one treatment works for all women, and you may find that a combination of treatments works best for you. It may take weeks or

---

PREVENTION TIP

To reduce your chances of getting genital warts or other sexually transmitted infections (STIs), you need to practice safe sex. Aside from abstinence, having a monogamous partner who has no sexually transmitted infections is the surest way to protect yourself. Using condoms is the next best thing. However, condoms aren't foolproof against disease.

even months for a new treatment regimen to noticeably improve your symptoms. Available options may include:

- **Medications.** Tricyclic antidepressants that can help lessen chronic pain include amitriptyline, desipramine (Norpramin) and nortriptyline (Pamelor). Other medications for chronic pain, such as duloxetine (Cymbalta) and pregabalin (Lyrica) may also lessen the pain, as may anticonvulsants such as gabapentin (Neurontin). Antihistamines, such as hydroxyzine, can reduce itching.
- **Biofeedback therapy.** This therapy can help reduce pain by teaching you how to control specific body responses. The goal of biofeedback is to help you enter a relaxed state in order to decrease pain sensation. To cope with vulvodynia, biofeedback can teach you to relax your pelvic muscles, which can contract in anticipation of pain and actually cause chronic pain itself.
- **Physical therapy.** A physical therapist with experience treating vulvar pain can help identify problems in your pelvic floor that may be contributing to your symptoms. Physical therapy techniques used for vulvodynia include massage, transcutaneous electrical nerve stimulation (TENS) therapy and exercises to relax your pelvic floor muscles. Other approaches include therapeutic ultrasound and trigger point pressure, in which hard, painful knots in your muscles are released.
- **Local anesthetics.** Medications, such as lidocaine ointment, can provide temporary symptom relief. Your doctor may recommend applying lidocaine a few minutes before sexual intercourse to reduce your discomfort. Your partner may experience temporary numbness after sexual contact, but this can be avoided with condom use or

by wiping away excess lidocaine before sexual activity.

Genital warts

Signs and symptoms
- Tiny pink or white nodules in your genital area

Genital warts (venereal warts or condyloma acuminata) are caused by the human papillomavirus (HPV) but not the same types of HPV that are associated with cervical cancer. You can get them from direct sexual contact with someone who has them. The incubation period is one to six months.

In women, these warts can grow on the vulva, the walls of the vagina, the cervix or around the anus. In men, they may be found on the shaft of the penis, the scrotum or around the anus. They can also develop on the mouth or in the throat of a person who has had oral sex with an infected person.

Diagnosis
A doctor usually can diagnose genital warts by their appearance. However, because you can acquire other sexually transmitted infections, such as chlamydia or the human immunodeficiency virus (HIV), from the same sexual exposure that caused the warts, you may need to be tested for other infections. Sometimes, a doctor will do a biopsy, in which a tissue sample is taken from the area in question and sent to a laboratory for analysis to rule out cancer.

How serious are genital warts?
By themselves, genital warts are mainly a nuisance. They have a tendency to recur.

Treatment
Whether genital warts are treated and how depends on their size and location. Some genital warts, such as smaller ones, may resolve on their own without any treatment.

Medication
Medications are available that can

be applied directly to the skin. These topical treatments include imiquimod (Aldara, Zyclara), trichloroacetic acid, podophyllin and podofilox (Condylox) and sinecatechins (Veregen). Don't use over-the-counter wart removers. They aren't intended for the genital area.

Other therapies
Warts may also be removed with laser surgery or by freezing with liquid nitrogen (cryosurgery) or burning (electrocautery). Sometimes, surgery is necessary to remove large warts or those that don't respond to treatment.

Prevention
While they won't completely prevent genital warts or cervical cancer, HPV vaccines protect against the most dangerous types of HPV — the virus that causes a majority of cervical cancers — as well as the types of HPV that cause most genital warts.

The national Advisory Committee on Immunization Practices recommends HPV vaccination for girls and boys ages 11 and 12, although it can be given as young as 9 years old. The vaccination is also recommended for girls and women ages 13 to 26 and boys and men ages 13 to 21 if they haven't received the vaccine already. The vaccine is most effective if given earlier in the recommended age range rather than waiting until later.

Bartholin's abscess

Signs and symptoms
- A hot, tender, swollen lump in the labia majora

Bartholin's glands, named for Danish anatomist Caspar T. Bartholin, are situated at the entrance to your vagina toward the back, one on each side. A gland or the duct on the organ's surface can become swollen and inflamed. If the opening to the gland becomes blocked and the accumulated fluid becomes infected, an abscess results.

Diagnosis

Your doctor will likely perform a pelvic examination, examine the lump and possibly order laboratory tests to check for sexually transmitted infections (STIs). The abscess itself generally requires surgical treatment. Sometimes, a chronic Bartholin's cyst forms afterward and may need to be removed surgically.

Treatment

Treatment generally involves draining the abscess, which may occur in an office or day surgery setting.

Vaginitis

Signs and symptoms

- Unusual vaginal discharge
- Itching and irritation in the vaginal area
- Pain during intercourse
- An unpleasant odor from the vaginal area

Vaginitis is an inflammation of your vagina, usually caused by an infection. A vaginal infection can be sexually transmitted; however, most vaginal infections aren't the result of a sexually transmitted infection (STI).

Most vaginal infections are common and treatable, but those resulting from an STI may be more serious. It's possible to have an infection but no symptoms.

Common types

Common causes of vaginitis are yeast infections (candidiasis), bacterial vaginosis and trichomoniasis.

Yeast infection

The main symptom of a yeast infection is itchiness in the vaginal area, but you may also have a white discharge that resembles cottage cheese. You're more likely to develop a yeast infection if you're pregnant or if you're taking antibiotics, corticosteroid medications or birth control pills.

Bacterial vaginosis

This type of vaginitis occurs when there's a disruption in the normal bacteria in the vagina. It's not caused by catching a bacterial infection. Signs and symptoms include a white or grayish, fishy-smelling vaginal discharge.

Trichomoniasis

This type of infection is caused by a parasite. You may have no symptoms, or you may develop a smelly, greenish-yellow, sometimes frothy discharge. Most of the time, trichomoniasis is contracted through intercourse.

Diagnosis

Your doctor will take a medical history and do a pelvic examination. He or she may take a sample of the discharge to identify the cause. Vaginitis is common and, because it tends to recur, can be annoying.

Treatment

Treatment depends on the type of vaginitis you have. Doctors usually treat trichomoniasis with oral metronidazole and yeast infections with antifungal creams, suppositories or pills. For bacterial vaginosis, your doctor may prescribe oral or vaginal metronidazole or oral or vaginal clindamycin.

Genitourinary syndrome of menopause

Signs and symptoms

- Soreness, burning or itching in your vagina
- Bleeding after intercourse
- Painful intercourse
- Thin, watery vaginal discharge

Genitourinary syndrome of menopause (GMS) is an inflammation of the vagina caused by thinning of vaginal tissue. This condition is most likely to develop after menopause, although it can occur during breast-feeding. In both situations, estrogen production is decreased, and the walls of the vagina may become drier, thinner, less elastic and more prone to bleeding.

Diagnosis

A pelvic examination may be all that's necessary to diagnose the problem, although your doctor may order some tests if it appears that you have a vaginal infection. Genitourinary syndrome of menopause isn't serious, but it can interfere with sexual intercourse and therefore may require treatment.

Treatment

In breast-feeding women, the problem is temporary. If you're past menopause, it's not.

Your doctor may prescribe menopausal hormone therapy, or you can apply low-dose vaginal estrogen — available as a cream, ring or tablet — directly to your vagina. If the primary problem is painful intercourse, using a lubricant also may help.

To help maintain vaginal moisture more generally, over-the-counter moisturizers can be used every two to three days on a regular basis.

Vaginal cysts

Signs and symptoms

- Small swellings in the walls of your vagina
- A lump that bulges out of your vaginal opening

Several types of noncancerous (benign) cysts can develop in your vagina. The most common are inclusion cysts and Gartner's cysts. Inclusion cysts are caused by trauma, such as an operation or childbirth. Gartner's cysts are remains of a duct that serves a purpose during fetal development and then disappears. Sometimes, a Gartner's cyst enlarges enough to poke through your vaginal opening.

Diagnosis

A doctor can identify most cysts during a pelvic examination. A cyst generally isn't a problem unless it's so large that it interferes with intercourse.

Kegel Exercises

Your pelvic floor muscles — those that surround your anus and vagina — are called the pubococcygeal muscles. In the 1950s, a physician by the name of A.H. Kegel developed an exercise regimen that may be helpful in strengthening these muscles:

- **Find the right muscles.** This is very important. Imagine that you're trying to stop urinating. When you use the correct muscles, you'll have a pulling feeling.
- **Pull in the pelvic muscles.** Hold them for a count of three and then relax for a count of three. Work up to 10 to 15 repetitions at a time, for a total of 50 to 60 minutes daily.
- **Repeat the exercise at least three times a day.** You can exercise the muscles most anytime — while lying down, sitting in your car or standing in your kitchen. Using different positions makes the muscles strongest.

As the tone in your pubococcygeal muscles gradually improves, you'll likely have better pelvic support. Be patient. You may not feel the improvement for up to six weeks. As a bonus, many women find that they're also more responsive sexually.

Treatment

If it's not bothering you, you may ignore a vaginal cyst. If a cyst causes discomfort, a doctor can remove it surgically.

Loss of pelvic support

Signs and symptoms
- A bulge in the walls of your vagina
- A feeling of fullness and discomfort when you bear down, sometimes with backache
- Difficulty defecating
- Pelvic pressure when lifting or when you stand for a long time

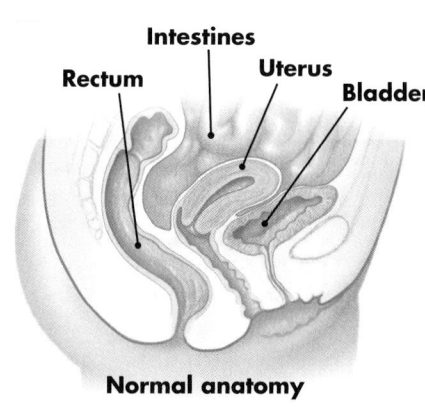

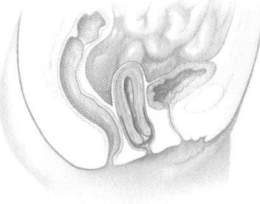

Uterine prolapse involves the uterus

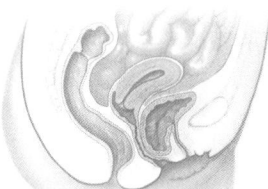

Cystocele involves the bladder

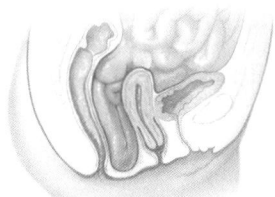

Enterocele involves the intestines

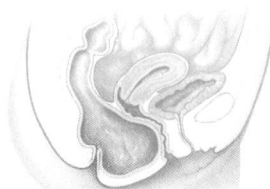

Rectocele involves the rectum

One or more female pelvic organs may be affected by pelvic floor muscle weakness. This weakness can cause prolapse of the uterus (uterine prolapse), bladder (cystocele), intestines (enterocele) or lower rectum (rectocele).

- Seeing or feeling tissue at or beyond the vaginal opening

Your pelvic floor consists of a sheet of muscles and ligaments that support the organs — such as your bladder, uterus, colon and small intestine — that fill the pelvic cavity. These muscles and ligaments also help close off your urethra where it leaves your bladder.

The muscles and ligaments can become stretched or slack from childbirth, aging or increased body weight or because of a hereditary weakness. When that happens, some of your internal organs may sink lower in your body (prolapse). Prolapse is more likely to develop in older women and in those who've given birth to several children.

Sometimes, weakened pelvic muscles allow your uterus to drop downward into your vagina. In extreme cases, your cervix may actually protrude from your vaginal opening. When your bladder prolapses, it produces a bulge in the front wall of the vagina. A bulge in the back wall typically means that the tissue between the anus and rectum have weakened, causing the bulge. Rarely, this may be due to the small intestine protruding between the rectum and vagina.

Diagnosis
Telltale bulges in your vaginal wall usually make prolapses easy to diagnose during a pelvic examination. Minor prolapses are common, especially in older women. They're not serious if they don't cause too much discomfort. If your

bulge symptoms are bothersome and are keeping you from doing normal activities, you should see your doctor. There are both surgical and nonsurgical treatment options for this condition.

Treatment

Treatment depends on the severity of the prolapse and how bothered you are by the bulge. Prolapse may be associated with urinary incontinence or urinary tract infections. These symptoms will be assessed during your visit to your doctor. He or she will discuss both surgical and nonsurgical treatment options for your condition and whether or not the prolapse is impacting urinary symptoms.

Self-care

Sometimes, simple exercises called Kegel exercises are the only treatment you need. If you're overweight, losing weight also may improve your symptoms. Eating high-fiber foods also helps by allowing you to have bowel movements without straining.

Devices

If self-help measures aren't beneficial and an operation is undesired, your doctor can fit you with a vaginal pessary, a silicone device that is placed in the vagina to support the prolapse. You'll have to remove it regularly to clean it.

Surgery

During surgery, a surgeon elevates your prolapsed organ or organs back into place and tightens the muscles and ligaments of your pelvic floor. Surgery may be performed vaginally, laparoscopically or through an abdominal incision. Vaginal approaches utilize sutures and your own tissues to repair the various defects, while abdominal approaches use a synthetic material to repair the prolapse. Whether or not the uterus will also be removed (hysterectomy) depends on what part of the vagina is involved with the prolapse.

Cervical, Uterine and Fallopian Tube Disorders

Your womb (uterus) is the organ that shelters the fetus when you're pregnant. The uterus is shaped like an upside-down pear. The narrower end, the cervix, extends into the vagina.

The fallopian tubes are connected to the uterus, one on each side of its broad top. Each tube extends from the interior of your uterus to a location close to each ovary. Once a month, one of the ovaries releases an egg that travels down a fallopian tube to the uterus.

Developmental disorders

Signs and symptoms
- Inability to begin menstruating at puberty
- An inability to conceive or to carry a pregnancy to term
  Because of genetic problems or because something goes wrong during fetal development, some women are born with abnormalities of the cervix, uterus or fallopian tubes. These can range from a near total absence of female reproductive organs to minor abnormalities that make it difficult to conceive or carry a pregnancy to term.

For instance, in a female fetus, an internal duct called the mullerian duct normally develops into fallopian tubes, a uterus and the upper portion of the vagina. If something interferes with this process, the baby may be born with a short or absent vagina and an absent uterus or a uterus in altered shape. This condition is known as mullerian agenesis.

Because most of these abnormalities are internal, there may be no indication of the problem until she reaches puberty and fails to menstruate.

Diagnosis

If your doctor suspects a developmental disorder, he or she may order a type of X-ray called a hysterosalpingogram. Because soft tissues can't be seen on an X-ray, this procedure uses a special dye that registers on the film. The dye is injected into your uterine cavity and travels up your fallopian tubes and into your abdominal cavity, where your body absorbs it. While the dye is spreading, a radiologist takes a series of X-rays.

Other diagnostic procedures may include ultrasound or magnetic resonance imaging (MRI), especially for adolescents. In some cases, laparoscopic surgery may be performed to get a direct view of the internal organs.

How serious are developmental disorders?

Although generally not life-threatening, these disorders can be emotionally difficult. Girls who have mullerian agenesis may not be able to carry a pregnancy. However, they can have genetic offspring — children of their own — carried by a surrogate.

Treatment

Treatment varies depending upon the abnormality and its cause. Surgery can sometimes correct a cervix that's unable to sustain a pregnancy to term and fix certain structural problems of the uterus and vagina.

Cervical polyps

Signs and symptoms
- Bleeding after intercourse, between periods or after menopause
- Watery, bloody discharge from your vagina
  Cervical polyps are growths that look similar to small grapes. They generally protrude from the opening of your cervix. You may have one polyp or a cluster. They're common, often occurring during pregnancy or in perimenopause.

Diagnosis

A doctor can often detect cervical polyps during a pelvic examination. He or she may also remove the growths.

How serious are cervical polyps?

They're almost never cancerous. A small polyp may produce no symptoms and may not be detected until your doctor finds it during a routine pelvic examination. Large polyps can cause bleeding.

Treatment

Your doctor may remove a single polyp in a brief office procedure. If you have many large polyps, you may need an operation, although this is rarely necessary.

Cervicitis

Signs and symptoms

- Vaginal discharge that's grayish or yellow
- Pain during intercourse
- Bleeding after intercourse

Cervicitis is an inflammation of your cervix. Most often, there are no symptoms and the condition is discovered as a result of a cervical cancer screen or a biopsy done for another condition. Common sexually transmitted infections (STIs), as well as exposure to certain bacteria, can cause cervicitis.

Diagnosis

Your doctor will likely take samples of cervical secretion with a swab to be analyzed in a laboratory.

Treatment

If the cause of the inflammation is an STI, both you and your sexual partner may require treatment. You may not need treatment if you have only a minor inflammation that isn't caused by an STI.

Nabothian cyst

Signs and symptoms

- A fluid-filled lump on your cervix that you're not likely to feel

A Nabothian cyst is named for German anatomist Martin Naboth. It forms when a mucus gland on your cervix becomes obstructed. These are more common with age. A doctor generally can diagnose a Nabothian cyst during a routine pelvic examination. A cyst may also be detected incidentally during a pelvic ultrasound or magnetic resonance imaging (MRI).

Treatment

The condition rarely requires treatment.

Uterine fibroids

Signs and symptoms

- Heavy or prolonged menstrual periods
- Pain or pressure in your lower abdomen or lower back

Emergency signs and symptoms

- Sudden sharp pain low in your abdomen

A fibroid is a noncancerous (benign) tumor that develops within your uterine wall or is attached to it. Also called leiomyomas, myomas or fibromyomas, fibroids are extremely common, particularly by the time a women reaches the age of 50. In many cases, women with fibroids have no symptoms.

Rather than a single fibroid, you're more likely to have several. They can be as small as a pea or larger than a grapefruit. Normally, fibroids grow slowly, but can grow rapidly. After menopause, these tumors usually shrink and no longer cause symptoms.

Diagnosis

Uterine fibroids often are detected during a pelvic examination. If there's any question about what they are, an ultrasound exam may be performed. In another procedure called hysteroscopy, a small scope is inserted into the uterus, allowing your doctor to look for fibroids.

How serious are uterine fibroids?

Fibroids can cause your menstrual periods to become very heavy, which could result in iron deficiency anemia. They can also make conception difficult, and they can cause miscarriage or interfere with delivery. Fibroids can lead to pelvic pressure, painful menses and pain during intercourse. If fibroids grow large enough, they can put pressure on the bladder, increasing urinary frequency.

Rarely, a fibroid attached to your uterine wall becomes twisted, cutting off its blood supply. If that happens, then you may feel a sudden, sharp pain in your lower abdomen. This situation requires surgery to remove the fibroid. Uterine fibroids very rarely become cancerous.

Treatment

If your fibroids don't cause symptoms, your doctor may suggest a wait-and-see approach. Your doctor may want to monitor you for symptoms and perform an ultrasound exam if you start to have heavy bleeding or pain. If you do develop symptoms, your doctor may recommend medication or surgery.

Medication

Most medical therapies are aimed at treating the symptoms of fibroids, such as heavy menstrual bleeding. Oral contraceptives and intrauterine devices (IUDs) can be effective at controlling bleeding. Nonhormonal options to reduce heavy bleeding include tranexamic acid and nonsteroidal anti-inflammatory drugs (NSAIDs).

Medications known as gonadotropin-releasing hormone (Gn-RH) agonists, such as leuporlide (Lupron), may help shrink fibroids by reducing the amount of estrogen and progesterone in your body. This form of drug therapy isn't a long-term solution, but it may be used as a preparation for surgery.

Unfortunately, Gn-RH agonists cause all of the symptoms of menopause, including hot flashes, mood swings, headaches, vaginal dryness and bone loss. If you need prolonged treatment, your doctor may use other medications to reduce menopausal symptoms. A new class of medications (selective progesterone receptor modulators) are undergoing clinical trials in the U.S. but are available in Europe and Canada. They shrink the fibroids and reduce bleeding but don't have the menopausal side effects, offering a promising new option for women with fibroids.

Hysterectomy

This operation — the removal of the uterus — remains the only proven permanent solution for uterine fibroids. But hysterectomy is major surgery. It ends your ability to bear children, and if you elect to also have your ovaries removed, it brings on menopause and the question of whether you'll take menopausal hormone therapy.

Myomectomy

In this surgical procedure, your surgeon removes the fibroids, leaving the uterus in place. If you want to bear children, you might choose this option. With myomectomy, as opposed to a hysterectomy, there is a risk of fibroid recurrence.

There are several ways a myomectomy can be done:

- **Abdominal myomectomy.** If you have multiple fibroids, very large or very deep fibroids, your doctor may use an open abdominal surgical procedure to remove the fibroids.
- **Laparoscopic myomectomy.** If the fibroids are few in number and distort the outside of the uterus, you and your doctor may opt for a laparoscopic procedure, which uses slender instruments inserted through small incisions in your abdomen to remove the fibroids from your uterus. Your doctor views your abdominal area on a remote monitor via a small camera attached to one of the instruments. A new technique uses a low-energy type of

radiation (radiofrequency) to destroy (ablate) and shrink the fibroids during a laparoscopic procedure.

- **Hysteroscopic myomectomy.** This procedure may be an option if the fibroids are contained inside the uterus (submucosal fibroids). A long, slender scope (hysteroscope) is passed through your vagina and cervix and into your uterus. Your doctor can see and remove the fibroids through the scope. This procedure is best performed by a doctor experienced in this technique.

Variations of myomectomy — in which uterine fibroids are destroyed without actually removing them — include:

- **Myolysis.** In this laparoscopic procedure, an electric current destroys the fibroids and shrinks the blood vessels that feed them.
- **Cryomyolysis.** In a procedure similar to myolysis, cryomyolysis uses liquid nitrogen to freeze the fibroids.

The safety, effectiveness and associated risk of fibroid recurrence after myolysis and cryomyolysis have yet to be determined.

- **Endometrial ablation.** This treatment, performed with a hysteroscope, uses heat to destroy the lining of your uterus, either ending menstruation or reducing your menstrual flow. Endometrial ablation is effective in stopping abnormal bleeding, but doesn't affect fibroids outside the interior lining of the uterus.

Uterine artery embolization

Small particles injected into the arteries supplying the uterus cut off blood flow to fibroids, causing them to shrink. This technique is proving effective in shrinking fibroids and relieving the symptoms they can cause. Advantages over surgery include not having to have an incision and a shorter recovery time.

Complications may occur if the blood supply to your ovaries or other organs is compromised.

Focused ultrasound surgery

MRI-guided focused ultrasound surgery (FUS) is another option for women with fibroids. Unlike other fibroid treatment options, FUS is noninvasive and preserves your uterus.

This procedure is performed while you're inside a specially crafted MRI scanner that allows doctors to visualize your pelvic organs, and then locate and destroy (ablate) fibroids inside your uterus without making an incision. Focused high-frequency, high-energy sound waves are used to target and destroy the fibroids. A single treatment session is done in an on- and off-again fashion, sometimes spanning several hours.

Initial results with this technology are promising, and it appears to be similar in effectiveness to uterine artery embolization.

Endometrial polyps

Signs and symptoms

- Spotting between menstrual periods
- Pelvic cramps
- Heavy or prolonged periods

Endometrial polyps are small, soft growths in the lining of your uterus (endometrium). You may have one polyp or a cluster of them.

Many endometrial polyps produce no symptoms and are discovered during an evaluation or screening for other conditions. For women who do experience symptoms, bleeding is the most common one. The polyps may also protrude into your vagina, causing cramps as they impinge on the opening of your cervix.

Diagnosis

Sometimes the growths can be detected by ultrasound. Most often a procedure called hysteroscopy is used. A small scope is inserted into the uterus to look for polyps. At the same time, instruments can be inserted into the scope to remove the growths.

Treatment

The polyps may be removed by hysteroscopy or a procedure called dilation and curettage (D&C), a minor operation in which your doctor scrapes the lining of your uterus. After removal, your doctor will likely have the polyps analyzed to be sure they're not cancerous (malignant). On occasion, the polyps may recur.

Endometrial hyperplasia

Signs and symptoms
- Bleeding between menstrual periods
- Heavy or prolonged menstrual periods

Endometrial hyperplasia occurs when the uterine lining (endometrium) grows too thick as a result of estrogen stimulation. Women with irregular menstrual cycles who don't ovulate are most apt to have this problem.

Diagnosis

If your doctor suspects endometrial hyperplasia, he or she will likely do an endometrial biopsy to remove a small sample of your endometrium for laboratory analysis. This may be done during a pelvic exam with a procedure called hysteroscopy, in which a small scope with attached instruments is inserted into the uterus or a procedure called dilation and curettage (D&C), in which tissue is scraped from your uterine lining.

How serious is endometrial hyperplasia?

It isn't serious as long as a tissue analysis reveals no precancerous (atypical) cells. It may indicate a hormone imbalance, which should be corrected. If precancerous cells are found, the condition is known as atypical hyperplasia. Atypical hyperplasia may be a precursor to endometrial (uterine) cancer.

Treatment

Treatment is fairly simple for hyperplasia without atypical cells.

Taking birth control pills or progesterone medications for a few months will often correct the problem. If a biopsy indicates atypical hyperplasia, you may be advised to have a hysterectomy.

Hydatidiform mole

Signs and symptoms
- During pregnancy, a uterine growth that grows quickly
- Vaginal bleeding
- Severe nausea and vomiting
- No fetal movement
- Passage of grape-like tissue from your vagina
- High blood pressure

A rare noncancerous (benign) growth called hydatidiform mole sometimes develops at the beginning of pregnancy from tissue surrounding the fertilized egg that would normally produce a placenta. Because of this condition, the fetus never forms.

The tumor grows quickly and can become large. Although most of these moles are benign, 15 to 20 percent develop into a condition called invasive mole. This mole, though still benign, reaches so deeply into your uterine wall that it can cause a hemorrhage and other serious problems. Rarely, a mole becomes a choriocarcinoma, a fast-growing cancerous (malignant) tumor that soon spreads to other parts of the body. Hydatidiform mole, invasive mole and choriocarcinoma are all gestational trophoblastic diseases.

Gestational trophoblastic diseases are more common in older women. According to the American Cancer Society, gestational trophoblastic disease occurs in about 1 out of every 1,000 pregnancies in the United States, with most cases being hydatidiform moles. More rare is choriocarcinoma, which affects 2 to 7 of every 100,000 pregnancies in the United States.

Diagnosis

The condition is most often detected during an ultrasound exam. Because hydatidiform moles produce quantities of human chorionic gonadotropin, a hormone that can be detected in blood or urine, your doctor may order a blood test to check for the condition.

How serious is a hydatidiform mole?

A noninvasive mole can be removed, and invasive moles and malignant tumors are treatable if caught early. Even for choriocarcinoma, the overall cure rate is 80 to 90 percent.

Treatment

A noninvasive mole can be removed surgically. If it's invasive or malignant, treatment may include chemotherapy.

Surgery

Your doctor may remove the mole in a procedure called dilation and curettage (D&C), in which tissue is scraped from your uterine lining. Afterward, he or she will likely monitor your level of human chorionic gonadotropin, which should return to normal. If they don't, you may have developed an invasive mole or choriocarcinoma. Rarely, a doctor will recommend a hysterectomy.

Chemotherapy

For both invasive moles and choriocarcinoma, chemotherapy is the treatment of choice. Pregnancy is possible after these diseases, but there's a risk of recurrence.

Endometriosis

Signs and symptoms
- Painful periods, sometimes with pain before and several days after the start of your period
- Heavy periods
- Pain during intercourse
- Infertility
- Pain when straining to have a bowel movement

Endometriosis occurs when bits of the tissue that lines your uterus (endometrium) become implanted

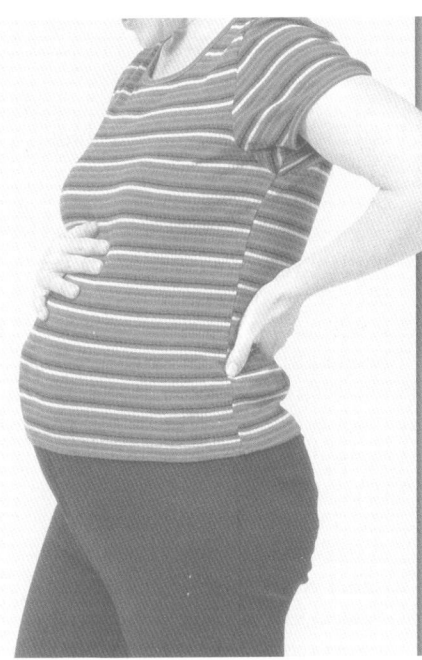

Endometriosis and Pregnancy

If you have early-stage endometriosis, your doctor may suggest that you try to become pregnant as soon as it's appropriate if you want to have children. It may become more difficult to conceive later on. During pregnancy, endometriosis implants generally shrink and the symptoms may disappear. However, endometriosis increases your risk of having an ectopic pregnancy, in which the fertilized egg implants itself outside of your uterus.

on pelvic organs. Some experts believe the implants are a result of menstrual flow that backs up into the fallopian tubes and spills into the pelvic cavity, but that may be just one factor. Most often, the implants develop on the outside of the ovaries, fallopian tubes, or the uterus or its supporting ligaments.

These cells cause bleeding as menstruation begins. Because the implants are embedded within other tissue, there's nowhere for the blood to go. Blood irritates the surrounding tissue, which may lead to the development of cysts. The cysts, in turn, may form a scar that binds organs together (adhesion). Scars and adhesions on your ovaries or fallopian tubes can prevent pregnancy.

Experts estimate that approximately 11 percent of American women have endometriosis. Most have no symptoms and require no treatment, but for some, endometriosis is a progressive disease that becomes more painful and debilitating with time. The condition, which may run in families, usually is detected between the ages of 25 and 40 and is more common in women who haven't had children.

Menopause cures endometriosis. Very rarely, menopausal hormone therapy may reactivate it.

Diagnosis

A doctor may be able to feel nodules of endometriosis during a pelvic examination, but a surgical procedure called laparoscopy can confirm the diagnosis. A laparoscope is a slim instrument equipped with a light. It's inserted into your abdomen through a small incision. Your doctor looks through the scope to examine your pelvic organs. Laparoscopy may be done with either local or general anesthesia, often on an outpatient basis.

How serious is endometriosis?

Endometrial implants aren't cancerous (malignant), but they're frequently associated with infertility. Although symptoms may wax and wane, they often worsen with time.

Treatment

Treatment for endometriosis focuses on relieving symptoms and, if you want to have a child, making it possible for you to conceive and carry the pregnancy to term. Although there's no one treatment option that works for everyone, most women who seek help for endometriosis find some, if not complete, relief from their symptoms.

Finding a doctor with whom you feel comfortable is crucial in managing and treating endometriosis.

Medication

Your doctor may recommend that you take over-the-counter pain relievers to help ease painful menstrual cramps. However, if you find that you're taking more than the recommended dose, it may be a sign that you need to try another treatment approach to manage your symptoms.

Hormone medications are very effective at reducing or eliminating the pain of endometriosis. That's because the rise and fall of hormones during the menstrual cycle causes endometrial implants to thicken, break down and bleed. Hormone therapies used to treat endometriosis include:

- **Birth control pills.** Birth control pills help control hormones responsible for the buildup of endometrial tissue each month. Taking the pill long term can reduce or eliminate the pain of endometriosis. Most women also experience lighter and shorter menstrual flow when taking the pill. Women over the age of 35 who smoke are generally advised not to take the pill because of a risk of blood clots.
- **Gonadotropin-releasing hormone (Gn-RH) agonists and antagonists.** These drugs block the production of ovarian-stimulating hormones. This prevents menstruation, which helps shrink endometrial implants. Gn-RH agonists and antagonists can force endometriosis into remission during the time of treatment and sometimes for months or years afterward.
- **Danazol.** Danazol blocks the production of ovarian-stimulating hormones, preventing menstruation and the symptoms of endometriosis. Danazol may not be the first choice because it can cause annoying side effects, such as acne and facial hair.

- **Medroxyprogesterone.** This injectable drug sold under the brand name Depo-Provera is effective at halting menstruation and the growth of endometrial implants, relieving symptoms of endometriosis. Its side effects include weight gain and depressed mood.

Surgery

Although hormone therapies are effective at relieving or eliminating symptoms of endometriosis, they prevent pregnancy. If you have endometriosis and are trying to become pregnant, surgery to remove implants may increase your chances of success. If you have severe pain from endometriosis, you may also benefit from surgery:

- **Conservative surgery.** Conservative surgery refers to removal of endometrial growths, scar tissue and adhesions without removing reproductive organs. The procedure may be accomplished laparoscopically or through traditional abdominal surgery. In laparoscopic surgery, a slender viewing instrument (laparoscope) is inserted through a small incision near your bellybutton. The laparoscope is equipped with a laser, a cautery — an instrument that destroys tissue with heat — or small surgical instruments. If surgery is ineffective at improving fertility, other procedures, such as in vitro fertilization techniques, may help.
- **Hysterectomy.** In severe cases of endometriosis, surgery to remove some or all of the female reproductive organs (hysterectomy) may be the best treatment. But this type of surgery is typically considered a last resort, especially for women still in their reproductive years.

Self-care

If pain persists or it takes a while for you and your doctor to find a treatment that works, try measures at home to relieve your discomfort. Warm baths and a heating pad can help relax pelvic muscles, reducing cramping and pain.

Regular exercise may reduce the symptoms of premenstrual syndrome and take the edge off endometriosis symptoms. Some women find that giving up or cutting back on caffeine, sugar and alcohol helps their symptoms.

Adenomyosis

Signs and symptoms

- Menstrual cramps that last throughout a period and worsen as you grow older
- Prolonged, excessive menstrual bleeding

In adenomyosis, some of the endometrial tissue that lines your uterus begins to grow within its muscular walls. This is most likely to happen late in your childbearing years and after you've had children. Some women with adenomyosis have no symptoms.

Diagnosis

During a pelvic examination, your doctor may discover that your uterus is enlarged and tender. This, along with prolonged painful cramps and excessive menstrual bleeding, suggests adenomyosis. Ultrasound and magnetic resonance imaging (MRI) may be helpful in making a diagnosis.

Treatment

Adenomyosis usually resolves after menopause, so treatment may depend on how close you are to that stage of life. If you're nearing menopause, your doctor may prescribe painkillers and suggest no other treatment. If your pain is severe or menopause is years away, your doctor may suggest a hysterectomy.

Pelvic inflammatory disease

Signs and symptoms

- Severe pain in your lower abdomen

Pelvic Pain

Anytime you have pain in your pelvic region that lasts longer than a few hours, recurs, or is accompanied by fever or vaginal bleeding, see your doctor. He or she will want to know if your pain is new or if it's a condition that's been with you for a while (chronic). If it's chronic, your doctor will want to know if it comes and goes (episodic) or is continuous.

Your doctor may also ask other questions about your pain, such as if it's associated with your menstrual periods, is related to bowel or bladder habits, or occurs with intercourse or physical activity.

- Mild, recurrent pain in your lower abdomen, perhaps with backache and irregular menstrual periods
- Infertility
- Pain during intercourse
- Irregular bleeding
- Vaginal discharge
- Emergency signs and symptoms
- Severe pain low in your abdomen
- Nausea and vomiting
- Temperature above 102 F

Every year, about 1 million American women develop pelvic inflammatory disease (PID), an infection of the pelvic organs that can cause scarring. Some women have no symptoms and are never diagnosed; some develop a low-level, long-lasting (chronic) infection. Still others have a severe and sudden (acute) attack. After treatment, about 15 to 25 percent of women develop PID again.

Usually, you acquire the organisms responsible for pelvic inflammatory disease through sexual intercourse. PID develops in almost 15 percent of women with gonorrhea. Chlamydia is an even more frequent cause.

If your partner uses a condom, you're somewhat protected from PID. If you have PID, your sexual partner should seek treatment, too, even if he has no symptoms. If he is infected, he may reinfect you.

Diagnosis

During a pelvic examination, your doctor may take samples of the discharge from your vagina and cervix for laboratory analysis to determine what organism is causing the infection. Blood tests also are helpful. If there's any question about the diagnosis or about how widespread the infection is, your doctor may do a surgical procedure known as laparoscopy. It involves inserting a thin, lighted instrument through a small incision in your abdomen and viewing your pelvic organs.

How serious is pelvic inflammatory disease?

Left untreated, PID can be serious. An abscess may develop on your fallopian tubes or ovaries, creating an emergency if it perforates. Your tubes or ovaries may be damaged or scarred, causing infertility.

PID can also lead to an inflammation of the membrane that lines your abdominal cavity (peritonitis). Peritonitis is always serious and needs intensive treatment with antibiotics. In rare cases, bacteria may invade your bloodstream, leading to blood poisoning (septicemia) and infection in your joints.

Long-term consequences of PID include chronic pelvic pain and tubal (ectopic) pregnancy, in which the fetus grows outside your uterus, usually in one of your fallopian tubes.

Treatment

Treatment may consist of medication, rest and possibly surgery.

Medication

Your doctor may prescribe a combination antibiotic and pain reliever.

Rest

Your doctor may recommend bed rest. You may even be hospitalized for a short time if you have a severe case or if your condition doesn't respond quickly to medication.

Surgery

Surgery is rarely necessary. However, if an abscess ruptures or threatens to rupture, it may require drainage or removal. Removal may mean that a fallopian tube or an ovary or both also be removed. Occasionally, total hysterectomy is necessary.

Chronic pelvic pain

Signs and symptoms

- Persistent pain in your pelvic region
- Painful intercourse
- Pain with bowel movements or urination

Chronic pelvic pain can take many forms: It can be steady or intermittent. It can be a dull ache, a sharp pain, cramping, or an overall feeling of pressure or heaviness deep in your abdomen. The pain may be worse when you sit or stand and better when you lie down.

Determining the cause can be difficult, if not impossible. Possible causes of chronic pelvic pain include:

- Endometriosis (see page 1214)
- Adenomyosis (see page 1216)
- Pelvic inflammatory disease (see page 1216)
- Myofascial pelvic pain syndrome (see below)
- Pelvic congestion syndrome resulting from varicose-type veins around the ovaries that cause pooling of blood
- A piece of ovary left after hysterectomy (ovarian remnant) that develops tiny, painful cysts
- Uterine fibroids (see page 1212)

If you're depressed, experience chronic stress, or have been sexually or physically abused, you may be more likely to experience chronic pelvic pain. Emotional distress makes pain worse and, likewise, living with chronic pain makes emotional distress worse. The two often get locked in a vicious cycle.

In some women with chronic pelvic pain, a condition known as central sensitization may develop. It involves changes to the central nervous system that can cause oversensitivity of nerves, resulting in persistent or increased pain, even when the original source or cause of pain is no longer present.

Diagnosis

Diagnosis may require a pelvic exam and various tests to try to identify the cause of the pain. Your health care team will try to identify causes of your pain and whether you have signs of central sensitization.

How serious is chronic pelvic pain?

Chronic pelvic pain can be a debilitating, long-term condition that sometimes results in the loss of reproductive function.

Treatment

Treatment is dependent on the cause, but it often requires a

Myofascial Pelvic Pain Syndrome

Myofascial pelvic pain syndrome is a type of pelvic pain that typically occurs because the pelvic muscles are in a chronically contracted state and spasm easily or do not fully relax. Myofascial pelvic pain syndrome may develop after pelvic surgery or childbirth, after repeated urinary tract or vaginal infections, in association with other pain conditions such as endometriosis or interstitial cystitis, or after sexual trauma. Treatment for myofascial pelvic pain usually involves pelvic floor physical therapy, often in conjunction with other treatments, such as sex therapy or individual counseling, and possibly medications, depending on your situation.

multidisciplinary approach. If the source of the pain is found, treatment focuses on that cause. If no cause can be found, treatment focuses on managing the pain. Medical professionals from several specialties may be consulted or involved in your care.

Medication

Antibiotics may be prescribed to treat pelvic inflammatory disease (PID), and hormones to suppress ovulation may be used to treat endometriosis or adenomyosis. Antidepressants and other medications may help manage chronic pelvic pain, even in women who aren't depressed, by decreasing the sensitivity of the nerves that are perpetuating the pain.

Self-care

Stress management and relaxation techniques, such as meditating, listening to music and practicing yoga, may help with some forms of chronic pelvic pain.

Physical therapy

Working with a physical therapist, you can learn how to relax and gently stretch your pelvic floor muscles if those muscles are causing the pain.

Complementary therapies

Other therapies that may help you manage your pain include acupuncture and biofeedback. For more information on these therapies, see Chapter 38, "Integrative Medicine."

Devices

An ultrasound device can apply soothing heat to your pelvic floor muscles and help relieve spasms.

Surgery

Surgery — sometimes a hysterectomy — may be used to treat endometriosis. PID and fibroids also may require a hysterectomy. Surgery may also be necessary to remove ovarian remnants.

Ovarian Disorders

Each of your two ovaries is about the size of an almond. The ovaries are situated in your abdomen, above and to the side of your uterus and about 4 to 5 inches below your waist. At birth, a female has roughly 1 million eggs (ova) stored in her ovaries, each egg housed in its own follicle.

Every month, from the time of puberty until menopause, one egg grows until rupture of its follicle releases it. The egg moves through the fallopian tube into your uterus.

Your ovaries also produce the female sex hormones estrogen and progesterone, which regulate your menstrual cycle. During the first half of the cycle, your ovaries secrete estrogen. The outer cells of the single follicle where the egg is growing manufacture most of it. Estrogen causes your uterine lining to thicken in preparation for receiving a fertilized egg.

Just before ovulation, the same follicle begins to produce tiny amounts of progesterone. After the egg is released, the follicle — at this stage, it's called the corpus luteum — expands rapidly and steps up production of both progesterone and estrogen.

These hormones act together to complete the development of your uterine lining. If pregnancy occurs, hormones secreted by the corpus luteum help to sustain the pregnancy. Otherwise, the corpus luteum begins to shrink, and levels of estrogen and progesterone decrease. Your uterus then sheds its lining, resulting in menstruation.

Ovarian cysts and noncancerous tumors

Signs and symptoms

- A dull ache, pressure or fullness in your abdomen
- Pain during intercourse
- Frequent urination
- Abrupt onset of sharp pain in your lower abdomen
  Emergency signs and symptoms
- Sudden, severe abdominal pain and perhaps vomiting

A cyst is a sac filled with fluid. Most ovarian cysts are harmless and disappear of their own accord. Often, they're noncancerous (benign) and don't cause symptoms. Other types of cysts warrant attention. Cysts are commonly seen on pelvic imaging ordered for other purposes. Those that develop after menopause are somewhat more likely to be an indicator of ovarian cancer.

In women who haven't gone through menopause, the ovaries normally grow cystlike structures called follicles each month. Follicles are little "chemical factories" that produce the hormones estrogen and progesterone and release an egg (ovum) when you ovulate.

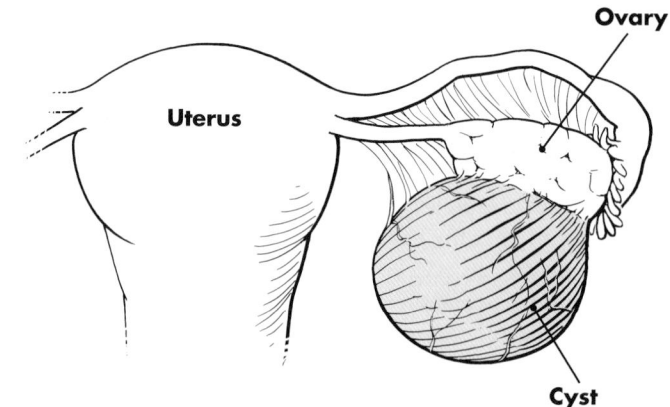

An ovarian cyst may be detected during a routine pelvic examination.

Sometimes, a normal monthly follicle just keeps growing. When that happens, it becomes what's called a functional cyst. This means it started during the normal function of your menstrual cycle. There are two types of functional cysts:

- **Follicular cyst.** A follicular cyst begins when a hormone called luteinizing hormone (LH) doesn't surge as it should during ovulation. The result is that the follicle holding your egg doesn't rupture or release the egg. Instead it grows and grows until it becomes a cyst. Follicular cysts are usually harmless, rarely cause pain, and often disappear on their own within two or three menstrual cycles.
- **Corpus luteum cyst.** If LH does surge and your egg is released, the follicle produces large quantities of estrogen and progesterone. At this stage, the follicle is called the corpus luteum. Sometimes, after the egg's release, the corpus luteum expands into a cyst. Although this cyst usually disappears on its own in a few weeks, it can grow to almost 4 inches in diameter and has the potential to bleed into itself or twist the ovary, causing pelvic or abdominal pain. If it fills with blood, the cyst may rupture, causing internal bleeding and sudden, sharp pain.

A tumor is a solid lump. Benign tumors don't invade neighboring tissue or spread to other parts of the body. Cancerous (malignant) tumors may do both.

However, if a benign tumor or ovarian cyst is large, it can cause abdominal discomfort. In some cases, it may interfere with production of ovarian hormones and result in irregular vaginal bleeding or an increase in body hair. If a large tumor or cyst presses on your bladder, you may need to urinate more frequently because your bladder's capacity is diminished.

If a tumor or cyst becomes twisted, you may experience spasms of pain. Sudden or sharp pain

may mean a cyst has ruptured. If you have severe abdominal pain, fever and vomiting, or signs and symptoms such as dizziness, cold, clammy skin and rapid breathing, seek immediate medical help.

Diagnosis

If during a pelvic examination your doctor detects something that feels like an ovarian cyst or tumor, he or she will likely order additional tests. These may include:

- **Pregnancy test.** A positive pregnancy test may suggest that your cyst is a corpus luteum cyst, which can develop when the ruptured follicle that released your egg reseals and fills with fluid.
- **Pelvic ultrasound.** In this procedure, a wandlike device (transducer) is used to send and receive high-frequency sound waves (ultrasound). The transducer can be moved over your abdomen and inside your vagina, creating an image of your uterus and ovaries. This image can then be photographed and analyzed by your doctor to confirm the presence of a cyst, help identify its location, and determine whether it's solid, filled with fluid or mixed.
- **Laparoscopy.** Using a laparoscope — a slim, lighted instrument inserted into your abdomen through a small incision — your doctor can see your ovaries and remove the ovarian cyst.
- **CA 125 blood test.** Blood levels of a protein called cancer antigen 125 (CA 125) often are elevated in women with ovarian cancer. If you develop an ovarian cyst that is partially solid and you are at high risk of ovarian cancer, your doctor may test the level of CA 125 in your blood to determine whether your cyst could be cancerous. Elevated CA 125 levels can also occur in noncancerous conditions, such as endometriosis, uterine fibroids and pelvic inflammatory disease.

Treatment

Treatment depends on your age, the type and size of your cyst, and your symptoms. Your doctor may suggest:

Watchful waiting

You can wait and be re-examined in one to three months if you're in your reproductive years, you have no symptoms and an ultrasound shows you have a simple, fluid-filled cyst. Your doctor will likely recommend that you get a follow-up pelvic ultrasound to see if your cyst has changed in size.

Watchful waiting, including regular monitoring with ultrasound, is also a common treatment option recommended for postmenopausal women if a cyst is filled with fluid and is less than 2 centimeters in diameter.

Birth control pills

Your doctor may recommend birth control pills to reduce the chance of new cysts developing in future menstrual cycles. Oral contraceptives offer the added benefit of reducing your risk of ovarian cancer — the risk decreases the longer you take birth control pills.

Surgery

Your doctor may suggest removal of a cyst if it is large, doesn't look like a functional cyst, is growing or isn't resolving on its own. Cysts that cause pain or other symptoms may be removed.

Some cysts can be removed without removing the ovary in a procedure known as a cystectomy. Your doctor may also suggest removing the affected ovary and leaving the other intact in a procedure known as oophorectomy. Both procedures may allow you to maintain your fertility if you're still in your childbearing years. Leaving at least one ovary intact also has the benefit of maintaining a source of estrogen production and improving longevity.

If a cystic mass is cancerous, however, your doctor will likely advise removal of both ovaries, the uterus and any visible tumor outside the ovaries. Your doctor will also evaluate the degree to which the tumor has spread to determine appropriate therapy. After menopause, the risk of a newly found cystic ovarian mass being cancerous increases. As a result, doctors more commonly recommend surgery when a cystic mass develops on the ovaries after menopause.

Hysterectomy

A hysterectomy is the removal of your uterus. A hysterectomy is most often performed for the following reasons:
- Endometrial (uterine) cancer
- Severe endometriosis or fibroids
- Severe, uncontrollable uterine bleeding
- Protrusion of the uterus from the vagina (uterine prolapse)

Hysterectomies aren't all alike. A supracervical hysterectomy leaves your cervix in place. In a total hysterectomy, the entire uterus, including the cervix, is removed. A bilateral salpingo-oophorectomy is the removal of your fallopian tubes and both ovaries. It may be performed at the same time as a hysterectomy. A radical hysterectomy, usually performed for cancer of the cervix, extends even further to include additional tissue around the cervix and the removal of the upper part of your vagina.

In performing a hysterectomy, a surgeon may remove the uterus vaginally, with an abdominal incision or laparoscopically, using a robotic system. Or a combination of methods may be used. The approach to surgery depends on the disease being treated, expertise of the surgeon and factors such as prior vaginal delivery and uterine size. In case of a large ovarian or uterine tumor, a surgeon will usually use the abdominal approach. For uterine prolapse, the vaginal approach often is preferred. Recovery generally takes several weeks, depending on the type of surgery performed.

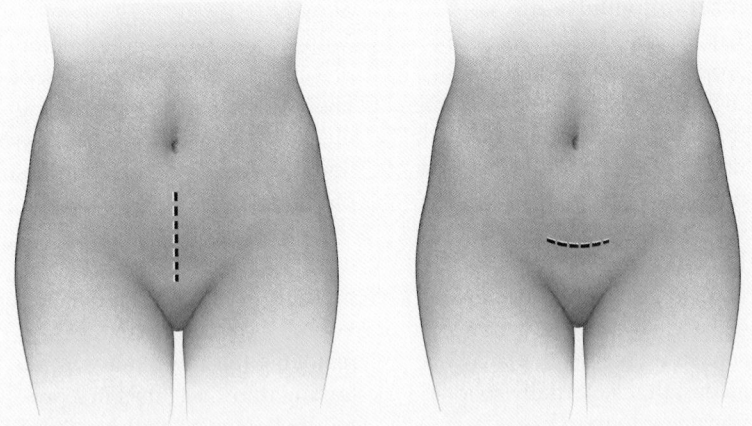

In an abdominal hysterectomy, the uterus is removed through an incision in your lower abdomen. The type of incision — vertical or horizontal bikini line — is dependent on several factors.

Possible complications of a hysterectomy include pelvic infections, kidney and bladder infections, and hemorrhage. After you get home, you'll have to forgo intercourse and lifting heavy objects for a time. For six to eight weeks, you can't engage in active sports.

Cancers of the Reproductive Tract

Cancer can develop in the fallopian tubes, uterus, ovaries, cervix, vagina and vulva. The chance of a successful outcome depends on which organ is involved and how early the cancer is diagnosed.

Endometrial cancer

Signs and symptoms
- Vaginal bleeding after menopause
- Before menopause, heavy periods or bleeding between periods
- A pink or watery discharge from your vagina
- Pelvic pain
- Unintended weight loss

Although the diagnosis of endometrial cancer is difficult to receive, the good news is that this type of cancer is often found at its earliest, most treatable stage.

Endometrial cancer, one of the most common cancers in American women, begins in the cells of the endometrium, the lining of your uterus — a hollow, pear-shaped pelvic organ where fetal development occurs. Endometrial cancer is sometimes called uterine cancer, but there are other cells in the uterus that can become cancerous — such as muscle or myometrial cells. These form much less common cancers called sarcomas.

In endometrial cancer, abnormal cells develop in the lining of the uterus. Why the cancer cells develop isn't entirely known. However, estrogen that isn't balanced with progestin can play a role in the development of some endometrial cancers. Factors that change this hormone balance and other risk factors for the disease have been identified and continue to emerge. In addition, ongoing research is devoted to studying changes in certain genes that may cause the cells in the endometrium to become cancerous.

Factors that increase the risk of endometrial cancer include:

- **Many years of menstruation.** If you started menstruating at an early age — before age 12 — or you began menopause later, you're at greater risk of endometrial cancer than is a woman who menstruated for fewer years.
- **Never having been pregnant.** Pregnancy decreases the risk of endometrial cancer. Pregnancy and lactation reduce the number of normal menstrual cycles, which provides some protection against cancer. Women may not become pregnant due to irregular ovulation and menses, which increases the risk. Hormonal contraception also reduces the risk of endometrial cancer, especially when used for a longer duration.
- **Irregular ovulation.** The monthly release of an egg from an ovary in menstruating women (ovulation), is regulated by hormones. Menstrual cycles without ovulation may fail to shed all of the uterine lining (endometrium) on a regular basis, increasing the risk of precancerous and cancerous endometrium forming. Ovulation irregularities have many causes, including obesity and a condition known as polycystic ovary syndrome (PCOS). With

PCOS, hormonal imbalances prevent regular ovulation and menstruation. Treating obesity and managing the symptoms of PCOS can help restore monthly menstruation cycles, decreasing the risk of endometrial cancer.

- **Obesity.** Ovaries aren't the only source of estrogen. Fat tissue can produce estrogen. Therefore, being obese can increase the level of estrogen in your body that is not balanced by progestin, putting you at a higher risk of endometrial cancer. Obese women have three times the risk of endometrial cancer, and overweight women have twice the risk, according to the American Cancer Society. However, women who are normal weight or underweight can also develop endometrial cancer.
- **A high-fat diet.** This type of diet may add to your risk of endometrial cancer by promoting obesity. In addition, fatty foods can directly affect estrogen metabolism, further increasing your risk of endometrial cancer.
- **Diabetes.** Endometrial cancer is more common in women with diabetes, possibly because obesity and type 2 diabetes often go hand in hand. However, even women with diabetes who aren't obese have a greater risk of endometrial cancer.

- **Estrogen-only hormone therapy.** Estrogen stimulates growth of the endometrium. Therefore, replacing estrogen alone after menopause in women with a uterus may increase their risk of endometrial cancer. Taking a form of the hormone progesterone with estrogen causes the lining of the uterus to thin and sometimes to shed and actually lowers the risk of endometrial cancer.
- **Ovarian tumors.** Some tumors of the ovaries may themselves produce estrogen, increasing estrogen levels.

Diagnosis

Your gynecologist or your primary care doctor will conduct a complete medical history and perform a physical and pelvic examination. During the pelvic examination, the doctor feels for any lumps or changes in the shape of the uterus that may indicate a problem.

Diagnosis may or may not involve these other tests:

- **Transvaginal ultrasound.** Your doctor may recommend a transvaginal ultrasound to look at the thickness and texture of the endometrium and help rule out other conditions. In this procedure, a wandlike device (transducer) is inserted into the vagina. The transducer uses sound waves to create a video image of your uterus. This test evaluates for ovarian tumors and can indicate if an endometrial biopsy is needed in postmenopausal women.
- **Endometrial biopsy.** To get a sample of cells from inside your uterus, you may undergo an endometrial biopsy. This involves removing tissue from your uterine lining for laboratory analysis. This may be done in your doctor's office and usually doesn't require anesthesia. Because of the increased risk, women who have HNPCC mutations should talk with their doctors about yearly

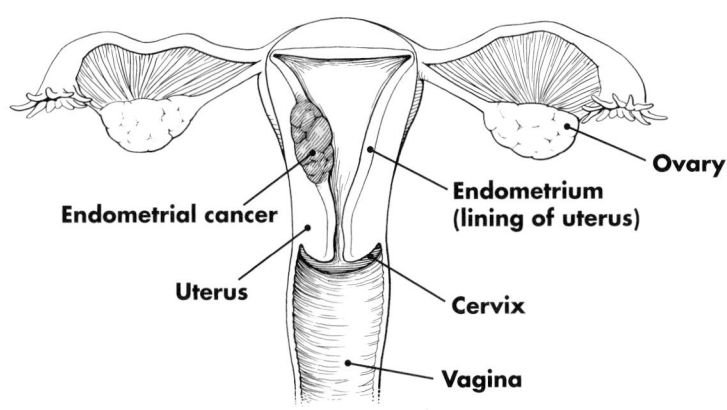

Endometrial (uterine) cancer develops in the lining of your uterus (endometrium). Treatment is usually very successful if the cancer is diagnosed early.

endometrial biopsies beginning around age 35.

- **Hysteroscopy, dilation and curettage (D&C), or both.** If enough tissue can't be obtained during a biopsy or if the biopsy suggests possible cancer, you'll likely need to undergo a D&C with or without hysteroscopy. During hysteroscopy, which can take place in a doctor's office or a day surgery setting, a small scope is placed into the uterine cavity to look for abnormalities. A direct biopsy of specific abnormalities may be performed for microscopic analysis. During a D&C, tissue is also obtained for microscopic analysis but is not focused on a specific area of concern.

- **Cervical cancer screen.** Your doctor takes a sample of cells from the cervix to detect another type of cancer — cervical cancer. Because endometrial cancer begins inside your uterus, it's rarely detectable by a cervical cancer screen.

If endometrial cancer is found, you may need more tests to deter-

Cervical Cancer Screen

Since the early 1940s, the death rate of women with cervical cancer has decreased dramatically, largely because so many women have Pap test screening. In women who develop cervical cancer, most have never been screened or don't have regular screenings.

Although not infallible, the cervical cancer screen detects most cervical cancers and, more importantly, detects precancerous conditions that are virtually 100 percent curable. Occasionally, a cervical cancer screen will also detect evidence of endometrial cancer.

A cervical cancer screen is performed during a pelvic examination. At most, it causes slight discomfort. Using a plastic spatula or brush, your doctor gently samples the surface of your cervix to gather cells and also inserts a brush into your cervical canal to sample its cells. The cells are sent to a laboratory for analysis. Based on your age, your doctor also may use a lab test called a high-risk HPV test to determine whether you have been infected with any of the 13 types of human papillomavirus (HPV) that are most likely to lead to cervical cancer. Like the cervical cancer screen, the high-risk HPV test involves collecting cells from the cervix for lab testing. HPV testing reduces the risk of missing precancerous cells and allows for less frequent cervical cancer screens.

Negative results mean your risk of cervical cancer in the next years is very low. Advances in the understanding of cervical cancer and its testing have led to recommendations for less frequent testing in women at low cancer risk who might not benefit from additional testing and procedures.

A positive result indicates the need for further testing to determine if abnormal cervical cells are present, but it doesn't prove that you have cancer or dysplasia, a precancerous condition.

You should have your first cervical cancer screen at age 21, with repeat testing every few years if results are normal. After age 30, testing may occur every five years if both HPV tests and cervical cancer screens are normal. The recommended time between normal tests may change as testing changes and more information about cervical cancer development is discovered. Ask your doctor about what's appropriate for you.

If you're in a high-risk group due to recent abnormal results, treatment for severe dysplasia, or reduced immunity due to disease or medical treatments, you'll likely require more-frequent testing than other women.

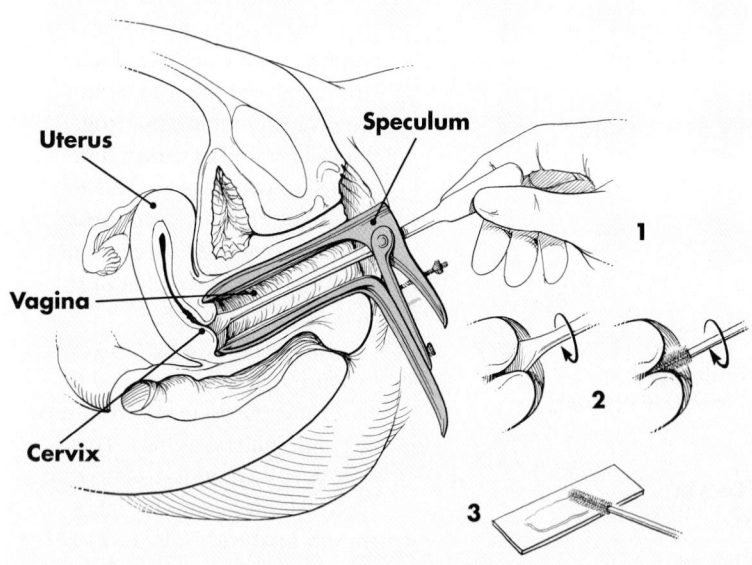

With a speculum in place, your doctor rotates a spatula and then a brush to remove a sample of cells (1 and 2). The cells are then placed in a bottle of solution or on a glass slide for evaluation (3).

mine if the cancer has spread (metastasized) to other parts of your body. These tests may include a chest X-ray, a computerized tomography (CT) scan and some blood tests.

How serious is endometrial cancer?

Because this type of cancer causes abnormal vaginal bleeding, it's often discovered at an early stage, when it's still localized. Therefore, treatment is successful in many cases. Rarely, the tumor is a faster growing, more aggressive type, and it may be more likely to recur after treatment.

Treatment

Depending on how aggressive the cancer is and whether it has spread, treatment may require just one or a combination of therapies. Women diagnosed with endometrial cancer have better outcomes when evaluated and treated by a gynecologic oncology expert.

Surgery

Surgery is the most common treatment for endometrial cancer.

Most doctors recommend either the surgical removal of the uterus alone (hysterectomy) or, more likely, the surgical removal of the uterus, fallopian tubes and ovaries (hysterectomy with bilateral salpingo-oophorectomy). Lymph nodes in the area also may be removed during surgery along with other tissue samples. A surgeon removes as much cancer as possible and helps determine what further treatment, if any, is needed.

Other therapies

If you have an aggressive form of endometrial cancer or the cancer has spread to other parts of your body, you may need additional treatments. These may include:

- **Radiation.** If your doctor believes you're at high risk of cancer recurrence, he or she may suggest that you have radiation therapy after a hysterectomy. Your doctor may also recommend radiation therapy if the cancerous tumor is fast growing, invades deeply into the muscle of the uterus or involves blood vessels. Radiation therapy involves the use of high-dose X-rays to kill cancer cells. When done from outside the body, it's called external beam radiation therapy. Brachytherapy is another form of radiation that involves the internal application of radiation, usually to the upper portion of the vagina.

- **Hormone therapy.** If the cancer has spread to other parts of your body, treatment with a form of the hormone progesterone may stop it from growing. The progesterone used in treating endometrial cancer is administered in higher doses than is used in hormone therapy for menopausal women. Other medications may be used as well. Hormone therapy may be an option for certain women with early endometrial cancer who want to have children and, therefore, don't want a hysterectomy. However, this approach is not without the risk that the cancer will return.

- **Chemotherapy.** It involves the use of drugs to kill cancer cells. Often, chemotherapy drugs are used in combination to increase their efficacy. Generally, women with more-aggressive tumor types or stage III or stage IV endometrial cancer will be offered chemotherapy as part of their treatment regimen. You may receive chemotherapy drugs by pill (orally) or through your veins (intravenously). These drugs enter your bloodstream and then travel through your body, killing cancer cells outside the uterus.

Each type of treatment for endometrial cancer can have side effects. Ask your doctor what side effects you can expect and what can be done to manage them.

Cervical dysplasia

Cervical dysplasia is an abnormality of the cells at the surface of the cervix. Doctors refer to these abnormal cells as lesions. This condition isn't cancer, but it may progress to

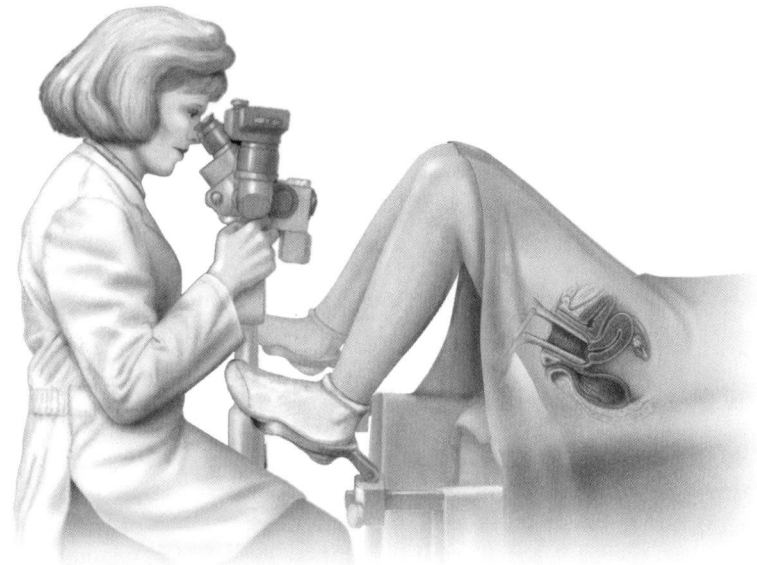

During a colposcopic examination, your doctor uses a device called a colposcope to view your cervix. The scope contains a bright light and a magnifying lens.

cancer over a period of years if it doesn't resolve on its own.

Cervical dysplasia is detected by means of a cervical cancer screen, high-risk HPV testing or both. The condition can occur at any age but is rarely associated with a risk of cancer while women are in their early 20s. It's strongly linked to a virus called the human papillomavirus. Dysplasia is more likely to occur in someone who began sexual intercourse as a teenager or has had multiple sexual partners.

Diagnosis

If your cervical cancer screen or high-risk HPV testing reveals dysplasia, you will likely need further diagnostic testing, including an additional cervical cancer screen or HPV test or a colposcopy. A colposcope is an instrument equipped with a magnifying lens and a light. A doctor uses it to examine the cervix.

If your doctor spots an abnormality, he or she may remove a tissue sample (biopsy) to send for laboratory analysis to confirm the dysplasia and its severity.

Depending on the results of your tests, your doctor may recommend treatment or monitoring of the condition.

How serious is cervical dysplasia?

While low-grade lesions (mild dysplasia) commonly resolve over a few years, some progress to high-grade lesions (severe dysplasia). When high-grade lesions are left untreated, the condition could lead to cancer.

Treatment

Doctors may treat cervical dysplasia with a variety of procedures:
- **Observation.** This involves repeat cervical cancer screens and high-risk HPV tests over several years to see if the body will "clear" the problem on its own.
- **LEEP.** During this procedure, known as loop electrosurgical excision procedure (LEEP), a doctor removes abnormal tissue using a thin wire loop and a carefully controlled electric current.
- **Cryocautery.** Cryocautery involves freezing the cervix to destroy abnormal tissue.
- **Conization.** For deeper or more worrisome dysplasias, a portion of the cervix is removed.

Cervical cancer

Signs and symptoms
- Bleeding from your vagina after intercourse, between periods or after menopause
- In advanced stages, a dull backache
- Pelvic pain or pain during intercourse

Cervical cancer has decreased markedly in American women who undergo screening. Unfortunately many underscreened women are still at risk. Various strains of the human papillomavirus (HPV), a sexually transmitted infection, play a role in causing most cases of cervical cancer.

When exposed to HPV, the body's immune system typically prevents the virus from doing harm. In a small group of women, however, the virus survives for years or decades, often undetected, before it eventually converts some cells on the surface of the cervix into cancer cells. Most cases of cervical cancer occur in women between the ages of 20 and 50.

Cervical cancer most commonly begins in the thin, flat cells that cover the cervix (squamous cells). Squamous cell carcinomas account for most cervical cancers. Other cervical cancers can occur in the glandular cells that line the upper portion of the cervix. These less common types of cervical cancers are called adenocarcinomas. Sometimes both types of cells are involved in cervical cancer. Very rare cancers can occur in other cells in the cervix.

HPV plays a role in the development of nearly all cervical cancers. While most sexually active women are exposed to HPV during their lifetimes, most never develop cervical cancer. This means other risk factors, such as your genetic makeup, your environment, or your lifestyle choices and whether you've been screened and treated for precancerous changes, also affect whether you'll develop cervical cancer.

Factors that may increase your risk of cervical cancer include:
- **Many sexual partners.** The greater your number of sexual partners — and the greater each partner's number of sexual partners — the greater your chance of acquiring HPV.
- **Early sexual activity.** Having sex before age 18 increases your risk of HPV. Immature cells seem to be more susceptible to the precancerous changes that HPV can cause.
- **Other sexually transmitted infections (STIs).** If you have other STIs — such as chlamydia, gonorrhea, syphilis or HIV/AIDS — you have a greater chance of also having acquired HPV.
- **A weak immune system.** Most women who are infected with HPV never develop cervical cancer. However, if you have an HPV infection and your immune system is weakened by another health condition or medical therapy, you may be more likely to develop cervical cancer.
- **Cigarette smoking.** The exact mechanism that links cigarette smoking to cervical cancer isn't known, but tobacco use increases the risk of precancerous changes as well as cancer of the cervix. Smoking and HPV infection may work together to cause cervical cancer.

Diagnosis

This type of cancer is generally screened for using a cervical cancer screen, sometimes in conjunction with high-risk HPV testing. If the test results come back abnormal, your doctor may also perform a colposcopy exam and biopsy for diagnosis of cancer. A colposcope is an instrument with a magnifying lens that permits a close look at the cervix. A biopsy is a procedure in which your doctor removes specimens of tissue from your cervix for microscopic study to determine if the tissue is cancerous (malignant).

How serious is cervical cancer?

Thanks largely to cervical cancer screening, the death rate from cervical cancer has decreased greatly over the last 50 years. Still, every year more than 12,000 women in the United States are diagnosed with invasive cervical cancer, and more than 4,000 die of cervical cancer, according to the American Cancer Society.

Treatment

Whether treatment is required depends on the severity of the abnormal cells found on the surface of the cervix (cervical dysplasia). Doctors refer to these abnormal cells as lesions. With low-grade lesions (mild dysplasia), no treatment is needed. Low-grade lesions commonly resolve over a few years, although some progress to high-grade lesions (severe dysplasia). Your doctor may recommend a follow-up in a year to check for additional changes.

High-grade lesions are unlikely to resolve on their own and have the potential to develop into cancer. Treatment to remove the abnormal cells, such as surgery or other procedures, may be required.

Treatment for dysplasia that has progressed to cervical cancer depends on several factors, such as the stage of the cancer, the type of cervical cancer, fertility desires, other health problems you may have and your own preferences about treatment. Options include the following:

Hysterectomy

Surgery to remove the uterus (hysterectomy) is typically used to treat cervical cancer that can be completely removed with surgery. Cervical cancer that has spread beyond the cervix requires different therapy. A simple hysterectomy involves the removal of the cancer, the cervix and the uterus. Simple hysterectomy is typically an option only when the cancer is in the very early stages. A radical hysterectomy — removal of the cervix and nearby tissue, the uterus, and part of the vagina, along with nearby lymph node sampling or removal — is the standard surgical treatment when the disease is confined close to the cervix and hasn't spread.

Hysterectomy can cure early-stage cervical cancers, but the absence of the uterus prevents the individual from carrying a pregnancy. However, women of reproductive age may be candidates for techniques that preserve fertility. Recovery time for a hysterectomy is about six weeks. Temporary side effects of radical hysterectomy include pelvic pain and difficulty with bowel movements and urination.

Radiation

Radiation therapy uses high-powered energy to kill cancer cells. Radiation therapy can be given externally using external beam radiation or internally (brachytherapy) by placing devices filled with radioactive material near your cervix. Radiation therapy may be used alone or with chemotherapy before surgery to shrink a tumor or after surgery to kill any remaining cancer cells.

Both methods of radiation therapy can be combined. Radiation therapy can be used alone, with chemotherapy, before surgery to shrink a tumor or after surgery to kill any remaining cancer cells. Side effects of radiation to the pelvic area include upset stomach, nausea, diarrhea, bladder irritation and narrowing of your vagina, which can make intercourse difficult. Premenopausal women may stop menstruating as a result of radiation therapy and begin menopause.

Chemotherapy

Chemotherapy uses strong anti-cancer chemicals to kill cancer cells. Chemotherapy drugs can be

Gene Mutations and Ovarian Cancer

While the vast majority of women who develop ovarian cancer don't have an inherited gene mutation, the most significant risk factor for ovarian cancer is having an inherited mutation in one of two genes called breast cancer gene 1 (BRCA1) and breast cancer gene 2 (BRCA2). These genes were originally identified in families with multiple cases of breast cancer, which is how they got their names, but people with these mutations also have a significantly increased risk of ovarian cancer.

Women with the BRCA1 mutation have a 35 to 70 percent higher risk of ovarian cancer than do women without this mutation. For women with a BRCA2 mutation, the risk is between 10 and 30 percent higher. For most women, the overall lifetime risk is about 1.5 percent, according to the American Cancer Society. You're at particularly high risk of carrying these types of mutations if you're of Ashkenazi Jewish descent.

Another known genetic link involves an inherited syndrome called hereditary nonpolyposis colorectal cancer (HNPCC). Women in HNPCC families are at increased risk of cancers of the uterine lining (endometrium), colon, ovary and stomach. Risk of ovarian cancer associated with HNPCC is lower than is that of ovarian cancer associated with BRCA mutations.

used alone or in combination with each other. They travel throughout your body killing quickly growing cells, including cancer cells. Low doses of chemotherapy are often combined with radiation therapy, since chemotherapy may enhance the effects of the radiation. Higher doses of chemotherapy are used to control advanced cervical cancer that may not be curable. Side effects of chemotherapy depend on the drugs being administered, but generally include diarrhea, fatigue, nausea and hair loss. Certain chemotherapy drugs may cause infertility and early menopause in premenopausal women.

Prevention

HPV vaccines offer protection from the most dangerous types of HPV — the virus that causes most cervical cancers — as well as the types of HPV that most commonly cause genital warts. The national Advisory Committee on Immunization Practices recommends HPV vaccination for both girls and boys ages 11 and 12, although it can be given as young as 9 years old.

The vaccination is also recommended for girls and women ages 13 to 26 and boys and men ages 13 to 21 if they haven't received the vaccine already. The vaccine is most effective in preventing cancer if given earlier in the range of recommended ages rather than waiting until later.

Women who are vaccinated still require cervical cancer screening because the vaccine will not prevent all cancers. However, screening recommendations for vaccinated women are evolving and may change in the future.

Ovarian cancer

Signs and symptoms
- Abdominal pressure, fullness, swelling or bloating
- Urinary symptoms such as urgency
- Persistent indigestion, gas or nausea

- Pelvic discomfort or pain
- Unexplained changes in bowel habits, such as constipation
- Loss of appetite or quickly feeling full
- Increased abdominal girth or clothes fitting tighter around your waist
- Pain during intercourse (dyspareunia)
- A persistent lack of energy
- Low back pain
- Changes in menstruation

Until recently, ovarian cancer was known as a silent killer because it usually wasn't found until it had spread to other areas of the body. But new evidence shows that most women may have symptoms even in the early stages, although typical symptoms of early ovarian cancer are most commonly due to other causes. Awareness of these symptoms may lead to earlier detection.

Early detection is ideal; still, only about 20 percent of ovarian cancers are found before tumor growth has spread beyond the ovaries. The chance of surviving ovarian cancer is better if the cancer is found early.

Women have two ovaries, one on each side of the uterus. Each, about the size of an almond, produces eggs (ova) as well as the female sex hormones estrogen and progesterone. An ovarian tumor is a growth of abnormal cells that may be either noncancerous (benign) or cancerous (malignant).

Although benign tumors are made up of abnormal cells, these cells don't spread to other body tissues (metastasize). Ovarian cancer cells metastasize in one of two ways. Generally, they spread directly to adjacent tissue or organs in the pelvis and abdomen. They can also spread through your bloodstream or lymph channels to other parts of your body.

Three basic types of ovarian tumors exist, designated by where they form in the ovary:
- **Epithelial tumors.** About 85 to 90 percent of ovarian cancers de-

velop in the thin layer of tissue that covers the ovaries (epithelium), according to the American Cancer Society.
- **Germ cell tumors.** These tumors occur in the egg-producing cells of the ovary and generally occur in younger women.
- **Stromal tumors.** These tumors develop in the estrogen- and progesterone-producing tissue that holds the ovary together.

Causes
The exact cause of ovarian cancer remains unknown. Some researchers believe it has to do with the tissue repair process that follows the monthly release of an egg through a tiny tear in an ovarian follicle (ovulation) during a woman's reproductive years. The formation and division of new cells at the rupture site may set up a situation in which genetic errors occur. Others propose that the increased hormone levels before and during ovulation may stimulate the growth of abnormal cells. Research also suggests that many ovarian cancers may begin in the fallopian tubes rather than the ovaries.

Factors that may increase your risk of ovarian cancer include:
- **Inherited gene mutations.** Certain genetic abnormalities are known to increase your risk of ovarian cancer.
- **Family history.** Sometimes, ovarian cancer occurs in more than one family member but isn't the result of any known inherited gene alteration. Women with a family history of ovarian cancer or certain genetic mutations, such as BRCA 1 and 2, are at increased risk of the disease.
- **A history of breast cancer.** Women with breast cancer who have a BRCA mutation also have an increased risk of ovarian cancer.
- **Age.** Ovarian cancer most often develops after menopause. Your risk of ovarian cancer increases with age through your late 70s.

- **Childbearing status.** Women who have had at least one pregnancy have a lower risk of developing ovarian cancer. Similarly, the use of oral contraceptives appears to offer some protection against ovarian cancer.
- **Infertility.** If you've had trouble conceiving, you may be at increased risk. Although the link is poorly understood, studies indicate that infertility increases the risk of ovarian cancer, even without use of fertility drugs. Some research has also suggested that taking fertility drugs, such as clomiphene (Clomid), for more than one year may increase your risk of ovarian cancer, but it's not clear whether the increased risk actually comes from the drug or from the infertility.
- **Lack of prior hormonal contraceptive use.** The use of an oral contraceptive is associated with a reduced risk of ovarian cancer, a reduction that is more favorable with duration of use.
- **Obesity.** Women who are obese have a greater risk of ovarian cancer. Obesity may also be linked to more-aggressive ovarian cancers.
- **Menopausal hormone therapy.** There are no convincing findings that menopausal hormone therapy causes the development of ovarian cancer. Some studies have suggested that prolonged use of menopausal hormone therapy may be associated with an increased risk of ovarian cancer. However, research indicates that if such a link exists, the overall risk is slight.

Diagnosis

If your doctor suspects your symptoms suggest the presence of ovarian cancer, he or she may recommend one or more of the following tests to diagnose ovarian cancer:

- **Pelvic examination.** Your doctor examines your vagina, uterus, rectum and pelvis, including your ovaries, for masses or growths.
- **Ultrasound.** Ultrasound uses high-frequency sound waves to produce images of the inside of the body. Pelvic ultrasound provides a safe, noninvasive way to evaluate the size, shape and configuration of the ovaries. If a mass is found, however, ultrasound can't reliably differentiate a cancerous growth from one that's not cancerous. Ultrasound also can detect fluid in your abdominal cavity (ascites), a possible sign of ovarian cancer. Ascites develops in many conditions other than ovarian cancer, so its presence necessitates more testing.
- **CA 125 blood test.** CA125 is a protein made by your body in response to many different conditions. Many women with ovarian cancer have abnormally high levels of CA 125 in their blood. However, a number of noncancerous conditions also cause elevated CA 125 levels, and many women with early-stage ovarian cancer have normal CA 125 levels. Because of this lack of specificity, the CA 125 test isn't used for routine screening in average-risk women and is of uncertain benefit in high-risk women.

Other diagnostic tests may include computerized tomography (CT) and magnetic resonance imaging (MRI), which both provide detailed, cross-sectional images of the inside of your body. Your doctor may also order a chest X-ray to determine if cancer has spread to the lungs or to the pleural space surrounding the lungs, where fluid can accumulate.

How serious is ovarian cancer?

Early detection is very important. Only about 20 percent of ovarian cancers are found before tumor growth has spread beyond the ovaries. Your chance of surviving ovarian cancer is better if the cancer is found early.

Treatment

Treatment for ovarian cancer usually involves a combination of surgery and chemotherapy.

Surgery

Generally, women with ovarian cancer require an extensive operation that includes removing both ovaries, fallopian tubes and the uterus as well as nearby lymph nodes and a fold of fatty abdominal tissue (omentum), where ovarian cancer often spreads.

During this procedure, your surgeon removes as much cancer as possible from your abdomen (surgical debulking) — ideally, leaving less than a total of 1 cubic centimeter of abdominal cavity after surgery (optimal debulking). This may involve removing part of your intestines.

In addition, the surgeon takes samples of tissue and fluid from your abdomen to examine for cancer cells. This evaluation is critical in identifying the stage of your disease and determining if you need additional therapy.

If you want to preserve the option to have children and if your tumor is discovered early, your surgeon may be able to remove only the involved ovary and its fallopian tube. But, subsequent chemotherapy may cause infertility. However, in some cases, it is possible to successfully bear children after treatment. Be sure to discuss your desire to have children with your doctor.

Chemotherapy

After surgery, you'll most likely be treated with chemotherapy — drugs designed to kill any remaining cancer cells. The initial regimen for ovarian cancer usually includes the combination of carboplatin and the drug paclitaxel (Taxol) injected into the bloodstream (intravenous administration). Clinical trials have found this combination is effective, though researchers are continually looking for ways to improve on it.

A more intensive regimen has recently been shown to improve survival in women with advanced ovarian cancer by combining standard intravenous chemotherapy with chemotherapy injected directly into the abdominal cavity through a catheter placed at the time of the initial operation. This intra-abdominal infusion exposes hard-to-reach cancer cells to higher levels of chemotherapy than can be reached intravenously.

Side effects — including abdominal pain, nausea and vomiting — may leave many women unable to complete a full course of treatment or others to forgo treatment entirely. But even an incomplete course of this treatment may help women live longer.

Other treatments being explored include new chemotherapy drugs, vaccines, gene therapy and immunotherapy, which boosts the immune system to help combat cancer. The newest option, if standard chemotherapy fails, is a drug called bevacizumab (Avastin). It works by disrupting the blood supply to the tumor, possibly causing it to shrink.

Radiation

While a mainstay in the treatment of some other cancers, radiation generally isn't considered effective for ovarian cancer. Sometimes, your doctor may recommend radiation therapy to treat the symptoms of advanced cancer.

Vulvar cancer

Signs and symptoms

- A small, hard lump that may itch in the skin of the vulva
- An ulcer on the vulva with raised edges that may bleed or seep fluid

Vulvar cancer is a very uncommon cancer of the outer surface area of the female genitalia. The exact cause of vulvar cancer isn't known. As many as 60 percent of vulvar cancers have been linked to the sexually transmitted human papillomavirus (HPV) infection. Many times women with vulvar cancer have a precancerous skin condition called vulvar intraepithelial neoplasia in more than one area of the vulva before developing cancer.

Vulvar cancers that occur in older women that aren't linked to HPV infection may be related to a mutation or defect in the p53 tumor suppressor gene. This gene plays a role in keeping cells from becoming cancerous. This type of cancer may also be seen in women with lichen sclerosus — a condition that causes the vulvar skin to become thin and itchy.

Diagnosis

To check for vulvar cancer, your doctor will first conduct a physical examination, including a pelvic exam. If your doctor finds any irregularities, you'll likely need further testing, including a colposcopy and biopsy of the suspicious tissue.

How serious is vulvar cancer?

With effective treatment, and depending on the extent of the disease at diagnosis, there's a good chance of full recovery.

Treatment

Treatment options for vulvar cancer depend on the type and stage of cancer and include surgical removal of the tumor, radiation therapy, chemotherapy or a combination of these. The more advanced a vulvar cancer is, the more tissue that may need to be surgically removed.

Vaginal cancer

Signs and symptoms

- Persistent, localized itching on part of the vulva
- Watery discharge from your vagina
- Bleeding after intercourse or a pelvic examination
- Pain during intercourse
- A frequent or urgent need to urinate
- Painful bowel movements

Vaginal cancer is a rare cancer that occurs in your vagina — the muscular tube that connects your uterus with your outer genitals. Vaginal cancer most commonly occurs in the cells that line the surface of your vagina, which is sometimes called the birth canal. Factors that may increase the risk of vaginal cancer include being over the age of 60, having atypical vaginal cells (vaginal intraepithelial neoplasia), being exposed to the drug diethylstilbestrol for the prevention of miscarriage, having the human papillomavirus (HPV) and having previous gynecologic cancer, especially cervical cancer.

Diagnosis

If you have any signs and symptoms, your doctor may conduct a pelvic exam and a cervical cancer screen to check for abnormalities that may indicate vaginal cancer. Additionally, your doctor may conduct other procedures to determine whether you have vaginal cancer, such as colposcopy and a biopsy. Colposcopy is an examination of your vagina with a special lighted microscope called a colposcope. Biopsy is a procedure to remove a sample of tissue to test for cancer cells.

How serious are vaginal cancers?

They're rare but they can be deadly, especially if not detected and treated early.

Treatment

Because vaginal cancer is rare, no standard treatment guidelines have been developed. You and your doctor work together to determine what treatments are best for you based on your goals of treatment and the side effects you're willing to endure. Treatment for vaginal cancer typically includes radiation and surgery, although surgery is primarily used for early-stage vaginal cancer that is limited to the vagina. ■

Men's Health

The main biological function of the male reproductive system is to produce sperm cells and transport them to the female reproductive system. Unlike a woman, whose reproductive ability usually comes to a halt in midlife, a man is capable of reproducing well into old age. Once a male reaches sexual maturity, he produces sperm constantly.

Each time a man ejaculates, millions of sperm are propelled in the semen. Whether one sperm finds its way to an egg (ovum) and fertilizes it depends on several factors, including the number and quality of the sperm and there being no physical barriers during the sperm's trip from the penis into a woman's vagina and fallopian tubes. Fertilization depends also on whether the woman has recently released an egg from her ovaries (ovulated).

As with females, there's some overlap in function between the reproductive and urinary systems, with some organs used in each. Although uncommon, a genital disorder may cause urinary symptoms, and vice versa.

Reproductive Organs

The male reproductive organs include the penis, testicles, sac of skin that holds the testicles (scrotum), tubes through which semen passes (epididymides and vasa deferentia), prostate gland and seminal vesicles.

The penis has a sexual function and a urinary function. Urine and ejaculated semen both leave the body by way of the urethra, which runs through the length of the penis. The two can't, however, use this pathway at the same time. Just before ejaculation, the bladder squeezes shut at the bladder neck, preventing semen from going backward into the bladder.

The penis is made up of soft, spongy tissues. But when a man is sexually aroused, these tissues become engorged with blood, causing an erection. The penis becomes firm and gets longer and wider. With sufficient stimulation, the man ejaculates, sending semen through the urethra and out the opening in the head (glans) of the penis.

Semen is the ejaculated fluid that contains sperm. It's produced by the prostate gland and seminal vesicles. The amount produced depends to some extent on the amount of time between ejaculations. The average amount of semen ejaculated varies from $1/3$ to $1\frac{1}{2}$ teaspoons. This white, sticky fluid helps the sperm survive inside the vagina. The average ejaculation contains about 255 million sperm.

Sperm are produced in the testicles, two oval-shaped organs about 2 inches long. They're contained in a pouch of skin called the scrotum, which hangs below the abdomen and behind the penis. Each testicle contains a tightly packed mass of coiled tubes in which sperm are produced.

A human sperm is made up of a head — which contains the genetic material of the cell — a body and a tail. Sperm are microscopically small. It would take about 600 of them lined up end to end to measure an inch.

When a boy reaches puberty, his testicles begin to produce sperm cells. This process continues throughout his life. In addition to producing sperm cells, the testicles secrete the male hormone testosterone. Other hormones — chemical messengers — are produced in other parts of the body.

Testosterone plays an important role in the development and maintenance of masculine physical characteristics, such as facial hair, greater muscle mass and strength, and a deeper voice. It also influences body shape, sex drive and the ability to have an erection.

Inside the testicles are the cells that make sperm. These cells are extremely sensitive to temperature. Sperm production only takes place at a temperature that's lower than the normal temperature within the rest of the body. That's why the testicles are located outside the abdominal cavity.

Male Genital Organs

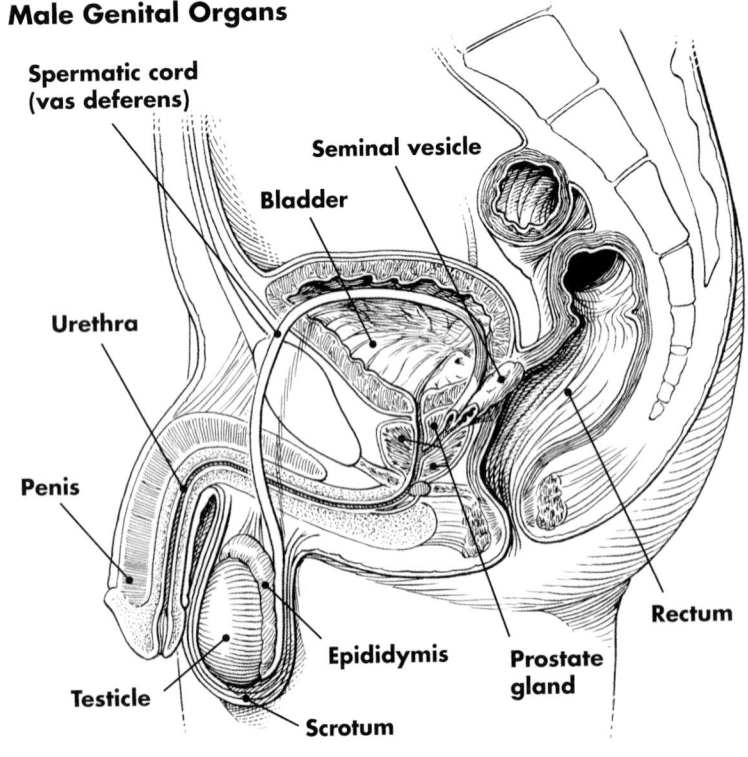

Spermatic cord (vas deferens)

Seminal vesicle

Bladder

Urethra

Penis

Testicle

Epididymis

Scrotum

Prostate gland

Rectum

1230　**PART IV: Diseases and Disorders**

The scrotal sac acts as a highly efficient thermostat, maintaining the temperature of the testicles slightly below the normal internal body temperature. When a man is cold, muscles in the scrotum contract to raise the testicles closer to the body to maintain adequate heat. When he's hot, the scrotum becomes larger and flaccid to expose more area for heat loss.

After being produced in a testicle, sperm travel to the

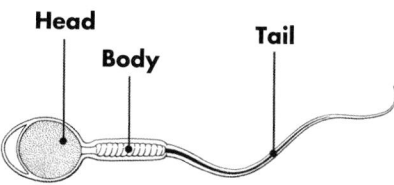

Head   **Body**   **Tail**

About ¹/₆₀₀ of an inch long, a human sperm is made up of a head — which contains the nucleus, or center, of the cell — a body and a tail to propel it.

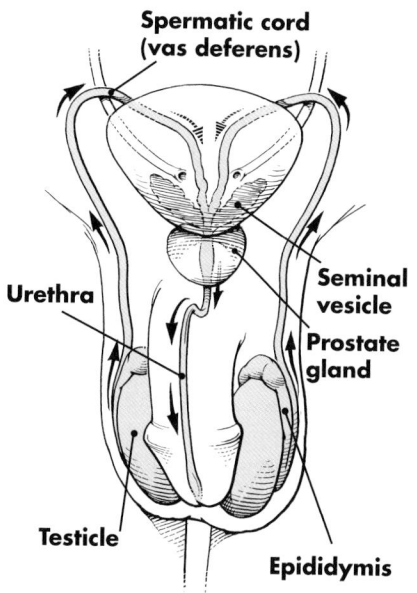

Spermatic cord (vas deferens)

Urethra

Seminal vesicle

Prostate gland

Testicle

Epididymis

From the testicle, sperm move by contractions through the epididymis and vas deferens. Fluids are added by the seminal vesicle and prostate gland. Semen is a combination of these fluids and sperm. Following sufficient sexual stimulation, a man ejaculates, sending semen through the urethra inside the penis and out the opening in the head of the penis.

epididymis, where they continue to mature and are stored. The epididymis is a long, coiled tube. A man has two of these organs, one attached to the top of each testicle. When sperm are ready, they're propelled by contractions out of these tubes and into the vasa deferentia.

The vasa deferentia are the conduits that carry sperm from the scrotum to the urethra. They're each about 18 inches long and run from the upper scrotum into the urethra at the base of the prostate. Millions of sperm enter the vasa deferentia every day.

The prostate gland surrounds the urethra. The prostate gland and seminal vesicles produce fluids that mix with sperm before ejaculation to make semen. After the semen is ejaculated from a man's penis into a woman's vagina, sperm cells search for a woman's egg to fertilize. The tail on the sperm whips to propel it. A sperm can travel an inch in four to 16 minutes in the vagina, depending on whether the female's cervical mucus is watery or thick. For pregnancy to occur, one sperm must penetrate an egg.

Preventing Pregnancy

Throughout history, men and women have tried — and not always successfully — to prevent pregnancy.

More than 1,500 years ago, a collection of Jewish writings known as the Talmud recommended that couples drink a beverage derived from roots to prevent pregnancy. Some American Indians brewed a special tea for those who wished to avoid conception.

And as early as the 1500s, Arabs were inserting into the vaginas of female camels an early version of today's intrauterine device in an effort to prevent an unwanted increase in the number of animals in the herd.

Today, many couples in the United States use some form of birth control (contraception). Some contraceptive methods depend on the actions of the woman. Three depend primarily on the actions of the man — a condom, withdrawing the penis from the vagina before ejaculation (*coitus interruptus*) and a vasectomy.

The Reproductive Process

The first step in reproduction is sexual arousal, which is regulated by a combination of psychological factors, sex hormones and physical stimulation. When a man is sexually stimulated, he gets an erection. During sexual intercourse he inserts his erect penis into a woman's vagina, and sexual excitement intensifies to the point of orgasm. It's usually during orgasm that ejaculation occurs. Muscles that surround the prostate gland and the seminal vesicles go through a series of involuntary contractions that suddenly propel the sperm-saturated semen through the urethra. This fluid traverses the length of the penis and is released into the vagina.

The vagina is flooded with millions of sperm swimming in all directions in search of an egg to fertilize. Most sperm die within the vagina and never even reach the woman's cervical canal — the opening between the vagina and uterus. Of those that make it to the 1-inch cervical canal, most never make it any farther. Only a few sperm reach the uterus and successfully make the journey midway down one of the fallopian tubes, where an egg is located if it's the time of the month when the woman has released an egg from an ovary (ovulated). When a sperm finds and penetrates an egg, fertilization has occurred and a pregnancy has begun. The sperm that fertilizes an egg has overcome enormous odds.

Condoms

About 10 to 15 percent of all couples practicing birth control use condoms. A condom is a thin sheath, usually made of latex (rubber), that's placed over the man's erect penis just before sexual intercourse. When the man ejaculates, the semen remains inside the condom and doesn't enter the vagina.

When used correctly, condoms are about 96 percent effective in preventing pregnancy. An added benefit is that condoms, if used properly, can help to protect against the spread of many sexually transmitted infections (STIs).

One reason condoms are so popular is that they're easy to buy. Condoms are available without a prescription in many stores. You can also buy them from vending machines in some restrooms. They come with or without a lubricant, are packaged in small or large quantities, and are available in several sizes.

They also come in various materials, including plastic and lambskin. Latex condoms offer the best protection from leakage and sexually transmitted infections. Packaged condoms are good for at least two to five years if they're kept in a cool, dry environment.

The proper use of a condom

If you decide to use a condom, make sure that as you unroll it onto the penis, you leave room at the tip for semen to collect. If you're uncircumcised, also make sure to pull back the foreskin before you put on the condom.

After intercourse, withdraw the penis from the vagina while holding the base of the condom so that the condom doesn't come off before your penis is out of the vagina. Then remove the condom and dispose of it.

Condom accidents can occur during intercourse, usually as a result of the condom breaking. The chance of such an accident can be reduced by:

- Allowing extra room at the condom's tip for semen to collect.
- Applying a water-based lubricant such as K-Y jelly on the condom after you've put it on, especially if your partner's vagina seems dry. An oil-based lubricant such as petroleum jelly or baby oil may weaken the latex material.

Using a condom with a spermicide gives you added protection against pregnancy. A spermicide is a sperm-killing cream that's inserted into the vagina before intercourse or used as a lubricant on the condom.

Withdrawal before ejaculation

Coitus interruptus means withdrawing the penis from the vagina before ejaculation. It's probably the oldest method of birth control — and one of the least effective. Although some couples have used *coitus interruptus* effectively, the overall failure rate is high, and most doctors don't recommend it. Aside from being frustrating for both partners, *coitus interruptus* requires that the man maintain stringent control. Even with excellent control and no ejaculation into the vagina, often small discharges of semen are released into the vagina, which can cause pregnancy.

Vasectomy

When couples make the decision not to have any more children — or not to have any children — they often consider sterilization. Either the man or the woman may be sterilized. The procedure in men is called a vasectomy. Compared with female sterilization (tubal ligation), a vasectomy is less physically traumatic and less expensive.

A vasectomy is an operation that can be done in an outpatient surgical setting. The procedure involves cutting and sealing the vasa deferentia, the two tubes that carry sperm from the testicles to the urethra. The procedure in no way interferes with your ability to maintain an erection or reach orgasm. The only change is that the transport of sperm has been interrupted, preventing it from mixing with semen.

In most cases, a man continues to ejaculate about the same amount of semen because sperm account for only a tiny part of the ejaculate. Sperm continue to be produced, but at a slower rate. The sperm are broken down and reabsorbed in the epididymis and a portion of the vas deferens.

How it's done

Before a vasectomy, you're given an injection of local anesthetic in the scrotum to numb the area. After your doctor locates the vasa deferentia, an opening is made in the skin of the scrotum. Each vas deferens is pulled through one of the openings until it forms a loop.

The two ends are separated using one of several techniques: removing a segment of the vas deferens, clipping the tubes, tying the vas deferens with a suture, cauterizing the ends, or sewing a layer of tissue between them.

The procedure takes about 20 to 40 minutes,

A Male Birth Control Pill?

Research into the use of hormonal and nonhormonal contraceptives for men has found the products to be highly effective. However, the entrance of male contraceptives into the marketplace has been stymied by costs, perceived regulatory obstacles and limited delivery methods. Still, many researchers believe reversible male contraception will become a reality in the future.

after which you may be asked to stay for a short time for observation. After a vasectomy, refrain from any strenuous activity for at least two days. If your work doesn't involve physical labor, you may be able to return to your job as soon as you feel able to.

You may notice some swelling, bruising and minor discomfort in your scrotum for several weeks. If the pain becomes severe or if you develop a fever, call your doctor. This may indicate an infection.

The failure rate for a vasectomy is less than 1 percent. But keep in mind that your vasectomy isn't an instant guarantee against pregnancy. That's because afterward you'll still have some sperm stored beyond the point where the vasa deferentia were severed.

In most men, the semen becomes sperm-free after eight to 10 ejaculations following the vasectomy. Your doctor will want to test your ejaculate for sperm a few weeks after the procedure. Until your doctor has determined that your ejaculate doesn't contain sperm, continue to use contraception.

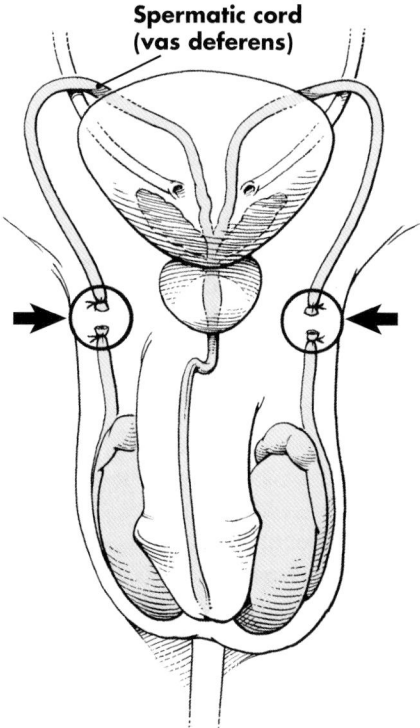

Spermatic cord (vas deferens)

In a vasectomy, the doctor severs and seals the spermatic cords (vasa deferentia), closing off the sperm's only paths to the outside.

Infertility

Doctors generally use the term *infertility* to describe the inability of a couple to conceive after a year of frequent sexual intercourse without using contraception. Infertility isn't the same as sterility, which means the inability to conceive a child under any circumstances. With infertility, the possibility of conceiving a child isn't ruled out.

Infertility is a common problem. Fortunately, major advances in treatment have made it a condition that can be overcome. Infertility may stem from problems with the sperm or egg or from difficulties in their union.

Ten to 15 percent of couples are infertile. Of such couples, the man is the infertile partner in about 30 percent of cases and contributes to the infertility problem in an additional 20 percent of cases. In both men and women, various factors can account for infertility.

Inadequate sperm

Forty percent of infertile couples have more than one cause of their infertility. Because of this, your doctor may begin a comprehensive infertility examination of both partners. The most common diagnostic test for men is semen analysis. Other tests may involve determining the man's level of testosterone and other hormones.

For a man to be fertile, his testicles must produce enough sperm, the sperm must be able to reach the seminal vesicles and the sperm must be ejaculated effectively into the woman's vagina. Male infertility tests attempt to determine if any of these steps are impeded.

The first step of your fertility evaluation is a general physical examination. This includes examination of the genitals and questions about your medical history, illnesses or disabilities, medications, and sexual habits. Your doctor may ask you for a specimen of ejaculated semen. To obtain this you masturbate or interrupt intercourse, and ejaculate semen into a container.

The fresh semen is analyzed in a laboratory. Technicians evaluate its quantity and color and search for evidence of infection or blood. Mainly, they analyze the sperm,

Reversing a Vasectomy

A vasectomy is done for permanent sterilization, but in most cases it is reversible. The success rate of a reversal procedure depends on several factors, the key factor being the duration of time that has passed since the vasectomy.

In some procedures, the two cut ends of the vas deferens are reattached (vasovasostomy). In other cases, the vasa deferentia need to be attached to the epididymis (vasoepididymostomy or epididymovasostomy). These procedures can take several hours, can be expensive and require the skill of a trained surgeon.

About 80 to 90 percent of men who have their vasectomies reversed do ejaculate semen that contains sperm. Pregnancy rates after reversal, however, range from 0 to 60 percent and depend on several factors, including the female partner's age, fertility and prior pregnancies, in addition to the number of healthy sperm produced and ejaculated by the male.

Consult your family doctor or a urologist — a specialist who treats urinary and male genital problems — for referral to a surgeon experienced in this procedure.

determining the concentration of sperm present in the ejaculate, their shape and their activity (motility). Sperm disorders include:

- **Azoospermia.** Azoospermia is the complete absence of sperm in the semen, generally due to a disorder of the testicles or a blockage in the passage leading from the testicles.
- **Oligospermia.** In this condition sperm are present in the semen but in smaller numbers, which may reduce the likelihood of fertilization.

Other causes

Sometimes the problem isn't one of infertility but a more general sexual problem. For example, you may be fertile but have erectile dysfunction — an inability to obtain an erection sufficient to have intercourse.

Premature ejaculation — ejaculation during foreplay or before the penis is very far into the vagina — also greatly reduces the chances of a sperm meeting an egg. In some men, sperm production is perfectly normal, but the sperm are ejaculated backward into the bladder rather than out the penis, called retrograde ejaculation (see page 1240). Or, no ejaculation occurs despite having an orgasm.

Another cause of male infertility is a varicocele, a swelling of the scrotum caused by enlarged (varicose) veins surrounding the testicle. The enlarged veins impair sperm production.

Several other problems with the testicles also can be responsible for infertility. Klinefelter syndrome is a relatively common genetic condition that affects the testes, impairing sperm production. Men who are carriers of the cystic fibrosis gene or who have cystic fibrosis may be missing one or more of the vasa, epididymides or seminal vesicles. Sexually transmitted infections (STIs) or other infections can block the passageways through which sperm travel, or they can injure or destroy sperm. Mumps and other infections can cause inflammation of one or both testicles that can permanently impair or prevent sperm production in the affected testicle.

In a small percentage of infertile men, the cause is a problem with the pituitary gland. The pituitary gland makes hormones that stimulate the testes to make sperm and testosterone. Abnormal production of these hormones can cause infertility.

Some medications can impair fertility, including some antihypertensive, psychotherapeutic and hormonal medications, in addition to some antibiotic, gastric and immunosuppressive drugs.

Substances such as marijuana and cocaine can reduce fertility, as can some products designed to build muscle. Alcohol and tobacco have milder impairments.

Treatment

Infertility can be treated in many ways. The type of treatment your doctor recommends will depend on what's causing the infertility. Improved therapies have increased the number of once infertile couples who are able to achieve pregnancy. Some causes of infertility can't be corrected, but even then, various means of insemination may be possible so that the woman can still become pregnant.

When the source of infertility is the man's sperm — or a lack of sperm — restoring or initiating fertility is sometimes possible. For example, a varicocele can be corrected surgically. Problems with the testicles, prostate gland, seminal vesicles and urethra also may be successfully treated.

In the rare instance when sperm production is impaired because of a pituitary gland problem, the hormones human chorionic gonadotropin and human follicle stimulating hormone have been helpful.

In some cases of abnormal sperm production, medications may be prescribed to improve the number and quality of sperm. Sometimes, however, too few sperm are produced and assisted reproductive technologies (ARTs)

Loss of Sexual Desire

Men can experience various physical problems that make it difficult to have sexual intercourse. But what if the urge to have sex goes away?

It's unusual for a man to have no sexual desire at all. But it's common for men to experience reduced desire. With increasing age most men experience somewhat diminished sexual desire, although this can vary greatly from one man to another.

The first cause to consider is a physical ailment. Illnesses that cause persistent pain, weakness or fatigue tend to reduce your sexual desire. So do emotional problems such as depression or difficulty dealing with stress. Antihormonal medications can reduce sexual desire. In addition, low testosterone levels can play a role. A blood test can measure testosterone levels.

Lack of enthusiasm from you or from your sexual partner also can lead to dampened desire. Or, you may experience a loss of desire because you don't tell your partner what arouses you or what stops your arousal. Also, your timing may be off. For example, you want to have intercourse when you or your partner is tired.

Loss of desire often can be cured. If you experience a continuing loss of sexual desire, don't assume that this is the natural course of events. Seek help from your doctor to search for the cause. You may benefit from counseling, changes in medication or other forms of therapy.

may be required. These include intrauterine insemination and in vitro fertilization with or without intracytoplasmic sperm injection (ICSI). ICSI involves injecting a single sperm directly into an egg to achieve fertilization.

Sexual Dysfunction

Sexual dysfunction refers to problems encountered during sexual intercourse that may be experienced by either the man or woman. For men, the most common problems are erection abnormalities and premature ejaculation.

The solution to sexual problems in either partner requires understanding and cooperation from both partners. One of the first steps in solving sexual problems in men is understanding the male sexual sequence and how it can be interrupted. The sequence involves:

- Stimulation
- Erection
- Orgasm with ejaculation
- Loss of erection

For men, the ability to function sexually depends on psychological, hormonal, neurologic and vascular factors. That's because the ability to have an erection is controlled by both the nervous system and vascular system, and sexual arousal is governed by a variety of hormones and psychological factors. If a man's hormone levels are low or if he is under a lot of emotional stress, he may lose interest in sex.

Ejaculation is controlled by the nervous system. The normal loss of an erection after sex is controlled by the neurological and vascular systems. Some neurological disorders and diseases of the urinary and reproductive systems directly interfere with sexual performance. Many other chronic diseases, such as diabetes and cancer, can impede a man's ability

to perform sexually because of their debilitating effect on overall health. Diabetes can also damage nerves that control an erection, as well as blood vessel function, blood supply and smooth muscle in the penis. The use of alcohol or some other drugs also may impair sexual function.

The good news is that effective treatments are available for most of the common causes of male sexual dysfunction.

Erectile dysfunction

Erectile dysfunction is a persistent inability to obtain an erection or to keep it long enough for sexual intercourse. Erectile dysfunction is commonly referred to as ED.

Diminished sexual desire or even the loss of sexual desire isn't the same as erectile dysfunction. ED refers to the inability to use the penis for sexual activity even when desire and opportunity are present.

It's important to realize that an occasional episode of erectile dysfunction happens to most men and is nothing to worry about. When it becomes a persistent problem, ED can hurt a man's self-image as well as his sex life. Erectile dysfunction is very common and it becomes increasingly common with age.

Sometimes, especially in younger men not affected by psychological factors, ED may signal a larger vascular health issue. It may indicate an increased risk of early heart disease, stroke or a related event.

The biology of an erection
To deal with ED, it's important to understand how an erection occurs. The penis has two cylindrical, sponge-like structures that run along its length. When a man is sexually aroused, nerve impulses cause the arteries in the penis to open larger and relaxed muscles cause more blood to enter. This sudden influx of blood expands the sponge-like structures and enlarges, straightens and stiffens

the penis, producing an erection. Continued sexual arousal maintains the higher rate of blood flow and closes the valves that would allow blood to drain from the penis, which maintains the erection.

After ejaculation, or when the sexual excitement passes, the excess blood drains out of the spongy tissue, and the penis returns to its nonerect size and shape.

Three important steps are necessary to produce the erection. The first is sexual arousal, which can come from the senses of sight, touch, hearing, taste and smell and

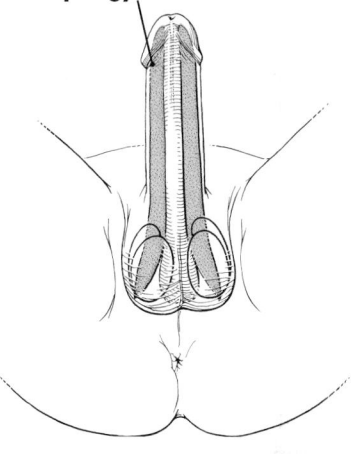

Spongy erectile tissue

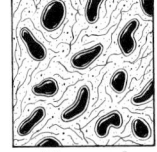
Normal tissue cells

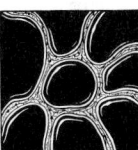
Engorged tissue cells

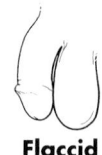
Flaccid

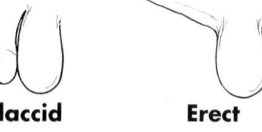
Erect

When a man is sexually aroused, two cylindrical, sponge-like erectile structures become engorged with blood. Veins that normally drain blood from the penis clamp down, keeping extra blood in the penis and maintaining the erection. After orgasm the excess blood drains from the spongy tissue, leaving the penis flaccid.

from thoughts. The second step is communication of the sexual arousal from nerves in the brain to nerves in the penis. The third step is a relaxing action of the smooth muscle in the penis and increased flow from blood vessels that supply the penis. If something affects any of these steps, ED can result.

Causes

Some causes of ED aren't physical. The most common nonphysical causes are stress and anxiety. If you can't relax and focus on the sexual situation, or if you're overwhelmed or confused by life circumstances, it's difficult for the three-stage erection process to take place. This happens to almost every man at some time.

ED is also an occasional side effect of psychological disorders such as depression. Other contributing factors include negative feelings toward the sexual partner, or expressed by the sexual partner, such as resentment, hostility or lack of interest.

The important thing is not to assume that an episode of ED means that you have a permanent problem and that you should expect it to happen repeatedly. The best thing to do if you experience an episode of ED is to treat it as something that happens once in a while to all men, and to expect a more successful experience at another time. ED isn't reflective of your self-worth or masculinity.

Physical conditions that account for most cases of ED include:
- Diabetes
- Vascular disorders
- Some prescription medications
- Surgery or radiation in the pelvic area, such as for prostate cancer
- A spinal cord injury
- Multiple sclerosis
- Hormone disorders
- Alcoholism and other forms of drug abuse
- Sleep apnea
- Normal aging

Physical and nonphysical causes can work together to trigger ED.

For example, a minor physical problem that slows sexual response might cause anxiety about attaining an erection, and the anxiety worsens the ED.

Diagnosis

If you experience recurring episodes of ED, consult your doctor. If your doctor suspects a nonphysical cause, he or she may ask if you get erections in other circumstances, such as during masturbation or while you're asleep. Most men experience many erections — without remembering them — during sleep.

If your doctor suspects a physical cause, you may have some blood tests. Your doctor may also want to measure hormone levels in your blood. Occasionally, additional tests such as an ultrasound exam may be performed. If your doctor suspects a prescription drug may be responsible for your ED, you may be prescribed a different medication.

Treatment

A variety of options exist for treating erectile dysfunction. These options range from medications and simple mechanical devices to surgery and psychological counseling. The cause and severity of your condition are important factors in determining the best treatment or combination of treatments for you.

You and your partner also may want to talk with your doctor about to what extent you're willing to go to improve your erections, including giving yourself injections in the penis or surgery.

Although the costs of treatments for ED vary, many mediations have generic alternatives available. If you find you're spending a significant amount of money on these therapies, talk to your doctor about less expensive alternatives. Insurance coverage varies. Treatments for erectile dysfunction may or may not be covered by your health insurance policy.

Oral medications

Oral medications are a successful erectile dysfunction treatment for many men. They include:
- Sildenafil (Viagra)
- Tadalafil (Adcirca, Cialis)
- Vardenafil (Levitra, Staxyn)
- Avanafil (Stendra)

All four medications enhance the effects of nitric oxide — a natural chemical your body produces that relaxes muscles in the penis. This increases blood flow and allows you to get an erection in response to sexual stimulation.

Taking one of these drugs won't automatically produce an erection. Sexual stimulation is needed first to cause the release of nitric oxide from your penile nerves. The medications amplify that signal, allowing some men to function normally.

Oral erectile dysfunction medications vary in dosage, how long they work and side effects. Possible side effects include flushing, nasal congestion, headaches, visual changes, backaches and stomach upset.

Your doctor will consider your particular situation to determine which medication might work best. The medications might not treat your erectile dysfunction immediately. You may need to work with your doctor to find the right medication and dosage for you.

Before taking any medication for erectile dysfunction, including over-the-counter supplements and herbal remedies, get your doctor's OK. Medications for erectile dysfunction don't work in all men and might be less effective in certain circumstances, such as after prostate cancer treatment or if you have diabetes. Some medications may also be dangerous if you:
- Take nitrate drugs — commonly prescribed for chest pain (angina) — such as nitroglycerin (Minitran, Nitro-Dur, Nitrostat, others), isosorbide mononitrate (Monoket) and isosorbide dinitrate (Dilatrate-SR, Isordil)
- Have severe heart disease or heart failure

Oral medications don't cure erectile dysfunction. Rather, they treat the symptoms. Often, they need to be taken from 30 to 60 minutes before anticipating intercourse and some of them should be taken on an empty stomach.

Prostaglandin E (alprostadil)
Two treatments involve using a drug called alprostadil. Alprostadil is a synthetic version of the hormone prostaglandin E. The hormone helps relax muscle tissue in the penis, which enhances the blood flow needed for an erection.

There are two ways to use alprostadil:

- **Self-administered intraurethral therapy (Muse).** This treatment involves using a disposable applicator to insert a tiny alprostadil suppository, about half the size of a grain of rice, into the tip of your penis. The suppository, placed about two inches into your urethra, is absorbed by erectile tissue in your penis, increasing the blood flow that causes an erection. Although needles aren't involved, you may still find this method painful or uncomfortable. It's also less effective than needle injection therapy. Side effects may include pain, minor bleeding in the urethra, dizziness and formation of fibrous tissue.
- **Needle-injection therapy.** With this method, you use a fine

Be Wary of 'Herbal Viagra'

After the medication Viagra was introduced in the late '90s, it quickly gained a reputation as an effective treatment for erectile dysfunction. A number of nonprescription products claiming to be "herbal Viagra" soon followed. Many of these products contain unknown quantities of potent ingredients similar to those in prescription medications, which can cause dangerous side effects. Some actually contain the real drug that should be given by prescription only. Although the Food and Drug Administration has banned several of these products, a number of other potentially dangerous erectile dysfunction remedies remain on the market.

Just because a product claims to be natural doesn't mean it's safe. Like prescription medications, many herbal remedies can cause side effects and dangerous interactions when taken with certain medications. Talk to your doctor before you try an herbal treatment for erectile dysfunction — especially if you're taking medications or you have any chronic health problems such as heart disease.

needle to inject medication into the base or side of your penis. The medication can be a single therapy such as alprostadil (Caverject Impulse, Edex), or it may be combined with other medications such as papaverine and phentolamine. Often these combination medications are known as bimix (if two medications are included) or trimix (if three are included).

Each injection is dosed to create an erection lasting no longer than an hour. Because the needle used is very fine, pain from the injection site is usually minor.

Side effects can include mild bleeding from the injection, prolonged erection (priapism) and, rarely, formation of fibrous tissue at the injection site.

Hormone replacement therapy
For men who have testosterone deficiency, testosterone replacement therapy may be an option.

Penis pumps
This treatment involves the use of a hollow tube with a hand-powered or battery-powered pump. The tube is placed over the penis, and then the pump is used to suck out the air. This creates a vacuum that pulls blood into the penis. Once you achieve an adequate erection, you slip a tension ring around the base of your penis to maintain the erection. You then remove the vacuum device. The erection typically lasts long enough for a couple to have sex. You remove the tension ring after intercourse.

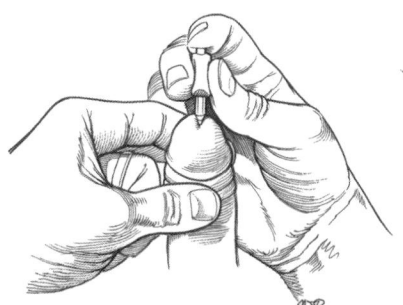

One therapy for impotence involves inserting a tiny suppository into the tip of your penis to help relax muscle tissue and increase blood flow to the penis.

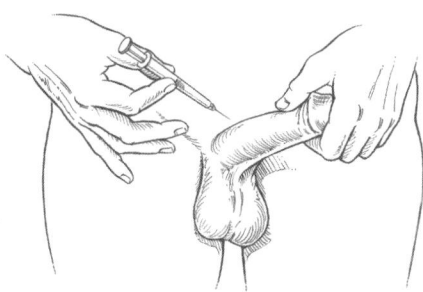

Self-injection therapy involves injecting medication directly into a specific area of the penis to increase blood flow and cause an erection.

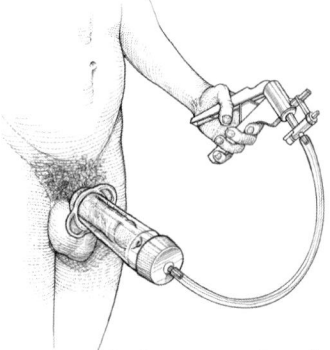

A vacuum device uses a hand pump to draw blood into the penis, creating an erection. An elastic ring placed at the base of the penis keeps it erect.

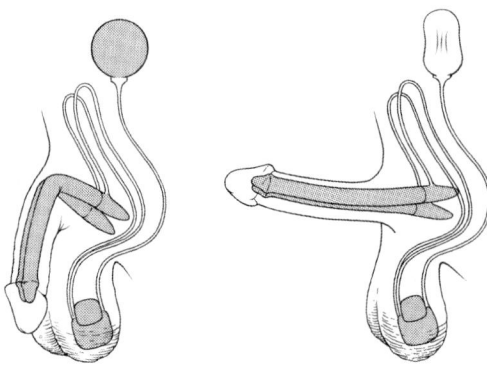

With some inflatable implants, you squeeze a pump located in the scrotum, causing fluid from a reservoir to fill inflatable cylinders in the penis and produce an erection. When an erection isn't wanted, the fluid is directed back to the reservoir.

Penile implants

This treatment involves surgically placing a device into the two sides of the penis, allowing an erection to occur as often and for as long as desired. These implants consist of either an inflatable device or semirigid rods made from silicone or polyurethane. The inflatable device allows you to control when and how long you have an erection, the semirigid rods keep the penis in a rigid state all the time. This treatment usually isn't recommended until other methods have been considered or tried first. As with any surgery, there is a small risk of complications such as an infection.

Psychological counseling and sex therapy

If stress, anxiety or depression is the cause of your erectile dysfunction, your doctor may suggest that you, or you and your partner, visit a psychologist or counselor with experience in treating sexual problems. Even if it is caused by something physical, erectile dysfunction can create stress and relationship tension. Counseling can help, especially when your partner participates.

Peyronie's disease

Peyronie's disease involves a curvature of the penis during an erection, which can be painful. The name comes from the French physician who first described the disorder.

Peyronie's disease occurs most often between the ages of 40 and 60 and can make sexual intercourse difficult or impossible. The disease is caused by scar tissue that forms inside the penis for unknown reasons. Sometimes, this tissue calcifies into hard lumps. The scar tissue and lumps are dense and firm and contract the adjacent lining of the penis. This may result in curvature, indentation or other deformities.

Peyronie's disease isn't related to any infection, tumor or contagious disease. Some researchers speculate that the problem might begin with mild trauma to the penis or from regular wear and tear on the penis that occurs with intercourse in men who are genetically susceptible. The condition is more common in men with ED, diabetes, or following prostate surgery or radiation.

How serious is Peyronie's disease?

The condition can prevent a man from having sex or might make it difficult to get or maintain an erection (erectile dysfunction). For many men, Peyronie's disease also causes stress, anxiety and depression.

In a small percentage of men, Peyronie's disease improves over time. But in most cases, it will remain stable or worsen.

Treatment

Treatment options include:

Medication

One medication has been approved by the Food and Drug Administration for the treatment of Peyronie's disease. It's called Clostridium histolyticum collagenase (Xiaflex). This medicine is approved for use in men with a palpable lump from plaque in the penis that causes a curvature of at least 30 degrees during erection.

The treatment works by breaking down the buildup of collagen that causes penile curvature. It involves a series of in-office injections, directly into the penile lump, as well as penile modeling — brief exercises to gently stretch and straighten the penis.

In clinical trials, collagenase therapy significantly reduced curvature and bothersome symptoms associated with Peyronie's disease in many participants. Discuss potential side effects of this medication with your doctor, as some of them can be serious.

Nondrug treatments

With several nondrug treatments for Peyronie's disease there's some evidence of improvements in penile curvature and length. This includes devices that stretch the penis (penile traction therapy) and vacuum devices. The therapies are likely most effective when used early in the course of the disease. More study is needed to know how effective they are after the disease is established.

Surgery

Surgery generally isn't recommended in the early phase of Peyronie's disease. Surgery may be an option if the deformity is severe or especially bothersome, or prevents you from having sex.

Surgical methods include:
- **Suturing (plicating).** A variety of procedures can be used to suture (plicate) the longer side of the penis (the side without

scar tissue). This can straighten the penis, but it might result in actual or perceived penile shortening. In some cases, plication procedures may worsen erectile function or penile sensation.

- **Incision or excision and grafting.** This procedure is used for more severe cases of Peyronie's disease. It's also like penile plication in that it may also reduce penile sensation and perceived penile size. A surgeon makes one or more cuts in the scar tissue, sometimes removing some of that tissue, allowing the sheath to stretch out and the penis to straighten. The surgeon may sew in a piece of tissue (graft) to cover openings within the penis.
- **Penile implants.** Penile implants might be considered if you have both Peyronie's disease and erectile dysfunction. The implants might be semirigid — manually bent down most of the time and bent upward for sexual intercourse. Another type of implant is inflated with a pump implanted in the scrotum.

Priapism

Priapism is a condition in which you have a sustained, often painful, erection that occurs without sexual stimulation. The term *priapism* comes from the Latin name for a male fertility god in ancient mythology, Priapus. The condition occurs most often as a reaction to injection therapies used to create an erection or to certain antidepressants or antipsychotic medications, but it may also occur as a result of a spinal cord disorder, leukemia, sickle cell anemia or inflammation of the urethra.

In one form of priapism the penile shaft is firm, but the head of the penis is soft. The penis becomes filled with blood as during a normal erection, but the blood doesn't drain out, and the erection doesn't go away as it normally should after sexual stimulation ceases.

How serious is priapism?
If an erection continues for several hours, blood trapped inside the penis may become thick because of oxygen loss. This can damage penile tissue.

If you have a painful erection that doesn't go away, seek medical help. Prompt treatment is necessary to preserve the ability of your penis to have a normal erection.

Treatment
Should you experience a prolonged erection, placing a towel-covered ice pack over the penis usually stops the erection. Taking an over-the-counter decongestant, such as pseudoephedrine (Sudafed, SudoGest, others) that causes your blood vessels to shrink also may relieve the condition. If these methods don't help and the erection continues for more than four hours, call your doctor or go to an emergency department. Blood may be with-

Blood in Semen

Blood in semen (hemospermia) alarms most men but is seldom something to worry about.

The color of semen in men with this condition ranges from pink to red. If you or your partner notice blood in your ejaculated semen but you have no other symptoms, the blood is usually nothing to worry about. If the bleeding continues or it comes back repeatedly, talk to your doctor. Your doctor may perform a thorough exam of your genital area, including your prostate gland and testicles. Other more extensive testing is rarely done.

Blood in semen can occur after a prostate biopsy. It usually clears after four to five ejaculations. If the source of blood in semen isn't clear, it probably comes from vessels lining the seminal vesicles and may be the result of harmless inflammation.

drawn from the penis using a needle.

If the erection recurs, other medications, such as adrenaline (epinephrine) can be used to constrict the blood vessels. In rare cases, a surgical procedure to allow blood to drain from the penis may be necessary. The longer you wait before seeking treatment, the greater the risk that damage may be done to the penile tissue.

Premature ejaculation

Premature ejaculation refers to ejaculation that occurs during foreplay with a sexual partner or soon after penetration. The only thing wrong with premature ejaculation is its timing — which is too soon, before either partner has had an opportunity to enjoy the sex act fully. In rare cases, merely touching a partner is enough to bring about ejaculation.

Premature ejaculation is a common sexual problem. It may be lifelong or something that's more recent. Premature ejaculation isn't necessarily a disease or disorder. It's only treated if the symptoms are distressing to you or your partner, or if you don't feel that you can control the condition.

Premature ejaculation and erectile dysfunction often occur together. When both are present, seek treatment for erectile dysfunction first, as this will often treat premature ejaculation.

Treatment
Common treatment options for premature ejaculation include behavioral techniques, condoms, medications and counseling. Behavioral treatment plus drug therapy is the most effective course.

Behavioral techniques
In some cases, therapy for premature ejaculation might involve taking simple steps, such as masturbating an hour or two before intercourse so that you're able to delay ejaculation during sex. Your

doctor also might recommend you and your partner use a method called the pause-squeeze technique. You begin sexual activity as usual, including stimulation of the penis, until you feel almost ready to ejaculate. At that time, have your partner squeeze the end of your penis, at the point where the head (glans) joins the shaft, and maintain the squeeze for several seconds, until the urge to ejaculate passes. Repeat the squeeze process as many times as necessary until you reach the point of entering your partner without ejaculating. After some practice sessions, the feeling of knowing how to delay ejaculation might become a habit, no longer requiring the pause-squeeze technique.

Condoms

Condoms might decrease penis sensitivity, which can help delay ejaculation. "Climax control" condoms available over the counter contain numbing agents or are made of thicker latex to delay ejaculation. Examples include Trojan Extended, Durex Performax Intense and Lifestyles Everlast Intense.

Medications

Anesthetic creams and sprays that contain a numbing agent, such as benzocaine, lidocaine or prilocaine, are sometimes used to treat premature ejaculation. These products are applied to the penis 10 to 15 minutes before sex to reduce sensation and help delay ejaculation.

Many medications might delay orgasm. Although none are specifically approved by the Food and Drug Administration to treat premature ejaculation, some are used for this purpose, including antidepressants and certain analgesics. These medications might be prescribed for on-demand or daily use, and might be used alone or in combination with other treatments.

Counseling

This approach involves talking with a mental health provider about your relationships and experiences. Sessions can help you reduce performance anxiety and find better ways of coping with stress. Counseling is most likely to help when it's used in combination with drug therapy.

Retrograde ejaculation and anejaculation

In retrograde ejaculation, little or no semen is ejaculated from the penis during a sexual climax. Instead, it travels backward into the bladder during ejaculation.

The word *retrograde* refers to the backward direction of the semen. Retrograde ejaculation is harmless. Semen that enters the bladder is simply expelled during urination. Retrograde ejaculation does, however, prevent fertility if no semen exits the penis. And it diminishes fertility if a decreased quantity of semen emerges.

Sometimes you can tell you have retrograde ejaculation by observing the urine that you void. If retrograde ejaculation has occurred, your urine will look cloudy because of the semen in it.

Retrograde ejaculation may occur with conditions such as diabetes or as a function of aging, or after certain prostate treatments to improve urine flow.

Anejaculation is similar to retrograde ejaculation in that you may not see anything when you ejaculate. It's often related to nerve damage to the organs that cause ejaculation and may occur with diabetes, spinal cord injury, pelvic surgery (including prostate surgery), or with certain medications used to improve urine flow or treat high blood pressure.

Treatment

Medications might work for retrograde ejaculation or anejaculation caused by nerve damage. These medications help keep the bladder neck muscle closed during ejaculation. Drugs generally won't help if the problem is due to surgery that causes permanent physical changes of your anatomy, such as prostate or bladder neck surgery.

If retrograde ejaculation or anejaculation stems from medication you're taking, switching to a different medication may solve the problem.

Infertility due to retrograde ejaculation that doesn't respond to medications may be managed with assisted reproductive techniques. Sperm may be retrieved directly from the testicles or from the bladder by way of a catheter immediately after ejaculation.

Testicular Injury

Because the testicles are located outside the abdomen, they're vulnerable to injury. Pain caused by striking the testicles is often severe.

Fortunately most injuries are minor. The sponginess of testicular tissues and the flexibility of their location generally enable them to absorb considerable shock without permanent harm.

If your testicles have been injured by a blunt object or in a fall and the pain and swelling of the scrotum go away within about an hour, there's probably no serious damage. If the scrotum remains swollen or is bruised or if the pain persists, seek prompt medical care. Untreated testicular injury can have serious complications, such as infertility or the loss of a testicle. If the scrotum has been penetrated by a sharp object, seek emergency care.

The same precautions apply to male babies and children. Persistent pain, swelling or bruising signal the need to see a doctor promptly. A young male can become infertile from an untreated testicular injury even though he hasn't reached sexual maturity.

Testicular and Scrotal Disorders

The testicles play two main roles. They produce sperm for reproduction, and they make hormones, such as testosterone, needed to generate and maintain masculine features.

The location of the testicles within the scrotum keeps them at a temperature slightly lower than inside your abdominal cavity — a requirement for healthy sperm. This relatively exposed location makes the testicles vulnerable to injury, but it also makes them easy to examine.

Sharp or sudden pain in your testicles can be a symptom of a serious condition, such as an infection or testicular torsion. See a doctor if the pain doesn't go away in 15 minutes or if it subsides but returns.

Testicular torsion

Signs and symptoms
- Sudden, severe pain in one testicle
- Elevation of one testicle within the scrotum

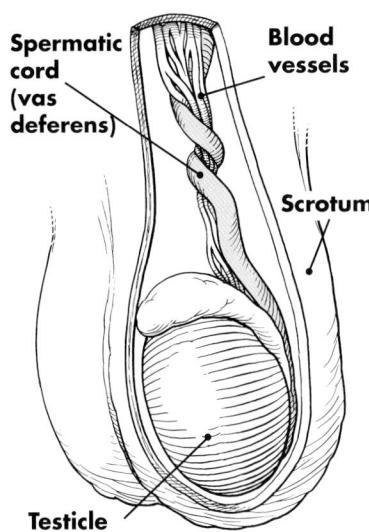

In testicular torsion, the testicle twists on its spermatic cord, cutting off the blood supply and producing sudden, severe pain.

- Swelling of a testicle
- Nausea and vomiting
- Faintness
- Fever

Each testicle is suspended in the scrotum on a spermatic cord that contains the vas deferens and blood vessels supplying the testicle. In a condition called testicular torsion, the testicle twists on its spermatic cord, closing off the blood supply to the testicle. Testicular torsion may occur without any apparent cause, even during sleep. At other times it happens after strenuous physical activity.

Diagnosis
To distinguish testicular torsion from other conditions affecting the testicles, your doctor may order an ultrasound examination of the testicle. Or you may need surgery to confirm the diagnosis.

How serious is testicular torsion?
If testicular torsion isn't corrected within a few hours — often by an operation — the testicle can be permanently damaged from a lack of blood supply and may even have to be removed. Severe pain in a testicle for no apparent reason or after strenuous physical activity requires prompt medical attention.

Treatment
Even if your doctor is able to manipulate the twisted testicle back to its normal position, you may need an operation to secure the testicle and prevent a recurrence. During surgery, the surgeon anchors the testicle in its normal position. The other testicle also may be anchored to prevent possible torsion of that testicle.

Testicular failure

Signs and symptoms
- Erectile dysfunction
- A lack of sex drive
- A delay of or the absence of puberty

- Loss of masculine characteristics
- Difficulty putting on muscle
- Increased fat mass
- Diabetes
- Osteoporosis
- Infertility
- Anemia
- Fatigue
- Concentration impairment

The term *testicular failure* refers to the inability of the testicles to produce sperm and, in some cases, male hormones. This condition may stem from chromosome abnormalities present before birth, problems involving sexual maturation, or damage to normally developed testicles from disease, drugs or injury.

If testicular failure occurs in childhood, sexual maturation may be delayed or absent. In adults, testicular failure can cause a variety of conditions or disorders.

Diagnosis
Testicular failure is one of many possible causes of infertility. To find out if a couple's infertility is caused by testicular failure, your doctor will likely interview and examine both sexual partners and perform blood and semen tests.

The diagnosis may be revealed by the history gathered during the interview. In addition, it may emerge after a physical examination and other tests.

How serious is testicular failure?
Testicular failure isn't immediately life-threatening. However, it can cause a variety of conditions that can contribute to emotional problems and can shorten your lifespan in the long term.

Treatment
If you have testicular failure, administering testosterone can often help treat symptoms that you may be experiencing. Testosterone won't restore fertility, but other medications that boost testosterone by other means may be used to improve fertility.

Epididymitis

Signs and symptoms
- Pain in the scrotum, generally severe, which develops gradually over several hours or days
- Pain, often limited to one testicle
- Fever
- Swelling of a testicle
- Pain during urination

At the top and rear of each testicle is a coiled tube called the epididymis, which transports sperm to the vas deferens. Epididymitis is an inflammation of this tube.

The swollen area will feel hot and sausage-shaped to the touch. Bacteria can cause epididymitis, but often the cause is unknown.

Diagnosis
Your doctor may take a urine sample and a sample of prostate gland secretions in an attempt to identify an infecting organism.

How serious is epididymitis?
Epididymitis usually comes on suddenly and can be corrected with medication. In some cases, epididymitis can lead to a blockage of sperm and impair fertility on the side where it occurs. Occasionally, long-lasting (chronic) epididymitis develops. Surgical treatment is rarely necessary with chronic epididymitis.

Treatment
If bacteria are the culprits, antibiotics are prescribed to treat the infection. Additional treatment may include bed rest, application of ice packs to the scrotum, elevation of the scrotum and over-the-counter anti-inflammatory medication. Because your sex partner may be infected with the same bacteria, treatment of your partner may be recommended as well.

Scrotal masses

Signs and symptoms
- A lump or swelling in the scrotum
- Local pain or tenderness

A lump in the scrotum can stem from any number of problems, including a tumor, physical injury, cyst, infection or inguinal hernia. The tumors may be noncancerous (benign) or cancerous (malignant). A tumor growing inside a testicle is most often cancerous. Those located elsewhere in the scrotum are generally noncancerous.

A common type of painless, benign cyst is a spermatic cyst (spermatocele). It's located in the epididymis, near the top of a testicle. Other benign sources of scrotal swelling include hydroceles, hematoceles and varicoceles.

A hydrocele is a collection of watery fluid. A hematocele is a pocket of blood caused by physical injury to the scrotum or a testicle. A varicocele is a swelling in the scrotum caused by enlarged (varicose) veins. With an inguinal hernia, a section of intestine can sometimes drop into the scrotum and appear as a scrotal mass.

Diagnosis
Every scrotal mass should be evaluated. Tests such as an ultrasound examination help to distinguish the many harmless causes of scrotal masses from serious tumors. Sometimes holding a light next to the scrotum can aid in diagnosis. If the light shines through, the mass is probably not cancerous but something less serious, such as a hydrocele. A mass within the testicle usually must be removed surgically before an accurate diagnosis can be made.

How serious are scrotal masses?
Cancerous tumors are serious and can be fatal. For more on testicular cancer, see page 1244.

Treatment
Many scrotal masses don't require any treatment unless they cause discomfort. Some problems require surgery. Testicular cancer requires surgical removal of the entire testicle and possibly additional treatment as well. Inguinal

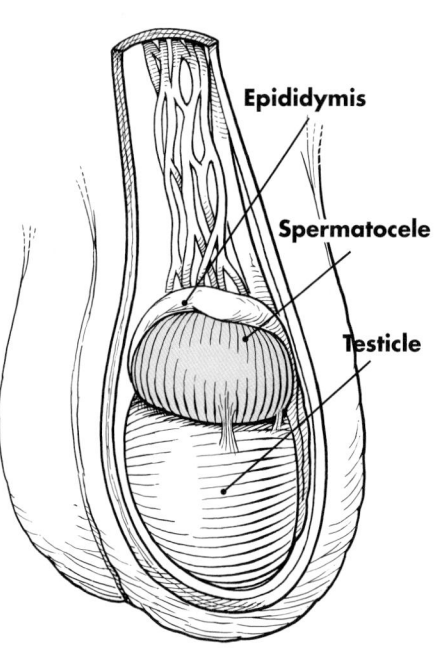

A painless, noncancerous, fluid-filled enlargement above the testicle is called a spermatic cyst (spermatocele).

hernias also generally require surgical repair.

Hydrocele

Signs and symptoms
- Soft, usually painless, swelling in the scrotum

The term *hydrocele* comes from the Greek terms *hydro* for "water" and *cele* for "tumor" or "cavity." A testicular hydrocele is a collection of watery fluid in the sheath around the testicle. Normally, this sheath contains a tiny amount of fluid. An excessive amount, which produces the hydrocele, develops because your genital area produces too much fluid due to trauma, because it doesn't absorb enough fluid or because the sac surrounding the testicle is too big.

Hydroceles are a common cause of scrotal swelling, and they may occur on one or both testicles. Hydroceles can occur at any age but are most common in young boys and older men.

Diagnosis
To help differentiate a hydrocele from a tumor or another source

of swelling, your doctor will feel the swollen area. An ultrasound examination also may be done.

How serious are hydroceles?
Hydroceles aren't serious. Treatment usually isn't required unless the scrotum is so swollen that it's uncomfortable.

Treatment
If the size of the hydrocele is large enough that it's impacting your quality of life, you may wish to seek treatment. Treatment generally involves a surgical procedure where the sac surrounding the testicle is reduced in size. Possible complications of surgery include infection, recurrence of the fluid or minor bleeding.

Varicocele

Signs and symptoms
- Painless swelling in the scrotum, usually on the left side
- An area of the scrotum that feels like a bag of worms — a sensation that may nearly disappear when you lie down

A varicocele is a swelling in the scrotum caused by enlarged (varicose) veins. Due to a problem with tiny valves inside the veins, blood backs up in the veins that lead from the testicles.

Diagnosis
Your doctor will examine the swollen scrotum. On occasion an ultrasound examination may be performed, especially if the condition develops rapidly.

How serious is a varicocele?
In most instances, a varicocele isn't a dangerous condition. But in some cases, it can signify something more serious taking place, such as a kidney or abdominal tumor or a blood clot.

Treatment
Unless a varicocele is associated with infertility or causes pain or one of the testicles is significant-

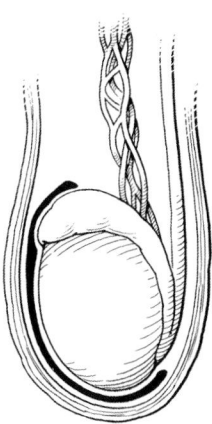 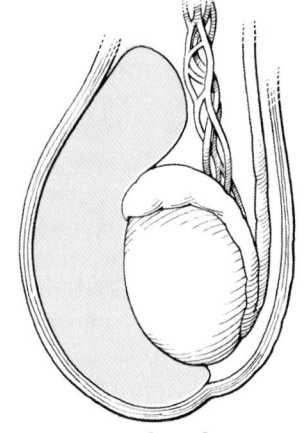 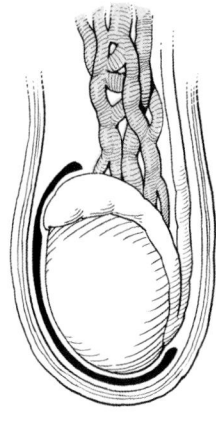

| Normal testicle | Hydrocele | Varicocele |

A hydrocele (middle) is a harmless but abnormal accumulation of watery fluid within the scrotum. It usually requires no treatment. Varicocele (right) is a swelling in the scrotum due to enlarged (varicose) veins. This condition may require treatment to prevent infertility.

ly smaller, treatment is rarely necessary. When infertility occurs, surgery to tie off the enlarged veins may be necessary. Another treatment, which is less successful, involves making an incision and inserting a tiny blocking object directly into a vein to cut off an excessive flow of blood.

Orchitis

Signs and symptoms
- Pain in a testicle
- Swelling, generally on one side of the scrotum only
- A heavy feeling in the scrotum

Orchitis is an inflammation of the testicle, usually due to a bacterial infection or the mumps virus. Orchitis may also develop if you have an infection of the prostate gland or epididymis.

Diagnosis
Your doctor will likely examine your scrotum. Because symptoms of orchitis are similar to those of epididymitis and other conditions affecting the testicles, your doctor may take a urine sample and perform other tests to identify associated infections.

How serious is orchitis?
Orchitis can permanently dam-

age one or both testicles, possibly resulting in infertility or reduced testicular size.

Treatment
Orchitis caused by a bacterial infection is treated with antibiotics. Orchitis associated with mumps or other viral infections is usually treated with rest and medication to relieve pain and reduce inflammation.

Undescended testicle

Before birth the testicles develop inside the male infant's abdomen. About a month before birth, the testicles usually move into their permanent place in the scrotum.

A small percentage of male infants, however, are born with one or both testicles undescended. In most of these babies, the testicles descend into the scrotum during the first few months of life, without any medical intervention. If the testicle hasn't moved into the scrotum by the time your son is 4 months old, the problem probably won't correct itself.

Diagnosis
Your doctor can confirm the absence of or stunted development of a testicle by feeling the scrotum.

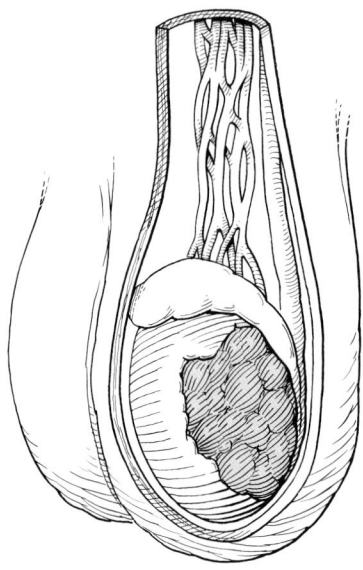

A lump in a testicle may indicate cancer.

Other tests may be required before determining the appropriate action for correcting the condition.

How serious is an undescended testicle?

A testicle that remains undescended might not produce sperm later in life, and the normally descended testicle also may have impaired sperm production. An undescended testicle — even one that has been corrected naturally or surgically — is more vulnerable to cancer than is a normal testicle.

Treatment

An undescended testicle is usually corrected with surgery. The surgeon carefully manipulates the testicle into the scrotum and stitches it into place (orchiopexy). When your son has surgery will depend on a number of factors, such as his health and how difficult the procedure might be. The surgeon will likely recommend doing the procedure when your son is about 6 months old and before he is 12 months old. Early surgical treatment appears to lower the risk of later complications.

Testicular cancer

Signs and symptoms
- A lump in a testicle
- Swelling of a testicle
- A heavy feeling in a testicle

Cancer of a testicle often begins in the cells that produce sperm. In its early stages, this type of cancer has no symptoms. The first noticeable sign is often a hard lump in a testicle. Most men discover the lump themselves during a self-examination.

Generally, testicular cancer affects only one testicle. It's more common among men ages 15 to 35, and it's more common in white men than in black men. If one or both testicles are undescended at birth, the risk of cancer in either testicle is increased. If testicular cancer is detected and treated early, it often can be cured.

Diagnosis

A self-examination can often detect the presence of a growth or tumor within the scrotum. An ultrasound examination may be performed to help in the diagnosis. A tumor in the testicle is almost always cancerous, but other conditions affecting the testicles and scrotum can produce a lump that feels quite similar.

How serious is testicular cancer?

The most common type of testicular cancer, seminoma, can be cured in nearly all cases if it's discovered and treated early. When all types of testicular cancers are considered, including cancers discovered at a late stage, about 90 percent of men with this condition will live for five years or more after treatment.

Treatment

Surgical removal of a cancerous testicle is necessary. Blood tests, computerized tomography (CT) scans and other tests may be necessary to determine if the cancer has spread to other parts of the body.

Removing a testicle doesn't cause any loss of virility because the remaining healthy testicle can maintain the body's normal sexual and hormone-producing functions. If both testicles are lost, infertility will result, but replacement of male hormones can maintain normal sexual function.

Chemotherapy, radiation and additional surgery may be advised to

Sexually Transmitted Infections

Sexually transmitted infections (STIs) are diseases that are passed on by contact with an infected person through vaginal intercourse, anal intercourse or oral sexual activity. In the case of human immunodeficiency virus (HIV) and AIDS, possible additional routes of transmission include infected semen and blood and needles shared for illegal intravenous (IV) drug use.

Symptoms of sexually transmitted infections may not develop immediately, and the course and consequences of the infections vary. For more information on STIs, see Chapter 16, "Infectious Diseases."

Proper use of a condom during sexual activity offers protection against acquiring or passing along an STI. But condoms don't provide foolproof protection. You can avoid STIs by being abstinent or engaging in sexual activity only with a noninfected partner. AIDS and HIV can be avoided by not sharing needles used for inappropriate use of drugs.

Testicular Self-Examination

Cancer of the testicles is a potential killer. But if detected early, it can usually be treated successfully. A simple self-examination that takes only one or two minutes can detect a growth in the testicles in its early stages. Like the breast self-examination for women, self-examination of the testicles is important. Because cancer of the testicles often occurs in younger men, monthly self-examination of the testicles should begin in the teen years.

Perform the examination after a warm shower or bath, when the skin of the scrotum is loose and relaxed. Examine one testicle at a time. Grasp the testicle and roll it gently between your thumb and forefinger. As you do so, feel for any lump on the surface of the testicle. Also notice if the testicle is enlarged, hardened or, if you've done a self-exam before, somehow different than it was during your last examination. If you feel a lump on a testicle or any change in the testicle, you don't necessarily have cancer. However, do see your doctor about it as soon as possible.

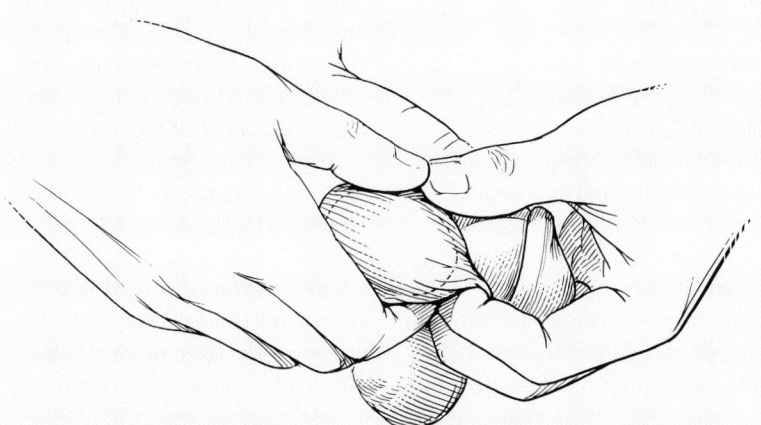

Grasp and roll the testicle between your thumb and forefinger, feeling for lumps, swelling, hardness or other changes.

prevent the spread of cancer or treat it if it has already migrated to other parts of the body. Even with cancer that has spread, chemotherapy can be very effective in destroying the cancer. For more information on radiation and chemotherapy, see Chapter 15, "Cancer."

Penile Disorders

The penis is both a sexual organ and urinary tract organ. Infections and other conditions can sometimes interfere with its functions, causing a variety of signs and symptoms.

Penile warts

Signs and symptoms
• Warts on the penis
Warts on the penis are similar to those found elsewhere on the body. All warts, including penile warts, are caused by viruses. This means that penile warts are contagious and may be transmitted during sexual activity. If you have penile warts, you and your sexual partner may require treatment.

Diagnosis
Penile warts are diagnosed on the basis of their appearance. Sometimes, however, a growth on the penis that looks like a wart may instead be a sign of another sexually transmitted infection or even a cancerous tumor. Warts that aren't visible may become visible when they're dabbed with vinegar (acetic acid), showing up as a white patch. Your doctor may use this procedure to help find warts that aren't easily seen otherwise.

How serious are penile warts?
Penile warts can spread to a sexual partner and can proliferate on your penis. Women are at increased risk of cervical cancer when exposed to the virus that causes penile warts. Vaccines are currently available against many of the viruses that cause penile warts and cervical cancer.

Treatment
Your doctor may prescribe a preparation that's applied to the warts to remove them. Other treatments include laser surgery, freezing the warts or destroying the warts with electrical current. These procedures may require local or general anesthesia.

Balanitis

Signs and symptoms
• Irritation and redness of the head of the penis
Balanitis is an inflammation of the head of the penis. It's a fairly common genital problem, especially in uncircumcised males whose foreskin is narrowed so that it can't be easily pulled back for cleaning.

Balanitis has many causes, including yeast or bacterial infection, reaction to contraceptive creams, and irritation from clothing that rubs against the penis or from chemicals used in the cleaning or manufacturing of clothing. Men with diabetes are especially prone to balanitis, although it's unclear why.

Diagnosis

If you have an inflammation of the penis that doesn't go away in a week or so, see your doctor or a urologist — a specialist who treats urinary and male genital problems. He or she will examine your penis and may perform some tests to help establish the cause of the inflammation.

Treatment

Antibiotics or antifungal agents are used to cure bacterial or yeast infections responsible for the inflammation. In an uncircumcised man whose foreskin doesn't easily retract, circumcision may be necessary to cure balanitis and prevent its recurrence.

Phimosis

Phimosis is a condition in which the uncircumcised foreskin covers the penis so tightly around its head that the foreskin can't be pulled back to expose and clean it. Sometimes this condition can interfere with urination and sexual activity.

Phimosis is fairly common in newborn boys. The foreskin normally loosens up in time, without treatment. In older boys and men, the foreskin may shrink or tighten because of an inflammation. Sometimes this requires circumcision.

Paraphimosis

Paraphimosis occurs when tight foreskin of an uncircumcised penis is pulled back and can't be returned over the head of the penis. This can cause painful swelling at the tip of the penis. If you experience severe swelling in the end of the penis, seek emergency medical help.

Surgical treatment by circumcision or partial circumcision may be necessary to release the foreskin. If treatment is prompt, permanent damage to the penis generally can be prevented.

Cancer of the penis

Signs and symptoms

- A painless ulcer, nodule or wart-like bump on the penis

Cancer of the penis is rare. When it occurs it's almost always in uncircumcised males. In its early stages, small, painless growths occur on the penis, usually near its tip. As the cancerous (malignant) growth progresses, you may experience pain and bleeding.

Diagnosis

Through examination, testing and possible surgical removal of the growth, your doctor can determine if it's malignant. If it is, more tests can determine if the cancer has spread to other parts of your body.

How serious is cancer of the penis?

Like any other cancer, penile cancer can be life-threatening. The earlier it's detected and treated, the better your chances of recovery.

Treatment

Removal of the malignant growth, and possibly of portions of the penis surrounding the growth, will likely be necessary. Often, enough of the penis can be left to allow for sexual activity and normal urination. Surgery, chemotherapy or radiation therapy may be used to prevent or control the spread of the disease to other parts of the body. For more information on chemotherapy and radiation therapy, see Chapter 15, "Cancer."

Prostate Gland Disorders

The prostate is a walnut-sized gland located in the pelvic area, just below the outlet of the bladder. Present only in males, the prostate gland surrounds the urethra, the tube that carries urine from your bladder out your penis. The prostate gland plays an important role in the reproductive process, producing the majority of the fluid that blends with sperm to create semen.

Prostatitis

Signs and symptoms

- Pain in the lower back and area between the rectum and scrotum
- Pain or a burning sensation while urinating
- Frequent and difficult urination
- An urgent need to urinate
- A sudden moderate to high fever
- Chills
- Occasionally, blood in urine

Prostatitis is an inflammation of the prostate gland. The inflammation may be due to an infection or another factor that's irritating the gland. Although many things are unclear about the disease, an accurate diagnosis is crucial to successfully treating it. Prostatitis is classified into four categories:

Acute bacterial prostatitis

Acute bacterial prostatitis is the most severe form of the disease. It results from an infection in the prostate gland that produces severe and often sudden symptoms. Bacteria found in the urinary tract or large intestine are often responsible for this type of infection.

Chronic bacterial prostatitis

Chronic bacterial prostatitis also results from a bacterial infection. Unlike acute bacterial prostatitis, its symptoms typically develop more slowly, and they're often less severe. The cause of the infection usually isn't clear. It may result from bacteria in your urinary tract, a bladder infection or a blood infection. The infection may also follow trauma to your urinary tract or insertion of an instrument such as a catheter or cystoscope.

Chronic nonbacterial prostatitis

Chronic nonbacterial prostatitis is the most common form of

prostatitis. Unfortunately, it's also the most difficult to diagnose and treat. Symptoms tend to be similar to those of chronic bacterial prostatitis, but one distinguishing factor separates the two. With nonbacterial prostatitis there's no evidence of bacteria in your urine or in fluid from the prostate gland, but white blood cells identified in urine specimens may signal the presence of inflammation.

Prostatitis vs. Painful Prostate

Sometimes men who see a doctor for what appears to be prostatitis may actually have a condition called painful prostate (prostatodynia, or prostatalgia). Men with this condition often refer to their symptoms as pain "down there," meaning anywhere in the genital (perineal) area. Symptoms typically mimic those of chronic nonbacterial prostatitis. The difference is that with prostatodynia, urine and prostate fluid samples show no evidence of infection or inflammation. Bacteria or white blood cells aren't detectable in the samples.

Rather than being a problem with your prostate gland, prostatodynia may instead stem from your pelvic floor muscles. When you're under stress, you may not completely relax the pelvic floor muscles supporting your bladder and urethra, causing urination difficulties. Many men with prostatodynia tend to be hard driven, tense and stressed. Prostatodynia also seems to occur more frequently among marathon runners, bicyclists, weightlifters and truck drivers.

Treatment for prostatodynia is similar in many ways to treatment for chronic nonbacterial prostatitis. Your doctor may also recommend physical therapy to help you relax your pelvic floor muscles and stress management to help you prevent and cope with stress.

Possible causes include other infectious agents, heavy lifting, occupations or hobbies that irritate the gland, interstitial cystitis (see page 915), or structural abnormalities of the urinary tract.

Asymptomatic inflammatory prostatitis
It's usually found during examination done for another reason. It often doesn't require treatment.

Diagnosis
Prostatitis is generally diagnosed by feeling the prostate gland. To do this your doctor inserts a gloved finger into your rectum and feels the outside wall of the gland. An inflamed prostate usually feels enlarged and tender. You may also need to provide urine and semen samples to check for bacteria that may be causing the infection.

How serious is prostatitis?
Left untreated, acute bacterial prostatitis can cause serious problems, including an inability to urinate. Chronic prostatitis tends to be more frustrating and debilitating. Without treatment, chronic bacterial prostatitis can lead to serious infection.

Treatment
Antibiotics are used to treat bacterial prostatitis caused by bacteria.

Some doctors prescribe antibiotics for chronic nonbacterial prostatitis to see if symptoms improve. For unknown reasons, some men with this condition seem to benefit from a continuous low dose of an antibiotic. If you're having difficulty urinating, your doctor may also prescribe an alpha blocker to help relax the bladder muscle. Muscle relaxants may be prescribed if your prostatitis is accompanied by pelvic muscle spasms.

In some men, certain pelvic exercises and relaxation techniques can improve symptoms of prostatitis, perhaps because tight or irritated muscles can contribute to the condition. Only in very severe cases when other treatments don't work, a doctor might consider surgical removal of the prostate.

Benign prostatic hyperplasia

Signs and symptoms
- Frequent or urgent need to urinate
- Difficulty starting urination
- Weak urine stream that stops and starts
- Increased frequency of urination at night (nocturia)
- Dribbling at the end of urination

Emergency signs and symptoms
- An inability to urinate

The prostate gland tends to enlarge with age. Enlargement

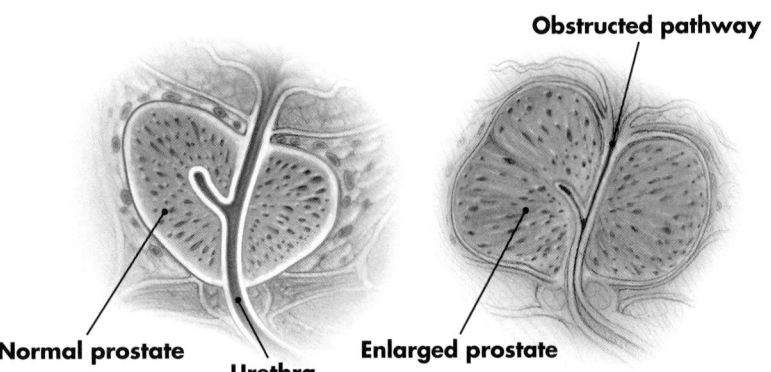

Obstructed pathway

Normal prostate

Urethra

Enlarged prostate

The urethra, the tube that drains the bladder, is surrounded by the prostate gland. Benign prostatic hyperplasia (BPH) results when tissues in the center of the prostate gland enlarge and press on the urethra, obstructing normal urine flow.

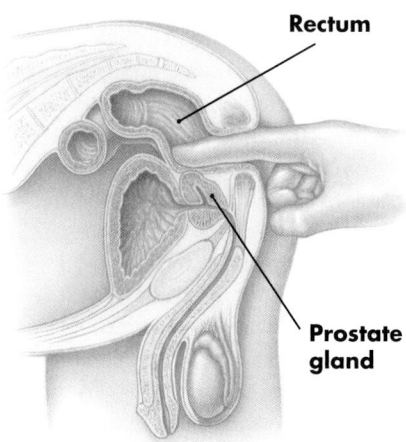

During a digital rectal exam, your doctor inserts a gloved, lubricated finger into your rectum and feels the back wall of the prostate gland for enlargement, tenderness, lumps or hard spots.

usually begins around age 50. In some men it may not occur until their 70s or 80s.

Noncancerous enlargement of the prostate is called benign prostatic hyperplasia (BPH). The word *benign* distinguishes this condition from prostate cancer. *Hyperplasia* means an increase in size.

Most men have continued prostate growth throughout their lives. In many men, the continued growth enlarges the prostate enough to cause urinary symptoms, which may require treatment.

Symptoms vary in severity from slight to severe. At first the symptoms tend to be only annoying. As the prostate continues to grow, they gradually worsen.

Diagnosis

Your doctor will likely ask about your prostate symptoms. He or she will likely also examine your prostate gland by inserting a gloved finger into your rectum and feeling the size and firmness of the gland. You might also be given a test to determine the strength of your urine flow and a prostate-specific antigen (PSA) blood test. The test assesses the possibility that cancer of the prostate is contributing to your symptoms.

How serious is BPH?

BPH isn't life-threatening unless symptoms become severe, making it difficult or impossible to urinate. Retention of urine increases your risk of developing urinary tract infections, which may damage your kidneys.

Treatment

Treatment for BPH depends on its severity and your personal preferences. Possible options include:

Watchful waiting

If your symptoms are mild and you're not bothered by them, you and your doctor may decide that watchful waiting is appropriate. Your doctor should periodically evaluate your symptoms to see if they stay the same or worsen.

Medication

Medication is the most common treatment for mild to moderate symptoms of prostate enlargement. The options include:
- **Alpha blockers.** These medications relax bladder neck muscles and muscle fibers in the prostate, making urination easier. Alpha blockers — which include alfuzosin (Uroxatral), doxazosin (Cardura), tamsulosin (Flomax) and silodosin (Rapaflo) — usually work quickly in men with relatively small prostates. Side ef-

fects might include dizziness and a harmless condition in which semen goes back into the bladder instead of out the tip of the penis (retrograde ejaculation).
- **5-alpha reductase inhibitors.** These medications shrink your prostate by preventing hormonal changes that cause prostate growth. These medications — which include finasteride (Proscar) and dutasteride (Avodart) — might take up to six months to be effective. Side effects include retrograde ejaculation.
- **Combination drug therapy.** Your doctor might recommend taking an alpha blocker and a 5-alpha reductase inhibitor at the same time if either medication alone isn't effective.
- **Tadalafil.** Studies suggest tadalafil (Cialis), which is often used to treat erectile dysfunction, can also treat prostate enlargement. However, this medication isn't routinely used for BPH and is generally prescribed only in men who also experience erectile dysfunction.

Minimally invasive therapies

There are several types of minimally invasive or surgical therapy.
- **Transurethral resection of the prostate (TURP).** A lighted scope is inserted into your urethra, and the surgeon removes all but the

INTEGRATIVE MEDICINE

Many herbal products are marketed to relieve common prostate problems. One that has shown some positive outcomes in treating benign prostatic hyperplasia (BPH) is saw palmetto (*Serenoa repens*).

Saw palmetto likely works in the same manner as the medications Proscar and Avodart, by blocking the enzyme that converts testosterone to dihydrotestosterone (DHT). DHT is very potent in stimulating prostate growth.

Saw palmetto is slow-acting. Most men who see an improvement in their urinary symptoms do so within one to three months. If after three months you haven't noticed any benefit from the product, then it may not work for you. Possible effects from long-term use are unknown.

One drawback of this herb is that it may suppress prostate-specific antigen (PSA) levels in your blood. This action can interfere with the effectiveness of the PSA test to screen for prostate cancer. If you take saw palmetto, it's important to tell your doctor before having a PSA test.

Screening for Prostate Cancer

A prostate checkup usually includes a digital rectal exam. Many doctors recommend that men age 50 and older have a yearly digital rectal exam. For this exam, you're asked to bend over — perhaps leaning on an examination table — while your doctor gently inserts a lubricated, gloved finger into your rectum. Because the prostate gland is located just in front of the rectum, your doctor can feel the gland for lumps or hard spots in the part where most cancerous tumors develop.

Another component of a prostate checkup is the prostate-specific antigen (PSA) blood test. PSA is naturally produced by your prostate gland to help liquefy semen. A small amount of it, though, enters your bloodstream and circulates in your blood. If a higher than normal level of PSA is detected in your blood, it could indicate prostate inflammation, enlargement or cancer.

The American Cancer Society recommends prostate cancer screening for men who have a life expectancy of greater than 10 years beginning at age 50. Screening may begin earlier if you have a family history of prostate cancer. However, using the PSA test as a screening tool for prostate cancer is controversial. The test cannot distinguish between cancer and other diseases. As a result, some men who don't have cancer undergo additional tests, such as a needle biopsy to remove tissue samples from the gland, to rule out cancer.

Some doctors feel that because prostate cancer is generally so slow in developing, the PSA test leads to some men undergoing unnecessary surgery or radiation to treat a form of cancer that might not have caused any health problems if left alone. Other doctors strongly support regular use of the PSA test because it's the best tool currently available for detecting prostate cancer in its early stages, and it's especially beneficial for younger men with treatable cancers.

Many urologists — specialists who treat urinary and male genital problems — recommend an annual PSA test beginning at age 50, unless you're at high risk of the disease, in which case they suggest that you begin testing sooner. A baseline PSA for men in their 40s also can help predict who is at risk for subsequent development of aggressive prostate cancer. Once life expectancy is less than 10 years, a yearly PSA test may no longer be necessary. Men who develop prostate cancer late in life generally die of causes other than the cancer.

---

outer part of the prostate. TURP generally relieves symptoms quickly, and most men have a stronger urine flow soon after the procedure. After TURP you might need a catheter temporarily to drain your bladder, and you can only do light activity until you've healed.

- **Transurethral incision of the prostate (TUIP).** A lighted scope is inserted into your urethra, and the surgeon makes one or two small cuts in the prostate gland — making it easier for urine to pass through the urethra. This surgery might be an option if you have a small or moderately enlarged prostate gland, especially if you have health problems that make other surgeries too risky.
- **Transurethral microwave thermotherapy (TUMT).** Your doctor inserts a special electrode through your urethra into your prostate area. Microwave energy from the electrode destroys the inner portion of the enlarged prostate gland, shrinking it and easing urine flow. This surgery is generally used only on small prostates in special circumstances because retreatment might be necessary.
- **Transurethral needle ablation (TUNA).** In this procedure, a scope is passed into your urethra, allowing your doctor to place needles into your prostate gland. Radio waves pass through the needles, heating and destroying excess prostate tissue that's blocking urine flow. This procedure might be a good choice if you bleed easily or have other health problems. Like TUMT, TUNA might only partially relieve your symptoms and it might take some time before you notice results.
- **Laser therapy.** A high-energy laser destroys or removes overgrown prostate tissue. Laser therapy generally relieves symptoms right away and has a lower risk of side effects than does surgery. Laser therapy might be used in men who shouldn't have other prostate procedures because they take blood-thinning medications.

Ablative laser procedures vaporize obstructive prostate tissue to increase urine flow. Examples include photoselective vaporization of the prostate (PVP) and holmium laser ablation of the prostate (HoLAP). Enucleative procedures, such as holmium laser enucleation of the prostate (HoLEP), generally remove all the prostate tissue blocking urine flow and prevent regrowth of tissue.

- **Prostate lift.** In this experimental transurethral procedure, special tags are used to compress the sides of the prostate to increase the flow of urine. Long-term data on the effectiveness of this procedure aren't available.
- **Embolization.** In this procedure, which also is experimental, the blood supply to or from the prostate gland is selectively blocked, causing the prostate to decrease in size. Long-term data on its effectiveness aren't available.

Surgery

In an open or robot-assisted prostatectomy, a surgeon makes an incision in your lower abdomen to reach the prostate and remove tissue. An open prostatectomy is generally done if you have a very large prostate, bladder damage or other complicating factors. The surgery usually requires a short hospital stay and is associated with a higher risk of needing a blood transfusion.

After prostate surgery and some minimally invasive procedures it's common for semen to enter the bladder during ejaculation (retrograde ejaculation) rather than being ejaculated through the penis. There's no harm in this, and the semen is eventually voided with the urine. However, retrograde ejaculation can cause infertility because no semen reaches the vagina.

Prostate cancer

Signs and symptoms

- Often none
- Trouble urinating
- Starting and stopping while urinating
- Decreased force in the stream of urine
- Blood in urine
- Blood in semen
- Painful ejaculation
- Pain in the lower back, hips or upper thighs
- Loss of weight and appetite

Prostate cancer is the most common cancer in American men (excluding skin cancer). About 1 man in 7 will be diagnosed with prostate cancer during his lifetime. The cancer is rarely detected before age 50 and the risk of finding prostate cancer increases with age.

Prostate cancer is the second-leading cause of cancer deaths in American men — not because it's so deadly but because it's so common. You're more likely to die *with* prostate cancer than you are to die *of* it. Typically, prostate cancer grows slowly and remains confined to the prostate gland,

where it doesn't cause any serious harm. But not all cancers act the same. Some forms of prostate cancer can be extremely aggressive and quickly spread to other parts of the body.

It isn't known what causes prostate cancer and why some types of prostate cancer behave differently than others. Research suggests a combination of factors may play a role, including family history, race, ethnicity, hormones, diet and environment.

Diagnosis

Prostate cancer may not cause any symptoms at first. The first indication of a problem may come during a routine screening test, such as:

- **Digital rectal exam (DRE).** During a DRE, your doctor inserts a gloved, lubricated finger into your rectum to examine your prostate, which is adjacent to the rectum. If your doctor finds any abnormalities in the texture, shape or size of your gland, you may need more tests.
- **Prostate-specific antigen (PSA) test.** A blood sample is drawn from a vein and analyzed for PSA, a substance that's naturally produced by your prostate gland to help liquefy semen. It's normal for a small amount of PSA to enter your bloodstream. However, if a higher than normal level is found, it may be an indication of prostate infection, inflammation, enlargement or cancer.
- **Prostate biopsy.** If initial test results suggest prostate cancer, your doctor may recommend a biopsy. To do a prostate biopsy, your doctor inserts a small ultrasound probe into your rectum. Guided by images from the probe, your doctor uses a fine, spring-propelled needle to retrieve several very thin sections of tissue from your prostate gland. A pathologist who specializes in diagnosing cancer and other tissue abnormalities

evaluates the samples. From those, the pathologist can tell if the tissue removed is cancerous and estimate how aggressive your cancer is.

Determining if cancer has spread
Once a cancer diagnosis has been made, you may need further tests to help determine if or how far the cancer has spread. Many men don't require additional testing and can directly proceed with treatment based on the characteristics of their tumors and the results of their pre-biopsy PSA tests.

- **Bone scan.** A bone scan takes a picture of your skeleton in order to determine whether cancer has spread to the bone. Prostate cancer can spread to any bones in your body, not just those closest to your prostate, such as your pelvis or lower spine.
- **Computerized tomography (CT) scan.** A CT scan produces

Mayo Clinic's PSA Standards

Mayo Clinic urologists who treat urinary and male genital problems use the following age-adjusted scale to determine whether the prostate-specific antigen (PSA) level in your blood is within a normal range.

Age	Normal PSA range
<40	0 to 2.0 ng/mL
40-49	0 to 2.5 ng/mL
50-59	0 to 3.5 ng/mL
60-69	0 to 4.5 ng/mL
70-79	0 to 6.5 ng/mL
≥80	0 to 7.2 ng/mL

Measurements are in nanograms per milliliter (ng/mL), based on the test used at Mayo Clinic.

cross-sectional images of your body. CT scans can identify enlarged lymph nodes or abnormalities in other organs.

- **Magnetic resonance imaging (MRI).** This type of imaging produces detailed, cross-sectional images of your body using magnets and radio waves. An MRI can help detect evidence of the possible spread of cancer to lymph nodes and bones. It also provides detailed imaging of the prostate gland, which can be helpful for determining the location and extent of the tumor and the potential involvement of the adjacent seminal vesicles.
- **Lymph node biopsy.** If enlarged lymph nodes are found by a CT scan or an MRI, a lymph node biopsy can determine whether cancer has spread to nearby lymph nodes. During the procedure, some of the nodes near your prostate are sampled and examined under a microscope to determine if cancerous cells are present.

Grading

When a biopsy confirms the presence of cancer, the next step, called grading, is to determine how aggressive the cancer is. The cancer cells are compared with healthy prostate cells. The more the cancer cells differ from the healthy cells, the more aggressive the cancer and the more likely it is to spread quickly.

Cancer cells may vary in shape and size. Some cells may be aggressive, while others aren't. The pathologist identifies the two most aggressive types of cancer cells when assigning a grade. The most common scale used to evaluate prostate cancer cells is called a Gleason score. Based on the microscopic appearance of cells, individual ratings from 1 to 5 are assigned to the two most common cancer patterns identified. These two numbers are then added together to determine your

overall score. Scoring ranges from 2 (nonaggressive cancer) to 10 (very aggressive cancer), although the vast majority of contemporary scores range between 6 and 10.

Staging

After the level of aggressiveness of your prostate cancer is known, the next step, called staging, determines if or how far the cancer has spread. Your cancer is assigned one of four stages, based on its spread. Stages II through IV have subgroups.

- **Stage I.** It signifies very early cancer that's confined to the prostate gland. It includes a Gleason score of 6 or less and a PSA level of less than 10.
- **Stage II.** The cancer is confined to the prostate gland with a Gleason score of 6 and a PSA level between 10 and 20, or a Gleason score greater than 6, or a PSA greater than 10.
- **Stage III.** The cancer has spread beyond the prostate gland to the seminal vesicles or other nearby tissues, but has not spread to the lymph nodes or bone.
- **Stage IV.** The cancer has spread to lymph nodes, bones, lungs

or other organs, or it's locally advanced and it has spread to organs adjacent to the prostate gland, such as the bladder or rectum.

How serious is prostate cancer?

Prostate cancer is the second-leading cause of cancer deaths in American men, following lung cancer. But if found early — when the cancer is confined to the prostate gland — prostate cancer often can be cured. It's after the cancer has spread to nearby organs that treating the disease becomes more difficult, but not impossible.

Treatment

There's more than one way to treat prostate cancer. For some men a combination of treatments — such as surgery followed by radiation or radiation paired with hormone therapy — works best.

The treatment that's best for you depends on several factors. These include how fast your cancer is growing, how much it has spread, your age and life expectancy, as well as the benefits and the potential side effects of the treatment.

Watchful waiting

The PSA blood test can help detect prostate cancer at a very early stage. This allows many men to choose watchful waiting as a treatment option. In watchful waiting (also known as observation, expectant therapy or deferred therapy), regular follow-up blood tests, rectal exams and possibly biopsies may be performed to monitor progression of the cancer. Watchful waiting may be an option if your cancer isn't causing symptoms, is expected to grow very slowly, and is small and confined to one area of your prostate.

Watchful waiting may be appropriate if you have very early-stage prostate cancer or if you're elderly, in poor health or both. Many of these men will live out their normal life spans without treatment and without the cancer causing other problems.

External beam radiation therapy

External beam radiation therapy (EBRT) uses high-powered X-rays to kill cancer cells. This type of radiation is effective at destroying cancerous cells, but it can also scar adjacent healthy tissue.

The first step is to map the precise area of your body that needs to receive radiation. Computer-imaging software helps your doctor find the best angles to aim the beams of radiation. Precisely focused radiation kills cancer in your prostate while minimizing harm to surrounding tissue.

Treatments are generally given five days a week for about eight weeks. Each treatment appointment takes about 10 minutes. However, much of this is preparation time and the radiation is received for only about one minute. You don't need anesthesia with external beam radiation, because the treatment isn't painful.

You'll be asked to arrive for therapy with a full bladder. This will push most of your bladder out of the path of the radiation beam. A body supporter holds you in the same position for each treatment. Ink marks on your skin help guide the radiation beam, and small gold markers may be placed in your prostate gland to ensure the radiation hits the same targets each time. Custom-designed shields help protect nearby normal tissue, such as your bladder, erectile tissues, anus and rectal wall.

EBRT can cause mild side effects, but in most cases they disappear shortly after your course of treatment is finished. Side effects may include urinary problems, loose stools, rectal bleeding, discomfort during bowel movements and possible sexual problems.

Radioactive seed implants

Radioactive seeds implanted into the prostate have gained popularity in recent years as a treatment for prostate cancer. The implants, also known as brachytherapy, deliver a higher dose of radiation than do external beams, but over a substantially longer period of time. The therapy is generally used in men with smaller or moderate-sized prostates with small and lower-grade cancers.

During the procedure, between 40 and 100 rice-sized radioactive seeds are placed in your prostate through ultrasound-guided needles. The implant procedure typically lasts one to two hours and is done during general anesthesia — which means you won't be awake. Most men can go home the day of the procedure. Sometimes, hormone therapy is used for a few months to shrink the size of the prostate before seeds are implanted. The seeds may contain one of several radioactive isotopes — including iodine and palladium. These seeds don't have to be removed after they stop emitting radiation. Iodine and palladium seeds generally emit radiation that extends only a few millimeters beyond their location. This type of radiation isn't likely to escape your body in significant doses. However, doctors recommend that for the first few months you stay at least 6 feet away from children and pregnant women, who are especially sensitive to radiation. All radiation inside the pellets is generally exhausted within a year.

Side effects of radioactive seed implants can include urinary problems, loose stools, discomfort during bowel movements and sexual problems. Some men experience erectile dysfunction.

Radical prostatectomy

Surgical removal of your prostate gland, called a radical prostatectomy, is used to treat cancer that's confined to the prostate gland (see the illustration on page 377). During this procedure, your surgeon uses special techniques to completely remove your prostate and nearby lymph nodes. This surgery can affect muscles and nerves that control urination and sexual function. Two surgical approaches are commonly used for a prostatectomy — open retropubic surgery and robotic laparoscopic surgery.

- **Open retropubic surgery.** In this surgery the gland is taken out through an incision in your lower abdomen that typically runs from just below the navel to an inch above the base of the penis. Your surgeon can use the same incision to remove pelvic lymph nodes, which are tested to determine if the cancer has spread.

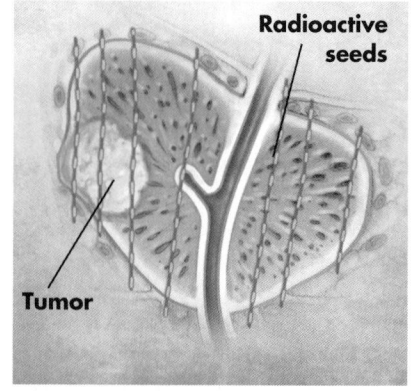

Rice-sized radioactive seeds are inserted into the prostate gland. The seeds emit radiation designed to destroy the cancer.

During the operation, a catheter is inserted into your bladder through your penis to drain urine from the bladder during your recovery. The catheter will likely remain in place for one to two weeks after the operation while the urinary tract heals.

A side effect of a radical prostatectomy is bladder control problems (urinary incontinence). Symptoms can last for weeks or even months, but most men eventually regain bladder control. Many men experience stress incontinence, meaning they're unable to hold their urine flow when their bladders are under increased pressure. This can happen when you sneeze, cough, laugh or lift something heavy. In some men, urinary incontinence doesn't get better and surgery is needed to help correct the problem.

Another common side effect of a radical prostatectomy is erectile dysfunction because nerves on both sides of your prostate that control erections may be damaged or removed during surgery. Most men younger than age 60 who have nerve-sparing surgery are able to achieve erections afterward, and even some men in their 70s are able to maintain normal sexual functioning. Men who had trouble achieving or maintaining an erection before surgery have a higher risk of being impotent after the surgery.

- **Robot-assisted laparoscopic radical prostatectomy.** This procedure became more popular in the mid-2000s and is now the most common way to remove prostate cancer. In a robot-assisted laparoscopy, six small incisions are made in the abdomen through which the doctor inserts tube-like instruments, including a long, slender tube with a small camera on the end (laparoscope). This creates a magnified view of the surgical area. The instruments are attached to

a mechanical device, and the surgeon sits at a console and guides the instruments through a viewing device to perform the surgery. Studies show that traditional open prostatectomies and robotic prostatectomies have had similar outcomes related to cancer-free survival rates, urinary continence and sexual function one year after surgery. One benefit of the robot-assisted laparoscopic approach is less blood loss on average and a quicker recovery.

Discuss with your doctor which type of surgery is best for your specific situation.

Hormone therapy

Hormone therapy involves trying to stop your body from producing the male sex hormone testosterone, which can stimulate the growth of cancer cells. This type of therapy can also block hormones from getting into cancer cells. Sometimes doctors use a combination of drugs to achieve both. In most men with advanced prostate cancer, this form of treatment is effective in helping to both shrink the cancer and slow the growth of tumors. Hormone therapy may be used in early-stage cancers to shrink large tumors so that surgery or radiation therapy can remove or destroy them more easily. In some cases, hormone therapy is used in combination

with radiation therapy or surgery. After these treatments, the drugs can slow the growth of any stray cancer cells left behind.

Hormone therapy options include the following:
- **Medications that stop your body from producing testosterone.** Medications known as luteinizing hormone-releasing hormone (LH-RH) agonists or antagonists prevent the testicles from receiving messages to make testosterone. Drugs typically used in this type of hormone therapy include leuprolide (Lupron, Eligard), goserelin (Zoladex), triptorelin (Trelstar), degarelix (Firmagon) and histrelin (Vantas). Other drugs sometimes used include ketoconazole and abiraterone (Zytiga).
- **Medications that block testosterone from reaching cancer cells.** Medications known as antiandrogens prevent testosterone from reaching your cancer cells. Examples include bicalutamide (Casodex), flutamide, and nilutamide (Nilandron). The drug enzalutamide (Xtandi) may be an option when other hormone therapies are no longer effective.

Simply depriving prostate cancer of testosterone usually doesn't kill all of the cancer cells. Within a few years, the cancer often learns to thrive without testosterone. Once this happens, hormone therapy is less likely to

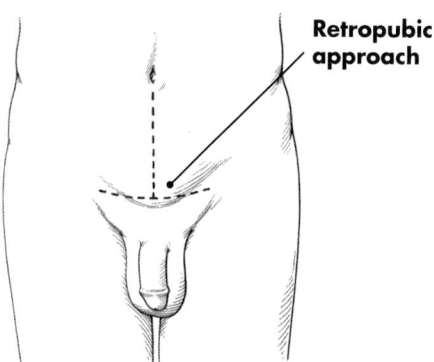

Retropubic approach

With open retropubic surgery, the prostate gland is removed through an incision in the lower abdomen.

be effective. However, several treatment options still exist. To avoid such resistance, intermittent hormone therapy programs have been developed. During this type of therapy, the hormonal drugs are stopped after your PSA drops to a low level and remains steady. You will need to resume taking the drugs if your PSA level rises again.

Side effects of hormone therapy can include breast enlargement (gynecomastia), reduced sex drive, erectile dysfunction, hot flashes, weight gain, and reduction in muscle and bone mass. Long-term hormone therapy can put you at risk of osteoporosis, so supplementing your diet with vitamin D and calcium are recommended.

Reports have shown that men who undergo hormone therapy for prostate cancer may have a higher risk of having a heart attack in the first year or two after starting hormone therapy. So your doctor should carefully monitor your heart condition and aggressively treat any other conditions that may predispose you to a heart attack, such as high blood pressure, high cholesterol or smoking.

Surgery to remove the testicles, which produce most of your testosterone, is as effective as other forms of hormonal therapy. Many men are not comfortable with the idea of losing their testicles, so they opt for other methods of lowering testosterone in the body. However, removing the testicles has the advantage of not having to have an injection of medication every three or four months and can be less expensive. The surgery can be done on an outpatient basis using a local anesthetic.

Chemotherapy

This type of treatment uses chemicals that destroy rapidly growing cells. Chemotherapy can be quite effective in treating prostate cancer, but it can't cure it. Because it has more side effects than hormone therapy does, chemotherapy is generally reserved for men who have hormone-resistant prostate cancer that has spread to other parts of the body. However, recent studies have shown that in men with widespread bone metastases at diagnosis, early use of chemotherapy can improve survival.

Cryotherapy

This treatment is used to destroy cells by freezing tissue. Original attempts to treat prostate cancer with cryotherapy often resulted in damage to tissue around the bladder and long-term complications such as injury to the rectum or the muscles that control urination.

Smaller probes and more-precise methods of monitoring the temperature in and around the prostate have been instituted. These advances may decrease the complications associated with cryotherapy, making it a more effective treatment option for prostate cancer. However, more time is still needed to determine how successful cryotherapy is as a prostate cancer treatment. ■

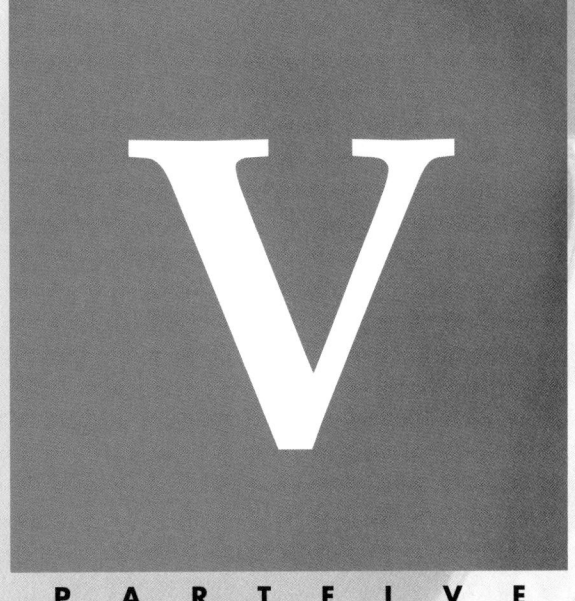

Tests and Treatments

Tests and Procedures

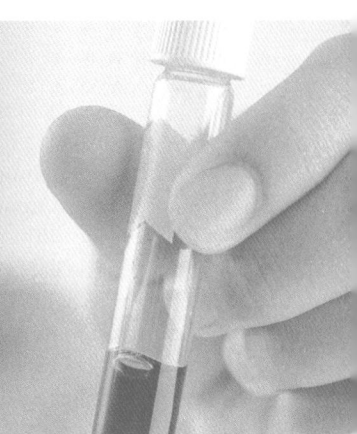

The purpose of this chapter is to provide some basic information about commonly used tests and procedures in the hope that the information may help answer a few of your questions. Following is a list of some of the most frequently used tests and procedures, listed alphabetically. The list is not intended to be all-inclusive.

Keep in mind that technology is ever changing. New tests and procedures are continually being developed, and some older tests are no longer used. For additional information regarding a particular test or procedure, check within specific chapters in the book or visit our online website *www.MayoClinic.org*. You can also talk with your doctor or another member of your health care team.

A

A1C blood test

The A1C test is a common blood test used to diagnose type 1 and type 2 diabetes and then to gauge how well you're managing your diabetes. The A1C test goes by many other names, including glycated hemoglobin, glycosylated hemoglobin, hemoglobin A1C and HbA1c. A1C test results reflect your average blood sugar level for the past two to three months. Specifically, the A1C test measures what percentage of your hemoglobin is coated with sugar. Hemoglobin is a protein in red blood cells that carries oxygen. The higher your A1C level, the poorer your blood sugar control and the higher your risk of diabetes complications.

Abdominal ultrasound

An abdominal ultrasound is performed to evaluate abdominal structures, including the abdominal aorta. This test may be used to check for a number of conditions. It's often the screening method of choice for detecting an abdominal aortic aneurysm, a weakened, bulging spot in your abdominal aorta, the artery that runs through the middle of your abdomen and supplies blood to the lower half of your body.

Ablation therapy

Ablation therapy is a minimally invasive procedure doctors use to destroy abnormal tissue that occurs with many conditions. For example, a doctor might use an ablation procedure to treat a small kidney tumor or to destroy (ablate) a small amount of heart tissue that's causing an abnormal heart rhythm. The abnormal tissue is injured or destroyed with heat, extreme cold, lasers or a chemical.

Allergy skin tests

During allergy skin testing, your skin is exposed to suspected allergy-causing substances (allergens) and is observed for signs of an allergic reaction. Along with your medical history, allergy tests may be used to confirm whether a particular substance you touch, breathe or eat is causing your symptoms.

Arthroscopy

Arthroscopy is a procedure for diagnosing and treating joint problems. During the procedure, a surgeon inserts a narrow tube attached to a fiber-optic video camera through a small incision in your skin — about the size of a buttonhole. The view inside your joint is transmitted to a high-definition video monitor. Arthroscopy allows a surgeon to see inside your joint without making a large incision. Surgeons can even repair some types of joint damage during arthroscopy, with pencil-thin surgical instruments that are inserted through additional small incisions.

B

Barium enema

A barium enema is an X-ray examination that can detect changes or abnormalities in the large intestine (colon). The procedure is also called a colon X-ray. To begin the procedure, liquid containing a metallic substance (barium) is injected into your rectum through a small tube. The liquid coats the lining of the colon, resulting in a relatively clear silhouette of the colon. During the procedure, air may be pumped into the colon. The air expands the colon and improves the quality of images. This is called an air-contrast (double-contrast) barium enema.

Bilirubin blood test

Bilirubin testing checks for levels of bilirubin in your blood. Bilirubin is an orange-yellow substance made during the normal breakdown of red blood cells. Bilirubin passes through your liver and is eventually excreted out of your body. Higher than normal levels of bilirubin may indicate different types of liver problems. Sometimes, higher bilirubin levels may indicate an increased rate of destruction of red blood cells (hemolysis).

Blood pressure test

A blood pressure test measures the pressure in your arteries. You might have a blood pressure test as a part of a routine doctor's appointment or as a screening for high blood pressure (hypertension). Systolic pressure — the top number of your blood pressure reading — is the pressure of the blood flow when your heart muscle contracts, pumping blood. Diastolic pressure — the bottom number of your blood pressure reading — is the pressure measured between heartbeats. Blood pressure is measured in millimeters of mercury, which is abbreviated mm Hg.

Bone density test

A bone density test determines if you have osteoporosis — a disease that causes bones to become more fragile and more likely to break. A bone density test uses X-rays to measure how many grams of calcium and other bone minerals are packed into a segment of bone (see page 955). The bones that are most commonly tested are those in the spine, hip and forearm.

Bone scan

A bone scan is a nuclear imaging test that helps diagnose and track several types of bone disease. For the test, tiny amounts of radioactive materials (tracers) are injected in a vein and taken up at different sites in the body. Your doctor may order a bone scan if you have unexplained skeletal pain, a bone infection or a bone injury that can't be seen on a standard X-ray. A bone scan is also an important tool for helping to detect cancer that has spread (metastasized) to the bone from the tumor's original location, such as the breast or prostate.

Breast biopsy

A breast biopsy is a procedure in which a small sample of breast tissue is removed for laboratory testing (see the illustration on page 807). A biopsy is typically performed to evaluate a suspicious area in your breast to determine whether the area is breast cancer. A breast biopsy provides a sample of tissue that doctors use to identify and diagnose abnormalities in the cells that make up breast lumps, other unusual breast changes, or suspicious or concerning findings on a mammogram or ultrasound. The lab report from a breast biopsy can help determine whether you need additional surgery or other treatment.

Bronchoscopy

Bronchoscopy is a procedure that lets doctors look at your lungs and air passages. During bronchoscopy, a thin tube (bronchoscope) is passed through your nose or mouth, down your throat, and into your lungs. Common reasons for needing the procedure are a persistent cough, infection, or something unusual seen on a chest X-ray or other test. Bronchoscopy can also be used to obtain samples of mucus or tissue, or to remove foreign bodies or other blockages from the airways or lungs.

C

Cardiac catheterization

Cardiac catheterization is a procedure used to diagnose and treat heart conditions. During cardiac catheterization, a long thin tube called a catheter is inserted in an artery or vein in your groin, neck or arm and threaded through your blood vessels to your heart. Using the catheter, doctors can perform diagnostic tests for heart disease, including identifying narrowed or blocked blood vessels. Cardiac catheterization also may be used to treat some heart conditions, such as stenting a narrowed artery or repairing a small defect in a heart chamber or a leaky valve.

Cardiac stress test

A cardiac stress test, also called an exercise stress test, gathers information about how your heart works during physical activity. Because exercise makes your heart pump harder and faster than usual, an exercise stress test can reveal heart problems that might not be otherwise noticeable. The test usually involves walking on a treadmill or riding a stationary bike while your heart rhythm, blood pressure and breathing are

monitored (see the photo on page 718). Your doctor may recommend an exercise stress test if he or she suspects you have coronary artery disease or an irregular heart rhythm (arrhythmia). If you're unable to exercise (for instance because of severe arthritis), an injected medication may be used to simulate exercise.

Cardioversion

Cardioversion is a medical procedure that restores a normal heart rhythm in people with certain types of abnormal heartbeats (arrhythmias). Cardioversion is usually done by sending electric shocks to your heart through electrodes placed on your chest. It's also possible to do cardioversion with medication.

Chest X-ray

Chest X-rays produce images of your heart, lungs, blood vessels, airways, and the bones of your chest and spine. Chest X-rays can also reveal fluid in or around your lungs or air surrounding a lung. A chest X-ray is a common way to diagnose disease. It can also be used to tell whether a certain treatment is working.

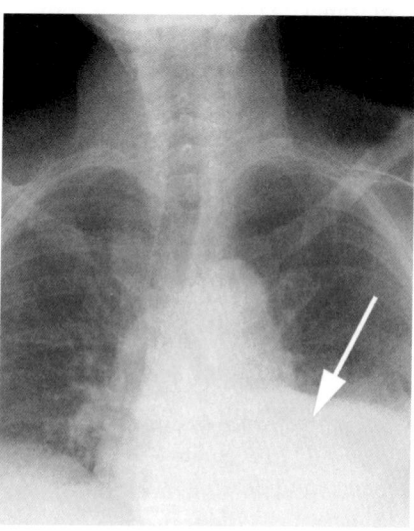

This chest X-ray shows a collection of fluid (pleural effusion) in the left lung.

Cholesterol blood test

A complete cholesterol test — also called a lipid panel or lipid profile — is a blood test that measures the amount of cholesterol and triglycerides in your blood. Cholesterol is a waxy, fat-like substance found in all of your body's cells. Triglycerides are a type of fat found in your blood.

Colonoscopy

A colonoscopy is an exam used to detect changes or abnormalities in the large intestine (colon) and rectum. During a colonoscopy, a long, flexible tube (colonoscope) is inserted into the rectum. A tiny video camera at the tip of the tube allows a doctor to view the inside of the entire colon (see page 858). If necessary, polyps or other types of abnormal tissue can be removed through the scope during a colonoscopy. Tissue samples (biopsies) can be taken during a colonoscopy as well. The samples are sent to a laboratory for testing.

Colposcopy

Colposcopy is a procedure to closely examine your cervix, vagina and vulva for signs of disease. During colposcopy, a doctor uses a special instrument called a colposcope. Your doctor may recommend colposcopy if your Pap test result is abnormal. If an unusual area of cells is detected during the exam, a sample of tissue can be collected for laboratory testing (biopsy).

Complete blood count (CBC)

A complete blood count is a blood test used to evaluate your overall health and detect a wide range of disorders, including anemia, infection and leukemia. A complete blood count test measures several components and features of your blood, including:

- Red blood cells, which carry oxygen
- White blood cells, which fight infection
- Hemoglobin, the oxygen-carrying protein in red blood cells
- Hematocrit, the proportion of red blood cells to the fluid component, or plasma, in your blood
- Platelets, which help with blood clotting

Coronary angiogram

A coronary angiogram is a procedure that uses X-ray imaging to see your heart's blood vessels. Coronary angiograms are part of a general group of procedures known as heart (cardiac) catheterizations. A coronary angiogram is the most common type of cardiac catheterization procedure. For the procedure, a type of dye that's visible by an X-ray machine is injected into the blood vessels of your heart. An X-ray machine rapidly takes a series of images (angiograms), offering a look at your blood vessels (see page 718). If necessary, a doctor can open clogged heart arteries (angioplasty and stenting) during a coronary angiogram.

Cortisone shot

A cortisone shot is an injection that may help relieve pain and inflammation in a specific area of your body. Cortisone is most commonly injected into joints — such as your ankle, elbow, hip, knee, shoulder, spine and wrist. Even the small joints in your hands and feet might benefit from a cortisone shot. The injections usually include a corticosteroid medication and a local anesthetic. Because of potential side effects, the number of cortisone shots you can receive in one year often is limited.

C-reactive protein blood test

The level of C-reactive protein (CRP), which can be measured in your blood, increases when there's inflammation in your body. Your doctor may check your C-reactive protein level for infections or for other medical conditions. A simple blood test measures C-reactive protein.

Creatinine test

A creatinine test reveals important information about your kidneys. Creatinine is a chemical waste product produced by normal muscle breakdown and to a smaller extent by eating meat. Healthy kidneys filter creatinine and other waste products from your blood. The waste products leave your body in your urine. If your kidneys aren't functioning properly, creatinine may accumulate in your body. A serum creatinine test measures the level of creatinine in your blood and provides an estimate of how well your kidneys are filtering waste (glomerular filtration rate). A creatinine urine test measures creatinine in your urine.

CT scan

A computerized tomography (CT) scan combines a series of X-ray images taken from different angles and computer processing to create cross-sectional images of the bones, blood vessels, organs and soft tissues inside your body. CT scan images provide more detailed information than do plain X-rays. A CT scan has many uses, but is particularly well-suited to quickly examine people who may have internal injuries. A CT scan can be used to diagnose disease or injury as well as to plan medical, surgical or radiation treatment. During a CT scan you're briefly exposed to a small amount of radiation.

Cystoscopy

Cystoscopy is a procedure that allows your doctor to examine the lining of your bladder and

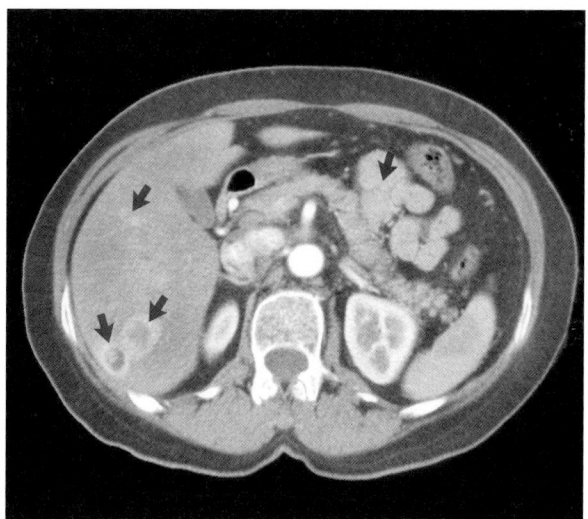

This CT scan reveals tumors in the pancreas and liver (see arrows).

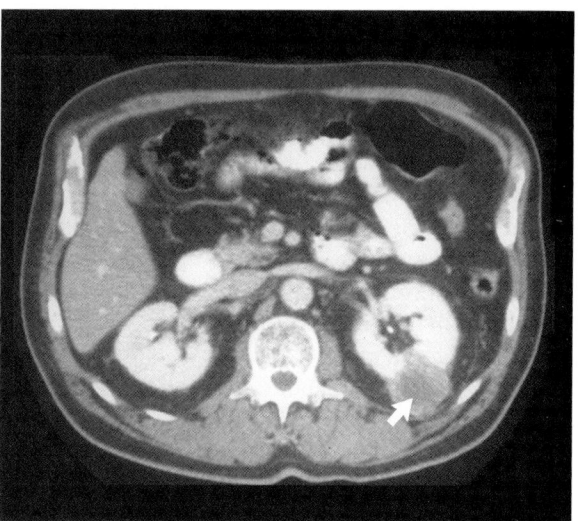

This CT scan shows a kidney tumor (see arrow).

the tube that carries urine out of your body (urethra). A hollow tube (cystoscope) equipped with a lens is inserted into your urethra and slowly advanced into your bladder. Abnormal findings can be biopsied for diagnosis through the cystoscope.

D

D&C

Dilation and curettage (D&C) is a procedure to remove tissue from inside a woman's uterus. A doctor may perform dilation and curettage to diagnose and treat certain uterine conditions — such as heavy bleeding — or to clear the uterine lining after a miscarriage.

E

Echocardiogram

An echocardiogram uses sound waves to produce images of your heart (see page 742). This commonly used test allows a doctor to see your heart beating and pumping blood. Your doctor can use the images from an echocardiogram to identify heart disease.

Electrocardiogram (ECG)

An electrocardiogram records the electrical signals in your heart. It's a common test used to detect heart rhythm problems and monitor the heart's status in many situations. An ECG is a noninvasive, painless test with quick results. During an ECG, sensors (electrodes) that can detect the electrical activity of your heart are attached to your chest and sometimes your limbs. The sensors are usually left on for just a few minutes.

Electroencephalogram (EEG)

An electroencephalogram (EEG) is a test that detects electrical activity in your brain using small, flat metal discs (electrodes) attached to your scalp. Your brain cells communicate via electrical impulses and are constantly active, even when you're asleep. This activity shows up as wavy lines on an EEG recording. An EEG is one of the main diagnostic tests for epilepsy and may also play a role in diagnosing other brain disorders.

Electromyography (EMG)

Electromyography is a diagnostic procedure used to assess the health of your muscles and the nerve cells that control them (motor neurons). Motor neurons transmit electrical signals that cause your muscles to contract. An EMG translates these signals into graphs, sounds or numerical values. During a needle EMG, a needle electrode inserted directly into a muscle records the electrical activity in that muscle. A nerve conduction study, another part of an EMG exam, uses electrodes taped to the skin to measure the speed and strength of signals traveling between two or more points. EMG results can reveal nerve dysfunction, muscle dysfunction or problems with nerve-to-muscle signal transmission.

EP heart study

An electrophysiology (EP) study is a test used to understand and map the electrical activity within your heart. An EP study may be performed on people with heart rhythm disorders (arrhythmias) and other heart problems. An EP study involves placing diagnostic catheters within your heart and running specialized tests to map the electrical currents.

Esophageal manometry

Esophageal manometry is a test that shows whether your esophagus is working properly. The test measures the rhythmic muscle contractions that occur in your esophagus when you swallow. It also measures the coordination and force exerted by the muscles of your esophagus. During esophageal manometry, a thin, flexible tube (catheter) that contains sensors is passed through your nose, down your esophagus and into your stomach. Esophageal manometry can be helpful in diagnosing certain disorders that may affect your esophagus.

F

Fecal occult blood test

A fecal occult blood test is a laboratory test used to check stool samples for hidden (occult) blood. Occult blood in stool may indicate the presence of colon cancer or polyps in the colon or rectum — however, not all cancers or polyps bleed. If blood is detected through a fecal occult blood test, additional tests may be needed to determine the source of the bleeding.

Ferritin blood test

A ferritin test measures the amount of ferritin in your blood. Ferritin is a blood cell protein that contains iron. A ferritin test helps your doctor understand how much iron your body is storing. If a ferritin test reveals that your blood ferritin level is lower than normal, you may have iron deficiency. If a ferritin test shows higher than normal levels, you have a condition that causes your body to store too much iron.

Flexible sigmoidoscopy

A flexible sigmoidoscopy is an exam used to evaluate the lower part of the large intestine (colon). During flexible sigmoidoscopy, a thin, flexible tube (sigmoidoscope)

is inserted into the rectum. A tiny video camera at the tip of the tube allows the doctor to view the inside of the rectum and most of the sigmoid colon — about the last 2 feet of the large intestine. If necessary, tissue samples (biopsies) can be taken through the scope during a flexible sigmoidoscopy exam.

G

General anesthesia

Under general anesthesia, you're completely unconscious and unable to feel pain during medical procedures. When your brain is anesthetized, it doesn't respond to pain signals or reflexes. General anesthesia usually uses a combination of intravenous drugs and inhaled gases (anesthetics).

Genetic testing

Genetic testing involves examining specific components of your DNA, the chemical database that carries instructions for your body's functions. Genetic testing can reveal changes (mutations) in your genes that may cause illness or disease.

Glucose tolerance test

The glucose tolerance test measures your body's response to sugar (glucose). This test can be used to screen for type 2 diabetes. You drink a sugary solution and two hours later your blood glucose level is measured.

H

Hysteroscopy

Hysteroscopy is a procedure that allows your doctor to look inside your uterus in order to diagnose

and treat causes of abnormal bleeding. Hysteroscopy is done using a hysteroscope, a thin, lighted tube that's inserted into the vagina to examine the cervix and the inside of the uterus. If necessary, a biopsy can be performed during this procedure.

I

Intravenous pyelogram

An intravenous pyelogram, also called an excretory urogram, is an X-ray exam of your urinary tract that may be used to diagnose disorders such as kidney stones, bladder stones, enlarged prostate, kidney cysts or urinary tract tumors. During the procedure, an X-ray dye (iodine contrast solution) is injected into a vein in your arm. The dye flows into your kidneys, ureters and bladder, outlining each of these structures. X-ray pictures are taken at specific times during the exam, so your doctor can see your urinary tract and assess how well it's working.

L

Liver function blood tests

Liver function tests are blood tests that are used to help diagnose and monitor liver disease or damage. The tests measure the levels of certain enzymes and proteins in your blood. Some tests measure how well the liver is performing its normal functions of producing protein and clearing bilirubin, a blood waste product. Other liver function tests measure enzymes that liver cells release in response to damage or disease. Liver function tests may be used to screen for liver infection, monitor liver disease progression or monitor possible side effects of certain medications.

Lumbar puncture

Lumbar puncture (spinal tap) is performed on your lower back, in the lumbar region. During a lumbar puncture, a needle is inserted between two lumbar bones (vertebrae) to remove a sample of cerebrospinal fluid — the fluid that surrounds your brain and spinal cord to protect them from injury. A lumbar puncture can help diagnose serious infections and other disorders of the central nervous system. Sometimes doctors use a lumbar puncture to inject anesthetic medications or chemotherapy drugs into the cerebrospinal fluid.

M

Mammogram

A mammogram is an X-ray image of your breasts used to screen for breast cancer. During a mammogram, your breasts are compressed between two firm surfaces to spread out the breast tissue. An X-ray then captures black-and-white images of your breasts, which are displayed on a computer screen and examined by a doctor who looks for signs of cancer. A mammogram can be used for screening or for diagnostic purposes.

Microalbumin urine test

A urine microalbumin test can detect very small levels of a blood protein (albumin) in your urine. A microalbumin test is used to detect early signs of kidney damage in people at risk of developing kidney disease. Healthy kidneys filter waste from your blood and hang on to the healthy components, including proteins such as albumin. Kidney damage can cause proteins to leak through your kidneys and exit your body in your urine. Albumin is one of the first proteins

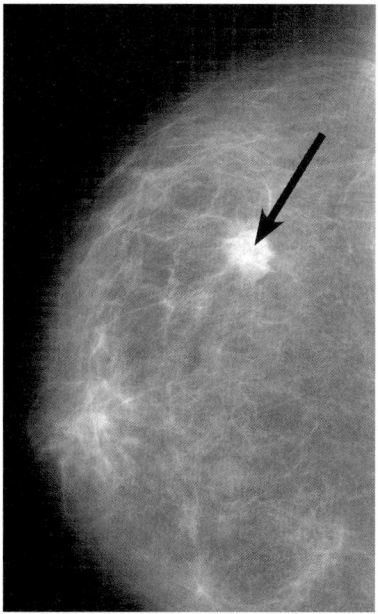

This X-ray of the breast (mammogram) shows a large tumor in the breast (see arrow).

to leak when kidneys become damaged.

Molecular breast imaging

Molecular breast imaging uses a radioactive tracer and special camera to detect breast cancer. The procedure creates pictures that show differences in tissue activity within the breast. Tissue that contains cells that are rapidly growing and dividing, such as cancer cells, appears brighter than less active tissue. During molecular breast imaging, a small amount of radioactive tracer is injected into a vein in your arm. The tracer attaches to breast cancer cells, which are identified using a camera that detects gamma radiation released by the tracer (gamma camera).

MRI

Magnetic resonance imaging (MRI) uses a magnetic field and radio waves to create detailed images of the organs and tissues within your body. Most MRI machines are large, tube-shaped magnets. When you lie inside the machine, the magnetic field temporarily realigns hydrogen atoms in your

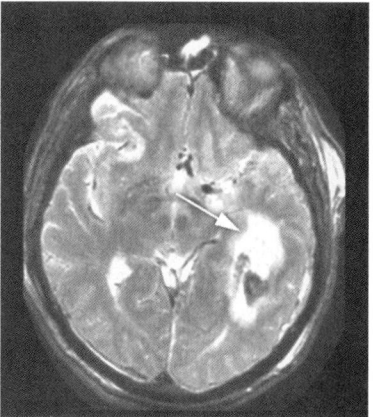

The arrow on this magnetic resonance image (MRI) points to an area of bleeding in the brain (brain hemorrhage).

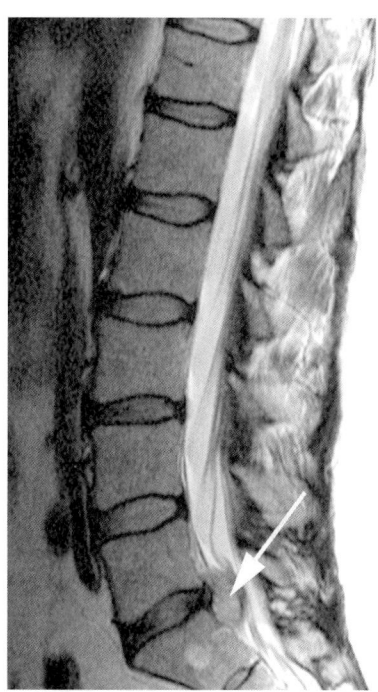

An MRI reveals compression of the spinal canal from a herniated disk (see arrow).

body. Radio waves cause the realigned atoms to produce very faint signals. A computer converts the signals into cross-sectional or 3-D images that may be viewed from many different angles. MRI is a noninvasive way to examine your organs, tissues and skeletal system. It's particularly useful for imaging the brain. MRI doesn't expose you to radiation associated with many other imaging studies. However, it can trigger feelings of claustrophobia in some people.

N

Needle biopsy

A needle biopsy is used to obtain a sample of cells from your body for laboratory testing. Common needle biopsy procedures include fine-needle aspiration and core needle biopsy. Needle biopsy may be used to take tissue or fluid samples from muscles, bones, and other organs, such as the liver or lungs. A doctor may suggest a needle biopsy to help diagnose a medical condition or to rule out a disease or condition.

Nuclear cardiac stress test

A nuclear stress test measures blood flow to your heart at rest and while it's working hard, as a result of exertion or medication. For a nuclear stress test, radioactive dye is injected into your bloodstream. Images provided by the test can show areas of low blood flow through the heart and damaged heart muscle. The test may be done if your doctor suspects you have coronary artery disease or if a routine stress test didn't pinpoint the cause of symptoms such as chest pain or shortness of breath. A nuclear stress test may also be used to guide your treatment if you've been diagnosed with a heart condition.

P

Pap test

A Pap test, also called a Pap smear, is a procedure to test for cervical cancer in women. The test involves collecting cells from the cervix — the lower, narrow end of the uterus located at the top of the vagina. A Pap test can also detect changes in cervical cells that suggest cancer may develop in the future.

Peak flow meter

A peak flow meter is a portable device that measures how well your lungs are able to expel air. By blowing hard through a mouthpiece on one end, a peak flow meter can measure the force of air in liters per minute and give you a reading on a built-in numbered scale. If you have asthma, your doctor may recommend that you use a peak flow meter to help track your asthma control.

PET scan

A positron emission tomography (PET) scan is an imaging test that helps reveal how your tissues and organs are functioning. A PET scan uses a radioactive drug (tracer) to show this activity. The tracer may be injected, swallowed or inhaled, depending on which organ or tissue is being studied. The tracer collects in areas of your body that have higher levels of chemical activity, which often correspond to areas of disease. On a PET scan, these areas show up as bright spots. Often, PET images are combined with CT or MRI scans to create special views.

Polysomnography

Polysomnography, also called a sleep study, is a test used to diagnose sleep disorders. Polysomnography records your brain waves, the oxygen level in your blood, your heart rate and breathing, as well as eye and leg movements. This test usually is performed in a sleep disorders unit within a hospital or at a sleep center.

Prothrombin time blood test

A prothrombin time test, sometimes called a PT or pro time test, uses a sample of your blood to measure how quickly your blood clots. Prothrombin is a protein produced by your liver. It's one of

many factors in your blood that help it to clot appropriately. If you take a blood-thinning medication such as warfarin (Coumadin), your prothrombin time test results will be expressed as a ratio called the international normalized ratio (INR).

PSA test

The PSA test is a blood test that's used primarily to screen for prostate cancer. The test measures the amount of prostate-specific antigen (PSA) in your blood. PSA is a protein produced by both cancerous and noncancerous tissue in the prostate gland. PSA is mostly found in semen, but small amounts also circulate in blood. A PSA test can reveal high levels of PSA that may indicate the presence of prostate cancer. However, many other conditions, such as an enlarged or inflamed prostate, can also increase PSA levels. PSA testing is controversial. Discuss the issue with your doctor to decide whether to have a PSA test.

Pulmonary function tests

Pulmonary function tests are a broad range of tests that measure how well your lungs take in and exhale air and how efficiently they transfer oxygen in the blood. The tests measure lung volume, capacity, rates of flow and gas exchange.

R

Regional anesthesia

Regional anesthesia is a form of anesthesia in which only part of your body is made numb (anesthetized). Regional anesthesia allows a procedure to be performed on a region of the body, such as your upper or lower extremities, while you remain conscious. Sometimes a sedative is administered intravenously to relax you. For regional anesthesia, the anesthetic is injected close to a nerve, a bundle of nerves or the spinal cord.

Rheumatoid factor test

A rheumatoid factor test measures the amount of rheumatoid factor in your blood. Rheumatoid factors are proteins produced by your immune system that can attack healthy tissues. High levels of rheumatoid factor in the blood are most often associated with autoimmune diseases, such as rheumatoid arthritis and Sjogren's syndrome. However, high rheumatoid factor levels may occur in healthy people, and some people with autoimmune diseases have normal levels of rheumatoid factor.

S

Sed rate

Sed rate, or erythrocyte sedimentation rate (ESR), is a blood test that can reveal inflammatory activity in your body. When your blood is placed in a tall, thin tube, red blood cells (erythrocytes) gradually settle to the bottom. Inflammation can cause the cells to clump. Because these clumps are denser than individual cells, they settle to the bottom more quickly. The sed rate test measures the distance red blood cells fall in a test tube in one hour. The farther the red blood cells have descended, the higher the number reported on the test and the greater the inflammatory response of your immune system.

Spirometry

Spirometry is a common test used to assess how well your lungs work by measuring how much air you inhale, how much you exhale and how quickly you exhale. Spirometry is used to diagnose asthma, chronic obstructive pul-

monary disease (COPD) and other conditions that affect breathing.

Stool DNA test

The stool DNA test is a noninvasive laboratory test that identifies DNA changes in the cells of a stool sample. The test specifically looks for DNA alterations associated with colon polyps and colon cancer. You receive a test kit for collecting and submitting the stool sample. The kit includes a container that attaches to the toilet and a preservative solution that is added to the stool sample before sealing the container. After the stool sample is collected, it can be returned to your doctor's office or sent by mail to the laboratory.

T

Tilt table test

A tilt table test is used to evaluate the cause of unexplained fainting (syncope). For this test, you begin by lying flat on a table. Straps are secured around your body to hold you in place. After about 15 minutes of lying flat, the table is quickly tilted to raise your body to an upright position — simulating a change in position from lying down to standing up. The table remains upright for several minutes, while your heart rate and blood pressure are monitored. This allows doctors to evaluate your body's cardiovascular response to the change in position.

Throat culture

A throat culture is most often performed when a doctor notices redness or pus on your tonsils or tissues in the back of your throat. To determine if a virus or a bacterium may be causing the inflammation or infection, your doctor rubs a sterile swab over the tissues to gather a sample of the secretions.

The swab is sent to a laboratory where the swab contents are placed in a medium to see if any of the contents grow. If the contents do grow, they are then analyzed. A throat culture is often performed to detect strep throat, which can often be diagnosed quickly with a DNA test for strep.

U

Ultrasound

Ultrasound, also called sonography, uses high-frequency sound waves to produce images of structures within your body. The images can provide valuable information for diagnosing and treating a variety of diseases and conditions. Most ultrasound examinations are done using a sonar device outside your body. A technician (sonographer) presses a small, hand-held device (transducer) against your skin over the area being examined. The transducer sends sound

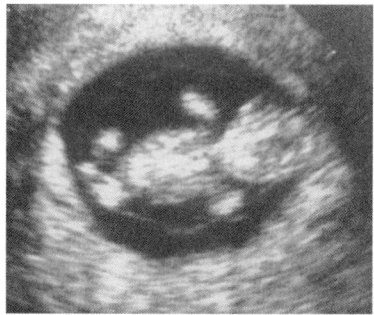

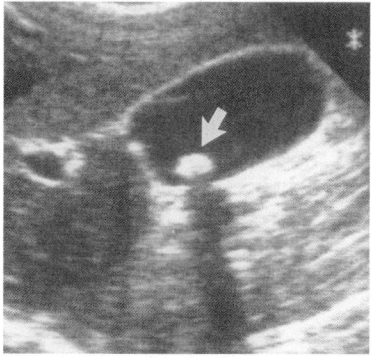

The ultrasound scan on top shows a fetus in the uterus. The scan on the bottom reveals a gallstone (see arrow).

waves into your body, collects sound waves that bounce back and sends them to a computer, which creates the images. Some ultrasounds are performed inside your body. For internal exams, a transducer is attached to a probe that's inserted into a natural opening in your body.

Upper endoscopy

Upper endoscopy is a procedure used to visually examine your upper digestive system. A tiny camera is attached to the end of a long, flexible tube that's inserted through your mouth and down your esophagus. Endoscopy is often used to diagnose and, sometimes, treat conditions that affect the esophagus, stomach and the beginning of the small intestine (duodenum).

Urinalysis

For a urinalysis, you provide a sample of your urine, which is examined in a laboratory. A urinalysis involves checking the appearance, concentration and content of urine. Abnormal urinalysis results may point to a disease or illness. For example, a urinary tract infection can make urine look cloudy instead of clear. Increased levels of protein in urine can be a sign of kidney disease.

Urine cytology

Urine cytology is a test to look for abnormal cells in your urine. Urine cytology is most often used to diagnose bladder cancer, though it may also detect cancers of the kidney, prostate, ureter and urethra.

X

X-ray

An X-ray is a quick, painless test that produces images of the struc-

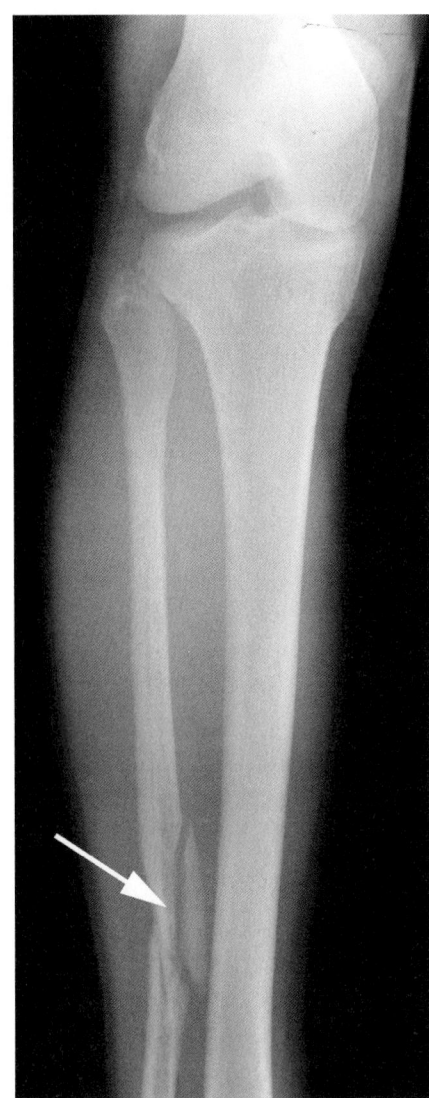

This X-ray shows a fractured bone (fibula) in a leg (see arrow).

tures inside your body — particularly your bones. X-ray beams pass through your body and are absorbed in different amounts depending on the density of the material they pass through. Dense materials, such as bone and metal, show up as white on X-rays. The air in your lungs shows up as black. Fat and muscle appear as shades of gray. For some types of X-ray tests, a contrast medium — such as iodine or barium — is introduced into your body to provide greater detail on the images. ∎

Medications Guide

Medications can be a marvel. When used properly they may soothe minor aches and pains, downshift a rapidly progressing disease into slow motion, improve your quality of life, or mean the difference between life and death.

But almost anything with the power to heal also carries the power to harm if used incorrectly. And many Americans *do* use medications incorrectly. In one study, researchers found numerous problems with use of both prescription and over-the-counter drugs. These problems included taking a different dose than recommended, not taking a medication or taking an inappropriate medication.

As helpful as medications can be, they can also be dangerous and even deadly if used inappropriately. This chapter will help you understand:

- How medications work
- Why two people can be affected by the same medication in different ways
- How to take your medications safely and avoid harmful interactions with other drugs or certain foods
- The potential advantages and drawbacks of generic drugs and brand-name medications
- How to make sure you're taking the right medications at the right time

At the end of the chapter, you'll find an overview of many common medications.

How Medications Work

Given the wide variety of medications and the different forms in which you can take them — tablets, capsules, lozenges, syrups, suppositories, suspensions, elixirs, creams, ointments, pastes, sprays, patches, inhalers, drops and injections — it's impossible to sum up exactly how they work in a sentence or two.

In general, the most common medications are in pill form and are absorbed into your bloodstream through the lining of your gastrointestinal tract. Once in the bloodstream, the medication is carried to your liver, your body's chemical processing center. Some medications aren't affected by the liver, but many are. The liver converts some medications into a chemically active form. These active chemicals are then distributed throughout your body, including the site where the medication is needed. The kidneys inactivate some medications and excrete many medications.

Means of delivery

The most common methods of administering medications are as follows:

- Swallowed as a liquid, tablet or capsule
- Chewed and swallowed
- Placed under the tongue
- Sprayed into the mouth or nose
- Inhaled
- Injected into a vein, muscle or under the skin
- Dropped into or applied to an eye
- Dropped into an ear
- Inserted into the rectum
- Inserted into the vagina
- Applied to the skin

Oral medications

Swallowing a tablet or capsule and drinking a liquid are the most common methods of taking medication. They're convenient, non-invasive, painless and inexpensive methods of getting medication into your body.

When swallowed, the medication travels down your esophagus to your stomach and eventually reaches your small intestine, where it's absorbed into your bloodstream and distributed throughout your body. Sometimes, though, a tablet or capsule may stick to the inner lining of your esophagus. If it dissolves there — instead of inside your stomach or intestines — it may cause irritation, which could lead to vomiting or chest pains.

Here are some ways to help your medications make it to their destination:

- Before swallowing a pill, sip a little water to lubricate your esophagus.
- Swallow the pill with a mouthful of water.
- Drink the rest of the water to wash the medication down.
- Drink at least half of an 8-ounce glass of water to help flush the pill into your stomach.
- Don't lie down when taking the pill. Stand up or sit up straight.
- Stay upright for at least a minute or two after you swallow the pill. Some pills may require you to stay upright longer or drink more water. Be sure to read the information that comes with your medication and consult your pharmacist.

If you have trouble swallowing pills, ask your doctor or pharmacist if the drug is available in liquid form. Another option is to take the pill with a soft, bulky food, such as a banana. The food will pass down your esophagus, carrying the pill with it. You can also try taking the pill with applesauce, perhaps crushing it if necessary. But check with your doctor or pharmacist first because crushing a pill can disrupt the timed release of some medications and damage the protective coating.

For medication in liquid form, shake the solution before taking a dose. Measure the dose with the measuring device that comes with the medicine. Don't use a kitchen teaspoon or tablespoon. Follow the directions on the label for storage. Some liquid medications must be refrigerated while others should remain at room temperature.

Some medications are placed between your gums and cheek (buccal administration). Allow this type of medicine to dissolve slowly. Don't bite or chew it. Other medicines are taken under the tongue (sublingual administration) as tablets, films or sprays. These medicines must also be allowed to dissolve without biting or chewing them. Don't swallow the medication whole unless your doctor has told you to.

Taking a medication under the tongue will allow the drug to bypass the stomach and directly enter the bloodstream. However, not all medicine can be taken this way. Only use this method if your doctor has instructed you to do so.

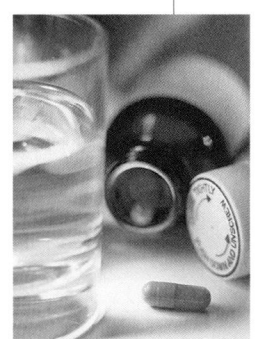

Inhalers

A variety of inhalers are available, but basically they fall into two categories — metered dose and dry powder. To use a metered dose inhaler, shake the inhaler vigorously five or six times immediately before using it. Remove the cap from the mouthpiece. If the cap wasn't on while you were carrying the inhaler, check the mouthpiece for dirt and foreign objects before using it.

If the inhaler hasn't been used for several days, do a test spray into the air. If your inhaler doesn't have a spacer built into it, attach a spacer to the nozzle end. A spacer is a 4- to 8-inch length of tubing that helps get more of the medication deep into your lungs. Without a spacer, medication is deposited in the back of your throat, which can lead to harmful side effects. You can buy a spacer or make your own out of a cardboard, plastic or paper tube.

Hold your head erect and sit up straight or stand. Breathe in and out normally once, then stop for a moment. Don't try to push all

of the air from your lungs. Close your mouth around the end of the spacer. Squeeze the inhaler once as you breathe in slowly. Keep inhaling even after finishing the squeeze. Continue inhaling for five to seven seconds. This process mixes the medication with the incoming air and pulls it into your lungs slowly.

After inhaling, remove the spacer from your mouth and hold your breath for 10 seconds. Then slowly exhale through your mouth. Wait a minute before taking your next inhalation. If you've been directed to take two doses at a time, breathe normally four or five times and repeat the process just described, beginning with shaking the inhaler. When you're done, gargle or brush your teeth and spit out the water.

Dry powder inhalers (DPI) may vary slightly but they typically need to be "loaded," or prepared for inhalation. To use a dry powder inhaler, turn your head to the side and exhale. Next, place your mouth around the mouthpiece without using a spacer and inhale strongly and steadily. Hold your breath for 10 seconds. Then take the inhaler away from your mouth and exhale slowly. When you're done, close the inhaler as directed.

Nasal sprays

Before you use a nasal spray, blow your nose to clear your nostrils. Shake the sprayer gently. Tilt your head forward. Close one nostril by pressing a finger against it. Insert the sprayer tip about a half-inch into your other nostril, with the tip pointing toward the side of your nose — away from the center of your nose. Squeeze the sprayer and sniff at the same time. Repeat these steps with the opposite nostril.

Try not to blow your nose for a couple of minutes to allow time for the medication to be absorbed into the blood vessels in your nose.

Clean the sprayer tip with warm water and dry it. Put the cap over the tip to keep it clean.

Nebulizers

Nebulizers are devices that turn a liquid into a fine mist that's then breathed into the lungs. To use a nebulizer, put the medicine in the nebulizer's medicine cup and turn on the device. Use a mouthpiece or mask and breathe slowly and deeply through your mouth until the medication is gone.

Topical medications

Creams, gels, ointments and sprays that you put directly on your skin can deliver medication directly to the site that needs it. Wash your hands before and after applying the medication. With creams, gels and ointments, apply the prescribed amount onto the center of the affected area and spread it out into a thin layer. Don't cover the area with gauze or other material unless instructed to by your doctor. With sprays, shake the can and hold the nozzle at least 6 inches from the skin, unless otherwise directed.

As with other forms of medications, more isn't better. An overdose of some topical medications, such as the steroid hydrocortisone, can affect other parts of your body and cause serious side effects.

Eye ointments

Always wash your hands before and after applying an eye ointment. Next, lie down, sit or stand with your head tilted back. Draw the lower eyelid down, look upward and place approximately a half-inch-long bead of the ointment along the inside margin of your lower eyelid. Don't touch your eye or eyelid with the tube because doing so can contaminate the medication in the tube. Close your eye and roll it around to distribute the ointment across the surface of the eye. With a tissue, gently remove any excess ointment from your eyelashes.

Eyedrops

Wash your hands, tilt your head back, draw the lower eyelid down and look upward. Place the drops in the pocket formed between your lower eyelid and eye. Close your eye and press a finger against the inner corner of the eye. Avoid putting drops directly on the cornea and don't touch the dropper to your eye. This could contaminate the rest of the eyedrops. Close your eye and use a tissue to gently remove any excess solution from your eyelashes or eyelid.

Eardrops

Tilt your head so that the affected ear is angled up. Straighten the ear canal to receive the medication. For kids, draw the earlobe down and back. For adults draw it up and back. Then deliver the prescribed number of drops into your ear. Try to avoid touching your ear canal with the dropper to prevent it from becoming contaminated. Keep your head tilted for a few minutes to allow the medication to drain deep into the ear.

Injections

Injections can be subcutaneous or intramuscular. Subcutaneous injections are often given in the abdomen, while intramuscular injections might be given in the thigh, buttocks or arms. Before giving yourself either kind of injection, clean the injection site with an alcohol swab.

For a subcutaneous injection, pinch up the skin and tissue slightly and insert the needle. Slowly press the plunger or button down. If you're using a pen, leave the needle in place for a few seconds before removing.

For an intramuscular injection, inject directly into the muscular region. There's no need to pinch up the skin.

Some injectable medications come in pre-filled syringes with a needle that retracts after the injection is given. Whatever type of needle you have, it's important to

dispose of it in a sharps container to avoid needle sticks and injury. You can purchase these containers at a pharmacy or online, or you can use a hard plastic container like an empty milk jug or laundry detergent jug.

Skin patches

Another way to deliver medication is through a patch worn on your skin. Patches can be filled with many medications, from fentanyl, which helps control severe pain, to estrogen, which helps reduce symptoms of menopause. Patches release a steady flow of medication until it's exhausted.

Your doctor will tell you where to place the patch on your body and when to change it. This information is also available in the instructions that come with the medication. To help avoid skin irritations, rotate where you place the patches. If you still experience skin irritation, tell your doctor. Don't cut the patches unless your doctor directs you to do so. In addition, follow your doctor's advice about how to discard a patch.

When it's time to put on a new patch, make sure to remove the old one first.

Rectal suppositories

Before inserting a rectal suppository, put on latex gloves. To make the suppository easier to insert, coat it with a lubricant such as petroleum jelly. Remove the foil or plastic packaging first, then lie on your side and insert the suppository, pointed end first, as far as possible into the rectum. Push the bottom of the suppository sideways to be sure that some portion of it touches the bowel wall.

If you have trouble keeping the suppository inside your rectum, you may not have inserted it far enough. You may also find it helpful to hold your buttocks together for a short while after inserting the suppository. When finished, dispose of the gloves and wash your hands.

Vaginal medications

Most vaginal medications, such as those for yeast infections, come in the form of creams, gels, foams and suppositories. Wash your hands before and after applying the medication. Lie down on your back or side and insert the medication as directed, typically a few inches inside the vagina. Don't insert a tampon afterward because it will absorb some of the medication. Wearing a panty liner will help protect your clothes from medication that may leak out.

Safety

To make sure your medication works as it's supposed to, take it as instructed. To ensure your safety, take the following steps:

Communicate

Share all medical information with your doctor and pharmacist so that he or she can ensure the most appropriate medication and dose for your individual needs. This includes letting him or her know about all medications (prescription and over-the-counter) and nutritional supplements that you're taking and any medical conditions you may have, such as high blood pressure or glaucoma. Ask questions if you don't understand why you're being prescribed a particular medication. Share any adverse effects you think you may be having from the medications you're taking.

Be sure to talk with your doctor or pharmacist before stopping any medications. Abruptly stopping certain medications may cause severe adverse effects.

Read the instructions

Before taking any new medication, read the label and any accompanying information to learn all you can about it. If you have unanswered questions, check with your pharmacist, doctor or other health care professional. For example, the label may contain directions about usage or information about side effects that you didn't know or weren't told about.

The label on the container of a prescription medication should bear your first and last name, the name of the person who prescribed it, the pharmacy address and telephone number, the prescription number, the date of dispensing, the name of the medication, the directions for its use and, in some states, a description of the medication in the container. An expiration date may be given and there may also be information on proper storage and proper disposal.

All of this information is important in identifying your medications and using them properly. Don't remove the label from a container and keep accompanying paperwork, which often contains more-detailed information that you can refer back to if needed.

Keep medication in its original containers whenever possible. Original containers are usually childproof, protect the medication from light and prevent members of your family from mixing up medications. If a label gets separated from its container and you're not sure of the contents, discard the medication or call your pharmacist, who may be able to help you identify the medication.

Don't share medications

A medication that calms your throbbing headache may not help a friend or relative in the same way. In fact, the medication could cause a life-threatening allergic reaction or other complications. Allergies, age, sex, race, weight, genetic factors and the general status of your health all can affect your reaction to medication.

Even if someone uses the same type of prescription medication as you, his or her prescription may be of a different strength or a different preparation. The pills may look the same, and the labels may appear to match, but that doesn't mean your medication is safe for that person.

In determining what's best for you, your doctor takes into consideration what other medications you're taking, your health, your age, and any drug allergies or sensitivities that you may have. Keeping these factors in mind, your doctor determines the appropriate medication, the appropriate dose and the duration of treatment.

Store your medications properly and securely

Having a designated area for medications that you take regularly can help you keep them organized, easy to find and out of the reach of children. Consider the following tips:

- Don't store your medications in humid places. Heat, moisture and direct light can change a medication's effectiveness. For these reasons, don't leave your medication on a windowsill or in a car.
- Store your medications in a dark, dry, cool place.
- Keep liquid medications from freezing.
- Don't store medication in the refrigerator unless directed to do so.

Regardless of where you keep your medications, they should be out of the reach of children, pets or anyone who should not have access to them. Even if visits from youngsters are rare, take precautions. Cabinet and dresser drawer locks are a good idea for keeping toddlers away from medications inside. Child-resistant caps provide a second line of defense.

It can be tempting to leave medication on a kitchen counter or bedside table for the sake of convenience. But because young children may find the bright colors irresistible, it's important to avoid the habit of leaving medications out. If you have medication that must be refrigerated, put it on a high shelf so that young children can't reach it, or in a place where it's not visible.

If you have teenagers at home, consider keeping prescription medications in a secure location that only you know about. A majority of teens who abuse prescription medicine tend to get it from family and other people they know.

If you're concerned about possible poisoning from medication, call the American Association of Poison Control Centers at 800-222-1222 or call your regional poison control center. Poison control centers are excellent resources for poisoning information and, in many situations, may advise that in-home observation is all that's needed.

Check for expired medications

Periodically go through your medications. Get rid of unused, outdated prescription drugs. Medication deteriorates over time — even sooner than the printed expiration date if it hasn't been stored properly. If the expiration date isn't listed, the general rule is to discard the medication a year after it was dispensed.

If you develop the same health problem you had several years ago, don't take leftover medication.

Dispose of medications safely

Always dispose of unused or expired drugs around your home so that no one accidentally takes a medication or intentionally misuses it. Check the label or patient information guide for disposal instructions or ask your pharmacist for advice on disposal.

Medicine take-back programs are a convenient way to dispose

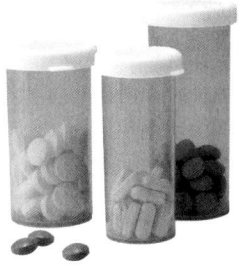
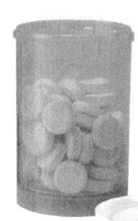

of unneeded medicines. Check with your local law enforcement agency to find out if one of these programs exists in your community. Some pharmacies are also authorized to collect unwanted medications. To find out if there's such a pharmacy in your area, visit the U.S. Drug Enforcement Administration's official website.

If a prescription drug label has no instructions for disposal and a medicine take-back program isn't nearby, you can throw unneeded medications in your trash. However, the Food and Drug Administration (FDA) recommends that you take these precautions:

1. Take the medicine out of its original container and mix it with something inedible such as dirt, kitty litter or used coffee grounds.
2. Place the mixture in a sealed bag and throw it into the trash.
3. Scratch out any personal information on the prescription label before disposing of the original container.

Have an emergency preparedness plan

Severe weather and other unexpected events may disrupt your daily routine and affect your care. It's important to have a plan in place so that you're prepared with the medications and supplies you need. As part of your plan, keep an up-to-date list of all of your medications and supplies. List the doctor who prescribed them and the pharmacy where you bought them. Also keep your prescription benefit card in a safe place.

Whenever possible, keep at least five to seven days' worth of medication and supplies on hand. Have extra batteries on hand for meters, hearing aids, or other medical equipment that you use. Store water to drink and to take your medications with and keep a supply of nonperishable foods for medicines that must be taken with food. If you have diabetes, include a quick-acting source of glucose.

For common injuries and emergencies, keep at least one well-stocked first-aid kit in your home and one in your car. Store your kits someplace easy to get to and out of the reach of young children. Make sure children who are old enough to understand the purpose of the kits know where they're stored. Periodically check the kit for expired or used supplies that need to be replaced.

You can buy first-aid kits at many drugstores or assemble your own (see page 31). You may want to tailor your kit based on your activities and needs.

If a disaster does happen, check your medications afterward. Moisture, light and excessive temperatures can damage medication. Be sure your medications are OK to use. Contact your pharmacist if you're not sure whether your medication is still good.

If you missed doses of medication during a disaster, follow the instructions the pharmacy gives about missed doses. Contact a pharmacist or doctor if you're not sure about what to do. Never take additional doses to make up for those you've missed. Talk first with your doctor.

Be prepared when traveling

Before traveling, pack extra medication in case you need to be away from home longer than expected. Follow these additional suggestions when preparing for travel.

Travel by plane

If you're traveling by plane with prescription medications, check the Transportation Security Administration's (TSA) website for medication guidelines. Bring medications in their original containers so that security personnel can easily verify that they're prescribed to you by a doctor. If you're traveling internationally, you may need to show a copy of the actual prescription from your doctor. Ask for this from your pharmacy ahead of time.

Carry your medications on the plane. Don't pack them in your luggage. Although you're allowed to bring only a limited amount of liquid medication on the plane, do not transfer liquid medication into a smaller container without a prescription label. Check with the TSA if you have a large amount of liquid medication you need to bring with you.

If you have a medical device, ask your doctor for a letter that explains the need for the device. Show the letter to airport security officials if they have questions during the screening process.

If you receive medication through a pump, such as insulin, there's a chance the pump motor may not work if it goes through a full-body scanner, X-ray machine or other imaging equipment. Remove your pump before going through a full-body scanner or ask to have a different screening process, such as a hand-wand inspection.

Travel by car

If traveling by car, bring medications in their original containers unless you use a pill box. Pack your medications in easy-to-reach places and avoid leaving them in extreme temperatures.

Watch for drug interactions

If you take more than one medication, you want to avoid potentially dangerous interactions. Two or more drugs taken together can produce an interaction that makes you feel worse instead of better — or

Common Drug Interactions

Here are some examples of drugs that can cause interactions. Many others that aren't listed here also can cause interactions. It's important to talk with your doctor or pharmacist before taking any new medication.

Type of medication	Talk to your doctor or pharmacist if you:
Antacids	• Take a prescription drug • Have kidney disease
Antihistamines	• Take sedatives or tranquilizers • Take a prescription drug for high blood pressure or depression • Have a breathing problem, such as emphysema, asthma or chronic bronchitis • Have glaucoma • Have difficulty urinating due to an enlarged prostate gland
HMGCoA reductase inhibitor (statin)	• Take gemfibrozil for high triglycerides • Eat grapefruit or drink grapefruit juice • Are prescribed certain antifungal medications • Take warfarin to prevent blood clots • Take antiretroviral medications for HIV infection
Inhalers (bronchodilators)	• Have heart disease, high blood pressure, thyroid disease or diabetes • Take prescription drugs for asthma or have ever been hospitalized for asthma
Nasal decongestants	• Have heart disease, high blood pressure, thyroid disease or diabetes • Have difficulty urinating due to an enlarged prostate gland
Nicotine replacement products	• Have high blood pressure not controlled by medication • Have heart disease or an irregular heartbeat or have had a recent heart attack • Take a prescription non-nicotine stop-smoking drug
Sleep medications	• Take prescription sedatives or tranquilizers • Consume alcohol • Have a breathing problem, such as emphysema, asthma or bronchitis • Have glaucoma
Pain relievers	• Consume three or more alcoholic beverages a day • Have kidney or liver disease • Take prescription drugs

Based on Food and Drug Administration data, 2013

may decrease the effectiveness of one or both drugs. Work with your doctor and pharmacist to ensure your medications don't clash.

Drug interactions become an increasing problem as you age because older adults tend to take more medications. They also don't eliminate the medication from their bodies as quickly as someone younger. Take the following precautions to prevent such adverse drug reactions from both prescription and over-the-counter drugs:

- Bring a list of all of the medications you're taking and their dosages to each medical appointment. Make sure to include nonprescription medications, including herbal supplements.
- Have all of your prescriptions filled at the same pharmacy, if possible. Having a pharmacist who can help you keep track of your medications and explain their proper use may prevent an adverse reaction.
- Talk to your doctor or pharmacist about possible drug interactions before taking any nonprescription medication.

Signs of drug interactions

During an office visit your doctor might notice signs of a possible drug interaction, such as an abnormal heart rhythm or changes in the results of your laboratory tests. But you may spot signs of potential problems even sooner. If you experience any of the following signs and symptoms after you start a new medication, contact your doctor right away:

- Skin rashes
- Change in bowel habits
- Continuing heartburn
- Dizziness
- Confusion
- Persistent nausea and vomiting
- Extreme fatigue

Watch for food and drug interactions

When you mix certain foods and drugs, you can end up with differ-

What You Should Know About Aspirin

Aspirin is a powerful medication with a wide range of uses, yet it's often taken for granted as a mere fever reducer, headache tamer or arthritis soother.

Aspirin can also help prevent a heart attack and stroke. According to the American Heart Association, chewing an aspirin at the first sign of a heart attack, such as chest pain, could save 5,000 to 10,000 lives each year. Because aspirin makes your blood less likely to clot, it lowers your risk of a blood clot obstructing a coronary artery. Chewing the aspirin gets the medicine into your bloodstream faster.

What is aspirin?

Aspirin is acetylsalicylic acid. This natural substance comes from the bark of willow trees. Aspirin is referred to in medical terms as an analgesic (pain reliever) and a nonsteroidal anti-inflammatory drug (NSAID).

Side effects

With its many benefits, aspirin also carries some potentially serious side effects: stomach irritation, gastrointestinal bleeding and urinary tract bleeding. In children, it can cause Reye's syndrome. If you take aspirin regularly, talk to your doctor about ways to reduce its side effects.

ent results than if you had taken them separately. In most cases, the interaction decreases how much the drug is absorbed into the bloodstream. But in some cases, it blocks the breakdown of the drug, causing buildup of the drug in your bloodstream.

Like many people, you might enjoy grapefruit or grapefruit juice at breakfast. But if you also take prescription drugs, the combination could result in a higher blood level of the medication than intended.

Researchers first discovered an interaction between grapefruit juice and felodipine, a drug used to treat cardiovascular disease. Later studies revealed that grapefruit juice alters the effects of many other medications as well.

Among juices made from citrus fruits, grapefruit juice is unique. Chemicals in this juice interfere with certain enzymes in your liver that break down many prescription drugs. This can result in high-

er blood levels of the drug than your doctor intended, even if you take the drug several hours after consuming grapefruit. If you take any medications, ask your doctor or pharmacist whether it's safe to eat grapefruit or drink grapefruit juice.

Here are some other effects of combining certain foods and drugs:

- Consuming variable amounts of leafy vegetables, green tea, and other foods or drinks that contain vitamin K can decrease the effect of warfarin, an anticoagulant medication, thereby increasing the risk of clotting.
- The antibiotic tetracycline may not be fully absorbed if taken with dairy products.

Watch for herb and drug interactions

Although herbal supplements are considered "natural," many contain active ingredients that

What is Pharmacogenomic Testing?

Your body is made up of thousands of genes that you inherited from your parents. Some of these genes are responsible for how your body processes medications. A form of testing called pharmacogenomics can determine how your genes may affect your response to drugs, including whether a medication may be an effective treatment for you or whether you may experience side effects to a specific drug.

The need for pharmacogenomic testing is determined on an individual basis. Currently, only certain medications can be tested, such as codeine, the blood thinning drug warfarin (Coumadin), the statin simvastatin (Zocor) and some antidepressants. Your doctor can determine whether a pharmacogenomic test is warranted before beginning a specific treatment.

don't safely mix with prescription or over-the-counter medications. Therefore, it's important to let your doctor know about any herbal supplements you take.

Following are some commonly used herbs and listings of prescription and over-the-counter drugs that you shouldn't mix them with:

Feverfew, garlic, ginger, ginkgo
These herbs may augment the anticoagulant effect of the following drugs and may cause spontaneous and excessive bleeding:
• Aspirin (Bayer, Bufferin, others)
• Clopidogrel (Plavix)
• Warfarin (Coumadin)

St. John's wort
St. John's wort has been shown to increase the body's breakdown of the following drugs. Many other medications also may be affected.
• Antidepressants
• Many chemotherapy drugs
• Digoxin (Lanoxin)
• Theophylline
• Cyclosporine (Neoral, Sandimmune)
• Warfarin (Coumadin)

The combination of St. John's wort and some antidepressant medications may cause an excess of the chemical serotonin (serotonin syndrome). Typical symptoms of serotonin syndrome include a headache, stomach upset, fever and restlessness.

Ginseng
Avoid mixing ginseng with:
• Warfarin (Coumadin)
• Phenelzine (Nardil)
• Digoxin (Lanoxin)

Taken with warfarin, ginseng can increase the risk of bleeding. Used with phenelzine, it may cause a headache, trembling and mania. Used with digoxin, it may interfere with the drug's intended action.

Melatonin
Combined with the following drugs, melatonin can produce deep sedation:
• Sedatives
• Antipsychotics
• Alcohol
• Drugs used to treat anxiety or Parkinson's disease

Echinacea
Echinacea can be toxic to the liver and shouldn't be combined with other medications that can cause liver damage. Because this herb stimulates the immune system, it can also interfere with the effects of some immunosuppressant medications. Avoid mixing echinacea with the following:
• Anabolic steroids
• Methotrexate
• Amiodarone (Pacerone)
• Ketoconazole (Nizoral)
• Cyclosporine (Neoral, Sandimmune)

Mixing Alcohol and Medication

Alcohol can change how some medications work. If you drink alcohol while you're on medication, you're putting yourself at risk of illness, injury and death. Because alcohol is sedating, this danger is especially true of drugs that tend to make you sleepy, such as many antihistamines and medications used to treat anxiety, depression, pain and muscle spasms. You could end up with two sedatives instead of one — an overdose.

Individuals who drink moderate to excessive amounts of alcohol on a regular basis (chronic drinkers) and who take acetaminophen (Tylenol) — even at the standard dose — are at increased risk of liver damage. In addition, ibuprofen (Advil, Motrin IB, others) and naproxen sodium (Aleve), like alcohol, can irritate your stomach. When taken with alcohol, they can cause stomach ulceration and bleeding. Consuming excessive amounts of alcohol while taking the anticoagulant drug warfarin (Coumadin) may enhance its effect, increasing your risk of life-threatening bleeding.

If you take medication regularly and wonder if it's OK to have an occasional alcoholic drink, ask your doctor.

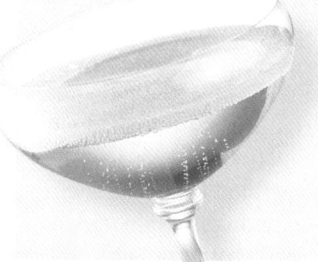

Gluten in Medication

In some medications, the inactive ingredients that bind together the contents of the pills or tablets contain gluten. If you have celiac disease, it's important to read the labels of any supplements or over-the-counter medications you purchase. Look for ingredients associated with gluten, especially wheat, wheat starch and other modified starches that aren't derived from corn or other gluten-free sources.

In addition, make sure to let your pharmacist know that you can't take prescription medications that contain gluten. If you switch from a brand medication to a generic drug or from one generic drug to a different generic made by a different manufacturer, you'll need to recheck that the medication doesn't contain gluten.

Gluten in medications may also be a concern for Jewish people during Passover (Pesach). It's recommended that you consult your rabbi regarding the permissibility of medicines during Pesach and throughout the year.

Cayenne

Cayenne may increase the absorption and impact of the following drugs:

- Angiotensin-converting enzyme (ACE) inhibitors, used for heart failure, high blood pressure, kidney disease
- Theophylline, an asthma medication

Cayenne may also increase the likelihood of developing a cough when it's taken with an ACE inhibitor.

Avoid the sun, if so instructed

Some medications can make your skin more sensitive to ultraviolet rays in sunlight. If you take such a medication, even slight sun exposure can result in skin redness, itching, swelling and blisters. This is known as a photosensitivity reaction, or photoreaction.

Medications that can produce this reaction include:

- Certain nonsteroidal anti-inflammatory drugs (NSAIDs), such as naproxen sodium (Aleve)
- Some types of antibiotics, such as tetracycline, sulfa drugs or quinolones
- The high blood pressure medication hydrochlorothiazide (Microzide, others)
- Some birth control pills
- Anti-nausea medications
- Tricyclic antidepressants
- Phenothiazines, taken for nausea and some psychological disorders
- Some chemotherapy drugs
- Some diabetes medications, such as glyburide
- The heart drug amiodarone (Pacerone)
- Tretinoin, used in prescription antiwrinkle creams and acne medications
- The acne medication isotretinoin (Claravis, Myorisan)

Anyone can have a photoreaction to a medication. Some reactions are mild, while others can be quite severe. If the combination of sun and your medication seems to be causing a photoreaction, talk to your doctor about steps that you can take to protect against future reactions.

Brand-Name vs. Generic Drugs

When a new drug is developed, the pharmaceutical company that developed the drug generally gets 20-year patent rights to it — meaning that during this time, the developer is the only company that can sell the drug. This allows the pharmaceutical company to recoup money spent on research, development, promotion and marketing of the drug.

Extensions and new patents are sometimes granted, but once a patent expires, other pharmaceutical companies are free to produce and sell their own version of the drug. This generic form of a drug must meet the same Food and Drug Administration (FDA) standards established for the original drug.

Because companies that produce generic drugs don't incur the large expenses in research and development, they can offer the drug at a much lower price than the brand-name drug. Generics get their name from the fact that when a drug is discovered or produced in a laboratory, it's first given a generic name that's designated by governmental agencies. This name identifies the drug as unique, and it distinguishes the drug from all others. The generic name is nonproprietary, meaning it's not owned by anyone.

When the drug receives approval for sale to the public, it's usually given another name (a brand name) by the original manufacturer. Other pharmaceutical companies that decide to produce their own version of the drug after the patent expires often market the drug under its generic name, or under their own brand name. In either case, it's usually less expensive than the original brand.

Generics are available for many medications now on the market. Aside from the name, price and inactive ingredients — such as dyes, fillers and coatings — there's typically little difference between a generic drug and its brand-name counterpart. The FDA mandates that generic and brand-name drugs have the same clinical effect.

What should I do if I forget to take my medication?

You want to take your medication on schedule, but sometimes you may simply forget to do so or an unexpected event may disrupt your routine. If you're an hour or two late and you're not scheduled to take the medication again for several more hours, it's usually best to go ahead and take it right away. If, however, you're more than several hours late and you're getting close to your next scheduled dose, wait until the next time you're scheduled to take the drug.

If you miss a dose, don't take a double dose the next time that you're scheduled to take the drug. Consult your doctor or pharmacist if you have questions.

Health Claims on Supplement Labels

Some dietary supplements have nutritional value that may be beneficial to your health. However, certain supplements claim to provide big benefits that go beyond nutritional value. The natural products industry refers to these items as nutraceuticals. These products may claim to boost your immune system, relieve memory loss, cure impotency or prevent any number of diseases. The claims are often unproved or fraudulent.

Be suspicious of products that promise to cure one or multiple conditions, help you lose weight effortlessly, or shrink tumors. Look out for any supplement that promotes itself as a scientific breakthrough, miracle cure or ancient remedy. Don't be fooled by the use of medical jargon and scientific terminology, which can often be misleading. Other signs of fraudulent health claims include excessive testimonials from patients or doctors, limited-time offers, and money-back guarantees.

Managing Your Medications

One of the most important steps you can take to get the most from your medications is to take an active role in your health care. Medical professionals will work with you, but you're ultimately responsible for your own health.

Be informed

Key to successfully managing your medications is to make sure that you and your doctor and pharmacist know:
- What medications you're taking
- Why you're taking them
- How you're taking them

Know the medications you're taking

Find out the exact name of each medication you take — both the generic name and the brand name. Write the names down in a personal medication record that you update at least once a year, or whenever you change a medication. Next to each drug listed, identify the name of the doctor who prescribed it.

PREVENTION TIP

Take these precautions to guard against food and drug interactions:
- Follow instructions from your doctor or pharmacist on how and when to take your medications.
- Don't take medications at the same time that you take vitamin or mineral supplements. Some supplements, especially calcium, can bind with many medications and impair their absorption.
- If you're instructed to take a drug on an empty stomach, take it at least an hour before or two hours after eating.
- Don't stir your medication into food.
- Don't mix medications into hot beverages. Heat can change or destroy some drug ingredients.

Know why you're taking each medication

Some people take so many medications that they find it hard to remember why they're taking some of them. Keep tabs on how each medication fits into your treatment plan.

Make sure you're taking each medication correctly

That means reviewing the dosages, the time of day you take the drugs and how you take them — on an empty stomach or with food.

Use only one pharmacy

A pharmacist is an important member of your health care team. In addition to performing traditional services, such as dispensing medications, your pharmacist can help you understand your medications and how to take them safely and effectively. Your pharmacist keeps a history of all medications

What are Biosimilars?

Many of today's newer medicines are made from living organisms, such as human or animal tissue, bacteria, or yeast. These medications are known as biologics. In contrast, conventional drugs are made of pure chemical substances, with structures that can be copied to produce an identical "generic" medicine. Because biologics are created from living organisms, an identical generic can't simply be created. That's where biosimilars come in.

Biosimilar agents are biologics with a molecular structure that's highly similar to, but not an exact match with, the original biologic product. The FDA will only approve a biosimilar product if it has the same mechanism of action, route of administration, dosage form and strength as the original biologic product. The biosimilar is expected to have no clinically meaningful difference in terms of safety, purity and potency. A pharmacist or doctor may substitute a biosimilar for the original biologic product, in the same way that a generic medication is used to replace the original drug.

that you have received from that pharmacy. Getting your medications at different pharmacies prevents your pharmacist from being able to check new medications against other medications you have received for drug interactions.

Because a pharmacist can play a vital role in protecting and improving your health, find a pharmacy that you feel comfortable with, whose staff are willing to assist you with your questions and concerns.

Other issues to consider include:
- Are you able to talk to a pharmacist without other people hearing you?
- Can a pharmacist be reached in case of an emergency?
- Does the pharmacy accept your prescription insurance plan?

If you change to a new pharmacy that doesn't have access to your medication records, it's important that you inform the pharmacists there about your medical history and the medications you're taking, including over-the-counter medications and dietary and herbal supplements.

A pharmacist can also help you select the appropriate medication. Many medications are available from more than one manufacturer.

Their effects may be the same, but their costs may be different.

Your insurance company, HMO or other third-party payer may reimburse you for only certain brands or for only part of their costs. A pharmacist can often help you determine which medications are covered by your medical payment plan and which cost less.

Review your medications with a pharmacist

During a medication therapy management (MTM) consultation, a pharmacist meets with you to discuss all of your medications, including prescriptions, over-the-counter drugs, vitamins, and dietary and herbal supplements. The pharmacist then examines each medication individually to determine possible side effects, negative interactions and unnecessary dosages. If medication issues are detected, the pharmacist will work with your health care providers to make beneficial changes to your medication regimen.

Develop a routine

If it would be helpful, use reminders to make sure that you take your medication at the right time.

Possibilities include:
- **Pillbox reminders.** Once a week or once a day, fill each compartment with the pills you need to take. Ask your pharmacist or doctor if it's OK to use a pillbox for your medications. Some pills, such as nitroglycerin, should be kept in their original container.
- **Medication containers with alarms.** Use a medication container that has a timer built into it. The timer can be set to sound an alarm or flash a small light when it's time to take your medication.
- **Cellphone alarms.** Set a timer on your phone to help you remember to take your medication each day.
- **Charts and calendars.** Develop a chart or calendar that lists your medication schedule. Keep it near your medications and each time you take a drug, check it off the list.

Common Medications

The purpose of this section is to provide some basic information about commonly used medications in the hope that the information may help answer some of your questions. Following is a list of some of the most frequently used medications and their functions. It's not intended to be an all-inclusive listing of medications in each class or an exhaustive list of medications available to treat a certain medical condition.

Medications are listed by body system, with included conditions listed in alphabetical order. We've included products available by prescription as well as some that are sold without a prescription.

The availability of medications is subject to change. New medications are continuously being developed, and some brand-name

Common Myths About Generics

You've taken the brand-name medication for years. Now your pharmacist says you have a choice — a generic drug is available too. Is what you've heard about generics true?

Myth: Generic drugs aren't as strong, effective or safe as brand-name drugs.
Fact: Generics are required by the Food and Drug Administration (FDA) to have the same quality, strength, purity, stability and effectiveness as their brand-name counterparts. And because generics have the same active ingredients, generics have the same risks and benefits as their brand-name counterparts.

Myth: Generic drugs don't act as quickly in the body.
Fact: A generic drug must deliver the same amount of active ingredient in the same amount of time as the original brand-name drug.

Myth: Generic drugs have more side effects.
Fact: A generic drug has the same active ingredient as its brand-name counterpart, therefore it has the same side effect risk.

Myth: Generics are often made in substandard facilities.
Fact: The FDA conducts thousands of inspections each year to ensure that the manufacturing facilities of both brand-name and generic drugs meet government standards. In fact, about half of all generics are produced by brand-name firms that make copies of their own or other brand-name drugs.

medications may be discontinued. For additional information regarding a particular medication, talk with your pharmacist or other member of your health care team.

Cardiovascular medications

Angina medications

Nitrates
Generic and common brand names
- Isosorbide dinitrate (Isordil, others)
- Isosorbide mononitrate
- Sublingual nitroglycerin (NitroMist, Nitrostat, others)

Action
Dilate your blood vessels, increasing blood and oxygen to your heart and reducing your heart's workload. Also dilate the veins, reducing the return of blood to the heart.

Note
These medications are used for relief of acute chest pain. Keep sublingual nitroglycerin in the original bottle and put that bottle in a container or location that protects it from sunlight. Replace the drug every three to six months to ensure a fresh supply. When taking sublingual nitrates, always be seated and don't attempt to drive or operate dangerous equipment because fainting is possible. Call for emergency help if your symptoms persist after three doses of sublingual nitroglycerin. If you've had a heart attack in the past, call if your symptoms persist after just one dose.

Arrhythmia medications

Anti-arrhythmics
Generic and common brand names
- Amiodarone (Pacerone)
- Dofetilide (Tikosyn)
- Flecainide
- Propafenone (Rythmol SR)

Action
Delay electric impulses through the nerves and muscle of the heart, helping to restore and maintain normal heart rate and rhythm.

Note
These drugs are used to correct irregular or rapid heartbeats (arrhythmias). Amiodarone can be associated with thyroid, liver and lung dysfunction, therefore, it's important to see a doctor regularly if taking these medications. In addition, several medications may interact with antiarrhythmics. Don't take a new medication before talking to your doctor or a health care professional.

Blood clot prevention medications

Anticoagulants (injected)
Generic and common brand names
- Dalteparin (Fragmin)
- Enoxaparin (Lovenox)
- Heparin

Action
Prevent the activation of clotting factors, proteins that are essential for normal blood clotting. Injected anticoagulants work more quickly than oral anticoagulants.

Note
These medications are used to treat circulatory disorders such as deep vein thrombosis. They're also commonly used after surgery or during hospitalization to prevent blood clotting. Low molecular weight heparin (dalteparin, enoxaparin) may be prescribed on an outpatient basis for certain individuals who have blood clots in the leg (deep vein thrombosis) and are capable of giving themselves daily injections of the drug.

Anticoagulants (oral)
Generic and common brand names
- Warfarin (Coumadin)

Action

Decrease the formation of clotting factors, proteins that are essential for normal blood clotting. Often referred to as blood thinners, though they don't actually thin the blood.

Note

These medications help to reduce the risk of a heart attack and stroke in people with artificial heart valves, irregular heart rhythms and blood-clotting disorders. Make sure to check with your doctor before taking other medications, including aspirin and NSAIDs, to avoid potentially harmful interactions. It's important to check your blood regularly to make sure you're getting the right dose.

Anti-platelet drugs

Generic and common brand names
• Aspirin (Bayer, Bufferin, others)
• Clopidogrel (Plavix)

Action

Reduce blood clotting by inhibiting the ability of platelets to cross-link, forming blood clots.

Note

These medicines help prevent blood clots, reducing your risk of a heart attack and stroke. Talk with your doctor or pharmacist before you take aspirin or any other NSAID.

Direct thrombin inhibitors

Generic and common brand names
• Dabigatran (Pradaxa)

Action

Reduces the risk of blood clots by blocking the action of thrombin, a substance that leads to clotting in the blood.

Note

Dabigatran is also used to treat blood clots and prevent them from happening again. This medication helps decrease the chance of developing blood clots. Among

Over-the-Counter vs. Prescription Medications

Over-the-counter, or nonprescription, medications can be purchased without a prescription. Innumerable over-the-counter medications, including aspirin, cough syrups and laxatives, are sold in drugstores, groceries, discount stores and convenience stores. In recent years, a number of prescription-strength medications have become available for over-the-counter use. These include certain nasal steroids, antihistamines, proton pump inhibitors and nicotine patches, gum and lozenges, as well as products for congestion, coughs, heartburn and acne.

Prescription medications, meanwhile, can be purchased only from a licensed pharmacy and with a written prescription from your doctor. These include an array of drugs from antibiotics to painkillers.

Some medications are available both over-the-counter and by prescription. The over-the-counter version may not contain the same amount of drug as its prescription counterpart, so be sure to check with your pharmacist if you have questions about what dose is appropriate.

Even nonprescription medications can cause side effects and be dangerous if misused. Read the product label before taking any over-the counter medication. The label lists important information, including the active ingredient or ingredients, the medication's uses (sometimes called indications), warnings, directions and inactive ingredients. If you still have questions after reading the label, talk to your doctor or pharmacist.

Be especially careful to check the active ingredients when taking medications for a fever, flu, cold or pain relief. Because many of these medicines contain acetaminophen, it's easy to accidentally take too much of this drug. Avoid using more than one acetaminophen-containing product at a time, regardless of whether it's nonprescription or prescription. Taking too much acetaminophen can lead to severe liver damage.

people with atrial fibrillation, it may reduce the risk of experiencing a stroke.

Factor Xa inhibitors

Generic and common brand names
• Apixaban (Eliquis)
• Edoxaban (Savaysa)
• Rivaroxaban (Xarelto)

Action

Reduce the risk of blood clots by stopping the formation of thrombin, a substance that leads to clotting in the blood.

Note

These drugs are used to treat blood clots. Some are also used to prevent

blood clots following surgery or in people with atrial fibrillation.

Blood pressure medications

Alpha blockers

Generic and common brand names
• Doxazosin (Cardura)
• Terazosin

Action

Block the stimulation of muscles that constrict smaller arteries and raise blood pressure.

Note

The drugs may also be used to treat symptoms of benign prostatic hyperplasia (BPH).

Ordering Drugs by Mail

Ordering medications by mail has become a common way for people to obtain prescriptions. You may choose a mail-order pharmacy rather than a local pharmacy for a number of reasons:

- **Convenience.** You don't have to go farther than your mailbox to get your medications.
- **Price.** Depending on your prescription coverage, mail-order pharmacies may be less expensive or allow higher quantities to be dispensed than what you'd receive at a local pharmacy.
- **Availability.** Some limited-distribution medications are only available through select specialty pharmacies.

One trade-off when using mail-order services is that you don't have a local pharmacist who knows you. Make sure the mail-order pharmacy you use sends you information on the medications you are receiving and has a toll-free number that you can call to speak with a pharmacist if you have questions.

Another thing to keep in mind is time lag. It can take up to 10 days to get drugs by mail, so it's imperative that you order medications far enough in advance to not run out of them. Because of this wait time, mail service is most appropriate for long-term-maintenance prescription drugs. Prescriptions for medications that are needed immediately or needed only once — such as an antibiotic for an infection — should be filled at your local pharmacy.

Mail-order prescriptions usually arrive in an unmarked package. After the medication is delivered, it's important to retrieve the package in a timely manner to prevent prolonged exposure to extreme temperatures. Many mail-order pharmacies will provide tracking numbers or shipping information to let patients know when an item is delivered.

Angiotensin-converting enzyme (ACE) inhibitors

Generic and common brand names
- Benazepril (Lotensin)
- Enalapril (Vasotec)
- Lisinopril (Prinivil, Zestril)
- Ramipril (Altace)

Action

Block production of a substance called angiotensin II, which narrows your blood vessels and causes you to retain salt and fluids, increasing blood pressure. The medications also enhance the action of a compound called bradykinin, which opens blood vessels.

Note

Notify your doctor immediately if you notice swelling in your face or lips. Don't take these medications if you're pregnant or plan to become pregnant because they can cause serious birth defects. Some ACE inhibitors are also used to treat congestive heart failure or kidney disease and to prevent recurrent heart attacks and strokes. These medications also help prevent or reduce complications of diabetes. In some people, these drugs can cause a dry cough.

Angiotensin II receptor blockers

Generic and common brand names
- Candesartan (Atacand)
- Losartan (Cozaar)
- Valsartan (Diovan)

Action

Prevent angiotensin II from binding to tissues, inhibiting blood vessel narrowing and retention of salt and fluids.

Note

These medications have less of a tendency to cause coughing compared with ACE inhibitors. Don't take these drugs if you're pregnant or planning to become pregnant because they can cause birth defects. Some of the drugs in this class may also be used to treat kidney disease and congestive heart failure and to prevent stroke.

Beta blockers

Generic and common brand names
- Atenolol (Tenormin)
- Carvedilol (Coreg)
- Metoprolol (Lopressor, Toprol XL)
- Propranolol (Inderal LA)

Action

Block the action of adrenaline and similar substances, helping to dilate blood vessels and slow the rate and intensity of the heartbeat.

Note

Some beta blockers are also used to treat a heart attack, heart arrhythmia and angina and to prevent a heart attack, heart failure and migraines.

Calcium channel blockers

Generic and common brand names
- Amlodipine (Norvasc)
- Diltiazem (Cardizem, Tiazac)
- Nifedipine (Adalat CC, Procardia, others)
- Verapamil (Calan, Verelan)

Action

Prevent calcium from flowing through muscle cell channels. This decreases the intensity with which your heart beats and relaxes the smooth muscles of the blood vessels.

Note

Some calcium channel blockers are also used to treat chest pain (angina) and heart arrhythmias. Don't eat grapefruit or drink grapefruit juice with some of these medications. A substance in the juice reduces your liver's ability to eliminate the medications from your body, potentially allowing them to accumulate to toxic levels.

Central-acting agents
Generic and common brand names
- Clonidine (Catapres)
- Methyldopa

Action
Prevent your brain from sending signals to your nervous system to speed up your heart rate and narrow your blood vessels.

Note
Abruptly stopping some of these drugs can cause your blood pressure to rise to dangerously high levels very quickly.

Diuretics
Generic and common brand names
Loop diuretics
- Furosemide (Lasix)
- Torsemide (Demadex)

Potassium-sparing diuretics
- Spironolactone (Aldactone)
- Triamterene (Dyrenium)

Thiazide diuretics
- Chlorthalidone
- Hydrochlorothiazide (Dyazide, Microzide, others)
- Indapamide
- Metolazone

Action
Cause your kidneys to excrete more sodium than usual. The sodium takes with it water from your blood. Less blood volume reduces blood pressure. Each class of diuretics works on a different part of your kidney.

Note
These drugs may also be used to reduce swelling caused by accumulation of fluid (edema). Thiazide and loop diuretics can decrease potassium in your body. Therefore, use of these medications may require potassium supplementation.

Cholesterol and triglyceride medications

Bile acid sequestrants

Generic and common brand names
- Cholestyramine (Prevalite)
- Colesevelam (Welchol)

Action
Lower cholesterol in your blood by binding with bile acids in your small intestine. This action ties up the acids and forces your liver to make more bile acids. Bile acids are made from cholesterol.

Note
To avoid drug interactions, inform your doctor of all other medications you take. Since bile acid sequestrants can bind to other medications, they must be taken at different times than other medicines.

Ezetimibe
Brand name
- Zetia

Managing the Cost of Medications

With the price of many prescription drugs in the United States steadily increasing, certain strategies can help make medications more affordable.

Talk to your doctor
Your doctor may be able to suggest generic drugs that are as effective as the brand-name medications you're currently taking (see page 1276). If a generic drug isn't available, your doctor may recommend a less-expensive brand-name medication. You can also ask your doctor if there's a cheaper over-the-counter medicine that is similar to your prescription.

For some medicines, the cost of a pill is the same regardless of the dose. Discuss with your doctor whether it's safe and cost-effective to prescribe a pill at twice the strength that you can split in half.

If you see more than one doctor for different conditions, bring a list of all the medicines you're taking to your appointment. Sometimes different doctors will unknowingly prescribe duplicate medicines that treat the same problem. It may be possible to eliminate one of them.

Check with your insurance plan
Most health insurance options, including Medicare, offer one or more prescription coverage plans. Ask your insurer for the list of medicines (formulary) that each prescription plan covers, along with the different co-pay levels for various medications. If any of your medications are subject to limitations or a high co-pay, contact your insurance company. An insurer may be able to suggest covered alternatives that you can discuss with your doctor.

Search for savings opportunities
Many pharmacies have savings programs that offer low costs on certain generic drugs. Some drug manufacturers also offer co-pay assistance cards or discount cards, which can reduce the co-pay or co-insurance of a brand-name medication. In addition, you may find that you can save money by ordering certain medications by mail instead of purchasing them from a local pharmacy.

Ask for help
If you don't have health insurance or can't afford your co-pay, talk with your pharmacist about options for making a medication more affordable.

Action
Reduces the amount of cholesterol your body absorbs from your diet.

Fibric acid
Generic and common brand names
- Fenofibrate (Antara, Tricor)
- Gemfibrozil (Lopid)

Action
Alters the synthesis of blood fats, lowering triglycerides and raising high-density lipoprotein (HDL, or "good") cholesterol. Also lowers total cholesterol levels.

Note
This medication lowers triglyceride levels in people with too much of this type of blood fat. Contact your doctor promptly if you experience unexplained muscle pain, tenderness or weakness.

Nicotinic acid (niacin)
Brand names
- Niaspan
- Niacor

Action
Lower triglyceride levels in blood and raise levels of high-density lipoprotein (HDL, or "good") cholesterol.

Note
These medications can occasionally cause drug-induced hepatitis (liver inflammation).

Statins
Generic and common brand names
- Atorvastatin (Lipitor)
- Rosuvastatin (Crestor)
- Simvastatin (Zocor)

Action
Decrease cholesterol synthesis and improve removal of low-density lipoprotein (LDL, or "bad") cholesterol from blood.

Note
Notify your doctor if you experience severe muscle pain, tenderness or weakness. These can be signs of a serious muscle condition.

Heart failure medications

Angiotensin-converting enzyme (ACE) inhibitors
See blood pressure medications on page 1281.

Angiotensin II receptor blockers
See blood pressure medications on page 1281.

Beta blockers
See blood pressure medications on page 1281.

Digitalis
Generic and common brand names
- Digoxin (Lanoxin)

Action
Increase the force of your heart muscle contractions and delay electric impulses through the nerves and muscle of your heart.

Note
It's important that this medication be taken exactly as recommended by your doctor. Stopping its use suddenly can cause a serious change in heart function. This medication also treats atrial fibrillation.

Diuretics
See blood pressure medications on page 1282.

Central nervous system medications

Alzheimer's disease medications

Cholinesterase inhibitors
Generic and common brand names
- Donepezil (Aricept)
- Galantamine (Razadyne)
- Rivastigmine (Exelon)

Action
Slow the breakdown of the brain chemical acetylcholine. Loss of acetylcholine is thought to be associated with Alzheimer's disease.

Note
These medications won't cure Alzheimer's disease or stop it from getting worse, but they may improve some of the cognitive symptoms. The drug rivastigmine is also available as a patch.

NMDA receptor antagonists
Generic and common brand names
- Memantine (Namenda)

Action
Reduce the actions of chemicals in the brain that may contribute to the symptoms of Alzheimer's disease.

Note
These medications are also available in combination with the medication donepezil. The combination drug won't cure Alzheimer's disease or stop it from getting worse, but it may improve some cognitive symptoms.

Antipsychotics and mood stabilizers

Antipsychotics
Generic and common brand names
- Aripiprazole (Abilify)
- Olanzapine (Zyprexa)
- Quetiapine (Seroquel)
- Risperidone (Risperdal)
- Ziprasidone (Geodon)

Action
Block the effects of the brain chemical dopamine, which is associated with psychosis.

Note
These medications are used to treat psychotic mental illnesses, such as schizophrenia, some forms of manic-depressive illness and severe depression.

Mood stabilizers
Generic and common brand names
- Lithium (Lithobid)

Action
Produces brain chemical changes that help curb mania, ease sadness and prevent extreme mood changes.

Note

This medication treats bipolar disorder. A test that measures the amount of lithium in your blood can help determine the right dose for you.

Depression and anxiety medications

Anxiolytics
Generic and common brand names
- Alprazolam (Xanax)
- Clonazepam (Klonopin)
- Lorazepam (Ativan)

Action

Slow down (sedate) the central nervous system by increasing the activity of the neurotransmitter gamma-aminobutyric acid (GABA).

Note

These medications treat anxiety and may also be referred to as benzodiazepines. Some anxiolytics may be taken for short periods to help promote sleep or they may be used for the acute treatment of seizures. Prolonged use isn't recommended because it can lead to dependence on the medication. Alcohol can magnify the sedating effects of the medication and should be avoided while taking anxiolytics.

Monoamine oxidase inhibitors
Generic and common brand names
- Phenelzine (Nardil)
- Selegiline (Emsam)

Action

Block the action of enzymes inside nerve cells that break down the brain chemicals norepinephrine and serotonin.

Note

Monoamine oxidase inhibitors may take two to three weeks or longer to begin working. Food and drug interactions are a serious concern. Foods that contain a high level of the amino acid tyramine, such as cheese and wine, can interact with monoamine oxidase inhibitors to cause a severe increase in blood pressure.

Selective serotonin reuptake inhibitors (SSRIs)
Generic and common brand names
- Citalopram (Celexa)
- Escitalopram (Lexapro)
- Fluoxetine (Prozac)
- Paroxetine (Paxil)
- Sertraline (Zoloft)

Action

Increase levels of the brain chemical serotonin.

Note

These medications are taken to treat depression, anxiety and obsessive-compulsive disorder. It may take two to three weeks or longer for the medication to begin working.

Tricyclic and tetracyclic antidepressants
Generic and common brand names
- Amitriptyline
- Duloxetine (Cymbalta)
- Nortriptyline (Pamelor)

Action

Increase levels of the brain chemicals noradrenaline and serotonin, among multiple other actions.

Note

Some of these medications are also used to treat anxiety and obsessive-compulsive disorder. It may take two to three weeks or longer for the medication to begin working.

Others
Generic and common brand names
- Bupropion (Wellbutrin XL, Wellbutrin SR)
- Desvenlafaxine (Pristiq)
- Trazodone
- Venlafaxine (Pristiq, Effexor XR)

Action

Increase the levels of several brain chemicals in which low levels are thought to be associated with depression.

Note

It may take two to three weeks, or possibly longer, for these medications to begin working. Bupropion is also used in smoking cessation therapy (Zyban).

Insomnia medications

Sleep-onset medications
Generic and common brand names
- Zolpidem (Ambien)
- Zaleplon (Sonata)
- Lorazepam (Ativan)

Sleep-maintenance medications
Generic and common brand names
- Eszopiclone (Lunesta)
- Zolpidem controlled release (Ambien CR)
- Temazepam (Restoril)

Action

Bind to various GABA receptors to promote sleep onset, prolong total sleep time or both.

Note

Don't consume alcohol while taking insomnia medications. Sedative effects can impair decision-making if you wake up before a full eight hours of rest. Only take these medications if you're able to devote eight hours to sleep. These medications should be used with caution in older adults.

Migraine medications

Preventive therapies
Anti-seizure medications
Generic and common brand names
- Divalproex (Depakote)
- Gabapentin (Neurontin)

Action

Unclear. May affect the actions of nerve fibers and brain transmitters.

Note

It may take two to three weeks before you begin to notice benefits from these drugs. Maximal benefits may not be evident for two to three months. Divalproex is also used in the treatment of seizure disorders, while gabapentin may be used in the treatment of seizures or nerve pain or both.

Beta blockers
Generic and common brand names
• Atenolol (Tenormin)
• Metoprolol (Lopressor, Toprol XL)

Action
Unclear how their action prevents migraines.

Note
These medications are used to treat migraines, high blood pressure and other cardiovascular conditions. They will slow your heart rate.

Tricyclic antidepressants
Generic and common brand names
• Amitriptyline
• Nortriptyline (Pamelor)

Action
Unclear. May modify brain chemicals that play a role in headaches.

Note
It may take several weeks before you begin to notice the benefits of these medications. These drugs are also used to treat depression.

Abortive therapies
Ergot derivatives
Generic and common brand names
• Dihydroergotamine (D.H.E. 45)
• Ergotamine (Ergomar)

Action
Interact with serotonin receptors and, possibly, constrict blood vessels in the outer area of your brain and scalp to relieve migraines.

Note
Alcohol counteracts the effects of these medications.

Triptans
Generic and common brand names
• Naratriptan (Amerge)
• Rizatriptan (Maxalt)
• Sumatriptan (Imitrex)

Action
Mimic the brain chemical serotonin to deactivate nerves and decrease swollen blood vessels.

Note
These medications are used only to treat, not to prevent, migraines. Using these medications too frequently can cause "rebound headaches."

Muscle relaxants

Generic and common brand names
• Baclofen (Lioresal)
• Cyclobenzaprine
• Tizanidine (Zanaflex)

Action
Act on your central nervous system, causing your muscles to relax.

Note
Alcohol dramatically increases the side effects of these medications and should be avoided while taking them.

Pain and inflammation relievers

Acetaminophen
Brand name
• Tylenol

Action
Blocks the effects of pyrogens, which are natural fever inducers, along with substances that lead to pain.

Note
This medicine is also used to treat fever. Avoid alcohol while taking acetaminophen. If you regularly combine even usual amounts of acetaminophen with alcohol, your chances for liver damage are increased.

Corticosteroids (oral)
Generic and common brand names
• Dexamethasone
• Hydrocortisone (Cortef)
• Methylprednisolone (Medrol)
• Prednisone (Rayos)

Note
These medications also treat a wide variety of allergic and inflammatory conditions, such as asthma, skin disorders and arthritis. After prolonged use of one of these medications, sudden withdrawal from it can be dangerous. Consult your doctor or pharmacist for direction on how to wean off of these medications.

COX-2 inhibitors
Generic and common brand names
• Celecoxib (Celebrex)

Action
Inhibits an enzyme in your body called cyclooxygenase-2 (COX-2). This enzyme makes hormone-like substances called prostaglandins, which are involved in the development of inflammation and pain.

Note
This medication may be less damaging to the stomach than aspirin and other NSAIDs.

Narcotics (opiates and opioids)
Generic and common brand names
• Fentanyl (Actiq, Duragesic)
• Hydrocodone and acetaminophen
• Hydromorphone (Dilaudid)
• Morphine (MS Contin)
• Oxycodone (OxyContin, Roxicodone)

Action
Decrease the brain's perception of pain.

Note
Don't take these medications with alcohol because both act as depressants. Tolerance can develop if the medication is taken for a lengthy period. The drugs can also become habit-forming (see page 1305). Consult your doctor or pharmacist for more information.

Nonsteroidal anti-inflammatory drugs (NSAIDs)
Generic and common brand names
• Aspirin (Bayer, Bufferin, others)

- Ibuprofen (Advil, Motrin IB, others)
- Indomethacin (Indocin)
- Naproxen (Naprosyn), naproxen sodium (Aleve)

Action

Relieve pain by blocking an enzyme called cyclooxygenase-2 (COX-1 and COX-2), which stimulates production of substances called prostaglandins, which are involved in inflammation and pain.

Note

These medicines can also be used to reduce fever. Aspirin may be taken to prevent the formation of blood clots, reducing the risk of a heart attack and stroke. NSAIDs can cause gastrointestinal irritation and bleeding with regular use. Many nonprescription pain relievers contain NSAIDs. Talk with your doctor or pharmacist to make sure you aren't double dosing. The risk of side effects increases with age, especially among women. Some NSAIDs are not appropriate for all ages. For example, aspirin shouldn't be taken by children.

Tramadol
Brand name
- Ultram

Action

Interferes with the transmission of pain signals and triggers the release of the brain chemicals noradrenaline and serotonin, both of which help reduce pain.

Parkinson's disease medications

Amantadine
Brand name
- Gocovri

Action

Causes complex actions within the brain, including increasing the release of the brain chemical dopamine. Blocks some actions of another brain chemical called glutamate, which may be benefi-

cial in the treatment of Parkinson's disease.

Note

This medication helps control involuntary movements (dyskinesias) caused by another Parkinson's disease drug, levodopa. Amantadine may also be used to treat the flu (influenza).

Anticholinergics
Generic and common brand names
- Benztropine (Cogentin)
- Trihexyphenidyl

Action

Block the action of the brain chemical acetylcholine.

Note

These medications are only mildly beneficial, and the benefits are often offset by side effects. The medications may make you sweat less, causing your body temperature to increase. Take care to avoid becoming overheated during hot weather and exercise.

COMT inhibitors
Generic and common brand names
- Entacapone (Comtan)
- Tolcapone (Tasmar)

Note

These medications are used in combination with another medication containing levodopa.

Dopamine agonists
Generic and common brand names
- Pramipexole (Mirapex)
- Ropinirole (Requip)

Action

Mimic the action of the brain chemical dopamine.

Note

These medications can cause dizziness, fatigue and confusion. If you're taking one of these medications, make sure you know how your body reacts to it before driving or operating equipment.

Levodopa and carbidopa
Generic and common brand names
- Levodopa and carbidopa (Sinemet)

Action

Increases amounts of the brain chemical dopamine. Levodopa is a natural substance that the brain transforms into dopamine. Carbidopa, used in combination with levodopa, helps reduce nausea and enhances levodopa's effects.

Note

This medication is the most potent and effective treatment for Parkinson's disease. An extended release version of levodopa and carbidopa is sold under the brand name Rytary.

Selegiline
Brand name
- Eldepryl

Action

Inhibits the enzyme that breaks down dopamine in the brain.

Seizure medications

Generic and common brand names
- Carbamazepine (Carbatrol, Tegretol)
- Divalproex (Depakote)
- Gabapentin (Neurontin)
- Lamotrigine (Lamictal)
- Levetiracetam (Keppra)
- Phenytoin (Dilantin, Phenytek)
- Pregabalin (Lyrica)
- Topiramate (Topamax)
- Valproic acid (Depakene)

Note

These medications can be used to prevent seizures. It may take two to three weeks before you can see the benefits of the drug. Some antianxiety medications may be used to treat seizures. The medications divalproex and gabapentin may also be used to treat migraines. Carbamazepine and gabapentin may be prescribed for trigeminal neuralgia and painful peripheral neuropathy.

Stimulants

Generic and common brand names
- Dextroamphetamine and amphetamine (Adderall)
- Lisdexamfetamine (Vyvanse)
- Methylphenidate (Concerta, Ritalin)
- Modafinil (Provigil)

Action
Stimulate cells in the brain and spinal cord (central nervous system), increasing alertness and concentration.

Note
These medications are used to treat narcolepsy and attention deficit/hyperactivity disorder (ADHD).

Dermatology medications

Acne medications

Anti-infectives
Generic and common brand names
Topical medications
- Azelaic acid (Azelex)
- Benzoyl peroxide (Benzac, others)
- Clindamycin (Cleocin T, others)
- Erythromycin (Erygel, others)

Oral medications
- Doxycycline (Doryx, Vibramycin)
- Minocycline (Minocin)

Action
Stop growth and reproduction of microorganisms that cause infection.

Note
Some topical medications are available in combination with another agent from this class of drugs or in a retinoid medication.

Retinoids
Generic and common brand names
Topical medications
- Adapalene (Differin)
- Tazarotene (Tazorac, others)
- Tretinoin (Avita, Retin-A, others)

Oral medications
- Isotretinoin (Absorica, Claravis, others)

Action
Help regulate skin cell growth.

Note
Retinoids can cause birth defects if used during pregnancy. Take precautions to avoid pregnancy while using isotretinoin.

Keratolytic agents
Generic and common brand names
- Salicylic acid (Clean & Clear, Stridex, others)

Action
Promotes shedding of dead skin cells.

Contact dermatitis medications

Topical corticosteroids
Generic and common brand names
- Desonide (DesOwen)
- Fluocinonide
- Hydrocortisone (Cortizone-10)
- Triamcinolone

Action
Reduce inflammation by slowing the reaction of cells to substances that trigger inflammation.

Note
Apply a thin film to your skin sparingly. Avoid putting the medication in sensitive areas, such as your eyes, mucous membranes, groin and armpits. Hydrocortisone is available without a prescription.

Eczema medications

Calcineurin inhibitors
Generic and common brand names
- Pimecrolimus (Elidel)
- Tacrolimus (Protopic)

Action
The medications work on certain areas of your immune system that may be involved in the development of eczema.

Note
These drugs have a black box warning about a potential cancer risk, but the American Academy of Allergy, Asthma & Immunology has concluded the risk-to-benefit ratios of topical pimecrolimus and tacrolimus are similar to those of other conventional treatments for persistent eczema.

Topical corticosteroids
See contact dermatitis medications on this page.

Psoriasis medications

Anthralin
Brand name
- Dritho-Scalp, Zithranol-RR

Action
The medication helps slow skin cell growth and can remove scales.

Note
It can irritate the skin, and it stains most everything it comes in contact with. It's usually applied for a short time then washed off.

Calcineurin inhibitors
Generic and common brand names
- Pimecrolimus (Elidel)
- Tacrolimus (Prograf)

Action
The medications reduce inflammation and plaque buildup.

Note
The medications aren't recommended for long-term use because of the potential for serious side effects.

Topical corticosteroids
See contact dermatitis medications on this page.

Topical retinoids
Generic and common brand names
- Tazarotene (Avage, Tazorac)

Action
These are vitamin A derivatives that decrease inflammation.

Note

Tazarotene isn't recommended for women who are pregnant or intend to become pregnant or are breast-feeding.

Vitamin D analogues

Generic and common brand names

- Calcipotriene (Dovonex)
- Calcitriol (Vectical)

Action

The medications slow skin cell growth.

Ear and eye medications

Ear medications

Antibiotic and steroid combinations

Generic and common brand names

- Ciprofloxacin and dexamethasone (Ciprodex)
- Ciprofloxacin and hydrocortisone (Cipro HC)
- Neomycin, polymyxin B and hydrocortisone

Action

The antibiotic destroys bacteria that cause ear infections and the steroid reduces swelling and inflammation.

Note

These medications are used to treat infections of the outer ear canal. To keep the medicine germ-free, don't touch the eardropper to any surface, including the ear canal.

Antibiotics

Generic and common brand names

- Ofloxacin

Action

Destroys bacteria that cause external ear infection.

Note

This medication is used to treat infections of the outer ear canal. To keep the medicine germ-free, don't touch the eardropper to any surface, including the ear canal.

Eye medications

Allergy medications

Antihistamines

Generic and common brand names

- Azelastine
- Ketotifen (Alaway)
- Olopatadine (Patanol, Pataday)

Action

Block histamine release, reducing itchy eyes.

Note

These medications are used to treat itchy eyes associated with allergies. Don't wear contact lenses when your eyes are itching and irritated.

Mast cell stabilizers

Generic and common brand names

- Cromolyn sodium
- Lodoxamide (Alomide)
- Nedocromil (Alocril)

Action

Act on certain inflammatory cells (mast cells) to prevent them from releasing substances that cause itching eyes.

Note

These medications are used to treat itchy eyes associated with allergies. Try not to wear contact lenses when your eyes are itching and irritated.

Anti-infectives

Generic and common brand names

- Ciprofloxacin (Ciloxan)
- Erythromycin
- Gentamicin (Genoptic, others)
- Moxifloxacin (Vigamox)
- Ofloxacin (Ocuflox)
- Polymyxin B-Trimethoprim (Polytrim)

Action

Kill the bacteria that cause eye infections.

Note

To avoid contaminating the medication, wash your hands before using the product, and don't touch the applicator tip to your hands or eye.

Dry or irritated eye medications

Artificial tears

Generic and common brand names

- Carboxymethylcellulose (Refresh Celluvisc, Refresh Plus, others)
- Hydroxypropyl methylcellulose (Isopto Tears, Nature's Tears)

Action

Lubricate dry eyes with substances similar to natural tears.

Note

These medications relieve dryness and irritation caused by reduced tear flow. To keep the medicine as germ-free as possible, don't touch the applicator tip to your hands or eye.

Immunologic agents

Generic and common brand names

Cyclosporine (Restasis)

Action

Increases tear production associated with ocular inflammation.

Note

Remove contact lenses before using this medication. After using the medication, wait 15 minutes before reinserting your contact lenses.

Vasoconstrictors

Generic and common brand names

- Naphazoline (Clear Eyes Redness Relief, others)
- Tetrahydrozoline (Murine Tears Plus, Visine, others)

Action

Constrict the blood vessels of the eye, reducing redness.

Note

These medications should be used only to relieve redness due to minor irritations, such as irritation caused by allergies, dust, smoke and wind. Don't use them for more than three days at time.

It's also recommended that you avoid these medications if you have glaucoma.

Glaucoma medications

Adrenergic agonists

Generic and common brand names
- Apraclonidine (Iopidine)
- Brimonidine (Alphagan P)

Action
Reduce the production of aqueous humor, which lowers pressure in the eye.

Beta blockers

Generic and common brand names
- Betaxolol (Betoptic S)
- Levobunolol (Betagan)
- Timolol (Betimol, Istalol, others)

Action
Reduce the production of aqueous humor, which lowers pressure in your eye.

Carbonic anhydrase inhibitors

Generic and common brand names
- Brinzolamide (Azopt)
- Dorzolamide (Trusopt)

Action
Reduce the secretion of fluid inside the front of the eyeball (aqueous humor), lowering pressure inside the eye.

Miotics

Generic and common brand names
- Pilocarpine (Isopto Carpine)

Action
Constricts the pupil and increases the outflow of aqueous humor to decrease intraocular pressure.

Prostaglandin agonists

Generic and common brand names
- Latanoprost (Xalatan)
- Travoprost (Travatan Z)

Action
Increase the outflow of fluid inside the front of the eyeball (aqueous humor), reducing pressure inside the eye.

Note
Latanoprost can cause your iris to darken and your eyelashes to become thicker and darker. These changes may be permanent.

Endocrine medications

Diabetes medications

Alpha-glucosidase inhibitors

Generic and common brand names
- Acarbose (Precose)

Action
Blocks the action of enzymes in your digestive tract that break down carbohydrates into sugar, delaying the digestion of carbohydrates. Sugar is absorbed into your bloodstream more slowly.

Note
This medication reduces blood sugar (glucose) in people with type 2 diabetes. Starting with a low dose and gradually increasing the dose usually minimizes side effects.

Amylin analogs

Generic and common brand names
- Pramlintide (Symlin)

Action
Slows the rate at which food is released from the stomach, lessening the rapid rise in glucose usually seen after eating.

Note
This medication treats type 1 and type 2 diabetes. Because it's given in addition to insulin, there's an increased risk of severely low blood sugar.

Biguanides

Generic and common brand names
- Metformin (Fortamet, Glucophage, others)

Action
Reduce the amount of sugar your liver produces and the amount the intestine absorbs. They also increase insulin sensitivity.

Note
These medications control blood sugar (glucose) in people with type 2 diabetes.

Dipeptidyl peptidase-4 inhibitor

Generic and common brand names
- Saxagliptin (Onglyza)
- Sitagliptin (Januvia)

Action
Slow the breakdown of incretin hormones. Incretin stimulates beta cells in your pancreas to produce and secrete more insulin.

Note
These medications are used to treat type 2 diabetes. The medications need to be monitored if you have kidney disease. Rarely, the medicines may cause acute pancreatitis. See your doctor right away if you experience severe stomach pain, nausea or vomiting.

Incretin mimetic agents

Generic and common brand names
- Dulaglutide (Trulicity)
- Exenatide (Byetta)
- Liraglutide (Saxenda, Victoza)

Action
Stimulate beta cells in your pancreas to produce and secrete more insulin. They also slow the rate at which food is released from the stomach, lessening the rapid rise in glucose that occurs after eating.

Note
These medications are used to treat type 2 diabetes. Rarely, they may cause acute pancreatitis. See your doctor right away if you experience severe stomach pain, nausea or vomiting.

Insulin

Generic and common brand names
- Insulin isophane suspension (Humulin N, Novolin N)
- Insulin isophane suspension with regular insulin injection (Humulin 70/30, Novolin 70/30)
- Regular insulin, human (Humulin R, Novolin R, others)

Action

Transport sugar from your bloodstream into individual cells, where it's used as a source of energy.

Note

Insulin is used to treat type 1 and type 2 diabetes. Rotate the injection sites to prevent skin side effects.

Insulin analogues

Generic and common brand names

Short-acting

- Insulin aspart (NovoLog)
- Insulin glulisine (Apidra)
- Insulin lispro (Humalog)

Long-acting

- Insulin detemir (Levemir)
- Insulin glargine (Lantus, Toujeo, others)

Action

Transport sugar from your bloodstream into individual cells, where it's used as a source of energy. The onset and duration of these newer types of insulin more closely resemble those of natural insulin.

Note

These medications are used to treat type 1 and type 2 diabetes.

Meglitinides

Common brand names

- Nateglinide (Starlix)
- Repaglinide (Prandin)

Action

Stimulate a rapid, short-lived release of insulin by the pancreas.

Note

These medications reduce blood sugar (glucose) levels in people with type 2 diabetes.

Sodium-glucose co-transporter-2 inhibitors

Generic and common brand names

- Canagliflozin (Invokana)
- Dapagliflozin (Farxiga)

Action

Inhibit the reabsorption of blood sugar (glucose) in the kidneys so that some excess glucose can be removed through the urine.

Note

These medications are used to treat type 2 diabetes.

Sulfonylureas

Generic and common brand names

- Glimepiride (Amaryl)
- Glipizide (Glucotrol)
- Glyburide (Glynase)

Action

Stimulate beta cells in your pancreas to release more insulin.

Note

These medications reduce blood sugar (glucose) levels in people with type 2 diabetes.

Thiazolidinediones

Generic and common brand names

- Pioglitazone (Actos)
- Rosiglitazone (Avandia)

Action

Make body tissues more receptive to insulin and increase glucose disposal by the liver.

Note

These medications reduce blood sugar (glucose) levels in people with type 2 diabetes. A rare but serious side effect of thiazolidinediones is liver injury. Have your liver enzymes checked before starting these medications. These drugs can also cause fluid retention, which can worsen or lead to heart failure.

Osteoporosis medications

Bisphosphonates

Generic and common brand names

- Alendronate (Fosamax)
- Ibandronate (Boniva)
- Risedronate (Actonel)

Action

Help preserve bone mass by preventing excess breakdown of bone.

Note

Take oral bisphosphonates with a full glass of water to protect against irritation of the esophagus. Take your dose 30 minutes before eating or drinking any beverage other than water. Don't lie down for 30 minutes after taking the drug. Let your dentist know if you're taking one of these medications.

Calcitonin

Generic and common brand names

- Calcitonin (Miacalcin)

Action

Helps maintain bone density and prevent bone loss. Available as a nasal spray.

Note

Blow your nose gently before using the spray and don't inhale while spraying.

Calcium supplements

Generic and common brand names

- Calcium carbonate (Caltrate, Os-Cal, others)
- Calcium citrate (Citracal)

Action

Help maintain bone density and prevent bone loss.

Note

These products are available without a prescription. Calcium carbonate is absorbed better when taken with food.

Thyroid medications

Hyperthyroidism medications

Generic and common brand names

- Methimazole (Tapazole)

Action

Interferes with iodine, which is required to produce thyroid hormone, to prevent excessive amounts of thyroid hormone in the body.

Note

This medication is used to treat

an overproductive thyroid gland (hyperthyroidism). It may take several days or weeks for the medication to work.

Hypothyroidism medications
Generic and common brand names
- Levothyroxine (Levoxyl, Synthroid, Tirosint, others)
- Liothyronine (Cytomel)
- Thyroid

Action
Increase thyroid hormone in the bloodstream.

Note
These medications are used to restore thyroid hormone levels to normal if the thyroid gland doesn't produce enough of this hormone. The drugs are also used for thyroid hormone replacement after removal or destruction of the thyroid gland. Treatment is generally lifelong. Blood tests can confirm the appropriate dose.

Gastrointestinal medications

Constipation medications

Laxatives and stool softeners
Generic and common brand names
- Bisacodyl (Dulcolax, Fleet, others)*
- Docusate sodium (Colace Clear, Diocto, others)
- Methylcellulose (Citrucel, Benefiber, others)
- Polyethylene glycol (Miralax)
- Psyllium (Metamucil, others)
- Senna (Ex-Lax, others)*
*stimulants

Action
Some of these products soften stool by helping fat and liquids mix with the stool or by providing bulk to help the stool pass more easily. Others stimulate bowel muscles to contract and move the stool out.

Note
Ask your doctor for advice before taking a laxative. Even some nonprescription laxatives may be harmful. Long-term use of stimulant laxatives may lead to dependency and severe constipation.

Diarrhea medications

Anti-diarrheals
Generic and common brand names
- Bismuth subsalicylate (Pepto-Bismol, Kaopectate)
- Diphenoxylate-Atropine (Lomotil)
- Loperamide (Imodium)

Action
Some decrease intestinal secretions, others absorb intestinal secretions and still others decrease contraction of your intestinal muscles, reducing cramping and diarrhea.

Note
Bismuth subsalicylate also helps relieve nausea. Don't take bismuth subsalicylate if you're allergic to aspirin. Children should also avoid these medications due to the risk of Reye's syndrome.

Gastroesophageal reflux disease (GERD) medications

Acid blockers (histamine blockers)
Generic and common brand names
- Famotidine (Pepcid)
- Ranitidine (Zantac)

Action
Interfere with the ability of the chemical histamine to stimulate your stomach to release acid.

Note
These medications may also be used in the treatment of ulcers.

Proton pump inhibitors
Generic and common brand names
- Lansoprazole (Prevacid)
- Omeprazole (Prilosec)
- Pantoprazole (Protonix)

Action
Block acid secretion by inhibiting an enzyme system in your stomach lining called the proton pump.

Note
These medications are most effective when taken on an empty stomach before meals. The medications may also be used to treat ulcers.

Heartburn medications

Antacids
Generic and common brand names
- Aluminum hydroxide
- Calcium carbonate (Rolaids, Tums)
- Magnesium hydroxide (Milk of Magnesia)

Action
Neutralize stomach acid.

Note
Several products are available that combine antacid ingredients. Other products add an additional ingredient, simethicone, to help with gas relief. If you take some antacids with certain medications, they may reduce the absorption of those medications.

Motility medications

Generic and common brand names
- Dicyclomine (Bentyl)
- Hyoscyamine (Anaspaz, Levsin, others)

Action
Relax intestinal muscles and relieve spasms.

Note
These medications, known as antispasmodics, can be used in people with irritable bowel syndrome and other gastrointestinal (GI) disorders to relieve cramps and spasms of the stomach, small intestine and colon.

Ulcer medications

Acid blockers
See acid blockers under the heading

gastroesophageal reflux disease (GERD) medications located on page 1291.

Ulcer-protective agents
Generic and common brand names
- Misoprostol (Cytotec)
- Sucralfate (Carafate)

Action
Misoprostol protects the stomach lining by stimulating mucus and bicarbonate production, forming an alkaline barrier or coating over the lining. Sucralfate coats an ulcer, providing a barrier against stomach acid.

Note
Don't take antacids 30 minutes before or after taking sucralfate. They may keep the medication from working properly. Misoprostol can cause birth defects or miscarriage if taken during pregnancy. Take precautions to avoid pregnancy.

Ulcerative colitis medications

Aminosalicylates
Generic and common brand names
- Balsalazide (Colazal)
- Mesalamine (Asacol HD, Pentasa, Rowasa)
- Sulfasalazine (Azulfidine)

Action
Reduce inflammation in the small and large intestines by blocking production of certain inflammatory substances.

Note
Some of these medications are taken by mouth. Others are administered rectally as an enema or suppository.

Infection medications

Antibiotics

Aminoglycosides
Generic and common brand names
- Amikacin
- Neomycin

Action
Bind with the bacteria's microscopic building blocks (ribosomes), interfering with the bacteria's growth process and thereby eliminating bacterial cells.

Note
These drugs are available in oral, topical, intravenous or inhaled forms, depending on the condition being treated.

Cephalosporins
Generic and common brand names
- Cefadroxil
- Cefdinir
- Cephalexin (Keflex)

Note
These medications treat many bacterial infections, especially of the skin, soft tissues and respiratory tract. Inform your doctor of any drug allergies, especially to penicillin, before taking these drugs. People with serious allergic reactions to penicillin may also be allergic to these medications.

Fluoroquinolones
Generic and common brand names
- Ciprofloxacin (Cipro)
- Levofloxacin (Levaquin)
- Moxifloxacin (Avelox)

Action
Block bacterial DNA enzyme needed for reproduction and repair, stopping growth of the bacteria.

Note
The medications treat bacterial infections in adults that affect the urinary tract, prostate, sinuses and lungs, as well as gonorrhea and chlamydial infections and complicated skin, soft tissue and bone infections. Don't take multivitamins containing minerals or antacids containing aluminum or magnesium at the same time you take these medications.

Macrolides and ketolides
Generic and common brand names

- Azithromycin (Zithromax)
- Clarithromycin (Biaxin)
- Erythromycin (Ery-Tab, E.E.S., others)

Action
Interfere with bacteria's formation of essential proteins, preventing growth and multiplication of cells.

Note
These medications treat bacterial infections, such as certain respiratory infections and some sexually transmitted infections (STIs). Azithromycin may also be used to treat traveler's diarrhea.

Metronidazole
Generic and common brand names
- Metronidazole (Flagyl)

Action
Destroys bacteria or protozoa causing an infection.

Note
This medication treats certain sexually transmitted infections (STIs) and some gastrointestinal, skin and gynecologic infections. If you experience stomach upset with an oral form of this medication, try taking it at mealtime. Refrain from using alcohol or alcohol-containing products while taking oral metronidazole.

Penicillins
Generic and common brand names
- Amoxicillin (Amoxil, Moxatag)
- Amoxicillin and clavulanate (Augmentin)
- Penicillin V

Action
Kill many bacteria by interfering with cells' ability to produce protective cell walls as they grow.

Note
These drugs treat many bacterial infections, including those of the skin and soft tissues and upper and lower respiratory tract (strep throat, ear infections, pneumonia and sinusitis).

Sulfonamides

Generic and common brand names
- Trimethoprim and sulfamethox-azole (Bactrim)

Action
Stop growth and reproduction of microorganisms by interfering with formation of folate, an essential nutrient for these organisms.

Note
These medications treat urinary tract infections, sinusitis, ear infections and, in some individuals, respiratory infections. Some of these drugs may increase your sensitivity to sunlight and may produce allergic reactions.

Tetracycline

Generic and common brand names
- Doxycycline (Doryx, Vibramycin)
- Minocycline (Minocin)
- Tetracycline

Action
Interfere with production of proteins needed for replication of certain microorganisms.

Note
These medications treat a variety of infections, such as respiratory tract infections, skin infections, chlamydial infections and tick-borne diseases. Doxycycline may be prescribed to travelers to prevent malaria. Antacids, calcium and dairy products can decrease absorption of tetracyclines and shouldn't be taken at the same time as these medications.

Antifungals

Generic and common brand names
- Fluconazole (Diflucan)
- Ketoconazole
- Terbinafine (Lamisil)
- Voriconazole (Vfend)

Action
Kill fungi by damaging cell walls and blocking enzymes necessary for growth and reproduction.

Note
These medications treat serious fungal infections as well as fungal nail disease and yeast infections.

For treatment of nail infections, you may need to take the medication for months. Some antifungals may require laboratory monitoring or may interact with other medications. Consult with your doctor or pharmacist before taking any new drug.

Antivirals

Generic and common brand names
- Acyclovir (Zovirax)
- Famciclovir
- Oseltamivir (Tamiflu)
- Valacyclovir (Valtrex)

Action
Block viruses from entering cells and inhibit viruses from replicating.

Note
The drugs treat infections caused by certain viruses, such as shingles, flu (influenza), hepatitis, herpes and cytomegalovirus.

HIV and AIDS medications

Cellular chemokine receptor antagonist

Generic and common brand names
- Maraviroc (Selzentry)

Action
Blocks the HIV virus from entering the cell.

HIV protease inhibitors

Generic and common brand names
- Atazanavir (Reyataz)
- Darunavir (Prezista)
- Ritonavir (Norvir)
- Ritonavir and lopinavir (Kaletra)

Action
Block the HIV enzyme (protease) to keep the virus from maturing.

Note
It's critical that you take doses precisely as scheduled. Several of these medications may interact with other drugs. Talk with your doctor or pharmacist before taking any new medications.

Integrase inhibitor

Generic and common brand names
- Raltegravir (Isentress)

Action
Inhibits an HIV enzyme that's required for the HIV virus to replicate.

Note
To get the maximum benefit, take the doses precisely as scheduled.

Non-nucleoside reverse transcriptase inhibitors

Generic and common brand names
- Delavirdine (Rescriptor)
- Efavirenz (Sustiva)
- Etravirine (Intelence)
- Nevirapine (Viramune)

Action
Interrupt an early stage of HIV replication, reducing the severity and extent of HIV infection.

Note
To get the full effect of the medication, it's important that you take doses precisely as scheduled.

Nucleoside reverse transcriptase inhibitors

Generic and common brand names
- Abacavir/Lamivudine/Zidovudine (Trizivir)
- Lamivudine (Combivir)
- Abacavir/Lamivudine (Epzicom)
- Emtricitabine/Tenofovir (Truvada)

Action
Block an enzyme that is needed for the virus to replicate.

Note
To get the full effect of the medication, it's important that you take doses precisely as scheduled.

Nucleoside analogue reverse transcriptase inhibitors

Generic and common brand names
- Abacavir (Ziagen)
- Emtricitabine (Emtriva)
- Lamivudine (Epivir)

Action
Interrupt an early stage of HIV replication to limit the severity and extent of HIV infection.

Note
To get the maximum benefit from the medication, it's critical that you take doses precisely as scheduled. Lamivudine is also used to treat hepatitis B infections.

Nucleotide reverse transcriptase inhibitor
Generic and common brand names
- Tenofovir (Viread)

Action
Reduces the amount of HIV in the body by interfering with the ability of the virus to multiply.

Note
To get the full effect of the medication, take doses precisely as scheduled.

Men's and women's health medications

Erectile dysfunction medications

Intracavernosal agents
Common brand names
- Alprostadil (Caverject, Muse)

Action
Relax smooth muscle tissue in the penis, increasing blood flow to the penis. Caverject is available as an injection, while Muse is an intracavernous suppository.

Note
Both medications require manual dexterity for their appropriate use.

Oral phosphodiesterase type 5 inhibitors
Common brand names
- Sildenafil (Viagra)

- Tadalafil (Cialis)
- Vardenafil (Levitra)

Action
Delay the action of an enzyme called phosphodiesterase, which works on the penis.

Note
Some of these medications may also be used in the treatment of pulmonary arterial hypertension or prostate gland enlargement, known as benign prostatic hyperplasia (BPH). These medications shouldn't be taken by men who take nitroglycerine-types of medication or who have significant coronary artery disease. Seek medical attention if you experience sudden loss of vision or if an erection lasts four hours or longer.

Menopausal hormone therapy

Generic and common brand names
- Conjugated estrogens (Premarin)
- Estradiol (Estrace, Vivelle-Dot, Climara)
- Estropipate (Ogen 5)

Action
Mimic actions of naturally produced female estrogen hormones. Estrogens prevent the excess breakdown of bone that occurs after menopause.

Note
These medications are used to help prevent osteoporosis in postmenopausal women and to reduce symptoms of menopause. Medications in this class are available as a tablet, vaginal cream, patch or injection.

Estrogens
Generic and common brand names
- Conjugated estrogens (Premarin)
- Estradiol (Estrace, Estring, Vagifem, Vivelle-Dot, others)

Action
Mimic the action of the natural female sex hormone estrogen.

Note
These medications provide additional estrogen when your body isn't able to produce enough. They're used in women to treat hot flashes and vaginal dryness and to prevent osteoporosis. Discuss the benefits and risks of estrogen hormones with your doctor.

Progestins
Generic and common brand names
- Medroxyprogesterone (Provera)
- Progesterone (Prometrium)

Action
Mimic the action of the natural female sex hormone progesterone.

Note
These medications regulate the menstrual cycle, help maintain an existing pregnancy, or treat endometriosis or abnormal uterine bleeding. Some progestins are used to treat cancers of the breast, kidney and uterus.

Overactive bladder medications

Generic and common brand names
- Oxybutynin (Ditropan XL, Gelnique, others)
- Tolterodine (Detrol, Detrol LA)
- Trospium
- Solifenacin (Vesicare)

Action
Reduce bladder contractions, decreasing the urgency and frequency of urination.

Note
Common side effects of these medications include dry mouth and dry eyes.

Prostate medications

Alpha blockers
Generic and common brand names
- Alfuzosin (Uroxatral)
- Doxazosin (Cardura)
- Tamsulosin (Flomax)

Action
Relax certain smooth muscles in

the urinary tract, making it easier to urinate.

Note

Some of these medications may also be used to treat high blood pressure.

Androgen hormone inhibitors
Generic and common brand name
• Dutasteride (Avodart)
• Finasteride (Proscar)

Action

Shrink prostate gland tissue by inhibiting conversion of testosterone to dihydrotestosterone.

Note

It often takes six months to a year for the drug to produce its full effect. A weaker version of Finasteride (Propecia) may also be used to prevent male pattern baldness.

Anti-androgens
Generic and common brand names
• Bicalutamide (Casodex)

Action

Stops production of most, but not all, male sex hormones that nourish the prostate gland and cancerous tumors of the prostate.

Note

This drug can be used alone or in combination with another medication.

Gonadotropin-releasing hormone agonists
Generic and common brand names
• Goserelin (Zoladex)
• Leuprolide (Lupron)

Action

Decrease estrogen and testosterone in the blood.

Note

These medications treat a number of medical problems, including prostate cancer in men and breast cancer and endometriosis in women. In rare instances, these medications can cause chest pain.

See a doctor immediately if this occurs.

Sex hormones

Androgens
Generic and common brand names
• Danazol
• Testosterone (AndroGel, Testim)

Action

Mimic the action of natural male sex hormones (androgens).

Note

These medications provide additional male sex hormones when a man is unable to produce enough (hypogonadism). They also are used to treat hereditary angioedema and certain types of breast cancer in females. These medications are available in many forms, including tablets, creams, gels, ointments, patches, and injections.

Respiratory medications

Allergy medications

Antihistamines
Generic and common brand names
Oral medications
• Cetirizine (Zyrtec Allergy)
• Diphenhydramine (Banophen, Benadryl, Genahist)
• Fexofenadine (Allegra)
• Loratadine (Alavert, Claritin)

Nasal spray
• Azelastine (Astepro)

Action

Block histamine from binding to its receptors, thereby preventing a runny nose, itchy and watery eyes, and sneezing due to an allergy.

Corticosteroids (nasal sprays)
Generic and common brand names
• Budesonide (Rhinocort)
• Fluticasone (Flonase Allergy Relief, others)
• Mometasone (Nasonex)

Action

Reduce inflammation by slowing the

reaction of individual cells to substances that trigger inflammation.

Note

Many of these medications are now available without a prescription.

Leukotriene receptor antagonists
Generic and common brand names
• Montelukast (Singulair)

Action

It works by blocking substances in the body called leukotrienes. These chemicals cause swelling in your lungs and tightening of the muscles around your airways. Blocking leukotrienes improves asthma and allergic rhinitis.

Note

This medication is also used to treat asthma.

Mast cell stabilizers
Generic and common brand names
• Cromolyn sodium

Action

Acts on specific cells called mast cells, preventing them from releasing histamine and other substances that cause allergic reactions.

Note

It may take a couple of weeks before the full effects of the medication become noticeable. The medication can cause burning, stinging or irritation of nasal membranes and increased sneezing.

Asthma medications

Beta agonists
Generic and common brand names
Short-acting
• Albuterol (Proventil-HFA, Ventolin HFA)
• Ipratropium (Atrovent)

Long-acting
• Formoterol (Foradil)
• Salmeterol (Serevent)

Action

Relax muscles in the bronchial

tubes, increasing the size of the airways.

Note
These medications may also be used to treat chronic obstructive pulmonary disease (COPD). Don't take salmeterol or formoterol for asthma emergencies because they're slow-acting bronchodilators.

Corticosteroids
Generic and common brand names
Inhalers
- Budesonide (Pulmicort)
- Flunisolide (Aerospan HFA)

Oral medications
- Methylprednisolone (Medrol)
- Prednisone

Action
Reduce inflammation and swelling of airways. Corticosteroid inhalers are slow acting and must be used on a regular basis. Oral medications (prednisone, prednisolone) generally are prescribed only for severe attacks of asthma.

Note
Rinse your mouth after each use of a corticosteroid inhaler to prevent a yeast infection. Don't suddenly stop taking oral corticosteroids. Their use needs to be tapered. Oral corticosteroids may also be used to treat rheumatoid arthritis.

Combination inhalers
Generic and common brand names
- Fluticasone and salmeterol (Advair HFA, Airduo Respiclick)
- Budesonide and formoterol (Symbicort)

Action
These are combination medications containing a corticosteroid and beta agonist. The corticosteroid reduces airway inflammation and swelling while the beta agonist opens up lung airways.

Note
Don't take these medications to relieve an asthma attack that has already started. These drugs may also be used to treat chronic obstructive pulmonary disease (COPD).

Leukotriene blockers
Generic and common brand names
- Montelukast (Singulair)
- Zafirlukast (Accolate)
- Zileuton (Zyflo)

Action
Keep airways open by blocking the action or formation of leukotrienes, a substance involved in inflammation.

Mast cell stabilizers
Generic and common brand names
- Cromolyn sodium

Action
Blocks the release of histamine and other mast cell chemicals that cause swelling and narrowing of bronchial tubes.

Note
This medication may be used to treat mild to moderate asthma and to prevent exercise-induced bronchospasms. Don't use this medication in emergency situations.

Methylxanthines
Generic and common brand names
- Theophylline

Action
Stimulates respiration and relaxes bronchial muscles, relieving bronchospasms and increasing lung capacity.

Note
A test that measures the amount of theophylline in your blood can help determine the right dose for you.

Monoclonal antibodies
Generic and common brand names
- Omalizumab (Xolair)

Action
Binds to substances in the body involved in the allergic response, inhibiting their action.

Note
This medication relieves moderate to severe persistent asthma in certain individuals. It should only be administered in a medical setting.

Chronic obstructive pulmonary disease (COPD) medications

Anticholinergics
Generic and common brand names
Short acting
- Ipratropium (Atrovent)

Long acting
- Aclidinium (Tudorza Pressair)
- Tiotropium (Spiriva)
- Umeclidinium (Incruse Ellipta)

Action
Reduce smooth muscle contraction and mucus secretion to open the airways.

Note
Tiotropium is available as a nebulized solution and as a capsule to be used with an inhaler. The capsule shouldn't be swallowed.

Beta agonists
Generic and common brand names
Short acting
See asthma medications on page 1295.

Long acting
- Aformoterol (Brovana)
- Indacaterol (Arcapta Neohaler)
- Olodaterol (Striverdi Respimat)

Action
Relax muscles in the bronchial tubes, increasing the size of the airways.

Note
Long-acting medications shouldn't be used to treat an acute attack of shortness of breath. Some of these medicines are available in combination with a long-acting beta agonist.

Corticosteroids
See entry under asthma medications on this page.

Selective phosphodiesterase 4 inhibitors
Generic and common brand names
• Roflumilast (Daliresp)

Action
Not well-defined but works to decrease the risk of COPD exacerbations.

Note
This medication shouldn't be taken for acute attacks of shortness of breath.

Cold medications

Cough suppressants (antitussives)
Generic and common brand names
• Benzonatate (Tessalon)
• Dextromethorphan (Delsym, Robitussin DM)
• Codeine

Action
Relieve coughs in different ways: The medications may act directly on the lungs and breathing passages; they may act on the cough center in your brain; and they may thin the mucus in your lungs to help your lungs clear it out.

Note
If your cough lingers for more than a week, see your doctor. Drink lots of fluids, especially if you're taking an expectorant, such as guaifenesin.

Decongestants
Generic and common brand names
Oral medications
• Oxymetazoline (Afrin, Dristan)
• Phenylephrine (Sudogest PE, others)
• Pseudoephedrine

Nasal sprays
• Oxymetazoline (Afrin, Dristan)
• Phenylephrine (Neo-Synephrine, Sinex Nasal Spray, others)

Action
Narrow the blood vessels in your nose and sinuses to relieve pressure and decrease congestion.

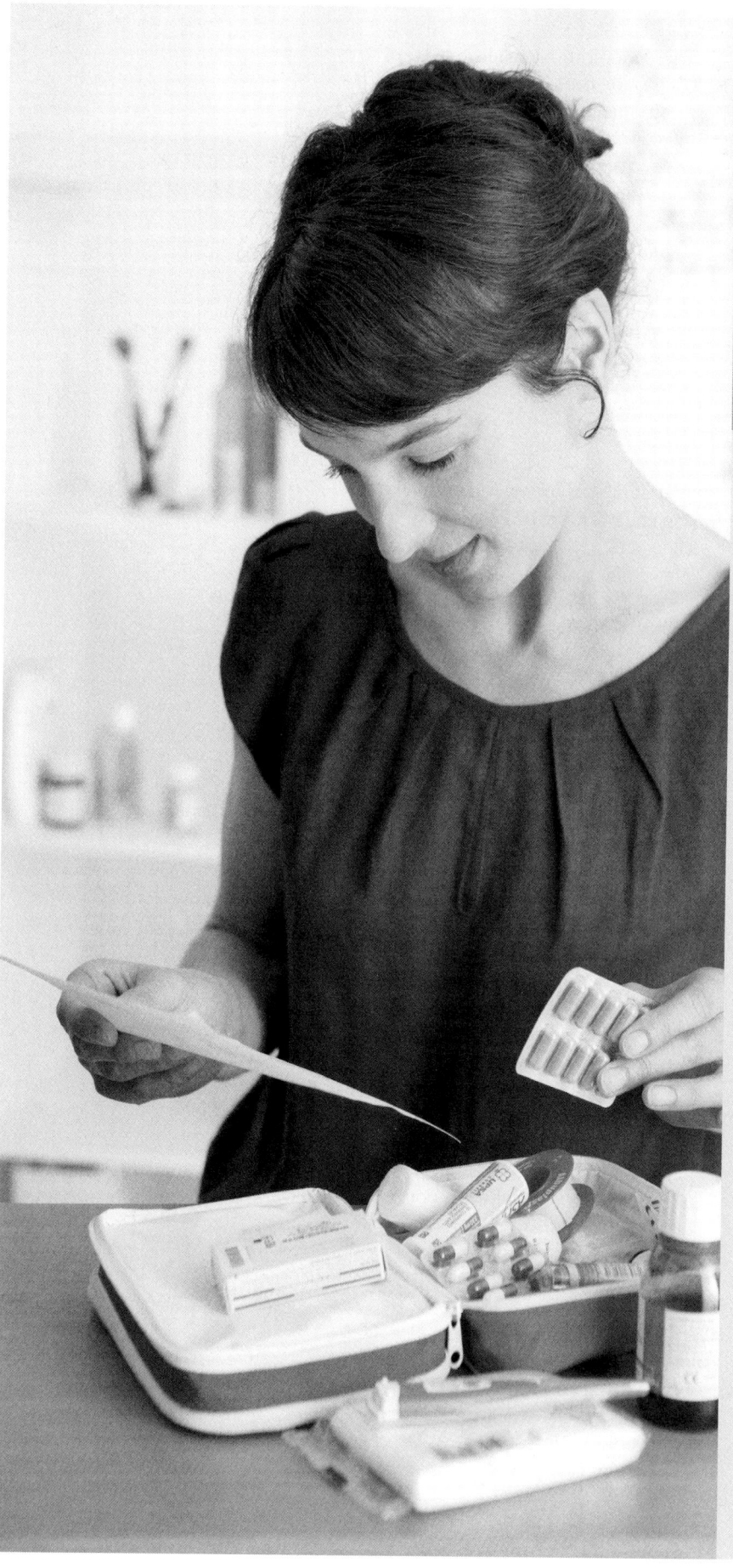

Note

These medications relieve nasal congestion caused by a cold, the flu (influenza), allergies or a sinus infection. They may be combined with an antihistamine to further relieve symptoms. Don't regularly take a decongestant nasal spray for more than three days or you may experience rebound congestion.

Expectorants

Generic and common brand names
- Guaifenesin (Mucinex, Tussin, others)

Action

Help thin and loosen mucus, making coughs more productive.

Note

Drink plenty of fluids, especially water, when using these medications.

Smoking cessation medications

Generic and common brand names
- Bupropion (Zyban)
- Nicotine gum (Nicorette)
- Nicotine inhaler (Nicotrol)
- Nicotine nasal spray (Nicotrol)
- Nicotine transdermal system patch (Nicoderm CQ, others)
- Varenicline (Chantix)

Action

Deliver controlled amounts of nicotine to your brain via your bloodstream. Bupropion is thought to raise the level of the brain chemical dopamine, the same chemical affected by nicotine. Varenicline partially blocks nicotine receptors and displaces nicotine at its sites of action in the brain.

Note

These medications reduce the symptoms of nicotine withdrawal. If not used as directed, nicotine replacement products can cause a nicotine overdose. Follow the directions carefully. ■

Pain Management

Physical pain is a part of life. That's why store shelves are stacked high with a variety of pain relievers. And, chances are, you've had to purchase some, at least from time to time.

There are times when pain can be helpful. Perhaps you've grabbed a hot iron skillet with a bare hand or stubbed your toe on a dresser. Like a blaring alarm, pain screams its urgent warning that something is wrong and that you need to tend to the problem.

But other pain — the day-after-day ache of arthritis or the constant throbbing of a headache — serves no useful purpose. You already know that something is wrong, and you're doing everything that you can to treat the problem. Relentless pain like this can be overwhelming.

Pain is also unique. Two people injured in much the same way may experience radically different levels of discomfort and react quite differently. Each individual's pain tolerance is the result of a variety of factors, including his or her biological, psychological and cultural makeup.

Strategies on how best to manage pain continue to evolve. For acute pain, such as that after surgery or an accident, medication can often alleviate the pain while the injury heals. For persistent pain — commonly called chronic pain — medication alone isn't always adequate

or the best form of treatment. A comprehensive approach that includes exercise, relaxation techniques and behavior changes may improve pain control.

People today are living longer, but often with disease that causes pain. That makes successful approaches for managing pain important.

How You Feel Pain

Understanding how your body feels pain can help you appreciate how unique your pain experiences are. It can also help you better understand why chronic pain is often difficult to treat.

Pain basically results from a series of electrical and chemical exchanges involving three major components: your peripheral nerves, spinal cord and brain.

Peripheral nerves

Your peripheral nerves encompass a network of nerve fibers that branch throughout your body, all the way down to your fingers and toes. Attached to some of these sensory fibers are special nerve endings that detect an unpleasant stimulus, such as a cut, burn or painful pressure. These nerve end-

ings are called nociceptors, which comes from the Latin, *noci*, for "hurt."

You have millions of nociceptors in your skin, bones, joints and muscles and in the protective membranes around your internal organs. You can't feel pain in your internal organs themselves. Nociceptors are concentrated in areas more prone to injury, such as your fingers and toes. That's why a splinter in your finger hurts more than one in your thigh or shoulder.

There may be as many as 1,300 nociceptors in just a single square inch of skin. Muscles, protected beneath your skin, have fewer nerve endings. And organ membranes, protected by skin, muscle and bone, have fewer still.

Some nociceptors sense sharp blows; others sense heat. One type senses pressure, temperature and chemical changes. Nociceptors are more active during inflammation caused by injury, disease and infection. This is why ice or anti-inflammatory drugs help relieve pain.

When nociceptors detect a harmful stimulus, they relay the pain messages — in the form of electrical impulses along a peripheral sensory nerve — to your spinal cord and brain. The speed at which the messages travel can vary, even if they're related to the same stimulus. For example, if you hit your finger with a hammer, you first feel a fast and sharp localized pain and then, more slowly, a dull and diffuse aching sensation.

Spinal cord

When pain messages reach your spinal cord, they're adjusted (modulated) within a network of neural connections. Depending on the circumstances, this modulation may either decrease or increase the rate at which the signals are relayed to the brain.

For severe pain that's linked to an immediate danger, such as when you touch a hot stove, the

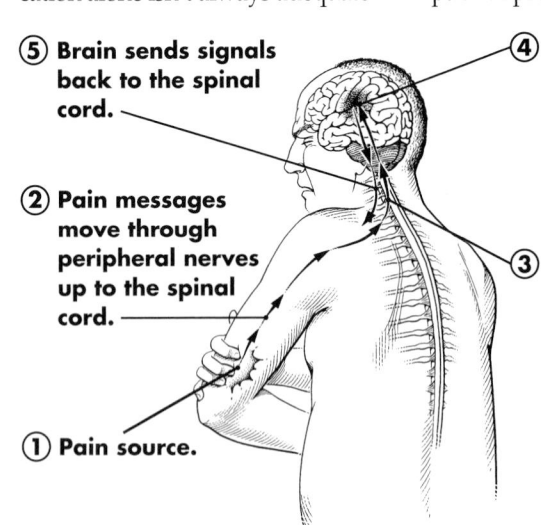

(5) **Brain sends signals back to the spinal cord.**

(2) **Pain messages move through peripheral nerves up to the spinal cord.**

(1) **Pain source.**

(4) **Your brain interprets the messages as pain, including its location, intensity and nature (burning, aching, stinging).**

(3) **Spinal cord filters and modulates signals, then sends them to the brain.**

messages take an express route to your brain. Nerve cells in your spinal cord also respond to these urgent warnings by triggering action in other parts of the spinal cord, such as your motor nerves. Motor nerves can signal your muscles to contract and pull your hand away from the burner, even before your brain is aware of the pain. Weaker pain signals, though, such as from a scratch, may not even be passed on to the brain.

Within your spinal cord, the messages can change in other ways. Other sensations may overpower and diminish the pain messages. This happens when you massage or apply pressure to the injured area. The result is that the warnings sent by your peripheral nerves are downgraded to a lower intensity, or filtered out entirely.

Brain signals can also modulate pain downward within the brain and spinal cord. Morphine and other opioid medications taken to relieve pain act on this same circuit, as do certain antidepressants. In contrast, the spinal cord is also where pain up-regulation, or windup, can occur, such as increased pain in response to chronic nociception.

Brain

When pain messages reach your brain, they arrive at the thalamus, a sorting and switching station located deep inside your brain. The thalamus quickly forwards them simultaneously to both the thinking part of your brain, called the cerebral cortex, and to your brain's limbic center.

The limbic center produces the emotions that often accompany pain, such as anxiety, fear and frustration. It's at this point that you actually begin to feel pain.

Your cerebral cortex reacts to the pain messages by locating the source of the injury, assessing the damage and determining a course of action, such as ordering you to take pressure off your foot if you've sprained your ankle.

The cerebral cortex processes additional key messages. An example is, *What is the meaning of the pain?* This determines if the brain responds in an up-regulation or down-regulation manner. In the case of down-regulation, the brain then dispatches the release of pain-suppressing chemicals and sends stop-pain messages to the spinal cord.

Pain response

When pain messages reach your brain, two components determine how you respond to the pain: the physical sensation and your personal makeup.

Physical sensation

Pain comes in many forms: sharp, jabbing, throbbing, burning, stinging, tingling, nagging, dull and aching. Sharp and jabbing pain generally produces greater discomfort than does dull, aching pain. It's also more likely to make you anxious or fearful.

Pain also varies from mild to severe. Severe pain grabs your attention more quickly, and it generally produces a greater physical and emotional response than does mild pain. Severe pain can incapacitate you, making it difficult or impossible to sit or stand.

The location of your pain also can affect your response to it. A headache that interferes with your ability to work or concentrate may be more bothersome, and therefore receive a stronger response, than may arthritic pain in your knee or a cut to your finger.

Personal makeup

Your emotional and psychological state, memory of past painful experiences, upbringing, and attitude also affect how you interpret pain messages and tolerate pain. For example, a minor sensation that would barely register as pain, such as a dentist's probe, can actually produce exaggerated pain for someone who has never been to the dentist but has heard horror stories of what it's like.

But your emotions can also work in your favor by reducing even major pain messages. For example, athletes can condition themselves to endure pain that would incapacitate others. In addition, if you're brought up in a home or culture that teaches "Grin and bear it," "No pain, no gain" or "Bite the bullet," you may experience less discomfort than do people who focus on their pain or are more prone to complain.

Acute vs. Chronic Pain

The two main types of pain are acute and chronic. Acute pain is usually short term and useful because it alerts you to a physical problem that you need to address. Chronic pain is long term, and instead of being helpful, it's often debilitating.

Acute pain

You probably already know about acute pain from firsthand experience. Acute pain is triggered by tissue damage. It's the type of pain that generally accompanies an injury or surgery. When you have acute pain, you usually know exactly where it hurts. In fact, the word *acute* comes from the Latin word for "needle," referring to a sharp pain.

Pain might be mild and last just a moment, such as from a pinch. Or it might be severe and last for months, such as from a burn, pulled muscle or broken bone. Examples of acute pain include a toothache from a cavity, a burning elbow from a scrape and a sore throat from having your tonsils removed.

With acute pain, doctors can generally figure out what the problem is and fix it. The goal of treatment is to manage the pain over the short term until healing occurs — when the cavity is filled, the skins grows back or the incision heals.

Some acute pain, though, is more difficult to link to its cause. For example, your left arm may hurt when you're having a heart attack, or you may have generalized abdominal pain with acute appendicitis. This is called *referred pain*.

Chronic pain

Chronic pain is pain that hangs on even after an injury has healed, seemingly unaffected by the passing of time. Chronic pain can also result from progressive injury that doesn't heal, such as from arthritis and some cancers. This is reflected in the word itself: *Chronic*, like *chronology*, comes from the Greek word for "time."

Like acute pain, chronic pain can span the full range of sensations and intensity. It can be dull or sharp, and it can tingle, jolt or burn. The pain may remain constant, or it can come and go.

Sometimes, the cause of chronic pain can't be determined. Other times, doctors are able to identify the cause.

Often, chronic pain results from one of the following three broad types of injury:

Joint and bone injury
Chronic conditions such as osteoarthritis, rheumatoid arthritis, degenerative disk disease and spinal stenosis are common causes of chronic bone and joint pain. Osteoporosis, a chronic bone disorder that's common among women older than 45, causes porous and weak bones. It can result in an increased risk of fractures, which can be painful, especially compression fractures of the vertebrae.

Tissue injury
Damage to tendons or muscles is another common cause of chronic pain. Conditions such as tendinitis or bursitis can produce persistent aching.

Nerve injury
Chronic pain may stem from an accident, infection or surgery that damages a peripheral or spinal nerve. The damaged nerve continues to cause pain even after the injury has seemingly healed. This type of nerve pain is called neuropathic pain. Sciatica is an example of neuropathic pain. This type of pain can also result from diseases that damage nerves, such as diabetes or shingles (herpes zoster). Some chemotherapy medications also can damage nerves.

Once damaged, the nerve may send pain messages that are unwarranted. For example, an increased blood sugar level from diabetes can damage the small nerves in your hands and feet, leaving you with a painful burning sensation in your fingers and toes.

When a nerve cell is damaged, the ends of surviving fibers can sprout a tangle of unorganized nerve fibers (neuroma). This bundle of nerve tissue may start sending warnings of injuries that don't exist. Damaged nerves may be more sensitive to external stimuli or fire more vigorously than they should. Or they may send signals spontaneously in the absence of painful stimuli.

The chronic pain challenge

Acute pain tends to be easier to treat than does chronic pain. It often responds well to medication, and with time — a few days to a few weeks — it begins to subside.

Chronic pain can be difficult to treat. For some types of chronic pain, medication or injections are beneficial. But these measures don't always work, or their effects are short-lived. Infrequently, surgery may cure or reduce the pain.

When the cause of the pain can't be cured, treatment often centers on ways to live with the pain, reducing its intensity and its effect on daily life. Learning to cope with chronic pain has a lot to do with attitude and lifestyle. People who can approach their condition with a positive attitude and a willingness to change their lifestyle to prevent or reduce pain triggers are often the most successful in coping with pain.

Methods for Treating Pain

When it comes to controlling pain, the first thing most people think of is medication. That's understandable. Medication is the most common method for treating pain. But it's not the only method. A variety of methods can be used to relieve pain, or to reduce its sting:
- Medications, ranging from over-the-counter to prescription analgesics and neuromodulating medications
- Mechanical therapies, such as ice, heat, massage and TENS units
- Invasive therapies, including injections and spinal cord stimulation
- Behavior therapies, such as exercise, relaxation and stress management
    Often, a combination of therapies provides the best approach for managing pain and reducing unwanted side effects.

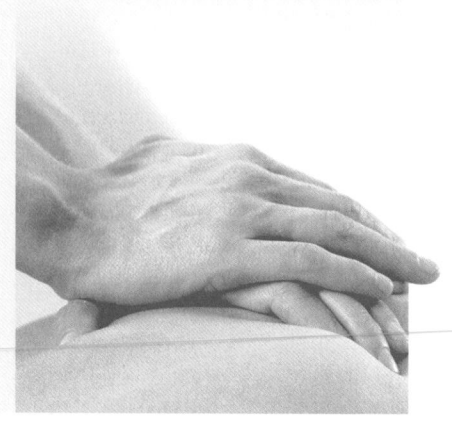

Pain Medications

Pain relievers (analgesics) are the most widely used medication for controlling pain. They control pain by interfering with the development of pain messages, their frequency, their path or how they're interpreted. Many types of over-the-counter and prescription pain relievers are available.

Acetaminophen

Acetaminophen is most effective for mild to moderate pain that isn't accompanied by inflammation. Acetaminophen doesn't interfere with the enzyme in your body that serves as a catalyst for inflammation. But this drug is often effective at controlling other types of pain.

Over-the-counter generic products are available. Brands of pain medication with acetaminophen include:
- Anacin Aspirin Free
- Excedrin Tension Headache
- Tylenol

When taken as recommended, acetaminophen is generally safe. But if you take more of the medication than recommended on the product label, it could lead to liver damage. Alcohol appears to enhance this risk.

Acetaminophen is sometimes combined with other drugs to provide stronger pain relief. Be sure to include these other sources of acetaminophen when calculating your daily dose. Adults should take no more than 4,000 milligrams of acetaminophen daily.

Nonsteroidal anti-inflammatory drugs

Nonsteroidal anti-inflammatory drugs, or NSAIDs, are most effective for mild to moderate pain that's accompanied by swelling and inflammation. These drugs relieve pain by inhibiting production of pain-intensifying chemicals activated by tissue damage.

NSAIDs are especially helpful for arthritis and pain resulting from muscle sprains, strains, back and neck injuries, or cramps.

Over-the-counter NSAIDs include:
- Ibuprofen (Advil, Motrin IB, others)
- Naproxen sodium (Aleve)

NSAIDs available by prescription include:
- Diclofenac sodium (Voltaren)
- Etodolac (Etodolac)
- Fenoprofen calcium (Fenoprofen calcium, Nalfon)
- Indomethacin (Indocin)
- Ketorolac (Ketorolac Tromethamine)
- Meloxicam (Mobic)
- Nabumetone
- Naproxen (Naprosyn)
- Oxaprozin (Daypro)
- Piroxicam (Feldene)
- Sulindac

When taken occasionally and as directed, NSAIDs are usually safe. But if you take them regularly for months or years, or if you take more than the recommended dosage, NSAIDs might cause nausea, stomach pain, stomach bleeding and ulcers.

Large doses of NSAIDs can also lead to kidney problems, fluid retention and heart failure. The risk of these conditions increases with age, especially among women. If you regularly take NSAIDs, talk to your doctor about monitoring potential side effects.

NSAIDs can also have a ceiling effect. Beyond a certain dosage, they don't provide additional pain relief benefits.

COX-2 inhibitors

NSAIDs relieve pain by inhibiting enzymes in your body called cyclooxygenase (COX). These enzymes make hormone-like substances called prostaglandins, which are involved in the development of pain and inflammation.

Traditional NSAIDs work against two versions of cyclo-oxygenase present in your body: COX-1 and COX-2. However, there's evidence that suppressing COX-1 can cause stomach and bleeding problems because COX-1 is the enzyme that protects your stomach lining and allows platelets to form blood clots.

COX-2 inhibitors primarily suppress COX-2 enzymes. Because they don't affect COX-1 as much, the drugs are considered less harmful to your digestive system. However, COX-2 inhibitors don't protect against blood clots, like aspirin and NSAIDs do — an important point for people with cardiovascular disease.

Celecoxib (Celebrex) is the only COX-2 inhibitor on the market today. Other brands were taken off the market because of potentially serious side effects.

In studies of COX-2 inhibitors, participants reported significantly less pain without common side effects associated with traditional NSAIDs. COX-2 inhibitors are usually more expensive than traditional NSAIDs.

Possible side effects of COX-2 inhibitors include abdominal pain, nausea and indigestion. The risk of adverse cardiac side effects, including heart attacks and worsening heart failure, are similar between selective and non-selective NSAIDs.

Neuromodulating medications

Some of the most effective medications to control chronic pain are medications that affect nerve conduction and modulation within pain pathways. These medications are termed "neuromodulating" medications.

Most of these drugs were initially developed for other conditions. Antidepressants and anti-seizure medications are the two main groups of medications that may be used to control chronic pain.

When Is It Addiction?

Chemical dependency can manifest itself in three ways: increased tolerance, physical dependence and addiction. People often lump all three forms under the term *addiction*, but addiction has a very specific meaning. Although addiction poses serious health risks, the other two forms of dependency aren't necessarily "bad."

Increased tolerance

As your body becomes accustomed to a drug, the medication can lose its effectiveness. To receive the same degree of relief, you may have to take higher doses. Don't increase your dosage unless you're under the supervision of a doctor and he or she recommends that you do so.

Physical dependence

To control your pain, you rely on receiving your medication at regular intervals. When use of the drug is abruptly stopped or its dosage substantially reduced, you experience physical withdrawal symptoms. Withdrawal can be avoided by tapering the medication dosage gradually. If you take opioid (narcotic) medications regularly, ask your doctor for guidance before decreasing the dosage.

Addiction

Addiction involves both physical and psychological dependence on a drug. You can develop this dependence with a prescription medication, nicotine, alcohol and illegal drugs, such as marijuana and cocaine. In cases of psychological dependence, you crave the psychological effects of the medication, leading to loss of control over its use. You take the drug even though it isn't helping you, and, in fact, the habit leads to harm — professionally, socially and psychologically.

These prescription medications are initiated by a doctor. Often, they're started at a low dose and increased to a dose that's been shown to improve pain. Once the effective dose is reached, it may take several weeks for pain improvement to occur.

Antidepressants

Tricyclic antidepressants (TCAs)

Tricyclic antidepressants are often used to relieve pain. They include:
- Amitriptyline
- Imipramine (Tofranil)
- Clomipramine (Anafranil)
- Nortriptyline (Pamelor)
- Desipramine (Norpramin)
- Doxepin

Tricyclic antidepressants seem to work best for pain that's caused by or associated with:
- Arthritis
- Nerve damage from diabetes (diabetic neuropathy)
- Nerve damage from shingles (postherpetic neuralgia)
- Nerve damage from other causes (peripheral neuropathy, spinal cord injury, stroke, radiculopathy)
- Tension headache
- Migraine
- Fibromyalgia
- Low back pain
- Facial pain
- Pelvic pain

The painkilling mechanism of these medications is still not fully understood. Tricyclic antidepressants appear to increase neurotransmitters in the spinal cord that reduce pain signals. But they don't work immediately. You may have to take a tricyclic antidepressant for several weeks before it starts reducing your pain.

Side effects of tricyclic antidepressants are usually mild and they may include drowsiness, dry mouth, constipation, weight gain, difficulty with urination and changes in blood pressure.

To reduce or prevent side effects, your doctor will likely start you at a low dose and slowly increase the amount. Most people are able to take tricyclic antidepressants, particularly in low doses, with only mild side effects. The doses that are effective for pain are typically lower than the doses used for depression.

Serotonin and norepinephrine reuptake inhibitors (SNRIs)

SNRIs that are commonly used for chronic pain include the following:
- Duloxetine (Cymbalta)
- Venlafaxine (Effexor)
- Milnacipran (Savella)
- Levomilnacipran (Fetzima)
- Desvenlafaxine (Pristiq, Khedezla)

These medications can be useful in many chronic pain conditions, specifically the following:
- Nerve damage for injury, surgery, diabetic neuropathy or postherpetic neuralgia
- Fibromyalgia
- Chronic musculoskeletal and arthritic pain

Similar to TCAs, SNRIs increase neurotransmitters in the brain and spinal cord to suppress pain signals. Side effects tend to be similar but less common compared to TCAs.

Anti-seizure medications

Developed mainly to reduce or control epileptic seizures, anti-seizure medications also may help control the stabbing, shooting or jabbing pain that can accompany nerve damage. The drugs seem to work by slowing or preventing damaged nerves from sending uncontrolled pain signals.

Anti-seizure medications used for chronic pain include:
- Carbamazepine (Carbatrol, Tegretol, others)
- Gabapentin (Neurontin, Gralise)
- Pregabalin (Lyrica)
- Oxcarbazepine (Trileptal)
- Phenytoin (Dilantin)
- Valproic acid (Depakene)

Although these medications can cause dizziness, confusion or swelling in the feet and legs, most people who take them are bothered only minimally by these side effects.

To reduce your risk of side effects, your doctor may start you on a small amount of the drug and gradually increase the dose over a period of several weeks — possibly monitoring you with blood tests during that time.

Opioids

Some opioids are natural compounds derived from the opium poppy plant. Others are synthetic medications that work in a similar fashion. These potent painkillers, often called narcotics, interfere with the transmission of pain signals and are taken most often to relieve pain following surgery or a traumatic injury or in people with cancer or a terminal illness.

Opioids include the following — those marked with an asterisk are multi-ingredient:

- Butorphanol (Butorphanol Tartrate)
- Codeine (aspirin with codeine*, acetaminophen with codeine*)
- Fentanyl (Actiq, Duragesic)
- Hydrocodone (Norco, Reprexain, others)
- Hydromorphone (Dilaudid, Hydromorphone HCL, others)
- Meperidine (Demerol)
- Methadone (Dolophine, Methadone HCL, others)
- Morphine (MS Contin, Kadian, others)
- Oxycodone (OxyContin, Percocet*, others)

Short-term use of opioids can cause several side effects, such as headache, nausea, vomiting, constipation, dizziness, drowsiness, fatigue and unclear thinking. In addition, an opioid can lose its effectiveness as your body develops a tolerance to it.

The biggest concern with opioids is the risk of addiction. The drugs can become habit-forming, and that's why doctors generally limit their use to acute pain.

Several studies indicate that most people who regularly take an opioid over a long period of time become physically dependent on the drug and experience some minor withdrawal symptoms if they abruptly stop using it. Although addiction is a serious problem, physical dependence itself may not result in serious problems, provided the medication is taken as directed.

The potential risks associated with long-term use of opioids make it difficult to justify the use of these medications for many forms of chronic pain. Long-term use of opioids should be done with a number of safety measures and under the care of a doctor who specializes in pain medicine.

Tramadol

Tramadol (Ultram, ConZip, others) is a prescription pain medication that works in two ways. It interferes with the transmission of pain signals, like an opioid, and it triggers the release of the brain neurotransmitters norepinephrine

Pain-Relieving Creams

Some pain relievers come in the form of a cream or gel. The medication is absorbed through your skin. Pain relief creams and gels can occasionally help relieve pain and inflammation just below your skin, such as pain from arthritis or nerve damage or pain near a surgical incision. Side effects tend to be limited to the site of application.

Here are four different types of pain-relieving creams and how they work.

EMLA

EMLA is a prescription pain-relieving cream made from two topical anesthetics: lidocaine and prilocaine. Your skin becomes numb within an hour after application, and the benefits are greatest two to three hours after application. EMLA is commonly used — especially on children — to reduce pain before a shot, drawing blood, inserting an intravenous line or treating a wart.

Capsaicin

Capsaicin (Qutenza) is a topical nonprescription cream made from the seeds of hot chili peppers. It's thought to work by depleting nerve cells of a chemical involved in transmitting pain messages. You rub the cream on your skin three or four times a day. Capsaicin cream initially causes an intense burning sensation. As you use it over time you become used to it in the same fashion that you become used to eating hot, spicy food. It usually takes one to two weeks before capsaicin's effects become noticeable. Maximum effects are often achieved after several weeks.

Capsaicin is most effective for temporary relief of arthritic pain in joints close to the skin, such as your fingers, knees and elbows. It's also used to help relieve skin sensitivity from shingles, pain resulting from nerve damage, pain that follows a mastectomy and chronic pain near healed surgical scars.

Methyl creams

Nonprescription, multi-ingredient medications such as Biofreeze, Bengay and Icy Hot use heat or cold to cover up the pain. These creams may relieve occasional, mild muscle aches, but they're not effective for most forms of chronic pain.

Aspirin-like creams

Nonprescription trolamine creams such as Aspercreme, Sportscreme and Myoflex contain a chemical that's similar to aspirin.

and serotonin, which suppress pain signaling.

Tramadol is used mainly to relieve mild to moderate acute pain. Side effects from tramadol can include dizziness, drowsiness, headache, nausea, constipation and seizures.

Mechanical Therapies

Pain-relief methods that target muscles and connective tissues involved in an injury are called mechanical therapies. Mechanical therapies for pain relief include cold therapy, heat therapy, exercise, massage, chiropractic care and ultrasound therapy.

Cold

Ice decreases pain by numbing the affected area. It works best for muscle spasms, swelling and joint pain. Ice decreases pain and swelling by temporarily reversing the blood vessel changes associated with inflammation. Early in the course of an injury, when inflammation is present, applying cold is best.

Ice massage
To give yourself an ice massage, gently rub a piece of ice over the affected area for five to seven minutes, until it becomes slightly numb. Watch for color changes in your skin. If you notice your skin losing its underlying red tone, stop immediately because it could indicate frostbite. If your skin becomes more than slightly numb during the ice massage, end the treatment.

Cold packs
To use a cold pack, wrap an ice pack or a bag of frozen vegetables in cloth. Hold it on the sore area for 15 minutes and repeat every two to three hours.

Heat

Heat increases blood flow and nutrients to painful muscles and joints. This helps the healing process and can improve flexibility. As an injury heals and after the inflammation is gone, heat is best.

Hot packs
To treat your pain with a hot pack, place several towels over the painful area. Lay a hot pack on top. Cover the pack with more towels for insulation. Add or remove towels between your skin and the pack to vary the heat. Check your skin every 15 minutes. If you see red and white blotches, stop the treatment at once to prevent a burn.

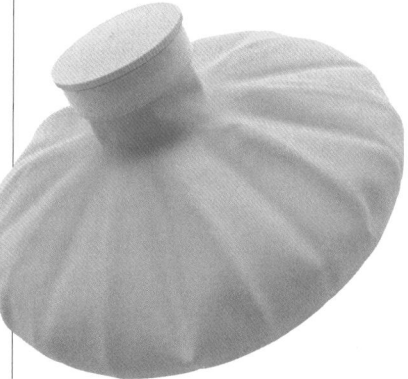

Heating pads
To treat your pain with an electric heating pad, first place a towel over the painful area. Then put the pad on top of the towel. Limit your use of a heating pad to 25 minutes at a time. Check occasionally for red and white blotches — signs that you've made the area too hot.

Heat lamps
A heat lamp produces infrared rays that warm your skin, which in turn increases blood circulation. Use a 250-watt reflector heat bulb. Position the lamp 18 to 20 inches from your skin. To decrease the heat intensity, move the lamp farther away.

Apply heat to the sore area for no longer than 20 minutes. If you think you might fall asleep while under the lamp, use an alarm clock or timer.

Baths and hot tubs
A 20-minute hot bath can be just as effective as a hot tub in relieving muscle and joint pain. Don't get the water too hot. If you have a hot tub, limit its use to no more than 30 minutes at a time.

Ultrasound

Ultrasound can do more than allow doctors to see inside your body. Physical therapists use ultrasound to treat painful injuries and to speed the healing process. Ultrasound acts as a deep-heating tool, warming tissue below the surface of the skin.

The heating effects — which you can't feel — are especially helpful in treating injured muscles, tendons and ligaments. They can also help relieve the pain associated with these injuries.

Exercise

A common misconception is that exercise increases pain. Actually, exercise can help reduce it. During physical activity, your body releases chemicals called endorphins and enkephalins that block pain signals from reaching your brain. These chemicals also help alleviate anxiety and depression, conditions that can make your pain more difficult to control.

Additionally, regular light exercise is a key treatment to certain chronic pain syndromes, such as chronic myofascial pain and fibromyalgia.

It's important, however, to distinguish between delayed muscle soreness after exercise, which is a normal sign that your muscles are growing stronger, and acute pain during exercise, which is a warning sign and means you should moderate your activity or stop.

A regular exercise program that includes flexibility, aerobic and strengthening exercises has many benefits. It can improve your overall fitness and help to control your pain. In addition, regular exercise can:

- Increase your energy and improve sleep
- Promote weight loss, reducing stress on your joints
- Increase bone mass, reducing your risk of injury

It's important to play it safe when it comes to exercise:

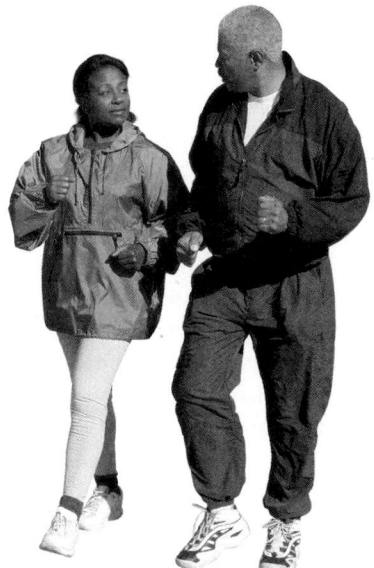

- If you've recently suffered an injury or haven't exercised in the past, consult a doctor before beginning an exercise program.
- Get advice on choosing the exercises best for you.
- Don't overdo it. Start out slowly, and gradually increase the time and pace of your exercise.

Find tips for getting and staying active in Chapter 9, "Fitness."

Invasive Therapies

Invasive therapies range from simple injections to surgical implants. They can also be an option when medications or mechanical approaches don't produce satisfactory results.

Injections

A shot (an injection) is most effective for nerve, joint or muscle pain that's confined to a specific location. The injections may include an anesthetic to control the pain, a steroid to reduce inflammation or a combination of the two.

The benefit of injections is that the medication works primarily on the painful area and doesn't spread throughout your body. This reduces potential side effects from the drug. The disadvantage of injections is that many times their effects are only temporary. In addition, there's a limit as to how often you can receive an injection, depending on the injection site and the type of medication used.

The two classes of injections are diagnostic and therapeutic. Diagnostic injections are used to test where the pain is coming from. Therapeutic injections are used to help provide long-term relief of symptoms. Sometimes the two are combined.

Injections generally aren't a cure, but they can help some people through an initial period of intense pain or a severe flare-up. The three general types of pain management injections are joint, soft tissue and nerve block.

Joint injection

If you're experiencing inflammation and pain caused by bone rubbing against bone, your doctor may recommend an injection near or into the affected joint. The joint is generally injected with a preparation of a local anesthetic to numb the area and then a medication.

The two main types of medication used for joint injections are corticosteroids and hyaluronic acid.

Corticosteroids
Corticosteroids suppress inflammation. They often begin working in one to two weeks and may offer pain relief for several months. When used for many months to years, they become less effective.

Hyaluronic acid
Hyaluronic acid is used to treat osteoarthritis of the knee and may be used for other joints. Hyaluronic acid is a substance found in normal joint fluid, which acts as a lubricant. It helps relieve pain by substituting for hyaluronic acid. Often, a local anesthetic is administered first, to relieve pain from the injections. Relief may last for up to six months.

What's the difference between a pain clinic and an interdisciplinary pain rehabilitation program?

Usually, a pain clinic offers a narrower range of services than does an interdisciplinary pain rehabilitation program.

A pain clinic is typically a facility with one or more doctors who specialize in the treatment of one or several painful conditions. For example, the doctors may specialize in the treatment of back pain or headache pain.

An interdisciplinary pain rehabilitation program is generally composed of a multidisciplinary group of doctors who specialize in the comprehensive treatment of pain. Their collective expertise allows for the management of a wide variety of pain problems.

Frequently, an interdisciplinary pain rehabilitation program does research and participates in the training of pain specialists.

The goal of this type of program is to improve quality of life and reduce distress for its participants. Research shows that this type of program is the most clinically effective and cost-effective way to treat chronic pain in adults.

Soft tissue injection

When a specific body part, such as a muscle or tendon, is inflamed or painful, an injection can be given directly into the surrounding soft tissue.

Trigger point injection

Trigger points are areas where your muscles and nearby tissues underneath your skin are sensitive to touch or movement. These areas are generally in the upper and lower back muscles. A trigger point injection — usually a preparation of a local anesthetic and a corticosteroid — is used to treat such an area. Depending on the medication used, a trigger point injection can reduce pain in a muscle, reduce inflammation, relax a muscle or increase movement.

Botulism toxin injections (Botox)

A small dose of botulism toxin can be injected in a muscle to cause muscle relaxation. This can be useful for chronic muscle spasms or certain types of headaches. For example, Botox injections have FDA approval for certain refractory chronic migraine headaches.

Bursa injection

Bursae are tiny, fluid-containing sacs that lubricate and cushion pressure points between your bones and the tendons or muscles near your joints. They help you move without pain. When a bursa becomes inflamed (bursitis), move-

ment or pressure may cause pain. Bursitis most often affects a shoulder, elbow or hip joint. An injection of a corticosteroid may be given to reduce inflammation in the bursa.

Nerve block injection

A nerve block procedure involves injecting an anesthetic around a nerve's fibers, preventing pain messages from traveling along that nerve pathway to your brain. Nerve blocks are used most often to relieve pain for a short period until other therapies or medications can take effect. They're also used to provide regional anesthesia for surgery or to control labor pain.

There are three main types of nerve blocks:

Peripheral

With a peripheral nerve block, an anesthetic is injected at a particular location, near specific nerves, to reduce pain in that area.

Spinal

Spinal nerve blocks are most often used for pain that affects a broader area, such as your lower back or a leg. An injection directly into the spinal fluid is called an intrathecal injection. This type of injection is often used during surgery on the abdomen or lower extremities.

If the injection isn't into the spinal fluid, it's called an epidural injection. Epidurals are the most common type of spinal injection. The needle is inserted between the

back bones into the epidural space that surrounds the spinal cord and spinal nerves. Epidural injections may be given in the neck (cervical), midback (thoracic) and low back (lumbar). The medication coats the nerves in the location where it's injected, relieving pain.

Epidurals are often used to relieve the pain of childbirth and sometimes are given to relieve back or extremity pain.

Sympathetic

Some forms of chronic pain, such as complex regional pain syndrome, may result from abnormally increased activity of your sympathetic nervous system. Your sympathetic nerves, part of your autonomic nervous system, control circulation and perspiration. To prevent messages produced by your sympathetic nerves from reaching the affected area of the body, an anesthetic may be injected near the sympathetic nerves. These injections are done in the neck for pain in the arms and in the low back for pain in the legs.

This type of injection can be done without causing numbness or weakness, allowing you to participate in physical therapy.

Spinal cord stimulation

A spinal cord stimulator is a small device that's surgically implanted, usually in your lower back. It's wired to your spinal cord to deliver electric pulses that block pain messages to your brain. The device is battery powered, much like a pacemaker, and is controlled by an external programming unit that turns the stimulator on and off and adjusts the level of the electric pulse. Some people who use this device say the pulse causes a tingling sensation.

Spinal cord stimulation is usually used only after other treatments have failed. However, studies indicate that it can provide substantial pain relief. The procedure is used for a variety of pain, including back and extremity pain not relieved by surgery and pain from nerve injury.

Pain pumps

For some people with excruciating pain that isn't helped by other measures, one option to control the pain is a pain pump. A small device is surgically implanted in the lower abdomen, where it provides a steady infusion of medication — typically an opioid — into the cerebrospinal fluid, which is the primary site of action for these medications. Sometimes, the medication is a combination of drugs, such as an opioid and local anesthetic.

Pain pumps are used most often to control pain associated with terminal illness. Because the medication is delivered to its site of action, medication side effects such as nausea and fatigue are less common.

Integrative Therapies

Integrative therapies combine the best of conventional medicine and evidence-based complementary treatments. Integrative therapies are used with conventional medi-

cine to treat a variety of ailments. Here are four of the many integrative therapies that show effectiveness in managing chronic pain:

Acupuncture

Acupuncture is based on the Chinese belief that within the human body are multiple pathways, called meridians. Through these pathways flows *qi* (pronounced CHEE), the Chinese word for "life force" or "life energy." When the flow of qi is obstructed, illness or pain results. By inserting needles into specific points along these meridians, acupuncture practitioners believe that your energy flow will re-balance.

Research shows that acupuncture is effective in treating chronic neck pain, chronic and acute low-back pain, knee pain, dental pain, osteoarthritis, labor pain, menstrual cramps, and headaches, including migraine headaches.

During acupuncture, an acupuncturist inserts anywhere between five and 20 hair-thin needles into your skin for 15 to 20 minutes. The acupuncturist may also manipulate the needles or apply electrical stimulation or heat to the needles.

Side effects from acupuncture are rare, but they can occur. Make sure your acupuncturist is trained and certified or licensed and follows good hygiene practices, including the use of disposable needles.

Massage

Massage is one of the oldest methods of therapy that's still practiced. It involves the use of different manipulative techniques to move your body's muscles and soft tissues.

A massage therapist primarily uses his or her hands to manipulate muscles and tissues. However, the therapist sometimes may use his or her forearms, elbows or feet.

Massage therapy is based on the belief that when muscles are overworked, waste products accumu-

late in them, causing soreness and stiffness. The therapy aims to improve circulation in the muscles, increasing the flow of nutrients and removing waste products.

Massage can relax your muscles, improve the range of motion in your joints and increase production of your body's natural painkillers. It may also help relieve stress and anxiety. Avoid massage if you have open sores, acute inflammation or circulatory problems.

Chiropractic

Chiropractic care is based on the idea that your body's structure — nerves, bones, joints and muscles — and its capacity for healthy function are closely intertwined. By aligning and balancing your body's structure, chiropractic treatment is intended to support the body's natural ability to heal itself. Adjustment is one form of therapy chiropractors use to treat spinal mobility. The goal is to restore spinal movement and, as a result, improve function and decrease back pain.

Chiropractic care is not appropriate for people who have severe osteoporosis, numbness, tingling, or loss of strength in an arm or leg, cancer in your spine, or an increased risk of stroke.

Transcutaneous electrical nerve stimulation (TENS)

TENS units are battery-powered devices that deliver painless continuous electrical impulses over an area of pain. These impulses are thought to improve pain by interfering with peripheral pain signaling.

Over-the-counter and prescription options are available. TENS units are safe and noninvasive, but should not be used over open skin or sores, or in people who have a pacemaker.

Learn more about integrative medicine in Chapter 38, "Integrative Medicine."

Cancer Pain

In the United States, millions of people live with cancer. Although not all people with cancer experience pain, as many as half do. Cancer pain can't always be eliminated, but it frequently can be controlled to lessen its impact on normal daily activities.

Treatment of cancer pain

Cancer-related pain can be treated in many different ways. The ideal method is to remove the source of the pain if possible, for example, through surgery, chemotherapy, radiation or some other form of treatment. Unfortunately, some cancer treatments themselves also can produce pain.

The type of medication used to control cancer pain depends on the severity of the pain. Sometimes, over-the-counter and prescription-strength pain relievers, such as aspirin, acetaminophen (Tylenol, others) and ibuprofen (Advil, Motrin IB, others) are helpful. Other times a stronger pain reliever is needed. This may include a weak opioid (narcotic), such as codeine, or a strong opioid, such as morphine. To provide more consistent pain control, opioids are often prescribed in a sustained-release formulation. You take the long-acting medication on a scheduled, regular basis. Your doctor may also prescribe a shorter-acting opioid for intermittent use to control breakthrough pain. If swallowing pills is difficult, opioids can be given in patch form, where they're absorbed through the skin. Other routes of delivery include transmucosal (lollipop), inhaled, intravenous, subcutaneous, spinal and rectal.

For some types of cancer, such as pancreatic cancer, a nerve block may effectively control the pain. During this procedure a doctor injects medication into the major nerves around the affected area to prevent the nerves from sending pain signals to the brain.

Undertreatment of cancer pain

Unfortunately, cancer pain often isn't adequately controlled. One reason has to do with doctors' knowledge of pain and their ability to evaluate and treat pain. Some doctors and other health care professionals may not specifically ask about pain, which should be a normal part of every cancer checkup.

A second factor is reluctance on the part of the person with cancer. Some people fear that pain means that their cancer is getting worse, or they worry that their doctor may think of them as weak if they complain of pain. Many people feel they're supposed to have pain with cancer and that they should be able to deal with it on their own. This simply isn't true.

Some people worry that taking medications, such as morphine, may shorten their lives. If the medication is dosed properly, it shouldn't shorten life or cause other severe side effects. Many people taking opioids still remain active.

A team approach

Inform your doctor if you're experiencing pain, and work together on a pain management plan. Set a main goal, such as keeping the pain at a level with which you're comfortable. If you aren't achieving that goal, keep working with your doctor. You might also ask to consult a pain specialist. Many medical facilities, especially major medical centers, have pain centers or pain clinics in which medical personnel are trained in a variety of pain management techniques. Hospice may also be a helpful option. Among its services, hospice provides pain control that helps the people who receive it to be comfortable and stay in control of and enjoy their lives.

Cognitive Behavioral Therapy

The goal of cognitive behavioral therapy is to identify and modify your pain triggers and reactions and adjust your lifestyle to better manage your pain.

Simple things, such as how you organize your day, can have a significant effect on your ability to manage your pain. If you overdo it to meet a deadline or overcommit yourself so that you're running from one activity to the next, fatigue sets in and your pain increases. The opposite — avoiding all activities and lying around the house — isn't any better. The isolation can cause you to focus only on your pain. Cognitive behavioral therapy is about finding a healthy balance of work, recreation and relaxation.

Time management

For many people, an important step to balancing their day is learning to use time more efficiently. Juggling work, household tasks and social activities can consume large amounts of your day. Procrastination, perfectionism or overcommitting yourself can make time management even more difficult. Try these strategies for using your time more wisely:

Plan

Schedule your day so that you have time for the things you must do and those you want to do. Start by writing down all of your activities in a daily planner. Then frequently refer to your planner to make sure you stay on track.

Placing a central calendar near your telephone where you mark down all of your events and appointments also can be helpful. By doing this, all of your appointments will be in one place, so that they don't come as a surprise and to avoid becoming overcommitted.

Identify

Notice when you waste time and avoid these time wasters. If you can't avoid them, try to make them productive. For example, while waiting for a doctor's appointment or during your daily train commute, listen to a relaxation tape or balance your checkbook.

Prioritize

If you're involved in too many activities that are competing for your time, decide which are the most important and let go of the rest. Your health needs should come before the wants of others. Not taking care of yourself can lead to increased pain and fatigue.

Delegate

On days when you have more to do than you can comfortably handle, seek help from others. Ask your spouse, son or daughter to do the laundry or prepare dinner.

Evaluate

Think about your day. Do you have realistic expectations regarding the number of tasks that you can complete in a day?

Educate

Discuss your time needs with those who rely on you the most. If family members, friends or co-workers make unreasonable demands on your time, explain to them that you need to pace yourself.

Organizational skills

Becoming more organized can save you time so that you can incorporate more activities into your day. Organization also helps conserve energy by eliminating wasted steps and unnecessary motions.

Think before you act

Before you begin a task, gather all of the items you need or make a list of what needs to be done. For example, keep all of your cleaning supplies in one container to avoid multiple trips up and down the stairs. Before you run errands, list all of the things you need to do to avoid a second trip later on.

Keep items accessible

Organize your work areas at home and at your job so that items you use frequently are close at hand. This can save you unnecessary bending or reaching.

Reduce clutter

Searching for items takes both time and energy. Organize your counters, cabinets, closets and drawers so that you can easily find what you need.

Moderation skills

Moderation involves how much, how long or how fast you do things to avoid overdoing or underdoing your day. Moderation helps you avoid large swings in your pain level so that at the end of each task, your pain is near the same level as when you began. To practice moderation:

Break apart lengthy tasks

Lengthy activities often sap your energy and may increase your pain. Instead of spending all day planting your garden, spend an hour or two a day in the garden for three or four days. Spread out a 10-hour car trip to visit friends or relatives over two days.

Alternate activities

Mix activities that require a lot of effort with those that require little energy. After vacuuming one room of the house, sit down and read or pay some bills. Then do a load of laundry. Note times of the day when you have the most energy and the least pain. Plan your priority tasks during these times.

Rest periodically

How often you should take a break depends on the activity. You may find that you can do some activities, such as word processing, for 30 minutes to an hour before you need a break. More-strenuous tasks, such as mowing the lawn, may require a break every 10 to 20 minutes.

Pace yourself

Instead of rushing to complete a task, work at a comfortable speed — a pace at which you feel like you're exerting yourself but not overdoing it. You expend twice as much energy when you work at a fast pace than you do at a moderate one. It may take you a little longer to get the job done, but in the end you'll feel better.

Stress management

Pain and stress go hand in hand. When you're in pain, you're less able to handle everyday stressors. Common hassles turn into major obstacles. Stress also causes you to do things that intensify your pain, such as tense your muscles, grit your teeth and stiffen your shoulders. In short, pain causes stress, and stress intensifies pain.

The first step in breaking this pain-stress cycle is to realize that stress is your response to an event, not the event itself. It's something you can control. That's why events that are stressful for some people aren't for others.

For example, your morning commute may leave you anxious and tense because you use it as worry time. A co-worker, however, may find the same commute relaxing. She may enjoy her time alone, perhaps listening to music or a book on tape.

Understanding that you have control over your stress helps you develop strategies for dealing with it. For information on stress management techniques, see Chapter 10, "Stress."

Treatment for depression and anxiety

As many as half the people with chronic pain experience mild to severe depression and anxiety. It's natural to feel down, frustrated or anxious when the pain first develops or for short periods afterward.

Your pain itself may cause signs or symptoms associated with depression, such as slowed movements or loss of energy. If your symptoms linger for several months or they become severe, you may be experiencing depression or anxiety.

Depression and anxiety are complex conditions that can make your pain worse. That's because it's difficult to separate your mood from the intensity of your pain. People who are depressed or anxious often report stronger, longer lasting and more severe pain than do people who aren't depressed. They're less able to tolerate pain.

Depression and anxiety should be treated. With appropriate treatment most people show improvement, usually in a matter of weeks. For information on these conditions, see Chapter 31, "Mental Health."

Common Chronic Conditions

Chronic pain can strike just about any part of your body, from your head to your toes, from your skin to your well-protected internal organs. Arthritis pain, back pain and headaches are among the most common types of chronic pain. But chronic pain can occur in many forms and for many reasons.

Your pain may be related to an existing illness or stem from an accident or injury. Perhaps your pain is linked to a condition that

doctors don't fully understand. Or maybe it has no apparent cause.

This section briefly reviews common types of chronic pain.

Bone and joint disorders

There are many painful disorders of the bones and joints, but the most common is arthritis — osteoarthritis, specifically. The word *arthritis* means "joint inflammation." Although people often talk about arthritis as one disease, it's not. It takes many forms. Some forms appear gradually. Others appear suddenly and then disappear, only to return again later.

The disease can strike any joint in your body and may be triggered by various causes, including an injury, lack of physical activity, natural wear on your joints and genetic disease. The two most common forms of arthritis are osteoarthritis and rheumatoid arthritis.

Osteoarthritis
Osteoarthritis affects more than 30 million Americans. This common condition results when cartilage that cushions the ends of bones in your joints starts to deteriorate. If the cartilage wears down completely, you may be left with bone rubbing against bone, irritating the joint and producing pain.

Your body tries to repair the damage, but often the repairs are unsuccessful, even resulting in growth of new bone along the sides of existing bone. The new bone may produce bony lumps, most noticeably in your hands and feet, and especially at the middle joints or ends of your fingers and toes. These lumps, some of which are called spurs, may or may not produce pain and tenderness.

Osteoarthritis can develop anywhere in your body, but it tends to be most common in your hands and feet and in major joints in your hands, knees, hips and spine. Initially, arthritis pain may be minor and hurt only when you use the affected joint. But in time, the pain can intensify and occur even when you're not using the joint.

Although there's no known cure for osteoarthritis, in recent years treatments to reduce pain and maintain joint movement have improved. Pain management generally includes a combination of medication, self-care and physical therapy, including daily exercise.

Medications include both topical medications, such as creams and gels that temporarily relieve the pain, and oral medications, such as NSAIDs. Over-the-counter medications may be sufficient for mild osteoarthritis. For moderate

Normal Spine

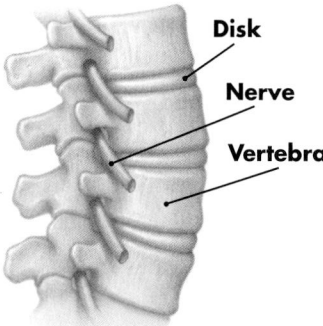

Disk

Nerve

Vertebra

Osteoarthritis

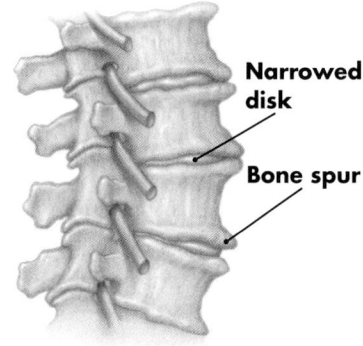

Narrowed disk

Bone spur

In a normal spine, your vertebrae are cushioned by elastic structures called disks, which help to keep the spine flexible. When you have osteoarthritis in the spine, the disks narrow, leading to bony lumps along the sides of vertebrae. Pain and stiffness may occur where bone surfaces rub together.

to severe disease, you may need a stronger, prescription medication.

The dietary supplements glucosamine and chondroitin sulfate are popular integrative treatments for osteoarthritis, but so far, research hasn't confirmed that the supplements can actually prevent cartilage loss. Some research shows that glucosamine and chondroitin can help decrease pain and improve joint function in people who have osteoarthritis. But other research suggests that glucosamine and chondroitin aren't any more effective in treating pain than was a placebo.

Glucosamine and chondroitin appear to be safe and to produce few side effects. However, if you're allergic to shellfish, you should avoid them. And be cautious if you take an anticoagulant drug, such as warfarin, since glucosamine may increase the risk of bleeding.

Rheumatoid arthritis

Unlike osteoarthritis, rheumatoid arthritis is thought to stem from an immune system disorder that causes your immune system to inappropriately attack the lining of your joints, just as it appropriately attacks invading viruses or bacteria.

White blood cells designed to destroy viruses and bacteria move into joint tissues, producing inflammation and pain. Swelling of the tissues triggers the release of natural chemicals that eventually dissolve cartilage and damage tendons and ligaments in the joint. Gradually, the joint becomes deformed. Rheumatoid arthritis most often affects joints in your wrists, hands, feet and ankles.

NSAIDs can often help ease pain and reduce inflammation associated with rheumatoid arthritis. Over-the-counter NSAIDs may be sufficient for mild pain. Disease-modifying antirheumatic drugs (DMARDs) can slow the progression of rheumatoid arthritis and save the joints and other tissues from permanent damage.

Connective tissue disorders

Your muscles help you move. Each skeletal muscle is attached to bones by fibrous bands called tendons. Muscles and tendons work with other soft tissues, such as ligaments, to enable you to run, walk or climb stairs. Damage to connective tissues can make movement painful. Common connective tissue disorders include sprains, strains, bursitis, tendinitis and fibromyalgia.

Low back pain

Four out of 5 adults have back pain at least once in their lives. Millions of Americans experience back pain on a frequent basis.

Most back pain occurs in your lower back (lumbar area), which bears most of your weight. Your lower back also serves as your body's pivot point, allowing you to bend forward and backward and twist sideways.

Acute back pain often stems from an injury or overuse. Sometimes, back pain can occur for no specific reason and frequently recur. Oftentimes, back pain is related to:

- Muscle strain and spasm
- Nerve irritation or compression
- Herniated disk
- Arthritis

For more on these conditions, see Chapter 27, "Bones, Joints and Muscles."

Treatment for low back pain often includes moderation of activities, NSAIDs, exercise, and heat and cold therapy. If these measures don't work, other options may include other types of prescription medications, therapeutic injections or spinal cord stimulation. A number of integrative therapies, such as chiropractic care, acupuncture, massage and yoga may be helpful, as well.

Bursitis

You have more than 150 bursae in your body. These tiny, fluid-con-

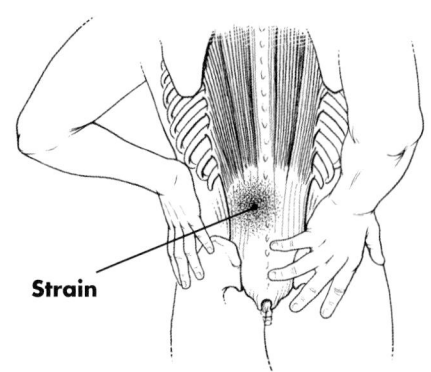

Strain

Your lower back, a pivot point for turning at your waist, is vulnerable to muscle strains.

taining sacs lubricate and cushion pressure points between your bones and the tendons and muscles near your joints. They help you move without pain. When they become inflamed — often through overuse or an injury — movement or pressure is painful.

Most often, bursitis affects the shoulder, elbow or hip joint. It can also affect your knee, heel and even the base of your big toe. With proper treatment, bursitis pain usually goes away within a week or so, but return flare-ups are common.

An injection of a steroid into the bursa may help relieve the inflammation. Often an anesthetic is included to relieve pain. Other options include an over-the-counter medication, such as ibuprofen (Advil, Motrin IB, others) or naproxen sodium (Aleve, others) to help relieve pain and inflammation. Other self-care measures include applying ice to reduce swelling, cushioning your knees if you sleep on your side by placing a small pillow between your legs, and avoiding leaning or placing your weight on your elbows when you rise from a lying position.

Tendinitis

Tendinitis is inflammation or irritation of a tendon — a thick, fibrous cord that attaches muscles to bone. Although tendinitis can be caused by a sudden injury, the condition is much more likely to stem from the repetition of a particular movement over time. The condition generally causes tenderness and stiffness near a joint that's aggravated by movement. Most often, tendinitis develops in a shoulder, elbow (tennis elbow) or knee, wrist or heel.

If tendinitis is severe and causes a rupture of a tendon, you may need to have the tendon repaired surgically. In many cases, though, rest and medications to reduce pain and inflammation may be the only treatment you need. Sometimes, a doctor may inject a steroid into tissue around the tendon to relieve the inflammation.

Fibromyalgia

Fibromyalgia is a disorder that targets your muscles, tendons and ligaments. It differs from arthritis in that the pain is in nearby tissues instead of the joints themselves. Also unlike arthritis, it doesn't cause inflammation — just pain.

The main symptoms of fibromyalgia are disturbed sleep, fatigue, aching all over, and brain fog. The pain may be a deep ache or a burning sensation. Symptoms of fibromyalgia may flare and subside, but they usually don't disappear completely.

In general, fibromyalgia may be treated with some medications, such as antidepressants or anticonvulsants, as well as lifestyle changes that include decreasing isolation, improving sleep, exercise and relaxation strategies. The emphasis is on minimizing symptoms and improving general health and functioning. Medications often include over-the-counter or prescription pain relievers. Antidepressants may be prescribed to help promote sleep and relieve pain. Medications are often combined with behavior therapies, including stress management and daily exercise.

Nerve disorders

Pain from nerve damage or disorders can be among the most difficult to treat. Your body's

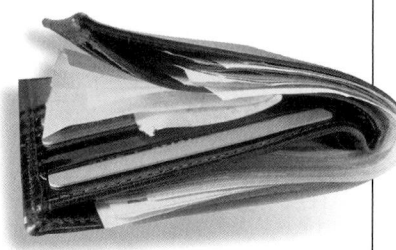
intricate network of nerves is what controls pain messages sent to your brain. When nerves don't work properly, they can cause a variety of symptoms that can be difficult to control. Here are several examples of common nerve disorders.

Diabetic neuropathy

High blood sugar characteristic of diabetes can be associated with damage to delicate peripheral nerves in your feet and hands. About 60 percent of people with diabetes experience this kind of nerve damage, which can be painful and disabling. Most commonly, nerves in the feet are affected, and less often, nerves in the fingers. Peripheral neuropathy may produce a tingling sensation, numbness, pain or a combination of all these.

Medications that tend to provide the greatest relief of nerve pain include anti-seizure or antidepressant medications. Another option is the cream capsaicin, made from hot chili pepper extract. When you rub it over the painful area, the extract helps block pain sensations. It can take one to four weeks for the cream to become effective.

Other therapies that may be beneficial include acupuncture, biofeedback and spinal cord stimulation.

Shingles and pain after shingles

Shingles (herpes zoster) can result in acute pain and also in persistent nerve pain known as postherpetic neuralgia.

Shingles is the re-emergence of the virus that caused an earlier case of chickenpox. The virus reactivates after lying dormant for years within your nerve cells. When it reactivates, the virus typically causes pain or tingling in a limited area, usually on part of one side of your body or face. As

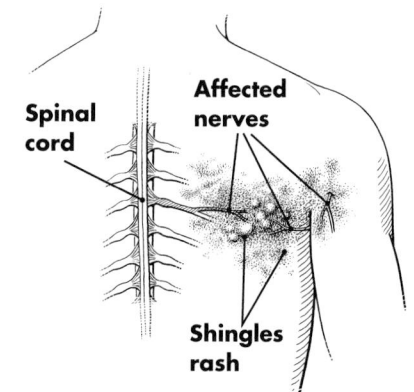

Shingles (herpes zoster) is a rash associated with an inflammation of nerves beneath the skin. Damage to the nerves may produce pain even after the rash has healed (postherpetic neuralgia).

the virus travels along a nerve that spreads outward from your spine or face, this pain or tingling can continue for several days or longer. Subsequently, a rash with small blisters typically appears. (For more information on shingles, and how to prevent it, see page 1097.)

Most people with shingles have pain requiring treatment with pain relievers, even prescription opioids. Antiviral medications, such as valacyclovir (Valtrex) and famciclovir, can hasten healing of skin lesions and reduce the severity of some complications caused by shingles.

If pain persists after the rash heals, it's known as postherpetic neuralgia. This chronic pain results from damage to nerve fibers from the shingles infection. Postherpetic neuralgia can be treated with tricyclic antidepressants and antiseizure drugs, among other medications. Some people are helped most by these drugs, which help suppress pain messages from damaged nerves.

Other steps that may reduce the pain include applying an anesthetic lidocaine patch (Lidoderm) or capsaicin cream.

Steroid injections near the affected nerves or in the epidural space may be beneficial, especially in the early stages of postherpetic neuralgia. Persistent pain that does not respond to less invasive treatments may respond to spinal cord stimulation.

The best way to prevent shingles and, thus, postherpetic neuralgia is to receive the shingles (herpes zoster) vaccination (Zostavax). This is recommended by the CDC for people age 60 years and older, who are not at risk of complications from the vaccination. The vaccine may be given to some individuals as early as age 50 if the benefits of receiving the vaccine outweigh the risks.

Radicular pain

Nerve inflammation or compression of a nerve root in your neck or lower back can cause pain that travels down your arm or leg in a specific location that corresponds to a specific nerve. This is called radicular pain. You may feel the pain radiating from your back through your buttock to your lower leg. Tingling, numbness or muscle weakness also can occur.

An example is sciatica — pain that radiates along the path of the sciatic nerve, which branches from your lower back through your hips and buttocks and down each leg. Typically, sciatica affects only one side of your body.

Radicular pain usually goes away on its own within four to six weeks, but severe nerve compression can cause progressive muscle weakness and continued pain.

Your doctor may recommend hot and cold compresses to relieve inflammation around the nerve. An NSAID also may reduce swelling and pain. If these don't work, other therapies may be beneficial. An injection of a corticosteroid near the spinal column also may be used. Back surgery to relieve pressure on the nerve is generally a last resort.

Headaches

Headaches represent a common type of pain that most people can have experienced. Nearly everyone gets a headache at one time or another. Headaches can range from fleeting annoyances to those that put you flat on your back. There are several types of headaches. Most fall into one of two categories.

Tension

This is the most common type of headache. The cause of tension headaches is not known. Experts used to think tension headaches stemmed from muscle contractions in the face, neck

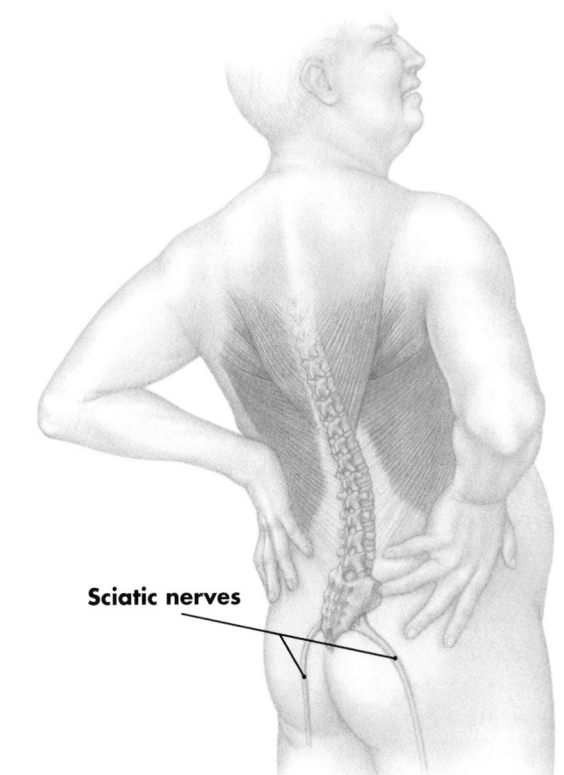

Sciatic nerves

Nerve irritation in your lower back can cause sciatica — pain that radiates from your back through your buttock to your lower leg.

and scalp, perhaps as a result of heightened emotions, tension or stress. But research suggests this isn't the cause. The most common theory supports a heightened sensitivity to pain in people who have tension headaches. Increased muscle tenderness, a common symptom of tension headaches, may result from a sensitized pain system.

A variety of medications, both over-the-counter (OTC) and prescription, are available for treating tension headaches. You may find fast, effective relief by taking pain relievers such as aspirin, ibuprofen (Advil, Motrin IB, others) or acetaminophen (Tylenol, others).

People with severe or chronic tension headaches may require preventive medications to reduce the frequency and severity of head pain. Which drug works best varies from one person to another. For more information on tension headaches and their treatment, see page 518.

Migraine

This type of headache not only gets your attention, but can put your life on hold. Migraines generally produce a throbbing pain on one side of your head — often your temple or forehead. The pain can range from moderate to severe. Migraine attacks can cause significant pain for hours to days.

Experts believe that migraines may be caused by changes in the brainstem and its interactions with the trigeminal nerve, a major pain pathway. Imbalances in brain chemicals — including serotonin, which helps regulate pain in your nervous system — also may be involved. Genetics and environmental factors also appear to play a role.

Treatment options for migraines have expanded greatly in the last decade — giving you more choices than ever for keeping migraine disruption to a minimum. Some of the drugs used for migraines today were originally designed to treat other conditions, such as epilepsy or hypertension. Migraine medications can be divided into two broad categories:

- Acute, to be taken only when you have a migraine
- Preventive, to be taken every day to ward off migraines

For more information on migraines and their treatment, see page 520.

Pain of Unknown Cause

Sometimes, chronic pain develops for no apparent reason. Despite repeated tests, your doctor isn't able to link it to an identifiable physical cause or condition. This doesn't mean that the pain doesn't exist. It simply means that your pain may be associated with factors that are difficult to diagnose.

Years of research have been spent on chronic pain syndromes that seem to lack a physical cause or a rational explanation. One explanation for pain that occurs without ongoing tissue damage is a syndrome called central sensitization.

To understand central sensitization, here's a little background. Tiny sensor cells throughout your body help you hear, see, taste, and feel sensations, such as pain. These sensors send information to your brain. Your brain interprets the information from the sensors and directs your body how to respond to it. You read about this process at the beginning of this chapter.

In central sensitization, the signals sent to your brain are strengthened, or turned up, causing the sensors to operate in overdrive. Sounds can seem louder, lights can seem brighter, movement can hurt more and pain can feel more intense.

Symptoms of central sensitization may include pain, numbness or tingling, headaches, chronic pelvic pain, fatigue, restless legs symptoms, sleep problems, dizziness and lightheadedness, weakness, brain fog, depression and anxiety, and sensitivities to a variety of things, such as food, medication or something in your environment.

Central sensitization has been linked to several painful conditions, including fibromyalgia, irritable bowel syndrome and temporomandibular disorder.

While it's not medically possible to completely shut off the brain signals that can lead to central sensitization, it is possible to "turn down" the line of communication that's producing these symptoms. To do so, you want to take the same steps that you would to manage other types of chronic pain.

In addition to moderating daily activity and getting good-quality sleep, daily exercise is important. This includes relaxation exercises that help loosen tense muscles, prevent muscle spasms and relieve stress. Exercises that may be particularly beneficial include relaxed breathing, progressive muscle relaxation and visualization.

For more information about relaxation exercises, see Chapter 10, "Stress." Other therapies such as meditation, yoga and tai chi also may be helpful. Biofeedback is another relaxation technique that may help. It teaches you how to control your body's functions, such as your heart rate and breathing. For some people, medications also may be beneficial.

Interdisciplinary pain rehabilitation centers provide many tools for helping people with chronic pain implement lifestyle changes to help improve their symptoms.

The bottom line with central sensitization, as with other types of chronic pain, is that a combination of therapies is often necessary to enjoy an active and fulfilling life. ■

Integrative Medicine

Whether it be herbs to battle a cold, dietary supplements to help reduce high blood pressure or acupuncture to control pain, Americans both young and old are increasingly turning to health and healing practices outside of mainstream medicine.

Known collectively as integrative medicine, these therapies are new to some people — but many of them have been used for thousands of years.

Put simply, integrative medicine is the practice of integrating the best of conventional medicine and evidence-based complementary treatments. The idea is to use conventional and complementary treatments in a unified approach to optimize health and wellness.

Once considered "unorthodox" or "alternative," these therapies were renamed as "complementary and alternative medicine," or CAM, in the 1990s. Today, CAM therapies that have been studied and found to be effective are integrated into conventional care, hence the term "integrative medicine."

Does this mean that all forms of complementary and alternative medicine are OK to use? No. Some carry significant risks, and others simply don't work. It does indicate, though, that certain therapies do have merit and can aid in health and healing.

Guiding Principles

Most products, practices and therapies are based around a few common principles:

- **Prevention.** One of the main philosophies of integrative medicine is to take preventive steps to promote good health.
- **Natural healing.** Your body has the ability to heal itself. The purpose of treatment is to encourage the natural healing process.
- **Active learning.** CAM practitioners see themselves as facilitators — teachers who offer guidance. You're the one who actually produces the healing.
- **"Holistic" care.** The focus is on treating the whole person — addressing physical, emotional, social and spiritual needs.

What to Watch For

People who do exhaustive research before deciding on a new car or appliance often don't approach health care in the same way. Cliché or not, knowledge is power. If you're considering an integrative treatment, find out all you can about it. In the interest of protecting your health and your

wallet, evaluate the benefits and risks — especially the risks. "Natural" doesn't mean harmless.

The difference between integrative practices and conventional medicine is scientific evidence of safety and effectiveness. For that, doctors rely on research, and they would advise you to do the same.

Ask your doctor for information on research results to help you make an informed decision about any treatment you're considering. Or, dig up the information on your own, keeping in mind that not all research meets the same exacting standards for credibility. It's important for you to understand the quality of the studies you're reading.

Pay attention to the terms

Here are several terms used to describe different types of research:

- **Clinical studies.** These studies involve research on people, rather than animals. Clinical studies, or trials, are usually preceded by studies that demonstrate the safety and effectiveness of the treatment in animals.
- **Randomized, controlled trials.** Participants are usually divided into two or more groups. One group receives the treatment under investigation. Another is a control group — the people in this group receive standard treatment, no treatment or an inactive substance called a placebo. Participants are assigned randomly to these groups to help prevent bias and ensure that the groups are similar in makeup.
- **Double-blind studies.** Here, neither the researchers nor the human subjects know who receives the active treatment and who gets the placebo.
- **Prospective studies.** These studies are forward looking. Researchers establish criteria for study participants to follow and then measure or describe the results. Information from these studies is usually more reliable than retrospective studies.

Integrative vs. Alternative: What's the Difference?

Integrative medicine combines conventional medical treatment with complementary therapies that have scientific evidence indicating they're safe to use, and they've been shown to be effective. An example of an integrative therapy is using acupuncture to help lessen nausea that can occur after surgery.

Alternative medicine, on the other hand, refers to treatment that's used in place of conventional medicine. An example would be an individual who chooses a special diet to treat his or her cancer instead of undergoing treatment such as surgery, radiation or drug therapy recommended by a conventional doctor.

- **Retrospective studies.** They involve looking at past data — for example, asking participants to recall information — which leaves more room for bias and errors in interpretation.
- **Peer-reviewed medical journals.** These journals publish only articles that have been reviewed by an independent panel of medical experts. The review is usually anonymous, and the reviewers typically aren't paid. Learn if a journal is peer-reviewed by visiting its homepage. There, look for the terms "peer-reviewed" and "acceptance rate." A medical journal that is peer-reviewed and has an acceptance rate below 20 percent offers the best-quality information.

Rely on the best studies

Now that you know the terms, here's what to look for: prospective, double-blind studies that have been controlled, randomized and published in peer-reviewed journals. They're considered the gold standard of medical research. If they involve large numbers of people (several hundred or more) who have been studied over several years, then they gain even more credibility.

In addition, doctors like studies that are replicated by different investigators who end up with similar results.

Much of the early research involving integrative treatments failed to meet these rigorous standards. Instead, what was most available consisted of anecdotal reports from practitioners and people who have undergone the treatments, inconclusive data and opinion — from opponents as well as proponents.

However, thanks to leadership at the National Center for Complementary and Integrative Health (NCCIH) and to researchers at academic institutions, the quality of research is improving rapidly.

A number of integrative therapies are being shown to be both safe and effective. As this occurs, the therapies are more often being combined with conventional care.

Herbal Preparations

The Food and Drug Administration (FDA) classifies herbal supplements, along with vitamins and minerals, as dietary supplements. Used for centuries for healing, herbs such as St. John's wort and echinacea have evolved from folk remedies into a multibillion-dollar industry in the United States.

Millions of Americans use herbal supplements. Because herbs are derived from plants, many people consider them "natural" and therefore, they assume they're safe. That's not necessarily so. Research has identified a number of herbal substances, such as ephedra, that can cause harmful, even deadly, effects. In addition, the effectiveness of many herbal preparations hasn't been established.

Regulation

One area of concern that is being addressed by the FDA is the question of quality of herbal products sold in the United States.

Prior to 2007, regulation of the quality and purity of dietary supplements in the United States was sporadic at best. Numerous reports made headlines when herbs sold in the United States were found to be contaminated with

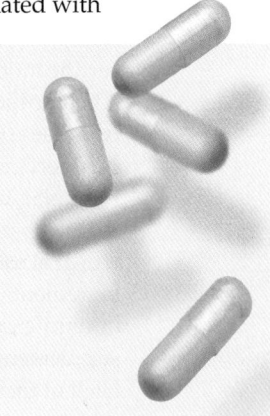

Common Categories

Hundreds of integrative therapies are available. Most can be classified into the following five major groups:

- Herbal preparations
- Manipulation and touch
- Mind-body interventions
- Natural energy restoration
- Complete medical systems

heavy metals or when analysis of specific herbal products showed that they didn't contain any of the herb they claimed on the bottle.

Fortunately, this has changed. Today, thanks to rules implemented in 2010 called Good Manufacturing Practices (GMPs), all supplements sold in the U.S. are now mandated to contain exactly what's stated on the label. However, some supplements still fall through the cracks. That's why despite GMPs, it's important that you know what to look for to ensure that you're purchasing good-quality products.

Of all of the unconventional treatments, herbal preparations may present the greatest potential for serious harm, so it's important to learn all that you can about any product you're using — or considering using.

Safety

If you decide to use an herbal preparation, exercise as much caution as you would with any prescription or over-the-counter medication with these tips.

Read the label
The quality and strength of an herbal preparation can vary greatly by brand. When considering an herbal preparation, look for these certifications or quality measures:
- Current Good Manufacturing Practices from the FDA
- International Organization for Standardization (ISO) 9000 or 9001
- European Union (EU) certification
- AUS certification, which comes from the Australian government
- NSF certification, which comes from NSF International
- A DNA barcoding program, which is used to identify herbal ingredients and to detect impure or unsafe ingredients in a dietary supplement

Each of these certifies that the product meets a certain standard.

Follow directions
Don't exceed recommended dosages. In addition, some herbs can be harmful if taken for too long a time. Get advice from your doctor and other reputable resources.

Tell your doctor what you're taking
Many people don't tell their doctors they take herbal remedies because they think their doctors will disapprove, they think it doesn't matter or the doctors don't ask. Tell your doctor what you're taking. Some herbs can interfere with the action of prescription or over-the-counter drugs or have other harmful effects. In addition, if you're taking an herbal preparation to treat a symptom, the symptom could signal that you have an underlying medical condition that requires treatment.

Keep track of what you take
Keep a record of what you take, the dosage and how it makes you feel. Note any side effects, such as drowsiness, sleeplessness, headaches or nausea.

Check where it's manufactured
Some herbal supplements manufactured in China, India and other countries have contained toxic ingredients — including lead, mercury and arsenic — and prescription drugs, such as prednisone.

Avoid herbs considered harmful
Herbs the FDA has determined to be harmful include belladonna, scotch broom, comfrey, lobelia and pennyroyal. Goldenseal and ephedra also are controversial herbs that can cause serious side effects. And kava, an herb used to treat anxiety, reportedly has been associated with liver damage in some people. Overdoses of any of these herbs can be fatal. But avoiding these herbs isn't the only thing you need to do to stay safe. Keep in mind that any herb — even ones deemed safe — can be dangerous if used incorrectly.

Avoid herbs if you're pregnant or breast-feeding
Herbal preparations may harm your baby or cause you to miscarry. Avoid them if you're pregnant or breast-feeding.

10 popular herbs

People take herbs for a host of reasons. Here's a look at some of the most popular ones, what they claim to do and what the research says about them.

Black cohosh (Cimicifuga racemosa)
With some effects similar to the female hormone estrogen, black cohosh is used to relieve menstrual cramps, painful periods and hot flashes, anxiety and depression associated with menopause.

Some research suggests that black cohosh may improve menopausal symptoms, but there isn't enough evidence to make a definitive recommendation. Study results are mixed, with some trials finding encouraging results, and others failing to return promising data.

Echinacea (Echinacea purpurea, Echinacea pallida)
Derived from the purple coneflower, echinacea is used to prevent colds and the flu. However, studies show that while echinacea may possibly shorten the duration of colds and the flu, it likely doesn't keep you from getting them.

Some researchers have raised concerns about the potential of this herb to be toxic to the liver. Don't take it for more than eight weeks at a time. Echinacea affects your immune system, so some medical professionals advise against its use if you have diabetes, or an autoimmune disease such as multiple sclerosis, lupus or rheumatoid arthritis.

Garlic (Allium sativum)
Some people believe that garlic can lower cholesterol and blood

pressure and keep blood clots from forming. Studies suggest that garlic and garlic supplements may help lower low-density lipoprotein (LDL, or "bad") cholesterol, and contribute to heart health. The supplements appear to be of low risk, except in individuals taking certain medications.

If you take garlic tablets, make sure they contain allicin, garlic's active ingredient. Odor-free preparations may not include allicin.

Garlic is supposedly more effective if eaten raw and in large amounts — five or more cloves a day. But eating that much can irritate your stomach, not to mention affect your breath and body odor.

Because garlic can have blood-thinning properties, don't use it if you're taking anti-clotting drugs such as warfarin (Coumadin). And before combining garlic with a daily dose of aspirin, talk to your doctor.

Ginger (*Zingiber officinale*)

The root of the ginger plant is used to relieve nausea and indigestion. Studies show it may be effective for preventing nausea associated with motion sickness and pregnancy. Ginger is generally considered safe when taken in small amounts and for a short time. High doses can cause abdominal discomfort.

A limited number of studies suggest that ginger may help ease nausea from pregnancy when used for short periods. However, talk to your doctor before taking ginger if you're pregnant.

The benefits of ginger for treating nausea following anesthesia or chemotherapy are unclear.

Ginkgo (*Ginkgo biloba*)

Ginkgo is used to increase blood flow to the brain in an effort to ease symptoms such as short-term memory loss, dizziness, ringing in the ears and headaches. It's also taken to treat activity-related leg pain caused by poor circulation in the legs (claudication). Evidence shows that ginkgo has a mild positive effect on claudication and on memory, and it's being studied to determine whether it can slow the progression of Alzheimer's disease. But more research on the herb is needed. Don't use ginkgo if you're taking anti-clotting medication or a thiazide diuretic.

Ginseng (*Panax ginseng, Panax quinquefolius*)

Some people use ginseng to boost mood, increase sexual stamina, treat heart disease and improve exercise performance. Evidence suggests that short-term use of ginseng may improve mental performance. And Mayo Clinic research shows that American ginseng can help relieve cancer-related fatigue. It produces few side effects when taken as directed.

Don't use ginseng for more than six months or exceed the recommended maximum dose. Also, Asian ginseng may affect blood sugar and blood pressure. If you have diabetes or high blood pressure, talk to your doctor before using Asian ginseng.

St. John's wort (*Hypericum perforatum*)

St. John's wort is used to treat mild to moderate depression. Some studies suggest that St. John's wort may work as well as some antidepressant drugs for mild depression, and with fewer side effects. It hasn't been shown to be effective in treating major depression.

A major concern is that the herb can dangerously alter the effects of a number of prescription drugs, including other antidepressants, birth control pills, anticoagulant drugs, certain asthma medications and steroids. Until more is known, a good rule of thumb is to not mix St. John's wort with any medication. It's also important to talk with your doctor before taking St. John's wort.

Saw palmetto (*Serenoa repens*)

Some research indicates that saw palmetto may improve urine flow and bladder emptying in men with noncancerous enlargement of the prostate gland (benign prostatic hyperplasia). More research is needed to determine the herb's

Too Good to Be True?

The Food and Drug Administration recommends that you watch for the following claims or practices, which can be warning signs of potentially fraudulent products or treatments:

- The advertisements or promotional materials include words such as *breakthrough, magical* or *new discovery*. If the product were in fact a cure, then it would be widely reported in the media, and your doctor would recommend it.
- The promotional materials include pseudomedical jargon such as *detoxify, purify* or *energize*. Such claims are difficult to define and measure.
- The manufacturer claims that the product can treat a wide range of symptoms or cure or prevent a number of diseases. No single product can do that.
- The product is supposedly backed by scientific studies, but the references aren't provided or they're limited or outdated.
- The product promotion mentions no negative effects, only benefits.
- The manufacturer of the product accuses the government or medical profession of suppressing important information about the product's health benefits. There's no reason for the government or medical profession to withhold information that could help people.

effectiveness. However, saw palmetto is generally safe when used as directed, and side effects are rare.

Turmeric (*Curcuma longa*)

While turmeric has been used for thousands of years in India and Asia, little scientific study has been conducted on its use for health conditions. Some studies suggest that turmeric — and, more specifically, a chemical found in turmeric called curcumin — may be effective for pain, inflammation, high cholesterol and other conditions, but more research is necessary.

For most adults, turmeric is safe to use. Side effects are usually mild, though high doses or long-term use may cause indigestion, nausea or diarrhea. Ask your doctor about taking turmeric if you have gallbladder disease (since it may worsen the condition) or if you take an anticoagulant medication, such as warfarin (since turmeric may increase the risk of bleeding).

Valerian (*Valeriana officinalis*)

Valerian is a tall, flowering grassland plant that has long been used to treat insomnia and anxiety. Products such as teas are made from the plant's roots.

Results from several small or short-term studies indicate that valerian may help you fall asleep and may improve sleep quality. Valerian may also reduce the symptoms of anxiety, but this requires further research. Don't take valerian for more than a few weeks at a time.

Manipulation and Touch

If you've ever had a massage, not to mention a hug from a friend or loved one, then you know how comforting human touch can be. Touch and manipulation of body tissues are at the core of several complementary and alternative treatments. These treatments are sometimes referred to as hands-on therapies.

Spinal manipulation

Spinal manipulation is based on the premise that health and disease are directly related to the functioning of the body's neuro-musculoskeletal system, and with proper alignment of your bones, joints, muscles and associated nerves come health and healing.

Spinal manipulation — sometimes called spinal adjustment — is practiced by chiropractors, doctors of osteopathic medicine and physical therapists. It's been shown to be effective in treating certain musculoskeletal conditions. Studies have found spinal manipulation to be an effective treatment for uncomplicated low back pain, especially if it has been present for less than four weeks. For this condition, short-term use of spinal manipulation has become an accepted practice and is no longer considered alternative. But there's little evidence

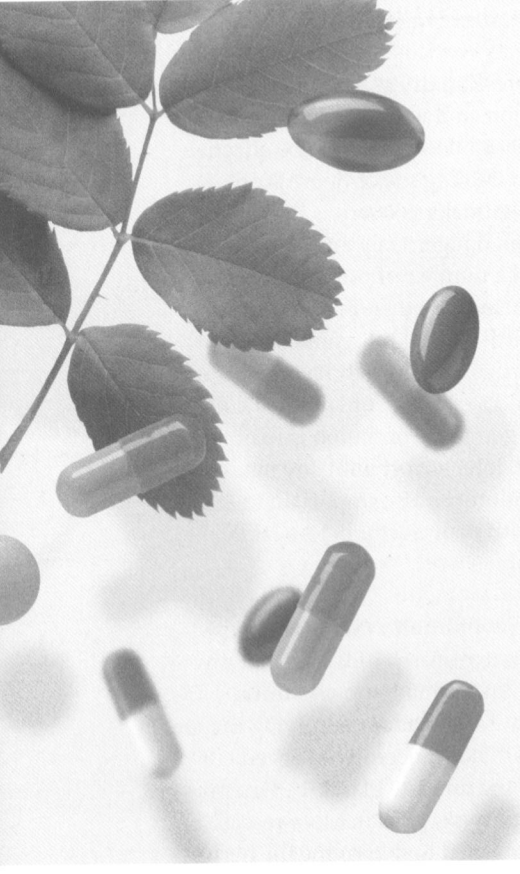

Avoiding Dangerous Interactions

Some herbal supplements contain ingredients that may not be taken safely with prescription or over-the-counter medications. Certain medical problems also may increase your risk of adverse effects from taking herbal products.

Talk to your doctor before taking any herbal products, especially if you're pregnant or nursing or if you regularly take prescription or over-the-counter medications.

Also talk to your doctor about herbal supplements if you have any of the following conditions:

- High blood pressure
- A history of stroke
- Blood-clotting problems
- Thyroid problems
- Diabetes
- Cardiovascular disease
- Epilepsy
- Glaucoma
- An enlarged prostate gland
- Human immunodeficiency virus (HIV), AIDS or other diseases of the immune system
- Depression or other psychiatric problems

Some herbal supplements also can be dangerous when combined with anesthesia. If you're having surgery, tell your doctor about any medications, including herbal supplements, that you're taking. Stop taking herbal supplements at least two to three weeks before surgery to allow them to clear from your body. If this isn't possible, then bring the herbal product in its original container to the hospital so that the anesthesiologist knows what you're taking.

About Chiropractic Treatment

Chiropractic treatment is based on the concept that restricted movement in the spine may lead to pain and reduced function. Spinal adjustment (manipulation) is one form of therapy chiropractors use to treat restricted spinal mobility. During an adjustment, chiropractors use their hands to apply a controlled, sudden force to a joint. This maneuver often results in a cracking sound made by the separation of the joint surfaces — not, as many people think, by "cracking joints." Chiropractors may also use massage and stretching to relax muscles that are shortened or in spasm. Many use other treatments as well, such as exercise, ultrasound and electrical muscle stimulation.

When limited to low back pain, chiropractic adjustment has few risks. However, manipulation of the neck has been associated with injury to the blood vessels supplying the brain. Rarely, neck manipulation may cause a stroke.

With increasing interest in integrative medicine, it's becoming more common to see chiropractors practicing alongside other medical providers. As with any medical specialist, select a chiropractor who's willing to work with other members of your health care team. And make sure you're comfortable with your chiropractor's recommendations.

that long-term treatment is more effective than other therapies.

Studies also suggest spinal manipulation may be effective for headaches and other spine-related conditions, such as neck pain. There's no evidence, though, to support the belief by some that spinal manipulation can cure whatever ails you.

Spinal manipulation is generally considered to be safe, but it's not appropriate if you have osteoporosis or symptoms of nerve damage, such as numbness, tingling or loss of strength in a limb, hand or foot. In addition, be cautious about spinal manipulation if you:

- Have a history of spinal surgery. Check with your surgeon before treatment.
- Have had a stroke related to vascular disease of neck arteries.
- Have back pain accompanied by fever, chills, sweats or unintentional weight loss. See a doctor to rule out the possibility of an infection or tumor.

Massage

You might think of massage as a luxury found in exotic spas and upscale health clubs. You may not know that massage — when combined with traditional medical treatments — is used to reduce stress and promote healing in people with certain health conditions.

Massage involves manipulation of your body's soft tissues — your skin, muscles and tendons. The type of manipulation — including its rhythm, intensity, rate and direction — varies with the type of massage, from the traditional kneading and rubbing in Swedish massage to the use of pressure at acupuncture points in shiatsu massage.

Almost everyone feels better after a massage. Massage has been shown to help relieve pain and soreness and reduce anxiety. Massage can also cause your body to release natural painkillers, and it may boost your immune system.

Mayo Clinic has conducted several studies on the most effective uses of massage therapy. Researchers have found that massage helps reduce pain and decrease anxiety in people undergoing certain types of surgery and procedures. As a result of this research, all patients at Mayo Clinic can

choose to include massage therapy as part of their hospital care.

If a massage causes discomfort, immediately inform the person who's performing it. If you've been injured, consult your doctor before getting a massage. While generally safe, there are some instances in which a massage may not be recommended. These include having conditions such as burns or open wounds, a recent heart attack, deep vein thrombosis, unhealed fractures, and severe osteoporosis.

Reflexology

The theory behind reflexology is that specific areas on the soles of your feet correspond to other parts of your body — such as your head or neck or your internal organs.

Reflexologists apply varying amounts of manual pressure to specific areas of the feet in an effort to influence a problem elsewhere in the body. The practice is sometimes combined with other hands-on therapies and may be offered by chiropractors or physical therapists.

There's little risk involved, and massaging the soles of your feet can feel good. While reflexology may promote relaxation, there's not much evidence to indicate it can treat disease.

Mind-Body Interventions

Your mind and body are inextricably linked, so your thoughts and emotions affect your body. That's the premise behind mind-body interventions.

Traditional medicine has long concentrated on the biology of the body and brain. But that's changing. Over the past few decades, researchers and doctors have focused more attention on the effects the mind has on the body, particularly for diseases that appear to be brought on or exacerbated by stress, such as cancer, heart disease and asthma.

Practitioners of mind-body therapies believe that negative thoughts and feelings may produce bodily symptoms. They use a number of relaxation techniques aimed at calming the mind.

Biofeedback

Biofeedback teaches you to control your body's functions, such as your heart rate. It's been shown to be effective in helping treat many medical conditions, as well as promote relaxation and relieve stress.

With biofeedback, you're connected to electrical sensors that help you receive information about your body. This feedback helps you focus on making subtle changes in your body, such as relaxing certain muscles, to achieve the results you want, such as reducing tension or relieving pain.

You can receive biofeedback training in physical therapy clinics, medical centers and hospitals, but biofeedback devices and programs are available for use at home, as well. Some of these are hand-held portable devices, while others connect to your computer.

Researchers have found that biofeedback helps control your rate of breathing and improve your focus on positive emotion. They have found that biofeedback is helpful for managing stress in many ways.

If you're interested in trying biofeedback to help manage stress, HeartMath or Relaxing Rhythms are two biofeedback tools you can try on your own.

Progressive muscle relaxation

Progressive muscle relaxation is designed to reduce the tension in your muscles. It's easy to do and can be practiced just about anywhere.

Progressive muscle relaxation offers a way to reduce stress and clear the mind within just a few minutes. You can use it after a difficult meeting, or to unwind at the end of the day. You can practice muscle relaxation by itself or combine it with another mind-body approach, such as meditation.

Studies suggest that progressive muscle relaxation is helpful in the treatment of anxiety and stress, headaches and high blood pressure.

To perform progressive muscle relaxation, first find a quiet place where you can sit or lie down. Then, loosen any tight clothing and get comfortable. Beginning with your feet and working up through your body to your head and neck, tense each muscle group to the count of eight and then relax the muscles for up to 30 seconds. Repeat before moving to the next muscle group.

Hypnotherapy

Hypnotherapy is a technique that induces a state of deep relaxation while keeping your mind alert and open to suggestion. No one knows for sure how it works, but experts believe it alters your brain-wave patterns in much the same way as do other relaxation techniques.

Some individuals are more susceptible to hypnotism than are others. Whether hypnotherapy can work for you depends on the expertise of the practitioner and your desire to cooperate. If you're using hypnotherapy to give up a bad habit, such as smoking or taking drugs, then you need to be strongly motivated to change for it to help.

Hypnotherapy may help relieve pain associated with a number of disorders, including cancer. It is also used in treating many behavioral problems. In addition, it may be used to reduce anxiety before a medical or dental procedure.

Hypnotherapy can be an effective method for coping with stress and anxiety. In particular,

---

Finding a Yoga Class and Teacher

If you decide to give yoga a try, your best bet is to learn in a class. But first you have to pick the style that's right for you. Basic hatha yoga is a gentle form that combines breathing techniques with a series of postures, called asanas.

Here's a rundown of variations of hatha yoga:

- *Iyengar yoga* is the most widely practiced type of yoga in the Western world. Focused on alignment, this style of yoga often includes breathing techniques. Postures can be matched to fitness level and ability.
- *Ashtanga yoga* — often known as power yoga — teaches asanas connected in a flowing, coordinated series combined with deep, rhythmic breathing. It also offers aerobic benefits.
- *Bikram yoga* is a system of 26 poses performed in the same sequence every time. It's designed to warm and stretch your muscles, ligaments and tendons, as well as rid the body of toxins through sweat.
- *Kripalu yoga* places minimal stress on your joints, so it's less strenuous than other forms of yoga. It stretches muscles and improves flexibility, while also helping reduce stress.

Yoga classes are generally easy to find in larger cities. Check with local health clubs, YMCAs, YWCAs, churches and community education centers.

There's no certification for yoga instructors, so look for one with a serious interest in yoga who has studied and practiced for years. Observe the class before you sign up to make sure it's right for you.

it can reduce stress and anxiety before a medical procedure, such as a breast biopsy. It has also been studied for many other conditions, including pain associated with cancer, irritable bowel syndrome, fibromyalgia, temporomandibular joint (TMJ) problems, dental procedures and headaches; symptoms of hot flashes associated with menopause. Hypnotherapy is also used to treat insomnia and bet-wetting; aid in smoking cessation; and help people lose weight and overcome phobias.

Be sure you carefully choose a therapist or health care professional to perform hypnotherapy. Get a recommendation from someone you trust. Learn as much as you can about any therapist you're considering.

Yoga

Yoga is an ancient practice that aims to induce physical, mental and spiritual well-being through a combination of postures (asanas), breathing techniques and meditation. It's increasingly popular among people seeking relaxation, a spiritual path or improvements in flexibility, coordination, balance, strength and endurance.

According to current research, yoga may help reduce low back pain, lessen stress, lower blood pressure, and help relieve anxiety, stress, depression and insomnia. It can also help improve overall physical fitness, strength and flexibility. Yoga has even been shown to potentially help pregnant women during labor.

At the very least, yoga can relax you, and some forms may improve your physical conditioning. If you find an experienced instructor who adapts postures to your levels of flexibility, yoga is likely to help you and unlikely to be harmful. But yoga isn't easy. It requires discipline and concentration.

Meditation

Spending time each day trying to quiet your mind with meditation can help you relax, slow your breathing and heart rate, and decrease muscle tension.

Meditation can lessen your body's response to the chemicals it produces when you're stressed, such as adrenaline, which can raise your blood pressure and make your blood more likely to clot — both of which raise your risk of heart disease.

Meditation helps you enter a deeply restful state in which you become very relaxed. The relaxation can help you manage pain and reduce stress and anxiety.

During meditation, you sit still and make an effort to focus on a single thing, such as a particular word, phrase or sound. When your thoughts wander — as they inevitably do — you bring your focus back to where it was.

How to Meditate

You don't have to twist your legs into a pretzel or spend your life at an ashram to learn to meditate. All you need to do is find a quiet place where you won't be disturbed. Sit or lie in a comfortable position and determine a focus for your mind. Here are a few to consider:

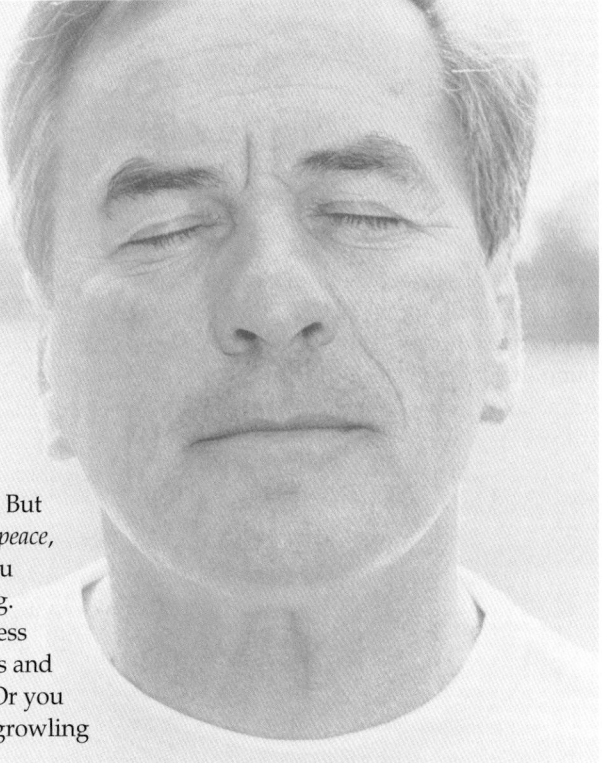

- *Focus on your breath.* Breathe in and out through your nose and pay attention to some aspect of your breathing, such as the pause between breaths or the sensation of air leaving your nostrils.
- *Focus on a word, phrase or prayer.* In Transcendental Meditation you mentally repeat a mantra, usually a Sanskrit word or sound assigned by your instructor. But you can choose your own mantra, such as the word *peace*, or you can count from one to four over and over. You can also coordinate your mantra with your breathing.
- *Focus on the moment.* This is also known as mindfulness meditation. You become aware of sensations, sounds and thoughts. You simply notice them and let them go. Or you may notice the sensations in your body — stomach growling or thigh cramping.

Many people meditate with their eyes closed. Others prefer to keep their eyes partially open with a soft focus. It doesn't matter whether you lie down or sit on the floor, a chair, a meditation cushion or a bench, as long as you're comfortable. But keep your spine straight and don't get so comfortable that you fall asleep. Start with five-minute meditation sessions once or twice a day and work up to 20-minute sessions.

A related practice is called guided imagery, in which someone's voice — whether taped or live — directs you through a visualization exercise. Once you reach a state of deep relaxation — most likely through meditation — you conjure up a visual image of whatever the person directing the exercise suggests. Perhaps it's a peaceful place, such as in a colorful garden or on a sandy beach, where you feel calm and safe. If you have an illness, you may be asked to visualize healthy cells attacking the disease.

Brain studies show that visualizing or imagining something stimulates the same parts of your brain that are stimulated during the actual experience. If sitting by the ocean relaxes you, you may achieve the same level of relaxation by visualizing yourself by the ocean.

Various types of meditation are used to treat anxiety and stress. Meditation is also used to help reduce high blood pressure and improve symptoms of fibromyalgia. For most conditions, better research is needed to produce more conclusive results about the possible benefits of meditation. However, the practice is considered safe.

Natural Energy Restoration

Natural energy techniques are based on the idea that the energy that flows through your body, or the field of energy that supposedly surrounds your body, can be disturbed or blocked and needs to be restored. Although many of the mind-body practices are based on the same premise, these energy-based techniques differ greatly from one another.

Acupuncture Tips

If you seek acupuncture, here's what you can expect:

- From 1 to 20 or more hair-thin needles are inserted under your skin.
- How deeply the needles are inserted depends on where they're placed in your body and what the treatment is for. Others are placed superficially.
- The needles usually are left in for 15 to 30 minutes.
- You should feel little or no pain from insertion. Significant pain is a sign that the procedure is being done improperly.
- Once inserted, the needles may be moved gently by hand or stimulated with an electrical current or heat.
- You'll probably have several sessions. You may not get relief from the first one, but if nothing's happening after six or eight sessions, then acupuncture probably isn't for you.
- If you feel some relief, give it a chance to work. It could take months to alleviate your pain.

There should be little or no pain from the insertion of the needles. Some people even find it relaxing.

Benefits of Focused Attention

Focused attention is an important part of meditation. At Mayo Clinic, focused attention is a skill taught in the Stress Management and Resiliency Training (SMART) program. Participants in the program learn how to train their attention so that they're more able to focus on the present moment.

The program has been tested in more than 20 completed research studies in and outside of Mayo Clinic, with the results showing a decrease in stress and anxiety and an improvement in positive health behaviors. Researchers have found that the skills taught in this program reduce stress and anxiety and increase well-being, resilience, self-regulation, mindfulness, happiness, and positive health behavior.

Acupuncture

A component of Chinese traditional medicine, acupuncture has existed for at least 2,500 years. The Eastern philosophy behind it is that health depends on a vital energy called *qi* (pronounced CHEE) that flows through your body along pathways called meridians. According to this ancient theory, if your qi is out of balance, you develop pain and disease. Inserting needles into specific points along the meridians unblocks the energy flow and restores your body's healthy balance.

Acupuncture has been used at Mayo Clinic since the mid-1990s in a variety of treatment settings. When performed properly by trained practitioners, acupuncture has proved to be an effective therapy for:

- *Pain,* including chronic neck pain, chronic and acute low-back pain, knee pain, dental pain, osteoarthritis, labor pain, menstrual cramps, and headaches.
- *Nausea and vomiting* in people who are receiving chemotherapy. And although it isn't completely proved, some women find that acupuncture helps relieve morning sickness during pregnancy.

Acupuncture is not suitable for everyone. You may be at risk of complications if you have a bleeding disorder, have a pacemaker or are pregnant.

The risks of acupuncture are low if you're working with a competent, certified acupuncture practitioner. The most common possible side effects include soreness or minor bleeding or bruising where the needles were inserted.

Tai chi

An ancient Chinese tradition, tai chi is based on a series of slow, flowing movements that resemble a dance. It's designed to foster the free flow of energy that practitioners believe is necessary for good health.

Today's practitioners use tai chi to gain emotional and physical balance, reduce stress, and strengthen muscles and joints. Because it can help you feel both alert and tranquil, some people use it as a form of moving meditation.

Tai chi comprises hundreds of combinations of continuous movements that require concentration, balance and grace. When combined with deep, rhythmic breathing, these movements can increase your circulation, relax your mind and body, and ease chronic pain. Practicing tai chi has also been shown to improve balance, reducing the risk of falling.

Healing touch

Advocates of therapeutic touch subscribe to the notion that your body is its own form of energy, surrounded by a field of energy. Disturbances to the surrounding energy field can lead to illness.

Some practitioners of therapeutic touch move their hands over a person's body in the belief that they can get rid of the disturbance and transfer healing energy from their hands to the individual who's ill. The benefits of therapeutic touch aren't supported by solid research.

Complete Medical Systems

Some practices derive from whole systems that combine treatments. They tend to take a variety of approaches to healing.

Homeopathy

Developed in Germany more than 200 years ago, homeopathy is a controversial treatment based on two beliefs — the law of similars and the law of infinitesimals.

Law of similars
The law of similars is the idea that any substance — plant, animal or mineral — that can produce certain symptoms in a healthy person can, when given in very small doses, cure similar symptoms that occur in an ill person.

Law of infinitesimals
The word *infinitesimal* means "too small to be measured." Homeopathy claims that the more dilute a substance, as long as it has been prepared by a series of shakings called succession, the more potent the medicine. This idea is called the law of infinitesimals.

Many practitioners of conventional medicine dismiss homeopathy as ineffective. Conventional doctors generally find it difficult to believe that homeopathic substances, which often are diluted in distilled water or alcohol to the point where there may be no active molecules left, could be beneficial.

Rigorous clinical trials and systematic analyses of research on homeopathy show that there's little evidence to support the idea that homeopathy can effectively treat any specific condition. Most doctors remain skeptical of both the studies and practice of homeopathy.

Ayurveda

Ayurveda is one of the oldest systems of medicine still practiced today. Hindu in origin, *ayurveda* means "the science of life." It begins with the premise that people differ from one another physically and psychologically, so treatments must take those differences into account.

According to ayurveda, people are made up of three types of energy (doshas). In most people one dosha is dominant. The different combinations of doshas create different metabolic types. Each dosha represents a pair of elements.

- *Vata.* The vata dosha controls movement and essential body processes such as cell division, the heart, breathing and the mind. It can be thrown off balance by things such as staying up late at night.
- *Pitta.* The pitta dosha is believed to control the body's hormones and digestive system. When it's out of balance, a person may experience negative emotions or digestive symptoms.
- *Kapha.* The kapha dosha is thought to help maintain strength and immunity and control growth. People with kapha as their main dosha are thought to be vulnerable to diabetes, cancer, obesity and respiratory illnesses, such as asthma.

According to ayurveda theory, when the energies get out of balance, such as through diet or stress, illness results. Ayurveda is best known for prevention of illness by promoting balance through nutrition, exercise, herbs, meditation and other treatments.

Naturopathy

Based on their belief in the healing power of nature, early naturopaths recommended soaking in hot springs, walking barefoot through streams and using other water-related activities to treat illness and maintain good health.

Today's naturopaths employ a combination of therapies, including nutrition, herbs, acupuncture and massage. They also use techniques from homeopathy, ayurveda, Chinese medicine and conventional treatments.

The main emphasis of naturopathy is on prevention of illness through a healthy lifestyle, including fresh air, clean water and exercise. ■

Is Integrative Medicine Right for You?

When considering integrative treatments, it's important to keep an open, albeit skeptical, mind. Steer a middle course between uncritical acceptance and outright rejection. Do your homework. Seek out trusted and credible information by using the tips you read about earlier in this chapter.

After you've done your homework, take the next step. Together with your health care team, discuss the information you've found, talk about your health history, and decide if the therapy makes sense and is safe for you.

During the conversation with your doctor, be honest. Answer his or her questions truthfully so that he or she can accurately monitor your health, assess any potential health risks and get you off to a good start. As part of your discussion, your doctor can:

- Inform you if a treatment has potentially dangerous side effects
- Tell you if a product may interact with a medication you use
- Help you determine the correct dosage
- Confirm that the therapy seems appropriate for you and your needs
- Put you in touch with someone who performs the therapy

you're interested in, or who can teach you how to do it

When seeking out an integrative health practitioner, be as thorough as you were when searching for your primary care physician. Take these steps:

- Check with your health care team for recommendations
- Learn as much as you can about a practitioner's education, training, licensing and certifications
- Choose a practitioner who will work with your health care team
- Find out if the practitioner's training and experience align with your goals for treatment

Some integrative treatments are less expensive than conventional health care. Others are very costly. Most integrative therapies aren't covered by health insurance. Find out what the treatment you're considering will cost you. Get it in writing, if possible. Then check with your insurance company to see if it's covered.

Finally, work in partnership with everyone on your health care team — conventional and integrative practitioners. Take responsibility for your own health by keeping up with health information and making healthy choices. Eating well, exercising, not smoking, managing stress and taking safety precautions — such as using your car's seat belt — will go a long way toward helping you live a longer, healthier life.

Glossary

The language of medicine is rich with specialized words. This wealth of vocabulary is a mixed blessing. Your doctor can use precise terminology to describe conditions, signs and symptoms to you and his or her colleagues, yet in some cases that same terminology can be confusing, worrisome or incomprehensible to the uninitiated listener.

Whenever possible, we've tried to use language familiar to the layperson to enhance the readability and utility of this book. In most cases, when a medical term is introduced, we define it, give the common term for it and put the medical term in parentheses. This glossary includes many of those terms, along with a wide range of other commonly used medical terms.

Given the limitations of space, this glossary doesn't include most of the conditions discussed in the book. Those are defined in entries devoted to them in the text and can be found by using the index. In addition, you can find testing procedures in Chapter 35, "Tests and Procedures" and drug terms in Chapter 36, "Medications Guide."

A

ablation. Elimination or removal.

abrasion. An area rubbed bare of skin or mucous membrane. Or, the normal wear of tooth enamel by chewing.

abscess. A localized formation of pus in a cavity, caused by the disintegration or displacement of tissue due to bacterial infection.

acetylcholine (ACh). A chemical in the body that carries electric messages between nerves and muscles; a neurotransmitter.

acuity. The sharpness or clarity with which you can see something. Someone with normal visual acuity is said to have 20/20 vision, which means that he or she can see objects clearly from 20 feet away that most people with normal sight are able to see clearly from 20 feet away.

acute. A term used to describe disorders, signs or symptoms that occur abruptly or that run a short course; the opposite of chronic.

addiction. Physical or emotional dependence on a substance — most often alcohol or another drug. Usually causes the user to require increasing amounts of the substance to achieve the same effect.

adenocarcinoma. A form of cancer arising from glands or glandular tissue.

adhesion. Tissue joining two surfaces, as in a healing wound.

adjunct therapy. Additional therapy used in the treatment of cancers. If surgical removal of the tumor is the primary therapy, then chemotherapy or radiation therapy is considered adjunct therapy.

adrenal glands. Endocrine glands that produce a range of hormones, including adrenaline (epinephrine), norepinephrine and corticosteroids.

adrenaline. A naturally occurring hormone that increases heart rate and blood pressure and affects other body functions. Also called epinephrine.

advance directive. A legal document that specifies the types of medical care you do or don't want to receive if you lose mental capacity or are unable to communicate your wishes.

adventitia. The outer layer of an organ.

aerobic. Requiring the presence of oxygen. Aerobic exercise, for example, is performed at an intensity level that allows oxygen intake from breathing to keep up with the body's use of oxygen in the chemical reaction that releases energy in muscles. *See also* anaerobic.

afterbirth. The placenta and membranes discharged from the uterus after childbirth.

agnosia. Loss of ability to interpret stimuli, usually classified according to the sense or senses affected.

albumin. A protein found in animal and plant tissues. Its presence in the urine is one sign of kidney disease.

aldosterone. An adrenal hormone that affects the body's handling of sodium, chloride and potassium.

allergen. Any substance that produces an allergic reaction. Common allergens include cat dander, dust mites, pollen and certain foods.

allergic reaction. An exaggerated immune system response to an allergen. The reaction results from the release of histamine or histamine-like substances in affected cells. Sign and symptoms include rashes, nasal congestion, asthma and, occasionally, shock. *See also* histamine.

alveoli. Microscopic air sacs in the lungs where gases are exchanged. Or, tooth sockets.

ambulatory. Able to walk.

amino acid. A nitrogen-containing component of protein. The body produces many amino acids. Those it needs but can't synthesize are known as essential amino acids and must be obtained through the diet.

amnesia. Loss of memory.

amniotic fluid. The protective liquid surrounding the fetus in the womb.

amputation. The act of cutting off or removing a limb or other body part.

amylase. A digestive enzyme made by the pancreas and salivary glands.

anaerobic. Able to live without oxygen, as do certain bacteria. Or, exercise in which the activity level is vigorous enough that the body uses oxygen faster than it can take it in, limiting the length of time the activity can be continued. *See also* aerobic.

analgesic. An agent that reduces pain.

anaphylaxis. An immediate and sometimes life-threatening allergic hypersensitivity reaction. Signs and symptoms include shock, breathing difficulty, itching, hives, convulsions and coma. *See also* shock.

androgen. A hormone such as testosterone or androsterone that's responsible for the development and maintenance of masculine physical characteristics. Produced in the testicles in males. Also produced in small amounts in females.

anemia. A condition characterized by a reduced number of red blood cells or a reduced amount of hemoglobin or blood.

anesthesia. Partial or complete loss of feeling or sensation. May be brought about by various anesthetics. Sometimes accompanied by loss of consciousness. Local anesthesia is confined to a particular region of the body. General anesthesia affects the whole body.

anesthetics. Substances used to induce anesthesia.

aneurysm. The localized enlargement of a blood vessel, usually an artery, that forms a bulge or sac.

angina pectoris. Episodic pain in the chest caused by a temporary decrease in blood flow to the heart.

angioedema. Allergic swelling of mucous membranes, tissues beneath the skin or in an internal organ.

angiogram. An X-ray picture produced by angiography.

angiography. A method for taking X-ray images of blood vessels after injecting contrast dye into a blood vessel.

angioplasty. A procedure for dilating a narrowed or blocked part of a blood vessel.

annulus. The ring around a heart valve where the valve leaflet merges with the heart muscle.

anorexia nervosa. An eating disorder characterized by a lack of appetite for food and caused by an emotional disturbance. It most often affects females in their teens and 20s and can result in severe loss of weight and even death.

anosmia. Loss of the sense of smell.

anterior chamber. The space in the eye between the iris and cornea filled with a fluid called aqueous humor.

antibodies. Immune system proteins that counteract or eliminate foreign substances known as antigens.

anticoagulant. A medication that keeps blood from clotting. Also called a blood thinner.

antidote. A substance that neutralizes the effects of a poison.

anti-emetic. A medication that prevents or alleviates nausea and vomiting.

antigens. Substances foreign to the body that cause antibodies to form.

anus. The outlet of the rectum, through which fecal waste passes.

aorta. The largest artery in the body. It carries blood from the heart's left ventricle and distributes it throughout the body.

aortic valve. The valve between the left ventricle and aorta. A normal aortic valve has three leaflets.

Apgar score. A rating given to a newborn at one and five minutes after birth, based on skin color, heart rate, muscle tone, respiration and reflexes. Zero to 2 points is given for each sign. Scores close to 10, the highest rating, are desirable.

aphasia. Loss of ability to speak or to understand speech because of brain damage.

aplastic. Arrested development of tissue or an organ.

apnea, sleep. Temporary cessation of breathing during sleep.

aqueous humor. A clear fluid that fills the anterior chamber of the eye. It nourishes the cornea and lens and helps maintain the internal pressure of the eye.

areola. The circular, pigmented area around the nipple of the breast.

arrhythmia. An abnormal heartbeat.

arteriole. A tiny artery that joins a larger artery to a capillary.

arteriosclerosis. A condition in which the walls of arteries become hard and thick, sometimes interfering with blood circulation.

arteritis. Inflammation of arteries.

artery. A blood vessel that carries blood from the heart to other tissues of the body.

arthritis. Inflammation of a joint.

arthroplasty. Surgical replacement or repair of a joint.

ascites. The accumulation of fluid in the abdominal cavity.

asphyxia. Suffocation caused by insufficient oxygen intake.

aspiration. Removal of fluids by suction, as from the nose, throat or lungs. Or, the inhalation into the lungs of fluids, such as water in drowning and stomach contents in vomiting.

asthma. A condition characterized by narrowing of the bronchial tubes, causing wheezing, coughing and difficulty breathing.

astigmatism. A focusing problem that occurs when your cornea is not curved evenly in all directions. Typically, what you see is distorted more in one direction than in others.

asymptomatic. Without symptoms.

ataxia. Incoordination of voluntary muscle movements.

atherectomy. A method for shaving or removing, with a specially designed catheter, atherosclerotic plaques from inside arteries.

atherosclerosis. A condition in which plaques accumulate in the lining of the arteries, resulting in narrower, less flexible pathways for the blood.

atopic dermatitis. *See* eczema.

atresia. Congenital absence of an opening, duct or canal in the body, as in the intestines or esophagus.

atria. Cavities or chambers, such as the upper chambers of the heart, that receive blood from veins and pass it to the ventricles. Singular form is atrium.

atrioventricular. Involving both atria and ventricles.

atrioventricular block. A blocking of the electric signal between the atria and ventricles. Varies in severity from first, second to third degree (complete heart block).

atrioventricular (AV) node. A cluster of cells that slows the flow of electric signals as they pass from the atria to the ventricles.

atrophy. Shrinking (wasting) of tissue or an organ due to disease or lack of use.

aura. A sensation felt before the onset of a convulsion or migraine.

auscultation. The act of listening to the sounds of various organs.

autograft. A surgical operation in which one of your body parts is used to repair another part, as when a pulmonary valve replaces the aortic valve.

autoimmune disease. A disease that occurs when antibodies react against the body's own tissues.

autoimmune response. A reaction by the body to one or some of its own tissues it perceives as foreign substances, resulting in production of antibodies against those tissues.

autologous transfusion. A transfusion of one's own blood previously donated in anticipation of surgery.

autonomic nervous system. The portion of the nervous system that regulates involuntary body functions.

autopsy. An examination of tissues and organs of the body after death.

avulsion. Forced tearing away of a body part or structure, such as a limb or tooth.

B

bacteria. Single-celled microorganisms, some of which cause disease and some of which are beneficial to biological processes.

barrel chest. An altered shape of the chest cage, as seen in some people with emphysema.

basal cell carcinoma. The most common form of skin cancer, often associated with sun exposure. This tumor can be locally invasive but rarely spreads.

B cell. A type of lymphocyte that works as part of the immune system by producing antibodies to fight infection.

benign. Harmless, not progressive or recurrent, non-cancerous.

bile. Bitter-tasting fluid produced by the liver and temporarily stored in the gallbladder before discharge into the small intestine. Bile facilitates the digestion of fats in the small intestine.

bilirubin. Orange or yellowish pigment that's the result of the breakdown of red blood cells. Excess bilirubin in the blood produces jaundice.

biofeedback. A behavior-training program that teaches a person how to control autonomic reactions such as heart rate, blood pressure, skin temperature and muscular tension.

biopsy. To take a sample of tissue for laboratory examination.

birth defect. Any of various congenital disorders, from a minor cosmetic irregularity to a life-threatening disorder.

bladder. A membranous sac that holds secretions, most commonly the sac that collects urine before its elimination.

blepharitis. An inflammation along the edge of the eyelid that can cause irritation and itching.

blood pressure. The force placed on the inner walls of the arteries. *See also* diastole; systole.

bone marrow. Soft material found inside bone cavities where blood cells are formed.

bone marrow transplant. A procedure in which a person's bone marrow is destroyed by chemotherapy or radiation or both and replaced with either donated bone marrow or the person's own marrow that was collected and stored before chemotherapy or radiation.

bowel. The small or large intestine. The large intestine is sometimes called the colon.

bradycardia. A slow heartbeat.

brainstem. The portion of the brain that connects with the spinal cord. The stem consists of the medulla oblongata, pons and midbrain.

Braxton Hicks contractions. Irregular uterine contractions that occur during pregnancy. Sometimes, they're referred to as false labor.

breech presentation. Positioning of the fetus during labor with feet or buttocks toward the cervix.

bronchial tubes. The two main breathing tubes leading from the windpipe (trachea) to the lungs.

bronchiectasis. Abnormal enlargement of the bronchial tubes caused by chronic infection.

bronchiole. One of the subdivisions of a bronchial tube.

bronchitis. Inflammation of the bronchial tubes.

bronchodilator. Medicine used to open (dilate) the airways.

bronchogenic. Arising from a bronchial tube.

bronchoscopy. A procedure in which an instrument is passed into the airway to look at the lung structures or obtain specimens.

bruises. Injuries in which blood vessels are broken and blood escapes beneath the skin, producing a discolored area.

bruit. Sound produced by the flow of blood through a narrowed vessel.

bundle branch block. A condition in which portions of the heart's conduction system become defective and unable to conduct electric signals normally. You can have right or left bundle branch block.

bursa. A fluid-filled sac near or involving a joint or bony prominence that helps to reduce friction between a tendon and bone or between bone and skin.

bypass. *See* cardiopulmonary bypass; coronary artery bypass graft.

C

cachexia. Malnutrition and wasting due to chronic illness.

café au lait spots. Coffee-colored areas of pigmentation.

calcitonin. A hormone, produced by the thyroid gland, that affects the amount of calcium in the blood.

calcium. A mineral important for strong teeth and bones and for muscle and nerve function. Dairy products are good sources of calcium.

calculus. An accumulation of mineral salts in various parts of the body or on the teeth.

callus. An area of thickened skin.

calorie. The amount of heat needed to raise the temperature of 1 gram of water by 1 degree Celsius.

cancer. A group of diseases characterized by abnormal growth of cells, resulting in the formation of malignant tumors in various parts of the body. *See also* benign; malignant

candida. A species of yeastlike fungi.

canines. The four teeth situated between a premolar and an incisor. Also called cuspids.

capillaries. Minute blood vessels connecting the smallest arteries to the smallest veins.

caput succedaneum. Swelling of a baby's scalp during labor.

carbohydrates. Compounds composed of starches or sugars and found primarily in breads, cereals, fruits and vegetables.

carcinogens. Cancer-causing agents.

carcinoid tumor. A specific type of tumor that arises in the intestines or a bronchial tube. It typically produces a chemical called serotonin, which can cause flushing, low blood pressure and diarrhea.

carcinoma. A form of cancer made up of epithelial cells. Epithelial cells line body cavities, cover internal organs and line the internal portions of organs.

cardiac. Pertaining to the heart.

cardiac arrest. Sudden cessation of heartbeats.

cardiac catheterization. A procedure in which a catheter is introduced into a blood vessel and guided into the heart in order to measure blood flow and evaluate structural defects.

cardiac cycle. The period from the beginning of one heartbeat to the beginning of the next.

cardiac output. The amount of blood the heart pumps through the circulatory system in one minute.

cardiomyopathy. A heart muscle disease that impairs the ability of the heart to pump.

cardiopulmonary. Pertaining to the heart and lungs.

cardiopulmonary bypass. A method by which a machine takes over the function of the heart and lungs during heart surgery.

cardiopulmonary resuscitation (CPR). A technique for reviving a person whose heart and breathing have stopped.

cardiovascular. Pertaining to the heart and blood vessels.

cardiovascular system. The circulatory system, including the heart, arteries, veins and lymphatic system.

cardioversion. Electric shock applied to the chest to convert an abnormal heartbeat to normal.

caries. Decayed areas of tooth or bone due to bacteria. Also known as cavities.

carotid arteries. The principal arteries of the neck that carry blood to the head and brain.

carrier. One who carries and may transmit an infectious agent or genetic defect but doesn't experience the signs and symptoms of conditions caused by that agent or defect.

cartilage. Dense, fibrous connective tissue located throughout the body, including the joints, nose and ears.

catabolism. The breakdown of body tissues as a source of calories.

cataract. A clouding of the normally clear lens of the eye.

catheter. A small, flexible tube that's inserted into a body part to inject or remove liquid.

catheterization. A procedure in which a catheter is inserted into the body.

cc Cubic centimeter, a unit of volume measurement. Thirty cubic centimeters (30 cc) equals 1 ounce.

cephalhematoma. A bruised area beneath the outer layer of the skull, usually in a newborn.

cephalopelvic disproportion. A circumstance in which a baby's head is too large to pass through the mother's pelvis.

cerclage. A surgical procedure in which stitches (sutures) are made around the cervix in an attempt to prevent premature birth.

cerebellum. The portion of the brain responsible for balance and coordination.

cerebral embolism. A blood clot that travels through arteries from the site where it formed and blocks blood flow in the brain.

cerebral hemorrhage. Bleeding in the brain.

cerebral vascular accident. *See* stroke.

cerebrovascular. Pertaining to the blood vessels of the brain.

cerebrum. The largest portion of the brain, containing the two hemispheres. It's responsible for speech, memory, vision, personality and muscle control in certain parts of your body.

cervical cap. A contraceptive device that fits over the cervix to help prevent sperm from entering the uterus.

cervical incompetence. A condition in which the cervix begins to open before pregnancy has come to term, causing miscarriage or preterm labor.

cervix. The neck of an organ, such as the neck of the uterus.

cesarean section. Surgical removal of a baby from the womb through an incision in the abdomen and the wall of the uterus.

chalazion. A relatively painless swelling on the eyelid caused by blockage of a small oil gland.

chemotherapy. The use of medications that have a direct effect on a disease-causing organism or abnormal cells. Widely used in the treatment of cancer.

chloasma. A mild darkening of the facial skin. Often called the mask of pregnancy.

cholesterol. A fat-like substance synthesized in the liver and found in the blood, brain, liver and bile and as deposits in the walls of blood vessels. Found in foods of animal sources and thought to contribute to heart disease in people who eat large quantities of it over a long period of time.

chordae tendineae. Strong cords that stretch from the edges of the tricuspid and mitral valves to the heart muscle and restrict how far the valve leaflets swing when they close.

chorionic villus sampling. A procedure in which a small sample of cells is removed from the placenta where it joins the uterus. Used to test for chromosome abnormalities such as Down syndrome.

choroid. A thin layer of arteries and veins sandwiched between the retina and sclera of the eye. The choroid plays an important role in nourishing the retina.

chromosome. One of 46 rod-shaped structures in the nucleus of each cell. Carries hereditary information.

chronic. Referring to long-lasting diseases or conditions.

chyme. The mixture of partly digested food and digestive secretions found in the stomach.

cilia. The eyelashes. Or, smaller hairlike projections lining the bronchial tubes and upper respiratory tract.

circumcision. Removal of the foreskin from the penis.

claudication. Activity-induced muscle pain produced by inadequate arterial blood flow.

clinical. Pertaining to information gathered from working with people, as distinct from laboratory findings.

clinical trial. An experiment designed to test the effectiveness and possible side effects of a treatment in humans.

clitoris. The small, erectile organ of the external female genitals.

clot. Coagulated blood.

coagulate. To solidify or change from a liquid to a semisolid, as when blood clots.

coccyx. The tailbone.

cochlea. The snail-shaped tube of the inner ear that's the receptor for sound vibrations.

cognitive. Pertaining to the mental process of thought, including perception, reasoning, intuition and memory.

coitus. Sexual intercourse between a male and female in which the male inserts his penis into the female's vagina.

colic. Pain in the abdomen produced by intermittent spasms of the intestines. In infants it may be manifested by episodes of crying, a distended abdomen and legs drawn up to the chest.

collagen. Fibrous protein found in connective tissues such as skin, ligaments and cartilage.

collateral vessels. Small branches of arteries and veins that develop to bypass narrowed or blocked segments.

colon. The large intestine, extending from the end of the small intestine to the anus. It's responsible for extracting water from undigested food particles and storing the waste, which is eliminated in bowel movements.

colorectal. Pertaining to the colon and rectum.

colostomy. A surgical procedure in which a section of colon is pulled through an opening (stoma) created in the abdominal wall, allowing for the passage of stool into a small bag securely fastened over the opening.

colostrum. The thin, lemon-colored liquid produced by a mother's breasts in the first day or so after giving birth. Its antibodies are beneficial to the infant.

coma. An abnormal state of deep unconsciousness due to illness or accident.

compensatory pause. In the heart, a slight delay that occurs after a premature contraction before the next heartbeat.

complex carbohydrates. Substances, such as starch, composed of several sugars linked together.

computerized tomography (CT). An X-ray technique that uses a computer to construct images of the body.

conception. Fertilization of an egg (ovum) by a sperm.

concussion. A temporary disturbance of brain function due to a head injury.

condom. A sheath that fits over an erect penis to catch semen during ejaculation.

conduction system. Special muscle fibers that conduct electric impulses throughout the muscle of the heart.

cones. Light-sensitive cells of the retina that provide your central vision and allow you to see fine detail and color.

congenital. Present at birth. Usually used in reference to an abnormality.

congestion. The presence of excessive blood or fluid, such as mucus, in an organ or tissue.

congestive heart failure. A condition in which the heart is unable to pump enough blood to meet the needs of the body. Characterized by fluid collecting in parts of the body, such as the legs, lungs and liver. Also called heart failure.

conjunctiva. A thin, moist, clear membrane that covers the exposed front portion of the sclera and lines the inside of your eyelids.

conjunctivitis. An inflammation of the conjunctiva, giving your eye a reddish or pinkish coloration.

contraception. Measures taken to prevent pregnancy.

contraction. The shortening and thickening of a muscle fiber or a muscle in action.

contracture. Permanent tightness or shortening of a muscle due to disease or injury.

contrast agent. A liquid dye, opaque to X-rays, that's taken into the gastrointestinal tract or injected into a blood vessel or the fluid-filled space around the spinal cord to permit X-ray visualization of structures of the body that couldn't otherwise be seen by X-ray.

contusions. Bruises.

convulsion. A sudden attack commonly characterized by a loss of consciousness and severe, sustained, rhythmic contractions of some or all voluntary muscles. Convulsions are most often a manifestation of a seizure disorder (epilepsy).

cord compression. A condition that prevents proper blood flow through the umbilical cord. Or, pressure on the spinal cord.

cornea. A domed layer of clear tissue at the front of the eye. It helps focus light entering the eye.

coronary. Pertaining to arteries that supply blood to the heart muscle.

coronary angiography. A diagnostic test in which dye is injected into a coronary artery and then an X-ray is taken to detect disease or blockage.

coronary arteries. The arteries that supply blood to the heart muscle.

coronary artery bypass graft. An operation that reroutes the blood supply by bypassing blocked or narrowed coronary arteries.

coronary artery disease. Narrowing or blockage of one or more of the coronary arteries, resulting in decreased blood supply (ischemia) to the heart muscle.

coronary insufficiency. An inability of the coronary arteries to provide enough oxygen to meet the needs of the heart muscle.

coronary occlusion. An obstruction in a coronary artery, interrupting blood flow to the heart muscle.

coronary sinus. The main vein that drains blood into the right atrium from the heart muscle.

corpus luteum. A small, hormone-producing structure that develops in the ovary where an egg had previously matured (the empty follicle).

corticosteroids. Hormones produced by the cortex of the adrenal glands. Or, a class of such hormones used as medications.

cortisol. A hormone produced by the adrenal glands.

cranium. The portion of the skull that houses the brain.

creatinine. A substance excreted in urine that's measured to help evaluate kidney function.

crowning. The appearance of the top of a baby's head at the vaginal opening during labor.

curettage. Scraping of a cavity, such as the uterus.

cusp. A segment of a heart valve.

cyanosis. Bluish discoloration of the skin due to a lack of oxygen in the blood.

cyanotic heart disease. Birth defects of the heart that permit oxygen-depleted (blue) blood to circulate in the body without passing through the lungs.

cyst. A closed sac or cavity filled with a fluid, gas or semisolid substance.

cystic fibrosis. A genetic disorder affecting the respiratory and digestive systems. Most commonly found among whites of Northern European descent.

cystitis. An inflammation of the urinary bladder, usually from a bacterial infection.

cystoscopy. A procedure in which a small instrument (cystoscope) is passed through the urethra to allow for direct examination of the urethra, bladder and, in men, prostate gland.

cytology. The study of cells, often used to identify the presence of cancer.

D

debility. A state of physical weakness.

debulking. The surgical removal of the major portion of a tumor mass when a tumor can't be completely removed.

decubitus ulcer. An open sore that forms in the skin because of prolonged pressure. Also called a bedsore.

deep vein thrombosis. A blood clot in the deep veins of the leg.

defibrillation. Electric shock applied to the heart to return an irregular heartbeat to normal.

dehydration. The result of excessive loss of body fluids or inadequate fluid consumption.

delirium. A state of mental confusion, sometimes characterized by disordered speech and often accompanied by hallucinations.

delusion. A firmly held belief with no basis in reality.

dementia. Mental deterioration due to organic causes.

dentin. The tissue of a tooth beneath the enamel and enclosing the pulp cavity.

deoxyribonucleic acid (DNA). A substance found in the nucleus of cells that carries hereditary information.

depression. A feeling of extreme sadness and discouragement. Signs and symptoms include disruption of sleeping and eating patterns and lack of energy.

dermatitis. Inflammation of the skin, often characterized by itching and redness.

dermatochalasis. An age-related drooping of the eyelid skin. The upper eyelid may sag over your eyelashes and interfere with your vision.

dermis. The layer of skin beneath the epidermis.

detoxification. The process of cleansing the body of a drug or toxin, such as alcohol.

dextrose. A simple sugar that's found in the blood. It's also a main component of honey and corn syrup. Also called glucose.

diabetes mellitus. A disorder characterized by high levels of sugar (glucose) in the blood. Diabetes mellitus may be caused by a failure of the pancreas to produce sufficient insulin or by resistance of the body to the action of insulin. Also called diabetes.

diabetic ketoacidosis. A serious condition that may develop in people with diabetes. Due to insufficient insulin, the body begins breaking down fat, producing an increased level of acids (ketones) in the blood.

diabetic retinopathy. A complication of diabetes that damages the tiny blood vessels that nourish the retina. Diabetic retinopathy is brought on by high blood sugar levels.

diagnosis. Identification of a disease or disorder by a health care professional.

dialysis. A technique for removing waste and toxins from the blood. Used primarily when the kidneys fail or in cases of overdose of a drug. Includes hemodialysis and peritoneal dialysis.

diaphragm. The muscle that separates the abdomen from the chest. Or, a contraceptive device that fits over the cervix to help prevent sperm from entering the uterus.

diastole. The period during the heart cycle in which the muscle relaxes, followed by contraction of the heart muscle (systole).

diastolic pressure. The lowest blood pressure reached during the relaxation of the heart. Recorded as the second number in a blood pressure measurement.

digestion. The breakdown of food in the digestive system so that its nutrients can be absorbed by the body and its indigestible parts can be excreted as waste.

digit. A finger or toe.

dilate. To expand or open a structure such as the pupil of the eye or a passageway such as an artery.

diplopia. Double vision.

disk. A platelike structure such as the cartilage cushion found between every two vertebrae.

dislocation. Displacement of a bone from its normal position at a joint.

diuretics. Drugs that increase the flow of urine. They're often used to treat conditions involving excess body fluid, such as high blood pressure and congestive heart failure. Also called water pills.

diverticulosis. Pouchlike bulges in the wall of the intestine.

DNA. *See* deoxyribonucleic acid.

dominant. A mode of inheritance in which a gene for a particular trait is required from only one parent for that trait to appear in his or her offspring. *See also* recessive.

drusen. Clumps of waste deposit that form under the retinal pigment epithelium. They appear as yellow dots behind the retina in the back of the eye. An early sign of macular degeneration.

duodenum. The section of the small intestine closest to the stomach.

dura mater. The tough outer membrane covering the spinal cord and brain.

dysphagia. Difficulty swallowing or an inability to swallow.

dysplasia. Abnormal development of tissue.

dyspnea. Shortness of breath.

dystocia. Difficult labor usually due to an abnormal position or size of the fetus.

E

echocardiography. A test in which pulses of sound are sent into the chest. The echoes returning from the heart produce images that are recorded as echocardiograms.

eclampsia. A serious complication of pregnancy manifested by convulsions and loss of consciousness, including coma.

ectopic. Abnormal placement, such as a pregnancy that occurs outside the uterus (tubal pregnancy).

ectropion. A condition that develops when the eyelid sags outward from the eye.

eczema. An acute or chronic inflammatory condition of the skin characterized by itching and scaling. Also called atopic dermatitis or dermatitis.

edema. Swelling of body tissues due to accumulation of excess fluid.

effusion. An accumulation of fluid in body cavities or joints.

ejaculation. The ejection of semen that occurs during male orgasm.

ejection fraction. The portion of blood that's pumped out of a filled ventricle. Normal ejection fraction is 50 percent or more.

electrocardiogram (ECG). A recording of the electric activity of the heart.

embolism. A blood clot, air bubble, fat deposit or other foreign substance that moves from the site where it formed and blocks a blood vessel.

embryo. The human organism from the time of implantation in the uterus to about the 10th to 12th week after conception.

emission. The discharge of fluid.

emphysema. A disease in which the walls of the air sacs (alveoli) of the lungs are weakened or destroyed. This results in lungs that can't empty air normally and can't transfer oxygen efficiently into the bloodstream.

endarterectomy. The surgical removal of material from inside an artery, such as atherosclerotic plaques.

endocarditis. An inflammation of the membrane that lines the chambers and valves of the heart, usually caused by infection.

endocardium. The thin, inner membrane that lines the cavities of the heart.

endocrine gland. An organ or tissue that releases a substance to be used elsewhere in the body.

endoscope. An illuminated optical instrument used to visualize the inside of a hollow organ or cavity.

endothelium. A layer of cells on the inner surface of blood vessels.

endotracheal tube. A tube inserted into the windpipe (trachea) to allow breathing with a ventilator.

enema. Introduction of fluid into the rectum and colon to induce a bowel movement or to introduce a contrast agent for a diagnostic procedure.

enzyme. A complex protein that acts as a catalyst for chemical reactions.

epicardium. The thin membrane that covers the surface of the heart muscle.

epidemiology. The study of disease in human populations.

epidermis. The outer layer of skin.

epiglottis. The flap of cartilage that covers the voice box (larynx).

epinephrine. *See* adrenaline.

episiotomy. A surgical incision to enlarge the vaginal opening during childbirth.

erection. The swelling and stiffening of the penis during sexual arousal.

erythema. An area of reddened skin due to dilated capillaries.

erythrocytes. Red blood cells, which transport oxygen.

esophagus. The muscular tube that connects the throat (pharynx) with the stomach.

estrogen. A hormone produced primarily in females that contributes to the development and maintenance of feminine physical characteristics, cyclic changes such as menstruation, and changes related to pregnancy. The hormone is also produced in small quantities in males.

eustachian tube. The tube connecting the middle ear to the throat (pharynx).

excisional biopsy. An attempt to remove an abnormal growth in its entirety.

expiration. Letting a breath out; exhalation.

extrasystole. A premature heartbeat.

F

faint. A brief loss of consciousness resulting from insufficient blood to the brain.

fallopian tubes. Tubes located on each side of a woman's uterus that convey eggs from the ovaries to the cavity of the uterus.

false labor. Irregular uterine pains and contractions that may occur during pregnancy. Also called Braxton Hicks contractions.

familial hypercholesterolemia. An inherited form of high blood cholesterol levels.

farsightedness. A focusing problem in which you can see faraway objects clearly, but nearby objects appear blurry. Also called hyperopia.

fats. Organic compounds composed of fatty acids. Fats are either saturated or unsaturated. Unsaturated fats are further classified as either monounsaturated or polyunsaturated.

febrile. Feverish.

feces. Body waste such as food residue discharged from the bowels.

femur. The thighbone.

fertility. The ability to reproduce.

fertilization. The process of conception in which a sperm penetrates an egg (ovum), usually in the fallopian tube.

fetal distress. A situation in which a fetus is in potential jeopardy. Indications include a change in fetal activity or heartbeat and meconium-stained amniotic fluid.

fetus. The human being from about the 10th to 12th week after conception until delivery.

fiber. A food substance that resists chemical digestion and passes through the system essentially unchanged.

fibrillation. Quivering or uncontrollable contraction of muscles. Fibrillation in the cardiac muscle causes an irregular heartbeat.

fibrocystic breasts. A benign condition of the breasts characterized by lumps that vary with the menstrual cycle. Also called benign breast disease.

fibroid. A benign tumor of connective and muscular tissue, usually of the uterus. Also called fibroma.

fibula. The smaller of the two bones that run from the knee to the ankle.

flaccid. Soft, limp, without tone.

flatulence. Excessive gas in the stomach and intestines.

floater. A small bit of debris floating in the vitreous that can look like a spot, hair or string before your eye. What you're seeing is the shadow that this material casts on your retina.

fluoride. An element found in nature that helps prevent tooth decay and possibly strengthens bone.

fluoroscopy. Use of X-rays to produce images on a screen rather than on X-ray film.

flutter. Very rapid, regular beating of a heart chamber.

follicle. A small, tubular gland or sac in the skin or ovary. Or, an aggregation of cells in a lymph node.

follicle-stimulating hormone. A hormone that stimulates the development of eggs (ova) in the ovaries.

fontanel. A soft spot atop an infant's head where the bones of the skull have yet to join.

forceps. A surgical instrument used for grasping or compressing tissue.

foreskin. The skin covering the end of an uncircumcised penis. Also called the prepuce.

fovea. A small depression in the center of the macula that contains only cone cells and provides your sharpest vision.

fracture. To break or crack a bone. Or, a break or crack in a bone.

fraternal twins. Twins developing from two separate, fertilized eggs (ova). Also called nonidentical twins.

fundal height. The distance from the top of the pregnant uterus to the pubic bone. This measurement is used in estimating fetal age.

fungus. An organism of plant origin that lacks chlorophyll. Some fungi cause disease.

G

gallbladder. A sac, located under the liver, that stores bile secreted from the liver and releases it into the small intestine during digestion.

gametes. The cells of reproduction — sperm (spermatozoa) and eggs (ova).

gamma globulin. A protein found in the blood that helps fight infection.

ganglion. A mass of nerve tissue made up mostly of nerve cell bodies. Or, a cyst in a tendon sheath.

gangrene. Death and decay of body tissue, usually due to a lack of blood supply. The tissue shrinks and turns black.

gastric. Pertaining to the stomach.

gastroenteritis. An inflammatory condition of the stomach and intestines leading to nausea, vomiting, abdominal pain and diarrhea. Usually of bacterial or viral origin.

gastrointestinal tract. The stomach and intestines.

gene. A structure, within a chromosome, that's responsible for inheritance of a particular characteristic.

general anesthesia. A state of unconsciousness induced by a medication that eliminates sensation.

generic drug. The nontrademark name of a drug.

genetic. Associated with genes and heredity.

genetic engineering. The manufacture, alteration or repair of genetic material by artificial means.

genetic marker. An identifiable substance that's associated with a normal or an abnormal gene.

genital herpes. A viral infection spread by sexual contact and marked by inflammation and blisters in the infected area.

genitals. Internal and external reproductive organs.

genome. The entire collection of genes of an organism.

geriatrics. The branch of medicine that specializes in the care of diseases and problems related to aging.

germ. A microorganism. Some may cause disease.

gestation. The period of time from conception to birth.

gestational diabetes. Diabetes that develops during pregnancy, resulting in improper regulation of sugar (glucose) levels in the blood.

gigantism. A disorder caused by an overproduction of growth hormone by the pituitary gland. It results in excessive body height and size. Also known as giantism.

gland. Any organ or tissue that releases a substance to be used elsewhere in the body. Endocrine glands release hormones directly into the bloodstream.

glaucoma. A group of eye conditions resulting in abnormally high pressure inside the eyeball. This pressure causes extensive damage to the optic nerve and loss of peripheral vision.

globulin. A category of blood proteins from which antibodies are formed.

globus. A sensation of a lump in your throat in the absence of a physical abnormality. May be related to stress.

glomeruli. Microscopic clusters of blood vessels in the kidneys. Responsible for filtering waste from the blood.

glucagon. A pancreatic hormone that releases the body's stored sugar (glycogen) from the liver into the blood.

glucose. Blood sugar. Also known as dextrose.

gluten. Plant proteins found in grains such as wheat, rye, oats and barley.

glycogen. Stored sugar (glucose) in the liver.

goiter. An enlargement of the thyroid gland.

gonadotropin. A hormone that stimulates the gonads (ovaries and testicles).

gonads. *See* ovaries; testicles.

gonorrhea. A bacterial disease spread by sexual contact.

gout. A condition in which excess uric acid leads to arthritis and kidney stones.

grading. The process of assigning a number to a cancerous tumor based on pathological evidence of its aggressiveness.

grand mal. A term used to describe a generalized convulsion accompanied by a loss of consciousness.

granulocytes. White blood cells (leukocytes) manufactured in the bone marrow and containing granules. They digest and destroy bacteria.

groin. The lower abdominal area where the trunk and thighs meet.

H

halitosis. Bad breath.

hallucination. A false perception with no basis in reality. May be seen, heard or smelled.

hamstrings. The muscles at the back of the thigh. The tendons of the hamstring muscles can be felt at the back of the knee.

hardening of the arteries. *See* arteriosclerosis.

HDL cholesterol. High-density lipoprotein cholesterol. A type of cholesterol thought to help protect against atherosclerosis. Also known as the "good" cholesterol.

heart attack. A myocardial infarction. Death of an area of heart muscle caused by blockage of one or more of the coronary arteries that results in sudden interruption of bloodflow to a part of the heart.

heart block. *See* atrioventricular block.

heartburn. A burning sensation beneath the breastbone (sternum) resulting from regurgitation of gastric juices (reflux) from the stomach into the esophagus.

heart catheterization. A diagnostic test in which a catheter is placed into the heart.

heart failure. *See* congestive heart failure.

heart murmur. An abnormal sound heard during the heartbeat. The condition can be a sign of a diseased heart valve or other abnormality.

heart rate. The number of contractions of the heart in one minute.

Heimlich maneuver. Abdominal thrusts applied manually to dislodge an object blocking the airway.

hemangioma. A benign tumor of dilated blood vessels.

hematemesis. Vomiting of blood.

hematoma. A blood-filled swelling beneath the skin or in an organ, due to injury to a blood vessel.

hematuria. Blood or blood clots in the urine.

hemiplegia. Paralysis of one side of the body.

hemochromatosis. A defect in iron metabolism with buildup of iron in the body.

hemodialysis. A mechanical technique for removing chemical waste and toxins from the blood. Also called dialysis.

hemoglobin. An iron-containing protein found in red blood cells. Hemoglobin transports oxygen to body tissues.

hemophilia. An inherited bleeding disorder in which blood clotting is abnormal.

hemoptysis. Coughing or spitting up of blood that comes from bleeding in the voice box (larynx), windpipe (trachea) or lungs.

hemorrhage. Internal or external bleeding.

hemorrhoid. A swollen vein in or around the anus that may bleed.

hepatic. Pertaining to the liver.

hepatitis. Inflammation of the liver.

heredity. The transmission of genetic traits from parent to child.

hernia. Protrusion of an organ or structure into surrounding tissues. Commonly called a rupture.

high blood pressure. A condition in which the blood is pumped through the body under increased pressure. Also called hypertension.

hirsutism. Excessive growth of body or facial hair.

histamine. A body chemical in tissues that stimulates production of gastric acid for digestion. Or, the active agent of allergic reactions that result when excessive amounts of histamine are released to combat a perceived invader (allergen).

histology. The study of the microscopic appearance of tissues.

HIV. Human immunodeficiency virus. The virus that causes AIDS and related conditions.

hives. Eruption of welts on the skin. Thought to result from the release of histamine and other chemicals into the bloodstream.

homograft. A surgical procedure in which a body part is replaced or repaired using sterilized human tissue, as when the aortic valve is replaced.

hormone. A substance secreted by an endocrine gland and carried through the bloodstream to regulate various body functions.

human immunodeficiency virus (HIV). The virus that causes AIDS and related conditions.

humerus. The bone of the upper arm.

humoral. Pertaining to body fluids.

hydramnios. An excess of amniotic fluid.

hydrocephalus. Increased size of the fluid-filled cavities (ventricles) of the brain.

hydrogenation. The process of changing an unsaturated fat to a more solid, saturated one.

hymen. A membrane partially covering the opening to the vagina.

hymenoptera. The order of insects that includes bees, wasps and ants.

hyperactivity. A condition of behavior characterized by constant overactivity, distractibility, impulsiveness, an inability to concentrate and aggressiveness.

hypercholesterolemia. An elevated level of cholesterol in the blood.

hyperglycemia. Excess sugar (glucose) in the bloodstream.

hyperlipidemia. The presence of excess fats (lipids) in the bloodstream.

hyperopia. *See* farsightedness.

hyperplasia. Excess number of cells in tissue.

hypertension. *See* high blood pressure.

hypertrophic cardiomyopathy. An overgrowth of heart muscle that may impede blood flow into and out of the heart.

hyperventilation. Rapid or deep breathing in excess of that needed to supply oxygen to the body.

hypochondria. Excessive concern about health.

hypoglycemia. A condition in which sugar (glucose) in the bloodstream falls below normal levels.

hypotension. Low blood pressure.

hypothalamus. A portion of the brain partly responsible for basic functions such as appetite, sleep, body temperature and procreation.

hypoxia. Decreased concentration of oxygen in the blood.

I

iatrogenic disease. A disorder or disease that's a side effect of a prescribed treatment.

identical twins. Twins arising from a single fertilized egg (ovum).

idiopathic. Pertaining to a condition or disease of unknown cause.

ileostomy. A surgical procedure in which a section of the small intestine is brought out through an opening (stoma) created in the abdominal wall, allowing for the passage of stool into a small bag fastened over the opening.

ileum. The lower portion of the small intestine.

ilium. The upper portion of the hipbone.

immobilize. To make a limb or other body part immovable in order to aid healing.

immune system. The system that protects the body from invasion by foreign substances such as bacteria, viruses, parasites and fungi.

immunity. Resistance to a disease, particularly an infectious one.

immunization. The introduction of antigens into the body in very small quantities in order to stimulate the development of immunity.

immunoglobulin. A protein that can act as an antibody.

impacted. Pressed firmly together so as to be immovable.

impotence. The inability of a man to achieve or keep an erection and engage in sexual intercourse.

incision. A cut made with a knife.

incisors. The eight front teeth, four in the upper jaw and four in the lower jaw.

incontinence. An inability to control the release of urine or feces.

indigestion. Incomplete or abnormal digestion.

infarct. An area of tissue that dies because of blockage of its blood supply.

infection. A condition in which the body or a part of it is invaded by a microorganism.

infectious. Disease-causing.

inferior vena cava. The large vein returning blood from the legs and abdomen to the heart.

infertility. An inability to reproduce.

inflammation. Body tissue's reaction to injury from infection, physical injury or irritation, resulting in swelling, pain, heat and redness.

inguinal. Pertaining to the groin area.

insemination. Insertion of semen into the vagina. May result in fertilization of an egg (ovum).

insomnia. The inability to sleep.

inspiration. Taking in a breath; inhalation.

insulin. The pancreatic hormone that enables the body to regulate the amount of sugar (glucose) in the bloodstream. *See also* diabetes mellitus.

insulin reaction. A condition in people who take insulin, resulting in low blood sugar (hypoglycemia) due to excess insulin or reduced carbohydrate intake.

intermittent claudication. Discomfort in the leg muscles brought on by walking and relieved by rest. Produced by inadequate blood flow.

interstitial cystitis. A chronic inflammation of the bladder wall, leading to frequent, painful urination.

intestines. The portion of the digestive tract extending from the stomach to the anus. Responsible for much of the absorption of nutrients.

intolerance. An inability to tolerate pain, a drug therapy, or substances such as sugar (glucose) and lactose.

intracranial. Within the skull.

intraocular pressure. Pressure inside the eyeball that's maintained by the aqueous humor. Elevated intraocular pressure can signal glaucoma.

intravenous. Within or into a vein.

intravenous (IV) catheter. A hollow tube inserted into a vein for administration of fluids or medications.

intrinsic factor. A substance found in the gastric juices that allows for the absorption of vitamin B-12 from the intestines.

involuntary. Can't be controlled through will.

iris. The colored part of the eye. The iris contains a ring of muscle fibers that can expand or contract the size of the pupil.

ischemia. Deficiency of blood within an organ or part of an organ. Often refers to the situation in which an artery is narrowed or blocked and can't deliver sufficient blood to the organ it supplies.

isometric. Contracting a muscle against resistance without changing its length.

isotonic. Muscular work that produces motion of a body part.

isotope. A form of a chemical element that has similar structure but a different mass. Some isotopes are radioactive.

IUD. Intrauterine device. A contraceptive device, made of plastic or metal, that's inserted into the uterus.

J

jaundice. Yellowing of the eyes and skin caused by excess bilirubin. This excess results from blockage of bile passages or from the liver's inability to metabolize bilirubin.

jejunum. The portion of the small intestine located between the duodenum and ileum.

joint. The point of juncture between two or more bones where movement occurs.

jugular veins. The veins, one on each side of the neck, that carry blood from the brain and head to the heart.

K

Kegel exercises. Exercises done to strengthen the muscles that control urinary incontinence in females.

keloid. An abnormally thick scar that can form after surgery or an injury.

keratin. A protein found in hair, nails and the outer layers of skin.

ketoacidosis. A complication of type 1 diabetes (formerly called juvenile or insulin-dependent diabetes) that results from too little insulin. It can cause loss of consciousness (diabetic coma) and death.

ketones. Acidic substances produced when the body must use fat for energy.

kidneys. The two bean-shaped organs located in the back portion of the upper abdomen, one on each side of the spine. Responsible for the formation and excretion of urine and the regulation of the water, electrolyte and acid-alkaline content of blood.

Korotkoff sounds. Sounds heard when blood pressure is taken.

kyphosis. Excessive curvature of the spine, resulting in humpback, hunchback or rounding of the shoulders. May result from osteoarthritis, rheumatoid arthritis, osteoporosis, rickets, a compression fracture, a congenital abnormality, or other diseases and conditions.

L

labia. Two sets of liplike genital organs in females. The labia majora are two folds of skin and fatty tissue that protect the vulva. The labia minora are smaller folds inside the labia majora.

labor. The process of uterine muscle contractions that opens the cervix and moves the baby through the birth canal.

labyrinth. The portion of the inner ear responsible for balance.

laceration. A wound caused by tearing of tissue.

lacrimal glands. The tear-producing glands. Located under each brow bone, just above your eye.

lactation. The production and secretion of milk from the breasts.

lactose. Sugar found naturally in milk.

Lamaze method. A program of physical and emotional preparation of mothers for childbirth.

laparoscopy. Examination of the inside of the abdominal cavity by means of a laparoscope, a viewing instrument inserted through a small incision.

larynx. The voice box. It's composed of cartilage housing the vocal cords and the muscles and ligaments used to produce sound.

LDL cholesterol. Low-density lipoprotein cholesterol. Necessary for body functions, but in excessive amounts it tends to accumulate in artery walls. The "bad" cholesterol.

leaflet. The part of a heart valve that opens and closes so that blood flows in one direction.

lens. A clear, elliptical structure located behind the iris and pupil. It works with the cornea to focus light entering the eye. The ability of the lens to thin or thicken allows it to change its focusing power.

lesion. An area of tissue either injured (as in a wound, abscess or a sore) or altered (as in a tumor, mole or cyst).

leukemia. A malignant disease of the blood-forming organs. It results in the uncontrolled production of abnormal white blood cells.

leukocytes. White blood cells. They fight infection.

libido. Sexual drive.

ligament. Strong, fibrous connective tissue resembling a band or sheet that connects one bone to another.

ligature. A synthetic or natural filament for tying off blood vessels during surgery to keep the vessels from bleeding. The procedure itself is called ligation.

lightening. The repositioning of a baby lower in the pelvis that usually occurs several weeks before the onset of labor.

lipids. Fats or fat-like substances in the blood, such as cholesterol.

lipoproteins. Proteins combined with lipids to make them dissolve in blood.

liposuction. The process of removing fat deposits from beneath the skin by using a suction device.

liver. The largest internal organ in the body. It's the site of many metabolic functions, including secreting bile, neutralizing poisons, synthesizing proteins, and storing glycogen and certain minerals and vitamins.

lobe. A well-defined portion of an organ.

localized. Limited to a discrete area, as in an infection or disease. *See also* systemic.

lordosis. An exaggerated curvature of the lower portion of the spine, causing swayback.

lower esophageal sphincter. A circular band of muscle where the esophagus joins the stomach.

low vision. Any eye problem that can't be corrected by standard eyeglasses, contact lenses or surgery. It's often the result of eye diseases such as macular degeneration, glaucoma and diabetic retinopathy.

lumbar. Pertaining to the lower back.

lungs. The two cone-shaped, spongy organs of respiration located around the bronchial tubes and their branches.

lung scan. An imaging procedure used to assess blood flow through the lungs.

lymph. Clear fluid present in lymphatic vessels.

lymphatic vessels. Structures throughout the lymphatic system that contain and convey lymph.

lymph nodes. Small (from pinhead-sized to olive-sized) structures found throughout the body that produce white blood cells called lymphocytes and monocytes. These white blood cells help protect the body from invasion by bacteria and other organisms.

lymphocytes. Disease-fighting white blood cells made in the lymph nodes and distributed throughout the body by way of lymphatic fluid and blood.

lymphoma. A type of cancer that begins in lymphatic tissue and may spread to other areas of the body.

M

maceration. Softening and breaking apart of tissue due to soaking it in liquid.

macrophages. Cells found throughout the body, particularly in the spleen, that have the ability to ingest other substances, such as worn-out red blood cells.

macula. A dark reddish patch at the center of your retina that's densely packed with cone cells. The macula is essential to your central vision and allows you to see fine detail.

macular degeneration. A condition that occurs when tissue in the macula deteriorates.

magnetic resonance imaging (MRI). An imaging procedure that uses strong magnetic fields to visualize body structures.

malabsorption. Inadequate absorption of nutrients from the small intestine. Signs and symptoms of malabsorption include loose, fatty stools, diarrhea, weight loss, weakness and anemia.

malaise. A general feeling of illness, discomfort and uneasiness, often a symptom of infection.

male factor infertility. Infertility caused by abnormalities of the semen or sperm.

malignant. A term used to describe cancerous tumors that can grow uncontrollably and spread to other areas of the body (metastasize).

malnutrition. Deficiency of nourishment in the body due to a lack of healthy food or improper digestion and distribution of nutrients.

malpresentation. Abnormal position of the fetus during labor, making normal vaginal delivery difficult or impossible.

mammary gland. A compound gland of the breast that secretes milk.

mandible. The lower jaw.

mania. A mental disorder characterized by an intense feeling of elation and excitability, often accompanied by increased activity.

mastectomy. The surgical removal of a breast.

masticate. To chew.

mastoid process. A round, honeycombed bone mass located behind the ear.

maxilla. The upper jaw.

meconium stool. A newborn's first bowel movements, composed of intestinal secretions and amniotic fluid, usually dark green.

medulla. The center of an organ, gland or bone.

melanin. Pigment that provides dark color to hair, skin and the choroid of the eye.

melanoma. A pigmented tumor of the skin and, in rare cases, of the mucous membranes. A malignant melanoma tumor may be invasive and spread to lymph nodes and other sites more frequently than do other skin cancers.

membrane. A thin, soft layer of tissue that lines, separates or covers an organ or structure.

meninges. The membranes that cover the spinal cord and brain.

meningitis. Inflammation of the membranes that cover the brain or spinal cord, usually caused by infection.

menopause. The gradual cessation of menstrual cycles, at the end of which a female is no longer able to become pregnant.

menstruation. The monthly shedding of blood and tissue from the lining of the uterus during a female's reproductive years.

mesentery. A fold in the abdominal lining that connects the intestines to the back of the abdominal wall and contains the arteries and veins that supply the intestines.

metabolism. The process in living things by which food is transformed into forms that can be used by organisms, energy is derived and tissues are broken down into waste products.

metastasis. The spreading of a disease from one part of the body to another, usually by movement of cells (as in cancer), or infection through the lymphatic system or bloodstream.

microbes. One-celled organisms such as bacteria, many of which cause disease.

milia. Pinpoint-sized white spots on a newborn's nose and cheeks. The spots eventually disappear and need no treatment.

miosis. Pupil contraction. Abnormal contraction is often a sign of a disease or disorder.

miscarriage. The premature, spontaneous termination of a pregnancy before the fetus can survive outside the womb. Also called spontaneous abortion.

mitosis. A type of cell division in which new cells have the same number of chromosomes as the parent cell.

mitral valve. The heart valve that allows blood to move into the left ventricle from the left atrium and prevents reverse flow.

mitral valve prolapse. A bulging of the leaflets of the mitral valve into the left atrium during the heart's contraction.

mm Hg. Millimeters of mercury. The unit of measurement used in taking blood pressure.

molars. The 12 grinding or chewing teeth, located at the back of both jaws.

mongolian spots. A type of birthmark with large, blue-gray spots resembling bruises. More common in dark-skinned babies, these marks usually disappear later in childhood. Also called blue spot or mongolian macula.

monoclonal. Derived from a single cell or clone of cells.

monocytes. Disease-fighting white blood cells made in the lymph nodes and distributed throughout the body by way of lymphatic fluid and the bloodstream.

motility. The ability to move.

motor development. The increasing ability to use muscles.

mucous membranes. Thin, moist membranes that line passages and cavities in contact with air, such as the nose, mouth and eyes.

multiple myeloma. A type of blood cancer that begins in bone marrow. Multiple myeloma may cause bone pain, anemia and hypercalcemia.

murmur. A sound made by turbulent blood moving through the chambers and valves of the heart or through the blood vessels near the heart. May signify a structural defect in the heart or valves.

muscle. Tissue that produces movement by its ability to contract.

musculoskeletal. Pertaining to the muscles and the skeleton.

mutation. A disorder leading to a change that may result from alterations of genetic material.

myalgia. Muscle tenderness or pain.

myelin. A white, fat-like substance that forms a sheath around some nerve fibers.

myelodysplastic disorders. Disturbances of the cells that form a type of white blood cell.

myocardial infarction. Heart attack. Death of an area of heart muscle due to a lack of blood supply.

myocarditis. Inflammation of the heart muscle.

myocardium. The heart muscle. *See also* endocardium and epicardium.

myopathy. Any disease of a muscle.

myopia. *See* nearsightedness.

N

narcosis. A state of stupor, often induced by drugs or other agents.

nares. The nostrils.

natal. Pertaining to birth.

nausea. A sensation of stomach sickness, often followed by vomiting.

nearsightedness. A focusing problem in which you can see nearby objects clearly, but faraway objects appear blurry. Also called myopia.

necrosis. Changes due to the death of cells or organs.

neonatal. Pertaining to a newborn up to age 4 weeks old.

neoplasm. New and abnormal growth that may be benign or malignant. A tumor.

neovascularization. The abnormal formation and growth of blood vessels, such as that which occurs under the retina when you have wet macular degeneration, and in the vitreous when you have proliferative diabetic retinopathy.

nephrectomy. The surgical removal of a kidney.

nephritis. Inflammation of a kidney.

nephrons. Structures of the kidney that remove waste and form urine.

nerve. A bundle of fibers that connects the brain and spinal cord with various parts of the body and through which impulses pass.

neuralgia. A sharp pain along the course of a nerve or in its area of distribution.

neural tube. A structure in early fetal life that develops into the brain, spinal cord, spinal nerves and spine.

neural tube defect. A birth defect resulting in improper development of the brain or spinal cord.

neurofibromatosis. A genetic condition that affects the nervous system, muscles, bones and skin.

neurogenic bladder. Loss of normal bladder function due to damage of the nervous system.

neurogenic bowel. Loss of normal bowel function due to damage of the nervous system.

neuromuscular. Pertaining to the nerves and muscles.

neuron. A nerve cell.

neuropathy. Disease of the nerves.

neurotransmitters. Nerve cell chemicals that act as messengers in the brain and nervous system.

nicotine. An addictive chemical found in tobacco.

node. A small, round or egg-shaped tissue or structure.

noradrenaline. A naturally occurring hormone that increases heart rate and blood pressure and affects other body functions. Also called norepinephrine.

norepinephrine. *See* adrenaline; noradrenaline.

nucleus. The center portion of most plant and animal cells. Essential for cell growth, nourishment and reproduction.

nutrients. Substances in food that provide nourishment for the body.

nutrition. A combination of processes by which the body receives and uses substances necessary for daily function, energy, growth and repair.

nystagmus. A repetitive, abnormal movement of the eyeballs.

O

obesity. Above normal body weight, usually defined as more than 20 percent above what's considered healthy for people of your age, height and bone structure.

occipital. Pertaining to the back of the head.

occipital lobe. An area at the back of the brain that receives and processes visual information.

occlusion. Closure of a passage such as ducts or blood vessels. In dentistry, the alignment of upper and lower teeth when the jaws are closed.

occult. Obscure; concealed.

ocular. Pertaining to the eye.

olfactory. Pertaining to the sense of smell.

oncogenes. Genes present in normal cells that, upon exposure to cancer-inducing factors, may lead to development of tumors.

oncology. The study of tumors.

opportunistic infection. An infection caused by microorganisms that usually aren't harmful in healthy people but can be extremely dangerous in people with suppressed immune systems.

optic disk. The location where the optic nerve forms at the back of the eyeball. It's visible on the retina as a yellowish circle.

optic nerve. A bundle of nerve fibers that carries the visual information gathered by your retina to the visual cortex of your brain.

orbit. The socket that protects and cradles your eyeball. It's formed by a structure of bone that includes the cheekbone, forehead bone, temple bone and bridge of your nose.

orgasm. The climax of sexual intercourse or stimulation of sexual organs. In males, it's associated with the ejaculation of semen, and in females, with contractions of the vagina.

orthopnea. Difficulty breathing except in an upright position.

orthostatic hypotension. A drop in blood pressure upon standing. May cause lightheadedness or fainting.

osseous. Pertaining to bones.

osteogenic. Derived from bone.

osteopathy. Any bone disease.

ostomy. A surgically created opening in which a portion of the urinary tract or bowel is brought to the abdominal surface. A generic word for all types of ostomies, such as colostomy and ileostomy.

ova. The female cells of reproduction. After fertilization by a sperm, an egg (ovum) is capable of developing into a zygote, an embryo, a fetus and then a baby.

ovaries. Gonadal organs in the female that produce eggs (ova) for reproduction and the female sex hormones estrogen and progesterone.

over-the-counter (OTC). A term used to describe medications sold without a prescription.

ovulation. The monthly discharging of an egg (ovum) from an ovary. It occurs approximately 14 days before the onset of the next menstrual period.

oxytocin. The pituitary hormone in adult females that stimulates the release of breast milk.

P

pacemaker. A group of cells located in the atrium of the heart that regulate the heart's rate and rhythm. Or, an electric device used to simulate the natural process by generating electric impulses. Termed an artificial cardiac pacemaker, this device can be placed outside or inside the chest.

palate. The hard roof of the mouth.

palliative. Treatment undertaken not to cure but to improve a problem or condition.

pallor. Paleness.

palpation. A method of examining by touch.

palpitation. A sensation felt as a result of a fluttering or rapid, forceful beating of the heart.

palsy. Paralysis.

pancreas. A gland that produces enzymes essential to the digestion of food. It contains the islets of Langerhans, which secrete insulin into the blood.

papilla. A nipplelike protuberance.

paralysis. An inability to move a part of the body. Slight or partial paralysis is known as paresis.

paranoia. A mental disorder characterized by suspicion, delusions of persecution and jealousy.

paraparesis. Weakness below the waist, including the legs.

paraplegia. Paralysis below the waist, including both legs.

parasite. An organism that lives on or within another organism at the expense of the host.

parathyroid glands. Endocrine glands located beneath the thyroid gland that help regulate the level of calcium in the blood.

parenteral. A term that describes methods of administering medication, fluid or nutrition other than swallowing, including intravenous (IV), subcutaneous and intramuscular.

parietal lobe. An area of the brain that lies in front of the occipital lobe. Important in processing information from the sense of touch and bringing together sensory information.

paroxysm. A sudden attack, such as a spasm or convulsion. Or, recurrence of symptoms of a disease.

paroxysmal nocturnal dyspnea. Episodic shortness of breath at night.

patella. The kneecap.

pathogen. A disease-producing microorganism.

pathology. The study of the cause and nature of diseases.

pectoral. Pertaining to the chest.

pelvic floor muscles. A group of muscles at the base of the pelvis. They help support the bladder, urethra, rectum and, in women, the vagina and uterus.

pelvis. The basin-shaped bone structure connecting the spine with the legs.

penis. The male organ for urination and sexual intercourse.

pepsin. The main enzyme in the digestive juices of the stomach.

peptic. Pertaining to digestion or the enzyme pepsin.

percussion. A method of examination by tapping the fingertips over various areas of the body to determine the position, size and consistency of a structure beneath the skin.

percutaneous transluminal coronary angioplasty. A procedure that uses balloon catheters to reopen narrowed coronary arteries. Also called balloon angioplasty or percutaneous coronary intervention.

perforation. The process of making a hole, or the hole itself.

pericardiectomy. Removal of the pericardium.

pericarditis. Inflammation of the pericardium.

pericardium. The membranous sac enclosing the heart.

perinatal. Referring to the time just before, during and immediately after birth.

perineum. The external area between the vulva and anus in a female or between the scrotum and anus in a male.

periodontal. Pertaining to the area immediately around a tooth.

periosteum. Leatherlike tissue that encases bone.

peristalsis. The wavelike motion of muscles, particularly in the digestive system, that forces food or food residue through the digestive tract.

peritoneum. The membrane lining the abdominal cavity.

peritonitis. Inflammation or infection of the peritoneum.

pernicious. Destructive, sometimes fatal. Pernicious anemia is a particular form of anemia caused by an inability to absorb vitamin B-12 from the intestinal tract.

perspiration. Sweat. The salty fluid excreted from the sweat glands of the skin.

pessary. A device inserted into the vagina to support the uterus or to prevent conception.

petechiae. Small hemorrhages that appear in the skin and mucous membranes.

petit mal. A term used to describe a mild form of epileptic attack, characterized by a blank stare and temporary cessation of activity.

pH. A measure of the acidity or alkalinity of a substance.

pharmacology. The study of drugs and their effects.

pharynx. Upper portion of the throat. The passageway for air from the nose to the voice box (larynx) and for food from the mouth to the esophagus.

phenylketonuria. A congenital condition in which the body lacks a specific enzyme. This causes abnormal metabolism that may result in brain damage.

phlebitis. Inflammation of a vein.

phlegm. Thick mucus, especially from the sinuses or respiratory tract.

phobia. A persistent, irrational fear.

phototherapy. Treatment by exposure to light.

pica. An uncommon urge to eat nonfood material such as dirt, baking powder or frost from a freezer.

pigment. Coloring matter.

pineal body. A small, cone-shaped gland in the brain, the function of which is unclear.

pinna. The exterior, easily visible part of the ear.

pituitary gland. An endocrine gland that produces a range of hormones to help control the body's long-term growth, day-to-day functioning and reproductive capabilities. Sometimes called the master gland.

placebo. A nondrug substance that has no specific pharmacological activity against illness. Sometimes called a sugar pill.

placenta. The spongy uterine structure, developed during pregnancy, through which the fetus takes nourishment and discards waste by way of the umbilical cord. The placenta is shed after delivery, at which point it's known as the afterbirth.

placental abruption. Separation of the placenta from the uterine wall.

placenta previa. An abnormal location of the placenta in which it partially or completely covers the cervical opening.

plague. A term previously used to describe any deadly contagious epidemic disease. Now used primarily to describe infection by *Yersinia pestis* that causes bubonic plague and pneumonic plague.

plaque. A film or deposit of bacteria and other material located on the surface of a tooth that may lead to tooth decay or periodontal disease. Or, one of many fatty deposits that accumulate in the lining of the arteries, resulting in narrower, less flexible pathways for the blood.

plasma. The fluid part of the blood and lymph.

platelets. Microscopic-sized disks found in blood. Also known as thrombocytes, platelets are necessary for the clotting of blood.

pleura. The membrane that covers both lungs and lines the chest cavity.

point of focus. The location within the eyeball where visual information is most sharply focused by the cornea and lens. The best sight occurs when the point of focus is directly on the retina.

polyp. A protruding growth, often on a stalk.

positron emission tomography (PET). An imaging technique used for measuring blood flow and the metabolism of body tissues, including the heart and brain.

postpartum. Pertaining to the time after childbirth.

preeclampsia. A condition that can occur during pregnancy. It's marked by pregnancy-induced high blood pressure, protein in the urine and swelling. Also called toxemia.

premolars. Eight teeth in the adult mouth having two points.

prepuce. The foreskin over the glans of an uncircumcised penis.

presbyopia. A problem that occurs when your lens loses its elasticity and ability to thicken or thin. This condition makes it difficult for you to focus on nearby objects.

primary care physician. The doctor responsible for providing or coordinating your general health care.

primary tumor. The site of origin of a cancerous tumor. If the cancer metastasizes to another site, it's called a secondary tumor.

progesterone. A female sex hormone responsible for, among other things, the thickening of the uterine lining in preparation for conception and implantation of a fertilized egg (ovum).

prognosis. A prediction of the course or outcome of a disease.

prolactin. A pituitary hormone that stimulates the breasts to produce milk.

prolapse. Displacement of an organ or a structure, such as the uterus or bladder, by dropping down or protruding.

prophylaxis. A term that refers to prevention of disease or its spread by following certain rules or taking specific precautions.

prostaglandins. A group of extremely active substances that affect many organs. Certain prostaglandins have a role in stimulating the uterine contractions of labor.

prostate gland. A gland located at the base of the bladder in males.

prostate-specific antigen (PSA). A protein, produced by the prostate gland, that can be measured in blood. PSA can be increased by a variety of abnormal conditions in the prostate, including but not limited to prostate cancer.

prosthesis. An artificial substitute for a missing body part, such as an arm or leg.

protein. Complex nitrogen-containing compounds composed of amino acids. Essential for the growth and repair of tissue.

prothrombin. A component of circulating blood that interacts with calcium salts to form thrombin, a step in the process of blood clotting.

prothrombin time. A test that measures the activity of certain clotting factors. It's often used to determine whether a person is receiving the correct dose of an anticoagulant.

pruritus. Itching.

psychogenic. Originating in the mind. Or, pertaining to the development of the mind.

psychomotor. Pertaining to voluntary physical movement.

psychosis. A mental disturbance of serious magnitude that's characterized by a loss of contact with reality. Delusions and hallucinations are often present.

psychosomatic. Pertaining to the relationship of the mind and body. Psychosomatic illnesses are those in which a physical disorder is caused or aggravated by emotional factors.

ptosis. A condition that causes the upper eyelid to droop over your eye and partially block your vision.

ptyalin. An enzyme in saliva that helps break down starch into sugars.

puberty. A period of rapid change in boys and girls during which sex characteristics mature. In girls (usually between 9 and 16 years) it's marked by the beginning of menstruation (menarche), and in boys (usually between 9 and 14 years) it's marked by discharge of semen and deepening of the voice.

pudendal block. A local anesthetic injection used to ease the pain of the last part of labor and for an episiotomy.

pulmonary. Pertaining to the lungs.

pulmonary artery. A blood vessel that carries oxygen-depleted blood from the right ventricle of the heart to the lungs.

pulmonary embolism. A condition in which a clot or other substance lodges in a lung artery.

pulmonary function test. A test used to measure the ability of the lungs to exchange air.

pulmonary valve. The valve between the right ventricle and the pulmonary artery.

pulmonary veins. Those blood vessels that carry newly oxygenated blood from the lungs back to the heart.

pupil. The dark area in the center of your iris through which light passes into your eye.

purpura. A condition characterized by hemorrhages of tiny blood vessels, causing patches on the skin or on mucous membranes. The patches begin as red, change to purple and then to brownish-yellow before disappearing.

purulent. Forming or containing pus.

pus. Thick, whitish-yellow fluid containing leukocytes and bacteria, formed at the site of certain kinds of infections.

pyloric stenosis. An obstruction at the outlet of the stomach.

pylorus. The opening at the stomach outlet into the duodenum.

pyrexia. Fever.

Q

quadriparesis. Weakness of all four limbs.

quadriplegia. Complete paralysis of all four limbs.

quickening. The first perception of fetal movements, usually between 16 and 20 weeks of pregnancy.

R

radial pulse. The pulse felt at the wrist.

radiation therapy. The use of high-energy waves to treat disease such as cancer. Sources of radiation include X-ray, cobalt and radium.

radius. The smaller of the two bones in the lower arm. It connects to the base of the thumb.

rales. Abnormal breathing sounds, sometimes indicating fluid in the air sacs (alveoli) of the lungs.

rash. Eruption on the skin, usually temporary.

recessive. A mode of inheritance in which a gene for a particular trait must be inherited from both parents in order for that trait to appear in their offspring. *See also* dominant.

rectum. The lowest portion of the large intestine. Stores stool until it's expelled.

reflex. An involuntary response to a stimulus.

reflux. Backflow or regurgitation.

refraction. The bending of light waves by the cornea and lens as light passes into the eyeball. Refraction allows images to be sharply focused and clear.

refractory. A temporary condition that resists treatment or a nerve or muscle that resists stimulation.

regurgitation. Backflow.

rejection. Refusal to accept, as with a transplanted organ.

relapse. Recurrence of disease after apparent recovery.

remission. Abatement of signs and symptoms.

REM sleep. Rapid eye movement sleep. The period of sleep when dreaming occurs and the eyes move cyclically even though closed.

renal. Pertaining to the kidneys.

renal failure. The inability of the kidneys to excrete wastes, concentrate urine and maintain electrolyte balance.

renin. A hormone released by the kidneys that affects blood pressure.

reperfusion. Resumption of blood flow.

resection. The surgical removal of an organ or tissue.

respiration. Breathing.

resuscitation. The restoration of breathing or a heartbeat after cardiac arrest.

retina. A thin layer of tissue on the inside back wall of your eyeball that receives and organizes visual information. The retina is connected to the brain by the optic nerve.

retinal detachment. Separation of the retina from the choroid. If untreated this condition almost always leads to visual loss.

retinal pigment epithelium. A layer of tissue forming the outermost surface of the retina. Deterioration of the retinal pigment epithelium plays an important role in macular degeneration.

retinopathy. An abnormality of the retina that may cause deterioration of eyesight.

Rh factor. Rhesus factor. A protein found in the blood serum of people who are Rh positive.

rhinovirus. A large subgroup of viruses that cause the common cold.

right heart failure. Decreased function of the right ventricle, resulting in swelling in the legs and abdominal organs, especially the liver. *See also* congestive heart failure.

risk factors. Conditions that increase chances of a disease developing. Such factors can be chemical, physiological, behavioral, psychological, genetic or environmental, among others.

rods. Light-sensitive cells of the retina that provide your peripheral vision and allow you to see in dim light. Or, rod-shaped bacteria.

root canal. The space in the root of the tooth that contains nerves.

roughage. Indigestible fiber of fruits, vegetables and cereals that aids in the evacuation of waste.

rupture. The tearing or bursting of tissue or an organ.

S

sacroiliac joint. The juncture between the sacrum and ilium. Not a true joint because this point has no movement.

sacrum. The triangular bone at the base of the spine just above the coccyx. Composed of five fused vertebrae and part of the bony pelvis.

saline. Salt (sodium chloride) solution.

saliva. Fluid secreted by the salivary glands that moistens food and begins the process of digestion.

saphenous vein. A large vein in the leg.

sarcoma. A malignant tumor originating in connective tissue or bone.

scabies. A skin disorder caused by a mite. Characterized by redness, itching and swelling of the involved area.

scapula. The shoulder blade.

Schlemm's canal. An open channel behind the trabecular meshwork that allows aqueous humor to drain from the eye.

sciatic nerve. The largest nerve in the body, formed by the motor and sensory nerves to and from the legs and feet. It begins at the base of the spinal cord as a number of roots and passes through the pelvis, down the back of each thigh to the heel.

sclera. A tough, white, leathery coating that forms the circular eyeball shape and protects the internal structures of the eye. Also known as the white of your eye.

sclerosis. The hardening or thickening of an organ or tissue, usually due to abnormal or excessive growth of fibrous tissue.

scrotum. The skin sac that holds the testicles.

sebaceous glands. Oil glands of the skin.

sebum. A fatty substance secreted by the sebaceous glands to lubricate the skin.

secretion. The process of producing materials by glands. Also, the substance produced.

seizure. A sudden attack, often including convulsions. If recurrent, often referred to as a seizure disorder or as epilepsy.

semen. Thick, whitish fluid containing reproductive cells (spermatozoa) and other fluids, discharged through the male urethra at ejaculation.

seminal vesicles. Saclike structures located behind the bladder in the male, which secrete fluid that's part of the composition of semen.

seminoma. A type of malignant tumor of the testicle.

sepsis. The state of being infected with disease-causing microorganisms in the bloodstream.

septal defect. A hole in the wall of the heart separating the two atria or the two ventricles.

septicemia. Another term for sepsis.

septum. A wall dividing two cavities or compartments of the body.

serum. Watery fluid left after coagulation of the blood to form a clot. Serum containing antibodies to a specific disease may be injected into a person to give temporary resistance to that disease. This is called passive immunity. *See also* vaccine.

shock. A clinical condition in which the body reacts to injury or severe pain by dilation or relaxation of blood vessels, producing what can be called circulatory failure. Signs and symptoms include rapid pulse and breathing, very low blood pressure, pallor, clammy skin, and, sometimes, unconsciousness.

shunt. A passage that diverts blood flow from one main route to another. Often constructed artificially.

sick sinus syndrome. A failure of the sinus node to properly regulate the heartbeat. It may result in periods of either fast or slow heartbeat.

side effects. Unwanted changes produced by medication or other treatment, ranging from trivial and transient (minor headache or dry mouth) to more serious (asthma, gastrointestinal bleeding).

silent ischemia. An insufficient supply of blood and oxygen to the heart muscle without signs and symptoms.

sinuses. Empty spaces or cavities within bone structure. Most commonly, the several sets of cavities adjacent to and connected to the nose by small openings.

sinus node. The heart's natural pacemaker.

sodium. A mineral that's essential in maintaining the fluid balance of the body. Table salt (sodium chloride) is nearly half sodium.

somatostatin. A hormone that helps regulate the body's production and release of the pancreatic hormones insulin and glucagon. It's also found in other tissues of the body, where it may have other functions.

sonogram. *See* ultrasound scan.

spasm. An involuntary movement produced by a muscular contraction.

speculum. A device used to examine a body opening such as the nose or vagina.

spermatozoa. The male cells of reproduction. When one such cell combines with an egg (ovum), fertilization has occurred. Produced by the testicles and transmitted in semen. Also referred to as sperm.

spermicide. A birth control agent used to kill sperm cells by contact.

sphincter. A circular muscle at an opening that can contract and expand to close and open it. The body has several sphincter muscles, including those at the anus, bladder, stomach and esophagus.

sphygmomanometer. A device used to measure blood pressure.

spinal canal. The space that contains the spinal cord and is protected by vertebrae of the backbone.

spinal column. The bony assemblage of vertebrae; spine.

spinal cord. A lengthy, cordlike bundle of nerves that links nerves in the trunk and extremities with the brain.

spleen. The organ, located to the left and just in front of the stomach, that stores and at times manufactures blood cells.

spontaneous abortion. A miscarriage.

sprain. Ligament damage, usually in the ankles and knees.

sputum. The fluid produced by coughing. If certain disorders or infections are suspected, the sputum may be examined in a laboratory.

squamous cell carcinoma. A malignant tumor arising from cells known as squamous epithelium.

stable angina. A predictable pattern of cardiac pain caused by ischemia.

staging. The process of categorizing the extent or spread of cancer for the purpose of planning treatment.

stenosis. The abnormal narrowing or closure of an opening or passageway in the body.

stenosis, aortic. Narrowing of the valve opening between the left ventricle and aorta.

stenosis, mitral. Narrowing of the valve opening between the left atrium and ventricle.

stent. A device, implanted during surgery, that helps keep tissues in place, as when a tubular, meshlike material is placed inside a blood vessel to keep it open.

sterilization. The process by which all microorganisms, such as bacteria, viruses and parasites, are removed from a substance or item, such as surgical instruments, to prevent infection. Or, the process, usually surgical, of rendering a male or female incapable of reproduction.

sternum. The breastbone, in the upper central portion of the chest and abutted by the ends of the clavicle and the ribs.

steroids. *See* corticosteroids.

stethoscope. A device for listening to sounds produced in the body.

stillborn. A term that refers to a fetus dead at birth.

stomach. The saclike organ to which food is delivered by the esophagus.

stomatitis. Inflammation of the mucous membranes of the mouth. May occur as a complication of chemotherapy or radiation therapy.

stool. Body waste, such as food residue, evacuated from the large bowel.

strain. Muscular injury produced by abuse or overuse of a muscle.

strep throat. Streptococcal infection of the throat.

striae. Streaks or stripes.

stroke. A condition produced by obstruction of an artery that blocks the flow of blood to a portion of the brain or by bleeding into the brain.

stupor. A state of reduced consciousness in which responsiveness and feeling are lessened.

sty. A painful, red lump, resembling a boil or pimple, on the eyelid. It's caused by a bacterial infection.

subacute. A term used to distinguish the intermediate duration of a disease that's neither chronic nor characteristically of brief duration.

subcutaneous. Beneath the skin.

sudden infant death syndrome (SIDS). The sudden, unexplained death of an infant.

sunblock. An over-the-counter preparation applied to the skin to limit damage from the rays of the sun.

superior vena cava. The large vein returning blood from your head and arms to your heart.

supine. Lying on the back.

suppository. A pharmaceutical preparation in a solid form, intended to be inserted into a passage such as the rectum or vagina.

suppuration. The formation and discharge of pus from an injury or infection.

suture. The process of joining two surfaces by stitching. Or, the surgical stitch itself.

synapse. The junction between two nerve cells (neurons).

syncope. Fainting.

syndrome. A collection of signs and symptoms that characterize an ailment.

synovial fluid. The clear, fluid lubricant in a joint.

syringe. An instrument for injecting or withdrawing fluids.

systemic. Affecting or pertaining to several areas of the body rather than one of its parts.

systole. The period during the heart cycle in which the heart muscle contracts, followed by relaxation (diastole).

systolic pressure. The highest blood pressure produced by the contraction of the heart. Recorded as the first number in a blood pressure measurement.

T

tachycardia. An abnormally rapid heart rate.

tachypnea. Rapid breathing.

tamponade. Compression of an organ, such as pericardial tamponade, in which pericardial fluid compresses the heart.

tartar. Plaque deposits on the teeth.

T cell. A type of white blood cell (lymphocyte) that's part of the body's immune system.

temporal lobes. Areas located on each side of the brain that are important in processing memory.

temporomandibular joint (TMJ). The joint between the lower jaw and the temporal bone of the skull.

tendon. Cordlike tissue that connects muscles to bones.

testicles. The male gonads that produce sperm for reproduction and the male sex hormone testosterone. Also called testes.

testosterone. A male sex hormone produced in the testicles.

thalassemia. Inherited anemias found predominantly among people of Mediterranean descent.

thoracic. Having to do with the chest (thorax).

thorax. The chest.

thrills. Vibrations due to abnormal blood flow.

thrombin. An enzyme that's part of the process of blood coagulation.

thrombocyte. Blood platelet, essential to the clotting process.

thrombolysis. The dissolution of blood clots.

thrombophlebitis. Clotting of blood and inflammation in a vein.

thrombus. A blood clot.

thrush. A fungal infection of the mouth.

thymus. A gland located in the upper chest that produces T cells, which are essential to developing the body's immune response.

thyroid gland. An endocrine gland that helps control the body's rate of function and contributes to maintaining a balance between the calcium in the blood and bones through production of the hormones thyroxine and calcitonin.

thyroxine. A thyroid hormone that controls the pace of chemical activity (metabolism) in the body.

TIA. *See* transient ischemic attack.

tibia. The shinbone. The larger of the two bones in the lower leg.

tic. An involuntary muscle spasm, usually of the face, head, neck or shoulder. A twitch.

tincture. A medication that's an alcoholic solution of a vegetable or animal extract or a chemical substance.

tissue. A collection of similar cells that, taken together, form a body structure.

tocolytic medications. Medications used to inhibit labor.

tonsils. Two masses of lymph tissues, located on each side of the back of the throat, that help filter out unwanted bacteria.

topical. Pertaining to the surface of the body.

tourniquet. A device tightened over an extremity to stop bleeding.

toxemia. A condition in which toxins circulate throughout the body via the blood. *See also* preeclampsia.

toxic. Poisonous.

toxin. A poisonous substance.

toxoid. A biological toxin treated so that it's no longer dangerous but upon injection into the body will induce antibodies to form. For example, tetanus toxoid.

toxoplasmosis. An infectious disease caused by a microscopic parasite found in infected cat feces and undercooked meat.

trabecular meshwork. A sievelike system of spongy tissue through which aqueous humor passes before draining from the eye through Schlemm's canal.

trachea. The tube that connects the throat to bronchial tubes in the lungs. Also called the windpipe.

traction. A treatment of some fractures and dislocations involving mechanical pulling on a body part.

tranquilizer. A medication used to reduce tension and anxiety.

transducer. A device that translates pressure, temperature, pulse or sound into an electric signal.

transfusion. The delivery of blood or a blood component into the bloodstream.

transient ischemic attack (TIA). A disorder caused by temporary lack of circulation to a part of the brain. It differs from a stroke in that the signs and symptoms generally disappear completely within 24 hours.

transplantation. The surgical transfer of an organ or tissue from one position or person to another.

transvaginal. Through the vagina, such as a transvaginal ultrasound.

tremor. An involuntary shaking that can result from a disease or a nervous disorder, as a side effect of a medication, or from some other cause.

triceps. A muscle in the arm that upon contraction extends the arm at the elbow.

tricuspid valve. The heart valve between the right atrium and right ventricle.

trigeminal nerve. The nerve that delivers sensory stimuli to the brain from the face, teeth and tongue.

triglyceride. A form of fat that the body makes from sugar, alcohol or excess calories.

trimester. One of the three periods of pregnancy, each lasting about three months.

truncal obesity. Fat deposited in the thorax and abdomen instead of the hips and thighs.

truss. A device worn externally to hold a hernia or organ in place.

tubal ligation. A sterilization procedure in the female in which the fallopian tubes are tied and cut.

tubules. Small tubes or canals, such as those located in the kidneys.

tumor. An abnormal growth of tissue. The tumor may be malignant or benign.

tumor markers. Substances circulating in the blood that are produced by tumors. The level of the tumor marker may reflect the activity or extent of the tumor.

tympanic membrane. The eardrum.

U

ulcer. An open sore on the skin or a mucous membrane.

ulcerative colitis. A disease characterized by inflammation of the lining of the colon and rectum.

ulna. The larger of the two bones in the forearm.

ultrasound scan. A technique that uses very high frequency sound waves to produce images of the inside of the body. Also known as ultrasonography.

umbilical cord. The structure that transports nutrients and oxygen from the placenta to the fetus and carries away fetal waste.

umbilical hernia. A bulge caused by stretched tissue around the umbilicus.

umbilicus. The navel. The scar that's formed by removal of the umbilical cord from the newborn following birth.

undescended testicle. Failure of a testicle to enter the scrotum.

unicuspid. A heart valve with one leaflet.

unstable angina. New or increasing chest pain caused by decreased blood flow to the heart.

urea. The principal waste product in urine. A nitrogen-containing product of protein metabolism. Its concentration in blood may be used as a measure of kidney function.

uremia. The buildup of urea in the bloodstream.

ureter. The tube that delivers urine from the kidney to the bladder.

urethra. The tube draining the bladder to outside of the body. In males, this canal is also the passage for semen.

uric acid. A waste byproduct of metabolism. When too little is excreted or too much is produced, the buildup can lead to the development of gout.

urination. The act of voiding fluid wastes (urine).

urine. Fluid waste produced in the kidneys, stored in the bladder and released through the urethra.

urticaria. *See* hives.

uterus. The female organ in which the fetus develops. Also called the womb.

uvula. The pendulous tissue at the back of the palate.

V

vaccination. Injection of a vaccine to create immunity.

vaccine. Weakened or killed microorganisms or viruses of a specific disease introduced into the body in order to stimulate immunity.

vagina. The passage connecting the female external genitalia with the uterus. Also called the birth canal.

vaginitis. Infection of the vagina.

vagus nerve. The nerve that serves the esophagus, voice box (larynx), stomach, intestines, lungs and heart.

variant angina. Chest pain caused by a spasm of the coronary arteries.

varicose veins. Dilated and distended veins due to defective valves in the veins.

vascular. Pertaining to blood vessels.

vas deferens. One of the two ducts that transport sperm to the urethra.

vasectomy. A sterilization procedure in the male involving tying and cutting the vas deferens to prevent sperm from entering the semen.

vasodilators. Medications that widen or dilate blood vessels.

vasovagal syncope. Simple faint.

vegans. People who don't eat food of animal origin.

vein. A blood vessel that returns blood to the heart.

venous. Pertaining to veins.

ventilation. The exchange of air in and out of the lungs.

ventilator. A machine that assists or controls breathing; a respirator.

ventricles. The two main pumping chambers of the heart. The left ventricle pumps blood to the body, and the right ventricle pumps blood to the lungs. Or, the fluid-filled cavities of the brain.

venule. A small vein.

verruca. A wart.

vertebra. Any of the 33 bones that make up the spine.

vertigo. Dizziness accompanied by the illusion of motion.

vesicle. A small sac containing a liquid.

viral. Pertaining to or caused by a virus.

virulent. Highly poisonous or infectious.

virus. Microscopic infectious agents that reproduce only in host cells.

viscera. The internal organs, especially those within the abdominal cavity.

visual field. The area in front of you that you can see at a given moment without moving your eyes. It's made up of your central and peripheral vision.

vital signs. Respiration, heart rate and body temperature.

vitamins. Organic substances essential for most metabolic functions of the body.

vitreous. A clear, gelatinous substance that fills the vitreous cavity. It helps maintain the shape of the eyeball and its internal pressure. Also called vitreous humor.

vitreous cavity. A chamber inside the eyeball extending from the back of the lens to the retina. It's filled with vitreous.

vomit. The ejection of partially digested matter from the stomach through the mouth. Or, the matter itself.

vulva. The external female genitals, including the clitoris and labia.

W

wart. A harmless skin growth produced by a virus.

wen. A cyst that develops in a sebaceous gland.

wheezing. A whistling sound produced during breathing.

withdrawal. The experience of stopping the use of a substance to which you're addicted, such as a medication, an illegal drug or alcohol. Signs and symptoms may be physiological, psychological or both.

womb. *See* uterus.

X

X-rays. Electromagnetic waves that penetrate most solid matter. Used in X-ray machines to produce images of internal structures of the body. Or, the photographs made using this diagnostic technique.

Z

zygote. The egg (ovum) after it's fertilized by a sperm.

Index

fine-needle aspiration biopsy, 807, 810
fingernails. *See* nails
first-aid supplies, 31
first trimester
    baby's development, 115–16
    cell division, 115
    changes in you, 114–15
    ectopic pregnancy and, 116, 117–18
    eight weeks illustration, 115
    fertilization, 114, 115
    miscarriage and, 116–17
    organ formation, 115–16
    overview, 114
    possible problems, 116–18
    vaginal bleeding or bloody
        discharge, 116
    See also pregnancy
first trimester screen, 110
fish, 98, 265
FISH (fluorescence *in situ*
    hybridization), 113
fitness
    age and, 283
    benefits of, 282–83
    everyday, 283–84
    family, 284–86
    "sitting disease" and, 283
fitness program
    activity planning, 287–91
    aerobic exercises, 287
    doctor consultation and, 286
    getting and keeping going, 296–97
    goals, identifying, 286–87
    goals, setting, 296
    making it fun and, 296
    progress, tracking, 296–97
    stability exercises, 289, 291
    strength exercises, 287–90
    stretching and flexibility exercises,
        290, 291
5-alpha reductase inhibitors, 1248
5-HTP, 1148
flatfeet, 204, 942–43
fleas, 463, 464–65
flexible sigmoidoscopy, 1262
floaters, 615
flossing teeth, 661–62, 676–77
flu (influenza)
    diagnosis, 447
    immunization, 149, 235, 237, 335,
        447
    signs and symptoms, 447
    treatment, 447–48
fluorescein angiography, 588–89
fluorescence *in situ* hybridization
    (FISH), 113
fluoride, 669
fluoroquinolones, 1292
folic acid, 95, 1045
folic acid deficiency anemia, 1042
follicular cyst, 1219
folliculitis
    deep, 1093

signs and symptoms, 1092
superficial, 1092–93
treatment, 1093–94
visual guide, 398
food allergies
    diagnosis, 507
    intolerance versus, 508
    signs and symptoms, 506–7
    treatment, 507–8
foodborne illness
    bacteria types, 55
    defined, 54, 262–63
    prevention, 56, 263–64
    signs and symptoms, 54
    treatment, 54–56
food intolerance, 508
food labels, 255–56
food poisoning, 837
food safety
    drinking water, 265
    foodborne illness and, 262–64
    safe-cooking temperatures and, 265
foot care, 1001
foot pain, 75
foot problems
    Achilles tendinitis, 938
    bunions, 942–43
    burning feet, 941
    corns and calluses, 942
    diabetes and, 1001
    flatfeet, 942–43
    foot ulcer, 943–44
    hammertoe and mallet toe, 942
    heel pain, 938–40
    ingrown toenail, 941
    metatarsalgia, 940–41
    Morton's neuroma, 941
    shoes and, 940
    swelling of feet, 82–83
foot ulcer, 943–44
foreign bodies
    in ears, 62–63, 627
    in eyes, 61–62, 595
    in nose, 63
    in skin, 64
    swallowed, 63, 825
    in windpipe or lungs, 63
fractures
    amputation and, 39
    arm, 38
    casts, 923
    closed, 36
    Colles', 922
    comminuted, 36
    complete, 36
    displaced, 36
    hip, 40, 923–25
    immobilizing, 37
    incomplete, 36
    jaw, 681
    leg, 38
    open, 36
    osteoporotic compression, 76

overview, 921–22
pain, 75
pelvic, 40
rib, 76
seriousness of, 922
signs and symptoms, 37, 921
skull, 42–43
slings and, 37
spinal compression, 956
spinal injuries, 39–40
splints, 38–40, 923
stress, 922
treatment, 37–38, 922–23
types of, 36
Friedreich's ataxia, 566–68
frontotemporal dementia, 553
frostbite, 65–66
frozen shoulder
    overview, 984–85
    prevention, 986
    signs and symptoms, 984
    treatment, 985–86
full-body skin exam, 242–43
fungal infections
    athlete's foot, jock itch and
        ringworm, 1098–99
    candida infections, 1099, 1100
    nails, 1116–17
    signs and symptoms, 1098
    tinea versicolor, 1099, 1100
    treatment, 1099–100
    visual guide, 398
fungal lung diseases
    coccidioidomycosis, 774–75
    cryptococcosis, 774
    histoplasmosis, 773–74
fungal meningitis, 540
fungi, 444
funnel chest, 173
fusion inhibitors, 482

G

gag and blink reflexes, 152
gait, posture, coordination and
    balance, 515
galactorrhea, 799–800
galactosemia, 142
gallbladder, 358, 818, 867
gallbladder and bile duct disorders,
    866–70
gallbladder attack, 74
gallstones
    as bile duct obstruction, 868
    defined, 866
    diagnosis, 867
    as overweight health effect, 269
    signs and symptoms, 866
    surgery, 867
    treatment, 867–68
    types of, 866

L

risk of becoming cancerous, 1102–3
skin cancer and, 1105
treatment, 1103
visual guide, 394
molluscum contagiosum, 396, 1098
Mongolian spots, 1072
monoamine oxidase inhibitors, 1284
monoclonal antibodies, 426, 814, 1296
monounsaturated fats, 249, 702
moodiness, as suicidal warning sign, 70
mood stabilizers, 1141–42, 1283–84
moral behavior, 186
moral reasoning, 213–14
morning sickness, 99
Morton's neuroma, 75, 941
motility medications, 1291
motion sickness, 339
mouth
adult, illustrated, 660
dry, 690–92
routine examination of, 688
See also oral infections/diseases
MRI. *See* magnetic resonance imaging
MS. *See* multiple sclerosis
MSG intolerance, 508
MSUD (maple syrup urine disease), 142
mucothermal method, 1184
mucus-thinning drugs, 781
multicystic dysplasia, 889
multiple endocrine neoplasia syndromes, 1029–30
multiple myeloma, 1036–37
multiple pregnancies, 117
multiple sclerosis (MS)
defined, 562
diagnosis, 563
myelin sheath and, 563
overview, 562–63
seriousness of, 563
signs and symptoms, 562
treatment, 563–64
mumps, 150, 236–37, 457–58
muscle, tendon and soft tissue disorders, 961–70
muscle and joint pain, 87
muscle cramp, 932
muscle relaxants, 1285
muscle relaxation, 521
muscles
illustrated, 920
overview, 921
visual guide, 356–57
muscle strains
heat vs. cold and, 929
overview, 928
pain, 75
prevention, 928
signs and symptoms, 927–28
treatment, 928–29
muscular dystrophy, 969–70
myasthenia gravis, 568

mycobacterium avium complex (MAC), 479
mycoplasma, 767
myelodysplastic syndrome, 1034–35
myelogram, 950
myelomeningocele, 575–76
myocardial infarction. *See* heart attack
myocardial ischemia, 717
myocarditis, 751–52
myofascial pelvic pain syndrome, 1217
myomectomy, 1213

N

nails
care of, 1117
discoloration or deformity, 1115
fungal infection and, 1116–17
illness and, 1115
illustrated, 1068
ingrown, 1117
overview, 1068
paronychia and, 1115–16
production of, 1114
toughening up, 1117
naps, 1162
narcissistic personality disorder, 1141
narcolepsy
defined, 1165
diagnosis, 1166
overview, 1165–66
self-care, 1167
signs and symptoms, 1165
treatment, 1166–67
nasal atropine, 489
nasal cavity, 369
nasal congestion
flying and, 629
as sign or symptom, 80, 87
nasal corticosteroids, 488, 494, 1295
nasal decongestant irritation, 651
nasal lavage, 490
nasal obstruction, 646–47
nasal polyps, 388
nasal continuous positive airway pressure (CPAP) device, 1164, 1165
nasal sprays, 1269
natural energy restoration, 1326–27
natural family planning, 1183–84
naturopathy, 1328
nausea, cancer treatment and, 428
nearsightedness, 584, 607
nebulizers, 1269
neck mass, 657–58
neck pain, 80, 931
necrotizing subcutaneous infection, 460
needle biopsy, 1264
neonatal lupus, 987
neonatal pimples, 1072
nephrotic syndrome, 908–9

nerve blocks, 431, 525, 1308
nerve stimulation, 915, 916, 918
nervous system
AIDS and, 543
autonomic, 513
disorders, alcohol and, 319
illustrated, 513
infections, 540–45
peripheral, 513
structures of, 513–14
visual guide, 367
See also central nervous system
neuroblastoma, 549–50
neurodermatitis, 1071
neurological examination, 515
neuromodulating medications, 1303–4
neutrophils, 443
newborn genetic screening, 412
newborn screening tests
biotinidase deficiency, 142
blood glucose, 143
congenital adrenal hyperplasia, 142
congenital hypothyroidism, 141–42
cystic fibrosis, 142
galactosemia, 142
hearing, 143–44
lysosomal storage disorders (LSD), 143
MCAD deficiency, 142–43
MSUD, 142
overview, 141
PKU, 141
sickle cell disease, 142
vision, 143
X-ALD, 143
nicotine patches, 848
nicotine replacement therapy, 314–15
nightmares, 192–93, 1169
night terrors, 192–93
nipple disorders, 176, 799
nipple-sparing mastectomy, 812
nitrates, 1279
NMDA receptor antagonists, 1283
nodular melanoma, 1109
noise, dangerous, 636
noise-induced hearing loss, 635
nonalcoholic steatohepatitis, 877
nonallergic drug reactions, 509
noncancerous skin tumors, 1101–4
nonfunctioning pituitary tumors, 1011–12
non-Hodgkin lymphoma, 480, 1054–55
nonproliferative diabetic retinopathy, 620
nonsteroidal anti-inflammatory drugs (NSAIDs)
action plan, 1286
frozen shoulder and, 985
generic and brand names, 1285–86
juvenile idiopathic arthritis and, 978
lupus and, 987
menorrhagia and, 1200

pseudomonas folliculitis (hot tub folliculitis), 1093–94
psoralen plus ultraviolet A (PUVA), 1079–80, 1086
psoriasis
  causes of, 1077
  dry skin and, 1083
  light therapy (phototherapy), 1079–80
  medications, 1287–88
  oral/injected medications, 1080
  self-care, 1080
  signs and symptoms, 1077
  topical treatments, 1077–79
  treatment, 1077–80
  visual guide, 392
psoriatic arthritis, 980
psychiatrists, 1147
psychodynamic psychotherapy, 1141, 1152
psychologists, 1147
psychotherapy
  adult ADHD and, 1135
  anxiety disorders and, 1134
  defined, 1151
  depression and, 1130
  eating disorders, 1139
  personality disorders and, 1141
  somatic symptom disorder and, 1146–48
  types of, 1151–52
psychotic depression, 1128
psychotic disorders
  brief psychotic disorder, 1145
  defined, 1142
  schizophrenia, 1143–45
  signs and symptoms, 1142–43
  substance-induced psychotic disorder, 1145–46
  types of, 1143–46
PTSD (post-traumatic stress disorder), 1134
puberty, premature, 206
pulmonary alveolar proteinosis, 768
pulmonary edema, 731
pulmonary embolism
  chest pain, 26, 76
  defined, 26
  diagnosis, 792
  overview, 792
  prevention, 793
  signs and symptoms, 26, 792
  treatment, 792–93
pulmonary function tests, 776, 779, 1264
pulmonary hypertension, 794
pulmonary stenosis, 168
pulmonary valve problems, 745–46
punch biopsy, 1112
pupil, 582
PUVA (psoralen plus ultraviolet A), 1079–80, 1086
pyloric stenosis, 169–70

Q

quadriplegia, 570
quad screen, 110

R

rabies
  prevention, 337–38
  risk of, 57
  seriousness of, 458
  signs and symptoms, 458
  travel and, 336
  treatment, 458
race
  as diabetes risk factor, 998
  as glaucoma risk factor, 607
  as high blood pressure risk factor, 709
radiation esophagitis, 822
radiation therapy
  acute lymphocytic leukemia and, 1051
  bladder cancer and, 905
  brain tumor and, 549
  breast cancer and, 812–13
  cancer and, 425
  cervical cancer and, 1225
  colorectal cancer and, 860
  defined, 425
  Hodgkin lymphoma and, 1054
  kidney cancer and, 902
  liver cancer and, 882
  lung cancer and, 786–87
  neuroblastoma and, 550
  non-Hodgkin lymphoma and, 1055
  oral cancer and, 690
  ovarian cancer and, 1228
  overview, 425
  pancreatic cancer and, 873
  pregnancy and, 106–7
  skin cancer and, 1108
  throat cancer and, 657
  thyroid cancer and, 1021
radical prostatectomy, 1252–53
radicular pain, 1315
radioactive iodine, 1017, 1021
radioactive seed implants, 1252
radiofrequency ablation, 881–82
radiosurgery, 549
rashes
  baby, 156–58
  in children, 199–200, 1081
  drug, 1087–88
  See also specific rashes
Raynaud's disease, 759–60
reactive arthritis, 980
recombinant DNA technology, 420
reconstruction, breast, 812

rectal bleeding, 30, 861
rectal suppositories, 1270
red blood cells
  blood transfusion, 1060
  count, 1033
  deficiency, 1047
  defined, 1032
  function of, 1033
  sickled, 1044
  size and shape, 1033
red cell antigen incompatibility, 112
reflexes, infant, 151–52
reflexology, 1323
refraction assessment, 587
refractive surgery
  benefits and disadvantages of, 594
  illustrated, 594
  LASIK surgery, 594
  overview, 593–94
  photorefractive keratectomy, 594
  surgeon selection, 595
  See also vision correction
regional anesthesia, 1264–65
relaxation techniques
  cancer and, 434
  muscle relaxation, 521
  osteoarthritis and, 974
  stress and, 308
relaxed breathing, 308
REM sleep, 1157
REM sleep behavior disorder, 1170
renal artery stenosis, 892–93
renal tubular acidosis, 891
renal tubular defects, 891
renal vein thrombosis, 893
renin inhibitors, 713
reproduction, successful, 1172
reproductive chromosome mutations, 410
reproductive organs
  female, 1172
  male, 1230–31
reproductive process, 1231
reproductive tract cancers
  cervical cancer, 1222, 1224–26
  endometrial cancer, 1220–23
  ovarian cancer, 1226–28
  vaginal cancer, 1228
  vulvar cancer, 1228
residential treatment programs, 1153–54
resistance training, 294–95
resistant hypertension, 713
respiratory allergies
  animal dander, mold and dust, 491–93
  chronic sinusitis and nasal polyps, 493–94
  hay fever (allergic rhinitis), 490
  pollen and, 491
  See also allergies
respiratory distress syndrome, 164–65
respiratory infections

infestations and bites, 397
insect bites, 1100
itching, 1079
lichen planus, 1080–81
lichen sclerosis, 1081–83
lymphadenitis and lymphangitis, 1096
methicillin-resistant *Staphylococcus aureus*, 1095
molluscum contagiosum, 1098
noncancerous tumors, 1101–4
oral disorders, 400
photosensitivity, 1088–89
pigmentary changes, 393, 1085–87
pityriasis rosea, 1083
Portuguese man-of-war stings, 1100–1101
precancerous skin lesions and, 1105
pregnancy and, 103
psoriasis, 392, 1077–80
rosacea, 1075–77
senile skin, 1089
shingles, 1097–98
sunburn, 1088
sun-damaged skin, 1089
xanthelasma and xanthoma, 1089–90
skin grafting, 759, 1086–87
skin infections, 1092–94
skin patches, 1270
skin protection, 439
skin resurfacing, 1084, 1118–19
skin-sparing mastectomy, 811
skin tags, 394, 1103
skull fractures, 42–43
sleep
    aging and, 1158
    are you getting enough? 1156
    back problems and, 949
    as basic necessity, 1156
    children and, 191–93
    cycles, 1157
    infants, 141, 160–61
    integrative medicine and, 1162
    naps and, 1162
    NREM, 1157
    patterns, 1157–59
    pregnancy and, 100
    REM, 1157
    shift workers and, 1160
    snoring and, 1165
    tips, 1161
    types and stages, 1157
    women and, 1158
sleep apnea
    dangers, 1163–64
    diagnosis, 1164
    illustrated, 1163
    overview, 1162–63
    as overweight health effect, 269
    risk factors, 1163
    signs and symptoms, 1163
    treatment, 1164–65
sleep centers, 1167

sleep problems
    insomnia, 1159–62
    menopause and, 1202–3
    narcolepsy, 1165–67
    nightmares, 1169
    overview, 1156
    periodic limb movement disorder, 1168–69
    REM sleep behavior disorder, 1170
    restless legs syndrome, 1167–68
    sleep apnea, 1162–65
    sleep terrors, 1169
    sleepwalking, 1169–70
    teeth grinding, 1170
sleep terrors, 1169
sleepwalking, 193, 1169–70
sleeve gastrectomy, 280
sling procedure, 915
slipped capital femoral epiphysis, 958–59
slit-lamp examination, 588
small intestine
    overview, 816–17
    parts of, 816–17
    tumors of, 855
    visual guide, 358
    wall illustration, 834
smallpox, 457
SMART goals, 277
smell, loss of sense of, 648
smokeless products, 689, 691
smoking
    as cervical cancer risk factor, 1224
    cholesterol and, 702
    cigarette alternatives and, 312–13
    COPD and, 310, 777
    disease and, 310–11
    genetics and, 777
    GERD and, 819
    gum disease and, 676
    high blood pressure and, 712
    lung cancer and, 784
    lung damage and, 777
    oral cancer and, 688
    pregnancy and, 106
    quitting, 313–16
    reasons for, 311–12
    secondhand smoke and, 313
    skin and, 1068
    as stroke risk factor, 533
    teenage, 225–26, 312
    women and, 311
    See also tobacco use disorder
smoking cessation
    aids, 437
    benefits of, 316
    in cancer prevention, 437, 438
    cardiovascular disease and, 698
    counseling, 315
    lapses, coping with, 313
    medications, 314–15, 1298
    menopause and, 1204
    nicotine replacement therapy, 314–15

as overweight risk factor, 268
    plan development, 313–14
    self-help, 314
    strategies, 314–15
    what to expect and, 316
snakebites, 60–61
snoring, 1165
SNRIs (serotonin and norepinephrine reuptake inhibitors), 1149–50
social anxiety disorder, 1133
social skills, children and, 186
sodium
    high blood pressure and, 709, 712
    reducing intake, 710–12
sodium-glucose co-transporter 2 inhibitors, 1290
soft spots (fontanels), 157
soft tissue fillers, 1075, 1084, 1119
soft tissue injection, 1308
solar lentigines, 393
solitary kidney, 888
solvent and fuels nephropathy, 907
somatic symptom disorder
    defined, 1146
    diagnosis, 1146
    self-care, 1148
    signs and symptoms, 1146
    treatment, 1146–48
sonohysterogram, 1199–200
sore throat
    as adult sign or symptom, 82
    as child sign or symptom, 87
    overview, 652
    treatment, 653
sound wave therapy, 858, 900
specialists, when to see, 245–46
special needs children
    autism, 184
    coping strategies, 208
    intellectual disability, 183–84
    taking time for oneself and, 184
speech therapy, 565
sperm
    illustrated, 1231
    inadequate, 1233–34
    overview, 1230
spider bites. *See* insect and spider bites and stings
spider veins, 1085
spina bifida, 166
spinal compression fractures, 956
spinal cord
    in feeling pain, 1300–1301
    stimulation, 1308–9
spinal cord injury
    diagnosis, 569–70
    emergency signs and symptoms, 569
    overview, 569
    rehabilitation, 570
    risk, reducing, 569
    seriousness of, 570
    treatment, 570–71
spinal disorders, visual guide, 373

U

ulcerative colitis
  anti-inflammatory drugs and, 847
  immune system suppressors and, 847–48
  medications, 1292
  nicotine patches and, 847–48
  seriousness of, 846–47
  signs and symptoms, 846
  surgery and, 848–49
  treatment, 847–49
  visual guide, 386
  See also inflammatory bowel disease
ulcers
  foot, 943–44
  GERD and, 820
  medications, 1291–92
  peptic, 828–31
  visual guide, 386
ulnar nerve dysfunction, 965
ultrasound
  defined, 1265–66
  fetal, 108–9
  in fracture treatment, 923
  illustrated, 1265
  transvaginal, 1221
ultrasound of abdominal aorta, 242
umbilical hernia, 158, 865–66
unconscious person, clearing airway of, 17
undescended testicle, 175, 1243–44
unhealthy behaviors
  alcohol use disorder, 316–24
  substance use disorders, 324–30
  tobacco use disorder, 310–16
  unsafe sex, 330–32
unstable angina, 722
upper endoscopy, 1266
upper extremity disorders, 171–72
upper gastrointestinal bleeding, 83
upper tract urothelial cancer, 902–3
urethra, injury of, 905–6
urethral infection, 909–10
urethral stricture, 918, 1206
urge incontinence, 912
urinalysis, 912, 1266
urinary disorders
  chronic urethral infection, 915
  interstitial cystitis, 915–17
  items contributing to bladder problems and, 916
  overactive bladder, 917–18
  urethral stricture, 918
  urinary incontinence, 911–15
  UTIs, 909–11
  visual guide, 389
urinary incontinence
  behavioral techniques, 913–14
  in children (bed-wetting), 912
  defined, 911

diagnosis, 912–13
electrical stimulation and, 914
interventional therapies, 914–15
medications, 914
menopause and, 1203
signs and symptoms, 911
stress incontinence, 912
surgery and, 915
treatment, 913–15
types of, 912
urge incontinence, 912
urinary problems
  as adult sign or symptom, 83
  as child sign or symptom, 87
urinary tract cancer, 424
urinary tract infections (UTIs)
  acute kidney infection, 910–11
  bladder infection, 909
  in children, 202
  in men, 911
  overview, 909
  sexual intercourse and, 910
  in teenagers/preteens, 217–18
  urethral infection, 909–10
urine, blood in, 31, 890
urine cytology, 1266
urine microalbumin test, 1010
urodynamic testing, 912
urothelial carcinoma, 903
USDA MyPlate, 256–57
uterine artery embolization, 1213
uterine fibroids, 1198, 1212–13
uterus, 1172
UTIs. *See* urinary tract infections
UVB phototherapy, 1079
uveitis, 605

V

vaccines
  additives, 147, 234
  for bacterial meningitis, 541
  benefits of, 145–47, 233–34
  effectiveness, 146, 233
  how they work, 144–45, 232–33
  HPV, for adolescents and teens, 216
  illustrated, 144
  immunity, 145, 232–33
  immunotherapy, 426
  multiple, at once, 151
  post-exposure immunity, 145
  reduction in suffering and, 233, 246
  safety, 146, 233
  severe reaction from, 235
  side effects of, 147, 234
  signs of a severe reaction, 147
  types of, 145, 233
  when to avoid, 146, 238
  See also immunizations
vagal maneuvers, 737
vagina, 1206

vaginal and vulvar disorders
  Bartholin's abscess, 1208–9
  developmental disorders, 1206–7
  genital warts, 1208
  genitourinary syndrome of menopause, 1209
  loss of pelvic support, 1210–11
  vaginal cysts, 1209–10
  vaginitis, 1209
  vulvar dystrophy, 1207
  vulvitis, 1207
  vulvodynia, 1207–8
vaginal bleeding, 30–31, 206
vaginal cancer, 1228
vaginal cysts, 1209–10
vaginal estrogen, 1204
vaginal ring, 1180–81
vaginismus, 1191
vaginitis, 1209
vagus nerve stimulation, 528, 531, 1153
valerian, 1322
valley fever, 982
valvular heart diseases, 733
variant angina, 722
varicocele, 1243
varicose veins, 100, 757–58
vascular dementia
  defined, 557
  overview, 552, 557
  seriousness of, 557–58
  signs and symptoms, 557
  treatment, 557
vascular problems of the bowel, 854–55
vascular skin ulcers, 758–59
vasculitis, 989
vasectomy, 132, 1232–33
vasoconstrictors, 1288–89
vasodilators, 713
vasomotor rhinitis, 648–49
vegetarian diet pyramid, 258
vegetarian diets, pregnancy and, 97
vein stripping, 758
vein surgery, 1118
venous bleeding, 27
venous ulcers, 759
ventricular aneurysm surgery, 738
ventricular fibrillation, 733, 735
ventricular septal defect, 167
ventricular tachycardia, 735
vertebroplasty, 956–57
vesicoureteral reflux, 887
vestibular nerve section, 642
vibrio vulnificus, 55
viral hepatitis, 479
viral meningitis, 540
virilization, 1029
viruses, 444
vision
  age and, 586
  astigmatism, 585–86
  common problems, 584–86
  double, 603

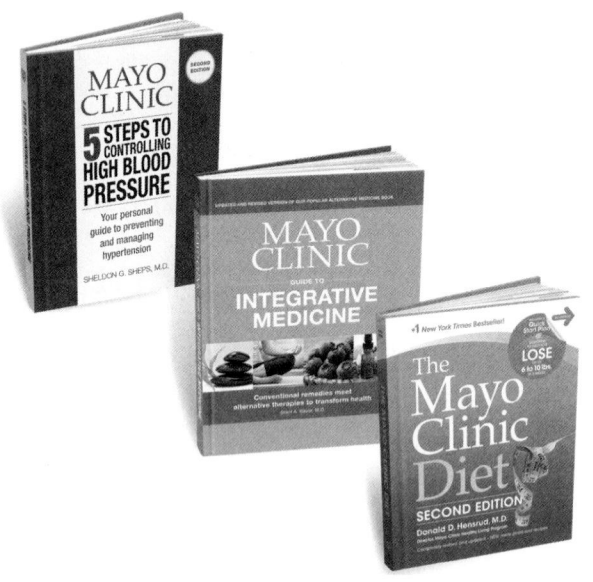
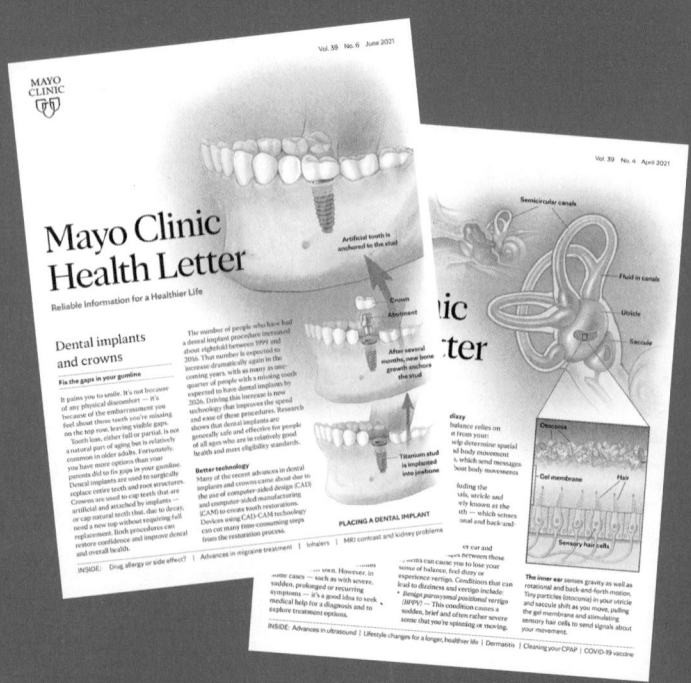